THE LIVER

Biology and Pathobiology

Fourth Edition

THE LIVER

BIOLOGY AND PATHOBIOLOGY

FOURTH EDITION

Editor-in-Chief
IRWIN M. ARIAS, M.D.

Professor and Chair
Department of Physiology
Tufts University
Boston, Massachusetts

Associate Editors

JAMES L. BOYER, M.D.

Director, Liver Center
Yale University School of Medicine and
Yale New Haven Hospital
New Haven, Connecticut

FRANCIS V. CHISARI, M.D.

Professor and Head
Department of Molecular & Experimental Medicine
The Scripps Research Institute
La Jolla, California

NELSON FAUSTO, M.D.

Professor and Chair
Department of Pathology
University of Washington School of Medicine
Seattle, Washington

DAVID SCHACHTER, M.D.

Professor
Departments of Physiology and Cellular Biophysics
Columbia University College of Physicians and Surgeons
New York, New York

DAVID A. SHAFRITZ, M.D.

Director, Marion Bessin Liver Research Center
Albert Einstein College of Medicine
Bronx, New York

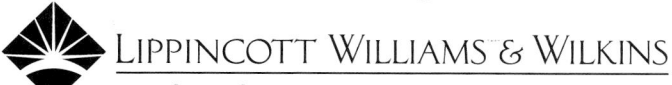
LIPPINCOTT WILLIAMS & WILKINS
A **Wolters Kluwer** Company
Philadelphia · Baltimore · New York · London
Buenos Aires · Hong Kong · Sydney · Tokyo

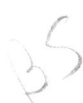

Acquisitions Editor: Beth Barry
Developmental Editor: Tanya Lazar
Production Editor: Jonathan Geffner
Manufacturing Manager: Benjamin Rivera
Cover Designer: Christine Jenny
Compositor: Lippincott Williams & Wilkins Desktop Division
Printer: Courier Westford

© 2001 by LIPPINCOTT WILLIAMS & WILKINS
530 Walnut Street
Philadelphia, PA 19106 USA
LWW.com

Printed in the USA

Library of Congress Cataloging-in-Publication Data

The liver: biology and pathobiology / editor-in-chief, Irwin M. Arias, associate editors,
    James L. Boyer ... [et al.].–4th ed.
        p. ; cm.
    Includes bibliographical references and index.
    ISBN: 0-7817-2390-6
    1. Liver–Physiology.   2. Liver–Pathophysiology.   I. Arias, Irwin M.   II. Boyer,
        J.L. (James L.), 1936–
    [DNLM: 1. Liver–pathology.   2. Liver–physiology. WI 702 L7845 2001]
QP185+
612.3'5–dc21
                                                                        00-0690996

Care has been taken to confirm the accuracy of the information presented and to describe generally accepted practices. However, the authors, editors, and publisher are not responsible for errors or omissions or for any consequences from application of the information in this book and make no warranty, expressed or implied, with respect to the currency, completeness, or accuracy of the contents of the publication. Application of this information in a particular situation remains the professional responsibility of the practitioner.

The authors, editors, and publisher have exerted every effort to ensure that drug selection and dosage set forth in this text are in accordance with current recommendations and practice at the time of publication. However, in view of ongoing research, changes in government regulations, and the constant flow of information relating to drug therapy and drug reactions, the reader is urged to check the package insert for each drug for any change in indications and dosage and for added warnings and precautions. This is particularly important when the recommended agent is a new or infrequently employed drug.

Some drugs and medical devices presented in this publication have Food and Drug Administration (FDA) clearance for limited use in restricted research settings. It is the responsibility of the health care provider to ascertain the FDA status of each drug or device planned for use in their clinical practice.

10 9 8 7 6 5 4 3 2 1

We dedicate this edition to the memory of Charles Sprecher Davidson—an inspiring teacher who stimulated three generations of students, basic scientists, and clinicians to apply fundamental biology to our understanding of liver disease. Dr. Davidson was one of the founders of modern hepatology as well as the American Association for the Study of Liver Diseases. In addition, he served as Director of the Harvard Medical Services at the Boston City Hospital from 1944 to 1973. It was there that he created one of the first liver research units in the United States. A quiet and modest man, he taught by example, provoked the intellect, guided the training of many leaders in hepatology worldwide, and coupled the highest professional standards with loyalty and friendship.

CONTENTS

CONTRIBUTING AUTHORS

Guy R. Adami, Ph.D. Assistant Professor, Department of Oral Medicine and Diagnostic Services, University of Illinois at Chicago, College of Dentistry, 801 South Paulina Street, Chicago, Illinois 60612

Gianfranco Alpini, Ph.D. Associate Professor, Department of Internal Medicine and Medical Physiology, Texas A&M University System Health Science Center, 702 Southwest H.K. Dodgen Loop, Room 316B, Temple, Texas 76504

Miriam J. Alter, Ph.D. Chief, Epidemiology Section, Hepatitis Branch, Centers for Disease Control & Prevention (MS G37), 1600 Clifton Road, Atlanta, Georgia 30333

Nancy C. Andrews, M.D., Ph.D. Associate Professor, Department of Pediatrics, Harvard Medical School; Associate Investigator, Associate in Medicine, Howard Hughes Medical Institute; Department of Pediatrics (Hematology/Oncology), Children's Hospital, 300 Longwood Avenue, Boston, Massachusetts 02115

Irwin M. Arias, M.D. Professor and Chair, Department of Physiology, Tufts University School of Medicine, 136 Harrison Avenue, Boston, Massachusetts 02111

Beth P. Bell, M.D., M.P.H. Deputy Chief, Epidemiology Section, Hepatitis Branch, Centers for Disease Control and Prevention, MS G37, 1600 Clifton Road Northeast, Atlanta, Georgia 30333

Bruce Beutler, Ph.D. Professor, Department of Immunology, The Scripps Research Institute, 10550 North Torrey Pines Road, IMM-31, La Jolla, California 92037

Johannes G. Bode, M.D. Research Fellow, Department of Internal Medicine, Division of Gastroenterology, Hepatology and Infectiology, Heinrich-Heines University, Düsseldorf, Universitätstrasse 1; Clinical Resident, Department of Internal Medicine, Division of Gastroenterology, Hepatology and Infectiology, Medical Institutes of the Heinrich-Heine University, Düsseldorf, Moorenstrasse 5, Düsseldorf 40225, Germany

James L. Boyer, M.D. Ensign Professor of Medicine, Director, Liver Center, Yale University School of Medicine, 333 Cedar Street, P.O. Box 208019, RM LMP 1080, New Haven, Connecticut 06520-8019; Attending Physician, Department of Medicine, Yale New Haven Hospital, 789 Howard Avenue, New Haven, Connecticut 06510

Filip Braet, Ph.D. Postdoctoral Researcher of the Fund for Scientific Research-Flanders, Laboratory for Cell Biology and Histology, Free University of Brussels, Laarbeeklaan 103, 1090 Brussels, Belgium

Christian Bréchot, PU-PH Professor of Cell Biology and Hepatology, Faculte Necker E-M, Inserm U370, 156 Rue De Vaugirard; Head, Hepatology Department Necker E-M Hospital, 149 Rue de Sèvres, 75730 Paris Cedex 15, France

Roger F. Butterworth, Ph.D., D.Sc. Professor, Department of Medicine, University of Montreal; Director, Neuroscience Research Unit, L'Hopital St. Luc (CHUM), 1058 St. Denis Street, Montreal, Quebec H2X 3J4, Canada

Francis V. Chisari, M.D. Professor, Department of Molecular and Experimental Pathology, The Scripps Research Institute, 10550 North Torrey Pines Road, La Jolla, California 92037

Rial A. Christensen, Ph.D. Research Assistant Professor, Department of Medicine, Center for Biomedical Research, St. Elizabeth's Medical Center, 736 Cambridge Street, Boston, Massachusetts 02135

Mark G. Clemens, Ph.D. Professor and Chair, Department of Biology, University of North Carolina at Charlotte, 9201 University City Boulevard, Charlotte, North Carolina 28223

Robert H. Costa, Ph.D. Professor, Department of Molecular Genetics, University of Illinois at Chicago, 900 South Ashland Avenue (M/C 669), Chicago, Illinois 60607-7170

David F. Crawford, M.D., Ph.D. Instructor, Departments of Pediatrics and of Cell Biology and Physiology, Washington University School of Medicine; Instructor, Department of Pediatrics, St. Louis Children's Hospital, One Children's Place, St. Louis, Missouri 63110

Mariana D. Dabeva, M.D., Ph.D. Assistant Professor, Department of of Medicine, Liver Research Center, Albert Einstein College of Medicine, 1300 Morris Park Avenue, Bronx, New York 10461

Sophie Dahan, Ph.D. Postdoctoral Research Fellow, Department of Biochemistry and Molecular Biology, Mayo Foundation, 200 First Street Southwest, Rochester, Minnesota 55905

Patricia A. D'Amore Professor, Departments of Ophthalmology and Pathology, Boston, Massachusetts 02115; Senior Scientist, Schepens Eye Research Institute, 20 Staniford Street, Boston, Massachusetts 02114

Isabel De Aós Scherpenseel, Ph.D. Research Fellow, Department of Medicine, St. Elizabeth's Medical Center, 736 Cambridge Street, Boston, Massachusetts 02135

Maria de Fatima Leite, Ph.D. Associate Professor, Department of Physiology and Biophysics, Federal University of Minas Gerais, Av. Antonio Carlos 6627, Belo Horizonte, MG, Brazil

Marie C. DeFrances, M.D., Ph.D. Assistant Professor, Department of Pathology, University of Pittsburgh, 200 Lothrop Street, Pittsburgh, Pennsylvania 15261

Maria A. Della Fazia, Ph.D. Researcher Scientist, Institute of General Pathology, University of Perugia, Policlinico Monteluce, Via Brunamonti 51, 06100 Perugia, Italy

Ronald A. DePinho, M.D. American Cancer Society Research Professor and Professor of Medicine and Genetics, Departments of Adult Oncology, Medicine and Genetics, Dana Farber Cancer Institute, Harvard Medical School, 44 Binney Street, Boston, Massachusetts 02115

Valeer J. Desmet, M.D. Emeritus Professor of Histology and Pathology, Department of Pathology, Catholic University of Leuven, Minderbroedersstraat 12, B-3000 Leuven, Belgium

J. Fred Dice, Ph.D. Department of Physiology, Tufts University School of Medicine, 136 Harrison Avenue, Boston, Massachusetts 02111

Anna Mae Diehl, M.D. Professor, Department of Medicine, Johns Hopkins University School of Medicine, 912 Ross Research Building, 720 Rutland Avenue; Staff, Department of Medicine, Division of Gastroenterology and Hepatology, Johns Hopkins Hospital, 600 North Wolfe Street, Baltimore, Maryland 21205

Michel Dominguez, Ph.D Postdoctoral Research Fellow, Mayo Foundation, 200 First Street Southwest, Rochester, Minnesota 55905

Heather S. Duffy, Ph.D. Department of Neuroscience, Albert Einstein College of Medicine, 1410 Pelham Parkway South, Bronx, New York, 10461

John H. Exton, M.D., Ph.D. Professor, Department of Molecular Physiology and Biophysics, Vanderbilt University, Light Hall, Room 831, Nashville, Tennessee 37232-4381

Deborah N. Farlow, Ph.D. Scientist II, Department of Immunology, Millennium Pharmaceuticals, Inc., 75 Sidney Street, Cambridge, Massachusetts 02139

Nelson Fausto, M.D. Professor and Chair, Department of Pathology, University of Washington School of Medicine, Box 357470, K078 Health Sciences Building, Seattle, Washington 98195-7705

Carlo Ferrari, M.D. Director, Department of Infectious Diseases, University Hospital of Parma, Via Gramsci 14, 43100 Parma, Italy

Marxa L. Figueiredo, B.S., Ph.D. Candidate, Department of Pathobiological Sciences, University of Wisconsin–Madison, 2015 Linden Drive West, Madison, Wisconsin 53706

J. Gregory Fitz, M.D. Professor, Department of Medicine, Division of Gastroenterology and Hepatology, University of Colorado Health Sciences Center, Campus Box B158, Room 6412, Denver, Colorado 80262

Mark D. Fleming, M.D., D.Phil. Assistant in Pathology, Department of Pathology, Children's Hospital, 300 Longwood Avenue; Assistant Professor, Department of Pathology, Harvard Medical School, Boston, Massachusetts 02115

Scott L. Friedman, M.D. Professor, Department of Medicine/Liver Diseases, Mount Sinai School of Medicine, 1425 Madison Avenue, Room 11-70F; Attending Physician, Division of Liver Diseases, Mount Sinai Hospital, 1 Gustave Levy Place, New York, New York 10029

Paolo Gentilini, M.D. Professor, Chief, Department of Internal Medicine, Università degli Studi di Firenze, Viale Morgagni 85, 50134 Florence, Italy

Jonathan D. Gitlin, M.D. Helene B. Roberson Professor of Pediatrics, Washington University School of Medicine, McDonnell Pediatric Research Building, 660 South Euclid Avenue, St. Louis, Missouri 63110

Patricia Greenwel, Ph.D. Assistant Professor, Department of Biochemistry and Molecular Biology, Mount Sinai School of Medicine, One Gustave Levy Place, New York, New York 10029

Marcus Grompe, M.D. Professor, Department of Molecular and Medical Genetics, Oregon Health Science University, 3181 Southwest Sam Jackson Park Road, Portland, Oregon 97201

Roberto J. Groszmann, M.D. Professor of Medicine, Department of Internal Medicine/Digestive Diseases, Yale University School of Medicine/1080 LMP, 333 Cedar Street, New Haven, Connecticut 06520; Chief, Digestive Diseases Section, Veteran's Administration CT Healthcare System/111H, 950 Campbell Avenue, West Haven, Connecticut 06516

José Carlos Gutiérrez-Ramos, Ph.D. Vice President, Immunology and Hematology, Department of Immunobiology and Inflammation, Millennium Pharmaceuticals, Inc., 75 Sidney Street, Cambridge, Massachusetts 02139

Iqbal Hamza, Ph.D. Postdoctoral Research Associate, Department of Pediatrics, Washington University School of Medicine, 660 South Euclid Avenue, St. Louis, Missouri 63110

Peter C. Heinrich, Ph.D. Professor and Chairman, Department of Biochemistry, University of the RWTH Aachen, Pauwelsstrasse 30, D-52074 Aachen, Germany

Ira M. Herman, Ph.D. Professor, Department of Cell and Molecular Physiology, Tufts University School of Medicine, 136 Harrison Avenue, Boston, Massachusetts 02111

Hector J. Hernandez, Ph.D. Research Associate, Department of Pathology, Tufts University School of Medicine, 136 Harrison Avenue, MV717, Boston, Massachusetts 02111

Richard J. Hift, M.B.Ch.B.,Ph.D. Department of Medicine, University of Cape Town, K-Floor, Old Groote Schuur; Senior Specialist, Department of Medicine (Liver), Groote Schuur Hospital, Observatory, Cape Town 7925, South Africa

Ai-Xuan Le Holterman, M.D. Assistant Professor, Department of Surgery, Division of Pediatric Surgery, University of Illinois at Chicago, 840 South Wood Street, M/C 958, Chicago, Illinois 60612

Ann L. Hubbard, Ph.D. Professor, Department of Cell Biology and Anatomy, Johns Hopkins University, School of Medicine, 725 North Wolfe Street, Baltimore, Maryland 21205-2196

Phillip B. Hylemon, Ph.D. Professor, Departments of Microbiology and Immunology, Medical College of Virginia, Virginia Commonwealth University, Medical Science Building, Room 515, 1217 East Marshall Street, Richmond, Virginia 23298

Masayasu Inoue, M.D., Ph.D. Chairman and Professor, Departments of Biochemistry and Molecular Pathology, Osaka City University Medical School, 1-4-3 Asahimachi, Abeno, Osaka 545-8585, Japan

Lee M. Kaplan M.D., Ph.D. Assistant Professor, Department of Medicine, Harvard Medical School, 25 Shattuck Street, Boston, Massachusetts 02115; Associate Chief for Research, Gastrointestinal Unit, Massachusetts General Hospital, 32 Fruit Street, Boston, Massachusetts 02114

Dietrich Keppler, M.D. Professor and Head, Department of Tumor Biochemistry, Germany Cancer Research Center, Im Neuenheimer Feld 280, D-69120 Heidelberg, Germany

Helmut Kipp, Ph.D. Research Fellow, Department of Physiology, Tufts University School of Medicine, 136 Harrison Avenue, Boston, Massachusetts 02111

Ralph E. Kirsch, M.D. Professor and Head, Department of Medicine, Executive Director, Medical Research Council/University of Cape Town Liver Research Centre, University of Capetown, Medical School; Chief, Department of Medicine, Groote Schuur Hospital, Observatory, Capetown 7925, South Africa

Takashi Kojima, D.V.M., Ph.D. Assistant Professor, Department of Pathology, Sapporo Medical University School of Medicine, S-1, W-17, Chuo-ku Sapporo 060-8556, Japan

Jörg König, Ph.D. Division of Tumor Biology, Germany Cancer Research Center, Im Neuenheimer Feld 280, D-69120 Heidelberg, Germany

Peter H. Krammer Head of Division, Department of Immunogenetics, Germany Cancer Research Center, Im Neuenheimer Feld 280, D-69120 Heidelberg, Germany

Betsy T. Kren Department of Medicine, GI Division, University of Minnesota Medical School, 420 Delaware Street Southeast, Minneapolis, Minnesota 55455

Giacomo Laffi, M.D. Professor, Department of Internal Medicine, University of Florence; Chief U.O. Patologia Medica I, Azienda Ospedaliera Careggi, Viale G. Pieroccini, 18, 50139 Florence, Italy

Michael M. C. Lai, M.D., Ph.D. Distinguished Professor, Department of Molecular Microbiology and Immunology, University of Southern California, Keck School of Medicine, 2011 Zonal Avenue, HMR-401, Los Angeles, California 90089-9094

Robert Langer, Sc.D. Kenneth J. Germeshauser Professor of Chemical and Biomedical Engineering, Department of Chemical Engineering, Harvard–MIT Division of Health Science and Technology, Massachusetts Institute of Technology, 45 Carleton Street, E25-342, Cambridge, Massachusetts 02139

Lucia R. Languino, Ph.D. Associate Professor, Department of Pathology, Yale University School of Medicine, 310 Cedar Street, New Haven, Connecticut 06510

Nicholas F. La Russo, M.D. Chairman, Department of Medicine, Mayo Medical School, Clinic, and Foundation, 200 First Street, Southwest, Rochester, Minnesota 55905

Giorgio La Villa, M.D. Professor, Department of Internal Medicine, University of Florence, Viale Morgagni 85, I-50134 Florence, Italy

John J. Lemasters, M.D., Ph.D. Professor, Department of Cell Biology and Anatomy, University of North Carolina School at Chapel Hill, CB# 7090, 236 Taylor Hall, Chapel Hill, North Carolina 27599

Dan Li, M.D. Senior Resrach Fellow, Department of Medicine, Division of Liver Diseases, Mount Sinai School of Medicine, 1425 Madison Avenue, New York, New York 10029

Jennifer Lippincott-Schwartz, Ph.D. Head, Section of Organelle Biology, Cell Biology and Metabolism Branch, National Institute of Child Health and Human Development, National Institutes of Health, Building 18T–Room 101, Bethesda, Maryland 20817

Stephen Locarnini, M.D., Ph.D. Associate Professor, Research and Molecular Development, Victorian Infectious Diseases Reference Laboratory, 10 Wreckyn Street, North Melbourne 3051, Australia

José M. Lora, Ph.D. Scientist II, Millennium Pharmaceuticals, Inc., 75 Sidney Street, Cambridge, Massachusetts 02139

Mauricio R. Loureiro-Silva, M.D. Postdoctoral Fellow, Department of Medicine (Digestive Diseases), Yale University School of Medicine, 333 Cedar Street, New Haven, Connecticut 06520; Section of Digestive Diseases, VA Medical Center, 950 Campbell Avenue, 111J, West Haven, Connecticut 06516

Lina Lu, M.D. Associate Professor, Department of Surgery, University of Pittsburgh Medical Center, 200 Lothrop Street, Pittsburgh, Pennsylvania 15213

Timothy T. Lu MSTP Student (for M.D./Ph.D), Department of Pharmacology, University of Texas Southwestern Medical Center, 5323 Harry Hines Boulevard, Dallas, Texas 75390-9041

Dianzhong Luo, M.D., Ph.D. Postdoctoral Researcher, Laboratory for Cell Biology and Histology, Free University of Brussels, Laarbeeklaan 103, 1090 Brussels, Belgium; Pathologist, Department of Pathology, First Affiliated Hospital, Guangxi Medical University, 6 Binhu Road, Nanning 530021, Guangxi, China

Makoto Makishima, M.D., Ph.D. Research Associate, Department of Pharmacology, Howard Hughes Medical Institute, University of Texas Southwestern Medical Center, 5323 Harry Hines Boulevard, Dallas, Texas 75390-9050

David J. Mangelsdorf, Ph.D. Professor, Department of Pharmacology, Howard Hughes Medical Institute, 5323 Harry Hines Boulevard, Dallas, Texas 75390-9050

William S. Mason, Ph.D. Senior Member, Basic Science Division, Fox Chase Cancer Center, 7701 Burholme Avenue, Philadelphia, Pennsylvania 19111

Mark A. McNiven, Ph.D. Associate Professor, Center for Basic Research in Digestive Diseases, Mayo Clinic, 200 First Street Southwest, Rochester, Minnesota 55905

Peter N. Meissner, B.Sc., Ph.D. Associate Professor and Wellcome Senior Fellow, Department of Medicine, University of Cape Town; Head, Lennox Eales Porphyria Laboratory, Medical Research Council/University of Cape Town Liver Center, K-Floor, Old Groote Schuur, Observatory, Cape Town 7925, South Africa

M. Dodson Michael, Ph.D. Senior Biologist, Department of Endocrine Research, Eli Lilly and Company, Lilly Corporate Center, Indianapolis, Indiana 46285

George K. Michalopoulos, M.D., Ph.D. Chairman, Department of Pathology, University of Pittsburgh, S410 BST, School of Medicine, Pittsburgh, Pennsylvania 15261

Suniti Misra, Ph.D. Research Assistant Professor, Department of Physiology, Tufts University School of Medicine, 136 Harrison Avenue, Boston, Massachusetts 02111

Martina Müller, M.D. Senior Physician, Department of Internal Medicine IV, Hepatology and Gastroenterology, University Hospital, Bergheimerstrasse 58, 69115 Heidelberg, Germany

Michael H. Nathanson, M.D., Ph.D. Associate Professor of Medicine and Cell Biology, Department of Internal Medicine, Yale University School of Medicine, 333 Cedar Street, P.O. Box 208019, New Haven, Connecticut 06520-8019; Associate Professor of Medicine, Department of Internal Medicine, Yale–New Haven Hospital–Yale University School of Medicine, 20 York Street, New Haven, Connecticut 06511

Uma Narayanasami, M.D. Assistant Professor, Departments of Hematology and Oncology, New England Medical Center, 750 Washington Street, Boston, Massachusetts 02111

Anne T. Nies, Ph.D. Division of Tumor Biochemistry, Germany Cancer Research Center, Im Neuenheimer Feld 280, D-69120 Heidelberg, Germany

Martin A. Nowak, Ph.D. Head, Institute for Advanced Study, Einstein Drive, Princeton, New Jersey 08540

William M. Pandak, Jr., M.D. Professor, Department of Medicine, Division of Gastroenterology, Medical College of Virginia/Virginia Commonwealth University, P.O. Box 980711, Richmond, Virginia 23298; Department of Medicine, Veteran's Affairs Medical Center, 1801 Broad Rock Boulevard, Richmond, Virginia 23249

David H. Perlmutter, M.D. Donald Strominger Professor of Pediatrics, Professor of Cell Biology and Physiology, Washington University School of Medicine, 660 South Euclid Avenue; Director, Division of Gastroenterology and Nutrition, St. Louis Children's Hospital, 1 Children's Place, St. Louis, Missouri 63110

Massimo Pinzani, M.D. Professor, Department of Internal Medicine, Università degli Studi di Firenze, Viale Morgagni 85, 50134 Florence, Italy

Helen Piwnica-Worms, Ph.D. Professor/Investigator-HHMI, Department of Cell Biology and Physiology, Washington University School of Medicine, 660 South Euclid Avenue, Box 8228, St. Louis, Missouri 63100-1093

Richard T. Prall, M.D. Instructor of Internal Medicine, Fellow, Division of Gastroenterology and Hepatology, Mayo Clinic and Foundation, 200 First Street Southwest, Rochester, Minnesota 55905

Shiguang Qian, M.D. Thomas E. Starzl Transplantation Institute, University of Pittsburgh, 200 Lothrop Street, Pittsburgh, Pennsylvania 15213

Richard A. Rachubinski, Ph.D. Professor, Department of Cell Biology, University of Alberta, Medical Sciences Building 5-14, Edmonton, Alberta T6G 2H7, Canada

Francisco M. Rausa, M.S. Department of Molecular Genetics, University of Illinois at Chicago, 900 South Ashland Avenue, Chicago, Illinois 60607

Joyce J. Repa, Ph.D. Research Associate, Department of Pharmacology, Howard Hughes Medical Institute, University of Texas Southwestern Medical Center, 5323 Harry Hines Boulevard, Dallas, Texas 75390-9050

Marcos Rojkind, M.D., Ph.D. Professor, Department of Medicine and Pathology, Marion Bessin Liver Research Center, Albert Einstein College of Medicine, 1300 Morris Park Avenue, Bronx, New York 10461

Richard M. Roman, M.D. Assistant Professor, Department of Medicine, University of Colorado Health Sciences Center, Campus Box B158, Room 6412, Denver, Colorado 80262

Jayanta Roy Chowdhury, M.D. Professor, Department of Medicine and Molecular Genetics, Albert Einstein College of Medicine, Liver Center, 1300 Morris Park Avenue; Attending Physician, Department of Medicine, Jack D. Weiler Hospital of Albert Einstein College of Medicine, 1825 Eastchester Road, Bronx, New York 10461

Namita Roy Chowdhury, Ph.D. Professor, Department of Medicine and Molecular Genetics, Albert Einstein College of Medicine, 1300 Morris Park Avenue, Bronx, New York 10461

Karl Lenhard Rudolph, M.D. Research Associate, Department of Gastroenterology and Hepatology, Medical School Hannover, 1 Carl-Neuberg-Str, 30623 Hannover, Germany

Neil B. Ruderman, M.D., Professor, Departments of Medicine and Physiology, Boston University School of Medicine; Director, Diabetes Unit, Department of Medicine (Endocrinology), Boston Medical Center, 650 Albany Street, Boston, Massachusetts 02118

Eric P. Sandgren, V.M.D., Ph.D. Department of Pathobiological Sciences, School of Veterinary Medicine, University of Wisconsin–Madison, 2015 Linden Drive West, Madison, Wisconsin 53706

Ram Sasisekharan, Ph.D. Associate Professor, Division of Bioengineering, Massachusetts Institute of Technology, 77 Massachusetts Avenue, Cambridge, Massachusetts 02139

Paolo Sassone-Corsi, Ph.D. Professor, Director of Research, Institute of Genetics and Molecular and Cell Biology, CNRS, Louis Pasteur University, 1, rue Laurent Fries, 67404 Illkirch-Strasbourg, France

Peter Satir, Ph.D. Professor and Chairman, Department of Anatomy and Structural Biology, Albert Einstein College of Medicine, 1300 Morris Park Avenue, Bronx, New York 10461-1602

Norimasa Sawada, M.D., Ph.D. Professor and Chief, Department of Pathology, Sapporo Medical University School of Medicine, S-1, W-17, Chuo-ku Sapporo 060-8556, Japan

David Schachter, M.D. Professor, Department of Physiology and Cellular Biophysics, Columbia University, 630 West 168th Street, New York, New York 10032

Giuseppe Servillo, M.D., Ph.D. Institute of General Pathology, University of Perugia, Policlinico Monteluce, Via Brunamonti 51, 06100 Perugia, Italy

David A. Shafritz, M.D. Professor, Departments of Medicine and of Cell Biology and Pathology, Director, Marrion Bessin Liver Research Center, Liver Research Center, Albert Einstein College of Medicine, 1300 Morris Park Avenue, Bronx, New York 10461

Zachary Shriver, Ph.D. Division of Bioengineering and Environmental Health, Massachusetts Institute of Technology, 77 Massachusetts Avenue, Cambridge, Massachusetts 02139

Francis R. Simon, M.D. Professor, Department of Medicine, University of Colorado Health Sciences Center, 4200 East Ninth Avenue; Physician, Department of Medicine, Denver Veterans Affairs Medical Center, Denver, Colorado 80262

Jennifer J. Smith, Ph.D. Postdoctoral Fellow, Institute for Systems Biology, 4225 Roosevelt Way Northeast, Suite 200, Seattle, Washington 98105-6099

Ilan Spector, Ph.D. Department of Physiology and Biophysics, Health Science Center, State University of New York at Stony Brook, Nicolls Road, Stony Brook, New York 11794-8661

David C. Spray, Ph.D. Professor of Neuroscience and Medicine, Department of Neuroscience, Albert Einstein College of Medicine, 1300 Morris Park Avenue, Bronx, New York 10461

Miguel J. Stadecker, M.D., Ph.D. Professor, Department of Pathology, Tufts University School of Medicine, 136 Harrison Avenue; Pathologist, Department of Pathology, New England Medical Center, 750 Washington Street, Boston, Massachusetts 02111

Clifford J. Steer, M.D. Professor, Departments Medicine and Genetics, Biology, and Development, University of Minnesota Medical School, MMC 36, Mayo Building, Room A536, 420 Delaware Street Southeast, Minneapolis, Minnesota 55455

Antonia E. Stephen, M.D. Research Fellow, Laboratory of Tissue Engineering and Organ Fabrication, Harvard Medical School, Boston, Massachusetts 02115; Resident, Department of Surgery, Massachusetts General Hospital, 55 Fruit Street, Boston, Massachusetts 02114

Richard J. Stockert, Ph.D. Professor, Department of Medicine, Albert Einstein College of Medicine, 1300 Morris Park Avenue, Bronx, New York 10461

Kevin Strange, Ph.D. Professor, Department of Anesthesiology and Pharmacology, Vanderbilt University, Nashville, Tennessee 37232

Sandra S. Strantnieks, Ph.D. Research Fellow, Department of Child Health, Guy's King's & St. Thomas' School of Medicine, King's College Hospital, Denmark Hill, London SE5 9RS, United Kingdom

Frederick J. Suchy, M.D. Professor and Chair, Department of Pediatrics, Mount Sinai School of Medicine; Pediatrician-in-Chief, Mount Sinai Hospital, 1 Gustave Levy Place, P.O. Box 1198, New York, New York 10029

Richard Thompson, M.D., Ph.D. Wellcome Advanced Fellow, Department of Child Health, Guy's and King's & St. Thomas' School of Medicine; Pediatric Liver Service, King's College Hospital, Denmark Hill, London SE5 9RS, United Kingdom

Angus W. Thomson, Ph.D., D.Sc. Professor, Department of Surgery, University of Pittsburgh, W1544 Biomedical Science Tower, 200 Lothrop Street, Pittsburgh, Pennsylvania 15213

Snorri S. Thorgeirsson, M.D., Ph.D. Chief, Laboratory of Experimental Carcinogenesis, National Cancer Institute–National Institutes of Health, 37 Convent Drive MSC 4255, Building 37, Room 3C28, Bethesda, Maryland 20892-4255

Joseph Torresi, M.B.B.S., Ph.D. Lecturer, Department of Medicine, University of Melbourne; Physician, Victorian Infectious Diseases Service, Royal Melbourne Hospital, Grathan Street, Parkville 3050, Victoria, Australia

Ming-Hung Tsai, M.D. Postdoctoral Fellow Yale University School of Medicine, 333 Cedar Street, New Haven, Connecticut 06520; Postdoctoral Fellow, Section of Digestive Diseases, Veterans Administration Medical Center, West Haven, 950 Campbell Avenue, West Haven, Connecticut 06516

Pamela L. Tuma, Ph.D. Postdoctoral Fellow, Department of Cell Biology and Anatomy, Johns Hopkins University School of Medicine, 725 North Wolfe Street, Baltimore, Maryland 21205

Peter Ujházy, M.D., Ph.D. Research Fellow, Department of Physiology, Tufts University School of Medicine, 136 Harrison Avenue, Boston, Massachusetts 02111

Joseph P. Vacanti, M.D. John Homans Professor of Surgery, Department of Pediatric Surgery, Harvard Medical School; Visiting Surgeon, Department of Pediatric Surgery, Massachusetts General Hospital, 55 Fruit Street, Boston, Massachusetts 02114

Lyuba Varticovski, M.D. Associate Professor, Department of Medicine and Physiology, Tufts School of Medicine, 136 Harrison Avenue, M&V 704, Boston, Massachusetts 02115; Staff, Hematology & Oncology, Department of Medicine, St. Elizabeth Medical Center, 736 Cambridge Street CBR 419, Boston, Massachusetts 02135

Ganesh Venkataraman, Ph.D. Research Engineer, Division of Bioengineering, Massachusetts Institute of Technology, 77 Massachusetts Avenue, Cambridge, Massachusetts 02139

David Vermijlen Bioengineer, Research Assistant, Laboratory of Cell Biology and Histology, Free University of Brussels, Laarbeeklaan 103, 1090 Brussels, Belgium

[1]**Z. Reno Vlahcevic, M.D.** Professor of Medicine, Division of Gastroenterology, P.O. Box 980711, Richmond, Virginia 23298-0711

Yoshiyuke Wakabayashi, Ph.D. Research Fellow, Department of Physiology, Tufts University School of Medicine, 136 Harrison Avenue, Boston, Massachusetts 02111

Nadine S. Weich, Ph.D. Director, Department of Inflammation, Millennium Pharmaceuticals, Inc., 75 Sidney Street, Cambridge, Massachusetts 02139

Rebecca G. Wells, M.D. Assistant Professor, Departments of Medicine and Pathology, Yale University School of Medicine, 333 Cedar Street; Physician, Department of Medicine, Yale New Haven Hospital, New Haven, Connecticut 06520

Eddie Wisse, M.D. Chairman, Department of Cell Biology and Histology, Free University of Brussels, Laarbeeklaan 103, 1090 Brussels, Belgium

Allan W. Wolkoff, M.D. Professor, Department of Medicine and of Anatomy and Structural Biology, Albert Einstein College of Medicine, 1300 Morris Park Avenue, Bronx, New York 10461-1602

Kenneth S. Zaret, Ph.D. Senior Member, Program Leader, Cell and Developmental Biology Program, Fox Chase Cancer Center, 7701 Burholme Avenue, Philadelphia, Pennsylvania 19111

Reza Zarnegar, Ph.D. Department of Pathology, University of Pittsburgh, 200 Lothrop Street, Pittsburgh, Pennsylvania 15261

---

[1]Deceased.

PREFACE

Predictions stated in the 1982, 1988, and 1994 editions of *The Liver: Biology and Pathobiology* have consistently come to pass at a faster rate than had been anticipated. Major advances in genetics, immunology, virology, chemistry, biophysics, and structural, molecular, and cellular biology increasingly affect our understanding of liver function and disease. The near future promises additional developments resulting from the sequencing of the human genome and advances in combinatorial chemistry, micro-imaging, stem-cell biology, and other areas of research.

The challenge addressed by this book has not changed since the Preface to the First Edition was written in 1982:

> The amazing advances in fundamental biology that have occurred within the past two decades have brought hepatology and other disciplines into new, uncharted and exciting waters. The dramatic changes in biology will profoundly influence our ability to diagnose, treat, and prevent liver disease. How can a student of the liver and its disease maintain a link to these exciting advances? Most physicians lack the time to take postgraduate courses in basic biology; most basic researchers lack an understanding of liver physiology and disease. This book strives to bridge the ever-increasing gap [between the amazing advances in basic biology and their application to liver structure, function, and disease].

A problem arises. How can a new edition remain reasonable in cost and size and still present essential background information, which has not changed since the last edition, as well as the panoply of major new contributions to our understanding of liver disease? We have attempted a novel solution. The present edition emphasizes exciting important information acquired within the past five years as well as rapidly developing concepts and discoveries. Appropriate background information and references, which comprise the Third Edition (1994), are provided on a web site (URL http://liver.med.tufts.edu), to which the contents have been cross-referenced in the new text. The chapters are designated by 🖥 and web site chapter numbers W-1 through W-42 when cited in the text. Therefore, readers can obtain new information in the printed Fourth Edition and background information through the web site.

The Fourth Edition includes 28 new chapters that present major progress as achieved in the laboratory and clinic. All other chapters either have been completely revised or appear in the web site. Frank Chisari has become an Associate Editor and edited four new chapters concerning viral hepatitis. Previous editions included a section entitled "Horizons," which presented advances of extraordinary nature in areas of potentially major importance to the liver. Virtually all of these fields have rapidly expanded and become topics for future chapters. Eleven new "Horizons" are presented in this edition. One may safely predict that their impact on hepatology will also be considerable.

As stated in the Preface to the Third Edition:

> The amazing advance in science proceeds at an ever-increasing pace...The implications for students of liver disease are considerable. The authors and editors will have achieved our goals if the reader finds within this volume glimpses into the current state and future direction of our discipline and perspectives that lead to better understanding of liver function and disease.

Irwin M. Arias, Editor
James L. Boyer, Associate Editor
Francis V. Chisari, Associate Editor
Nelson Fausto, Associate Editor
David Schachter, Associate Editor
David A. Shafritz, Associate Editor

ACKNOWLEDGMENTS

We thank the distinguished authors for their expertise and enthusiastic participation and for their patience in responding to editorial suggestions. Appreciation is also acknowledged for the administrative and editorial assistance of Charlotte White and Karen Hatch at Tufts University School of Medicine and to the staff at Lippincott Williams & Wilkins, particularly Tanya Lazar.

THE LIVER

Biology and Pathobiology

Fourth Edition

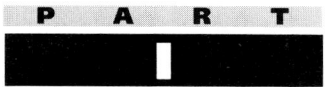

P A R T

I

INTRODUCTION

1

ORGANIZATIONAL PRINCIPLES

VALEER J. DESMET

> Nothing is as simple as it seems.
> *A. Einstein*

ANATOMY

The liver is the largest solid organ of the body, constituting approximately 2% to 5% of body weight in the adult and 5% in the neonate. Classic anatomy distinguishes two main (right and left) and two accessory (quadrate and caudate) lobes according to peritoneal attachments and surface fissures. However, today's hepatobiliary surgeons pay more attention to the functional vascular anatomy of the liver (1) already studied by Francis Glisson in 1654 (2). The organ is divided into sectors and segments with independent afferent and efferent blood supply and biliary channels without collateral circulation between the segments. The latter were described by Couinaud and numbered clockwise from II to VIII, with the caudate lobe as an autonomous part or segment I (3).

The structural organization of the liver reflects its remarkable functions.

This eight-segmented organ, unique in the body and endowed with specific functions, is interposed as a guardian between the digestive tract (and spleen) and the rest of the body. Because of its interposition, the liver is provided with a dual blood supply: it receives blood from the portal vein in addition to its vascularization by the hepatic artery. These channels import a large variety of endobiotics and xenobiotics, including nutrients as well as toxic substances derived from the digestive system. Hence, a major function of the liver involves efficient uptake of amino acids, carbohydrates, lipids, and vitamins and their subsequent storage, metabolic conversion, and release into the blood and bile. Equally important is hepatic biotransformation, which converts hydrophobic substances into water-soluble derivatives that can be excreted into bile or urine. Although biotransformation is a function of some other organs like the kidney and the gut, the liver takes the major share, rendering it the most "capitalistic" organ of the body (4). Because of its countless metabolic functions and secretions into the blood, the liver qualifies as a metabolic, and on occasion even as an endocrine, gland. At the same time, its bile production and secretion impose the organizational principles of an exocrine gland.

In addition, the liver is integrated into the body's complex system of defense against foreign macromolecules and particles such as bacteria. Accordingly, the cells of the hepatic capillary bed (see Sinusoidal Lining Cells, below) are quantitatively the most effective site of phagocytosis of particulate material (5). Further, the sponge-like structure

V. J. Desmet: Department of Pathology, Catholic University of Leuven, B-3000 Leuven, Belgium.

of the liver with large vascular capacity serves as a reservoir in the regulation of blood volume and flow through the body (6).

To meet specific demands, six specific principles govern the structure and function of the liver (5):

1. A double blood supply, mentioned above, including the portal system between two capillary beds (intestinal and hepatic). The liver-specific supply of splanchnic blood allows for the establishment of enterohepatic circulation of biliary solutes.
2. A unique architectural arrangement of hepatic parenchymal cells to facilitate maximal exchange between the blood and the hepatocytes (see Histology, below).
3. A peculiar texture of the perihepatocellular space, to optimize further metabolic exchange between blood and hepatocytes (see Extracellular Matrix in the Disse Space, below).
4. Specific biochemical composition and functional properties of hepatocellular organelles and plasma membranes, allowing for specific functions and interactions with blood and neighboring cells and matrix components.
5. Combined expression of exocrine secretory and metabolic functions in the same hepatic parenchymal cell.
6. Separation of a biliary compartment from the "milieu interne" to ensure an exocrine pathway.

These organizational principles result in the creation of a unique organ composed of a unique cell type with complex secretory polarity (see Hepatocyte, below).

PHYLOGENESIS

Both the structural principles and the unique demands made on the liver are reflected in hepatic phylogenesis and ontogenesis (5). Phylogenetically the liver is a very old organ, first appearing in Coelenterates (e.g., sea anemones), as a regional thickening of the entoderm or primordial gut serving metabolism and storage (7,8).

The liver developed into a morphologically identified organ, designated as midgut gland, when aquatic animals became terrestrial. The lack of an aquatic milieu, which facilitates exchanges, made homeostasis a problem, biotransformation essential, and immunologic reactivity more sophisticated (5). The liver became the central homeostatic organ for the main extracellular compartment of adult vertebrates (9).

An intriguing variability in liver structure, cell composition, and ultrastructural details is found between different animal species (10). In teleost fishes, the liver organ also comprises the pancreas arranged in strands within the portal tracts (hepatopancreas), with small acini emptying into the bile ducts (2,10). It is of interest that in higher vertebrates in which liver and pancreas are separate organs of common embryonic origin, under certain conditions the liver retains the capacity to form pancreatic tissue (11) and the pancreas to give rise to hepatocytes (12), and that peribiliary glands in human liver share with the pancreas the secretion of amylase and trypsin (13). Bile-secreting livers are present only in vertebrates (14).

EMBRYOLOGY (ALSO SEE CHAPTER 2)

In embryonal development, the yolk sac fulfills the early function of the liver; hence, the liver is a substitute yolk sac (2) and in every vertebrate, the liver develops in close association with the yolk sac.

A battery of liver-enriched transcription factors is expressed prior to the emergence of cells recognized to be committed to liver lineages and prior to liver organogenesis, suggesting a role for the expression of these genes in the determination of early liver cells (15).

In the human embryo, the liver bud or hepatic diverticulum arises on the 18th day of gestation as a thickening of the endoblastic epithelium in the ventral wall of the foregut (16). At this very early stage α-fetoprotein messenger RNA (mRNA) is expressed, indicating the commitment of this part of the ventral foregut to the lineage of liver cells and justifying their indication with the term *hepatoblasts* (17). The caudal part of the hepatic diverticulum gives rise to the common bile duct and gallbladder; the cranial part gives off irregular outgrowths of hepatoblasts that invade the septum transversum, a sheet of mesenchyme that separates the developing heart from the yolk sac. The liver precursor cells grow between small endothelium-lined spaces that connect with the capillary plexus of the vitelline (or omphalomesenteric) veins, thus establishing the basic architecture of liver parenchyma: parenchymal cords and plates alternating with hepatic sinusoids.

In the rat, translation of α-fetoprotein mRNA into the protein product is first detected when liver cords are being formed while albumin mRNA is detected 1 day later (17). Some controversy exists as to the arrangement of hepatoblasts in tubules or in several cell thick plates ("muralium multiplex") (18,19). The early hepatoblasts in humans are characterized by the expression of cytokeratins 8, 18, and 19, and have at least two developmental options (bipotential progenitor cells) (15,20).

The majority embarks upon the hepatocytic differentiation pathway and gradually loses cytokeratin 19 (21). Intercellular bile canaliculi, initially lined by several cells, appear from 7 to 8 weeks of gestation. Bile acid synthesis begins near week 12 (22). Bile acid transport capacity appears late in fetal development and increases dramatically in direct relationship with the expression of a 49-kd Na^+-dependent bile acid transport protein (23). In the initial phase hepatocyte-specific gene expression is subject to a complex regulation at the transcriptional and translational level (24), and is modulated by interactions between hepatoblasts and mesenchyme (25). For most enzymes, the heterogeneity between periportal and pericentral hepatocytes (see Parenchymal Heterogeneity, below) only gradually develops during early postnatal life. However, enzymes such as carbamoylphosphate synthetase and arginase reveal a heterogeneity related to the vascular architecture as early as 6 days before birth in the rat (26).

A minor part of the primitive hepatoblasts commits itself to the bile duct cell lineage. During the first 7 weeks of embryonic life, there are no intrahepatic bile ducts. The intrahepatic biliary tree develops in close association with the developing portal vein, starting around its largest branches close to the liver hilum. The hepatoblasts in contact with the mesenchyme that surrounds the portal vein ramifications develop into bile duct type cells, with increased expression of cytokeratins 8, 18, and 19, later on expression of cytokeratin 7, and additional biliary phenotypic markers (18,19). The initial cylinder of bile duct epithelium surrounding the portal vein (the ductal plate) is gradually remodeled into tubular ducts that become incorporated into the mesenchyme (27). The remodeling of the ductal plate starts near the hilum of the liver, and gradually extends toward the periphery as more peripheral ramifications of the portal vein with their surrounding ductal plates are formed. Preliminary evidence suggests an important role of the mesenchymal sleeve around the portal vein (the future portal tract) for the induction of biliary differentiation in the hepatoblasts of the ductal plate and its subsequent remodeling into tubular ducts (18,19). Lack of remodeling of the ductal plate results in the persistence of an excess of embryologic bile duct structures in ductal plate configuration. Such ductal plate malformation constitutes a basic structural component of all congenital diseases of intrahepatic bile ducts (28).

In short, intrahepatic bile ducts develop from hepatoblasts in contact with periportal mesenchyme during the whole period of fetal development, starting at the liver hilum, and extending toward the liver periphery. Complete maturation of the finest bile duct ramifications is not fully achieved at the time of birth, and requires some additional weeks during postnatal life in humans (27).

Initial hepatic sinusoids are lined by endothelium. Other cell types become identifiable during the third month of gestation. Kupffer cells appear to originate from primitive macrophages derived from the yolk sac that colonize the liver or may develop *in loco* from hematopoietic stem cells. Hepatic stellate cells (Ito cells) appear from 6 to 8 weeks' gestation (18).

The afferent vitelline veins eventually become the portal vein. The sinusoidal network is drained by confluent venous branches that develop into the hepatic veins. According to the hemodynamic theory (29) the portal and hepatic venous channels are induced by the flow of blood through the hepatic sinusoids. Intrahepatic lymphatics develop from the 15th week of gestation (30).

The embryonic liver is a hematopoietic organ. In human liver hematopoiesis starts at 5 to 6 weeks of gestation, reaches its maximum toward the 6th to 7th month, and then regresses to cease completely during the first week after birth (18,19). However, pluripotent hematopoietic stem cells may persist in the adult liver, as demonstrated in the mouse (31). There exists an intriguing relationship between hematopoietic stem cells and presumed hepatic progenitor cells (see Liver Stem Cells, below).

HISTOLOGY

At birth, the liver parenchymal cells are arranged in two-cell-thick plates (muralium duplex), which after the age of 5 years are converted in cell plates only one cell thick (muralium simplex) (2). Such arrangement maximizes contact between blood and hepatocytes.

In the past, several concepts of parenchymal architecture have prevailed. Gerlach proposed an arrangement in liver cords (cylinders formed of double rows of cells) in 1849. Modifications to accommodate kinks in canaliculi were those of Stöhr and Schultze in 1918, Braus in 1924, and McIndoe in 1928 (2). In 1866, Hering had proposed a continuous mass of liver cell plates, but his discovery remained ignored, until Elias rediscovered the hepatic muralium in 1948 (2). Since then, the muralium concept became universally accepted and beautifully confirmed by scanning electron microscopy (32,33).

The muralium simplex builds a sponge-like network of hepatocellular plates that anastomoses at different angles and surrounds the hepatic lacunae that harbor the sinusoids. The cell mass is traversed by two tracts of connective tissue that ramify within the liver. The wider one represents the portal tracts that carry afferent blood vessels, bile ducts, lymphatics, and nerves. The narrower one surrounds tributaries of draining hepatic veins. The two tracts interdigitate but do not connect (34), albeit with some portohepatic crossovers (35). In this way, the terminal branches of the afferent vessels are separated from hepatic vein tributaries by hepatic parenchyma and sinusoids.

Parenchymal blood flow depends in part on the pressure gradient between the terminal portal vein (estimated at 50 mL water) and the initial hepatic vein (approximately 10 mL water). Structural adaptations are present at many levels in the blood channels of the liver to constantly receive and release a large volume of circulating blood at low pressure. These histoarchitectonics provide hepatic hemodynamics with high capacitance and high compliance properties (35). Studies evaluating hepatic microcirculation by intravital microscopy suggest that hepatic stellate cells (HSCs) may be involved in the regulation of sinusoidal tone in normal liver (36) in spite of the fact that contractility is a feature of "activated," myofibroblast-like HSCs rather than quiescent HSCs of normal liver, which have a "storing" phenotype (35,37). This apparent paradox has been explained as follows. It appears that sinusoidal blood pressure normally distends the sinusoidal wall, which can recoil when the pressure drops. Presumably HSCs are responsible for this reaction (38). The direct targets of the hepatic artery are not the liver cells, but stromal compartments corresponding to the peribiliary vascular plexus, the portal tract interstitium, the portal vein vasa vasorum, the liver capsule, and the vasa vasorum of the draining hepatic veins (35,39).

HEPATOCYTE

The muralium simplex is built up by polygonal parenchymal cells or hepatocytes, which enclose a chicken-wire–like network of bile canaliculi in the central plane, and are flanked by sinusoids on both sides of the muralium (40). The equivalent of an apical pole for the exocrine secretion of bile by the hepatocyte corresponds to the canalicular membrane, which surrounds the parenchymal cell periphery in a belt-like fashion. This structural organization implies that the biliary secretory polarity of the hepatocyte is oriented toward a peripheral ring around the middle of the parenchymal cell. In contrast, metabolic uptake (and secretions) occur at (or toward) the surfaces facing the sinusoids, implying a bidirectional metabolic secretory activity. This complex secretory polarity requires a well-organized intracellular system for adequate and correct addressing of secretory products toward their respective destinations (41,42). As a metabolically highly active cell, the hepatocyte contains huge numbers of a vast array of organelles: 15% of the cell volume is for endoplasmic reticulum; it contains over 1,000 mitochondria, about 300 lysosomes, equal numbers of peroxisomes, some 50 Golgi complexes per cell (6,43), and a typically organized cytoskeleton (44). Liver parenchymal cells are not all equal to each other; but reveal considerable heterogeneity (see Parenchymal Heterogeneity, below).

A highly specific component of the liver parenchymal cell is its plasma membrane, which guarantees its separation from and at the same time its link with the environment of cells and matrix.

HEPATOCELLULAR PLASMA MEMBRANE (SEE CHAPTERS 6–8, 11, AND 26)

Three morphologically distinct and functionally different areas can be recognized in the hepatocellular plasma membrane: (a) the sinusoidal domain in contact with the space of Disse and indirectly with the bloodstream (37% of the parenchymal cell surface); (b) the intercellular domain or the hepatocyte-to-hepatocyte contact area (50% of the surface); and (c) the bile canalicular domain or the bile secretory pole ("apical" pole) of the hepatocyte (13% of the surface) (45).

The sinusoidal domain features irregular microvilli that increase the surface area of the cell available for exchange with the bloodstream (see Chapters 6 and 7). The microvilli are surrounded by the fluid and the matrix components of the space of Disse, and have easy access to the sinusoidal blood because of the peculiarities of the sinusoidal lining (see Sinusoidal Lining Cells, below). The sinusoidal membrane domain represents a cellular frontier with incredibly busy traffic of molecules from and toward the sinusoidal blood. It is the site of the sodium pump and organic ion and drug transporters (see Chapter 7) Receptors for glycoproteins, immunoglobulin A, asialoglycoprotein, various peptides and hormones, and growth factors are located in the sinusoidal domain; it is the site for fluid phase- and receptor-mediated endocytosis and transmembrane proteins ("integrins") which recognize specific matrix components laminin, collagen, and fibronectin. The $\alpha_3\beta_1$ integrin is a critical mediator of the hepatocellular differentiation response to the extracellular matrix (46) (see Chapter 34).

The intercellular domain is a region specialized in intercellular adhesion and intercellular communication. Intercellular attachment is assured by junctional complexes, comprising the tight junction, intermediate junction, and desmosomes. Intercellular communication occurs via gap junctions (see Chapter 3).

The parenchymal cell tight junctions are of particular interest with regard to bile secretion. They constitute the delicate canaliculo-sinusoidal barrier and represent part of the paracellular pathway in bile secretion, functioning as a bioelectrical barrier with selective permeability for cations (see Chapter 26).

The canalicular domain of the hepatocyte's plasma membrane has its own morphologic hallmarks and specialized functions (see Chapters 25 and 26). It is the seat of recently identified adenosine triphosphate (ATP)-dependent export pumps that assure unidirectional and concentrative transport, including the canalicular bile salt transporter (cBST), a multispecific canalicular organic anion transporter (cMOAT or isoform 2 of multidrug resistance protein, MRP2), the multidrug resistance protein MDR3, and the multidrug resistance protein 1 MDR1 (or P glycoprotein) (see Chapters 26–28 and 48).

With its highly specific domains, the hepatocellular plasma membrane reflects the polarity of the parenchymal cell (see Chapters 8 and 25). This polarity is disturbed in cholestasis, with shift of the bile salt export carrier to the basolateral membrane, and is decreased in case of chronic bile drainage.

The expression of various adhesion molecules on the hepatocellular membrane is markedly changed in inflammatory conditions (see Chapters 54 and 56). The phenotypic shift in hepatocellular expression of adhesion molecules and the secretion of (chemotactic) cytokines indicates that the parenchymal cell is not merely a passive target in cell-mediated immunologic target cell killing; instead, it seems to acquire the capacities of an antigen-presenting and immunomodulating cell (47).

Attention has been drawn to the cell volume as a new principle for control of hepatocellular metabolic functions and exocrine biliary secretion. Alterations in cell volume act like a second or third messenger mediating hormone effects (see Chapter 14).

SINUSOIDAL LINING CELLS (SEE CHAPTERS 30 AND 31)

The sinusoids are lined by a specific and characteristic set of cells, including sinusoidal endothelial cells, Kupffer cells, hepatic stellate cells, and Pit cells. In rat liver, also immune-associated (Ia) antigen–expressing dendritic cells were described.

The main structural characteristic of *sinusoidal endothelial cells* is the occurrence of fenestrae of about 1,000 Å diameter, grouped together in sieve plates (see Chapter 30). The diameter of the fenestrae, which controls the interchange between blood and perisinusoidal space, is influenced by endobiotics (hormones, neurotransmitters) and xenobiotics (ethanol, drugs), apparently via contraction of cytoskeletal components (48). Normal fenestral density and porosity require a complex perisinusoidal matrix containing basement membrane components, not provided by an interstitial collagen matrix and the presence of nearby parenchymal cells. Blood cells passing through the sinusoids may influence exchange through endothelial massage and forced sieving.

Endothelial cells were found to have numerous functions in various biologic reactions, including active transport, coagulation, fibrinolysis, inflammation, immune responses, regulation of blood pressure, angiogenesis, lipid metabolism, and synthesis of stromal components, similar to vascular endothelial cells in general (see Chapter 30). Nevertheless, liver sinusoidal endothelial cells differ from vascular endothelial cells (e.g., portal vein, central vein) in different respects (49).

Kupffer cells are stellate in shape and attached to the sinusoidal wall, but possibly migrating along the lumen (50). They function as a waste receptacle for all kinds of old, unnecessary, damaged, altered, or foreign material. Upon activation (e.g., zymosan or endotoxin uptake) they secrete a number of products with potent biologic effects, including proteases and cytokines with influence on parenchymal and other sinusoidal lining cells. The relationship between Kupffer cells and immunologically involved dendritic cells requires further clarification.

Hepatic stellate cells (HSCs) were originally identified by Von Kupffer in the 1870s, rediscovered by Ito and Nemoto in 1952, and confirmed in electron microscopy by Yama-

gishi in 1959 (see Chapter 32). The term *hepatic stellate cells* is a consensus term to replace the confusing terminology of the past (para- or perisinusoidal cells, Ito cells, fat storing cells, vitamin A storing cells, lipocytes, etc.). *Arachnocytes* is a later proposed competing term (35).

HSCs occupy a perisinusoidal location, with cytoplasmic extensions wrapped around the sinusoidal endothelial lining, comparable to pericytes in other locations. They represent the largest pool of retinol (retinyl esters) in the body. They transform via an intermediate phenotype into myofibroblast-like cells, expressing desmin and α-smooth muscle actin under a variety of stimuli. Quiescent HSCs *in vitro* undergo migration, augmented by their activation, and influenced by chemokines such as monocyte chemotactic protein-1. HSCs and their activated derivatives express neuroendocrine markers, including glial fibrillary acidic protein, neural cell adhesion molecule, the class VI intermediate filament protein nestin (51), and synaptophysin (52). Such characteristics raise the question of a possible neural crest origin of HSCs.

HSCs play a role in the maintenance of the extracellular matrix (ECM) by synthesis and secretion of its normal components and their degradation by proteases. Thus HSCs have four major functions in a normal liver: (a) production and maintenance of the ECM; (b) control of microvascular tone; (c) storage of retinoids; and (d) a role in the control of regeneration in the normal liver and in response to necrosis.

Together with other mesenchymal cells, HSCs are the main producers of ECM in hepatic fibrosis and cirrhosis, and may modulate chronic inflammation by secretion of cytokines and chemokines. They are capable of fine-tuning the wound-healing response in the liver, according to the duration, the type, and the amount of damage.

Pit cells, located on the endothelial lining, correspond to large granular lymphocytes with natural killer (NK) activity. They are well placed to play defensive roles against viral infection and tumor metastasis. The liver contains several unusual subtypes of T lymphocytes and NK-T cells, rendering the liver a unique immunologic environment and a tolerogenic organ where peripheral deletion of T lymphocytes occurs (53).

EXTRACELLULAR MATRIX IN THE DISSE SPACE (SEE CHAPTER 33)

The space of Disse is the perisinusoidal cleft between the sinusoidal lining and the liver cell plates. Its oldest known components are reticulin fibers, nerves, and HSCs. Transmission electron microscopy fails to identify a basement membrane, except in the liver of some species such as sheep. However, immunohistochemical investigations revealed a variety of matrix components in the space of Disse. Rather than being an empty space, it contains collagens type I, III,

IV, VI, fibronectin, undulin, trace amounts of collagen V and laminin, tenascin, proteoglycans, and the recently discovered nonfibrillar collagen XVIII (54). These matrix components are essential in maintaining the specific phenotype and function of hepatocytes and sinusoidal lining cells, and in modulating the activities of bound growth factors (55).

Newer technologies revealed that the reticulin fiber demonstrated by empiric silver impregnation correspond to collagen type III with attached fibronectin and glycoprotein, with collagen type I forming hybrid fibrils with type III. The proteoglycan components of the liver matrix form orderly three-dimensional supramolecular complexes with other matrix components.

STRUCTURAL AND FUNCTIONAL LIVER UNITS

Most glands are composed of repetitive units of glandular tissue. The quest for the grail of the structural/functional unit of the liver has continued for over 300 years, since Wepfer described the first liver units in 1664 (56). Based on his studies on the pig's liver, Kiernan described the classic hepatic lobule as the unit of liver tissue, with portal tracts in its periphery and the hepatic vein tributary in its center (the centrolobular vein) (57). However, typical lobules delineated by connective tissue septa are only found in adult (not suckling) pigs, polar bears, racoons, and, to a lesser degree, camels.

Brissaud and Sabourin (58) discovered in 1888 that, in the liver of the seal, a lobulation prevails in which liver cell plates and sinusoids radiate from the portal canals. Impressed by this observation, Mall (59) proposed his "portal" lobule as the basic structural unit of the liver, centered by a portal tract with draining hepatic vein tributaries at the periphery.

On the basis of vascular injection studies, Rappaport et al. (60) described his concept of the "liver acinus," with a hierarchic order of simple acini, complex acini, and acinar agglomerates. The simple acinus is defined as the clump of liver parenchyma vascularized by a terminal, distributory branch of the portal vein. The merit of Rappaport et al.'s concept lies in the fact that it draws attention to the terminal, distributory afferent vessels that branch off from the vessels in the preterminal portal tracts. The liver acinus has the terminal afferent vessels in its center; its sinusoids are drained by neighboring terminal hepatic venules. According to its proximity to the afferent vessels, the acinar parenchyma was arbitrarily divided into three zones: acinar zone 1 surrounding the afferent vessels in a bulb-like fashion and receiving blood rich in oxygen and nutrients, itself surrounded by an intermediate acinar zone 2, in turn surrounded by the acinar zone 3 or the microcirculatory periphery. The complex acinus of Rappaport is essentially a

refinement and modification of the portal lobule proposed by Mall. Although the acinar concept has gained wide popularity and features in most of today's textbooks, critical voices continued to be raised, emphasizing a hepatic lobular type of unit.

A more restricted area of hepatic tissue has been proposed as the functional unit by Bloch (56). This unit comprises an individual sinusoid with its contiguous hepatic tissue and its immediate afferent and efferent vascular, biliary, lymphatic, and neural connections. However, this unit is probably too restricted, since not all sinusoids receive direct connections from the hepatic artery, and the periphery of the unit would bisect parenchymal cells in mammals with one-cell-thick parenchymal plates. A somewhat comparable unit is the "perisinusoidal functional unit" of David and Reinke with the Disse space as the central playground.

Based on detailed angioarchitectural studies, another structural and functional unit of the liver was proposed by Matsumoto and Kawakani (61): the primary lobule. It can be viewed as a refinement of the classic hepatic lobule of Kiernan. Six to eight cone-shaped primary lobules make up one secondary lobule, corresponding to the classic lobule of Kiernan, whereby the inflow-fronts of the primary lobules are combined to form a closed surface covering the classic lobule. The inflow-fronts are formed by the terminal ("septal") ramifications of the afferent vessels, which empty into a labyrinthic network of sinusoids (the vascular septum); the latter extends between two adjacent preterminal (or conducting) portal tracts, appears as a sickle-shaped area on cross section, comprises a portal and a septal part, and creates an equipotential surface from which radial sinusoids run into a tributary of the hepatic vein.

The concept of the primary lobule received support from more recent histochemical studies, resulting in the "metabolic lobulus" (62). The essence of the concept implies—in contrast to Rappaport's acinar concept—that the periportal domains form a three-dimensional continuity, whereas the pericentral domains represent discrete branches. The metabolic lobular concept specifically applies to physiologic conditions, whereas in certain pathologic states the acinar concept seems to better delineate the boundaries of hepatic units.

A functional unit of liver tissue, proposed from the viewpoint of bile secretory function, is the choleon, which comprises the group of hepatocytes and their canaliculi, drained by a single ductule, in analogy with the glomerulus and tubuli that constitute the nephron in the kidney (63).

Ekataksin and Wake (64) demonstrated that the most terminal portal vessels (inlet venules) perfuse a preferred column of sinusoids that can be visualized as a conical structure, with a broader base at the lobular perimeter and a pointed end tapering toward the central vein. This pyramidal group of sinusoids is termed the hepatic microcirculatory subunit (HMS). These authors further showed that the first segment of the biliary passages (the canal of Her-

ing) and the inlet venule colocalize at the lobular periphery, and hence that the territory of intralobular bile canaliculi extending through the canal of Hering (a choleon) overlaps spatially with the corresponding HMS. The subpopulation of liver cells associated with an HMS is therefore equipped with all of the elementary structures that a liver unit needs to perform its dual exocrine-endocrine functions. Hence, this configuration was designated as the choleohepaton, to represent the most elementary morphofunctional unit of the liver: the smallest group of cells and sinusoids performing the endocrine (metabolic) duties of the liver, and at the same time the smallest group of hepatocytes secreting bile drained by a single canal of Hering. The choleohepaton is to be viewed as a subunit of the primary lobule; it has no clear anatomic borders and can only be visualized by meticulous investigation. For the histopathologist, the most important discussion about unit concepts concerns the classic lobule of Kiernan (or the secondary lobule according to Matsumoto) versus the acinus concept of Rappaport.

Studies in later years on angioarchitecture, three-dimensional reconstruction (65), histochemistry (62), and gradients in hepatic gene expression (66) all favor the lobular concept. The most important structural feature of Matsumoto's secondary lobule (or Kiernan's classic lobule) is that the central vein represents its longitudinal axis while the terminal branches of the portal vein form its periphery (67).

It is a sobering thought that after more than three centuries the debate on hepatic structural–functional units is still ongoing!

The human liver has no clear-cut boundaries delineating well-defined structural units, neither lobular (hepatic, portal, primary) nor acinar. The liver is an indivisible continuum that shows no anatomically definable units.

Nevertheless, hepatic angioarchitecture determines regional directions of blood flow and gradients in oxygen and nutrients in defined territories throughout the parenchymal continuum, resulting in metabolic heterogeneity of parenchymal cells with variability in the size of the "metabolic zones," which is pathway specific. It hence follows that angioarchitectural units are helpful in explaining the function of the organ including the reciprocity of antagonistic metabolic engagements of different parenchymal territories.

PARENCHYMAL HETEROGENEITY

Liver parenchymal cells, primarily responsible for hepatic metabolism, appear homogeneous only at a superficial glance through the light microscope. Closer analysis, and even more, histochemical, ultrastructural, and morphometric investigations reveal a striking heterogeneity. Originally merely descriptive, this heterogeneity received more functional interpretation in later years (68).

Heterogeneity of liver units can be demonstrated in different ways: zonality (nonhomogeneous characteristics along the portal–central axis); regionality [differences according to septal (interportal) or portal regions]; locality (referring to lobular shape variations according to subcapsular or deep locations); and laterality (indicating asymmetrical features of the left and right lobe of the liver).

The heterogeneity that has been most studied concerns zonality, and, to a lesser extent regionality, which have been recently summarized (69).

Hepatocytes reveal a remarkable heterogeneity along the portal–central axis of the lobule with respect to ultrastructure and enzyme activities, resulting in different cellular functions in different lobular zones. This resulted in the concept of "metabolic zonation," originally proposed for carbohydrate metabolism, and implying that opposite metabolic pathways such as gluconeogenesis and glycolysis are carried out simultaneously by hepatocytes in the periportal and centrolobular region, respectively. This solved the "glucose paradox" and makes the liver function as the "glucostat" of the organism.

Analogous reciprocal localizations in different lobular territories are observed for the enzymes of ammonia metabolism, with carbamoyl phosphate synthetase in the periportal zone and glutamine synthetase in a very narrow ring of centrolobular hepatocytes (70).

It appears that the concept of metabolic zonation is applicable to virtually all liver functions (e.g., xenobiotic metabolism; bile secretion; etc.) and reflects an interesting level of metabolic control. The topic has been reviewed elsewhere (71). Two types of zonal patterns of gene expression in the liver have been recognized: a gradient versus a compartment type zonation, and a dynamic versus stable type of zonation (72).

The mechanisms underlying heterogeneous gene expression are not well elucidated. Several hypotheses have been proposed to account for restrictions in the spectrum of genes that can be expressed: the differentiation hypothesis, the "streaming liver" hypothesis (now largely contradicted), and the cell-matrix hypothesis. However, at present, there is no evidence in favor of a restriction of the gene spectrum that can be expressed in one or another zone; instead, all hepatocytes appear to retain the capacity to express the same spectrum of genes. During liver development, the emergence of zonality is linked to the establishment of a lobular architectural framework.

Heterogeneity originates within the liver, probably produced by the hepatocytes themselves. The phenotype of upstream, periportal hepatocytes appears to be determined by the concentration of regulatory signals in the afferent blood, whereas the phenotype of the downstream, centrolobular hepatocytes is, additionally, determined by changes in blood composition as a result of metabolic and/or biosynthetic activity of the upstream hepatocytes (the upstream-downstream hypothesis). Among the circulating signals, oxygen is of special importance; it modulates hepatic metabolism acutely and gene expression chronically (73).

Teutsch et al. (65) have emphasized the importance of considering three-dimensionality for an adequate functional interpretation of the metabolic heterogeneity of hepatocytes, in order to avoid underestimation of periportal changes and overestimation of centrolobular events.

Parenchymal heterogeneity appears to be required for the regulatory "altruistic" functions of the organ as a metabolitostat. Loss of heterogeneity in cirrhotic nodules has been interpreted as a first step in the direction of "autistic" malignancy.

Not only parenchymal cells, but also sinusoids and their lining cells show zonal variations. Sinusoids in the lobular periphery are more narrow and tortuous with frequent intersinusoidal anastomoses, whereas they are of broader diameter, straighter course, and with less intersinusoidal sinusoids in midzonal and centrolobular territories. Furthermore, there are differences between portal and septal sinusoids according to Matsumoto's primary lobule.

Endothelial cells possess larger and more numerous pores in the centrolobular zone, assuring higher endothelial porosity in that area (see Chapter 30); they display differences in lectin-binding patterns and in production of reactive oxygen metabolites according to lobular zonation (74) and also differ in the expression of endothelial markers.

Kupffer cells are larger and more numerous and provided with larger lysosomes in the periportal area, corresponding with higher phagocytic potential and activity, whereas in the centrolobular areas they are smaller and more involved in cytokine production and cytotoxicity (75).

The perisinusoidal HSCs display marked heterogeneity in their zonal and regional distribution. Their desmin immunoreactivity and vitamin A content is higher in the periportal zone, whereas their thornlike microprojections prevail in the centrolobular area (76).

Also the biomatrix in the space of Disse reveals zonal variation (see Chapters 32 and 33). There is a shift from collagens type IV and V in the periportal to fibrillar collagens type I, III, and VI in the centrolobular zone. Periportally one finds laminin and heparan sulfate proteoglycan, whereas fibronectin, chondroitin sulfate, and dermatan sulfate proteoglycans prevail in the center of the lobule. In the latter zone, the matrix chemistry (fibrillar collagens, fibronectin, and proteoglycans) is similar to that typically produced by mesenchymal cells.

BILE DUCT EPITHELIAL CELLS

Bile duct epithelial cells (BECs) have long been the neglected party in the liver, only receiving appropriate attention after many years of primary interest in hepatocytes and sinusoidal lining cells; today, they represent a new chapter in cell biology (77) (see Chapter 29). The exocrine secretion of the hepatocytes (bile) is drained by a system of channels that starts inside the parenchymal lobules with the canals of Hering followed by the finer and larger branches of the intrahepatic and extrahepatic portions of the bile draining system or the biliary tree (78). The channels are lined by bile duct epithelial cells. Although derived from common embryologic progenitor cells, the BECs differ from hepatocytes in phenotype and function.

The most striking differences with hepatocytes include smaller numbers of mitochrondria and less extensive endoplasmic reticulum, a more strongly developed network of intermediate cytoskeletal filaments (cytokeratins), and the presence of a basement membrane. BECs are characterized by the expression of several molecules that are absent in parenchymal liver cells, and that are used as "markers" of BECs. The most popular markers at present include cytokeratins 7 and 19, epithelial membrane antigen, carcinoembryonic antigen, carbonic anhydrase, and γ-glutamyltranspeptidase. It is of interest that BECs do not constitute a homogeneous cell population. They reveal marked heterogeneity along the course of the biliary passageways from the finest intrahepatic branches down to the larger extrahepatic ducts (79).

Although BECs represent only a minority (3% to 5%) of the total cell population of the liver, they subserve important physiologic functions. BECs modify the composition of bile by secretion of water, proteins, and bicarbonate, and reabsorption of glucose, glutamate, anions, and proteins (80). They are the site of bile acid uptake with associated cholehepatic cycling, resulting in choleresis and bicarbonate secretion after injection of dihydroxy bile acids.

BECs exhibit a lack of cytochrome P-450–dependent monooxygenase activities, but possess a number of distinct phase II conjugating enzymes; this "resistance phenotype" would provide BECs with survival advantage in hepatotoxic or hepatocarcinogenic environments.

BECs are the targets of autoimmune inflammatory destruction, and actively participate in the immune response by the expression of adhesion molecules and secretion of cytokines (81,82).

An important aspect of BECs is their role in fibrogenesis during chronic cholestatic liver diseases, as has been emphasized for many years. The contribution of BECs to periductular and periportal fibrosis is gradually becoming detailed by their synthesis of collagens type IV and V, laminin, integrins, syndecans, inhibitors of proteases, expression of transforming growth factors β_1 and β_2 (83), and chemotactic attraction of HSCs by their secretion of chemokine MCP-1 (84).

The interlobular bile ducts are surrounded by a single- or double-layered peribiliary capillary plexus derived from the hepatic artery, and draining into adjacent sinusoids and interlobular branches of the portal vein. Both routes warrant the designation of "peribiliary portal system," and presumably allow BEC-derived products to reach and influence the downstream hepatocytes and nonparenchymal cells.

The development of more refined techniques for isolation and culture is opening new perspectives for detailed study of the physiology and pathophysiology of BECs (see Chapter 29).

LIVER STEM CELLS

A most intriguing aspect of BECs is that they appear to harbor a compartment of stem cells for the liver, presumably located within the most terminal bile duct ramifications or canals of Hering, with a phenotype resembling small cholangiocytes (85) (see Chapter 29). The liver stem cell concept implies that putative progenitor cells may become activated to proliferate and differentiate along different lineages (e.g., hepatocyte, biliary epithelial cell, intestinal cell, pancreatic acinar cell) (86).

The concept still raises debate, since there is no obvious need for liver stem cells, as differentiated hepatocytes [especially smaller ones (87)] can swiftly assure regeneration after partial hepatectomy or pathologic tissue loss. Transplanted hepatocytes can cycle sufficient times (at least 100 rounds) to repopulate the organ (88). Therefore, the concept has been redefined as "facultative stem cells," taking over the task of liver regeneration in case of paralysis of hepatocellular division. The concept arose mainly from studies in carcinogenic and noncarcinogenic damage to rodent livers in which these so-called oval cells are repeatedly found to co-proliferate with HSC, apparently mutually interacting through reciprocal growth factors and growth factor receptors.

However, there is a growing body of evidence that the concept may also apply to human liver (see Chapters 42 and 61). Of interest is the observation that reactive bile ductules proliferating in cholestatic liver disease and in submassive liver necrosis exhibit a neuroendocrine phenotype, including electron-dense cored vesicles at ultrastructural investigation. They show immunoreactivity for parathyroid hormone–related peptide, a factor influencing growth and differentiation. Furthermore, a novel epithelial cell type with close resemblance to oval cells in rats, and with apparent differentiation options into parenchymal and biliary type cells, was detected by ultrastructural investigation in human liver specimens, and may be at the origin of rare tumors with progenitor cell phenotype and rapidly fatal evolution (89).

Definite confirmation of a progenitor cell in human liver, and knowledge of the factors governing its proliferation and differentiation commitments along parenchymal and biliary lineages, will be of paramount importance for the elucidation of basic biologic processes like regeneration and neoplasia (see Chapter 68).

It is further possible that such cells, located in a periportal niche, in or near canals of Hering, play some still unrecognized role in normal function and homeostasis of the liver, a concept supported by emerging insights into the paracrine functions of stem-like cells of other tissues (15).

The stem cell story took a surprising turn in recent years. Remarkably, a set of hematopoietic precursor markers (c-Kit, CD33, CD34, and Thy-1) appear to be shared by embryonic bile duct precursor cells (90,91), whereas rat oval cell antigens (OC2 and OC3) were also found on hematopoietic precursor cells (92), suggesting a close relationship between hepatic and hematic precursors.

Later studies added a new dimension by demonstrating that bone marrow–derived progenitor cells may give rise to hepatocytes (93,94) suggesting the existence of additional sources of hepatic stem cells outside the canals of Hering: the adult liver retains remnants of a hematopoietic environment from embryonic times, and bone marrow itself may be a site of liver progenitor cells (95).

Alchemists of olden times would jubilate when reading present-day reports on turning blood into liver (95) and brain into blood (96).

The new turn in the hepatic stem cell saga tells us that the differentiation potential of stem cells in adult tissues is much broader than thought by traditional dogma. Such reactivation of dormant genetic programs is complementary to the demonstration of conserved genomic totipotentiality in adult somatic cells (96) as shown by the cloning of an adult ewe (97).

The discovery that tissue resident stem cells are endowed with the appropriate machinery for expressing an otherwise silent genomic potentiality in response to an appropriate pattern of stimulation has promising implications for new treatments of human disease (95,96).

BIOECOLOGY AND SOCIOLOGY OF LIVER CELLS

The unique juxtaposition of diverse cell populations and matrix components in harmony with the angioarchitecture results in a delicate bioecologic system. Hepatologic research of recent years has provided and continues to provide amazing new insights into the interactions and feedback loops between the different cell types and matrix components of the organ, building up a new science of hepatic bioecology and sociology of liver cells. Examples include multiple metabolic interactions and numerous cytokine networks, and the diversity and complexity of parenchymal and nonparenchymal cell interactions.

Well-coordinated interactions between hepatocytes include (a) the reciprocal pathways localized in different lobular territories for carbohydrate and ammonia metabolism; (b) the cell-to-cell communication via gap junctions, assuring teamwork among hepatocytes; for instance, a complex interaction between gap junctional coupling, sufficient agonist stimulation of each hepatocyte, and individual cell uniqueness in response rate (promoting different hepatocytes to "pacemakers" for various agonists) provides the liver lobule with a "collective intelligence" allowing it to assure a unified response to a hormonal stimulus (98,99); and (c) the intercellular signals through surface molecules (100).

Hepatocyte–Kupffer cell interactions are so manifold that entire volumes are devoted to this subject (101). Notorious examples include vitamin A metabolism, the acutephase reaction, activation of hepatic stellate cells, and hepatocyte proliferation control by cytokines produced by nonparenchymal cells (Kupffer cells and/or endothelial and/or HSC).

Hepatocyte–endothelial interactions involve modulation of the sinusoidal endothelial phenotype by hepatocytes and endothelial production of prostaglandins, endothelin, interleukin-6, and hepatocyte growth factor (HGF). Hepatocyte–HSC signaling comprises peptides released from parenchymal cells (hepitoin) that stimulate HSCs, and cytokines from HSCs that inhibit hepatocellular proliferation (transforming growth factor-β) as well as cytokines that stimulate parenchymal proliferation (HGF) (see Chapters 40 and 41). Transforming growth factor-β_1 may be the elusive hepatic chalone. There may be mutual dialogue between hepatocytes and HSCs. Insulin-like growth factor-I (IGF-I) and IGF-I–independent factors from hepatocytes can stimulate HGF production by HSCs, and thus hepatocyte-derived factors may indirectly affect hepatocytes via a paracrine loop.

Hepatocyte-matrix interactions rely on adhesion molecules and on integrin and nonintegrin matrix receptors, on the propensity of the matrix to act as a reservoir and presenter of cell growth factors and cytokines, and on matrix turnover and its modification (be it by hepatocytes or other liver cells) (see Chapters 32 and 33). Particular integrins, like the laminin receptor $\alpha_3\beta_1$ integrin, may play a predominant role in hepatocellular differentiation.

Kupffer cells adhere to endothelial cells through the endothelial surface molecules CD4 and intercellular adhesion molecule-1 (ICAM-1) and initiate activation of HSCs.

Endothelial cells produce the endogenous signaling molecule nitric oxide (NO) by their endothelial constitutive NO synthase (eNOS), thereby contributing to sinusoidal perfusion and providing antiinflammatory and antithrombotic effects (see Chapter 31). The inducible or inflammatory nitric oxide synthase (iNOS), increased in response to inflammation and oxidative stress, is expressed not only in endothelial cells, but also in hepatocytes, HSCs, and cholangiocytes, resulting in chaotic quantities of NO that may be injurious to hepatic cells (see Chapter 31).

HSCs play a primordial role in liver fibrogenesis, and are modulated in this cascade-like progressive process by damaged hepatocytes, Kupffer cells, endothelial cells, platelets, and inflammatory cells. HSCs interact with inflammatory cells through expression of adhesion molecules, secretion of chemokines and cytokines, and hence play regulatory roles in liver inflammation. It looks as if HSCs first participate in the recruitment of inflammatory cells, and then predominantly contribute to the reparative phase of wound healing through extracellular matrix production, assuring a finetuning of the wound-healing response according to the duration, the type, and the amount of damage. A newly described function of HSCs is their role in liver morphogenesis through a morphogenic protein termed epimorphin (102).

The matrix in the space of Disse influences the phenotype and function of endothelial cells, HSCs, and hepatocytes (see Chapters 32 and 33). Laminin, for instance, induces tube formation in cultured endothelial cells. Furthermore, the composition of the matrix at specific points is crucial for finer modulation of intercellular signaling. The extracellular matrix is fundamental in hepatic development, regeneration, and maintenance of the liver architecture in the normal differentiated state (103,104).

Nerve fibers contact virtually every parenchymal cell and influence its metabolic activity (105). Metabolites, hormones, and cytokines from the sinusoidal blood influence parenchymal and sinusoidal cell activity, according to lobular gradients and density of cellular receptors.

Bile duct epithelial cells (BECs) or cholangiocytes are influenced by hepatocytes in a downstream paracrine fashion; adenosine nucleotides, apparently of hepatocellular origin, are present in bile, and BECs lining the bile ducts carry apical purinergic receptors (see Chapter 28).

BECs may also influence differentiated hepatocellular function through direct contact, through the peribiliary portal system, through cholehepatic cycling, and through release of interleukin-6, tumor necrosis factor-α, and hepatocyte growth factor (see Chapter 29).

Each cell type of the liver interacts with all the others and with the extracellular matrix, so that the functional activity of each cell is constantly influenced by the metabolic activity of the others. At the end, liver function is the result of a great number of complex interactions. If any cell fails, the performance of the others is affected. For this reason, the liver is to be considered as a bioecologic system, in which the components maintain homeostasis through constant mutual communication.

Pathologic conditions such as fibrosis and cirrhosis reflect disturbances in the harmonious equilibrium of the innumerable cellular interactions and cytokine networks, whereas uncontrolled cell growth in neoplasia reflects a breakdown of liver cell sociology.

In pathologic conditions, liver cell death occurs in different ways, with mitochondria as the integrators of signals for life or death, with as possible options for dying conspicuous murder (necrosis) or discreet suicide (apoptosis) (see Chapter 13). Imaginative scientists recognize in drug-induced liver disease: "euthanasia" of hepatocytes by cytotoxic lymphocytes, altruistic suicide of potential murderers carrying DNA mutations, and fratricidal killing of hepatocytes in case of oxidative stress.

The known repertoire of liver cell activities collectively termed "liver function" is unbelievably complex. Nonetheless, additional surprises still cause wonderment today. Recently, homeostatic control of angiogenesis was suggested as a newly identified function of the liver (106). Of interest is the "tinkerer" aspect of the story, in that degradation fragments of well-known liver proteins (plasminogen and collagen XVIII) perform the job as biologic response modifiers (angiostatin, endostatin) endowed with functions that appear to be completely different from those of the parent molecule. For sure, the liver holds still more surprise in petto!

Impressive progress has been achieved in recent years in liver physiology, pathology, and therapy. Biology and pathobiology of the liver benefit from the startling progress in molecular biology.

The third millennium starts with the imminent completion of the Human Genome Project, 20th century biology's equivalent of Mendeleyev's periodic table, with genomics and proteinomics realizing breathtaking progress in biologic sciences (107,108). The actual discovery of this genetic "terra incognita" has jolted biology much as the discovery of America jolted Europe 500 years ago, showing us how much of the world is still beyond the frontier—mysterious, tantalizing, and unexplored (109).

The next great challenge is to convert data into information and information into knowledge (110) and to discern the underlying order (108).

With the introduction of sophisticated laboratory instrumentation, robotics, and large, complex data sets, biomedical research is increasingly becoming a cross-disciplinary endeavor requiring the collaboration of biologists, engineers, software and database designers, physicists, and mathematicians (110). The centrifugal explosion of subdisciplines generating their own concepts, languages, and idioms increases the risk of a scientific Tower of Babel.

In hepatology, and medicine in general, there is a growing need to bridge the gap between basic science and clinical practice. This book serves just that purpose, conscious of the fact that "Vieles ist bekannt, aber leider in verschiedenen Köpfen" (W. Kollath) ("Much is known, but unfortunately in different heads").

REFERENCES

1. Bismuth H. Surgical anatomy and anatomical surgery of the liver. In: Blumgart LH, ed. *Surgery of the liver and biliary tract.* Edinburgh: Churchill Livingstone, 1988:1–9.
2. Elias H, Sherrick JC, eds. *Morphology of the liver.* New York: Academic Press, 1969.
3. Dawson JL, Tan KC. Anatomy of the liver. In: Millward-Sadler GH, Wright R, Arthur MJP, eds. *Wright's liver and biliary disease. Pathophysiology, diagnosis and management,* 3rd ed, vol 1. London: WB Saunders, 1992:3–11.
4. Berk PD, Potter BJ, Stremmel W. The sinusoidal surface of the hepatocyte: a dynamic plasma membrane specialized for high volume molecular transit. In: Reutter W, Popper H, Arias IM, et al., eds. *Modulation of liver cell expression.* Lancaster: MTP Press, 1987:107–125.
5. Popper H. Introduction: organizational principles. In: Arias IM, Jakoby WB, Popper H, et al., eds. *The liver: biology and pathobiology,* 2nd ed. New York: Raven Press, 1988:3–6.
6. Miyai K. Structural organization of the liver. In: Meeks RG, Harrison SD, Bull RJ, eds. *Hepatotoxicology.* Boca Raton: CRC Press, 1991:1–65.
7. Popper H. Hepatology in the next seventy-five years. In: Berk PD, Chalmers TC, eds. *Frontiers in liver disease.* New York: Thieme Stratton, 1981:336–339.
8. Cornelius CE. Hepatic ontogenesis. *Hepatology* 1985;5: 1213–1221.
9. Schreiber G, Aldred AR. Gene activity and regulation. In: Le Bouton AV, ed. *Molecular and cell biology of the liver.* Boca Raton: CRC Press, 1993:3–29.
10. Beresford WA, Henninger JM. A tabular comparative histology of the liver. *Arch Histol Jpn* 1986;49:267–281.
11. Rao MS, Bendayan M, Kimbrough RD, Reddy JK. Characterization of pancreatic-type tissue in the liver of rat induced by polychlorinated biphenyls. *J Histochem Cytochem* 1986;34: 197–201.
12. Rao MS, Dwivedi RS, Yeldandi AV, et al. Role of periductal and ductular epithelial cells of the adult rat pancreas in pancreatic hepatocyte lineage. A change in the differentiation commitment. *Am J Pathol* 1989;134:1069–1086.
13. Terada T, Nakanuma Y. Immunohistochemical demonstration of pancreatic alpha-amylase and trypsin in intrahepatic bile ducts and peribiliary glands. *Hepatology* 1991;14:1129–1135.
14. Vassy J, Kraemer M. Fetal and postnatal growth. In: Le Bouton AV, ed. *Molecular and cell biology of the liver.* Boca Raton: CRC Press, 1993:265–307.
15. Coleman WB, Grisham JW. Epithelial stem-like cells of the rodent liver. In: Strain A, Diehl AM, eds. *Liver growth and repair.* London: Chapman & Hall, 1998:50–99.
16. Dubois AM. The embryonic liver. In: Rouiller C, ed. *The liver.* New York: Academic Press, 1963:1–39.
17. Shiojiri N, Lemire JM, Fausto N. Cell lineages and oval cell progenitors in rat liver development. *Cancer Res* 1991;51: 2611–2620.
18. Desmet VJ. Embryology of the liver and intrahepatic biliary tract, and an overview of malformations of the bile duct. In: Bircher J, Benhamou J-P, McIntyre N, et al., eds. *Oxford textbook of clinical hepatology.* 2nd ed, vol. 1. Oxford: Oxford University Press, 1999:51–61.
19. Roskams T, Van Eyken P, Desmet V. Human liver growth and development. In: Strain A, Diehl AM, eds. *Liver Growth and Repair.* London: Chapman & Hall, 1998:541–557.
20. Marceau N, Blouin MJ, Noël M, et al. The role of bipotential progenitor cells in liver ontogenesis and neoplasia. In: Sirica AE, ed. *The role of cell types in hepatocarcinogenesis.* Boca Raton: CRC Press, 1992:121–149.
21. Desmet VJ, Van Eyken P, Sciot R. Cytokeratins for probing cell lineage relationships in developing liver. *Hepatology* 1990;12: 1249–1251.
22. Suchy FJ, Bucuvalas JC, Novak DA. Determinants of bile formation during development: ontogeny of hepatic bile acid metabolism and transport. *Semin Liver Dis* 1987;7:77–84.
23. Von Dippe P, Levy D. Expression of the bile acid transport protein during liver development and in hepatoma cells. *J Biol Chem* 1990;265:5942–5945.
24. Van Roon MA, Aten JA, Van Oven CH, Charles R, Lamers WH. The initiation of hepatocyte-specific gene expression within embryonic hepatocytes is a stochastic event. *Dev Biol* 1989;136:508–516.
25. Reif S, Terranova VP, El-Bendary M, Lebenthal E, Petelll JK. Modulation of extracellular matrix proteins in rat liver during development. *Hepatology* 1990;12:519–525.

26. Gaasbeek JW, Westenend PJ, Charles R, et al. Gene expression in derivatives of embryonic foregut during prenatal development of the rat. *J Histochem Cytochem* 1988;36:1223–1230.

27. Van Eyken P, Sciot R, Callea F, et al. The development of the intrahepatic bile ducts in man: a keratin-immunohistochemical study. *Hepatology* 1988;8:1586–1595.

28. Desmet VJ. Congenital diseases of intrahepatic bile ducts: variations on the theme "ductal plate malformation." *Hepatology* 1992;16:1069–1083.

29. Lassau JP, Bastian D. Organogenesis of the venous structures of the human liver: a hemodynamic theory. *Anat Clin* 1983;5:97–102.

30. Verbeke C, Buyssens N. Intrahepatic lymphatics in the human fetus. *Lymphology* 1990;23:36–38.

31. Taniguchi T, Toyoshima T, Fukao K, et al. Presence of hematopoietic stem cells in the adult liver. *Nat Med* 1996;2:198–203.

32. Grisham JW, Nopanitaya W, Compagno J. Scanning electron microscopy of the liver: a review of methods and results. In: Popper H, Schaffner F, eds. *Progress in liver diseases*, vol. 5. New York: Grune and Stratton, 1976:1–23.

33. Motta P. The three dimensional microanatomy of the liver. *Arch Histol Jpn* 1984;47:1–30.

34. Takahashi T. Lobular structure of the human liver from the viewpoint of hepatic vascular architecture. *Tohoku J Exp Med* 1970;101:119–140.

35. Ekataksin W, Kaneda K. Liver microvascular architecture: an insight into the pathophysiology of portal hypertension. *Semin Liver Dis* 1999;19:359–382.

36. Clemens MG, Zhang JX. Regulation of sinusoidal perfusion: in vivo methodology and control by endothelins. *Semin Liver Dis* 1999;19:383–396.

37. Pinzani M, Gentilini P. Biology of hepatic stellate cells and their possible relevance in the pathogenesis of portal hypertension in cirrhosis. *Semin Liver Dis* 1999;19:397–410.

38. McCuskey RS. Morphological mechanisms for regulating blood flow through hepatic sinusoids. *Liver* 2000;20:3–7.

39. Ekataksin W. The isolated artery: an intrahepatic arterial pathway that can bypass the lobular parenchyma in mammalian livers. *Hepatology* 2000;31:269–279.

40. Desmet VJ. Anatomy I: hepatocyte—canaliculus. In: Bianchi L, Gerok W, Sickinger K, eds. *Liver and Bile*. Lancaster: MTP Press, 1977; 3–31.

41. Desmet VJ. The hepatocyte: structural specialization and functional integration. In: Molino G, Avagnina P, eds. *Systematic and quantitative hepatology. Pathophysiological and methodological aspects*. Milano: Masson, 1990:43–50.

42. Desmet VJ. Modulation of the liver in cholestasis. *J Gastroenterol Hepatol* 1992;7:313–323.

43. Reddy JK, Rao MS. Hepatic ultrastructure and adaptation. In: Farber E, Phillips MJ, Kaufman N, eds. *Pathogenesis of liver diseases*. Baltimore: Williams and Wilkins, 1987:11–42.

44. Feldmann G. The cytoskeleton of the hepatocyte. Structure and functions. *J Hepatol* 1989;8:380–386.

45. Weibel ER, Stäubli W, Gnägi HR, et al. Correlated morphometric and biochemical studies on the liver cell. I. Morphometric model, stereologic methods, and normal morphometric data for rat liver. *J Cell Biol* 1969;42:68–91.

46. Lora JM, Rowader KE, Soares L, et al. Alpha (3) beta (1)-integrin as a critical mediator of the hepatic differentiation response to the extracellular matrix. *Hepatology* 1998;28:1095–1104.

47. Adams DH. Lymphocyte-endothelial cell interactions in hepatic inflammation. *Hepatogastroenterology* 1996;43:32–43.

48. Arias IM. The biology of hepatic endothelial cell fenestrae. In: Popper H, Schaffner F, eds. *Progress in liver diseases*, vol 9. Philadelphia: WB Saunders, 1990:11–26.

49. Yokota S. Functional differences between sinusoidal endothelial cells and intralobular or central vein endothelium in rat liver. *Anat Rec* 1985;212:74–80.

50. MacPhee PJ, Schmidt EE, Groom AC. Evidence for Kupffer cell migration along liver sinusoids, from high-resolution in vivo microscopy. *Am J Physiol* 1992;236:G17–G23.

51. Niki T, Pekny M, Hellemans K, et al. Class VI intermediate filament protein nestin is induced during activation of rat hepatic stellate cells. *Hepatology* 1999;29:520–527.

52. Cassiman D, Van Pelt J, De Vos R, et al. Synaptophysin: a novel marker for human and rat hepatic stellate cells. *Am J Pathol* 1999;155:1831–1839.

53. Crispe IN. The liver: a unique immunologic environment. In: Boyer JL, Ockner RK, eds. *Progress in liver diseases*, vol 15. Philadelphia: WB Saunders, 1997:109–124.

54. Musso O, Rehn M, Saarela J, et al. Collagen XVIII is localized in sinusoids and basement membrane zones and expressed by hepatocytes and activated stellate cells in fibrotic human liver. *Hepatology* 1998;28:98–107.

55. Schuppan D, Schmid M, Somasundaram R, et al. Collagens in the liver extracellular matrix bind hepatocyte growth factor. *Gastroenterology* 1998;114:139–152.

56. Bloch EH. The termination of hepatic arterioles and the functional unit of the liver as determined by microscopy of the living organ. *Ann NY Acad Sci* 1970;170:78–87.

57. Kiernan F. The anatomy and physiology of the liver. *Philos Trans R Soc Lond* 1833;123:711–770.

58. Brissaud E, Sabourin C. Sur la constitution lobulaire du foie et les voies de la circulation sanguine intra-hépatique. *C R Soc Biol* 1888;40:757–762.

59. Mall FP. A study of the structural unit of the liver. *Am J Anat* 1906;5:227–308.

60. Rappaport AM, Borowy ZJ, Lougheed WM, et al. Subdivision of hexagonal liver lobules into a structural and functional unit. Role in hepatic physiology and pathology. *Anat Rec* 1954;119:11–34.

61. Matsumoto R, Kawakami M. The unit-concept of hepatic parenchyma—a re-examination based on angioarchitectural studies. *Acta Pathol Jpn* 1982;32:285–314.

62. Lamers WH, Hilberts A, Furt E, et al. Hepatic enzymic zonation: a reevaluation of the concept of the liver acinus. *Hepatology* 1989;10:72–76.

63. Hofmann AF. The cholehepatic circulation of unconjugated bile acids: an update. In: Paumgartner G, Stiehl A, Gerok W, eds. *Bile acids and the hepatobiliary system. From basic science to clinical practice*. Dordrecht: Kluwer Academic Publishers, 1993:143–160.

64. Ekataksin W, Wake K. New concepts in biliary and vascular anatomy of the liver. In: Boyer JL, Ockner RK, eds. *Progress in liver diseases*, vol. XV. Philadelphia: WB Saunders, 1997:1–30.

65. Teutsch HF, Schuerfeld D, Groezinger E. Three-dimensional reconstruction of parenchymal units in the liver of the rat. *Hepatology* 1999;29:494–505.

66. Lamers WH, Geerts WJC, Jonker A, et al. Quantitative graphical description of porto-central gradients in hepatic gene expression by image analysis. *Hepatology* 1997;26:398–406.

67. Saxena R, Theise ND, Crawford JM. Microanatomy of the human liver—exploring the hidden interfaces. *Hepatology* 1999;30:1339–1346.

68. Jungermann K, Katz N. Functional specialization of different hepatocyte populations. *Physiol Rev* 1989;69:708–764.

69. Vidal-Vanaclocha F, ed. *Functional heterogeneity of liver tissue: from cell lineage diversity to sublobular compartment-specific pathogenesis*. Austin: R.G. Landes, 1997.

70. Häussinger D. Nitrogen metabolism in liver: structural and functional organization and physiological relevance. *Biochem J* 1990;267:281–290.

71. Kietzmann T, Jungermann K. Metabolic zonation of liver parenchyma and its short-term and long-term regulation. In: Vidal-Vanaclocha F, ed. *Functional heterogeneity of liver tissue.* Austin: R.G. Landes, 1997:1–42.

72. Christoffels VM, Sassi H, Ruijter JM, Moorman AFM, Grange T, Lamers WH. A mechanistic model for the development and maintenance of portocentral gradients in gene expression in the liver. *Hepatology* 1999;29:1180–1192.

73. Jungermann K, Kietzmann T. Oxygen: modulator of metabolic zonation and disease of the liver. *Hepatology* 2000;31:255–260.

74. Vidal-Vanaclocha F. The hepatic sinusoidal endothelium: functional aspects and phenotypic heterogeneity. In: Vidal-Vanaclocha F, ed. *Functional heterogeneity of liver tissue.* Austin: R.G. Landes, 1997:69–107.

75. Laskin DL. Role of hepatic macrophages in inflammation and tissue injury. In: Vidal-Vanaclocha F, ed. *Functional heterogeneity of liver tissue.* Austin: R.G. Landes, 1997:161–176.

76. Wake K. Sinusoidal structure and dynamics. In: Vidal-Vanaclocha F, ed. *Functional heterogeneity of liver tissue.* Austin: R.G. Landes, 1997:57–67.

77. Alvaro D. Biliary epithelium: a new chapter in cell biology. *Ital J Gastroenterol Hepatol* 1999;31:78–83.

78. Desmet VJ, Roskams T, De Vos R. Normal Anatomy. In: Feldman M, ed. *Gastroenterology and hepatology: the comprehensive visual reference: vol. 6: gallbladder and bile ducts,* LaRusso N, ed. Philadelphia: Current Medicine, 1997:1.1–1.29.

79. Lakehal F, Wendum D, Barbu V, et al. Phase I and phase II drug-metabolizing enzymes are expressed and heterogeneously distributed in the biliary epithelium. *Hepatology* 1999;30:1498–1506.

80. Baiocchi L, Le Sage G, Glaser S, et al. Regulation of cholangiocyte bile secretion. *J Hepatol* 1999;31:179–191.

81. Adams DH. Biliary epithelial cells: innocent victims or active participants in immune-mediated liver disease? *J Lab Clin Med* 1996;128:528–530.

82. Vierling JM. Immunology of acute and chronic hepatic allograft rejection. *Liver Transplant Surg* 1999;5 (suppl 1):S1–S20.

83. Desmet VJ, Roskams T, Van Eyken P. Pathology of the biliary tree in cholestasis: ductular reaction. In: Manns MP, Boyer JL, Jansen PLM, et al., eds. *Cholestatic liver diseases.* Lancaster: Kluwer Academic, 1998:143–154.

84. Morland CM, Fear J, McNab G, Joplin R, et al. Promotion of leukocyte transendothelial cell migration by chemokines derived from human biliary epithelial cells in vitro. *Proc Assoc Am Physicians* 1997;109:1–11.

85. Theise ND, Saxena R, Portmann BC, et al. The canals of Hering and hepatic stem cells in humans. *Hepatology* 1999;30:1425–1433.

86. Grisham JW, Thorgeirsson SS. Liver stem cells. In: Potten CS, ed. *Stem cells.* London: Academic Press, 1997:233–282.

87. Tateno C, Takai-Kajihara K, Yamasaki C, et al. Heterogeneity of growth potential of adult rat hepatocytes in vitro. *Hepatology* 2000;31:65–74.

88. Grompe M, Laconi E, Shafritz DA. Principles of therapeutic liver repopulation. *Semin Liver Dis* 1999;19:7–14.

89. Robrechts C, De Vos R, Van den Heuvel M, et al. Primary liver tumour of intermediate (hepatocyte-bile duct cell) phenotype: a progenitor cell tumor? *Liver* 1998;18:288–293.

90. Blakolmer K, Jaskiewicz K, Dunsford HA, Robson SC. Hematopoietic stem cell markers are expressed by ductal plate and bile duct cells in developing human liver. *Hepatology* 1995; 21:1510–1516.

91. Petersen BE, Goff JP, Greenberger JS, et al. Hepatic oval cells express the hematopoietic stem cell marker Thy-1 in the rat. *Hepatology* 1998;27:433–445.

92. Sigal SH, Brill S, Reid LM, et al. Characterization and enrichment of fetal rat hepatoblasts by immunoadsorption ("panning") and fluorescence-activated cell sorting. *Hepatology* 1994; 19:999–1006.

93. Petersen BE, Bowen WC, Patrene KD, et al. Bone marrow as a potential source of hepatic oval cells. *Science* 1999;284: 1168–1170.

94. Theise ND, Badve S, Saxena R, et al. Derivation of hepatocytes from bone marrow cells in mice after radiation-induced myeloablation. *Hepatology* 2000;31:235–240.

95. Strain AJ. Changing blood into liver: adding further intrigue to the hepatic stem cell story. *Hepatology* 1999;30: 1105–1107.

96. Bjornson CRR, Rietze RL, Reynolds BA, et al.. Turning brain into blood: a hematopoietic fate adopted by adult neural stem cells in vivo. *Science* 1999;283:534–536.

97. Wilmut I, Schnieke AE, McWhir J, et al.. Viable offspring derived from fetal and adult mammalian cells. *Nature* 1997; 385:810–813.

98. Burgstahler A, Nathanson MH. Coordination of calcium waves among hepatocytes: teamwork gets the job done. *Hepatology* 1998;27:634–635.

99. Suresh KJ. Making waves: regulation of inositol triphosphate receptors and propagation of calcium signals in the liver. *Hepatology* 1997;26:799–801.

100. Zaret KS. The touch that hepatocytes seem to like. *Hepatology* 1992;15:1204–1205.

101. Billiar TR, Curran RD, eds. *Hepatocyte and Kupffer cell interactions.* London: CRC Press, 1992.

102. Hirose M, Watanabe S, Oide H, et al. A new function of Ito cells in liver morphogenesis: evidence using a novel morphogenic protein, epimorphin, in vitro. *Biochem Biophys Res Commun* 1996;225:155–160.

103. Roskelley CD, Srebrow A, Bissell MJ. A hierarchy of ECM-mediated signalling regulates tissue-specific gene expression. *Curr Opin Cell Biol* 1995;7:736–747.

104. Martinez-Hernandez A, Amenta PS. The extracellular matrix in hepatic regeneration. *FASEB J* 1995;9:1401–1410.

105. Tiniakos DG, Lee JA, Burt AD. Innervation of the liver: morphology and function. *Liver* 1996;16:151–160.

106. Clément B, Musso O, Liétard J, et al. Homeostatic control of angiogenesis: a newly identified function of the liver? *Hepatology* 1999;29:621–623.

107. Lander ES. The new genomics: global views of biology. *Science* 1996;274:536–539.

108. Lander ES. Array of hope. *Nat Genet* 1999;21:3–4.

109. Brown PO, Botstein D. Exploring the new world of the genome with DNA microarrays. *Nature Genet* 1999;21:33–37.

110. Basset DEJ, Eisen MB, Boguski MS. Gene expression informatics—it's all in your mind. *Nature Genet* 1999;21:51–55.

The Liver: Biology and Pathobiology, Fourth Edition, edited by I. M. Arias, J. L. Boyer, F. V. Chisari, N. Fausto, D. Schachter, and D. A. Shafritz. Lippincott Williams & Wilkins, Philadelphia © 2001.

EMBRYONIC DEVELOPMENT
OF THE LIVER

KENNETH S. ZARET

The liver is one of the first organs to develop in the embryo and it rapidly becomes one of the largest organs in the fetus. The most essential function of the fetal liver is to provide a site for hematopoiesis. The early dependence of the fetus on its own blood cell supply makes embryonic liver growth and viability a sensitive phenotypic indicator for gene inactivation studies. From an experimental perspective, the developing liver is relatively easy to study, and new insights have emerged from recent work on genetically modified mice and explants of embryonic tissues. Many genes that control early liver development have been identified. Although less is known about how gene function is orchestrated to control tissue morphogenesis, the depth of understanding in this area has established liver development as a paradigm for the genesis of other gut-derived tissues. Also, understanding the mechanisms that govern liver development should provide insight into future therapies for liver diseases. Examples of such applications include new approaches to activating stem cells in the adult liver (see Chapter 61, and website chapter 🖳 W-31), replenishing diseased livers with cells from embryonic liver, trans-differentiating cells from different organs, and reconstituting proper liver morphology and function. This chapter highlights ways in which understanding embryonic development of the liver can impact these goals. This review spans from the initial specification of the liver and morphogenesis of the hepatic bud to the stage of hematopoietic cell invasion of the nascent organ. The reader is referred to other reviews for summaries of the

mid- and late-fetal stages of liver development (1–4) (see Chapter 2).

ACQUISITION OF HEPATIC DEVELOPMENTAL COMPETENCE WITHIN THE ENDODERM

The liver, lung, pancreas, thyroid, and gastrointestinal tract are derived from the definitive endoderm, the latter being one of the three germ layers that arise during gastrulation. Initially, the endoderm is an epithelial sheet that lines the ventral surface of the embryo. Infolding of the sheet at the anterior and posterior of the embryo generates the foregut and hindgut. When these morphogenetic movements reach the middle of the embryo, the gut tube closes off. During gut tube formation, different tissues are specified along the anterior-posterior and dorsal-ventral axes of the embryo, with the liver arising from the prospective ventral endoderm domain of the foregut (Fig. 2.1). It is important to note that the definitive endoderm is different from the primitive endoderm, or embryonic yolk sac, which expresses many serum proteins in common with the liver (5–7) but is an extraembryonic tissue unrelated to the liver lineage (8).

Several questions need to be answered with regard to the specification of the liver hepatocytes and other cell types in the endoderm. Are there "pre-patterns" or local domains of endoderm that are competent to differentiate into a subset of the gut-derived tissues, such as the liver? What are the molecular signals that cause a local domain of endoderm to develop into the liver? The answers to these questions may ultimately

K. S. Zaret: Cell and Developmental Biology Program, Fox Chase Cancer Center, Philadelphia, Pennsylvania 19111.

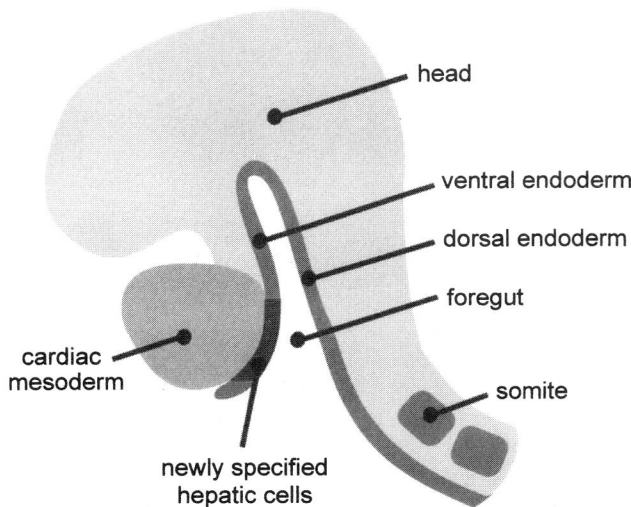

FIGURE 2.1. Parasagittal diagram of an embryo at the time of hepatic specification.

lead to strategies for redirecting healthy, nonliver cells to the hepatic phenotype in order to repair diseased livers.

Evidence of a prepattern for the liver comes from tissue explant studies of chick endoderm. LeDouarin (9) found that only the prospective anterior-ventral domain of endoderm had the capacity to develop into the liver, when this tissue was transplanted from an early somite stage chicken embryo into another embryo (10). More recent studies with mouse embryos and more sensitive assays of gene expression reveal that whereas the prospective dorsal endoderm (Fig. 2.1) does not normally activate liver genes or become liver in a tissue explant assay, the dorsal endoderm cells can initiate liver gene expression (11). Further studies found that mesoderm and ectoderm from the dorsal domain of the embryo actively inhibit the liver program in the dorsal endoderm (11,12). Although the molecular signals involved in the repression of liver genes in the dorsal endoderm are unknown, these studies show that, as initially established in more genetically tractable organisms such as *Drosophila* (13), other germ layers (typically mesoderm) have a major role in regulating domains of developmental competence within the endoderm.

The ability of the dorsal endoderm to activate early liver genes may be an evolutionary remnant of the primordial gut, which performed diverse functions that are presently distributed to different organs. However, since the dorsal endoderm apparently lacks the potential for the terminal hepatic differentiation exhibited by the ventral endoderm (9,10), the ventral endoderm appears to be prepatterned differently. The diverse developmental potential of gut-derived cells is also revealed in certain experimental models, in which diet-induced damage to the liver or pancreas induces the appearance of intestinal cells or hepatocytes, respectively (14,15).

Another approach to understand how the endoderm gains the competence to develop into the liver is to determine whether regulatory factors that are known to be important for liver differentiation are expressed in prehepatic endoderm, prior to hepatic specification. Such factors could operate by helping to open up chromatin structure for genes that need to be transcribed during liver differentiation (16). Two transcription factors that are expressed in the prehepatic domain of ventral foregut endoderm, and later in the liver, are HNF3β (17–20) and GATA-4 (21–24). Indeed, gene inactivation studies have shown that both of these factors are essential for development of the foregut endoderm itself (25–29). The requirement of these factors for endoderm development precludes a direct genetic analysis of their roles in hepatogenesis and awaits conditional gene knockout mutations in which the liver phenotypes can be assessed after the time of foregut formation. The divergent homeobox transcription factor Hex is also expressed in the endoderm, prior to liver development (30), as well as in mature liver (31). Therefore, Hex may also be involved in priming or specification of the hepatic lineage.

The role of these transcription factors can be discerned by understanding how the factors function in a chromatin context. DNA binding by both HNF3 and GATA factors is required for the activity of a transcriptional enhancer of the serum albumin gene (12,32), the latter being one of the earliest genes to be activated in hepatic development (11). Analysis of the DNA binding sites for HNF3β and GATA-4 by "*in vivo* footprinting" (33) showed that both sites are occupied on the albumin gene enhancer in the endoderm (Fig. 2.2) prior to transcriptional activation or hepatic commitment (11,12). Further analysis showed that as long as the HNF3 and GATA factor binding sites

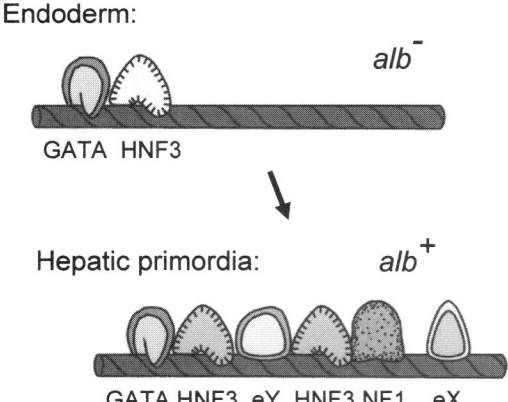

FIGURE 2.2. Transcriptional competence factors in the endoderm. DNA binding sites for GATA and HNF3 transcription factors are occupied on the albumin gene prior to albumin expression or hepatic commitment. During hepatic specification, other transcription factors bind DNA at adjacent sites and the albumin gene becomes active.

remain occupied in endodermal development, the endoderm remains competent to express liver genes, even in domains of endoderm that do not normally become the liver (12). Once hepatic specification has occurred, adjacent binding sites for a variety of other transcription factors become occupied and the albumin gene becomes active (Fig. 2.2). These data indicate that genetic activation of hepatogenesis is "primed" by transcription factors before cell type differentiation. In the future, directed expression of these and other transcription factors in nonhepatic cells might endow the cells with the potential to initiate hepatic differentiation under appropriate growth conditions.

SIGNALS THAT SPECIFY THE EMBRYONIC LIVER

What causes the liver to be specified from the ventral foregut endoderm? Again, embryo tissue transplant and explant studies have been illuminating, whereas directed gene inactivation studies in mice have yet to reveal rate-limiting genes. Morphologically, the prospective ventral foregut endoderm comes in contact with the cardiac mesoderm prior to emergence of the liver (Fig. 2.1). LeDouarin (34) showed that when ventral foregut endoderm from chick embryos, prior to the five-somite stage, is transplanted to another embryo, it fails to develop into liver. But if cardiac mesoderm is transplanted with the ventral endoderm, liver development ensues in the latter. Similar results have been obtained with ventral foregut endoderm from the mouse (11), which confirms that the cardiac mesoderm is the general inducer of the liver in the vertebrate endoderm. In both systems, close proximity of the cardiac mesoderm is required to impart a hepatic fate to the endoderm.

Further studies with embryonic explants cultured *in vitro* reveal that fibroblast growth factor signaling from the cardiac mesoderm induces the liver in the endoderm. There are at least 18 genes for fibroblast growth factors (FGFs) and four genes for FGF receptors (FRs) (35,36). Each FGF receptor has different binding specificities for FGFs, and the existence of multiple spliced isoforms of the receptors provides further complexity to the receptor–ligand relationship. FGF binding induces tyrosine phosphorylation activity by the cytoplasmic domain of the receptors, resulting in activation of mitogen-activated protein kinase signaling pathways within cells (36,37). At the time of hepatic induction, the cardiac mesoderm expresses at least FGF-1, FGF-2, and FGF-8 (38–40) and the ventral foregut endoderm expresses FGF receptors 1 and 4 (41,42). Inactivation of the genes for FGF-8 and FR-1 are embryonic lethal prior to hepatic development (43–45) and inactivation of the genes for FGF-1, FGF-2, or FR-4 have minimal embryologic phenotype (46–49),

suggesting functional redundancy. In an embryonic tissue explant system, purified FGF-1 or FGF-2 can efficiently activate liver gene expression within the isolated ventral foregut endoderm, whereas FGF-8 is inefficient (40). In addition, antagonists to FGF signaling suppress liver gene induction when the cardiac mesoderm is proximal to the endoderm. Together, these results show that FGF signaling from the cardiac mesoderm is necessary and sufficient to induce hepatic gene activity within the endoderm, in an explant assay. Compound null and conditional mutations of FGF signaling components in mice will be necessary to assess the hepatogenic role of FGF signaling in the intact embryo.

Interestingly, ectopic expression of an FGF family member in the adult pancreas of transgenic mice induces appearance of hepatocytes in the pancreas (50). It is not known whether the target of transgenic FGF signaling in this instance is pancreatic ductular cells (51), endocrine cells, or another cell type. The result emphasizes how FGF signaling in the embryo may be recapitulated in the adult to redirect organ differentiation.

MORPHOGENESIS OF THE LIVER BUD

Within half a day of liver gene activation in the endoderm, the newly specified hepatic cells begin to proliferate. It seems likely that the initial signals for enhanced proliferation of the hepatic endoderm are either coincident in time with, or closely follow the signals for, hepatic specification. As the hepatic endoderm cells multiply, the endoderm layer thickens (Fig. 2.3C). The cells then emerge from the epithelium and begin to migrate into the loose mesenchymal cell environment of the septum transversum (Fig. 2.3C). Presumably, the cell migration is accompanied by major remodeling of the extracellular matrix surrounding the hepatic cells. During this period, the entire ventral foregut domain extends toward the midgut, bringing the liver region with it (Fig. 2.3A,B). The mass of cells emerging from the endoderm and concentrating in the septum transversum is referred to as the liver bud.

At least two growth signals control development of the liver bud. Experiments with embryonic tissue explants showed that an FGF signal distinct from FGF-1 and FGF-2, probably FGF-8, works in conjunction with other as yet unidentified signals to promote outgrowth of the newly specified hepatic endoderm (40). The existence of these signals is inferred from experiments in which an FGF inhibitor blocked morphogenetic outgrowth response of the endoderm to cardiac mesoderm and septum transversum mesenchyme. The inhibition could be overcome by the addition of excess FGF-8, but FGF-8 treatment alone, in the absence of mesoderm cells, failed to promote endoderm outgrowth (40). Thus, FGF-8 must work with other factors.

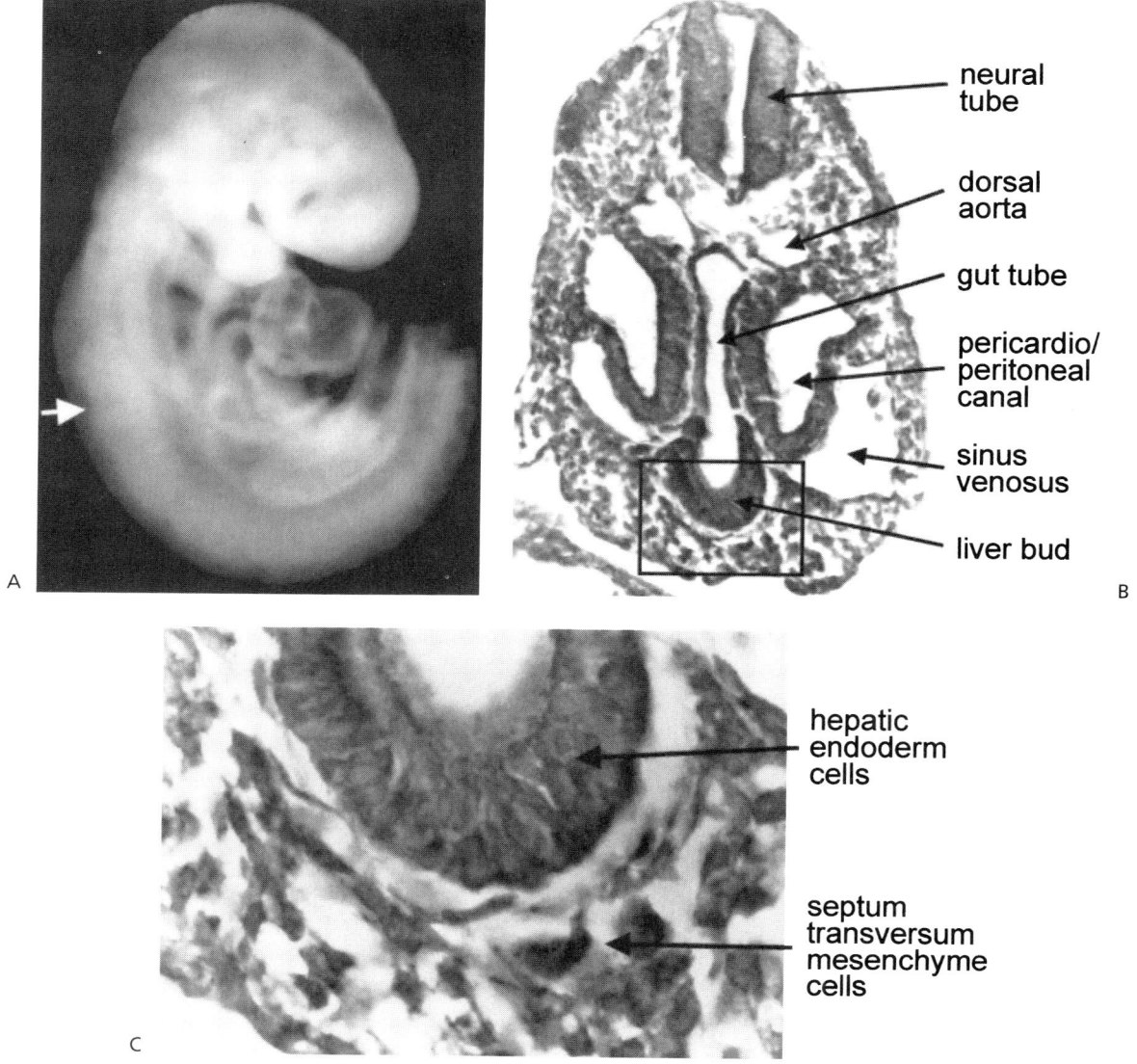

FIGURE 2.3. The beginning of liver development. **A:** Mouse embryo, 9 days' gestation. Tail is removed; *arrow* indicates plane of section in panel **B**. **B:** Original magnification 100× of transverse section. Note the thickening of the endodermal epithelium of the gut tube at the region of the liver bud. Boxed area is magnified to 400× in panel **C.** *Arrows* depict the liver bud and other landmarks of the embryo. (Photographs courtesy of J. Rossi.)

CELL INTERACTIONS THAT PROMOTE ORGAN FORMATION FROM THE LIVER BUD

The complex signals that cause emergence of the liver bud are followed closely by distinct signals required to grow the bud into the liver organ. During this period, the hepatic endoderm cells are quite immature in terms of function and morphology; consequently they are often referred to as hepatoblasts. The hepatoblasts differentiate into both hepatocytes and biliary cells as the liver organ forms (52–54). Cells that are slightly caudal to the liver bud, or within the caudal portion of the liver bud itself, give rise to the common bile duct and gallbladder. Studies in which hepatic endoderm cells are individually marked and followed in development are required to establish lineage relationships. If such studies are sustained into the adult and coupled with experimental models for repair of chronic liver damage, it should be possible to identify the embryologic cell type(s) that gives rise to liver stem cells.

As the hepatoblasts in the liver bud migrate away from the cardiac region, the surrounding septum transversum cells (Fig. 2.3C) promote further hepatic differentiation, even in the absence of cardiac tissue (9,55). In the septum transversum, the hepatoblasts are exposed to a new extracellular matrix (ECM) environment (56). This probably helps promote the hepatoblasts' differentiation, given the powerful influence that the ECM exerts on adult hepatocyte differentiation (57,58). Consistent with this possibility, β_1 integrin, a prominent ECM receptor subunit, is essential early for hepatocyte growth (59) and the expression of other integrins in liver development is highly dynamic (60) (also see Chapter 33).

Mouse genetic studies show that extensive interactions between hepatoblasts and mesenchyme cells in the septum transversum are critical for hepatic development. In the absence of the Hlx homeobox transcription factor in the mesenchyme cells, hepatocyte proliferation is greatly impaired (61). Also, mesenchymal cell expression of hepatocyte growth factor (HGF), together with hepatocyte expression of the HGF receptor, c-*met* is critical for early liver growth (62,63). HGF or c-*met* inactivation results in apoptosis of hepatocytes, but Hlx inactivation does not, suggesting the existence of distinct mesenchymal-hepatocyte interactions for liver growth. Additional mesenchymal signaling is implicated by a hepatic growth requirement for the stress signaling kinase SEK1/MKK4 (64). Although SEK1 activation results in activation of the c-*jun* transcription factor (65) and c-*jun* is also required for early liver growth (66), the SEK1 liver defect is manifest earlier in gestation than is the c-*jun* defect, indicating that other critical downstream targets exist for SEK1. In summary, a multitude of signaling events from the mesenchyme cells promote hepatic growth.

Other cell types contribute to the embryonic liver mass, including endothelial cells that surround the hepatic sinusoids (67). Veins anastomose near the liver bud (Fig. 2.3B) to form a capillary bed that becomes interspersed within the migrating hepatoblasts. These transitions establish the liver's sinusoidal architecture, which is critical for organ function and sets the stage for the liver to support fetal hematopoiesis.

Hematopoietic cells migrate to the early liver first from the yolk sac (68) and later from the aorta–gonad–mesonephros region (69). Proper intermediate filament expression is critical for blood cell homing, as erythrocytes accumulate excessively in the fetal liver of keratin 8 mutants (70). However, embryos deficient in the heavy metal-responsive transcription factor MTF-1 exhibit reduced cytokeratin expression as well as enlarged sinusoids, and dissociated epithelial cells, but not anemia (71). The primary defect in MTF-1–deficient embryos appears to be failure to control metal homeostasis and the oxidation-reduction state in hepatocytes at mid-gestation.

Both hematopoietic and endothelial cells provide differentiating signals to the hepatoblasts, because heterogeneity in hepatic gene expression is related to the vascular architecture of the fetal liver (72). More specifically, mouse gene inactivation studies have shown that oncostatin M signaling from hematopoietic cells to hepatocytes

is critical for liver growth (73). Impaired hematopoietic cell proliferation in c-*myb* mutant embryos (74) or impaired erythrocytic cell proliferation in retinoblastoma gene (*Rb*) mutant embryos (75,76) also results in impaired liver growth. The failure of hematopoietic cells to migrate to the liver in β_1 integrin-null embryos, therefore, is also thought to contribute to the liver developmental defect in the β_1 mutants (59,77).

During this period of organogenesis, the liver capsule forms and the organ continues to grow at a rapid rate. N-*myc* gene expression in the capsule and *jumonji* gene expression in the hepatic stromal cells help promote growth during mid-gestation (78–80). Although many of the genes that affect hepatoblast proliferation are probably most important during the initial transition from the liver bud to the organ stage, inactivation of these genes usually manifests itself as a hematopoietic defect well after the organ is formed. In these cases, a liver capsule develops and hematopoietic cells migrate to the liver, but the paucity of hepatoblasts leads to a defect in the hematopoietic environment and, conseqently, embryonic lethality. Furthermore, mutations of several liver regulatory factors yield a fetal liver growth defect due to apoptosis of the hepatoblasts. These proteins include c-jun (66,81), IKK2 (82), RelA (83), and XBP-1 (84).

The mesenchymal cell population of the nascent liver has considerable morphogenetic potential, because the hepatic mesenchyme can develop into a liver-like structure in the apparent absence of hepatoblasts (9). This observation, based on tissue manipulation studies in chick embryos, is consistent with the observation that a significant liver structure develops in mice that are homozygous mutant for many of the aforementioned genes, which are required for hepatoblast proliferation. Based on these considerations, cell-based and artificial organ therapies for liver disease would benefit from a better understanding of the signaling, cell structure, and ECM components provided by the embryonic hepatic mesenchyme.

HEPATOCYTE DIFFERENTIATION IN THE EARLY LIVER

As mentioned above, newly specified hepatoblasts express very few liver-specific genes; these include α-fetoprotein, serum albumin, and transthyretin (11,52,56,85–87). Shortly after formation of the liver organ, the activity of these genes increases dramatically (56,88,89) and a variety of other liver-specific genes are activated. In addition, the hepatoblasts rapidly acquire the signal transduction pathways to induce the carbamoylphosphate synthetase and phosphoenolpyruvate carboxykinase genes in response to amino acid and hormone levels (90,91). Morphogenetic development of the liver lobule structure is also important for hepatoblast differentiation into hepatocytes (92).

Gene inactivation studies in mice have shown that different transcription factors control different groups of liver genes. For example, HNF4, a member of the nuclear hormone receptor family (93), is required for early liver expression of various apolipoproteins, metabolic enzymes, serum factors, and other transcription factors such as HNF1α (94,95) and PXR In turn, HNF1α, a homeobox transcription factor, regulates the phenylalanine hydroxylase gene in mice (96). The limited apparent role of HNF1α based on gene inactivation studies in animals contrasts sharply with ectopic and overexpression studies in cultured hepatic cell lines, which suggest that HNF1α is critical for the expression of a wide variety of liver-specific genes (97). Such distinctions indicate how strongly the mechanisms of gene regulation are influenced by whole animal physiology, beyond simple notions of gene redundancy (e.g., 98,99). Indeed, for future studies, identification of target genes is perhaps best guided by phenotypic expression changes in gene knockout studies (see Chapter 63). For example, gene expression array analysis of embryos that were homozygous mutant for the basic-leucine zipper transcription factor XBP-1 revealed hepatic defects in β1-antitrypsin expression, and the XBP-1 protein was then found to bind and activate the β1-antitrypsin gene promoter (84). Although many other liver-enriched transcription factors are expressed early in liver development, their inactivation does not yield an embryonic defect (100). When compound gene inactivation studies are performed with these regulatory factor genes, however, many early developmental roles are likely to be discovered. Such studies will reveal how signaling pathways coordinately promote early liver differentiation and morphogenesis.

PERSPECTIVES

This chapter has highlighted ways that our understanding of embryonic liver development may yield new insights into therapies for liver disease. Other approaches to cell-based therapies are discussed in Chapters 61 and 62. The application of concepts from liver development is new because only recently have we become aware of molecules and signaling systems that control the key aspects of hepatogenesis. However, given the large number of proteins that were discovered in studies of adult liver and yet result in embryonic liver phenotypes when deleted in mice, there is a measure of confidence that many of these proteins' functions in the adult recapitulate activities in the embryo. Thus, continued investigation of embryonic liver development is certain to be instructive about the function, regeneration, and repair of the adult liver, and seems likely to provide new sources of cells and molecules for combating liver disease. Further refinements in the ability to inactivate genes in the early liver and better methods of embryo tissue culture are needed to advance the analysis of liver development. Such

advances may come from adaptations of methodology for other endoderm-derived organ systems (101). In addition, relevant new genes will emerge from studies of model organisms in which genetic screens can be coupled with knowledge of genomic sequences and interrelationships of protein function. Considering that our mechanistic understanding of liver development has emerged in just the past few years, the prospects are bright for much deeper knowledge and new applications for liver therapies.

ACKNOWLEDGMENTS

Thanks to Pascale Bossard, Dina Chaya, and Jennifer Rossi for comments on the manuscript and Sarah Costello-Berman for help in its preparation. The author's research on liver development is supported by a grant from the National Institutes of Health (GM36477).

REFERENCES

1. Elias H. Origin and early development of the liver in various vertebrates. *Acta Hepat* 1955;3:1–57.
2. Du Bois AM. The embryonic liver. In: Rouiller CH, ed. *The Liver*, vol 1. New York: Academic Press 1963:1–39.
3. Severn CB. A morphological study of the development of the human liver. *Am J Anat* 1968;133:85–108.
4. Zaret KS. Molecular genetics of early liver development. *Annu Rev Physiol* 1996;58:231–251.
5. Meehan RR, Barlow DP, Hill RE, et al. Pattern of serum protein gene expression in mouse visceral yolk sac and fetal liver. *EMBO J* 1984;3:1881–1885.
6. Thomas T, Southwell BR, Schreiber G, et al. Plasma protein synthesis and secretion in the visceral yolk sac of the fetal rat: Gene expression, protein synthesis and secretion. *Placenta* 1990;11:413–430.
7. Duncan SA, Nagy A, Chan W. Murine gastrulation requires HNF-4 regulated gene expression in the visceral endoderm: tetraploid rescue of Hnf-4(−/−) embryos. *Development* 1997;124:279–287.
8. Lawson KA, Pedersen RA. Cell fate, morphogenetic movement and population kinetics of embryonic endoderm at the time of germ layer formation in the mouse. *Development* 1987;101:627–652.
9. LeDouarin NM. An experimental analysis of liver development. *Med Biol* 1975;53:427–455.
10. Fukuda-Taira S. Hepatic induction in the avian embryo: specificity of reactive endoderm and inductive mesoderm. *J Embryol Exp Morph* 1981;63:111–125.
11. Gualdi R, Bossard P, Zheng M, et al. Hepatic specification of the gut endoderm *in vitro*: cell signalling and transcriptional control. *Genes Dev* 1996;10:1670–1682.
12. Bossard P, Zaret K. GATA transcription factors as potentiators of gut endoderm differentiation. *Development* 1998;125:4909–4917.
13. Hoch M, Pankratz MJ. Control of gut development by fork head and cell signaling molecules in Drosophila. *Mech Dev* 1996;58:3–14.
14. Elmore LW, Sirica AE. Sequential appearance of intestinal mucosal cell types in the right and caudate liver lobes of furan-treated rats. *Hepatology* 1992;16:1220–1226.

15. Rao MS, Dwivedi RS, Yelandi A, et al. Role of periductal and ductalar epithelial cells of the adult rat pancreas in pancreatic hepatocyte lineage: a change in the differentiation commitment. *Am J Pathol* 1989;134:1069–1086.

16. Zaret K. Developmental competence of the gut endoderm: genetic potentiation by GATA and HNF3/fork head proteins. *Dev Biol* 1999;209:1–10.

17. Sasaki H, Hogan BLM. Differential expression of multiple fork head related genes during gastrulation and pattern formation in the mouse embryo. *Development* 1993;118:47–59.

18. Ang S-L, Wierda A, Wong D, et al. The formation and maintenance of the definitive endoderm lineage in the mouse: involvement of HNF3/forkhead proteins. *Development* 1993;119:1301–1315.

19. Monaghan AP, Kaestner KH, Grau E, et al. Postimplantation expression patterns indicate a role for the mouse forkhead/HNF-3α, β, and γ genes in determination of the definitive endoderm, chordamesoderm and neuroectoderm. *Development* 1993;119:567–578.

20. Ruiz i Altaba A, Prezioso VR, Darnell JE, et al. Sequential expression of HNF-3α and HNF-3β by embryonic organizing centers: the dorsal lip/node, notochord, and floor plate. *Mech Dev* 1993;44:91–108.

21. Laverriere AC, MacNeill C, Mueller C, et al. GATA-4/5/6, a subfamily of three transcription factors transcribed in developing heart and gut. *J Biol Chem* 1994;269:23177–23184.

22. Arceci R, King AAJ, Simon MC, et al. Mouse GATA-4: a retinoic acid-inducible GATA-binding transcription factor expressed in endodermally derived tissues and heart. *Mol Cell Biol* 1993;13:2235–2246.

23. Suzuki E, Evans T, Lowry J, et al. The human GATA-6 gene: structure, chromosomal location, and regulation of expression by tissue-specific and mitogen-responsive signals. *Genomics* 1996;38:283–290.

24. Gao X, Sedgwick T, Shi YB, et al. Distinct functions are implicated for the GATA-4, -5, and -6 transcription factors in the regulation of intestine epithelia cell differentiation. *Mol Cell Biol* 1998;18:2901–2911.

25. Ang S-L, Rossant J. HNF-3β is essential for node and notochord formation in mouse development. *Cell* 1994;78:561–574.

26. Weinstein DC, Ruiz i Altaba A, Chen WS, et al. The winged-helix transcription factor HNF-3β is required for notochord development in the mouse embryo. *Cell* 1994;78:575–588.

27. Dufort D, Schwartz L, Harpal K, et al. The transcription factor HNF3β is required in visceral endoderm for normal primitive streak morphogenesis. *Development* 1998;125:3015–3025.

28. Kuo CT, Morrisey EE, Anandappa R, et al. GATA4 transcription factor is required for ventral morphogenesis and heart tube formation. *Genes Dev* 1997;11:1048–1060.

29. Molkentin JD, Lin Q, Duncan SA, et al. Requirement of the transcription factor GATA4 for heart tube formation and ventral morphogenesis. *Genes Dev* 1997;11:1061–1072.

30. Thomas PQ, Brown A, Beddington RSP. Hex: a homeobox gene revealing peri-implantation asymmetry in the mouse embryo and an early transient marker of endothelial cell precursors. *Development* 1998;125:85–94.

31. Hromas R, Radich J, Collins S. PCR cloning of an orphan homeobox gene (PRH) preferentially expressed in myeloid and liver cells. *Biochem Biophys Res Commun* 1993;195:976–983.

32. Liu J-K, DiPersio CM, Zaret KS. Extracellular signals that regulate liver transcription factors during hepatic differentiation *in vitro*. *Mol Cell Biol* 1991;11:773–784.

33. Mueller PR, Wold B. *In vivo* footprinting of a muscle specific enhancer by ligation mediated PCR. *Science* 1989;246:780–786.

34. LeDouarin N. Etude expérimentale de l'organogenèse du tube digestif et du foie chez l'embryon de poulet. *Bull Biol Fr Belg* 1964;98:543–676.

35. McKeehan WL, Wang F, Kan M. The heparan sulfate-fibroblast growth factor family: diversity of structure and function. *Prog Nucleic Acid Res Mol Biol* 1998;59:135–176.

36. Szebenyi G, Fallon JF. Fibroblast growth factors as multifunctional signaling factors. *Int Rev Cytol* 1999;185:45–106.

37. Wang J-K, Gao G, Goldfarb M. Fibroblast growth factor receptors have different signaling and mitogenic potentials. *Mol Cell Biol* 1994;14:181–188.

38. Zhu X, Sasse J, McAllister D, et al. Evidence that fibroblast growth factors 1 and 4 participate in regulation of cardiogenesis. *Dev Dyn* 1996;207:429–438.

39. Crossley PH, Martin GR. The mouse *Fgf8* gene encodes a family of polypeptides and is expressed in regions that direct outgrowth and patterning in the developing embryo. *Development* 1995;121:439–451.

40. Jung J, Zheng M, Goldfarb M, et al. Initiation of mammalian liver development from endoderm by fibroblasts growth factors. *Science* 1999;284:1998–2003.

41. Stark KL, McMahon JA, McMahon AP. FGFR-4, a new member of the fibroblast growth factor receptor family, expressed in the definitive endoderm and skeletal muscle lineages of the mouse. *Development* 1991;113:641–651.

42. Sugi Y, Lough J. Activin-A and FGF-2 mimic the inductive effects of anterior endoderm on terminal cardiac myogenesis *in vitro*. *Dev Biol* 1995;168:567–574.

43. Sun X, Meyers EN, Lewandoski M, et al. Targeted disruption of Fgf8 causes failure of cell migration in the gastrulating mouse embryo. *Genes Dev* 1999;13:1834–1846.

44. Meyers EN, Lewandowski M, Martin GR. An *Fgf8* mutant allelic series generated by Cre- and Flp-mediated recombination. *Nat Genet* 1998;18:136–141.

45. Ciruna BG, Schwartz L, Harpal K, et al. Chimeric analysis of fibroblasts growth factor receptor-1 (Fgfr-1) function: a role for FGFR1 in morphogenetic movement through the primitive streak. *Development* 1997;124:2829–2841.

46. Ortega S, Ittmann M, Tsang SH, et al. Neuronal defects and delayed wound healing in mice lacking fibroblast growth factor 2. *Proc Natl Acad Sci USA* 1998;95:5672–5677.

47. Dono R, Texido G, Dussel R, et al. Impaired cerebral cortex development and blood pressure regulation in FGF-2–deficient mice. *EMBO J* 1998;17:4213–4225.

48. Weinstein M, Xu X, Ohyama K, et al. FGFR-3 and FGFR-4 function cooperatively to direct alveogenesis in the murine lung. *Development* 1998;125:3615–3623.

49. Miller DL, Ortega S, Bashayan O, et al. Compensation by fibroblast growth factor 1 (FGF1) does not account for the mild phenotypic defects observed in FGF2 null mice. *Mol Cell Biol* 2000;20:2260–2268.

50. Krakowski ML, Kritzik MR, Jones EM, et al. Pancreatic expression of keratinocyte growth factor leads to differentiation of islet hepatocytes and proliferation of duct cells. *Am J Pathol* 1999;154:683–691.

51. Dabeva MS, Hwang SG, Vasa SR, et al. Differentiation of pancreatic epithelial progenitor cells into hepatocytes following transplantation into rat liver. *Proc Natl Acad Sci USA* 1997;94:7356–7361.

52. Shiojiri N. Enzymo- and immunocytochemical analyses of the differentiation of liver cells in the prenatal mouse. *J Embryol Exp Morph* 1981;62:139–152.

53. Shiojiri N. Analysis of differentiation of hepatocytes and bile duct cells in developing mouse liver by albumin immunofluorescence. *Dev Growth Differ* 1984;26:555–561.

54. Germain L, Blouin MJ, Marceau N. Biliary epithelial and hepa-

tocytic cell lineage relationships in embryonic rat liver as determined by the differential expression of cytokeratins, a-fetoprotein, albumin, and cell surface-exposed components. *Cancer Res* 1988;48:4909–4918.

55. Houssaint E. Differentiation of the mouse hepatic primordium. I. An analysis of tissue interactions in hepatocyte differentiation. *Cell Differ* 1980;9:269–279.

56. Cascio S, Zaret KS. Hepatocyte differentiation initiates during endodermal-mesenchymal interactions prior to liver formation. *Development* 1991;113:217–225.

57. Maher JJ, Bissell DM. Cell-matrix interactions in liver. *Semin Cell Biol* 1993;4:189–201.

58. Stamatoglou SC, Hughes RC. Cell adhesion molecules in liver function and pattern formation. *FASEB J* 1994;8:420–427.

59. Fässler R, Meyer M. Consequences of lack of b1 integrin gene expression in mice. *Genes Dev* 1995;9:1896–1908.

60. Couvelard A, Bringuier AF, Dauge MC, et al. Expression of integrins during liver organogenesis in humans. *Hepatology* 1998;27:839–847.

61. Hentsch B, Lyons I, Ruili L, et al. Hlx homeo box gene is essential for an inductive tissue interaction that drives expansion of embryonic liver and gut. *Genes Dev* 1996;10:70–79.

62. Schmidt C, Bladt F, Goedecke S, et al. Scatter factor/hepatocyte growth factor is essential for liver development. *Nature* 1995;373:699–702.

63. Bladt F, Riethmacher D, Isenmann S, et al. Essential role for the c-met receptor in the migration of myogenic precursor cells into the limb bud. *Nature* 1995;376:768–772.

64. Nishina H, Vaz C, Billia P, et al. Defective liver formation and liver cell apoptosis in mice lacking the stress signaling kinase SEK1/MKK4. *Development* 1999;126:505–516.

65. Rodrigues GA, Park M, Schlessinger J. Activation of the JNK pathway is essential for transformation by the Met oncogene. *EMBO J* 1997;16:2634–2645.

66. Hilberg F, Aguzzi A, Howells N, et al. c-Jun is essential for normal mouse development and hepatogenesis. *Nature* 1993;365:179–181.

67. Medlock ES, Haar JL. The liver hemopoietic environment: I. Developing hepatocytes and their role in fetal hemopoiesis. *Anat Rec* 1983;207:31–41.

68. Johnson GR, Moore MA. Role of stem cell migration in initiation of mouse foetal liver haemopoiesis. *Nature* 1975;258:726–728.

69. Medvinsky A, Dzierzak E. Definitive hematopoiesis is autonomously initiated by the AGM region. *Cell* 1996;86:897–906.

70. Baribault H, Price J, Miyai K, et al. Mid-gestational lethality in mice lacking keratin 8. *Genes Dev* 1993;7:1191–1202.

71. Günes C, Heuchel R, Georgiev O, et al. Embryonic lethality and liver degeneration in mice lacking the metal-responsive transcriptional activator MTF-1. *EMBO J* 1998;17:2846–2854.

72. Gaasbeek Janzen JW, Westenend PJ, Charles R, et al. Gene expression in derivatives of embryonic foregut during prenatal development of the rat. *J Histochem Cytochem* 1988;36:1223–1230.

73. Kamiya A, Kinoshita T, Ito Y, et al. Fetal liver development requires a paracrine action of oncostatin M through the gp130 signal transducer. *EMBO J* 1999;18:2127–2136.

74. Mucenski ML, McLain K, Kier AB, et al. A functional c-myb gene is required for normal murine fetal hepatic hematopoiesis. *Cell* 1991;65:677–689.

75. Jacks T, Fazeli A, Schmitt EM, et al. Effects of an *Rb* mutation in the mouse. *Nature* 1992;359:295–300.

76. Lee EY, Chang CY, Hu N, et al. Mice deficient for Rb are non-viable and show defects in neurogenesis and haematopoiesis. *Nature* 1992;359:288–294.

77. Hirsch E, Iglesias A, Potocnik AJ, et al. Impaired migration but not differentiation of haematopoietic stem cells in the absence of beta1 integrins. *Nature* 1996;380:171–175.

78. Sawai S, Shimono A, Wakamatsu Y, et al. Defects of embryonic organogenesis resulting from targeted disruption of the N-*myc* gene in the mouse. *Development* 1993;117:1445–1455.

79. Giroux S, Charron J. Defective development of the embryonic liver in N-myc-deficient mice. *Dev Biol* 1998;195:16–28.

80. Motoyama J, Kitajima K, Kojima M, et al. Organogenesis of the liver, thymus and spleen is affected in *jumonji* mutant mice. *Mech Dev* 1997;66:27–37.

81. Eferl R, Sibilia M, Hilberg F, et al. Functions of c-Jun in liver and heart development. *J Cell Biol* 1999;145:1049–1061.

82. Li Q, Antwerp DV, Mercurio F, et al. Severe liver degeneration in mice lacking the lkB kinase 2 gene. *Science* 1999;284:321–325.

83. Beg AA, Sha WC, Bronson RT, et al. Embryonic lethality and liver degeneration in mice lacking the RelA component of NF-KB. *Nature* 1995;376:167–170.

84. Reimold AM, Etkin A, Clauss I, et al. An essential role in liver development for transcription factor XBP-1. *Genes Dev* 2000;14:152–157.

85. Schmid P, Schulz WA. Coexpression of the C-MYC protooncogene with a-fetoprotein and albumin in fetal mouse liver. *Differentiation* 1990;45:96–102.

86. Shiojiri N, Lemire JM, Fausto N. Cell lineages and oval cell progenitors in rat liver development. *Cancer Res* 1991;51:2611–2620.

87. Makover A, Soprano DR, Wyatt ML, et al. An in situ-hybridization study of the localization of retinol-binding protein and transthyretin messenger RNAs during fetal development in the rat. *Differentiation* 1989;40:17–25.

88. Tilghman SM, Belayew A. Transcriptional control of murine albumin/a-fetoprotein locus during development. *Proc Natl Acad Sci USA* 1982;79:5254–5257.

89. Moorman AF, De Boer PA, Evans D, et al. Expression patterns of mRNAs for a-fetoprotein and albumin in the developing rat: the ontogenesis of hepatocyte heterogeneity. *Histochem J* 1990;22:653–660.

90. Lamers WH, Zonneveld D, Charles R. Inducibility of carbamoylphosphate synthetase (ammonia) in cultures of embryonic hepatocytes: ontogenesis of the responsiveness to hormones. *Dev Biol* 1984;105:500–508.

91. Lamers WH, van Roon M, Mooren PG, et al. Amino acid environment determines expression of carbamoylphosphate synthetase and phosphoenolpyruvate carboxykinase in embryonic rat hepatocytes. *In Vitro Cell Dev Biol* 1985;21:606–611.

92. Notenboom RG, de Boer PA, Moorman AF, et al. The establishment of the hepatic architecture is a prerequisite for the development of a lobular pattern of gene expression. *Development* 1996;122:321–332.

93. Sladek FM, Zhong W, Lai E, et al. Liver enriched transcription factor HNF-4 is a novel member of the steroid hormone receptor superfamily. *Genes Dev* 1990;4:2353–2364.

94. Li J, Ning G, Duncan SA. Mammalian hepatocyte differentiation requires the transcription factor HNF-4α. *Genes Dev* 2000;14:464–474.

95. Kuo CJ, Conley PB, Chen L, et al. A transcriptional hierarchy involved in mammalian cell-type specification. *Nature* 1992;355:457–461.

96. Pontoglio M, Barra J, Hadchouel M, et al. Hepatocyte nuclear factor 1 inactivation results in hepatic dysfunction, phenylketonuria, and renal Fanconi syndrome. *Cell* 1996;84:575–585.

97. Tronche F, Bach I, Chouard T, et al. Hepatocyte nuclear factor 1(HNF1) and liver gene expression. In: Tronche F, Yaniv M, eds. *Liver gene expression.* Austin, TX: R.G. Landes, 1994:155–182.

98. Cereghini S, Ott M-O, Power S, et al. Expression patterns of vHNF1 and HNF1 homeoproteins in early postimplantation embryos suggest distinct and sequential developmental roles. *Development* 1992;116:783–797.

99. Barbacci E, Reber M, Ott MO, et al. Variant hepatocyte nuclear factor 1 is required for visceral endoderm specification. *Development* 1999;126:4795–4805.

100. Cereghini S. Liver-enriched transcription factors and hepatocyte differentiation. *FASEB J* 1996;10:267–282.

101. Wells JM, Melton DA. Vertebrate endoderm development. *Annu Rev Cell Dev Biol* 1999;15:393–410.

The Liver: Biology and Pathobiology, Fourth Edition, edited by I. M. Arias, J. L. Boyer, F. V. Chisari, N. Fausto, D. Schachter, and D. A. Shafritz. Lippincott Williams & Wilkins, Philadelphia © 2001.

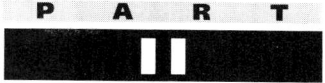

THE CELLS

GAP AND TIGHT JUNCTIONS IN LIVER: COMPOSITION, REGULATION, AND FUNCTION

TAKASHI KOJIMA
NORIMASA SAWADA
HEATHER S. DUFFY
DAVID C. SPRAY

STRUCTURE OF JUNCTIONS IN THE LIVER

Coordinated function of the liver depends on both long- and short-range signaling among the numerous cell types that comprise hepatocytes, Ito cells, cholangiocytes, and endothelial cells. Such signaling is accomplished by hormones and transmitters moving through the extracellular space as well as by direct intercellular diffusion of ions and messenger molecules. Elaborate junctional complexes decorate the appositional surfaces of hepatocytes, separating apical from basolateral membrane domains and directly linking the cytoplasm of one cell with that of its neighbors. The junctional types that are the subject of this chapter are tight junctions, or *zonula occludens*, which separate extracellular bulk fluid phases and maintain the segregation between apical and basolateral domains of the plasma membrane, and gap junctions or *macula communicans*, which function in direct intercellular communication from a cell to its direct neighbors. This chapter is an update that integrates new

findings on both junctional types; for more detailed historical background on gap junctions in particular, the reader is referred to the previous edition (1).

Thin sections and freeze-fracture images of the junctions between dissociated hepatocytes reveal structures that are similar to those seen *in vivo* (Fig. 3.1). In vertebrates, tight junctions play a central role in regulating the movement of solutes, ions, and water through the extracellular space in epithelial or endothelial sheets. Tight junctions between hepatocytes surround the bile canaliculi, where they seal the paracellular spaces between hepatocytes and maintain cellular polarity. By contrast, gap junctions control cell-to-cell movement of solutes, ions, and water, providing an intercellular pathway not accessible to dilution by extracellular fluid. In the hepatic acinus, bile flow in hepatocyte canaliculi is thought to require the organized and periodic contraction of bile canaliculi, where cell-to-cell spread of contraction occurs through signaling via gap junction channels (2). In perfused rat liver, bile secretion induced by glucagon or vasopressin has been shown to be modulated by gap junction communication (3).

Gap junctions occupy a large fraction, as much as 3%, of the total surface area of hepatocytes (4,5). In stained thin sections of liver tissue (6) and of hepatocyte cell pairs, gap

T. Kojima and N. Sawada: Department of Pathology, Sapporo Medical University School of Medicine, Sapporo 060-8556, Japan.
H. S. Duffy and D. C. Spray: Department of Neuroscience, Albert Einstein College of Medicine, Bronx, New York 10461.

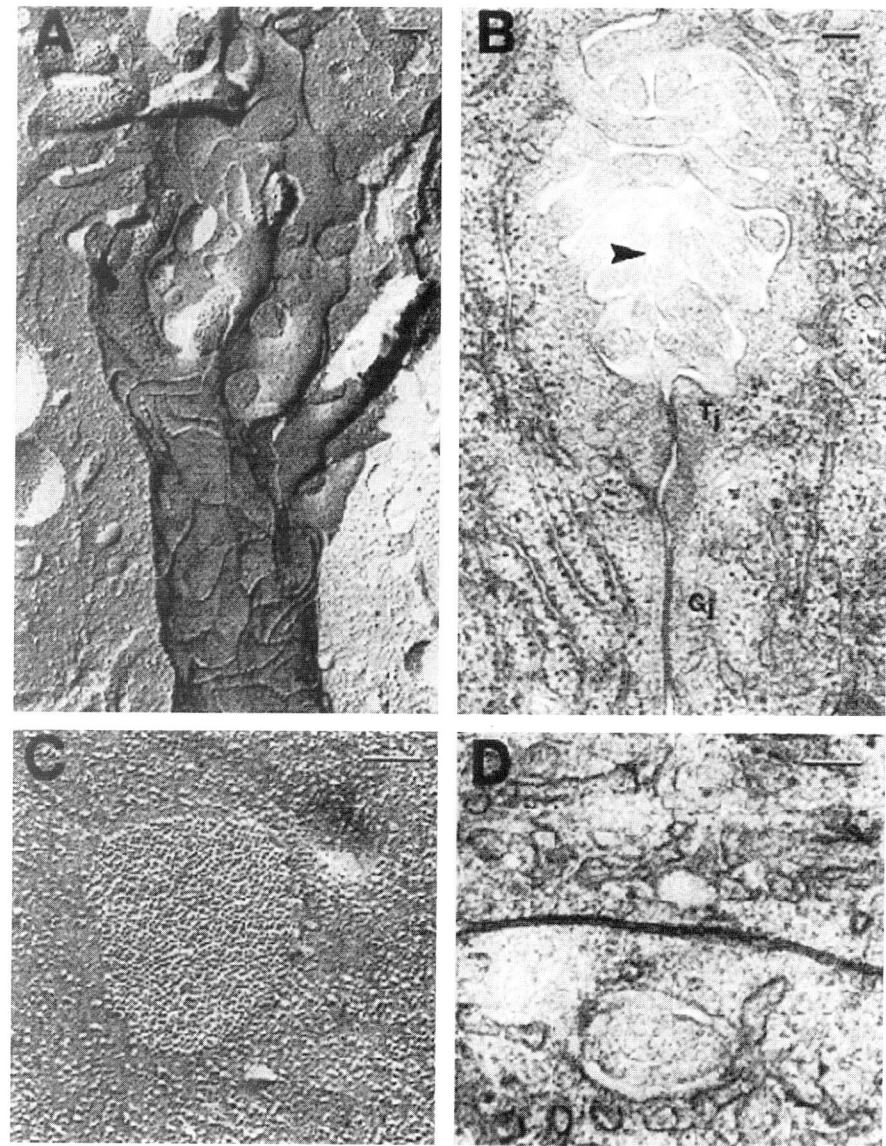

FIGURE 3.1. Fine structure of appositional membranes between rat hepatocytes. **A,C:** Freeze fracture. **B,D:** Thin sections. **A:** Below the bile canaliculi, tight junction webs seen in this freeze-fracture electron micrograph seal off the canalicular surfaces from the rest of the appositional membrane. **B:** Thin-section micrograph illustrates tight junctions (T_j) sealing the canaliculus (*arrowhead*) and a large gap junction (G_j) below it. Freeze-fracture **(C)** and thin-section **(D)** views show larger gap junctions below and in isolation from tight junctional strands. *Bars* = 0.1 nm (From Spray DC, Saez JC, Hertzberg EL, et al. Gap junctions in liver: Composition, function and regulation. In: Arias I, Boyer JL, Fausto N, et al., eds. *The Liver: Biology and Pathobiology.* Third edition. New York: Raven Press, 1994:951–967, with permission.)

junctions are recognized as septilaminar linear membrane appositions separated by an extracellular gap (Fig. 3.1C, D). The seven laminae are the transparent extracellular gap sandwiched on either side by each cell's membrane, consisting of two stained and thus electron-opaque lipid head groups on each side of the electron-lucent membrane interior. The overall thickness of this double membrane specialization is approximately 15 to 18 nm, and the extracellular space in the region of gap junctional contact is approximately 2 to 4 nm wide.

In freeze-fracture images, gap junctions of liver and hepatocyte cell pairs are recognizable as arrays or plaques of approximately 8- to 9-nm intramembranous particles present in the P-fracture face in vertebrate tissues; complementary pits appear on the E-fracture face. These plaques are generally round or oval and can be quite large in hepatocytes (Fig. 3.1C,D), commonly exceeding 1 mm in diameter and containing more than 10,000 particles. The particles seen in freeze-fracture replicas and the bridges across the extracellular space in thin section are believed to represent channels with hydrophilic walls extending from the cytoplasmic aspect of one cell to that of another (Fig. 3.2A).

High-resolution ultrastructural studies on isolated liver gap junctions using techniques of x-ray diffraction and low-angle scattering have added detail to the model of the gap junction channel (7–11). It is now generally accepted that liver gap junction channels are composed of 12 subunits, six of which are contributed by each cell; the assemblage of the six subunits contributed by each cell has been termed a connexon or hemichannel (Fig. 3.2A). The subunits are radially symmetric around the central pore, and each is tilted slightly relative to the plane of the membrane. Recent

cryoelectron microscopy and computer modeling have provided evidence that the formation of rat liver gap junctions requires a 30-degree rotation between hemichannels for proper docking (12).

The ultrastructure of tight junctions is quite different from that of gap junctions. In freeze fracture, tight junctions appear as a set of continuous, anastomosing strands in the P-fracture face (Fig. 3.1A), with complementary grooves in the E-face; in thin section, they appear as very close membrane appositions (13,14). The role of tight junctions is to provide a high-resistance barrier to leakage of water and solutes into and from the bile canaliculus [the resistance to current flow has been measured as approximately 50 kO by insertion of a microelectrode into the canalicular space (15)]. The number of tight junctional strands encircling the bile canaliculus is normally high,

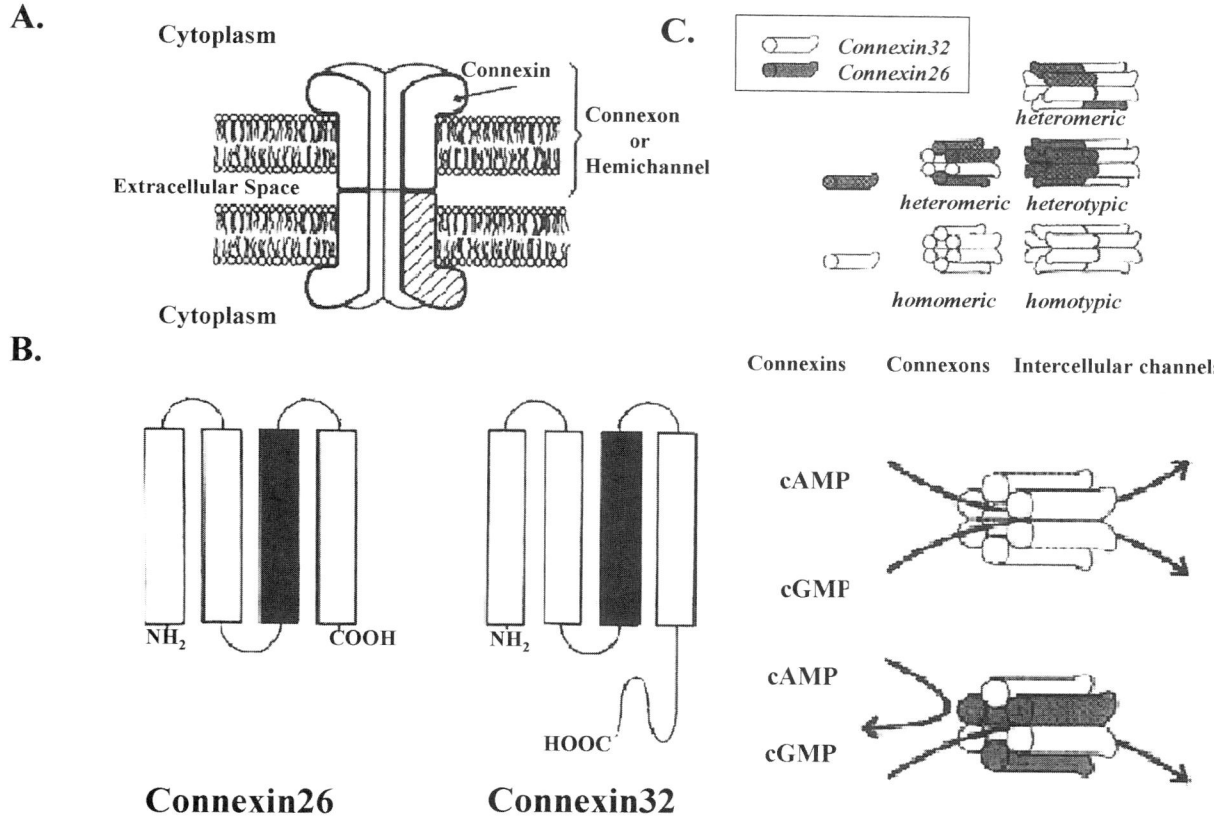

FIGURE 3.2. Molecular components of liver gap junction channels. **A:** Each gap junction channel consists of two connexons or hemichannels, each containing six protein subunits (connexins, one of which is shaded in cross section). These connexons pair across extracellular space, forming the walls of the gap junction channel. **B:** Membrane topologies of the two liver gap junction proteins Cx26 and Cx32. Note four transmembrane domains (*open rectangles*), the third of which (*filled rectangles*) is the most amphipathic and thought to line the pore, extracellular loops with symmetrical sulfhydryl groups (SH), which are believed to play a role in channel formation, and the cytoplasmic location of amino and carboxy termini. **C:** Organization of connexins into connexons and intercellular gap junction channels. Connexin proteins are oligomerized into connexons that are termed homomeric if they have one type of connexin or heteromeric if they contain multiple connexins. Different types of connexons give rise to either homotypic, heterotypic, or heteromeric intercellular channels (Modified from Spray DC, Saez JC, Hertzberg EL, et al. Gap junctions in liver: Composition, function and regulation. In: Arias I et al., Boyer JL, Fausto N, eds. *The Liver: Biology and Pathobiology.* Third edition. New York: Raven Press, 1994:951–967, with permission).

indicating a tight permeability barrier (16). As a consequence, the composition of the canalicular fluid can be quite different from that of the other pericellular fluid, allowing the accumulation of high concentrations of preferentially secreted organic anions within this intercellular compartment (2,15,17).

MOLECULAR COMPONENTS OF GAP AND TIGHT JUNCTIONS

Gap Junctions

The first gap junction protein isolated from detergent solubilized gap junctions displayed an apparent molecular weight of 27 kd, although a 21-kd protein was also detected (for historical overview, see ref. 1). Cloning of the cDNA encoding the 27-kd protein (18,19) indicated that its predicted molecular weight is about 32,000 and is generally referred to as connexin32 (Cx32; in an alternative nomenclature this gap junction protein is referred to as β1; see ref. 20). The cDNA encoding the 21-kd protein was subsequently cloned and found to encode a protein of predicted molecular weight of 26,000 (21); this connexin is now termed Cx26 (or β2).

Cx32 and Cx26, the components of hepatocyte gap junctions, are also found in a variety of other cell types (for review, see ref. 20); moreover, another gap junction protein, Cx43 (or α1) is prominent between other liver cell types, including Ito cells and endothelium. The connexin gene family now comprises at least 20 proteins in vertebrates; connexins are apparently absent in invertebrates, where gap junction channels are formed by a separate gene family encoding innexin proteins (22).

Hydropathy plots, confirmed by protease cleavage and epitope mapping studies, indicate that connexins are tetraspan membrane proteins with a very high degree of homology in extracellular and transmembrane domains (Fig. 3.2B). Homologous extracellular domains are thought to account for the ability of many connexins to form heterotypic channels (i.e., that cells expressing one type of connexin can often form gap junctions with cells expressing a different connexin). The greatest dissimilarities among connexins occur in the sequence and length of the C-terminus, which is thought to play a major role in regulation of gap junction channels. It is within this region of the proteins that most of the potential phosphorylation sites are found and against which most of the useful connexin-specific antibodies have been raised.

Most cells express more than one type of connexin, leading to the possibility that both homomeric and heteromeric connexons may exist *in vivo* (Fig. 3.2C). The existence of heteromeric connexons in the liver has been supported by biochemical experiments that have fractionated detergent-solubilized gap junctions (23) and electrophysiologic properties on hepatocytes isolated from Cx32-deficient and wild-type mice (24). Experiments examining the movement of ions and dyes between cells coupled by different connexins have revealed that there are connexin-dependent differences in the permeation of intercellular channels (25–27). One striking example of possible importance to hepatocytes is that homomeric connexons made of Cx32 are permeable to both 3′,5′-cyclic adenosine monophosphate (cAMP) and 3′,5′-cyclic guanosine monophosphate (cGMP), whereas heteromeric connexons composed of Cx32 and Cx26 lose permeability to cAMP but not to cGMP (Fig. 3.2C) (28).

Characterization of the genomic sequence corresponding to Cx32 defined a gene structure (29) that is common to almost all other members of the connexin gene family. The Cx32 coding sequence is included within one open reading frame on a single exon, which is separated from a tiny upstream exon [100 base pair (bp)] by about 6 kilobase (kb) of intervening intronic sequence. Promoter mapping in the human liver-derived HuH-7cell line localized a minimal basal promoter within a 70-bp region immediately upstream of the messenger RNA (mRNA) start sites and DNAase hypersensitive sites 1.2 kb downstream of the Cx32 open reading frame (30,31). More recent experiments have identified positive and negative regulatory domains of the Cx32 promoter and nuclear proteins [hepatocyte nuclear factor-1 (HNF-1)]that bind to them from experiments performed on MH1C1 rat hepatoma cells (32).

The other hepatocyte gap junction protein, Cx26, has been proposed to be a tumor suppressor gene, on the basis of subtractive hybridization using normal and malignant human mammary epithelial cells (33). Cx26 expression in human mammary epithelial cells induced by 12-O-tetradecanoylphorbol-13-acetate (TPA) treatment is controlled at the level of transcriptional modification (34). Kiang et al. (35,36) have cloned and sequenced the 5′ portion of human Cx26 gene, revealing that the promoter region contains six GC boxes, two GT boxes, a TTAAAA box, and a TPA-induced DNase I hypersensitivity region, providing a site by which TPA may exert transcriptional control over Cx26. Nevertheless, induction of exogenous Cx26 in neuroblastoma cells by TPA treatment appears to be controlled by posttranslational mechanisms (37).

Tight Junctions

Tight junctions have a complex molecular composition that is only recently beginning to be clarified in detail (Table 3.1). The integral membrane components of tight junctions include occludin (38) (See Fig. 3.6A on page 39), the claudin family (39,40), and the junctional adhesion molecule (JAM) (41).

The claudin family at present consists of 18 members, including several previously identified junction-associated proteins such as RVP1 (claudin-3) (42), CPE-R (claudin-4) (43), TMVCF (claudin-5) (44), and OSP (claudin-11) (45).

TABLE 3.1. TIGHT JUNCTION–ASSOCIATED PROTEINS

Protein Name	M_r (kd)	Localization/Type	Reference
Occludin	65–82	Integral membrane	38
Claudins	23	Integral membrane	39,40
JAM	36–41	Integral membrane	41
Zonula occludens-1 (ZO-1)	220–225	Peripheral	51
Zonula occludens-2 (ZO-2)	160	Peripheral	52
Zonula occludens-3 (ZO-3)	130	Peripheral	53
7H6	155–175	Peripheral	54
Cingulin	140–160	Peripheral	55
Symplekin	150	Peripheral	56
Rab3B	25	Peripheral	57
AF-6	180–195	Peripheral	58
ASIP	150, 180	Peripheral	59

ASIP, atypical protein kinase C interacting protein; JAM, junctional adhesion molecule; M_r, relative molecular mass.

Two or more distinct claudins are generally coexpressed in single cells of various tissues (14,39,46); for example, claudin-1, -2, and -3 are expressed in the bile canaliculus region of mature mouse hepatocytes (47). By contrast, only a single occludin transcript has been described, although an alternatively spliced form of occludin (termed occludin 1B) has been reported recently (48).

As with the connexins, the major tight junction components occludin and the claudins are tetraspan proteins with intracellular amino and carboxyl termini. Recent detailed analyses of the manner of interaction of heterogeneous claudin species within and between tight junction strands suggest that distinct species of claudins are copolymerized linearly to form tight junction strands as homopolymers or heteropolymers and that the claudins interact between each of the paired strands in a homophilic or heterophilic manner, including both other claudins and/or occludin (47). Loss of claudins has been shown to cause the disruption of tight junctions *in vitro*, where selective downregulation of Cln-4 resulting from treatment with Clostridium toxin led to a loss of complex tight junction formation, although rudimentary tight junctions remained (49). In contrast, *in vivo* deletion of another claudin, Cln-11, has been shown to cause complete loss of tight junctions in specific cell types (50).

Several cytoplasmic proteins, including ZO-1 (51), ZO-2 (52), ZO-3 (53), 7H6 antigen (54), cingulin (55), symplekin (56), Rab3B (57), Ras target AF-6 (58), and ASIP (an atypical protein kinase C interacting protein) (59), have been reported to be associated with tight junctions, and some of these are believed to play roles in signal transduction. The cytoplasmic domains of occludin and claudins are reported to bind to ZO-1, ZO-2, and ZO-3 (53,60–62), forming a macromolecular complex at cell membranes. ZO-1, ZO-2, and ZO-3 are members of the membrane-associated guanylate kinase (MAGUK) family of proteins displaying a characteristic multidomain structure composed of SH3, guanylate kinase-like (GUK), and multiple PDZ (PSD95-Dlg-ZO1) domains (63).

Interaction Between Gap and Tight Junctions

In hepatocytes, ZO-1 is detected not only in the tight junction zone but also at the adherens junction, whereas in intestinal epithelial cells bearing well-developed tight junctions, cadherins and ZO-1 are clearly segregated into adherens and tight junctions, respectively (64). Recently, it has become established that Cx43 interacts with ZO-1 in Cx43 transfectants, in normal fibroblasts, and in cardiac myocytes (65,66). This interaction is direct, through binding of the extreme carboxyl terminus of Cx43 and the second PDZ domain of ZO-1 (65,66). Furthermore, small gap junction plaques are associated with tight junction strands in some cell types including hepatocytes (Fig. 3.3A,B). In primary cultured rat hepatocytes, Cx32 was partly colocalized with occludin and claudin-1, in which form tight junction structures (Fig. 3.3C, See Fig. 3.6A on page 39). To examine roles of gap junctions in regulating expression and structure of tight junctions, we transfected human Cx32 cDNA into immortalized mouse hepatocytes (CHST8 cells) that lack endogenous Cx32 and Cx26 (67). In Cx32 transfectants, induction of tight junction strands and the integral tight junction proteins occludin and claudins were observed, and small gap junction plaques appeared within the induced tight junction strands. The induced endogenous occludin protein in the transfectants was found to bind to the exogenously expressed Cx32 protein. These results indicate that gap junction and tight junction expression are closely correlated in hepatocytes, and we speculate that through this association gap junction expression may play a crucial role in the establishment of cell polarity via regulation of tight junction proteins. This

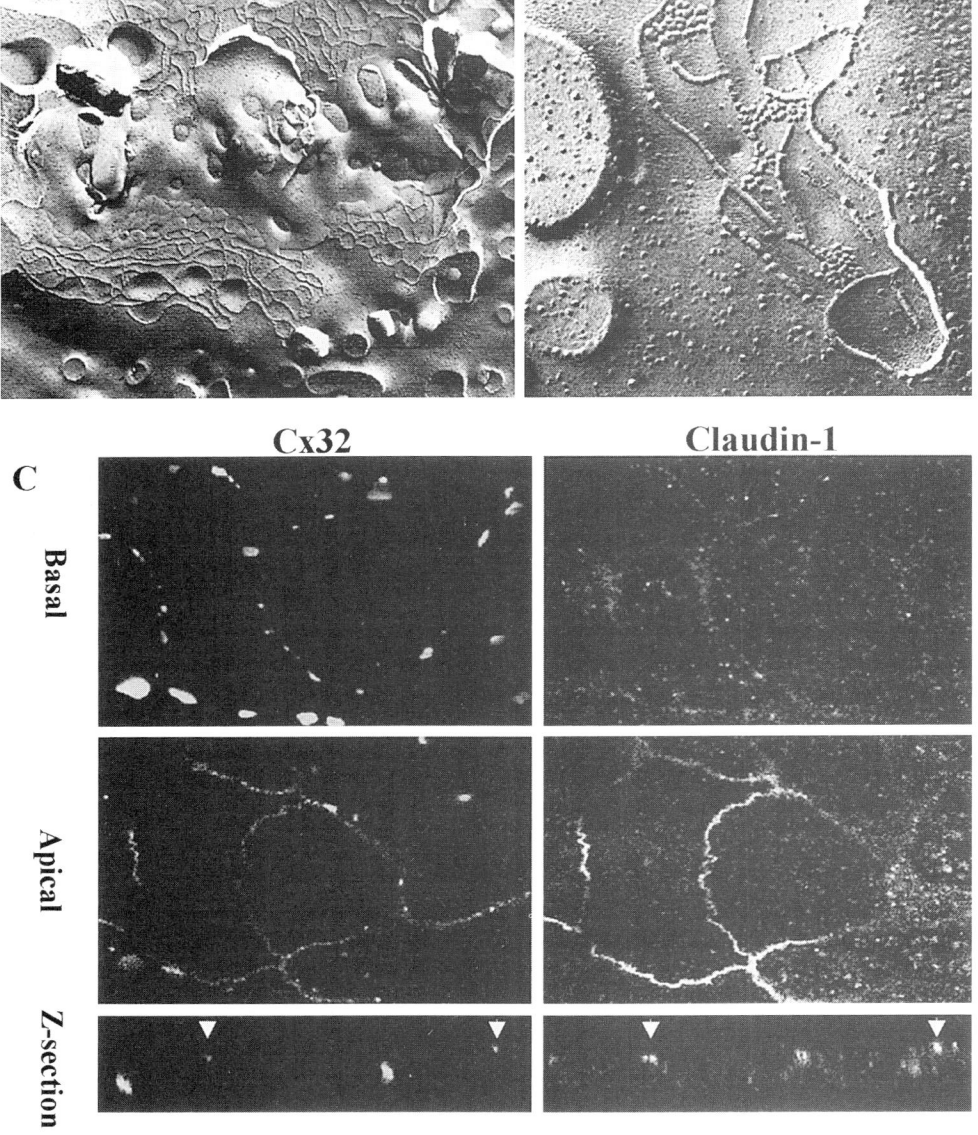

FIGURE 3.3. Interaction between gap junctions and tight junctions in primary cultured rat hepatocytes. **A, B:** Freeze fracture. **C:** Double staining of Cx32 and claudin-1. In freeze fracture analysis of the adluminal plasma membrane, tight junction strands form well-developed networks **(A)** and many small gap junction plaques were observed peripherally or within the tight junction network **(B)**. Cx32-immunoreactive lines were observed on the most subapical plasma membrane at cell borders, while Cx32-positive spots could be observed on the basolateral membrane **(C)**. Claudin-1–immunoreactive lines were observed on the most subapical plasma membrane of the cell borders and were colocalized with Cx32-immunoreactive lines (*arrowheads* in **C**).

finding supports previous studies in which gap junctions have been associated with other components of intercellular junctional components. More importantly, however, the present demonstration of a direct linkage between occludin and Cx32 and previous studies showing high-affinity interactions between ZO-1 and Cx43 (65,66) indicate that connexins may form selective association with specific compo-

nents of adhesive or occluding junctions. Through binding of these proteins to cytoskeletal, adhesion, and signaling proteins, we have proposed that different connexins may promote the aggregation of connexin-specific scaffolds at junctional regions, providing not only intercellular signaling but also sites where intracellular signaling is transduced (67,68).

FUNCTIONS OF GAP JUNCTIONS IN THE LIVER

Signaling

Gap junctions are found between each of the cell populations of the liver, where the type of connexin expressed is cell-type and region specific (Fig. 3.4). For example, the cells of the liver capsule, Ito (fat-storing) cells, cholangiocytes, and endothelial cells lining the venules express Cx43 as a major gap junction protein (69–71), whereas hepatocytes express only Cx26 and/or Cx32 (10,72).

Physiologic consequences of the high level of gap junction expression between hepatocytes appear to include signal transfer and growth control. The relay of metabolic signals is important not only because of the anatomic arrangement of the hepatic acini but also because certain phenotypic features of hepatocytes are graded from periportal regions (characterized by the portal triad that includes the terminal portal venule) to pericentral regions (surrounding the terminal hepatic venule). For example, hepatocytes with higher glucogenic activity are found periportally rather than pericentrally (73,74). Nevertheless, the

strong electrical coupling mediated by gap junctions between hepatocytes serves to equilibrate the membrane potentials among hepatocytes (75,76). In isolated rat liver, perfusion with glucagon leads to hyperpolarization of all hepatocytes across the hepatic acinus. However, in the presence of octanol, a gap junction blocker, glucagon-induced hyperpolarization is higher in periportal than in pericentral hepatocytes (77). Furthermore, heptanol blockade of gap junctions has been shown to abolish metabolic and hemodynamic effects of nerve stimulation within the liver (78). These findings are consistent with the notion that gap junctions play important functional roles during responses of liver cells to agents affecting the metabolic state of this organ.

An unresolved question is the identity of the molecule(s) that provide gap-junction–mediated signaling. Gap junction channels are permeable to solutes up to a molecular weight cutoff of about 1 kd (Fig. 3.5A), allowing possible involvement of both ions and second messengers in intercellular signaling. Imaging studies on hepatocyte pairs demonstrated that injection of Ca^{2+} into one cell leads to diffusional spread to the adjacent cell (79). This intercellu-

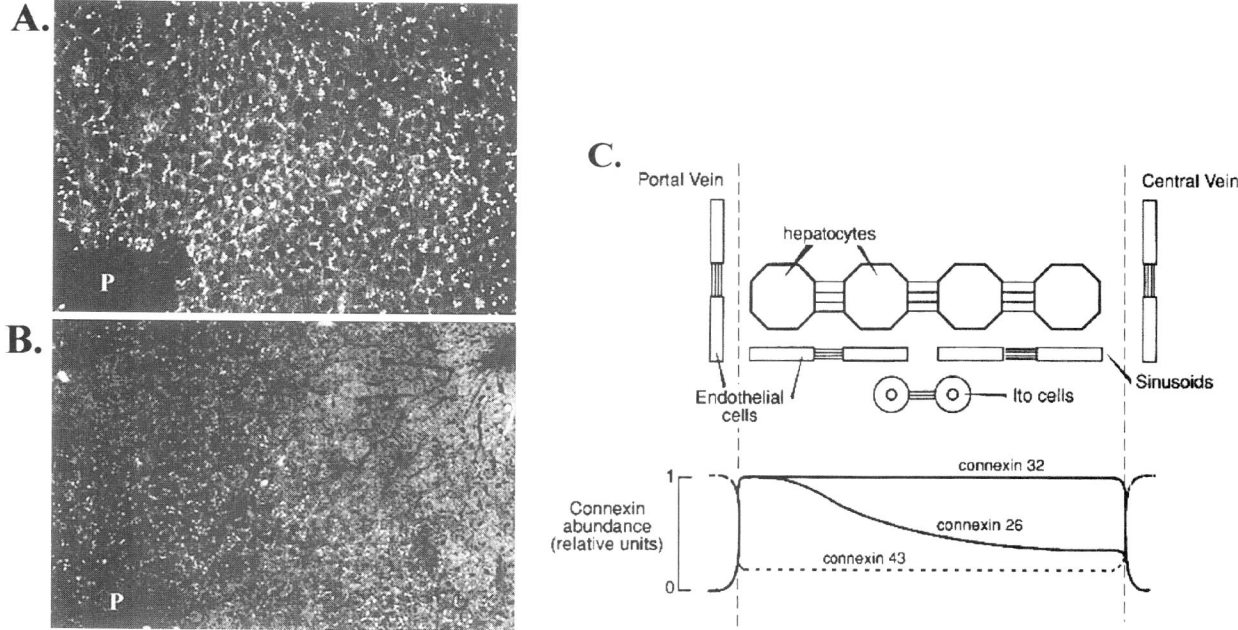

FIGURE 3.4. Communication compartments in liver. **A:** Cx32 staining in rat liver. **B:** Cx26 staining in rat liver. (Central vein in upper right corner; *P*, periportal vein at lower left). Cx32-positive spots are constant across the acinar unit, while Cx26-positive spots decrease in a gradient from high levels periportally to low levels pericentrally. **C:** The major hepatic cell type is the parenchymal cell or hepatocyte, which extends in branched arrays from the portal triad to the central vein. Each hepatocyte is coupled to all adjacent hepatocytes by generally massive gap junction plaques consisting of Cx32 and Cx26. In the rodent liver, Cx32 expressions is constant across the acinar unit, while Cx26 expression decreases in a gradient from high levels periportally to low levels pericentrally (graphed schematically in the *lower* portion of the figure). Other cell types in the liver include endothelial cells, which line the portal vein and sinusoids, as well as fat-storing Ito cells. Both of these cell populations express Cx43, with the most intense staining within the portal triad (distribution graphed below the diagram).

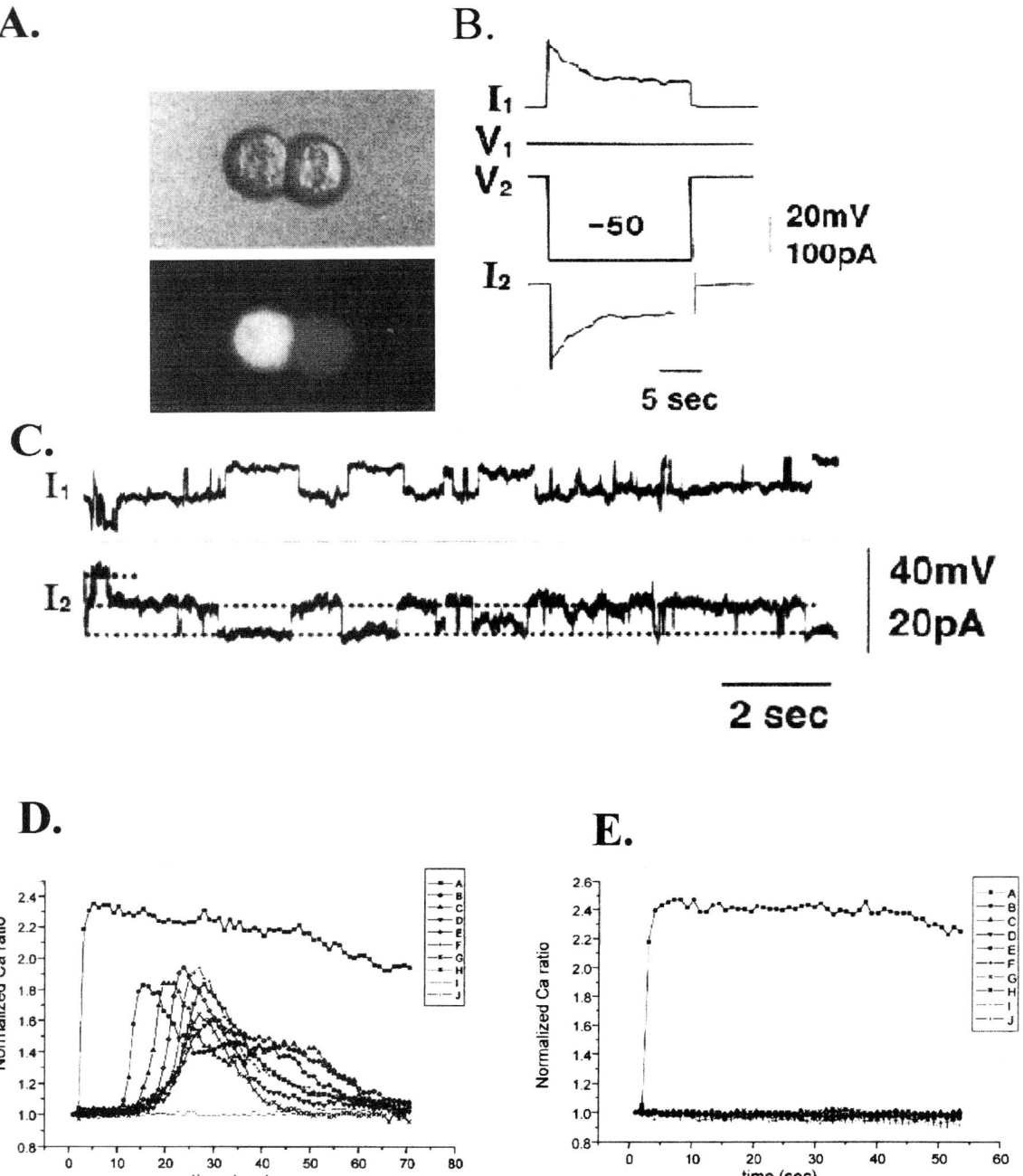

FIGURE 3.5. Communication through gap junction channels. **A:** Light and epifluorescence photos showing that Lucifer yellow CH (5% wt/vol) injected iontophoretically into one cell of a pair of hepatocytes passes detectably to a coupled neighboring cell within 30 seconds. **B:** Voltage-clamp experiment on a pair of hepatoma cells stably transfected with Cx32. A 50-mV hyperpolarization (*V2*) of one cell produces an initial current in the other cell (*I1*), which decreases over a period of seconds. This voltage sensitivity is characteristic of liver gap junction channels. **C:** Single gap junction channel openings and closures can be seen in this example of a high-gain recording from a poorly coupled pair of SKHep1 cells transfected with rat Cx32. In response to a driving force of 50 mV, channels continuously open and close, as indicated by abrupt transitions of equal size but opposite polarity recorded in each cell's voltage-clamp circuit. In these initial studies (81), unitary conductance of Cx32 channels was calculated as about 120 pS; more recent studies in N2A cells transfected with human Cx32 or Cx26 revealed channels of about 55 and 135 pS (107), which are consistent with conductances recorded from hepatocytes obtained from wildtype and Cx32 knockout mice (41). **D:** Mechanical induced Ca^{2+} wave propagation in mouse hepatocyte cell line stable transfected with Cx32. Ca^{2+} is measured in fluorescence of cells loaded Indo-1-AM (10 µM) and the changes in $[Ca^{2+}]_i$ are indicated by the pseudocolored images. **Upper and bottom of left figures** are fluorescence ratio images at 0 and 20 seconds after a single cell was mechanically stimulated **(A)**. *Upper and bottom of right graphs* are time course of changes of fluorescence rations in the cells untreated or treated with gap junction blocker (18β-glycyrrhetinic acid).

lar spread was blocked by treatment of the cells with the gap junction inhibitor heptanol, indicating that movement is by way of gap junction channels. Intracellularly injected inositol 1,4,5-triphosphate (IP$_3$) leads to localized rises in intracellular Ca^{2+} in the injected cell and in its coupled partner. Because the Ca^{2+} rise in the recipient cell can occur far from the junctional region, diffusion is likely to be IP$_3$ or its metabolite, but not of Ca^{2+} itself. This study and others in which synchronous Ca^{2+} oscillations occur in hepatocyte couplets (80) indicate that intercellular diffusion of Ca^{2+} and IP$_3$ can lead to regenerative Ca^{2+} release within hepatocytes. Such regenerative Ca^{2+} elevations may serve the role of long-range signaling in propagation of canalicular contractions (2).

Intercellular Ca^{2+} signaling is commonly used by cells to coordinate and regulate a wide range of cellular functions including cell growth and differentiation (81,82). Ca^{2+} waves may also closely contribute to the various functions of liver and occur in the intact liver, following vasopressin stimulation (83,84). Ca^{2+} wave signaling among cultured hepatocytes may use two parallel pathways (Fig. 3.5D) (85–88). One is of these is the intercellular propagation of Ca^{2+} waves initiated by the generation of IP$_3$, which diffuses to adjacent neighboring cells via gap junctional channels and were inhibited by gap junction blocker (Fig. 3.4D). The other pathway involves extracellular Ca^{2+} wave propagation to both adjacent and nonadjacent cells, through the activation of purinergic receptors by adenosine triphosphate (ATP) released from the stimulated cell and was inhibited by purinergic receptor blockade (84–86). Furthermore, when Ca^{2+} wave propagation after injection of IP$_3$ into HeLa cells transfected with murine Cx26, Cx32, or Cx43 was measured, the Ca^{2+} wave propagation in Cx32 transfectants was increased by a larger amount than in Cx26 or Cx43 transfectants (88). Intercellular Ca^{2+} wave propagation using the multiplets of connected hepatocytes and the perfused liver may be useful as models in which to study coordination and regulation of the cellular functions via gap junctional channels.

Growth Control

As in many other cell types, one of the roles that has long been proposed for gap junctions lies in the control of normal tissue growth (89). Evidence supporting this association includes reduced gap junction expression in hepatomas compared with that in adjacent normal tissue (90), inhibition of growth of tumors constitutively expressing Cx32 (91), and stimulation of hepatocyte growth by tumor promoters that reduce functional coupling, including TPA, phenobarbital (92), benzoyl peroxide, DDT, lindane (93), arachidonic acid, and prostaglandins (94). Furthermore, the liver tumor promoters phenobarbital, PCB, DDT, and clofibrate decrease dye coupling in rat liver slices *in vivo* (95). These changes appear to involve aberrant expression

or function of gap junction proteins, as searches for linkage between Cx32 mutations and hepatocarcinogenesis have been largely unsuccessful (96).

Models that have been useful for clarifying the association between gap junction expression and growth control in liver include the regeneration of this tissue following surgical or chemical insults. Following partial hepatectomy, gap junctions between cells in the undamaged liver disappear over a time course of approximately 24 hours (4,5). Cells then undergo mitosis as the tissue regenerates and gap junctions reappear, all within 48 to 72 hours after injury. Electrical measurements from the tissue suggest that junctional conductance changes with a similar time course, although increased nonjunctional resistance partially compensates in electrical coupling measurements (97). Using immunoblot techniques, Klaus Willecke's group demonstrated that the total amount of Cx32 in livers following partial hepatectomy underwent a similar cycle of decrease that coincided with time of maximal DNA synthesis and then reappearance (98); Cx26 was regulated in parallel (99,100). At times after partial hepatectomy or bile duct ligation when levels of gap junction protein in plasma membranes are reduced to the lowest levels, Cx26 and Cx32 expression may be regulated by posttranscriptional modification (98,101). Parallel measurements of steady-state Cx32 mRNA and protein levels and junctional conductance show that partial hepatectomy and acute hepatotoxicity cause similar changes (102,103). However, Cx26 mRNA was selectively increased before the onset of the S-phase after partial hepatectomy and after bile duct ligation (104,105).

By means of double-immunolabeling using the nucleotide analogue bromodeoxyuridine as an S-phase marker, Dermietzel et al. (106) showed a reciprocal correlation between the expression of Cx32 and the mitotic activity of hepatocytes during liver regeneration. The conclusion reached by this work indicated a significant reduction of Cx32 expression in S-phase cells. From these findings it seems reasonable to conclude that quantitative changes in gap junction expression play an important role in the control of proliferation in liver (107,108). Studies on chemically induced rat hepatocarcinomas also revealed a dramatic reduction in Cx32 expression under proliferative conditions (109). It is plausible that the partial loss of gap junctions provides a selective advantage for those preneoplastic liver cells that develop into rapidly proliferating tumor cells.

Dissociated hepatocytes undergo changes in gap junction, gap junction protein, and electrical coupling that are temporally similar to those following tissue injury *in situ*; gap junctions initially disappear and then reappear over a time course of days (110). The disappearance of gap junctions can be delayed by treatment with cAMP or glucagon or with protein synthesis inhibitors indicating that mRNA stability may be responsible (110). The reexpression phase of gap junctions in cell culture is associated with renewed synthesis of gap junction mRNA and recovery of gap junction protein levels and electrotonic coupling. Transcription of tissue-specific mRNA including Cx32 was enhanced when hepatocytes were cultured in hormonally defined medium (HDM) in combination with certain glycosaminoglycans (GAGs) and proteoglycans (PGs) (111). Moreover, Cx32 reexpression in primary cultured rat hepatocytes was dramatically enhanced in medium containing epidermal growth factor (EGF) and 2% dimethylsulfoxide (DMSO) (112), and Cx26 could also be induced when glucagon was added together with 2% DMSO (113,114). These latter studies suggest that expression of gap junctions in hepatocytes may be closely related to oxidative stress such that oxygen radical scavengers such as DMSO or melatonin might be important inducing substances (115,116).

Properties of Cx32-Deficient (Cx32 KO) Mouse Liver

A human genetic disease, the X-linked form of Charcot–Marie–Tooth disease (CMTX), involves more than 100 distinct mutations of Cx32 (117,118). In an attempt to mimic CMTX disease in a rodent model, Cx32-deficient [Cx32 knockout (KO)] mice were generated through homologous recombination (119). Although these mice did demonstrate progressive demyelination typical of the human disease, they also showed two deficiencies that have not been observed in CMTX patients. First, liver function was compromised, as evidenced by reduced glucose release from intact liver in response to sympathetic nerve stimulation (119) or induction by hormones (120). Furthermore, in Cx32 KO livers, Cx26 levels were decreased compared to wild types (119), and electrophysiologic properties and permeability to IP$_3$ in Cx32 KO hepatocytes were decreased compared to wild types (24,27,120,121). Second, proliferation rate of Cx32 KO hepatocytes *in vivo* was high, and spontaneous and chemically induced liver tumors were more prevalent in Cx32 KO than wild-type livers (122,123). Furthermore, when we have compared cultured hepatocytes from Cx32 KO and wild type mice using serum free medium, proliferation rate of Cx32 KO hepatocytes was markedly higher than of wild-type *in vitro* (124). Interestingly, however, the proliferation rate of Cx32 KO hepatocytes after partial hepatectomy was reported to be significantly lower than in wild types (125). The Cx32 KO mouse model thus is extraordinarily promising for understanding various functions of liver gap junctions during cell growth and differentiation.

REGULATION OF COUPLING BETWEEN HEPATOCYTES

The extent to which signals spread in the liver depends on the number of open gap junction channels. Gap junction channels between hepatocytes are closed by cytoplasmic

acidification, cell injury, exposure of the cytoplasmic aspect to very high Ca^{2+} concentrations, CCl$_4$, and certain alcohols, and by large voltage gradients imposed across the junctional membrane (126–128). Sensitivity of hepatocyte gap junctions to cytoplasmic acidification is low to near-normal pH$_i$, but becomes profound at acidic pH$_i$ values (126). Strong impermeant acids and buffers do not act on conductance of the junctional membrane when applied to the cell exterior, indicating that the gating domain is on the cytoplasmic aspect of the channel. Treatments that elevate cytoplasmic free Ca^{2+} have long been known to decrease intercellular coupling, but sensitivity of gap junctional membranes to calcium is actually very low (79,129). In hepatocytes, elevating cytoplasmic calcium to levels adequate to contract the bile canaliculus (2) does not block electrical or dye coupling. Moreover, the gap junction–mediated diffusion of calcium ions demonstrated in hepatocytes (79) limits the role of Ca^{2+} in closing liver gap junctions to gross tissue insult involving exposure of cytoplasmic aspects of the gap junction to extracellular Ca^{2+} concentrations.

Modulation of signal spread through gap junction protein phosphorylation may be a common type of regulation in the liver and elsewhere. Connexin32 is phosphorylated on SER233 in the cytoplasmic tail of this protein by cAMP-dependent protein kinase, which is correlated with increased conductance (130,131). Numerous other protein kinases are found in liver, including protein kinase C, Ca^{2+}-calmodulin–dependent kinase, as well as several tyrosine kinases (including the insulin and epidermal growth factor receptors). Ca^{2+}-calmodulin–dependent protein kinase II and protein kinase C phosphorylate Cx32 in isolated junctions, producing tryptic fingerprints distinct from those obtained with cAMP-dependent protein kinase (131), but their relevance has not yet been shown *in vivo*. Although in other cell types inhibition of junctional communication has been associated with the expression of tyrosyl kinases, Cx32 in isolated rat liver gap junctions is not phosphorylated by purified pp60v-src tyrosine kinase or the insulin receptor (131), and the functional state of exogenously expressed Cx32 channels in *Xenopus* oocytes is not affected by the expression of pp60v-src (132). Recent evidence indicates that EGF stimulates phosphorylation of Cx32 on at least one tyrosine residue and that EGF receptor tyrosine kinase directly phosphorylates Cx32 (133).

Cx26 has the shortest carboxyl tail of all the connexins thus far sequenced and is not phosphorylated (24). On the basis of experiments performed in cell-free systems, it has been proposed that Cx26 can insert into membranes post-translationally, whereas Cx32 is believed to insert cotranslationally (134). Rapid specific appearance of Cx26 in the plasma membrane after perfusion of female rat liver without an increase in total protein or mRNA levels was reported (135). Furthermore, brefeldin A, a drug that disrupts the Golgi network, had minimal effects on trafficking of Cx26 to the plasma membrane in contrast to its disruption of Cx32 trafficking (136), which suggests that the formation of Cx26 homotypic channels on the membranes may follow an alternative nonclassic trafficking pathway bypassing the Golgi system, in contrast to the classic trafficking pathway [endoplasmic reticulum (ER)-Golgi-plasma membrane] followed by Cx32.

FUNCTION AND REGULATION OF TIGHT JUNCTIONS

Tight junctions, the most apically located of the intercellular junctional complexes, inhibit solute and water flow through the paracellular space (termed the "barrier" function; 137,138). They also separate the apical from the basolateral cell surface domains to establish cell polarity (termed the "fence" function; 139,140). To investigate the barrier function of tight junctions, three approaches are commonly used to evaluate the permeability of the paracellular pathway to ions and uncharged hydrophilic macromolecules: passage of electron-dense dyes, transepithelial electrical resistance (TER), and transepithelial flux of substances lacking affinity for membrane transporters (141). Barrier function can be visualized by the ability of tight junctions to block the passage of electron dense molecules, such as ruthenium red, lanthanum (Fig. 3.6B), and cationic ferritin (142). A modification of this method combining biotinylated compounds and fluorescence microscopy has been used (143). Measurement of TER is the simplest and most rapid method, in which electrodes placed on opposite sides of an epithelial sheet are used to pass current pulses and measure resultant voltage deflections (67,144,145). The third approach to determining paracellular permeability is to measure the passive movement of flux of hydrophilic uncharged molecules, commonly radioactively labeled D-mannitol, raffinose, polyethylene glycol, and various methylated dextrans across an epithelial sheet as a function of time (146). To investigate the fence function of tight junctions, fluorescent lipid probes (such as BODIPY-sphingomyelin) are inserted into the outer leaflet of the plasma membrane and the ability of the tight junction to restrict the dye localization to the cell surface domain is examined (Fig. 3.7D,E) (145,147).

Using electron microscopy, actin filaments have been localized near the cytoplasmic side of tight junctions (Fig. 3.7B) and some integral or peripheral tight junction proteins that bind to actin filaments have been seen (61,148,149). ZO-1 and ZO-2 also bind to actin filaments (61,149), suggesting a role of tight junctions in the organization of the actin cytoskeleton. Disruption of actin filaments deteriorates barrier function of tight junctions, though the protein interaction among tight junction proteins has not fully clarified. Polarized epithelial cells, such as Madin-Darby canine kidney (MDCK), Caco-2, and T84 cell lines, have been successfully exploited to study the reg-

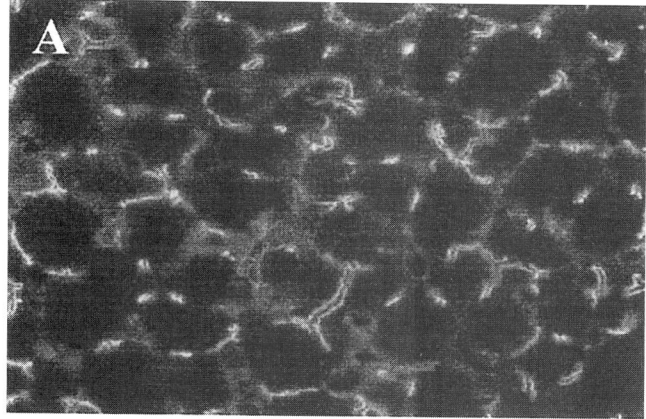
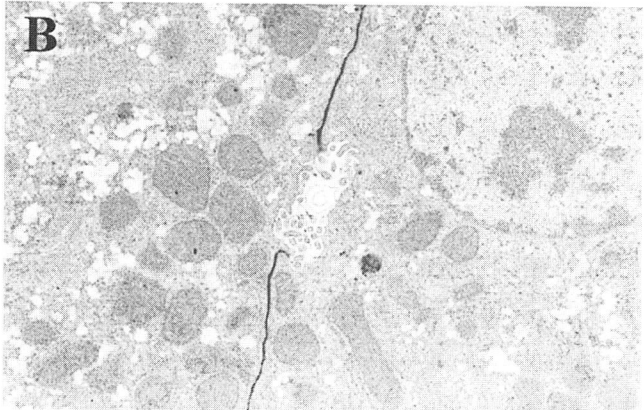

FIGURE 3.6. Tight junctions in rat liver *in vivo*. **A:** Distribution of occludin in rat liver. Occludin is observed in bile canalicular regions. **B:** Thin-section image in which the tight junctions can be seen flanking the microvillus-filled canaliculus. Lanthanum was introduced into the extracellular spaces via the vascular system and is seen to penetrate the extracellular spaces but is denied access to the canalicular lumen by the tight junctions.

ulation of tight junctions *in vitro*. However, because hepatocytes display a complex polarity and deliver apical proteins via an indirect route, *in vitro* studies have been hampered by lack of well-polarized hepatic cell lines, although it has been reported that phalloidin and vasopressin induce dysfunction of tight junctions and the cytoskeleton of rat hepatocyte couplets (150,151). Recently, in primary rat hepatocytes cultured with DMSO/glucagon, tight junction strands formed well-developed networks in freeze fracture at the adluminal plasma membrane (Fig. 3.7A), circumferential actin filaments were observed near the tight junction regions (Fig. 3.7B) (152,153), and occludin, claudin-1, ZO-1, and ZO-2 immunoreactive lines were strongly observed on the most subapical plasma membrane of the cell borders (Fig. 3.7C). The fence function of tight junctions in the cells, as examined by diffusion of labeled sphingomyelin, was well maintained (Fig. 3.7D,E). Treatment of the cells with the actin polymerizing drug mycalolide B caused disappearance of both the circumferential actin fila-

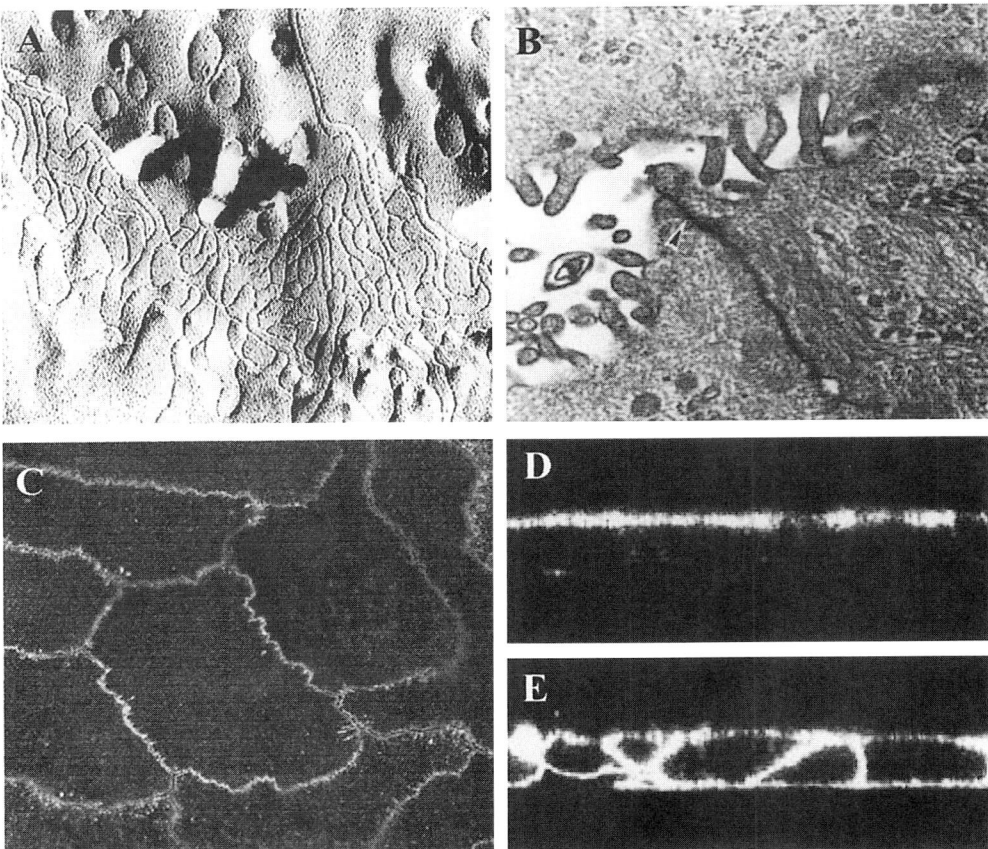

FIGURE 3.7. Tight junctions in primary cultured rat hepatocytes *in vitro* in the presence of dimethylsulfoxide (DMSO)/glucagon medium. **A:** In freeze fracture of the adluminal plasma membrane, tight junction strands form well-developed networks. **B:** Thin-section image in which the tight junctions can be seen with circumferential actin filaments. **C:** Occludin-immunoreactive lines are observed on the most subapical plasma membranes at cell borders. **D, E:** Fence function images of tight junctions. The hepatocytes are labeled with BODIPY-sphingomyelin. The fluorescent probe was effectively retained in the apical domain **(D)**. In the hepatocytes treated with 3 mM ethyleneglycoltetraacetic acid (EGTA) for 5 minutes, the probe diffused through the tight junction, labeling the basolateral face and therefore appeared to penetrate the cells **(E)**.

ments and occludin, while tight junction strands remained virtually intact, leading to the hypothesis that occludin, but not other transmembrane proteins, play a role in the linkage between the actin cytoskeleton and tight junctions in hepatocytes (154). Furthermore, changes of tight junction strands and occludin expression are observed during DNA synthesis and redifferentiation in the cultured hepatocytes (155,156). Because tight junctions in these differentiated cultured hepatocytes assume the distribution seen in simple polarized epithelial cells, this culture system may provide a useful model in which to study hepatocyte tight junctions.

A role for tight junctions in intracellular signaling has been proposed. To elucidate the mechanisms of signal transmission required for the regulation of the tight junction, researchers have recently examined the effect of signaling pathways such as mitogen-activated protein (MAP) kinase and PI$_3$ kinase on the regulation of tight junctions (157–161). The paracellular permeability is influenced by

the state of perijunctional actin (162). Treatment of cultured epithelial cells with the actin disrupters cytochalasin and mycalolide B decreased the barrier function of tight junctions, as assayed by TER and tracer flux studies (145,163–166). Furthermore, a number of signaling molecules have been associated with the regulation of tight junctions, including tyrosine kinases, cAMP, Ca^{2+}, protein kinase C (PKC), heteromeric G proteins, and phospholipase C (167–169). The use of switching between Ca^{2+}-containing and Ca^{2+}-free solutions has demonstrated that in monolayers incubated in low-calcium medium, tight junction proteins are disassembled and dephosphorylated, and they are less tightly associated with actin filaments (154,169,170). This indicates that the function of tight junctions may be locally regulated by signaling events within the tight junction plaque or may regulate some aspect of intracellular signaling. Phosphorylation of the tight junction proteins may also be important to coordinate tight junction assembly or regulate tight junction function (171).

It is also thought that cytoplasmic signaling pathways can affect the barrier function of tight junctions. ATP depletion experiments resulted in altered tight junction structure, decreased TER, and an increased association of tight junction proteins with the actin filaments (169,172, 173). The PKC-activating phorbol esters induce a rapid decrease in tight junction permeability and alter perijunctional actomyosin (174,175). Changes in paracellular permeability induced by the *Vibrio cholerae* toxin zonula occludens toxin (ZOT) are also associated with a reorganization of perijunctional actin (176). The small guanosine triphosphate (GTP)-binding protein rho regulates actin filament organization and influences the organization and permeability of associated tight junctions (177,178).

Because hepatocyte tight junctions are the only intercellular barrier between the sinusoidal and canalicular spaces, major consequences of liver disease may be due to the disturbance of tight junctions. In thin section, the tight junctions of hepatocytes can be seen to block access of the experimentally administered extracellular tracer (lanthanum) to the canalicular lumen (Fig. 3.6B); irregularities in the structure and distribution of tight junctions, accompanied by increased permeability, have been observed during extrahepatic cholestasis after common bile duct ligation, intrahepatic choleostasis after ethinyl estradiol treatment (179–182), partial hepatectomy (183–185), and hepatocyte injury repair following hepatotoxic drug administration or experimental colitis (186–188). Loss of gap junctions, leaky tight junctions, and disorganized actin bundles may be sufficient aberrations to cause cholestasis and eventual development of jaundice.

PROSPECTS AND PERSPECTIVES

The two most prominent junctional types in liver are gap junctions, which provide direct intercellular communication, and tight junctions, which partition membrane domains of individual cells and occlude extracellular space, restricting pericellular diffusion. The integral membrane proteins of vertebrate gap junctions, the connexins, are well characterized and bind to cytoplasmic proteins, suggesting that the connexins may be a nucleation site for intracellular as well as intercellular signaling molecules. In contrast, peripheral proteins associated with the tight junction were identified before integral membrane proteins were discovered. A finding of current interest is the participation of a novel family of integral membrane proteins, the claudins. Although gap and tight junctions perform different functions, there are numerous points at which functional studies overlap. Indeed, traditionally tight junction-associated protein ZO-1 also binds to a connexin, and occludin is colocalized with Cx32 in transfectants, indicating the pos-

sibility for coordinate or reciprocal regulation of macromolecular complexes containing gap and tight junction proteins. Studies of protein–protein interactions and of coordinate and subordinate regulation of gene families are expected to disclose the intricacies of inter- and intracellular signaling and growth control at gap junctions and the regulatory mechanisms of the "blood–biliary barrier" formed by tight junctions.

ACKNOWLEDGMENTS

The authors thank Dr. Y. Mochizuki, Dr. Y. Kokai, Dr. Y. Takakuwa (Sapporo Medical University, Japan), and Dr. M. Yamamoto (Kurume University, Japan). The research by our laboratories is largely supported by National Institutes of Health grant DK-41918.

REFERENCES

1. Spray DC, Saez JC, Hertzberg EL, et al. Gap junctions in liver: Composition, function and regulation. In: Arias I, Boyer JL, Jakoby N, et al., eds. *The Liver: Biology and Pathobiology.* Third edition. New York: Raven Press, 1994:951–967.
2. Watanabe S, Phillips MJ. Ca^{2+} causes active contraction of the bile canaliculi: direct evidence from microinjection studies. *Proc Natl Acad Sci USA* 1984;81:6164–6165.
3. Nathanson MH, Rios-Velez L, Burgstahler AD, et al. Communication via gap junctions modulates bile secretion in the isolated perfused rat liver. *Gastroenterology* 1999;116:1176–1183.
4. Yee AG, Revel JP. Loss and reappearance of gap junctions in regenerating liver. *J Cell Biol* 1978;78:554–564.
5. Yancey SB, Easter E, Revel JP. Cytological changes in gap junctions during liver regeneration. *J Ultrastruct Res* 1979;67: 229–242.
6. Revel JP, Karnovsky MJ. Hexagonal array of subunits in intercellular junctions of the mouse heart and liver. *J Cell Biol* 1967; 33:C7–C12.
7. Unwin PNT, Zampighi G. Structure of the junction between communicating cells. *Nature* 1980;283:545–549.
8. Unwin PNT, Ennis PD. Calcium-mediated changes in gap junction structure: evidence from the low angle x-ray pattern. *J Cell Biol* 1983;97:1459–1466.
9. Unwin PNT, Ennis PD. Two configuration of a channel-forming membrane protein. *Nature* 1984;307:609–613.
10. Makowski L. Structural domains in gap junctions; implications for the control of intercellular communication. In: Bennett MVL, Spray DC, eds. *Gap junctions.* New York: Cold Spring Harbor, 1985:5–12.
11. Makowski L, Casper DLD, Phillips WC, et al. Gap junction structures: VI. Variation and conservation in connexon conformation and packing. *Biophys J* 1984;45:208–218.
12. Perkins GA, Goodenough DA, Sosinsky GE. Formation of the gap junction intercellular channel requires a 30 degree rotation for interdigitating two apposing connexons. *J Mol Biol* 1998; 277:171–177.
13. Easter DW, Wade JB, Boyer JL. Structural integrity of hepatocyte tight junctions. *J Cell Biol* 1983;96:745–749.
14. Tsukita S, Furuse M. Occludin and claudins in tight-junction strands: leading or supporting players? *Trends Cell Biol* 1999;9: 268–273.

15. Graf J, Gautam A, Boyer JL. Isolated rat hepatocyte couplets: a primary secretory unit for electrophysiologic studies of bile secretory function. *Proc Natl Acad Sci USA* 1984;81:6516–6520.

16. Claude P, Goodenough DA. Fracture faces of zonulae occludentes from "tight" and "leaky" epithelia. *J Cell Biol* 1973;58:390–400.

17. Barth CA, Schwartz LR. Transcellular transport of fluorescein in hepatocyte monolayers: evidence for functional polarity of cells in culture. *Proc Natl Acad Sci USA* 1982;79:4985–4987.

18. Paul D. Molecular cloning of cDNA for rat liver gap junction protein. *J Cell Biol* 1986;103:123–134.

19. Kumar NM, Gilula NB. Cloning and characterization of human and rat cDNAs coding for a gap junction protein. *J Cell Biol* 1986;103:767–776.

20. Kumar NM, Gilula NB. The gap junction communication channel. *Cell* 1996;84:381–388.

21. Zhang JT, Nicholson BJ. Sequence and tissue distribution of a second protein of hepatic gap junctions, Cx26, as deduced from its cDNA. *J Cell Biol* 1989;109:3391–3401.

22. Phelan P, Bacon JP, Davies JA, et al. Innexins: a family of invertebrate gap-junction proteins. *Trends Genet* 1998;14:348–349.

23. Stauffer KA. The gap junction proteins beta 1-connexin (connexin-32) and beta 2-connexin (connexin-26) can form heteromeric hemichannels. *J Biol Chem* 1995;270:6768–6772.

24. Valiunas V, Niessen H, Willecke K, et al. Electrophysiological properties of gap junction channels in hepatocytes isolated from connexin32-deficient and wild-type mice. *Pflugers Arch* 1999;437:846–856.

25. Elfgang C, Eckert R, Lichtenberg-Fraté H, et al. Specific permeability and selective formation of gap junction channels in connexin-transfected HeLa cells. *J Cell Biol* 1995;129:805–817.

26. Cao F, Eckert R, Elfgang C, et al. A quantitative analysis of connexin-specific permeability differences of gap junctions expressed in HeLa transfectants and *Xenopus* oocytes. *J Cell Sci* 1998;111:31–43.

27. Niessen H, Willcke K. Strongly decreased gap junctional permeability to inositol 1,4,5-trisphosphate in connexin32 deficient hepatocytes. *FEBS Lett* 2000;146:112–114.

28. Bevans CG, Kordel M, Rhee SK, et al. Isoform composition of connexin channels determines selectivity among second messengers and uncharged molecules. *J Biol Chem* 1998;273:2808–2816.

29. Miller T, Dahl G, Werner R. Structure of gap junction gene: rat connexin32. *Biosci Rep* 1988;8:455–461.

30. Bai S, Spray DC, Burk RD. Identification of proximal and distal regulatory elements of the connexin32 gene. *Biochim Biophys Acta* 1993;1216:197–204.

31. Bai S, Schoenfeld A, Píetrangelo A, et al. Basal promoter of the rat connexin 32 gene: identification and characterization of an essential element and its DNA-binding protein. *Mol Cell Biol* 1995;15:1439–1445.

32. Piechocki MP, Toti RM, Fernstrom MJ, et al. Liver cell-specific transcriptional regulation of connexin32. *Biochim Biophys Acta* 2000;1491:107–122.

33. Lee SW, Tomasetto C, Paul D, et al. Transcriptional downregulation of gap junction proteins blocks junctional communication in human mammary tumor cell line. *J Cell Biol* 1992;118:1213–1221.

34. Li GY, Lin HH, Tu ZJ, et al. Gap junction Cx26 gene modulation by phorbol esters in benign and malignant human mammary cells. *Gene* 1998;209:139–147.

35. Kiang DT, Tu ZJ, Lin HH. Upstream genomic sequence of the human connexin 26 gene. *Gene* 1997;199:165–171.

36. Tu ZJ, Kiang DT. Mapping and characterization of the basal promoter of human connexin 26 gene. *Biochim Biophys Acta* 1998;1443:169–181.

37. Kojima T, Srinivas M, Fort A, et al. TPA induced expression and function of human connexin 26 by post-translational mechanisms in stably transfected neuroblastoma cells. *Cell Struct Funct* 1999;24:435–441.

38. Furuse M, Hirase T, Itoh M, et al. Occludin: a novel integral membrane protein localizing at tight junctions. *J Cell Biol* 1993;123:1777–1788.

39. Furuse M, Fujita K, Hiiragi T, et al. Claudin-1 and -2: novel integral membrane proteins localizing at tight junctions with no sequence similarity to occludin. *J Cell Biol* 1998;141:1539–1550.

40. Morita K, Furuse M, Fujimoto K, et al. Claudin multigene family encoding four-transmembrane domain protein components of tight junction strands. *Proc Natl Acad Sci USA* 1999;96:511–516.

41. Martin-Padura I, Lostaglio S, et al. Junctional adhesion molecule, a novel member of the immunoglobulin superfamily that distributes at intercellular junctions and modulates monocyte transmigration. *J Cell Biol* 1998;142:117–127.

42. Briehl MM, Miesfeld RL. Isolation and characterization of transcripts induced by androgen withdrawal and apoptotic cell death in the rat ventral prostate. *Mol Endocrinol* 1991;5:1381–1388.

43. Katahira J, Inoue N, Horiguchi Y, et al. Molecular cloning and functional characterization of the receptor for *Clostridium perfringens* enterotoxin. *J Cell Biol* 1997;136:1239–1247.

44. Sirotkin H, Morrow B, Saint-Jore B, et al. Identification, characterization, and precise mapping of a human gene encoding a novel membrane-spanning protein from the 22q11 region deleted in Velo-Cardio-Facial syndrome. *Genomics* 1997;42:245–251.

45. Bronstein JM, Popper P, Micevych PE, et al. Isolation and characterization of a novel oligodendrocyte-specific protein. *Neurology* 1996;47:772–778.

46. Simon DB, Lu Y, Choate KA, et al. Paracellin-1, a renal tight junction protein required for paracellular Mg2+ resorption. *Science* 1999;285:103–106.

47. Furuse M, Sasaki H, Tsukita S. Manner of interaction of heterogenous claudin species within and between tight junction strands. *J Cell Biol* 1999;147:891–903.

48. Muresan Z, Paul DL, Goodenough DA. Occludin1B, a variant of the tight junction protein occludin. *Mol Biol Cell* 2000:627–634.

49. Sonoda N, Furuse M, Sasaki H, et al. *Clostridium perfringens* enterotoxin fragment removes specific claudins from tight junction strands: evidence for direct involvement of claudins in tight junction barrier. *J Cell Biol* 1999;147:195–204.

50. Gow A, Southwood CM, Li JS, et al. CNS myelin and Sertoli cell tight junction strands are absent in Osp/claudin-11 null mice. *Cell* 1999;99:649–659.

51. Stevenson BR, Siliciano JD, Mooseker MS, et al. Identification of ZO-1: a high molecular weight polypeptide associated with the tight junction (zonula occludin) in a variety of epithelia. *J Cell Biol* 1986;103:755–766.

52. Jesaitis LA, Goodenough DA. Molecular characterization and tissue distribution of ZO-2, a tight junction protein homologous to ZO-1 and the *Drosophila* discs—large tumor suppressor protein. *J Cell Biol* 1994;124:949–961.

53. Haskins J, Gu L, Wittchen ES, et al. ZO-3, a novel member of the MAGUK protein family found at the tight junction, interacts with ZO-1 and occludin. *J Cell Biol* 1998;141:199–208.

54. Zhong Y, Saitoh T, Minase T, et al. Monoclonal antibody 7H6 reacts with a novel tight junction-associated protein distinct from ZO-1, cingulin and ZO-2. *J Cell Biol* 1993;120:477–483.

55. Citi S, Sabanay H, Jakes R, et al. Cingulin, a new peripheral component of tight junctions. *Nature* 1988;333:272–275.
56. Keon BH, Schafer S, Kuhn C, et al. Symplekin, a novel type of tight junction plaque protein. *J Cell Biol* 1996;134:1003–1018.
57. Weber E, Berta G, Tousson A, et al. Expression and polarized targeting of a rab3 isoform in epithelial cells. *J Cell Biol* 1994;125:583–594.
58. Yamamoto T, Harada N, Kano K, et al. The Ras target AF-6 interacts with ZO-1 and serves as a peripheral component of tight junctions in epithelial cells. *J Cell Biol* 1997;139:785–795.
59. Izumi Y, Hirose T, Tamai Y, et al. An atypical PKC directly associates and colocalizes at the epithelial tight junction with ASIP, a mammalian homologue of *Caenorhabditis elegans* polarity protein PAR-3. *J Cell Biol* 1998;143:95–106.
60. Furuse M, Itoh M, Hirase T, et al. Direct association of occludin with ZO-1 and its possible involvement in the localization of occludin at tight junctions. *J Cell Biol* 1994;127:1617–1626.
61. Itoh M, Morita K, Tsukita S. Characterization of ZO-2 as a MAGUK family member associated with tight as well as adherens junctions with a binding affinity to occludin and alpha catenin. *J Biol Chem* 1999;274:5981–5986.
62. Itoh M, Furuse M, Morita K, et al. Direct binding of three tight junction-associated MAGUKs, ZO-1, ZO-2, and ZO-3, with the COOH termini of claudins. *J Cell Biol* 1999;147:1351–1363.
63. Anderson JM. Cell signaling: MAGUK magic. *Curr Biol* 1996;6:382–384.
64. Itoh M, Nagafuchi A, Yonemura S, et al. The 220-kD protein colocalizing with cadherins in non-epithelial cells is identical to ZO-1, a tight junction-associated protein in epithelial cells: cDNA cloning and immunoelectron microscopy. *J Cell Biol* 1993;121:491–502.
65. Giepmans BNG, Moolenaar WH. The gap junction protein connexin43 interacts with the second PDZ domain of the zona occludens-1 protein. *Curr Biol* 1998;8:931–934.
66. Toyofuku T, Yabuki M, Otsu K, et al. Direct association of the gap junction protein connexin-43 with ZO-1 in cardiac myocytes. *J Biol Chem* 1998;273:12725–12731.
67. Kojima T, Sawada N, Chiba H, et al. Induction of tight junctions in human connexin 32 (hCx32)-transfected mouse hepatocytes: connexin 32 interacts with occludin. *Biochem Biophys Res Commun* 1999;266:222–229.
68. Spray DC, Duffy HS, Scemes E. Gap junctions in glia: types, roles and plasticity. The function of glial cells in health and disease: dialogue between glia and neurons. *Adv Exp Med Biol* 1999;468:339–359.
69. Rojkind M., Novikoff PM, Grenwel P, et al. Characterization and functional studies on rat liver fat-storing cell line and freshly isolated hepatocyte co-culture system. *Am J Pathol* 1995;146:1508–1520.
70. Sáez JC, LaRusso NF. Intrahepatic bile duct epithelial cells are functionally coupled by connexin 43–enriched gap junctions. *Gastroenterology* 1993;104:A983.
71. Berthoud VM, Ivanij V, Garcia AM, et al. Connexins and glucagon receptors during development of the rat hepatic acinus. *Am J Physiol* 1992;263:G650–G658.
72. Traub O, Look J, Dermietzel R, et al. Comparative characterization of the 21-kD and 26-kD gap junction protein in murine liver and cultured hepatocytes. *J Cell Biol* 1989;108:1039–1051.
73. Jungerman K, Kats K. Functional specialization of different hepatocyte populations. *Physiol Rev* 1989;69:708–761.
74. Gumusio JJ, Miller DL. Functional implications of liver cell heterogeneity. *Gastroenterology* 1981;80:393–403.
75. Penn RD. Ionic communication between liver cells. *J Cell Biol* 1966;29:171–174.
76. Graf J, Petersen OH. Cell membrane and resistance in liver. *J Physiol Lond* 1978;284:105–126.
77. Lee S-M, Clemens MG. Subacinar distribution of hepatocyte membrane potential response to stimulation of gluconeogenesis. *Am J Physiol* 1992;263:G319–G326.
78. Seseke FG, Gardeman A, Jungermann K. Signal propagation via gap junctions, a key step in the regulation of liver metabolism by the sympathetic hepatic nerves. *FEBS Lett* 1992;301:265–270.
79. Sáez JC, Connor JA, Spray DC, et al. Hepatocyte gap junctions are permeable to the second messengers inositol 1, 4, 5-trisphosphate and calcium ions. *Proc Natl Acad Sci USA* 1989;86:2708–2712.
80. Nathanson MH, Burgstahler AD. Coordination of hormone-induced calcium signals in isolated rat hepatocyte couplets: demonstration with confocal microscopy. *Mol Biol Cell* 1992;3:113–121.
81. Bootman MD, Berridge MJ. The elemental principles of calcium signaling. *Cell* 1995;83:675–678.
82. Clapham DE. Calcium signaling. *Cell* 1995;80:259–268.
83. Nathanson MH, Burgstahler AD, Mennone A, et al. Ca^{2+} waves are organized among hepatocytes in the intact organ. *Am J Physiol* 1995;269:G167–G171.
84. Robb-Gaspers LD, Thomas AP. Coordination of Ca^{2+} signaling by intercellular propagation of Ca2+ waves in the intact liver. *J Biol Chem* 1995;270:8102–8107.
85. Schlosser SF, Burgstahler AD, Nathanson MH. Isolated rat hepatocytes can signal to other hepatocytes and bile duct cells by release of nucleotides. *Proc Natl Acad Sci USA* 1996;93:9948–9953.
86. Tordjmann T, Berthon B, Claret M, et al. Coordinated intercellular calcium waves induced by noradrenaline in rat hepatocytes: dual control by gap junction permeability and agonist. *EMBO J* 1997;16:5398–5407.
87. Scemes E, Suadicani SO, Spray DC. Intercellular calcium wave communication via gap junction-dependent and independent mechanisms. In: Peracchia C, ed. *Current topics in membranes*, vol 49. San Diego: Academic Press, 2000:145–173.
88. Niessen H, Harz H, Bedner P, et al. Selective permeability of different connexin channels to the second messenger inositol 1,4,5-triphosphate. *J Cell Sci* 2000;113:1365–1372.
89. Loewenstein WR, Rose B. The cell-cell channel in the control of growth. *Semin Cell Biol* 1992;3:59–79.
90. Yamasaki H, Hollstein M, Mesnil M, et al. Selective lack of intercellular communication between transformed and non-transformed cells as a common property of chemical and oncogene transformation of BALB/c 3T3 cells. *Cancer Res* 1987;47:5658–5664.
91. Eghbali B, Kessler JA, Reid LM, et al. Involvement of gap junctions in tumorigenesis: transfection of hepatoma cells with connexin32 cDNA retards growth in vivo. *Proc Natl Acad Sci USA* 1991;88:10701–10705.
92. Armato U, Andreis PG, Romano F. The stimulation by the tumor promoters 12-O-tetradecanoyl-phorbol-13-acetate and phenobarbital of the growth of primary neonatal rate hepatocytes. *Carcinogenesis* 1985;6:811–821.
93. Armato U, Andreis PG, Romano F. Exogenous Cu Zu superoxide dismutase suppresses the stimulation of neonatal rat hepatocytes growth by tumor promoters. *Carcinogenesis* 1984;5:1547–1555.
94. Andreis PG, Whitfield JF, Armato U. Stimulation of DNA synthesis and mitosis of hepatocytes in primary cultures of neonatal rat liver by arachidonic acid and prostaglandins. *Exp Cell Res* 1981;134:265–272.
95. Krutovskikh VA, Mesnil M, Mazzoleni G, et al. Inhibition of rat liver gap junction intercellular communication by tumor-

promoting agents in vivo. Association with aberrant localization of connexin proteins. *Lab Invest* 1995;72:571–577.

96. Omori Y, Krutovskikh V, Mironov N, et al. Cx32 gene mutation in a chemically induced rat liver tumour. *Carcinogenesis* 1996;17:2077–2080.

97. Meyer DJ, Yancey SB, Revel JP, et al. Intercellular communication in normal and regenerating rat liver: a quantitative analysis. *J Cell Biol* 1981;91:505–523.

98. Traub O, Druge PM, Willecke K. Degradation and resynthesis of gap junction protein in plasma membrane regenerating liver after partial hepatectomy or cholestasis. *Proc Natl Acad Sci USA* 1983;80:755–759.

99. Traub O, Jansen-Timmen U, Druge P, et al. Immunological properties of gap junction protein from mouse liver. *J Cell Biochem* 1982;19:27–44.

100. Willecke K, Traub O, Look J, et al. Different protein components contribute to the structure and function of hepatic gap junctions. In: Hertberg EL, Johnson RG, eds. *Gap junctions*. New York: Alan R. Liss, 1988:41–52.

101. Kren BT, Kumar NM, Wang S, et al. Differential regulation of multiple gap junction transcripts and proteins during rat liver regeneration. *J Cell Biol* 1993;123:707–718.

102. Kojima T, Sawada N, Zhong Y, et al. Sequential changes of intercellular junctions in hepatocytes during the course of acute liver injury and restoration after thioacetamide treatment. *Virchows Arch* 1994;425:407–412.

103. Gingalewski C, Wang K, Clemens MG, et al. Posttranscriptional regulation of connexin 32 expression in liver during acute inflammation. *J Cell Physiol* 1996;166:461–467.

104. Neveu MJ, Hully JR, Babcock KL, et al. Proliferation-associated differences in the spatial and temporal expression of gap junction genes in rat liver. *Hepatology* 1995;22:202–212.

105. Fallon MB, Nathanson MH, Mennone A, et al. Altered expression and function of hepatocyte gap junctions after common bile duct ligation in the rat. *Am J Physiol* 1995;268:C1186–C1194.

106. Dermietzel R, Yancey SB, Traub O, et al. Major loss of the 28 kDa protein of gap junction in proliferating hepatocytes. *J Cell Biol* 1987;105:1928–1934.

107. Fladmark KE, Gjertsen BT, Molven A, et al. Gap junctions and growth control in liver regeneration and isolated rat hepatocytes. *Hepatology* 1997;25:847–855.

108. Kojima T, Yamamoto M, Mochizuki C, et al. Different changes in expression and function of connexin 26 and connexin 32 during DNA synthesis and redifferentiation in primary rat hepatocytes using a DMSO culture system. *Hepatology* 1997;26:585–597.

109. Janssen-Timmen U, Traub O, Dermietzel R, et al. Reduced number of gap junctions in rat hepatocarcinomas detected by monoclonal antibody. *Carcinogenesis* 1986;7:1475–1482.

110. Saez JC, Gregory WA, Watanabe T, et al. cAMP delays disappearance of gap junctions between pairs of rat hepatocytes in primary cultures. *Am J Physiol* 1989;26:C1–C11.

111. Fujita M, Spray DC, Choi H, et al. Glycosaminoglycans and proteoglycans induce gap junction expression and restore transcription of tissue-specific mRNAs in primary liver cultures. *Hepatology* 1987;7:1S–9S.

112. Kojima T, Mitaka T, Paul D, et al. Reappearance and long-term maintenance of connexin 32 in proliferated adult rat hepatocytes: use of serum-free L-15 medium supplemented with EGF and DMSO. *J Cell Sci* 1995;108:1347–1357.

113. Kojima T, Mitaka T, Shibata Y, et al. Induction and regulation of connexin 26 by glucagon in primary cultures of adult rat hepatocytes. *J Cell Sci* 1995;108:2771–2780.

114. Kojima T, Yamamoto M, Tobioka H, et al. Changes in cellular distribution of connexin 32 and 26 during formation of gap junctions in primary cultures of adult rat hepatocytes. *Exp Cell Res* 1996;223:314–326.

115. Kojima T, Mitaka T, Mizuguchi T, et al. Effects of oxidant radical scavengers on connexins 32 and 26 expression in primary cultures of adult rat hepatocytes. *Carcinogenesis* 1996;17:537–544.

116. Kojima T, Mochizuki C, Mitaka T, et al. Effects of melatonin on proliferation, oxidative stress and Cx32 gap junction protein expression in primary cultures of adult rat hepatocytes. *Cell Struct Funct* 1997;22:347–356.

117. White TW, Paul DL. Genetic diseases and gene knockouts reveal diverse connexin functions. *Annu Rev Physiol* 1999;61:283–310.

118. Bergoffen J, Scherer SS, Wang S, et al. Connexin mutation in X-linked Charcot-Marie-Tooth disease. *Science* 1993;262:2039–2042.

119. Nelles E, Butzler C, Jung D, et al. Defective propagation of signals generated by sympathetic nerve stimulation in the liver of connexin32-deficient mice. *Proc Natl Acad Sci USA* 1996;93:9565–9570.

120. Stumpel F, Ott T, Willcke K, et al. Connexin32 gap junctions enhance stimulation of glucose output by glucagon and noradrenaline in mouse liver. *Hepatology* 1998;28:1616–1620.

121. Niessen H, Willcke K. Strongly decreased gap junctional permeability to inositol 1,4,5-triphosphate in connexin32 deficient hepatocytes. *FEBS Lett* 2000;466:112–114.

122. Temme A, Buchmann A, Gabriel HD, et al. High incidence of spontaneous and chemically induced liver tumors in mice deficient for connexin32. *Curr Biol* 1997;7:713–716.

123. Moennikes O, Buchmann A, Ott T, et al. The effect of connexin32 null mutation on hepatocarcinogenesis in different mouse strains. *Carcinogenesis* 1999;20:1379–1382.

124. Kojima T, Fort A, Tao M, et al. Gap junction expression and function in primary cultures of Cx32 deficient (KO) mouse hepatocytes. *Am J Physiol (in press)*.

125. Temme A, Ott T, Dombrowski F, et al. The extent of synchronous initiation and termination of DNA synthesis in regenerating mouse liver is dependent on connexin32 expressing gap junctions. *J Hepatol* 2000;32:627–635.

126. Spray DC, Ginzberg RD, Morales EA, et al. Physiological properties of dissociated rat hepatocytes. *J Cell Biol* 1986;103:135–144.

127. Moreno AP, Eghbali B, Spray DC. Connexin32 gap junction channels in stably transfected cells: equilibrium and kinetic properties. *Biophys J* 1991;60:1267–1277.

128. Sáez JC, Bennett MVL, Spray DC. Carbon tetrachloride at hepatotoxic levels blocks reversibly gap junctional communication between rat hepatocytes. *Science* 1987;23:967–969.

129. Spray DC, Stern JH, Harris AL, et al. Comparison of sensitivities of gap junctional conductance to H and Ca ions. *Proc Natl Acad Sci USA* 1982;79:441–445.

130. Sáez JC, Spray DC, Nairn A, et al. cAMP increases junctional conductance and stimulates phosphorylation of the 27 kDa gap junction polypeptide. *Proc Natl Acad Sci USA* 1986;83:2473–2477.

131. Sáez JC, Nairn AC, Czernik AJ, et al. Phosphorylation of connexin32, a hepatocyte gap-junction protein by cAMP-dependent protein kinase, protein kinase C and Ca^{2+}/calmodulin-dependent protein kinase II. *Eur J Biochem* 1991;192:263–273.

132. Swenson KI, Piwnica-Worms H, McNamee H, et al. Tyrosine phosphorylation of the gap junction protein connexin43 is required for the pp60v-src induced inhibition of communication. *Cell Regul* 1991;1:989–1002.

133. Díez JA, Elvira M, Villalobo A. The epidermal growth factor receptor tyrosine kinase phosphorylates connexin32. *Mol Cell Biol* 1998;187:201–210.

134. Zhang JT, Chen M, Foote CI, et al. Membrane integration of

in vitro-translated gap junctional proteins: co-and post-translational mechanisms. *Mol Biol Cell* 1996;7:471–482.

135. Kojima T, Sawada N, Oyamada M, et al. Rapid appearance of connexin 26–positive gap junctions in centrilobular hepatocytes without induction of mRNA and protein synthesis in isolated perfused liver of female rat. *J Cell Sci* 1994;107:3579–3590.

136. Evans WH, Ahmad S, Diez J, et al. Trafficking pathways leading to the formation of gap junctions. *Novartis Found Symp* 1999;219:44–54.

137. Gumbiner B. Breaking through the tight junction barrier. *J Cell Biol* 1993;123:1631–1633.

138. Schneeberger EE, Lynch RD. Structure, function, and regulation of cellular tight junctions. *Am J Physiol* 1992;262:L647–L661.

139. van Meer G, Simon K. The function of tight junctions in maintaining differences in lipid composition between the apical and basolateral cell surface domains of MDCK cells. *EMBO J* 1986;5:1455–1464.

140. Cereijido M, Valdés J, Shoshani L, et al. Role of tight junctions in establishing and maintaining cell polarity. *Annu Rev Physiol* 1998;60:161–177.

141. Yap AS, Mullin JM, Stevenson BR. Molecular analyses of tight junction physiology: insight and paradoxes. *J Membr Biol* 1998;163:159–167.

142. Mullin JM, Marano CW, Laughlin KV, et al. Different size limitations for increased transepithelial paracellular solute flux across phorbol ester and tumor necrosis factor-treated epithelial cell sheets. *J Cell Physiol* 1997;171:226–233.

143. Chen Y-H, Merzdorf C, Paul DL, et al. COOH terminus of occludin is required for tight junction barrier function in early *Xenopus* embryos. *J Cell Biol* 1997;138:891–899.

144. Claude P. Morphological factors influencing transepithelial permeability: a model for the resistance of the zonula occludens. *J Membr Biol* 1978;39:219–232.

145. Takakuwa R, Kokai Y, Kojima T, et al. Uncoupling of gate and fence functions of MDCK cells by the actin depolymerizing reagent mycalolide B. *Exp Cell Res* 2000;157:238–244.

146. Madara JL, Parkos C, Colgan S, et al. The movement of solutes and cells across tight junctions. *Ann NY Acad Sci* 1992;664:47–60.

147. Balda MS, Whitney JA, Flores C, et al. Functional dissociation of paracellular permeability and transepithelial electrical resistance and disruption of the apical-basolateral intramembrane diffusion barrier by expression of a mutant tight junction membrane protein. *J Cell Biol* 1996;134:1031–1049.

148. Madara JL. Intestinal absorptive cell tight junctions are linked to the cytoskeleton. *Am J Physiol* 1987;253:C171–C175.

149. Wittchen ES, Haskins J, Stevenson BR. Protein interactions at the tight junction. Actin has multiple binding partners, and ZO-1 forms independent complexes with ZO-2 and ZO-3. *J Biol Chem* 1999;274:35179–35185.

150. Nathanson MH, Gautam A, Oi Cheng NG, et al. Hormonal regulation of paracellular permeability in isolated rat hepatocyte couplets. *Am J Physiol* 1992;262:G1079–G1086.

151. Roma MG, Stone V, Shaw R, et al. Vasopressin-induced disruption of actin cytoskeletal organization and canalicular function in isolated rat hepatocyte couplets: possible involvement of protein kinase C. *Hepatology* 1998;28:1031–1041.

152. Kojima T, Yamamoto M, Tobioka H, et al. Changes in cellular distribution of connexin 32 and 26 during formation of gap junctions in primary cultures of adult rat hepatocytes. *Exp Cell Res* 1996;223:314–326.

153. Kojima T, Mochizuki C, Tobioka H, et al. Formation of actin filament networks in cultured rat hepatocytes treated with DMSO and glucagon. *Cell Struct Funct* 1997; 22:269–278.

154. Kojima T, Sawada N, Yamamoto M, et al. Disruption of circum-

ferential actin filament causes disappearance of occludin from the cell borders of rat hepatocytes in primary culture without distinct changes of tight junctions. *Cell Struct Funct* 1999;24:11–17.

155. Kojima T, Yamamoto M, Mochizuki C, et al. Different changes in expression and function of connexin 26 and connexin 32 during DNA synthesis and redifferentiation in primary rat hepatocytes using a DMSO culture system. *Hepatology* 1997;26:585–597.

156. Kojima T, Sawada N, Kokai Y, et al. Occludin expression and tight junction strand formation during replicative DNA synthesis in primary cultures of rat hepatocytes. *Med Electron Microsc* 1998;31:169–176.

157. Potempa S, Ridley AJ. Activation of both MAP kinase and phosphatidylinositide 3-kinase by ras is required for hepatocyte growth factor/scatter-induced adherens junction disassembly. *Mol Biol Cell* 1998;9:2185–2200.

158. Woo PL, Ching D, Guan YI, et al. Requirement for ras and phosphatidylinositide 3-kinase signaling uncouples the glucocorticoid-induced junctional organization and transepithelial electrical resistance in mammary tumor cells. *J Biol Chem* 1999;274:32818–32828.

159. Li D, Mrsny RJ. Oncogenic raf-1 disrupts epithelial tight junctions via downregulation of occludin. *J Cell Biol* 2000;148:791–800.

160. Chen Yh, Lu Q, Schneeberger EE, et al. Restoration of tight junction structure and barrier function by down-regulation of the mitogen-activated protein kinase pathway in ras-transformed Madin-Darby canine kidney cells. *Mol Biol Cell* 2000;11:849–862.

161. Kinugasa T, Sakaguchi T, Gu X, et al. Claudins regulate the intestinal barrier in response to immune mediators. *Gastroenterology* 2000;118:1001–1011.

162. Yeaman C, Grindstaff KK, Hansen MD, et al. Cell polarity: versatile scaffolds keep things in place. *Curr Biol* 1999;9:R515–R517.

163. Bentzel CJ, Hainau B, Edelman A, et al. Effects of plant cytokinins on microfilaments and tight junction permeability. *Nature* 1976;264:666–668.

164. Madara JL, Barenberg D, Carlson S. Effects of cytochalasin D on occluding junctions of intestinal absorptive cells: further evidence that the cytoskeleton may influence paracellular permeability and junctional charge selectivity. *J Cell Biol* 1986;102:2125–2136.

165. Madara JL, Stafford J, Barenberg D, et al. Functional coupling of tight junctions and microfilaments in T84 monolayers. *Am J Physiol* 1988;254:G416–G423.

166. Stevenson BR, Begg DA. Concentration-dependent effects of cytochalasin D on tight junctions and actin filaments in MDCK epithelial cells. *J Cell Sci* 1994;107:367–375.

167. Balda MS, Gonzalez-Mariscal L, Macias-Silva M, et al. Assembly and sealing of tight junctions: possible participation of G-proteins, phospholipase C, protein kinase C and calmodulin. *J Membr Biol* 1991;122:193–202.

168. Anderson JM, Van Itallie CM. Tight junctions and the molecular basis for regulation of paracellular permeability. *Am J Physiol* 1995;269:G467–G475.

169. Denker BM, Nigam SK. Molecular structure and assembly of the tight junction. *Am J Physiol* 1998;274:F1–F9.

170. Sakakibara A, Furuse M, Saitou M, et al. Possible involvement of phosphorylation of occludin in tight junction formation. *J Cell Biol* 1997;137:1393–1401.

171. Gonzalez-Mariscal L, Betanzos A, Avila-Flores A. MAGUK proteins: structure and role in tight junctions. *Semin Cell Devel Biol* 2000;11:315–324.

172. Zhong Y, Enomoto K, Isomura M, et al. Localization of the 7H6 antigen at tight junctions correlates with the paracellular barrier function of MDCK cells. *Exp Cell Res* 1994;214:614–620.

173. Tsukamoto T, Nigam SK. Tight junction proteins form large complexes and associate with the cytoskeleton in an ATP depletion model for reversible junction assembly. *J Biol Chem* 1997; 272:16133–16139.

174. Hecht G, Robinson B, Koutsouris A. Reversible disassembly of an intestinal epithelial monolayer by prolonged exposure to phorbol ester. *Am J Physiol* 1994;266:G214–G221.

175. Turner JR, Angle JM, Black ED, et al. PKC-dependent regulation of transepithelial resistance: roles of MLC and MLC kinase. *Am J Physiol* 1999;277:C554–C562.

176. Fasano A, Fiorentini C, Donelli G, et al. Zonula occludens toxin (ZOT) modulates tight junctions through protein kinase C-dependent actin reorganization in vitro. *J Clin Invest* 1995; 96:710–720.

177. Nusrat A, Giry M, Turner JR, et al. Rho protein regulates tight junctions and perijunctional actin organization in polarized epithelia. *Proc Natl Acad Sci USA* 1995;92:10629–10633.

178. Jou T-S, Schneeberger EE, Nelson WJ. Structural and functional regulation of tight junctions by RhoA, and Rac1 small GTPases. *J Cell Biol* 1998;142:101–115.

179. Metz J, Aoki A, Merio M, et al. Morphological alterations and functional changes of interhepatocellular junctions induced by bile duct ligation. *Cell Tissue Res* 1977;182:299–310.

180. Fallon MB, Mennone A, Anderson JM. Altered expression and localization of the tight junction protein ZO-1 after common bile duct ligation. *Am J Physiol* 1993;264:C1439–C1447.

181. Rahner C, Stieger B, Landmann L. Structure–function correlation of tight junctional impairment after intrahepatic and extrahepatic cholestasis in rat liver. *Gastroenterology* 1996;110: 1564–1578.

182. Kawaguchi T, Sakisaka S, Sata M, et al. Different lobular distributions of altered hepatocyte tight junctions in rat models of intrahepatic and extrahepatic chalestasis. *Hepatology* 1999;29: 205–216.

183. Yee G, Revel J. Loss and reappearance of gap junctions in regenerating liver. *J Cell Biol* 1978;78:554–564.

184. Poucell S, Hardison WGM, Miyai K. Regenerative stimulus increases hepatocyte tight junctional permeability. *Hepatology* 1992;16:1061–1068.

185. Fujimoto K, Nagafuchi A, Tsukita S, et al. Dynamics of connexins, E-cadherin and alpha-catenin on cell membranes during gap junction formation. *J Cell Sci* 1997;110:311–322.

186. Robenak H. Themann H, Ott K. Carbon tetrachloride induced proliferation of tight junctions in the rat liver as revealed by freeze-fracturing. *Eur J Cell Biol* 1979;20:62–70.

4

MOTOR MOLECULES

PETER SATIR

In the sense to be discussed here, motor molecules are proteins that utilize adenosine triphosphate (ATP) to produce mechanical work. The motors act by generating a force to move elements within the cytoplasm in relationship to each other in conjunction with the cytoskeleton, to cause motility or positional change of the cell with respect to its surrounding, or of cytoskeletal elements with respect to one another, or of organelles with respect to their position in the cytoplasm. Since this topic was reviewed in the last edition of this volume (1) it has become obvious that epithelial cells, such as the hepatocyte, are endowed with a great variety of motor molecules in three known superfamilies: the myosins, the dyneins, and the kinesins. These motor molecules operate to specify molecular, organelle, and cytoskeletal distributions and trafficking within the differentiated cell, and are the basis for mitosis and cytokinesis in a dividing cell. Each superfamily of motors seems to act differentially with specific major components of the cytoskeleton—myosins with actin filaments and dyneins and kinesins with microtubules—but cross-reactivity with both cytoskeletal systems and also with the intermediate filament cytoskeleton is already evident in a few instances, and will probably prove to be relatively common.

It is instructive to begin the discussion of motor molecule function within the hepatocyte with a general picture of cytoskeletal and membrane distribution in the nondividing cell (Fig. 4.1) (see website chapter 🖳 W-3). Kinesins and cytoplasmic dynein are critical in spindle assembly and chromosome movement during mitosis (2) and myosin II is essential for normal cytokinesis (3); how-ever, this chapter focuses primarily on motors in the interphase differentiated cell. Figure 4.1 is loosely extrapolated from detailed information from Novikoff et al. (4) on the arrangement of the microtubule and actin cytoskeleton in primary cultured rat hepatocytes (see also website chapters 🖳 W-1 and W-2). The actin cytoskeleton exists primarily in the region immediately subjacent to the cell membrane, as the microvillar core filaments in the bile canaliculus and in adherens junctions encircling the canaliculus. Membrane trafficking to and from the cell membrane necessitates contact with and transfer through the actin-rich layer. Within the cytoplasm proper, there are few actin filaments per se, but short actin filaments are probably found in the membrane skeleton of vesicular membranes within the cell as part of the dynactin complex (see below). The major cytoskeletal components that fill the cytoplasm are microtubules (MTs) and intermediate filaments; the distribution of the former has been well studied. MTs emanate from the cell center or centrosome, containing a pair of centrioles. In the hepatocyte, many MTs run close together in a parallel bundle near the centrosome, and then splay out as they approach the cell surface. As they near the cell surface, they turn and run parallel to the cell membrane, just below the actin rich cortex. The effect, looking from a cell surface toward the centrosome, is like an umbrella whose ribs are the MTs. The membrane-bound cellular organelles, particularly the endoplasmic reticulum and the Golgi apparatus, but also mitochondria, are positioned by interactions with the MT cytoskeleton. Certain protein or riboprotein complexes also interact with the microtubules. The positioning and the dynamic changes in position seen with these organelles and nanomachines depend on motor molecule interactions.

P. Satir: Department of Anatomy and Structural Biology, Albert Einstein College of Medicine, Bronx, New York 10461-1602.

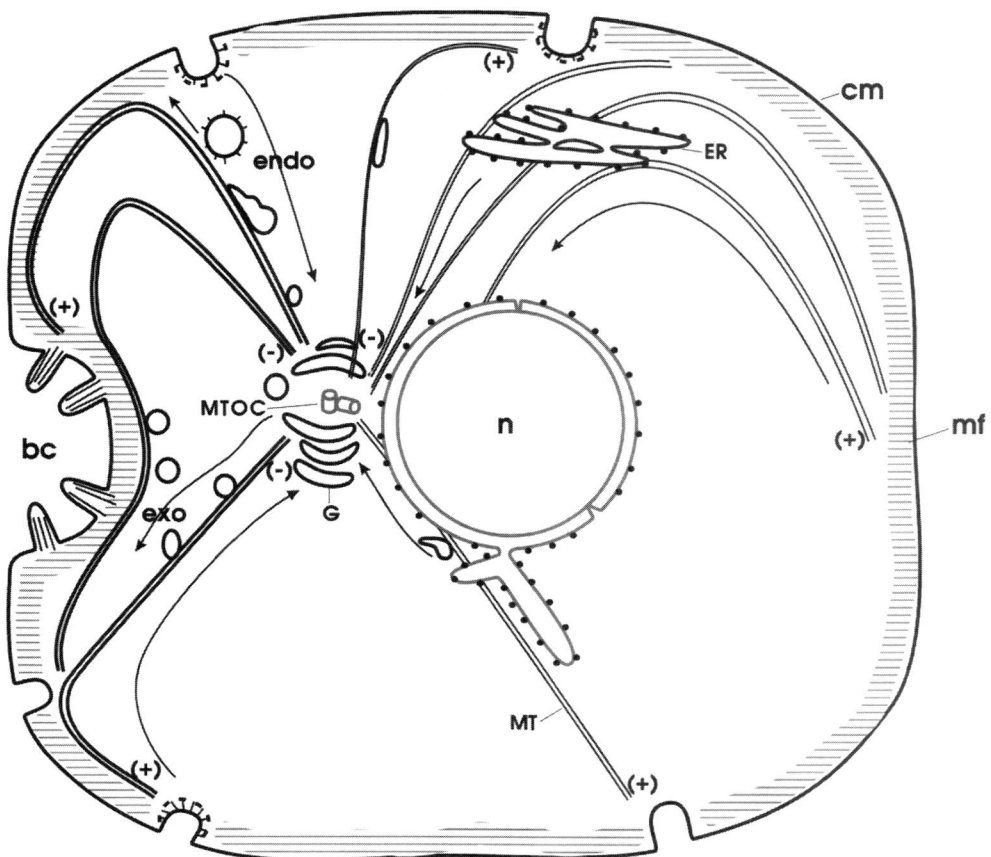

FIGURE 4.1. Organization of a hepatocyte in primary culture. Actin microfilaments (*mf*) are primarily part of microvilli at the bile canaliculus (*bc*) and the membrane skeleton and adherens junction lying beneath the cell membrane (*cm*). Microtubules (*MT*) are nucleated at their (–) ends and radiate out toward the cell surface from an organizing center (*MTOC*) around which the Golgi apparatus (*G*) is located, with their (+) ends lying just below the mf-rich layer. The endoplasmic reticulum (*ER*), the Golgi apparatus, and probably the nucleus (*n*) maintain their relative positions on the MT cytoskeleton in part by countervailing molecular motor activity (see text). Vesicular trafficking pathways along MTs from ER to Golgi and for exocytosis (*exo*) and receptor-mediated endocytosis (*endo*) are illustrated by *arrows*.

An important feature of the motor molecules that helps to determine organelle positioning, membrane trafficking direction, and other characteristics of cell organization is polarity. The cytoskeletal polymers—actin microfilaments and tubulin-based MTs—are built of polarized subunits, such that the two ends of the polymer are not equivalent. Studies by x-ray diffraction, nuclear magnetic resonance (NMR), and cryoelectromicroscopy have defined the structure of the actin-filament (5,6) and the MT (7) at atomic resolutions. These structures have been combined with images of motor molecules to match decoration patterns of actin with S1 heads of myosin II (8,9) and MTs decorated with several different kinesin motors (see ref. 10). As is well known, the decoration of actin filaments yields arrowheads in negative stain; the barbed end of the filament at the cell membrane is the fast polymerizing (+) end; the arrowhead or pointed end extending into the cytoplasm is the slow-

growing (–) end. The barbed end is usually capped by a protein—Cap Z—that prevents depolymerization; the pointed end may be capped by a dimer of actin-related proteins Arp2/3 or by tropomodulin. For MTs, a similar picture has emerged. MTs are nucleated at the centrosome in conjunction with a γ-tubulin complex or ring and then they polymerize with their fast-growing (+) end pushing into the cytoplasm. This polarity has been demonstrated in cultured hepatocytes (WIF-B cells) (11). The (–) end often remains capped at its origin, but some MTs are released and migrate outward with free (–) ends. Because MTs are composed of heterodimers of α- and β-tubulin, the two ends have different tubulins exposed. The slow polymerizing (–) end is terminated by α-tubulin (and then γ-tubulin and other proteins at the centrosome); the (+) end is terminated by β-tubulin, with a β-tubulin–guanosine triphosphate (GTP) cap and perhaps additional stabilizing proteins.

TABLE 4.1. MOLECULAR MOTORS OF THE HEPATOCYTE

Molecular Motor		Reference
Myosins		
I	Myr 1—130 kd	Coluccio and Geeves (60)
	Myr 2—110 kd	Coluccio (16)
	Myr 3	Stoffler and Bahler (61)
II		Phillips (14)
V	Myr 6	Cheney (21)
VIIA	(Embryo liver)	Sahly et al. (59)
X	Myr 5 (Rho-GAP)	Chieregatti et al. (62)
Kinesins		
(Uncharacterized + end motor)		Komatsu et al. (47)
KIF 1B		Hirokawa (53)
KIF C		Bananis et al. (57)
Cytoplasmic dynein		
DHC 1a	(MAP1C)	Collins and Vallee (58)
DHC 1b		Criswell et al. (24)

DHC, dynein-heavy chain; GAP, guanosine triphosphatase (GTPase)-activating protein; KIF, kinesin (super) family protein; MAP, microtubule-associated protein; MV, myosin V.

Consider now the movement of secretory (exocytic) or endocytic vesicles through the cell. Although in small cells, such as yeast, vesicles may move mainly via diffusion, arriving at their destinations in sufficiently high numbers per unit time, in larger cells, such as the hepatocyte, diffusion is unreliable and most vesicles move along directed cytoskeletal pathways using molecular motors. For example, vesicles bud from the rough endoplasmic reticulum and move along MTs toward the Golgi apparatus situated near the centrosome. Such motion requires a (−) end directed MT motor. From the *trans*-Golgi network, vesicles exit and traffic along MTs toward the cell surface. Such motion requires a (+) end directed MT motor. For exocytosis, the vesicle transfers from the MT cytoskeleton to move through the actin cytoskeleton, probably requiring a (+) end directed myosin. For endocytosis, movement through the actin-rich layer, especially where there are microvilli, may require a (−) end directed myosin; in the absence of microvilli, this distance is perhaps small enough that a microfilament motor may not be necessary. The endosome continues on its way by attaching to MTs for sorting and fission, which may require both (−) end directed motors for ligand-enriched endosomes moving onward after fission toward fusion with Golgi or lysosomal membranes and (+) end directed motors for receptor-recycling to the cell membrane.

A list of molecular motors currently described for the hepatocyte is given in Table 4.1. As will be discussed, some classes of motors are not well characterized and the list is likely to be incomplete. The physiologic roles for molecular motors in the differentiated nondividing hepatocyte are based on the polarity mentioned above (see also ref. 12). For each motor, polarity and cellular localization must be defined. Physiologic function depends in some measure on the biophysical and biochemical properties of the motor including its three-dimensional configuration and its constituent protein chains, the amount of force produced by one cycle of the motor, the cycle time, and the distance along the cytoskeletal microfilament or MT that the motor moves, its duty cycle, and processivity. These characteristics are listed in Table 4.2 and are worked out to some extent for major members of each motor class—myosins, kinesins,

TABLE 4.2. GENERAL PROPERTIES OF SOME TYPICAL MOLECULAR MOTORS

	Myosin II	Conventional Kinesin	Dynein[a]
Duty phase ratio[b]	0.05	0.85	0.01
Force per ATP	5–8 pN	5–8 pN	~5 pN
Cytoskeletal partner	Actin microfilament	MT	MT
Step size	4–5 nm	8 nm	16 nm? (8–40)
Speed *in vitro*[b]	0.25–8 μms^{-1}	0.8 μms^{-1}	1.25 μms^{-1}
Polarity	+ end	+ end	− end

[a]Values except speed *in vitro* for axonemal 22S dynein.
[b]Duty phase ratio is time of strong attachment and force generating phase (t_s) divided by total time of one mechanochemical cycle (t_c). Speed *in vitro* taken from Howard (49).
ATP, adenosine triphosphate; MT, microtubule.

and dyneins—but the variations within each motor super-family are incompletely explored. Since many different motor molecules are present in a single cell, such as the hepatocyte, and they must perform different functions at different times, there must be various mechanisms by which the motor molecules are under cellular controls. First, there must be targeting information so that the proper motor is linked to the proper cargo in a specific location. As part of the targeting mechanism, the cell must have ways of turning specific motors on and off. Motor switching is probably extremely important in the zone just below the terminal

web or membrane skeleton in epithelial cells, including hepatocytes, where organelles move from actin to MT-rich zones. As a finer control, the mechanochemistry of the motor may be altered to speed up or slow down a particular process.

THE MYOSINS

There are now at least 15 classes of myosin, 14 of which are diagrammed in Fig. 4.2. There are at least 26 myosin

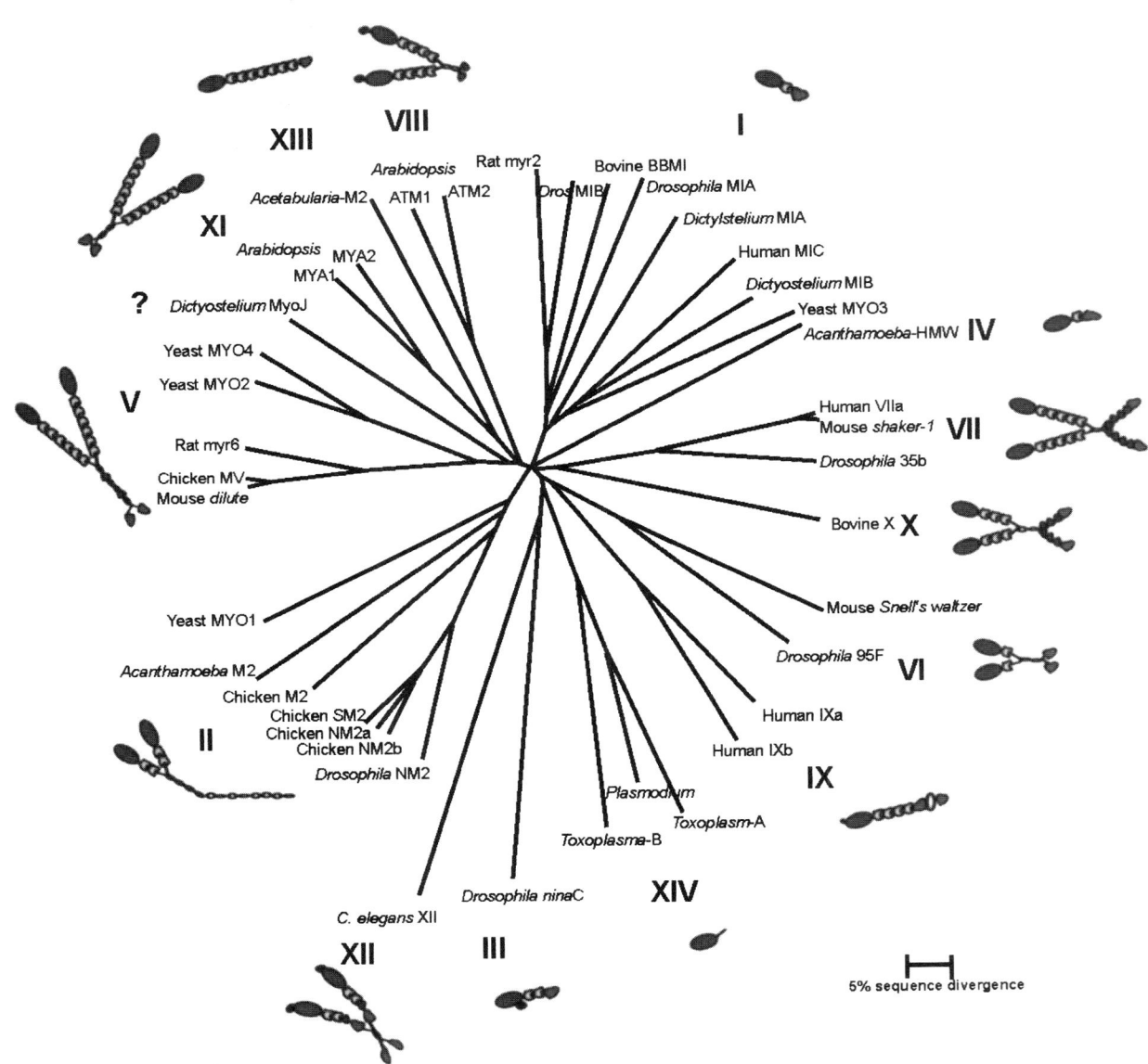

FIGURE 4.2. The myosin superfamily of molecular motors. This is an unrooted phylogenetic tree based on head domain protein sequences with myosin classes shown in roman numerals and corresponding drawings of each class inferred from images of isolated molecules and sequence homologies. (From Mermall V, Post PL, Mooseker MS. Unconventional myosins in cell movement, membrane traffic and signal transduction. *Science* 1998;279:527–533, with permission.)

genes in seven classes in mouse. Conventional myosin, the myosin present in striated muscle, is myosin II. It consists of two heavy (H) chains, each with a motor domain that binds to actin filaments and hydrolyzes ATP, a flexible neck, and a long α-helical tail. The two H chain tails form a coiled coil, and are responsible for polymerization into thick filaments. The neck region of each H chain binds two light chains, orthologs of calmodulin, in a region containing several IQ motifs (13). Light chains (LCs) regulate the activity of myosin via their phosphorylation. There are two human myosin II H chain genes, encoding slightly different isoforms that are found in varying amounts in various nonmuscle cells, including hepatocytes.

Myosin II, like all known myosins except those in class VI, is a (+) end directed motor, whose mechanochemical properties are well studied. Its two isoforms have different biochemical properties, different cellular localizations, and presumably different functions. Under appropriate conditions, nonmuscle myosin II tails self-assemble into short bipolar filaments, which are responsible for the sliding of actin filaments in the contractile ring at cytokinesis. In nondividing hepatocytes, myosin II localized to the actin belt supporting the bile canaliculus is responsible for bile canalicular contraction (14) and perhaps aspects of cortical extension or microvillar growth. About half the classes of myosins, including classes IX and VII found in hepatocytes, yield molecules with dimeric H chains. The other classes of myosin, notably myosin I, are single chains. All classes have motor domains that resemble myosin II. Their LC-binding domains tend to be more extensive than those of myosin II; some LCs are calmodulin itself, suggesting that activation is Ca^{2+}-regulated. Following the motor and LC domains, the two-headed molecules contain a coiled-coil domain responsible for dimerization. Other interesting recognizable heavy-chain (HC) domains include pleckstrin homology (PH) domains, talin-binding domains, SH3 and membrane-binding domains, a domain in myosin V that binds a 8-kd dynein light chain, and domains in myosin XI that bind Zn^{2+} and rho, the small G protein. This variety of myosin HC domain constructs suggests that the various myosins additional to myosin II perform many different functions in the cell, including organelle transport and interaction with a variety of signal transduction and other cytoskeletal systems. We now consider some of these roles in more detail, with relevance to the hepatocyte.

Myosin I

There are at least three different myosin class I molecules in hepatocytes, products of the *myr1, myr2,* and *myr3* genes. All are single chains with the conserved motor domain at their N-termini, a neck with a number of LC-binding IQ motifs, and a C-terminal rich in basic residues, the polybasic domain. This domain can bind to membranes or to

phospholipid vesicles *in vitro*. One of these molecules, myosin Iα, is involved in endocytosis.

Raposo et al. (15) have shown that myosin 1α associates with tubulovesicular endosomes and that the delivery of fluid-phase markers from late endosomes to lysosomes is inhibited when myosin 1α function is impaired. A close relative of myosin Iα, myr2, or myosin Iβ, is brush-border myosin I, a 110-kd protein well characterized in rat liver (16). In addition to attachments between the actin microvillar core and the microvillar membrane, this class of myosins is present on Golgi-derived vesicles in some cells, and could play a role in actin-dependent transport of vesicles to the cell surface. Myr3 (17), which contains an SH3 domain, is thought to stabilize adherens junctions and might be involved in "purse string" contractions at the bile canaliculus.

Myosin V and VI

These two-headed myosins are the basic myosins involved in organelle transport in animal cells (cf. ref. 18). There is considerable evidence that myosin V is a processive (+) end motor with a high duty ratio that can tether organelles (19), effecting short-range actin-based motility in axons and pigment cells, probably in conjunction with kinesin-based or dynein-based microtubule movement, perhaps in the zone of transfer from MT-based transport deeper in the cell to actin-based transport at the periphery. Myosin Va and non-neural kinesin have been shown to interact (20), and myosin Va and dynein share a common 8-kd light chain. A variant of this molecule (myr 6) is probably present in liver (cf. ref. 21). In hepatocytes, myosin V would be valuable in effecting constitutive exocytosis or perhaps mitochondria or organelle placement.

The class VI myosins, present in intestinal epithelium and probably in liver, are so far unique in that they are (−) end microfilament motors (22). They too seem to be involved in organelle trafficking. In *Drosophila*, myosin VI interacts with CLIP-170 and dynactin—two molecules that tether vesicles to MTs. CLIP-170, dynactin, and dynein lie in an appropriate position to move endosomes centipetally from the (+) end of MTs. Myosin VI would be valuable in delivering endosomes through the actin cortex into this region; in differentiated epithelia it is localized in the terminal web, the appropriate position for this function.

Myosin VIIA and Myosin IX

Myosin VIIA is a two-headed myosin containing IQ, myth 4, and talin domains, which may serve as phospholipid-binding sites. It is detected in embryonic liver and other epithelial cells, such as retinal pigment epithelia. A role in organelle transport in connection with actin-rich regions has been suggested. Myosin IX is probably a single-headed class of myosins that contain a tail domain with homology to the guanosine triphosphatase (GTPase)-activating proteins (GAPs) of the Rho subfamily of small G proteins. The rat protein myr 5 is a negative regulator of Rho, converting the active molecule to its inactive guanosine diphosphate (GDP) state. Active Rho is located on membranes. It would seem that myosin IX is involved in attaching to actin microfilaments and organizing them and their relationships to membranes under specific signal transduction conditions. It will be instructive to study the location and function of these myosins in the hepatocyte further in relation to liver cell physiology.

CYTOPLASMIC DYNEIN

Cytoplasmic dynein is a complex molecule composed of two homodimeric ca. 500-kd HCs, responsible for adenosine triphosphatase (ATPase) activity and force generation, two ca. 74-kd intermediate chains (ICs), containing WD repeats, light intermediate chains (55 to 57 kd), and a number of LCs (8 to ca. 21 kd) (23). Cytoplasmic dynein is readily detected in hepatocytes; at least two homologous forms of the HC motor domain have been reported, DHCla or MAP1C and DHC1b (24); both homologues probably participate in intercellular trafficking. Moreover, two IC genes apparently code for six cytoplasmic dynein IC isoforms, so the molecular diversity of cytoplasmic dyneins may be considerable. The specific composition of cytoplasmic dyneins associated with physiologic events such as endocytosis or endoplasmic reticulum (ER)-Golgi trafficking has not been identified. Cytoplasmic dynein is usually depicted in isolated form as a two-headed bouquet (Fig. 4.3) with the motor domains protruding from a base containing the ICs, but the *in vivo* form of the molecule may be somewhat more compact, as is the case for axonemal dynein (25).

Some LCs associate with the HCs heads, while others associate with the IC base. The LCs are responsible for regulation of activity of the molecule, presumably by altering its mechanochemical or binding properties.

Some LCs have been characterized with interesting properties (26). LC 8, which is the common stoichiometric LC of cytoplasmic dynein and myosin V, has a direct association with a form of nitric oxide synthase (NOS). Other cytoplasmic dynein LCs are members of the Tctex 1 family, a group of proteins first identified in mice where they are encoded by the *t* locus. Immunolocalization and fractionation studies suggest that different members of the Tctex-1 family are associated with different populations of cytoplasmic dynein. Another ca. 12-kd LC is related to the *Drosophila* protein roadblock. One unidentified hepatocyte LC is probably homologous to *Paramecium* p29, a molecule that binds to a specific HC whose phosphorylation increases the activity of 22S axonemal dynein (27). Other LCs of interest, characterized for certain axonemal dyneins,

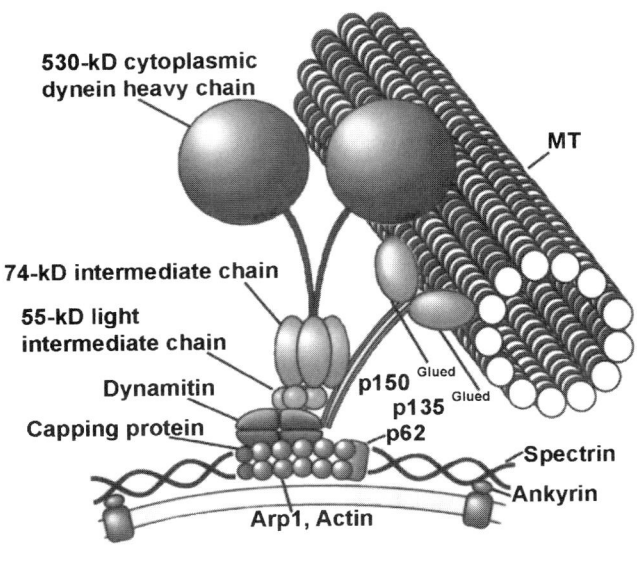

FIGURE 4.3. Proposed organization of cytoplasmic dynein and dynactin in relation to vesicle trafficking. In this model, the actin base of dynactin is integrated into the membrane skeleton of the vesicle; dynein binds to the dynamitin subunits of dynactin and both dynactin and a dynein-heavy chain (DHC) interact with the microtubule (*MT*) track along which the vesicle moves, permitting processivity. (Modified from Hirokawa N. Kinesin and dynein superfamily proteins and the mechanism of organelle transport. *Science* 1998;279:519–526.)

which could be present in some cytoplasmic dyneins, are Ca^{2+}-binding EF hand, calmodulin-related protein, and thioredoxin, which could regulate dynein in relation to redox state and disulfide bond formation.

Cytoplasmic dynein is a (−) end motor, with a low duty ratio, perhaps about 0.01 (Table 4.2), which implies that the HCs are detached from MTs and not force generating for about 99% of their mechanochemical cycle. Since cytoplasmic dynein seems to be involved in organelle and nanomachine transport, as will be indicated shortly, and only a few copies of the molecule can attach to a vesicle or ribonucleoprotein (RNP) particle, this poses a problem. The problem was solved by the discovery of dynactin (28,29).

Dynactin is a 20S protein complex that binds to and colocalizes with cytoplasmic dynein and can be demonstrated to be essential for the function of dynein in organelle transport. Its subunit composition and ultrastructure are well characterized (Fig. 4.3). Each molecule contains an extended subunit of M_r 150 kd, now called p150^Glued after the *Drosophila* gene product, attached to a short filament of actin-related subunits (Arp1) and possibly authentic actin, and capped at both ends, the barbed end by [capping protein (Cap Z)], and the pointed end by p62. The Arp1 filament interacts with or perhaps forms part of an ankyrin spectrin-actin membrane skeleton around vesicular cargo (30). At its projecting head end, p150[Glued] binds to MTs, possibly in a phosphorylation-dependent manner, while the coiled-coil region of the protein interacts with the 74-kd LC of cytoplasmic dynein. A protein of M_r ca. 50 kd (p50), called dynamitin, connects the p150[Glued] arm to the Arp1 filament; overexpression of p50 disrupts the binding of dynactin-dynein to its cargo (31–33).

Dynactin also contains several ca. 24-kd (p24, p25, p27) accessory chains that may regulate attachment. Whereas it does not radically alter the ATPase activity, dynactin increases the processivity of cytoplasmic dynein, that is, the distance a dynein molecule will remain moving along a MT before falling off (34). Together with dynactin, cytoplasmic dynein maintains the Golgi apparatus, late endosomes, and lysosomes in their positions draped around the centrosome, near the (−) ends of MTs, in most epithelial cells (33,35,36), and drives ER to Golgi transport in the face of (+) end directed MT motors. Disruption by dynamitin produces Golgi, lysosome, and late endosome dispersion to the cell periphery (35,36) and disrupts ER to Golgi transport (37), but does not affect early endosomes or receptor recycling (36). This work confirms the findings of Goltz et al. (38) and Oda et al. (39) using *in vitro* assays, where ligand-containing postsegregation late endosomes from overnight cultured hepatocytes become bound to MTs in an ATP-sensitive manner and coimmunoprecipitate with cytoplasmic dynein. It seems likely that cytoplasmic dynein attached to late endosomes by dynactin is responsible for trafficking of the endosomes to lysosomes in the hepatocyte.

Cytoplasmic dynein is also the motor for RNP transport along MTs, which is important during embryonic development and cell differentiation (40,41). It is not yet known whether RNP transport is also dynactin-dependent or whether there are other molecules that modify dynein processivity in this process.

KINESIN

A recent version of some of the extended superfamily of kinesins and kinesin related proteins in shown in Fig. 4.4 (42). The globular motor domains of all members of the superfamily are similar, but the position of the motor domain in the molecule varies. Conventional kinesin (KHC subfamily), the first kinesin to be identified, is a dimeric molecule with an N-terminal motor domain. It was identified as the (+) end motor anterograde transporter of vesicles along axonal MTs. Targeting of kinesin to particular vesicles is thought to occur via a ca. 64-kd light chain (KLC) associated with each 120-kd heavy chain (KHC) in the dimer, in some cases possibly involving specific receptors such as kinectin. There are at least three conventional kinesins in mouse and many other kinesin related proteins (cf. ref. 43). In epithelial cells, kinesin is often localized to the area of the Golgi apparatus. A role for conventional kinesin as a (+) end MT motor in Golgi to ER recycling and lysosomal secretion or other exocytic events has been proposed (44). Kinesin is also associated with mitochondrial movement. Gyoeva and Gelfand (45) showed that vimentin intermediate filaments attach to microtubules by kinesin, and Prahlad et al. (46) have shown that such intermediate filaments are transported along MTs by kinesin, which suggests that kinesin is involved in overall cytoskeletal organization in

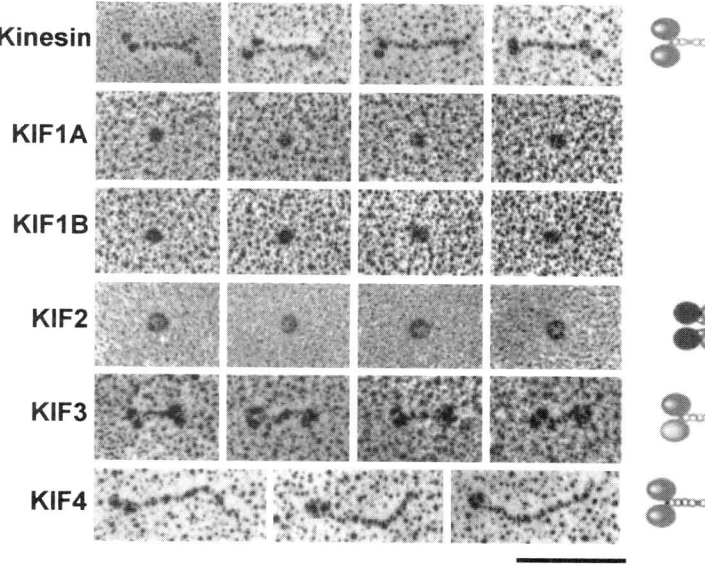
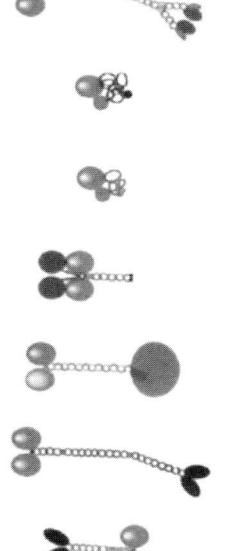

FIGURE 4.4. The kinesin superfamily of molecular motors: representative examples. Rotary shadowed panels of individual molecules and interpretative diagrams are shown. All except KIFC2 are (+) end directed MT motors. *Scale bar* 100 nm. (From Hirokawa N. Kinesin and dynein superfamily proteins and the mechanism of organelle transport. *Science* 1998;279:519–526.)

cells as well as in membrane trafficking, as the opposite number to cytoplasmic dynein.

Most studies of kinesin rely on features of the motor domain, and specific members of the kinesin superfamily, so far uncharacterized, could be associated with the specific cellular processes described above. This is likely to be true for the hepatocyte, where only a seemingly conventional kinesin has been isolated and partly characterized (47,48), but there are probably many different types of kinesin present in the cytoplasm (see also below).

Conventional kinesin, like cytoplasmic dynein, is an MT-activated ATPase. However, kinesin differs from cytoplasmic dynein not only in the direction of force generation along the MT, but also in its duty ratio and processivity (Table 4.2). The mechanochemical cycle of kinesin is such that the molecule remains attached to the MT for over 80% of a cycle (cf. ref. 49); effectively dimeric kinesin almost never detaches completely from the tubulin lattice, and there is no need for a dynactin-like component. Kinesin walks along a single tubulin protofilament in the MT for about 100 steps at a time in a straight line with a step size of 8 nm. It remains to be determined whether this is a feature of all members of the superfamily.

Consider now what would happen if kinesin and dynein both worked on the same MT. Vale et al. (50) has shown that *in vitro* MTs will translocate first one way, then the other. When movement occurs with the (−) end of the MT leading, the kinesins are active, the dynein inactive; when movement occurs with the (+) end of the MT leading, the opposite is true. Switching between directions occurs randomly, but for equal timing in both directions there needs to be about an order of magnitude more dynein on the substratum than kinesin. For vesicular trafficking, this difference might be largely overcome by dynactin, so that a vesicle with only a few kinesins and a few dyneins could potentially move along MTs in either a (+) or a (−) direction, depending on which motor was active; if both motors actively balanced each other, the vesicle would essentially jog in position.

Movement by kinesin is largely inhibited by 1 mM adenosine monophosphate (AMP-PNP), but little affected by 5 (μM vanadate, while movement by cytoplasmic dynein is largely unaffected by AMP-PNP but stopped by vanadate (51). Although most kinesins are (+) end motors, one class of the subfamily has its motor domain at the C terminus. These kinesins, of which the best studied is the *Drosophila* gene product Ncd, are (−) end motors. C-type kinesins are associated with spindle dynamics in mitosis, but it is likely that members of this class are also associated with some vesicle movements in epithelial cells, including hepatocytes (see below); three C-type kinesins have been identified in mouse brain. One C-type kinesin, KIFC2, seems to move multivesicular body-like membrane-bounded vesicles in dendrites (42); another, KICFC3, is cytoplasmic or membrane-bound in different cell types (52). Kinesins that have their motor domain in the central position of the molecule, the so-called Kin1 or KIF2 family of motors, are (+) end directed motors that affect MT assembly during mitosis. Bipolar kinesins and chromokinesins are also mainly known for their effects on mitosis.

Two other subfamilies of kinesin are noteworthy here: monomeric kinesins and heterotrimeric kinesins.

Monomeric Kinesin

These kinesins consist of a single motor domain that acts as a (+) end motor to transport vesicles and/or mitochondria, mainly in neurons. KIF 1B is a ubiquitously expressed globular protein found in liver that colocalizes with mitochondria (53).

Heteromeric or Heterotrimeric Kinesin

These kinesins are (+) end motors consisting of two different KHCs that dimerize together; they are usually capped at their tail end by another larger, nonmotor globular subunit. In ciliated cells, they are responsible for anterograde (tip-directed) interflagellar transport. This transport involves the movement of nonvesicular protein rafts along MTs (54,55). Heterotrimeric kinesins may also be involved in vesicular transport along MTs in certain cells, such as melanocytes. In neurons and other cells, presumably including hepatocytes, (+) end directed motors are responsible for moving nonvesicular protein complexes and certain messenger RNAs (mRNAs) (56) along MTs through the cytoplasm. Heterotrimeric kinesins are candidate molecules for such motors.

Kinesins and Liver Endosomal Trafficking

Murray et al. (51) have extended the *in vitro* endocytosis assays described previously for dynein using video microscopy and a purified population of liver endosomes containing fluorescently labeled asialo-orosomucoid (ASOR). They observed endosome motility directly on polarity-labeled MTs. About one third to one quarter of endosomes attached to MTs move in the presence of ATP at average rates of roughly 0.7 μms^{-1}, with oscillatory variations; about half the endosomes move toward the (−) and half toward the (+) end of the MTs. Motility is unaffected by the exogenous addition of a preparation of motor molecules, suggesting that the purified endosomes are saturated with motor proteins and that only small numbers of motors are required for motility. Continuing such studies, Bananis et al. (57) have demonstrated the presence of receptor in essentially all the ligand-containing endosomes originally bound to the MTs in the Murray et al. preparations, indicating that the population represents early, presegregation, endosomes. Moreover, careful observation revealed that in the presence of 50 µM ATP about 10% of the moving endosomes undergo fission (Fig. 4.5), which results in segregation of ligand and receptor in the two daughter vesicles, such that one daughter is enriched severalfold in ligand relation to receptor and one is enriched in receptor, containing approximately 80% of the original receptor. Fission absolutely requires ATP-dependent endosome motility on the MT, and unattached endosomes never move or split.

Movement is again unbiased, as about 50% of vesicles move toward the (+) end of polarity-labeled MTs. Both (+) end directed and (−) end directed movement, and all fission events, are abolished by AMP-PNP even at high ATP concentrations but unaffected by vanadate, suggesting that movement and fission of early endosomes depend on kinesins rather than cytoplasmic dynein, which is also supported by the results of Valetti et al. (36). In further support of this conclusion, antibodies to the motor domain of kinesin colocalize with most of the ligand-containing MT-bound presegregation endosomes, while cytoplasmic dynein localizes only to a few bound early endosomes. Evidently, presegregation endosomes bind to MTs and activate their attached kinesin motors to cause endosome splitting. It seems likely that the molecular motor contributes the force to pull the splitting vesicles apart. One or more plus end kinesin is probably responsible for (+) end directed endosomal movement and receptor recycling, while one or more (−) end kinesin participates in

(−) end directed movement during fission. As the endosome matures, perhaps through multiple rounds of fission, dynein attached to the ligand-containing daughter becomes activated and completes movement toward the lysosome. Motor attachment, selectivity, and activation become important for endosomal processing throughout the cell.

CONCLUSION

The variety of molecular motors within the hepatocyte and other differentiated cells is unexpected, and independent of the complexity of motors governing mitotic events. It indicates that important aspects of cell organization are controlled at least in part by specific motors. These aspects include membrane and organelle placement, membrane trafficking in endo- and exocytosis, organization of the intermediate filament cytoskeleton, sites of mRNA localization, protein synthesis, and protein delivery for specific assembly. As indicated above, membrane and organelle placement is probably the result of countervailing forces, where (+) end MT motors, often specific kinesins with N-terminal motor domains, balance (−) end motors, often cytoplasmic dyneins, but sometimes kinesins with C type motor domains. Examples include Golgi placement near the cell center and peripheral mitochondrial distribution in the cytoplasm. One zone of particular interest is the cytoplasm lying just below the membrane skeleton, where

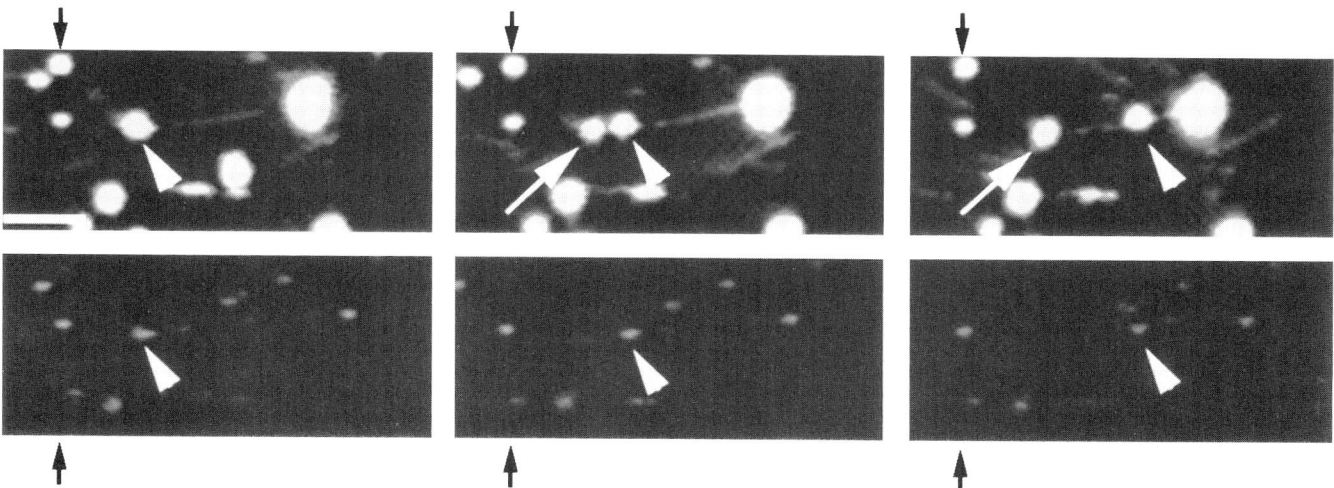

FIGURE 4.5. Microtubule and motor-dependent endosome segregation *in vitro*. A series of frames showing fission of an early endosome (*arrowhead*) as it moves along a MT. **Upper panels:** Texas red labeled MTs. **Lower panels:** Cy2 secondary antibody labeling primary antibody to receptor. *Scale bar* 10 µm. *Black arrows* indicate alignment of panels. At zero time, when adenosine triphosphate (ATP) is added (**right panels**) the endosome contains ligand and receptor. Ten seconds later (**middle panels**) a dumbbell has formed where one daughter contains most of the receptor (*arrowhead*), while the other daughter contains virtually only ligand (*white arrow*). By 30 seconds the daughters have separated, as one daughter moves away along the MT. (From Bananis E, Murray JW, Stockert RJ, et al. Microtubules and motor dependent endocytic vesicle sorting in vitro. *J Cell Biol* 2000;151:179–186, with permission.)

events such as endosome delivery and sorting or secretory vesicle storage occur. Here the organelle positioning occurs at the point where the actin cytoskeleton effectively ends and the MT-intermediate filament cytoskeleton begins. As Fig. 4.6 indicates, one might anticipate a rich series of transitions of active motors in this region, and this is suggested

by present *in vitro* analysis. A strong suggestion from this analysis is that many different types of motors are bound to any given organelle; for countervailing force these may all be active, but for directed movement and membrane trafficking, the motors will be segregated and specifically activated or turned off, probably in response to signaling events

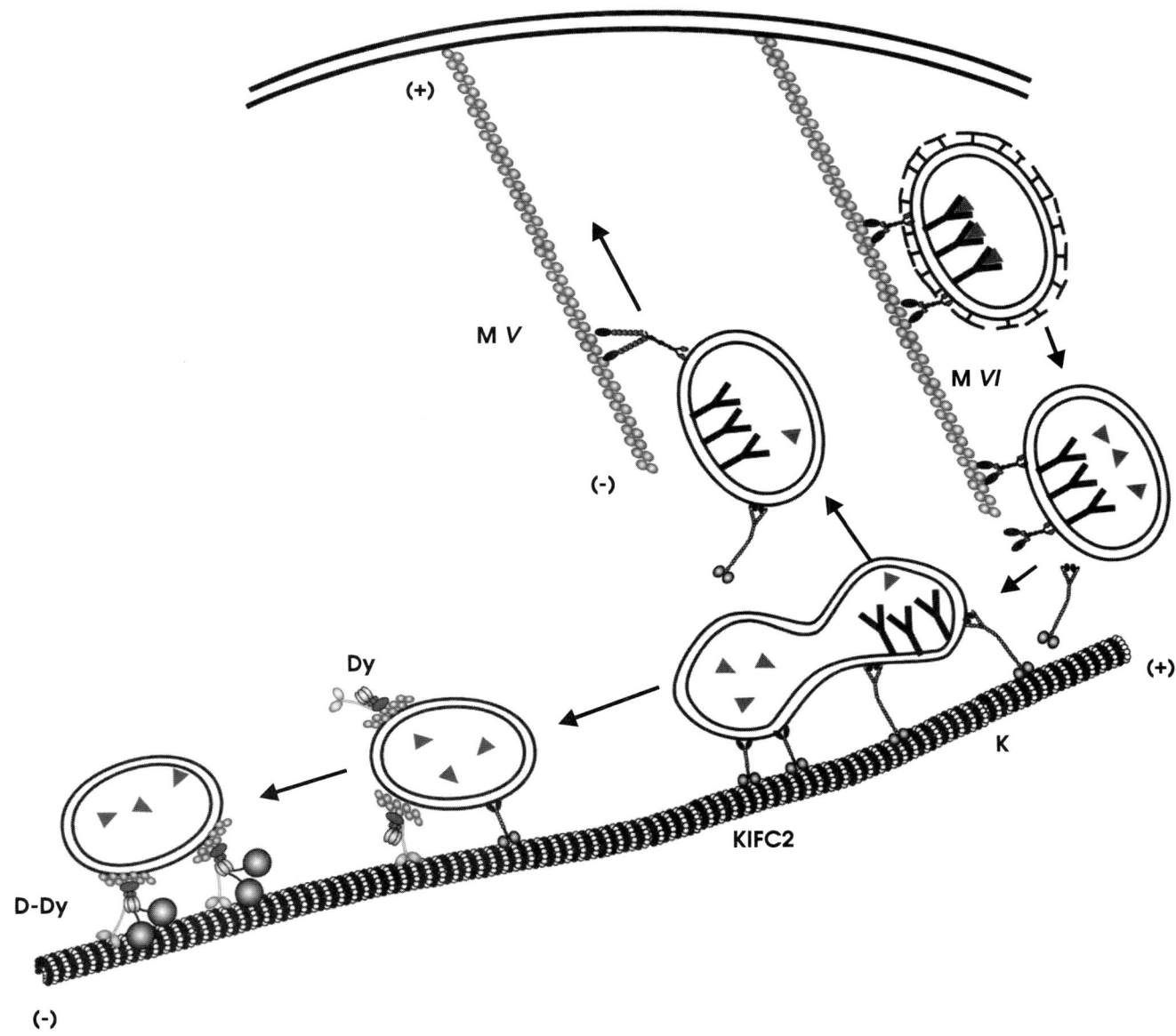

FIGURE 4.6. A proposed model of motor-involvement in receptor mediated endocytosis in the hepatocyte. Movement of the clathrin-coated vesicle through the actin-rich belt might require Myosin VI (*MVI*); the uncoated acidified vesicle would reach the MT cytoskeleton, attach, and begin to undergo fission, using a (+) end directed kinesin (*K*), perhaps conventional kinesin, and a (−) end kinesin, possibly KIFC2, attached to the receptor-rich daughter to begin recycling. After repeated fissions, the ligand-containing late endosome would bind dynactin (*Dy*) and then cytoplasmic dynein (*D*) for a journey toward the lysosome. The recycling vesicle would pass through the actin belt aided by myosin V (*MV*). The endosomal pathway therefore requires multiple specific motors. In this cartoon, they generally attach sequentially to the vesicle, but in some instances several types of motors may be present simultaneously, with differential activity controlled by cell signal pathways, including phosphorylation.

within the cytoplasm. We can begin to picture specific processes within the hepatocyte in these terms, which add a mechanistic dimension to the cell biologic events of hepatocyte differentiation and function.

ACKNOWLEDGMENTS

I thank Allan Wolkoff for helpful discussion and M. Ann Holland for assistance with the preparation of the manuscript. I am grateful to Charles Guerra for help in producing the figures; his computer skills were invaluable. This work was supported by grants DK 41918-09 and DK 41296-12 from The National Institutes of Health.

REFERENCES

1. Satir P. Motor molecules of the cytoskeleton: possible functions in the hepatocyte. In: Arias I, Boyer JL, Fausto N, et al., eds. *The liver: biology and pathology*, 3rd ed. New York: Raven Press, 1994:45–52.
2. Hirokawa N, Noda Y, Okada Y. Kinesin and dynein superfamily proteins in organelle transport and cell division. *Curr Opin Cell Biol* 1998;10:60–73.
3. Field C, Rong L, Oegama K. Cytokinesis in eukaryotes: a mechanistic comparison. *Curr Opin Cell Biol* 1999;11:68–80.
4. Novikoff P, Cammer M, Tao L, et al. Three-dimensional organization of rat hepatocyte cytoskeleton: relation to the asialoglycoprotein endocytosis pathway. *J Cell Sci* 1996;109:21–32.
5. Lorenz M, Popp D, Holmes KC. Refinement of the F-actin model against x-ray fiber diffraction data by use of a directed mutation algorithm. *J Mol Biol* 1993;234:826–836.
6. Hanein D, Matsudeira P, DeRosier DJ. Evidence for a conformational change in actin induced by fimbrin (N375) binding. *J Cell Biol* 1997;139:387–396.
7. Nogales E, Whittaker M, Milligan RA, et al. High-resolution model of the microtubule. *Cell* 1999;96:79–88.
8. Rayment I, Holden HM, Whittaker M., et al. Structure of the actin-myosin complex and its implications for muscle contraction. *Science* 1993;261:58–65.
9. Volkmann N, Hanan D. Quantitative fitting of atomic models into observed densities derived by electron microscopy. *J Struct Biol* 1999;125:176–184.
10. Mandelkow E, Hoenger A. Structures of kinesin and kinesin-microtubule interactions. *Curr Opin Cell Biol* 1999;11:34–44.
11. Mead T, Schroer TA. Polarity and nucleation of microtubules in polarized epithelial cells. *Cell Motil Cytoskeleton* 1995;32:273–288.
12. Hamm-Alvarez SF, Sheetz MP. Microtubule-dependent vesicle transport: modulation of channel and transporter activity in liver and kidney. *Physiol Rev* 1998;78:1109–1129.
13. Cheney RE, Mooseker MS. Unconventional myosins. *Curr Opin Cell Biol* 1992;4:27–35.
14. Phillips MJ. Biology and pathobiology of actin in the liver. In: Arias I, Boyer JL, Fausto N, et al., eds. *The liver: biology and pathology*, 3rd ed. New York: Raven Press, 1994:19–32.
15. Raposo G, Cordonnier MN, Tenza D, et al. Association of myosin1 alpha with endosomes and lysosomes in mammalian cells. *Mol Biol Cell* 1999;10:1477–1494.
16. Coluccio LM. Differential calmodulin binding to three myosin I isoforms from liver. *J Cell Sci* 1994;107:2279–2284.
17. Wu X, Jing G, Hammer JA III Function of unconventional myosin. *Curr Opin Cell Biol* 2000;12:42–51.
18. Mermall V, Post PL, Mooseker MS. Unconventional myosins in cell movement, membrane traffic and signal transduction. *Science* 1998;279:527–533.
19. Mehta AD, Rock RS, Rief M, et al. Myosin V is a processive actin-based motor. *Nature* 1994;400:590–593.
20. Huang JD, Brady ST, Richards BW, et al. Direct interaction of microtubule and actin-based transport motors. *Nature* 1999;397:267–270.
21. Cheney RE. Myosin V. In: Kreis T, Vale R, eds. *Guidebook to the cytoskeletal and motor proteins*, 2nd ed. Oxford: Oxford University Press, 1999:440–444.
22. Wells AL, Lin AW, Chen LQ, et al. Myosin VI is an actin-based motor that moves backwards. *Nature* 1999;401:505–508.
23. Vallee R. Dynein, cytoplasmic. In: Kreis T, Vale R, eds. *Guidebook to the cytoskeletal and motor proteins*, 2nd ed. Oxford: Oxford University Press, 1999:386–389.
24. Criswell PS, Ostrowski LE, Asai DJ. A novel cytoplasmic dynein heavy chain: expression of DHC1b in mammalian ciliated epithelial cells. *J Cell Sci* 1996;109:1891–1898.
25. Barkalow K, Avolio J, Holwill MEJ, et al. Structural and geometrical constraints on the outer dynein arm *in situ*. *Cell Motil Cytoskeleton* 1994;27:299–312.
26. King SM. The dynein microtubule motor. *Biochim Biophys Acta* 2000;1496:60–75.
27. Wang H, Satir P. The 29 kDa light chain that regulates axonemal dynein activity binds to cytoplasmic dynein. *Cell Motil Cytoskeleton* 1998;39:1–8.
28. Gill SR, Schroer TA, Szilak I, et al. Dynactin, a conserved, ubiquitously expressed component of an activator of vesicle motility mediated by cytoplasmic dynein. *J Cell Biol* 1991;115:1639–1650.
29. Schafer DA, Gill SR, Cooper JA, et al. Ultrastructural analyses of the dynactin complex: an actin-related protein is a component of a filament that resembles F-actin. *J Cell Biol* 1994;126:403–412.
30. Holleran EA, Tokito MK, Karki S. Centractin (ARP1) associates with spectrin revealing a potential mechanism to link dynactin to intracellular organelles. *J Cell Biol* 1996;135:1815–1829.
31. Lippincott-Schwartz J. Cytoskeletal proteins and Golgi dynamics. *Curr Opin Cell Biol* 1998;10:52–59.
32. Paschal BM, Holzbaur EL, Pfister KK, et al. Characterization of a 50 kDa polypeptide in cytoplasmic dynein preparations reveals a complex with p150^{Glued} and a novel actin. *J Biol Chem* 1993;268:15318–15323.
33. Burkhardt JK, Echeverri CJ, Nilsson T, et al. Over expression of the dynamitin (p50) subunit of the dynactin complex disrupts dynein-dependent maintenance of membrane organelle distribution. *J Cell Biol* 1997;139:469–484.
34. King SJ, Schroer TA. Dynactin increases the processivity of the cytoplasmic dynein motor. *Nature Cell Biol* 2000;2:20–24.
35. Harada A, Takai Y, Kanai Y, et al. Golgi vesiculation and lysosome dispersion in cells lacking cytoplasmic dynein. *J Cell Biol* 1998;141:51–59.
36. Valletti C, Wetzel DM, Schrader M, et al. Role of dynactin in endocytic traffic: effects of dynamitin overexpression and co-localization with CLIP-170. *Mol Biol Cell* 1999;10:4107–4120.
37. Presley JF, Zaal KJM, Schroer TA, et al. ER to Golgi transport visualized in living cells. *Nature* 1997;389:81–85.
38. Goltz JS, Wolkoff AW, Novikoff P, et al. A role for microtubules in sorting of endocytic vesicles in rat hepatocytes. *Proc Natl Acad Sci USA* 1992;89:7026–7030.
39. Oda H, Stockert RJ, Collins C, et al. Interaction of the microtubule cytoskeleton with endocytic vesicles and cytoplasmic dynein in cultured rat hepatocytes. *J Biol Chem* 1995;270:15242–15249.

40. Oleynikov Y, Singer RH. RNA localization: different zip codes, same postman? *Trends Cell Biol* 1998;8:381–383.

41. Hays T, Karess R. Swallowing dyneins. A missing link in RNA activation? *Nature Cell Biol* 2000;2:60–62.

42. Hirokawa N. Kinesin and dynein superfamily proteins and the mechanism of organelle transport. *Science* 1998;279:519–526.

43. Vale RD. Kinesin, conventional. In: Kreis T, Vale R, eds. *Guidebook to the cytoskeletal and motor proteins*, 2nd ed. Oxford: Oxford University Press, 1999:398–402.

44. Lippincott-Schwartz J, Cole NB, Masotta A, et al. Kinesin is the motor for microtubule-mediated Golgi to ER membrane traffic. *J Cell Biol* 1995;128:293–306.

45. Gyoeva F, Gelfand V. Coalignment of vimentin intermediate filaments with microtubules depends on kinesin. *Nature* 1991;353:445–448.

46. Prahlad V, Yoon M, Moir RD, et al. Rapid movements of vimentin on microtubule tracks: kinesin-dependent assembly of intermediate filament networks. *J Cell Biol* 1998;143:159–170.

47. Komatsu M, Nakajima K, Goto M, et al. Isolation of kinesin from rat liver. *Gastroenterol Jpn* 1992;27:793.

48. Marks DL, Larkin JM, McNiven MA. Association of kinesin with the Golgi apparatus in rat hepatocytes. *J Cell Sci* 1994;107:2417–2426.

49. Howard J. Molecular motors: structural adaptations to cellular functions. *Nature* 1997;389:561–567.

50. Vale RD, Malik F, Brown D. Directional instability of microtubule transport in the presence of kinesin and dynein, two opposite polarity motors. *J Cell Biol* 1992;119:1589–1596.

51. Murray JW, Bananis E, Wolkoff AW. Reconstitution of ATP-dependent movement of endocytic vesicles along microtubules *in vitro*: an oscillatory bidirectional process. *Mol Biol Cell* 2000;11:419–433.

52. Endow SA. Kinesins, C-terminal motor domain. In: Kreis T, Vale R, eds. *Guidebook to the cytoskeletal and motor proteins*, 2nd ed. Oxford: Oxford University Press, 1999:403–408.

53. Hirokawa N. Kinesin, monomeric. In: Kreis T, Vale R, eds. *Guidebook to the cytoskeletal and motor proteins*, 2nd ed. Oxford: Oxford University Press, 1999:415–417.

54. Kozminski KG, Beech PL, Rosenbaum JL. The *Chlamydomonas* kinesin-like protein FLA10 is involved in motility-associated with the ciliary membrane. *J Cell Biol* 1995;131:1517–1527.

55. Signor D, Wedaman KP, Rose LS, et al. Two heterotrimeric kinesin complexes in chemosensory neurons and sensory cilia of *Caenorhabditis elegans. Mol Biol Cell* 1999;10:345–360.

56. Bassell GJ, Oleynikov Y, Singer RH. The trails of RNA through all cells large and small. *FASEB J* 1999;13:447–454.

57. Bananis E, Murray JW, Stockert RJ, et al. Microtubules and motor dependent endocytic vesicle sorting in vitro. *J Cell Biol* 2000;151:179–186.

58. Collins CA, Vallee RB. Preparation of microtubules from rat liver and testes: cytoplasmic dynein is a major microtubule-associated protein. *Cell Motil Cytoskel* 1989;14:491–500.

59. Sahly I, El-Amraqui A, Abitbol M, et al. Expression of myosin VIIA during mouse embryogenesis. *Anat Embryol* 1997;196:159–170.

60. Coluccio LM, Geeves MA. Transient kinetic analysis of the 130 kDa myosin I (MYR-1 gene product) from rat liver. A myosin I designed for maintenance of tension? *J Biol Chem* 1999;274:21575–21580.

61. Stoffler HE, Bahler M. The ATPase activity of Myr3, a rat myosin I, is allosterically inhibited by its own tail domain and by Ca2+ binding to its light chain calmodulin. *J Biol Chem* 1998;273:14605–14611.

62. Chieregatti E, Gartner A, Stoffer HE, et al. Myr7 is a novel myosin IX-Rho GAP expressed in rat brain. *J Cell Sci* 1998;111:3597–3608.

5

GENE REGULATION AND *IN VIVO* FUNCTION OF LIVER TRANSCRIPTION FACTORS

ROBERT H. COSTA
AI-XUAN LE HOLTERMAN
FRANCISCO M. RAUSA
GUY R. ADAMI

R. H. Costa: Department of Molecular Genetics, College of Medicine, University of Illinois at Chicago, Chicago, Illinois 60607-7170.

A.-X. Le Holterman: Department of Molecular Genetics, College of Medicine, Department of Surgery, Division of Pediatric Surgery, University of Illinois at Chicago, Chicago, Illinois 60612.

F. M. Rausa: Department of Molecular Genetics, College of Medicine, University of Illinois at Chicago, Chicago, Illinois 60607-7170.

G. R. Adami: Department of Oral Medicine and Diagnostic Sciences, University of Illinois at Chicago College of Dentistry, Chicago, Illinois 60612.

MECHANISM OF HEPATOCYTE-SPECIFIC GENE TRANSCRIPTION

Hepatocyte Transcription Factor Families

The liver performs essential functions in the body by uniquely expressing hepatocyte-specific genes encoding plasma proteins, and enzymes involved in gluconeogenesis, glycogen storage, glucose metabolism, cholesterol homeostasis, and synthesis of bile salts (1). Functional analysis of numerous hepatocyte-specific promoter and enhancer regions reveals that they are composed of multiple *cis*-acting DNA sequences that bind different families of hepatocyte nuclear factors (HNFs) (2). Although none of these transcriptional regulatory factors is entirely liver-specific, the requirement for combinatorial protein interactions to achieve high transcriptional levels plays an important role in maintaining hepatocyte-specific gene expression (2,3). Isolation of the complementary DNA (cDNA) clones encoding these transcription factors facilitated the identification of their DNA binding and transcriptional activation domains. On the basis of homology within DNA binding domains, the transcription factors were grouped into related protein families, which include the winged helix HNF-3α,

-3β, and -3γ proteins (4,5); the cut-homeodomain HNF-6 (OC-1) and one cut-2 (OC-2) proteins (6–10), the orphan steroid hormone receptors HNF-4α (11), and fetoprotein transcription factor (FTF) proteins (12,13), the POU-homeodomain HNF-1α and vHNF-1 proteins (14–16), and the nkx homeodomain nkx-2.8 protein (17), the basic region leucine zipper (bZIP) CCAAT/enhancer binding proteins (C/EBPs) (18,19), and the related bZip family member albumin D-site–binding protein (DBP), which contains an additional proline and amino acid–rich (PAR) region in the DNA-binding domain (20–22).

Transthyretin DNA Control Region as a Model for Hepatocyte-Specific Gene Regulation

We have utilized the DNA regulatory regions of the transthyretin (TTR) gene, which encodes the serum carrier protein of thyroxine and vitamin A (23), as a model to understand hepatocyte-specific gene transcription. Studies of TTR suggest that hepatocyte-specific gene transcription is dependent on combinatorial interactions of multiple DNA binding sites by several distinct families

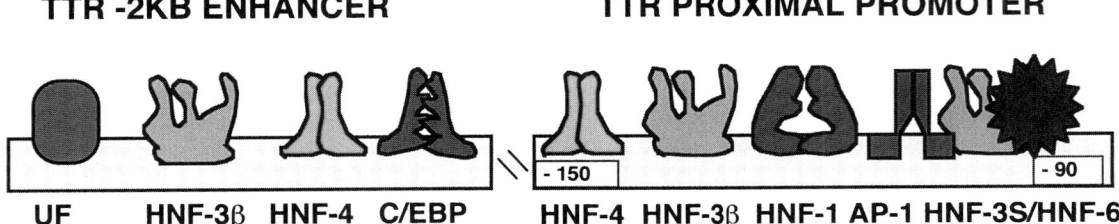

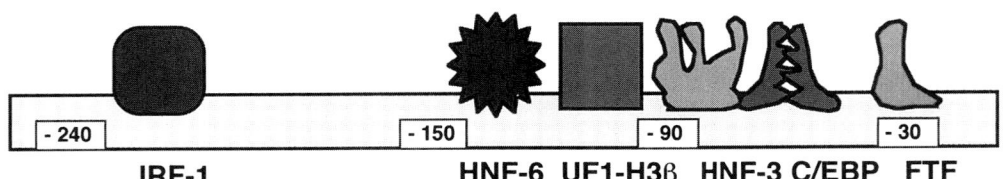

FIGURE 5.1. Transcription factors that regulate expression of the transthyretin (TTR) and hepatocyte nuclear factor (HNF)-3β genes and their binding sites. Schematically shown are the HNF-3β and TTR promoter constructs and their corresponding transcription factors. The TTR regulatory regions are bound by members of four different liver-enriched transcription factors HNF-1, HNF-3, HNF-4, HNF-6 and C/EBP (10,24,29,31) and the growth factor inducible AP-1 protein (30). The strong affinity HNF-3 binding site (HNF-3S) overlaps with the HNF-6 binding site in the TTR promoter (10). The TTR enhancer is also recognized by an uncharacterized ubiquitous factor (UF) and contains one HNF-3 binding site which is selectively recognized by the HNF-3β isoform (31). The HNF-3β promoter is regulated by three liver and pancreas transcription factors: HNF-3 and HNF-6 as well as by the C/EBP family (9). A third liver and pancreas-restricted orphan receptor family member fetoprotein transcription factor (FTF) (12,13) recognizes a sequence that is identical to the HNF-3β UF2-H3β promoter-binding site (130). Two additional binding sites are recognized by generally expressed factors, UF1-H3β (130) and the interferon (IFN) response factor-1 (IRF-1), which is activated in response to IFN-γ (127,131).

of liver-enriched transcription factors (Fig. 5.1). This assembly of numerous liver transcription factors is a regulatory feature found in most hepatocyte-specific genes and is required to achieve high levels of expression (2). The TTR regulatory region is composed of a proximal promoter region and a distal 100-nucleotide enhancer region located 2 kb from the transcriptional initiation site, which is sufficient to elicit hepatocyte expression in transgenic mice and in hepatoma cell (HepG2) transfections (24–28). This enhancer region provides a five- to tenfold stimulation in proximal TTR promoter expression (25,27). Transfection analysis of mutations in the TTR proximal promoter region allowed the identification of binding sites for the transcription factors HNF-3

TABLE 5.1. KNOWN AND POTENTIAL HEPATOCYTE NUCLEAR FACTOR-3 (HNF-3) TARGET GENES

Target Gene[a]	Genbank	Position	Sequence
Rat hepatocyte nuclear factor-3β (HNF-3β)	U50407	−97/−86	c c T G T T T G T T T T
Rat hepatocyte nuclear factor-3α	U86584	−466/−477	T T T G T T T A C a a A
Rat hepatocyte nuclear factor-1α	X63959	−21/−32	c A T A T T T A T c C G
Human insulin-like growth factor-I (IGF-I)	S85346	−180/−169	T c T G T T T G C T a A
Mouse annexin V promoter A	g4007573	−21/−32	T T T G T T T A T a T c
Rat IGF binding protein-1 (IGFBP-1)	M84484	−166/−176	T A T G T T T G T c C T
Rat IGFBP-2	M58560	−860/−872	A T T A T T G A C T c c
Human IGFBP-3	M35878	−1,537/−1,526	T T T A T T T A T T T A
Mouse transthyretin (TTR)	M19524	−95/−106	A T T A T T G A C T T A
Human thyroxine-binding globulin	X64171	−131/−120	A A T A T T T A C T a T
Human retinol-binding protein (RBP)	X02775	−547/−558	A A T A T T T G T T C T
Mouse albumin enhancer	U04199	533/522	A A T G T T T G T T C T
Rat α-fetoprotein (AFP)	M18351	−6,091/−6,102	T T T A T T G A C T T A
Mouse transferrin (TFN)	M30819	−73/−84	T g T G T T T G C g C A
Human apolipoprotein B	M19808	+892/+903	A A T A c T G A C T T T
Human apolipoprotein AI/CIII	J00098	−535/−546	T g T G T T T A C T C A
Human protein C	U47685	−15/−26	A A T A T T T G C T T G
Human clotting factor IX	X75349	−372/−383	T T T A T T G A T T T c
Rat α-fibrinogen	X02922	−892/−903	A A T A T T G A T g T A
Human clotting factor VIII	U24224	−900/−911	T T T A T T T A T T T T
Human clotting factor VII	U14580	−392/−381	A A T A T T T A C a T c
Mouse complement component C5	M64852	−656/−645	T T T G T T T G T T T T
Mouse plasminogen activator inhibitor-3	U67877	−910/−921	T A T G T T T A T c C T
Human glucokinase	M90297	−797/−784	A c T A T T G A C T g A
Rat phosphoenolpyruvate carboxykinase	K02299	−247/−258	T T g A T T G A C T a A
Rat glucose-6-phosphatase	U57552	−356/−366	T g T A T T T G T T T G
Rat 6-phosphofructo-2-kinase	M26261	−26/−37	A A T A T T T A T T C c
Rat tyrosine aminotransferase	M34257	−3,788/−3,777	c T T G T T T G C T C T
Rat glycogen phosphorylase	M85280	+304/+315	T g T A T T T G T T C T
Rat carbamoylphosphate synthetase I	X90476	−125/−114	A g T G T T T G C T C T
Rat α-amylase (Amy-1)	M14152	−72/−61	T T T A T T G A T T c A
Rat catalase	M25669	−250/−239	c T T A T T T A T T T G
Rat arginase	M17924	−42/−53	T c T G T T T A T c C A
Human tyrosinase	g37506	−484/−495	T T T G T T T A T T T T
Rat cytochrome P-450 CYP2C12	M33544	−49/−38	A A T A T G A T T T T
Rat cytochrome P-450 CYP2C13	X79810	−53/−42	A A T A T G A T T c T
Rat cytochrome P-450e	Y00410	−229/−218	T c T G T T T A C T T A
Human cytochrome P-450 CYP2C18	L16869	−692/−703	A A T G T T T A T c C T
Human cholesterol 7α-hydroxylase	M89647	−290/−279	T T T A T T T G T T C T
Rat sodium-taurocholate cotransporter protein (Ntcp)	L76612	−758/−769	T T T A T T G A C T g T
Mouse P-glycoprotein mdr2	M74151	−752/−741	T T T A T T T A T T T T
Mouse organic cation transporter-2	AJ006037	−144/−125	T g T G T T T A T T g T
HNF-3 consensus[b]			W W T R T T T R Y T Y D
			W W T A T T G A Y T T W

[a]Shown are the name of the putative HNF-3 target gene, GenBank accession number, position in the gene, and the HNF-3 binding consensus sequence (10,150).
[b]Nucleotide abbreviations in the HNF-3 DNA binding consensus sequence are as follows: W = A or T, R = G or A, Y = C or T, and D is not C.
Lower case letters represent nucleotides that deviate from the HNF-3 binding consensus sequence.

(−106 to −94 bp) and HNF-4 (−151 to −140 bp) (25). Additional binding sites for hepatocyte transcription C/EBP, HNF-1, HNF-3, and HNF-4 were found in these regulatory regions as well as sites recognized by other widely distributed transcription factors (4,11,25,29–31). Interestingly, two of the HNF-3 binding sites in the TTR control regions are recognized by only the HNF-3β pro-

tein, suggesting that a subset of hepatocyte-specific genes may be regulated by a distinct HNF-3 isoform (5,31). In the presence of the TTR enhancer region, TTR promoter expression was abolished with a site-directed mutation that disrupted the strong affinity HNF-3 binding site (HNF-3S) and an overlapping HNF-6 recognition sequence (−106 to −94) (10,25,26). HepG2 transfection

TABLE 5.2. KNOWN AND POTENTIAL HEPATOCYTE NUCLEAR FACTOR (HNF-6) TARGET GENES

Target Gene[a]	Genbank	Position	Sequence
Rat hepatocyte nuclear factor-3β (HNF-3β	U50407	−139/−127	G A T A T T G A T T T T T
Mouse hepatocyte nuclear factor-4α	S77762	−363/−375	A T c A T T G A C T T c T
Human growth hormone receptor	AJ131868	−913/−925	T T c A T T G A T T T A T
Human insulin-like growth factor-I (IGF-I)	S85346	−289/−301	G T T A T T G A g T A A G
Rat IGF binding protein-1 (IGFBP-1)	M84484	−278/−266	G C c t T T G A T T T c T
Rat IGFBP-2	M58560	−860/−872	A T T A T T G A C T c c T
Human IGFBP-3	M35878	−1,507/−1,429	G A a A T T G A T c T T T
Human IGFBP-4	Y12508	−2,063/−2,051	G T T A c T G A T T A T T
Human IGFBP-5	U20271	−457/−469	G C a A T T G A C T g T A
Mouse transthyretin (TTR)	M19524	−95/−107	A T T A T T G A C T T A G
Human thyroxine-binding globulin	X64171	−101/−113	c A c A T T G A T T A A T
Human retinol-binding protein (RBP)	X02775	−552/−540	A A T A T T G A C c A g A
Mouse albumin enhancer	U04199	624/636	T g T A T T G A T c A g T
Rat α-fetoprotein (AFP)	M18351	−6,091/−6,102	T T T A T T G A C T T A G
Rat ceruloplasmin	M80529	−483/−471	T T T A T T G A C T A C T
Human protein C	U47685	−692/−704	T C c A T T G A T T g c A
Human clotting factor IX	X75349	−372/−384	T T T A T T G A T T T c A
Rat α-fibrinogen	X02922	−892/−9,034	A A T A T T G A T g T A T
Human β-fibrinogen	X05018	−470/−458	A C T A T T G A T T T T A
Human Apolipoprotein AI/CIII	J00098	−811/−799	A A c A T T G A T c A A G
Human Apolipoprotein B	M19808	+892/+904	A A T A C T G A C T T T A
Mouse α₁-antitrypsin		−195/−184	T C c A T T G A T T T A G
Rat α₂-macroglobulin	M23567	−442/−454	G g T A T T G A C T T T A
Human glucokinase	M90297	−797/−78	A c T A T T G A C T g A G
Rat phosphoenolpyruvate carboxykinase	K02299	−247/−259	T T g A T T G A C T A A A
Rat glucose-6-phosphatase	U57552	−547/−359	A A T A T T G A T T T T T
Rat 6-phosphofructo-2-kinase	M26261	−200/−212	G A A A T T G A T T T c A
Rat tyrosine aminotransferase	M34257	−776/−764	T Tg A T T G A T T A T T
Rat tryptophan oxygenase	X05145	−220/−208	T C T A T T G A T T T A T
Human ornithine transcarbamylase	D00221	−314/−302	T C A A T T G A T T T T G
Rat α-amylase (Amy-1)	M14152	−72/−60	T T T A T T G A T T c A A
Rat catalase	M25669	−836/−824	c C T A T T G A T T A A A
Rat arginase	M17924	−231/−243	A C A A T T G A C A A T T
Rat serine dehydratase (SDH2)	J03864	−655/−643	T A c A T T G A T T T g G
Rat cytochrome P-450 CYP2C12	M33544	−49/−37	A A T A T T G A T T T T T
Rat cytochrome P-450 CYP2C13	X79810	53/−41	A A T A T T G A T T c T G
Human cytochrome P-450 CYP2C9	L16877	−95/−107	T A a A T T G A C c A A T
Human cytochrome P-450 CYP2C18	L16869	−927/−915	c A T A T T G A T T T A T
Human alcohol dehydrogenase-2	M24308	−150/−162	A A T A T T G A C T T C C
Human cholesterol 7α-hydroxylase	M89647	−1,370/−1,392	T A T A T T G A a T A T G
Rat sodium-taurocholate cotransporter protein (Ntcp)	L76612	−758/−770	T T T A T T G A C T g T T
Mouse P-glycoprotein mdr2	M74151	−877/−889	c C T A T T G A C T g T G
HNF-6 DNA binding consensus sequence[b]			D H W A T T G A Y T W W D

[a]Shown are the name of the putative HNF-6 target gene, GenBank accession number, position in the gene, and the HNF-6 DNA binding consensus sequence (10).
[b]Nucleotide abbreviations in the HNF-6 DNA binding consensus sequence are as follows: D is not C, H is not G, W = A or T, and Y = C or T. Lower case letters represent nucleotides that deviate from the HNF-6 DNA binding consensus sequence.

of TTR promoter constructs that altered the HNF-3S (HNF-3S/HNF-6; −106 to −94) sequence so that it bound either HNF-3 or HNF-6 resulted in a 30% reduction in TTR promoter activity, suggesting that normal TTR gene transcription requires binding of both transcription factors (10). It is interesting to note that HNF-3 and HNF-6 potentially regulate expression of similar set of hepatocyte-specific target genes (Tables 5.1 and 5.2). Mutations in the other proximal HNF-binding sites elicited a 40% to 60% reduction in promoter activity, whereas in the absence of the TTR enhancer region these promoter mutations eliminated TTR transcriptional activity (26). These studies suggest that a minimal number of hepatocyte-enriched transcription factors are required to occupy promoter sites to achieve transcriptional activity.

PHYSIOLOGIC ROLE OF HNF-3 IN MOUSE LIVER AND PANCREATIC FUNCTION

Transcriptional Activity of the HNF-3 Proteins

The HNF-3 proteins are members of a growing family of transcription factors that play important roles in the differentiation of distinct cellular lineages in *Caenorhabditis elegans, Drosophila*, rodents, and humans (32). These transcription factors share homology in the winged helix DNA-binding domain that consists of a modified helix turn helix motif, which allows binding to DNA as a monomer (33–35). Amino acid sequences located at both the amino and carboxyl terminus of the HNF-3 winged helix DNA-binding domain are sufficient to mediate nuclear localization (36), suggesting that the winged helix motif also evolved with a nuclear translocation function (36–38). The HNF-3β protein is a potent activator of gene expression through transcriptional activation domains located at the amino and carboxyl terminus (36,39). HNF-3 proteins may also play a role in hepatocyte differentiation because induction of albumin transcription during hepatic specification coincides with *in vivo* footprinting of HNF-3–binding sites in the albumin enhancer region (40). Moreover, HNF-3 proteins are involved in organizing the nucleosome architecture of the −10-kilobase (kb) albumin enhancer sequences (41–43), and HNF-3 protein exhibited more stable binding to the nucleosome assembled DNA albumin enhancer templates (44). Consistent with the ability of HNF-3 to position nucleosome core particles, *in vitro* transcription studies using nucleosome associated α-fetoprotein (AFP) promoter templates demonstrated that HNF-3 binding diminishes chromatin-mediated transcriptional repression of the AFP expression (45).

Potential HNF-3 Target Genes in the Liver

The rodent HNF-3 proteins regulate expression of numerous genes critical for liver function [reviewed in refs. 2 and 3) (Table 5.1)]. These hepatocyte genes include the serum carrier proteins albumin, AFP, apolipoprotein AI, and transferrin (46–50); the cholesterol 7α-hydroxylase (Cpy7A) enzyme involved in bile acid synthesis (51–53), and the glucose metabolism enzymes L-type 6-phosphofructo-2-kinase (PFK-2), aldolase B, and glucose-6-phosphatase (54–56). HNF-3 is an important regulator of angiotensinogen, the precursor of the vasoregulator angiotensin II (57), the anticoagulation protein C (58,59) and coagulation factors (Table 5.1) and the cytochrome P-450 enzymes [(CYP2C6) (60); for others see Table 5.1)]. HNF-3 proteins also recognize the insulin response elements of phosphoenolpyruvate carboxykinase (PEPCK), aspartate aminotransferase, and insulin-like growth factor binding protein-1 (IGFBP-1) promoter regions (61–63) and participate in growth hormone activation of the insulin-like growth factor-I (IGF-I) gene expression (64). In support of HNF-3's role in regulating transcription of hepatocyte-specific genes, a hepatoma cell line that expresses a dominant negative HNF-3 mutant specifically extinguished transcription of numerous HNF-3 target genes, specifically albumin, TTR, transferrin, PEPCK, and aldolase B (65).

Cellular Expression Pattern of HNF-3 Isoforms in Mouse Development and Adult Organs

In the mouse embryo, HNF-3β expression initiates during gastrulation [day 6.5 postcoitus (pc)] in the node, notochord mesoderm, floor-plate neuroepithelium, and in visceral, definitive endoderm and gut endoderm (66–69). HNF-3α expression initiates 1 day later during mouse gastrulation in the definitive endoderm, the anterior notochord, and the entire gut endoderm and the midbrain floor plate (67–69). During organogenesis, HNF-3α and HNF-3β genes are expressed in epithelial cells of the developing liver, esophagus, trachea, salivary gland, lung, pancreas, intestine, and stomach (66–69) (Table 5.3). Furthermore, HNF-3α is expressed in epithelial cells of the renal pelvis, prostate gland, bladder, and urinary tract (70), and its transcription in the prostate gland is testosterone-dependent (71). Furthermore, retinoic acid–mediated differentiation of F9 embryonic stem cells toward visceral endoderm induces HNF-3α transcription (72), whereas expression of HNF-3β is delayed (73). In contrast to the other HNF-3 isoforms, HNF-3γ expression is absent from the lung, trachea, or esophagus (67), but its expression is restricted to the pancreas, stomach, gut, testis, and ovaries (74).

TABLE 5.3. EXPRESSION PATTERNS OF HEPATOCYTE TRANSCRIPTION FACTORS

Gene	DNA Binding	Mouse Embryonic Expression Pattern	Adult Expression
Hnf3β	Winged helix domain (monomer)	Gastrulation (6.5–8.5 days pc): Definitive, visceral, gut endoderm, notochord, floor plate of neurotube Organogenesis (9–18 days pc): Endoderm-derived epithelial cells of liver, pancreas, lung, intestine, stomach, esophagus, tongue trachea, floor plate, and midbrain	Hepatocytes, epithelial cells of pancreas (acinar and β cells), lung, stomach and large intestine, intestinal crypt
Hnf3α	Winged helix domain (monomer)	Gastrulation (7.5–8.5 days pc): Similar to *Hnf3β* except *Hnf3α* expression initiates 1 day later in development Organogenesis (9–18 days pc): Similar to *Hnf3β*	Similar to *Hnf3β* except *Hnf3α* is also expressed in epithelial cells of intestinal villus, renal pelvis, prostate and urinary tract
Hnf3γ	Winged helix domain (monomer)	(8.5 days pc): Foregut and hindgut endoderm Organogenesis (9–18 days pc): Gut endoderm-derived epithelial cells of liver, pancreas, intestine, and stomach; visceral endoderm of yolk sac, testis, and ovaries	Hepatocytes, pancreas, stomach, small intestine, large intestine, testes, and ovaries
Hnf6	One cut-homeodomain (monomer)	Organogenesis (9–18 days pc): Gut endoderm-derived epithelial cells of liver, bile duct, gallbladder, pancreas, and intestine; neural crest cells of dorsal root ganglia and marginal layer and ganglion of retina	Hepatocytes, and epithelial cells of intrahepatic bile duct, common bile duct, gallbladder, pancreatic ducts, and exocrine acinar cells
Ftf	Zinc finger orphan steroid hormone receptor (monomer)	Gastrulation (8 days pc): Visceral endoderm of yolk sac, branchial arch, and neurocrest cells Organogenesis (9–18 days pc): Endoderm-derived epithelial cells of liver, pancreas, and intestine; neural crest cells of marginal layer and in rib primordium	Hepatocytes and pancreatic acinar and ductal epithelial cells; restricted to the epithelial cells of the intestinal crypts
Hnf4α	Zinc finger orphan steroid hormone receptor (dimer)	Blastocyst (4.5 days pc): Primary endoderm Gastrulation (5.5–8.5 days pc): Extraembryonic visceral endoderm cells of the yolk sac Organogenesis (9–18 days pc): Endoderm-derived epithelial cells of liver, pancreas, intestine, and stomach; in mesonephric and metanephric tubules of kidney	Hepatocytes, and epithelial cells of pancreas, kidney, intestine, and skin
Hnf1α LFB1	POU-homeodomain (dimerization uses DCoH)	Organogenesis (9–18 days pc): Gut endoderm-derived epithelial cells of liver, pancreas, intestine, and stomach; extraembryonic yolk sac endoderm; polarized epithelium of kidney following appearance of three nephrons	Hepatocytes, and epithelial cells of pancreas, intestine, stomach, and proximal and distal tubules of kidney
C/EBPα	Basic domain leucine zipper domain (bZIP) (dimer)	Organogenesis (13–18 days pc): Hepatocytes of liver, hippocampus (CA1–CA4 and dentate gyrus), Purkinje cells of cerebellum, neurons of midbrain and forebrain	Hepatocytes and adipocytes; epithelial cells of intestine, pancreas, lung, and skin; adrenal gland, placenta, and myeloid cells
C/EBPβ	bZIP domain (dimer)	Organogenesis (9–18 days pc): Similar to *C/EBPα* except *C/EBPα* is expressed earlier than *C/EBPβ* during hepatic development	Hepatocytes, adipocytes; epithelial cells of intestine, lung, skin, and mammary gland; myeloid cells, testis, ovaries; hippocampus.

Expression references: *Hnf3α,β,γ* (5,9,66–71,74,83,141,151); *Hnf6* (7,9); fetoprotein transcription factor (FTF) (13); HNF-4 (11,104,152); HNF-1 (14,111); *C/EBPα,β* (115,117,121,153–164). pc, postcoitus.

The *HNF-3*β Gene Is Critical for Early Embryonic Development

HNF-3β is known to regulate notochord transcription of the sonic hedgehog (SHH) gene, which is required for inductive signaling during the formation of the neurotube (75,76). Moreover, ectopic expression of HNF-3β in the hindbrain/midbrain region of day 8.5 transgenic mouse embryos changes the cellular fate of the dorsal neurotube and converts it to floor-plate neuroepithelium, resulting in severe defects in skull, midbrain, colliculi, and cerebellum formation (77). Homozygous null *Hnf3*β embryos die *in utero* because of defective formation of the node, notochord, and visceral endoderm, which are required for development of the primitive streak during gastrulation (78,79). Tetraploid rescue of the visceral endoderm defect in *Hnf3*β −/− embryos restored normal primitive streak morphogenesis, but the embryos failed to undergo proper gastrulation because they were still missing the node and notochord and did not develop foregut and midgut endoderm (80). This *Hnf3*β −/− embryo defect has thereby precluded examination of *in vivo* function of HNF-3β in the regulation of its hepatocyte target genes.

Elevated Levels of HNF-3β in Mouse Hepatocytes Influence Expression of Genes Involved in Bile Acid and Glucose Homeostasis

In recent studies, we have increased hepatocyte HNF-3β levels in transgenic mice using the −3 kb TTR promoter region to assess the role of HNF-3β in hepatocyte-specific gene regulation (81). We found that increased hepatocyte expression of the rat HNF-3β transgene protein disrupted the normal hepatic levels of the endogenous mouse HNF-3α,-3β, -3γ, and HNF-6 transcription factors. Moreover, we found that diminished hepatic expression of the endogenous mouse HNF-3 and HNF-6 genes were specific because the transgenic livers exhibited normal expression of the HNF-1α, HNF-4α, C/EBPα, and C/EBPβ transcription factors. Postnatal transgenic mice exhibit growth retardation, depletion of hepatocyte glycogen storage and elevated serum levels of bile acids. The retarded growth phenotype is likely due to a 20-fold increase in hepatic expression of IGFBP-1, which limits the biologic availability of IGFs required for postnatal growth. The defects in glycogen storage and serum bile acids coincide with diminished postnatal expression of hepatocyte genes involved in gluconeogenesis (PEPCK) and sinusoidal bile acid uptake [sodium-taurocholate cotransporter protein (Ntcp)] respectively. These transgenic studies represent the first *in vivo* demonstration that the HNF-3β transcriptional network regulates expression of hepatocyte-specific genes required for bile acid and glucose homeostasis as well as postnatal growth.

Targeted Disruption of the Mouse *Hnf3* Genes Demonstrates that They Regulate Expression of Genes Required for Glucose Homeostasis

Use of *Hnf3*β −/−—deficient embryonic stem (ES) cells to form embryoid bodies (EBs) for *in vitro* differentiation toward visceral (yolk sac) endoderm demonstrates that HNF-3β is involved in cross-regulating the transcription of the *Hnf3*α, *Hnf1*α, and *Hnf4*α genes and is required for expression of apolipoproteins, aldolase B, pyruvate kinase, TTR, and albumin (82). Furthermore, using the EB differentiation system, Duncan and co-workers (82) demonstrated that HNF-3β expression is increased in the presence of insulin, which is consistent with HNF-3β's role in regulating glucose homeostasis genes. Surprisingly, expression of these HNF-3 target genes is upregulated in *Hnf3*α-deficient embryoid bodies, suggesting that HNF-3α negatively regulates the transcription of these genes and opposes the transcriptional stimulatory activity of HNF-3β protein (82). In contrast, these target genes were normally expressed in *Hnf3*α −/− livers, suggesting that hepatocytes and visceral endoderm exhibit differences in HNF-3α regulatory pathways (83,84). The *Hnf3*α −/− mice fail to thrive, are hypoglycemic, and display reduced pancreatic islet expression and secretion of glucagon (83,84). The hypoglycemic phenotype is likely due to a decrease in pancreatic α-cell expression of glucagon, which is required to mobilize hepatic glycogen (Table 5.4). These results suggest that Hnf3α plays an important role in regulating pancreatic transcription of the glucagon gene, which is critical in mobilizing hepatic glycogen stores for serum glucose homeostasis. The *Hnf3*γ −/− mice displayed no morphologic defects in the intestine, liver, pancreas, and testis, which normally express abundant levels of Hnf3γ (85). Hepatocytes deficient in the *Hnf3*γ gene display a 50% reduction in expression of several HNF-3 target genes including PEPCK, transferrin, tyrosine aminotransferase (TAT), and a compensatory increase in the level of *Hnf3*α and *Hnf3*β expression (Table 5.4). These results suggest that the *Hnf3*γ isoform is required to regulate a specific subset of hepatocyte-specific genes, several of which are involved in glucose homeostasis.

PHYSIOLOGIC ROLE OF HNF-6 IN LIVER AND PANCREATIC FUNCTION

Potential HNF-6 Target Genes in the Liver

Functional analysis of the TTR and HNF-3β promoter regions enabled us to identify a cut-homeodomain transcription factor, HNF-6, which is also involved in regulating the expression of numerous hepatocyte-specific genes required for liver function (10) (Table 5.2). The HNF-6 cDNA was isolated by biochemical purification using a

TABLE 5.4. PHENOTYPE OF HEPATOCYTE TRANSCRIPTION FACTOR HOMOZYGOUS NULL OR KNOCKOUT MICE

Gene	General Phenotype of Homozygous Null (–/–) Mouse	Liver Phenotype of Homozygous Null (–/–) Mouse
Hnf3β–/– mice	Hnf3β–/– embryos die *in utero* by day 10 because they fail to undergo gastrulation; lack formation of node, notochord, visceral endoderm, foregut, and midgut, and exhibit defects in neurotube	Unknown because of Hnf3β–/– early embryonic lethal phenotype
Hnf3β–/– EB	Use of null Hnf3β–/– embryonic stem (ES) cells to form embryoid bodies (EB) *in vitro*, which differentiate toward visceral endoderm (VE)	Decreased VE expression of Hnf3α, Hnf4α, Hnf1α, apolipoproteins (Apo A1, A2, A4, B, C2), aldolase-B, pyruvate kinase, transthyretin (TTR), and albumin
Hnf3α–/– mice	All Hnf3α–/– mice die 4 weeks postnatally and exhibit growth retardation and hypoglycemia caused by decreased in pancreatic expression of glucagon, which is required to mobilize hepatic glycogen; increased expression of hexokinase and IGFBP-1 in postnatal gut	No liver phenotype was noted, which is possibly due to compensation by the Hnf3β and Hnf3γ isoforms but their expression are not elevated in the Hnf3α–/– hepatocytes
Hnf3α–/– EB	Use of null Hnf3α–/– ES cells to form EB *in vitro*, which differentiate toward VE	Increased VE expression of Hnf3β target genes; no change in Hnf3β expression
Hnf3γ–/– mice	Deficient Hnf3τ–/– embryos and adult mice display no morphologic defects	50% reduction in expression of several hepatocyte genes: tyrosine aminotransferase, PEPCK, transferrin (TFN); compensatory increased expression of Hnf3β and Hnf3α.
Hnf6–/– mice	70% of Hnf6–/– mice die 2 weeks postnatally from diabetes mellitus exhibiting low serum insulin levels; no ventral pancreas and delay in formation of pancreatic islets, but glucagon producing cells in these regenerated islets are not appropriately organized	Hnf6–/– mice lack a gallbladder and show perturbed differentiation of intrahepatic bile ducts, which is associated with a cholestatic syndrome; intrahepatic bile duct regenerates in the liver of 30% of Hnf6–/– mice that survive the postnatal insulin and cholestasis crisis
Hnf4α–/– mice	Hnf4α–/– embryos die *in utero* by day 6.5 with defects in visceral endoderm (yolk sac), which is essential for ectoderm survival and gastrulation; tetraploid rescue of visceral endoderm defect in Hnf4α–/– embryos restores gastrulation and allows formation of embryonic liver	In tetraploid rescued day 12 Hnf4α–/– fetal livers—diminished expression of pregnane-X-receptor (PXR), Hnf1α, albumin, α-fetoprotein (AFP), TFN, Apo A1, A4, B, C3, C2, phenylalanine hydroxylase (PAH), L-type fatty acid binding protein, erythropoietin, and retinol-binding protein (RBP)
Hnf1α–/– mice	Hnf1α–/– mice die around weaning after massive urinary loss of glucose and amino acids (Fanconi syndrome) caused by renal proximal tubular dysfunction; defective glucose-mediated insulin secretion from pancreatic β cells leading to elevated serum glucose	Hepatic expression of phenylalanine hydroxylase is totally silent in Hnf1α–/– liver leading to phenylketonuria; Hnf1α–/– mice exhibit diminished hepatic expression of albumin, α₁-antitrypsin, and β-fibrinogen, and compensatory increase in hepatic levels of vHNF1
C/EBPα–/– mice	C/EBPα–/– mice die from hypoglycemia within 8 hours after birth, fail to store hepatic glycogen; hepatocytes and adipocytes do not store lipid; defects in lung, neutrophils, and eosinophils	Increased hepatocyte proliferation and diminished postnatal hepatic expression of glycogen synthase, gluconeogenic enzymes PEPCK and glucose-6-phosphatase
C/EBPα–/– adult mice	LoxP targeted C/EBPα gene locus allowed disruption of C/EBPα gene in the adult liver using tail vein injection of adenovirus expressing the Cre recombinase gene (95% of adenovirus infects the liver)	In addition to hepatic glucose homeostasis genes listed above, C/EBPα–/– liver exhibits diminished expression of bilirubin UDP-glucuronosyl-transferase (jaundiced phenotype) and factor IX

Homozygous null (–/–) mice: Hnf3β (78–80); Hnf3β and Hnf3α deficient embryoid bodies (EB) (82); Hnf3α (83,84); Hnf3γ (85); Hnf4α (105–107); Hnf1α (109–111); C/EBPα (117,119,121,165,166); and adult C/EBPα (124).
IGFBP, insulin-like growth factor binding protein; PEPCK, phosphoenolpyruvate carboxykinase.

functional element from the PFK-2 promoter (8) and the yeast one hybrid selection method using the HNF-6 site from the HNF-3β promoter region (9). Northern blot analysis demonstrates that HNF-6 expression is restricted to adult liver and pancreas and that it is 9 kb in length. The cut-homeodomain HNF-6 protein is a member of the one-cut family of transcription factors, which binds to the DNA recognition sequence as a monomer using both cut and homeodomain protein motifs (6,7,9). HNF-6 potentially regulates numerous hepatocyte genes including serum carrier proteins, clotting factors, cytochrome P-450, and detoxifying proteins and those involved in glucose and amino acid homeostasis and in bile acid synthesis and transport (Table 5.2). Furthermore, HNF-6 inhibits glucocorticoid-mediated activation of PFK-2 and PEPCK in hepatoma cell transcription, suggesting that it plays a role in regulating glucose homeostasis (86). Moreover, hypophysectomized rats exhibited significant reductions in hepatic HNF-6 messenger RNA (mRNA), and its normal expression was restored following 1 week of growth hormone treatment (87). Consistent with this notion, growth hormone activates the signal transducer and activator of transcription 5 (STAT5) protein, which binds to and mediates induction of HNF-6 promoter expression (88). These studies indicate that HNF-6 transcription is regulated by the growth hormone signaling pathway.

Cellular Expression Pattern of HNF-6 in Mouse Development and Adult Organs

In day 9 pc mouse embryos, the one-cut-homeodomain HNF-6 transcription factor is expressed at the onset and during morphogenesis of the liver, gallbladder, and pancreas (7,9). Later in mouse development, HNF-6 mRNA levels are observed in the neurocrest cells of the dorsal root ganglia, marginal layer, and nuclei of the mesencephalon and pons as well as the ganglion cells of the retina (7,9). In the developing liver, HNF-6 is expressed in hepatocytes and in the epithelial cells of the intrahepatic and extrahepatic bile ducts (Table 5.3). HNF-6 expression continues in the developing epithelial cells of the pancreatic ducts and endocrine and exocrine cells of the mouse embryo. At 18 days pc of mouse pancreatic development, HNF-6 expression diminishes in the pancreatic endocrine cells when the definitive islets of Langerhans first begin to be organized (9). This suggests that terminal differentiation of the pancreatic endocrine cells requires the cessation of HNF-6 expression.

Persistent Expression of HNF-6 in Mouse Islet Endocrine Cells Causes Disrupted Islet Architecture and Diabetes

To examine whether the reduction in islet expression of HNF-6 is critical for proper pancreatic function, we generated transgenic mice in which the islet-specific regulatory element from the *pancreatic/duodenal homeobox (pdx1)* gene drives persistent expression of HNF-6 in pancreatic islets (89). In these mice, the HNF-6 expressing islet cells were hyperplastic and have aberrant islet organization with an increase in the number of α, β, and PP (secretes pancreatic polypeptide) cells. The transgenic pancreatic islets fail to express the *glucose transporter 2 (glut2)* gene, which is essential for insulin secretion from pancreatic β cells. The transgenic mice are therefore diabetic and are unable to secrete insulin in response to a glucose challenge. These deficits reveal that downregulation of HNF-6 expression during pancreatic islet cell ontogeny is critical for normal organiza-

tional development of the pancreatic islet cells and for transcriptional regulation of the glut2 gene, which is necessary to regulate β-cell secretion of insulin.

Targeted Disruption of the Mouse *Hnf6* Gene Causes Diabetes and Defects in Gallbladder and Intrahepatic Bile Duct Formation

Consistent with this important role of HNF-6 in pancreatic function, the *Hnf6 –/–* mice display severe defects in pancreatic islet formation and do not form the ventral pancreas during development (90). The *Hnf6*-deficient mice are diabetic and most of them do not survive postnatal development (Table 5.4). *Hnf6 –/–* mice do not develop a gallbladder and develop cholestasis from disrupted intrahepatic bile duct formation. Approximately 30% of the postnatal *Hnf6 –/–* mice survive these pancreatic defects and form aberrant pancreatic islets displaying abnormal organization of glucagon-producing α cells. The surviving *Hnf6 –/–* mice are also able to regenerate intrahepatic bile ducts and thus partially restore normal biliary function. These genetic studies indicate that HNF-6 expression is critical for the formation of pancreatic endocrine cells, intrahepatic bile ducts, and gallbladder.

FUNCTIONAL ROLE OF HEPATIC HNF-1 AND HNF-4 USING HOMOZYGOUS NULL MICE

Human Autosomal-Dominant Form of Non–Insulin-Dependent Diabetes Is Caused by Mutations in the *Hnf1*α and *Hnf4*α Genes

In the adult mouse, the POU-Homeodomain HNF-1α and steroid hormone receptor HNF-4α transcription factors are expressed in the hepatocytes and epithelial cells of the pancreas, intestine, stomach, and kidney (Table 5.3). The HNF-1α protein binds to its DNA recognition sequence as a dimer using a myosin-like dimerization domain located at the amino terminus of the protein (14,15). HNF-1α dimers are stabilized through association with dimerization cofactor of HNF-1α (DcoH) protein, which is identical to the aromatic amino acid metabolizing enzyme 4α-carbinolamine dehydratase (91). HNF-1α will also form heterodimers with a related family member named vHNF-1 (16), whose expression is detected earlier than HNF-1α in the visceral endoderm of the yolk sac (Table 5.3). The steroid hormone family member HNF-4 protein utilizes a zinc finger domain to recognize DNA either as a homodimer or as heterodimer with retinoic X receptor α (92–94). Transcriptional activity of HNF-4 has been reported to be modulated through binding of the endogenous ligand fatty acyl–coenzyme A (CoA) thioesters (long chain) and through protein phosphorylation (11,95–97). Numerous hepatocyte-specific genes are known to be potentially regulated by the HNF-1 and HNF-4 transcription factors (98,99). The HNF-1α and HNF-4α genes are also mutated in pedigrees of human families suffering from a maturity onset diabetes of the young 3 (MODY-3) and MODY-1, respectively (100–103). These patients exhibit an autosomal-dominant form of early-onset non–insulin-dependent diabetes. Mutation of HNF-1α and HNF-4α transcription factors cause non–insulin-dependent diabetes, which indicates that they regulate expression of genes critical for glucose homeostasis.

Targeted Disruption of the Mouse *Hnf4*α Gene Identifies Glucose Homeostatic Target Genes

In mouse development, *Hnf4*α is expressed in the primary and extraembryonic visceral endoderm prior to gastrulation (104). During organogenesis, it is expressed in epithelial cells at the onset of liver, pancreas, and intestine formation. Consistent with its early embryonic expression pattern, *Hnf4*α –/– embryos exhibited a severe visceral endoderm defect preventing gastrulation and they fail to develop past day 6.5 pc (105). Use of *Hnf4*α null ES cells to form EB *in vitro* to differentiate toward the visceral endoderm cell lineage revealed decreased expression of glucose transporter 2, the glycolytic enzymes aldolase B and glyceraldehyde-3-phosphate dehydrogenase, and liver pyruvate kinase, substantiating the role of HNF-4α in regulating genes involved in glucose homeostasis (101). *Hnf4*α-deficient visceral endoderm displays reduced expression of *Hnf1,*α, AFP, transferrin (TFN), several of the apolipoproteins (Apo), TTR, and retinol-binding protein (RBP) (106). Tetraploid rescue of the visceral endoderm defect in *Hnf4*α –/– embryos restores gastrulation and allowed formation of the liver and other organs to proceed. At day 12.5 pc, *Hnf4*α –/– fetal liver exhibits diminished expression of the steroid hormone family member *pregnane-X-receptor (PXR)* and *Hnf1*α genes, the latter of which substantiates its role in cross-regulation of hepatic HNF-1α expression (107). The disruption of this liver transcriptional regulatory pathway resulted in diminished expression of albumin, AFP, TFN, several distinct apolipoproteins, phenylalanine hydroxylase (PAH), L-type fatty acid binding protein, erythropoietin, and RBP (Table 5.4). In summary, HNF-4 is not required for liver specification but it regulates hepatocyte-specific genes essential for liver function.

Targeted Disruption of the Mouse *Hnf1*α Gene Causes Non–Insulin-Dependent Diabetes, Renal Dysfunction, and Phenylketonuria

In support of the previously mentioned *Hnf1*α MODY phenotype, *Hnf1*α –/– mice exhibit defective glycolytic signaling of pancreatic β cells, resulting in diminished insulin secretion in response to a glucose challenge (108–110). *Hnf1*α –/– mice died at the time of weaning from the severe wasting Fanconi syndrome (111), which is caused by renal proximal tubular dysfunction leading to massive uri-

nary loss of serum glucose and amino acids (Table 5.4). Hepatic expression of PAH is also completely extinguished in the *Hnf1*α –/– mice and resembles the human disease phenylketonuria (109,111). Interestingly, inactivation of the *Hnf1*α gene eliminated liver-specific DNase I hypersensitive sites within the PAH promoter region, suggesting that this transcription factor is involved in chromatin remodeling of the PAH regulatory locus (112). *Hnf1*α –/– mice also exhibited diminished hepatic expression of albumin, α₁-antitrypsin, and fibrinogen, and compensatory increase in vHNF-1 levels (109,111). In another knockout mouse study, the LoxP *Hnf1*α targeted locus was mated to an EIIa promoter driven Cre recombinase transgenic mouse to elicit an early embryonic removal of the selectable neomycin gene and first *Hnf1*α exon sequences. These *Hnf1*α –/– mice were viable and exhibited minimal renal dysfunction (109). It was noted that the *Hnf1*α –/– mice displayed non–insulin-dependent diabetes and diminished hepatic expression of IGF-I and IGF-II, leading to a significant reduction in postnatal growth (109). The HNF-1α protein is involved in transcriptional activation of genes critical for hepatocyte and pancreatic β-cell function but it was not required for specification of these cellular lineages.

Targeted Disruption of the Mouse *vHnf1* Gene Demonstrates Its Essential Role in Visceral Yolk Sac and Gut Endoderm Formation

Consistent with an earlier expression pattern of vHNF1 in the visceral endoderm, disruption of the *vHnf1* gene resulted in an embryonic lethal phenotype due to disorganization of the visceral yolk sac endoderm, which prevented gastrulation (113). Tetraploid rescue of the visceral endoderm defect in *vHnf1* –/– embryos restores gastrulation and allows mouse embryos to develop until day 10 of gestation, but gut formation is impaired and the mouse embryo does not turn. Use of *vHnf1* –/– ES cells to form embryoid bodies demonstrates that *vHnf1* is required for visceral endoderm expression of *Hnf1*α, *Hnf4*α, AFP, *ApoA1*, *Apo A4*, and *TTR* genes and displays reduced expression of the HNF-3 isoforms, transferrin, and GATA-4 transcription factor (113). Taken together these studies indicate that *vHnf1* is critical for specification of the visceral yolk sac and gut endoderm.

C/EBPα REGULATES HEPATIC GENES CRITICAL FOR METABOLIC HOMEOSTASIS

Cellular Expression Pattern of C/EBPα in Mouse Development and in Adult Organs

The CCAAT/enhancer-binding proteins (C/EBP) utilize a basic leucine zipper (bZIP) bipartite DNA-binding domain consisting of a dimerization interface composed of heptad repeated leucine residues termed the "leucine zipper" and a DNA-binding interface consisting of basic amino acids

(114). In mouse development, hepatic expression of C/EBPα is observed by day 13 and significant mRNA levels are also observed in the hippocampus, Purkinje cells of the cerebellum, and neurons of midbrain and forebrain (115). In adult mice, C/EBPα is expressed in differentiated hepatocytes, adipocytes, keratinocytes, and myeloid cells as well as epithelial cells of the lung, intestine, adrenal gland, pancreas, and placenta (Table 5.3). A similar expression pattern is observed with the C/EBPβ isoform, except that C/EBPβ's expression initiates later in hepatic development and its levels are also found in epithelial cells of the mammary gland, testes, ovaries, as well as neurons of the hippocampus (Table 5.3). Furthermore, in regenerating and acute-phase liver a transient decrease in C/EBPα levels is observed with compensatory increase in hepatic expression of the C/EBPβ and C/EBPδ isoforms (116–119).

Targeted Gene Disruption of Mouse C/EBPα Gene Displays Diminished Expression of Hepatic Genes Critical for Glucose Homeostasis

Because C/EBP was expressed in tissues involved in lipid and glucose homeostasis, McKnight and co-workers (120) proposed over 10 years ago that the C/EBPα transcription factor regulates expression of genes involved in energy metabolism. In support of this hypothesis, *C/EBPα −/−* mice die from hypoglycemia within 8 hours postpartum due to a complete absence of hepatic glycogen storage and a failure to store lipid in hepatocytes and adipocytes (121). The hepatic glycogen storage defect is due to diminished postnatal expression of glycogen synthase and gluconeogenic enzymes PEPCK and glucose-6-phosphatase. Consistent with the antiproliferative activity of C/EBPα protein, *C/EBPα*-deficient liver shows increased hepatocyte proliferation and disruption of the normal liver and lung architecture (117,119). Further characterization of this aberrant proliferation in *C/EBPα*-deficient hepatocytes demonstrated that C/EBPα stabilizes the cyclin kinase inhibitor p21 protein to inhibit hepatocyte replication (122). Furthermore, C/EBPα regulates activity of a hepatic protease that is involved in generating a transcriptional repressor LIP (liver-enriched transcriptional inhibitory protein), an amino-terminal truncation of the normal C/EBPβ protein (123). Moreover, use of adenovirus delivery of cre recombinase to inactivate adult hepatic expression of a loxP targeted *C/EBPα* gene locus identified other target genes that were not discovered in the straight knockout due to its early postnatal lethality (124). In addition to the glucose homeostatic genes, *C/EBPα*-deficient adult liver exhibited diminished expression of the bilirubin uridine diphosphate (UDP) glucuronosyltransferase gene causing an increase in serum levels of unconjugated bilirubin leading to severe jaundice (124). Furthermore, the *C/EBPα −/−* adult hepatocytes exhibited decreased hepatic expression of the blood clotting factor IX gene (124), which was also observed in the homozygous null *C/EBPα −/−* mice (125). These stud-

ies demonstrate that C/EBPα regulates expression of genes involved in hepatic glucose and bilirubin homeostasis as well as hepatic and adipocyte lipid storage. Other studies identified C/EBPα as an important mediator of neutrophil and eosinophil development (Table 5.4).

EVIDENCE FOR CROSS-REGULATION OF LIVER TRANSCRIPTION FACTOR EXPRESSION

Accumulating evidence suggests that maintenance of hepatocyte-enriched expression of transcription factors involves cross-regulation by one or more unrelated liver-enriched transcription factors (7,9,10,13,70,82,106,107,126–128). Characterization of the HNF-3β promoter region has allowed the identification of three distinct DNA-binding sites that are essential for HNF-3β promoter activity and that are bound by the HNF-6, FTF, and C/EBP protein families (7,9,10,13,127). Hepatoma cell transfection studies have demonstrated that HNF-6 and FTF proteins potentiate expression of the HNF-3β promoter and that their embryonic expression pattern is consistent with the maintenance of HNF-3β transcription in the developing liver primordium (7,9,13). It is interesting to note that FTF exhibits an embryonic expression pattern identical to that of HNF-6 in the liver and pancreas (13). Based on these experiments, we propose that collaboration among HNF-6, FTF, and C/EBPβ is involved in maintaining HNF-3β promoter expression in embryonic hepatocytes (Fig. 5.2). Additional transcriptional

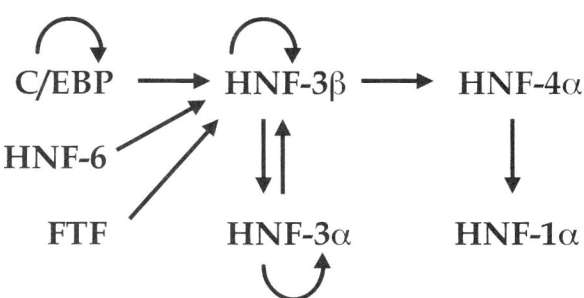

FIGURE 5.2. Cross-regulation of liver transcription factors. Schematically shown is the regulation of HNF-3β in which *arrows* indicate positive stimulation and *curved arrows* indicate autoregulation. This regulatory scheme is based on transfection data, *in vivo* expression patterns, and on knockout embryoid bodies and mice. We propose that maintenance of the HNF-3β promoter expression in embryonic and adult hepatocytes is due to collaboration among the cut-homeodomain HNF-6 protein (9,10), bZIP (C/EBPα and C/EBPβ) (127), and the orphan receptor family member FTF (12,13). Furthermore, the HNF-3β protein regulates its own expression (130) and cross-regulates the expression of other liver transcription factors including HNF-3α (70), HNF-1α (126), and HNF-4α (82). Hepatic expression of HNF-1α is cross-regulated by HNF-4α (107). Although the HNF-4α promoter contains HNF-1–binding sites (128), its expression was not affected in HNF-1α–deficient hepatocytes (109,111). Furthermore, normal hepatic expression of HNF-6 expression was observed in HNF-4α–deficient hepatocytes (107), even though an HNF-4–binding site was present in the HNF-6 promoter region (88).

activation of the HNF-3β promoter may involve the bZIP family members DBP and C/EBPα (127), whose hepatic expression is observed perinatally and at 13 days of gestation, respectively (115,129). Once HNF-3 is expressed, *in vitro* and *in vivo* studies suggest that an autoregulatory promoter site functions to further activate its own expression (Figs. 5.1 and 5.2) (77,130), which may also be cross-regulated by the other HNF-3 proteins (70). The HNF-3β promoter also contains functional binding sites for a widely expressed factor, UF1-H3β (130) and for the interferon regulatory factor-1 (IRF-1) protein (127). *In vitro* and *in vivo* studies demonstrated that the IRF-1 binding site in the HNF-3β promoter region mediated interferon-γ activation of HNF-3β expression (127,131).

OTHER TRANSCRIPTION FACTORS REQUIRED FOR LIVER FUNCTION AND DEVELOPMENT (SEE CHAPTER 1)

Tissue-Specific Transcription Factors Involved in Liver Development

In vivo footprinting studies by Zaret (40) have shown that GATA-4 and HNF3 binding sites in chromatin are occupied on the albumin enhancer region prior to hepatic specification, suggesting that the GATA-4 transcription factor may be involved in liver development. Consistent with this notion, in addition to the disruption of heart tube formation, GATA-4 deficient embryos exhibit severe defects in foregut morphogenesis, which gives rise to the presumptive liver (132,133).

Mesenchyme–epithelial interactions using paracrine and cell-cell contact play an important role in mediating organ morphogenesis. The homeodomain *Hlx* gene is expressed in the visceral mesenchyme of the developing liver, gallbladder, and intestine. Consistent with a role of Hlx in regulating genes mediating mesenchyme–epithelial morphogenic signaling, homozygous *Hlx* null mouse embryos die *in utero* and display severe inhibition in proliferative expansion during liver and intestine morphogenesis (134).

Proliferation-Specific Transcription Factors Involved in Liver Development

A number of proliferation-specific transcription factors and DNA repair enzymes play an important role in liver development. Mice deficient in *c-jun* display an embryonic lethal liver phenotype in which day 13 pc fetal livers exhibit extensive apoptosis of both hematopoietic cells and hepatoblasts (135). Liver degeneration and apoptosis were also observed in mouse embryos deficient in the *IκB* kinase-β gene, which encodes the kinase responsible for activation of NFκB through phosphorylation of IκB (136). Mouse embryo hepatocytes deficient in the XBP-1 transcription factor (bZIP family member) displayed significantly reduced growth rate and prominent apoptosis leading to an embryonic lethal phenotype (137). Targeted disruption of

the *heavy metal-responsive transcriptional activator (MTF-1)* gene, which encodes a transcription factor regulating basal and heavy metal-induced expression of metallothioneins leads to an embryonic lethal phenotype displaying impaired development of hepatocytes (138). Mouse hepatocytes that are disrupted in the *excision repair cross-complementing (ERCC)-1* gene are prematurely polyploid, and ultimately these knockout mice die perinatally from liver failure (139). Clevers and colleagues have shown aberrant embryonic polyploid phenotypes in cardiomyocytes and hepatocytes of mouse embryos deficient in the proliferation-specific winged helix transcription factor, HFH-11/Trident (140,141), and the mice die immediately after birth (142). These results indicate that loss of HFH-11/Trident function causes the uncoupling of DNA synthesis from mitosis and suggest that HFH-11/Trident may regulate genes involved in cell cycle checkpoint control. The fact that premature expression of HFH-11/Trident in regenerating liver accelerates the timing of both hepatocyte DNA replication and mitosis further supports its role in cell-cycle regulation (143).

Steroid Hormone Receptors Regulates Transcription of Cholesterol 7α-Hydroxylase Gene in Response to Cholesterol Metabolites (See Chapter 16)

The liver plays a central role in cholesterol synthesis via transcriptional regulation of key cholesterol biosynthetic genes by the sterol regulatory element binding proteins (SREBPs), which are membrane-bound transcription factors that are activated by proteolysis in response to diminished membrane cholesterol content (144). Hepatocytes also metabolize cholesterol into bile acids, which are released into the digestive tract for digestion of lipids and as the major pathway for eliminating cholesterol from the body (145). Cholesterol 7α-hydroxylase (Cyp7A) is the rate-limiting enzyme involved in hepatocyte-specific synthesis of bile acids from cholesterol, and its transcription is stimulated by cholesterol metabolites and repressed by bile acids (145). Recent studies demonstrated that the steroid hormone family members, liver X receptors (LXRs), are activated by oxysteroid ligands (oxidized derivatives of cholesterol) and that LXR transcriptionally activates Cyp7A promoter expression (146). Consistent with a critical role in cholesterol metabolism, LXR-deficient mice are unable to induce transcription of the Cyp7A gene in response to dietary cholesterol. The *LXR −/−* mice accumulate excessive amounts of cholesterol in the liver and develop impaired hepatic function (147). Conversely, bile acids function as endogenous ligands for the farnesoid X-receptor (FXR), which binds to the Cyp7A regulatory region and mediates its transcriptional repression in response to increased hepatic bile acid levels (148,149). Bile acid transcriptional control of the Cyp7A gene by FXR thereby mediates regulation of de novo hepatocyte synthesis of bile acid. These studies demonstrate that the steroid hormone receptors regulate transcription of the Cyp7A gene, which encodes the major enzyme involved in synthesis of bile acid from cholesterol, through ligand binding of metabolites of the cholesterol-bile acid metabolic pathway.

ACKNOWLEDGMENTS

Due to space limitations, we were unable to discuss mechanisms of transcriptional activation and coactivator recruitment by liver transcription factors. We also omitted reference to excellent studies on numerous liver promoter and enhancer regions, which form the basis for our understanding of liver gene regulation. We thank Pradip Raychaudhuri for critically reading this chapter and for many helpful discussions. This work was supported by Public Health Service grants R01 GM43241-11 and R01 DK54687-02 (R.H.C.) from the National Institute of General Medical Sciences and National Institute of Diabetes and Digestive and Kidney Diseases.

REFERENCES

1. Jungermann K, Katz N. Functional specialization of different hepatocyte populations. *Physiol Rev* 1989;69:708–764.
2. Cereghini S. Liver-enriched transcription factors and hepatocyte differentiation. *FASEB J* 1996;10:267–282.
3. Costa RH. Hepatocyte nuclear factor 3/fork head protein family: mammalian transcription factors that possess divergent cellular expression patterns and binding specificities. In: Tronche F, Yaniv M, eds. *Liver gene transcription.* Austin, TX: R. G. Landes, 1994:183–206.
4. Lai E, Prezioso VR, Smith E, et al. HNF-3A, a hepatocyte-enriched transcription factor of novel structure is regulated transcriptionally. *Genes Dev* 1990;4:1427–1436.
5. Lai E, Prezioso VR, Tao WF, et al. Hepatocyte nuclear factor 3α belongs to a gene family in mammals that is homologous to the Drosophila homeotic gene fork head. *Genes Dev* 1991;5: 416–427.
6. Jacquemin P, Lannoy VJ, Rousseau GG, et al. OC-2, a novel mammalian member of the ONECUT class of homeodomain transcription factors whose function in liver partially overlaps with that of hepatocyte nuclear factor-6. *J Biol Chem* 1999;274: 2665–2671.
7. Landry C, Clotman F, Hioki T, et al. HNF-6 is expressed in endoderm derivatives and nervous system of the mouse embryo and participates to the cross-regulatory network of liver-enriched transcription factors. *Dev Biol* 1997;192:247–257.
8. Lemaigre FP, Durviaux SM, Truong O. Hepatocyte nuclear factor 6, a transcription factor that contains a novel type of homeodomain and a single cut domain. *Proc Natl Acad Sci USA* 1996;93:9460–9464.
9. Rausa F, Samadani U, Ye H, et al. The cut-homeodomain transcriptional activator HNF-6 is coexpressed with its target gene HNF-3β in the developing murine liver and pancreas. *Dev Biol* 1997;192:228–246.
10. Samadani U, Costa RH. The transcriptional activator hepatocyte nuclear factor six regulates liver gene expression. *Mol Cell Biol* 1996;16:6273–6284.
11. Sladek FM, Zhong WM, Lai E, et al. Liver-enriched transcription factor HNF-4 is a novel member of the steroid hormone receptor superfamily. *Genes Dev* 1990;4:2353–2365.
12. Galarneau L, Pare JF, Allard D, et al. The α1-fetoprotein locus is activated by a nuclear receptor of the Drosophila FTZ-F1 family. *Mol Cell Biol* 1996;16:3853–3865.
13. Rausa FM, Galarneau L, Belanger L, et al. The nuclear receptor fetoprotein transcription factor is coexpressed with its target gene HNF-3beta in the developing murine liver intestine and pancreas. *Mech Dev* 1999;89:185–188.
14. Baumhueter S, Mendel DB, Conley PB, et al. HNF-1 shares three sequence motifs with the POU domain proteins and is identical to LF-B1 and APF. *Genes Dev* 1990;4:372–379.
15. Frain M, Swart G, Monaci P, et al. The liver-specific transcription factor LF-B1 contains a highly diverged homeobox DNA binding domain. *Cell* 1989;59:145–157.
16. Ott MO, Rey-Campos J, Cereghini S, et al. vHNF1 is expressed in epithelial cells of distinct embryonic origin during development and precedes HNF1 expression. *Mech Dev* 1991; 36:47–58.
17. Apergis GA, Crawford N, Ghosh D, et al. A novel nk-2–related transcription factor associated with human fetal liver and hepatocellular carcinoma. *J Biol Chem* 1998;273:2917–2925.
18. Landschulz WH, Johnson PF, Adashi EY, et al. Isolation of a recombinant copy of the gene encoding C/EBP. *Genes Dev* 1988;2:786–800.
19. Descombes P, Chojkier M, Lichtsteiner S, et al. LAP, a novel member of the C/EBP gene family, encodes a liver-enriched transcriptional activator protein. *Genes Dev* 1990;4:1541–1551.
20. Mueller CR, Maire P, Schibler U. DBP, a liver-enriched transcriptional activator, is expressed late in ontogeny and its tissue specificity is determined posttranscriptionally. *Cell* 1990;61: 279–291.
21. Haas NB, Cantwell CA, Johnson PF, et al. DNA-binding specificity of the PAR basic leucine zipper protein VBP partially overlaps those of the C/EBP and CREB/ATF families and is influenced by domains that flank the core basic region. *Mol Cell Biol* 1995;15:1923–1932.
22. Iyer SV, Davis DL, Seal SN, et al. Chicken vitellogenin gene-binding protein, a leucine zipper transcription factor that binds to an important control element in the chicken vitellogenin II promoter, is related to rat DBP. *Mol Cell Biol* 1991;11:4863–4875.
23. Dickson PW, Howlett GJ, Schreiber G. Rat transthyretin (prealbumin). Molecular cloning, nucleotide sequence, and gene expression in liver and brain. *J Biol Chem* 1985;260: 8214–8219.
24. Costa RH, Lai E, Grayson DR, et al. The cell-specific enhancer of the mouse transthyretin (prealbumin) gene binds a common factor at one site and a liver-specific factor(s) at two other sites. *Mol Cell Biol* 1988;8:81–90.
25. Costa RH, Grayson DR, Darnell JE Jr. Multiple hepatocyte-enriched nuclear factors function in the regulation of transthyretin and α1-antitrypsin genes. *Mol Cell Biol* 1989;9: 1415–1425.
26. Costa RH, Grayson DR. Site-directed mutagenesis of hepatocyte nuclear factor (HNF) binding sites in the mouse transthyretin (TTR) promoter reveal synergistic interactions with its enhancer region. *Nucleic Acids Res* 1991;19:4139–4145.
27. Costa RH, Van Dyke TA, Yan C, et al. Similarities in transthyretin gene expression and differences in transcription factors: liver and yolk sac compared to choroid plexus. *Proc Natl Acad Sci USA* 1990;87:6589–6593.
28. Yan C, Costa RH, Darnell JE Jr, et al. Distinct positive and negative elements control the limited hepatocyte and choroid plexus expression of transthyretin in transgenic mice. *EMBO J* 1990;9:869–878.

29. Costa RH, Grayson DR, Xanthopoulos KG, et al. A liver-specific DNA-binding protein recognizes multiple nucleotide sites in regulatory regions of transthyretin, α1-antitrypsin, albumin, and simian virus 40 genes. *Proc Natl Acad Sci USA* 1988;85:3840–3844.

30. Qian X, Samadani U, Porcella A, et al. Decreased expression of hepatocyte nuclear factor 3α during the acute-phase response influences transthyretin gene transcription. *Mol Cell Biol* 1995;15:1364–1376.

31. Samadani U, Qian X, Costa RH. Identification of a transthyretin enhancer sequence that selectively binds the hepatocyte nuclear factor-3β isoform. *Gene Expression* 1996;6:23–33.

32. Kaufmann E, Knochel W. Five years on the wings of fork head. *Mech Dev* 1996;57:3–20.

33. Clark KL, Halay ED, Lai E, et al. Co-crystal structure of the HNF-3/fork head DNA-recognition motif resembles histone H5. *Nature* 1993;364:412–420.

34. Marsden I, Jin C, Liao X. Structural changes in the region directly adjacent to the DNA-binding helix highlight a possible mechanism to explain the observed changes in the sequence-specific binding of winged helix proteins. *J Mol Biol* 1998;278:293–299.

35. Jin C, Marsden I, Chen X, et al. Dynamic DNA contacts observed in the NMR structure of winged helix protein-DNA complex. *J Mol Biol* 1999;289:683–690.

36. Qian X, Costa RH. Analysis of HNF-3β protein domains required for transcriptional activation and nuclear targeting. *Nucleic Acids Res* 1995;23:1184–1191.

37. Biggs WH 3rd, Meisenhelder J, Hunter T, et al. Protein kinase B/Akt-mediated phosphorylation promotes nuclear exclusion of the winged helix transcription factor FKHR1. *Proc Natl Acad Sci USA* 1999;96:7421–7426.

38. Hellqvist M, Mahlapuu M, Blixt A, et al. The human forkhead protein FREAC-2 contains two functionally redundant activation domains and interacts with TBP and TFIIB. *J Biol Chem* 1998;273:23335–23343.

39. Pani L, Overdier DG, Porcella A, et al. Hepatocyte nuclear factor 3β contains two transcriptional activation domains, one of which is novel and conserved with the Drosophila fork head protein. *Mol Cell Biol* 1992;12:3723–3732.

40. Zaret K. Developmental competence of the gut endoderm: genetic potentiation by GATA and HNF3/fork head proteins. *Dev Biol* 1999;209:1–10.

41. McPherson CE, Shim EY, Friedman DS, et al. An active tissue-specific enhancer and bound transcription factors existing in a precisely positioned nucleosomal array. *Cell* 1993;75:387–398.

42. Shim EY, Woodcock C, Zaret KS. Nucleosome positioning by the winged helix transcription factor HNF3. *Genes Dev* 1998;12:5–10.

43. Cirillo LA, McPherson CE, Bossard P, et al. Binding of the winged-helix transcription factor HNF3 to a linker histone site on the nucleosome. *EMBO J* 1998;17:244–254.

44. Cirillo LA, Zaret KS. An early developmental transcription factor complex that is more stable on nucleosome core particles than on free DNA. *Mol Cell* 1999;4:961–969.

45. Crowe AJ, Sang L, Li KK, et al. Hepatocyte nuclear factor 3 relieves chromatin-mediated repression of the α-fetoprotein gene. *J Biol Chem* 1999;274:25113–25120.

46. Auge-Gouillou C, Petropoulos I, Zakin MM. Liver-enriched HNF-3α and ubiquitous factors interact with the human transferrin gene enhancer. *FEBS Lett* 1993;323:4–10.

47. Harnish DC, Malik S, Kilbourne E, et al. Control of apolipoprotein AI gene expression through synergistic interactions between hepatocyte nuclear factors 3 and 4. *J Biol Chem* 1996;271:13621–13628.

48. Lee KC, Crowe AJ, Barton MC. p53-Mediated Repression of α-fetoprotein gene expression by specific DNA binding. *Mol Cell Biol* 1999;19:1279–1288.

49. Liu JK, DiPersio CM, Zaret KS. Extracellular signals that regulate liver transcription factors during hepatic differentiation in vitro. *Mol Cell Biol* 1991;11:773–784.

50. Millonig JH, Emerson JA, Levorse JM, et al. Molecular analysis of the distal enhancer of the mouse α-fetoprotein gene. *Mol Cell Biol* 1995;15:3848–3856.

51. Cooper AD, Chen J, Botelho-Yetkinler MJ, et al. Characterization of hepatic-specific regulatory elements in the promoter region of the human cholesterol 7alpha-hydroxylase gene. *J Biol Chem* 1997;272:3444–3452.

52. Molowa DT, Chen WS, Cimis GM, et al. Transcriptional regulation of the human cholesterol 7α-hydroxylase gene. *Biochemistry* 1992;31:2539–2544.

53. Wang DP, Stroup D, Marrapodi M, et al. Transcriptional regulation of the human cholesterol 7α-hydroxylase gene (CYP7A) in HepG2 cells. *J Lipid Res* 1996;37:1831–1841.

54. Lemaigre FP, Durviaux SM, Rousseau GG. Liver-specific factor binding to the liver promoter of a 6-phosphofructo-2-kinase/fructose-2,6-bisphosphatase gene. *J Biol Chem* 1993;268:19896–19905.

55. Lin B, Morris DW, Chou JY. The role of HNF1alpha, HNF3gamma, and cyclic AMP in glucose-6-phosphatase gene activation. *Biochemistry* 1997;36:14096–14106.

56. Raymondjean M, Pichard AL, Gregori C, et al. Interplay of an original combination of factors: C/EBP, NFY, HNF-3 and HNF-1 in the rat adolase B gene promoter. *Nucleic Acids Res* 1991;19:6145–6153.

57. Cui Y, Narayanan CS, Zhou J, et al. Exon-I is involved in positive as well as negative regulation of human angiotensinogen gene expression. *Gene* 1998;224:97–107.

58. Spek CA, Greengard JS, Griffin JH, et al. Two mutations in the promoter region of the human protein C gene both cause type I protein C deficiency by disruption of two HNF-3 binding sites. *J Biol Chem* 1995;270:24216–24221.

59. Tsay W, Lee YM, Lee SC, et al. Synergistic transactivation of HNF-1alpha, HNF-3, and NF-I contributes to the activation of the liver-specific protein C gene. *DNA Cell Biol* 1997;16:569–577.

60. Shaw PM, Weiss MC, Adesnik M. Hepatocyte nuclear factor 3 is a major determinant of CYP2C6 promoter activity in hepatoma cells. *Mol Pharmacol* 1994;46:79–87.

61. Beurton F, Bandyopadhyay U, Dieumegard B, et al. Delineation of the insulin-responsive sequence in the rat cytosolic aspartate aminotransferase gene: binding sites for hepatocyte nuclear factor-3 and nuclear factor I. *Biochem J* 1999;343:687–695.

62. O'Brien RM, Noisin EL, Suwanichkul A, et al. Hepatic nuclear factor 3– and hormone-regulated expression of the phosphoenolpyruvate carboxykinase and insulin-like growth factor-binding protein 1 genes. *Mol Cell Biol* 1995;15:1747–1758.

63. Unterman TG, Fareeduddin A, Harris MA, et al. Hepatocyte nuclear factor-3 (HNF-3) binds to the insulin response sequence in the IGF binding protein-1 (IGFBP-1) promoter and enhances promoter function. *Biochem Biophys Res Commun* 1994;203:1835–1841.

64. Nolten LA, Steenbergh PH, Sussenbach JS. The hepatocyte nuclear factor 3 stimulates the transcription of the human insulin-like growth factor I gene in a direct and indirect manner. *J Biol Chem* 1996;271:31846–31854.

65. Vallet V, Antoine B, Chafey P, et al. Overproduction of a truncated hepatocyte nuclear factor 3 protein inhibits expression of liver-specific genes in hepatoma cells. *Mol Cell Biol* 1995;15:5453–5460.

66. Ang SL, Wierda A, Wong D, et al. The formation and maintenance of the definitive endoderm lineage in the mouse: involvement of HNF3/forkhead proteins. *Development* 1993;119: 1301–1315.

67. Monaghan AP, Kaestner KH, Grau E, et al. Postimplantation expression patterns indicate a role for the mouse forkhead/ HNF-3α, β, and γ genes in determination of the definitive endoderm, chordamesoderm and neuroectoderm. *Development* 1993;119:567–578.

68. Ruiz i Altaba A, Prezioso VR, Darnell JE, et al. Sequential expression of HNF-3β and HNF-3α by embryonic organizing centers: the dorsal lip/node, notochord and floor plate. *Mech Dev* 1993;44:91–108.

69. Sasaki H, Hogan BL. Differential expression of multiple fork head related genes during gastrulation and axial pattern formation in the mouse embryo. *Development* 1993;118:47–59.

70. Peterson RS, Clevidence DE, Ye H, et al. Hepatocyte nuclear factor-3α promoter regulation involves recognition by cell-specific factors, thyroid transcription factor-1 and autoactivation. *Cell Growth Differ* 1997;8:69–82.

71. Kopachik W, Hayward SW, Cunha GR. Expression of hepatocyte nuclear factor-3α in rat prostate, seminal vesicle, and bladder. *Dev Dyn* 1998;211:131–140.

72. Jacob A, Budhiraja S, Qian X, et al. Retinoic acid-mediated activation of HNF-3α during EC stem cell differentiation. *Nucleic Acids Res* 1994;22:2126–2133.

73. Reichel RR, Budhiraja S, Jacob A. Delayed activation of HNF-3 b upon retinoic acid-induced teratocarcinoma cell differentiation. *Exp Cell Res* 1994;214:634–641.

74. Kaestner KH, Hiemisch H, Luckow B, et al. The HNF-3 gene family of transcription factors in mice: gene structure, cDNA sequence, and mRNA distribution. *Genomics* 1994;20: 377–385.

75. Chang BE, Blader P, Fischer N, et al. Axial (HNF3beta) and retinoic acid receptors are regulators of the zebrafish sonic hedgehog promoter. *EMBO J* 1997;16:3955–3964.

76. Epstein DJ, McMahon AP, Joyner AL. Regionalization of Sonic hedgehog transcription along the anteroposterior axis of the mouse central nervous system is regulated by Hnf3–dependent and -independent mechanisms. *Development* 1998;126: 281–292.

77. Sasaki H, Hogan BL. HNF-3β as a regulator of floor plate development. *Cell* 1994;76:103–115.

78. Ang SL, Rossant J. HNF-3β is essential for node and notochord formation in mouse development. *Cell* 1994;78:561–574.

79. Weinstein DC, Ruiz i Altaba A, Chen WS, et al. The winged-helix transcription factor HNF-3β is required for notochord development in the mouse embryo. *Cell* 1994;78:575–588.

80. Dufort D, Schwartz L, Harpal K, et al. The transcription factor HNF3 is required in visceral endoderm for normal primitive streak morphogenesis. *Development* 1998;125:3015–3025.

81. Rausa FM, Tan Y, Zhou H, et al. Elevated levels of HNF-3β in mouse hepatocytes influence expression of genes involved in bile acid and glucose homeostasis. *Mol Cell Biol* 2000;20: 8264–8282.

82. Duncan SA, Navas MA, Dufort D, et al. Regulation of a transcription factor network required for differentiation and metabolism. *Science* 1998;281:692–695.

83. Kaestner KH, Katz J, Liu Y, et al. Inactivation of the winged helix transcription factor HNF3α affects glucose homeostasis and islet glucagon gene expression in vivo. *Genes Dev* 1999;13: 495–504.

84. Shih DQ, Navas MA, Kuwajima S, et al. Impaired glucose homeostasis and neonatal mortality in hepatocyte nuclear factor 3α-deficient mice. *Proc Natl Acad Sci USA* 1999;96: 10152–10157.

85. Kaestner KH, Hiemisch H, Schutz G. Targeted disruption of the gene encoding hepatocyte nuclear factor 3γ results in reduced transcription of hepatocyte-specific genes. *Mol Cell Biol* 1998;18:4245–4251.

86. Pierreux CE, Stafford J, Demonte D, et al. Antiglucocorticoid activity of hepatocyte nuclear factor-6. *Proc Natl Acad Sci USA* 1999;96:8961–8966.

87. Lahuna O, Fernandez L, Karlsson H, et al. Expression of hepatocyte nuclear factor 6 in rat liver is sex-dependent and regulated by growth hormone. *Proc Natl Acad Sci USA* 1997;94: 12309–12313.

88. Lahuna O, Rastegar M, Maiter D, et al. Involvement of STAT5 (signal transducer and activator of transcription 5) and HNF-4 (hepatocyte nuclear factor 4) in the transcriptional control of the hnf6 gene by growth hormone. *Mol Endocrinol* 2000;14: 285–294.

89. Gannon M, Ray MK, Zee KV, et al. Persistent expression of HNF-6 in islet endocrine cells causes disrupted islet architecture and loss of β-cell function. *Development* 2000;127: 2883–2895.

90. Jacquemin P, Durviaux SM, Jensen JN, et al. Transcription factor hepatocyte nuclear factor 6 regulates pancreatic endocrine cell differentiation and controls expression of the proendocrine gene ngn3. *Mol Cell Biol* 2000;20:4445–4454.

91. Sourdive DJ, Transy C, Garbay S, et al. The bifunctional DCOH protein binds to HNF1 independently of its 4-α-carbinolamine dehydratase activity. *Nucleic Acids Res* 1997;25: 1476–1484.

92. Jiang G, Nepomuceno L, Hopkins K, et al. Exclusive homodimerization of the orphan receptor hepatocyte nuclear factor 4 defines a new subclass of nuclear receptors. *Mol Cell Biol* 1995; 15:5131–5143.

93. Jiang G, Lee U, Sladek FM. Proposed mechanism for the stabilization of nuclear receptor DNA binding via protein dimerization. *Mol Cell Biol* 1997;17:6546–6554.

94. Jiang G, Sladek FM. The DNA binding domain of hepatocyte nuclear factor 4 mediates cooperative, specific binding to DNA and heterodimerization with the retinoid X receptor α. *J Biol Chem* 1997;272:1218–1225.

95. Hertz R, Magenheim J, Berman I, et al. Fatty acyl-CoA thioesters are ligands of hepatic nuclear factor-4α. *Nature* 1998; 392:512–516.

96. Jiang G, Nepomuceno L, Yang Q, et al. Serine/threonine phosphorylation of orphan receptor hepatocyte nuclear factor 4. *Arch Biochem Biophys* 1997;340:1–9.

97. Ktistaki E, Ktistakis NT, Papadogeorgaki E, et al. Recruitment of hepatocyte nuclear factor 4 into specific intranuclear compartments depends on tyrosine phosphorylation that affects its DNA- binding and transactivation potential. *Proc Natl Acad Sci USA* 1995;92:9876–9880.

98. Sladek FM. Orphan receptor HNF-4 and liver-specific gene expression. *Receptor* 1994;4:64.

99. Tronche F, Ringeisen F, Blumenfeld M, et al. Analysis of the distribution of binding sites for a tissue-specific transcription factor in the vertebrate genome. *J Mol Biol* 1997;266:231–245.

100. Sladek FM, Dallas-Yang Q, Nepomuceno L. MODY1 mutation Q268X in hepatocyte nuclear factor 4α allows for dimerization in solution but causes abnormal subcellular localization. *Diabetes* 1998;47:985–990.

101. Stoffel M, Duncan SA. The maturity-onset diabetes of the young (MODY1) transcription factor HNF4α regulates expression of genes required for glucose transport and metabolism. *Proc Natl Acad Sci USA* 1997;94:13209–13214.

102. Yamagata K, Furuta H, Oda N, et al. Mutations in the hepatocyte nuclear factor 4α gene in maturity onset diabetes of the young (MODY1). *Nature* 1996;384:458–460.

103. Yamagata K, Oda N, Kaisaki PJ, et al. Mutations in the hepatocyte nuclear factor-1α gene in maturity onset diabetes of the young (MODY3). *Nature* 1996;384:455–458.

104. Duncan SA, Manova K, Chen WS, et al. Expression of transcription factor HNF-4 in the extraembryonic endoderm, gut, and nephrogenic tissue of the developing mouse embryo: HNF-4 is a marker for primary endoderm in the implanting blastocyst. *Proc Natl Acad Sci USA* 1994;91:7598–7602.

105. Chen WS, Manova K, Weinstein DC, et al. Disruption of the HNF-4 gene, expressed in visceral endoderm, leads to cell death in embryonic ectoderm and impaired gastrulation of mouse embryos. *Genes Dev* 1994;8:2466–2477.

106. Duncan SA, Nagy A, Chan W. Murine gastrulation requires HNF-4 regulated gene expression in the visceral endoderm: tetraploid rescue of Hnf-4(−/−) embryos. *Development* 1997;124:279–287.

107. Li J, Ning G, Duncan SA. Mammalian hepatocyte differentiation requires the transcription factor HNF-4α. *Genes Dev* 2000;14:464–474.

108. Dukes ID, Sreenan S, Roe MW, et al. Defective pancreatic β-cell glycolytic signaling in hepatocyte nuclear factor-1α-deficient mice. *J Biol Chem* 1998;273:24457–24464.

109. Lee YH, Sauer B, Gonzalez FJ. Laron dwarfism and non-insulin-dependent diabetes mellitus in the *Hnf-1α* knockout mouse. *Mol Cell Biol* 1998;18:3059–3068.

110. Pontoglio M, Sreenan S, Roe M, et al. Defective insulin secretion in hepatocyte nuclear factor 1 Hnf-1α-deficient mice. *J Clin Invest* 1998;101:2215–2222.

111. Pontoglio M, Barra J, Hadchouel M, et al. Hepatocyte nuclear factor 1 inactivation results in hepatic dysfunction, phenylketonuria, and renal Fanconi syndrome. *Cell* 1996;84:575–585.

112. Pontoglio M, Faust DM, Doyen A, et al. Hepatocyte nuclear factor 1 gene inactivation impairs chromatin remodeling and demethylation of the phenylalanine hydroxylase gene. *Mol Cell Biol* 1997;17:4948–4956.

113. Coffinier C, Thepot D, Babinet C, et al. Essential role for the homeoprotein vHNF1/HNF1beta in visceral endoderm differentiation. *Development* 1999;126:4785–4794.

114. Vinson CR, Sigler PB, McKnight SL. Scissors-grip model for DNA recognition by a family of leucine zipper proteins. *Science* 1989;246:911–916.

115. Kuo CF, Xanthopoulos KG, Darnell JE Jr. Fetal and adult localization of C/EBP: evidence for combinatorial action of transcription factors in cell-specific gene expression. *Development* 1990;109:473–481.

116. Diehl AM. Roles of CCAAT/enhancer-binding proteins in regulation of liver regenerative growth. *J Biol Chem* 1998;273:30843–30846.

117. Flodby P, Barlow C, Kylefjord H, et al. Increased hepatic cell proliferation and lung abnormalities in mice deficient in CCAAT/enhancer binding protein α. *J Biol Chem* 1996;271:24753–24760.

118. Poli V. The role of C/EBP isoforms in the control of inflammatory and native immunity functions. *J Biol Chem* 1998;273:29279–29282.

119. Soriano HE, Kang DC, Finegold MJ, et al. Lack of C/EBP α gene expression results in increased DNA synthesis and an increased frequency of immortalization of freshly isolated mice hepatocytes. *Hepatology* 1998;27:392–401.

120. McKnight SL, Lane MD, Gluecksohn-Waelsch S. Is CCAAT/enhancer-binding protein a central regulator of energy metabolism? *Genes Dev* 1989;3:2021–2024.

121. Wang ND, Finegold MJ, Bradley A, et al. Impaired energy homeostasis in C/EBPα knockout mice. *Science* 1995;269:1108–1112.

122. Timchenko NA, Harris TE, Wilde M, et al. CCAAT/enhancer binding protein α regulates p21 protein and hepatocyte proliferation in newborn mice. *Mol Cell Biol* 1997;17:7353–7361.

123. Welm AL, Timchenko NA, Darlington GJ. C/EBPα regulates generation of C/EBPβ isoforms through activation of specific proteolytic cleavage. *Mol Cell Biol* 1999;19:1695–1704.

124. Lee YH, Sauer B, Johnson PF, et al. Disruption of the *c/ebpα* gene in adult mouse liver. *Mol Cell Biol* 1997;17:6014–6022.

125. Davies N, Austen DE, Wilde MD, et al. Clotting factor IX levels in C/EBP α knockout mice. *Br J Haematol* 1997;99:578–579.

126. Kuo CJ, Conley PB, Chen L, et al. A transcriptional hierarchy involved in mammalian cell-type specification. *Nature* 1992;355:457–461.

127. Samadani U, Porcella A, Pani L, et al. Cytokine regulation of the liver transcription factor HNF-3β is mediated by the C/EBP family and interferon regulatory factor 1. *Cell Growth Differ* 1995;6:879–890.

128. Zhong W, Mirkovitch J, Darnell JE Jr. Tissue-specific regulation of mouse hepatocyte nuclear factor 4 expression. *Mol Cell Biol* 1994;14:7276–7284.

129. Nagy P, Bisgaard HC, Thorgeirsson SS. Expression of hepatic transcription factors during liver development and oval cell differentiation. *J Cell Biol* 1994;126:223–233.

130. Pani L, Qian XB, Clevidence D, et al. The restricted promoter activity of the liver transcription factor hepatocyte nuclear factor 3β involves a cell-specific factor and positive autoactivation. *Mol Cell Biol* 1992;12:552–562.

131. Magdaleno SM, Wang G, Jackson KJ, et al. Interferon-γ regulation of Clara cell gene expression: in vivo and in vitro. *Am J Physiol* 1997;272:L1142–L1151.

132. Kuo CT, Morrisey EE, Anandappa R, et al. GATA4 transcription factor is required for ventral morphogenesis and heart tube formation. *Genes Dev* 1997;11:1048–1060.

133. Molkentin JD, Lin Q, Duncan SA, et al. Requirement of the transcription factor GATA4 for heart tube formation and ventral morphogenesis. *Genes Dev* 1997;11:1061–1072.

134. Hentsch B, Lyons I, Li R, et al. Hlx homeobox gene is essential for an inductive tissue interaction that drives expansion of embryonic liver and gut. *Genes Dev* 1996;10:70–79.

135. Eferl R, Sibilia M, Hilberg F, et al. Functions of c-Jun in liver and heart development. *J Cell Biol* 1999;145:1049–1061.

136. Tanaka M, Fuentes ME, Yamaguchi K, et al. Embryonic lethality, liver degeneration, and impaired NF-κB activation in IKK-β-deficient mice. *Immunity* 1999;10:421–429.

137. Reimold AM, Etkin A, Clauss I, et al. An essential role in liver development for transcription factor XBP-1. *Genes Dev* 2000;14:152–157.

138. Gunes C, Heuchel R, Georgiev O, et al. Embryonic lethality and liver degeneration in mice lacking the metal-responsive transcriptional activator MTF-1. *EMBO J* 1998;17:2846–2854.

139. McWhir J, Selfridge J, Harrison DJ, et al. Mice with DNA repair gene (ERCC-1) deficiency have elevated levels of p53, liver nuclear abnormalities and die before weaning. *Nat Genet* 1993;5:217–224.

140. Korver W, Roose J, Clevers H. The winged-helix transcription factor Trident is expressed in cycling cells. *Nucleic Acids Res* 1979;25:1715–1719.

141. Ye H, Kelly TF, Samadani U, et al. Hepatocyte nuclear factor 3/fork head homolog 11 is expressed in proliferating epithelial and mesenchymal cells of embryonic and adult tissues. *Mol Cell Biol* 1997;17:1626–1641.

142. Korver W, Schilham MW, Moerer P, et al. Uncoupling of S phase and mitosis in cardiomyocytes and hepatocytes lacking the winged-helix transcription factor trident. *Curr Biol* 1998;8:1327–1330.

143. Ye H, Holterman A, Yoo KW, et al. Premature expression of the winged helix transcription factor HFH-11B in regenerating mouse liver accelerates hepatocyte entry into S-phase. *Mol Cell Biol* 1999;19:8570–8580.

144. Brown MS, Goldstein JL. The SREBP pathway: regulation of cholesterol metabolism by proteolysis of a membrane-bound transcription factor. *Cell* 1997;89:331–340.

145. Chiang JYL. Regulation of bile acid synthesis. *Front Biosci* 1998;3:D176–D193.

146. Lehmann JM, Kliewer SA, Moore LB, et al. Activation of the nuclear receptor LXR by oxysterols defines a new hormone response pathway. *J Biol Chem* 1997;272:3137–3140.

147. Peet DJ, Turley SD, Ma W, et al. Cholesterol and bile acid metabolism are impaired in mice lacking the nuclear oxysterol receptor LXRα. *Cell* 1998;93:693–704.

148. Makishima M, Okamoto AY, Repa JJ, et al. Identification of a nuclear receptor for bile acids. *Science* 1999;284:1362–1365.

149. Koopen NR, Wolters H, Voshol P, et al. Decreased Na+-dependent taurocholate uptake and low expression of the sinusoidal Na+-taurocholate cotransporting protein (Ntcp) in livers of mdr2 P-glycoprotein-deficient mice. *J Hepatol* 1999;30:14–21.

150. Overdier DG, Porcella A, Costa RH. The DNA-binding specificity of the hepatocyte nuclear factor 3/forkhead domain is influenced by amino-acid residues adjacent to the recognition helix. *Mol Cell Biol* 1994;14:2755–2766.

151. Zhou L, Lim L, Costa RH, et al. Thyroid transcription factor-1, hepatocyte nuclear factor-3β, surfactant protein B, C, and Clara cell secretory protein in developing mouse lung. *J Histochem Cytochem* 1996;44:1183–1193.

152. Taraviras S, Monaghan AP, Schutz G, et al. Characterization of the mouse HNF-4 gene and its expression during mouse embryogenesis. *Mech Dev* 1994;48:67–79.

153. Antonson P, Xanthopoulos KG. Molecular cloning, sequence, and expression patterns of the human gene encoding CCAAT/enhancer binding protein α (C/EBPα). *Biochem Biophys Res Commun* 1995;215:106–113.

154. Birkenmeier EH, Gwynn B, Howard S, et al. Tissue-specific expression, developmental regulation, and genetic mapping of the gene encoding CCAAT/enhancer binding protein. *Genes Dev* 1989;3:1146–1156.

155. Bossard P, McPherson CE, Zaret KS. In vivo footprinting with limiting amounts of embryo tissues: a role for C/EBPβ in early hepatic development. *Methods* 1997;11:180–188.

156. Cao Z, Umek RM, McKnight SL. Regulated expression of three C/EBP isoforms during adipose conversion of 3T3-L1 cells. *Genes Dev* 1991;5:1538–1552.

157. Darlington GJ, Ross SE, MacDougald OA. The role of C/EBP genes in adipocyte differentiation. *J Biol Chem* 1998;273: 30057–30060.

158. Lenny N, Westendorf JJ, Hiebert SW. Transcriptional regulation during myelopoiesis. *Mol Biol Rep* 1997;24:157–168.

159. Landschulz WH, Johnson PF, McKnight SL. The DNA binding domain of the rat liver nuclear protein C/EBP is bipartite. *Science* 1989;243:1681–1688.

160. Lekstrom-Himes J, Xanthopoulos KG. Biological role of the CCAAT/enhancer-binding protein family of transcription factors. *J Biol Chem* 1998;273:28545–28548.

161. Sterneck E, Tessarollo L, Johnson PF. An essential role for C/EBPβ in female reproduction. *Genes Dev* 1997;11: 2153–2162.

162. Seagroves TN, Krnacik S, Raught B, et al. C/EBPβ, but not C/EBPα, is essential for ductal morphogenesis, lobuloalveolar proliferation, and functional differentiation in the mouse mammary gland. *Genes Dev* 1998;12:1917–1928.

163. Robinson GW, Johnson PF, Hennighausen L, et al. The C/EBPbeta transcription factor regulates epithelial cell proliferation and differentiation in the mammary gland. *Genes Dev* 1998;12:1907–1916.

164. Yukawa K, Tanaka T, Tsuji S, et al. Expressions of CCAAT/ Enhancer-binding proteins β and δ and their activities are intensified by cAMP signaling as well as Ca2+/calmodulin kinases activation in hippocampal neurons. *J Biol Chem* 1998; 273:31345–31351.

165. Nerlov C, McNagny KM, Doderlein G, et al. Distinct C/EBP functions are required for eosinophil lineage commitment and maturation. *Genes Dev* 1998;12:2413–2423.

166. Zhang DE, Zhang P, Wang ND, et al. Absence of granulocyte colony-stimulating factor signaling and neutrophil development in CCAAT enhancer binding protein α-deficient mice. *Proc Natl Acad Sci USA* 1997;94:569–574.

The Liver: Biology and Pathobiology, Fourth Edition, edited by I. M. Arias, J. L. Boyer, F. V. Chisari, N. Fausto, D. Schachter, and D. A. Shafritz.
Lippincott Williams & Wilkins, Philadelphia © 2001.

THE HEPATOCYTE PLASMA MEMBRANE: ORGANIZATION, DIFFERENTIATION, BIOGENESIS, AND TURNOVER

DAVID SCHACHTER

This chapter presents background for subsequent chapters that detail specific advances in our understanding of the biology and pathobiology of the hepatocyte plasma membrane. (See also website chapter 🖳 W-4). Recent references may be found in Chapters 7, 8, and 24.

PRINCIPLES OF MEMBRANE ORGANIZATION

The hepatocyte plasma membrane separates the intracellular environment from the extracellular fluid and has evolved to perform essential *barrier functions*, which highly restrict random traffic; *transport functions*, which mediate and regulate transfer of specific substances and signals, and *integrative functions*, which coordinate ordered sequences of metabolic reactions. The fundamental structure evolved to fulfill these functions is the phospholipid bilayer, which is associated with other lipids and membrane proteins (1–3). The organizing principle of these components is "like seeks like," i.e., polar (hydrophylic) components seek to interact

with water molecules or other polar substances at the aqueous interfaces, whereas nonpolar (hydrophobic) components are constrained to minimize contact with water and to interact with each other. In the plasma membrane, therefore, the phospholipid polar head groups face the aqueous interfaces, whereas the nonpolar acyl chains are directed away from the interfaces. The hydrophobic cholesterol molecule is intercalated between the phospholipid acyl chains with its hydroxyl group positioned toward the aqueous interface. Membrane glycolipids are similarly oriented with their hydrophilic sugar residues toward the water. Maintenance of this membrane structure is dependent on the avidity of water molecules for interaction with each other and with other polar groups, an avidity that also repels and expels hydrophobic components from the aqueous medium. Thus the aqueous environment is essential for normal membrane structure and function, and nonpolar solvents disrupt biologic and artificial bilayer membranes.

ORGANIZATION OF MEMBRANE PROTEINS

Membrane proteins are categorized as intrinsic (integral) or extrinsic (peripheral). Extrinsic proteins are associated with

D. Schachter: Department of Physiology and Cellular Biophysics, Columbia University College of Physicians and Surgeons, New York, New York 10032.

aqueous interfaces of the membrane and relatively easily removed by changing the ionic composition or pH of the suspending medium or by treating with divalent cation chelators. Some extrinsic proteins can be removed by protease treatment to clip at an accessible anchoring site. Once free of the membrane, these proteins are usually soluble in aqueous media and contain no or little adherent lipid. In contrast, intrinsic membrane proteins contain stretches of hydrophobic amino acid residues that traverse the hydrophobic bilayer lipids. Drastic treatments with detergents or organic solvents are required to remove these proteins. Detergents are needed to maintain their solubility in aqueous media and they have a relatively high lipid content when isolated. Portions of intrinsic proteins within the nonpolar bilayer are generally rich in α-helical secondary structure inasmuch as the exclusion of water favors hydrogen bonding and stabilization of the α-helix. The amino acid sequences of the α-helical regions may be oriented with nonpolar residues toward the lipids and polar residues away from the lipids to form an aqueous microchannel pore for transmembrane transport of hydrophilic substances. Some membrane proteins are covalently bound to fatty acids via acylation of an amino terminus or formation of thioesters with cysteine (4–6). Covalent binding to membrane phosphatidylinositol anchors a variety of proteins, including alkaline phosphatase, acetylcholinesterase, 5'-nucleotidase, and thy 1 (7).

DYNAMICS OF MEMBRANE COMPONENTS

The major modes of motion of the bilayer phospholipids include *translational (lateral) diffusion* within each hemileaflet, *rotational diffusion* around an axis perpendicular to the plane of the membrane, and *transverse diffusion*, or "flip-flop," from one hemileaflet to the other. The last mode is relatively constrained and estimated to occur at 1/10,000 the rate of the other two modes. The freedom of the lipids to move, i.e., the "fluidity" of the membrane, is dependent on its biochemical composition. Lipid fluidity is decreased with increasing ratios of cholesterol/phospholipid, sphingomyelin/lecithin, and protein/lipid. The fluidity is enhanced by *cis*-unsaturation of the acyl chains, and it is greater at the midplane of the bilayer, i.e., at the methyl ends of the phospholipid acyl chains, and decreases toward the aqueous interfaces. Differentiation of the plasma membranes of polarized cells such as hepatocytes, intestinal enterocytes, and renal tubular cells is accompanied by characteristic differences in lipid composition and fluidity (8). In all three of these cell types the microvillus regions (the canalicular region in the hepatocyte) are less fluid than the opposite poles. Differences in fluidity between the hemileaflets of a given plasma membrane have been reported (9), and certain membrane proteins, such as the sodium- and potassium-dependent adenosine triphosphatase, are thought to exist in particularly fluid microdomains of the membrane. Plasma membranes are generally less fluid and contain higher amounts of cholesterol and sphingomyelin than intracellular organellar membranes.

The motions of membrane proteins can be constrained by protein-protein interactions, e.g., binding to cytoskeletal elements at the cytosolic membrane face. Proteins not so constrained are free to undergo translational (lateral) diffusion and rotational diffusion, the rates of which are 1/10 to 1/100 those of the membrane lipids. Protein motions are also dependent on the resistance to motion of the lipids, i.e., the lipid fluidity. Thus enzymatic and transport functions of intrinsic proteins of the hepatocyte plasma membrane are influenced by the fluidity and physical state of the lipids.

BIOCHEMICAL COMPOSITION OF THE HEPATOCYTE PLASMA MEMBRANE

Hepatocytes are estimated to account for over 90% by weight of the cells of the organ and contribute approximately 74% of the plasma membrane surface area (10). The hepatocyte plasma membrane is differentiated morphologically, functionally, and biochemically into three domains—sinusoidal, contiguous, and canalicular (11)—whose relative surface areas are 77%, 15%, and 13%, respectively (12). The sinusoidal domain is specialized functionally for hormone binding and the exchange of a wide variety of metabolites with sinusoidal blood. The contiguous domain separates adjacent hepatocytes, is responsible for intercellular communication, and contains gap junctions, tight junctions, and desmosomes. Tight junctions delimit the biliary canalicular membrane domain, which lines the terminal biliary canaliculus and is the port for bile secretion.

Biochemical analyses (13) of hepatocyte plasma membrane preparations not fractionated into the preceding domains yielded the following ranges of values: total lipid, 30.6% to 49.8% (dry weight); total protein, 50.2% to 69.4% dry weight); protein/lipid ratio, 1.01 to 2.27; cholesterol/phospholipid molar ratio, 0.38 to 0.81; sphingomyelin/phosphatidylcholine molar ratio, 0.41 to 0.81. The percentage of the total lipids contributed by individual lipids and classes in these studies ranged as follows: cholesterol, 12.9% to 21.2%, total phospholipids, 52.1% to 70.0%; phosphatidylcholine, 18.1% to 26.5%, sphingomyelin, 10.6% to 19.6%; phosphatidylethanolamine, 6.4% to 15.7%; phosphatidylserine, 3.5% to 9.2%; and phosphatidylinositol, 3.5% to 5.2%.

Differences in lipid composition between canalicular and sinusoidal membrane domains, respectively, are for cholesterol content (mg/mg protein), 0.17 to 0.25 versus 0.15; sphingomyelin content (mg/mg protein), 0.16 to 0.19 versus 0.09; molar ratio cholesterol/phospholipid, 0.54 to 0.70 versus 0.53; and molar ratio sphingomyelin/

phospholipid, 0.61 to 0.75 versus 0.27. These differences predict the observed lower lipid fluidity of canalicular compared to sinusoidal membranes (14).

PROTEINS OF HEPATOCYTE PLASMA MEMBRANE DOMAINS

In accord with their functional specialization, hepatocyte membrane domains contain specific enzymes, channels, and transporters (see Chapters 7, 8, and 24 and website chapter 🖥 W-4).

INFLUENCES OF DRUGS, CHEMICAL AGENTS, AND DIET

Various agents can influence hepatocyte plasma membrane proteins directly or indirectly via effects on membrane lipid composition and fluidity. For example, lipid-fluidizing agents increase, whereas rigidifying treatments decrease, the activities of intrinsic membrane proteins such as the (Na^+ + K^+)-dependent adenosine triphosphatase (ATPase) and adenylate cyclase. These effects are demonstrable on treating hepatocyte plasma membranes *in vitro* with the fluidizing agents benzyl alcohol and ethanol (15). Chronic administration of alcohol to rats, however, decreased lipid fluidity of synaptosomes and liver mitochondrial membranes, apparently owing to compensatory changes in lipid composition (16). Hepatocyte plasma membrane fluidity and (Na^+ + K^+)-dependent ATPase activity were increased by *in vivo* treatments of rats with S-adenosyl-L-methionine, propylene glycol, cortisone acetate, or 3,3',5-triodo-L-thyroxine. Decreases in hepatocyte plasma membrane fluidity and reductions in (Na^+ + K^+)-dependent ATPase have been reported on treating rats *in vivo* with ethinyl estradiol or chlorpromazine and certain of its metabolites.

Dietary regimens in the rat can alter hepatocyte plasma membrane lipid composition, fluidity, and intrinsic membrane protein activities. Thus a starve-refeed regimen, known to induce fatty acyl chain desaturases in rat liver endoplasmic reticulum, increased the content of monoenoic and polyenoic acyl chains, decreased the cholesterol/phospholipid molar ratio, enhanced the (Na^+ + K^+)-dependent ATPase activity (17) and partially restored bile flow in rats treated with ethinyl estradiol to induce cholestasis (18). These observations point to the possibility of regulating hepatocyte membrane functions by dietary means.

BIOGENESIS OF THE HEPATOCYTE PLASMA MEMBRANE

Knowledge of the molecular mechanisms responsible for the synthesis of plasma membrane proteins and lipids, their transport to the appropriate plasma membrane domains, and their turnover in those domains has increased markedly in recent years, along with an overall understanding of the routes of vesicular membrane trafficking between the plasma membrane and the cytosolic membrane organelles (19). In this section an overall description of these processes will be given to orient the reader. Details of specific molecular mechanisms are further elaborated in Chapters 7, 8, and 24 and website chapter 🖥 W-4).

The basic organization of the lipids and proteins of biologic membranes described above is characteristic of both the outer, plasma membrane and the inner, cytosolic membrane organelles. Indeed, the synthesis of new hepatocyte plasma membrane occurs on preexisting membrane templates in the endoplasmic reticulum (ER) and Golgi cytosolic organelles. Each of these organelles has the structure of a single, cytosolic, membrane-bounded compartment that is elaborately folded into sac-like and tubular elements. The lumen of each, i.e., the interior compartment delimited from the cytosol, is analogous to the extracellular space in relation to the cytosol. New membrane formed in the endoplasmic reticulum template buds off as vesicles (the interior of which corresponds to the extracellular space), which proceed to and fuse with the Golgi membrane. After alteration of the membrane components in the Golgi apparatus, a corresponding process of membrane vesicle formation by budding, vesicle transfer through the cytosol and fusion to an appropriate domain of the plasma membrane completes the synthetic pathway. In the steady state, addition of new plasma membrane via the synthetic pathway is balanced by removal of plasma membrane via vesicle formation, transfer through the cytosol, and fusion with additional cytosolic organelles, the endosomes and lysosomes (see Chapters 8 and 10 and website chapter 🖥 W-9). In common with many other cell types, vesicle addition and removal at the hepatocyte plasma membrane surface is in part constitutive, i.e., occurs continually, and allows the cell to take up extracellular medium, the process of *pinocytosis*.

Membrane Protein Formation in the Endoplasmic Reticulum

Cytosolic messenger RNA molecules encoding plasma membrane proteins contain specific signal sequences that are translated by ribosomes into *signal peptide* sequences that direct the emerging proteins into the cytosolic face of the ER membrane (see Chapters 9 and 10). The process of insertion into the ER occurs as the ribosome translates the messenger RNA (mRNA), i.e., cotranslationally. One signal category consists of N-terminal *signal peptides*, which initiate the insertions, and these peptides are usually cleaved from the maturing protein. A second category, termed *signal patches*, are specific internal sequences along the amino acid chain of the protein that act as start-insertion or stop-insertion signals. The sequential actions of start-insertion and stop-insertion signals accounts for the threading of certain intrinsic membrane proteins multiple times across the hydrophobic interior of the lipid bilayer.

The processes of cotranslation of mRNA by ribosomes and insertion into the ER are carried out by the integrated action of a number of protein components. A cytosolic *signal-recognition particle* (SRP) binds to the signal peptide as it is formed on the ribosome, temporarily pauses further translation of the mRNA, and docks the ribosomal complex to an SRP receptor protein in the ER membrane. Docked on the cytosolic face of the ER, the ribosomal complex is stabilized by the additional binding of the ribosome to a ribosomal receptor protein in the ER membrane. The SRP is then displaced to recycle and dock additional ribosomes, while protein formation continues in the docked ribosome. The emerging nascent protein is fed through the ER lipid bilayer by a protein translocation complex intrinsic to the ER membrane. The presence of multiple ribosomal complexes on the cytosolic face of the ER gives this region its characteristic microscopic appearance described as the *rough ER*.

Membrane Lipid Formation in the Endoplasmic Reticulum

Other regions of the ER lack bound cytosolic ribosomes and are termed *smooth ER*. These regions contain many enzymes necessary for lipid biosynthesis. The hepatocyte is particularly rich in smooth ER-containing enzymes responsible for the formation of lipoprotein particle lipids and for many detoxifying reactions, e.g., those carried out by the cytochrome P-450 enzymes. The biosynthesis of the membrane phospholipids occurs at the cytosolic face of the ER where the required cytosolic reactants are available. Phosphatidylcholine (PC), phosphatidylethanolamine, phosphatidylserine, and phosphatidylinositol are formed and incorporated into the cytosolic leaflet of the ER membrane. An ER "flippase" enzyme specific for PC moves some of these molecules by "flip-flop" to the luminal leaflet, whereas the other phospholipids remain mainly confined to the cytosolic leaflet, an asymmetric distribution that is preserved in the plasma membranes of hepatocytes and other cell types. The smooth ER is also the site of formation of cholesterol and ceramide. (In subsequent reactions in the Golgi apparatus, ceramide is used as a precursor of glycosphingolipids and, with PC, of sphingomyelin. These reactions occur in the luminal leaflet of the Golgi membrane, and the resulting lipids are thus eventually located in the exofacial leaflet of the plasma membrane.)

Vesicle Transfer to and Membrane Modification in the Golgi Organelle

The proteins and lipids synthesized in the ER are assembled into bilayer membranes in the smooth ER region and exported by budding into vesicles that translocate through the cytosol to the Golgi apparatus (see Chapters 9 and 10 for a detailed description of ER-Golgi trafficking). Here they fuse with the cis face of the organelle and may be further modified by luminal Golgi enzymes as they proceed sequentially through the cis, medial, and trans cysternae to the trans face. Transfer between the cysternae is believed to occur by vesicle formation, translocation, and subsequent fusion. Export to the cytosol occurs in the *trans*-Golgi network at the trans face of the organelle by formation of vesicles destined for the various domains of the plasma membrane or for other cytosolic organelles. Many membrane proteins bear carbohydrate residues, and this glycosylation is the result of enzymatic reactions in the ER and Golgi apparatus. It often begins in the ER by the covalent attachment of a specific oligosaccharide composed of 14 residues (nine mannose, three glucose, and two *N*-acetyl-glucosamines) to the amino group of the side chain of an asparagine residue in the protein. This reaction takes place at the luminal surface and results in an N-linked glycoprotein whose sugar residues will eventually face the extracellular fluid bordering the exofacial leaflet of the plasma membrane. While in the ER the oligosaccharide is usually processed by the removal of the three glucoses and one of the mannose residues. Further trimming occurs in the Golgi apparatus and often leaves a core of five residues, three mannose, and two *N*-acetyl-glucosamines. Various other modifications are mediated by Golgi membrane enzymes, including the following: addition of mannose residues to yield the high-mannose oligosaccharide glycoproteins; addition of *N*-acetylglucosamine, galactose, sialic acid, or fucose residues in various combinations to yield the complex oligosaccharide glycoproteins; linkage of sugar residues to OH groups of serine or threonine sidechains to form O-linked glycoproteins; and formation of proteoglycans, very heavily glycosylated proteins containing many sulfated sugar residues and thus large negative charges. In the plasma membrane the proteoglycans form the glycocalyx prominent in certain epithelial cells.

Export from the *trans*-Golgi network is by vesicle formation and translocation to the appropriate hepatocyte plasma membrane domains. What is known of the mechanisms responsible for the vesicular traffic patterns and the maintenance of different membrane proteins in the sinusoidal, contiguous, and canalicular domains of the hepatocyte plasma membrane is considered in Chapter 10. Fusion of the vesicles at the endofacial surface of the plasma membrane adds new lipids and proteins to the membrane, while soluble components within the vesicular lumen are discharged (secreted) into the extracellular medium, the process of exocytosis.

ENDOCYTOSIS, EXOCYTOSIS, AND PLASMA MEMBRANE TURNOVER

In the steady state the foregoing addition of new lipids and proteins to the plasma membrane by exocytosis is balanced by endocytosis, the removal of plasma membrane components by formation of vesicles at the cytosolic interface and their translocation to cytosolic organelles, the endosomes, and lysosomes. Balanced processes of endocytosis and exocytosis result in plasma membrane turnover and maintenance of a dynamic state. Endocytosis comprises both pinocytosis ("cell drinking") and receptor-mediated endocytosis. In pinocytosis small vesicles are constitutively and continually pinched off, thereby bringing extracellular water and solutes into the cell. Receptor-mediated endocytosis involves the binding of specific extracellular ligands, e.g., hormones, growth factors, lipoproteins, to exofacial membrane receptors, thereby greatly increasing the efficiency of uptake, followed by vesicle formation and translocation in the cytosol (see Chapter 10). Formation of endocytic vesicles occurs at differentiated regions of the plasma membrane visualized on electron microscopy as membrane evaginations into the cytosol covered by a basket-like cage of the protein clathrin. These clathrin-coated pits pinch off to form clathrin-coated vesicles, thereafter rapidly lose the clathrin coat, and translocate to cytosolic membrane sites, often the endosomes and lysosomes. The fates of the plasma membrane receptors and their ligands vary depending on their specific functional roles. In the endosomal compartment the ligand-receptor complex may be dissociated and the receptor recycled to the original domain of the plasma membrane, or translocated to another domain of the plasma membrane, a process termed transcytosis, or moved to the lysosomes for degradation (see Chapter 10 and website chapter 🖳 W-9). Directing membrane vesicles into their appropriate pathways is an important sorting function of the endosomal compartment. An example of how these traffic patterns subserve specific functions for the cell is the recycling of the plasma membrane transferrin receptor for uptake of iron. Transferrin loaded with iron in the extracellular fluid is bound to the plasma membrane transferrin receptor and the complex brought into the cytosol in a clathrin-coated vesicle. After shedding the clathrin coat, the vesicle is translocated to and fused with an endosomal compartment lying close to the plasma membrane ("early endosome"). Here the more acid environment of the endosomal lumen dissociates iron from the transferrin protein (apotransferrin), and the apotransferrin-receptor complex is recycled to the plasma membrane by vesicular transport. Once fused with the plasma membrane and exposed to the extracellular medium the apotransferrin dissociates from the receptor and is available to bind more iron for cellular uptake.

REFERENCES

1. Singer SJ. The molecular organization of membranes. *Annu Rev Biochem* 1974;43:805–833.
2. Marchesi BT, Furthmayr H, Tomita M. The red cell membrane. *Annu Rev Biochem* 1976;45:667–698.
3. Tanford C. *The hydrophobic effect: formation of micelles and biological membranes.* New York: John Wiley, 1980.
4. Schlesinger MJ. Proteolipids. *Annu Rev Biochem* 1981;50:193–206.
5. Schmidt MFG. Fatty acid binding: a new kind of posttranslational modification of membrane proteins. *Curr Top Microbiol Immunol* 1983;102:101–129.
6. Magee AI, Courtneidge SA. Two classes of fatty acid acylated proteins exist in eukaryotic cells. *EMBO J* 1985;4:1137–1144.
7. Low MG, Ferguson MAJ, Futerman AH, et al. Covalently attached phosphatidylinositol as a hydrophobic anchor for membrane proteins. *Trends Biochem Sci* 1986;11:212–215.
8. Schachter D. Lipid dynamics and lipid-protein interactions in intestinal plasma membranes. In: Watts A, De Pont JJHHM, eds. *Progress in protein interactions.* Amsterdam: Elsevier, 1985:231–258.
9. Wisnieski BJ, Iwata KK. Electron spin resonance evidence for vertical asymmetry in animal cell membranes. *Biochemistry* 1977;16:1321–1326.
10. Blouin A, Bolender RP, Weibel ER. Distribution of organelles and membrane between hepatocytes and nonhepatocytes in rat liver. *J Cell Biol* 1977;72:441–455.
11. Evans WH. A biochemical dissection of the functional polarity of the plasma membrane of the hepatocyte. *Biochim Biophys Acta* 1980;604:27–64.
12. Weibel ER. Stereological approach to the study of cell surface morphometry. Sixth European Congress on Electron Microscopy, Jerusalem, 1976:6–9.
13. Emmelot P, Bos CJ, Van Hoeven RP, et al. Isolation of plasma membranes from rat and mouse livers and hepatomas. *Methods Enzymol* 1974;31:230–239.
14. Storch J, Schachter D, Inoue M, et al. Lipid fluidity of hepatocyte plasma membrane subfractions and their differential regulation by calcium. *Biochim Biophys Acta* 1983;727:209–212.
15. Schachter D. Fluidity and function of hepatocyte plasma membranes. *Hepatology* 1984;4:140–151.
16. Rubin E, Rottenberg H. Ethanol-induced injury and adaptation in biological membranes. *Fed Proc* 1982;41:2465–2471.
17. Storch J, Schachter D. Dietary induction of acyl chain desaturases alters the lipid composition and fluidity of rat hepatocyte plasma membranes. *Biochemistry* 1984;23:1165–1170.
18. Storch J, Schachter D. A dietary regimen alters hepatocyte plasma membrane lipid fluidity and ameliorates ethinyl estradiol cholestasis in the rat. *Biochim Biophys Acta* 1984;798:137–140.
19. Zegers MMP, Hoekstra D. Mechanisms and functional features of polarized membrane traffic in epithelial and hepatic cells. *Biochem J* 1998;336:257–269

The Liver: Biology and Pathobiology, Fourth Edition, edited by I. M. Arias, J. L. Boyer, F. V. Chisari, N. Fausto, D. Schachter, and D. A. Shafritz.
Lippincott Williams & Wilkins, Philadelphia © 2001.

HEPATOCYTE BASOLATERAL MEMBRANE ORGANIC ANION TRANSPORTERS

ALLAN W. WOLKOFF
FREDERICK J. SUCHY

A major function of the liver is the removal from the circulation of various organic anionic compounds. These compounds include a class of organic anions represented by bilirubin and bromsulfophthalein (BSP) and another class of compounds represented by bile acids. These molecules have, in many cases, limited aqueous solubility, and circulate by virtue of their ability to bind to serum albumin. Despite being almost entirely protein bound, these organic anions are rapidly cleared from the circulation by the liver (1). There is no evidence that the albumin-organic anion complex is taken up by the hepatocyte. Rather, a number of studies indicate that the organic anion is extracted from its protein carrier during the uptake process (2,3). The liver is ideally designed for extraction of protein-bound molecules. Unlike most other organs, which have a tight capillary endothelium, the hepatic capillary (sinusoidal) endothelium is fenestrated. This permits direct interaction of large molecular complexes with the hepatocyte plasma membrane (4,5). Thus, although a particular organic anionic molecule may have lipophilic properties, its tight binding to albumin limits the extent of cellular uptake by simple dissolution across lipid bilayers. Although this process can occur (6), uptake of these compounds is facilitated by several recently described hepatocyte plasma membrane proteins that have been cloned and characterized.

HEPATOCYTE UPTAKE OF BILE ACIDS

Sodium-Dependent Bile Acid Uptake Across the Hepatocyte Basolateral Membrane

Uptake of conjugated bile acids from sinusoidal blood occurs against unfavorable electrical and chemical gradients and is mediated largely by a saturable, sodium-dependent symport system (7–9). The marked dependency of bile acid uptake on extracellular sodium has been demonstrated in multiple experimental models including the isolated, perfused rat liver, isolated and cultured hepatocytes, and basolateral plasma membrane vesicles (7,10,11). However, there is a substantial sodium-independent fraction of bile acid

A. W. Wolkoff: Departments of Medicine and Anatomy and Structual Biology, Albert Einstein College of Medicine, Bronx, New York 10461-1602.

F. J. Suchy: Department of Pediatrics, Mt. Sinai School of Medicine, New York, New York 10029.

uptake, representing approximately 20% to 25% of total uptake. The avid affinity of the hepatocyte for bile acids results in a high first-pass clearance from portal blood of as much as 90%. The driving force for this largely sodium-dependent process is the extracellular to intracellular sodium gradient that is maintained by the action of the basolateral sodium pump, Na$^+$-K$^+$–adenosine triphosphatase (ATPase). In several experimental models, sodium-dependent taurocholate transport had an apparent Michaelis' constant (K_m) of 6 to 56 μM, depending on the species and experimental system. Efficiency of bile acid transport is dependent on the position and number of hydroxyl groups on the steroid nucleus as well as the length and charge of the bile acid side chain (9,12,13); 6-hydroxylated bile acid derivatives are preferred substrates for the hepatic sodium-dependent bile acid transporter (14). In contrast, the 3α-hydroxy group present in all natural bile acids is not essential for high-affinity interaction with this transporter (15). Furthermore, Na$^+$ gradient-dependent sinusoidal uptake of taurocholate can be stimulated by low concentrations of albumin (16). The process is electrogenic based on electrophysiologic measurements of transport-associated currents, as well as direct measurement of fluorescent bile acid transport rates in voltage-clamped cells (17,18). These studies support a Na$^+$:bile acid coupling stoichiometry of 2:1.

Na$^+$/Taurocholate Cotransporting Polypeptide (ntcp)

The sodium-dependent bile acid transporter, now called the Na$^+$/taurocholate cotransporting polypeptide (ntcp), has been isolated by Hagenbuch and associates (19) by expression cloning in *Xenopus laevis* oocytes. Ntcp is part of a new family of mammalian sodium-dependent bile acid transporters that also includes the brush-border membrane transporter expressed in the ileum, renal proximal tubule cell, and cholangiocyte with which it shares approximately 35% amino acid sequence identity (20). The cloned transporter is strictly sodium dependent and can be inhibited by various non–bile-acid organic compounds. An open reading frame of 1,086 nucleotides was found on sequence analysis of the Ntcp complementary DNA (cDNA). These nucleotides encoded a protein of 362 amino acids (calculated molecular mass 39 kd) with five potential *N*-linked glycosylation sites and seven putative transmembrane domains. Membrane insertion scanning of the human ileal sodium/bile acid cotransporter, which is structurally related to ntcp, provides support for a transmembrane domain model with nine rather than seven integrated segments with an exoplasmic N-terminus and a cytoplasmic C-terminus (21). Northern blot analysis with the cloned ntcp probe revealed cross-reactivity with messenger RNA (mRNA) species from rat kidney and intestine as well as from liver tissues of mice, guinea pigs, rabbits, and humans. A 1,599–base pair (bp) cDNA encoding the human NTCP-was subsequently cloned and consists of 349 amino acids (calculated molecular mass of 38 kd) and exhibits 77% amino acid homology with the rat ntcp (22). *In vitro* translation experiments indicate that the transporter is glycosylated and that its polypeptide backbone has an apparent molecular mass of 33 to 35 kd. Kinetic studies indicated that the human NTCP has a higher affinity for taurocholate (apparent K_m = 6 μM) than the rat transporter (apparent K_m = 25 μM). Southern blot analysis of genomic DNA and immunofluorescence *in situ* hybridization have mapped the human NTCP gene to chromosome 14 and the rat ntcp gene to chromosome 2 (22,23).

Ntcp2, encoding a truncated 317 amino acid protein, has been cloned from mouse liver (24). It has a shorter C-terminal end and also mediates saturable Na$^+$-dependent transport of taurocholate when expressed in *Xenopus laevis*

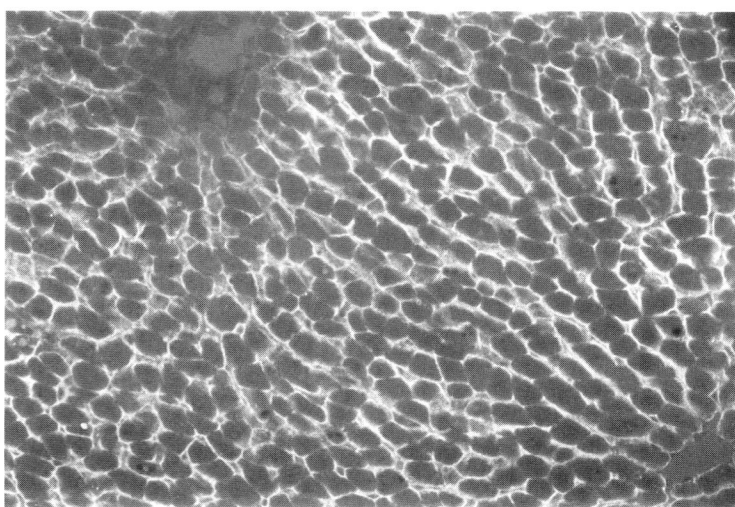

FIGURE 7.1. Immunofluorescence localization of ntcp in a section of rat liver. In this representative study, ntcp is seen localized to the sinusoidal (basolateral) plasma membrane domain of hepatocytes with no acinar gradient in the pattern of staining. There is no significant localization of ntcp in intracellular or bile canalicular (apical) membranes.

oocytes. Analysis of the gene revealed that Ntcp2 is produced by alternative splicing where the last intron is retained. Its functional importance and cellular localization are unknown.

Several studies have used antipeptide and antifusion protein antibodies to the COOH-terminal part of ntcp to further characterize its expression (25,26). On Western blot analysis, antisera but not preimmune serum specifically detected a protein of approximately 50 to 51 kd in isolated rat liver basolateral plasma membranes (BLPM). Deglycosylation of BLPM with *N*-glycanase followed by antibody probing led to decrease of the molecular mass to 34.5 kd, suggesting that the protein is *N*-glycosylated *in vivo*. Two-dimensional immunoblotting indicated that the ntcp protein had an isoelectric point of approximately 6.0. The antibody did not react with any proteins in rat ileal and kidney cortex brush-border membranes, human liver basolateral plasma membranes, or rat hepatoma tissue culture cell homogenates.

Immunofluorescence localization studies revealed specific staining of the sinusoidal membrane domain but not of intracellular or bile canalicular membranes (Fig. 7.1). Moreover, there was no acinar gradient in the pattern of staining. In short-term cultured hepatocytes, a positive surface immunoreaction with a COOH-terminal antibody was only obtained in detergent-permeabilized cell cultures, indicating that the C-terminal portion of the ntcp molecule is intracellular (26). In primary cultures of rat hepatocytes, ntcp expression is rapidly lost. However, culture of cells in a collagen sandwich reestablishes normal morphology and partially maintains bile acid uptake (27).

Phylogeny and Ontogeny of Ntcp

The phylogenic and ontogenic expression of mRNA for ntcp was studied further by Northern analysis (28); mRNA was detected in several mammalian species, including rats, mice, and humans, but could not be found in livers from nonmammalian species, including chicken, turtle, frog, and small skate. When expression of ntcp was studied in developing rat liver, mRNA was detected between 18 and 21 days of gestation, at the time when Na$^+$-dependent bile acid transport activity is first detected (29). The hepatoma cell lines HTC and HepG2, the latter of which is known to have lost the Na$^+$/bile acid cotransport system, also did not express mRNA for this transporter. Finally, when mRNA from the small skate was injected into *Xenopus*-oocytes, only sodium-independent, chloride-dependent bile acid uptake was expressed, consistent with prior functional studies of bile acid transport in this species. These findings establish that Na$^+$/bile acid cotransport is a property of the well-differentiated hepatocyte. mRNA is first transcribed in mammalian species, a process that is recapitulated late during mammalian fetal development in rat liver.

The mechanisms underlying ontogenic regulation of ntcp have been studied in detail (30). Steady-state mRNA levels for the basolateral transporter were less than 20% of adult values prior to birth, increased to 35% on the first postnatal day, and reached adult levels by 1 week of age. This was paralleled by transcription rates that were low prior to birth, reached 47% by day 1, and were maximal by 1 week of age. Surprisingly, the full complement of the ntcp protein was present well before adult levels of mRNA were reached. The basolateral protein was expressed at 82% of adult levels on the first day of life but was of lower apparent molecular mass (39 kd), a difference that persisted until 4 weeks of age. *N*-glycanase digestion suggested that this difference could be fully accounted for by differences in extent of N-linked glycosylation. These results indicate that ontogeny of ntcp is complex and appears to be regulated at transcriptional, translational, and posttranslational levels.

Ntcp Mediates Hepatocyte Uptake of Conjugated Bile Acids and Other Compounds

It is now clear that ntcp is a multispecific transporter with preference for bile salts and other anionic steroidal compounds (31). In primary cultured rat hepatocytes and Ntcp-transfected COS-7 (CV-l origin, SV40) cells, the Na$^+$-dependent uptake of taurocholate (TC) was inhibited by nine bile acids and five non–bile-acid organic anions in a concentration-dependent manner (32). BQ-123 (1 μM) and indomethacin (10 μM), both of which exhibit no ntcp-mediated transport, significantly inhibited the Na$^+$-dependent uptake of TC mediated by ntcp. The contribution of NTCP to the Na$^+$-dependent uptake of glycocholic acid into rat hepatocytes was approximately 80%, whereas that of cholic acid was 40%. In transfected Chinese hamster ovary (CHO) cells, saturable Na$^+$-dependent uptake of [^{3}H]taurocholate was strongly inhibited by all major bile salts, estrone 3-sulfate, bumetanide, and cyclosporin A (33). Sodium-dependent taurocholate uptake was also inhibited by addition of bumetanide, BSP, and oligomycin (34). In addition, the analysis indicated that the contribution of NTCP to the Na$^+$-dependent uptake of several ligands (ouabain, ibuprofen, glutathione-conjugate of BSP, glucuronide- and sulfate-conjugates of 6-hydroxy-5, 7-dimethyl-2-methylamino-4-(3-pyridylmethyl) benzothiazole) was negligible (35). Hepatic uptake of thyroid hormones and their metabolites is mediated at least in part by Ntcp and oatp1 (36).

Several Transcription Factors Are Critical to the Expression of Ntcp

The rat genomic DNA encoding ntcp has been cloned and several cis elements and *trans*-activating factors involved in expression of the gene have been identified (37). The rat ntcp gene is distributed over 16.5 kilobase (kb) pairs as five exons. Primer extension analysis revealed two closely spaced transcription initiation sites, 27 and 41 nucleotides downstream of a TATA sequence. A minimal promoter element, nucleotide −158 to +47, was investigated by transfection of primary rat hepatocytes with a series of 5′-deleted rat ntcp promoter-driven luciferase constructs (from approximately −6 kb pairs to −59 bp of upstream sequences, terminating at nucleotide +47). This minimal promoter was active in transfected HepG2, but inactive in NIH3T3, Caco-2, and Madin-Darby canine kidney (MDCK) cells, indicating that the determinants of hepatocyte-specific expression reside within this region. Three elements that direct the basal and tissue-restricted expression of the rat ntcp promoter have been found on deoxyribonuclease I footprint analysis, gel mobility shift assays, and expression of a series of 5′-deleted promoter-driven luciferase constructs: a TATA element, the liver-enriched transcription factor hepatocyte nuclear factor-1 (HNF-1), and an unknown liver-enriched factor that binds within a novel palindrome in footprint B. The divergent homeobox protein Hex has also been found to transcriptionally activate ntcp (38).

The ntcp footprint B binding site was recently found to have homology to a retinoid x receptor:retinoid α receptor (RXRα:RARα) consensus element (39). Retinoids were found to mediate transactivation of ntcp through the formation of retinoid x receptor and retinoid α receptor heterodimers. An adjacent binding site for CAAT/enhancer-binding proteins was required for maximal transactivation of the ntcp promoter by RXRα:RARα.

Prolactin (PRL) increases hepatic Na⁺/taurocholate cotransport activity and messenger RNA in the postpartum liver (40,41). In electrophoretic mobility gel shift assays, the transcription factor Stat5 exhibited specific DNA-binding to interferon-γ–activated sequence (GAS)-like elements (GLEs) in the ntcp promoter (42). Transient cotransfections in HepG2 cells revealed that long PRL inducibility required coexpression of the long form of the long PRL receptor (PRLRL) and Stat5. Deletion analysis mapped the PRL inducible region to −1237 to −758 bp of the ntcp promoter. Linking this 0.5-kb region to a heterologous thymidine kinase promoter, or linking multimerized ntcp GLEs either upstream of the ntcp minimal promoter (−158 to +47 bp) or the heterologous promoter, conferred dose-dependent PRL responsiveness. These results indicate that PRL acts via the PRLRL to facilitate Stat5 binding to ntcp-GLEs and to transcriptionally regulate ntcp (42).

Functional Activity of Ntcp Is Regulated by Cyclic AMP

Adenosine 3′,5′-cyclic monophosphate (cAMP) increases the V_{max} for Na⁺-taurocholate cotransport in hepatocytes (43). This effect is mediated via protein kinase A. It is potentiated, but not mediated, by Ca²⁺/calmodulin-depen-

dent processes, and may be downregulated by protein kinase C (44). Cycloheximide did not inhibit basal or cAMP-induced increases in taurocholate uptake in rat hepatocytes, indicating that cAMP does not stimulate transporter synthesis. Studies in plasma membrane vesicles showed that taurocholate uptake was not stimulated by the catalytic subunit of protein kinase A, but was higher when vesicles were prepared from hepatocytes that had been pretreated with cAMP. Immunoblot analysis showed that pretreatment of hepatocytes with cAMP increased ntcp content in plasma membranes but not in homogenates. This was attributed to reduced ntcp content of an endosomal fraction (45), suggesting that cAMP increases the V_{max} of Na⁺-dependent taurocholate transport at least in part by translocating ntcp from endosomes to plasma membranes. Subsequent immunoblot analysis with phosphoamino antibodies showed that ntcp is a serine/threonine, and not a tyrosine, phosphoprotein, and cAMP inhibited both serine and threonine phosphorylation (46). cAMP-mediated dephosphorylation of ntcp leads to an increased retention of ntcp in the plasma membrane. Addition of okadaic acid, an inhibitor of protein phosphatase PP2A, inhibits cAMP-mediated stimulation of Na⁺/taurocholate cotransport by reversing the ability of cAMP to increase cytosolic [Ca²⁺] and to induce ntcp dephosphorylation (47).

Ntcp Is Downregulated in Cholestasis

The effects of bile duct ligation and the administration of ethinyl estradiol or endotoxin on expression of ntcp have been recently studied (48–53). The function and expression of ntcp are rapidly downregulated in rat liver in models of experimental cholestasis including cholestasis induced by common bile duct ligation, estrogen, endotoxin, or cytokine treatment (54). The loss of transport activity is largely related to a marked decrease in transcription rates of the ntcp gene as well as a rapid reduction in ntcp mRNA and protein levels. Administration of endotoxin results in decreased binding activity of a critical nuclear transcription factor, HNF-1, required for basal Ntcp gene expression (55). The effects of endotoxin may in part be mediated by the release of several inflammatory cytokines since reductions in ntcp mRNA and protein also occur after the administration of tumor necrosis factor-α (TNF-α) and interleukin-1β (IL-1β). The cytokine IL-1β downregulates the ntcp promoter and does so by reducing the specific binding of the RXRα:RARα heterodimer to the ntcp retinoid-response element (39). There is limited information available about the effects of cholestasis on bile acid transporters in humans. However, NTCP mRNA levels are also markedly decreased in infants with biliary atresia and subsequently increase if biliary drainage is restored by portoenterostomy (56). Thus, data so far indicate that downregulation of ntcp is a secondary effect of cholestasis possibly aimed at protection of the hepatocyte against toxicity of high intracellular bile salt concentrations (57).

Expression of ntcp is reduced in various experimental models of cholestasis associated with increased plasma bile salt concentrations (see Chapter 46). Mdr2 P-glycoprotein–deficient mice lack biliary phospholipids and cholesterol but maintain biliary bile salt secretion and increased bile flow (58). In these mice, plasma bile salt concentrations are markedly increased. Kinetic analysis showed a twofold decrease in the V_{max} of Na$^+$-dependent taurocholate transport, with an unaffected K_m in (−/−) mice compared with (+/+) controls. Ntcp protein levels were four- to sixfold reduced in plasma membranes of (−/−) mice relative to sex-matched controls. However, hepatic ntcp mRNA levels were not significantly affected in the (−/−) mice. Thus, the reduced ntcp expression and transport activity observed in the mdr2 P-glycoprotein–deficient mice is due to posttranscriptional downregulation of ntcp (58).

Since expression and function of ntcp are downregulated in several models of experimental cholestasis, studies have defined whether retention and/or depletion of biliary constituents are involved in ntcp regulation (59). In choledochocaval fistula (CCF) rats, a model of bile acid retention, ntcp mRNA expression specifically and markedly declined after 1 and 3 days, respectively, but returned to control levels by 7 days. However, protein expression as assessed by Western blotting remained unchanged for up to 7 days of CCF. In rats with bile fistulas, a model of bile acid depletion, both ntcp protein and mRNA expression remained unaltered for up to 7 days. Infusion of either taurocholate or taurochenodeoxycholate for 12 hours also did not affect ntcp mRNA expression in intact animals, probably because of its inability to increase serum and intrahepatic bile acid levels. In rats with selective bile duct ligation, ntcp mRNA levels were downregulated by approximately 40% after 12 to 24 hours in ligated lobes, but mRNA levels returned to control values in these lobes after 2 and 4 days. Ntcp mRNA expression remained unchanged in the nonobstructed lobes at any time. Serum bile acids correlated linearly with ntcp mRNA over a 0 to 110 μmol/L range on analysis of data combined from choledochocaval fistula and selective bile duct ligation. These results indicate that ntcp is constitutively expressed and remains unaffected by either depletion with a bile fistula or increased flux of biliary constituents. However, retention of biliary constituents in choledochocaval fistula rats or after selective bile duct ligation results in rapid downregulation of ntcp mRNA, consistent with the concept that hepatocytes may be protected from bile acid toxicity during cholestasis by this mechanism (52,59). In long-term (8 days) bile-diverted rats, with a transhepatic bile salt flux of 0, and in streptozotocin-induced diabetic rats with a 2.5-fold increased bile salt flux (with a variation in hepatic bile salt flux from 0 to 250% of normal values in these models)

there was no effect on hepatic ntcp expression or taurocholate transport activity in basolateral plasma membrane vesicles (60). These studies are consistent with the notion that retention in, but not increased flux through, the hepatocyte alters the expression of Ntcp.

Ntcp Expression Is Downregulated During Hepatic Regeneration

Ntcp protein and mRNA were decreased by 50% to 90% 24 hours after partial hepatectomy (61,62) (see Chapter 42). *In vitro* transcription assays demonstrated that ntcp gene transcription was also markedly reduced. As noted below, the organic anion transporting polypeptides oatp1 and oatp2 were downregulated at both protein and steady-state mRNA levels by 50% to 60% of controls during early replicative stages of regeneration (12 hours to 2 days) (63). Expression of all basolateral transporters returned to control values by 4 days after partial hepatectomy. In contrast, hepatic Na$^+$,K$^+$–ATPase activity, protein expression, and gene expression were unaffected by partial hepatectomy (61). Protein and mRNA expression of both the canalicular adenosine triphosphate (ATP)-dependent bile salt export pump (bsep) and the multiorganic anion transporter mrp2 were also unchanged or were slightly increased during liver regeneration, but also returned to control values 7 to 14 days after partial hepatectomy (63). Preservation of bsep and mrp2 expression provides a potential molecular mechanism for regenerating liver cells to maintain or even increase bile secretion expressed per weight of remaining liver (62). However, downregulation of basolateral organic anion transporters might protect replicating liver cells by diminishing uptake of potentially hepatotoxic bile salts, because the remaining liver initially cannot cope with the original bile acid pool size.

Microsomal Epoxide Hydrolase

Levy and colleagues suggested that microsomal epoxide hydrolase (mEH) may also mediate basolateral sodium-dependent bile acid transport (64). They showed functional expression of sodium-dependent bile acid transport in the relatively well differentiated MDCK cell line that was transfected with mEH cDNA. They also provided evidence that mEH is inserted into the endoplasmic reticulum membrane with two topologic orientations, one of which is targeted to the plasma membrane (64). However, other investigators failed to show uptake of taurocholate following expression of mEH in *Xenopus laevis* oocytes and in a stably transfected fibroblast cell line (65). They also showed that mEH is expressed in hepatoma tumor cell lines that show no bile acid transport activity (65). Whether these results are due to failure to target mEH to the plasma membrane in these cells remains to be determined.

HEPATOCYTE UPTAKE OF NONBILE ACID ORGANIC ANIONS

Sodium-Independent Organic Anion Transport

Similar to hepatic uptake of bile acids, uptake of organic anions such as bilirubin and BSP is rapid and efficient, and has carrier-mediated kinetics (1). Studies performed in overnight cultured rat hepatocytes revealed saturable uptake of BSP that was inhibited by bilirubin (66,67). Ligand was taken up by cells, while albumin remained extracellular. Of interest was the finding that isosmotic substitution of NaCl in medium by sucrose resulted in an over 80% reduction of BSP uptake (66). This was not due to a requirement for extracellular Na^+, as has been described for Na^+-dependent bile acid transport; substitution of Na^+ by K^+, Li^+, or choline had no effect on BSP uptake by these cells. However, replacement of Cl^- by HCO_3^- or gluconate reduced BSP uptake by approximately 40% (66). Similar results were found for bilirubin uptake by cultured rat hepatocytes as well as by isolated perfused rat liver. The basis for this chloride dependency is not clear. Studies performed with ^{36}Cl revealed that BSP uptake requires the presence of external Cl^- and is not stimulated by unidirectional Cl^- gradients, suggesting that BSP transport is not coupled to Cl^- transport (67).

Searching for Sodium-Independent Organic Anion Transporters

The studies described above support the existence of a hepatocyte surface membrane organic anion transporter(s). The nature of this transporter has been the basis of much study and some controversy. In early studies, Berk's group (68) isolated a 55-kd protein that they termed a BSP/bilirubin binding protein. They reported that preincubation of rat hepatocytes with relatively high concentrations of polyclonal antibody to this protein partially inhibited the uptake of BSP and bilirubin (69,70). Wolkoff and Chung (71) identified a 55-kd protein (oabp) in preparations of basolateral liver cell plasma membrane on the basis of photoaffinity labeling by ^{35}S-BSP. However, the sequence of this cDNA was identical to the carboxyl 454 amino acids of the β-subunit of the inner mitochondrial membrane protein, F_1-ATPase (72). Interestingly, antigenic reactivity was present in both plasma membrane and mitochondrial domains as seen by immunocytochemical electron microscopy as well as by immunoprecipitation of surface-iodinated hepatocytes (72). Tiribelli and Sottocasa's group (73) isolated a 170-kd protein putative transport protein that they termed bilitranslocase. This protein is composed of 37- and 35.5-kd subunits. They reported that liposomes into which bilitranslocase was inserted were able to transport BSP. They also reported that antibody to this protein inhibited transport of BSP into liver cell plasma membrane vesicles. Bilitranslocase was cloned from a λgt11 rat liver library utilizing a monoclonal antibody (74). The sequence is available on the GenBank database (accession number Y12178). The derived protein sequence is unique and has been used in studies of potential bilirubin-binding sites (75). However, BLAST (Basic Local Alignment Search Tool) analysis reveals that the nucleotide sequence from which the protein sequence was derived is 93% identical to the inverse strand sequence of rat ceruloplasmin. This suggests that a cloning artifact likely occurred.

More recent studies used the uptake system described in cultured rat hepatocytes as an expression cloning transport assay in *Xenopus laevis* oocytes (76). Injection of oocytes with total rat liver poly-(A)$^+$ RNA resulted in the functional expression of chloride-dependent BSP extraction from albumin (76). Using a subselection cloning protocol, a single cDNA was isolated (77). The encoded protein was named organic anion transporting polypeptide 1 (oatp1). This protein mediates uptake of BSP and also mediates transport of various bile salts such as taurocholate in a Na^+-independent fashion (78). It is the first member of a new family of transport proteins that have now been identified in rats, mice, and humans (79–88). These proteins have overlapping substrate specificities and tissue distributions. Although their physiologic roles and relative importance in hepatocyte transport have not as yet been elucidated fully, a number of studies have defined intriguing biologic and biochemical characteristics.

Oatp Family Members in the Hepatocyte

The oatp family of proteins has been expanding greatly over the past year as additional members have been identified in humans, rats, and mice. These proteins are highly homologous and have amino acid identities ranging from 40% to 95%. Interestingly, they appear to be separate gene products that are encoded on multiple chromosomes. Their nomenclature has not as yet been standardized, and may pose some confusion. In the rat, oatp1 (77,89) (originally called oatp), oatp2 (80,90,91), and a newly described family member that has been termed rlst-1 are present in the liver (87). Three members of the oatp family have also been described as being present in human liver. These are OATP-A (86) (originally called OATP), OATP-C (88,92,93) (also known as OATP2 and LST-1), and OATP-8 (94). A murine member of the family that has been named oatp1 has recently been cloned (79). This protein, the mRNA of which is abundant in liver, is 81% identical to rat oatp1, 78% identical to rat oatp2, and 79% identical to rat oatp3 (a protein that is present in the cholangiocyte and other cells, but not the hepatocyte). All of these proteins have a high degree of overlap with respect to substrate specificities. Interestingly, none of these proteins has been described as mediating bilirubin transport, although most can transport BSP and bilirubin glucuronides. It has been believed that bilirubin and other organic anions such as BSP share a common uptake system. However, that their uptake systems are at least in part independent was suggested from studies performed in perfused livers that were obtained from rats following nafenopin treatment (95). Thus far there has been no way to estimate relative protein masses, and the contribution and importance of any one of these proteins to a specific transport process *in vivo* remains undefined. Rat oatp1 is one of the better characterized proteins of this family. It will be described in more detail below, with the expectation that results and insights obtained with this protein will have applicability to other members of the oatp family.

Subcellular Localization and Characterization of Oatp1

As described above, oatp1 was initially identified by application of an expression cloning strategy in which *Xenopus* oocytes were microinjected with mRNA derived from rat liver. This resulted in cloning of a cDNA with an open reading frame of 2,010 nucleotides, encoding a potential protein of 74 kd. Computer analysis indicated that the protein had a high degree of hydrophobicity and provided a topologic model consisting of 12 transmembrane domains and three potential *N*-glycosylation sites on the extracellular domain (78). Northern blot under conditions of high stringency indicates that oatp1 mRNA is limited to liver and kidney (89). Under conditions of lower stringency, there is hybridization to mRNA derived from many other tissues,

consistent with multiple other closely related proteins in this family (77). Interestingly, even under high stringency, there are multiple transcripts in liver and kidney that hybridize with an oatp1 probe, possibly related to heterogeneity in 5′ and 3′ untranslated regions of the mRNA.

Oatp1 (as well as the other members of this transporter family) has not been expressed in amounts sufficient for antibody production. Utilizing the theoretical sequence, synthetic oatp1 peptides of 13 to 15 amino acids in length were synthesized and linked to the haptenizing agent keyhole limpit hemocyanin (KLH) (89). Sera obtained from rabbits that were immunized with this material were screened for the presence of antibodies to oatp1. Initial screening was by Western blot utilizing rat liver homogenate as the antigen. No immunoreactivity was seen. However, following extraction of soluble and weakly membrane-associated proteins by 0.1M Na_2CO_3, a strongly immunoreactive 80-kd band was seen. When a purified preparation of sinusoidal but not canalicular plasma membrane was immunoblotted, an identical 80-kd band was seen, even in the absence of Na_2CO_3 treatment (89). The enzyme *N*-glycanase is known to remove N-linked carbohydrate chains from glycoproteins. Incubation of sinusoidal plasma membrane preparations with this enzyme resulted in a reduction of the apparent mass of oatp1 from 80 to 65 kd, consistent with removal of several carbohydrate chains (89). Using this antiserum, oatp1 was immunolocalized to the sinusoidal (basolateral) plasma membrane of the rat

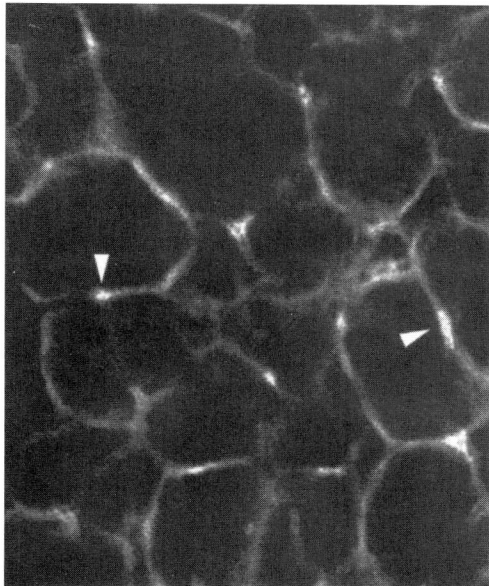 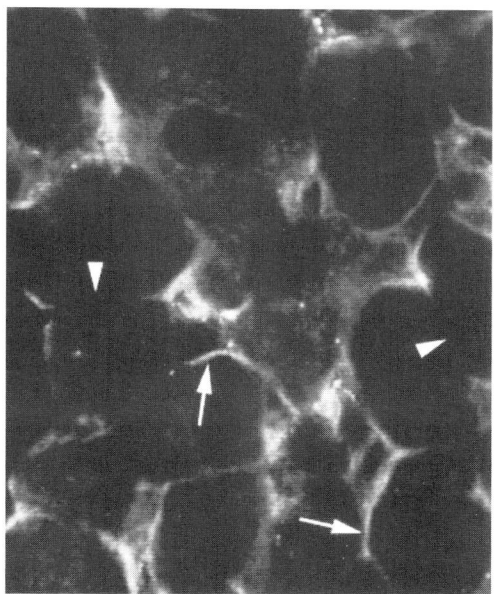

A   B

FIGURE 7.2. Localization of actin **(A)** and oatp1 **(B)** in a section of rat liver by confocal immunofluorescence microscopy. An aldehyde-fixed section of rat liver was exposed to rabbit oatp1 antiserum and to FITC-phalloidin. Anti-oatp1 distribution was visualized in the same section by Cy3-linked second antibody. **A:** Actin is especially abundant around the bile canaliculi (*arrowheads*). **B:** Oatp1 is present on the sinusoidal (basolateral) plasma membrane (*arrows*) and is not present in areas identified as bile canaliculi (*arrowheads*). (With acknowledgment to Dr. Phyllis M. Novikoff.)

hepatocyte (Fig. 7.2), and was seen to be evenly distributed across the lobule (89,96). Interestingly, in the kidney, oatp1 was localized to the apical plasma membrane of epithelial cells of the S_3 segment of the proximal tubule, located in the outer medulla (89). Immunoblot analysis reveals that renal oatp1 migrates slightly higher than the liver protein and is sensitive to reduction (89). Whether this renal protein is indeed oatp1 or represents a newly described related protein that has been termed oatp5 (accession number: AF053317), remains to be determined. Although oatp1 was not detected by Northern blot of mRNA obtained from whole brain, reverse-transcriptase polymerase chain reaction (RT-PCR) of mRNA obtained from the choroid plexus revealed its presence in that tissue that expresses numerous otherwise liver-specific proteins (97). Results were confirmed by *in situ* hybridization analysis of whole brain, and by immunoblot analysis of choroid plexus proteins (96,97). Other studies indicated that oatp2 is also present in the choroid plexus (98). Presumably, these proteins are involved in permeability of specific solutes across the blood–brain barrier.

Transport Function of Oatp1

Initial studies characterized transport function of oatp1 following its expression in *Xenopus* oocytes (77,99). Subsequently, studies were performed in HeLa cells transiently cotransfected with vaccinia virus and an oatp1 expression plasmid (100–102). These studies revealed a relatively broad range of substrates for oatp1-mediated transport that included BSP, taurocholate, and 17β-D-glucuronide. Intensive but unsuccessful efforts were made to establish a cell line that constitutively expressed active oatp1. Because of the possibility that expressed oatp1 could permit cells to take up potentially toxic amounts of constituents of the cell medium, HeLa cells were transfected with a plasmid in which oatp1 expression was under regulation of a metal-lothionein promoter (103). This led to establishment of cell lines in which oatp1 was not expressed unless cells were induced for 1 to 2 days with zinc. Cells in which oatp1 expression was not induced had essentially no uptake of taurocholate or BSP. In contrast, following zinc induction, uptake of these compounds was rapid. Studies in these cells showed that oatp1-mediated transport was Na⁺-independent, bidirectional, saturable, and of high affinity (103). Studies in hepatocytes suggested that BSP uptake might be associated with HCO_3^- exchange (67). This possibility was tested directly in the stably transfected cell system by examining the rates of taurocholate-dependent HCO_3^- efflux from alkali-loaded noninduced and induced cells that had been loaded with the pH sensitive dye BCECF (104). Addition of taurocholate to the outside of oatp1-expressing cells led to a rapid fall in intracellular pH, but had no effect on nonexpressing cells. These studies show directly that oatp1 is an ion exchanger. Subsequent studies performed in *Xenopus* oocytes that had been microinjected with oatp1 cDNA

showed that intracellular glutathione could also serve as an exchanged substrate (105). As glutathione concentrations are high within hepatocytes, this could serve as an important driving force for organic anion uptake. The prostaglandin transporter, pgt, another member of the oatp family, has also been shown to be an anion exchanger (106). A similar strategy for preparing CHO cells that stably express oatp1 has also been described (107). These transfected cells have a low level of oatp1 expression that can be increased considerably by addition of 5 mM butyrate to the cell medium for 24 hours.

As noted above, it is difficult to know the relative importance of any of the individual members of the oatp family on transport that are seen *in vivo*. An approach to answering this question was developed in a study in which antisense oligonucleotides to ntcp or oatp1 were co-injected into *Xenopus* oocytes along with total rat liver mRNA (108). The ntcp antisense oligonucleotide blocked the expression of Na⁺-dependent taurocholate uptake by approximately 95%. The oatp1 antisense oligonucleotide had no effect on Na⁺-dependent taurocholate uptake, but reduced Na⁺-independent taurocholate uptake by 80% and BSP uptake by 50%. Although these studies cannot be interpreted in a strictly quantitative way, they suggest that ntcp and oatp1 likely account for a substantial proportion of hepatocyte organic anion transport.

Modulation of Oatp1 Transport Activity

A number of physiologic perturbations have been associated with altered oatp1 expression and function. In regenerating liver following two-thirds partial hepatectomy, influx of bilirubin falls by approximately 50% within 6 hours of surgery and returns to normal by 4 days (109). Interestingly, hepatic oatp1 and oatp2 mRNA and protein levels show a similar pattern of expression during regeneration (63). As regenerating liver in many ways recapitulates ontogeny of liver development, studies were also performed in the developing rat liver. Uptake of BSP in hepatocytes prepared from 3-week-old animals was reduced by approximately 70% as compared to adults (96). There was little oatp1 expression in liver until animals were 1 month of age, and this correlated with mRNA expression (96,110). Of note is the fact that oatp1 protein in the choroid plexus of 1-day-old rats was essentially the same as in the adult, although examination of its subcellular distribution showed a major intracellular pool in contrast to an apical plasma membrane distribution in the adult choroid plexus (96). The large differences in oatp1 expression seen in choroid plexus and liver suggest the presence of potent organ-specific transcription factors (111).

Oatp1 expression is also modulated following endotoxin administration and during cholestatic events. Eighteen hours following endotoxin administration to rats, uptake of indocyanine green by their isolated perfused livers is reduced by 40% as compared to controls (112). Although oatp1 mRNA was unchanged, oatp1 protein expression was reduced by 50%. Following 3 to 7 days of bile duct ligation, oatp1 mRNA and protein expression are reduced by approximately 50% (113). Cholestasis due to administration of ethinyl estradiol for 5 days to rats was associated with an 80% to 90% reduction in expression of oatp1 mRNA and protein (114). The time course over which reduced oatp1 protein expression takes place during cholestasis is relatively long, and the mechanism by which it occurs is not known. As bile acids have been found to be noncompetitive inhibitors of BSP uptake by short-term cultured rat hepatocytes, even following acute exposure (115), it is reasonable to hypothesize that they may play a role in this process. A more rapid reduction in BSP transport was observed following exposure of hepatocytes to extracellular ATP (116). Uptake was reduced by 80% within minutes and evidence was presented that this effect was mediated by a unique hepatocyte cell surface purinergic receptor. Subsequent studies demonstrated that extracellular ATP reduces the V_{max} for transport of BSP by rat hepatocytes without altering K_m (117). Similar reduced transport also occurs within minutes following incubation of hepatocytes with the phosphatase inhibitors okadaic acid or calyculin A (117). Immunoprecipitation of biotinylated cell surface proteins demonstrated that oatp1 remains on the cell surface after incubation of hepatocytes in ATP or okadaic acid,

indicating that loss of transport activity under these conditions is not caused by removal of oatp1 from the cell surface. However, when hepatocytes were preloaded for 2 hours with inorganic ^{32}P, subsequent short-term incubation in extracellular ATP resulted in serine phosphorylation of oatp1 (Fig. 7.3) with the appearance of a single major tryptic phosphopeptide. This phosphopeptide comigrated with one of four phosphopeptides resulting from incubation of cells with okadaic acid. Phosphorylation of oatp1 does not occur in stably transfected HeLa cells, and transport of BSP by these cells is unaffected by incubation with extracellular ATP or phosphatase inhibitors, suggesting that they lack the kinase that mediates this effect. The physiologic consequences of downregulation of organic anion transport during cholestasis and with extracellular ATP are only speculative at this time. In conditions resulting in cellular injury, there may be local increases of extracellular ATP, reducing the ability of neighboring hepatocytes to extract organic anions from the blood. This could be a protective event, by keeping potentially toxic compounds from entering the cell, or it could exacerbate the consequences of an already reduced functional state. These studies indicate that the phosphorylation state of the transporter may be an important determinant of its function, and that simple quantitation of protein and mRNA expression may not be sufficient to explain all events in which organic anion transport is perturbed.

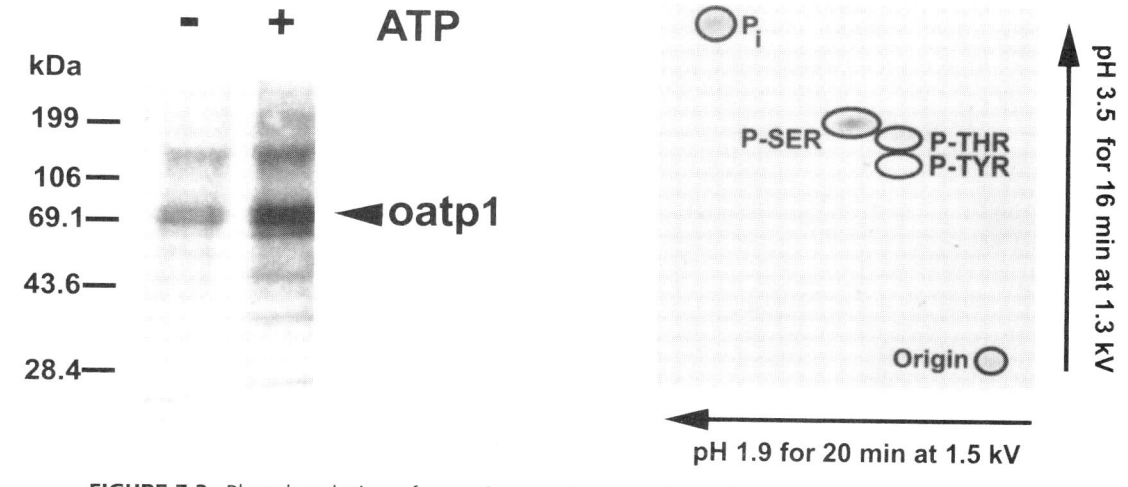

FIGURE 7.3. Phosphorylation of organic anion transporting polypeptide 1 (*oatp1*) following a 10-minute exposure of hepatocytes to extracellular adenosine triphosphate (*ATP*). **A:** Isolated rat hepatocytes were loaded for 2 hours with inorganic ^{32}P. Following an additional 10-minute exposure to buffer alone or buffer supplemented with 5 mM ATP, as indicated in the figure, cells were lysed and were subjected to immunoprecipitation using an oatp1-specific antibody. Following sodium dodecyl sulfate–polyacrylamide gel electrophoresis (SDS-PAGE), transfer to nitrocellulose, and radioautography, oatp1 was seen to have become phosphorylated. **B:** A nitrocellulose strip corresponding to immunoprecipitated oatp1 was excised and subjected to acid hydrolysis, two-dimensional electrophoresis, and radioautography. Migration of unlabeled amino acid standards was revealed by subsequent exposure of the plate to ninhydrin. As seen in the figure, oatp1 was phosphorylated exclusively on serine. (With acknowledgment to Drs. Joseph S. Glavy and George A. Orr.)

ACKNOWLEDGMENTS

The authors would like to acknowledge their support by National Institutes of Health grants DK 23026 (A.W.W.), DK 41296 (A.W.W.), and HD20632 (F.J.S.).

REFERENCES

1. Scharschmidt BF, Waggoner JG, Berk PD. Hepatic organic anion uptake in the rat. *J Clin Invest* 1975;56:1280–1292.

2. Stollman YR, Gartner U, Theilmann L, et al. Hepatic bilirubin uptake in the isolated perfused rat liver is not facilitated by albumin binding. *J Clin Invest* 1983;72:718–723.

3. Inoue M, Hirata E, Morino Y, et al. The role of albumin in the hepatic transport of bilirubin: Studies in mutant analbuminemic rats. *J Biochem* 1985;97:737–743.

4. Goresky CA. A linear method for determining liver sinusoidal and extravascular volumes. *Am J Physiol* 1963;204:626–640.

5. Grisham JW, Nopanitaya W, Compagno J, et al. Scanning electron microscopy of normal rat liver: the surface structure of its cells and tissue components. *Am J Anat* 1976;144:295–322.

6. Zucker SD, Goessling W, Gollan JL. Kinetics of bilirubin transfer between serum albumin and membrane vesicles. *J Biol Chem* 1995;270:1074–1081.

7. Boyer JL, Meier PJ. Characterizing mechanisms of hepatic bile acid transport utilizing isolated membrane vesicles. *Methods Enzymol* 1990;192:517–533.

8. Meier PJ. Molecular mechanisms of hepatic bile salt transport from sinusoidal blood into bile. *Am J Physiol* 1995;269: G801–G812.

9. Hagenbuch BM, Meier PJ. Sinusoidal (basolateral) bile salt uptake systems of hepatocytes. *Semin Liver Dis* 1996;16: 129–136.

10. Duffy MC, Blitzer BL, Boyer JL. Direct determination of the driving forces for taurocholate uptake into rat liver plasma membrane vesicles. *J Clin Invest* 1983;72:1470–1481.

11. Meier PJ, Boyer JL. Preparation of basolateral (sinusoidal) and canalicular plasma membrane vesicles for the study of hepatic transport processes. *Methods Enzymol* 1990;192:534–545.

12. Hardison WG, Bellentani S, Heasley V, et al. Specificity of an Na⁺-dependent taurocholate transport site in isolated rat hepatocytes. *Am J Physiol* 1984;246:G477–G483.

13. Hardison WG, Heasley VL, Shellhamer DF. Specificity of the hepatocyte Na(+)-dependent taurocholate transporter: influence of side chain length and charge. *Hepatology* 1991;13: 68–72.

14. Kramer W, Stengelin S, Baringhaus KH, et al. Substrate specificity of the ileal and the hepatic Na(+)/bile acid cotransporters of the rabbit. I. Transport studies with membrane vesicles and cell lines expressing the cloned transporters. *J Lipid Res* 1999; 40:1604–1617.

15. Baringhaus KH, Matter H, Stengelin S, et al. Substrate specificity of the ileal and the hepatic Na(+)/bile acid cotransporters of the rabbit. II. A reliable 3D QSAR pharmacophore model for the ileal Na(+)/bile acid cotransporter. *J Lipid Res* 1999;40: 2158–2168.

16. Blitzer BL, Lyons L. Enhancement of Na⁺-dependent bile acid uptake by albumin: Direct demonstration in rat basolateral liver plasma membrane vesicles. *Am J Physiol* 1985;249:G34–G38.

17. Lidofsky SD, Fitz JG, Weisiger RA, et al. Hepatic taurocholate uptake is electrogenic and influenced by transmembrane potential difference. *Am J Physiol* 1993;264:G478–G485.

18. Weinman SA. Electrogenicity of Na(+)-coupled bile acid transporters. *Yale J Biol Med* 1997;70:331–340.

19. Hagenbuch B, Stieger B, Foguet M, et al. Functional expression cloning and characterization of the hepatocyte Na⁺/bile acid cotransport system. *Proc Natl Acad Sci USA* 1991;88: 10629–10633.

20. Love MW, Dawson PA. New insights into bile acid transport. *Curr Opin Lipidol* 1998;9:225–229.

21. Hallen S, Branden M, Dawson PA, et al. Membrane insertion scanning of the human ileal sodium/bile acid co-transporter. *Biochemistry* 1999;38:11379–11388.

22. Hagenbuch B, Meier PJ. Molecular cloning, chromosomal localization, and functional characterization of a human liver Na⁺/bile acid cotransporter. *J Clin Invest* 1994;93:1326–1331.

23. Cohn MA, Rounds DJ, Karpen SJ, et al. Assignment of a rat liver Na⁺/bile acid cotransporter gene to chromosome 6q24. *Mamm Genome* 1995;6:60.

24. Cattori V, Eckhardt U, Hagenbuch B. Molecular cloning and functional characterization of two alternatively spliced Ntcp isoforms from mouse liver. *Biochim Biophys Acta* 1999;1445: 154–159.

25. Ananthanarayanan M, Ng OC, Boyer JL, et al. Characterization of cloned rat liver Na(+)-bile acid cotransporter using peptide and fusion protein antibodies. *Am J Physiol* 1994;267: G637–G643.

26. Stieger B, Hagenbuch B, Landmann L, et al. In situ localization of the hepatocytic Na⁺/taurocholate cotransporting polypeptide in rat liver. *Gastroenterology* 1994;107:1781–1787.

27. Liu X, Brouwer KL, Gan LS, et al. Partial maintenance of taurocholate uptake by adult rat hepatocytes cultured in a collagen sandwich configuration. *Pharm Res* 1998;15:1533–1539.

28. Boyer JL, Hagenbuch B, Ananthanarayanan M, et al. Phylogenic and ontogenic expression of hepatocellular bile acid transport. *Proc Natl Acad Sci USA* 1993;90:435–438.

29. Suchy FJ, Bucuvalas JC, Goodrich AL, et al. Taurocholate transport and Na⁺-ATPase activity in fetal and neonatal rat liver plasma membrane vesicles. *Am J Physiol* 1986;251: G665–G673.

30. Hardikar W, Ananthanarayanan M, Suchy FJ. Differential ontogenic regulation of basolateral and canalicular bile acid transport proteins in rat liver. *J Biol Chem* 1995;270: 20841–20846.

31. Meier PJ, Eckhardt U, Schroeder A, et al. Substrate specificity of sinusoidal bile acid and organic anion uptake systems in rat and human liver. *Hepatology* 1997;26:1667–1677.

32. Kouzuki H, Suzuki H, Stieger B, et al. Characterization of the transport properties of organic anion transporting polypeptide 1 (oatp1) and Na(+)/taurocholate cotransporting polypeptide (Ntcp): comparative studies on the inhibitory effect of their possible substrates in hepatocytes and cDNA-transfected COS-7 cells. *J Pharmacol Exp Ther* 2000;292:505–511.

33. Schroeder A, Eckhardt U, Stieger B, et al. Substrate specificity of the rat liver Na(+)-bile salt cotransporter in Xenopus laevis oocytes and in CHO cells. *Am J Physiol* 1998;274:G370–G375.

34. Platte HD, Honscha W, Schuh K, et al. Functional characterization of the hepatic sodium-dependent taurocholate transporter stably transfected into an immortalized liver-derived cell line and V79 fibroblasts. *Eur J Cell Biol* 1996;70:54–60.

35. Kouzuki H, Suzuki H, Ito K, et al. Contribution of sodium taurocholate co-transporting polypeptide to the uptake of its possible substrates into rat hepatocytes. *J Pharmacol Exp Ther* 1998;286:1043–1050.

36. Friesema EC, Docter R, Moerings EP, et al. Identification of thyroid hormone transporters. *Biochem Biophys Res Commun* 1999;254:497–501.

37. Karpen SJ, Sun AQ, Kudish B, et al. Multiple factors regulate the rat liver basolateral sodium-dependent bile acid cotransporter gene promoter. *J Biol Chem* 1996;271:15211–15221.

38. Denson LA, Jacobs HC, McClure MH, et al. A liver-enriched homeobox protein, hex, trans-activates the rat liver Na+/taurocholate transporter (ntcp) gene promoter and is downregulated by endotoxin and associated cytokines. *Hepatology* 1998;28:505A.

39. Denson LA, Auld KL, Schiek DS, et al. Interleukin-1beta suppresses retinoid transactivation of two hepatic transporter genes involved in bile formation. *J Biol Chem* 2000;275:8835–8843.

40. Ganguly TC, Liu Y, Hyde JF, et al. Prolactin increases hepatic Na+/taurocholate co-transport activity and messenger RNA post partum. *Biochem J* 1994;303:33–36.

41. Liu Y, Ganguly T, Hyde JF, et al. Prolactin increases mRNA encoding Na(+)-TC cotransport polypeptide and hepatic Na(+)-TC cotransport. *Am J Physiol* 1995;268:G11–G17.

42. Ganguly TC, O'Brien ML, Karpen SJ, et al. Regulation of the rat liver sodium-dependent bile acid cotransporter gene by prolactin. Mediation of transcriptional activation by Stat5. *J Clin Invest* 1997;99:2906–2914.

43. Botham KM, Suckling KE. The effect of dibutyryl cyclic AMP on the uptake of taurocholic acid by isolated rat liver cells. *Biochim Biophys Acta* 1986;883:26–32.

44. Grune S, Engelking LR, Anwer MS. Role of intracellular calcium and protein kinases in the activation of hepatic Na+/taurocholate cotransport by cyclic AMP. *J Biol Chem* 1993;268:17734–17741.

45. Mukhopadhayay S, Ananthanarayanan M, Stieger B, et al. cAMP increases liver Na+-taurocholate cotransport by translocating transporter to plasma membranes. *Am J Physiol* 1997;273:G842–G848.

46. Mukhopadhyay S, Ananthanarayanan M, Stieger B, et al. Sodium taurocholate cotransporting polypeptide is a serine, threonine phosphoprotein and is dephosphorylated by cyclic adenosine monophosphate. *Hepatology* 1998;28:1629–1636.

47. Mukhopadhyay S, Webster CR, Anwer MS. Role of protein phosphatases in cyclic AMP-mediated stimulation of hepatic Na+/taurocholate cotransport. *J Biol Chem* 1998;273:30039–30045.

48. Green RM, Beier D, Gollan JL. Regulation of hepatocyte bile salt transporters by endotoxin and inflammatory cytokines in rodents. *Gastroenterology* 1996;111:193–198.

49. Moseley RH, Wang W, Takeda H, et al. Effect of endotoxin on bile acid transport in rat liver: a potential model for sepsis-associated cholestasis. *Am J Physiol* 1996;271:G137–G146.

50. Gartung C, Ananthanarayanan M, Rahman MA, S et al. Down-regulation of expression and function of the rat liver Na+/bile acid cotransporter in extrahepatic cholestasis. *Gastroenterology* 1996;110:199–209.

51. Sturm E, Zimmerman TL, Crawford AR, et al. Endotoxin-stimulated macrophages decrease bile acid uptake in WIF-B cells, a rat hepatoma hybrid cell line. *Hepatology* 2000;31:124–130.

52. Trauner M, Meier PJ, Boyer JL. Molecular regulation of hepatocellular transport systems in cholestasis. *J Hepatol* 1999;31:165–178.

53. Trauner M, Fickert P, Stauber RE. Inflammation-induced cholestasis. *J Gastroenterol Hepatol* 1999;14:946–959.

54. Gartung C, Matern S. Molecular regulation of sinusoidal liver bile acid transporters during cholestasis. *Yale J Biol Med* 1997;70:355–363.

55. Trauner M, Arrese M, Lee H, et al. Endotoxin downregulates rat hepatic ntcp gene expression via decreased activity of critical transcription factors. *J Clin Invest* 1998;101:2092–2100.

56. Shneider BL, Fox VL, Schwarz KB, et al. Hepatic basolateral sodium-dependent-bile acid transporter expression in two unusual cases of hypercholanemia and in extrahepatic biliary atresia. *Hepatology* 1997;25:1176–1183.

57. Kullak-Ublick GA, Beuers U, Paumgartner G. Hepatobiliary transport. *J Hepatol* 2000;32:3–18.

58. Koopen NR, Wolters H, Voshol P, et al. Decreased Na+-dependent taurocholate uptake and low expression of the sinusoidal Na+-taurocholate cotransporting protein (Ntcp) in livers of mdr2 P-glycoprotein-deficient mice. *J Hepatol* 1999;30:14–21.

59. Gartung C, Schuele S, Schlosser SF, et al. Expression of the rat liver Na+/taurocholate cotransporter is regulated in vivo by retention of biliary constituents but not their depletion. *Hepatology* 1997;25:284–290.

60. Koopen NR, Wolters H, Muller M, et al. Hepatic bile salt flux does not modulate level and activity of the sinusoidal Na+-taurocholate cotransporter (ntcp) in rats. *J Hepatol* 1997;27:699–706.

61. Green RM, Gollan JL, Hagenbuch B, et al. Regulation of hepatocyte bile salt transporters during hepatic regeneration. *Am J Physiol* 1997;273:G621–G627.

62. Vos TA, Ros JE, Havinga R, et al. Regulation of hepatic transport systems involved in bile secretion during liver regeneration in rats. *Hepatology* 1999;29:1833–1839.

63. Gerloff T, Geier A, Stieger B, et al. Differential expression of basolateral and canalicular organic anion transporters during regeneration of rat liver. *Gastroenterology* 1999;117:1408–1415.

64. Zhu Q-S, von Dippe P, Xing W, et al. Membrane topology and cell surface targeting of microsomal epoxide hydrolase. *J Biol Chem* 1999;274:27898–27904.

65. Honscha W, Platte HD, Oesch F, et al. Relationship between the microsomal epoxide hydrolase and the hepatocellular transport of bile acids and xenobiotics. *Biochem J* 1995;311:975–979.

66. Wolkoff AW, Samuelson AC, Johansen KL, et al. Influence of Cl- on organic anion transport in short-term cultured rat hepatocytes and isolated perfused rat liver. *J Clin Invest* 1987;79:1259–1268.

67. Min AD, Johansen KJ, Campbell CG, et al. Role of chloride and intracellular pH on the activity of the rat hepatocyte organic anion transporter. *J Clin Invest* 1991;87:1496–1502.

68. Stremmel W, Gerber MA, Glezerov V, et al. Physicochemical and immunohistological studies of a sulfobromophthalein- and bilirubin-binding protein from rat liver plasma membranes. *J Clin Invest* 1983;71:1796–1805.

69. Stremmel W, Berk PD. Hepatocellular uptake of sulfobromophthalein and bilirubin is selectively inhibited by an antibody to the liver plasma membrane sulfobromophthalein/bilirubin binding protein. *J Clin Invest* 1986;78:822–826.

70. Berk PD, Potter BJ, Stremmel W. Role of plasma membrane ligand-binding proteins in the hepatocellular uptake of albumin-bound organic anions. *Hepatology* 1987;7:165–176.

71. Wolkoff AW, Chung CT. Identification, purification, and partial characterization of an organic anion binding protein from rat liver cell plasma membrane. *J Clin Invest* 1980;65:1152–1161.

72. Goeser T, Nakata R, Braly LF, et al. The rat hepatocyte plasma membrane organic anion binding protein is immunologically related to the mitochondrial F1 adenosine triphosphatase beta-subunit. *J Clin Invest* 1990;86:220–227.

73. Sottocasa GL, Baldini G, Sandri G, et al. Reconstitution in vitro of sulfobromophthalein transport by bilitranslocase. *Biochim Biophys Acta* 1982;685:123–128.

74. Battiston L, Passamonti S, Macagno A, et al. The bilirubin-binding motif of bilitranslocase and its relation to conserved motifs in ancient biliproteins. *Biochem Biophys Res Commun* 1998;247:687–692.

75. Battiston L, Macagno A, Passamonti S, et al. Specific sequence-

directed antibilitranslocase antibodies as a tool to detect potentially bilirubin-binding proteins in different tissues of the rat. *FEBS Lett* 1999;453:351–355.

76. Jacquemin E, Hagenbuch B, Stieger B, et al. Expression of the hepatocellular chloride-dependent sulfobromophthalein uptake system in Xenopus laevis oocytes. *J Clin Invest* 1991;88:2146–2149.

77. Jacquemin E, Hagenbuch B, Stieger B, et al. Expression cloning of a rat liver Na⁺-independent organic anion transporter. *Proc Natl Acad Sci USA* 1994;91:133–137.

78. Wolkoff AW. Hepatocellular sinusoidal membrane organic anion transport and transporters. *Semin Liver Dis* 1996;16:121–127.

79. Hagenbuch B, Adler I-D, Schmid W. Molecular cloning and functional characterization of the mouse organic-anion-transporting polypeptide 1 (oatp1) and mapping of the gene to chromosome X. *Biochem J* 2000;345:115–120.

80. Noé B, Hagenbuch B, Stieger B, et al. Isolation of a multispecific organic anion and cardiac glycoside transporter from rat brain. *Proc Natl Acad Sci USA* 1997;94:10346–10350.

81. Abe T, Kakyo M, Sakagami H, et al. Molecular characterization and tissue distribution of a new organic anion transporter subtype (oatp3) that transports thyroid hormones and taurocholate and comparison with oatp2. *J Biol Chem* 1999;273:22395–22401.

82. Saito H, Masuda S, Inui K-I. Cloning and functional characterization of a novel rat organic anion transporter mediating basolateral uptake of methotrexate in the kidney. *J Biol Chem* 1996;271:20719–20725.

83. Masuda M, Ibaramoto K, Takeuchi A, et al. Cloning and functional characterization of a new multispecific organic anion transporter, oat-k2, in rat kidney. *Mol Pharmacol* 1999;55:743–752.

84. Kanai N, Lu R, Satriano JA, et al. Identification and characterization of a prostaglandin transporter. *Science* 1995;268:866–869.

85. Lu R, Kanai N, Bao Y, et al. Cloning, in vitro expression, and tissue distribution of a human prostaglandin transporter cDNA (hPGT). *J Clin Invest* 1996;98:1142–1149.

86. Kullak-Ublick G-A, Hagenbuch B, Stieger B, et al. Molecular and functional characterization of an organic anion transporting polypeptide cloned from human liver. *Gastroenterology* 1995;109:1274–1282.

87. Kakyo M, Unno M, Tokui T, et al. Molecular characterization and functional regulation of a novel rat liver-specific organic anion transporter rlst-1. *Gastroenterology* 1999;117:770–775.

88. Abe H, Kakyo M, Tokui T, et al. Identification of a novel gene family encoding human liver-specific organic anion transporter LST-1. *J Biol Chem* 1999;274:17159–17163.

89. Bergwerk A, Shi X, Ford A, et al. Immunologic distribution of an organic anion transport protein in rat liver and kidney. *Am J Physiol* 1996;271:G231–G238.

90. Kakyo M, Sakagami H, Nishio T, et al. Immunohistochemical distribution and functional characterization of an organic transporting polypeptide 2 (oatp2). *FEBS Lett* 1999;445:343–346.

91. Reichel C, Gao B, VanMontfoort J, et al. Localization and function of the organic anion-transporting polypeptide oatp2 in rat liver. *Gastroenterology* 1999;117:688–695.

92. Hsiang B, Zhu Y, Wang Z, et al. A novel human hepatic organic anion transporting polypeptide (OATP2). *J Biol Chem* 1999;274:37161–37168.

93. Konig J, Cui Y, Nies AS, et al. A novel human hepatic organic anion transporting polypeptide localized to the basolateral hepatocyte membrane. *Am J Physiol* 2000;278:G156–G164.

94. Konig J, Cui Y, Nies AS, et al. Localization and genomic organization of a new hepatocellular organic anion transporting polypeptide. *J Biol Chem* 2000;in press:

95. Gartner U, Stockert RJ, Levine WG, et al. Effect of nafenopin on the uptake of bilirubin and sulfobromophthalein by isolated perfused rat liver. *Gastroenterology* 1982;83:1163–1169.

96. Angeletti R, Bergwerk A, Novikoff PM, et al. Dichotomous development of the organic anion transport protein in liver and choroid plexus. *Am J Physiol* 1999;275:C882–C887.

97. Angeletti R, Novikoff PM, Juvvadi S, et al. The choroid plexus epithelium is the site of the organic anion transport protein in the brain. *Proc Natl Acad Sci USA* 1997;94:283–286.

98. Gao B, Stieger B, Noé B, et al. Localization of the organic anion transporting polypeptide 2 (oatp2) in capillary endothelium and choroid plexus epithelium of rat brain. *J Histochem Cytochem* 1999;47:1255–1264.

99. Kullak-Ublick G-A, Hagenbuch B, Stieger B, et al. Functional characterization of the basolateral rat liver organic anion transporting polypeptide. *Hepatology* 1994;20:411–416.

100. Kanai N, Lu R, Bao Y, et al. Estradiol 17??D-glucuronide is a high-affinity substrate for oatp organic anion transporter. *Am J Physiol* 1996;270:F326–F331.

101. Kanai N, Lu R, Bao Y, et al. Transient expression of oatp organic anion transporter in mammalian cells: identification of candidate substrates. *Am J Physiol* 1996;270:F319–F325.

102. Cvetkovic M, Leake B, Fromm MF, et al. Oatp and p-glycoprotein transporters mediate the cellular uptake and excretion of fexofenadine. *Drug Metab Disp* 1999;27:866–871.

103. Shi X, Bai S, Ford AC, et al. Stable inducible expression of a functional rat liver organic anion transport protein in HeLa cells. *J Biol Chem* 1995;270:25591–25595.

104. Satlin LM, Amin V, Wolkoff AW. Organic anion transporting polypeptide mediates organic anion/HCO₃⁻ exchange. *J Biol Chem* 1997;272:26340–26345.

105. Li L, Lee TK, Meier PJ, et al. Identification of glutathione as a driving force and leukotriene C4 as a substrate for oatp1, the hepatic sinusoidal organic solute transporter. *J Biol Chem* 1998;273:16184–16191.

106. Chan BS, Satriano JA, Pucci M, et al. Mechanism of prostaglandin E2 transport across the plasma membrane of HeLa cells and Xenopus oocytes expressing the prostaglandin transporter "PGT." *J Biol Chem* 1998;273:6689–6697.

107. Eckhardt U, Schroeder A, Stieger B, et al. Polyspecific substrate uptake by the hepatic organic anion transporter oatp1 in stably transfected CHO cells. *Am J Physiol* 1999;276:G1037–G1042.

108. Hagenbuch B, Scharschmidt BF, Meier PJ. Effect of antisense oligonucleotides on the expression of hepatocellular bile acid and organic anion uptake systems in *Xenopus laevis* oocytes. *Biochem J* 1996;316:901–904.

109. Gartner U, Stockert RJ, Morell AG, et al. Modulation of the transport of bilirubin and asialoorosomucoid during liver regeneration. *Hepatology* 1981;1:99–106.

110. Dubuisson C, Cresteil D, Desrochers M, et al. Ontogenic expression of the Na⁺-independent organic anion transporting polypeptide (oatp) in rat liver and kidney. *J Hepatol* 1996;25:932–940.

111. Yan C, Costa RH, Darnell JEJ, et al. Distinct positive and negative elements control the limited hepatocyte and choroid plexus expression of transthyretin in transgenic mice. *EMBO J* 1990;9:869–878.

112. Lund M, Kang L, Tygstrup N, et al. Effects of LPS on transport of indocyanine green and alanine uptake in perfused rat liver. *Am J Physiol* 1999;277:G91–G100.

113. Dumont M, Jacquemin E, D'Hont C, et al. Expression of the liver Na⁺-independent organic anion transporting polypeptide

(oatp-1) in rats with bile duct ligation. *J Hepatol* 1997;27: 1051–1056.

114. Simon FR, Fortune J, Iwahashi M, et al. Ethinyl estradiol cholestasis involves alterations in expression of liver sinusoidal transporters. *Am J Physiol* 1996;271:G1043–G1052.

115. Ishii K, Wolkoff AW. Inhibition of rat hepatocyte organic anion transport by bile acids. *Am J Physiol* 1994;267:G458–G464.

116. Campbell CG, Spray DC, Wolkoff AW. Extracellular ATP^{4-} modulates organic anion transport by rat hepatocytes. *J Biol Chem* 1993;268:15399–15404.

117. Glavy JS, Wu SM, Wang PJ, et al. Down-regulation by extracellular ATP of rat hepatocyte organic anion transport is mediated by serine phosphorylation of oatp1. *J Biol Chem* 2000;275: 1479–1484.

The Liver: Biology and Pathobiology, Fourth Edition, edited by I. M. Arias, J. L. Boyer, F. V. Chisari, N. Fausto, D. Schachter, and D. A. Shafritz.
Lippincott Williams & Wilkins, Philadelphia © 2001.

8

THE HEPATOCYTE SURFACE: DYNAMIC POLARITY

PAMELA L. TUMA
ANN L. HUBBARD

The hepatocyte, the major epithelial cell of the liver, performs many crucial functions that stem largely from its strategic position between two different environments, the blood plasma and the bile. The functions carried out at the two fronts are distinct, which means that the hepatocyte surface is asymmetric or polarized.

Polarity is a fundamental characteristic of most eukaryotic cells, either as a transient phenomenon (e.g., in a moving fibroblast) or a permanent feature (e.g., of an epithelial layer) (1). In epithelial cells, polarity is evident at many levels. At the cell surface, the basolateral and apical membrane domains face different environments (internal and external, respectively) and each membrane contains a distinct set of proteins and lipids (2). The stereotypical locations of different organelles within a particular epithelial cell type are additional indicators of polarity. For example, the Golgi is positioned between the nucleus and apical surface in most epithelial cells; this relationship reflects the polarized organization of microtubules. Acquisition of the fully polarized phenotype requires coordination of multiple processes: cell-substrate and cell-cell adhesion; activation of multiple signal transduction pathways; reorganization of cytoskeletal elements; assembly of tight and adherens junctions; and

P. L. **Tuma** and A. L. **Hubbard:** Department of Cell Biology and Anatomy, Johns Hopkins University School of Medicine, Baltimore, Maryland 21205-2196.

polarized vesicle traffic. Furthermore, although the epithelial phenotype is temporally and spatially stable, its maintenance requires all of the above processes to be continuously "on," prompting the addition of "dynamic" to the title. (Ref. 3 has a fresh perspective on polarity.)

This chapter focuses on the pathways and mechanisms of plasma membrane (PM) biogenesis and turnover in polarized hepatocytes. These pathways include organelles of the cell's biosynthetic and endocytic pathways (see Chapters 10 and 11). After presenting selected features of hepatocyte organization, we describe several experimental systems used to study hepatocyte PM dynamics. We then present our current understanding of the pathways, sorting signals and targeting machinery used by these cells in the dynamic maintenance of their surface polarity. Vesicle formation and transport between successive compartments are essential features of the pathways and are covered elsewhere (see Chapters 9–11). Throughout, we raise unresolved issues to stimulate interest in solving them. We also draw on studies performed in different types of polarized epithelial cells. However, it is clear from research over the past decade that differences in the pathways and mechanisms of PM biogenesis and turnover exist between hepatocytes and simpler, bipolar epithelial cells. Thus, a full understanding will come only when comparable experiments are done on hepatocytes *in vivo*. Space limitations prevent us from citing all the work being done in this area; we cite reviews that we found particularly helpful and/or whose bibliographies were extensive. The reader is also directed to a review (4) and our 1994 chapter (5) (see website chapter 🖥 W-5).

HEPATOCYTE ORGANIZATION
Structural Aspects

Liver architecture, in which hepatocytes are arranged in cords, is unique among epithelial organs. An individual cell is polygonal and faces at least two blood sinusoids (the basal domain). A branched network of grooves between adjacent cells forms the bile canaliculus (apical domain), which in a single optical section can appear variously round or tubular (Fig. 8.1A,B). Such a polygonal shape means that hepato-

cytes do not have a single basolateral-to-apical axis as do the simple bipolar epithelial cells lining kidney tubules or the intestinal lumen. Moreover, hepatocyte organelles of the secretory and endocytic pathways must simultaneously serve these "fragmented" PM domains. The low magnification view of hepatocytes *in situ* (Fig. 8.1C) doesn't reveal many clues as to how this is accomplished. In fact, aside from the rough endoplasmic reticulum (ER), the major organelles (Golgi, secretory vesicles, endosomes, and lysosomes) composing the two pathways occupy a small fraction of the hepatocyte cytoplasm (Fig. 8.1D, shaded areas). Furthermore, the Golgi and lysosomes have seemingly paradoxical locations: they are concentrated around the apical pole despite the fact that they serve predominantly the sinu-

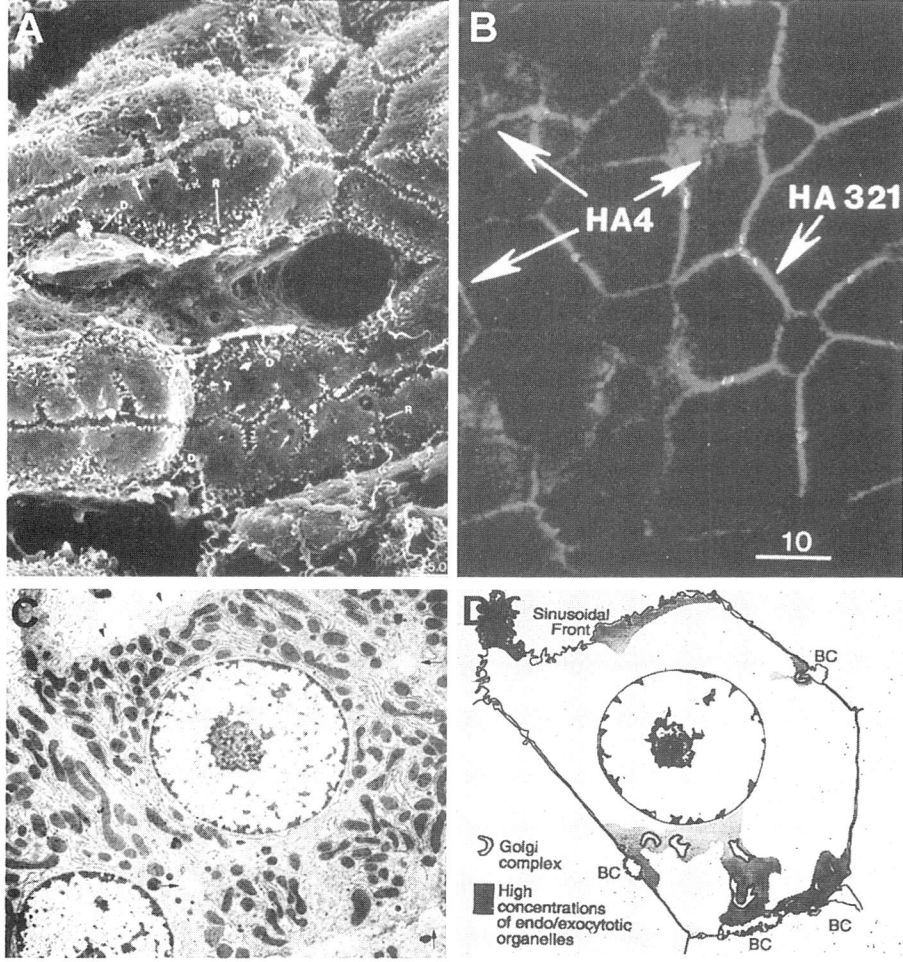

FIGURE 8.1. The architecture of the liver is unique. **A:** A scanning electron micrograph of a portion of a liver lobule. A continuous network of bile canaliculi (*BC*) runs along the exposed cell surfaces of the liver plate. **B:** The two distinct plasma membrane (PM) domains are visualized by immunofluorescence detection of the basolateral PM protein, HA321/BEN (*red*) and the apical PM protein, HA4/cell-CAM105/ecto-adenosine triphosphatase (ATPase) (*blue*). An electron micrograph of a hepatocyte **(C)** and a corresponding schematic drawing **(D)** highlight the "active zones" in vesicular trafficking. The major sorting organelles [*trans*-Golgi network (TGN) and endosomes] and transport vesicles are concentrated in small "clear" zones that are probably the most active in vesicle traffic. These zones are located between the Golgi and the apical PM and near the basolateral PM (the *shaded regions* in **D**). See Color Plate 1.

soidal pole. Most newly synthesized membrane and secretory proteins exiting the *trans*-Golgi network (TGN) are directed to the basolateral front, with less TGN-derived traffic directed to the apical front. Similarly, macromolecular cargo (including PM components) internalized at the sinusoidal front is delivered to lysosomes, the apical PM, or bile. Because we know that multiple vesicular steps in the biosynthetic and endocytic pathways rely on microtubules, this cytoskeletal system (and its associated motors) is strongly implicated as the link between the apical and basolateral regions of polarized epithelial cells (see Chapter 1 and website chapters 🖥 W-1 and W-2).

Molecular Aspects

The hepatocyte PM has long been studied as a biochemical entity, and the differences in the protein and lipid composition among the domains were appreciated early. Although disagreements about assignments for certain PM proteins continue, domain-specificity seems to be the general rule in hepatocytes and other epithelia. That is, in a particular cell type, an integral PM protein is restricted to a single PM domain (Fig. 8.1B). However, there is great plasticity in PM protein locations among epithelial cells in different organs; a basolateral PM protein in hepatocytes, e.g., NaK–adenosine triphosphatase (ATPase), might be apical in another organ, e.g., retinal pigment epithelial cells (6). The increasing number of examples of "protein location following function" has important implications for cell type-specific sorting and targeting mechanisms. Paradoxically, an important family of integral PM proteins involved in vesicle targeting, the t-SNAREs [target-soluble N-ethylmaleimide (NEM)–sensitive factor attachment protein (SNAP) receptors], do not conform to the general rule of domain specificity.

Although the PM lipids of epithelial cells do not show the same absolute domain specificity as do most classes of PM proteins, differences between the domains exist. In hepatocytes, as in most epithelial cells, sphingomyelin and cholesterol are relatively enriched in apical versus basolateral PM subcellular fractions. Additionally, 75% of the major hepatocyte gangliosides (GM$_1$ and GM$_2$) have been found in the PM, but individual domains have not been analyzed (7). Despite the apparent similarities with other epithelial cells, the lipid dynamics, if not the lipids themselves, of the hepatocyte apical PM must be unique since this PM functions as the site of bile secretion, which includes detergent-like bile salts, phosphatidylcholine (PC), and cholesterol (see Chapter 24). The fact that the PC present in the apical PM contains longer and more unsaturated fatty acyl chains than that in bile, which is predominantly sn1-16:0/sn2-18:1 or 2 (8), points to exquisite selectivity in the mechanisms for removal of PC from the apical PM. More detailed aspects of biliary transport of lipids are covered elsewhere (see Chapter 24). However, relevant to our discussion is the rate of PC release into bile, reported to be equivalent to 10% of the apical PM

outer (luminal) leaflet per minute *in vivo* (8). This extraordinary flux of lipid through the apical PM bilayer must place constraints on its physical structure.

Dynamic Aspects

The amount of traffic through the secretory and endocytic/transcytotic pathways of the hepatocyte is truly remarkable. In the secretory pathway, the quantity of plasma proteins made and shipped out each day by a single hepatocyte nearly equals the total cell content of protein (9); 120 × 10^3 albumin molecules are synthesized per minute per cell. Vesicles 200 to 400 nm in diameter deliver this and other secretory cargo to the basolateral PM, which increases its surface area by 0.5%/min/cell. Fluid phase endocytosis at the basolateral surface of hepatocytes is even more robust, with an estimated 8% of the PM domain surface area internalized per minute per cell (8). Despite this flux of membrane into and out of the basolateral PM, there is homeostasis in membrane surface area and identity. The dynamic nature of the apical PM is just as impressive. From studies of fluid phase transcytosis, 600 to 850 vesicles (100 nm in diameter) are estimated to fuse with the apical surface every minute (8). This means that the apical membrane surface area would double or triple every 20 minutes if there were no mechanism for removal of molecular components. Clearly, maintenance of the polarized phenotype is a continuous process.

EXPERIMENTAL SYSTEMS FOR STUDYING THE ITINERARIES OF PLASMA MEMBRANE PROTEINS AND LIPIDS
Cell Systems

There are advantages to studying PM dynamics in whole animals or the perfused liver: cell polarity and tissue architecture are maintained; and, since the liver is composed of 70% hepatocytes, organelles from a single cell type can be isolated in abundance and relative purity. Among the disadvantages are physiologic variation among animals; dilution of precursors, inhibitors, etc. throughout the whole body; and difficulties in quickly modulating experimental conditions (e.g., temperatures, inhibitors, etc.). Nonetheless, results from work in the whole organ have established the basic parameters of hepatocyte PM dynamics. This is important, since the fidelity and rates of many processes are much higher *in vivo* than they are in the *in vitro* cell systems so far examined (10).

Recent progress in understanding the molecular aspects of PM traffic in epithelial cells has come from the use of *in vitro* cell systems. Dissociation of liver tissue into isolated cells that were suitable for culture was first described over 25 years ago (5). However, the loss of structural polarity and mixing of membrane domains made them poor models for studies of polarity. The development of isolated couplets was a significant advance for short-term studies of polarized hepatocyte functions, such as transcytosis and bile formation (11). As the important role the extracellular matrix (ECM) plays in maintaining gene expression and promoting cell repolarization became apparent, investigators began culturing hepatocytes on different matrix components in various geometries and physical states. The most successful reconstitution of polarity has come from use of sandwiches of collagen gels or Matrigel (see refs. 12 and 13 and references therein). Despite these advances, the limited life span of primary hepatocytes and the difficulties in reproducibly obtaining such polarized cultures prompted many investigators to use secondary hepatocyte cell lines.

HepG2 Cells

The human hepatoma HepG2 is currently being used for studies of polarized membrane traffic. This line, which expresses many liver-specific genes, was generated in the late 1970s from liver tumor biopsies in which the histology presented as "well-differentiated hepatocellular carcinoma with a trabecular pattern (14)." In 1990 the existence of bile canalicular-like cysts within and between cultured HepG2 cells was reported (15); electron microscopy (EM) observations and one apical PM marker were used in this study. Unfortunately, little additional characterization has been reported, so the extent of polarity in the culture can only be estimated at 10%. Hoekstra and colleagues (16–18) have studied sphingolipid traffic in HepG2 cells.

WIF-B Cells

Cassio and colleagues (19,20) have generated many somatic cell hybrid lines in their studies of the genetic basis of liver-

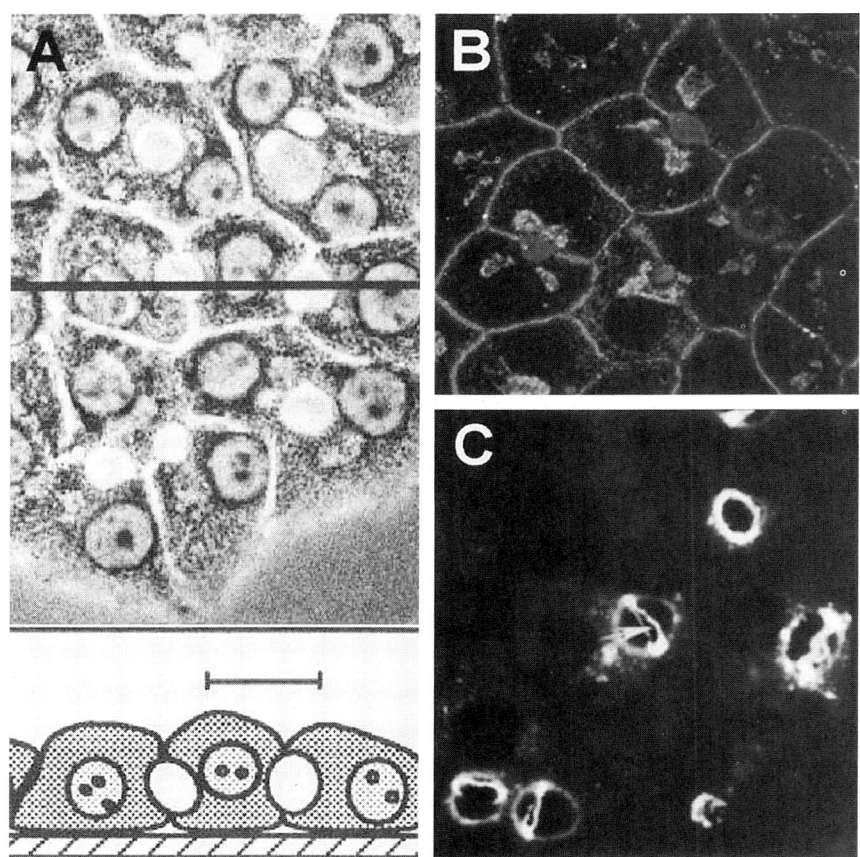

FIGURE 8.2. WIF-B cells are an *in vitro* model of polarized hepatocytes. **A:** The phase contrast morphology of living WIF-B cells is shown (**top**). The phase-lucent "blisters" between neighboring cells correspond to the "bile canalicular" or apical space. A cross-sectional "reconstruction" of the cell monolayer (**bottom panel**) taken along the line indicated in the **upper panel** shows that the bile canalicular spaces (BCs) are closed off from both the substrate and overlying medium. **B:** Triple immunofluorescence labeling of apical (*blue*), basolateral (*red*), and Golgi (*green*) proteins is shown in fully polarized WIF-B cells. The apical protein, HA4/ cell-CAM105/ecto–adenosine triphosphatase (ATPase), is localized to the membrane lining the dilated spaces, HA321/BEN is found along the basolateral surface, and albumin is concentrated at the Golgi. **C:** The tight junction protein, ZO-1 (*yellow*) marks the borders between the apical and basolateral domains. HA4/ cell-CAM105/ecto-ATPase is also labeled (*blue*) to mark the apical surface. See Color Plate 2.

specific gene expression. The WIF-B cells that we currently use were generated by fusion of the differentiated (i.e., expressing liver-specific genes) but unpolarized rat hepatoma cells (Fao) with human skin fibroblasts (WI-38 cells). Clonal selections ultimately yielded a polarized hepatic phenotype, the WIF12-1 cells, which exhibited a maximum apical polarity of 40%. That is, a maximum of 40% of cells in a mature culture formed apical poles (or cysts) with adjacent cells. In collaboration with Cassio, we performed further selections and generated the WIF-B cells, whose apical polarity index is 80% (21). Figure 8.2A presents a phase contrast image of mature WIF-B cells grown on plastic.

Before using these cells for membrane traffic studies, we characterized their mature phenotype, especially with regard to cell polarity (22). Most proteins show the same distribution as *in vivo* (Fig. 8.2B), as does microtubule organization, at least near the apical PM (23). Microtubules radiate from the BC membrane, with actin and foci of γ-tubulin also concentrated in this region. The presence of γ-tubulin leads us to conclude that the minus ends of polarized microtubules are closest to the underlying apical PM. We also explored the structural and functional properties of the tight junction boundary (22). Zonula occludens (ZO-1), the tight junction-associated protein, marks the boundary between the two PM domains (Fig. 8.2C). Using short chain lipid analogues in living cells, we established that the tight junctions were an effective "fence" prohibiting the lateral mixing of outer leaflet PM lipids. Surface labeling of living cells with sulfo-N-hydroxysulfosuccinimide-long chain (sNHS-LC)–biotin (557 d) indicated that small molecules had access to the entire PM, while streptavidin (60 kd) was restricted to only the basolateral domain, establishing that the tight junctions also provided an effective barrier to the diffusion of large molecules into the apical space.

Our careful characterization of the WIF-B cells convinced us that they were a suitable model for the study of membrane trafficking and targeting in hepatocytes. Nonetheless, *in vitro* models always have limitations that are important to be aware of, and the polarized WIF-B cells are no exception. To achieve maximal polarity, the cells require strict culture conditions. The presence of seven to nine human chromosomes (Chr 4, 5, 6, 8, 12, 18, and X) must be considered when identifying new gene products. Their "bile canaliculi (BC)" are spherical and closed, making difficult the types of experimentation performed in simpler, columnar epithelia where there is easy access to the apical PM. The extent to which this BC morphology reflects a cholestatic state is not known. Cassio's group (24) explored the development of hepatic polarity in a clonal derivative, the WIF-B9 cells. Prior to expressing the polygonal hepatic phenotype, the cells adopt a simple, bipolar organization, much like that of the well-studied epithelial Madin-Darby canine kidney (MDCK) cell line. For more details on WIF-B cells, see Chapter 24 and our Web site at www.bs.jhmi.edu/wifb.

Tools

Subcellular Fractionation

A crucial aspect of *in vivo* studies in which ^{35}S-metabolically labeled proteins are followed through the cell is the use of fractionation methods that yield quantitative information on the amounts of those molecules in the different subcellular compartments at different times after labeling. Several of the methods we use for studies *in vivo* are described on the Web site (5). With the increasing availability of antibodies to proteins present in different membrane compartments, immunoisolation provides a powerful method for more precise identification of organelles in a transport pathway and the molecules regulating traffic along that pathway (25,26).

Antibodies and Lipid Analogues as Surrogate Markers to Study Plasma Membrane Pathways

Antibodies have been effectively used as probes to visualize the trafficking behavior of many membrane proteins. We adapted this approach to our studies of basolateral-to-apical transcytosis of newly synthesized apical PM proteins in polarized WIF-B cells (27). Importantly, we found that although the vast majority of apical membrane proteins reside at the apical PM at steady state, the integrity of the tight junctions prohibited access of antibody to these molecules in living WIF-B cells.

The antibody trafficking method is simple. Cells are cooled to 4°C to stop all membrane traffic and incubated with antibody. After removing unbound antibody, cells are warmed to 37°C for various times, fixed, permeabilized, and the locations of the primary antibody detected with a fluorescently labeled secondary antibody. Alternatively, primary antibody can be directly labeled with a fluorophore and followed in living cells in real time.

The validity of the antibody trafficking method depends on the assumption that the antibodies are serving as faithful reporters of the membrane proteins to which they are bound, i.e., that the trafficking behavior is specific to a subset of membrane proteins and is not an antibody-induced phenomenon. To test this assumption, we conducted several control experiments, which are explained elsewhere (27), that included the use of Fab fragments, to test for possible cross-linking of the antigen by divalent immunoglobulin G (IgG); the use of antibodies to track proteins that have an intracellular itinerary different from the transcytosing apical PM proteins (e.g., to endosomes or lysosomes); and measurements of the stability of the trafficked antibodies to determine the extent of their degradation and/or release into the medium during the experiments.

The use of short chain, fluorescent lipid analogues to study membrane lipid pathways in eukaryotic cells was pioneered by Pagano and Sleight (28) and has given us important insights into the dynamics of different classes of membrane lipids. Because of the short C_6 acyl chain, nitroben-zoxadiazole (NBD)-lipids can diffuse through the aqueous medium and insert into the outer leaflet of the PM. Lipids with nonpolar head groups, such as C_6NBD-ceramide, can subsequently translocate across a bilayer and partition into intracellular membranes even at 4°C. Those lipid analogues with polar head groups, such as C_6NBD-sphingomyelin (C_6NBD-SM) and C_6NBD-glucosyl-ceramide (C_6NBD-Glc-Cer), are restricted at 4°C to the outer PM leaflet only and thus become internalized only when cells are warmed and membrane traffic resumes.

In lipid trafficking assays, cells are incubated at 4° to 10°C with the NBD analogue, which is usually bound to a carrier such as defatted albumin. After being rinsed and warmed to allow trafficking and/or metabolism to proceed (depending on the lipid analogue), the cells are cooled and an excess of albumin is added to the medium to remove lipid analogues from the external PM leaflet (called "back-exchange"). At this point, the intracellular locations of the fluorescent lipids can be visualized. In polarized WIF-B and HepG2 cells, whose tight junctions prohibit access of albumin (60 kd) to the outer leaflet of the apical PM, any lipid reaching the apical PM by vesicle transport will be protected from removal by back-exchange (22,29). Small molecules, such as the oxidizing agent dithionite (190 d), can penetrate the tight junctions and quench any fluorescent lipids they meet (30). However, this reagent must be used under strictly controlled conditions, because membranes are not totally impermeable to it.

What are the assumptions in this approach and the relevant controls to perform? Complete removal by back-exchange of any lipids in the external leaflet of the PM seems very important if one wants to conclude that subsequent fluorescent lipid dynamics reflect movements from intracellular and not PM lipid pools. Use of dithionite requires monitoring at the microscope to ensure that intracellular quenching is not occurring. Finally, the assumption that these unusual lipids are reporting the behavior of their endogenous counterparts is difficult to test but important to remember, since they are significantly less hydrophobic than biologic lipids.

Recombinant Proteins

Insights into the pathways and mechanisms of epithelial PM biogenesis and turnover have been aided enormously through the judicious use of recombinant proteins. Examples include expression of engineered mutants of PM proteins with the goal of identifying sorting signals and expression of mutant regulatory proteins to assess their effects on membrane dynamics. In all of these studies, the most essential requirement is to maintain cell polarity, but homogeneous and controlled expression are also important factors. Generally, these requirements have been met in stably transfected kidney cell lines but not routinely with polarized

intestinal or hepatic cells. In this regard, the report that stably transfected WIF-B cells express a green fluorescent protein (GFP, 27 kd)-tagged apical PM transporter is very encouraging (see below). We have successfully used a recombinant adenovirus to deliver genes to polarized WIF-B cells and hepatocytes *in vivo* (31). Although expression of the gene products is transient (4 days), it is high and reasonably uniform, and retention of polarity is excellent. There are caveats to the use of a recombinant protein approach. Since overexpression can lead to mislocalization of proteins (e.g., 32), it is important to know the levels and locations of endogenous protein in cells as well as those of the ectopically expressed protein for meaningful interpretations of results. However, overexpression can be exploited when the right question is asked. For example, saturation of the apical secretory pathway through protein overexpression in MDCK cells has indicated that recognition mechanisms with finite capacities exist (33).

PLASMA MEMBRANE BIOGENESIS: SIGNALS, SORTING MECHANISMS, DELIVERY SYSTEMS

The pathways and mechanisms of post-TGN membrane protein and lipid transport to the PM have been studied intensely (reviewed in refs. 34–38) (see Chapters 10 and 11). Work in simple epithelial cells, such as MDCK, Caco-2, and Lewis Lung Carcinoma–pig kidney 1 (LLC-PK1), has demonstrated that most newly synthesized PM proteins are sorted in the TGN into vesicles that deliver them directly to their appropriate PM destination. This has been called the "direct" route, which predicted that at least two PM-destined vesicles containing either basolaterally or apically directed cargo budded from the TGN in the same cell. This prediction was confirmed using ectopically expressed viral proteins in MDCK cells. In contrast, in studies conducted on hepatocytes *in vivo*, we reported that newly synthesized single-transmembrane domain (TMD) apical PM proteins took an "indirect" route via the basolateral PM before transcytosing across the cell (39). Subsequently, we showed that the glycosyl-phosphatidylinositol (GPI)-anchored apical protein, 5'-nucleotidase, followed the same indirect route (40). As in many simple epithelia, the basolateral PM proteins we examined took a "direct" route to the basolateral PM *in vivo*. At the same time, both direct and indirect routes to the apical surface were found to operate in the delivery of several single-TMD apical proteins in intestinal epithelial cells in culture and *in vivo* (41,42). At least one basolateral PM protein, the NaK-ATPase, may be delivered to all surfaces in MDCK cells, followed by retrieval and degradation of the apical cohort but stabilization of the basolateral cohort through association with the submembranous actin network (43; but see 44). As more epithelial cell types and classes of PM proteins are studied, an emerging theme is that the steady-state localizations can be accomplished in a variety of ways.

How do integral PM proteins delivered to a single PM domain find their way into the right intracellular path? Structural signals, such as amino acid sequences, conformations, or modifications, are on the protein itself. These specify a correct destination ("address") that can be read by a decoder (a recognition mechanism, the "post office") that will direct it into the appropriate carrier (vesicle/tubule, "post person's bag") for correct delivery.

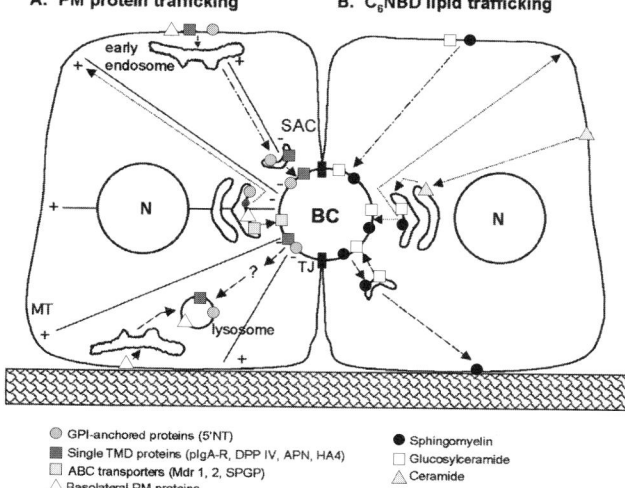

FIGURE 8.3. Protein and C₆-nitrobenzoxadiazole (*NBD*) lipid trafficking in polarized hepatocytes. **A:** Protein trafficking patterns of resident hepatic plasma membrane (*PM*) proteins are shown. Newly synthesized basolateral proteins are transported directly from the *trans*-Golgi Network (TGN) to the basolateral PM. In contrast, newly synthesized single-transmembrane domain (*TMD*) and glycosyl-phosphatidylinositol (*GPI*)-anchored proteins take the indirect route where they are transported from the TGN to the basolateral PM, selectively internalized and transcytosed to the apical PM. En route to the apical PM, they traverse at least two known compartments: the early endosome and the subapical compartment (*SAC*). Newly synthesized multispanning apical PM transporters are directly transported from the TGN to the apical PM. The life cycles of both resident apical and basolateral proteins likely end with degradation in lysosomes (see text for details). Although the apical PM proteins do not traverse the SAC en route to lysosomes, they may traverse an as yet unidentified compartment (*question mark*). **B:** Trafficking of C₆-NBD–labeled lipids in hepatocytes is indicated. Exogenously introduced ceramide is delivered to the Golgi where it is synthesized into sphingomyelin (SM) and glucosylceramide (GlcCer) at the TGN. These lipids are in turn, delivered to the apical or basolateral PM directly from the TGN. Basolaterally delivered or exogenously added SM and GlcCer are transcytosed to the apical PM, but whether they traverse the same compartments as transcytosing proteins, is not known. At 18°C, apically located SM and GlcCer recycle from the PM to a subapically located compartment. Whether this compartment is the SAC has not been clearly established. From this compartment, GlcCer is preferentially targeted back to the apical PM, whereas SM is preferentially targeted to the basolateral PM. *ABC*, adenosine triphosphate binding cassette; *APN*, aminopeptidase N; *DPP IV*, dipeptidylpeptidase IV; *Mdr*, multi-drug resistant protein; *5'NT*, 5' nucleotidase; *pIgA-R*, polymeric immunoglobulin A receptor; *SPGP*; sister of P-glycoprotein.

Multiple PM signals may be present on a single PM protein, but one will prevail in a particular location. The following sections discuss the current ideas about direct sorting of PM proteins from the TGN to the two major PM domains and indirect sorting from the basolateral to the apical PM. Although we focus on proteins, PM lipid sorting in hepatic cells has gained increasing attention. Figure 8.3 presents diagrams of known PM protein and lipid pathways in hepatic cells.

The *trans*-Golgi Network-to-Basolateral Pathway

The most obvious hepatocyte secretory cargo destined for the basolateral surface are very low density lipoproteins and albumin; they are easily detected in large, distinctive vesicles 200 to 400 nm in diameter. Do PM proteins travel with the secretory molecules to the basolateral PM? Few newly synthesized endogenous PM proteins have been seen inside hepatocytes *in situ*; because most are relatively long-lived, their rates of synthesis are consequently very low (45) and they are transported continuously to the basolateral surface without storage. The *in vivo* evidence suggests that the hepatic polymeric immunoglobulin A receptor (pIgA-R) and secretory proteins are sorted into separate classes of basolaterally destined vesicles, presumably at the TGN. In support of this result, Pous et al. (46) reported that the Mg salt of ilimaquinone, which specifically depolymerized dynamic microtubules in polarized WIF-B cells, slowed albumin's secretion but had no effect on the appearance of newly synthesized apical or basolateral PM proteins at the cell surface. (See ref. 47 for a different result in HepG2 cells.) Furthermore, two secretory molecules (albumin and ³⁵S-heparan sulfate proteoglycans) were found in different vesicle carriers isolated from primary hepatocytes (48). Unfortunately, integral PM proteins were not examined in this study and there has been no follow-up. In sum, it appears that at least two, and perhaps three, carriers with distinct basolateral cargoes exit the hepatocyte TGN.

The dynamics of membranes arising from the TGN and carrying transfected PM proteins tagged with GFP to the PM have been recorded in living, nonpolarized cells (49). The elements appeared tubular and contained the GFP-model PM glycoprotein of *v*esicular *s*tomatitis *v*irus (VSV-G). Since VSV-G is delivered to the basolateral PM in simple epithelial cells, this provocative result suggests that basolateral PM proteins may not be in carrier vesicles at all, but in carrier tubules (see Chapter 9 and website chapter 🖳 W-6).

Several different types of signals that are required for correct basolateral targeting and/or localization have been identified on PM proteins, and generally they reside in the cytoplasmic tails (reviewed in ref. 50). Most of the signals contain either a tyrosine in the context of a short degenerate sequence or a di-leucine motif. Some signals overlap with those used at the PM in receptor-mediated endocytosis, while other basolateral signals, such as that in the pIgA-R, are unique. Compelling *in vitro* evidence that these sorting signals are specifically recognized by the μ subunit of the Golgi tetrameric adaptor protein-1 (AP-1) (see Chapter 9) conflicts with the picture *in vivo*, in which the same proteins are *not* found in clathrin-coated buds in the TGN. Possibly, AP-1 proteins found in basolateral early endosomes (51) are the active sorting population, since two newly synthesized basolateral endocytic receptors, the H1 subunit of the human asialoglycoprotein receptor (ASGP-R) and the transferrin receptor (Tf-R), have been detected in endosomes prior to their appearance at the PM (52,53).

Identification of a new μ1 subunit, μ1B, that is restricted to epithelia (54) but absent from brain and liver has added yet another twist to basolateral sorting. μ1B appears to be dominant over μ1A in the recognition of basolateral signals in those epithelial cells that express both AP-1 isoforms, since kidney cells, LLC-PK1, which lack μ1B, fail to deliver the low-density lipoprotein receptor (LDL-R) and Tf-R with high fidelity to the basolateral PM (55). However, in liver, these same basolateral PM receptors are delivered directly and with high fidelity despite the absence of any μ1B. Even more intriguing is the fact that a recently generated μ1A knockout mouse, which is embryonic lethal (presumably because developing brain requires functional AP-1), shows only minimal disruption of intercellular associations between hepatocytes in the embryonic liver with an otherwise normal appearing organ (P. Schu, personal communication). The unanswered question is whether hepatocytes having no functional AP-1 complexes are nonetheless capable of basolateral PM protein delivery.

One basolateral PM protein, the cell adhesion molecule E-cadherin, achieves its destination via signals and mechanisms distinct from those described above and illustrates that we still have much to learn. Chen et al. (56) reported that newly synthesized E-cadherin must bind to a cytoplasmic chauffeur, β-catenin, to exit the ER, progress through the biosynthetic pathway, and reach the basolateral PM. Mutational analysis of E-cadherin indicates that the entire 150 amino acid tail is essential for β-catenin's binding and escort function. This mechanism has interesting implications for β-catenin's central role as a growth regulator in epithelial cells. If β-catenin is functioning in the nucleus and not available in the cytoplasm, E-cadherin will not reach the PM, its steady-state levels will fall, and cell-cell adhesion will be reduced, further enhancing cell growth. Thus, sorting of an important cell adhesion molecule is linked to growth regulation.

Finally, a newly found localization signal in basolateral and apical PM proteins consists of short degenerate sequences, often at the C-terminus, that are recognized by PDZ proteins. Members of the fast-growing PDZ protein family, named after the three founding members (*PSD-95*, *d*iscs large, and *ZO-1*, reviewed in ref. 57), all contain one or more globular PDZ motifs that are 80 to 100 amino acids in

length and are proposed to function as scaffolds in multiprotein complexes. The function of PDZ proteins that bind to PM proteins may be to retain the molecule once it has reached the basolateral PM rather than to sort it into basolaterally destined vesicles in the TGN (58). However, a targeting function has been ascribed to several artificial PDZ modules (59). Finally, PDZ proteins that bind apical PM proteins have also been identified (e.g., (60)), but whether they serve a sorting or retention function is not yet clear.

The Basolateral-to-Apical Pathway—Transcytosis

The basolateral-to-apical transcytotic pathway has been studied extensively in polarized hepatocytes because it comprises a retrieval system for circulating dimeric IgA (dIgA), an important component of the mucosal immune system. The hepatocyte pIgA-R on the basolateral surface binds circulating dimeric IgA, transports it across the cell, and releases it along with a proteolytic fragment of the receptor ectodomain (secretory component) into bile (reviewed in ref. 61). In rats, up to 15% of total daily dIgA is handled in this way, while in humans it is less. Early *in vivo* experiments identified clathrin-coated pits and vesicles as the entry sites for the ligand and receptor (62,63). Subsequently, both the ligand and receptor were found together with other receptor-mediated ligand systems (e.g., ASGP-R) in basolateral endosomes but only the pIgA-R and ligand were present in a subapical compartment before their release into the bile. Other internalized receptor proteins moved along one of two other arms of the endocytic pathway—to lysosomes or back to the basolateral PM.

Our initial discovery that single TMD and GPI-anchored PM proteins in hepatocytes *in vivo* were first delivered to the basolateral PM before they appeared in bona fide apical PM suggested to us that the transcytotic pathway taken by pIgA-R might also be used by these newly synthesized proteins (Fig. 8.3). We tested this hypothesis by ligating the bile duct of rats, a condition reported to perturb IgA transport across hepatocytes (64), then using immunofluorescence and immuno-EM to localize newly synthesized apical PM proteins and pIgA-R (65). We found that the proteins accumulated in a *subapical compartment* we have named SAC. We next applied pulse-chase metabolic labeling combined with subcellular fractionation, vesicle immunoisolation, and immunoprecipitation of apical PM proteins to obtain more quantitative information about this intracellular compartment (26). We found newly synthesized dipeptidyl peptidase IV (DPPIV), a single TMD apical PM protein, first in immunoisolated early endosomes and subsequently in isolated SAC. The high specific radioactivity of DPPIV (i.e., ^{35}S-DPPIV/immunoreactive DPPIV) in this latter vesicle fraction indicated that very little preexisting (unlabeled) DPPIV was present. This meant that recycling of resident apical PM proteins was either very limited or did not involve SAC (Fig. 8.3).

We turned to the WIF-B cells and an antibody trafficking approach to extend our *in vivo* findings (27). We were able to follow the apical PM proteins as well as endocytic receptors with different itineraries to determine where they became segregated. Our results suggest that in hepatocytes single TMD and GPI-anchored apical PM proteins and the pIgA-R use a transcytosis route that diverges early on from the major recycling pathways taken by the ASGP-R, Tf-R, or the late endosomal marker, mannose-6-phosphate receptor. Importantly, we found no recycling receptors in SAC at steady state or at any time during trafficking *in vitro*. Thus, SAC does not act as a major common sorting station for basolaterally internalized cargo in hepatocytes. Furthermore, the dynamic motile properties of SAC structures are quite distinct from those of kinetically early and late endocytic structures (Schroer et al., in preparation), again indicating divergence into separate pathways of the two classes of internalized molecules. However, the apical proteins we studied and pIgA-R showed significant colocalization in SAC and other intracellular structures by confocal microscopy. Thus, these molecules appeared to use the same transcytotic pathway, regardless of their different protein structures (GPI-linked or single TMD with short or long cytoplasmic tails).

Our EM data indicate that SAC in WIF-B cells consists of two types of subapical endomembranes: tubulovesicular and cup-shaped structures found within 1.5 μm of the apical PM (Fig. 8.4). These are reminiscent of subapical structures we identified in the livers of bile duct–ligated rats (65). We have not detected coats on SAC structures in intact cells or after isolation.

The transcytotic pathway taken by pIgA-R and ligand has also been studied intensively in the simpler, bipolar MDCK cells with the goal of identifying and characterizing all of the intracellular intermediates. Debate over nomenclature and the use of different experimental approaches that led to conflicting views of the pathway appears to have been resolved. Several recent reports (e.g., 66) establish that basolateral-to-apical transcytosis of dimeric IgA in MDCK cells involves at least four compartments, including basolateral "sorting" endosomes, a "common" endosome, transcytotic vesicles, and an apical recycling endosome. Compared to hepatocytes, there are more intracellular intermediates in the MDCK pathway. However, the apical recycling endosome is most similar to the hepatic SAC, in that both have a neutral pH (Schroer et al., in preparation), only membrane components destined for the apical PM pass through these compartments, and they are located closest to the apical PM. The major difference between them is the absence of recycling apical PM proteins in hepatic SAC and their presence in the MDCK apical recycling endosome.

One of the many unanswered questions regarding the transcytosis of hepatic apical PM proteins is how they are internalized at the basolateral surface. The cytoplasmic tails on several ectoenzymes that we have studied are very short (six to eight amino acids) or nonexistent (the GPI-anchored proteins), yet the proteins appear to be transported as rapidly as the pIgA-R (27). We have explored the possibility that caveolae are involved, but have no definitive results to date, although we know that expression of caveolin 1 is very low in liver and WIF-B cells (G. Ihrke, unpublished data).

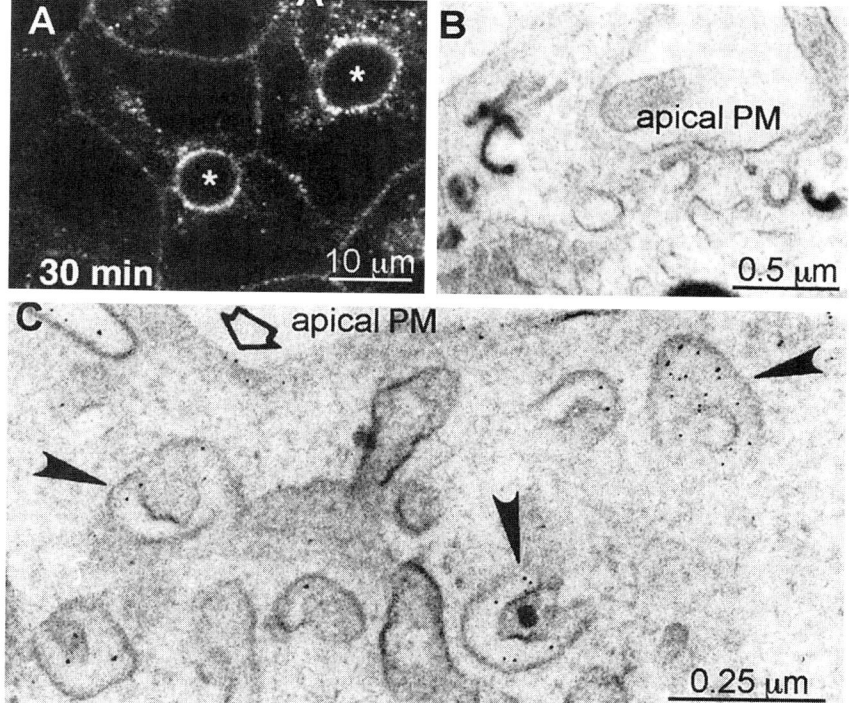

FIGURE 8.4. The subapical compartment (SAC) is an intermediate of the transcytotic pathway. Aminopeptidase N (APN) that was present at the basolateral plasma membrane (*PM*) was labeled with antibodies and chased to the apical surface for 30 minutes. Immunofluorescence detection of the antibody-antigen complexes reveals staining in a region just adjacent to the apical surface that corresponds to the SAC **(A)**. The SAC was visualized at the ultrastructural level using a similar assay, except trafficking antibodies were labeled with horseradish peroxidase **(B)** or 5 nm gold **(C)**. *Asterisks* in **A** indicate bile canalicular spaces in WIF-B cells. The *arrow* in **C** points to apical PM proteins present at the apical surface. *Arrowheads* point to the apical proteins in the SAC.

Hoekstra's group (29,30) reported that C_6-NBD-SM and -GlcCer, incorporated into the outer leaflet of the basolateral PM of HepG2 cells at 4°C, are transported via vesicles to the apical PM within 30 minutes at 37°C. Apparently, a subapical compartment such as SAC is not an intermediate in this pathway at 37°C, although puncta elsewhere in the cell are evident. However, in HepG2 cells transfected with the pIgA-R, these investigators observed partial overlap between transcytosing IgA ligand (presumed to be in SAC) and NBD-sphingolipids previously delivered to the apical PM at 37°C and then allowed to traffic at 18°C for 60 minutes (30). Curiously, basolateral-to-apical transcytosis of the membrane lipids is not inhibited by microtubule disruption, although their internalization at the basolateral PM is decreased by actin depolymerization (67). In contrast, we find that transcytosis of apical PM proteins transiently present in the basolateral PM of WIF-B cells is significantly inhibited by microtubule disruption. Thus, important differences exist between the trafficking of apical PM proteins and C_6-NBD-lipids.

The *trans*-Golgi Network-to-Apical Pathway

Until recently, there was no evidence of the existence of a direct TGN-to-apical route in hepatocytes. However, Arias's group (68,69; see Chapter 24) have made the exciting finding that several multispanning apical PM transporters take such a route in polarized WIF-B cells and *in vivo*. In WIF-B cells, they stably expressed a fusion protein of an adenosine triphosphate (*A*TP)-*b*inding *c*assette (ABC) protein, the multidrug resistance (MDR-1) transporter, with GFP attached at its C-terminus. At the light microscope level, the fluorescent structures arising from the Golgi region and moving toward the apical PM were predominantly tubular in shape. They seemed not to accumulate in any subapical compartment prior to their arrival at or near the apical surface. Biochemical confirmation of this direct route was also reported using *in vivo* pulse-chase metabolic labeling in combination with subcellular fractionation and immunoprecipitation of MDR1, MDR2, and sister of P-glycoprotein (SPGP), a related ABC transporter, which transports bile acids (see Chapter 24 for more details). Of importance is that MDR trafficked directly from Golgi to the apical membrane, whereas SPGP trafficked from Golgi into another hepatocellular pool(s) prior to transfer to the apical membrane (69). It is interesting that the ^{35}S-proteins differed in the rates at which they reached the apical PM, hinting at the existence of parallel pathways (carriers?) for their delivery. Identification of the relevant signals and sorting mechanisms is the next important step.

Given the existence of a direct pathway for at least one class of apical PM proteins in hepatocytes, why are single TMD and GPI-anchored apical PM proteins excluded from it? We know that the hepatic apical PM proteins contain sorting signals, because they are directly delivered to the apical PM when expressed in simple epithelial cells, such as

MDCK (70). Therefore, the relevant sorting mechanisms must be either absent from hepatocytes or present but not in the TGN. If present, the obvious compartment in which to look for them is the basolateral endosome. What might these mechanisms be?

Identification of apical PM protein recognition mechanisms has been difficult, because, with one exception, identification of the signals has been elusive. A GPI anchor is the clearest apical sorting signal, since its transfer onto a randomly secreted protein is sufficient to redirect the protein into the apical pathway of most cells (71). Aside from this class, the signals on integral apical PM proteins seem to be located either in the ectodomain or in the transmembrane domain (reviewed in ref. 50). The recognition mechanisms have been postulated to be lectins that bind to *N*-glycan signals, cholesterol-rich lipid "rafts," and/or a membrane proteolipid with which transmembrane domain signals interact. However, none of these mechanisms appears to be utilized universally, since exceptions to each have been reported (see ref. 50 for complete references).

A tetra-spanning TMD protein of 17 kd, first identified in myelin and lymphocytes, hence the name MAL, has been implicated by Puertollano et al (72) in the apical sorting of a single TMD apical protein surrogate, the influenza hemagglutinin (HA). MAL is expressed in many epithelial cells, where it is concentrated in the TGN region (73). Using an antisense approach to study the apical delivery of HA in MDCK cells lacking MAL, these investigators found HA's transport to be less efficient and less specific in the absence of MAL; the ectopic expression of human MAL rescued the defect. Therefore, it is intriguing that liver does not express MAL, a finding consistent with the absence of a direct apical delivery mechanism for the single-TMD class of apical PM proteins in hepatocytes.

Membrane domains, termed "rafts," that are enriched in glycolipids and cholesterol have been proposed as "platforms" upon which apical PM protein sorting occurs in MDCK cells (reviewed in refs. 74–76). The rafts are defined operationally as detergent-insoluble, lipid-containing complexes that float in sucrose density gradients (77). As some newly synthesized single TMD and GPI-anchored PM proteins move through the Golgi, they appear in such complexes. This behavior correlates with the efficiency of subsequent delivery to the apical PM. Lowering cholesterol levels through use of metabolic inhibitors and/or reagents that extract cholesterol acutely from living cells disrupts the rafts (i.e., decreases the detergent insolubility of the proteins) and also reduces the specificity of apical delivery of some proteins (78; but see 79). At present there is no information on the existence of "rafts" in the hepatocyte PM or Golgi.

A direct Golgi-to-apical PM pathway for fluorescent lipid analogues was identified in polarized HepG2 cells some time ago (80). Experimentally, C_6-NBD-ceramide was incubated with HepG2 cells at 4° then briefly (10 minutes) at 37°C, to allow de novo synthesis of C_6-NBD-SM and C_6-NBD-Glc-Cer, which occurs in the Golgi (81,82) (Fig. 8.3). Longer incubation of cells at 37°C allowed further membrane trafficking and the microtubule-dependent accumulation of fluorescence at the apical PM (67). As evidence that the apical PM signal was delivered from an intracellular site (the Golgi) and not the basolateral PM, albumin was included in the basal medium during the last 37°C incubation to extract any lipid transported to the basolateral PM, thereby preventing it from subsequently moving via transcytosis to the apical PM. This direct apical pathway could be similar to that recently identified for apical PM transporters (see above).

PLASMA MEMBRANE TARGETING MACHINERY

How do cargo-bearing vesicles deliver their contents to the correct target domain? Morphologic, biochemical, and genetic approaches have successfully identified many molecules involved in "vesicle targeting," a complex series of molecular events that minimally includes docking and fusion (see Chapter 10). These approaches indicate that the basic mechanisms are conserved among the membrane compartments throughout the biosynthetic and endocytic pathways and in organisms ranging from yeast to humans. The players so far identified fall into two broad categories: some are used repeatedly throughout the pathways, and others belong to discrete protein families, where one or a few members act at one or a few transport sites. Members of three protein families are central players in vesicle targeting and fusion (reviewed in refs. 83–86). They are (a) the SNAREs, which in general are a group of cytoplasmically oriented integral membrane proteins that are present on vesicles (v-SNAREs) or target membranes (t-SNAREs); (b) the Sec1/Munc18 proteins; and (c) small molecular weight guanosine triphosphate (GTP)-binding proteins, the rabs.

The SNARE hypothesis was originally proposed as a model to describe the mechanism by which the SNAREs promoted membrane docking and fusion through interactions with an ATPase, *N*-ethylmaleimide (NEM)–sensitive factor (NSF), and its receptor, α-SNAP (87). This hypothesis has undergone considerable revision as more is learned about these and other essential proteins and as the cyclical nature of the process is better appreciated (for an excellent discussion, see ref. 85). For vesicle trafficking to continue past one round, some machinery must continually cycle between vesicle and target membranes, making the order of events difficult to define. Also, the t- and v-SNAREs, whose pairwise coupling was originally thought to confer targeting specificity, show promiscuity in their binding *in vitro*, suggesting that other factors are required for the high fidelity of membrane targeting observed *in vivo*. Furthermore, the ATPase NSF, which was originally postulated to function in the fusion reaction itself, most likely functions as a chaperone to disassemble the SNARE pairs (84,88). Whether this occurs when the pairs are in "trans" (on the cognate membranes) or in "cis" (on the same membrane after vesicle consumption) may differ upon the cell type or transport step examined. Newer models have integrated the enormous and confusing body of information and have identified common steps in membrane targeting including: (a) SNARE activation (which likely involves NSF chaperone activity) and rab recruitment to proper organelle sites; (b) cognate membrane attachment; and (c) membrane fusion and bilayer mixing (85). The order of events and the mechanistic details are not clear, yet there is considerable evidence that the SNAREs, rabs, and Sec1/Munc18 proteins are key players in the process. Figure 8.5 depicts a simplified model of how these molecules might operate. The following sections discuss the possible roles of a few selected members of these families in regulating PM targeting in hepatocytes (Table 8.1).

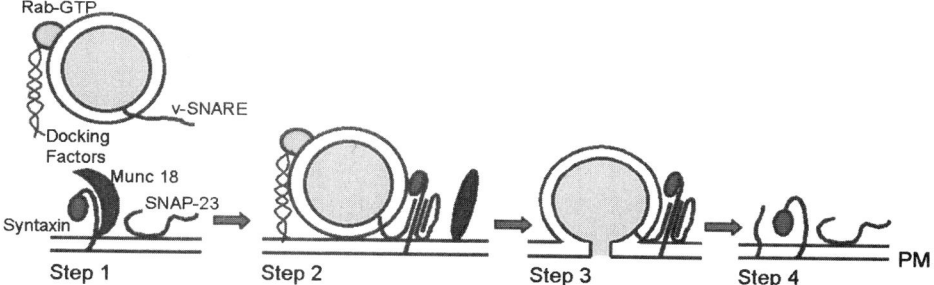

FIGURE 8.5. Hypothetical model for vesicle docking and fusion. *Step 1*: Rab proteins, in their active guanosine triphosphate (*GTP*)-bound conformations, bind transport vesicles and recruit effector molecules. In this case, coiled-coil docking factors are shown. At the plasma membrane (*PM*), syntaxin is bound to Munc18, thus preventing its association with SNAP-23 and subsequent ternary complex formation. *Step 2*: The vesicle is docked at the *PM* and the v- and t-SNAREs form the four-stranded, parallel, α-helical array central to ternary complex formation. Munc18 is dissociated from syntaxin to allow the complex to form. *Step 3*: The vesicle is shown fusing with the PM with the ternary complex still associated. Although this is portrayed as a single step, little is understood about the actual mechanism for fusion and bilayer mixing, which probably requires multiple steps. It is not known whether Munc18, rab proteins or docking factors are dissociated from the membrane at this step. *Step 4*: Vesicle consumption is complete and the ternary complex is dissociated likely through *N*-ethylmaleimide-sensitive factor (NSF) chaperone activity. We have not indicated the placement of the SNAP proteins (NSF receptors), but they are required for NSF activity. Also, it is not clear how v-SNAREs are internalized and targeted back to their proper transport vesicles.

TABLE 8.1. PUTATIVE REGULATORS OF PLASMA MEMBRANE (PM) TARGETING IN POLARIZED EPITHELIAL CELLS

Protein	Subcellular Location in Epithelial Cells Morphology (M)/Fractionation (F)	Epithelial Cells Examined	Evidence for Role in PM Targeting	References
t-SNAREs				
Syntaxin 2, 3, 4	Apical and/or basolateral PM (M, F)	Hepatocytes (M, F), pancreatic acinar and intestinal epithelial cells, kidney collecting duct, Caco-2, MDCK, WIF-B (M)	Location; syntaxin 3 overexpression and antibody sensitivity in MDCK cells	89–95
Syntaxin 8, 13	Endosomes?	N/D		85
Syntaxin 6, 10	TGN	N/D		85
SNAP-23	Apical and/or basolateral PM (M, F), endosomes (M,F)	Hepatocytes (F), MDCK, WIF-B (M), HepG2 (M)	Location; toxin and anti-SNAP-23 sensitivity in MDCK	91,95–101
v-SNAREs				
Cellubrevin/VAMP 3	Endosomes (M, F)	Hepatocytes (M, F)	Location	102
Endobrevin/VAMP 8	Early endosomes (F, M)	Hepatocytes (F), MDCK	Location	103
Ti-VAMP/VAMP 7	Subapical structures (M), apical PM (M)	Caco-2	Location	104
VAMP 2	Endosomes (F)	Gastric parietal cells, MDCK	Location; toxin sensitivity in MDCK	105, 106
Others				
NSF	Golgi (M, F), endosomes (F), coated vesicles (F)	Placenta, pinealocytes, MDCK	NEM- and anti-NSF sensitivity and mutational analysis in MDCK	96,97,106–108
Munc18-2	Apical PM (M)	Murine intestinal, lung, kidney, testis and spleen epithelia, MDCK	Location; epithelial-specific expression	109
α-SNAP	N/D	MDCK	Anti-α-SNAP sensitivity in MDCK	106,110
Rab Proteins				
Rab1 and 2	Golgi (F), transcytotic vesicles (F)	Hepatocytes (F)	Copurification with transcytotic vesicles	111
Rab3B	Tight junctions (M)	Intestinal and kidney epithelia, hepatocytes (M), HT-29, T84	Location	112
Rab3D	Apical PM (M)	Hepatocytes (M)	Location	113
Rab4 and 5	Early endosomes, apical and basolateral PM (M, F)	Kidney epithelia, hepatocytes (F), MDCK	Location; overexpression in MDCK	114,115
Rab6	Golgi	Hepatocytes (F)	Location; TGN budding assay	116
Rab8	Golgi, basolateral PM (M, F)	MDCK	Location; sensitivity to rab8 inhibitory peptides in MDCK cells	117
Rab11	Subapical structures (M, F)	Gastric parietal, pancreatic acinar and prostate epithelial cells, enterocytes, hepatocytes (F), MDCK	Location; change in distribution upon parietal cell activation; mutational analysis in gastric parietal and MDCK cells	118–120
Rab13	Tight junctions (M)	Small intestinal and kidney epithelia, hepatocytes (M), Caco-2, LLC-PK$_1$	Location	121
Rab17	Basolateral PM (M), apical vesicles and tubules (M), transcytotic vesicles (F)	Hepatocytes (F), kidney epithelia, MDCK, Eph4	Location; epithelial-specific expression; mutational analysis and overexpression in MDCK and Eph4 cells	111,122–125
Rab18	Basolateral PM (M), subapical tubules (M)	Kidney tubule epithelia	Location	126
Rab20	Subapical tubules (M)	Kidney tubule epithelia	Location	126
Rab25	Subapical structures (F, M)	Gastric parietal cells, MDCK	Location; mutational analysis in MDCK	105,119,120

LLC-PK, Lewis Lung Carcinoma–pig kidney; MDCK, Madin-Darby canine kidney; NEM, N-ethylmaleimide; NSF, NEM-sensitive factor; PM, plasma membrane; SNAP, sensitive factor attachment protein; SNARE, soluble NEM SNAP receptor; TGN, trans-Golgi network; VAMP, vesicle-associated membrane protein.

NEM-Sensitive Factor and α-SNAP

NSF was initially implicated as a regulator of polarized PM targeting from studies that examined the effects of NEM on protein transport. Addition of NEM reduced IgA transcytosis by 70% and its basolateral targeting by 90% in permeabilized MDCK cells (90,97). It also inhibited fusion (as assayed by pIgA-R processing) of transcytotic carrier vesicles with the apical PM in a hepatic cell free system reconstituting the final step of transcytosis (127). Since NSF ATPase activity is inhibited by alkylating agents (reviewed in ref. 128), it was the likely target for NEM. In support of that, addition of recombinant NSF restored much of the activity lost in MDCK cells or hepatic cell free systems treated with NEM or anti-NSF antibodies (90,97,106, 127). Interestingly, direct apical PM targeting was insensitive to NEM (90,106), indicating that it requires an unidentified NSF homologue or does not require NSF-like activity at all. Other key factors, the SNAP family of NSF receptors (α, β, and γ isoforms), recruit NSF to organelles and activate its ATPase activity (128). α-SNAP has been identified in polarized epithelial cells and its role in TGN to PM targeting examined in MDCK cells. Addition of α-SNAP antibodies and treatment of cells with botulinum E (an α-SNAP-specific toxin) inhibited direct transport to both domains (its role in transcytosis was not examined (97,106,110).

t-SNAREs and v-SNAREs

There are two families of t-SNARE proteins: the syntaxins and the SNAP-25 family. To date, at least 18 syntaxin family members have been identified in mammalian cells of which five (syntaxins 1A, 1B, 2, 3, and 4) are PM-specific isoforms (85). The SNAP-25 family is much smaller, with only three identified members: SNAP-25, -23, and -29 (85). Like the syntaxins, these proteins are relatively small (23 to 29 kd), cytoplasmically oriented molecules. Although not integral membrane proteins as are all PM syntaxins, SNAP-25 proteins associate with the bilayer through cysteine-linked palmitoyl chains located near the middle of the protein. Biochemically, SNAP-25 proteins bind PM-associated syntaxins and v-SNAREs *in vitro* to form the four-stranded α-helical ternary complexes required for vesicle docking and fusion (Fig. 8.5) (reviewed in ref. 85).

What about PM t-SNAREs in hepatocytes? We found that rat hepatocytes express three endogenous PM-associated syntaxin isoforms (syntaxins 2, 3, and 4) and SNAP-23 (94,95). Quantitative immunoblotting revealed that all four t-SNAREs are relatively abundant in liver (11 to 668 nM corresponding to 0.5 to 28×10^5 molecules/cell). Biochemically, each of the t-SNAREs was observed predominantly in hepatocyte PM sheets with overlapping but distinct expression patterns among the PM domains (Fig. 8.6).

Both syntaxin 4 and SNAP-23 are restricted to the basolateral PM while syntaxins 2 and 3 are more apically distributed, with greater enrichment of syntaxin 3 in this domain. Despite the biochemical abundance of the molecules, morphologic detection of the syntaxins in liver and WIF-B cells has been problematic. Furthermore, some distributions do not fit with our biochemical data. For example, syntaxin 4 and SNAP23 are localized to both PM domains in WIF-B cells, as is syntaxin 4 in liver sections, whereas both are basolateral in their biochemical distributions. Likewise, syntaxin 2 is restricted to the apical PM in WIF-B cells (Fig. 8.6C), less so in liver sections (Fig. 8.6A), and is distributed in both domains biochemically (Fig. 8.6, graph). These varied distributions likely reflect important differences in regulation of PM dynamics between the *in vivo* and *in vitro* systems and may point to interesting features of the cellular itineraries and functions of the t-SNAREs. Little is known about how these putative targeting molecules are themselves targeted to the correct PM domain, and once delivered, how and if they are retained there.

Interestingly, the PM syntaxins also display remarkable variability in their domain distributions in other polarized cells (Table 8.1). Only syntaxin 3 appears to be consistently at the apical PM in all polarized cells examined (90,92–94,129). SNAP-23 distributes to both PM domains in all but two epithelial cell types (Table 8.1). Since it is thought to be required for vesicle docking and fusion, SNAP-23's uniform PM distribution fits with the current model of its ubiquitous involvement in t- and v-SNARE ternary complex formation. However, its absence at the apical PM in hepatocytes and pancreatic cells is somewhat paradoxical. Either these cells have unique mechanisms for regulating transport at their apical surfaces or other SNAP-25 isoforms are yet to be identified.

To date, the roles of the t-SNAREs in polarized PM targeting have been tested directly only in MDCK cells that were stably expressing pIgA-R and overexpressing wild-type syntaxins 2, 3, or 4 (90). Neither transcytosis nor basolateral transport of pIgA-R was affected, suggesting that the syntaxins do not regulate these transport pathways or that other yet-to-be-identified isoforms are involved. Alternatively, overexpression was not high enough to be inhibitory or does not negatively regulate these processes. Overexpression of syntaxin 3 did slightly inhibit (20%) direct TGN to apical PM delivery of a chimeric pIgA-R molecule and IgA apical recycling (also 20%). Since anti–syntaxin 3 antibodies also inhibited the direct targeting, this isoform is important in apical vesicle delivery (110). In MDCK cells treated with SNAP-23/25–specific neurotoxins, basolateral to apical transport of pIgA was inhibited by 30% (97), as was its basolateral targeting, but the TGN to apical targeting of HA was not affected (97,106). More recent studies confirmed this result and found that toxin activity also impairs transferrin recycling (100).

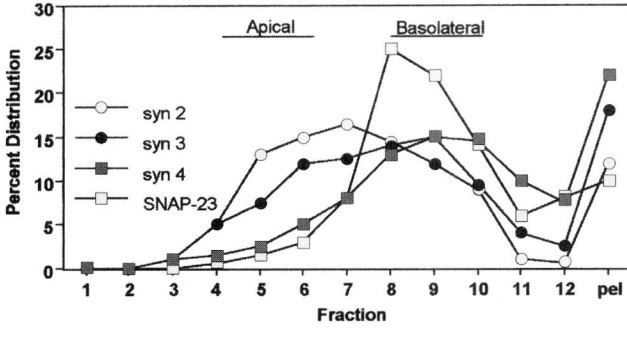

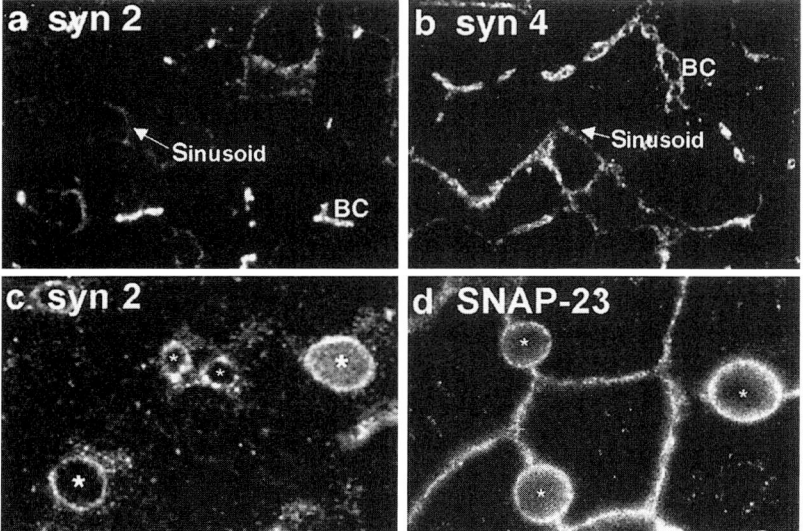

FIGURE 8.6. Hepatic t-SNAREs differentially distribute among the plasma membrane (PM) domains. **Upper panel:** Isolated hepatocyte PM sheets were vesiculated by sonication and applied to linear sucrose gradients. Fractions were analyzed by quantitative immunoblotting and the relative levels of each syntaxin (*syn*) and SNAP-23 were determined by densitometric analysis. Peak distributions of known resident apical (fractions 4–6) or basolateral PM proteins (fractions 8–10) are indicated. **Lower panels:** Rat liver semi-thin sections were stained for syntaxin 2 **(A)** or syntaxin 4 **(B)** and WIF-B cells stained for syntaxin 2 **(C)** or SNAP-23 **(D)**. *Arrows* in **A** and **B** are pointing to sinusoidal membranes, and the *asterisks* in **C** and **D** are marking bile canaliculi (*BCs*).

The direct involvement of v-SNARES in PM targeting has not been explored, but the obvious prediction is that they are required. Both visicle-associated membrane protein (VAMP) 1 and 2 and cellubrevin/VAMP 3 are ubiquitously expressed and the presence of cellubrevin on endosomal structures in hepatocytes has been reported (102). Endobrevin/VAMP 8 and TI-VAMP/ VAMP 7 may also function in apical PM targeting, since endobrevin is primarily associated with early endosomes (130) and TI-VAMP is localized both to the apical PM and in subapically located structures in CaCo-2 cells (104). Interestingly, TI-VAMP has a long N-terminal extension encoding a 30 amino acid sequence resembling a region in annexin XIIIb, another protein implicated in regulating apical vesicle delivery (131). This sequence encodes a lipid-binding domain in annexin XIIIb; whether TI-VAMP shares this property is not yet known.

Munc18

Munc18 homologues have been identified in systems from yeast to mammals and are thought to participate in multiple vesicle transport steps (reviewed in refs. 132 and 133). The 68-kd mammalian Munc18 proteins peripherally associate with the PM through interactions with syntaxins; *in vitro*, they bind syntaxins 1, 2, and 3 with nanomolar affinity. Interestingly, Munc18 binding to syntaxins cannot occur when the syntaxins are bound to SNAP-25 proteins, suggesting that the different complexes form reciprocally. Munc18 has been ascribed both positive and negative regulatory roles in PM targeting. Mutational analyses of related proteins in yeast, *Drosophila* and *Caenorhabditis elegans,* all implicate Munc18 species as positive regulators, while *in vitro* assays suggest the opposite (132,133). As for most of the SNARE molecules, no direct evidence for the involvement of Munc18 proteins in polarized PM targeting exists. However, Munc18-2 is primarily limited to polarized epithelial cells (109), and its expression seems restricted to the apical PM where it forms complexes with syntaxin 3 (134). This distribution and behavior suggest a unique function for Munc18-2 in vesicle delivery from the TGN to the apical PM.

The Rab Proteins

The rab proteins belong to the largest family of small molecular weight (20 to 30 kd) GTP-binding proteins. There are 11 known yeast isoforms and at least 40 rabs in mammalian cells (recently reviewed in refs. 116, 135, and 136). Examination of transfected cells overexpressing either wild-type or dominant negative mutant [usually the guanosine diphosphate (GDP)-bound conformer] forms of various rabs either stimulate or inhibit protein transport and in some cases alter organelle morphology. Although their precise roles are not known, they have been proposed to function in one of three ways: (a) facilitating vectorial traffic via associations with the cytoskeleton; (b) regulating vesicle docking by recruiting effector molecules, thereby promoting the formation of "molecular tethers"; and (c) "priming" docking and fusion by activating SNARE molecules (135,136).

Given the large number of mammalian rabs and their varied distributions, it is likely that polarized PM transport in hepatocytes is regulated by multiple isoforms, but which ones? Of the rab proteins identified in hepatocytes (Table 8.1), rabs 3B, 3D, 13, 17, and 25 and two others (rab18 and 20) are preferentially expressed in epithelial cells, suggesting a unique function in polarized membrane transport. Although expressed in nonpolarized cells, rabs 1, 2, 3D, 4, 5, 6, and 11 have also been identified in hepatocytes. Of these ten rabs, six have been localized to the apical pole: rab3D is at the apical PM, rabs 3B and 13 are at the tight junction, and rabs 17, 11, and 25 are found in subapical structures. Rabs 18 and 20, although not yet identified in hepatocytes, are also localized to subapical structures in kidney epithelia. The large number of different rab proteins in the apical region may point to the complexity of membrane transport events at this PM domain.

Although little direct evidence exists at present for a role for any rab isoform in PM targeting in hepatocytes, work from other cell types strongly implicates several isoforms, particularly rab5 (137). In all nonpolarized cells examined to date, rab5 is localized to the PM, clathrin-coated vesicles, and/or early endosomes. Overexpression of rab5 increased endocytic transport and stimulated early endosome fusion *in vitro*, whereas inhibition of rab5 led to the opposite effects. Recently, it was proposed that rab5 recruits early endosomal antigen 1 (EEA1) (one of its many effectors) to sites of endosome fusion, along with NSF and syntaxin 13, thus driving the formation of a large oligomeric complex that in turn may coordinate fusion pore assembly (138). This general role of rab5 in endocytosis strongly suggests its involvement in the early steps of the transcytotic pathway in hepatocytes, which is consistent with the report of rab5 on endocytic structures in hepatocytes (114). It has also been localized to early endosomes located near the apical and basolateral PM in mouse kidney epithelia and MDCK cells (115). When overexpressed in MDCK cells, increased rates of fluid phase internalization from the apical and basolateral PM were observed, suggesting a role for rab5a in endocytosis from both domains (115).

Recently, several studies have directly addressed rab17 function in transcytosis. In MDCK cells, the overexpression of wild-type rab17 impaired the basolateral to apical transcytosis of dIgA (139). Conversely, in Eph 4 cells expressing guanosine triphosphatase (GTPase)-deficient rab17 mutants, the basolateral-to-apical transcytosis of transferrin receptor, and a chimeric receptor was enhanced as well as apical recycling of the chimeric receptor (124). Rab17 has also been copurified with a population of transcytotic vesicles from rat liver, suggesting it is an important regulator of hepatic basolateral to apical transcytosis, too. Interestingly, both rab1 and 2 also copurified with the vesicles implicating them as additional regulators of transcytosis (111). Furthermore, the subapical location of rab17 in kidney-derived cells argues that apical endocytic structures are important intermediates in the transcytotic pathway. The next steps will be pinpointing the site of function in the transcytotic pathway, examining whether the role of rab17 is universal among epithelial cells, and identifying the cellular effectors that rab17 activity regulates.

Rab11 and rab25 have also been identified in subapical structures in many polarized epithelial cell types including hepatocytes (Table 8.1). Although their function in hepatocytes has not been established, roles for rab11 and 25 in apical PM targeting have been tested in gastric parietal cells and/or MDCK cells (118–120). Transfection of dominant-negative rab11 molecules into gastric parietal cells inhibited the hormone-stimulated recruitment of the H^+K^+–ATPase to the apical PM (118). In polarized MDCK cells, both rab11 and 25 were found to be associated with the apical recycling system (119). Further analysis of GTP-binding mutants (120) revealed that both of these rabs regulated the basolateral to apical transcytosis of IgA, although the activated form of rab25 inhibited transport more than the rab11 mutant. Since both mutants also inhibited the apical recycling of IgA, but not basolateral recycling of transferrin, the block in transcytosis was likely occurring at a transport step at or near the apical PM. The puzzle is why these rabs apparently regulate the same transport steps at the apical PM. Do the differential responses suggest separable roles in transport? Also, why is rab11 required for transferrin recycling in nonpolarized cells, but not in polarized cells? Clearly, additional careful examination of these rabs is required to understand their role in apical PM dynamics.

Surprisingly there is little direct evidence for the involvement of specific molecules in hepatic polarized PM targeting, although many promising candidates are emerging. However, a cautionary flag must be raised. Much of what we discussed is based on studies performed only in tissue culture models of polarized cells (especially MDCK cells) and has not yet been tested in a physiologic context. Furthermore, many of the *in vitro* studies have relied on transient overexpression of either wild-type or mutated proteins. We believe that careful enumeration and examination of endogenous molecules in a single cell type are required before a clear understanding of their roles in targeting will emerge. Finally, in many cases the inhibitory or stimulatory effects on PM targeting of transfection or pharmacologic agents have been small. What does this mean? Does the size of the response *in vitro* reflect loss of normal regulation that would be observed *in vivo* or does it represent fine-tuning regulation that may be critical for proper organ function? If it is the latter, what appears to be a minimal change *in vitro* may have a large impact on the overall homeostatic balance of the organism. Thus, physiologic studies are needed.

DYNAMIC RESIDENCE AND TURNOVER OF PLASMA MEMBRANE PROTEINS AND LIPIDS

Once a PM protein reaches the correct PM domain, its residence there will be dictated by many factors, most of which reside in the protein's sequence and structure. However, regional differences in cellular machinery and organization likely exist, because the mechanisms regulating internalization from the apical and basolateral domains differ in polarized epithelial cells (140–143). Every PM protein also has a finite life span that is determined by its physical properties, assembly status, etc. PM protein turnover in hepatocytes is known to occur through degradation in lysosomes, cleavage at the surface and solubilization from the membrane (5). We assume that the extent to which a particular degradation mechanism/site is used depends on a PM protein's specific degradation signals, its domain location and the physiological state of the cell.

There is abundant evidence in all epithelial cells that many basolateral PM components, especially endocytic proteins, recycle through intracellular endosomal compartments during their lifetime, with some probability of being diverted to and degraded in lysosomes. In hepatocytes as well as nonpolarized cells, the epithelium growth factor (EGF) receptor is downregulated upon ligand binding by selective diversion into the degradative arm of the endocytic pathway, sequestration in microvesicles that bud into the lumen of endosomes producing multivesicular endosomes, and subsequent degradation in lysosomes (144,145). It is assumed that constitutive degradation of basolateral PM proteins occurs in a similar manner, but randomly. At present we know very little about the dynamic behavior of specific basolateral PM proteins such as bile salt transporters (see Chapter 7), basal PM integrins, or E-cadherin, whose half-life in MDCK cells is quite short ($t^1/2$ 5 hours (146; but see 147). Although ubiquitin-proteosomal degradation has not been documented for basolateral PM proteins in hepatocytes, the Met tyrosine kinase receptor, which is expressed in liver, is reportedly downregulated via this mechanism in tissue culture cells (148).

The hepatocyte apical PM is another story. Very few studies have documented endocytosis at the apical PM, and

early models proposed that the detergent-like bile was responsible for the solubilization (i.e., loss) of both membrane lipids and proteins from the canalicular surface (reviewed in ref. 149). However, we found that a maximum of only 20% to 30% of the loss of resident apical PM proteins could be accounted for by passive solubilization (45). Thus, either endocytic retrieval or proteasome-mediated mechanisms must exist. In simple bipolar epithelial cells, endocytosis at the apical PM is less robust than that at the basolateral (150,151) and is subject to different regulation (140–143). However, we can infer the presence of apical PM retrieval mechanisms from studies examining the proteins in that domain. For example, pIgA-R is continuously synthesized—our estimates are 1×10^5 molecules per minute per cell (45)—and delivered to the apical domain by transcytosis. Once delivered, the receptor is cleaved, releasing the secretory component into the bile and leaving a 30-kd tail fragment anchored in the membrane. Only a small proportion of the tail has been detected in bile, suggesting that other mechanisms exist to rid the apical PM of the fragment.

Although examination of hepatic apical PM dynamics has been difficult, there are strategies available. We adopted a pharmacologic approach and documented for the first time the internalization of membrane proteins from the hepatic apical surface (152). Treatment of WIF-B cells with phosphoinositide-3 (PI-3)-kinase inhibitors wortmannin or LY294002 led to the accumulation of several apical PM proteins in lysosomal vacuoles. By monitoring the trafficking of antibody-labeled molecules, we determined that the apical proteins in vacuoles came from the apical PM; neither newly synthesized nor transcytosing apical proteins accumulated in vacuoles. These results confirm a long-held but unproven assumption that lysosomes are the final destination of apical PM proteins in hepatocytes. More recently, in collaboration with Backer we examined the role(s) played by specific PI-3-kinases (classes I and III) by microinjecting inhibitory antibodies and proteins into WIF-B cells. We have found that inhibition of a class III PI-3-kinase, Vps34p, recapitulated almost completely the wortmannin phenotype we initially observed. Therefore, we suggest that PI-3-P, the sole product of Vps34p, regulates endocytic trafficking of apical PM proteins from the apical surface. These new results confirm that lipid kinases (and their lipid products) are important modulators of membrane transport in polarized hepatocytes (see Chapter 24).

Hoekstra's group (29,30,153) studied lipid traffic from the apical surface of HepG2 cells and made several intriguing yet puzzling observations in light of our PM protein results. They found that C_6-NBD-SM and -Glc-Cer, which were initially located at the apical PM through basolateral-to-apical transport at 37°C followed by 4°C back-exchange, subsequently accumulated at 18°C in a subapical compartment they named SAC. Upon shift to 37°C, the SM analogue preferentially moves from the subapical compartment to the basolateral PM while the Glc-Cer analogue moves back to the apical PM (Fig. 8.3). Thus, these investigators view their subapical compartment as an apical endosome that receives membrane lipids from the apical PM. In contrast, we found that apically internalized PM proteins did not travel through SAC en route to lysosomal vacuoles in wortmannin-treated cells, supporting our hypothesis that SAC is not an apical endosome for proteins. Importantly, basolateral-to-apical transcytosing apical PM proteins continued to traverse the SAC in wortmannin-treated cells, suggesting that it remained functional (152). Thus, apically destined and apically located PM proteins and lipids behave oppositely, a puzzle that clearly needs resolution (Fig. 8.3).

CONCLUSION

We have learned much about the polarized hepatocyte PM since the last edition of this book; nevertheless, much remains mysterious. For example, the hepatocyte seems to be unique among epithelial cells in the relative paucity or downright absence of several molecules/mechanisms involved in the sorting and targeting of PM proteins. Yet its surface remains exquisitely polarized, even in the face of enormous flux into and out of the PM domains. How is this accomplished? What role do microtubules play in this specificity and fidelity? And, lastly, how might failure or dysregulation of the streamlined mechanisms maintaining surface polarity play out in malignant transformation? Perhaps there will be answers in the next edition.

ACKNOWLEDGMENTS

We thank Drs. Lita Braiterman and Janet Larkin for valuable comments and critical reading of this manuscript. Our work has been supported by National Institutes of Health grants DK44375 and GM29185 (A.L.H.) and fellowship DK09620 (P.L.T.).

REFERENCES

1. Drubin DG, Nelson WJ. Origins of cell polarity. *Cell* 1996;84: 335–344.
2. Simons K, Fuller SD. Cell surface polarity in epithelia. *Annu Rev Cell Biol* 1985;1:243–288.
3. Yeaman C, Grindstaff KK, Nelson WJ. New perspectives on mechanisms involved in generating epithelial cell polarity. *Physiol Rev* 1999;79:73–98.
4. Ihrke G, Hubbard AL. Control of vessicle traffic in hepatocytes. In: Boyer JL, Ockner RK, eds. *Progress in liver diseases*, vol 13. Philadelphia: WB Saunders, 1995:63–99.
5. Hubbard AL, Barr VA, Scott LJ. Hepatocyte Surface Polarity. In: Arias IM, Boyer JL, Fausto N, et al., eds. *The liver: biology and pathobiology*, 3rd ed. New York: Raven Press, 1994: 189–213.
6. Gundersen D, Orlowski J, Rodriguez-Boulan E. Apical polarity of Na,K-ATPase in retinal pigment epithelium is linked to a reversal of the ankyrin-fodrin submembrane cytoskeleton. *J Cell Biol* 1991;112:863–872.
7. Matyas GR, Morre DJ. Subcellular distribution and biosynthesis of rat liver gangliosides. *Biochim Biophys Acta* 1987;921: 599–614.
8. Crawford JM. Role of vesicle-mediated transport pathways in hepatocellular bile secretion. *Semin Liver Dis* 1996;16: 169–189.
9. Glaumann H, Peters T Jr, Redman C, eds. In: Glaumann H, Peters T Jr, Redman C, eds. *Plasma protein secretion by the liver*. London: Academic Press, 1983.
10. Burgess L, Kelly RB. Constitutive and regulated secretion of proteins. *Annu Rev Cell Biol* 1987;3:243–293.
11. Boyer JL. Isolated hepatocyte couplets and bile duct units—novel preparations for the in vitro study of bile secretory function. *Cell Biol Toxicol* 1997;13:289–300.
12. Gomez-Lechon MJ, Jover R, Donato T, et al. Long-term expression of differentiated functions in hepatocytes cultured in three-dimensional collagen matrix. *J Cell Physiol* 1998;177:553–562.
13. Liu X, Brouwer KL, Gan LS, et al. Partial maintenance of taurocholate uptake by adult rat hepatocytes cultured in a collagen sandwich configuration. *Pharm Res* 1998;15:1533–1539.
14. Aden DP, Fogel A, Plotkin S, et al. Controlled synthesis of HBsAg in a differentiated human liver carcinoma-derived cell line. *Nature* 1979;282:615–616.
15. Chiu JH, Hu CP, Lui WY, et al. The formation of bile canaliculi in human hepatoma cell lines. *Hepatology* 1990;11:834–842.
16. Hoekstra D, Kok JW. Trafficking of glycosphingolipids in eukaryotic cells; sorting and recycling of lipids. *Biochim Biophys Acta* 1992;1113:277–294.
17. Hoekstra D, Zegers MM, van Ijzendoorn SC. Membrane flow, lipid sorting and cell polarity in HepG2 cells: role of a subapical compartment [In Process Citation]. *Biochem Soc Trans* 1999; 27:422–428.
18. Hoekstra D, van Ijzendoorn SC. Lipid trafficking and sorting: how cholesterol is filling gaps [In Process Citation]. *Curr Opin Cell Biol* 2000;12:496–502.
19. Cassio D, Weiss MC. Expression of fetal and neonatal hepatic functions by mouse hepatoma-rat hepatoma hybrids. *Somat Cell Genet* 1979;5:719–738.
20. Cassio D, Hamon-Benais C, Guerin M, et al. Hybrid cell lines constitute a potential reservoir of polarized cells: isolation and study of highly differentiated hepatoma-derived hybrid cells able to form functional bile canaliculi in vitro. *J Cell Biol* 1991; 115:1397–1408.
21. Shanks MS, Cassio D, Lecoq O, et al. An improved rat hepatoma hybrid cell line. Generation and comparison with its hepatoma relatives and hepatocytes in vivo. *J Cell Sci* 1994;107: 813–825.
22. Ihrke G, Neufeld EB, Meads T, et al. WIF-B cells: an in vitro model for studies of hepatocyte polarity. *J Cell Biol* 1993;123: 1761–1775.
23. Meads T, Schroer TA. Polarity and nucleation of microtubules in polarized epithelial cells. *Cell Motil Cytoskeleton* 1995;32: 273–288.
24. Decaens C, Rodriguez P, Bouchaud C, et al. Establishment of hepatic cell polarity in the rat hepatoma-human fibroblast hybrid WIF-B9. A biphasic phenomenon going from a simple epithelial polarized phenotype to an hepatic polarized one. *J Cell Sci* 1996;109:1623–1635.
25. Howell KE, Gruenberg J, Ito A, et al. Immuno-isolation of subcellular components. *Prog Clin Biol Res* 1988;270:77–90.

26. Barr VA, Scott LJ, Hubbard AL. Immunoadsorption of hepatic vesicles carrying newly synthesized dipeptidyl peptidase IV and polymeric IgA receptor. *J Biol Chem* 1995;270:27834–27844.

27. Ihrke G, Martin GV, Shanks MR, et al. Apical plasma membrane proteins and endolyn-78 travel through a subapical compartment in polarized WIF-B hepatocytes. *J Cell Biol* 1998;141:115–133.

28. Pagano RE, Sleight RG. Defining lipid transport pathways in animal cells. *Science* 1985;229:1051–1057.

29. van Ijzendoorn SC, Zegers MM, Kok JW, et al. Segregation of glucosylceramide and sphingomyelin occurs in the apical to basolateral transcytotic route in HepG2 cells. *J Cell Biol* 1997;137:347–357.

30. van Ijzendoorn SC, Hoekstra D. (Glyco)sphingolipids are sorted in sub-apical compartments in HepG2 cells: a role for non-Golgi-related intracellular sites in the polarized distribution of (glyco)sphingolipids. *J Cell Biol* 1998;142:683–696.

31. Bastaki M, Braiterman LT, Chen Y, et al. Indirect transport of apical single transmembrane domain (TMD) proteins in hepatocytes. *Mol Biol Cell* 2000;[abstract]311a.

32. Fullekrug J, Scheiffele P, Simons K. VIP36 localisation to the early secretory pathway. *J Cell Sci* 1999;112:2813–2821.

33. Marmorstein AD, Csaky KG, Baffi J, et al. Saturation of, and competition for entry into, the apical secretory pathway. *Proc Natl Acad Sci USA* 2000;97:3248–3253.

34. Matter K, Mellman I. Mechanisms of cell polarity: sorting and transport in epithelial cells. *Curr Opin Cell Biol* 1994;6:545–554.

35. Ikonen E, Simons K. Protein and lipid sorting from the trans-Golgi network to the plasma membrane in polarized cells. *Semin Cell Dev Biol* 1998;9:503–509.

36. van Meer G, Holthuis JC. Sphingolipid transport in eukaryotic cells. *Biochim Biophys Acta* 2000;1486:145–170.

37. Mostov KE, Verges M, Altschuler Y. Membrane traffic in polarized epithelial cells [In Process Citation]. *Curr Opin Cell Biol* 2000;12:483–490.

38. Mostov KE, Cardone MH. Regulation of protein traffic in polarized epithelial cells. *BioEssays* 1995;17:129–138.

39. Bartles JR, Feracci HM, Stieger B, et al. Biogenesis of the rat hepatocyte plasma membrane in vivo: comparison of the pathways taken by apical and basolateral proteins using subcellular fractionation. *J Cell Biol* 1987;105:1241–1251.

40. Schell MJ, Maurice M, Stieger B, et al. 5′ nucleotidase is sorted to the apical domain of hepatocytes via an indirect route. *J Cell Biol* 1992;119:1173–1182.

41. Maroux S, Coudrier E, Feracci H, et al. Molecular organization of the intestinal brush border. *Biochimie* 1988;70:1297–1306.

42. Hauri H-P, Sterchi EE, Bienz D, et al. Expression and intracellular transport of microvillus membrane hydrolases in human intestinal epithelial cells. *J Cell Biol* 1985;101:838–851.

43. Hammerton RW, Krzeminski KA, Mays RW, et al. Mechanism for regulating cell surface distribution of Na+,K+-ATPase in polarized epithelial cells. *Science* 1991;254:847–850.

44. Dunbar LA, Roush DL, Courtois-Coutry N, et al. Sorting of ion pumps in polarized epithelial cells. *Ann NY Acad Sci* 1997;834:514–523.

45. Scott LJ, Hubbard AL. Dynamics of four rat liver plasma membrane proteins and polymeric IgA receptor. Rates of synthesis and selective loss into the bile. *J Biol Chem* 1992;267:6099–6106.

46. Pous C, Chabin K, Drechou A, et al. Functional specialization of stable and dynamic microtubules in protein traffic in WIF-B cells. *J Cell Biol* 1998;142:153–165.

47. Strous GJ, Lodish HF. Intracellular transport of secretory and membrane proteins in hepatoma cells infected by vesicular stomatitis virus. *Cell* 1980;22:709–717.

48. Nickel W, Huber LA, Kahn RA, et al. ADP ribosylation factor and a 14-kD polypeptide are associated with heparan sulfate-carrying post-trans-Golgi network secretory vesicles in rat hepatocytes. *J Cell Biol* 1994;125:721–732.

49. Hirschberg K, Miller CM, Ellenberg J, et al. Kinetic analysis of secretory protein traffic and characterization of Golgi to plasma membrane transport intermediates in living cells. *J Cell Biol* 1998;143:1485–1503.

50. Aroeti B, Okhrimenko H, Reich V, et al. Polarized trafficking of plasma membrane proteins: emerging roles for coats, SNAREs, GTPases and their link to the cytoskeleton. *Biochim Biophys Acta* 1998;1376:57–90.

51. Stoorvogel W, Oorschot V, Geuze HJ. A novel class of clathrin-coated vesicles budding from endosomes. *J Cell Biol* 1996;132:21–33

52. Leitinger B, Hille-Rehfeld A, Spiess M. Biosynthetic transport of the asialoglycoprotein receptor H1 to the cell surface occurs via endosomes. *Proc Natl Acad Sci USA* 1995;92:10109–10113.

53. Futter CE, Connolly CN, Cutler DF, et al. Newly synthesized transferrin receptors can be detected in the endosome before they appear on the cell surface. *J Biol Chem* 1995;270:10999–11003.

54. Ohno H, Tomemori T, Nakatsu F, et al. Mu1B, a novel adaptor medium chain expressed in polarized epithelial cells. *FEBS Lett* 1999;449:215–220.

55. Folsch H, Ohno H, Bonifacino JS, et al. A novel clathrin adaptor complex mediates basolateral targeting in polarized epithelial cells [see comments]. *Cell* 1999;99:189–198.

56. Chen YT, Stewart DB, Nelson WJ. Coupling assembly of the E-cadherin/beta-catenin complex to efficient endoplasmic reticulum exit and basal-lateral membrane targeting of E-cadherin in polarized MDCK cells. *J Cell Biol* 1999;144:687–699.

57. Fanning AS, Anderson JM. Protein modules as organizers of membrane structure. *Curr Opin Cell Biol* 1999;11:432–439.

58. Perego C, Vanoni C, Villa A, et al. PDZ-mediated interactions retain the epithelial GABA transporter on the basolateral surface of polarized epithelial cells. *EMBO J* 1999;18:2384–2393.

59. Schneider S, Buchert M, Georgiev O, et al. Mutagenesis and selection of PDZ domains that bind new protein targets [see comments]. *Nat Biotechnol* 1999;17:170–175.

60. Rashbass P, Skaer H. Cell polarity: nailing crumbs to the scaffold. *Curr Biol* 2000;10:R234–236.

61. Mostov KE. Transepithelial transport of immunoglobulins. *Annu Rev Immunol* 1994;12:63–84.

62. Geuze HJ, Slot JW, Strous GJ, et al. Intracellular receptor sorting during endocytosis: comparative immunoelectron microscopy of multiple receptors in rat liver. *Cell* 1984;37:195–204.

63. Hoppe CA, Connolly TP, Hubbard AL. Transcellular transport of polymeric IgA in the rat hepatocyte: biochemical and morphological characterization of the transport pathway. *J Cell Biol* 1985;101:2113–2123.

64. Larkin JM, Palade GE. Transcytotic vesicular carriers for polymeric IgA receptors accumulate in rat hepatocytes after bile duct ligation. *J Cell Sci* 1991;98:205–216.

65. Barr VA, Hubbard AL. Newly synthesized hepatocyte plasma membrane proteins are transported in transcytotic vesicles in the bile duct-ligated rat. *Gastroenterology* 1993;105:554–571.

66. Wang E, Brown APS, Aroeti B, et al. Apical and basolateral endocytic pathways of MDCK cells meet in acidic common endosomes distinct from a nearly neutral apical recycling endosome. *Traffic* 2000;1:480–493.

67. Zegers MM, Zaal KJ, van Ijzendoorn SC, et al. Actin filaments and microtubules are involved in different membrane traffic pathways that transport sphingolipids to the apical surface of polarized HepG2 cells. *Mol Biol Cell* 1998;9:1939–1949.

68. Sai Y, Nies AT, Arias IM. Bile acid secretion and direct targeting of mdr1-green fluorescent protein from Golgi to the canalicular membrane in polarized WIF-B cells. *J Cell Sci* 1999; 112:4535–4545.

69. Kipp H, Arias IM. Newly synthesized canalicular ABC transporters are directly targeted from the Golgi to the hepatocyte apical domain in rat liver. *J Biol Chem* 2000;275: 15917–15925.

70. Casanova JE, Hubbard AL, Mishumi Y, et al. Direct apical sorting of rat liver dipeptidylpeptidase IV expressed in Madin-Darby canine kidney cells. 1991;266:24428–24432.

71. Lisanti MP, Caras IW, Davitz MA, et al. A glycophospholipid membrane anchor acts as an apical targeting signal in polarized epithelial cells. *J Cell Biol* 1989;109:2145–2156.

72. Puertollano R, Martin-Belmonte F, Millan J, et al. The MAL proteolipid is necessary for normal apical transport and accurate sorting of the influenza virus hemagglutinin in Madin-Darby canine kidney cells. *J Cell Biol* 1999;145:141–151.

73. Kim T, Fiedler K, Madison DL, et al. Cloning and characterization of MVP17: a developmentally regulated myelin protein in oligodendrocytes. *J Neurosci Res* 1995;42:413–422.

74. Brown DA, London E. Functions of lipid rafts in biological membranes. *Annu Rev Cell Dev Biol* 1998;14:111–136.

75. Edidin M. Lipid microdomains in cell surface membranes. *Curr Opin Struct Biol* 1997;7:528–532.

76. Harder T, Simons K. Caveolae, DIGs, and the dynamics of sphingolipid-cholesterol microdomains. *Curr Opin Cell Biol* 1997;9:534–542.

77. Brown DA, London E. Structure and function of sphingolipid- and cholesterol-rich membrane rafts. *J Biol Chem* 2000;275: 17221–17224.

78. Keller P, Simons K. Cholesterol is required for surface transport of influenza virus hemagglutinin. *J Cell Biol* 1998;140: 1357–1367.

79. Hannan LA, Edidin M. Traffic, polarity, and detergent solubility of a glycosylphosphatidylinositol-anchored protein after LDL-deprivation of MDCK cells. *J Cell Biol* 1996;133: 1265–1276.

80. Zaal KJ, Kok JW, Sormunen R, et al. Intracellular sites involved in the biogenesis of bile canaliculi in hepatic cells. *Eur J Cell Biol* 1994;63:10–19.

81. Futerman AH, Stieger B, Hubbard AL, et al. Sphingomyelin synthesis in rat liver occurs predominantly at the cis and medial cisternae of the Golgi apparatus. *J Biol Chem* 1990;265: 8650–8657.

82. Futerman AH, Pagano RE. Determination of the intracellular sites and topology of glucosylceramide synthesis in rat liver. *Biochem J* 1991;280:295–302.

83. Pfeffer Scheller R. Transport vesicle docking: SNAREs and associates. *Annu Rev Cell Dev Biol* 1996;12:441–461.

84. Hay JC, Scheller RH. SNAREs and NSF in targeted membrane fusion. *Curr Biol* 1997;9:505–512.

85. Jahn R, Sudhof TC. Membrane fusion and exocytosis. *Annu Rev Biochem* 1999;68:863–911.

86. Johannes T, Galli T, Ludger J. Exocytosis: SNAREs drum up! *Eur J Neurosci* 1998;10:415–422.

87. Sollner T, Whiteheart SW, Brunner M. SNAP receptors implicated in vesicle targeting and fusion. *Nature* 1993;362: 318–324.

88. Hass A. NSF—fusion and beyond. *Trends Cell Biol* 1998;8: 471–473.

89. Mandon B, Chou CL, Nielsen S, et al. Syntaxin-4 is localized to the apical plasma membrane of rat renal collecting duct cells: possible role in aquaporin-2 trafficking. *J Clin Invest* 1996;98: 906–913.

90. Low SH, Chapin SJ, Wimmer C, et al. The SNARE machinery is involved in apical plasma membrane trafficking in MDCK cells. *J Cell Biol* 1998;141:1503–1513.

91. Gaisano HY, Sheu L, Grondin G, et al. The vesicle-associated membrane protein family of proteins in rat pancreatic and parotid acinar cells. *Gastroenterology* 1996;111:1661–1669.

92. Peng X-R, Yao X, Chow D-C, et al. Association of syntaxin 3 and vesicle-associated membrane protein (VAMP) with H^+/K^+-ATPase-containing tubulovesicles in gastric parietal cells. *Mol Biol Cell* 1997;8:399–407.

93. Delgrossi MH, Breuza L, Mirre C, et al. Human syntaxin 3 is localized apically in human intestinal cells. *J Cell Sci* 997;110: 2207–2214.

94. Fujita H, Tuma PL, Finnegan CM, et al. Endogenous syntaxins 2, 3 and 4 exhibit distinct but overlapping patterns of expression at the hepatocyte plasma membrane. *Biochem J* 1998;329: 527–538.

95. Tuma P, Yi JH, Hubbard AL. Endogenous SNAP-23, ARF6 and syntaxins 1,2,3, and 4 exhibit overlapping patterns of expression at the hepatocyte plasma membrane. *Mol Biol Cell* 1997;8:88a.

96. Low SH, Roche PA, Anderson HA, et al. Targeting of SNAP-23 and SNAP-25 in polarized epithelial cells. *J Biol Chem* 1998;273:3422–3430.

97. Apodaca G, Cardone MH, Whiteheart SW, et al. Reconstitution of transcytosis in SLO-permeabilized MDCK cells: existence of an NSF-dependent fusion mechanism with the apical surface of MDCK cells. *EMBO J* 1996;15:1471–1481.

98. Inoue T, Nielsen S, Mandon B, et al. SNAP-23 in rat kidney: colocalization with aquaporin-2 in collecting duct vesicles. *Am J Physiol* 1998;275:F752–760.

99. Banerjee A, Shih T, Alexander EA, et al. SNARE proteins regulate H(+)-ATPase redistribution to the apical membrane in rat renal inner medullary collecting duct cells. *J Biol Chem* 1999; 274:26518–26522.

100. Leung SM, Chen D, DasGupta BR, et al. SNAP-23 requirement for transferrin recycling in sreptolysin-O-permeabilized Madin-Darby canine kidney cells. *J Biol Chem* 1998;273: 17732–17741.

101. Chen D, Whiteheart SW. Intracellular localization of SNAP-23 to endosomal compartments. *Biochem Biophys Res Commun* 1999;255:340–346.

102. Calvo M, Pol A, Lu A, et al. Cellubrevin is present in the basolateral endocytic compartment of hepatocytes and follows the transcytotic pathway after IgA internalization. *J Biol Chem* 2000;275:7910–7917.

103. Wong PP, Daneman N, Volchuk A, et al. Tissue distribution of SNAP-23 and its subcellular localization in 3T3-L1 cells. *Biochem Biophys Res Commun* 1997;230:64–68.

104. Galli T, Zahraoui A, Vaidyanathan VV, et al. A novel tetanus neurotoxin-insensitive vesicle-associated membrane protein in SNARE complexes of the apical plasma membrane of epithelial cells. *Mol Biol Cell* 1998;9:1437–1448.

105. Calhoun BC, Goldenring JR. Two Rab proteins, vesicle-associated membrane protein 2 (VAMP-2) and secretory carrier membrane proteins (SCAMPs), are present on immunoisolated parietal cell tubulovesicles. *J Biochem* 1997;325:559–564.

106. Ikonen E, Tagaya M, Ullrich O, et al. Different requirements for NSF, SNAP, and Rab proteins in apical and basolateral transport in MDCK cells. *Cell* 1995;81:571–580.

107. Mastick CC, Falick AL. Association of N-ethylmaleimide sensitive fusion (NSF) protein and soluble NSF attachment proteins-alpha and -gamma with glucose transporter-4–containing vesicles in primary rat adipocytes. *Endocrinology* 1997;138: 2391–2397.

108. Moriyama Y, Yamamoto A, Tagaya M, et al. Localization of N-ethylmaleimide-sensitive fusion protein in pinealocytes. *Neuroreport* 1995;6:1757–1760.

109. Riento K, Jantti J, Jansson S, et al. A Sec1-related vesicle-transport protein that is expressed predominantly in epithelial cells. *Eur J Biochem* 1996;239:638–646.

110. Lafont F, Verkade P, Galli T, et al. Raft association of SNAP receptors acting in apical trafficking in Madin-Darby canine kidney cells. *Proc Natl Acad Sci USA* 1999;96:3734–3738.

111. Jin M, Saucan L, Farquhar MG, et al. Rab1a and multiple other Rab proteins are associated with the transcytotic pathway in rat liver. *J Biol Chem* 1996;271:30105–30113.

112. Weber E, Berta G, Tousson A, et al. Expression and polarized targeting of a Rab3 isoform in epithelial cells. *J Cell Biol* 1994;125:583–594.

113. Larkin JM, Woo B, Balan V, et al. Rab3D, a small GTP-binding protein implicated in regulated secretion, is associated with the transcytotic pathway in rat hepatocytes. *Hepatology* 2000; 32:348–356.

114. Juvet LK, Berg T, Gjoen T. The expression of endosomal rab proteins correlates with endocytic rate in rat liver cells. *Hepatology* 1997;25:1204–1212.

115. Bucci C, Wandinger-Ness A, Lutcke A, et al. Rab5a is a common component of the apical and basolateral endocytic machinery in polarized epithelial cells. *Proc Natl Acad Sci USA* 1994;91:5061–5065.

116. Martinez O, Goud B. Rab proteins. *Biochim Biophys Acta* 1998; 1404:101–112.

117. Huber LA, Pimplikar S, Parton RG. et al. Rab8, a Small GTPase Involved in Vesicular Traffic between the TGN and the Basolateral Plasma Membrane. *J Cell Biol* 1993;123:35–45.

118. Duman JG, Tyagarajan K, Kolsi MS, et al. Expression of rab11a N124I in gastric parietal cells inhibits stimulatory recruitment of the H+-K+-ATPase [see comments]. *Am J Physiol* 1999;277: C361–372.

119. Casanova JE, Wang X, Kumar R, et al. Association of Rab25 and Rab11a with the apical recycling system of polarized Madin-Darby canine kidney cells. *Mol Biol Cell* 1999;10: 47–61.

120. Wang X, Kumar R, Navarre J, et al. Regulation of vesicle trafficking in MDCK cells by Rab11a and Rab25. *J Biol Chem* 2000;275:29138–29146.

121. Zahraoui A, Joberty G, Arpin M, et al. A small rab GTPase is distributed in cytoplasmic vesicles in non polarized cells but colocalizes with the tight junction marker ZO-1 in polarized epithelial cells. *J Cell Biol* 1994;124:101–115.

122. Lutcke A, Jansson S, Parton RG, et al. Rab17, a novel small GTPase, is specific for epithelial cells and is induced during cell polarization. *J Cell Biol* 1993;121:553–564.

123. Hunziker W, Peters PJ. Rab17 localizes to recycling endosomes and regulates receptor-mediated transcytosis in epithelial cells. *J Biol Chem* 1998;273:15734–15741.

124. Zacchi P, Stenmark H, Parton RG, et al. Rab17 regulates membrane trafficking through apical recycling endosomes in polarized epithelial cells. *J Cell Biol* 1998;140:1039–1053.

125. Hansen GH, Niels-Christiansen LL, Immerdal L, et al. Transcytosis of immunoglobulin A in the mouse enterocyte occurs through glycolipid raft- and rab17-containing compartments. *Gastroenterology* 1999;116:610–622.

126. Lutcke A, Parton RG, Murphy C, et al. Cloning and subcellular localization of novel rab proteins reveals polarized and cell type-specific expression. *J Cell Sci* 1994;107:3437–3448.

127. Sztul E, Colombo M, Stahl P, et al. Control of protein traffic between distinct plasma membrane domains. *J Biol Chem* 1993;268:1876–1885.

128. Whiteheart SW, Kubalek EW. SNAPs and NSF: general members of the fusion apparatus. *TICB* 1995;5:64–68.

129. Gaisano HY, Ghai M, Malkus PN, et al. Distinct cellular locations of the syntaxin family of proteins in rat pancreatic acinar cells. *Mol Biol Cell* 1996;7:2019–2027.

130. Wong SH, Zhang T, Xu Y, et al. Endobrevin, a novel synaprobrevin/VAMP-like protein preferentially associated with the early endosome. *Mol Biol Cell* 1998;9:1549–1563.

131. Fiedler K, Lafont F, Parton RG, et al. Annexin XIIIb: a novel epithelial specific annexin is implicated in vesicular traffic to the apical plasma membrane. *J Cell Biol* 1995;128:1043–1053.

132. Pevsner J. The role of Sec1p-related proteins in vesicle trafficking in the nerve terminal. *J Neurol Res* 1996;45:89–95.

133. Halachmi N, Lev Z. The Sec1 family: a novel family of proteins involved in synaptic transmission and general secretion. *J Neurochem* 1996;66:889–897.

134. Riento K, Kauppi M, Keranen S, et al. Munc18-2, a functional partner of syntaxin 3, controls apical membrane trafficking in epithelial cells. *J Biol Chem* 2000;275:13476–13483.

135. Schimmoller F, Simon I, Pfeffer SR. Rab GTPases, directors of vesicle docking. *J Biol Chem* 1998;273:22161–22164.

136. Gonzalez L, Scheller RH. Regulation of membrane trafficking: structural insights from a Rab/effector complex. *Cell* 1999;96: 755–758.

137. Rodman JS, Wandinger-Ness A. Rab GTPases coordinate endocytosis. *J Cell Sci* 2000;113:183–192.

138. McBride HM, Rybin V, Murphy C, et al. Oligomeric complexes link Rab5 effectors with NSF and drive membrane fusion via interactions between EEA1 and syntaxin 13. *Cell* 1999;98: 377–386.

139. Hunziker W, Kraehenbuhl J-P. Epithelial transcytosis of immunoglobulins. *J Mammary Gland Biol Neoplasia* 1998;3: 287–302.

140. Gottlieb TA, Ivanov IE, Adesnik M, et al. Actin microfilaments play a critical role in endocytosis at the apical but not the basolateral surface of polarized epithelial cells. *J Cell Biol* 1993;120: 695–710.

141. Shurety W, Bright NA, Luzio JP. The effects of cytochalasin D and phorbol myristate acetate on the apical endocytosis of ricin in polarised Caco-2 cells. *J Cell Sci* 1996;109:2927–2935.

142. Llorente A, Garred O, Holm PK, et al. Effect of calmodulin antagonists on endocytosis and intracellular transport of Ricin in polarized MDCK cells. *Exp Cell Res* 1996;227:298–308.

143. Holm PK, Eker P, Sandvig K, et al. Phorbol myristate acetate selectively stimulates apical endocytosis via protein kinase C in polarized MDCK cells. *Exp Cell Res* 1995;217:157–168.

144. Renfrew CA, Hubbard AL. Sequential processing of epidermal growth factor in early and late endosomes of rat liver. *J Biol Chem* 1991;266:4348–4356.

145. Futter CE, Pearse A, Hewlett LJ, et al. Multivesicular endosomes containing internalized EGF-EGF receptor complexes mature and then fuse directly with lysosomes. *J Cell Biol* 1996; 132:1011–1023.

146. Shore EM, Nelson WJ. Biosynthesis of the cell adhesion molecule uvomorulin (E-cadherin) in Madin-Darby canine kidney epithelial cells. *J Biol Chem* 1991;266:19672–19680.

147. Le TL, Yap AS, Stow JL. Recycling of E-cadherin: a potential mechanism for regulating cadherin dynamics. *J Cell Biol* 1999; 146:219–232.

148. Jeffers M, Taylor GA, Weidner KM, et al. Degradation of the Met tyrosine kinase receptor by the ubiquitin-proteasome pathway. *Mol Cell Biol* 1997;17:799–808.

149. Oude Elferink RPJ, Meijer DKF, Kuipers F, et al. Hepatobiliary secretion of organic compounds: molecular mechanisms of membrane transport. *Biochim Biophys Acta* 1995;1241: 215–268.

150. Naim HY, Dodds DT, Brewer CB, et al. Apical and basolateral coated pits of MDCK cells differ in their rates of maturation

into coated vesicles, but not in the ability to distinguish between mutant hemagglutinin proteins with different internalization signals. *J Cell Biol* 1995;129:1241–1250.

151. Bomsel M, Prydz K, Parton RG, et al. Endocytosis in filter-grown Madin-Darby canine kidney cells. *J Cell Biol* 1989;109:3243–3258.

152. Tuma PL, Finnegan CM, Yi JH, et al. Evidence for apical endocytosis in polarized hepatic cells: phosphoinositide 3-kinase inhibitors lead to the lysosomal accumulation of resident apical plasma membrane proteins. *J Cell Biol* 1999;145: 1089–1102.

153. van Ijzendoorn SC, Hoekstra D. Polarized sphingolipid transport from the subapical compartment: evidence for distinct sphingolipid domains. *Mol Biol Cell* 1999;10:3449–3461.

The Liver: Biology and Pathobiology, Fourth Edition, edited by I. M. Arias, J. L. Boyer, F. V. Chisari, N. Fausto, D. Schachter, and D. A. Shafritz. Lippincott Williams & Wilkins, Philadelphia © 2001.

THE ENDOPLASMIC RETICULUM AND GOLGI COMPLEX IN SECRETORY MEMBRANE TRANSPORT

JENNIFER LIPPINCOTT-SCHWARTZ

The secretory pathway is responsible for the regulated delivery of newly synthesized proteins, carbohydrate, and lipids to the surface of eukaryotic cells. It is composed of membrane-bound structures, including the endoplasmic reticulum (ER), Golgi complex, and vesicles/tubule transport intermediates that function in the processing, assembly, and plasma membrane delivery of secretory cargo that is synthesized in the ER (Fig. 9.1). Upon cotranslational insertion into the ER, newly synthesized cargo molecules are processed and assembled into transport competent forms. The cargo molecules are then packaged into vesicle/tubules that bud off the ER and translocate to the Golgi complex. In the Golgi complex, released cargo undergoes further processing before being sorted into transport intermediates that are destined for the cell surface. The directional flow of secretory cargo from ER to Golgi to plasma membrane is balanced by retrieval pathways that bring membrane and selected proteins back to the ER. Selective trafficking and retention of specific protein and lipid species within the secretory pathway allows cells to modify newly synthesized secretory products in a series of controlled steps, store molecules as needed, and then deliver them to specific cell surface domains. In this way, cellular growth and homeostasis are regulated.

Understanding the molecular basis for the organization and functioning of the secretory pathway and its selective

membrane transport is a major goal of cell biologic research. This chapter summarizes our current knowledge of this subject, and focuses on the functions of the ER and Golgi complex in secretory traffic, as well as the pathways connecting these organelles and the plasma membrane (see Chapters 8, 10, 11, and 24 and website chapter 🖥 W-6).

ENDOPLASMIC RETICULUM

Morphology and Organization

The ER is the port of entry of cargo into the secretory pathway, and is composed of an extensive array of interconnecting membrane tubules and cisternae. It is the largest compartment within the cell, occupying an extremely large surface area. In rat hepatocytes, for example, the ER occupies approximately 63,000 μm^2 per cell or about 38 times the surface area of the plasma membrane (1). The morphology of the ER includes cisternae, which are large, flat, sheet-like structures localized near the cell center, and tubules that extend off cisternae and interconnect as an elaborate network (Fig. 9.2). Lipophilic, cationic, fluorescent dyes, such as $DiOC_6$ (2), which selectively stain the ER, as well as proteins fused to green fluorescent protein (GFP) (3), have been used to study the dynamics of ER membranes in living cells (4,5). Polygonal-shaped ER networks form by extension, branching, and fusion of tubules (2). Branching and extension of free-ended ER tubules often occur along microtubules, which radiate out from the centrosomal region of the cell to

J. Lippincott-Schwartz: Section on Organelle Biology, Cell Biology and Metabolism Branch, National Institute of Child Health & Human Development, National Institutes of Health, Bethesda, Maryland 20817.

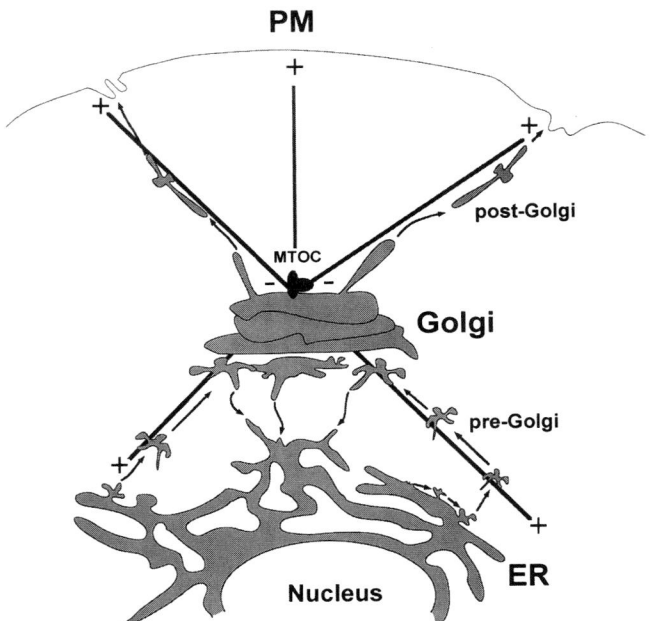

FIGURE 9.1. Diagram of the secretory membrane system. Newly synthesized proteins are synthesized in the endoplasmic reticulum (*ER*) and are packaged into transport intermediates that bud off from multiple sites of the ER. The pre-Golgi transport intermediates track into the Golgi region along microtubules, which extend plus-end–directed out from the microtubule organizing center (*MTOC*). Pre-Golgi intermediates fuse with the Golgi complex whereupon cargo undergoes processing by the variety of enzymes localized in the Golgi. Cargo is then packaged into post-Golgi transport intermediates that move plus-end–directed along microtubule tracks to reach the plasma membrane (*PM*) where they fuse and deliver their contents. The forward flow of cargo through the secretory pathway is balanced by retrieval pathways that bring selected membrane components back to the ER.

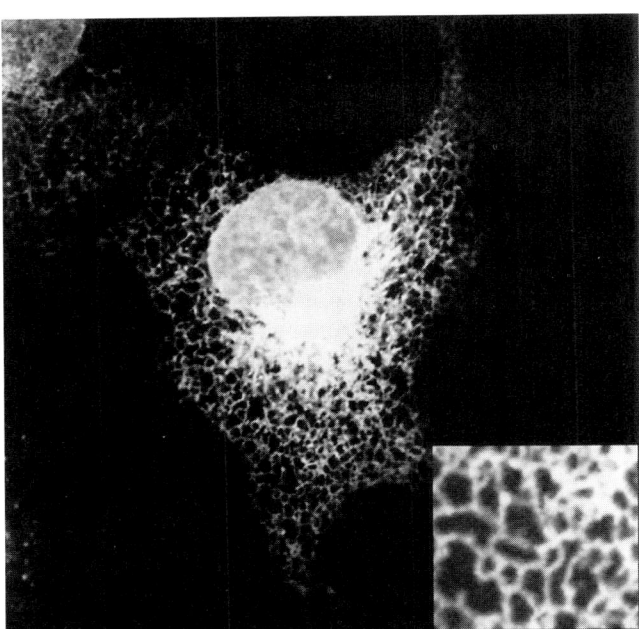

FIGURE 9.2. Morphology of the endoplasmic reticulum (ER) labeled with the cargo protein vesicular stomatitis virus tagged with green fluorescent protein (VSVG-GFP) retained in the ER at its restrictive temperature of 40°C. See Color Plate 3.

the periphery. The dynamic movements of ER tubules are thought to distribute ER membranes throughout the cytoplasm so it can take part in coordinating processes over large regions of the cytoplasm (2).

As a consequence of its tubular morphology, the ER is extensively disrupted by gentle homogenization. ER fragments generated during this procedure are called microsomes, whose closed vesicular morphology (approximately 100 nm diameter) is vastly different from that of the intact ER, which exists as a single interconnected network. Biochemical studies using ER-derived microsomal vesicles have been important for investigating the molecular composition, symmetry, distribution, and function of specific proteins associated with the ER.

The ER is generally subdivided into rough and smooth domains (called RER and SER, respectively) depending on whether ribosomes are associated with the cytoplasmic surfaces of the membrane. The RER is the site of synthesis and cotranslational membrane translocation of proteins, and is composed of flat cisternae and tubules studded with ribo-

somes. By contrast, the SER is composed of an irregular network of smooth-surfaced tubules with diverse functions including lipid biosynthesis, detoxification, and calcium regulation. These functions are not restricted to the SER, but also occur at some level in the RER. The ratio of RER/SER varies considerably among cells depending on the level of protein synthesis and other activities. For example, cells that synthesize large amounts of secretory proteins (i.e., plasma cells and acinar cells of the pancreas) lack distinct SER, while cells specialized in steroid biosynthesis (i.e., ovary, testis, and adrenal cortex cells) have mostly smooth ER. In rat hepatocytes approximately 60% of the ER is RER that is arranged in parallel arrays of broad flattened cisternae (1).

In addition to the SER and RER, there are many other morphologically distinct domains of the ER including nuclear envelope, transitional elements (where membrane exits the ER), crystalloid ER, and luminal ER bodies that contain protein aggregates (6). Each of these domains is enriched in specific proteins and perform different functions. These functions include lipid biosynthesis and metabolism; detoxification; protein synthesis, folding assembly, degradation, and transport; nuclear compartmentalization; glycogen mobilization; and calcium homeostasis. The spatial extension of the ER and the fact that its membranes and luminal spaces are continuous (so proteins can diffuse freely throughout) enables the ER to coordinate these diverse sets of functions.

Protein Folding, Processing, and Degradation

A major function of the ER is the processing and folding of newly synthesized proteins. When newly synthesized proteins emerge from ribosomes in the cytoplasm, they are targeted to the ER via a complex machinery, including signal recognition particle (SRP) and SRP receptor, that recognizes hydrophobic signal sequences on the peptide and then transports the ribosome-peptide complex to sites on the ER where translocation into the ER lumen can occur (7). Upon insertion into the ER lumen or membrane, newly synthesized proteins encounter the luminal environment of the ER, which is enriched in folding enzymes and chaperones (8,9). Folding reactions by ER chaperones are necessary for converting newly synthesized proteins from low-energy, monomeric forms to higher-energy multimeric complexes that function in various final destinations within cells. Proteins that are unable to fold and assemble correctly in the ER are degraded (10). In this way, the ER serves as a quality control system for ensuring that only correctly folded molecules enter the secretory pathway (11).

As a protein folding environment, the ER exhibits unique properties. These include the generation of oxidizing conditions to facilitate disulfide bond formation, the presence of chaperones to facilitate folding [i.e., BiP, oligosaccharide transferase, calnexin, calreticulin, and protein disulfide isomerase (PDI)], and maintenance of ionic conditions (i.e., high free calcium concentrations) appropriate for the folding process (9). Many resident proteins of the ER (including PDI, GRP94, and GRP74) exist in very high concentrations in the ER lumen and are thought to form a proteinaceous network with a gel-like consistency (12). Studies measuring the diffusional mobility of noninvasive probes in the ER lumen showed that they diffused 9 to 18 times slower than in water, demonstrating that the ER lumen is a highly viscous environment (5). This characteristic of the ER lumen could facilitate the processes whereby newly synthesized proteins continuously fold, unfold, and refold into their proper conformation prior to entry into the secretory pathway.

Proper folding of proteins synthesized in the ER occurs in stages, beginning as the nascent protein enters the ER cotranslationally. The polypeptide moiety first translocated into the ER lumen, usually the N-terminus, frequently starts to fold before the entire molecule has been translocated (7). Folding is facilitated by several processes (9), including (a) removal of the signal sequence of the polypeptide by signal peptidase, (b) addition of carbohydrate chains, (c) catalyzed isomerization of prolines by *cis-trans* proline isomerase, and (d) association with folding chaperones like BiP and/or calnexin.

The formation of disulfide bonds plays a crucial role in the folding of newly synthesized proteins (13–16). Not only do disulfide bonds give extra stability to the folded state, but the orderly formation of disulfide cross-links may limit the number of conformations that a polypeptide undergoes during folding and therefore direct the folding process toward one final direction. The abundant ER protein, PDI, is the enzyme primarily involved in disulfide bond formation (14). Its active sites can act as a reductase, an isomerase, or oxidase depending on the redox conditions in the ER (14).

The addition of carbohydrate to newly synthesized proteins within the ER plays an additional role in the folding process and is believed to increase the solubility of folding intermediates, perhaps by counteracting the propensity of partially folded polypeptides to aggregate (17,18). When glycosylation is inhibited, many proteins misfold in the ER, acquiring aberrant intermolecular disulfide bonds and becoming transport incompetent (17,19). These proteins lacking glycosylation have been shown in biochemical and diffusional mobility experiments to form large immobile aggregates (4,17).

The most common type of glycosylation occurring within the ER is N-linked glycosylation of proteins involving the addition of oligosaccharides to the amino group of asparagine residues (18). The core carbohydrate moiety used in this process is assembled on a common dolicol pyrophosphate molecule. This requires the translocation of lipid-linked oligosaccharides and nucleotide sugars across the ER membrane, which is mediated by specific translocases and nucleotide sugar transporters (20). The enzyme oligosaccharide transferase then transfers the core sugars as preassembled 14-saccharide units ($GlcNAC_2$-Man_9Glc_3) to a specific consensus sequence (Asn-X-Ser/Thr) on the polypeptide.

Many proteins while in the ER proceed to assemble into homo- or hetero-oligomeric structures. The oligomeric state of these proteins has been shown to be crucial in controlling both their functional properties as well as their intracellular transport and distribution within cells. Misfolded and unassembled polypeptides, for example, are usually retained in the ER and are frequently degraded there (10). Oligomer formation can arise either from polypeptides that are synthesized separately and then assembled or by posttranslational proteolytic cleavages of precursor polypeptides. Whatever mechanisms by which they are generated, the individual subunits first fold independently before being assembled (9). Stabilization of the oligomeric state is achieved primarily by extensive noncovalent interactions, although some have interchain disulfide bonds (8,9). Once assembled correctly, these molecules are rapidly and selectively exported from the ER.

Individual subunits of multimeric complexes often are synthesized in the ER at different rates, leading to an excess of some chains (10). Since most of these unassembled or incompletely assembled subunits cannot exit the ER, a mechanism for preventing their accumulation is required. For many proteins that fail to assemble properly in the ER, a selective degradation process is the mechanism for their removal (10,21). Degradation is thought to occur through a process involving retrograde translocation of the proteins across the ER membrane back into the cytosol where they are degraded by proteosomes (22). Thus, inhibitors of proteosomal function block degradation of these ER proteins. Examples of multimeric complexes whose unassembled subunits are retained in the ER and then undergo rapid degradation include T-cell antigen receptor (TCR) α, β, γ, and δ chains, mutated immunoglobulin chains, and the H2 α-subunit of the asialoglycoprotein receptor (10).

Extensive research has been devoted to understanding what structural features of a protein and its environment determine whether it is retained or degraded in the ER. For the TCR α-subunit, a mutational analysis revealed two residues, arg and lys, in its transmembrane domain as crucial for the degradation phenotype (21). Transfer of this sequence to other proteins resulted in rapid degradation of the chimeric proteins in the ER. Similar observations for other rapidly degraded ER membrane proteins have led to the idea that there exists a consensus motif for degradation, which is a predominantly hydrophobic sequence containing one or two potentially charged amino acid residues.

Studies examining the diffusional mobility of fluorescently tagged reporter proteins have addressed whether misfolded proteins are retained in the ER by being immobilized or aggregated in this compartment. In one study (4), a comparison of the diffusional mobility using fluorescence recovery after photobleaching (FRAP) was made of misfolded and correctly folded forms of the temperature sensitive variant (ts045) of vesicular stomatitis virus tagged with GFP (VSVG-GFP), which has been used as a model protein for analyzing protein folding and transport. No difference was observed in the diffusional mobility and mobile fraction of ER-localized VSVG-GFP when it was misfolded at the restrictive temperature or when it was correctly folded at the permissive temperature. This indicates that misfolded VSVG complexes are not retained in the ER as a result of forming immobilized aggregates or by tethering to a rigid meshwork. Rather, retention of these molecules, and possibly other misfolded proteins, appears to result from their failure to interact with ER export machinery, which prevents them from being exported out of this compartment.

ENDOPLASMIC RETICULUM-TO-GOLGI TRAFFICKING

Transport from the ER to the Golgi complex involves a series of steps whereby transport intermediates form, bud off from the ER, and move to the Golgi complex. This involves three fundamental processes: (a) sorting and concentration for exit out of the ER, (b) differentiation and translocation of membrane-bound transport intermediates, and (c) regulated fusion of transport intermediates with tar-

get membranes. As discussed below, a wide variety of approaches have been used to gain insight into how these processes occur and what molecular machinery controls them.

Endoplasmic Reticulum Export and the Role of Coat Protein Complexes

The formation of vesicles/tubules that bud off from the ER is the first step in delivery of newly synthesized cargo to the Golgi complex. This process occurs within specialized regions of the ER that are devoid of ribosomes and are adjacent to clusters of elaborate membrane tubules/vesicles called pre-Golgi intermediates (23), vesicular tubule clusters (VTCs) (24), or the intermediate compartment (25). ER exit sites are sometimes localized to discrete regions of the ER, as in differentiated muscle cells, where they localize along the nuclear envelope. In other cell types, they are distributed throughout the ER. In all cases, they comprise relatively large domains (1 to 2 μm diameter) that contain multiple budding profiles (23,24). Small 50- to 90-nm vesicles are thought to bud off from these sites and then to fuse locally to form pre-Golgi intermediates, which subsequently translocate through the cytoplasm to fuse with the Golgi complex. Because ultrastructural studies sometimes show direct membrane connections between ER exit sites and pre-Golgi intermediates (26), it is possible that the tubule clusters comprising pre-Golgi intermediates directly bud off from ER exit sites without the use of small vesicles.

Two sets of soluble protein complexes or coats, COPII and COPI, are thought to underlie sorting and concentration of secretory cargo at ER exit sites (27,28). COPII complexes assemble onto these sites first and are thought to initiate the concentration of cargo. Assembly of COPII originates with Sec12p-mediated nucleotide exchange of guanosine triphosphate (GTP) for guanosine diphosphate (GDP) on the small guanosine triphosphatase (GTPase) Sar1p (27). Cargo molecules are thought to trigger Sar1p activation to the GTP-bound form. Following activation of Sar1, the Sec 23p/Sec24p and Sec13p/31p complexes of COPII are recruited to the cytoplasmic leaflet of the ER and are thought to transform these membranes into buds and vesicles (Fig. 9.3). Electron microscopy studies have shown that when COPII assembles onto the surface of ER exit sites they form a hexagonal array that could provide the mechanical force necessary for creating a bud (24). Events triggering coat disassembly are unknown, but might be coupled to fission of COPII coated structures that have budded out from the ER.

The essential role of COPII in protein exit out of the ER has been demonstrated both in yeast and mammalian cells (27,29). Temperature-sensitive Sec23p (the GTPase activating protein, GAP, for Sar1p) mutants in yeast show a complete lack of protein exit from the ER and dominant-negative forms of Sar1p, as well as anti-Sar1p antibodies,

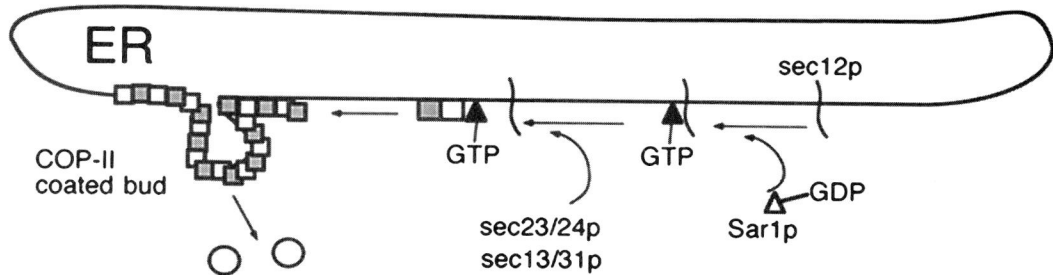

FIGURE 9.3. Model for COPII-mediated membrane budding at endoplasmic reticulum (*ER*) exit sites. *GDP*, guanosine diphosphate; *GTP*, guanosine triphosphate.

prevent exit of cargo from the ER in mammalian cells. In addition, COPII is thought to play a direct role in the concentration of cargo at ER exit sites, since the cytoplasmic domains of numerous transmembrane proteins, several of which are putative cargo receptors, have been shown to bind Sec23p *in vitro* (29).

While the activity of Sar1p/COPII appears to be crucial for initiating the organization of ER exit sites and leads to selective concentration of cargo, because it acts only at this location, Sar1p/COPII is insufficient to complete the job of membrane transport and organellogenesis. For this, surface-destined membrane components must be selectively retained within forward moving membrane domains as transport machinery necessary for ER export recycles back to the ER system (30). Growing evidence indicates that COPI helps to perform this job. The COPI coat is composed of seven subunits of a cytosolic protein complex called coatomer and is localized on pre-Golgi intermediates, along the cis face of the Golgi and associated with the rims of subsequent cisternae (31). COPI binding to membrane requires activation of ADP ribosylation factor 1 (ARF1) GTPase, analogous to the dependence of SAR1 GTPase for COPII binding. Sequential binding of COPII followed by COPI at ER exit sites (32–34) indicates that association of COPI to membranes arises after these membranes have been first differentiated by the activity of COPII. COPI binding appears to play a critical role in the further differentiation of these sites. Not only are additional proteins recruited to ER exit sites upon COPI binding, but as pre-Golgi intermediates mature into Golgi elements, retention of the concentrated assembly of proteins within these structures is critically dependent on COPI binding (30). This view is based on *in vivo* studies that have shown that cargo proteins such as VSVG fail to efficiently cluster into ER exit sites or concentrate in pre-Golgi intermediates in cells where COPI is prevented from binding to membranes (e.g., in cells expressing ARF dominant-negative mutants and in cells treated with the drug brefeldin A) even though COPII still associates with membranes (35–37). Additionally, *in vitro* studies reconstituting ER-to-Golgi transport have

shown that inhibitory mutants of ARF1 block ER-to-Golgi traffic, as do temperature sensitive mutants of COPI subunits (38,39).

Pre-Golgi Intermediates

The pre-Golgi transport intermediates generated by the sequential activities of COPII and COPI have only a transient existence before they translocate to and fuse with the Golgi complex. Time-lapse imaging studies using GFP-tagged cargo to label pre-Golgi intermediates have shown that they translocate through the cytoplasm as large structures using microtubules to track inward to the Golgi complex (32,40) (Fig. 9.4). During movement toward the Golgi complex, the pre-Golgi intermediates often deform in shape, extending long tubular processes. They also sort and recycle selected components back to the ER (41). COPI association with pre-Golgi intermediates is thought to play a key role in regulating this retrograde transport back to the ER, although exactly how is controversial (30,42). COPI subunits can bind to dilysine motifs, which are found on the C-terminus of several proteins that constitutively cycle between the Golgi and ER (43,44). This has led to the proposal that upon binding dilysine-containing proteins, COPI assembles retrograde transport vesicles (45). If COPI mediates retrograde transport in this fashion, however, ARF inhibition (which blocks COPI association with membranes) should block retrograde transport. In fact, ARF inhibition enhances retrograde traffic and leads to a block in protein export out of the ER (36–39). An alternative role of COPI, therefore, is in sorting/retention of molecules within pre-Golgi and Golgi structures (30). This activity could serve to limit the type and extent of retrograde traffic back to the ER. In so doing, it would allow pre-Golgi intermediates to differentiate and mature.

Pre-Golgi intermediates undergo homotypic fusion with each other and Golgi elements as they track down into the Golgi region (40). Specificity of fusion is ensured by a number of different factors including small GTPases of the Rab family and various tethering factors in combination with SNARE (soluble *N*-ethylmaleimide–sensitive factor attach-

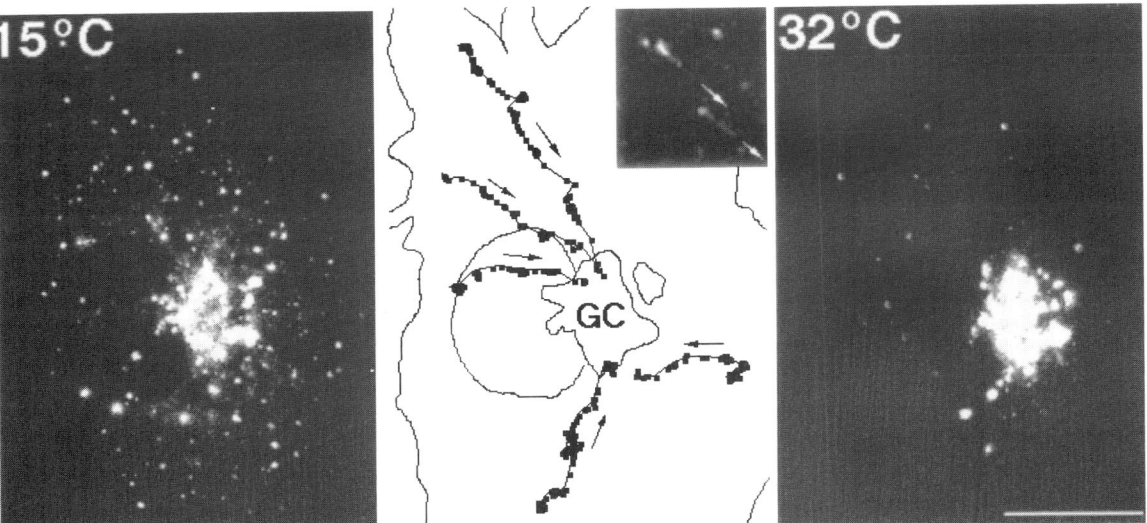

FIGURE 9.4. Translocation of pre-Golgi intermediates through the cytoplasm to the Golgi complex (*GC*) Pre-Golgi intermediates were loaded with vesicular stomatitis virus tagged with green fluorescent protein (VSVG-GFP) at 15°C. Cells were then warmed to 32°C to allow the pre-Golgi structures to track into the Golgi region. The **camera-lucent drawing** shows the microtubule-dependent paths followed by individual structures over a 10-minute interval after warm-up (see ref. 40).

ment protein receptor) proteins (28). The SNAREs are a family of membrane proteins that include vesicular (v)-SNAREs and target (t)-SNAREs that when brought in close proximity form complexes upon activation by the ATPase NSF (*N*-ethylmaleimide–sensitive factor) and subsequently drive fusion (28). These complexes can form on the same membrane or between SNAREs in different membranes. Tethering factors play a key role in assisting the targeting specificity of t- and v-SNAREs. In yeast, these factors include Uso1p, a homodimeric molecule with two heads and a long coiled-coil tail, Sec35p, and Sly1p (46,47). Ypt1p, a Rab-GTPase, is thought to coordinate the upstream events involved in membrane tethering and downstream SNARE-mediated functions. A large 800-kd protein complex of ten subunits termed TRAPP has also been proposed to function in membrane tethering events related to ER-Golgi trafficking (48).

GOLGI COMPLEX

Because pre-Golgi intermediates undergo maturation (by recycling of selected components back to the ER), are capable of homotypic fusion, and track into the Golgi region, it is generally thought that they are the direct precursors of Golgi elements, with Golgi cisternae formed by continuous maturation/differentiation of pre-Golgi intermediates. The Golgi complex, under this view, represents a dynamic steady-state system of ER-derived membranes undergoing maturation, recycling, and transport steps that give rise to selective enrichment in the Golgi of a variety of different

proteins and lipids (30,49). Among the proteins that are enriched in Golgi membranes are enzymes involved in glycosylation that orchestrate carbohydrate addition and remodeling of protein and lipid moving through the secretory pathway. There are an estimated 100 to 200 different glycosyltransferase enzymes distributed throughout the Golgi stack (50). These proteins are involved in the ordered remodeling of N-linked oligosaccharide side chains and the addition of O-linked glycans and oligosaccharide portions of proteoglycans and glycolipids. Collectively, they represent the major proportion of resident Golgi membrane proteins. Other Golgi components associated with this glycosylation machinery include nucleotide sugar transporters to transfer nucleotide sugars (which are the substrates for glycosyltransferases) from cytosol to Golgi lumen, and nucleoside diphosphatases, which are required to convert the nucleoside diphosphates to monophosphates (20). Besides proteins involved in carbohydrate modification, there are resident Golgi proteins that participate in membrane transport and the recycling of ER proteins. In addition, there are Golgi resident proteins involved in maintenance of the structural organization of the Golgi complex and its association with the cytoskeleton.

Golgi Compartmentalization and Function

Given the diversity of Golgi resident components, it is not surprising that this organelle has multiple cellular functions. These include receipt and recycling of membrane and soluble components arriving from the ER; glycosylation and processing of glycoproteins and glycolipids; and sorting of membrane and soluble components for delivery to the plasma membrane, lysosomes, or secretory granules (49,51). How does Golgi structure facilitate these diverse functions? The details of Golgi morphology vary between different cell types, but the classic image is of a set of three to ten flattened cisternae (1 µm diameter) with dilated rims arranged as a stack near the microtubule organizing center (26,49) (Fig. 9.5). Associated with this stack-like structure

are an array of small vesicles and a network of tubules that are believed to be involved in the transport of components into, out of, and within the Golgi. Newly synthesized membrane and secretory components first enter the Golgi complex at the *cis*-Golgi network (CGN), where pre-Golgi intermediates fuse. They then traverse through the Golgi stacks where they are sequentially modified by a variety of processing enzymes. Exit out of the Golgi occurs from the opposite face of the Golgi complex known as the *trans-*

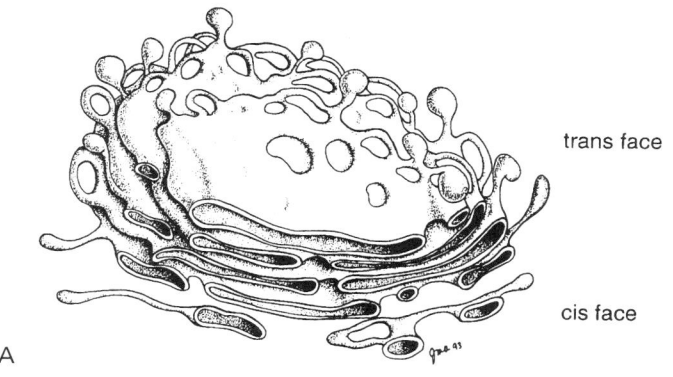

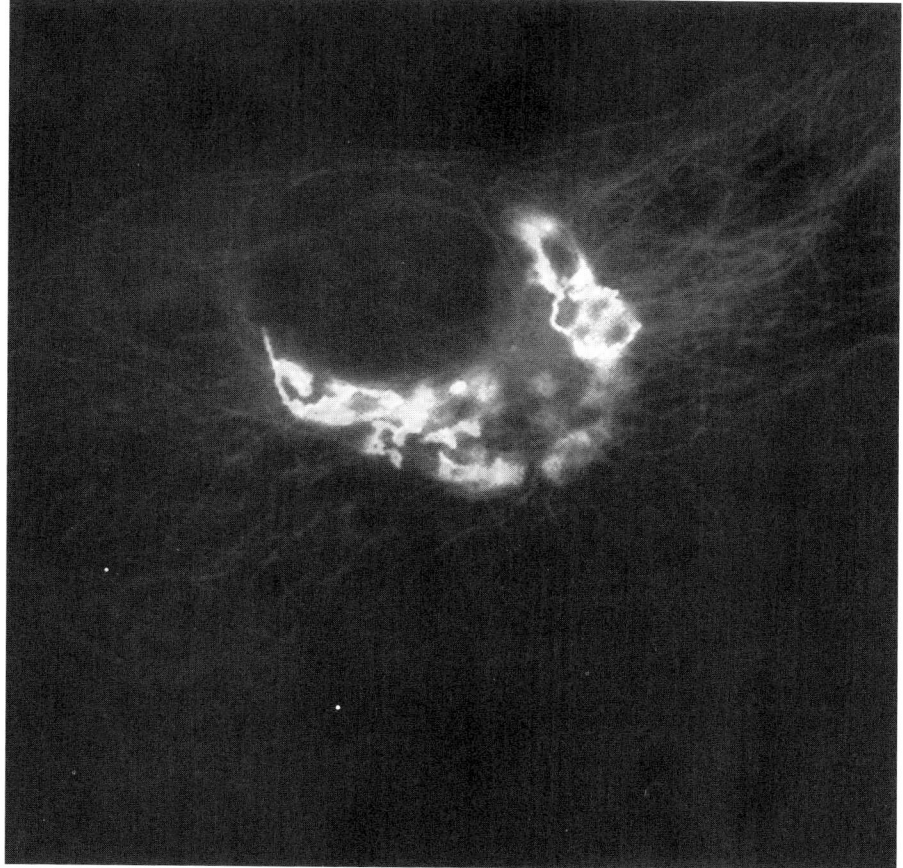

FIGURE 9.5. A: Three-dimensional structure of the Golgi complex. **B:** Localization of the Golgi complex in mammalian cell. *Green* is antibody labeling of tubulin, and *yellow* is antibody staining to the Golgi enzyme mannosidase II. See Color Plate 4.

Golgi network (TGN), which is the subcompartment where membrane and secretory components are sorted to different final cellular sites.

The polarized, compartmental view of the Golgi complex described above is supported by immunocytochemical and fractionation studies (localizing different Golgi proteins to different regions of the Golgi complex) and is reflected in the functions of the Golgi complex, which are associated with different domains of this organelle (49) (Table 9.1). The CGN, for example, not only serves as the site of entry into the Golgi complex but also functions in recycling of protein and lipid components back into the ER. Recycling of membrane and protein back into the ER is crucial for maintaining the surface area of the ER in the face of continuous outward flow of membrane (31). In addition, it might serve as a retrieval mechanism to prevent loss of ER resident proteins into the secretory pathway. Such a retrieval process is thought to underlie ER retention of soluble ER proteins containing the C-terminal tetrapeptide sequence KDEL (or HDEL) (51). Selective recycling of components back to the ER might also provide a quality control for transport of molecules out of the ER-Golgi system as has been suggested for newly synthesized heavy and light chains of major histocompatibility complex class 1 (MHC-1) in certain mutant cells that fail to assemble properly (52). These molecules constitutively cycle between the ER and Golgi instead of being transported to the plasma membrane. The membranes of the CGN are selectively stained after prolonged osmification and are enriched in several proteins including ERGIC53, KDELR, and Rab 2 (53,54). Since these proteins also are found in transitional elements and pre-Golgi intermediates, they are not resident CGN components, but probably constitutively cycle between the ER and Golgi. Only a limited population of molecules that enter the CGN appear to recycle back to the ER in this manner. The CGN, therefore, is the site of sorting of these molecules from the bulk of membrane and content moving through the secretory pathway.

In contrast to the CGN, which has only a limited role in carbohydrate-processing events, the Golgi stacks are where the bulk of the protein and lipid modifications occur within the Golgi complex. Remodeling of protein and lipid moving through the Golgi stacks proceeds in an ordered and efficient manner owing to the polarized distribution and high degree of specificity of the glycosidases and glycosyltransferases involved. The cisternal stack-like appearance of the Golgi stacks also is likely to enhance the efficiency of glycosylation by minimizing luminal volume and increasing membrane surface area.

One common posttranslational sugar modification occurring within the Golgi stacks is the remodeling of N-linked glycoproteins (Fig. 9.6). High-mannose N-linked glycoproteins are initially generated in the ER. In the Golgi stacks they are radically remodeled to complex structures owing to both sugar removal by specific glycosidases and terminal sugar addition (18). The majority of these glycosylation reactions occur at the luminal face of the membranes of the Golgi with several discrete enzymes (including mannosidase I, mannosidase II, and galactosyltransferase) acting sequentially to modify the precursor (20). Specific translocator proteins for UDP-N-acetylglucosamine, UDP-galactose, and CMP-N-acetylneuramic acid have been identified and have been shown to act as antiports, exchanging nucleotide sugars for nucleoside monophosphates formed during glycosyl transfer (20).

An additional set of processing reactions occurring in the Golgi stacks is the initiation and extension of O-linked glycan chains of glycosaminoglycans (55). During this process a specific tetrasaccharide composed of xylose, two residues of galactose, and glucuronic acid is added to selected serine and threonine residues on the polypeptide. Repeating disaccharides with their polypeptide backbones are then added

TABLE 9.1. GOLGI SUBCOMPARTMENTS

Subcompartment	Function	Markers
CGN	Receive components leaving ER	p53, p58, rab2
	Selective recycling to ER	OsO$_4$ reduction
Golgi stacks	Processing of N-linked and O-linked glycoproteins	Mannosidase II
	Phosphorylation of glycoproteins	Galactosyl transferase
	Elongation of GAGs and glycolipids	NADPase
	Addition of lipid to secretory lipoproteins	TPPase
		C$_{16}$-NBD-ceramide
TGN	Terminal glycosylation events	TGN38
	Tyrosine sulfation	WGA
	Proteolytic cleavages	Sialyltransferase
	Sorting to lysosomes and plasma membrane	TPPase
	Concentration of content	C$_{16}$-NBD-ceramide

CGN, *cis*-Golgi network; ER, endoplasmic reticulum; GAG, glycosaminoglycan; NADPase, nicotinamide adenine dinucleotide phosphatase; NBD, nitrobenzoxadiazole; TGN, *trans*-Golgi network; TPPase, thiamine pyrophosphatase; WGA, wheat germ agglutinin.

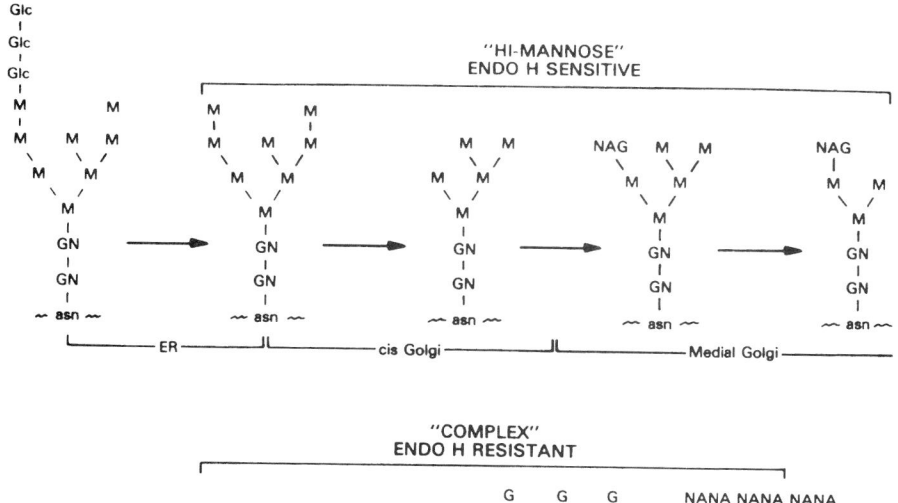

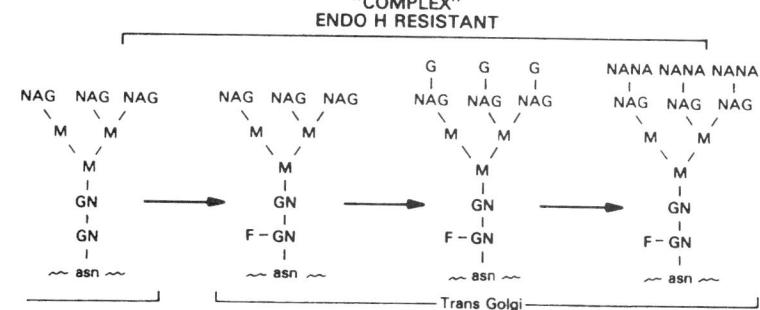

FIGURE 9.6. Pathway for processing of N-linked oligosaccharides in glycoproteins within the endoplasmic reticulum and Golgi complex.

as the molecule moves through the Golgi stacks. These units then undergo sulfation before exiting the Golgi complex in the TGN.

Phosphorylation of selected N-glycan chains on proteins and their modification to mannose-6-phosphate units also occurs within the Golgi stacks (56). This modification enables the terminal glycan unit to interact with mannose-9-phosphate receptors (M6PRs), which are concentrated in the TGN and are crucial for targeting lysosomal acid hydrolases to lysosomes (56). Failure to add these phosphate units results in mistargeting of lysosomal hydrolases to the medium and the inability of lysosomes to degrade substrates. Lysosomes then become engorged with indigestible materials leading to cell and tissue abnormalities. This occurs in the fatal human disease mucolipidosis II (I syndrome), in which mannose-6-phosphate units are not added to newly synthesized lysosomal hydrolases.

The Golgi stacks are also responsible for the massive noncovalent addition of lipids to secretory lipoproteins (55). This includes the low- and high-density lipoproteins secreted by liver cells to which extensive cores of cholesterol and phospholipids are added. Furthermore, Golgi stacks are the major site of sphingolipid synthesis, whose precursor ceramide is produced in the ER (57). In the Golgi, ceramide is utilized in the biosynthesis of glycosylceramide or sphingomyelin. Various studies have indicated that sphingomyelin and cholesterol concentrations increase in

the *cis-* to *trans*-Golgi direction. This change in concentration has led to the idea that preferential partitioning of proteins into domains that are more or less enriched in sphingomyelin and cholesterol underlies sorting within the Golgi (58). The ability of the Golgi to drive glycosphingolipid synthesis, therefore, contributes to its function as a membrane sorting station.

The most distal subcompartment of the Golgi complex, the TGN, mediates the sorting and final exit of membrane and protein from the Golgi (59). Morphologically, it appears as a sacculotubular network near the trans face of the Golgi stacks. The TGN can be identified using the vital dye C_6-NBD-ceramide (60), with the lectin wheat germ agglutinin (WGA) (61), with antibodies to TGN proteins, including TGN 38 (62), or probes to cargo molecules after incubation of cells at 20°C (59).

Although the main function of the TGN is to sort proteins and lipids to different post-Golgi compartments, the TGN also functions in certain protein modifications, including galactose α2,6-sialyation, tyrosine sulfation, and proteolytic cleavage of dibasic residues on prohormones (50). In addition, the TGN is also involved in the process of condensation of macromolecular luminal content, which can be observed in cells producing secretion granules. This process is thought to involve charge neutralization, protein aggregation, and active ion extrusion (63,64).

The TGN normally communicates with the endosomal system, receiving membrane traffic from this system. During brefeldin A (BFA) treatment, for example, the TGN appears to mix with the endosomal system unlike other Golgi compartments, which redistribute into the ER (65). Constitutive cycling of endosomal membrane through the TGN has been suggested normally to play a role in remodeling of surface markers as well as in the processing of components internalized from the extracellular space (59,66).

Transport, Recycling, and Sorting Within the Golgi Complex

Given this organization of the Golgi complex, how does the Golgi maintain its structural integrity in the face of extensive membrane trafficking through the secretory pathway? Membrane recycling pathways play a key role in maintaining the organization of the Golgi complex by enabling Golgi membranes to become selectively enriched in certain proteins and lipids. The mechanism of recycling is still unclear but is likely to be regulated and to involve lipid partitioning to segregate recycling components from forward-moving cargo (30). The Golgi is known to be a major site of lipid transition within cells. Its lipid composition is intermediate between that of the ER (whose lipids are enriched in glycerophospholipids) and the plasma membrane (whose lipids are enriched in cholesterol and glycosphingolipids) (57). Changes in lipid composition across the Golgi complex have been proposed to underlie sorting of proteins, with Golgi membrane proteins partitioning into thinner regions of the membrane bilayer due to the thinness of their transmembrane domains and excluded from thicker regions that are enriched in sphingolipid and sterols destined for the plasma membrane (67). The finding that shortening the transmembrane domain of VSVG leads to its localization within the Golgi where it undergoes constitutive cycling between the ER and Golgi is consistent with this model (68).

How does secretory cargo pass through the Golgi complex? Traditional models, which assume that maintenance of functionally discrete Golgi subcompartments requires vesicle budding and fusion, provide two alternatives (31,69,70). In the vesicle transport model, vesicles carrying secretory cargo bud off from one cisternae and fuse with the next in a series of budding and fusion steps that occur in a cis to trans direction across the Golgi stack (31). In this model Golgi cisternae are considered to be relatively stable structures containing a specific set of Golgi enzymes. In the alternative cisternal progression model, transport of secretory cargo through the Golgi stack does not involve the formation of transport vesicles, but is mediated by the cisternae themselves through cisternal progression (70). The resident distribution of enzymes within the Golgi stack in this view arises through the activity of retrograde vesicles that bud and fuse in a trans to cis direction across the Golgi stack.

Recent studies visualizing Golgi resident enzymes tagged with GFP in living cells have shown that they are highly mobile in Golgi membranes with no constraints to their lateral diffusion (71). Other studies have further shown that Golgi enzymes and lipid readily move between Golgi stacks through dynamic tubule connections (72). An alternative possibility for intra-Golgi trafficking, therefore, is that cargo diffuses across the Golgi system via the extensive tubule connections between stacks (26,69). Golgi enzymes could diffusively self-organize within this system since substrates for early acting enzymes are available upon entry into the Golgi and substrates for later acting enzymes arise later when cargo has diffused deeper into Golgi stacks. In this way, the process of sequential processing of forward moving cargo by Golgi enzymes would drive the spatial organization of Golgi enzymes within Golgi membranes.

Whatever model for intra-Golgi trafficking proves to be correct, it must be able to explain why virtually all conditions that interfere with delivery of proteins from the ER to the Golgi complex, including treatments with BFA and okadaic acid, and overexpression of particular Rab mutants and Sar1 and ARF1 mutants, result in Golgi dispersal and redistribution of Golgi proteins to the site where membrane traffic is inhibited (30). For example, microtubule disruption, which prevents peripheral pre-Golgi intermediates from tracking into the Golgi region, causes Golgi proteins to reversibly redistribute to ER exit sites (73), while blocking ER export with Sar1p mutants leads to the redistribution of Golgi proteins into the ER (74). These results underscore the Golgi's dynamic nature and imply that a constant influx of membrane from the ER is required to maintain Golgi structure and that Golgi proteins undergo constitutive cycling to and from the ER.

GOLGI-TO-PLASMA MEMBRANE TRANSPORT

Once the dynamic steady-state flux of proteins through forward and recycling pathways of the Golgi complex become established, glycoprotein and glycolipid processing reactions become efficient, and give rise to highly processed and complex protein and lipid products. These products, in turn, are packaged into transport intermediates that bud off the trans face of the Golgi complex, translocate through the cytoplasm, and fuse with the plasma membrane or other final destinations.

The mechanisms and carriers involved in exocytic transport from Golgi to plasma membrane have recently been clarified using GFP imaging techniques (75–78). Such work has revealed that post-Golgi carriers are large, pleomorphic structures rather than small vesicles and that they fuse with the plasma membrane without intersecting other membrane pathways in the cell (Fig. 9.7). Fluorescently labeled secretory cargo leaving the Golgi complex was found to first concentrate in discrete domains that lacked TGN resident proteins such as furin. These domains then elongated into tubules before detaching from the Golgi. Severing of these structures from Golgi membranes is likely to involve dynamin-2, a TGN localized GTPase and mechanoenzyme, as well as the actin cytoskeleton, since inhibitors of dynamin-2 activity or actin depolymerization interfere with the process(es) whereby cargo-enriched carriers detach from the Golgi (75,79,80).

After detaching as tubules from the Golgi complex, the post-Golgi carriers often undergo dramatic shape changes as they track out to the cell periphery along microtubules. Correlative light-electron microscopy, which examines structures at both the light and electron microscope level, has revealed that these carriers can be as large as half the size of Golgi cisternae and that they often exist as tubular-saccular structures (77). They move along microtubule tracks to the cell periphery where they fuse and integrate their membrane with the cell surface (81,82).

CONCLUSION

Our understanding of the ER and Golgi complex in secretory trafficking to the plasma membrane has evolved from a variety of morphologic-, biochemical-, and genetic-based studies that have elucidated the distinct structures, functions, and interdependence of these organelles. Proper functioning of the ER and Golgi complex and the pathways that connect them has been shown to be fundamental to the generation, maintenance, and control of secretory membrane and protein traffic within cells. The ER exists as an extensive array of interconnecting tubules that radiate out from the nuclear envelope to the cell periphery. Its structural differentiation and dynamic morphology are ideal for coordinating lipid and protein biogenesis as well as membrane transport. The Golgi complex, by contrast, is localized at the cell center as a discrete set of flattened cisternae and functions to receive, process, and sort molecules exported from the ER. Future work in this system will continue to focus on understanding the mechanisms controlling membrane traffic between the ER, Golgi, and plasma membrane, and the distinct mechanisms for sorting and

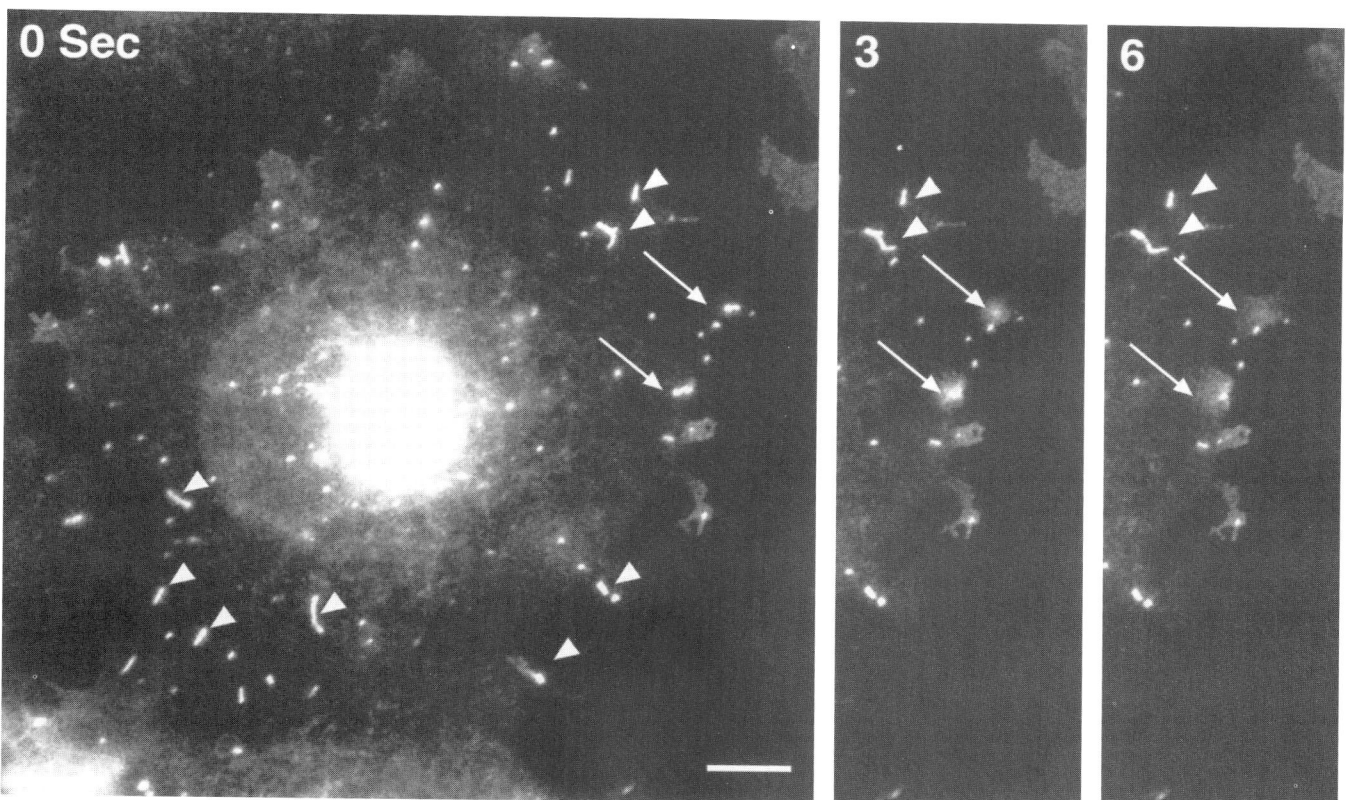

FIGURE 9.7. Golgi-to-plasma membrane transport intermediates in a cell expressing green fluorescent protein–tagged VSVG protein 60 minutes after shift to permissive temperature. *Arrowheads* indicate post-Golgi carriers; *arrows* indicate post-Golgi carriers that are fusing with the plasma membrane. *Scale bar* represents 5 μm.

retaining the variety of membrane and luminal components moving between them.

REFERENCES

1. De Pierre JW, Andersson G, Dallner G. Endoplasmic reticulum and Golgi complex. In: Arias IM, Jakoby WB, Popper H, et al., eds. *The liver: biology and pathobiology.* New York: Raven Press, 1988:165–188.
2. Terasaki M, Chen LB, Fujiwara K. Microtubules and the endoplasmic reticulum are highly interdependent structures. *J Cell Biol* 1986;103:1557–1568.
3. Tsien RY. The green fluorescent protein. *Annu Rev Biochem* 1998;67:509–544.
4. Nehls S, Snapp EL, Cole NB, et al. Protein retention in the endoplasmic reticulum: diffusional mobility of folded and misfolded proteins. *Nat Cell Biol* 2000;2:288–295.
5. Dayel MJ, Hom EF, Verkman AS. Diffusion of green fluorescent protein in the aqueous-phase lumen of endoplasmic reticulum. *Biophys J* 1999;76:2843–2851.
6. Sitia R, Meldolesi J. Endoplasmic reticulum: a dynamic patchwork of specialized subregions. *Mol Biol Cell* 1993;3:1067–1072.
7. Walter P, Lingappa VR. Mechanism of protein translocation across the endoplasmic reticulum membrane. *Annu Rev Cell Biol* 1986;2:499–516.
8. Hurtley SM, Helenius A. Protein oligomerization in the endoplasmic reticulum. *Annu Rev Cell Biol* 1989;5:277–307.
9. Helenius A, Marquardt T, Braakman I. The endoplasmic reticulum as a protein-folding compartment. *Trends Cell Biol* 1992;2: 227–231.
10. Bonifacino JS, Lippincott-Schwartz J. Degradation of proteins within the endoplasmic reticulum. *Curr Opin Cell Biol* 1991;3: 592–600.
11. Hammond C, Helenius A. Quality control in the secretory pathway. *Curr Opin Cell Biol* 1995;7:525–539.
12. Koch GLE. Reticuloplasmins: a novel group of proteins in the endoplasmic reticulum. *J Cell Sci* 1987;87:491–492.
13. Braakman I, Helenius J, Helenius A. The role of ATP and disulfide bonds during folding in the endoplasmic reticulum. *Nature* 1992;356:260–262.
14. Freedman R. Protein disulfide isomerase: multiple roles in the modification of nascent secretory proteins. *Cell* 1990;57: 1069–1072.
15. Braakman I, Helenius J, Helenius A. Manipulating disulfide bond formation and protein folding in the endoplasmic reticulum. *EMBO J* 1992;11:1717–1722.
16. Gething M-J, Sambrook J. Protein folding in the cell. *Nature* 1992;355:33–45.
17. Gibson RS, Schlesinger S, Kornfeld S. The nonglycosylated glycoprotein of vesicular stomatitis virus is temperature sensitive and undergoes intracellular aggregation at elevated temperatures. *J Biol Chem* 1979;254:3600–3607.
18. Kornfeld R, Kornfeld S. Assembly of asparagine-linked oligosaccharides. *Annu Rev Biochem* 1985;54:631–664.
19. Leavitt R, Schlesinger S, Kornfeld S. Impaired intracellular migration and altered solubility of nonglycosylated glycoproteins of vesicular stomatitis virus and Sindbis virus. *J Biol Chem* 1977;252:9018–9023.
20. Hirschberg CB, Snider MD. Topography of glycosylation in the rough endoplasmic reticulum and Golgi apparatus. *Annu Rev Biochem* 1987;56:63–87.
21. Bonifacino JS, Suzuki CK, Klausner RD. A peptide sequence confers retention and rapid degradation within the endoplasmic reticulum. *Science* 1990;247:79–82.
22. Shamu CE, Story CM, Rapoport TA, et al. The pathway of US11–dependent degradation of MHC class I heavy chains involves a ubiquitin-conjugated intermediate. *J Cell Biol* 1999; 147:45–58.
23. Saraste J, Svensson K. Distribution of the intermediate elements operating in ER to Golgi transport. *J Cell Sci* 1991;100: 415–430.
24. Bannykh SI, Rowe T, Balch WE. The organization of endoplasmic reticulum export complexes. *J Cell Biol* 1996;135:19–35.
25. Hauri H-P, Schweizer A. Relationship of the ER-Golgi intermediate compartment to endoplasmic reticulum and Golgi apparatus. *Curr Opin Cell Biol* 1992;4:600–608.
26. Clermont Y, Rambourg A, Hermo L. Connections between the various elements of the cis- and mid- compartments of the Golgi apparatus of early rat spermatids. *Anat Rec* 1994;240:469–480.
27. Schekman R, Orci L. Coat proteins and vesicle budding. *Science* 1996;271:1526–1533.
28. Rothman JE, Wieland FT. Protein sorting by transport vesicles. *Science* 1996;272:227–234.
29. Barlowe C. COPII and selective export form the endoplasmic reticulum. *Biochim Biophys Acta* 1998;1404:67–76.
30. Lippincott-Schwartz J, Cole NB, Donaldson JG. Building a secretory apparatus: role of ARF1/COPI in Golgi biogenesis and maintenance. *Histochem Cell Biol* 1998;109:449–462.
31. Rothman JE. Mechanisms of intracellular protein transport. *Nature* 1994;372:55–63.
32. Scales SJ, Pepperkok R, Kreis TE. Visualization of ER-to-Golgi transport in living cells reveals a sequential mode of action for COPII and COPI. *Cell* 1997;90:1137–1148.
33. Aridor M, Bannykh WI, Rowe T, et al. Sequential coupling between COPII and COPI vesicle coats in endoplasmic reticulum to Golgi transports. *J Cell Biol* 1995;131:875–893.
34. Barlowe C, Orci L, Yeung T, et al. COPII: a membrane coat formed by sec proteins that drive vesicle budding from the endoplasmic reticulum. *Cell* 1994;77:895–907.
35. Lippincott-Schwartz J, Donaldson JG, Schweizer A, et al. Microtubule-dependent retrograde transport of proteins into the ER in the presence of brefeldin A suggests an ER recycling pathway. *Cell* 1990;60:821–836.
36. Dascher C, Balch WE. Dominant inhibitory mutants of ARFI block endoplasmic reticulum to Golgi transport and trigger disassembly of the Golgi apparatus. *J Biol Chem* 1994;269: 1437–1448.
37. Peters PJ, Hsu VW, Ooi CE, et al. Overexpression of wild-type and mutant ARFI and ARF6: distinct perturbations of non-overlapping membrane compartments. *J Cell Biol* 1995;128: 1003–1017.
38. Guo Q, Vasile E, Krieger M. Disruptions in Golgi structure and membrane traffic in a conditional lethal mammalian cell are corrected by ε-COP. *J Cell Biol* 1994;125:1213–1224.
39. Gaynor EC, Chen CY, Emr SD, et al. ARF is required for maintenance of yeast Golgi and endosome structure and function. *Mol Biol Cell* 1998;9:653–670.
40. Presley JF, Cole NB, Schroer TA, et al. ER-to-Golgi transport visualized in living cells. *Nature* 1997;389:81–85.
41. Tang BL, Low SH, Hauri H-P, et al. Segregation of ERGIC53 and the mammalian KDEL receptor upon exit from the 150C compartment. *Eur J Cell Biol* 1995;68:398–410.
42. Lowe M, Kreis TE. Regulation of membrane traffic in animal cells by COPI. *Biochim Biophys Acta* 1998;1404:53–66.
43. Letourneur F, Gaynor EC, Hennecke S, et al. Coatomer is essential for retrieval of dilysine-tagged proteins to the endoplasmic reticulum. *Cell* 1994;79:1199–1207.
44. Nilsson T, Jackson B, Peterson PA. Short cytoplasmic sequences serve as retention signals for transmembrane proteins in the endoplasmic reticulum. *Cell* 1989;58:707–718.

45. Pelham HRB. About turn for the COPS? *Cell* 1994;79: 1125–1127.
46. Cao X, Ballew, N, Barlowe C. Initial docking of ER-derived vesicles requires Uso1p and Ypt1p but is independent of SNARE proteins. *EMBO J* 1998;17:2156–2165.
47. Van Rheenen SM, Cao X, Lupashin VV, et al. Sec 35p, a novel peripheral membrane protein, is required for ER to Golgi vesicle docking. *J Cell Biol* 1998;141:1107–1119.
48. Sacher M, Jiang Y, Barrowman J, et al. TRAPP, a highly conserved novel complex on the cis-Golgi that mediates vesicle docking and fusion. *EMBO J* 1998;17:2494–2503.
49. Mellman I, Simons K. The Golgi complex: in vitro veritas? *Cell* 1992;68:829–840.
50. Gleeson P. Targeting of proteins to the Golgi apparatus. *Histochem Cell Biol* 1998;109:517–532.
51. Pelham HRB. The retention signal for luminal ER proteins. *Trends Biochem Sci* 1990;15:483–486.
52. Hsu VW, Yuan LC, Nuchtern JG, et al. A recycling pathway between the endoplasmic reticulum and the Golgi apparatus for retention of unassembled MHC class I molecules. *Nature* 1991; 352:441–444.
53. Schweizer A, Fransen JAM, Matter K, et al. Identification of an intermediate compartment involved in protein transport from endoplasmic reticulum to Golgi apparatus. *Eur J Cell Biol* 1990; 53:185–196.
54. Chavier P, Parton RG, Hauri H-P, et al. Localization of low molecular weight GTP binding proteins to exocytic and endocytic compartments. *Cell* 1990;62:317–329.
55. Tartakoff AM, Turner JR. The Golgi complex. In: *Fundamentals of medical cell biology, vol. 4, membranology and subcellular organelles.* Greenwich, UK: JAI Press, 1992:283–304.
56. Kornfeld S. Trafficking of lysosomal enzymes in normal and disease states. *J Clin Invest* 1986;77:1–6.
57. Fang M, Rivas MP, Bankaitis VA. The contribution of lipids and lipid metabolism to cellular functions of the Golgi complex. *Biochim Biophys Acta* 1998;1404:85–100.
58. Simons K, Ikonen E. Functional rafts in cell membranes. *Nature* 1997;387:569–572.
59. Griffiths G, Simons K. The trans Golgi network: sorting at the exit site of the Golgi complex. *Science* 1986;234:438–443.
60. Pagano RE, Sepanski MA, Martin OC. Molecular trapping of a fluorescent ceramide analogue at the Golgi apparatus of fixed cells: interaction with endogenous lipids provides a trans-Golgi marker for both light and electron microscopy. *J Cell Biol* 1989;113:1267–1279.
61. Virtanen I, Ekblom P, Laurila P. Subcellular compartmentalization of saccharide moieties in cultured normal and malignant cells. *J Cell Biol* 1980;85:429–434.
62. Humphrey JS, Peters PJ, Yuan LC, et al. Localization of TGN 38 to the trans-Golgi network: involvement of a cytoplasmic tyrosine-containing sequence. *J Cell Biol* 1993;12:1123–1135.
63. Huttner WB, Baeuerle PA. Protein sulfation on tyrosine. *Mod Cell Biol* 1988;6:97–140.
64. Sossin WS, Fisher JM, Scheller RH. Sorting within the regulated secretory pathways occurs in the trans-Golgi network. *J Cell Biol* 1990;110:1–12.
65. Lippincott-Schwartz J, Yuan KL, Tipper C, et al. Brefeldin A's effects on endosomes, lysosomes and TGN suggest a general mechanism for regulating organelle structure and membrane traffic. *Cell* 1991;67:601–616.
66. Farquhar MG. Protein traffic through the Golgi complex. In: Steer CJ, Hanover JA, eds. Intracellular trafficking of proteins. Cambridge: Cambridge University Press, 1991:431–471.
67. Bretscher MS, Munro S. Cholesterol and the Golgi apparatus. *Science* 1993;261:1280–1281.
68. Cole NB, Ellenberg J, Song J, et al. Retrograde transport of Golgi-localized proteins to the ER. *J Cell Biol* 1998;140:1–15.
69. Mironov AA, Weidman P, Luini A. Variations on the intracellular transport theme: maturing cisternae and trafficking tubules. *J Cell Biol* 1997;138:481–484.
70. Glick BS, Elston T, Oster G. A cisternal maturation mechanism can explain the asymmetry of the Golgi stack. *FEBS Lett* 1997; 414:177–181.
71. Cole NB, Smith CL, Sciaky N, et al. Diffusional mobility of Golgi proteins in membranes of living cells. *Science* 1996;273: 797–801.
72. Sciaky N, Presley J, Smith C, et al. Golgi tubule traffic and the effects of Brefeldin A visualized in living cells. *J Cell Biol* 1997; 139:1137–1155.
73. Cole NB, Sciaky N, Marotta A, et al. Golgi dispersal during microtubule disruption: Regeneration of Golgi stacks at peripheral endoplasmic reticulum exit sites. *Mol Biol Cell* 1996;7: 631–650.
74. Zaal KJM, Smith CL, Polishchuk RS, et al. Golgi membranes are absorbed into and reemerge from the ER during mitosis. *Cell* 1999;99:589–601.
75. Hirschberg K, Miller CM, Ellenberg J, et al. Kinetic analysis of secretory protein traffic and characterization of Golgi to plasma membrane transport intermediates in living cells. *J Cell Biol* 1998;143:1485–1503.
76. Nakata T, Terada S, Hirokawa N. Visualization of the dynamics of synaptic vesicle and plasma membrane proteins in living axons. *J Cell Biol* 1998;140:659–674.
77. Polishchuk RS, Polishchuk EV, Marra P, et al. Correlative light-electron microscopy reveals the tubular-saccular ultrastructure of carriers operating between Golgi apparatus and plasma membrane. *J Cell Biol* 2000;148:45–58.
78. Toomre D, Keller P, White J, et al. Dual-color visualization of trans-Golgi network to plasma membrane traffic along microtubules in living cells. *J Cell Sci* 1999;112:21–33.
79. Kreitzer G, Marmorstein A, Okamoto P, et al. Kinesin and dynamin are required for post-Golgi transport of a plasma-membrane protein. *Nat Cell Biol* 2000;2:125–127.
80. Cao H, Thompson HM, Krueger EW, et al. Disruption of Golgi structure and function in mammalian cells expressing a mutant dynamin. *J Cell Sci* 2000;113:1993–2002.
81. Schmoranzer J, Goulian M, Axelrod D, et al. Imaging constitutive exocytosis with total internal reflection fluorescence microscopy. *J Cell Biol* 2000;*in press.*
82. Toomre DK, Steyer JA, Almers W, et al. Observing fusion of constitutive membrane traffic in real time by evanescent wave microscopy. *J Cell Biol* 2000;149:33–40.

The Liver: Biology and Pathobiology, Fourth Edition, edited by I. M. Arias, J. L. Boyer, F. V. Chisari, N. Fausto, D. Schachter, and D. A. Shafritz.
Lippincott Williams & Wilkins, Philadelphia © 2001.

10

MOLECULAR MECHANISMS OF HEPATOCELLULAR VESICLE FORMATION

SOPHIE DAHAN
MICHEL DOMINGUEZ
MARK A. MCNIVEN

One of the major functions of the hepatocyte is the synthesis, packaging, and directed transport of multiple plasma proteins into the sinusoidal space. Conversely, the hepatocyte also performs regulated endocytic uptake of various proteins and lipids from the blood sinusoid for subsequent processing and transport into bile (Fig. 10.1). These processes depend on a complex, yet highly organized, vesicle trafficking machinery that requires the coordinated synergistic action of scores of enzymes, cytoskeletal proteins, molecular motors, and coat proteins. Through the combination of conventional biochemical and molecular methods, the utilization of genetic model organisms, and the recent advancements of live cell imaging, much has been learned about these trafficking pathways in the hepatocyte and other epithelial cells. This review will provide an in-depth focus on the initial step of these transport processes, mainly, the formation and liberation of distinct populations of vesicle carriers from membranous compartments of the endocytic and secretory pathways.

VESICLE FORMATION IN THE ENDOCYTIC PATHWAY

The endosomal apparatus is a heterogenous population of membrane-bound structures involved in the uptake of exogenous substances into cells. Internalization of materials is nonselective in macropinocytosis where cells take up small droplets of fluid nonspecifically, or it is selective in receptor-mediated endocytosis where specific soluble molecules are internalized.

Endocytosed materials are accepted to be translocated from a peripheral to a perinuclear location as they progress from early to late endosomes. The translocation of internalized cargo proteins from the cell surface to the early endosome, and the subsequent delivery of lysosomally destined components to late endosomes and lysosomes, however, involve multiple vesicular trafficking events in which endosomal compartments are thought to undergo maturation to temporally later compartments. In this model, clathrin-coated vesicles derived from the plasma membrane lose their coat and fuse together to assemble an early endosome which undergoes a gradual remodeling and transformation to give rise to late endosomes and eventually dense lysosomes.

S. Dahan: Department of Biochemistry and Molecular Biology, Center for Basic Research in Digestive Diseases, Mayo Clinic and Foundation, Rochester, Minnesota 55905.

M. Dominguez: Department of Biochemistry Molecular Biology, Thoracic Diseases Research Unit, Mayo Clinic and Foundation, Rochester, Minnesota 55905.

M.A. McNiven: Department of Biochemistry and Molecular Biology, Center for Basic Research in Digestive Diseases, Mayo Clinic and Foundation, Rochester, Minnesota 55905.

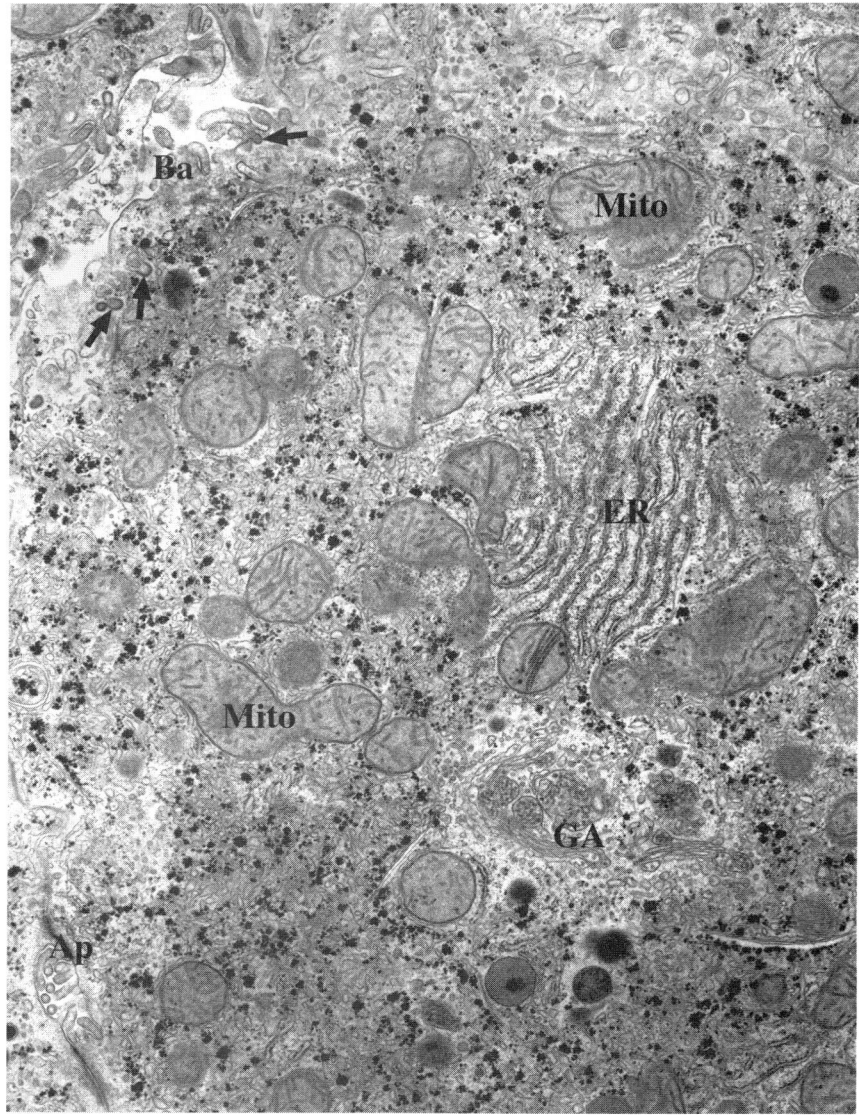

FIGURE 10.1. Elaborate vesicular processes in the hepatocyte. This is a thin-section electron micrograph of a rat liver hepatocyte taken from original collections of Dr. Keith Porter, circa 1962. On the sinusoidal membrane (*Ba*), small invaginations with an electron-dense coat, likely clathrin-coated vesicles (*arrows*), are clearly visualized between the microvilli. Deeper into the cytoplasm, parallel cisternae of the endoplasmic reticulum (*ER*) appear to lead into the flattened stacked saccules of the Golgi apparatus (*GA*). Scores of small vesicular profiles can be seen in the Golgi region, as well as larger lipoprotein-filled secretory vesicles budding from the *trans* side of the Golgi. Specific coats, accessory proteins and address tags are known to characterize many of these vesicles. *Ap*, apical membrane; *Mito*, mitochondria.

Clathrin-Coated Vesicles

Coated Pits/Vesicles and Receptor-Mediated Endocytosis

Clathrin-coated pits mediate the initial steps in receptor-mediated endocytosis (RME). In these cell surface microdomains, itinerant membrane proteins are segregated from resident plasma membrane proteins, and are internalized into the cell (Fig. 10.2). That coated pits act as molecular filters was first demonstrated by Bretscher and colleagues (1) when they showed that Thy1, a resident plasma membrane protein with a glycolipid anchor, was excluded from coated regions of the membrane. Ligands and membrane proteins are therefore selectively taken up while other portions of the plasma membrane are prevented from being internalized in the endocytic flow.

Coated pits are relatively uniform in size in any one cell type; that is, 100 to 150 nm profile diameter (Fig. 10.2D). They were first observed by Roth and Porter, who noted that the endocytosis of yolk protein into the oocyte of the

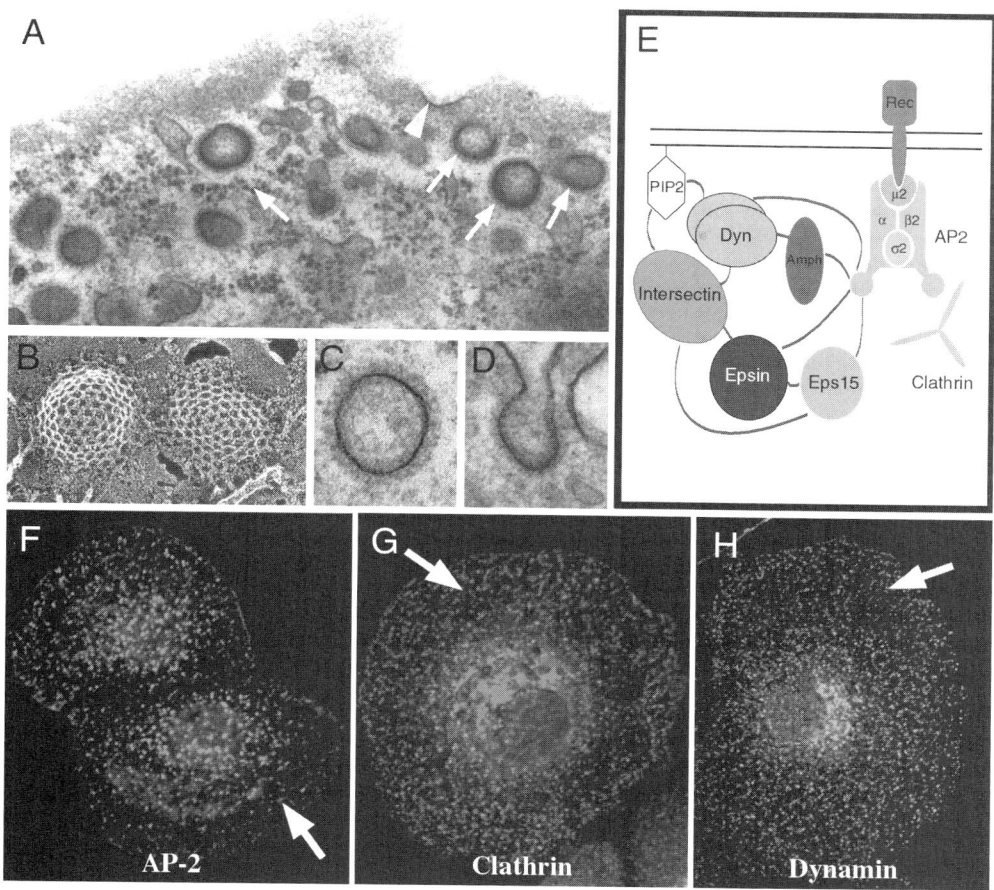

FIGURE 10.2. Clathrin-coated vesicle formation at the plasma membrane. **A:** Thin-section electron micrograph of a rat hepatocyte taken from original collections of Dr. Keith Porter. Numerous electron-dense bristle coats are found to line the cytosolic side of cell surface invaginations (*arrowhead*) and small internalized vesicles (*arrows*). **B:** Electron micrographs showing an intracellular view of clathrin-coated pits in fibroblasts. Clathrin lattices are clearly visualized in these replicas. (From Heuser J. Effects of cytoplasmic acidification on clathrin lattice morphology. *J Cell Biol* 1989;108:401–411, with permission.) **C and D:** Clathrin-coated vesicle and clathrin-coated pit in rat liver hepatocyte micrographs from Dr. Keith Porter. **E:** Clathrin-coated vesicle formation involves clathrin and a number of accessory proteins that are known to interact with each other via specific protein:protein interaction domains (see text) and in this way effect a regulatory role on coated vesicle biogenesis. **F–H:** Immunofluorescence images of plasma membrane adaptor complex, adaptor protein 2 (*AP2*), clathrin, and the molecular pinchase dynamin in clone 9 cultured rat hepatocytes reveal a punctate pattern of labeling at the cell surface (*arrows*). In double-labeling experiments, these three clathrin-coated pit components are found to colocalize. (Images from Dr. Hong Cao, Mayo Clinic.). See Color Plate 5.

mosquito was associated with a marked increase in invaginations of the oocyte cell membrane which were coated on the cytoplasmic face with what those authors termed a *bristle coat* (2). Soon thereafter, the major protein component of the coat was identified as clathrin (3), and the concentration of a specific ligand in coated pits followed by its internalization was demonstrated using ferritin–low-density lipoprotein (LDL) on cultured fibroblasts (4).

The number of coated pits and vesicles at the plasma membrane as well as the dynamics of their formation have been estimated by several investigators. Coated pits have been found to occupy 1.2 to 2% of the cell surface area, based on calculations on human fibroblasts (4), rat hepatocytes (5) and other cells (6,7). They assemble and bud with a half-time of approximately 5 minutes in broken A-431 cells (8) and in K^+-depleted fibroblasts that are incubated in the presence of KCl (9). Morphometric quantitation of the number of coated pits at the plasma membrane in Baby Hamster Kidney cells estimated the lifetime of coated pits to be 1 to 2 minutes (6), and while earlier estimates from quantitative ligand (α_2-MG) uptake suggest that each coated pit may be able to transfer ligands into endocytic vesicles every 20 seconds at 37°C (10), biochemical analyses of receptor internalization kinetics in rat liver parenchyma demonstrate that following ligand stimulation, receptors (epidermal growth factor receptor and insulin receptor) known to utilize the coated pit pathway are rapidly lost from the plasma membrane ($t_{1/2}$ approximately 1 minute) (11,12).

In addition to soluble ligands, many viruses enter cells by way of coated pits. These include adenovirus, vesicular stomatitis virus (VSV), Rous sarcoma virus, and Semliki forest virus. Viruses possessing a lipid membrane that surrounds the nucleocapsid contain glycoproteins involved in receptor recognition and virus entry into cells (13).

Clathrin-coated vesicles are also found at the level of the Golgi apparatus, where they mediate (a) the transport of lysosomal enzymes from the *trans*-Golgi network to the endosomal apparatus, (b) the formation of regulated secretory granules in regulated secretory cells, and (c) the maturation of immature zymogen granules to mature secretory granules (see Vesicle Formation in the Secretory Pathway below).

Coated Pit Ultrastructure and Coat Proteins

The structure of coated pits and vesicles as well as the molecular nature of the clathrin coat and regulatory mechanisms have been elucidated in great detail using both biochemical and ultrastructural techniques. The purification of coated vesicles has allowed the major structural units of the coat, namely clathrin triskelions and adaptors, to be identified (14). The characteristic ultrastructural honeycomb lattice of coats (15) as visualized by quick-freeze, deep-etch rotary shadowing, is made up of clathrin (Fig. 10.2B), while the inner shell of the coat consists of adaptor proteins. The adaptors are thought to interact with the cytoplasmic domains of plasma membrane receptors clustered in the pit/vesicle or may be recruited to bud sites by accessory proteins (see Accessory Proteins in Clathrin-Mediated Endocytosis below) (Fig. 10.2E, Table 10.1).

The first class of coat proteins are the clathrin triskelions. They have a flexible design that allows them to pack together to form polyhedral lattices (16). Each triskelion is a three-legged structure consisting of three heavy chains and three associated light chains. Each leg of the triskelion consists of three distinct regions (a C-terminal proximal domain, followed by a distal domain and a globular domain at the N-terminus). The recent elucidation of crystal structures of two domains of the clathrin heavy chain, a fragment in the proximal domain and the N-terminal domain, has led to important insights into how clathrin coats might assemble (see Coated Pit/Vesicle Formation and Associated Factors, below).

The adaptor proteins (AP) are the second major type of coat proteins. Four structurally related classes of APs are known and all are ubiquitously expressed. By freeze-etch electron microscopy (rotary shadowing), adaptors appear as barrel-shaped molecules flanked by two smaller appendages (17). The best characterized of these are AP-2, the plasma membrane coated pit adaptor, and AP-1, the Golgi-associated coated pit adaptor (reviewed in ref. 17). AP-3 is localized to the Golgi region and peripheral membranes, some of which may be endosomal in nature (17), and AP-4 has been demonstrated to be associated with non–clathrin-coated vesicles in the region of the *trans*-Golgi network (TGN) (18). Each adaptor protein consists of a complex of four subunits: two heavy chains ($\gamma/\alpha/\delta/\epsilon$ and $\beta1/\beta2/\beta3/\beta4$ of 90 to 140 kDa), one medium chain ($\mu1/\mu2/\mu3/\mu4$ of approximately 50 kDa) and one light chain ($\sigma1/\sigma2/\sigma3/\sigma4$ of 20 kDa). Sequence data have shown that particular subunits are closely related to each other (19) and likely have similar roles in protein sorting. For example, for adaptor complexes AP-1, AP-2, and AP-3, the μ chain specifically interacts with tyrosine- and leucine-based sorting signals (20–23), the two most common sorting signals within cytoplasmic tails of integral membrane proteins. The μ chain of AP-4 has recently been demonstrated to interact specifically with a tyrosine-based internalization signal (18). The β chains of AP-1, AP-2, and AP-3 interact with the clathrin heavy chain (24–26). The AP-2 α chain and the AP-1 γ chain have been shown to bind to various accessory proteins which may be involved in the regulation of vesicle formation (see Accessory Proteins in Clathrin-Mediated Endocytosis, below).

Coated Pit/Vesicle Formation and Associated Factors

Although the specific function(s) of APs *in vivo* has yet to be established, a working model for their role in coated pit assembly, budding, and receptor sorting has emerged from the large amount of information on their biochemical and functional properties *in vitro*. APs bind to the N-terminal domains of clathrin heavy chains and thereby mediate the attachment of clathrin to membrane. The recent determination of the crystal structure of parts of the clathrin heavy chain has revealed that the N-terminal domains project into the inside of the clathrin cage, thereby providing multiple binding sites for AP-2. Notably, a set of adaptor proteins termed *arrestins* has been shown to also bind clathrin with high affinity (27).

APs are thought to initiate coated pit assembly on the membrane, regulate coated pit growth, and mediate receptor sorting into coated pits by binding directly or indirectly to the cytoplasmic tails of receptor molecules (17). Purified ^{125}I-labeled AP-2 complexes, but not AP-1, were retained on an LDL receptor–tail affinity matrix column. This binding could be inhibited by soluble cytoplasmic tails of cation-independent mannose-6-phosphate receptor (CI-MPR) and the polymeric immunoglobulin receptor (pIg-R). The ligand-regulated receptor EGF-R was shown to interact with adaptors *in vivo*, by coimmunoprecipitation of plasma membrane adaptors and EGF-Rs in EGF-treated cells (28). Remarkably, in the G-protein coupled receptor system, arrestin APs have been shown to bind to the cytoplasmic tails of activated/phosphorylated receptors, attenuate receptor

TABLE 10.1. COAT AND VESICLE-ASSOCIATED PROTEINS

Clathrin-coated Vesicles

	Subunits	Function	Domain Features	Binding Partners
Coat Proteins				
Clathrin heavy chain		Triskelion assembly thought to shape membrane into buds		AP-2, AP-1, arrestins
Clathrin light chain		Regulates clathrin lattice assembly		
Accessory Proteins				
AP-2	α			Clathrin, amphiphysin, eps15, epsin, AP180
	β_2	Concentrate receptors in coated pits		Clathrin
	μ_2			Tyrosine-based internalization motifs found in receptor tails
	σ_2			
Dynamin		Vesicle scission	GTPase, CC, PH, PRD	Amphiphysin, endophilin, AP-2, intersectin, Dap160, profilin, cortactin, synapsin, syndapin
Eps15		Required for vesicle formation	EH, CC, repeated DPF motifs	AP-2 (α-adaptin), eps15R, epsin, synaptojanin, intersectin
Epsin		Required for vesicle formation	ENTH, repeated DPW motifs	AP-2, eps15, eps15R, intersectin, Ese1 and Ese2 (vertebrate homologues of Dap160)
Intersectin (short form)		Component of endocytic machinery	EH, CC, SH3	
Intersectin (long form)		Component of endocytic machinery	EH, CC, SH3, DH, PH, C2	Dynamin, synaptojanin, eps15, eps15R, epsin
Amphiphysin		Required for vesicle formation	SH3	Synaptojanin, endophilin, dynamin
Synaptojanin		inositol 5-phosphatase	PRD	Amphiphysin, Grb2, endophilin, syndapin, Eps15
Syndapin		Actin-binding protein	CC, NPF motifs, SH3	Dynamin, synaptojanin, synapsin, N-WASP

Caveolae

	Subunits	Function	Domain Features	Binding Partners
Coat Proteins				
Caveolin		Promotes caveolae formation		
		Regulates cell signalling by sequestering signal molecules	Caveolin-scaffolding domain	$G\alpha s$, c-Src, EGF receptor, cNOS, PKCα, phospholipase D1, MEK/ERK, Ha-Ras
		Internalization of cholera toxin, GPI-anchored proteins		
Accessory Proteins				
Dynamin		Caveolae scission	GTPase, CC, PH, PRD	Amphiphysin, endophilin, AP-2, intersectin, Dap160, profilin, cortactin, synapsin, syndapin

COPI-coated Vesicles

	Subunits	Function	Domain Features	Binding Partners
Coat Proteins				
COPI coatamer	α-COP		WD-40 repeats	β'-COP, ϵ-COP
	β-COP	COPI coat components recruited from the cytosol believed to shape membranes into buds	WD-40 repeats	δ-COP, ARF1
	β'-COP			α-COP
	γ-COP			ζ-COP, ARF1, KKXX motifs, p24 family
	δ-COP			β-COP
	ϵ-COP			α-COP
	ζ-COP			γ-COP
ARF1		GTPase regulating recruitment of COPI to membranes	GTPase	β-COP, γ-COP
Accessory Proteins				
ARF-GAP		GAP activity towards ARF		KDEL-receptor
P619		Putative ARF-GEF		

(Continued)

TABLE 10.1. *Continued*

COPII-coated Vesicles

	Subunits	Function	Domain Features	Binding Partners
Coat Proteins				
Sec13 complex	hSec13p	COPII structural components	WD-40 repeats	
	hSec31p		WD-40 repeats	
Sec23 complex	hSec23p	GAP for Sar1p		p24
	hSec24p			
Accessory Proteins				
Sar1		Recruitment of COPII to membranes	GTPase	
Sec12p		ER membrane protein		
		GEF activity towards Sar1		
Sec16		Required for vesicle budding in vivo		Sec23, Sed4
p125		Possibly a phospholipid-modifying enzyme		Sec23

TGN-derived Vesicles

Clathrin-coated Vesicles	Subunits	Function	Domain Features	Binding Partners
Coat proteins				
	Clathrin Heavy Chain	Triskelion assembly thought to shape membrane into buds		AP-2, AP-1, arrestins
	Clathrin Light Chain	Regulates clathrin lattice assembly		
Accessory Proteins				
AP-1	γ	Selectively concentrates certain transmembrane proteins into forming vesicles		ARF, γ-synergin
	β_1	TGN/endosome to lysosomal trafficking		TGN38
	μ_1			
	σ_1	Regulated secretion		
AP-3	δ			
	β_3	TGN/endosome to lysosome vesicle trafficking		Tyrosine-based internalization motifs found in receptor tails
	μ_3			
	σ_3			
Dynamin		Vesicle scission	GTPase, CC, PH, PRD	Amphiphysin, endophilin, AP-2, intersectin, Dap160, profilin, cortactin, synapsin, syndapin
γ-synergin			EH	AP-1(γ)
ARF1		GTPase regulating membrane association of AP-1		

Non–Clathrin-coated Vesicles	Subunits	Function	Domain Features	Binding Partners
Vesicle-associated proteins				
p200/MyosinII vesicles		Possibly the main component of lace like coated vesicles		p62, rab6, TGN38
p230 vesicles		Non-clathrin coat on TGN vesicles		
Accessory Proteins				
Dynamin		Vesicle scission		
ARF1		GTPase regulating membrane association of AP1		

AP, adaptor protein; ARF, ADP ribosylation factor; cc, coiled coil; DH, Dbl homology; EH, Epsis homology; ER, endoplasmic reticulum; GAP, GTP-activating protein; GEF, GTP–GDP exchange factor; PH, pleckstrin homology; PRD, proline rich domain; SH3, src homology 3; TGN, *trans*-Golgi network.

activation, and mediate their sequestration in clathrin-coated pits for subsequent internalization and downregulation (29).

The process of coated pit formation involves the recruitment and assembly of clathrin and associated coat proteins and other factors at the plasma membrane to form a pit, which subsequently invaginates, buds, and produces a coated vesicle. Coat proteins assemble onto the cell surface as planar structures which later gain curvature forming invaginated pits (9,15). The light chains are believed not to be required for cage assembly in *in vitro* studies where intact, proteolytically truncated, or light chain-depleted triskelions were found to spontaneously self-assemble into "cages" virtually identical to the coat on a coated vesicle (30). However, based on their external position on the coat, as visualized in the vitreous ice cage structure (31), their possession of calcium binding sites (32) and phosphorylation sites (33), their interactions with uncoating ATPase (34), and the negative regulation of polymerization *in vitro*, it has been suggested that light chains participate in regulating clathrin assembly and disassembly *in vivo* by preventing cage assembly in the cytosol (35).

Clathrin triskelions can join together to form flat hexagonal lattices which gain curvature by the introduction of pentagons. This change in lattice arrangement appears not to be the sole driving force for membrane curvature; membrane lipid modifications have recently been suggested to be involved (see Lipid Regulators Involved in Vesicle Biogenesis, below). The budding process also has been suggested to be independent of clathrin, this protein postulated to have the role, together with adaptins, of holding endocytosing receptors in coated pits (36).

Initiation of coat protein assembly is believed to be mediated by at least two components: cargo receptor tails binding to AP-2 and an AP-2 "receptor" at the coated pit. In favor of the former component, increased receptor numbers (transferrin receptors in transfected cells) have been reported to promote clathrin lattice growth in the initial planar stage (37). Lattices containing α- and β-adaptins associate with integral membrane proteins only when they are on the cell surface (38), and therefore it has been suggested that a receptor protein in the plasma membrane acts as a nucleation site for adaptor complexes and that these complexes in turn recruit receptors with internalization signals (39). However, cell surface receptors may not be the only recruiting factors for AP-2.

Accessory Proteins in Clathrin-Mediated Endocytosis

A battery of accessory proteins (Epsin, Eps15, amphiphysin, and dynamin) involved in vesicle formation/scission and substrate recruitment have recently been identified in GST-α-appendage pulldown binding experiments. These proteins are known to also interact between themselves and other proteins via a number of specific protein binding sequence motifs including EH, coiled-coil, proline-rich and SH3 domains (reviewed in ref. 40) (Fig. 10.2E, Table 10.1).

A role for Eps15 and Epsin in coated pit assembly and endocytosis has been suggested from experiments in which their function was disrupted (by microinjection of neutralizing antibodies, or overexpression/microinjection of truncation mutants), leading to an inhibition of clathrin-mediated endocytosis (40–42). Functional studies remain to be conducted on intersectin; however, together with Eps15 and epsin, it has been found to colocalize with clathrin and/or coated vesicles at the plasma membrane in neuronal and nonneuronal cells (40,43). Interestingly, detailed electron microscopy (EM) immunolocalization studies on Eps15 in fibroblasts have revealed that while the AP-2 adaptor is distributed homogenously over the whole coated pit surface, Eps15 is restricted to the rim, or the growing part, of the budding coated pit (44), suggesting that Eps15 may dissociate from AP-2 during coat and vesicle formation. Clathrin appears to be a competing factor in the Eps15:AP-2 interaction and has been shown to release Eps15 from AP-2 during coated pit formation (45).

*E*pidermal growth factor receptor *p*rotein *s*ubstrate (Eps) *h*omology (EH) domains are protein:protein interaction domains originally identified as a repeated sequence present in the N-terminus of Eps15 and Eps15R (Eps15-*r*elated molecule). Eps15 is predominantly found complexed to AP-2 in the cell; binding to the α-appendage of this adaptor is via repeated DPF motifs in the C terminus of Eps15. Although the order of association of accessory proteins with the newly forming vesicle stills needs to be worked out, it appears that Eps15 recruitment to the plasma membrane is necessary for subsequent AP-2 association (41). AP-2 has been shown to interact with the central region of epsin (39), a protein also thought to have a role in clathrin-mediated endocytosis. At its C-terminal region, epsin harbors repeats of an EH domain binding consensus motif, NPF, which have been shown to interact with Eps15 and intersectin, another recently identified EH domain-containing family member (40). Intersectin also contains five SH3 domains (40), 50 to 70 amino acid modules through which it can bind to proline-rich ligands. All these protein:protein interaction domains allow intersectin to form various macromolecular complexes and bridges between proteins with binding regions for EH domains (e.g., NPF repeats in epsin) and SH3 domains (e.g., proline-rich domains in dynamin, a large GTPase involved in vesicle scission (see Coated Vesicle Scission and the Molecular Pinchase Dynamin, below), and synaptojanin, an inositol-5-phosphatase implicated in intracellular signaling and vesicular trafficking events). Indeed, intersectin is homologous to *Drosophila* Dap160, a protein known to associate with dynamin (dynamin-associated protein) (46). The long form of intersectin (which also exists in a short form due to alternative splicing) (47) also harbors a pleckstrin homology (PH) domain and a C2 domain, both of which can mediate the association of intersectin with membranes. This has led to the suggestion that intersectin may be one of the first accessory proteins to be recruited to a newly forming vesicle, further recruiting Eps15, and then AP-2 (48). Intersectin may also be recruited to clathrin-coated pits by intersectin-binding protein-2 (Ibp2), recently demonstrated to interact with the EH domains of intersectin, with the clathrin heavy chain, and with AP-2 (43,46). Eps15/Eps15R and epsins 1 and 2 have been shown to be expressed ubiquitously including in liver, albeit much lower than in brain extracts (42,49). Furthermore, although the long form of intersectin is expressed specifically in neurons, the short form is expressed in many nonneuronal cells (43).

The phosphorylation state of the accessory proteins appears to be a means by which vesicle formation is under regulatory control at the cell surface. Many of these [Eps15, epsin (50), dynamin, amphiphysin, and AP-2 (51)] are constitutively phosphorylated on serine and threonine residues. In neurons, upon a depolarization stimulus, these molecules are known to be dephosphorylated and thus activated (40). This allows them to be recruited to membranes from their predominantly cytosolic location (51) and to associate with the AP-2 adaptor (50).

Coated Vesicle Scission and the Molecular Pinchase Dynamin

Late stages in coated vesicle formation, namely invagination of coated pits and liberation of coated vesicles, appear to be mediated in large part by the large GTPase dynamin. Its role in vesicle scission could not be more graphic than in the images of presynaptic nerve terminals of *shibire*^{ts1} mutants of *Drosophila melanogaster* which express a temperature-sensitive mutation in the GTP-binding domain of the fly dynamin (52). At the restrictive temperature, the nerve terminals of these paralyzed flies were depleted of synaptic vesicles and appeared to accumulate "collared coated pits," profiles of invaginated pits with a bristle-like coat at the end portion and an electron-dense collar or ring at the neck of the pits, indicating that synaptic vesicle recycling was inhibited in these mutant flies. These ultrastructural alterations of the plasma membrane could also be seen in various epithelial cells of these flies and indicated a general block in endocytosis (52,53). Shortly thereafter, rat dynamin, isolated from calf brain on the basis that it could cross-link and bundle microtubules *in vitro*, was shown to share a high degree of sequence homology with the *shibire* gene product (54,55). Notably, receptor-mediated endocytosis, as evaluated by transferrin internalization, was demonstrated also to be inhibited in two mammalian cell lines (HeLa and COS7 cells) overexpressing dynamin with mutations similar to that in *Drosophila shibire*^{ts} (56,57). These studies indicated that receptor-mediated endocytosis via clathrin-coated pits requires a functional dynamin GTPase. Indeed, in cultured mouse hepatocytes, microinjection of inhibitory antibodies recognizing peptide sequences in the NH$_2$-terminal enzymatic domain of dynamin inhibited transferrin, and therefore clathrin-mediated, endocytosis (58). Most striking, however, are EM images of these hepatocytes which showed that microinjection of inhibitory dynamin antibodies induced the formation of long clathrin-coated pits that are continuous with the plasma membrane, as verified by ruthenium red staining of the outer leaflet of the plasma membrane (58). These observations were reminiscent of the plasmalemmal invaginations seen in the *shibire*^{ts1} mutant cells at the restrictive temperature. Furthermore, in the case of the cultured hepatocyte model, this implicated the ubiquitously expressed dynamin-2 isoform (59) (dynamin-1 being neuron-specific and dynamin-3 expressed only in testis, brain, and lung) (reviewed in ref. 60) in the formation of clathrin-coated vesicles. At least four alternatively spliced variants are encoded by the dynamin-2 gene; immunofluorescence studies of two of these spliced isoforms [Dyn2(aa) and Dyn2(ab)] in clone 9 rat hepatocytes have revealed colocalization of dynamin-2 with clathrin-coated structures at the plasma membrane and at the Golgi apparatus (61). Different dynamins as well as dynamin-like proteins are situated at distinct cellular locations and suggest roles aside from clathrin-mediated endocytosis, for the dynamin family of proteins (60).

Dynamin is believed to be a molecular motor which upon binding and hydrolyzing GTP induces the compression and severing of membrane tubules (reviewed in refs. 60, 62). For this reason, dynamin has also been referred to as a *pinchase* for the generation of discrete vesicles from invaginated coated pits. Dynamin, like clathrin, has been shown to self-assemble in the absence of nucleotide. Polymeric dynamin complexes have been visualized along lipid vesicles (63) and membrane tubules in rat brain synaptosomal membranes under specified conditions (64). In addition to dynamin 'rings' on the tubular invaginations, amphiphysin and endophilin [SH3 domain-containing accessory proteins that can bind to the proline-rich domain of dynamin (65)] were also reported on the membrane tubules (64,66). *In vitro* studies using phosphatidylserine liposomes have revealed that purified dynamin, in the absence of any nucleotide, can tubulate the originally spherical liposomes; in the presence of GTP (but not GTPγS or the use of purified GTPase-defective dynamin), the elongated tubules are constricted and fragmented into small vesicles (67). Dynamin-mediated tubulation and fragmentation events have also been reported with more physiological liposomes from total brain membranes (68,69). These and more recent studies have led to various models for dynamin function in vesicle formation (reviewed in ref. 60).

Regulators of Clathrin-Mediated Endocytosis and Vesicle Uncoating

The budding off of coated vesicles from plasma membrane coated pits may also be mediated by the actin cytoskeleton lining the cell membrane. Although most studies have been carried out in yeast, the role of actin in endocytosis in mammalian cells is in the process of being deciphered. Mutations in a yeast actin-binding protein, Sla2p, have also been shown to lead to altered endocytosis and actin cytoskeletal organization (70). A mammalian homologue of Sla2p, huntingtin interacting protein 1 (Hip1) has recently been demonstrated to colocalize with clathrin, AP-2, and endocytosed transferrin, suggesting that Hip is an integral component of clathrin-coated pits that could bridge the actin cytoskeleton to endocytosis (71). Other actin links to the endocytic machinery include actin-binding proteins, profilin, synapsin, syndapin, and cortactin. These are known binding partners of dynamin and have been shown to colocalize with this molecular pinchase (72–74, M. McNiven, L. Kim, E.W. Krueger et al., personal communication).

Many of the studies on the role of actin in clathrin-mediated endocytosis in mammalian cells have been conflicting, however. In polarized epithelial cells, disassembly of actin filaments with cytochalasin D was shown to result in a block in apical endocytosis while internalization from the basolateral domain was unaffected (75). Interestingly, regulation of clathrin-coated pit mobility within the plane of the plasma membrane, as evaluated using green fluorescent protein (GFP)-tagged clathrin light chain, was reported to be significantly enhanced in COS-1 cells in the presence of low concentrations of latrunculin B, an inhibitor of actin assembly. These results suggest that the actin cytoskeleton underneath the plasma membrane is involved in maintaining the cell surface arrangement of clathrin-coated pits (76).

Morphological studies have shown that once formed, coated vesicles uncoat rapidly (77) and fuse with each other or with peripheral endosomes (78). The half-life of a coated vesicle was reported to be less than 1 minute (78), while photobleaching studies following rhodamine–clathrin microinjection estimated the half-life of polymerized clathrin to be about 10 to 15 seconds (79). Using GFP-tagged clathrin light chain, it was proposed that coated vesicles release their coat very close to the coated pit (76). Both heavy and light chains of clathrin are released by uncoating ATPase, a member of the 70-kDa heat shock protein family (80).

Clathrin-Independent Endocytosis

Endocytosis of membrane and fluid also occurs through a pathway that is independent of clathrin. Internalization still continues after endocytosis from clathrin-coated pits is inhibited under conditions of incubation in hypertonic medium (81), potassium depletion (82), or acidification of the cytosol (83). Clathrin-independent endocytosis has been demonstrated in unperturbed cells and may contribute up to half of the total membrane and fluid-phase uptake of the cell (84). Caveolae have been classified as one kind of clathrin-independent endocytosis. While clathrin-mediated and caveolae-mediated endocytosis are inhibited under conditions of cholesterol depletion, endocytosis of

ricin has been demonstrated to occur (85), suggesting that there are other types of non–clathrin-mediated internalization. Although the membrane invaginations in clathrin-independent endocytosis are not fully characterized, vesicles produced by this process have been identified in Hep-2 cells. These vesicles have an average diameter of 95 nm (86), which is significantly smaller than the clathrin-coated vesicles formed in this cell type, and thus these invaginations may be caveolae. Ligands taken into Hep-2 cells by clathrin-independent endocytosis were shown to be targeted to the Tf-R-enriched early endosome, indicating that this pathway may merge with the clathrin-dependent pathway (87). It has been proposed that the coated pit and clathrin-independent pathway of EGF-R endocytosis can be distinguished by their kinetic characteristics (88–91), with rapid internalization occurring via the coated pit pathway (especially at low cell surface receptor occupancy) and slow (constitutive) internalization occurring via a clathrin-independent pathway in macropinocytosis. Clathrin-independent internalization is believed to be responsible for the uptake of molecules that do not utilize coated pits, such as GPI-anchored proteins (92) and cholera and tetanus toxins (93), and may play a role in the turnover of membrane proteins.

Caveolae

Endocytic Function of Caveolae

One type of clathrin-independent endocytosis is mediated by caveolae. This type of cell surface pit is flask-shaped, has a small diameter of 50 to 100 nm and has been reported on the surface of various cells including fibroblasts (94) (Fig. 10.3A), in different liver-derived cell lines (58,93) and in whole rat liver (95). Notably, smooth membrane microinvaginations in a cultured liver cell line, KLTRYPV, of about 60 to 70 nm in diameter, were described in classic studies by Lelio Orci's group as being involved in the initial binding of gold-labeled cholera and tetanus toxin, two known ligands of caveolar membrane glycolipids (93). Caveolae have a unique lipid makeup, and are often associated with a spiral coat on their cytoplasmic side consisting in part of the integral membrane protein caveolin (reviewed in ref. 96) (Fig. 10.3B). Caveolae and caveolin are also known to be important regulators of transmembrane signaling (96).

Due to their long half-life and to their never directly being observed detaching from the plasma membrane, caveolae were originally characterized as having a potocytosis function in which caveolae could transiently seal without scission from the plasma membrane to allow the transfer of bound ligand across the invaginated membrane; this was described especially for glycosylphosphotidylinositol (GPI)-anchored protein-mediated uptake of small metabolites (97). This process had placed in doubt whether caveolae

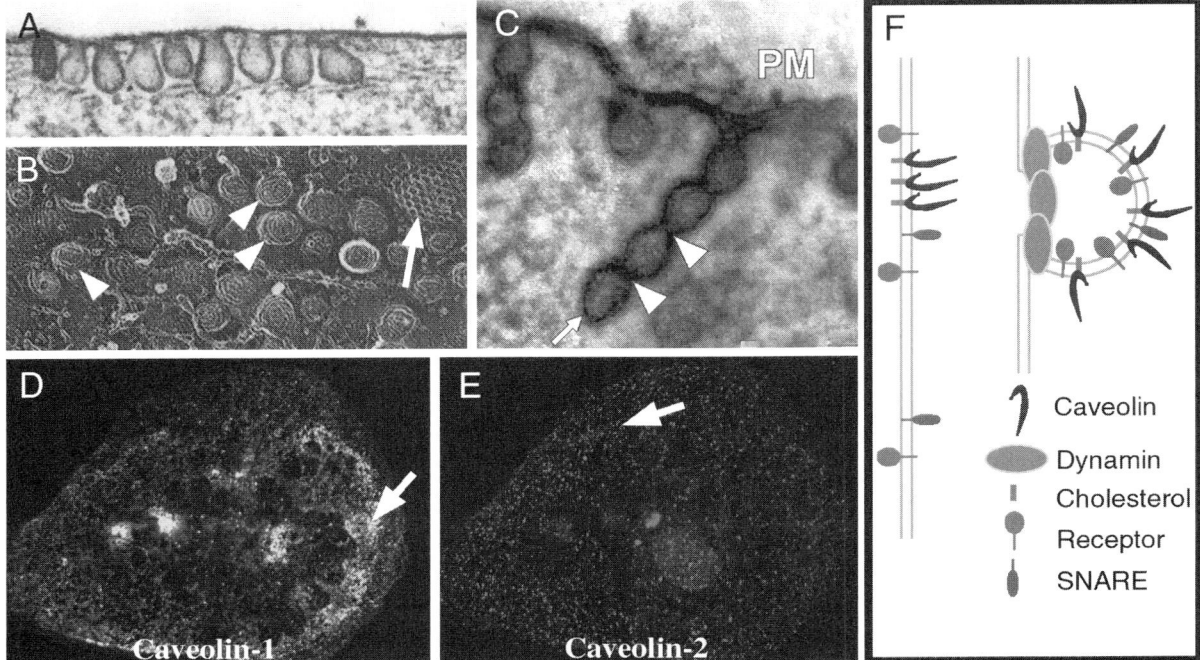

FIGURE 10.3. Caveolae and flask-shaped structures at the plasma membrane (*PM*). **A:** Thin-section electron micrograph showing homogenous small flask-shaped invaginations, caveolae, at the cell surface of human fibroblasts. (From Rothberg KG, Heuser JE, Donzell WC, et al. Caveolin, a protein component of caveolae membrane coats. *Cell* 1992;68:673–682, with permission.) **B:** Deep-etch intracellular view of caveolae (*arrowheads*) clearly showing the characteristic spiral coat distinct from the organized lattice coat structure of a clathrin coated pit (*arrow*). (From Rothberg KG, et al., as above.) **C:** Cultured hepatocytes microinjected with inhibitory dynamin antibodies exhibit accumulated chains of caveolae separated by constrictions still attached to the PM. This shows the key role of dynamin in caveolae scission (From Henley JR, Krueger EW, Oswald BJ, et al. Dynamin-mediated internalization of caveolae. *J Cell Biol* 1998;141:85–99, with permission.) **D** and **E:** Immunofluorescence images of caveolin-1 (as revealed by a GFP-tagged caveolin-1) and caveolin-2 demonstrate a patchy versus punctate cell surface distribution for these caveolin isoforms, respectively (Images from Dr. Hong Cao, Mayo Clinic.) **F:** Caveolae vesicle formation is known to involve the presence of caveolin-1, cholesterol, and dynamin. SNAREs are known to also be present in caveolae and are involved in addressing caveolae to their correct target membrane. See Color Plate 6.

could be considered a form of clathrin-independent endocytosis, since no free cytoplasmic vesicle is released into the cytoplasm under normal conditions. Internalization of caveolae has nevertheless has been demonstrated under experimental conditions of increased phosphorylation induced by phosphatase inhibition (98). It has clearly been shown that caveolae do pinch off (98); cholera toxin (99) and GPI-anchored folate receptors (100) could be found in early endosomes containing α_2-macroglobulin or transferrin, respectively, suggesting common endocytic compartments in clathrin-coated pit and caveolae internalization pathways.

Caveolae are known to mediate different vesicular transport processes including fluid-phase and receptor-mediated endocytosis and transcytosis of proteins and various molecules including toxins and viruses (reviewed in ref. 101). Cholera toxin, for example, makes use of the high content of GM$_1$ gangliosides in caveolae, binds to these lipid constituents, and is subsequently internalized in a pathway

involving the endosomal and Golgi compartments followed by retrograde transport to the ER.

Lipid Composition and Caveolar Ultrastructural Integrity

Characterized as unique lipid microdomains at the cell surface, caveolae are known to be enriched in cholesterol and sphingolipids, while the rest of the plasma membrane mainly consists of phospholipids. Local concentrations of cholesterol and sphingolipids which may or may not be associated with caveolae have also been referred to as detergent-insoluble glycolipid-enriched (DIG) domains due to their insolubility in Triton X-100 (reviewed in ref. 96). Whether these 'lipid rafts' truly exist *in vivo*, however, is still a matter of debate (102).

The lipid composition of caveolae appears to be important for both maintenance of caveolae structure and function. That a relationship between plasma membrane caveolae and cholesterol trafficking exists in cells was strongly suggested in studies in which cholesterol was demonstrated to efflux from fibroblasts via caveolae (103). Furthermore, perturbations in plasma membrane cholesterol by the sterol-binding agent, filipin (104) or the cholesterol sequestering drug, methyl-β-cyclodextrin (85), were shown to alter the ultrastructural integrity of caveolae and endocytosis through this microdomain. Transcytosis of insulin and albumin across cultured endothelial cell monolayers was significantly diminished when uncoated plasmalemmal vesicles were disassembled with filipin (104). At the electron microscope level, a complete loss of morphologically identifiable caveolae was reported in two epithelial cell lines [MDCK (105) and HEp-2 cells (85)] depleted of their cholesterol with methyl-β-cyclodextrin. Levels of caveolin protein in the MDCK cells were decreased 50% when in the presence of methyl-β-cyclodextrin (105), suggesting that a necessary steady-state balance exists between caveolin protein levels and cholesterol content in caveolae. Indeed, one of the isoforms of caveolin, caveolin-1 (see Protein Composition and Caveolae Biogenesis, below), can bind to cholesterol (106), and its expression was upregulated when levels of intracellular cholesterol were increased (105). Moreover, disruption of the cholesterol composition of the plasma membrane with cholesterol oxidase has been reported to lead to the rapid redistribution of caveolin from the plasma membrane to the Golgi region (107); at this site it was suggested that caveolin may bind cholesterol molecules and mediate their transport to caveolae at the cell surface.

Protein Composition and Caveolae Biogenesis

Although caveolae do not exhibit any visible coat by standard transmission electron microscopy, as do clathrin-coated pits, rapid-freeze, deep-etch replicas have revealed a distinct striated filamentous coat on the cytoplasmic surface of caveolae (108) (Fig. 10.3B). This coat has been shown to contain caveolin, a 21 kDa protein that has also been localized in post-Golgi vesicles where it has been referred to as vesicle integral protein of 21 kDa, or VIP21 (reviewed in ref. 96). Caveolin mRNA and protein levels were found to be most predominant in adipose, lung, and muscle tissues, and initially undetectable in liver (109). Recent studies, however, have verified that caveolin is indeed present in membrane fractions isolated from a normal mouse hepatocyte cell line (58) and rat liver (110).

Caveolin-1 is the best characterized of the three identified isoforms in the caveolin protein family (consisting of caveolin-1, -2, and -3) (96). While caveolin-1 and -2 are ubiquitously expressed, caveolin-3 is restricted to muscle. Notably, within frozen thick sections of rat liver, caveolin-1 was demonstrated to localize within the same plasma membrane domain as the asialoglycoprotein receptor (ASGP-R), a receptor protein exclusively expressed by hepatocytes in the liver, and not with RECA-1, an endothelial cell marker

(110). Although caveolin-1 and ASGP-R were localized mainly in "corner" regions between two hepatocytes, where most protein and membrane trafficking events are known to take place, they were distributed in different plasma membrane microdomains (110).

Unlike the clathrin light and heavy chains that are cytosolic proteins, caveolin-1 has been shown to be an integral membrane protein that forms a hairpin-like loop within the membrane. Thus, both the N- and C-terminal domains are cytosolically exposed. Regions in the N-terminal domain are known to be important for interaction between caveolin proteins in the formation of caveolin homooligomers and heterooligomers, resulting in high molecular weight multimers. Proximal to the transmembrane domain, a protein: protein interaction domain called the caveolin scaffolding domain, consisting of about 20 amino acids, mediates the association and sequestration of various caveolin-interacting proteins. G-protein-coupled receptors, many species of heterotrimeric G-proteins, various lipid-modified signaling accessory proteins [Src-like kinases, H-ras, nitric oxide synthase (NOS)], mitogen activated protein (MAP) kinase, and receptor tyrosine kinases have all been shown to be sequestered and inactivated within the caveolin scaffolding domain (reviewed in ref. 96).

Since the discovery of caveolin as a coat protein component of caveolae that can form homo- and heterooligomers, parallels have been attempted with the clathrin coat, and thus caveolin has been evaluated in terms of roles that it may have in caveolae formation at the plasma membrane. A key study in lymphocytes, which normally do not express any caveolin and which lack any morphologically identifiable caveolae, has shown that this is indeed the case (111). In these cells, transient expression of caveolin-1 resulted in the appearance of plasma membrane invaginations, reminiscent of caveolae, harboring caveolin-1. This suggested that caveolin-1 is an important structural component necessary for caveolar biogenesis. Similar results were obtained in two polarized epithelial cell lines, Caco-2 (112) and Fischer rat thyroid (FRT) (113) cells, which also are lacking in caveolae and caveolin-1 expression.

The questions of whether the only component in caveolae formation is caveolin and whether lipids are also involved in this process are still being evaluated. Caveolin is known to cycle between the plasma membrane and the ER/Golgi apparatus and is believed to supply cholesterol to caveolae to facilitate invagination of these microdomains (96). In support of this proposal, caveolin-1 has been localized to intracellular locations including the ER and *trans*-Golgi network (107) and recently within the lumen of secretory vesicles in pancreatic acinar cells (114), suggesting a mechanism by which caveolin might recycle between caveolae and the ER/Golgi apparatus. Because caveolin-1 oligomers can directly bind to cholesterol (106) and this may help stabilize oligomeric complexes, this has been proposed to be a driving force that may recruit caveolin to cholesterol-enriched domains, or caveolae, not only at the plasma membrane but also at the level of the Golgi apparatus. At this intracellular location, segregation of caveolins into lipid microdomains may initiate the biogenesis of caveolae for subsequent transport to the cell surface. Indeed, expression of recombinant caveolin-1 has been demonstrated to mediate the ER-to-plasma membrane intracellular movement of newly synthesized cholesterol (96).

Scission of Caveolae from the Plasma Membrane

Using cholera toxin as a ligand for caveolae, Parton and colleagues (98) clearly showed that caveolae could be internalized under certain experimental conditions and that subsequent to endocytosis, the toxin could be found in various endosomal compartments. This demonstrated an important parallel with clathrin-mediated endocytosis and sparked interest in evaluating the molecular mechanisms involved in vesiculation of plasmalemmal caveolae. It is now well established that the liberation of clathrin-coated vesicles from the plasma membrane is in large part mediated by the large GTPase, dynamin (see Coated Vesicle Scission and the Molecular Pinchase Dynamin, above), and thus this molecular pinchase was evaluated as a possible candidate mediating the internalization of caveolae. Two studies demonstrated that dynamin is indeed involved in the scission of caveolae from the plasma membrane (58,115). Fission of caveolae in bovine lung endothelial cells was shown to require wild-type cytosolic dynamin and GTP hydrolysis; overexpression of GTPase-deficient mutant dynamin abrogated caveolar budding and inhibited caveolae-mediated cholera toxin internalization (115). Furthermore, microinjection of inhibitory dynamin-2 antibodies in cultured mouse hepatocytes led to both the generation of long tubular invaginations of the plasmalemma with visible clathrin coats at their ends, and the accumulation of distinct, non–clathrin-coated, flask-shaped invaginations at the plasma membrane morphologically similar to caveolae (Fig. 10.3C). Cholera toxin internalization was also inhibited in these antibody-injected cells. Moreover, immunofluorescence and biochemical experiments have demonstrated that dynamin and caveolae colocalize within intracellular vesicular structures in mouse hepatocytes (58). Finally, EM immunogold labeling of lung endothelial cells revealed dynamin to be localized at the necks of caveolae where it is believed to mediate their scission from the plasma membrane.

VESICLE FORMATION IN THE SECRETORY PATHWAY

The basic structural framework of the secretory apparatus includes the endoplasmic reticulum (ER) and the Golgi apparatus. Usually located at the periphery of the cell, the ER is characterized by a network of interconnected, highly convoluted membranous cisternae. The Golgi apparatus, in contrast, is localized in the perinuclear region of cells and consists of organized stacks of flattened saccules and associated secretory vesicles. The *cis*- and *trans*-Golgi networks are membranous tubular reticulums at the entry and exit sides of the Golgi apparatus, respectively.

The ER and Golgi apparatus were analyzed extensively in exocrine pancreas and rat liver as the early hypotheses of protein secretion were being evaluated, owing to the ease of secretory product visualization in these models. These organelles were postulated to act sequentially in the synthesis, transport, and packaging of proteins destined for extracellular discharge by exocytosis.

Since these classic studies, the mechanism by which proteins are transported in an anterograde direction from the ER to the Golgi apparatus, and vectorially through the Golgi apparatus itself, is thought to involve in part, vesicular carriers. At the level of the ER, constituents of the COPII coat (see COPII-Coated Vesicles, below) are recruited to form buds and generate vesicles known as vesicular tubular clusters (VTC) which have been proposed to coalesce to form a complex network of tubules called the endoplasmic reticulum/Golgi intermediate compartment (ERGIC) (116). From the ERGIC, COPI coat (see COPI-Coated Vesicles, below) components are recruited and induce the formation of vesicles that mediate ERGIC-to-Golgi protein/membrane transport; COPI-coated vesicles are also thought to mediate retrograde transport of resident ER proteins and Golgi enzymes from the Golgi apparatus to the ERGIC and ER or to the *cis*-Golgi network, respectively. In addition to secretory proteins, membrane proteins and lysosomal enzymes also pass through the secretory apparatus to reach their final destinations, reflecting the important sorting role of the Golgi apparatus. This sorting function has been predominantly attributed to, and is best characterized for, the *trans*-Golgi network (TGN). At this site, several distinct vesicle types containing different cargo proteins and harboring particular coat proteins have been reported to arise. Noncoated secretory vesicles from the TGN are thought to transport constitutively secreted proteins to the cell surface.

Notably, the formation of COPI- and COPII-coated vesicles and TGN-derived vesicles require similar molecular components. In these vesicle populations, priming of vesicle budding is initiated by the binding of specific small GTPases (ADP ribosylation factor (ARF) for both COPI-coated vesicles and clathrin-coated AP-1-, p200-, or p230-positive vesicles, and Sar1 for COPII-coated vesicles) at the site of vesicle budding. Moreover, unique GTP–GDP exchange factors (GEFs) and GTP-activating proteins (GAPs) for each vesicle type activate the membrane binding and GTP hydrolysis activity of the GTPases, respectively. Once bound to the membrane, the GTPases induce the recruitment of COPI coat components, COPII, or the AP-1 complex in clathrin-coated vesicles. The coat proteins, as well as accessory factors, are necessary components for vesicle biogenesis from various compartments along the secretory pathway.

COPI-Coated Vesicles

COPI-Coated Vesicles and Protein Trafficking through the Endoplasmic Reticulum and Golgi Apparatus

Classic electron micrographs of Golgi regions in various cells have typically revealed the stacked cisternae of the Golgi complex and the ER–Golgi apparatus interface replete with numerous small vesicular and tubular profiles. How proteins get transported through the complex ultrastructure of the Golgi apparatus has always been a subject of intense study, even today. These small vesicles, because of their close proximity to Golgi stacks in the cell, were hypothesized in the mid-1980s to be the vehicles for intra-Golgi protein transport. This led to the designing of cell-free protein assays by Rothman and colleagues, which were instrumental in identifying many of the components involved in vesicle formation and protein transport through the secretory pathway. From this assay, which makes use of isolated Golgi membranes, those authors concluded that small vesicles of approximately 70 nm in diameter mediated the transport of a reporter glycoprotein, vesicular stomatitus virus G (VSV-G) protein, from a donor to an acceptor Golgi compartment (reviewed in ref. 117). Subsequent experiments demonstrated that when isolated Golgi membranes were treated with cytosol and GTPγS (a nonhydrolyzable analogue of GTP), this led to the generation of transport vesicles that had a cytoplasmic coat made up of a series of obtuse spikes, distinct from the bristled appearance of clathrin coats (118) (Fig. 10.4A and B). Because the coat was found to consist of multiple subunit proteins (117) (Table 10.1), the term coat protomer, or coatomer, was coined to describe this new coat. This coat protein however is mostly referred to as COP. As these vesicles were the first of two non–clathrin-coated vesicles to be discovered in the secretory pathway, they are referred to as COPI-coated vesicles.

Since the original *in vitro* assays, COPI-coated vesicles have been implicated in both anterograde and retrograde vesicular trafficking through the secretory pathway. By EM immunogold labeling of rat exocrine pancreas, COPI components were localized to the delimiting membrane of vesicles and buds in the Golgi region (119). Similar results were observed in β-cells of pancreatic islets where lateral terminal rims of cisternae and associated vesicles were seen to be labeled for two COPI coat components (120), implicating a role for COPI-coated vesicles in anterograde protein transport through the flattened stacked cisternae of the Golgi apparatus. However, because most of the Golgi-associated vesicular labeling was observed over vesicular profiles between the ER and Golgi apparatus, at the *cis*-side of the Golgi stack (119), this suggested that COPI-coated vesicles may also mediate protein

transport to and from the Golgi apparatus in addition to within the Golgi apparatus. Indeed, antibodies against coat proteins were shown to inhibit ER-to-Golgi apparatus transport of a temperature-sensitive version of VSV-G protein in permeabilized normal rat kidney (NRK) cells (121) or in Vero cells (also kidney cells) microinjected with the antibody (122). In support of these findings, when coat recruitment was inhibited with the fungal metabolite brefeldin A (BFA), secretion of various proteins was blocked at a pre-Golgi compartment in cultured rat hepatocytes (123,124).

More recently, COPI-coated vesicles have been implicated in the retrieval of escaped ER resident proteins, owing to the association of selected COPI subunits with dilysine amino acid motifs in the cytoplasmic domains of ER resident enzymes (125). Furthermore, several COPI temperature-sensitive mutants in yeast revealed defects in Golgi-to-ER protein transport but not ER-to-Golgi transport, at the restrictive temperature, further confirming this retrieval role for COPI coat proteins (126). At the level of the Golgi apparatus, separate populations of COPI-coated vesicles were shown to mediate anterograde protein cargo transport of pro-insulin for secretion, and retrograde transport of resident ER proteins utilizing the KDEL (single letter code for amino acids) receptor in a second set of vesicles (127). Interestingly, live cell imaging of GFP-tagged cargo protein moving from the ER to the Golgi apparatus put forth striking images of COPI coat proteins associated with cargo-containing transport intermediates only at a post-ER site, notably the ERGIC compartment; COPII vesicles (see COPII-Coated Vesicles, below) were found to colocalize with cargo proteins upon ER exit (128), implicating a sequential role of COPII followed by COPI in ER-to-Golgi protein trafficking. At the ERGIC, COPI was suggested to be involved in secretory protein cargo sorting (128,129), yet another role for this coat complex. Indeed, subsequent studies revealed a segregation of transport intermediates containing COPI coats from those containing cargo proteins (130,131). Other studies showing detailed EM images of the COPI compartment in exocrine pancreas and rat liver demonstrated that immunogold labeling for COPI coats could be seen over vesicular–tubular membrane profiles about the Golgi apparatus (130; S. Dahan, J. Gushue, M. Dominguez et al., unpublished data). A vesicular–tubular localization of COPI, plus the finding that this coat is present at peripheral rim bud sites of cisternae (119,120), have supported proposals for COPI coats in preventing nonspecific fusion of membranes in the secretory pathway (132,133).

COPI-coated Vesicle Protein Components and Vesicle Formation

The COPI coat proteins and associated factors were identified in the cell-free intra-Golgi transport assays making use of GTPγS to induce the accumulation of these transport vesicles (117). The coated vesicles were isolated and the proteins form-

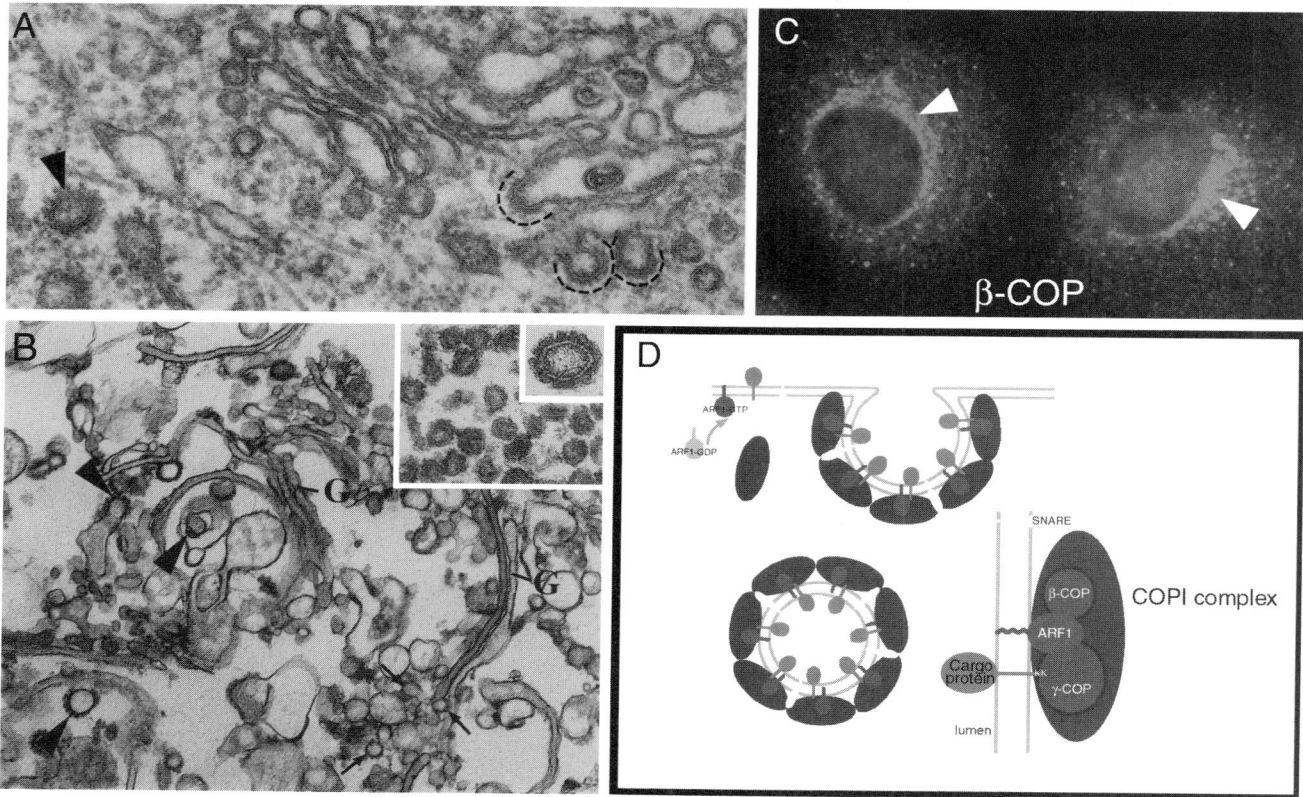

FIGURE 10.4. COPI-coated vesicles in protein trafficking through the secretory pathway. *A:* COPI-coated buds (*dotted lines*) on Golgi cisternae from Chinese Hamster Ovary (CHO) cells are distinct from the spiny coats of clathrin-coated vesicles (*arrowhead*) (From Orci L, Glick BS, Rothman JE. A new type of coated vesicular carrier that appears not to contain clathrin; its possible role in protein transport within the Golgi stack. *Cell* 1986;46:171–184, with permission.) **B:** An isolated rat liver Golgi fraction shows Golgi stacks of 2–3 flattened cisternae (*G*) and scores of vesicular and budding profiles. The bristle coat of clathrin on some of these profiles (*arrowheads*) is visibly different from the thin electron-dense coat of COPI buds and vesicles (*arrows*) (Images from Dr. John Bergeron, McGill University, Montreal, Canada.) **Inset:** Purified yeast COPI vesicles. (From Schekman R, Orci L. Coat proteins and vesicle budding. *Science* 1996;271:1526–1533, with permission.) **C:** Immunofluorescence labeling with antibodies against a COPI component, β-COP, reveals prominent perinuclear staining of cultured clone 9 rat hepatocytes. (Image from Dr. Yisang Yoon, Mayo Clinic.) **D:** COPI-coated vesicle formation is known to involve the COPI coatomer complex consisting of 7 subunit proteins. Two of these, β-COP and γ-COP, are known to mediate important interactions with the small GTP binding protein ARF1 and the cytosolic tails (specifically dilysine, or KK, motifs) of transmembrane proteins (such as p24 family members, see text). ARF–GDP/GTP exchange is one of the initial steps in the recruitment of the coatomer complex for COPI vesicle biogenesis. See Color Plate 7.

ing the coat were identified (Table 10.1). Thus, the COPI coat consists of seven coat proteins (α, β, β', γ, δ, ε, ζ COP) forming a complex of 680 kDa associated with the small GTP-binding protein ARF1. Sequence similarity between β-, δ-, ζ-COP and β, μ, σ adaptor subunits of the clathrin complex, respectively, have suggested that both sets of proteins originated from a common ancestor and might have analogous functions (132,134,135). In support of this proposal, both adaptor protein complexes (AP-1 and AP-3) and the COPI protein coat are known to require the GTP-binding protein ARF1 for coat recruitment stages of vesicle budding (136,137), and are able to bind to cytoplasmic tails of transmembrane proteins/receptors in the vesicles (138,139) (see below).

COPI bud formation is thought to be mediated by a cytoplasmic pool of coats recruited *en bloc* as a preassembled coat complex to budding regions on membranes, following initiation by GTP-ARF (140) (Fig. 10.4D). ARF is activated upon binding of GTP, catalyzed by the membrane-associated GTP-GDP exchange factor (GEF), which is sensitive to the fungal agent brefeldin A. GTP-ARF binds to Golgi membranes via its myristic moiety (141) and possibly via a specific receptor in the membrane as indicated by its binding saturability (142). Although ARF's mode of action in recruiting COPI molecules is still not well understood, ARF may induce the generation of membrane-associated phosphatidic acid [through activation of phospholipase D present in Golgi membranes (see Lipid Regulators Involved in Vesicle Biogenesis, below)], which has been shown to mediate the noncovalent membrane association of β-COP (143). Notably, antibodies to ζ-COP also have been shown to block ARF-dependent coatomer recruitment to the Golgi membrane (134), suggesting that an association of COPI molecules with ARF may exist. Indeed, the recruitment of the COPI complex to the membrane has been suggested to occur by interaction of WD40 motif repeats (a protein:protein interaction motif found in subunits of various heteromeric protein complexes) of α- and β-COP with ARF1 (144). Furthermore, using two ARF mutants containing photolabile amino acids, the direct interaction of ARF with β-COP was demonstrated both at the level of Golgi membranes and in isolated COPI-coated vesicles, indicating a direct binding of ARF and COPI during the vesicle coating process (145).

Recruitment of COPI coat proteins to target sites is thought to shape the membrane into buds (reviewed in refs. 117,146). When isolated Golgi membranes from Chinese Hamster Ovary (CHO) cells were incubated in the presence of ARF, purified coatomer proteins, and GTP, coated buds were seen to assemble on the membranes. The shape of the COPI-coated bud was suggested to be determined by the uniform organization of coatomer and ARF in their polymerized form. In support of these findings, membrane-mediated budding could not be observed if Golgi membranes were incubated with cytosol depleted of coatomer, suggesting that formation of the COPI coat is the driving force for budding (146). *In vitro* vesiculation budding assays using lipid bilayers have recently identified what the strict molecular requirements for vesicle biogenesis are. Formation of COPI-coated vesicles from liposomes having a similar lipid constitution as mammalian Golgi membranes only requires coatomer, ARF, GTP, and the cytoplasmic domains of p24 protein family members (147). The latter are known binding partners of COPI coat subunits (139), and have been shown to cycle between the ER and Golgi apparatus (139,148). Moreover, p24 family members have been suggested to have a role as putative cargo receptors and have been demonstrated to induce polymerization of the coatomer complex. If high concentrations of acidic and unsaturated phospholipids are utilized in these assays, it appears that the need for p24 transmembrane proteins can be bypassed. In support of these findings, original cell-free assays demonstrated a requirement for palmitoyl coenzyme A for the pinching of COPI-coated buds from Golgi membranes. From these *in vitro* findings, a model for COPI-coated vesicle formation has been proposed whereby a trimeric complex of coatomer, ARF, and a tetramer of p24 cytoplasmic tails is postulated to provide the vesicle budding machinery in the biogenesis of COPI vesicles (reviewed in ref. 137).

Hydrolysis of ARF-bound GTP initiates the uncoating of coated vesicles, which is critical for their fusion to the acceptor membrane. Once in a GDP-bound form, ARF dissociates from the membrane, causes coatomer to detach and yields uncoated vesicles. Notably, ARF-GAP, which is an activator of ARF GTP hydrolysis activity, has been shown to be recruited to membranes by interacting with the KDEL receptor, suggesting that this receptor tail may be regulating COPI coat assembly at the Golgi (137).

COPII-Coated Vesicles

COPII-Coated Vesicles and Endoplasmic Reticulum-to-Golgi Protein Trafficking

Protein transport from the ER to the Golgi complex is believed to be mediated by vesicular carriers originating from morphologically defined, specialized ribosome-free regions of the ER called transitional elements (149). ER buds and an abundance of small vesicular profiles at these sites could be clearly visualized in the classic electron micrographs from Jamieson and Palade of pancreatic acinar cells (150), and have always been characterized as being distinct from smooth ER. Studies involving live cell imaging have demonstrated these transitional areas to be transiently and randomly formed from the endoplasmic reticulum (129).

The cargo carriers that mediate ER-to-Golgi protein transport has been a subject of intense study, and like many of the protein trafficking steps along the secretory pathway, the answers arose from studies in yeast *Saccharomyces cerevisiae* conditional *sec* (for secretion) mutants. A series of SEC genes were found to have a role in ER-to-Golgi transport (reviewed in ref. 151), with subsequent genetic and morphological analyses revealing that one class of mutants exhibited defects in vesicle formation because these mutants were found to accumulate ER tubules when incubated at the restrictive temperature. In a second class of mutants, both ER tubules and small vesicles accumulated; thus, these mutants appeared to be defective in vesicle consumption. Using yeast membranes for ER vesicle budding *in vitro*, cell-free assays could be reconstituted. This led to isolation of ER-derived transport vesicles (Fig. 10.5A, bottom inset); these vesicles were 60 to 65 nm in diameter and exhibited a distinct electron-dense coat on their surface that was termed COPII (152). COPII coat components were identified from the purified vesicles and were revealed to be distinct from those of COPI coats (152).

At around the same time, COPII studies were being conducted in mammalian cells using reagents developed in the yeast experiments. Using antibodies to yeast COPII coat components, immunoreactivity could be detected throughout groups of vesicles about ER cisternae in pancreatic β-cells and acinar cells (153,154). These COPII-positive vesicular profiles were postulated to be anterograde transport carriers, owing to their ER-proximal location. Indeed, two independent studies, in normal rat kidney (NRK) cells

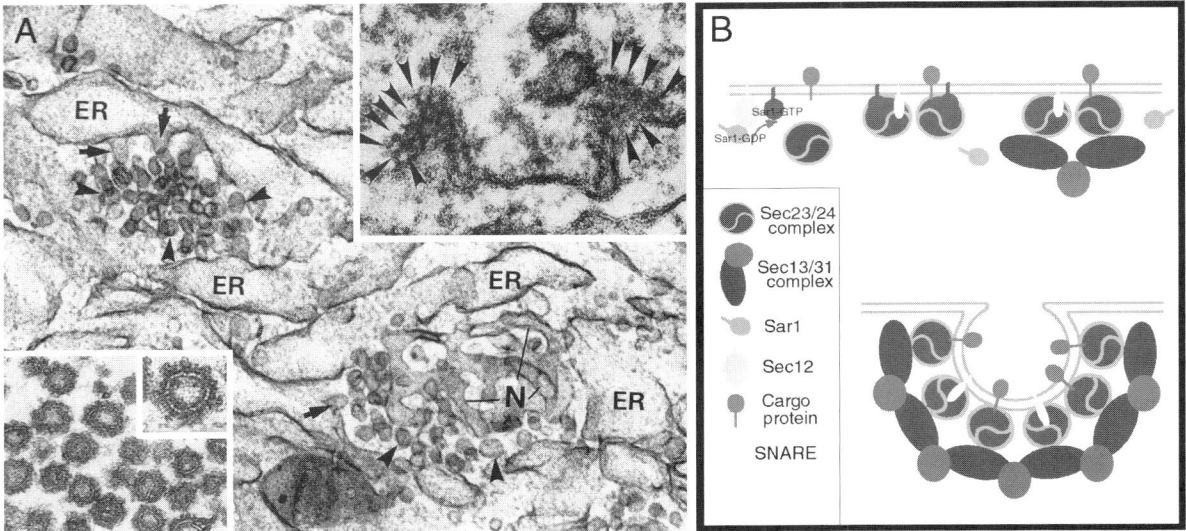

FIGURE 10.5. COPII-coated vesicles in endoplasmic reticulum (*ER*)-to-Golgi protein trafficking. **A:** Clusters of small vesicular profiles, likely representing COPII vesicles (*arrowheads*), can be seen to be closely surrounded by ER cisternae and budlike projections (*arrows*) in this electron micrograph of principal cells of the epididymal initial segment (From Hermo L, Green H, Clermont Y. Golgi apparatus of epithelial principal cells of the epididymal initial segment of the rat: structure, relationship with endoplasmic reticulum, and role in the formation of secretory vesicles. *Anat Rec* 1991;229:159–176, with permission.) **Top inset:** Honeycombed appearance of the coat (*arrowheads*) of COPII vesicles in rat basophilic leukemia cells (From Bannykh SI, Rowe T, Balch WE. The organization of endoplasmic reticulum export complexes. *J Cell Biol* 1996;135:19–35, with permission.) **Bottom inset:** Purified yeast COPII vesicles (From Schekman R, Orci L. Coat proteins and vesicle budding. *Science* 1996;271:1526–1533, with permission.) **B:** COPII-coated vesicle formation, like COPI, involves several protein complexes, and a small GTP-binding protein, Sar1, which is known to be one of the initiating factors in the generation of COPII vesicles. Membrane association of Sar1 is regulated by Sec12, GTPase-activating protein for Sar1. *N*, anastomosing network of tubules. See Color Plate 8.

(155) and in human hepatoma HepG2 cells (156) reported that cargo protein was present at bud sites upon ER exit and within small 40 to 80 nm carrier vesicles and tubules referred to as vesicular-tubular clusters (VTCs) (Fig. 10.5A), thus confirming the forward transport carrier role of these groups of vesicles. Subsequently, detailed thin serial sections of rat basophilic leukemia (RBL) cells demonstrated that the ER export sites were remarkably organized with ER cisternae arranged in a cuplike fashion around groups of VTCs (116). The ER cisternae around VTCs often exhibited budding profiles that were decorated with an electron-dense honeycomb patterned coat (Fig. 10.5A, top inset) that was identified to be COPII by immunogold labeling of normal rat kidney (NRK) cell sections with antibodies against COPII coat components.

In support of the functional yeast data on the role of COPII coats in ER-derived vesicle formation, COPII coat components were found to be recruited to isolated NRK microsomal membranes in a similar GTP-dependent fashion, requiring the COPII-specific GTPase Sar1p, but not COPI-specific ARF (157). Furthermore, export of cargo protein out of the ER, while enhanced when perforated NRK cells were incubated in the presence of GTP-restricted

Sar1p mutants (i.e., constitutively in the 'on' state), was blocked in the presence of Sar1p mutants restricted to the GDP-bound form (i.e., in the 'off' state) (157). Using the same GDP-restricted Sar1p mutant, but this time transiently expressed in intact HeLa cells, cargo protein transport from the ER to the Golgi apparatus was similarly inhibited (158). Furthermore, a role for COPI in ER vesicle budding was found to not be essential (157). These findings suggested that COPII-coated vesicles mediate anterograde transport out of the ER, while COPI coats on pre-Golgi intermediates mediate sorting of anterograde transported secretory cargo from ER resident and intermediate compartment proteins, which recycle between the ER and pre-Golgi intermediates. This was confirmed by live-cell imaging of GFP-tagged vesicular stomatitus virus G protein in Vero cells (128). Upon exiting the ER, COPII colocalized with GFP-VSV-G protein-containing structures, which assemble to form the intermediate compartment or transport complexes, as evaluated by the marker proteins ERGIC-53 and the KDEL receptor (see above sections on COPI-coated vesicles). Only COPI was found to be associated with these transport complexes as they subsequently migrated to the Golgi apparatus.

COPII-Coated Vesicle Protein Components and Vesicle Formation

The COPII coat components, distinct from the COPI coatomer, were postulated to induce vesicle budding of ER-derived transport vesicles, as only the GTPase Sar1p, the Sec13p complex, and the Sec23p complex were found to be necessary for the generation of COPII-coated vesicles from washed microsomes (152). The Sec13p complex consists of Sec13p and Sec31p proteins, and the Sec23p complex is made up of Sec23p and Sec24p proteins. These two protein complexes are recruited to the ER membrane, following the activation of the small GTPase Sar1, by transient binding of Sar1p to the N-terminal domain of Sec12p. Sec12p is a transmembrane protein localized to the ER that is a GTP-GDP exchange factor (GEF) for Sar1p. Because it is anchored to the ER donor compartment, Sec12p has been postulated to be a key indicator for sites of membrane budding at the ER (146). GTP-Sar1p binds to the ER membrane, and then mediates the recruitment of Sec13p and Sec23p complexes. Remarkably, COPII-coated vesicles can be generated from liposomes consisting of purified phospholipids (159). In the presence of acidic phospholipids, GTP-bound Sar1p was found to recruit the Sec23/24p complex to the liposome; together, the new Sar1p-Sec23/24p complex then recruits Sec13/31p (Fig. 10.5B). This sequential assembly of COPII components onto the liposomes was suggested to be the driving force that mediates vesicle budding and formation at the ER membrane *in vivo*. Binding proteins, including members of the p24 family of membrane proteins (139) and v-SNARE proteins (important for directing the newly formed vesicle to the correct target membrane) (160) have been proposed as well to possibly serve as nucleation sites on membranes for assembly of the COPII complex (137).

The presence of COPII-coated vesicles in mammalian cells and the role of the coat in vesicle formation were first demonstrated with the cloning and sequencing of two mammalian orthologues of SAR1 (Sar1a and Sar1b). GDP-restricted mutants of hSar1p (*h*uman Sar1p) inhibit the formation of ER buds and the export of cargo in mammalian cells (157,158). Using mammalian Sec23/24 and Sec13/31 complexes purified from rat liver and recombinant GST-tagged Sar1p, Aridor and colleagues (161) have demonstrated that, like in yeast, the Sar1-activation induced recruitment of the Sec23/24 complex to the ER membrane increased the GTP hydrolysis of Sar1p and led to the sorting of cargo protein into prebudding domains where ER resident proteins (ribophorin, calnexin, and BiP) were excluded. Subsequent addition of the Sec13/31 complex resulted in vesicle formation (161). These experiments seem to indicate that as in yeast, the Sar1–Sec23/24–Sec13/31 complex constitutes the minimal machinery needed for vesicle formation in mammalian cells. Notably, in mammalian cells, two functional homologues of Sec23p (hSec23A and

hSec23B) (162,163), a Sec13p orthologue (Sec13R) (164), four Sec24p orthologues (Sec24A, Sec24B, Sec24C, Sec24D) (165,166), and a mammalian orthologue of Sec31, p137 (167), have been identified.

Although the minimal requirements for *in vitro* vesicle biogenesis are the five molecules listed above, the essential gene product of SEC16 appears to be required for vesicle formation *in vivo* (146). Sec16p interacts on the vesicle with Sec23/Sec24p (146), Sec31p (162), and Sec4p, an ER membrane protein homologous to Sec12p. Sec16 likely plays a regulatory role, which is bypassed in *in vitro* experiments (146). In mammalian cells, GST-hSec23 binding columns allowed for the identification of a 250 kDa protein that could be detected by Western blotting using an antibody against yeast Sec16, indicating that Sec16 orthologues are also present in mammalian cells (168). Another protein isolated from the GST-hSec23 binding columns, p125, has recently been shown to likely be expressed in liver, as demonstrated in Northern blots (168), although the role of this protein in COPII vesicle formation remains to be elucidated. Nevertheless, amino acid analysis shows sequence homology between p125 and phosphatidic acid–preferring phospholipase A1, and seems to indicate the importance of phospholipid metabolism in vesicle formation (168). In the final stages of COPII vesicle biogenesis, the GTP used during vesicle formation is hydrolyzed by Sec23p, a Sar1p-specific GTPase-activating protein (GAP).

Trans-Golgi Network–Derived Vesicles

Protein Sorting and Trafficking Events at the TGN

The *trans*-Golgi network is a tubulovesicular network that acts primarily in sorting proteins to their final destination. Within this membranous reticulum, cargo proteins are efficiently segregated into distinct vesicles that will be targeted to various compartments, including the endosome/lysosome system, the apical or basolateral domains in polarized cells, and the secretory granule pool. In regulated secretory cells, this granule pool waits for the appropriate extracellular stimulus to exocytose its contents.

In hepatocytes, the proximity of endocytic vesicles to Golgi stacks and the TGN, all of which are loaded with lipoprotein, has made it difficult to distinguish between multivesicular endosomes and secretory vesicles. Furthermore, the elaborate ultrastructure of the TGN, and its morphological adjacency to the ER and lysosomes in hepatocytes, led it to be originally described as a specialized area of the ER known as GERL (*G*olgi, *E*R, *l*ysosome)(Fig. 10.6A). Interpreted as being another population of lipoprotein-containing cisternae and vacuoles apart from the Golgi apparatus proper (169), GERL is considered to be synonymous with TGN, as are all other names previously attributed to this sorting compartment (*trans*-tubular network, *trans*-

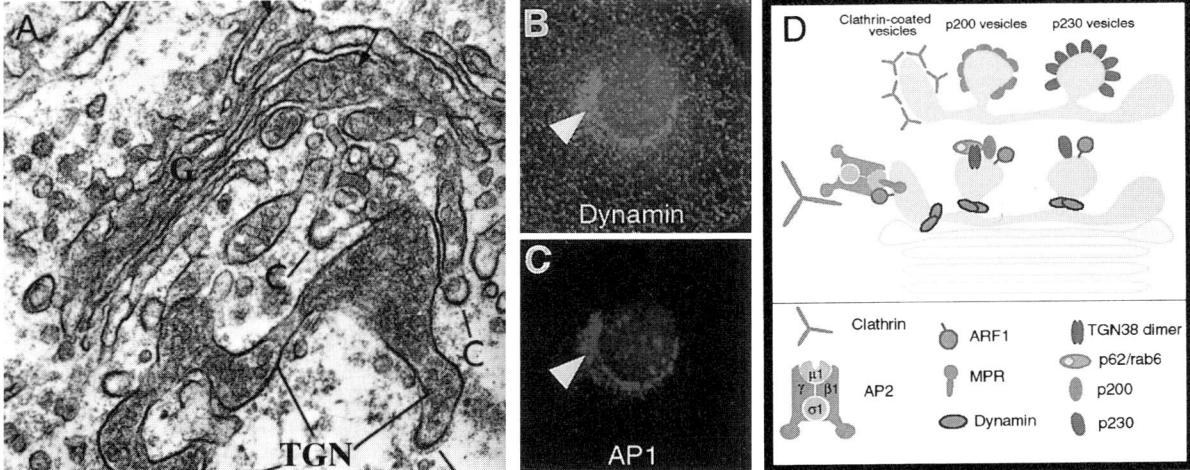

FIGURE 10.6. Secretory vesicles derived from the *trans*-Golgi network (*TGN*). **A:** Electron micrograph of a Golgi apparatus from a rat liver hepatocyte. The tubular network of the TGN is clearly visible in this micrograph as are uncoated and coated buds (*C*) (From Novikoff PM, Yam A. Sites of lipoprotein particles in normal rat hepatocytes. *J. Cell Biol.* 1978;76:1–11, with permission.) **B–C:** Immunofluorescence images of clone 9 cultured rat hepatocytes labeled for dynamin and AP1. These two accessory proteins involved in TGN-derived clathrin-coated vesicle formation are colocalized in a perinuclear location. (Images from Dr. Hong Cao, Mayo Clinic). **D:** Several vesicle types are known to arise from the TGN. Formation of clathrin-coated vesicles is known to involve membrane receptors [such as the mannose-6-phosphate receptor (*MPR*)], the Golgi adaptor protein complex, AP1, ARF1, which mediates AP1 membrane association, and the molecular pinchase dynamin. p200 vesicles are known to involve p62/rab6/TGN38. Notably, a lacelike coated vesicle population identified in normal rat kidney cells have been suggested to be coated by p200 (196). p230 vesicles are known to have a distinct coat from p200. Formation of non–clathrin-coated vesicles is known to require ARF1 and dynamin for vesicle release. See Color Plate 9.

reticular Golgi, and *trans*-Golgi reticulum). Experiments have shown that while the Golgi stack redistributes into the ER in the presence of the fungal metabolite BFA, the TGN fuses with the plasma membrane and/or the endosomal compartments, suggesting the existence of central and peripheral membrane systems (170). The TGN is thought to be a member of the latter system, where it is known to intimately and dynamically interact with the endosomal apparatus in events related especially to receptor recycling and endosomal maturation, and in the delivery of lysosomal enzymes (reviewed in ref. 171).

In polarized cells, the apical and basolateral plasma membranes are characterized by specific cell-surface components. This polarized distribution is achieved differently depending on cell type. Two routes are known to exist from the TGN to the cell surface domains (172). In MDCK cells and in fibroblasts (173), apically and basolaterally destined membrane proteins are packaged into distinct post-Golgi transport vesicles, and are transported directly to their final membrane destination. In hepatocytes, most proteins leaving the TGN are first delivered to the basolateral membrane, with apical membrane proteins sorted at that site and subsequently transported to the apical membrane by transcytosis. Interestingly, specific lumenal cargo proteins of rat liver hepatocytes have been reported to be concentrated in distinct secretory vesicles (174). Both routes, direct and indirect, are used by

Caco-2 cells and primary intestinal epithelial cells for delivery to the appropriate membrane domain (172).

Secretion in animal cells involves various types of vesicles that bud from the TGN and are required to follow distinct pathways. Due to the multitude of destinations for cargo proteins exiting the Golgi apparatus, vesicle trafficking from the TGN is quite a complex process. The list of exocytic secretory vesicles involved is far from being complete; however, they may be roughly classified into two categories, clathrin-coated and non–clathrin coated vesicles. The former are responsible for (a) concentrating newly synthesized lysosomal hydrolases for delivery to the endosomal apparatus and then lysosomes, and (b) for enzymes and hormones in the secretory granules of cells that have regulated secretory pathways (171,175). In contrast, non–clathrin coated vesicles are believed to mainly package cargo proteins that are constitutively secreted. Specific sets of proteins are associated with both types of vesicles, with some having been shown by various biochemical and *in vitro* TGN budding assays to be required for vesicle formation at this site.

Clathrin-Coated TGN-Derived Vesicles

Clathrin was the first coat to be visualized in the Golgi region of mammalian cells. An electron-dense spiked coat could clearly be seen on TGN membranes in the original micrographs of Novikoff and Yam (169) in liver hepato-cytes (Fig. 10.6A). Similar coats were visible on buds and vesicles of the TGN compartment in the principal epithelial cells of the epididymus (176), and clathrin patches have been reported along the delimiting membrane of secretory granules in regulated secretory cells (177). TGN-derived clathrin-coated vesicles are now known to have a coat composed of clathrin triskelions and adaptor protein complex AP-1 (made up of γ-, β1-, μ1, and σ1-adaptin subunits) and possibly the recently identified AP-3 adaptor protein complex (δ-, β3-, μ3-, and σ3-adaptin subunits) (178). Both AP-1 and AP-3 are predominantly found in vesicular structures in the Golgi region; however, an endosomal localization has also been reported (17).

Clathrin-coated vesicles generated from the TGN have been shown to be involved in the transport of newly synthesized lysosomal enzymes and, in regulated cells, in the formation of secretory granules. It now appears that these two functions of TGN-derived clathrin-coated vesicles may be linked, at least in regulated secretory cells. Newly synthesized soluble lysosomal enzymes are known to acquire mannose-6-phosphate residues at the *cis*-Golgi network that are recognized by the mannose-6-phosphate receptor (MPR) at the TGN (171). At this site, MPRs are known to bind to the AP-1 adaptor complex which then recruits clathrin for bud and vesicle formation. These clathrin-coated vesicles subsequently mediate the transport of the MPR-lysosomal enzyme complexes to endosomes (179). Notably, clathrin-coated vesicles originating from a post-Golgi compartment may also be involved in lysosomal protein sorting. In regulated secretory cells, although clathrin-coated regions on secretory granules have frequently been observed, the role of coated membranes at this site has largely been unknown. Small coated vesicles could be seen pinching off from secretory granule membranes in pancreatic acinar cells, hence it was thought that clathrin may be required to remove membrane in the form of small vesicles to mediate the concentration of secretory enzymes and the maturation of immature secretory granules to the typically smaller-sized mature granules (180). Because lysosomal enzymes have long been known to be present in secretory granules (181), a recent study has put forward the hypothesis that clathrin patches along secretory granule membranes may further enable secretory granule maturation by carrying out a function similar to that which it serves at the TGN and at the plasma membrane, namely, the sequestration of receptors and receptor-bound ligands that are destined to not be secreted by the cell.

A newly uncovered adaptor protein complex at the TGN, AP-3, may have a similar lysosomal protein sorting role. AP-3 is ubiquitously expressed, has been localized on buds/vesicles associated with the TGN (178), and can interact with clathrin (24) and with sorting signals in the cytoplasmic tails of lysosomal membrane proteins (21). The correct targeting of lysosomal-associated membrane pro-

tein, LAMP-1, and lysosomal integral membrane protein, LIMP-2, is mediated by the AP-3 adaptor complex (182). In support of these findings, LIMP-2 was found in a separate study to interact with AP-3, but not AP-1, indicating the specificity of recognition and sorting by the AP-3 complex (183). Furthermore, defective AP-3 results in a mistargeting of lysosomal proteins, CD63, LAMP-1, and LAMP-2 to the cell surface in fibroblasts from patients with Hermansky–Pudlak syndrome, a genetic disorder in which lysosome-related organelles are defective (184).

How are clathrin-coated vesicles formed at the TGN? Part of the answer lies in what is already known about clathrin coats at the plasma membrane. Adaptors at both the cell surface (AP-2) and at the Golgi apparatus (AP-1) are thought to initiate coat assembly by recruiting clathrin triskelia that polymerize to form the coat (17). As with the AP-2 adaptor at the plasma membrane, the AP-1 β1 subunit is known to promote clathrin cage assembly *in vitro* (26) and the μ1 subunit has been shown to associate with specific sorting motifs on cytosolic tails of MPR and TGN38 (a membrane protein predominantly localized to the TGN) (21). However, whether membrane receptors such as the MPR are the main factors involved in recruiting AP-1 to TGN membranes is still a matter of debate. Although the AP-1 adaptor complex is able to bind to MPR-negative TGN membranes (185), a separate study has demonstrated that the MPRs are required for the recruitment of AP-1, and that the amount of MPR on TGN membranes regulates TGN-derived vesicle formation, especially at low MPR expression levels (186).

In addition to the MPR, multiple factors are also likely to contribute to vesicle biogenesis at the TGN (Fig. 10.6D). It has been clearly demonstrated that like the COPI coatomer, AP-1 recruitment to TGN membranes is sensitive to BFA, and thus is regulated by ARF (see COPI-Coated Vesicles above) (187,188). Indeed, one of the minimal requirements for clathrin-coat assembly appears to be ARF1, since ARF-GTP was recently demonstrated to recruit both AP-1 and clathrin onto protein-free liposomes in the presence of other cytosolic factors (189). Thus like COPI-, COPII-, and AP-2-containing clathrin-coated vesicles on protein-free liposomes (68,159,190), integral membrane proteins appear not to be required for *in vitro* AP-1-mediated coat assembly.

Although the *in vivo* order of association of AP-1, MPR and ARF is still being deciphered, models have been proposed suggesting that ARF may (a) mediate the recruitment of AP-1 to ARF-activated MPRs or by generating other high-affinity AP-1 binding sites on TGN membranes (191), or (b) regulate ARF-GTP hydrolysis, and thus clathrin-coated vesicle formation, by interacting and recruiting an ARF GAP onto membranes, since it was indirectly shown that ARF-GTP hydrolysis is enhanced in MPR-positive Golgi membranes as compared to that in MPR-negative membranes (185). The latter proposal is supported by what is known about the formation of COPI-coated vesicles at the Golgi apparatus: the transmembrane receptor, ERD2 (i.e., the KDEL receptor involved in the retrieval of KDEL-containing soluble ER resident enzymes), interacts with and mediates the membrane association of ARF-GAP and in this way regulates the assembly of the COPI coat (192). Additional components may be involved in clathrin-coated vesicle formation at the TGN, especially following the identification and characterization of a large inventory of accessory proteins involved in clathrin-coated vesicle formation at the plasma membrane (40). In a study searching for analogous AP-1 binding partners implicated in clathrin-coated vesicle formation at the TGN, an Eps15 homology (EH) domain-containing protein, γ-synergin, was recently found to interact with the γ subunit of AP-1 on TGN membranes and in clathrin-coated vesicles (193). Besides, dynamin (see below), γ-synergin is the first accessory protein to be uncovered at the TGN, and it has been suggested that owing to its EH domain, γ-synergin may regulate clathrin-coated vesicle formation at the TGN by linking AP-1 to other regulatory proteins.

Non–Clathrin-Coated TGN-Derived Vesicles

Cell-free protein transport assays, successfully used in the characterization of key protein components involved in ER-to-Golgi and intra-Golgi protein transport, have also been instrumental in the primary identification of proteins, other than AP-1 and clathrin, which are involved in vesicle budding at the TGN. With the use of a purified rat liver stacked Golgi fraction immobilized on magnetic beads, vesicle budding was shown to be ATP-, cytosol-, and temperature-dependent (194). Vesicles purified from the budding fraction were between 50 and 200 nm in diameter and were found to be devoid of any visible coat. To determine which cytosolic protein components may be required for the generation of vesicles in this *in vitro* system, TGN38, a known transmembrane protein marker of the TGN which cycles between the TGN and the plasma membrane, was tested for a role in Golgi-to-plasma membrane vesicular trafficking and for potential cytosolic binding partners. In a CHAPS-solubilized stacked Golgi fraction, the cytosolic domain of TGN38 was found to associate with a cytoplasmic complex consisting of a 62 kDa protein (with homology to the phosphotidylinositol 3-kinase regulatory subunit), and a small 25 kDa GTP-binding protein suggested to be rab6 (195). Dissociation of the complex from TGN38 and the TGN membrane was also found to be regulated by p62 phosphorylation (195). The p62/rab6/TGN38 cytosolic domain complex was found to be essential for exocytic vesicle formation from the TGN; vesicle budding was inhibited when the assay was carried out with p62- or rab6-immunodepleted cytosol, or with cytosol containing competing peptides of either of those proteins or the cytosolic

tail of TGN38. In support of these findings, electroporation of NRK cells with antibodies against the TGN38 cytosolic tail was reported to lead to a significant decrease in protein secretion (196).

Another cytosolic protein recently found to be localized to vesicles in the TGN, p200, was found to bind selectively to Golgi membranes and to be involved in vesicle budding from the TGN upon activation of heterotrimeric G proteins, with GTPγS (a nonhydrolyzable analogue of GTP), AlF4⁻, or mastoparan (197). Notably, p200 was found to be localized to a subset of TGN38-containing vesicles in NRK cells by immunogold labeling (197), and it has been reported to bind to Golgi membranes via the p62 complex (196), although a direct interaction between these sets of molecules has not been demonstrated. Notably, protein secretion was decreased by 50% in cells electroporated with antibodies to p200, further supporting a role for this protein in exocytic membrane traffic. Due to its large size, p200 was suggested to be the structural coat protein of lace-like coated vesicles (196), originally visualized in a 3D-reconstruction study of the TGN compartment in NRK cells by high-voltage electron microscopy, and characterized by scallop-shaped subunits at their delimiting membrane (198). A complex consisting of p200, p62, a small GTP-binding protein and a dimer of TGN38 has been proposed to be involved in the formation of TGN-derived vesicles (Fig. 10.6D). Further characterization of p200 has revealed that it dissociates from membranes in the presence of brefeldin A, like the coatomer protein β-COP (199), although TGN vesicles bearing either of these coat proteins were seen to be distinct (197). It was discovered that the p200 protein is the heavy chain of nonmuscle myosin II, a protein demonstrated to be involved in the generation of constitutive transport vesicles containing vesicular stomatitus virus G protein from the TGN of polarized semiintact MDCK cells (200).

p230 is a peripheral membrane protein also shown to be localized on the TGN in HeLa cells, and appears to behave similarly to p200 in that its association with Golgi membranes is (a) enhanced in the presence of G protein activators, (b) disrupted by brefeldin A, and (c) localized to small coated vesicles distinct from clathrin-coated or p200-coated vesicles (201). Because p230 was found to recycle between the cytosol and TGN membrane buds and vesicles in a G protein-dependent fashion, it was suggested that this vesicle-associated protein may be involved in the formation of a specific set of non–clathrin-coated vesicles (Fig. 10.6D).

Scission of TGN-Derived Vesicles

Ever since the localization of the large GTPase dynamin on the Golgi apparatus was reported, in addition to its known cell surface distribution, it has been suggested that vesicle fission at the level of the Golgi apparatus may be mediated by this molecular pinchase. With the use of a battery of dynamin antibodies specific to the brain (DynI) (60) and ubiquitous (DynII) (202) isoforms in immunofluorescence analyses, dynamin was shown to be distributed as punctate spots at the plasma membrane and within the perinuclear area of cells, with both localizations largely overlapping with a clathrin antibody staining pattern. Dynamin's association with Golgi membranes was also demonstrated biochemically with specific antibodies detecting dynamin in immunoblots of purified rat liver Golgi fractions, and immunoisolating Golgi membranes on magnetic beads coated with those dynamin antibodies (202). Immunogold localization of DynII on the TGN of HeLa cells (203) and the Golgi distribution of various GFP-tagged dynamin isoforms [especially the DynII(aa)] (61), confirmed these findings. Remarkably, with the use of the *in vitro* TGN budding assay described above, dynamin was found to play a significant role in exocytic vesicle formation (204) (Fig. 10.6D). Generation of both clathrin-coated and non–clathrin-coated polymeric immunoglobulin A receptor-containing vesicles was decreased upon addition of dynamin-specific antibodies to the assay mixture, or by using cytosol immunodepleted of dynamin. Recently, Golgi-to-plasma membrane transport of basolaterally and apically targeted plasma membrane proteins was inhibited in cells transfected with a GTPase-defective DynII(aa) mutant (205,206). An 8- to 11-fold accumulation of nascent GFP-VSV-G-tsO45 in the Golgi apparatus of transfected BHK cells was observed, as was a hypertrophy of the TGN compartment, as evaluated by electron microscopy (205), suggesting that dynamin is likely required for TGN protein exit.

LIPID REGULATORS INVOLVED IN VESICLE BIOGENESIS

With the vast number of studies examining and reporting on the role of proteins in vesicle formation, it has often been assumed that the membrane lipids of a vesicle may not play an active role. More and more, however, it appears that lipids of the membrane bilayer are important mediators of both the budding and scission reactions in vesicle biogenesis. Indeed, studies in model membrane systems have revealed that budding can be facilitated if the lipid composition is modified to provide favorable membrane bending energy. Cone-shaped lipids influence negative curvature (if found in the inner membrane leaflet of a bud) or positive curvature (if found in the outer leaflet) of a membrane depending on whether they are right-side-up or inverted, respectively (reviewed in ref. 207). Also, drugs involved in changing the membrane lipid content or organization, such as the cholesterol chelator methyl β-cyclodextrin, have been shown to abrogate both clathrin-mediated and caveolae-mediated endocytosis at the vesicle budding stage (85).

To date, several lipids and membrane lipid-modifying proteins have been identified to have a regulatory role in vesicle formation. Most of these appear to be involved in the formation of several types of vesicles that bud from the Golgi apparatus, and it appears that phosphatidic acid (PA) is a key ingredient in the bilayer for membrane curvature.

As mentioned earlier in the section entitled COPI-Coated Vesicles, the small GTP-binding protein ARF mediates the recruitment of coat proteins that are thought to deform the membrane bilayer, resulting in a coated vesicle bud at the level of the compartments in the early secretory pathway. In addition, various lipid factors are known to regulate, and in turn be regulated by, ARF binding. Since phosphotidylinositol-4,5-bisphosphate (PtdIns(4,5)P$_2$) is a GTPase exchange factor (GEF) for ARF, it has been suggested that it may be involved in recruiting ARF to sites of vesicle formation (208). PtdIns(4,5)P$_2$ is known to be required for an ARF1 interaction with phospholipase D (PLD) (209,210), a protein with abundant activity in Golgi-enriched membranes (211). Together with activated ARF, PtdIns(4,5)P$_2$ has been shown to activate PLD1 to generate PA from phosphatidylcholine (PC). PA has been demonstrated to be required for the *in vitro* formation of coated vesicles from Chinese Hamster Ovary cell Golgi membranes (143), and has been suggested to be an important factor mediating a shape change in the lipid bilayer to facilitate invagination. So important is this requirement in fact that treating membranes with exogenous PLD can bypass the need for ARF in generating vesicles from this fraction (212). This reaction appears to be autoregulatory, since local membrane increases in PA can stimulate PtdIns(4)P-5 kinase, leading to the generation of more PtdIns(4,5)P$_2$, which may in turn increase the exchange reaction on ARF (213). However, PtdIns(4,5)P$_2$ and PA are also known to inactivate ARF by stimulating an ARF GTPase-activating protein (GAP) (210). Notably, PLD has been suggested to also be activated by protein kinase C to facilitate vesicle scission at the TGN. This is based on the findings that specific PKC isoforms (PKCα and PKCε) are localized to Golgi membranes (214,215). Furthermore, the role of PA in membrane curvature has also been shown in a recent study demonstrating the role of brefeldin A-ADP-ribosylated substrate (BARS) in inducing Golgi membrane fission by the selective acylation of lysophosphatidic acid with acyl CoA-generating PA (216). Both the formation of constitutive secretory vesicles and immature secretory granules from the TGN have been reported to be stimulated by the concerted action of phosphatidylinositol transfer protein (PITP) and PLD in a cell-free system using PC12 membrane fractions (217). This stimulatory effect is inhibited by geneticin, an antibiotic known to bind to phosphoinositides, demonstrating a role for phosphoinositides in promoting secretory vesicle formation downstream of PITP and PLD. PITP and PtdIns(3)kinase have also been shown to be essential components in the cell-free formation of polymeric immunoglobulin A receptor-containing exocytic vesicles from Golgi fractions isolated from rat liver (204).

Together, PITP and PtdIns(3)kinase lead to the generation of a pool of PtdIns(3)P, which has been suggested to be essential for vesicle formation from the TGN (204).

At the cell surface, the role of lipids in endocytosis is also becoming quite apparent. The role of PA in vesicle budding has been demonstrated again in a recent study examining the function of endophilin, a lysophosphatidic acid acyl transferase that catalyzes the conversion of lysophosphatidic acid to PA by the addition of arachidonic acid. Although, *in vitro* results evaluating the role of endophilin are conflicting (66,218), *in vivo* experiments in which endophilin antibodies were microinjected into lamprey synapses (66) revealed that this dynamin-, amphiphysin-, and synaptojanin-binding partner plays an essential role in clathrin-mediated synaptic vesicle recycling. Endophilin is proposed to introduce a favorable microenvironment at the synaptic membrane, possibly by inducing a lower membrane tension that would facilitate membrane curvature and subsequent tubulation and vesiculation by the pinchase dynamin (66). Vesicle membrane curvature has also been proposed to be facilitated by sphingomyelinase in an ATP-independent manner in macrophages (219), and at presynaptic terminals by specific interactions between cholesterol and synaptophysin in synapticlike microvesicles.

FUTURE DIRECTIONS

While a substantial amount of information has been gathered on the mechanisms of vesicle formation, many challenges still remain. We now have an extensive but continuously expanding list of protein and lipid components of the vesicle-forming machinery, yet not all of their functions have been determined. Moreover, new evidence indicates that selected steps in protein transport may not implicate vesicles, but rather continuous tubular compartments, maturation events or direct fusion between membranes (220–223). It will be important to understand how vesicle protein components interact in a regulated manner, to coordinate the sequestration of secretory and endocytic ligands, the deformation of specific membrane domains, coat assembly, and the final scission and targeting of the resulting vesicles. Insights into these processes will provide us with a better understanding of hepatocyte function.

ACKNOWLEDGMENTS

The authors wish to thank Dr. Molly Accola, and Noah Gray for critically reading the manuscript, Drs. Hong Cao, Yisang Yoon, and John J.M. Bergeron (McGill University, Montreal, Canada) for contributing valuable images, and Barbara Oswald and Eugene Krueger for assistance in preparing the schematic drawings. We apologize to authors whose work we did not refer to due to space restrictions. This chapter review is dedicated to the late Dr. Keith Porter.

REFERENCES

1. Bretscher MS, Thomson JN, Pearse BM. Coated pits act as molecular filters. *Proc Nat Acad Sci U S A* 1980;77:4156–4159.
2. Roth RI, Porter KR. Yolk protein uptake in the oocyte of the mosquito *Aedes aegypti* L. *J Cell Biol* 1964;20:313–332.
3. Pearse BM. Clathrin: a unique protein associated with intracellular transfer of membrane by coated vesicles. *Proc Nat Acad Sci U S A* 1976;73:1255–1259.
4. Anderson RG, Goldstein JL, Brown MS. Localization of low density lipoprotein receptors on plasma membrane of normal human fibroblasts and their absence in cells from a familial hypercholesterolemia homozygote. *Mol Cell Endocrin* 1976;73:2434–2438.
5. Carpentier JL, Fehlmann M, Van Obberghen E, et al. Redistribution of 125I-insulin on the surface of rat hepatocytes as a function of dissociation time. *Diabetes* 1985;34:1002–1007.
6. Griffiths G, Back R, Marsh M. A quantitative analysis of the endocytic pathway in baby hamster kidney cells. *J Cell Biol* 1989;109:2703–2720.
7. Pelchen-Matthews A, Armes JE, Griffiths G, et al. Differential endocytosis of CD4 in lymphocytic and nonlymphocytic cells. *J Exp Med* 1991;173:575–587.
8. Smythe E, Pypaert M, Lucocq J, et al. Formation of coated vesicles from coated pits in broken A431 cells. *J Cell Biol* 1989;108:843–853.
9. Larkin JM, Donzell WC, Anderson RG. Potassium-dependent assembly of coated pits: new coated pits form as planar clathrin lattices. *J Cell Biol* 1986;103:2619–2627.
10. Pastan IH, Willingham MC. Journey to the center of the cell: role of the receptosome. *Science* 1981;214:504–509.
11. Burgess JW, Bevan AP, Bergeron JJ, et al. Pharmacological doses of insulin equalize insulin receptor phosphotyrosine content but not tyrosine kinase activity in plasmalemmal and endosomal membranes. *Biochem Cell Biol* 1992;70:1151–1158.
12. Di Guglielmo GM, Baass PC, Ou WJ, et al. Compartmentalization of SHC GRB2 and mSOS and hyperphosphorylation of Raf-1 by EGF but not insulin in liver parenchyma. *EMBO J* 1994;13:4269–4277.
13. Marsh M, Helenius A. Virus entry into animal cells. *Adv in Virus Res* 1989;36:107–151.
14. Pearse BM. Coated vesicles from pig brain: purification and biochemical characterization. *J Mol Biol* 1975;97:93–98.
15. Heuser J. Three-dimensional visualization of coated vesicle formation in fibroblasts. *J Cell Biol* 1980;84:560–583.
16. Crowther RA, Pearse BM. Assembly and packing of clathrin into coats. *J Cell Biol* 1981;91:790–797.
17. Hirst J, Robinson MS. Clathrin and adaptors. *Biochim Biophys Acta* 1998;1404:173–193.
18. Hirst J, Bright NA, Rous B, et al. Characterization of a fourth adaptor-related protein complex. *Mol Biol Cell* 1999;10:2787–2802.
19. Ponnambalam S, Robinson MS, Jackson AP, et al. Conservation and diversity in families of coated vesicle adaptins. *J Biol Chem* 1990;265:4814–4820.
20. Dell'Angelica EC, Ohno H, Ooi CE, et al. AP-3: an adaptor-like protein complex with ubiquitous expression. *EMBO J* 1997;16:917–928.
21. Ohno HJ, Stewart MC, Fournier H, et al. Interaction of tyrosine-based sorting signals with clathrin-associated proteins. *Science* 1995;269:1872–1875.

22. Ohno H, Fournier MC, Poy G, et al. Structural determinants of interaction of tyrosine-based sorting signals with the adaptor medium chains. *J Biol Chem* 1996;271:29009–29015.
23. Hofmann MW, Honing S, Rodionov D, et al. The leucine-based sorting motifs in the cytoplasmic domain of the invariant chain are recognized by the clathrin adaptors AP1 and AP2 and their medium chains. *J Biol Chem* 1999;274:36153–36158.
24. Dell'Angelica EC, Klumperman J, Stoorvogel W. Association of the AP-3 adaptor complex with clathrin. *Science* 1998;280:431–434.
25. Ahle S, Ungewickell E. Identification of a clathrin binding subunit in the HA2 adaptor protein complex. *J Biol Chem* 1989;264:20089–20093.
26. Gallusser A, Kirchhausen T. The beta 1 and beta 2 subunits of the AP complexes are the clathrin coat assembly components. *EMBO J* 1993;12:5237–5244.
27. Goodman OB, Krupnick Jr JG, Santini F, et al. Beta-arrestin acts as a clathrin adaptor in endocytosis of the beta2-adrenergic receptor. *Nature* 1996;383:447–450.
28. Sorkin A, Carpenter G. Interaction of activated EGF receptors with coated pit adaptins. *Science* 1993;261:612–615.
29. Goodman OB, Krupnick Jr JG, Santini F, et al. Role of arrestins in G-protein-coupled receptor endocytosis. *Adv Pharmacol* 1998;42:429–433.
30. Schmid SL, Matsumoto AK, Rothman JE. A domain of clathrin that forms coats. *Proc Nat Acad Sci U S A* 1982;79:91–95.
31. Vigers GP, Crowther RA, Pearse BM. Three-dimensional structure of clathrin cages in ice. *EMBO J* 1986;5:529–534.
32. Nathke I, Hill BL, Parham P, et al. The calcium-binding site of clathrin light chains. *J Biol Chem* 1990;265:18621–18627.
33. Hill BL, Drickamer K, Brodsky FM, et al. Identification of the phosphorylation sites of clathrin light chain LCb. *J Biol Chem* 1988;263:5499–5501.
34. Schmid SL, Braell WA, Schlossman DM, et al. A role for clathrin light chains in the recognition of clathrin cages by `uncoating ATPase.' *Nature* 1984;311:228–231.
35. Ungewickell E,, Ungewickell H. Bovine brain clathrin light chains impede heavy chain assembly in vitro. *J Biol Chem* 1991;266:12710–12714.
36. Cupers P, Veithen A, Kiss A, et al. Clathrin polymerization is not required for bulk-phase endocytosis in rat fetal fibroblasts. *J Cell Biol* 1994;127:725–735.
37. Miller K, Shipman M, Trowbridge IS, et al. Transferrin receptors promote the formation of clathrin lattices. *Cell* 1991;65:621–632.
38. Peeler JS, Donzell WC, Anderson RG. The appendage domain of the AP-2 subunit is not required for assembly or invagination of clathrin-coated pits. *J Cell Biol* 1993;120:47–54.
39. Robinson PJ, Liu JP, Powell KA, et al. Phosphorylation of dynamin I and synaptic-vesicle recycling. *Trends Neurosci* 1994;17:348–353.
40. Santolini E, Salcini AE, Kay BK, et al. The EH network. *Exp Cell Res* 1999;253:186–209.
41. Benmerah A, Bayrou M, Cerf-Bensussan N, et al. Inhibition of clathrin-coated pit assembly by an Eps15 mutant. *J Cell Sci* 1999;112:1303–1311.
42. Rosenthal JA, Chen H, Slepnev VI, et al. The epsins define a family of proteins that interact with components of the clathrin coat and contain a new protein module. *J Biol Chem* 1999;274:33959–33965.
43. Hussain NK, Yamabhai M, Ramjaun AR, et al. Splice variants of intersectin are components of the endocytic machinery in neurons and nonneuronal cells. *J Biol Chem* 1999;274:15671–15677.
44. Tebar F, Sorkina T, Sorkin A, et al. Eps15 is a component of clathrin-coated pits and vesicles and is located at the rim of coated pits. *J Biol Chem* 1996;271:28727–28730.
45. Cupers P, Jadhav AP, Kirchhausen T. Assembly of clathrin coats disrupts the association between Eps15 and AP-2 adaptors. *J Biol Chem* 1998;273:1847–1850.
46. Yamabhai M, Hoffman NG, Hardison NL, et al. Intersectin a novel adaptor protein with two Eps15 homology and five Src homology 3 domains. *J Biol Chem* 1998;273:31401–31407.
47. Guipponi M, Scott HS, Chen H, et al. Two isoforms of a human intersectin (ITSN) protein are produced by brain-specific alternative splicing in a stop codon. *Genomics* 1998;53:369–376.
48. Ungewickell E. Wrapping the package. *Proc Nat Acad Sci U S A* 1999;96:8809–8810.
49. Chen H, Fre S, Slepnev VI. Epsin is an EH-domain-binding protein implicated in clathrin-mediated endocytosis. *Nature* 1998;394:793–797.
50. Chen H, Slepnev VI, Di Fiore PP, et al. The interaction of epsin and Eps15 with the clathrin adaptor AP-2 is inhibited by mitotic phosphorylation and enhanced by stimulation-dependent dephosphorylation in nerve terminals. *J Biol Chem* 1999;274:3257-3260.
51. Slepnev VI, Ochoa GC, Butler MH, et al. Role of phosphorylation in regulation of the assembly of endocytic coat complexes. *Science* 1998;281:821–824.
52. Kosaka T, Ikeda K. Reversible blockage of membrane retrieval and endocytosis in the garland cell of the temperature-sensitive mutant of Drosophila melanogaster shibirets1. *J Cell Biol* 1983;97:499–507.
53. Kosaka T, Ikeda K. Possible temperature-dependent blockage of synaptic vesicle recycling induced by a single gene mutation in Drosophila. *J Neurobiol* 1983;14:207–225.
54. Chen MS, Obar RA, Schroeder CC, et al. Multiple forms of dynamin are encoded by shibire a Drosophila gene involved in endocytosis. *Nature* 1991;351:583–586.
55. van der Bliek AM, Meyerowitz EM. Dynamin-like protein encoded by the Drosophila shibire gene associated with vesicular traffic. *Nature* 1991;351:411–414.
56. Herskovits JS, Burgess CC, Obar RA, et al. Effects of mutant rat dynamin on endocytosis. *J Cell Biol* 1993;122:565–578.
57. van der Bliek AM, Redelmeier TE, Damke H, et al. Mutations in human dynamin block an intermediate stage in coated vesicle formation. *J Cell Biol* 1993;122:553–563.
58. Henley JR, Krueger EW, Oswald BJ, et al. Dynamin-mediated internalization of caveolae. *J Cell Biol* 1998;141:85–99.
59. Cook TA, Urrutia R, McNiven MA. Identification of dynamin 2 an isoform ubiquitously expressed in rat tissues. *Proc Nat Acad Sci U S A* 1994;91:644–648.
60. McNiven MA, Cao H, Pitts KR, et al. The dynamin family of mechanoenzymes: pinching in new places. *Trends Biochem Sci* 2000;25:115–120.
61. Cao H, Garcia F, McNiven MA. Differential distribution of dynamin isoforms in mammalian cells. *Mol Biol Cell* 1998;9:2595–2609.
62. McNiven MA, Dynamin: a molecular motor with pinchase action. *Cell* 1998;94:151–154.
63. Tuma PL, Collins CA. Dynamin forms polymeric complexes in the presence of lipid vesicles. Characterization of chemically cross-linked dynamin molecules. *J Biol Chem* 1995;270:26707–26714.
64. Takei K, McPherson PS, Schmid SL, et al. Tubular membrane invaginations coated by dynamin rings are induced by GTP-gamma S in nerve terminals [see comments]. *Nature* 1995;374:186–190.
65. Ringstad N, Nemoto Y, De Camilli P. The SH3p4/Sh3p8/SH3p13 protein family: binding partners for synaptojanin and dynamin via a Grb2-like Src homology 3 domain. *Proc Nat Acad Sci U S A* 1997;94:8569–8574.

66. Ringstad N, Gad H, Low P, et al. Endophilin/SH3p4 is required for the transition from early to late stages in clathrin-mediated synaptic vesicle endocytosis. *Neuron* 1999;24:143–154.

67. Sweitzer SM, Hinshaw JE. Dynamin undergoes a GTP-dependent conformational change causing vesiculation. *Cell* 1998;93:1021–1029.

68. Takei K, Haucke V, Slepnev V, et al. Generation of coated intermediates of clathrin-mediated endocytosis on protein-free liposomes. *Cell* 1998;94:131–41.

69. Takei K, Slepnev VI, Haucke V, et al. Functional partnership between amphiphysin and dynamin in clathrin-mediated endocytosis. *Nat Cell Biol* 1999;1:33–39.

70. Holtzman DA, Yang S, Drubin DG. Synthetic-lethal interactions identify two novel genes SLA1 and SLA2 that control membrane cytoskeleton assembly in Saccharomyces cerevisiae. *J Cell Biol* 1993;122:635–644.

71. Engqvist-Goldstein AE, Kessels MM, Chopra VS, et al. An actin-binding protein of the Sla2/Huntingtin interacting protein 1 family is a novel component of clathrin-coated pits and vesicles. *J Cell Biol* 1999;147:1503–1518.

72. Witke W, Podtelejnikov AV, Di Nardo A, et al. In mouse brain profilin I and profilin II associate with regulators of the endocytic pathway and actin assembly. *EMBO J* 1998;17:967–976.

73. Foster-Barber A,, Bishop JM. Src interacts with dynamin and synapsin in neuronal cells. *Proc Nat Acad Sci U S A* 1998;95:4673–4677.

74. Qualmann B, Kelly RB. Syndapin isoforms participate in receptor-mediated endocytosis and actin organization. *J Cell Biol* 2000;148:1047–1061.

75. Gottlieb TA, Ivanov IE, Adesnik M. Actin microfilaments play a critical role in endocytosis at the apical but not the basolateral surface of polarized epithelial cells. *J Cell Biol* 1993;120:695–710.

76. Gaidarov I, Santini F, Warren RA, et al. Keen Spatial control of coated-pit dynamics in living cells. *Nat Cell Biol* 1999;1:1–7.

77. Petersen OW, van Deurs B. Serial-section analysis of coated pits and vesicles involved in adsorptive pinocytosis in cultured fibroblasts. *J Cell Biol* 1983;96:277–281.

78. Anderson RG, Brown MS, Goldstein JL. Role of the coated endocytic vesicle in the uptake of receptor-bound low density lipoprotein in human fibroblasts. *Cell* 1977;10:351–364.

79. Gruenberg J, Howell KE. Membrane traffic in endocytosis: insights from cell-free assays. *Ann Rev Cell Biol* 1989;5:453–481.

80. Heuser J, Steer CJ. Trimeric binding of the 70-kD uncoating. ATPase to the vertices of clathrin triskelia: a candidate intermediate in the vesicle uncoating reaction. *J Cell Biol* 1989;109:1457–1466.

81. Daukas G, Zigmond SH. Inhibition of receptor-mediated but not fluid-phase endocytosis in polymorphonuclear leukocytes. *J Cell Biol* 1985;101:1673–1679.

82. Larkin JM, Brown MS, Goldstein JL, et al. Depletion of intracellular potassium arrests coated pit formation and receptor-mediated endocytosis in fibroblasts. *Cell* 1983;33:273–285.

83. Sandvig K, Olsnes S, Petersen OW, et al. Acidification of the cytosol inhibits endocytosis from coated pits. *J Cell Biol* 1987;105:679–689.

84. Sandvig K, van Deurs B. Endocytosis without clathrin. *Cell Biol Int Rep* 1991;15:3–8.

85. Rodal SK, Skretting G, Garred O, et al. Extraction of cholesterol with methyl-beta-cyclodextrin perturbs formation of clathrin-coated endocytic vesicles. *Mol Biol Cell* 1999;10:961–974.

86. Hansen SH, Sandvig K, van Deurs B. The preendosomal compartment comprises distinct coated and noncoated endocytic vesicle populations. *J Cell Biol* 1991;113:731–741.

87. Hansen SH, Sandvig K, van Deurs B. Molecules internalized by clathrin-independent endocytosis are delivered to endosomes containing transferrin receptors. *J Cell Biol* 1993;123:89–97.

88. Wiley HS. Anomalous binding of epidermal growth factor to A431 cells is due to the effect of high receptor densities and a saturable endocytic system. *J Cell Biol* 1988;107:801–810.

89. Wiley HS, Herbst JJ, Walsh BJ, et al. The role of tyrosine kinase activity in endocytosis compartmentation and down-regulation of the epidermal growth factor receptor. *J Biol Chem* 1991;266:11083–11094.

90. Chen WS, Lazar CS, Lund KA, et al. Functional independence of the epidermal growth factor receptor from a domain required for ligand-induced internalization and calcium regulation. *Cell* 1989;59:33–43.

91. Lund KA, Opresko LK, Starbuck C, et al. Quantitative analysis of the endocytic system involved in hormone-induced receptor internalization. *J Biol Chem* 1990;265:15713–15723.

92. Deckert M, Ticchioni M, Bernard A. Endocytosis of GPI-anchored proteins in human lymphocytes: role of glycolipid-based domains actin cytoskeleton and protein kinases. *J Cell Biol* 1996;133:791–799.

93. Montesano R, Roth J, Robert A, et al. Non-coated membrane invaginations are involved in binding and internalization of cholera and tetanus toxins. *Nature* 1982;296:651–653.

94. Bretscher MS, Whytock S. Membrane-associated vesicles in fibroblasts. *J Ultrastruct Res* 1977;61:215–217.

95. Malaba L, Smeland S, Senoo H, et al. Retinol-binding protein and asialo-orosomucoid are taken up by different pathways in liver cells [published erratum appears in *J Biol Chem* 1995;270:27389]. *J Biol Chem* 1995;270:15686–15692.

96. Smart EJ, Graf GA, McNiven MA, et al. Caveolins liquid-ordered domains and signal transduction. *Mol Cell Biol* 1999;19:7289–7304.

97. Anderson RG, Kamen BA, Rothberg KG, et al. Potocytosis: sequestration and transport of small molecules by caveolae. *Science* 1992;255:410–411.

98. Parton RG, Joggerst B, Simons K. Regulated internalization of caveolae. *J Cell Biol* 1994;127:1199–1215.

99. Tran D, Carpentier JL, Sawano F, et al. Ligands internalized through coated or noncoated invaginations follow a common intracellular pathway. *Proc Nat Acad Sci U S A* 1987;84:7957–7961.

100. Mayor S, Sabharanjak S, Maxfield FR. Cholesterol-dependent retention of GPI-anchored proteins in endosomes. *EMBO J* 1998;17:4626–4638.

101. Anderson RG. The caveolae membrane system. *Ann Rev Biochem* 1998;67:199–225.

102. Jacobson K, Dietrich C. Looking at lipid rafts? *Trends Cell Biol* 1999;9:87–91.

103. Fielding PE, Fielding CJ. Plasma membrane caveolae mediate the efflux of cellular free cholesterol. *Biochemistry* 1995;34:14288–14292.

104. Schnitzer JE, Oh P, Pinney E, et al. Filipin-sensitive caveolae-mediated transport in endothelium: reduced transcytosis scavenger endocytosis and capillary permeability of select macromolecules. *J Cell Biol* 1994;127:1217–1232.

105. Hailstones D, Sleer LS, Parton RG, et al. Regulation of caveolin and caveolae by cholesterol in MDCK cells. *J Lipid Res* 1998;39:369–379.

106. Murata M, Peranen J, Schreiner R, et al. VIP21/caveolin is a cholesterol-binding protein. *Proc Nat Acad Sci U S A* 1995;92:10339–10343.

107. Smart EJ, Ying YS, Conrad PA, et al. Caveolin moves from caveolae to the Golgi apparatus in response to cholesterol oxidation. *J Cell Biol* 1994;127:1185–1197.

108. Rothberg KG, Heuser JE, Donzell WC, et al. Caveolin a protein component of caveolae membrane coats. *Cell* 1992;68:673–682.

109. Scherer PE, Lisanti MP, Baldini G, et al. Induction of caveolin

during adipogenesis and association of GLUT4 with caveolin-rich vesicles. *J Cell Biol* 1994;127:1233–1243.

110. Pol A, Calvo M, Lu A, et al. The "early-sorting" endocytic compartment of rat hepatocytes is involved in the intracellular pathway of caveolin-1 (VIP-21). *Hepatology* 1999;29:1848–1857.

111. Fra AM, Williamson E, Simons K, et al. De novo formation of caveolae in lymphocytes by expression of VIP21-caveolin. *Proc Nat Acad Sci U S A* 1995;92:8655–8659.

112. Vogel U, Sandvig K, van Deurs B. Expression of caveolin-1 and polarized formation of invaginated caveolae in Caco-2 and MDCK II cells. *J Cell Sci* 1998;111:825–832.

113. Lipardi C, Mora R, Colomer V, et al. Caveolin transfection results in caveolae formation but not apical sorting of glycosylphosphatidylinositol (GPI)-anchored proteins in epithelial cells. *J Cell Biol* 1998;140:617–626.

114. Liu PS, Li WP, Machleidt T, et al. Identification of caveolin-1 in lipoprotein particles secreted by exocrine cells. *Nat Cell Biol* 1999;1:369–375.

115. Oh P, McIntosh DP, Schnitzer JE. Dynamin at the neck of caveolae mediates their budding to form transport vesicles by GTP-driven fission from the plasma membrane of endothelium. *J Cell Biol* 1998;141:101–114.

116. Bannykh SI, Rowe T, Balch WE. The organization of endoplasmic reticulum export complexes. *J Cell Biol* 1996;135:19–35.

117. Rothman JE. Mechanisms of intracellular protein transport. *Nature* 1994;372:55–63.

118. Orci L, Glick BS, Rothman JE. A new type of coated vesicular carrier that appears not to contain clathrin: its possible role in protein transport within the Golgi stack. *Cell* 1986;46:171–184.

119. Oprins A, Duden R, Kreis TE, et al. Beta-COP localizes mainly to the cis-Golgi side in exocrine pancreas. *J Cell Biol* 1993;121:49–59.

120. Orci L, Palmer DJ, Ravazzola M, et al. Budding from Golgi membranes requires the coatomer complex of non-clathrin coat proteins. *Nature* 1993;362:648–652.

121. Peter F, Plutner H, Zhu H, et al. Beta-COP is essential for transport of protein from the endoplasmic reticulum to the Golgi in vitro. *J Cell Biol* 1993;122:1155–1567.

122. Pepperkok R, Scheel J, Horstmann H, et al. Beta-COP is essential for biosynthetic membrane transport from the endoplasmic reticulum to the Golgi complex in vivo. *Cell* 1993;74:71–82.

123. Misumi Y, Miki K, Takatsuki A, et al. Novel blockade by brefeldin A of intracellular transport of secretory proteins in cultured rat hepatocytes. *J Biol Chem* 1986;261:11398–11403.

124. Oda K, Hirose S, Takami N, et al. A arrests the intracellular transport of a precursor of complement C3 before its conversion site in rat hepatocytes. *FEBS Lett* 1987;214:135–138.

125. Cosson P, Letourneur F. Coatomer interaction with di-lysine endoplasmic reticulum retention motifs. *Science* 1994;263:1629–1631.

126. Letourneur F, Gaynor EC, Hennecke S, et al. Coatomer is essential for retrieval of dilysine-tagged proteins to the endoplasmic reticulum. *Cell* 1994;79:1199–1207.

127. Orci L, Stamnes M, Ravazzola M, et al. Bidirectional transport by distinct populations of COPI-coated vesicles. *Cell* 1997;90:335–349.

128. Scales SJ, Pepperkok R, Kreis TE. Visualization of ER-to-Golgi transport in living cells reveals a sequential mode of action for COPII and COPI. *Cell* 1997;90:1137–1148.

129. Presley JF, Cole NB, Schroer TA, et al. ER-to-Golgi transport visualized in living cells [see comments]. *Nature* 1997;389:81–85.

130. Martinez-Menarguez JA, Geuze HJ, Slot JW, et al. Vesicular tubular clusters between the ER and Golgi mediate concentration of soluble secretory proteins by exclusion from COPI-coated vesicles. *Cell* 1999;98:81–90.

131. Shima DT, Scales SJ, Kreis TE, et al. Segregation of COPI-rich and anterograde-cargo-rich domains in endoplasmic-reticulum-to-Golgi transport complexes. *Curr Biol* 1999;9:821–824.

132. Duden R, Griffiths G, Frank R, et al. Beta-COP a 110 kDa protein associated with non-clathrin-coated vesicles and the Golgi complex shows homology to beta-adaptin. *Cell* 1991;64:649–665.

133. Dominguez M, Fazel A, Dahan S, et al. Fusogenic domains of golgi membranes are sequestered into specialized regions of the stack that can be released by mechanical fragmentation. *J Cell Biol* 1999;145:673–688.

134. Kuge O, Hara-Kuge S, Orci L, et al. zeta-COP a subunit of coatomer is required for COP-coated vesicle assembly. *J Cell Biol* 1993;123:1727–1734.

135. Cosson P, Demolliere C, Hennecke S, et al. Delta- and zeta-COP two coatomer subunits homologous to clathrin-associated proteins are involved in ER retrieval. *EMBO J* 1996;15:1792–1798.

136. Ooi CE, Dell'Angelica EC, Bonifacino JS. ADP-Ribosylation factor 1 (ARF1) regulates recruitment of the AP-3 adaptor complex to membranes. *J Cell Biol* 1998;142:391–402.

137. Wieland F, Harter C. Mechanisms of vesicle formation: insights from the COP system. *Curr Opin Cell Biol* 1999;11:440–446.

138. Pearse BM. Receptors compete for adaptors found in plasma membrane coated pits. *EMBO J* 1988;7:3331–3336.

139. Dominguez M, Dejgaard K, Fullekrug J. gp25L/emp24/p24 protein family members of the cis-Golgi network bind both COP I and II coatomer. *J Cell Biol* 1998;140:751–765.

140. Hara-Kuge S, Kuge O, Orci L, et al. En bloc incorporation of coatomer subunits during the assembly of COP-coated vesicles [published erratum appears in *J Cell Biol* 1994 Jul;126:589]. *J Cell Biol* 1994;124:883–892.

141. Berger SJ, Resing KA, Taylor TC, et al. Mass-spectrometric analysis of ADP-ribosylation factors from bovine brain: identification and evidence for homogeneous acylation with the C14:0 fatty acid (myristate). *Biochem J* 1995;311:125–132.

142. Finazzi D, Cassel D, Donaldson JG, et al. Aluminum fluoride acts on the reversibility of ARF1-dependent coat protein binding to Golgi membranes. *J Biol Chem* 1994;269:13325–13330.

143. Ktistakis NT, Brown HA, Waters MG, et al. Evidence that phospholipase D mediates ADP ribosylation factor-dependent formation of Golgi coated vesicles. *J Cell Biol* 1996;134:295–306.

144. Harter C. COP-coated vesicles in intracellular protein transport. *FEBS Lett* 1995;369:89–92.

145. Zhao L, Helms JB, Brugger B, et al. Direct and GTP-dependent interaction of ADP ribosylation factor 1 with coatomer subunit beta. *Proc Nat Acad Sci U S A* 1997;94:4418–4423.

146. Schekman R, Orci L. Coat proteins and vesicle budding. *Science* 1996;271:1526–1533.

147. Bremser M, Nickel W, Schweikert M, et al. Coupling of coat assembly and vesicle budding to packaging of putative cargo receptors. *Cell* 1999;96:495–506.

148. Fiedler K, Veit M, Stamnes MA, et al. Bimodal interaction of coatomer with the p24 family of putative cargo receptors. *Science* 1996;273:1396–1399.

149. Lippincott-Schwartz J. Membrane cycling between the ER and Golgi apparatus and its role in biosynthetic transport. *Subcell Biochem* 1993;21:95–119.

150. Jamieson JD, Palade GE. Synthesis intracellular transport and discharge of secretory proteins in stimulated pancreatic exocrine cells. *J Cell Biol* 1971;50:135–158.

151. Barlowe C. COPII and selective export from the endoplasmic reticulum. *Biochim Biophys Acta* 1998;1404:67–76.

152. Barlowe C, Orci L, Yeung T, et al. COPII: a membrane coat formed by Sec proteins that drive vesicle budding from the endoplasmic reticulum. *Cell* 1994;77:895–907.

153. Orci L, Ravazzola M, Meda P, et al. Mammalian Sec23p homologue is restricted to the endoplasmic reticulum transitional cytoplasm. *Proc Nat Acad Sci U S A* 1991;88:8611–8615.

154. Orci L, Perrelet A, Ravazzola M, et al. Coatomer-rich endoplasmic reticulum. *Proc Nat Acad Sci U S A* 1994;91:11924–11928.

155. Balch WE, McCaffery JM, Plutner H, et al. Vesicular stomatitis virus glycoprotein is sorted and concentrated during export from the endoplasmic reticulum. *Cell* 1994;76:841–852.

156. Mizuno M, Singer SJ. A soluble secretory protein is first concentrated in the endoplasmic reticulum before transfer to the Golgi apparatus. *Proc Nat Acad Sci U S A* 1993;90:5732–5736.

157. Aridor M, Bannykh SI, Rowe T, et al. Sequential coupling between COPII and COPI vesicle coats in endoplasmic reticulum to Golgi transport. *J Cell Biol* 1995;131:875–893.

158. Kuge O, Dascher C, Orci L, et al. Sar1 promotes vesicle budding from the endoplasmic reticulum but not Golgi compartments. *J Cell Biol* 1994;125:51–65.

159. Matsuoka K, Orci L, Amherdt M, et al. COPII-coated vesicle formation reconstituted with purified coat proteins and chemically defined liposomes. *Cell* 1998;93:263–275.

160. Springer S, Schekman R. Nucleation of COPII vesicular coat complex by endoplasmic reticulum to Golgi vesicle SNAREs. *Science* 1998;281:698–700.

161. Aridor M, Weissman J, Bannykh S, et al. Cargo selection by the COPII budding machinery during export from the ER. *J Cell Biol* 1998;141:61–70.

162. Shaywitz DA, Orci L, Ravazzola M, et al. Human SEC13Rp functions in yeast and is located on transport vesicles budding from the endoplasmic reticulum. *J Cell Biol* 1995;128:769–777.

163. Paccaud JP, Reith W, Carpentier JL, et al. Cloning and functional characterization of mammalian homologues of the COPII component Sec23. *Mol Biol Cell* 1996;7:1535–1546.

164. Swaroop A, Yang-Feng TL, Liu W, et al. Molecular characterization of a novel human gene SEC13R related to the yeast secretory pathway gene SEC13 and mapping to a conserved linkage group on human chromosome 3p24-p25 and mouse chromosome 6. *Hum Mol Genet* 1994;3:1281–1286.

165. Pagano A, Letourneur F, Garcia D, et al. Sec24 proteins and sorting at the endoplasmic reticulum. *J Biol Chem* 1999;274: 7833–7840.

166. Tang BL, Kausalya J, Low DY, et al. A family of mammalian proteins homologous to yeast Sec24p. *Biochem Biophys Res Commun* 1999;258:679–684.

167. Shugrue CA, Kolen ER, Peters H, et al. Identification of the putative mammalian orthologue of Sec31P a component of the COPII coat. *J Cell Sci* 1999;112:4547–4556.

168. Tani K, Mizoguchi T, Iwamatsu A, et al. p125 is a novel mammalian Sec23p-interacting protein with structural similarity to phospholipid-modifying proteins. *J Biol Chem* 1999;274: 20505–20512.

169. Novikoff PM, Yam A. Sites of lipoprotein particles in normal rat hepatocytes. *J Cell Biol* 1978;76:1–11.

170. Luzio JP, Banting G. Eukaryotic membrane traffic: retrieval and retention mechanisms to achieve organelle residence. *Trends Biochem Sci* 1993;18:395–398.

171. Kornfeld S, Mellman I. The biogenesis of lysosomes. *Ann Rev Cell Biol* 1989;5:483–525.

172. Matter K, Mellman I. Mechanisms of cell polarity: sorting and transport in epithelial cells. *Curr Opin Cell Biol* 1994;6:545–554.

173. Yoshimori T, Keller P, Roth MG, et al. Different biosynthetic transport routes to the plasma membrane in BHK and CHO cells. *J Cell Biol* 1996;133:247–256.

174. Saucan L, Palade GE. Membrane and secretory proteins are transported from the Golgi complex to the sinusoidal plasmalemma of hepatocytes by distinct vesicular carriers. *J Cell Biol* 1994;125:733–741.

175. Bauerfeind R, Huttner WB. Biogenesis of constitutive secretory vesicles secretory granules and synaptic vesicles. *Curr Opin Cell Biol* 1993;5:628–635.

176. Hermo L, Green H, Clermont Y. Golgi apparatus of epithelial principal cells of the epididymal initial segment of the rat: structure relationship with endoplasmic reticulum and role in the formation of secretory vesicles. *Anat Rec* 1991;229:159–176.

177. Geuze JJ, Kramer MF. Function of coated membranes and multivesicular bodies during membrane regulation in stimulated exocrine pancreas cells. *Cell Tissue Res* 1974;156:1–20.

178. Simpson F, Bright NA, West MA, et al. A novel adaptor-related protein complex. *J Cell Biol* 1996;133:749–760.

179. Klumperman J, Hille A, Veenendaal T, et al. Differences in the endosomal distributions of the two mannose 6-phosphate receptors. *J Cell Biol* 1993;121:997–1010.

180. Beaudoin AR, St-Jean P, Grondin G. Pancreatic juice composition: new views about the cellular mechanisms that control the concentration of digestive and nondigestive proteins. *Dig Dis* 1989;7:210–220.

181. Taugner R, Buhrle CP, Nobiling R. Coexistence of renin and cathepsin B in epithelioid cell secretory granules. *Histochemistry* 1985;83:103–108.

182. Le Borgne R, Alconada A, Bauer U, et al. The mammalian AP-3 adaptor-like complex mediates the intracellular transport of lysosomal membrane glycoproteins. *J Biol Chem* 1998;273: 29451–29461.

183. Honing S, Sandoval IV, von Figura K. A di-leucine-based motif in the cytoplasmic tail of LIMP-II and tyrosinase mediates selective binding of AP-3. *EMBO J* 1998;17:1304–1314.

184. Dell'Angelica EC, Shotelersuk V, Aguilar RC, et al. Altered trafficking of lysosomal proteins in Hermansky–Pudlak syndrome due to mutations in the beta 3A subunit of the AP-3 adaptor. *Mol Cell* 1999;3:11–21.

185. Zhu Y, Traub LM, Kornfeld S. High-affinity binding of the AP-1 adaptor complex to trans-golgi network membranes devoid of mannose 6-phosphate receptors. *Mol Biol Cell* 1999;10:537–549.

186. Le Borgne R, Hoflack B. Mannose 6-phosphate receptors regulate the formation of clathrin-coated vesicles in the TGN. *J Cell Biol* 1997;137:335–345.

187. Stamnes MA, Rothman JE. The binding of AP-1 clathrin adaptor particles to Golgi membranes requires ADP-ribosylation factor a small GTP-binding protein. *Cell* 1993;73:999–1005.

188. Traub LM, Ostrom JA, Kornfeld S. Biochemical dissection of AP-1 recruitment onto Golgi membranes. *J Cell Biol* 1993;123: 561–573.

189. Zhu Y, Drake MT, Kornfeld S. ADP-ribosylation factor 1 dependent clathrin-coat assembly on synthetic liposomes. *Proc Nat Acad Sci U S A* 1999;96:5013–5018.

190. Spang A, Matsuoka K, Hamamoto S, et al. Coatomer Arf1p and nucleotide are required to bud coat protein complex I-coated vesicles from large synthetic liposomes. *Proc Nat Acad Sci U S A* 1998;95:11199–11204.

191. Ludwig T, Le Borgne R, Hoflack B. Roles for mannose 6-phosphate receptors in lysosomal enzyme sorting IGF-II binding and clathrin-coat assembly. *Trends Cell Biol* 1995;5:202–206.

192. Aoe T, Cukierman E, Lee A, et al. The KDEL receptor ERD2 regulates intracellular traffic by recruiting a GTPase-activating protein for ARF1. *EMBO J* 1997;16:7305–7316.

193. Page LJ, Sowerby PJ, Lui WW, et al. Gamma-synergin: an EH domain-containing protein that interacts with gamma-adaptin. *J Cell Biol* 1999;146:993–1004.

194. Salamero J, Sztul ES, Howell KE. Exocytic transport vesicles generated in vitro from the trans-Golgi network carry secretory and plasma membrane proteins. *Proc Nat Acad Sci U S A* 1990; 87:7717–7721.

195. Jones SM, Crosby JR, Salamero J, et al. A cytosolic complex of

p62 and rab6 associates with TGN38/41 and is involved in budding of exocytic vesicles from the trans-Golgi network. *J Cell Biol* 1993;122:775–788.

196. Wang J, Ladinsky MS, Howell KE. Molecules and vesicle coats involved in the budding of exocytotic vesicles from the trans-Golgi network. *Cold Spring Harb Symp Quant Biol* 1995;60: 139–146.

197. Narula N, Stow JL. Distinct coated vesicles labeled for p200 bud from trans-Golgi network membranes. *Proc Nat Acad Sci U S A* 1995;92:2874–2878.

198. Ladinsky MS, Kremer JR, Furcinitti PS, et al. HVEM tomography of the trans-Golgi network: structural insights and identification of a lace-like vesicle coat. *J Cell Biol* 1994;127:29–38.

199. Narula N, McMorrow I, Plopper G, et al. Identification of a 200-kD brefeldin-sensitive protein on Golgi membranes. *J Cell Biol* 1992;117:27–38.

200. Ikonen E, de Almeid JB, Fath KF, et al. Myosin II is associated with Golgi membranes: identification of p200 as nonmuscle myosin II on Golgi-derived vesicles. *J Cell Sci* 1997;110: 2155–2164.

201. Gleeson PA, Anderson TJ, Stow JL, et al. p230 is associated with vesicles budding from the trans-Golgi network. *J Cell Sci* 1996;109:2811–2821.

202. Henley JR, McNiven MA. Association of a dynamin-like protein with the Golgi apparatus in mammalian cells. *J Cell Biol* 1996;133:761–775.

203. Maier O, Knoblich M, Westermann P. Dynamin II binds to the trans-Golgi network. *Biochem Biophys Res Commun* 1996;223: 229–233.

204. Jones SM, Howell KE, Henley JR, et al. Role of dynamin in the formation of transport vesicles from the trans-Golgi network. *Science* 1998;279:573–577.

205. Cao H, Thompson HM, Krueger EK, et al. Distribution of Golgi structure and function in mammalian cells expressing a mutant dynamin. *J Cell Sci* 2000;113:1993–2002.

206. Kreitzer G, Marmorstein A, Okamoto P, et al. Kinesin and dynamin are required for post-Golgi transport of a plasma-membrane protein. *Nat Cell Biol* 2000;2:125–127.

207. Scales SJ, Scheller RH. Lipid membranes shape up. *Nature* 1999;401:123-4.

208. Roth MG, Bi K, Ktistakis NT, et al. Phospholipase D as an effector for ADP-ribosylation factor in the regulation of vesicular traffic. *Chem Phys Lipids* 1999;98:141–152.

209. Brown HA, Gutowski S, Moomaw CR, et al. ADP-ribosylation factor a small GTP-dependent regulatory protein stimulates phospholipase D activity [see comments]. *Cell* 1993;75: 1137–1144.

210. Randazzo PA, Kahn RA. GTP hydrolysis by ADP-ribosylation factor is dependent on both an ADP-ribosylation factor GTPase-activating protein and acid phospholipids [published erratum appears in *J Biol Chem* 1994 Jun 10;269(23):16519]. *J Biol Chem* 1994;269:10758–10763.

211. Ktistakis NT, Brown HA, Sternweis PC, et al. Phospholipase D is present on Golgi-enriched membranes and its activation by ADP ribosylation factor is sensitive to brefeldin A. *Proc Nat Acad Sci U S A* 1995;92:4952–4956.

212. Chen YG, Siddhanta A, Austin CD, et al. Phospholipase D stimulates release of nascent secretory vesicles from the trans-Golgi network. *J Cell Biol* 1997;138:495–504.

213. Liscovitch M, Cantley LC. Signal transduction and membrane traffic: the PITP/phosphoinositide connection. *Cell* 1995;81: 659–662.

214. Simon JP, Ivanov IE, Adesnik M, et al. The production of post-Golgi vesicles requires a protein kinase C-like molecule but not its phosphorylating activity. *J Cell Biol* 1996;135:355–370.

215. Lehel C, Olah Z, Jakab G, et al. Protein kinase C epsilon is localized to the Golgi via its zinc-finger domain and modulates Golgi function. *Proc Nat Acad Sci U S A* 1995;92:1406–1410.

216. Weigert R, Silletta MG, Spano S, et al. CtBP/BARS induces fission of Golgi membranes by acylating lysophosphatidic acid. *Nature* 1999;402:429–433.

217. Tuscher O, Lorra C, Bouma B, et al. Cooperativity of phosphatidylinositol transfer protein and phospholipase D in secretory vesicle formation from the TGN—phosphoinositides as a common denominator? *FEBS Lett* 1997;419:271–275.

218. Schmidt A, Wolde M, Thiele C, et al. Endophilin I mediates synaptic vesicle formation by transfer of arachidonate to lysophosphatidic acid [see comments]. *Nature* 1999;401: 133–141.

219. Zha X, Pierini LM, Leopold PL, et al. Sphingomyelinase treatment induces ATP-independent endocytosis. *J Cell Biol* 1998; 140:39–47.

220. Griffiths G. On vesicles and membrane compartments. *Protoplasma* 1996;195:37–58.

221. Hirschberg K, Miller CM, Ellenberg J, et al. Kinetic analysis of secretory protein traffic and characterization of golgi to plasma membrane transport intermediates in living cells. *J Cell Biol* 1998;143:1485–1503.

222. Allan BB, Balch WE. Protein sorting by directed maturation of Golgi compartments. *Science* 1999;285:63–66.

223. Polishchuk RS, Polishchuk EV, Marra P, et al. Correlative light-electron microscopy reveals the tabular-saccular ultrastructure of carriers operating between Golgi apparatus and plasma membrane. *J Cell Biol* 2000;148:45–58.

224. Heuser J. Effects of cytoplasmic acidification on clathrin lattice morphology. *J Cell Biol* 1989;108:401–411.

225. Alberts B, Bray D, Lewis J, et al. *Molecular Biology of the Cell.* 3rd ed, 1996. New York and London: Garland Publishing Inc.

The Liver: Biology and Pathobiology, Fourth Edition, edited by I. M. Arias, J. L. Boyer, F. V. Chisari, N. Fausto, D. Schachter, and D. A. Shafritz. Lippincott Williams & Wilkins, Philadelphia © 2001.

11

RECEPTOR-MEDIATED ENDOCYTOSIS

RICHARD J. STOCKERT

Endocytosis is a process by which the cell internalizes proteins and lipids from the plasma membrane, and trafficks through a variety of tubular–vesicular compartments. In its broadest sense, endocytosis can be viewed as a means either to acquire extracellular macromolecules or to establish unique plasma membrane domains. Receptor-mediated endocytosis is distinguished from other forms of endocytosis by the initial binding of ligand prior to sequestration through the formation of an endocytic vesicle. The itinerary and ultimate destination of the receptor and ligand vary with the particular species of internalized complex. The receptor may recycle back to the cell surface with or without its ligand, continue across the cell emerging at the opposite pole or be routed to lysosomes for degradation. In all cases, the receptor will traffick along an intracellular cytoskeleton network driven by a variety of molecular motors, the fidelity of the pathway being retained by the interaction of membrane and soluble proteins. This chapter attempts to summarize the current knowledge of the molecular basis of receptor-mediated endocytosis with an emphasis on the biochemical mechanisms that govern compartmentalization and vesicular trafficking (Fig. 11.1).

R. J. Stockert: Department of Medicine, Albert Einstein College of Medicine, Bronx, New York 10461.

CLATHRIN-DEPENDENT INTERNALIZATION

The most common and best described pathway of receptor ligand internalization is via clathrin-dependent endocytosis (1–3). While there is considerable overlap, receptors that enter the cell by this pathway can be functionally divided into three classes. There are those involved in the uptake and degradation of macromolecules to either supply the cell with needed nutrients or remove unwanted proteins from the circulation. Within this group, the most extensively studied are the low-density lipoprotein receptor (LDLR), the asialoglycoprotein receptor (ASGR) in hepatocytes, the transferrin receptor (TfR), and the mannose-6-phosphate receptor (also known as the insulin-like growth factor II receptor). Along with other such receptors, they enter the cell and recycle to back to the surface in a constitutive fashion with or without bound ligand (4,5). In contrast, the signal-transducing receptors that respond to various peptide hormones such as the insulin receptor (IR) and epidermal growth factor receptor (EGFR) that in addition to constitutive recycling (6–8) are rapidly cleared from the plasma membrane in response to agonist stimulation, ostensibly to desensitize the cell. The third class of clathrin-dependent endocytic receptors is exemplified by the polymeric immunoglobulin receptor (pIgR), which enters the cell at the basolateral membrane and trafficks to the apical aspect of polarized cells by a process known as transcytosis (9–12). While the consequence of receptor ligand association and ultimate itinerary varies for these three classes of receptors,

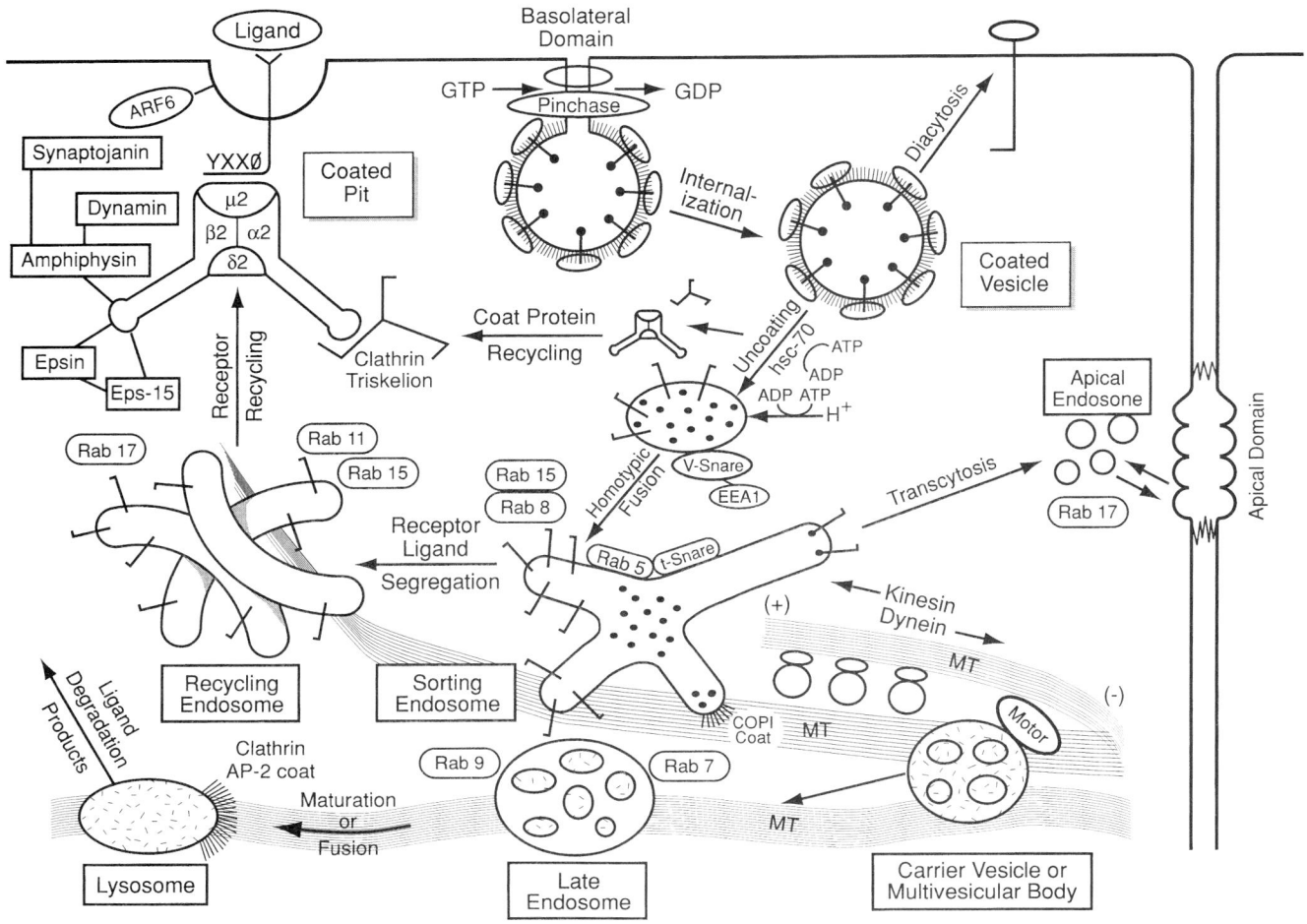

FIGURE 11.1. Transport intermediates in the endocytic pathway. Major routes of membrane transport are outlined, and transport intermediates are labeled. *Arrows* indicate the net direction of transport. The major scaffold and associated proteins required for clathrin coat and vesicle formation are indicated in the coated pit region. *MT*, microtubule.

the internalization of all three types have common molecular mechanisms of compartmentalization.

Electron microscopic (EM) studies provided the first insight into the mechanism of clathrin-dependent endocytosis. As early as 1964, Roth and Porter speculated that the electron-dense coated invaginations at the plasma membrane of mosquito oocyte that accumulated yoke proteins gave rise to endocytic vesicles (13). A morphological study of these so-called coated vesicles isolated from nerve ending led to the conclusion that the coat corresponded to a cage-like structure (14,15). The first detailed map of these cages, containing eight hexagons and 12 pentagons (36 triskelions) was provided by Pearse and co-workers (16,17). Coated vesicles were isolated from brain tissue, and the major coat protein was identified as clathrin. The main scaffold protein is the 190 kd clathrin heavy chain (18), which is associated with the 25 kd light chain. Trimers of these proteins associate to form the basic clathrin assembly unit (the triskelions) that can oligomerize, forming the

polygon seen at the EM level (19,20). Early studies that showed coated pits and vesicles to be enriched in receptor-bound LDL (21,22) and asialoglycoprotein (23) suggested that the formation of these structures plays a significant role in receptor-mediated endocytosis. Today it is well accepted that the formation of these clathrin-based structures is the initial step in the internalization of a wide variety of receptor-ligand complexes.

The essential events initiating the internalization process are the recruitment of soluble clathrin from the cytoplasm to the plasma membrane and the receptors to form a coated pit. Between clathrin and the lipid bilayer is a layer of clathrin adaptor protein (AP). AP promotes clathrin cage assembly, links clathrin to the lipid bilayer, and interacts with receptors that contain the appropriate sorting signals for inclusion within the coated pit (24–26). At present, four members of the AP protein family, that is, AP-1–4, have been identified in mammals (27,28). This heterotetrameric protein consists of two large α and β (100 kd) subunits, one medium σ (50 kd) subunit and one small μ (25 kd) subunit (19). Of the four, AP-2 alone appears to mediate the assembly of clathrin cages on the plasma membrane (29,30). The carboxy-terminal β₂ subunit of AP-2 interacts with the NH_2-terminal domain of the clathrin heavy chain (31), while the μ₂ subunit completes the bridge by binding with the receptor sorting motif (31–34). In addition to the clathrin–receptor interaction, nonscaffold proteins that bind to either AP-2 or clathrin participate in the nucleation of coat assembly, facilitating receptor sorting into the coated pit.

Perhaps the most significant of these nonscaffold proteins is dynamin, a cytoplasmic guanosine triphosphatase (GTPase) thought to be a major player in the conversion of the coated pit to a coated vesicle (35,36) (see Chapter 10). Of the isoforms of dynamin so far identified, dynamin-2 is most likely involved in receptor mediated endocytosis (37). The temperature-sensitive *Shibire* mutation of dynamin identified in *Drosophila melanogaster* provided the first indication of dynamin's unique role in coated vesicle formation (38). At the nonpermissive temperature when dynamin was inactive, endocytic defects observed at the EM level were interpreted as a failure in vesicle scission (39,40). Consistent with dynamin's proposed function to constrict the coated pit in the formation of a coated vesicle was its localization to the neck region of invagination (36). Formation of constricted pits requires that a collar of dynamin be recruited to the neck of the membrane invagination. Compelling evidence now suggests that the amphiphysins, a group of dynamin-binding proteins first identified in brain tissue, play a key role in this interaction (41–43). Disruption of the dynamin–amphiphysin association by transfection into COS-7 cells of the SH3 domain of amphiphysin, the proposed dynamin binding site, resulted in a potent inhibition of transferrin uptake and the recruitment of dynamin to coated pits. Two isoforms of amphiphysin have now been identified (44,45) and shown to form heterodimers via their coiled-coil regions (43). Both isoforms can simultaneously bind to clathrin (45) and AP-2 (46) through different domains, providing a potential bridge between dynamin and the coated pit. In what is surely an oversimplified model of dynamin function, dynamin is targeted to the coated pit in a GTP-dependent manner, and self-assembled into a helical collar around the necks of invaginated pits, followed by a coordinated GTP hydrolysis initiating a conformational change that tightens the collar (37).

It is evident from an ever increasing host of genetic, cell biological, and biochemical studies that additional components are required for clathrin coat and vesicle formation. Association of these proteins with the scaffold proteins is a dynamic process, and they often do not copurify with the coated vesicle, making their identification difficult. For the most part their various functions have been defined by the ability of isolated domains to act as dominant negative

inhibitors of endocytosis. The Eps15 (*E*GFR *p*athway *s*ubstrate 15) homology (EH) and SRC homology 3 (SH3) protein–protein binding domains appear to be elements common to most of the proteins so far identified (47,48). The EH domain is a site of protein–protein interaction that binds proteins containing the NPF (asparagines, proline, phenylalanine) sequence (49,50). Utilization of these sequences as "bait" in the yeast two-hybrid system has led to an ever increasing list of proteins with the potential to form different multivalent complexes regulating the sequential steps of clathrin-dependent receptor-mediated endocytosis. For example, the Eps15–EseI (also known as intersectin) complex (51) was identified as an analogue to the yeast Pan1p–End3p complex required for endocytosis and organization of the actin cytoskeleton (52). Formation of this complex utilizes both EH and SH3 domains to link dynamin and a presumed docking protein, synaptojanin (53), to other components of the endocytic machinery through an AP-2 binding protein, Epsin (54,55).

SORTING DETERMINANTS

The presence of sorting determinants that promote receptor clustering into the coated pits was first suggested by a naturally occurring mutation in the LDLR (22). A cysteine substitution for tyrosine on the cytoplasmic tail of the LDLR resulted in a randomized distribution of the receptor within the plasma membrane (56). The significance of tyrosine or another aromatic amino acid at this position was confirmed by site-directed mutagenesis. Using a similar approach and more recently the application of the yeast two-hybrid system, a large number of sorting or internalization signal motifs have been identified on the cytoplasmic tail of receptor proteins (57–59). Although heterogeneous, these short linear sequence motifs fall into two general classes. The most common is characterized by an essential tyrosine residue, as part of the tetrapeptide NPXY signal motif (X = any residue) as described for the LDLR (56) or in the context of YXXφ (where φ = a bulky hydrophobic residue: L, I, M, or P) for TfR (58,59). In rare instances, a phenylalanine can replace the tyrosine residue as is the case for ASGR (60). Many residues are permitted in the X position, although arginine and proline are favored at the second X position (34,61). Flanking residues have also been shown to play an important role in stabilizing the overall secondary structure of the internalization signal in a type I β turn or what has come to be known as the tight turn conformation (57). This extended conformation allows for the binding to AP μ₂ via separate hydrophobic pockets for the tyrosine and the φ residues (62). Resolution of the crystal structure of μ₂ in association with tyrosine-based motifs suggest that the strength and selectivity of receptor binding may be enhanced by their binding as dimers to dimeric μ subunits (31).

The second most common internalization motif that serve as a signal for coat pit uptake typically contain a dileucine sequence (25,63,64). In some instances, one of the leucines may be substituted by an isoleucine, valine, alanine, or methionine. CD3, CD4 and MHC class II are examples of receptors with dileucine internalization motifs (65,66). The independence of the two signal motifs was evidenced by the overexpression of a lysosomal protein bearing a tyrosine signal that saturated lysosomal sorting and internalization of tyrosine directed proteins without affecting those receptors with dileucine signals (67,68). Unlike the tyrosine-based internalization signals, little is known about the structural context that defines the functional relationship between the dileucine motif and the coated pit. The yeast two-hybrid system has failed to uncover interactions of AP-2 subunits with the dileucine-based motif; however, cross-linking studies have suggested that the AP-2 β subunit might be involved (69). It is interesting to note that both tyrosine and dileucine internalization motifs also serve as membrane targeting signals. This should not be surprising in light of the highly conserved sequences of the adaptor proteins involved in coated vesicle transport between various subcellular organelles of the biosynthetic and endocytic pathways.

The third major class of receptors that are internalized via the coat pit are the signaling receptors such as EGFR and IR. These receptors are more or less randomly distributed on the plasma membrane and migrate to the coat pit only after ligand binding (70). Their sequestration into coated pits and rapid endocytosis in response to ligand binding appears to be linked to their intrinsic kinase activity (71). In the case of the EGFR, this aggregation of receptor occurs rapidly, and receptors can be detected inside the cell within minutes after the association of ligand (72). Ligand binding and the presence of a functional kinase activity are necessary for the association of EGFR with the clathrin-AP-2 complex (73,74). Association of EGFR with AP-2 is through the μ_2 subunit via the receptor's FYRAL binding motif (75). In this instance, AP-2 is best viewed in the role of recruiter as opposed to mediator of internalization. Eps-1, which is phosphorylated in response to EGF (76), binds to the α_2 subunit of AP-2 in the coated pit (55) and could provide the link required for endocytosis. Both EGFR and IR are linked to the signal transduction machinery of the cell through a series of small GTP-binding proteins or G-proteins. Recent data suggest that one of these G-proteins, Ral, and its downstream partners Ral binding protein (RalBP1) and partner of RalB>P1 (POB1) are involved in the regulated internalization of EGFR and IR by transmitting the signal for rapid internalization to Epsin and Eps15 complex (77).

Current understanding of the "fine tuning" that confers specificity to sorting signals and their complex interaction with components of the coated pit remains limited. The high degree of degeneracy in the sorting signals could explain why the same motif directs internalization in one context and sorting to other subcellular organelles in another. Posttranslational modifications such as phosphorylation of acid clusters (78), fatty acid acylation (79,80), or ubiquitination (81,82) have all been suggested to play a role in directing endocytosis. In addition, the lipid composition of the membranes, especially phosphoinositides, has been proposed to direct receptor internalization and trafficking (83–85). At the extreme other end of the septum, an alternative model in which coated pit formation proceeds independently of any endocytic signal has been suggested (86).

SORTING ENDOSOME

Whatever the mechanisms are for receptor–ligand entry into the coated pit and coated vesicle formation, internalized receptor–ligand complexes first enter what is known as the early endosomal compartment. The first step required for entry into the early endosomal compartment is removal of the scaffold proteins, clathrin and AP-2. The release of clathrin from the coat vesicle is mediated by the ATP-dependent action of a heat shock protein (hsc70), allowing regeneration of the cytosolic pool of clathrin for additional rounds of endocytosis (87,88). Several laboratories have confirmed the original observation (89) that AP-2 remains associated with the vesicle after clathrin depletion (90,91). It was demonstrated that removal of the residual AP shell, a presumed barrier to membrane fusion, required additional unidentified cytosolic factors along with hsc70 and ATP and that prior removal of clathrin was not a prerequisite for the reaction (92). While the mechanism for AP release is still unresolved, the association of hsc70 with kinase activity (93,94) suggests that AP depletion is dependent on a selective phosphorylation reaction. The newly formed smooth vesicles or endosomes undergo a homotypic fusion, forming a tubular–vesicular system known as the early endosomal compartment localized just below the plasma membrane. This early endosomal compartment can be divided into two functionally and morphologically distinct vesicle populations, the sorting and recycling endosomes.

The sorting endosomes have a tubulovesicular morphology that has been suggested to play a significant role in their primary function, the physical separation of ligands from their receptors (95–97). Colocalization of ASGR and its fluorescent-labeled ligand within the sorting endosome, known at that time as CURL (*c*ompartment of *u*ncoupling of *r*eceptor and *l*igand), indicated that following dissociation, ligand would accumulate in the vesicular space and receptors would concentrate in the tubular extensions (98). The pinching off or budding of the tubular elements, giving rise to the recycling and the late endosomal compartments, could then complete the physical separation of the receptors from their ligands. The underlying assumption of this model is that tubular budding or pinching off is a rapid repetitive process occurring during the comparatively short half-life of the sorting endosome (99,100). This pure geometric model has gained support from numerous immunocytochemical and kinetic studies of ligand accumulation and exit from the sorting endosome population. Despite the elegant simplicity of the geometric model, the ability of receptors to concentrate in the tubular extensions suggests the existence of signal-based sorting. By analogy to coated vesicle formation, the presence of coated regions on the tubular extensions of sorting endosome support a potential role for signal-based sorting (101). Forces driving receptor clustering to these specialized regions have been suggested to be mediated by interactions with cytoskeleton-related elements (102–104).

Within 5 minutes of internalization, receptor and ligand complexes are localized to the sorting endosome (1). It is within these vesicles that the vast majority of receptors destined to recycle back to the plasma membrane dissociate from their ligands (56,105,106). Studies in a number of laboratories have established that the luminal pH of these vesicles become increasingly acidic over time (107–110). While the mechanism by which receptors dissociate from their ligand in the sorting endosome is still speculative, both *in vitro* and *in vivo* studies strongly suggest that a change in receptor conformation brought on by the reduction in endosomal pH is responsible for the decrease in the receptor's affinity for ligand (111,112). Vacuolar (H⁺)-ATPases or V-ATPases, associated with the coated vesicles and endosomes, are believed to be primarily responsible for acidification of these compartments (113). V-ATPase is a heterooligomeric complex composed of at least 13 unique subunits arranged into two domains, a peripheral V_1 and an integral membrane domain V_0 (114). The V_1 domain is responsible for ATP hydrolysis while the V_0 functions in proton transfer (113,115).

Early approaches to monitor endosomal pH took advantage of internalized fluoresce dyes that respond to hydrogen ion concentration (116,117). This technique was later refined by the application of digital image analysis limiting the recorded signal of pH-dependent fluorescent indicators to individual endosomes containing receptor–ligand complexes (118). By following the change in signal intensity at various times after internalization of fluorescent-labeled α_2-macroglobulin, it was possible to establish that an endosomal pH as low as 5.0 could be attended in a prelysosomal compartment (118). Extensive studies of the characteristic pH within the early endosome compartments indicated a more limited range of pH between 5.9 and 6.5 with the sorting endosome being most acidic (108,111). A pH just below 6.0 has been directly shown to be sufficient to dissociate ligands from receptors such as ASGR and LDLR (56,119). In addition to ligand dissociation, endosomal acidification appears to be required for the formation of carrier vesicles that function in the trafficking of ligand from the early to late endosomal compartment (120).

Treatment of cells with the proton ionophore monensin, which collapses the pH gradient of the endosome, has been used to confirm the pH sensitivity of various receptor–ligand complexes (119,121). Examples of recycling receptors that dissociate within the sorting endosome include the ASGR, LDLR, IR, and the α_2-macroglubolin receptor (5, 56,107,109). The one notable exception to the rule is the TfR. Unlike the vast majority of ligands, transferrin is not dissociated from its receptor at acidic pH (122). Following the pH-dependent release of iron, the newly formed apo-transferrin is more tightly bound to the TfR (123). The complex recycles back to the cell surface, where on exposure to a slightly alkaline pH the now iron-depleted transferrin is released back to the circulation to begin the cycle once again. *In vivo* and *in vitro* experiments have provided strong evidence that a large fraction of pH-sensitive receptors recycles back to the cell surface still associated with their ligand (22,121,124). This so-called diacytosis was assumed to occur before dissociation and therefore before acidification of the endosome. The origin of this rapid (1 to 2 minute) recycling compartment is still unclear, though it has been suggested that this recycling pathway is mediated by a more primitive class of receptors (125). A trafficking mutant (Trf1) isolated from the human hepatoma cell line HuH-7 confirmed the presence of this primitive class of ASGR at the genetic level and implicated both the TfR and mannose receptor as existing in two subpopulations (126).

RECYCLING ENDOSOME

Receptors that have dissociated from their ligands enter the recycling endosomal compartment. Because inhibition of protein synthesis has no effect on the rate of continuous endocytosis of asialoglycoproteins, it was assumed that ASGR recycled back to the cell surface to be reutilized (127). Selective alteration of ASGR ligand specificity provided additional evidence of a recycling pathway, since the same cell–surface receptors were used over and over again without dilution by the large intracellular pool of unmodified receptors (5). Dissociated ligands rarely appear in this compartment, indicating that sorting is substantially completed prior to receptor entry into the recycling endosome. In contrast to the peripheral localization of the sorting endosomal compartment, recycling endosomes may be localized throughout the cytoplasmin, as in nonpolarized CHO cells (97) or as a pericentriolar tubular compartment maintained by a microtubule network as seen in hepatocytes (100). There still exists some confusion as to whether the majority of recycling receptors enters a peripheral compartment and fuse directly with the plasma membrane or enters perinuclear-recycling vesicles prior to returning to the plasma membrane. However, there is little question that at least some if not all recycling receptors transiently accumulate in vesicles and tubular elements near the microtubule organizing center. Assuming that the TfR can be taken as a gauge of the intracellular pathway followed by all recycling receptors, then at any given time over 70% would be localized intracellularly and predominantly in the recycling endosome (128). The finding that the TfR recycled back to the basolateral membrane originates from two distinct endosomal populations (129) suggests that the accumulation of receptors within the recycling compartment represents a rate-limiting step in return to the plasma membrane. Whether one of these endosomal subpopulations is related to the diacytosis pathway described for ASGR has yet to be resolved.

By following the trafficking of fluorescent lipid analogues in conjunction with TfR in nonpolarized cells, it was concluded that recycling is not a signal-dependent event and should be considered a default pathway (97, 130). However, recent studies indicate that exit of the TfR from the recycling endosome in polarized cells such as hepatocytes depends on a hierarchy of sorting signals (78, 131). In hepatocytes, the presence in the recycling endosomes of proteins that follow a transcytosis pathway to the apical membrane, such as pIgR (132), provides additional evidence for a sorting function within this compartment. Since little if any of the TfR that accumulates within the recycling endosome is ever detected at the apical aspect of the liver cell, it must be assumed that a very effective sorting mechanism is operative within the recycling compartment. It would seem that recycling in nonpolarized cells or from the prerecycling endosomes of polarized cells occurs by default. However, sorting from the recycling endosomal compartment of polarized cells such as hepatocytes must be presumed to be signal-dependent (see Chapter 8 and website chapter 💻 W-5). A major limitation to describing trafficking between the sorting and recycling endosomal compartments and the plasma membrane has been the inability to fully resolve these vesicles into different fractions.

ENDOSOMAL CARRIER VESICLES

In contrast to the recycling pathway, transport to the late endosome of receptors and ligands destined for degradation is highly selective. Specific endosomal carrier vesicles that mediate transport from the early to the late endosomal compartment have been identified (133). These carrier vesicles often exhibit a multivesicular morphology and are commonly referred to as multivesicular bodies (134,135,136). *In vivo* and *in vitro* studies have shown that formation of these carrier vesicles involves the coatomer complex, COPI, which is usually associated with transport within the biosynthetic secretory pathway (137,138) (see Chapter 10). In the biosynthetic pathway, coatomer complex is formed by the association of seven unrelated polypeptides, α, β, β', γ, δ, ε, and ζ-COP. Neither γ-nor δ-COP have been detected associated with the endosomal compartment

(139). A working model for the membrane association of endosomal COPs has been developed (137,138). In this model, acidification of the endosome causes a conformational change in a putative transmembrane pH sensor protein, which allows recruitment of the cytosolic GTP-binding protein ARF-1. Association of β-COP with the newly recruited membrane ARF-1 promotes the formation of coatomer complex on the early endosome. Since all seven subunits are associated prior to membrane binding (140), it is assumed that γ- and δ-COP dissociate soon after coat formation. In addition to a potential role in the biogenesis of carrier endosomes, a link between COPI and the function of the early endosomal compartment was suggested by inhibition of TfR recycling in a temperature-sensitive mutant at the restrictive temperature (141).

LATE ENDOSOME/LYSOSOME

Although the early events of endocytosis have been reasonably well mapped out, trafficking within the late endosomal/lysosomal compartment is much less well characterized. Late endosomes, sometimes called prelysosomes, can be defined as vesicles that accumulate and concentrate internalized ligands on their way to the lysosome for degradation. Due to their lower density, late endosomes can be isolated from lysosomes by Percoll gradient centrifugation (106). The presence of lysosomal hydrolyses in this less dense vesicle population has been used as evidence to support bidirectional trafficking between the late endosomal and lysosomal compartments (142–144). Whether the mixing of contents is the result of vesicular transport between late endosome and lysosome or direct fusion of these compartments or both has not been resolved. It has been demonstrated in a cell-free system derived from rat hepatocytes that late endosomes can fuse directly with preexisting lysosomes giving rise to hybrid vesicles with an intermediate density (66,145). The physiological relevance of this cell-free system was evidenced by the requirement for proteins commonly associated with membrane fusion. Alternatively, acid hydrolyses and proteins characteristic of lysosomal membranes are accumulated during the maturation of the prelysosomal vesicle prior to its fusion with preexisting lysosomes (135,136,146). In support of the maturation model, it has been demonstrated in Hep-2 cells that mannose-6-phosphate receptor (M6PR)-acid hydrolase complexes are delivered to endocytic vesicles that still retain TfR and that both the M6PR and TfR recycle out of the maturing prelysosomal compartment (143).

Lysosomes have long been accepted as the end point of the endocytic pathway mediated by cargo-bearing receptors. Several independent lines of investigation have provided evidence for retrograde lysosomal transport. *In vitro* studies with purified lysosomes and semiintact cells demonstrated that AP-2 can initiate the assembly of clathrin coat formation on the surface of lysosomes similar to that seen at the cell surface (140,147,148). Recycling of membrane lipids and endocytosed proteins (149,150) from the lysosomal compartment through late endosomes has also been reported. It is becoming increasingly obvious that the relationship between the lysosome and late endosomal compartment is dynamic and that the lysosome should not be viewed in the simple context of an end of endocytosis, but rather as one of multiple compartments in a complex equilibrium.

APICAL ENDOSOME/TRANSCYTOSIS

The main feature of polarized epithelial cells is the compartmentalization of the plasma membrane into apical and basolateral domains separated by tight junctions (see Chapter 3). Newly synthesized apical ectoenzymes and an adhesion molecule, CCAMIOS, but not ABC transporters (see Chapters 8 and 24 and website chapter W-5) in the hepatocyte are first delivered to the basolateral membrane and subsequently transcytosed to the apical domain (151–155). These domains perform specialized functions and differ in their lipid protein composition (156,157). To maintain this compartmentalization, the lipids and proteins associated with apical and basolateral membranes must be appropriately sorted. The presence of an early endosomal population dedicated to the sorting and recycling of apical proteins is in question. Early endosome subpopulations unique to the apical aspect of Madin-Darby Canine Kidney (MDCK) cells (158) and rat intestine (159), from which these proteins could selectively sort, have been suggested by tracer studies. However, the presence of recycling transferrin within this compartment led to the suggestion that no domain-specific apical endosomal population exists (160). Indeed, it was previously shown in CaCo-2 cells that endosomes loaded from the basolateral membrane could be accessed from the apical aspect of the cell (161). The identification of endotubin, a glycoprotein highly enriched in a subset of endosomal tubules in rat ileum, is consistent with the presence of a subpopulation of early apical endosomes (162,163). The strongest support for an apical early endosomal compartment comes from studies using the WIF-B cell model of protein trafficking in the hepatocyte (164) (see Chapters 8 and 24). By following the itineraries of endogenous membrane proteins, a subapical compartment was identified as a secondary sorting site for proteins bound to the apical membrane. In addition, this compartment was capable of sorting membrane proteins to the lysosomes for degradation.

In hepatocytes, transcytosis of pIgR from the basolateral to the apical (bile canaliculi) membranes has provided much knowledge related to early apical endosomes. While pIgR is constitutively transcytosed in the absence of its ligand, rapid transcytosis to the apical domain in liver (11) and other polarized cells (132) is induced by pIgA binding.

Unlike the well established sorting determinants that are unresponsive to ligand binding, pIgA binding to pIgR appears capable of transducing a signal to intracellular sorting motifs that are superimposed on pIgR's common endocytic determinants (144). Whether the transcytotic pathway followed by pIgR in response to ligand binding is a true marker of the apical early endosomal compartment has been brought into question by the localization of the apical endosome structural protein, annexin VI, to a transferrin containing recycling vesicles devoid of immunodetectable pIgR (165).

ENDOSOME FUSION / THE SNARE HYPOTHESIS

From the previous description, it should be obvious that the pathways of receptor-mediated endocytosis are best portrayed as membrane compartments in a constant dynamic flux. Vesicles emerging from donor compartments are specifically targeted to acceptor compartments to which they fuse. Fusion requires that the lipid bilayer of the carrier vesicle becomes continuous with that of the acceptor membrane. The proper targeting of transport vesicles is achieved by highly conserved transmembrane and associated proteins that were identified in cell-free assays of membrane fusion (166). The N-ethylmaleimide-sensitive factor (NSF) was the first component of this system identified (167,168). NSF is a cytosolic protein possessing ATPase activity that regulates the formation and dissociation of membrane fusion complexes in conjunction with a second cytosolic protein, the soluble NSF attachment protein (SNAP) (169). Membrane components that determine the fidelity of vesicle docking and fusion events were identified by their ability to interact with SNAP (170). These SNAP receptors (SNAREs) are divided into two classes: those found on cargo-containing vesicles are known as v-SNAREs, and those present on target membranes are called t-SNAREs. The functional basis of the SNARE hypothesis is that v- and t-SNAREs residing in opposing membranes bind to each other in a cognate fashion, resulting in membrane fusion (166). A direct role for NSF and SNAPS in membrane fusion has come into question (171,172). NSF and SNAP act at a pre- or postfusion reaction, either to prime the SNAREs for docking or more likely to disassemble the complex once fusion has occurred (173). Nonhydrolyzable ATP stabilizes the NSF/SNAP/SNARE into a 20S complex that probably represents SNAREs in a pre- or postfusion state (174).

Since much of the present nomenclature arose from studies of synaptic fusion events, v-SNARES are often identified as members of the vesicle-associated membrane proteins (VAMPs) or synaptobrevins, while t-SNARES are members of the syntaxin and synaptosome-associated protein of 25 kd (SNAP-25) families. Of all the known SNAREs, only a v-SNARE (cellubrevin) and two t-SNAREs (syntaxin-7 and -12, presumed to be the same proteins as syntaxin-13 and -14) have been associated with the endosomal pathway (175–178). These numbers are sure to increase, as a recent search of the data base of mammalian-expressed sequence tags proposes at least 16 mammalian syntaxins. Along with NSF and SNAP, cellubrevin and syntaxin-12 appear to be localized to both the early and late endosomal compartments and have been suggested to function in docking and fusion between these two compartments (179). Functional studies in permeabilized PC12 cells support a role for syntaxin-12 (-13) in TfR recycling (180). If cognate v- and t-SNARES mediate fusion of the endocytic vesicles, their activity and or localization must account for the specificity within the trafficking pathway. Although the structure of the SNARE complex suggests that this specificity could arise from the pairing of specific helical bundles termed SNARE-pins, which drive the two membranes together (172), it has recently been shown that SNARE interactions are not selective (181). Therefore, the assembly of SNAREpins must be closely regulated by restraint and catalysis, or all the endocytic compartments would simply coalesce. Data from a number of *in vitro* experiments now suggest that additional components are required for the regulated membrane fusion necessary to maintain the organization of the endosomal pathway (182,183). The mechanisms by which SNAREs are localized are even less well understood. Although no experimental data exist to support this hypothesis, it has been suggested that each SNARE pair contains specific recognition motifs that direct binding to a particular adaptor protein (178).

SMALL GTPases

In recent years, a large number of small monomeric GTPases of the Rab family have been identified. Based on their restricted distribution on membranes and the phenotypes resulting from overexpression of wild-type and mutant proteins, it has been suggested that they play critical regulatory roles in vesicular transport (184). Rab5 localizes to the plasma membrane and the sorting endosomal compartment (185,186), where in conjunction with EEA1 it is presumed to regulate homotypic fusion of early endosomes (187). Rab4 is also associated with the sorting endosome membranes and is thought to regulate receptor recycling between the early sorting endosome and the pericentriolar recycling endosome (128,129). Rab7 and Rab9 are localized to the late endosomal compartment (188,189). Cells transfected with mutant Rab7 are unable to degrade LDL at the normal rate and accumulate the lysosomal enzyme, cathepsin D and the calcium-independent mannose phosphate receptor in the early endocytic compartment (190). This phenotype would suggest that Rab7 is involved in transport to the late endosome and from the late endosome to the lysosome. On the other hand, Rab9 appears to regulate transport from the late endosome to the *trans*-Golgi network (189,191). Rab15 codistributes with both Rab4 and Rab5 within the sorting endosome and with Rab11 on the pericentriolar recycling endosome (192,193). Functional studies suggest that Rab15 may play a role as an inhibitory GTPase in early endocytic trafficking (194). Another study suggests that Rab17 colocalizes with internalized transferrin within the perinuclear recycling endosome of BHK cells and with the apical recycling endosome in polarized cells (195). Although Rab22 and Rab24 have been localized to endocytic vesicles (196), no functional studies have defined their role in membrane trafficking.

Rabs regulate vesicle fusion events by recruitment of specific effector proteins involved in membrane tethering and docking in a GTP to GDP-dependent cycle (184,197). Newly synthesized Rabs are posttranslationally modified on their carboxy terminal cysteine residues with geranylgeranyl groups rendering the protein hydrophobic, allowing reversible membrane association necessary to their function (198,199). Rabs in their GDP-bound inactive form are delivered to the appropriate membranes associated with the Rab escort protein, REP (198). Following REP dissociation, Rab is converted to the GTP active form by the action of a GDP/GTP exchange factor (GEF) and its membrane association is stabilized by the interaction with effector proteins that presumably regulate the local concentration of v/t-SNARE complexes (200). Following vesicle fusion, GTP is hydrolyzed, accelerated by a GTPase-activating protein converting the Rab back to its GDP-bound conformation. In the case of Rab5, nucleotide exchange is an essential step in the cycle for endosome fusion, whereas GTP hydrolysis is not. Rab-GDP is then released from the membrane to the cytosol bound to a GDP dissociation inhibitor (GDI), which, like REP, escorts Rab-GDP to a new site of vesicle fusion initiated by the dissociation of GDI (201).

The best understood Rab effectors, Rabaptin-5 and Rabex-5, a Rab5 GEF, act in concert to maintain Rab5 in the active GTP conformation (202), modifying the timing of the GTP/GDP cycle (203). This shift in equilibrium in favor of an active Rab-GTP pool might serve to increase the number of productive docking and fusion events. Two additional Rab5 effectors have been identified, Rabaptin-5β (204) and EEA1 (205,206), previously identified as a marker of the early endosomal compartment. Much like Rabaptin-5, Rabaptin-5β is recruited to the endosome by Rab5 in a GTP-dependent manner and specifically interacts with Rabex-5 (207). Therefore, it is likely that recruitment of Rabaptin-5β is coupled to nucleotide exchange. EEA1 recruitment is dependent on active Rab5 and on the product of phosphatidylinositol-3-OH kinase, phosphatidylinositol-3-phosphate (PtdIns (3) P) (208). Inhibition of kinase activity with wortmannin or LY294002 induces a pronounced change in the morphology of the early endosomal compartment (209), interfering with endosome fusion. PtdIns(3)P binding to the carboxy terminus FYVE zinc finger domain of EEA1 appears to direct EEA1 targeting to the endosomal membrane (210). In addition to EEA1's interaction with Rab5, EEA1 has been shown to complex directly with the t-SNARE syntaxin-6 (211). It has been suggested that EEA1 interacts with other Rab5 complexes to regulate homotypic fusion in the early endosomal compartment (212).

In addition to the Rab GTPases, ADP-ribosylation factor (ARF) plays a significant role in receptor-mediated endocytosis. By analogy to Rabs, the discrete localization of ARF proteins to various vesicular compartments suggests that specific recognition motifs order their function. Of the six identified ARFs, ARF6, the least conserved member of the ARF family, is uniquely localized to the endocytic pathway. It appears to recycle between the plasma membrane and the recycling endosomes, depending upon its nucleotide status (213). A mutant of ARF6 defective in GTP hydrolysis remains associated with the plasma membrane, and its expression reduces the rate of transferrin uptake (214). In contrast, a mutant defective in GTP binding accumulates in the perinuclear recycling endosome, colocalizing with the TfR and the v-SNARE cellubrevin (215). As might be predicted, overexpression of this dominant negative mutant ARF protein interferes with TfR–transferrin recycling (214). These alterations in endocytic trafficking are accompanied by major structural changes in plasma membrane and endosomal morphology (216), potentially through the ability of ARF6 to stimulate cortical actin rearrangement (217). It is this interaction with the actin cytoskeleton that has led to the postulation that ARF6 links membrane traffic with actin microfilaments (217,218). Recent studies in polarized MDCK cells localized ARF6 to the apical membrane, suggesting a role in clathrin-mediated endocytosis at the apical surface of epithelial cells (219). A recently identified ARF6-specific GEF, EFA6 (220) links ARF6 to actin and receptor recycling.

Perhaps the least well understood of the small GTPases are the members of the Rho family (see Chapter 10). Although Rho family members modulate multiple endocytic pathways, up- or downstream effectors have yet to be established. Expression of a dominant negative RhoA in polarized MDCK cells disrupted basolateral transferrin recycling, increasing ligand release at the apical membrane (221). In addition, transcytosis of pIgA was severely impaired in these transfected cells. While no direct evidence has been provided for a role of RhoB in endocytosis, it has been localized to the early endosomal compartment. Overexpression of wild-type RhoD causes endosomal scattering, reducing their overall motility and dynamic properties (222,223). Consistent with the documented effects of Rho on the assembly/disassembly of the actin cytoskeleton (224), alterations in Rho expression appear to effect those steps in the endocytic pathway presumed to be directed along the actin microfilament network. In addition to Rho,

other members of the family (RacI and Cdc42) have been implicated in the regulation of actin organization (221, 225). It is clear from these few examples that recycling of small GTPases between the GTP and GDP bound conformations has the potential to provide molecular switches assembling multiprotein complexes necessary to regulate endosomal traffic.

CYTOSKELETON

Actin microfilaments and microtubules (MT) are dynamic polarized structures (see Chapter 4 and website chapters W-1 and W-2). Differential rates of subunit addition and subtraction are used to define the ends of the preformed structures. The relatively stable end is termed "minus," while the fast growing or contracting end is denoted as "plus." The uniform MT polarity in a minus-to-plus orientation radiating out from the centrosome to the cell periphery provides a directional network on which endosomes can be envisioned to traffic in an ordered fashion. Unlike MTs, actin filaments appear less organized, and it is unclear just how they might provide the necessary scaffolding for directional transport. Much of the evidence that efficient transport of cargo along the endocytic pathway and transcytosis in polarized epithelial cells is dependent on the association of transport vesicles with the cytoskeleton network has come from studies utilizing inhibitors of cytoskeleton polymerization such as nocodazole or colchicine (MT) and cytochalasin D (actin microfilaments).

A reevaluation of earlier work (226,227) in conjunction with recent confocal immunocytochemical analysis has led to the conclusion that actin microfilaments are involved in two separate steps of the lysosomal pathway (228,229). The distribution of transferrin and α2-macroglobulin after cytochalasin D treatment of a nonpolarized mouse hepatoma cell line, BWTG3, indicated that actin microfilaments were involved in ligand internalization via coated pit and transfer to the lysosome from the late endosomal compartment (230). Ultrastructural analysis suggests that actin filaments are required for late events in endocytic coated vesicle formation from the plasma membrane (231). In polarized MDCK cells, analysis of the effect of cytochalasin D on postendocytic traffic of IgA and transferrin revealed that the role of actin microfilaments may be limited to transcytosis from the early endosomal compartment to the apical recycling endosome (232). This limited role in polarized cells has been brought into question by the overexpression of a mutant Rho GTPase, a regulator of actin cytoskeleton function (233,224), shown to affect both basolateral recycling of transferrin and the degradation of internalized EGF as well as the transcytosis of pIgA in MDCK cells (221). Although the morphologic details and site of action may differ with cell type, all the findings are consistent with a significant role for actin microfilaments in the endocytic pathway.

In contrast to actin microfilaments, a role for MTs in various steps of the endocytic pathway is better established. Early studies using MT-disrupting drugs such as nocodazole and colchicine had already suggested that MTs participated in the sorting of receptors from their ligands (106, 234,235). One of the best characterized MT-dependent pathways in liver is the endocytosis of asialoglycoproteins (ASP) mediated by ASGR. Application of a monensin-based assay to measure retention within a common vesicle was one of the earliest studies to indicate that colchicine inhibits the segregation of ASP from ASGR (236). Consistent with this finding, resolution of endocytic compartments by density gradient centrifugation following vinblastine treatment of rat hepatocytes resulted in the localization of internalized ASP to early endosomal compartment (237). Retention of ASP in the early endosome in response to colchicine treatment was confirmed in hepatocyte couplets by direct visualization of labeled glycoprotein (238). At a more biochemical level, the affinity of vesicles labeled with ASP was probed by cosedimentation with MT (102,239). While all vesicles containing ASP and ASGR bound to purified MTs, the addition of ATP selectively released vesicles containing ASP. This finding was interpreted to indicate that movement along the MT network provided the force necessary to sort the receptor from its ligand (102).

In addition to inhibiting trafficking from the early to late endosome in the lysosomal pathway, disruption of the MT network in hepatocytes reduces transferrin uptake and recycling from early and late endosomal compartments (240, 241). Interestingly, this effect is mimicked by inhibitors of the serine–threonine protein phosphatase, PP2A, (242, 243). MTs play a critical role in the transcytosis of several proteins from the basolateral to the apical membrane. Nocodazole blocked transcytosis of pIgA at an early stage between basolateral early endosomes and apical recycling compartment (244,245). Fusion with the apical membrane and subsequent transfer of ligand may require interaction with both actin and MT.

It is evident that endocytic trafficking requires coordination between actin and MT cytoskeleton. Examination of the cytoarchitecture of the hepatocyte cytoskeleton underscores the spatial and potential functional relationship between the actin and microtubule-based systems of vesicle trafficking (104). ASP-containing endosomes were shown to be captured just below the actin layer at the cell periphery and transported centrally along the umbrella of MTs, so that the concentration of endosomes near the centrosome and subsequent efficient lysosomal degradation of ASP were consequences of the confluence of the MT array in this region. The molecular details of the actin–MT connections are beginning to emerge with the identification of cytoskeleton-associated proteins with the capacity to recognize actin microfilaments, MTs, and endosomes. The prototype of such a connector is a class of cytoplasmic linker proteins or CLIPs, which recruit motor proteins responsible for vesicle movement along the cytoskeleton pathways (246,247). Other cytoskeleton-associated proteins implicated in orchestration of the actin–MTs link include the GTP-binding protein subfamily, Rho (233), annexins (248), calmodulin, and calmodulin-binding proteins (249), all of which have been isolated from or localized to various endosomal compartments (250).

MOLECULAR MOTORS

There are three superfamilies of mechanochemical enzymes thought responsible for movement of endosomes along the cytoskeleton network, with ATP hydrolysis providing the chemical energy converted into mechanical force by induction of conformational changes in these "molecular motors" (251). Myosins are associated with the actin microfilaments; kinesin and dynein are associated with the MTs. Although a role for actin–myosin interactions are implied from various inhibition studies, direct evidence for the involvement of specific myosins in receptor-mediated endocytosis in vertebrate cells is sparse. Biochemical and immunomicroscopic studies have localized myosin I to both the endosomal and lysosomal compartments (252). Consistent with a role for actin in late endosome to lysosome transport, overproduction of mutant myosin I lacking either the ATP binding site or the motor domain in BWTG3 hepatoma cells resulted in dispersion of the perinuclear endosomal compartment throughout the cytoplasm and reduced α2-macroglobulin degradation (230). Much of the experimental data directly supporting an actin-motor in the early steps of endocytosis are presently limited to studies in yeast and *Dictyostelium*, in which mutations in myosin I interfere with ligand uptake (253,254).

Unlike the limited experimental evidence supporting myosins, there is little question that kinesin and dynein play a significant role in receptor-mediated endocytosis (255). Both kinesin and dynein have been identified in various endosomal fractions isolated from rat liver (250). At one time, it was assumed that kinesin directed motility to the plus end of the MTs toward the cell periphery and that dynein directed movement to the minus end toward the cell center in an independent fashion. These simple unidirectional lines of movement have become more defuse, especially in polarized epithelial cells in which ligand can be endocytosed from both the apical and basolateral domains. The convergence of endosomes originating from these domains appears to require both kinesin and dynein for a balance between plus end- and minus end-directed movement (256). The development of an *in vitro* assay to follow the movement of endosomes containing fluorescent-labeled asialoorosomucoid confirmed the bidirectional nature of movement along the MT network (257). More intriguing was the observation that these vesicles appeared to stretch along the MTs, leading to fission with the segregation of receptor from ligand. These findings raise the distinct possibility that interaction with the MT network and associated proteins provide the mechanical basis for receptor–ligand sorting.

CONCLUSION

By its very nature, the complexity of receptor-mediated endocytosis in polarized epithelial cells has opened lines of investigation into almost every area of cell biology. Although morphological studies have provided an outline of the pathways followed by receptors and ligands, the specific interactions between these dynamic compartments and the numerous molecules that regulate their flow have yet to be identified. The application of what is known and what is to be learned will surely provide new insights into liver biology and pathobiology.

REFERENCES

1. Mukherjee S, Ghosh RN, Maxfield FR. *Endocytosis Physiol Rev* 1997;77:759–803.
2. Mellman I. Endocytosis and molecular sorting. *Annu Rev Cell Dev Biol* 1996;12:575–625.
3. Schmid SL. Clathrin-coated vesicle formation and protein sorting: an integrated process. *Annu Rev Biochem* 1997;66:511–548.
4. Brown MS, Anderson RG, Goldstein JL. Recycling receptors: the round-trip itinerary of migrant membrane proteins. *Cell* 1983;32:663–667.
5. Stockert RJ, Morell AG, Scheinberg IH. Hepatic binding protein: the protective role of its sialic acid residues. *Science* 1977;197:667–668.
6. Pastan IH, Willingham MC. The internalization of insulin and other hormones by fibroblastic cells. *Diabetes Care* 1981;4:33–37.
7. Capeau J, Lascols O, Flaig-Staedel C, et al. Degradation of insulin receptors by hepatoma cells: insulin-induced down-regulation results from an increase in the rate of basal receptor degradation. *Biochimie* 1985;67:1133–1141.
8. Carpentier JL, Gazzano H, Van Obberghen E, et al. Intracellular pathway followed by the insulin receptor covalently coupled to 125I-photoreactive insulin during internalization and recycling. *J Cell Biol* 1986;102:989–996.
9. Mostov KE. Transepithelial transport of immunoglobulins. *Annu Rev Immunol* 1994;12:63–84.
10. Hemery I, Durand-Schneider AM, Feldmann G, et al. The transcytotic pathway of an apical plasma membrane protein (B10) in hepatocytes is similar to that of IgA and occurs via a tubular pericentriolar compartment. *J Cell Sci* 1996;109:1215–1227.
11. Sztul E, Kaplin A, Saucan L, et al. G. Protein traffic between distinct plasma membrane domains: isolation and characterization of vesicular carriers involved in transcytosis. *Cell* 1991;64:81–89.
12. Brown WR, Kloppel TM. The liver and IgA: immunological, cell biological and clinical implications. *Hepatology* 1989;9:763–784.
13. Roth TF, Porter KR. Yoke protein uptake in the oocytee of the mosquito *Aedes aegypti*. *J Cell Biol* 1964;20:313–332.
14. Heuser J. Three-dimensional visualization of coated vesicle formation in fibroblasts. *J Cell Biol* 1980;84:560–583.
15. Kanaseki T, Kadota K. The "vesicle in a basket." A morphological study of the coated vesicle isolated from the nerve endings of the guinea pig brain, with special reference to the mechanism of membrane movements. *J Cell Biol* 1969;42:202–220.
16. Pearse BM. Coated vesicles from pig brain: purification and biochemical characterization. *J Mol Biol* 1975;97:93–98.
17. Smith CJ, Pearse BM. Clathrin: anatomy of a coat protein. *Trends Cell Biol* 1999;9:335–338.
18. Marsh M, McMahon HT. The structural era of endocytosis. *Science* 1999;285:215–220.
19. Heuser JE, Keen J. Deep-etch visualization of proteins involved in clathrin assembly. *J Cell Biol* 1988;107:877–886.
20. Kirchhausen T, Harrison SC. Protein organization in clathrin trimers. *Cell* 1981;23:755–761.
21. Anderson RG, Brown MS, Goldstein JL. Role of the coated endocytic vesicle in the uptake of receptor-bound low density lipoprotein in human fibroblasts. *Cell* 1977;10:351–364.
22. Goldstein JL, Brown MS, Anderson RG, et al. Receptor-mediated endocytosis: concepts emerging from the LDL receptor system. *Annu Rev Cell Biol* 1985;1:1–39.
23. Haimes HB, Stockert RJ, Morell, LG, et al. Carbohydrate-specified endocytosis: localization of ligand in the lysosomal compartment. *Proc Natl Acad Sci U S A* 1981;78:6936–6939.
24. Heilker R, Manning-Krieg U, Zuber JF, et al. In vitro binding of clathrin adaptors to sorting signals correlates with endocytosis and basolateral sorting. *EMBO J* 1996;15:2893–2899.
25. Heilker R, Spiess M, Crottet P. Recognition of sorting signals by clathrin adaptors. *Bioessays* 1999;21:558–567.
26. Gallusser A, Kirchhausen T. The beta 1 and beta 2 subunits of the AP complexes are the clathrin coat assembly components. *EMBO J* 1993;12:5237–5244.
27. Mostov K, ter Beest MB, Chapin SJ. Catch the mu1B train to the basolateral surface [Comment]. *Cell* 1999;99:121–122.
28. Hirst J, Robinson MS. Clathrin and adaptors. *Biochim Biophys Acta* 1998;1404:173–193.
29. Haucke V, De Camilli P. AP-2 recruitment to synaptotagmin stimulated by tyrosine-based endocytic motifs. *Science* 1999;285:1268–1271.
30. Rapoport I, Miyazaki M, Boll W, et al. Regulatory interactions in the recognition of endocytic sorting signals by AP-2 complexes. *EMBO J* 1997;16:2240–2250.
31. Owen DJ, Vallis Y, Noble ME, et al. A structural explanation for the binding of multiple ligands by the alpha-adaptin appendage domain. *Cell* 1999;97:805–815.
32. Ahle S, Ungewickell E. Identification of a clathrin binding subunit in the HA2 adaptor protein complex. *J Biol Chem* 1989;264:20089–20093.
33. Morris SA, Ahle S, Ungewickell E. Clathrin-coated vesicles. *Curr Opin Cell Biol* 1989;1:684–690.
34. Boll W, Ohno H, Songyang Z, et al. Sequence requirements for the recognition of tyrosine-based endocytic signals by clathrin AP-2 complexes. *EMBO J* 1996;15:5789–5795.
35. Urrutia R, Henley JR, Cook T, et al. The dynamins: redundant or distinct functions for an expanding family of related GTPases? *Proc Natl Acad Sci U S A* 1997;94:377–384.
36. Warnock DE, Schmid SL. Dynamin GTPase, a force-generating molecular switch. *Bioessays* 1996;18:885–893.
37. Schmid SL, McNiven MA, De Camilli P. Dynamin and its partners: a progress report. *Curr Opin Cell Biol* 1998;10:504–512.
38. Grigliatti TA, Hall L, Rosenbluth R, et al. Temperature-sensitive mutations in Drosophila melanogaster. XIV. A selection of immobile adults. *Mol Gen Genet* 1973;120:107–114.
39. Koenig JA, Edwardson JM. Endocytosis and recycling of G protein-coupled receptors. *Trends Pharmacol Sci* 1997;18:276–287.
40. Kosaka T, Ikeda K. Reversible blockage of membrane retrieval and endocytosis in the garland cell of the temperature-sensitive

mutant of Drosophila melanogaster, shibirets1. *J Cell Biol* 1983; 97:499–507.

41. Wigge P, McMahon HT. The amphiphysin family of proteins and their role in endocytosis at the synapse. *Trends Neurosci* 1998;21:339–344.

42. Wigge P, Vallis Y, McMahon HT. Inhibition of receptor-mediated endocytosis by the amphiphysin SH3 domain. *Curr Biol* 1997;7:554–560.

43. Wigge P, Kohler K, Vallis Y, et al. Amphiphysin heterodimers: potential role in clathrin-mediated endocytosis. *Mol Biol Cell* 1997;8:2003–2015.

44. Butler MH, David C, Ochoa GC, et al. Amphiphysin II (SH3P9; BIN1), a member of the amphiphysin/Rvs family, is concentrated in the cortical cytomatrix of axon initial segments and nodes of ranvier in brain and around T tubules in skeletal muscle. *J Cell Biol* 1997;137:1355–1367.

45. Ramjaun AR, McPherson PS. Multiple amphiphysin II splice variants display differential clathrin binding: identification of two distinct clathrin-binding sites. *J Neurochem* 1998;70: 2369–2376.

46. Wang LH, Sudhof TC, Anderson RG. The appendage domain of alpha-adaptin is a high affinity binding site for dynamin. *J Biol Chem* 1995;270:10079–10083.

47. Sengar AS, Wang W, Bishay J, et al. The EH and SH3 domain Ese proteins regulate endocytosis by linking to dynamin and Eps15. *EMBO J* 1999;18:1159–1171.

48. Di Fiore PP, Pelicci PG, Sorkin A. EH: a novel protein-protein interaction domain potentially involved in intracellular sorting. *Trends Biochem Sci* 1997;22:411–413.

49. Salcini AE, Chen H, Iannolo G, et al. Epidermal growth factor pathway substrate 15, Eps15. *Int J Biochem Cell Biol* 1999 31:805–809.

50. Salcini AE, Confalonieri S, Doria M, et al. Binding specificity and in vivo targets of the EH domain, a novel protein-protein interaction module. *Genes Dev* 1997;11:2239–2249.

51. Yamabhai M, Hoffman NG, Hardison NL, et al. Intersectin, a novel adaptor protein with two Eps15 homology and five Src homology 3 domains. *J Biol Chem* 1998;273:31401–31407.

52. Wendland B, Emr SD, Riezman H. Protein traffic in the yeast endocytic and vacuolar protein sorting pathways. *Curr Opin Cell Biol* 1998;10:513–522.

53. McClure SJ, Robinson PJ. Dynamin, endocytosis and intracellular signalling (review). *Mol Membr Biol* 1996;13:189–215.

54. Chen H, Fre S, Slepnev VI, et al. Epsin is an EH-domain-binding protein implicated in clathrin-mediated endocytosis. *Nature* 1998;394:793–797.

55. Tebar F, Sorkina T, Sorkin A, et al. Eps15 is a component of clathrin-coated pits and vesicles and is located at the rim of coated pits. *J Biol Chem* 1996;271:28727–28730.

56. Davis CG, Goldstein JL, Sudhof TC, et al. Acid-dependent ligand dissociation and recycling of LDL receptor mediated by growth factor homology region. *Nature* 1987;326:760–765.

57. Collawn JF, Stangel M, Kuhn LA, et al. Transferrin receptor internalization sequence YXRF implicates a tight turn as the structural recognition motif for endocytosis. *Cell* 1990;63: 1061–1072.

58. Jing SQ, Spencer T, Miller K, et al. Role of the human transferrin receptor cytoplasmic domain in endocytosis: localization of a specific signal sequence for internalization. *J Cell Biol* 1990; 110:283–294.

59. McGraw TE, Maxfield FR. Human transferrin receptor internalization is partially dependent upon an aromatic amino acid on the cytoplasmic domain. *Cell Regul* 1990;1:369–377.

60. Stockert RJ. The asialoglycoprotein receptor: relationships between structure, function, and expression. *Physiol Rev* 1995; 75:591–609.

61. Ohno H, Aguilar RC, Yeh D, et al. The medium subunits of adaptor complexes recognize distinct but overlapping sets of tyrosine-based sorting signals. *J Biol Chem* 1998;273:25915–25921.

62. Ohno H, Fournier MC, Poy G, et al. Structural determinants of interaction of tyrosine-based sorting signals with the adaptor medium chains. *J Biol Chem* 1996;271:29009–29015.

63. Marks MS, Woodruff L, Ohno H, et al. Protein targeting by tyrosine- and di-leucine-based signals; evidence for distinct saturable components. *J Cell Biol* 1996;135:341–354.

64. Kil SJ, Hobert M, Carlin C. A leucine-based determinant in the epidermal growth factor receptor juxtamembrane domain is required for the efficient transport of ligand-receptor complexes to lysosomes. *J Biol Chem* 1999;274:3141–3150.

65. Miettinen HM, Rose JK, Mellman I. Fc receptor isoforms exhibit distinct abilities for coated pit localization as a result of cytoplasmic domain heterogeneity. *Cell* 1989;58:317–327.

66. Mullock BM, Perez JH, Kuwana T, et al. Lysosomes can fuse with a late endosomal compartment in a cell-free system from rat liver. *J Cell Biol* 1994;126:1173–1182.

67. Warren RA, Green FA, Stenberg PE, et al. Distinct saturable pathways for the endocytosis of different tyrosine motifs. *J Biol Chem* 1998;273:17056–17063.

68. Pelchen-Matthews A, Boulet I, Littman DR, et al. The protein tyrosine kinase p56lck inhibits CD4 endocytosis by preventing entry of CD4 into coated pits. *J Cell Biol* 1992;117: 279–290.

69. Rapoport I, Chen YC, Cupers P, et al. Dileucine-based sorting signals bind to the beta chain of AP-1 at a site distinct and regulated differently from the tyrosine-based motif-binding site. *EMBO J* 1998;17:2148–2155.

70. Lamaze C, Schmid SL. Recruitment of epidermal growth factor receptors into coated pits requires their activated tyrosine kinase. *J Cell Biol* 1995;129:47–54.

71. Avruch J, Zhang XF, Kyriakis JM. Raf meets Ras: completing the framework of a signal transduction pathway. *Trends Biochem Sci* 1994;19:279–283.

72. Herbst JJ, Opresko LK, Walsh BJ, et al. Regulation of postendocytic trafficking of the epidermal growth factor receptor through endosomal retention. *J Biol Chem* 1994;269:12865–12873.

73. Nesterov A, Kurten RC, Gill GN. Association of epidermal growth factor receptors with coated pit adaptins via a tyrosine phosphorylation-regulated mechanism. *J Biol Chem* 1995;270: 6320–6327.

74. Lamaze C, Fujimoto LM, Yin HL, et al. The actin cytoskeleton is required for receptor-mediated endocytosis in mammalian cells. *J Biol Chem* 1997;272:20332–20335.

75. Sorkin A, Mazzotti M, Sorkina T, et al. Epidermal growth factor receptor interaction with clathrin adaptors is mediated by the Tyr974-containing internalization motif. *J Biol Chem* 1996; 271:13377–13384.

76. van Delft S, Schumacher C, Hage W, et al. Association and colocalization of Eps15 with adaptor protein-2 and clathrin [published erratum appears in. *J Cell Biol* 1997;137:259]. *J Cell Biol* 1997;136:811–821.

77. Nakashima S, Morinaka K, Koyama S, et al. Small G protein Ral and its downstream molecules regulate endocytosis of EGF and insulin receptors. *EMBO J* 1999;18:3629–3642.

78. Matter K, Yamamoto E, Mellman I. Structural requirements and sequence motifs for polarized sorting and endocytosis of LDL and Fc receptors in MDCK cells. *J Cell Biol* 1994;126: 991–1004.

79. Roth MG, Bi K, Ktistakis NT, et al. Phospholipase D as an effector for ADP-ribosylation factor in the regulation of vesicular traffic. *Chem Phys Lipids* 1999;98:141–152.

80. Roth MG. Lipid regulators of membrane traffic through the Golgi complex. *Trends Cell Biol* 1999;9:174–179.

81. Govers R, ten Broeke T, van Kerkhof P, et al. Identification of a novel ubiquitin conjugation motif, required for ligand-induced internalization of the growth hormone receptor. *EMBO J* 1999;18:28–36.

82. Strous GJ, Govers R. The ubiquitin-proteasome system and endocytosis. *J Cell Sci* 1999;112:1417–1423.

83. Gaidarov I, Keen JH. Phosphoinositide-AP-2 interactions required for targeting to plasma membrane clathrin-coated pits. *J Cell Biol* 1999;146:755–764.

84. Gaidarov I, Krupnick JG, Falck JR, et al. Arrestin function in G protein-coupled receptor endocytosis requires phosphoinositide binding. *EMBO J* 1999;18:871–881.

85. Corvera S, D'Arrigo A, Stenmark H. Phosphoinositides in membrane traffic. *Curr Opin Cell Biol* 1999;11:460–465.

86. Santini F, Marks MS, Keen JH. Endocytic clathrin-coated pit formation is independent of receptor internalization signal levels. *Mol Biol Cell* 1998;9:1177–1194.

87. Chappell TG, Welch WJ, Schlossman DM, et al. Uncoating ATPase is a member of the 70 kilodalton family of stress proteins. *Cell* 1986;45:3–13.

88. Rothman JE, Schmid SL. Enzymatic recycling of clathrin rom coated vesicles. *Cell* 1986;46:5–9.

89. Schlossman DM, Schmid SL, Braell WA, et al. An enzyme that removes clathrin coats: purification of an uncoating ATPase. *J Cell Biol* 1984;99:723–733.

90. Greene LE, Eisenberg E. Dissociation of clathrin from coated vesicles by the uncoating ATPase. *J Biol Chem* 1990;265:6682–6687.

91. Buxbaum E, Woodman PG. Reaction mechanism of Hsc70. *Biochem Soc Trans* 1995;23:557S.

92. Hannan LA, Newmyer SL, Schmid SL. ATP- and cytosol-dependent release of adaptor proteins from clathrin-coated vesicles: A dual role or Hsc70. *Mol Biol Cell* 1998;9:2217–2229.

93. Wilde A, Brodsky FM. In vivo phosphorylation of adaptors regulates their interaction with clathrin. *J Cell Biol* 1996;135:635–645.

94. Pratt WB, Toft DO. Steroid receptor interactions with heat shock protein and immunophilin chaperones. *Endocr Rev* 1997;18:306–360.

95. Geuze HJ, Slot JW, Strous GJ, et al. The pathway of the asialoglycoprotein-ligand during receptor-mediated endocytosis: a morphological study with colloidal gold/ligand in the human hepatoma cell line, Hep G2. *Eur JCell Biol* 1983;32:38–44.

96. Gruenberg J. In vitro studies of endocytic membrane traffic. *Infection* 1991;19 [Suppl] 4:S210–S215.

97. Mayor S, Presley JF, Maxfield FR. Sorting of membrane components from endosomes and subsequent recycling to the cell surface occurs by a bulk flow process. *J Cell Biol* 1993;121:1257–1269.

98. Geuze HJ, Slot JW, Strous GJ, et al. Intracellular site of asialoglycoprotein receptor-ligand uncoupling: double-label immunoelectron microscopy during receptor-mediated endocytosis. *Cell* 1983;32:277–287.

99. Dunn KW, McGraw TE, Maxfield FR. Iterative fractionation of recycling receptors from lysosomally destined ligands in an early sorting endosome. *J Cell Biol* 1989;109:3303–3314.

100. Ghosh RN, Gelman DL, Maxfield FR. Quantification of low density lipoprotein and transferrin endocytic sorting HEp2 cells using confocal microscopy. *J Cell Sci* 1994;107:2177–2189.

101. Stoorvogel W, Oorschot V, Geuze HJ. A novel class of clathrin-coated vesicles budding from endosomes. *J Cell Biol* 1996;132:21-33.

102. Goltz JS, Wolkoff AW, Novikoff PM, et al. A role for microtubules in sorting endocytic vesicles in rat hepatocytes. *Proc Natl Acad Sci U S A* 1992;89:7026–7030.

103. Oda H, Stockert RJ, Collins C, et al. Interaction of the microtubule cytoskeleton with endocytic vesicles and cytoplasmic dynein in cultured rat hepatocytes. *J Biol Chem* 1995;270:15242–15249.

104. Novikoff PM, Cammer M, Tao L, et al. Three-dimensional organization of rat hepatocyte cytoskeleton: relation to the asialoglycoprotein endocytosis pathway. *J Cell Sci* 1996;109:21–32.

105. DiPaola M, Maxfield FR. Conformational changes in the receptors for epidermal growth factor and asialoglycoproteins induced by the mildly acidic pH found in endocytic vesicles. *J Biol Chem* 1984;259:9163–9171.

106. Wolkoff AW, Klausner RD, Ashwell G. Intracellular segregation of asialoglycoproteins and their receptor: a prelysosomal event subsequent to dissociation of the ligand-receptor complex. *J Cell Biol* 1984;98:375–381.

107. Ashwell G, Harford J. Carbohydrate-specific receptors of the liver. *Annu Rev Biochem* 1982;51:531–554.

108. Yamashiro DJ, Maxfield FR. Kinetics of endosome acidification in mutant and wild-type Chinese hamster ovary cells. *J Cell Biol* 1987;105:2713–2721.

109. Maxfield FR, Yamashiro DJ. Endosome acidification and the pathways of receptor-mediated endocytosis. *Adv Exp Med Biol* 1987;225:189–198.

110. Stevens TH, Forgac M. Structure function and regulation of the vacuolar (H+)-ATPase. *Annu Rev Cell Dev Biol* 1997;13:779–808.

111. Yamashiro DJ, Maxfield FR. Acidification of morphologically distinct endosomes in mutant and wild- type Chinese hamster ovary cells. *J Cell Biol* 1987;105:2723–2733.

112. Blumenthal R, Klausner RD, Weinstein JN. Voltage-dependent translocation of the asialoglycoprotein receptor across lipid membranes. *Nature* 1980;288:333–338.

113. Forgac M. Structure, function and regulation of the vacuolar (H+)-ATPases. *FEBS Lett* 1998;440:258–263.

114. Xu T, Vasilyeva E, Forgac M. Subunit interactions in the clathrin-coated vesicle vacuolar [H(+)]- ATPase complex. *J Biol Chem* 1999;274:28909–28915.

115. Forgac M. Structure and properties of the vacuolar (H+)-ATPases. *J Biol Chem* 1999;274:12951–12954.

116. Ohkuma S, Poole B. Fluorescence probe measurement of the intralysosomal pH in living cells and the perturbation of pH by various agents. *Proc Natl Acad Sci U S A* 1978;75:3327–3331.

117. Maxfield FR. Measurements of vacuolar pH and cytoplasmic calcium in living cells using fluoresence microscopy. *Methods Enzymol* 1989;173:745–771.

118. Tycko B, Maxfield FR. Rapid acidification of endocytic vesicles containing alpha 2- macroglobulin. *Cell* 1982;28:643–651.

119. Harford J, Bridges K, Ashwell G, et al. Intracellular dissociation of receptor-bound asialoglycoproteins in cultured hepatocytes. A pH-mediated nonlysosomal event. *J Biol Chem* 1983;258:3191–3197.

120. Clague M J, Urbe S, Aniento F, et al. Vacuolar ATPase activity is required for endosomal carrier vesicle ormation. *J Biol Chem* 1994;269:21–24.

121. Kaiser J, Stockert RJ, Wolkoff AW. Effect of monensin on receptor recycling during continuous endocytosis of asialoorosomucoid. *Exp Cell Res* 1988;174:472–480.

122. Ciechanover A, Schwartz A , Dautry-Varsat A, et al. Kinetics of internalization and recycling of transferrin and the transferrin receptor in a human hepatoma cell line. Effect of lysosomotropic agents. *J Biol Chem* 1983;258:9681–9689.

123. Klausner RD, Ashwell G, van Renswoude J, et al. Binding of apotransferrin to K562 cells: explanation of the transferrin cycle. *Proc Natl Acad Sci U S A* 1983;80:2263–2266.

124. Levy JR, Olefsky JM. The trafficking and processing of insulin and insulin receptors in cultured rat hepatocytes. *Endocrinology* 1987;121:2075–2086.

125. Weigel H, Oka JA. The dual coated pit pathway hypothesis: vertebrate cells have both ancient and modern coated pit pathways for receptor mediated endocytosis. *Biochem Biophys Res Commun* 1998;246:563–569.

126. Stockert RJ, Potvin B, Tao L, et al. Human hepatoma cell mutant defective in cell surface protein trafficking. *J Biol Chem* 1995;270:16107–16113.

127. Bridges K, Harford J, Ashwell G, et al. Fate of receptor and ligand during endocytosis of asialoglycoproteins by isolated hepatocytes. *Proc Natl Acad Sci U S A* 1982;79:350–354.

128. van der Sluijs P, Hull M, Webster P. The small GTP-binding protein rab4 controls an early sorting event on the endocytic pathway. *Cell* 1992;70:729–740.

129. Daro E, van der Sluijs P, Galli T, et al. Rab4 and cellubrevin define different early endosome populations on the pathway of transferrin receptor recycling. *Proc Natl Acad Sci U S A* 1996; 93:9559–9564.

130. Matlin KS. W(h)ither default? Sorting and polarization in epithelial cells. *Curr Opin Cell Biol* 1992;4:623–628.

131. Sheff DR, Daro EA, Hull M, et al. The receptor recycling pathway contains two distinct populations of early endosomes with different sorting functions. *J Cell Biol* 1999;145:123–139.

132. Barroso M, Sztul ES. Basolateral to apical transcytosis in polarized cells is indirect and involves BFA and trimeric G protein sensitive passage through the apical endosome. *J Cell Biol* 1994; 124:83–100.

133. Gu F, Gruenberg J. Biogenesis of transport intermediates in the endocytic pathway. *FEBS Lett* 1999;452:61–66.

134. Dunn WA, Connolly TP, Hubbard AL. Receptor-mediated endocytosis of epidermal growth factor by rat hepatocytes: receptor pathway. *J Cell Biol* 1986;102:24–36.

135. van Deurs B, Holm PK, Kayser L, et al. Multivesicular bodies in HEp-2 cells are maturing endosomes. *Eur J Cell Biol* 1993; 61:208–224.

136. Futter CE, Pearse A, Hewlett LJ, et al. Multivesicular endosomes containing internalized EGF-EGF receptor complexes mature and then fuse directly with lysosomes. *J Cell Biol* 1996; 132:1011–1023.

137. Aniento F, Gu F, Parton RG, et al. An endosomal beta COP is involved in the pH-dependent formation of transport vesicles destined for late endosomes. *J Cell Biol* 1996;133:29–41.

138. Gu F, Aniento F, Parton RG, et al. Functional dissection of COP-I subunits in the biogenesis of multivesicular endosomes. *J Cell Biol* 1997;139:1183–1195.

139. Kreis TE, Pepperkok R. Coat proteins in intracellular membrane transport. *Curr Opin Cell Biol* 1994;6:533–537.

140. Whitney JA, Gomez M, Sheff D, et al. Cytoplasmic coat proteins involved in endosome function [see comments]. *Cell* 1995;83:703–713.

141. Guo Q, Penman M, Trigatti BL, et al. A single point mutation in epsilon-COP results in temperature-sensitive, lethal defects in membrane transport in a Chinese hamster ovary cell mutant. *J Biol Chem* 1996;271:11191–11196.

142. Bright NA, Reaves BJ, Mullock BM, et al. Dense core lysosomes can fuse with late endosomes and are re-formed from the resultant hybrid organelles. *J Cell Sci* 1997;110:2027–2040.

143. Hirst J, Futter CE, Hopkins CR. The kinetics of mannose 6-phosphate receptor trafficking in the endocytic pathway in HEp-2 cells: the receptor enters and rapidly leaves multivesicular endosomes without accumulating in a prelysosomal compartment. *Mol Biol Cell* 1998;9:809–816.

144. Gibson A, Futter CE, Maxwell S, et al. Sorting mechanisms regulating membrane protein traffic in the apical transcytotic pathway of polarized MDCK cells. *J Cell Biol* 1998;143: 81–94.

145. Mullock BM, Bright N A, Fearon CW, et al. Fusion of lysosomes with late endosomes produces a hybrid organelle of intermediate density and is NSF dependent. *J Cell Biol* 1998;140: 591–601.

146. Griffiths G. On vesicles and membrane compartments. *Protoplasma* 1996;195:37–58.

147. Seaman MN, Ball C L, Robinson MS. Targeting and mistargeting of plasma membrane adaptors in vitro. *J Cell Biol* 1993;123: 1093–1105.

148. Traub LM, Bannykh SI, Rodel JE, et al. AP-2-containing clathrin coats assemble on mature lysosomes. *J Cell Biol* 1996; 135:1801–1814.

149. Forestier C, Moreno E, Pizarro-Cerda J, et al. Lysosomal accumulation and recycling of lipopolysaccharide to the cell surface of murine macrophages, an in vitro and in vivo study. *J Immunol* 1999;162:6784–6791.

150. Burd CG, Babst M, Emr SD. Novel pathways, membrane coats and PI kinase regulation in yeast lysosomal trafficking. *Semin Cell Dev Biol* 1998;9:527–533.

151. Bartles J R, Feracci H M, Stieger B, et al. Biogenesis of the rat hepatocyte plasma membrane in vivo: comparison of the pathways taken by apical and basolateral proteins using subcellular fractionation. *J Cell Biol* 1987;105:1241–1251.

152. Schell MJ, Maurice M, Stieger B, et al. 5'nucleotidase is sorted to the apical domain of hepatocytes via an indirect route [published erratum appears in J Cell Biol 1993 Nov;123(3)following 767]. *J Cell Biol* 1992;119:1173–1182.

153. Maurice M, Schell MJ, Lardeux B, et al. Biosynthesis and intracellular transport of a bile canalicular plasma membrane protein: studies in vivo and in the perfused rat liver. *Hepatology* 1994;19:648–655.

154. Barr VA, Scott LJ, Hubbard AL. Immunoadsorption of hepatic vesicles carrying newly synthesized dipeptidyl peptidase IV and polymeric IgA receptor. *J Biol Chem* 1995;270:27834–27844.

155. Barr VA, Hubbard AL. Newly synthesized hepatocyte plasma membrane proteins are transported in transcytotic vesicles in the bile duct-ligated rat [see comments]. *Gastroenterology* 1993; 105:554–571.

156. Rodriguez-Boulan E, Nelson WJ. Morphogenesis of the polarized epithelial cell phenotype. *Science* 1989;245:718–725.

157. Sargiacomo M, Lisanti M, Graeve L, et al. Integral and peripheral protein composition of the apical and basolateral membrane domains in MDCK cells. *J Membr Biol* 1989;107: 277–286.

158. Apodaca G, Katz LA, Mostov KE. Receptor-mediated transcytosis of IgA in MDCK cells is via apical recycling endosomes. *J Cell Biol* 1994;125:67–86.

159. Gonnella PA, Neutra MR. Membrane-bound and fluid-phase macromolecules enter separate prelysosomal compartments in absorptive cells of suckling rat ileum. *J Cell Biol* 1984;99: 909–917.

160. Odorizzi G, Pearse A, Domingo D, et al. Apical and basolateral endosomes of MDCK cells are interconnected and contain a polarized sorting mechanism. *J Cell Biol* 1996;135:139–152.

161. Hughson EJ, Hopkins CR. Endocytic pathways in polarized Caco-2 cells: identification of an endosomal compartment accessible from both apical and basolateral surfaces. *J Cell Biol* 1990;110:337–348.

162. Allen K, Gokay KE, Thomas MA, et al. Biosynthesis of endotubin: an apical early endosomal glycoprotein from developing rat intestinal epithelial cells. *Biochem J* 1998;330:367–373.

163. Wilson JM, Colton TL. Targeting of an intestinal apical endosomal protein to endosomes in nonpolarized cells. *J Cell Biol* 1997;136:319–330.

164. Tuma PL, Finnegan CM, Yi JH, et al. Evidence for apical endo-

cytosis in polarized hepatic cells: phosphoinositide 3-kinase inhibitors lead to the lysosomal accumulation of resident apical plasma membrane proteins. *J Cell Biol* 1999;145:1089–1102.

165. Ortega D, Pol A, Biermer M, et al. Annexin VI defines an apical endocytic compartment in rat liver hepatocytes. *J Cell Sci* 1998;111:261–269.

166. Rothman JE, Orci L. Molecular dissection of the secretory pathway. *Nature* 1992;355:409–415.

167. Block MR, Glick B S, Wilcox CA, et al. Purification of an N-ethylmaleimide-sensitive protein catalyzing vesicular transport. *Proc Natl Acad Sci U S A* 1988;85:7852–7856.

168. Malhotra V, Orci L, Glick BS, et al. Role of an N-ethyl-maleimide-sensitive transport component in promoting usion of transport vesicles with cisternae of the Golgi stack. *Cell* 1988; 54:221–227.

169. Clary DO, Griff IC, Rothman JE. SNAPs, a family of NSF attachment proteins involved in intracellular membrane fusion in animals and yeast. *Cell* 1990;61:709–721.

170. Sollner T, Whiteheart SW, Brunner M, et al. SNAP receptors implicated in vesicle targeting and fusion [see comments]. *Nature* 1993;362:318–324.

171. Hay JC, Scheller, RH. SNAREs and NSF in targeted membrane fusion. *Curr Opin Cell Biol* 1997;9:505–512.

172. Weber T, Zemelman BV, McNew JA, et al. SNAREpins: minimal machinery for membrane fusion. *Cell* 1998;92:759–772.

173. Gotte M, von Mollard GF. A new beat for the SNARE drum [see comments]. *Trends Cell Biol* 1998;8:215–218.

174. Ungermann C, Sato K, Wickner W. Defining the functions of trans-SNARE pairs. *Nature* 1998;396:543–548.

175. Link E, McMahon H, Fischer von Mollard G, et al. Cleavage of cellubrevin by tetanus toxin does not affect fusion of early endosomes. *J Biol Chem* 1993;268:18423–18426.

176. Wong SH, Xu Y, Zhang T, et al. Syntaxin 7, a novel syntaxin member associated with the early endosomal compartment. *J Biol Chem* 1998;273:375–380.

177. Tang BL, Tan AE, Lim LK, et al. Syntaxin 12, a member of the syntaxin family localized to the endosome. *J Biol Chem* 1998; 273:6944–6950.

178. Advani RJ, Bae HR, Bock JB, et al. Seven novel mammalian SNARE proteins localize to distinct membrane compartments. *J Biol Chem* 1998;273:10317–10324.

179. Robinson LJ Aniento F, Gruenberg J. NSF is required for transport from early to late endosomes. *J Cell Sci* 1997;110: 2079–2087.

180. Prekeris R, Klumperman J, Chen YA, et al. Syntaxin 13 mediates cycling of plasma membrane proteins via tubulovesicular recycling endosomes. *J Cell Biol* 1998;143:957–971.

181. Yang B, Gonzalez L, Jr, Prekeris R, et al. SNARE interactions are not selective. Implications for membrane fusion specificity. *J Biol Chem* 1999;274:5649–5653.

182. Bennett MK. SNAREs and the specificity of transport vesicle targeting. *Curr Opin Cell Biol* 1995;7:581–586.

183. Pfeffer SR. Motivating endosome motility. *Nat Cell Biol* 1999; 1:E145–E147.

184. Novick P, Zerial M. The diversity of Rab proteins in vesicle transport. *Curr Opin Cell Biol* 1997;9:496–504.

185. Bucci C, Parton RG, Mather IH, et al. The small GTPase rab5 functions as a regulatory factor in the early endocytic pathway. *Cell* 1992;70:715–728.

186. Gorvel JP, Chavrier P, Zerial M, et al. rab5 controls early endosome fusion in vitro. *Cell* 1991;64:915–925.

187. Mills IG, Jones AT, Clague MJ. Involvement of the endosomal autoantigen EEA1 in homotypic fusion of early endosomes. *Curr Biol* 1998;8:881–884.

188. Chavrier P, Parton RG, Hauri HP, et al. Localization of low

189. Lombardi D, Soldati T, Riederer MA, et al. Rab9 functions in transport between late endosomes and the trans Golgi network. *EMBO J* 1993;12:677–682.

190. Chavrier P, Goud B. The role of ARF and Rab GTPases in membrane transport. *Curr Opin Cell Biol* 1999;11:466–475.

191. Diaz E, Schimmoller F, Pfeffer SR. A novel Rab9 effector required for endosome-to-TGN transport. *J Cell Biol* 1997;138: 283–290.

192. Ullrich O, Reinsch S, Urbe S, et al. Rab11 regulates recycling through the pericentriolar recycling endosome. *J Cell Biol* 1996; 135:913–924.

193. Green EG, Ramm E, Riley NM, et al. Rab11 is associated with transferrin-containing recycling compartments in K562 cells. *Biochem Biophys Res Commun* 1997;239:612–616.

194. Zuk PA, Elferink LA. Rab15 mediates an early endocytic event in Chinese hamster ovary cells. *J Biol Chem* 1999;274: 22303–22312.

195. Zacchi P, Stenmark H, Parton RG, et al. Rab17 regulates membrane trafficking through apical recycling endosomes in polarized epithelial cells. *J Cell Biol* 1998;140:1039–1053.

196. Olkkonen VM, Dupree P, Killisch I, et al. Molecular cloning and subcellular localization of three GTP-binding proteins of the rab subfamily. *J Cell Sci* 1993;106:1249–1261.

197. Lazar T, Gotte M, Gallwitz D. Vesicular transport: how many Ypt/Rab-GTPases make a eukaryotic cell?. *Trends Biochem Sci* 1997;22:468–472.

198. Alexandrov K, Horiuchi H, Steele-Mortimer O, et al. Rab escort protein-1 is a multifunctional protein that accompanies newly prenylated rab proteins to their target membranes. *EMBO J* 1994;13:5262–5273.

199. Wilson AL, Sheridan KM, Erdman RA, et al. Prenylation of a Rab1B mutant with altered GTPase activity is impaired in cell-free systems but not in intact mammalian cells. *Biochem J* 1996; 318:1007–1014.

200. Pfeffer SR. Transport vesicle docking: SNAREs and associates. *Annu Rev Cell Dev Biol* 1996;12:441–461.

201. Mohrmann K, van der Sluijs P. Regulation of membrane transport through the endocytic pathway by rabGTPases. *Mol Membr Biol* 1999;16:81–87.

202. Stenmark H, Vitale G, Ullrich O, et al. Rabaptin-5 is a direct effector of the small GTPase Rab5 in endocytic membrane usion. *Cell* 1995;83:423–432.

203. Rybin V, Ullrich O, Rubino M, et al. GTPase activity of Rab5 acts as a timer for endocytic membrane fusion [see comments]. *Nature* 1996;383:266–269.

204. Gournier H, Stenmark H, Rybin V, et al. Two distinct effectors of the small GTPase Rab5 cooperate in endocytic membrane usion. *EMBO J* 1998;17:1930–1940.

205. Christoforidis S, McBride HM, Burgoyne RD, et al. The Rab5 effector EEA1 is a core component of endosome docking. *Nature* 1999;397:621–625.

206. Rubino M, Miaczynska M, Lippe R, et al. Selective membrane recruitment of EEA1 suggests a role in directional transport of clathrin-coated vesicles to early endosomes. *J Biol Chem* 2000; 275:3745–3748.

207. Horiuchi H, Lippe R, McBride HM, et al. A novel Rab5 GDP/GTP exchange factor complexed to Rabaptin-5 links nucleotide exchange to effector recruitment and function. *Cell* 1997;90:1149–1159.

208. Simonsen A, Lippe R, Christoforidis S, et al. EEA1 links PI(3)K function to Rab5 regulation of endosome fusion [see comments]. *Nature* 1998;394:494–498.

209. Nielsen E, Severin F, Backer JM, et al. Rab5 regulates motility

of early endosomes on microtubules. *Nat Cell Biolog* 1999;1: 376–382.

210. Stenmark H, Aasland R. FYVE-finger prote. *J Cell Sci* 1999; 112:4175–4183.

211. Simonsen A, Gaullier JM, D'Arrigo A, et al. The Rab5 effector EEA1 interacts directly with syntaxin-6. *J Biol Chem* 1999;274: 28857–28860.

212. Callaghan J, Nixon S, Bucci C, et al. Direct interaction of EEA1 with Rab5b. *Eur J Biochem* 1999;265:361–366.

213. Gaschet J, Hsu VW. Distribution of ARF6 between membrane and cytosol is regulated by its GTPase cycle. *J Biol Chem* 1999; 274:20040–20045.

214. D'Souza-Schorey C, Li G, Colombo MI, et al. A regulatory role for ARF6 in receptor-mediated endocytosis. *Science* 1995;267: 1175–1178.

215. D'Souza-Schorey C, van Donselaar E, Hsu VW, et al. ARF6 targets recycling vesicles to the plasma membrane: insights from an ultrastructural investigation. *J Cell Biol* 1998;140:603–616.

216. Peters PJ, Hsu VW, Ooi C E, et al. Overexpression of wild-type and mutant ARF1 and ARF6: distinct perturbations of nonoverlapping membrane compartments. *J Cell Biol* 1995; 128:1003–1017.

217. Radhakrishna H, Donaldson JG. ADP-ribosylation factor 6 regulates a novel plasma membrane recycling pathway. *J Cell Biol* 1997;139:49–61.

218. D'Souza-Schorey C, Boshans RL, McDonough M, et al. A role for POR1, a Rac1-interacting protein, in ARF6-mediated cytoskeletal rearrangements. *EMBO J* 1997;16:5445–5454.

219. Altschuler Y, Liu S, Katz L, et al. ADP-ribosylation factor 6 and endocytosis at the apical surface of Madin-Darby canine kidney cells. *J Cell Biol* 1999;147:7–12.

220. Franco M, Peters PJ, Boretto J, et al. EFA6, a sec7 domain-containing exchange factor for ARF6, coordinates membrane recycling and actin cytoskeleton organization. *EMBO J* 1999;18: 1480–1491.

221. Leung SM, Rojas R, Maples C, et al. Modulation of endocytic traffic in polarized madin-darby canine kidney cells by the small GTPase rhoA [In Process Citation]. *Mol Biol Cell* 1999;10: 4369–4384.

222. Adamson P, Paterson HF, Hall A. Intracellular localization of the P21rho proteins. *J Cell Biol* 1992;119:617–627.

223. Cussac D, Leblanc P, L'Heritier A, et al. Rho proteins are localized with different membrane compartments involved in vesicular trafficking in anterior pituitary cells. *Mol Cell Endocrinol* 1996;119:195–206.

224. Murphy C, Saffrich R, Grummt M, et al. Endosome dynamics regulated by a Rho protein. *Nature* 1996;384:427–432.

225. Kroschewski R, Hall A, Mellman I. Cdc42 controls secretory and endocytic transport to the basolateral plasma membrane of MDCK cells. *Nat Cell Biol* 1999;1:8–13.

226. Salisbury JL, Condeelis JS, Satir P. Role of coated vesicles, microfilaments, and calmodulin in receptor-mediated endocytosis by cultured B lymphoblastoid cells. *J Cell Biol* 1980;87: 132–141.

227. Salisbury JL, Condeelis JS, Maihle NJ, et al. Receptor-mediated endocytosis by clathrin-coated vesicles: evidence for a dynamic pathway. *Cold Spring Harb Symp Quant Biol* 1982;46:733–741.

228. Durrbach A, Louvard D, Coudrier E. Actin filaments facilitate two steps of endocytosis. *J Cell Sci* 1996;109:457–465.

229. van Deurs B, Holm PK, Kayser L, et al. Delivery to lysosomes in the human carcinoma cell line HEp-2 involves an actin filament-facilitated fusion between mature endosomes and preexisting lysosomes. *Eur J Cell Biol* 1995;66:309–323.

230. Durrbach A, Collins K, Matsudaira P, et al. Brush border myosin-I truncated in the motor domain impairs the distribution and the function of endocytic compartments in an

hepatoma cell line. *Proc Natl Acad Sci U S A* 1996;93: 7053–7058.

231. Snigirevskaya ES, Cottier H. Immunogold visualization of actin near the coated pits at the apical surface of human mammary epithelial cells. *Tsitologiia* 1999;41:586–589.

232. Maples CJ, Ruiz WG, Apodaca G. Both microtubules and actin filaments are required for efficient postendocytotic traffic of the polymeric immunoglobulin receptor in polarized Madin-Darby canine kidney cells. *J Biol Chem* 1997;272:6741–6751.

233. Hall A. Rho GTPases and the actin cytoskeleton. *Science* 1998; 279:509–514.

234. Oka JA, Weigel PH. Microtubule-depolymerizing agents inhibit asialo-orosomucoid delivery to lysosomes but not its endocytosis or degradation in isolated rat hepatocytes. *Biochim Biophys Acta* 1983;763:368–376.

235. Matteoni R, Kreis TE. Translocation and clustering of endosomes and lysosomes depends on microtubules. *J Cell Biol* 1987;105:1253–1265.

236. Harford J, Wolkoff AW, Ashwell G, et al. Monensin inhibits intracellular dissociation of asialoglycoproteins from their receptor. *J Cell Biol* 1983;96:1824–1828.

237. Holen I, Stromhaug PE, Gordon PB, et al. Inhibition of autophagy and multiple steps in asialoglycoprotein endocytosis by inhibitors of tyrosine protein kinases (tyrphostins). *J Biol Chem* 1995;270:12823–12831.

238. Harada M, Sakisaka S, Yoshitake M, et al. Role of cytoskeleton and acidification of endocytic compartment in asialoglycoprotein metabolism in isolated rat hepatocyte couplets. *Hepatology* 1995;21:1413–1421.

239. Satir P, Goltz JS, Wolkoff AW. Microtubule-based cell motility: the role of microtubules in cell motility and differentiation. *Cancer Invest* 1990;8:685–690.

240. Jin M, Snider MD. Role of microtubules in transferrin receptor transport from the cell surface to endosomes and the Golgi complex. *J Biol Chem* 1993;268:18390–18397.

241. Thatte HS, Bridges KR, Golan DE. Microtubule inhibitors differentially affect translational movement, cell surface expression, and endocytosis of transferrin receptors in K562 cells. *J Cell Physiol* 1994;160:345–357.

242. Runnegar M, Wei X, Berndt N, et al. Transferrin receptor recycling in rat hepatocytes is regulated by protein phosphatase 2A, possibly through effects on microtubule-dependent transport. *Hepatology* 1997;26:176–185.

243. Hamm-Alvarez SF, Wei X, Berndt N, et al. Protein phosphatases independently regulate vesicle movement and microtubule subpopulations in hepatocytes. *Am J Physiol* 1996;271: C929–C943.

244. Goldman IS, Jones AL, Hradek GT, et al. Hepatocyte handling of immunoglobulin A in the rat: the role of microtubules. *Gastroenterology* 1983;85:130–140.

245. Mullock BM, Jones RS, Peppard J, et al. Effect of colchicine on the transfer of IgA across hepatocytes into bile in isolated perfused rat livers. *FEBS Lett* 1980;120:278–282.

246. Vaughan KT, Tynan SH, Faulkner NE, et al. Colocalization of cytoplasmic dynein with dynactin and CLIP-170 at microtubule distal ends. *J Cell Sci* 1999;112:1437–1447.

247. Valetti C, Wetzel DM, Schrader M, et al. Role of dynactin in endocytic traffic: effects of dynamitin overexpression and colocalization with CLIP-170 [In Process Citation]. *Mol Biol Cell* 1999;10:4107–4120.

248. Burgoyne RD, Clague MJ. Annexins in the endocytic pathway. *Trends Biochem Sci* 1994;19:231–232.

249. Apodaca G, Enrich C, Mostov KE. The calmodulin antagonist, W-13, alters transcytosis, recycling, and the morphology of the endocytic pathway in Madin-Darby canine kidney cells. *J Biol Chem* 1994;269:19005–19013.

250. Pol A, Ortega D, Enrich C. Identification of cytoskeleton-associated proteins in isolated rat liver endosomes. *Biochem J* 1997; 327:741–746.

251. Lane J, Allan V. Corrigendum to "Microtubule-based membrane movement" [Biochimica Et biophysica acta, 1376 (1998) 27–55]1. *Biochim Biophys Acta* 1999;1422:205.

252. Raposo G, Cordonnier MN, Tenza D, et al. Association of myosin I alpha with endosomes and lysosomes in mammalian cells. *Mol Biol Cell* 1999;10:1477–1494.

253. Sutherland JD, Witke W. Molecular genetic approaches to understanding the actin cytoskeleton. *Curr Opin Cell Biol* 1999; 11:142–151.

254. Mermall V, Post PL, Mooseker MS. Unconventional myosins in cell movement, membrane traffic, and signal transduction. *Science* 1998;279:527–533.

255. Hirokawa N, Noda Y, Okada Y. Kinesin and dynein superfamily proteins in organelle transport and cell division. *Curr Opin Cell Biol* 1998;10:60–73.

256. Bomsel M, Parton R, Kuznetsov SA. Microtubule- and motor-dependent fusion in vitro between apical and basolateral endocytic vesicles from MDCK cells. *Cell* 1990;62: 719–731.

257. Murray JW, Bananis E, Wolkoff AW. Reconstitution of ATP-dependent Movement of Endocytic Vesicles Along Microtubules In Vitro: An Oscillatory Bidirectional Process. *Mol Biol Cell* 2000;11:419–433.

The Liver: Biology and Pathobiology, Fourth Edition, edited by I. M. Arias, J. L. Boyer, F. V. Chisari, N. Fausto, D. Schachter, and D. A. Shafritz.
Lippincott Williams & Wilkins, Philadelphia © 2001.

12

PEROXISOMAL ASSEMBLY, BIOLOGY, AND DISEASE RELATIONSHIP

JENNIFER J. SMITH
RICHARD A. RACHUBINSKI

Peroxisomes are members of the microbody family of organelles, along with the glyoxysomes of plants and the glycosomes of trypanosomes. They are found in organisms from yeasts to mammals and in most cell types (1,2). Peroxisomes were first identified in kidney and liver cells as small, electron-dense, membrane-enclosed vesicles (3). They are defined as containing at least one hydrogen peroxide-producing oxidase and catalase to decompose the hydrogen peroxide to water and molecular oxygen (4). Mature peroxisomes appear spherical in electron micrographs, with diameters between 0.5 and 1.0 micrometer (Fig. 12.1), although there is evidence that in some mammalian tissues, peroxisomes form a reticulum (5–7). Each peroxisome is delimited by a single unit membrane and contains a fine granular matrix and sometimes a paracrystalline core. Peroxisomes do not contain DNA (8) or an independent protein synthesis machinery, as do mitochondria or chloroplasts. Accordingly, all peroxisomal proteins are encoded by nuclear genes and synthesized on cytoplasmic polysomes (9,10). Peroxisomes are the site of diverse metabolic reactions that vary depending on the organism or the cell type. They perform a myriad of biochemical functions, including the β-oxidation of fatty acids (Fig. 12.2), bile acid synthesis, plasmalogen synthesis and cholesterol biosynthesis (1,11). In accordance with their functional diversity, the number, volume and protein composition of peroxisomes in a cell can dramatically change in response to developmental and environmental cues (1,12,13). The essential nature of peroxisomes for normal human development and physiology is underscored by the lethality of the

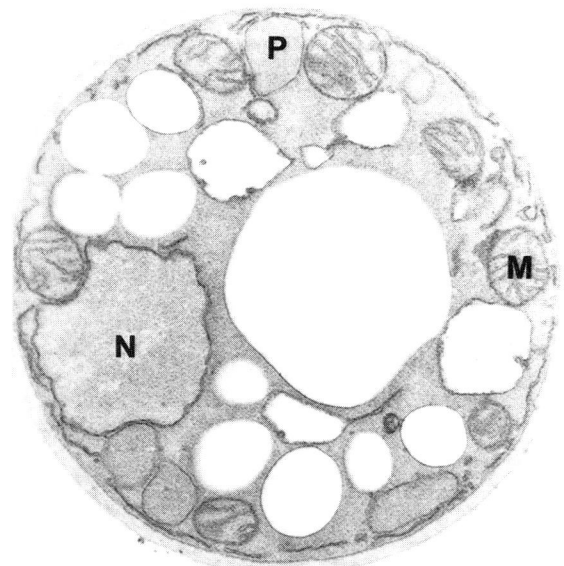

FIGURE 12.1. Electron micrograph of the yeast *Yarrowia lipolytica* grown in a peroxisome-proliferating medium containing oleic acid. *P*, peroxisome; *M*, mitochondrion; *N*, nucleus. *Bar* = 1 μm.

J. J. Smith and R. A. Rachubinski: Department of Cell Biology, University of Alberta, Edmonton, Alberta T6G 2H7, Canada.

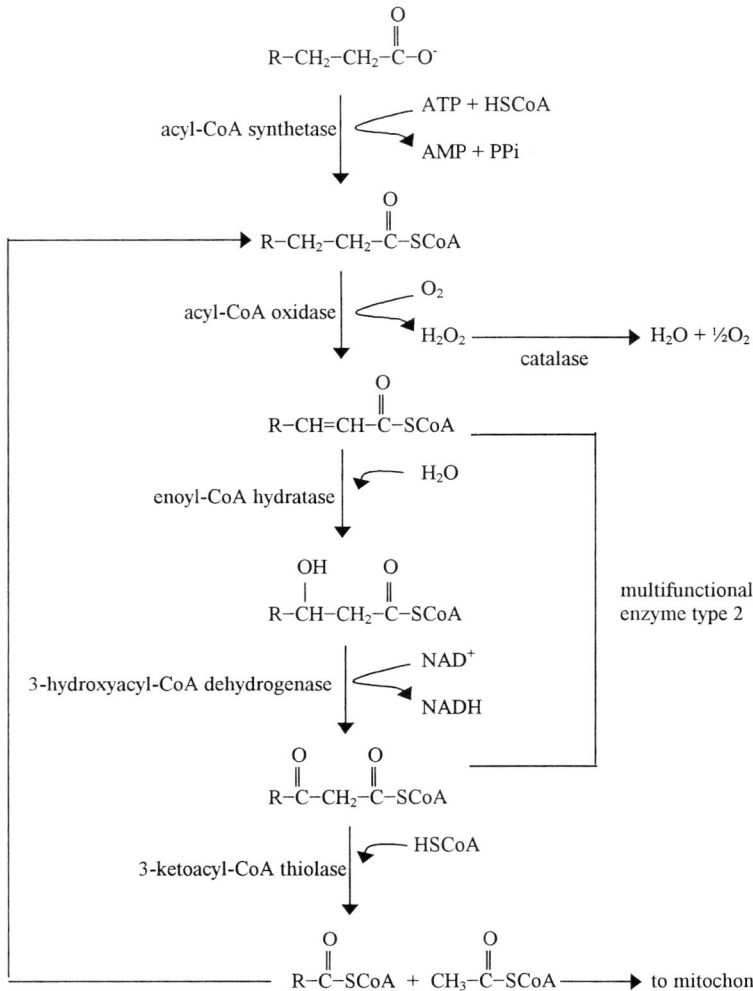

FIGURE 12.2. Peroxisomal β-oxidation.

peroxisome biogenesis disorders (PBDs), a group of autosomal recessive disorders that includes Zellweger syndrome, neonatal adrenoleukodystrophy and rhizomelic chondrodysplasia punctata, in which peroxisomes fail to assemble normally (14–16). Therefore, a great deal of attention has been paid to the molecular cascade of events involved in peroxisome assembly. This chapter will describe some of the molecular events and players involved in peroxisome assembly and their relationship to human disease (see also website chapter 💻 W-8).

PEROXISOMAL PROTEIN TARGETING AND IMPORT PATHWAYS

Similar to the sorting of proteins of other membrane compartments within the cell, the targeting of proteins to the peroxisome involves the specific interaction of peroxisomal targeting signals (PTSs) and their cognate receptors with the peroxisome-specific protein import machinery.

Matrix Proteins

There are two well defined PTSs involved in the translocation of proteins into the peroxisomal matrix (10,17,18). PTS1 is a carboxyl-terminal tripeptide of the sequence SKL, or conserved variants thereof conforming to the consensus sequence (S/A/C)(K/R/H)(L/I/M), which is found in the majority of mammalian peroxisomal matrix proteins (19–22). PTS2 is an amino-terminal or internal nonapeptide, $(R/K)(L/V/I)X_5$ (Q/H)(L/A), found in a small subset of matrix proteins, notably 3-ketoacyl-CoA thiolase, the final enzyme of the peroxisomal β-oxidation pathway (23,24). Both types of PTS have been conserved in evolution from yeasts to humans (25–27). Other PTSs have been reported that are internal to peroxisomal proteins and unrelated to either PTS1 or PTS2 (28,29), but these PTSs remain largely uncharacterized and the receptors that recognize them remain to be identified. The peroxin (protein required for peroxisome assembly) Pex5p is the receptor for PTS1 (30–32), while another peroxin, Pex7p, is the receptor for PTS2 (33–35). These peroxins will be discussed later in greater detail.

Membrane Proteins

The elucidation of the molecular events and players involved in the targeting of membrane proteins to peroxisomes has been much slower than for the peroxisomal matrix proteins, and our knowledge of how membrane proteins are targeted to peroxisomes and how peroxisomal membranes assemble remains rudimentary.

Peroxisomal membrane targeting signals, called mPTSs, have been defined in the most general of terms for a few peroxisomal membrane proteins of yeasts. The mPTSs that have been characterized show limited similarity one to another, although stretches of positively charged, basic amino acids appear to be important in the targeting of some proteins to the peroxisomal membrane (36,37). No receptors for the mPTSs and required for the specific targeting of peroxisomal membrane proteins have been conclusively demonstrated. The biogenesis of the peroxisomal membrane itself appears to be independent of the targeting and import of matrix proteins, as a number of mutants of peroxisome assembly in both lower and higher eukaryotes show evidence of so-called peroxisome "ghosts," which are vestigial structures containing peroxisomal membrane proteins but lacking peroxisomal matrix proteins (38).

GENETIC ANALYSIS OF PEROXISOME ASSEMBLY

PEX Genes and Their Encoded Proteins, the Peroxins

The discovery and definition of the different types of PTSs and the demonstration that the mechanism of peroxisome assembly has been essentially conserved from both lower eukaryotes such as yeast and higher eukaryotes including humans led to the exploitation of genetic systems in both yeast and cultured mammalian cells to identify proteins called peroxins that complement *pex* mutants that are compromised in peroxisome assembly. The identification of these *PEX* genes in model systems has subsequently led to the rapid identification of a number of human *PEX* genes whose mutations are responsible for many of the identified complementation groups of the PBDs. To date, 23 *PEX* genes have been identified that are required for peroxisomal protein import, biogenesis, proliferation, and inheritance (Table 12.1). These *PEX* genes encode peroxins that act as the PTS1receptor (Pex5p) (30–32), the PTS2 receptor (Pex7p) (33–35), docking factors for the PTS receptors (Pex13p and Pex14p) (39–43), AAA ATPases involved in

TABLE 12.1. PEROXINS

Peroxin	Characteristics	Subcellular Location	Human Ortholog Identified	PBD Known
Pex1p	contains AAA ATPase domains; sequence is similar to NSF	cytosol; peripheral association with vesicles	+	+ (CG 1)
Pex2p	contains RING-finger motif	PM (integral)	+	+ (CG 10)
Pex3p	contains mPTS	PM (integral)	+	
Pex4p	ubiquitin conjugating enzyme	PM (peripheral, cytosolic face)		
Pex5p	sequence is similar to Pex20p; contains TPR repeats	PM; cytosol; peroxisomal matrix	++	+ (CG 2)
Pex6p	contains AAA ATPase domains; sequence is similar to NSF	cytosol; peripheral association with vesicles	+	+ (CG 4)
Pex7p	contains WD-40 repeats	PM; cytosol; peroxisomal matrix	+	+ (CG 11)
Pex8p	contains PTS1 and PTS2	PM (peripheral, matrix face); peroxisomal matrix		
Pex9p	contains cysteine-rich region	PM (integral)		
Pex10p	contains RING-finger motif	PM (integral)	+	+ (CG 5,7)
Pex11p	homodimerizes	PM (integral; peripheral, matrix face)	++	
Pex12p	contains RING-finger motif	PM (integral)	+	+ (CG 3)
Pex13p	contains SH3 domain	PM (integral)	+	+ (CG 13)
Pex14p	phosphorylated	PM (peripheral, cytosolic face)	+	
Pex15p	phosphorylated; contains mPTS	PM (integral)		
Pex16p	glycosylated in *Y. lipolytica*	PM (integral; peripheral, matrix face)	+	+ (CG 9)
Pex17p		PM (integral; peripheral, cytosolic face)		
Pex18p	sequence is similar to Pex21p	cytosol		
Pex19p	farnesylated	PM (peripheral, cytosolic face); cytosol	+	+ (CG 14)
Pex20p	sequence is similar to Pex5p	PM (peripheral, cytosolic face); cytosol		
Pex21p	sequence is similar to Pex18p	cytosol		
Pex22p		PM (integral)		
Pex23p		PM (integral)		

The number of plus signs denotes the number of human orthologs or PBD complementation groups that have been identified. AAA, ATPases associated with diverse cellular activities; CG, complementation group; NSF, *N*-ethylmaleimide-sensitive factor; PBD, peroxisome biogenesis disorder; PM, peroxisomal membrane; SH3, Src homology 3; TPR, tetratricopeptide repeat.

peroxisomal membrane fusion (Pex1p and Pex6p) (44), proteins involved in peroxisome proliferation (Pex11p and Pex16p) (45–48), and additional functions as well.

Pex5p and Pex7p, the PTS Receptors, and Their Docking at the Peroxisomal Membrane

The PTS1 receptor is encoded by the *PEX5* gene. *PEX5* genes have been identified in a number of yeast species, as well as in mammalian cells, including those of humans (16,30–32,49–51). Pex5p is a member of the tetratricopeptide repeat (TPR) family of proteins. Pex5p receptors bind the PTS1 sequence directly through a limited number of their TPR repeats (31). Binding occurs whether the receptor is found in the cytosol or bound to peroxisomes. The same PTS1 receptor binds to the canonical SKL tripeptide and functional conserved variants thereof (51). The involvement of Pex5p in the import of peroxisomal matrix proteins has been demonstrated directly by the demonstration that antibodies to human Pex5p inhibit the import of PTS1-containing proteins in an *in vitro* import assay system using semi-permeabilized Chinese hamster ovary cells (49).

In mammalian cells, approximately 95% of the PTS1 receptor is cytosolic, while the remainder is associated with the peroxisome, principally on the cytosolic face of the peroxisomal membrane (50). This observation, combined with the fact that Pex5p recognizes and binds the PTS1 tripeptide in the absence of peroxisomes, led to the model in which the PTS1 receptor binds its cargo in the cytosol and then traffics along with its cargo to the surface of the peroxisome. The receptor then returns to the cytosol after delivering its cargo to initiate a further round of cargo recognition in the cytosol and delivery to the peroxisome (52).

The association of Pex5p with the surface of the peroxisomal membrane is mediated through the specific actions and interactions of docking proteins found at the peroxisomal membrane. The peroxin Pex13p appears to be the major docking protein for the PTS1 receptor (39–41), although interactions of Pex5p with other peroxisomal membrane proteins including Pex14p have been demonstrated (42,43). Pex13p is a peroxisomal integral membrane protein.

Interestingly, multiple locations have been reported for the PTS1 receptor in different organisms. Pex5p has been demonstrated to be primarily cytosolic, essentially on the cytosolic face of the peroxisome or even exclusively within the peroxisome (31,32,39,40). Apparently, the experimental determination of the location of the PTS1 receptor is very much dependent on the growth state of the cell and the biochemical and microscopical methods used to localize the receptor. The multiple locations found for the receptor have led to a model to explain the multiple locations of the PTS1 receptor (53). In this model, hypothetical proteins act either to obstruct the entry of receptors complexed with their cargo into the peroxisome or to help in returning the empty receptor to the

cytosol. Different physiological states of a cell affect the numbers of cargoes, receptors, docking proteins, and gatekeeper or recycler proteins, which in turn might affect the subcellular location of receptor molecules to primarily one particular subcellular compartment or another. The fate of the receptor in the peroxisome lumen, whether it is degraded or reported for another round of cargo import, is still unknown.

The PTS2 receptor is encoded by the *PEX7* gene. The *PEX7* gene has been identified in various yeast species (33–35,54,55), mice (56), and humans (55–57). Pex7p is a member of the WD repeat family of proteins. The receptor has been shown to bind the PTS2 sequence directly (34,35). The subcellular location of the PTS2 receptor has been the subject of some controversy. In both the yeast *Saccharomyces cerevisiae* (33) and in human cells (56), Pex7p has been reported to be primarily cytosolic, with a small amount of the receptor to be associated with the peroxisomal membrane. These observations have led to a model in which Pex7p, like the PTS1 receptor Pex5p, recruits cargo, shuttling it between the cytosol and the peroxisome surface. An alternative model proposes that Pex7p, at least in *S. cerevisiae*, is essentially intraperoxisomal and contains a PTS. Pex7p is purported to be first targeted to the peroxisomal matrix and there to act as a molecular ratchet, pulling PTS2-containing proteins into the organelle (35,58). The different locations found for the PTS2 receptor may again be the result of the different experimental conditions used or the different physiological states of the cells. Further investigation is required for an unambiguous localization of the PTS2 receptor. In the shuttling model of Pex7p, Pex7p interacts primarily with the docking protein Pex14p (42,43,59); however, Pex7p also interacts with Pex13p and Pex5p and modulates the import efficiency of PTS1 proteins (42,43,59,60). A model for matrix protein import is presented in Figure 12.3, and the web of peroxin interactions is presented in Figure 12.4.

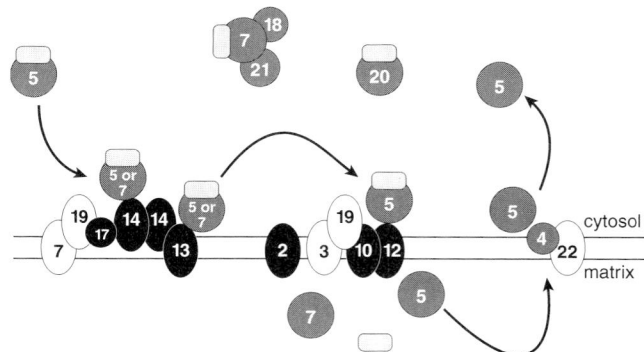

FIGURE 12.3. Model of peroxisomal matrix protein import. Cargo proteins are *black boxes*; peroxins involved in targeting are *black circles*; membrane-bound peroxins involved in import are *black ovals*; peroxins that interact with import components, but which have not been shown to have a direct role in import, are *white*. Physically interacting proteins are drawn connected.

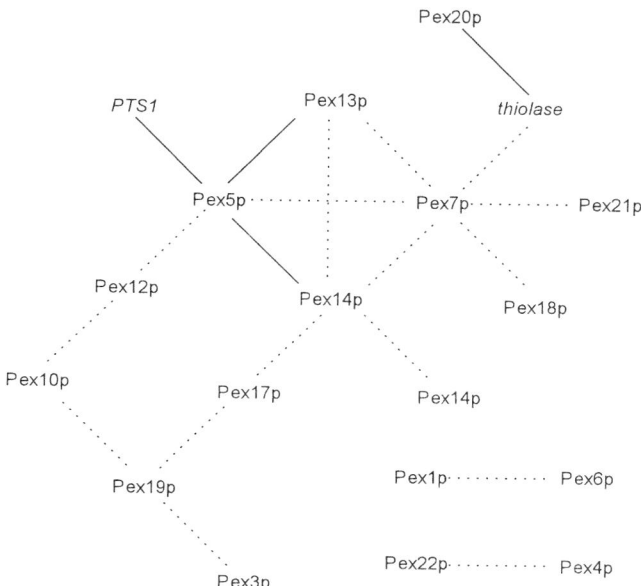

FIGURE 12.4. Physical interactions between peroxins. Interacting proteins that are not peroxins are *italicized*. Interactions that are direct (i.e., no intermediate bridging protein) are represented by *solid lines*. All other interactions are represented by *dotted lines*.

THE PEROXISOME BIOGENESIS DISORDERS

The PBDs are a genetically heterogenous set of autosomal recessive disorders that have as their defining characteristic multiple defects in peroxisome function (reviewed in refs. 14–16) (see also website chapter 🖥 W-8). The PBDs are classified into three groups. Group A is compromised of Zellweger syndrome, infantile Refsum disease and neonatal adrenoleukodystrophy and is characterized by severe neurological and hepatic dysfunction, craniofacial abnormalities and hypotonia. These extremely severe diseases occur at a frequency of 1 in 25,000 to 1 in 50,000 live births. Early death is common, usually before the age of ten years. Patients accumulate phytanic acid and very-long-chain fatty acids in the circulation and show low levels of plasmalogens, an ether lipid. Patients in Group B, which includes the disease rhizomelic chondrodysplasia punctata, display growth defects, rhizomelia, cataracts, epiphyseal calcifications and ichthyosis. Individuals in this group have higher levels of phytanic acid and normal levels of very-long-chain fatty acids, but they lack plasmalogens. Patients with Group C disorders show milder symptoms than those in Groups A and B. Most of the diseases in Group C are the result of mutations in single genes that compromise the activity or localization of single enzymes normally resident in the peroxisome, while the defects in Groups A and B affect the locations of multiple peroxisomal proteins. Group A disorders fall into twelve complementation groups, while the Group B disorders fall into essentially one complementation group, CG11.

The Protein Import Defects in the Peroxisome Biogenesis Disorders

Zellweger syndrome was first described in 1964. Work of Goldfischer and others in 1973 was the first to demonstrate that Zellweger syndrome was linked to peroxisomes (61) (see website chapter 🖥 W-8). They demonstrated that mature peroxisome profiles were absent in micrographs of cells of Zellweger patients. However, this link was ignored, since peroxisomes at that time were thought to have only a minor role in metabolism. Attention was turned back to peroxisomes after it was found that peroxisomes are indispensable for the β-oxidation of very-long-chain fatty acids (62,63) and the biosynthesis of plasmalogens (64,65). The link between Zellweger syndrome and peroxisome dysfunction was firmly established in the late 1980s when it became evident that many cell lines of Zellweger patients harbored peroxisome membrane "ghosts" that resembled peroxisomes but did not contain most matrix proteins (38,66–68). Subsequent work demonstrated that as for yeast *pex* mutants, human mutant cells deficient in peroxisome assembly could be divided into four groups: (a) those affected in PTS1 import only, (b) those affected in PTS2 import only, (c) those affected in both PTS1 and PTS2 import but not peroxisomal membrane protein biogenesis, and (d) those affected in PTS1 and PTS2 import, as well as in the biogenesis of the peroxisomal membrane.

Evolutionary Conservation of *PEX* Genes and Their Role in Human Disease

The demonstration that the molecular mechanisms of protein targeting to peroxisomes and of overall peroxisome assembly had been essentially conserved during evolution suggested that the search for human homologues of the yeast *PEX* genes would identify the genes compromised in the human PBDs. This link between human and yeast genes was firmly established by the identification of the human *PEX5* gene encoding the PTS1 receptor (49–51) by its homology with the *PEX5* gene of the methylotrophic yeast *Pichia pastoris* (30) and the demonstration that deficiency of import of PTS1-containing proteins observed in CG2 of the PBDs, which was similar to the defect observed in *pex5* mutants of *P. pastoris*, could be rescued by functional complementation with the human *PEX5* gene (49,50).

The rapid and continuing identification and characterization of *PEX* genes in different yeast species and the in silico identification of human Expressed Sequence Tags homologous to the yeast *PEX* genes has led to an unprecedented rapid identification of human genes compromised in the PBDs. To date, ten human *PEX* genes have been show to be mutated in different complementation groups of the PBDs (Table 12.1). Of particular note is that the *PEX7* gene encoding the PTS2 receptor is mutated in patients with rhizomelic chondrodysplasia punctata (CG11 of the PBDs, Table 12.1) (55–57) and that the *PEX1* and *PEX6* genes encoding AAA ATPases are mutated in approximately 80% of all Zellweger patients (CG1 and CG4), and disruption of the interaction between Pex1p and Pex6p is the most common cause of the PBDs (69). All the human genes affected in the PBDs have yeast homologues. Since to date 23 *PEX* genes have been identified in various yeast species (Table 12.1), and more are assuredly to be discovered and characterized in the near future with the rapid throughput analysis afforded by the new technologies of global genomics and proteomics, it can be anticipated that in the next few years, all of the genes involved in the human PBDs will be identified, cloned, and characterized. Given this fact, the future direction of research in regards to the PBDs will surely be to define the exact molecular event of peroxisome assembly that is compromised by a particular mutation in a particular *PEX* gene using a combination of in vitro systems that reconstitute peroxisome assembly (44) and transgenic animal models that mimic the PBD phenotype (70).

ACKNOWLEDGMENTS

This work was supported by operating grants from the Medical Research Council of Canada (MRC) to R.A.R. J.J.S. is the recipient of a Studentship from the MRC. R.A.R. is a Senior Scientist of the MRC and an International Research Scholar of the Howard Hughes Medical Institute.

REFERENCES

1. van den Bosch H, Schutgens RBH, Wanders RJA, et al. Biochemistry of peroxisomes. *Annu Rev Biochem* 1992;61:157–197.
2. Subramani S. Protein import into peroxisomes and biogenesis of the organelle. *Annu Rev Cell Biol* 1993;9:445–478.
3. Rhodin J. *Correlation of Ultrastructural Organization and Function in Normal and Experimentally Changed Proximal Convoluted Tubule Cells of the Mouse Kidney.* PhD. Karolinska Institute, Aktiebolaget Godvil, Sweden.
4. de Duve C, Baudhuin P. Peroxisomes (microbodies and related particles). *Physiol Rev* 1966;46:323–357.
5. Gorgas K. Peroxisomes in sebaceous glands V. Complex peroxisomes in the mouse preputial gland: serial sectioning and three-dimensional reconstruction studies. *Anat Embryol* 1984;169:261–270.
6. Gorgas K. Serial section analysis of mouse hepatic peroxisomes. *Anat Embryol* 1985;172:21–32.
7. Yamamoto K, Fahimi HD. Three-dimensional reconstruction of a peroxisomal reticulum in regenerating rat liver: evidence of interconnections between heterogeneous segments. *J Cell Biol* 1987;105:713–722.
8. Kamiryo T, Abe M, Okazaki K, et al. Absence of DNA in peroxisomes of *Candida tropicalis. J Bacteriol* 1982;152:269–274.
9. Lazarow PB, Fujiki Y. Biogenesis of peroxisomes. *Annu Rev Cell Biol* 1985;1:489–530.
10. Subramani S. Components involved in peroxisome import, biogenesis, proliferation, turnover, and movement. *Physiol Rev* 1998;78:171–188.
11. Lazarow PB, de Duve C. A fatty acyl-CoA oxidizing system in rat liver peroxisomes: enhancement by clofibrate, a hypolipidemic drug. *Proc Natl Acad Sci U S A* 1976;73:2043–2046.

12. Fujiki Y, Rachubinski RA, Lazarow PB. Synthesis of a major integral membrane polypeptide of rat liver peroxisomes on free polysomes. *Proc Natl Acad Sci U S A* 1984;81:7127–7131.
13. Reddy JK, Chu R. Peroxisome proliferator-induced pleiotropic responses: pursuit of a phenomenon. *Ann N Y Acad Sci* 1996;804:176–201.
14. Lazarow PB, Moser HW. Disorders of peroxisome biogenesis. In: Scriver CR, Beaudet AL, Sly WS, Valle D, eds. *The metabolic and molecular bases of inherited disease.* New York: McGraw-Hill, 1994;2287–2324.
15. Moser HW, Moser AB. Peroxisomal disorders: overview. *Ann N Y Acad Sci* 1996;804:427–441.
16. Wanders RJA. Peroxisomal disorders: clinical, biochemical and molecular aspects. *Neurochem Res* 1999;24:565–580.
17. de Hoop MJ, Ab G. Import of proteins into peroxisomes and other microbodies. *Biochem J* 1992;286:657–669.
18. Hettema EH, Distel B, Tabak HF. Import of proteins into peroxisomes. *Biochim Biophys Acta* 1999;1451:17–34.
19. Gould SJ, Keller G-A, Hosken N, et al. A conserved tripeptide sorts proteins to peroxisomes. *J Cell Biol* 1989;108:1657–1664.
20. Motley A, Lumb MJ, Oatey PB, et al. Mammalian alanine/glyoxylate aminotransferase 1 is imported into peroxisomes via the PTS1 translocation pathway. Increased degeneracy and context specificity of the mammalian PTS1 motif and implications for the peroxisome-to-mitochondrion mistargeting of AGT in primary hyperoxaluria type 1. *J Cell Biol* 1995;131:95–109.
21. Swinkels BW, Gould SJ, Subramani S. Targeting efficiencies of various permutations of the consensus C-terminal tripeptide peroxisomal targeting signal. *FEBS Lett* 1992;305:133–136.
22. Aitchison JD, Murray WW, Rachubinski RA. The carboxyl-terminal tripeptide Ala-Lys-Ile is essential for targeting *Candida tropicalis* trifunctional enzyme to yeast peroxisomes. *J Biol Chem* 1991;266:23197–23203.
23. Swinkels BW, Gould SJ, Bodnar AG, et al. A novel, cleavable peroxisomal targeting signal at the amino-terminus of the rat 3-ketoacyl-CoA thiolase. *EMBO J* 1991;10:3255–3262.
24. Glover JR, Andrews DW, Subramani S, et al. Mutagenesis of the amino targeting signal of *Saccharomyces cerevisiae* 3-ketoacyl-CoA thiolase reveals conserved amino acids required for import into peroxisomes *in vivo. J Biol Chem* 1994;269:7558–7563.
25. Gould SJ, Keller G-A, Schneider M, et al. Peroxisomal protein import is conserved between yeast, plants, insects and mammals. *EMBO J* 1990;9:85–90.
26. Gould SJ, Krisans S, Keller G-A, et al. Antibodies directed against the peroxisomal targeting signal of firefly luciferase recognize multiple mammalian peroxisomal proteins. *J Cell Biol* 1990;110:27–34.
27. Keller G-A, Krisans S, Gould SJ, et al. Evolutionary conservation of a microbody targeting signal that targets proteins to peroxisomes glyoxysomes and glycosomes. *J Cell Biol* 1991;114:893–904.
28. Small GM, Szabo LJ, Lazarow PB. Acyl-CoA oxidase contains two targeting sequences each of which can mediate protein import into peroxisomes. *EMBO J* 1988;7:1167–1173.
29. Kragler F, Langeder A, Raupachova J, et al. Two independent peroxisomal targeting signals in catalase A of *Saccharomyces cerevisiae. J Cell Biol* 1993;120:665–673.
30. McCollum D, Monosov E, Subramani S. The pas8 mutant of *Pichia pastoris* exhibits the peroxisomal protein import deficiencies of Zellweger syndrome cells—the PAS8 protein binds to the COOH-terminal tripeptide peroxisomal targeting signal, and is a member of the TPR protein family. *J Cell Biol* 1993;121:761–774.
31. Terlecky SR, Nuttley WM, McCollum D, et al. The *Pichia pastoris* peroxisomal protein PAS8p is the receptor for the C-terminal tripeptide peroxisomal targeting signal. *EMBO J* 1995;14:3627–3634.
32. Szilard RK, Titorenko VI, Veenhuis M, et al. Pay32p of the yeast *Yarrowia lipolytica* is an intraperoxisomal component of the matrix protein translocation machinery. *J Cell Biol* 1995;131:1453–1469.

33. Marzioch M, Erdmann R, Veenhuis M, et al. PAS7 encodes a novel yeast member of the WD-40 protein family essential for the import of 3-oxoacyl-CoA thiolase, a PTS2-containing protein, into peroxisomes. *EMBO J* 1994;13:4908–4918.
34. Rehling P, Marzioch M, Niesen F, et al. The import receptor for the peroxisomal targeting signal 2 (PTS2) in *Saccharomyces cerevisiae* is encoded by the PAS7 gene. *EMBO J* 1996;15:2901–2913.
35. Zhang JW, Lazarow PB. Peb1p (Pas7p) is an intraperoxisomal receptor for the NH$_2$-terminal, type 2, peroxisomal targeting signal of thiolase: Peb1p itself is targeted to peroxisomes by an NH$_2$-terminal peptide. *J Cell Biol* 1996;132:325–334.
36. McCammon D, McNew JA, Willy PJ, et al. An internal region of the peroxisomal membrane protein PMP47 is essential for sorting to peroxisomes. *J Cell Biol* 1994;124:915–925.
37. Dyer JM, McNew JA, Goodman JM. The sorting sequence of the peroxisomal integral membrane protein PMP47 is contained within a short hydrophilic loop. *J Cell Biol* 1996;133:269–280.
38. Santos MJ, Imanaka T, Shio H, et al. Peroxisomal membrane ghosts in Zellweger syndrome—aberrant organelle assembly. *Science* 1988;239:1536–1538.
39. Gould SJ, Kalish JE, Morrell JC, et al. Pex13p is an SH3 protein of the peroxisomal membrane and a docking factor for the predominantly cytoplasmic PTS1 receptor. *J Cell Biol* 1996;135:85–95.
40. Elgersma Y, Kwast L, Klein A, et al. The SH3 domain of the peroxisomal membrane protein Pex13p functions as a docking site for Pex5p, a mobile receptor for peroxisomal proteins. *J Cell Biol* 1996;135:97–109.
41. Erdmann R, Blobel G. Identification of Pex13p, a peroxisomal membrane receptor for the PTS1 recognition factor. *J Cell Biol* 1996;135:111–121.
42. Albertini M, Rehling P, Erdmann R, et al. Pex14p, a peroxisomal membrane protein binding both receptors of the two PTS-dependent pathways. *Cell* 1997;89:83–92.
43. Brocard C, Lametschwandtner G, Koudelka R, et al. Pex14p is a member of the protein linkage map of Pex5p. *EMBO J* 1997;16:5491–5500.
44. Titorenko VI, Chan H, Rachubinski RA. Fusion of small peroxisomal vesicles in vitro reconstructs an early step in the in vivo multistep peroxisome assembly pathway of *Yarrowia lipolytica. J Cell Biol* 2000;148:29–43.
45. Marshall PA, Krimkevich YI, Lark RH, et al. Pmp27 promotes peroxisomal proliferation. *J Cell Biol* 1995;129:345–355.
46. Erdmann R, Blobel G. Giant peroxisomes in oleic acid-induced *Saccharomyces cerevisiae* lacking the peroxisomal membrane protein Pmp27p. *J Cell Biol* 1995;128:509–523.
47. Eitzen GA, Szilard RK, Rachubinski RA. Enlarged peroxisomes are present in oleic acid-grown *Yarrowia lipolytica* overexpressing the *PEX16* gene encoding an intraperoxisomal peripheral membrane protein. *J Cell Biol* 1997;137:1265–1278.
48. South ST, Gould SJ. Peroxisome synthesis in the absence of pre-existing peroxisomes. *J Cell Biol* 1999;144:255–266.
49. Wiemer EA, Nuttley WM, Bertolaet BL, et al. Human peroxisomal targeting signal-1 receptor restores peroxisomal protein import in cells from patients with fatal peroxisomal disorders. *J Cell Biol* 1995;130:51–65.
50. Dodt G, Braverman N, Wong C, et al. Mutations in the PTS1 receptor gene, *PXR1*, define complementation group 2 of the peroxisome biogenesis disorders. *Nature Genet* 1995;9:115–125.
51. Fransen M, Brees C, Basumgart E, et al. Identification and characterization of the putative human peroxisomal C-terminal targeting signal import receptor. *J Biol Chem* 1995;270:7731–7736.
52. Dodt G, Gould SJ. Multiple *PEX* genes are required for proper

53. Rachubinski RA, Subramani S. How proteins penetrate peroxisomes. *Cell* 1995;83:525–528.
54. Nuttley WM, Szilard RK, Smith JJ, et al. The *PAH2* gene is required for peroxisome assembly in the methylotrophic yeast *Hansenula polymorpha* and encodes a member of the tetratricopeptide repeat family of proteins. *Gene* 1995;160:33–39.
55. Motley A, Hettema E, Hogenhout EM, et al. Rhizomelic chondrodysplasia punctata is a peroxisomal targeting disease caused by a non-functional PTS2 receptor. *Nature Genet* 1997;15:377–380.
56. Braverman N, Steel G, Obie C, et al. Human PEX7 encodes the peroxisomal PTS2 receptor and is responsible for rhizomelic chondrodysplasia punctata. *Nature Genet* 1997;15:369–376.
57. Purdue PE, Zhang JW, Skoneczy M, et al. Rhizomelic chondrodysplasia punctata is caused by deficiency of human Pex7p, a homologue of the yeast PTS2 receptor. *Nature Genet* 1997;15:381–384.
58. Zhang JW, Lazarow PB. PEB1 (PAS7) in *Saccharomyces cerevisiae* encodes a hydrophilic, intra-peroxisomal protein that is a member of the WD repeat family and is essential for the import of thiolase into peroxisomes. *J Cell Biol* 1995;129:65–80.
59. Shimizu N, Itoh R, Hirono Y, et al. The peroxin Pex14p. cDNA cloning by functional complementation on a Chinese hamster ovary cell mutant, characterization, and functional analysis. *J Biol Chem* 1999;274:12593–12604.
60. Girzalsky W, Rehling P, Stein K, et al. Involvement of Pex13p in Pex14p localization and peroxisomal targeting signal 2-dependent protein import into peroxisomes. *J Cell Biol* 1999;144:1151–1162.
61. Goldfischer S, Moore CL, Johnson AB, et al. Peroxisomal and mitochondrial defects in the cerebro-hepato-renal syndrome. *Science* 1973;182:62–64.
62. Brown FR, McAdams AJ, Cummins JW, et al. Cerebro-hepato-renal (Zellweger) syndrome and neonatal adrenoleukodystrophy: similarities in phenotype and accumulation of very long chain fatty acids. *Johns Hopkins Med J* 1982;151:344–351.
63. Singh I, Moser AE, Goldfischer S, et al. Lignoceric acid is oxidized in the peroxisome: implications for the Zellweger cerebro-hepato-renal syndrome and adrenoleukodystrophy. *Proc Natl Acad Sci U S A* 1984;81:4203–4207.
64. Hajra AK, Burke CL, Jones CL. Subcellular localization of acyl coenzyme A: dihydroxyacetone phosphate acyltransferase in rat liver peroxisomes (microbodies). *J Biol Chem* 1979;254:10896–10900.
65. Heymans HAS, Schutgens RBH, Tan R, et al. Severe plasmalogen deficiency in tissues of infants without peroxisomes (Zellweger syndrome). *Nature* 1983;306:69–70.
66. Wanders RJA, Schutgens RBH, Tager JM. Peroxisomal matrix enzymes in Zellweger syndrome: activity and subcellular localization in liver. *J Inher Metab Dis* 1985;8:151–152.
67. Schram AW, Strijland A, Hashimoto T, et al. Biosynthesis and maturation of peroxisomal B-oxidation enzymes in fibroblasts in relation to the Zellweger syndrome and infantile Refsum's disease. *Proc Natl Acad Sci U S A* 1986;83:6156–6158.
68. Santos MJ, Imanaka T, Shio H, et al. Peroxisomal integral membrane proteins in control and Zellweger fibroblasts. *J Biol Chem* 1988;263:10502–10509.
69. Geisbrecht BV, Collins CS, Reuber BE, et al. Disruption of a PEX1-PEX6 interaction is the most common cause of the neurologic disorders Zellweger syndrome, neonatal adrenoleukodystrophy, and infantile Refsum disease. *Proc Natl Acad Sci U S A* 1998;95:8630–8635.
70. Baes M, Gressens P, Baumgart E, et al. A mouse model for Zellweger syndrome. *Nature Genet* 1997;17:49–57.

The Liver: Biology and Pathobiology, Fourth Edition, edited by I. M. Arias, J. L. Boyer, F. V. Chisari, N. Fausto, D. Schachter, and D. A. Shafritz. Lippincott Williams & Wilkins, Philadelphia © 2001.

13

INTEGRATED CELL FUNCTION: APOPTOSIS

MARTINA MÜLLER
PETER H. KRAMMER

APOPTOSIS—HISTORICAL ASPECTS

Programmed cell death was discovered by C. Vogt in the middle of the 19th century (1) by the morphology of dying cells during the metamorphosis of amphibians. Before the term apoptosis was coined (2), the morphological appearance of this mode of cell death in the liver had been known as shrinkage necrosis, Councilman bodies (3), chromatolysis, acidophilic bodies, or eosinophilic single-cell necrosis, and apoptotic shrinkage of the chromatin, described as pyknosis (4–10). The earliest description of hepatic apoptosis dates back to 1890 with the characterization of histopathology due to yellow fever (3). Strong interest in hepatic apoptosis developed in the 1960s, and the state of the art at that time is compiled in the milestone review by Kerr (2). First evidence of intracellular mechanisms characteristic of apoptosis was found in 1970, when Williams described oligonucleosomal DNA fragmentation in embryonic liver (11).

APOPTOSIS—MORPHOLOGY

The apoptotic program is present in latent form in virtually all cell types throughout the body. A coordinated and inter-

M. Müller: Department of Internal Medicine IV, University Hospital, Hepatology and Gastroenterology, 69115 Heidelberg, Germany.

P. H. Krammer: Department of Immunogenetics, German Cancer Research Center, 69120 Heidelberg, Germany.

TABLE 13.1. HUMAN LIVER DISEASES IN WHICH DYSREGULATION OF APOPTOSIS OCCURS

Increased Apoptosis	Decreased Apoptosis
Viral hepatitis B, C, and D	Hepatocellular carcinoma
Alcohol-induced hepatitis	Cholangiocarcinoma
Autoimmune hepatitis	
Ischemia reperfusion injury	
Primary biliary cirrhosis	
Primary sclerosing cholangitis	
Wilson's disease	

nally programmed series of events takes place in cells doomed to die in a variety of biologically significant situations. Among these are the sculpting of tissues during development, endocrine-dependent atrophy, selection of specific immunologically competent subpopulations in both T- and B-cell lineages during the response to antigen, and cytotoxic T-lymphocyte killing. Identical changes are also observed in normal and tumor tissues exposed to low or moderate doses of chemotherapeutic agents or ionizing radiation. Apoptosis is involved in many physiological processes, and there is hardly any disease whose pathogenesis can be explained without apoptosis, either too much or too little of it (reviewed in ref.12)(13) (see Chapter 15). Human liver diseases in which dysregulation of apoptosis occurs are listed in Table 13.1.

Once triggered by a variety of physiologic or pathophysiologic signals, the apoptotic program unfolds in a defined series of steps. The morphological changes themselves include shrinkage of cell volume accompanied by dilatation of endoplasmic reticulum and convolution of the plasma

membrane. The cell breaks up into a series of membrane-bound, nearly spherical bodies containing structurally normal but compacted organelles, and the nucleus undergoes profound, initially discontinuous chromatin condensation around the nuclear periphery (12). The ultimate fate of apoptotic cells in tissues varies. Some are phagocytosed. Others lose contact with their neighbors and basement membrane and so float into adjacent spaces. There is no acute inflammatory reaction.

Almost all of this contrasts with the changes that occur in *necrosis* (Table 13.2). Necrosis is observed in acute, high-dose toxicological exposure or severe hypoxia. Here, the injured cells swell, their plasma membranes breaking to release proinflammatory material from the cell interior into the extracellular space. The term apoptosis was originally coined to emphasize the difference between the two modes of death and to point up the hypothesis that the stereotyped morphology of apoptosis represents a common underlying mechanism (2,12). The cellular and molecular events in apoptosis are the subject of the first part of this chapter. The existence of a common mechanism of death implies that defects in such a mechanism might lead to the inappropriate survival of damaged cells that could lead to diseases and to cancer. This is discussed in the latter part of the chapter.

DEATH RECEPTORS AND LIGANDS

The growing subfamily of death receptors is part of the TNF/NGF-receptor superfamily (Table 13.3). This receptor superfamily is characterized by a sequence of two to five cysteine-rich extracellular repeats. The death receptors have

TABLE 13.2. DISTINGUISHING FEATURES OF APOPTOSIS AND NECROSIS

	Apoptosis	Necrosis
Nucleus	Condensation of chromatin	Condensation (pyknosis) at initial stages
	Disintegration into sharply delineated spherical chromatin masses	Later disintegration (karyorrhexis) and dissolution (karyolysis)
Cytoplasm	Condensation of cytosol	Edematous swelling of organelles
	Packing of intact organelles	Rupture of intracellular membranes
	Pronounced autophagic vacuolization	
Tissue distribution	Mostly affecting scattered single cells	Contiguous groups of cells are affected
	Detachment of apoptotic cells from neighboring cells and rounding up	
Plasma membrane	Loss of microvilli	Blebbing, leading to rupture of plasma and spillage of intracellular contents
	Blebbing (zeiosis)	
	Rapid loss of lipid asymmetry	
DNA fragmentation	Characteristic high molecular weight DNA fragmentation into 50-kbp and 300-kbp fragments	Random DNA degradation
	Oligonucleosomal cleavage into n × 180-bp DNA fragments	
Phagocytosis	Removal by professional phagocytes and by neighboring cells	Removal of necrotic tissue by infiltrating phagocytes after disintegration of cells
Tissue reaction	Inconspicuous	Inflammatory response
	Often apoptosis necessary for tissue organization	Leukocyte infiltration

TABLE 13.3. THE TNF RECEPTOR SUPERFAMILY

Receptor	Alternative Nomenclature	Reference(s)
CD95	APO-1, Fas	161,162
TNF-R1	CD120a	163–165
TNF-R2	CD120b	166
CD40		167
CD30		168
CD27		169
OX-40		170
ILA	4-1BB	171
NGF-R		172
DR3	APO-3, Wsl, TRAMP, LARD	173–177
HVEM	ATAR, TR2	178–180
GITR		181
TACI		182
TRAIL-R1	DR4, APO-2	129,183
TRAIL-R2	DR5, KILLER, TRICK2	130,184–186
TRAIL-R3	DR6, DcR1, LIT, TRID	130,131,185,187,188
TRAIL-R4	DcR2, TRUNDD	176,189,190
DR6		191
RANK		192
TR6	DcR3	20,21
OPG		193
AITR		194
BCMA		195

an intracellular death domain (DD), which is essential for transduction of the apoptotic signal. Six members of this subfamily are known so far: TNF-R1 (CD120a), CD95 (APO-1/Fas), DR3 (APO-3, LARD, TRAMP, WSL1), TRAIL-R1 (APO-2, DR4), TRAIL-R2 (DR5, KILLER, TRICK2), and DR6 (14) (Table 13.3, Fig. 13.1). Among

these, CD95 is the best characterized death receptor (13,15).

Death receptors are activated through their natural ligands, which have coevolved as a death ligand family corresponding to the death receptors, called the TNF family (Table 13.4 and Fig. 13.1). Except for LTα, the death ligands are type II transmembrane proteins of which a soluble form can be generated by the activity of metalloproteases. Several groups reported activity of the soluble CD95L (13), whereas others ascribe the capacity to induce apoptosis to the membrane-bound form (16,17). The role of soluble and membrane bound CD95L remains to be shown *in vivo*.

Normally a ligand binds to its special receptor. For TRAIL, however, five receptors have been published so far. For TNF receptors, the situation is almost equally complex. The soluble forms of TNFα and LTα bind to both TNF receptors; the soluble TNFα, however, shows a higher affinity to TNF-R1 than the membrane form of TNFα to TNF-R2. Furthermore, LTα, in combination with transmembrane LTB, binds as a heterotrimer to the LTB-R (18,19).

Closely related to the death receptors are the so called "decoy" receptors (Table 13.3, Fig. 13.1). These are TRAIL-R3 (DcR-1, LIT, TRID), TRAIL-R4 (DcR-2, TRUNDD), OPG, and DcR-3 (TR6). DcR-3 (TR6) binds to CD95L and LIGHT (20,21), the others to TRAIL (22). So far, no correlation between expression of TRAIL-R3 or TRAIL-R4 and resistance to TRAIL-induced apoptosis has been shown (23,24). Thus, it remains to be elucidated whether these receptors really function as decoys.

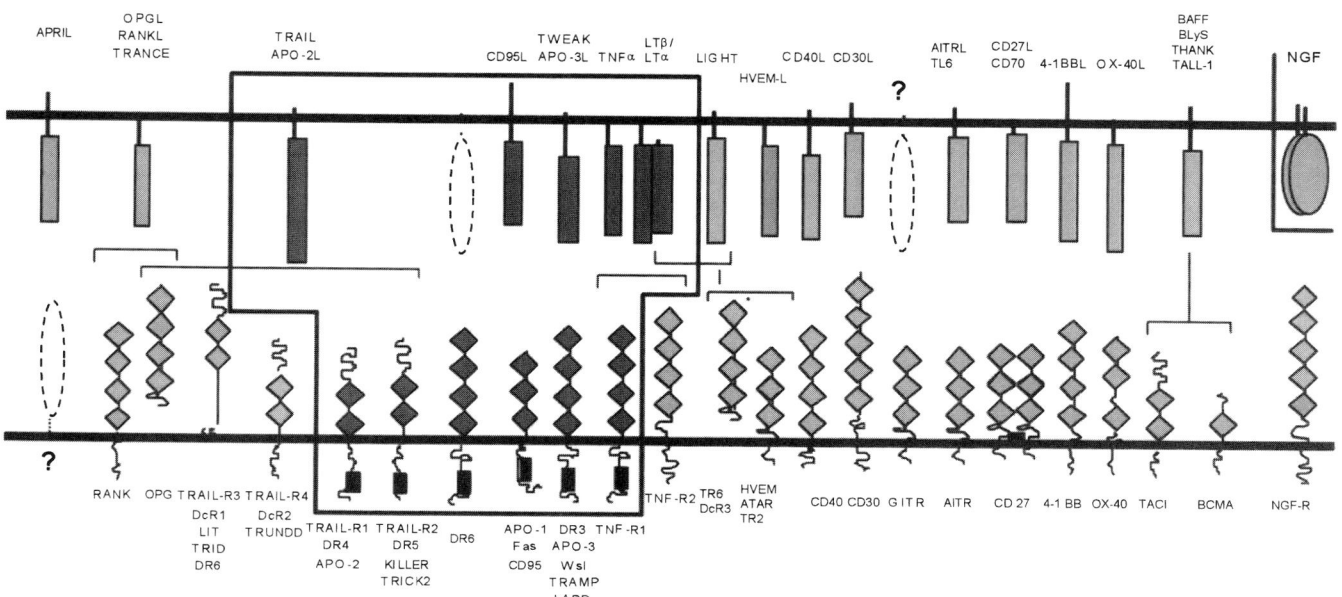

FIGURE 13.1. Death receptors and death ligands. Ligands are shown at the top, receptors at the bottom. Death receptors and death ligands are designated in *dark gray* and grouped in a box. Homologues, including decoy receptors, are shown in *light gray*.

TABLE 13.4. THE TNF FAMILY

Ligand	Alternative Nomenclature	Reference(s)
CD95L	FasL, APO-1L	196
TNFα	DIF Cachexin	197–199
LTα	TNFβ	200
LTβ		201
CD40L	TRAP, gp39	202–204
CD30L		205
CD27L	CD70	206
OX-40L	gp34, TXGP1	207
4-1BBL		208
TWEAK	APO-3L	209,210
LIGHT		211
TRAIL	APO-2L	125,137
RANKL	OPGL, TRANCE	192,212–214
APRIL		215
BAFF	TALL-1 THANK BLyS	216–218
HVEM-L		219
AITRL		194

TABLE 13.5. THE CASPASE FAMILY

Caspase	Alternative Nomenclature	Reference(s)
Caspase-1	ICE	220,211
Caspase-2	ICH-1, Nedd-2	222,223
Caspase-3	CPP-32, Yama, Apopain	224–226
Caspase-4	ICH-2, TX, ICE-rel-II	227–229
Caspase-5	ICE-rel-III, TY	229,230
Caspase-6	Mch2	231
Caspase-7	Mch3, ICE-LAP3, CMH-1	232–234
Caspase-8	FLICE, MACH, Mch5	75,76,235
Caspase-9	Mch6, ICE-LAP6	236,237
Caspase-10	Mch4, FLICE2	235,238
mCaspase-11	mICH-3, mCASP-11	239,240
mCaspase-12	mCASP-12	240
Caspase-13	ERICE	241
Caspase-14		61,242,243

CASPASES

Caspases are a growing family of cysteine proteases (Table 13.5, Fig. 13.2) (25). Caspases are crucial for execution of apoptosis, since inhibition of caspases by zVAD-fmk, a broad-spectrum caspase inhibitor, does not prevent death but results in necrosis rather than apoptosis (26). So far, 14 mammalian caspases are known which can be subdivided into three families based on their sequence homology and substrate specificity (27). Two "gatekeeper" caspases, caspase-8 and caspase-9, are activated by death receptors such as CD95 or by the cytochrome *c* released from mitochondria (see Role of Mitochondria, below). These proximal caspases trigger the activation of downstream effector caspases that execute the death program through selective destruction of subcellular structures and organelles, and of the genome.

Caspases are synthesized as proenzymes (zymogens) that are activated by proteolytic cleavage. The active enzyme is a heterotetrameric complex of two large subunits containing the active site and two small subunits, as deduced from the crystal structure of caspase-1 and caspase-3 (28–30). Activation of caspases has been reported for a variety of apoptotic stimuli, including signal transduction through the death receptors (13). A number of recent knockout mice have demonstrated the important role of caspases in apoptosis and development (31,32).

The activity of caspases characterizes the execution phase of apoptosis. Therefore, the search for substrates cleaved by caspases during apoptosis should provide insight into the more downstream events in apoptosis signaling. Several of these so-called "death substrates" are known (Table 13.6). First, caspases can cleave and activate other caspases as described earlier. Second, molecules involved in DNA repair, such as poly (ADP-ribose) polymerase (PARP) or the

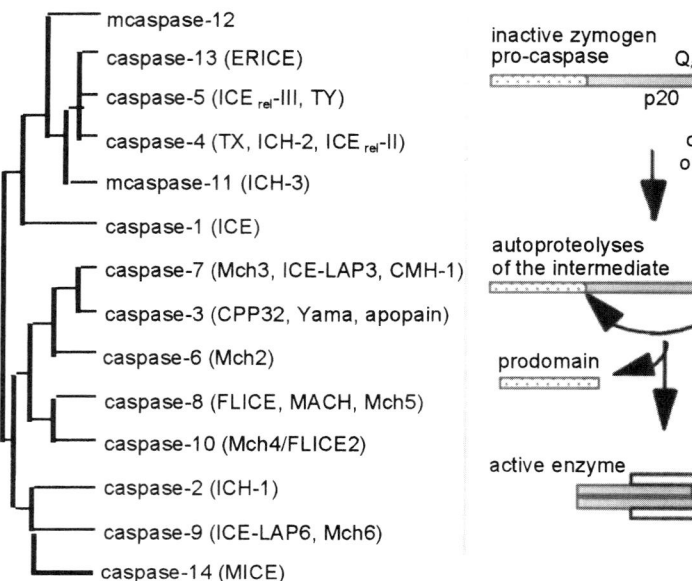

FIGURE 13.2. The caspase family. All known mammalian caspases are listed by numbers. Synonyms are indicated. Caspases are synthesized as proenzymes (zymogens) that are activated by proteolytic cleavage. The active enzyme is a heterotetrameric complex of two large subunits containing the active site and two small subunits.

TABLE 13.6. SELECTION OF CASPASE SUBSTRATES

Group	Substrate	Reference(s)
I	PARP	33
	DNA-PK	35
	U1-70kDa	37
	C1 and C2	39
II	PKCδ	42
	PAK2	244
	SREBP-1, SREBP-2	41
	cPLA$_2$	245
	PITSLRE kinase α2-1	46
III	Lamin A and B	47
		48
		49
	Fodrin	50
		51
	Gas2	52

catalytic subunit of the DNA-dependent protein kinase (DNA-PK), were described to be cleaved and thereby inactivated by downstream caspase-3-like caspases (33–36). Furthermore, the ribonucleoproteins U1-70kDa C1 and C2, components responsible for the splicing reaction of precursor mRNA, are inactivated by cleavage through caspases (37–39). Thus, caspases may inactivate cellular processes that prevent apoptosis from proceeding.

Another set of death substrates contains molecules that are involved in the regulation of other signaling processes. One example is the sterol regulatory element-binding proteins SREBP-1 and SREBP-2 that are cleaved by caspase-3 or -7 (40,41). The delta isoform of protein kinase C (PKCδ) is a target for caspases during CD95- or TNF-R-mediated apoptosis (42,43). The PISTLRE kinase, a member of a superfamily of cdc2-like kinases, is also cleaved by caspases during CD95-induced apoptosis. This is accompanied by increased activity of this kinase and may lead to apoptosis (44–46). Therefore, the cleavage of these signaling molecules may be involved in the downstream execution of apoptosis.

Another set of death substrates are structural proteins of the cell. Thus, lamin cleavage by caspase-6 may occur during TNF-R- and CD95-induced apoptosis (47–49). Similarly, α-fodrin is cleaved during apoptosis induced by CD95 or by TNF-R1 triggering (50,51). Gas2, a component of the microfilament system, was reported to be cleaved on induction of apoptosis (52). Therefore, cleavage of these structural proteins may account for some of the massive morphological changes such as membrane blebbing, nuclear fragmentation, and the formation of apoptotic bodies during apoptosis.

Taken together, the number of caspase substrates identified should increase in the future, and further studies are necessary to identify crucial targets for caspases that establish the link between caspase activation and more downstream events in apoptosis.

BCL-2 FAMILY

Bcl-2 family members can be divided into apoptotic proteins (e.g., Bcl-2 and Bcl-x$_L$) and proapoptotic proteins (e.g., Bax and Bak (Table 13.7)). The Bcl-2 family is characterized by different homologous α-helical amino acid stretches called Bcl-2 homology (BH) domains and known as BH1-4. The antiapoptotic group of proteins of the Bcl-2 family is characterized by the BH4 domain, whereas the BH3 domain is crucial for the induction of apoptosis. This is illustrated by a subgroup of the proapoptotic Bcl-2 family members, the BH3 domain-only proteins (e.g., Bid, Bad, and Bim) (53).

Although the impact of Bcl-2 family members on apoptosis is quite obvious, the biochemical mechanism of their function is unclear. Several models have been postulated to explain apoptosis promoting and inhibiting functions. The first model was based on the heterodimerization properties of the family members and suggested that the ratio between pro- and antiapoptotic family members determines cell fate (53). However, the scenario became more complex when mitochondria joined the apoptotic play. Some family members share a transmembrane domain (e.g., Bcl-2, Bcl-x$_L$, Bak, Bax) which targets these proteins to intracellular membranes like the endoplasmic reticulum, the nuclear envelope and the mitochondrium (see Role of Mitochondria, below). Research focuses on the latter. Bcl-2 family members can regulate opening of the so-called permeability transition (PT) pore. Bax and Bcl-2 interact with proteins of the PT pore complex (53). In addition, Bcl-x$_L$ and Bid are structurally similar to pore-forming bacterial toxins (54–58), and Bcl-2, Bcl-x$_L$, Bid, and Bax are able to form pores in artificial membranes (59,60). However, the connection between PT pore, loss of the mitochondrial transmembrane potential and the release of apoptogenic factors (see Role of Mitochondria, below) is not well defined.

Another hypothesis for the antiapoptotic function of Bcl-2 and Bcl-x$_L$ is the interaction with the so-called apoptosome. The active apoptosome consists of the adapter protein Apaf1, cytochrome *c*, and caspase-9. Apaf1 was shown to bind to Bcl-x$_L$ in overexpression systems (61,62). However, this issue is controversial and could not be confirmed with endogenous proteins (63).

TABLE 13.7. REGULATION OF APOPTOSIS BY THE BCL-2 FAMILY OF PROTEINS

Inhibit Apoptosis	Promote Apoptosis
Bcl-2	Bax
Bcl-x$_L$	Bak
Bcl-w	Bcl-x$_s$
Mcl-I	Bag
Bfl-I	Bid
Brag-I	Bik
AI	Hrk
	Bad
	Bim

ROLE OF MITOCHONDRIA

Many of the signals that induce apoptosis converge on the mitochondria. The regulatory mechanisms underlying apoptosis and necrosis partially overlap in that selective mitochondrial membrane permeabilization may constitute a common event of both death modalities (53,64–66). For mitochondrial membrane permeabilization, three phases of cell death can be distinguished: initiation, decision and degradation (Fig. 13.3). During the initiation phase, cells accumulate effector molecules which directly act on mitochondria to cause mitochondrial membrane permeabilization. The nature of these effectors depends on the death-inducing stimulus, implying a great diversity of mechanisms. During the decision phase, mitochondrial membrane permeabilization occurs, and determines the cell's fate. The metabolic consequences of mitochondrial membrane permeabilization as well as the leakage of proteins normally confined to mitochondria determine the features of cell death with irreversible loss of cellular functions and/or activation of nucleases and proteases (degradation).

Mitochondria are organelles with two well defined compartments: the matrix, surrounded by the inner membrane, and the intermembrane space, surrounded by the outer membrane. The inner membrane is folded into numerous christae, which greatly increase its surface area. It contains the protein complexes from the electron transport chain, the ATP synthase and the adenine nucleotide translocator. To function properly, the inner membrane is almost impermeable in physiological conditions, thereby allowing the respiratory chain to create an electrochemical gradient ($\Delta\Psi$). Apoptotic outer membrane permeabilization involves the release of proteins

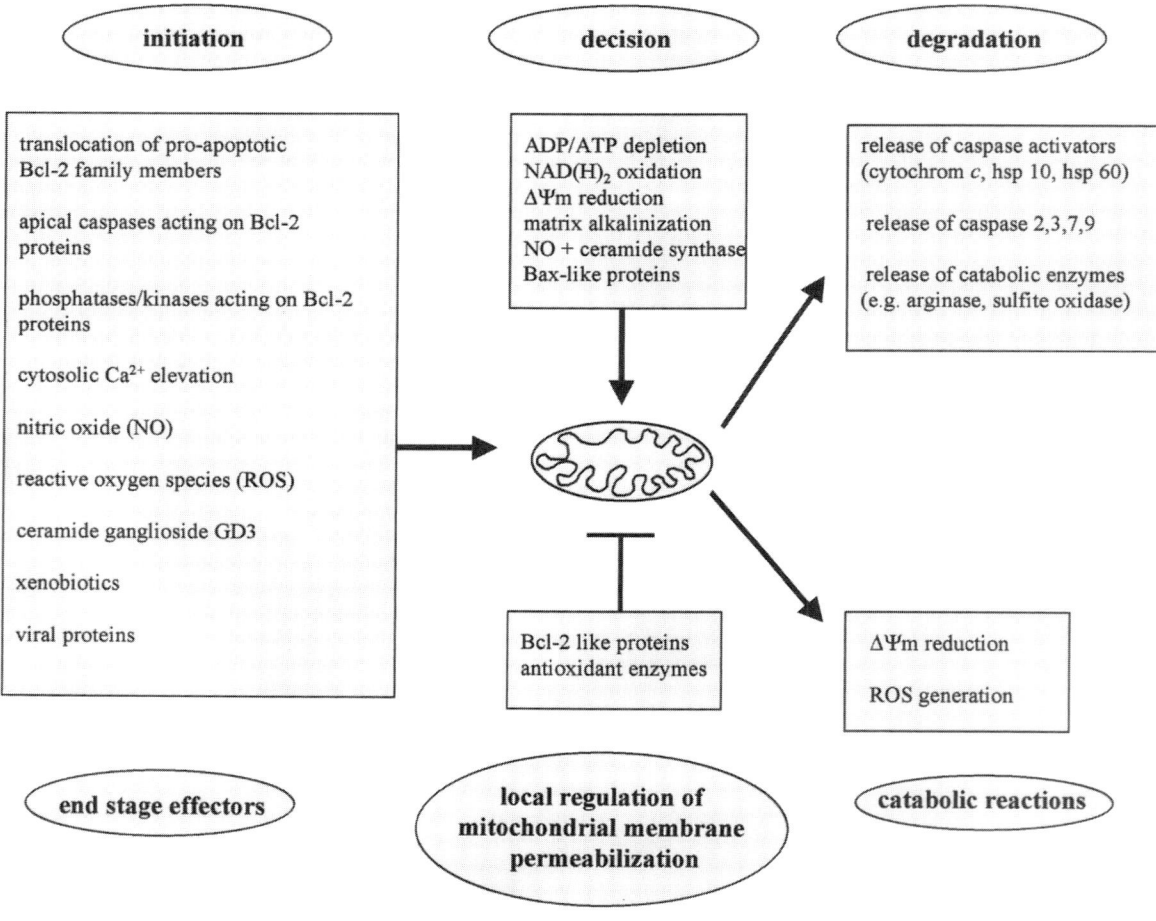

FIGURE 13.3. Involvement of mitochondria in cell death. For mitochondrial membrane permeabilization, three phases can be distinguished: initiation, decision and degradation (modified according to Kroemer G and Reed JC. Mitochondrial control of cell death. *Nature Medicine* 2000; 6:513, with permission). During the initiation phase, effector molecules act directly on mitochondria to cause mitochondrial membrane permeabilization. During the decision phase, mitochondrial membrane permeabilization occurs. This leads to loss of cellular functions and/or activation of nucleases and proteases (degradation).

which are normally confined to the intermembrane space of these organelles, including cytochrome *c*, certain pro-caspases, adenylate kinase 2, and apoptosis-inducing factor.

Permeabilization of the inner membrane leads to increasing permeability to solutes up to about 1,500 Da, and is manifested as a dissipation of the proton gradient responsible for the transmembrane potential ($\Delta\Psi_m$), an extrusion of small solutes (i.e., calcium and glutathione), or an influx of water and sucrose.

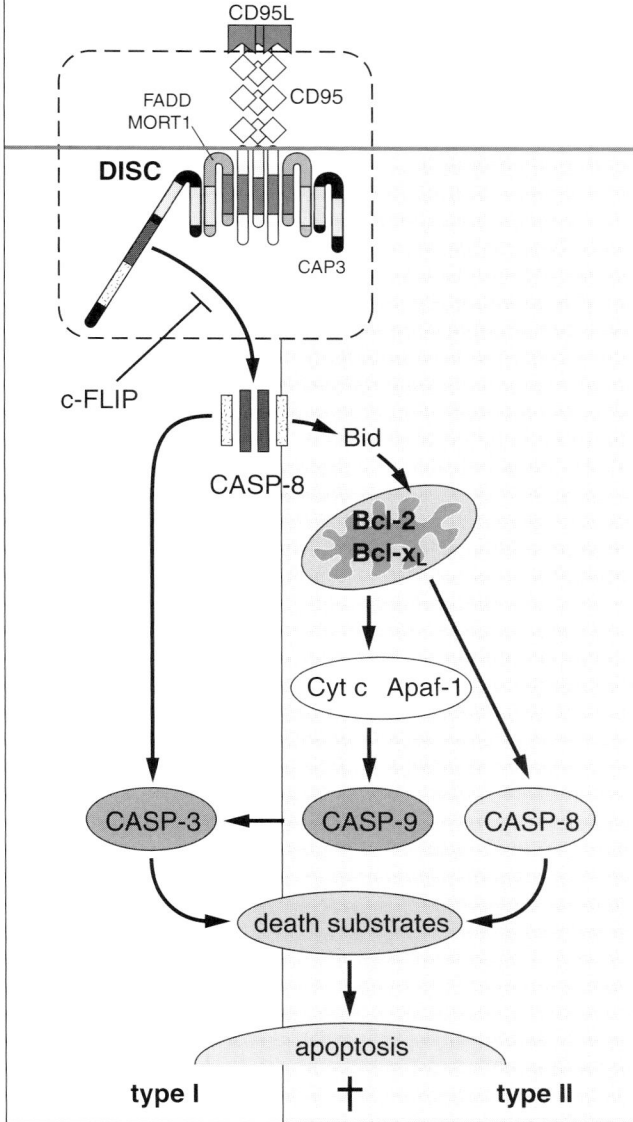

FIGURE 13.4. Two CD95 signaling pathways. Two cell types that each preferably use one of two different CD95 signaling pathways have been identified, termed type I and type II. In type I cells, the induction of apoptosis is accompanied by the activation of large amounts of caspase-8 by the DISC, followed by the rapid cleavage of caspase-3 prior to loss of mitochondrial transmembrane potential ($\Delta\Psi_m$), suggesting activation of a direct caspase cascade. In type II cells, DISC formation is strongly reduced and activation of caspase-8 and of caspase-3 occurs following the loss of $\Delta\Psi_m$.

Mitochondria manifest signs of outer membrane and/or inner membrane permeabilization when exposed to a variety of second messengers. Proapoptotic members of the Bcl-2 family of proteins act in part by governing mitochondrial death signaling. Induction of mitochondrial membrane permeabilization has been shown for Bax, Bak, and Bid (64) and probably, as discussed earlier, reflects a principal mechanism by which these proteins trigger cell death (67–71). For example, cytosolic Bid is cleaved by caspase-8, the apical caspase activated through ligation of tumor necrosis factor family death receptors (Fig. 13.4). The truncated cleavage product (tBid) translocates to mitochondrial membranes. Bid$^{-/-}$ mice are resistant to hepatocyte apoptosis induced by antibody against CD95, emphasizing the importance of this pathway for CD95/caspase-8 signaling in hepatocytes (72).

THE CD95 APOPTOSIS SYSTEM

Triggering of CD95 by either agonistic antibodies or CD95L leads to trimerization of CD95 receptors (Fig. 13.4). Subsequently, the adaptor molecule Fas-associated death domain (FADD)/Mort-1 (73,74), pro-caspase-8 (FLICE, MACH, MCH5) (75,76), and CAP3 (77), an as yet uncharacterized molecule, are recruited to oligomerized CD95, forming a death-inducing signaling complex (DISC) (77). Pro-caspase-8 is autoproteolytically cleaved at the DISC (57,78). Thereby, the active tetramer of caspase-8 is formed and the apoptosis signal is initiated.

Two cell types that each preferably use one of two different CD95 signaling pathways have been identified, termed type I and type II (79) (Fig. 13.4). In type I cells, the induction of apoptosis was accompanied by the activation of large amounts of caspase-8 by the DISC, followed by the rapid cleavage of caspase-3 prior to loss of mitochondrial transmembrane potential ($\Delta\Psi_m$), suggesting activation of a direct caspase cascade. In contrast, in type II cells DISC formation was strongly reduced and activation of caspase-8 and caspase-3 occurred following the loss of $\Delta\Psi_m$. Thus, in type II cell mitochondria are used as "amplifiers" to initiate the executionary apoptosis caspase cascade. It is still not completely clear how mitochondria are activated in both type I and type II cells. The BH3 domain-containing Bcl-2 family member Bid has been suggested to fulfill this function (80,81). Bid is a substrate of caspase-8 which is activated in low amounts at the DISC of type II cells. Cleaved and truncated Bid translocates to the mitochondria and induces loss of $\Delta\Psi_m$ and release of apoptogenic factors like cytochrome *c* (82–85). In the cytosol, cytochrome *c* binds to Apaf1, which then recruits caspase-9 (86,87). At this so-called "apoptosome" pro-caspase-9 is autocatalytically processed to the mature enzyme and initiates a caspase cascade downstream of the mitochondrium (88,89).

In both type I and type II cells, mitochondria were activated equally upon CD95 triggering. In both cell types, apoptogenic activities of mitochondria were blocked by Bcl-2 overexpression. However, in type II cells only, Bcl-2 overexpression blocked caspase-8 and caspase-3 activation as well as apoptosis. Thus, in type II cells, CD95-mediated apoptosis is dependent and in type I cells it is independent of mitochondrial activity.

Recent studies in genetically targeted mice support the possibility that the usage of type I and type II pathways is determined by tissue specificity. Hepatocytes from $Bid^{-/-}$ mice have been shown to be relatively resistant to CD95-mediated death, yet thymocytes from $Bid^{-/-}$ mice were shown in the same study to be sensitive to CD95-mediated cell death (72). This suggests that thymocytes use the type I pathway whereas hepatocytes utilize the type II pathway.

ROLE OF THE CD95/CD95L SYSTEM IN LIVER HOMEOSTASIS

CD95 is expressed in the developing (90) and the mature (91) liver. Primary hepatocytes from mice (92) and humans (93) were demonstrated to be sensitive toward CD95-mediated apoptosis *in vitro*. A physiological role of CD95 in maintaining liver homeostasis has been suggested as mice deficient in CD95 develop increased cellularity and substantial liver hyperplasia (94).

CD95 IN LIVER DISEASE

The striking finding of acute hepatic failure in mice on CD95 triggering (95) has stimulated general interest in the involvement of CD95-mediated apoptosis in human liver disease.

The liver is highly sensitive to induction of apoptosis by the agonistic antibody anti-APO-1. Mice injected intraperitoneally with 10 to 100 μg anti-Fas died within several hours (95). Biochemical, histologic, and electron microscopic analyses revealed severe liver damage by apoptosis as the most likely cause of death. Subsequent studies have confirmed and extended these data. Transgenic mice expressing human Bcl-2 were protected from CD95-mediated cytotoxicity (96), in contrast to their nontransgenic counterparts. Likewise, Bcl-2 expression under control of the α1-antitrypsin promoter prevented hepatic destruction after antibody treatment. However, it did not delay death of the animals, demonstrating involvement of other organs in addition to the liver in CD95-mediated death (97).

Recent experimental data point to the involvement of the CD95 system in toxic liver damage. In alcoholic cirrhosis, hepatocytes were demonstrated to produce high levels of CD95L mRNA. Since hepatocytes bear the CD95 and are highly sensitive to CD95 stimulation (93,95) one CD95L-expressing hepatocyte might kill the other by induction of apoptosis. Similar data have been obtained for cytostatic agents *in vitro* (98) but also for copper-loaded hepatocytes in Wilson disease (99). Furthermore, involvement of the CD95

system in viral liver disease was shown (93). Thus, activation of the CD95 receptor and ligand system might represent a universal response of hepatocytes to toxic injury, eventually resulting in removal of damaged cells by apoptosis.

REGULATION OF APOPTOSIS SIGNALING

Apoptosis can be modulated directly at the death receptor level. The glycosylation status of CD95 has been shown to modulate CD95-mediated apoptosis (100). Inside the cell, apoptosis can be modulated on different levels. So-called inhibitors of apoptosis (IAPs) directly inhibit caspases (101). Other intracellular regulators of apoptosis include FLICE-inhibitory proteins (FLIPs), chaperones, and related proteins and kinases.

FLIPs (FLICE-Inhibitory Proteins)

An entire family of death effector domain-containing proteins has been found in the data bases. Some of those proteins are encoded by class γ herpes viruses such as herpes virus Saimiri (HVS), by human herpes virus 8 (HHV 8), a Karposi sarcoma-associated herpes virus, and by moluscum contagiosum (102). The proteins have been called viral FLICE inhibitory proteins (v-FLIPs). v-FLIPs consist of two DEDs, and a biochemical analysis of v-FLIP-transfected cells showed that they bind to the CD95/FADD complex and thus inhibit the recruitment of caspase-8 and a functional DISC formation. In transfected cells, v-FLIP was capable of inhibiting apoptosis induced by several apoptosis-inducing receptors (CD95, TNF-R1, DR3, and TRAIL-R1). This suggests that these receptors use similar signaling pathways. A human homologue of v-FLIP is called c-FLIP/FLAME-1/I-FLICE/Casper/CASH/MRIT/CLARP/Usurpin. c-FLIP occurs in two forms, a short form and a long form. The short form structurally resembles v-FLIP. The long form contains domains similar to caspase-8 but an inactive enzymatic site and interferes with the generation of active caspase-8 subunits at the receptor level (103,104) (Fig. 13.5). In addition to CD95-mediated apoptosis, c-FLIP inhibits anti-CD3-induced cell death (105). It was suggested that resistance towards TRAIL-induced apoptosis in melanoma cell lines correlates with the expression of c-FLIP (23). However, this issue is controversial (24). In contrast to death receptor-mediated apoptosis, cell death induced by γ-irradiation, chemotherapeutic drugs, and perforin/granzyme B cannot be inhibited by c-FLIP (105).

Recent studies reveal that FLIPs might play a role in tumorigenesis. In Epstein–Barr virus, transformed B-cell resistance and sensitivity towards CD95-mediated death correlate with the ratio of c-FLIP and caspase-8 (106). Moreover, tumor cells transfected with human herpes virus 8-encoded v-FLIP or with murine c-FLIP$_{long}$ have a growth advantage *in vivo* (107,108).

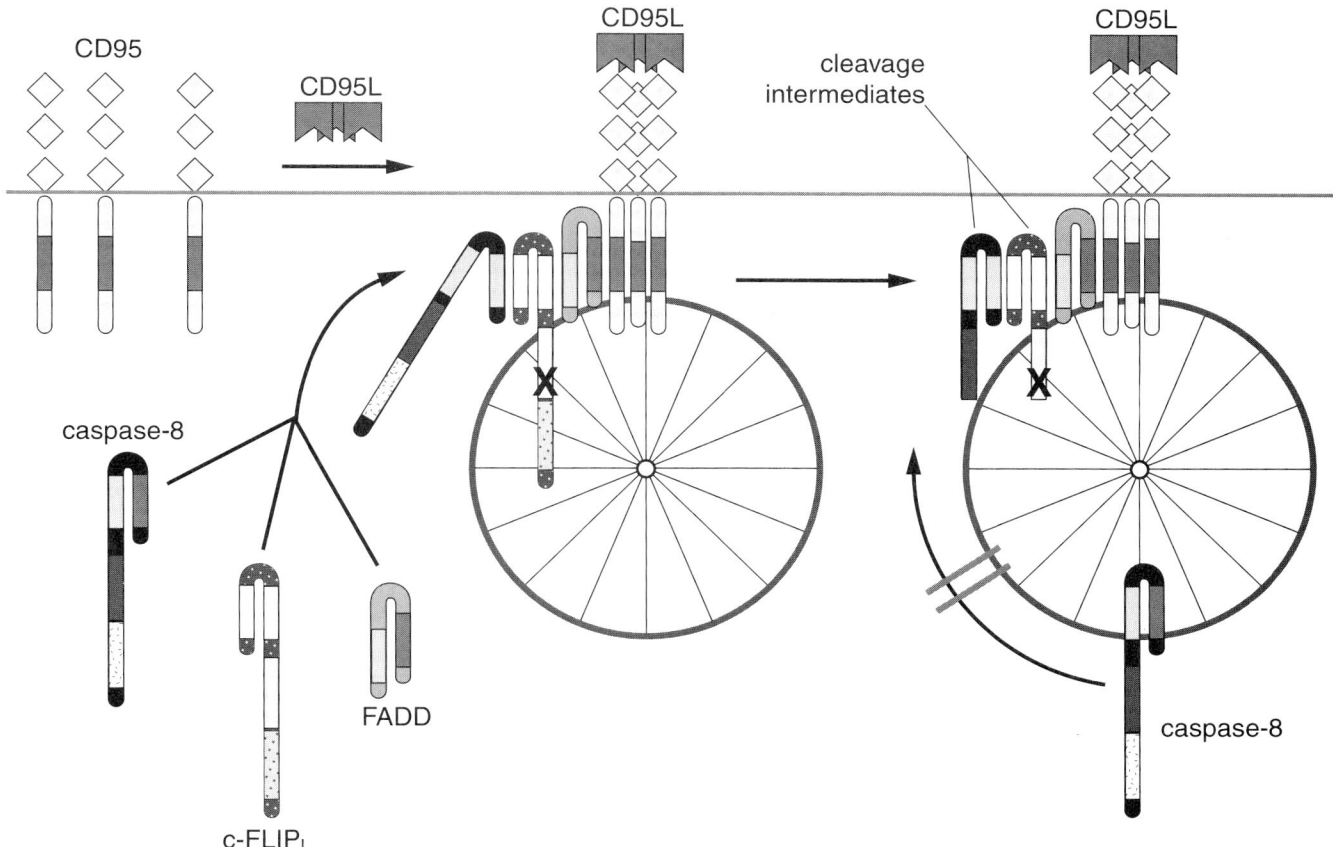

FIGURE 13.5. Inhibition of CD95-mediated apoptosis by c-FLIP$_L$. c-FLIP occurs in two forms, a short form and a long form. The short form structurally resembles v-FLIP. The long form has domains similar to those of caspase-8 but an inactive enzymatic site and interferes with the generation of active caspase-8 subunits at the receptor level in both CD95 type I and type II cells.

Chaperones and Related Proteins

Chaperones are proteins known to facilitate the correct folding of newly synthesized proteins (109). Recent findings suggest a role for chaperones in apoptosis signaling.

In a search for molecules associated with the death receptor DR3, a silencer of death domains (SODD) was found (110). SODD interacts with the DD of DR3 and TNF-R1 but not with other death receptors. SODD does not contain a death domain. However, binding of SODD to the death domain of a death receptor prevents binding of signaling molecules necessary for activation of caspases or the transcription factor NF-κB.

SODD is specific for DR3 and TNF-R1; homologous proteins may exist for other death receptors.

Kinases

Phosphoinositide 3-kinase (PI3-K) is a dual-specificity kinase with lipid and protein kinase activity. One of its targets is the protein kinase B (PKB or Akt) (111). Recently, molecular links between the PI3-K/PKB survival pathway

and apoptosis signaling have been reported. PKB phosphorylates and thereby inactivates apoptosis inducers; that is, Bad (112,113), caspases (114), and the transcription factors AFX and FKHRL1, which induce CD95L (115,116).

Mitogen-activated protein kinases (MAPK) are mediators of proliferation (117). MAPKs have been shown to mediate survival by transcription-dependent and -independent mechanisms (118,119). Transcription-dependent mechanisms might involve upregulation of c-FLIP (120). The transcription-independent mechanism may be due to a direct effect of MAPKs on the CD95 signaling pathway (121,122).

THE TRAIL APOPTOSIS SYSTEM

In 1995, the TNF-related apoptosis-inducing ligand, TRAIL, was identified purely on the basis of sequence homology to the other members of the TNF family (reviewed in ref. 123). The revealing homology resided within two short but highly conserved sequence motifs characteristic for TNF family members. Like CD95L, its closest homologue, TRAIL was indeed also capable of inducing apoptosis (124). Interestingly, however, TRAIL induced apoptosis in many tumor cell lines, yet normal cells were not killed.

TRAIL is expressed in many human tissues, although not in the liver and brain (125), which indicates that TRAIL does not have a cytotoxic effect on normal cells. In fact, many normal primary cells such as epithelial cells, fibroblasts, and skeletal muscle cells are resistant to TRAIL-induced apoptosis (126). Furthermore, hepatocytes from mouse and monkey are resistant to TRAIL (127).

TRAIL can bind to five different receptors (128–130). TRAIL can bind two apoptosis-inducing receptors, TRAIL-R1 (DR4) and TRAIL-R2 (Killer, DR5, Trick2), two additional cell-bound receptors incapable of transmitting an apoptotic signal, TRAIL-R3 (LIT, DcR1) and TRAIL-R4 (TRUNDD, DcR2), and a soluble receptor called osteoprotegerin (OPG). OPG binds not only to TRAIL but also to another member of the TNF family, the osteoclast differentiation factor (ODF, OPGL, RANKL) (128).

At first it seemed that the existence of these functionally so distinct receptors might provide an answer to the differential sensitivity to TRAIL observed between normal and transformed cells. The initial finding indicated that TRAIL-R3 and TRAIL-R4 may act as so-called "decoy receptors" by competing with TRAIL-R1 and TRAIL-R2 for binding of TRAIL (130,131). However, it was recently shown for various cellular systems that TRAIL resistance is controlled intracellularly rather than at the level of TRAIL-R3 and/or TRAIL-R4, the putative "decoy receptors." Thus, in melanoma cells, TRAIL-R expression levels did not correlate with sensitivity towards TRAIL. In addition, in primary versus transformed keratinocytes, the levels of c-FLIP inversely correlated with sensitivity to TRAIL and to TRAIL-R1/R2-specific antibodies, whereas TRAIL-R3 and -R4 were not involved (23,24,132). Thus, the "decoy" concept awaits confirmation, and the function of the non–apoptosis inducing receptors, TRAIL-R3, TRAIL-R4, and OPG, remains unsolved.

Biochemical Pathway of TRAIL-Induced Apoptosis

Soon after its discovery, TRAIL was shown to use a caspase-dependent pathway to kill its target cells (133). TRAIL-induced apoptosis involves early activation of caspase-8 and caspase-3 as well as induction of DNA fragmentation. Dissipation of mitochondrial membrane potential and cytochrome *c* release are late events during TRAIL-induced apoptosis. In addition, inhibition of caspase-8 but not caspase-9 or -3 prevents mitochondrial permeability transition and apoptosis. Various cell lines overexpressing the anti-apoptotic proteins Bcl-2 or Bcl-x_L are not or only marginally protected against TRAIL-induced apoptosis. Thus, TRAIL may induce apoptosis via a direct caspase signaling cascade that may bypass mitochondria (134). Analysis of

the TRAIL DISC under native conditions in analogy to studies of the CD95 DISC revealed that both FADD/Mort1 and caspase-8 are recruited to the TRAIL DISC in all cell lines tested (BJAB, BL60, CEM, and Jurkat) and that these two proteins constitute integral components of the TRAIL-R2 DISC (135). A recent report indicates that TRAIL induces the formation of a complex consisting of TRAIL-R1, TRAIL-R2, FADD, and caspase-8, also indicating that its apoptotic signal transduction pathway is similar to that used by CD95 and TNF-R1 (136).

Antitumor Potential of TRAIL

As initial studies indicated TRAIL induces apoptosis in tumor cells but not in normal cells, TRAIL was proposed as a potential cancer therapeutic agent (125,126,137). The other known apoptosis-inducing members of the TNF family, CD95L and TNF, are detrimental upon systemic administration.

Preclinical studies in mice and nonhuman primates have indicated that TRAIL produces little systemic toxicity (126,138). Thus, in contrast to its predecessors, TNF and anti-APO-1, TRAIL induced the *in vivo* regression of tumors without severe side effects. However, recent data now suggest that human primary hepatocytes are very sensitive towards TRAIL-induced apoptosis (127). This indicates that administration of TRAIL could cause severe side effects (e.g., substantial liver toxicity) if used in human cancer therapy. The possible side effects of TRAIL in the liver raise serious concerns about its potential use as a safe therapeutic agent.

TNF-R1, TNF-R2, AND TNF

While the main activity of CD95 is to trigger cell death, TNFR-1 can signal a diverse range of activities, including fibroblast proliferation, resistance to intracellular pathogens including chlamydiae, synthesis of prostaglandin E2, inflammation, tumor necrosis, differentiation, and apoptosis (139).

These responses are mediated by TNF-induced trimerization of two distinct cell surface receptors, TNF-R1 (p55) and TNF-R2 (p75), at least one of which is present in almost every cell (140,141). The structural similarity between the two TNF receptors is limited to their extracellular domains (140). The intracellular domains of TNF-R1 and TNF-R2 are completely different, suggesting that these two receptors are involved in distinctly different signaling pathways (142). The intracellular domain of TNF-R1 has a death domain, whereas TNF-R2 does not. The role of TNF-R2 in liver biology is less well defined. TNF-R1 is expressed in hepatocytes and Kupffer cells. TNF-R1-induced apoptosis has clinical relevance to the pathophysiology of many human liver diseases. The expression of TNF-R1 has been shown to be strongly enhanced in hepatitis B, hepatitis C, autoimmune hepatitis, and especially alcohol-induced hepatitis (143). TNF-R1 also plays a critical role in liver injury induced by concanavalin A, a model relevant to inflammatory liver injury (144–146).

TNF-R1 ligation, like CD95 stimulation, requires receptor oligomerization and can use the FADD-caspase-8 pathway, except that an additional adaptor, TNF-R1-associated death domain protein (TRADD), links TNF-R-1 to FADD. The association between the two molecules is mediated via the death domains of FADD and TRADD. TRADD has been shown to bind a number of signaling molecules, including FADD, TNF-R-associated factor 2 (TRAF2), and the serine/threonine kinase receptor–interacting protein (RIP). An alternative apoptosis pathway by this receptor involves the binding of RIP to TRADD. RIP appears to function as an adaptor protein recruiting RAIDD/CRADD (*RIP-a*ssociated *I*CM-1/CED-3-homologous protein with a *DD/C*aspase and *R*IP *a*daptor with a *DD*) to the receptor complex, which in turn mediates the binding and activation of caspase-2, resulting in a caspase-initiated death cascade. Thus, TNF-R1 appears to be able to cause cell death by a caspase-8- and/or caspase-2-sensitive mechanism. While FADD activates the apoptotic machinery, TRAF2 and also RIP mediate NF-κB activation. Furthermore, the Jun N-terminal kinase (JNK) signaling pathway participates in proapoptotic signals via TNF-R1 signaling; activation of this pathway is dependent on TRAF-2, but not RIP.

To summarize, the TNF-R1 signaling complex leads to activation of at least three effector functions: the protein kinase JNK, the transcription factor NF-κB, and induction of apoptosis. This multiplicity of effector functions can explain why TNF-R1 can transduce a large number of diverse biological functions (139,147–150).

TNF-α functions as a "two-edged sword" in the liver. TNF-α is required for normal hepatocyte proliferation during liver regeneration. It functions both as a co-mitogen and as an inducer of NF-κB, which mediates antiapoptotic effects. On the other hand, TNF-α is the mediator of hepatotoxicity in many animal models including concanavalin A and the endotoxin/galactosamine model. TNF-α has also been proposed as an important mediator in patients with alcoholic liver disease and viral hepatitis (reviewed in ref. 151).

HEPATOCELLULAR CARCINOMA

The possibility that apoptosis serves as a barrier to cancer was first raised in 1972, when Kerr, Wyllie, and Currie (2) described massive apoptosis in the cells populating rapidly growing hormone-dependent tumors following hormone withdrawal.

The current notion is that virtually all cancer cells harbor alterations that enable evasion of apoptosis. Resistance to apoptosis can be acquired by cancer cells through a variety of strategies.

CD95L and Immune Privilege

Tumors have developed multiple mechanisms to evade the attack of the immune system. These range from lack of expression of costimulatory or major histocompatibility complex (MHC) molecules to active strategies such as the production of immunosuppressive cytokines and other molecules. Based on early studies, it was hypothesized that expression of CD95L by tumor cells enabled them to counterattack the immune system, and that transplant rejection could be prevented by expressing CD95L on transplanted organs. However, experiments in which CD95L expression is induced in a tumor or tissue, either through use of transgenic mice or by transfection or transduction of transplanted cells, have shown that overexpression of CD95L on tumor cells or grafts does not confer immune privilege, but instead induces a granulocytic response that accelerates rejection. Thus, the *in vivo* consequences of CD95L expression on tumors and grafts are far from clear.

A number of studies suggested that counterattack was also operative *in vivo*. Apoptosis of tumor-infiltrating lymphocytes has been found *in situ* within CD95L-expressing hepatocellular carcinoma (152), human melanoma (153), gastric adenocarcinoma (154), and lymphoepithelioma-like cancer of the stomach (155).

Many studies on tumor counterattack have been published, but the results are contradictory and therefore it is not clear whether tumor counterattack is an immune escape mechanism active *in vivo*. No study has demonstrated that a tumor (or graft), by CD95L expression, deleted antitumor-specific lymphocytes, escaped the immune response, and thus had a growth advantage *in vivo*.

Downregulation of CD95

Downregulation of CD95 represents another mechanism resulting in the escape of tumor cells from immune surveillance. There have been observations that different tumors (including hepatocellular carcinoma) that had originated from tissues normally expressing CD95 might downregulate CD95 expression (91,156). Analysis of hepatocellular carcinomas revealed complete or partial loss of CD95 expression (152). Loss of CD95 may result in reduced sensitivity of the tumor cells towards CD95-mediated apoptosis, including cytotoxic action of antitumor T-lymphocytes.

p53

The most commonly occurring loss of a proapoptotic regulator through mutation involves the *p53* tumor suppressor gene. The resulting functional inactivation of its product, the p53 protein, is seen in greater than 50% of human cancers and results in the removal of a key component of the DNA damage sensor that can induce the apoptotic effector cascade (reviewed in ref. 157) (158).

The frequent occurrence of *p53* mutations in hepatocellular cancer provides further support for the hypothesis that a failure to trigger apoptotic pathways contributes to the pathogenesis of this disease. The p53 mutational spectrum of hepatocellular carcinoma is an example of a molecular linkage between carcinogen exposure and cancer. In liver tumors from persons living in geographic areas in which aflatoxin B_1 and hepatitis B virus are cancer risk factors, most p53 mutations are at the third nucleotide pair of codon 249 (reviewed in ref. 158). Expression of the 249_{ser} mutant p53 protein may provide a specific growth and /or survival advantage to liver cells.

Failure of normal p53-dependent apoptotic mechanisms to eliminate cells with oncogenic mutations might explain the strong association between *p53* mutations and hepatocellular carcinoma. The insensitivity of most hepatocellular cancers to traditional chemotherapeutic agents might partially be explained by the presence of *p53* mutations.

Numerous studies indicate that the proapoptotic activity of p53 plays a major role in mediating its tumor suppressor effects. In addition, the activity of p53 can affect not only the development of a tumor, but also its response to various types of anticancer treatments. p53 has been shown to play a role in promoting the apoptotic death of tumor cells upon treatment with DNA-damaging agents such as ionizing radiation and many types of chemotherapeutic drugs.

Chemotherapy, p53, and CD95 in Hepatocellular Carcinoma

Normal *p53* function is necessary for chemotherapy-induced apoptosis in some contexts. The CD95 system is involved in induction of cytotoxicity by anticancer drugs in hepatoma cells. Clinically relevant concentrations of diverse anticancer drugs induce CD95 expression in hepatoma cell lines, thereby increasing the sensitivity towards CD95-induced apoptosis (98). Thus, chemotherapy may sensitize tumor cells by upregulating expression of death regulators such as CD95. p53 has been shown to directly transactivate the CD95 gene in response to DNA damage by chemotherapeutic drugs (Fig. 13.6). Induction of CD95 gene transcription by p53 is mediated through a strong p53-responsive element, located within the first intron of the gene (98,159). The fact that wild-type p53 had a stimulatory effect on CD95 gene activity, whereas the mutant p53 proteins investigated were not able to activate the CD95 gene may explain why mutations in p53 contribute to tumor progression and to resistance of cancer cells to chemotherapy. Thus, the observation that p53-dependent cell death following DNA damage is mediated by TNF-R family members could have significant implications for manipulating apoptosis and therapy.

A critical question is whether p53-induced apoptosis is functionally dependent on the induction of the CD95 gene. With the identification of killer/DR5 (160) as

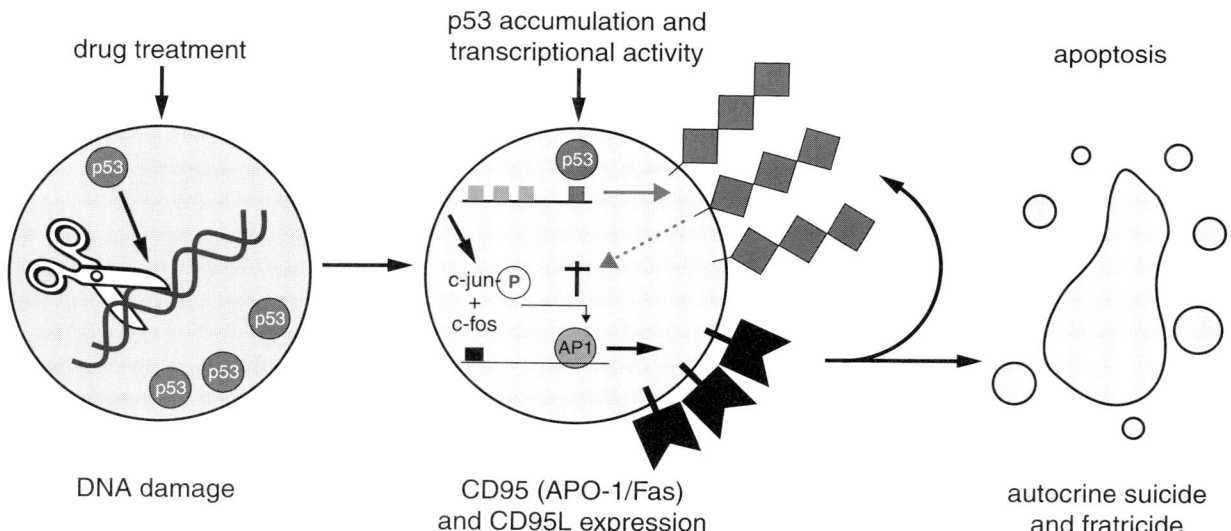

FIGURE 13.6. Molecular mechanisms of chemotherapy-induced apoptosis. p53 activates the CD95 gene in response to DNA damage by anticancer drugs. Induction of CD95 gene transcription by p53 is mediated through a p53-responsive element, located within the first intron of the gene. Furthermore, chemotherapeutic drugs induce upregulation of the CD95L in hepatoma cells. Cytostatic drugs engage the JNK/SAPK signaling pathway, leading to the activation of the transcription factor AP-1 (246). In turn, via an AP-1 site in the CD95L promoter, recognized by Jun/Fos heterodimers, CD95L expression is enhanced.

another pathway of p53-dependent apoptosis following DNA damage, it is evident that p53-dependent apoptosis is not solely mediated by the CD95 system.

Furthermore, additional effector pathways besides CD95/CD95L signaling may contribute to drug-induced apoptosis; that is, other death systems such as Trail-R2 and TNF-R1, cytochrome *c* release by mitochondria and activation of caspases.

There is obviously a diversity of death receptor/death ligand systems, and a diversity of parallel intracellular signaling pathways operating in drug-induced apoptosis. This diversity of regulatory and effector components in apoptotic signaling holds important implications for the development of novel types of antitumor therapy. Successful therapies will need to intervene very precisely in these pathways to avoid unrestricted cell killing.

ACKNOWLEDGMENTS

This work was supported by grants of the Deutsche Forschungsgemeinschaft, SFB 601 (Molekulare Pathogenese Hepato-gastroenterologischer Erkrankungen), by the Medizinische Forschungsförderung Heidelberg (317/99), the Tumorzentrum Heidelberg/Mannheim and the Forschungsschwerpunkt Transplantation to M.M. and P.H.K.

REFERENCES

1. Vogt C. 1842. Untersuchungen über die Entwicklungsgeschichte der Geburtshelferkröte.
2. Kerr JF, Wyllie AH, AR Currie. Apoptosis: a basic biological phenomenon with wide-ranging implications in tissue kinetics. *Br J Cancer* 1972;26:239.
3. Councilman WT. Report on the etiology and prevention of yellow fever. Sternberg, GM. 1328, 151–159. 1890. Government printing office, Washington DC, United States Marine Hospital Service, Treasury Department. Public health bulletin 2.
4. Biava C, Mukhlova-Montiel M. Changes in human liver cells: Electron microscopic observation on councilman-like acidophlic bodies and other forms of acidophililic changes in human liver cells. *Am J Pathol* 1965;46:775.
5. Miyai K, Slusser RJ, Ruebner BH. Viral hepatitis in mice: an electron microscopic study. *Exp Mol Pathol* 1962;2:464.
6. Moppert J, Ekesparre DV, Bianchi L. On the morphogenesis of eosinophilic single cell necrosis in the liver parenchyma of humans. Light and electron optical correlative studies. *Virchows Arch Pathol Anat Physiol Klin Med* 1967;342:210.
7. Kerr JF. Shrinkage necrosis: a distinct mode of cellular death. *J Pathol* 1971;105:13.
8. Klion FM, Schaffner F. The ultrastructure of acidophilic "councilman-like" bodies in the liver. *Am J Pathol* 1966;48:755.
9. Svoboda D, Nielson A, Werder A, et al. An electron microscopic study of viral hepatitis in mice. *Am J Pathol* 1962;41:205.
10. Child PL, Ruiz A. Acidophilic bodies. Their chemical and physical nature in patients with Bolivian hemorrhagic fever. *Arch Pathol* 1968;85:45.
11. Williamson R. Properties of rapidly labelled deoxyribonucleic acid fragments isolated from the cytoplasm of primary cultures of embryonic mouse liver cells. *J Mol Biol* 1970;51:157.
12. Wyllie AH. Apoptosis and carcinogenesis. *Eur J Cell Biol* 1997; 73:189.
13. Krammer PH. CD95(APO-1/Fas)-mediated apoptosis: live and let die. *Adv Immunol* 1999;71:163.
14. Schulze-Osthoff K, Ferrari D, Los M, et al. Apoptosis signaling by death receptors. *Eur J Biochem* 1998;254:439.
15. Nagata S. Apoptosis by death factor. *Cell* 1997;88:355.
16. Suda T, Hashimoto H, Tanaka M, et al. Membrane Fas ligand kills human peripheral blood T lymphocytes, and soluble Fas ligand blocks the killing. *J Exp Med* 1997;186:2045.
17. Schneider P, Holler N, Bodmer JL, et al. Conversion of membrane-bound Fas(CD95) ligand to its soluble form is associated with downregulation of its proapoptotic activity and loss of liver toxicity. *J Exp Med* 1998;187:1205.
18. Grell M, Douni E, Wajant H, et al. The transmembrane form of tumor necrosis factor is the prime activating ligand of the 80 kDa tumor necrosis factor receptor. *Cell* 1995;83:793.
19. Crowe PD, VanArsdale TL, Walter BN, et al. A lymphotoxin-beta-specific receptor [see comments]. *Science* 1994;264:707.
20. Pitti RM, Marsters SA, Lawrence DA, et al. Genomic amplification of a decoy receptor for Fas ligand in lung and colon cancer. *Nature* 1998;396:699.
21. Yu KY, Kwon B, Ni J, et al. A newly identified member of tumor necrosis factor receptor superfamily (TR6) suppresses LIGHT-mediated apoptosis. *J Biol Chem* 1999;274:13733.
22. Ashkenazi A, Dixit VM. Death receptors: signaling and modulation. *Science* 1998;281:1305.
23. Griffith TS, Chin WA, Jackson GC, et al. Intracellular regulation of TRAIL-induced apoptosis in human melanoma cells. *J Immunol* 1998;161:2833.
24. Zhang XD, Franco A, Myers K, et al. Relation of TNF-related apoptosis-inducing ligand (TRAIL) receptor and FLICE-inhibitory protein expression to TRAIL-induced apoptosis of melanoma. *Cancer Res* 1999;59:2747.
25. Alnemri ES, Livingston ES, Nicholson DJ, et al. ICE/CED-3 protease nomenclature. *Cell* 1996;87:171.
26. Hirsch T, Marchetti P, Susin SA, et al. The apoptosis-necrosis paradox. Apoptogenic proteases activated after mitochondrial permeability transition determine the mode of cell death. *Oncogene* 1997;15:1573.
27. Nicholson DW. Caspase structure, proteolytic substrates, and function during apoptotic cell death. *Cell Death Differ* 1999;6:1028.
28. Wilson KP, Black JA, Thomson JA, et al. Structure and mechanism of interleukin-1 beta converting enzyme [see comments]. *Nature* 1994;370:270.
29. Walker NP, Talanian RV, Brady KD, et al. Crystal structure of the cysteine protease interleukin-1 beta-converting enzyme: a (p20/p10)2 homodimer. *Cell* 1994;78:343.
30. Mittl PR, Di-Marco S, Krebs JF, et al. Structure of recombinant human CPP32 in complex with the tetrapeptide acetyl-Asp-Val-Ala-Asp fluoromethyl ketone. *J Biol Chem* 1997;272:6539.
31. Los M, Wesselborg S, Schulze OK. The role of caspases in development, immunity, and apoptotic signal transduction: lessons from knockout mice. *Immunity* 1999;10:629.
32. Zheng TS, Hunot S, Kuida K, et al. Caspase knockouts: matters of life and death. *Cell Death Differ* 1999;6:1043.
33. Lazebnik YA, Kaufmann SH, Desnoyers S, et al. Cleavage of poly(ADP-ribose) polymerase by a proteinase with properties like ICE. *Nature* 1994;371:346.
34. Gu Y, Sarnecki C, Aldape RA, et al. Cleavage of poly(ADP-ribose) polymerase by interleukin-1 beta converting enzyme

and its homologs TX and Nedd-2. *J Biol Chem* 1995;270: 18715.

35. Casciola RL, Anhalt GJ, Rosen A. DNA-dependent protein kinase is one of a subset of autoantigens specifically cleaved early during apoptosis. *J Exp Med* 1995;182:1625.

36. Song Q, Lees MS, Kumar S, et al. DNA-dependent protein kinase catalytic subunit: a target for an ICE-like protease in apoptosis. *EMBO J* 1996;15:3238.

37. Casciola RL, Miller DK, Anhalt GJ, et al. Specific cleavage of the 70-kDa protein component of the U1 small nuclear ribonucleoprotein is a characteristic biochemical feature of apoptotic cell death. *J Biol Chem* 1994;269:30757.

38. Tewari M, Beidler DR, Dixit VM. CrmA-inhibitable cleavage of the 70-kDa protein component of the U1 small nuclear ribonucleoprotein during Fas- and tumor necrosis factor-induced apoptosis. *J Biol Chem* 1995;270:18738.

39. Waterhouse N, Kumar S, Song Q, et al. Heteronuclear ribonucleoproteins C1 and C2, components of the spliceosome, are specific targets of interleukin 1 beta-converting enzyme-like proteases in apoptosis. *J Biol Chem* 1996;271:29335.

40. Wang X, Pai JT, Wiedenfeld EA, et al. Purification of an interleukin-1 beta converting enzyme-related cysteine protease that cleaves sterol regulatory element-binding proteins between the leucine zipper and transmembrane domains. *J Biol Chem* 1995; 270:18044.

41. Pai JT, Brown MS, Goldstein JL. Purification and cDNA cloning of a second apoptosis-related cysteine protease that cleaves and activates sterol regulatory element binding proteins. *Proc Natl Acad Sci U S A* 1996;93:5437.

42. Ghayur T, Hugunin M, Talanian RV, et al. Proteolytic activation of protein kinase C delta by an ICE/CED 3-like protease induces characteristics of apoptosis. *J Exp Med* 1996;184:2399.

43. Emoto Y, Manome Y, Meinhardt G, et al. Proteolytic activation of protein kinase C delta by an ICE-like protease in apoptotic cells. *EMBO J* 1995;14:6148.

44. Bunnell BA, Heath LS, Adams DE, et al. Increased expression of a 58-kDa protein kinase leads to changes in the CHO cell cycle [published erratum appears in *Proc Natl Acad Sci U S A* 1991;88:2612]. *Proc Natl Acad Sci U S A* 1990;87:7467.

45. Lahti JM, Xiang J, Heath LS, et al. PITSLRE protein kinase activity is associated with apoptosis. *Mol Cell Biol* 1995;15:1.

46. Beyaert R, Kidd VJ, Cornelis S, et al. Cleavage of PITSLRE kinases by ICE/CASP-1 and CPP32/CASP-3 during apoptosis induced by tumor necrosis factor. *J Biol Chem* 1997;272:11694.

47. Orth K, Chinnaiyan AM, Garg M, et al. The CED-3/ICE-like protease Mch2 is activated during apoptosis and cleaves the death substrate lamin A. *J Biol Chem* 1996;271:16443.

48. Neamati N, Fernandez A, Wright S, et al. Degradation of lamin B1 precedes oligonucleosomal DNA fragmentation in apoptotic thymocytes and isolated thymocyte nuclei. *J Immunol* 1995;154:3788.

49. Zhivotovsky B, Gahm A, Orrenius S. Two different proteases are involved in the proteolysis of lamin during apoptosis. *Biochem Biophys Res Commun* 1997;233:96.

50. Cryns VL, Bergeron L, Zhu H, et al. Specific cleavage of alpha-fodrin during Fas- and tumor necrosis factor-induced apoptosis is mediated by an interleukin-1beta-converting enzyme/Ced-3 protease distinct from the poly(ADP-ribose) polymerase protease. *J Biol Chem* 1996;271:31277.

51. Martin SJ, O'Brien GA, Nishioka WK, et al. Proteolysis of fodrin (non-erythroid spectrin) during apoptosis. *J Biol Chem* 1995;270:6425.

52. Brancolini C, Benedetti M, Schneider C. Microfilament reorganization during apoptosis: the role of Gas2, a possible substrate for ICE-like proteases. *EMBO J* 1995;14:5179.

53. Gross A, McDonnell JM, Korsmeyer SJ. BCL-2 family members and the mitochondria in apoptosis. *Genes Dev* 1999;13: 1899.

54. Muchmore SW, Sattler M, Liang H, et al. X-ray and NMR structure of human Bcl-xL, an inhibitor of programmed cell death. *Nature* 1996;381:335.

55. Sattler M, Liang H, Nettesheim D, et al. Structure of Bcl-xL-Bak peptide complex: recognition between regulators of apoptosis. *Science* 1997;275:983.

56. Aritomi M, Kunishima N, Inohara N, et al. Crystal structure of rat Bcl-xL. Implications for the function of the Bcl-2 protein family. *J Biol Chem* 1997;272:27886.

57. Chou JJ, Li H, Salvesen GS, et al. Solution structure of BID, an intracellular amplifier of apoptotic signaling. *Cell* 1999;96:615.

58. McDonnell JM, Fushman D, Milliman CL, et al. Solution structure of the proapoptotic molecule BID: a structural basis for apoptotic agonists and antagonists. *Cell* 1999;96:625.

59. Schendel SL, Xie Z, Montal MO, et al. Channel formation by antiapoptotic protein Bcl-2. *Proc Natl Acad Sci U S A* 1997;94: 5113.

60. Schendel SL, Montal M, Reed JC. Bcl-2 family proteins as ion-channels. *Cell Death Differ* 1998;5:372.

61. Hu S, Snipas SJ, Vincenz C, et al. Caspase-14 is a novel developmentally regulated protease. *J Biol Chem* 1998;273:29648.

62. Pan G, O'Rourke K, Dixit VM. Caspase-9, Bcl-XL, and Apaf-1 form a ternary complex. *J Biol Chem* 1998;273:5841.

63. Moriishi K, Huang DC, Cory S, et al. Bcl-2 family members do not inhibit apoptosis by binding the caspase activator Apaf-1. *Proc Natl Acad Sci U S A* 1999;96:9683.

64. Kroemer G, Reed JC. Mitochondrial control of cell death. *Nature Medicine* 2000;6:513.

65. Kroemer G, Dallaporta B, Resche RM. The mitochondrial death/life regulator in apoptosis and necrosis. *Annu Rev Physiol* 1998;60:619.

66. Green DR, Reed JC. Mitochondria and apoptosis. *Science* 1998;281:1309.

67. Jurgensmeier JM, Xie Z, Deveraux Q, et al. Bax directly induces release of cytochrome c from isolated mitochondria. *Proc Natl Acad Sci U S A* 1998;95:4997.

68. Marzo I, Brenner C, Zamzami N, et al. Bax and adenine nucleotide translocator cooperate in the mitochondrial control of apoptosis. *Science* 1998;281:2027.

69. Narita M, Shimizu S, Ito T, et al. Bax interacts with the permeability transition pore to induce permeability transition and cytochrome c release in isolated mitochondria. *Proc Natl Acad Sci U S A* 1998;95:14681.

70. Desagher S, Osen SA, Nichols A, et al. Bid-induced conformational change of Bax is responsible for mitochondrial cytochrome c release during apoptosis. *J Cell Biol* 1999;144:891.

71. Pastorino JG, Tafani M, Rothman RJ, et al. Functional consequences of the sustained or transient activation by Bax of the mitochondrial permeability transition pore. *J Biol Chem* 1999; 274:31734.

72. Yin XM, Wang K, Gross A, et al. Bid-deficient mice are resistant to Fas-induced hepatocellular apoptosis. *Nature* 1999;400: 886.

73. Boldin MP, Varfolomeev EE, Pancer Z, et al. A novel protein that interacts with the death domain of Fas/APO-1 contains a sequence motif related to the death domain. *J Biol Chem* 1995; 270:7795.

74. Chinnaiyan AM, O'Rourke K, Tewari M, et al. FADD, a novel death domain-containing protein interacts with the death domain of Fas and initiates apoptosis. *Cell* 1995;81:505.

75. Boldin MP, Goncharov TM, Goltsev YV, et al. Involvement of MACH, a novel MORT1/FADD-interacting protease, in Fas/APO-1- and TNF receptor-induced cell death. *Cell* 1996;85: 803.

76. Muzio M, Chinnaiyan AM, Kischkel FC, et al. FLICE, a novel FADD-homologous ICE/CED-3-like protease, is recruited to the CD95 (Fas/APO-1) death—inducing signaling complex. *Cell* 1996;85:817.

77. Kischkel FC, Hellbardt S, Behrmann I, et al. Cytotoxicity-dependent APO-1 (Fas/CD95)-associated proteins form a death-inducing siganling complex (DISC) with the receptor. *EMBO J* 1995;14:5579.

78. Medema JP, Scaffidi C, Kischkel FC, et al. FLICE is activated by association with the CD95 death-inducing signaling complex (DISC). *EMBO J* 1997;16:2794.

79. Scaffidi C, Fulda S, Srinivasan A, et al. Two CD95 (APO-1/Fas) signaling pathways. *EMBO J* 1998;17:1675.

80. Meinl E, Fickenscher H, Tho M, et al. Anti-apoptotic strategies of lymphotropic viruses. *Immunol Today* 1998;19:474.

81. Tschopp J, Irmler M, Thome M. Inhibition of fas death signals by FLIPs. *Curr Opin Immunol* 1998;10:552.

82. Liu X, Kim CN, Yang J, et al. Induction of apoptotic program in cell-free extracts: requirement for dATP and cytochrome c. *Cell* 1996;86:147.

83. Li H, Zhu H, Xu CJ, et al. Cleavage of BID by caspase 8 mediates the mitochondrial damage in the Fas pathway of apoptosis. *Cell* 1998;94:491.

84. Luo X, Budihardjo I, Zou H, et al. Bid, a Bcl2 interacting protein, mediates cytochrome c release from mitochondria in response to activation of cell surface death receptors. *Cell* 1998;94:481.

85. Gross A, Yin XM, Wang K, et al. Caspase cleaved BID targets mitochondria and is required for cytochrome c release, while BCL-XL prevents this release but not tumor necrosis factor-R1/Fas death. *J Biol Chem* 1999;274:1156.

86. Zou H, Henzel WJ, Liu X, et al. Apaf-1, a human protein homologous to *C. elegans* CED-4, participates in cytochrome c-dependent activation of caspase-3 [see comments]. *Cell* 1997;90:405.

87. Li P, Nijhawan D, Budihardjo I, et al. Cytochrome c and dATP-dependent formation of Apaf-1/caspase-9 complex initiates an apoptotic protease cascade. *Cell* 1997;91:479.

88. Srinivasula SM, Ahmad M, Fernandes AT, et al. Autoactivation of procaspase-9 by Apaf-1-mediated oligomerization. *Mol Cell* 1998;1:949.

89. Zou H, Li Y, Liu X, et al. An APAF-1.cytochrome c multimeric complex is a functional apoptosome that activates procaspase-9. *J Biol Chem* 1999;274:11549.

90. French LE, Hahne M, Viard I, et al. Fas and Fas ligand in embryos and adult mice: ligand expression in several immune-privileged tissues and coexpression in adult tissues characterized by apoptotic cell turnover. *J Cell Biol* 1996;133:335.

91. Leithäuser F, Dhein J, Mechtersheimer G, et al. Constitutive and induced expression of APO-1, a new member of the NGF/TNF factor receptor superfamily, in normal and neoplastic cells. *Lab Invest* 1993;69:415.

92. Ni R, Tomita Y, Matsuda K, et al. Fas-mediated apoptosis in primary cultured mouse hepatocytes. *Exp Cell Res* 1994;215:332.

93. Galle PR, Hofmann WJ, Walczak H, et al. Involvement of the APO-1/Fas (CD95) receptor and ligand in liver damage. *J Exp Med* 1995;182:1223.

94. Adachi M, Suematsu S, Kondo T, et al. Targeted mutation in the Fas gene causes hyperplasia in peripheral lymphoid organs and liver. *Nat Genet* 1995;11:294.

95. Ogasawara J, Watanabe Fukunaga R, Adachi M, et al. Lethal effect of the anti-Fas antibody in mice [published erratum appears in *Nature* 1993;365:568]. *Nature* 1993;364:806.

96. Lacronique V, Mignon A, Fabre M, et al. Bcl-2 protects from lethal hepatic apoptosis induced by an anti-Fas antibody in mice. *Nature Medicine* 1996;2:80.

97. Rodriguez I, Matsuura K, Khatib K, et al. A bcl-2 transgene expressed in hepatocytes protects mice from fulminant liver destruction but not from rapid death induced by anti-Fas antibody injection. *J Exp Med* 1996;183:1031.

98. Müller M, Strand S, Hug H, et al. Drug-induced apoptosis in hepatoma cells is mediated by the CD95 (APO-1/Fas) receptor/ligand system and involves activation of wild-type p53. *J Clin Invest* 1997;99:403.

99. Strand S, Hofmann WJ, Grambihler A, et al. Hepatic failure and liver cell damage in acute Wilson's disease involve CD95 (APO-1/Fas) mediated apoptosis. *Nat Med* 1998;4:588.

100. Keppler OT, Peter ME, Hinderlich S, et al. Differential sialylation of cell surface glycoconjugates in a human B lymphoma cell line regulates susceptibility for CD95 (APO-1/Fas)-mediated apoptosis and for infection by a lymphotropic virus. *Glycobiology* 1999;9:557.

101. Deveraux QL, Reed JC. IAP family proteins—suppressors of apoptosis. *Genes Dev* 1999;13:239.

102. Peter ME, Kischkel FC, Scheuerpflug CG, et al. Resistance of cultured peripheral T cells towards activation-induced cell death involves a lack of recruitment of FLICE (MACH/caspase 8) to the CD95 death-inducing signaling complex. *Eur J Immunol* 1997;27:1207.

103. Scaffidi C, Schmitz I, Krammer PH, et al. The role of c-FLIP in modulation of CD95-induced apoptosis. *J Biol Chem* 1999;274:1541.

104. Scaffidi C, Schmitz I, Zha J, et al. Differential modulation of apoptosis sensitivity in CD95 type I and type II cells. *J Biol Chem* 1999;274:22532.

105. Kataoka T, Schroter M, Hahne M, et al. FLIP prevents apoptosis induced by death receptors but not by perforin/granzyme B, chemotherapeutic drugs, and gamma irradiation. *J Immunol* 161:3936.

106. Tepper CG, Seldin MF. 1999. Modulation of caspase-8 and FLICE-inhibitory protein expression as a potential mechanism of Epstein-Barr virus tumorigenesis in Burkitt's lymphoma. *Blood* 1998;94:1727.

107. Djerbi M, Screpanti V, Catrina AI, et al. FLICE-inhibitory protein defines a new class of tumor progression factors [see comments]. *J Exp Med* 1999;190:1025.

108. Medema JP, de-Jong J, van-Hall T, et al. Immune escape of tumors in vivo by expression of cellular FLICE-inhibitory protein [see comments]. *J Exp Med* 1999;190:1033.

109. Bukau B, Horwich AL. The Hsp70 and Hsp60 chaperone machines. *Cell* 1998;92:351.

110. Tschopp J, Martinon F, Hofmann K. Apoptosis: Silencing the death receptors. *Curr Biol* 1999;9:R381.

111. Datta SR, Brunet A, Greenberg ME. Cellular survival: a play in three Akts. *Genes Dev* 1999;13:2905.

112. Datta SR, Dudek H, Tao X, et al. Akt phosphorylation of BAD couples survival signals to the cell-intrinsic death machinery. *Cell* 1997;91:231.

113. del-Peso L, Gonzalez GM, Page C, et al. Interleukin-3-induced phosphorylation of BAD through the protein kinase Akt. *Science* 1997;278:687.

114. Cardone MH, Roy N, Stennicke HR, et al. Regulation of cell death protease caspase-9 by phosphorylation. *Science* 1998;282:1318.

115. Brunet A, Bonni A, Zigmond MJ, et al. Akt promotes cell survival by phosphorylating and inhibiting a Forkhead transcription factor. *Cell* 1999;96:857.

116. Kops GJ, de-Ruiter ND, De-Vries-Smits AM, et al. Direct control of the Forkhead transcription factor AFX by protein kinase B. *Nature* 1999;398:630.

117. Seger R, Krebs EG. The MAPK signaling cascade. *FASEB J* 1995;9:726.

118. Nishina H, Fischer KD, Radvanyi L, et al. Stress-signalling kinase Sek1 protects thymocytes from apoptosis mediated by CD95 and CD3. *Nature* 1997;385:350.

119. Bonni A, Brunet A, West AE, et al. Cell survival promoted by the Ras-MAPK signaling pathway by transcription-dependent and -independent mechanisms [see comments]. *Science* 1999; 286:1358.

120. Yeh JH, Hsu SC, Han SH, et al. Mitogen-activated protein kinase kinase antagonized fas-associated death domain protein-mediated apoptosis by induced FLICE-inhibitory protein expression. *J Exp Med* 1998;188:1795.

121. Holmstrom TH, Chow SC, Elo I, et al. Suppression of Fas/APO-1-mediated apoptosis by mitogen-activated kinase signaling. *J Immunol* 1998;160:2626.

122. Holmstrom TH, Tran SE, Johnson VL, et al. Inhibition of mitogen-activated kinase signaling sensitizes HeLa cells to Fas receptor-mediated apoptosis. *Mol Cell Biol* 1999;19:5991.

123. Degli EM. To die or not to die—the quest of the TRAIL receptors. *J Leukoc Biol* 1999;65:535.

124. Wiley SR, Schooley K, Smolak PJ, et al. Indentification and characterization of a new member of the TNF family that induces apoptosis. *Immunity* 1997;3:673.

125. Wiley SR, Schooley K, Smolak PJ, et al. Identification and characterization of a new member of the TNF family that induces apoptosis. *Immunity* 1995;3:673.

126. Walczak H, Miller RE, Ariail K, et al. Tumoricidal activity of tumor necrosis factor-related apoptosis-inducing ligand in vivo [see comments]. *Nat Med* 1999;5:157.

127. Jo M, Kim TH, Seol DW, et al. Apoptosis induced in normal human hepatocytes by tumor necrosis factor–related apoptosis-inducing ligand. *Nat Med* 2000;6:564.

128. Emery JG, McDonnell P, Burke MB, et al. Osteoprotegerin is a receptor for the cytotoxic ligand TRAIL. *J Biol Chem* 1998; 273:14363.

129. Pan G, O'Rourke K, Chinnaiyan AM, et al. The receptor for the cytotoxic ligand TRAIL. *Science* 1997;276:111.

130. Sheridan JP, Marsters SA, Pitti RM, et al. Control of TRAIL-induced apoptosis by a family of signaling and decoy receptors [see comments]. *Science* 1997;277:818.

131. Pan G, Ni J, Wei YF, et al. An antagonist decoy receptor and a death domain-containing receptor for TRAIL [see comments]. *Science* 1997;277:815.

132. Leverkus M, Neumann M, Mengling T, et al.. Regulation of tumor necrosis factor-related apoptosis-inducing ligand sensitivity in primary and transformed human keratinocytes. *Cancer Res* 2000;60:553.

133. Mariani SM, Matiba B, Armandola EA, et al. Interleukin 1 beta-converting enzyme related proteases/caspases are involved in TRAIL-induced apoptosis of myeloma and leukemia cells. *J Cell Biol* 1997;137:221.

134. Walczak H, Bouchon A, Stahl H, Krammer PM. Tumor necrosis factor–related apoptosis-inducing ligand retains its apoptosis-inducing capacity on Bcl-2- or Bcl-xL-overexpressing chemotherapy-resistant tumor cells. *Cancer Res* 2000;60:3051.

135. Sprick MR, Weigand MA, Rieser E, et al. FADD/MORT1 and caspase-8 are recruited to TRAIL receptors 1 and 2 and are essential for apoptosis mediated by TRAIL receptor 2. *Immunity* 2000;12:599.

136. Bodmer JL, et al. Trail receptor-2 signals apoptosis through FADD and caspase-8. *Nat Cell Biol* 2000;2:241.

137. Pitti RM, Marsters SA, Ruppert S, et al. Induction of apoptosis by Apo-2 ligand, a new member of the tumor necrosis factor cytokine family. *J Biol Chem* 1996;271:12687.

138. Ashkenazi A, Pai RC, Fong S, et al. Safety and antitumor activity of recombinant soluble Apo2 ligand. *J Clin Invest* 1999; 104:155.

139. Liu ZG, Hsu H, Goeddel DV, et al. Dissection of TNF receptor 1 effector functions: JNK activation is not linked to apoptosis while NF-kappaB activation prevents cell death. *Cell* 1996; 87:565.

140. Tartaglia LA, Goeddel DV. Two TNF receptors. *Immunol Today* 1992;13:151.

141. Vandenabeele P, Declercq W, Beyaert R, et al. Two tumour necrosis factor receptors: structure and function. *Trends Cell Biol* 1995;5:392.

142. Tartaglia LA, Rothe M, Hu YF, et al. Tumor necrosis factor's cytotoxic activity is signaled by the p55 TNF receptor. *Cell* 1993;73:213.

143. Su F, Schneider RJ. Hepatitis B virus HBx protein sensitizes cells to apoptotic killing by tumor necrosis factor alpha. *Proc Natl Acad Sci U S A* 1997;94:8744.

144. Louis H, Le-Moine O, Peny MO, et al. Production and role of interleukin-10 in concanavalin A-induced hepatitis in mice. *Hepatology* 1997;25:1382.

145. Tagawa Y, Sekikawa K, Iwakura Y. Suppression of concanavalin A-induced hepatitis in IFN-gamma(−/−) mice, but not in TNF-alpha(−/−) mice: role for IFN-gamma in activating apoptosis of hepatocytes. *J Immunol* 1997;159:1418.

146. Iimuro Y, Gallucci RM, Luster MI, et al. Antibodies to tumor necrosis factor alpha attenuate hepatic necrosis and inflammation caused by chronic exposure to ethanol in the rat. *Hepatology* 1997;26:1530.

147. Lee SY, Choi Y. TRAF-interacting protein (TRIP): a novel component of the tumor necrosis factor receptor (TNFR)- and CD30-TRAF signaling complexes that inhibits TRAF2-mediated NF-kappaB activation. *J Exp Med* 1997;185:1275.

148. Natoli G, Costanzo A, Ianni A, et al. Activation of SAPK/JNK by TNF receptor 1 through a noncytotoxic TRAF2-dependent pathway. *Science* 1997;275:200.

149. Reinhard C, Shamoon B, Shyamala V, et al. Tumor necrosis factor alpha-induced activation of c-jun N-terminal kinase is mediated by TRAF2. *EMBO J* 1997;16:1080.

150. Yeh WC, Shahinian A, Speiser D, et al. Early lethality, functional NF-kappaB activation, and increased sensitivity to TNF-induced cell death in TRAF2-deficient mice. *Immunity* 1997;7: 715.

151. Plumpe J, Streetz K, Manns MP, et al. Tumour necrosis factor alpha-mediator of apoptosis and cell proliferation of hepatocytes. *Ital J Gastroenterol Hepatol* 1999;31:235.

152. Strand S, Hofmann WJ, Hug H, et al. Lymphocyte apoptosis induced by CD95 (APO-1/Fas) ligand-expressing tumor cells— a mechanism of immune evasion? [see comments]. *Nat Med* 1996;2:1361.

153. Hahne M, Rimoldi D, Schroter M, et al. Melanoma cell expression of Fas(Apo-1/CD95) ligand: implications for tumor immune escape [see comments]. *Science* 1996;274:1363.

154. Bennett MW, O'Connell J, O'Sullivan GC, et al. Expression of Fas ligand by human gastric adenocarcinomas: a potential mechanism of immune escape in stomach cancer. *Gut* 1999;44:156.

155. Kume T, Oshima K, Yamashita Y, et al. Relationship between Fas-ligand expression on carcinoma cell and cytotoxic T-lymphocyte response in lymphoepithelioma-like cancer of the stomach. *Int J Cancer* 1999;84:339.

156. Higaki K, Yano H, Kojiro M. Fas antigen expression and its relationship with apoptosis in human hepatocellular carcinoma and noncancerous tissues. *Am J Pathol* 1996;149:429.

157. Hanahan D, Weinberg RA. The hallmarks of cancer. *Cell* 2000; 100:57.

158. Harris CC. p53 tumor suppressor gene: from the basic research laboratory to the clinic—an abridged historical perspective. *Carcinogenesis* 1996;17:1187.

159. Müller M, Wilder S, Bannasch D, et al. p53 activates the CD95 (APO-1/Fas) gene in response to DNA damage by anticancer drugs. *J Exp Med* 1998;188:2033.

160. Wu GS, Burns TF, McDonald ER, et al. KILLER/DR5 is a DNA damage-inducible p53-regulated death receptor gene [Letter]. *Nat Genet* 1997;17:141.

161. Itoh N, Yonehara S, Ishii A, et al. The polypeptide encoded by the cDNA for human cell surface antigen Fas can mediate apoptosis. *Cell* 1991;66:233.

162. Oehm A, Behrmann I, Falk W, et al. Purification and molecular cloning of the APO-1 cell surface antigen, a member of the tumor necrosis factor/nerve growth factor receptor superfamily. Sequence identity with the Fas antigen. *J Biol Chem* 1992;267: 10709.

163. Loetscher H, Pan YC, Lahm HW, et al. Molecular cloning and expression of the human 55 kd tumor necrosis factor receptor. *Cell* 1990;61:351.

164. Schall TJ, Lewis M, Koller KJ, et al. Molecular cloning and expression of a receptor for human tumor necrosis factor. *Cell* 1990;61:361.

165. Smith CA, Davis T, Anderson D, et al. A receptor for tumor necrosis factor defines an unusual family of cellular and viral proteins. *Science* 1990;248:1019.

166. Dembic Z, Loetscher H, Gubler U, et al. Two human TNF receptors have similar extracellular, but distinct intracellular, domain sequences. *Cytokine* 1990;2:231.

167. Stamenkovic I, Clark EA, Seed B. A B-lymphocyte activation molecule related to the nerve growth factor receptor and induced by cytokines in carcinomas. *EMBO J* 1989;8:1403.

168. Durkop H, Latza U, Hummel M, et al. Molecular cloning and expression of a new member of the nerve growth factor receptor family that is characteristic for Hodgkin's disease. *Cell* 1992; 68:421.

169. Camerini D, Walz G, Loenen WA, et al. The T cell activation antigen CD27 is a member of the nerve growth factor/tumor necrosis factor receptor gene family. *J Immunol* 1991;147: 3165.

170. Mallett S, Fossum S, Barclay AN. Characterization of the MRC OX40 antigen of activated CD4 positive T lymphocytes—a molecule related to nerve growth factor receptor. *EMBO J* 1990;9:1063.

171. Kwon BS, Weissman SM. cDNA sequences of two inducible T-cell genes. *Proc Natl Acad Sci U S A* 1989;86:1963.

172. Radeke MJ, Misko TP, Hsu C, et al. Gene transfer and molecular cloning of the rat nerve growth factor receptor. *Nature* 1987;325:593.

173. Chinnaiyan AM, O'Rourke K, Yu GL, et al. Signal transduction by DR3, a death domain-containing receptor related to TNFR-1 and CD95. *Science* 1996;274:990.

174. Bodmer JL, Burns K, Schneider P, et al. TRAMP, a novel apoptosis-mediating receptor with sequence homology to tumor necrosis factor receptor 1 and Fas(Apo-1/CD95). *Immunity* 1997;6:79.

175. Kitson J, Raven T, Jiang YP, et al. A death-domain-containing receptor that mediates apoptosis. *Nature* 1996;384:372.

176. Marsters SA, Sheridan JP, Donahue CJ, et al. Apo-3, a new member of the tumor necrosis factor receptor family, contains a death domain and activates apoptosis and NF-kappa B. *Curr Biol* 1996;6:1669.

177. Screaton GR, Xu XN, Olsen AL, et al. LARD: a new lymphoid-specific death domain containing receptor regulated by alternative pre-mRNA splicing. *Proc Natl Acad Sci U S A* 1997;94:4615.

178. Montgomery RI, Warner MS, Lum BJ, et al. Herpes simplex virus-1 entry into cells mediated by a novel member of the TNF/NGF receptor family. *Cell* 1996;87:427.

179. Hsu H, Solovyev I, Colombero A, et al. ATAR, a novel tumor necrosis factor receptor family member, signals through TRAF2 and TRAF5. *J Biol Chem* 1997;272:13471.

180. Kwon BS, Tan KB, Ni J, et al. A newly identified member of the tumor necrosis factor receptor superfamily with a wide tissue distribution and involvement in lymphocyte activation. *J Biol Chem* 1997;272:14272.

181. Nocentini G, Giunchi L, Ronchetti S, et al. A new member of the tumor necrosis factor/nerve growth factor receptor family inhibits T cell receptor-induced apoptosis. *Proc Natl Acad Sci U S A* 1997;94:6216.

182. von-Bulow GU, Bram RJ. NF-AT activation induced by a CAML-interacting member of the tumor necrosis factor receptor superfamily. *Science* 1997;278:138.

183. Schneider P, Thome M, Burns K, et al. TRAIL receptors 1 (DR4) and 2 (DR5) signal FADD-dependent apoptosis and activate NF-kappaB. *Immunity* 1997;7:831.

184. Walczak H, Degli EM, Johnson RS, et al. TRAIL-R2: a novel apoptosis-mediating receptor for TRAIL. *EMBO J* 1997;16: 5386.

185. MacFarlane M, Ahmad M, Srinivasula SM, et al. Identification and molecular cloning of two novel receptors for the cytotoxic ligand TRAIL. *J Biol Chem* 1997;272:25417.

186. Screaton GR, Mongkolsapaya J, Xu XN, et al. TRICK2, a new alternatively spliced receptor that transduces the cytotoxic signal from TRAIL. *Curr Biol* 1997;7:693.

187. Degli EM, Smolak PJ, Walczak H, et al. Cloning and characterization of TRAIL-R3, a novel member of the emerging TRAIL receptor family. *J Exp Med* 1997;186:1165.

188. Mongkolsapaya J, Cowper AE, Xu XN, et al. Lymphocyte inhibitor of TRAIL (TNF-related apoptosis-inducing ligand): a new receptor protecting lymphocytes from the death ligand TRAIL. *J Immunol* 1998;160:3.

189. Degli EM, Dougall WC, Smolak PJ, et al. The novel receptor TRAIL-R4 induces NF-kappaB and protects against TRAIL-mediated apoptosis, yet retains an incomplete death domain. *Immunity* 1997;7:813.

190. Pan G, Ni J, Yu G, et al. TRUNDD, a new member of the TRAIL receptor family that antagonizes TRAIL signalling. *FEBS Lett* 1998;424:41.

191. Pan G, Bauer JH, Haridas V, et al. Identification and functional characterization of DR6, a novel death domain-containing TNF receptor. *FEBS Lett* 1998; 431:351.

192. Anderson DM, Maraskovsky E, Billingsley WL, et al. A homologue of the TNF receptor and its ligand enhance T-cell growth and dendritic-cell function. *Nature* 1997;390:175.

193. Simonet WS, Lacey DL, Dunstan CR, et al. Osteoprotegerin: a novel secreted protein involved in the regulation of bone density [see comments]. *Cell* 1997;89:309.

194. Kwon B, Yu KY, Ni J, et al. Identification of a novel activation-inducible protein of the tumor necrosis factor receptor superfamily and its ligand. *J Biol Chem* 1999;274:6056.

195. Madry C, Laabi Y, Callebaut I, et al. The characterization of murine BCMA gene defines it as a new member of the tumor necrosis factor receptor superfamily. *Int Immunol* 1998;10:1693.

196. Suda T, Takahashi T, Goldstein P, et al. Molecular cloning and expression of the Fas ligand, a member of the tumor necrosis factor family. *Cell* 1993;75:1169.

197. Pennica D, Nedwin GE, Hayflick JS, et al. Human tumour necrosis factor: precursor structure, expression and homology to lymphotoxin. *Nature* 1984;312:724.

198. Shirai T, Yamaguchi H, Ito H, et al. Cloning and expression in Escherichia coli of the gene for human tumour necrosis factor. *Nature* 1985;313:803.

199. Wang AM, Creasey AA, Ladner MB, et al. Molecular cloning of the complementary DNA for human tumor necrosis factor. *Science* 1985;228:149.

200. Gray PW, Aggarwal BB, Benton CV, et al. Cloning and expression of cDNA for human lymphotoxin, a lymphokine with tumour necrosis activity. *Nature* 1984;312:721.

201. Browning JL, Ngam eA, Lawton P, et al. Lymphotoxin beta, a novel member of the TNF family that forms a heteromeric complex with lymphotoxin on the cell surface. *Cell* 1993;72:847.

202. Gauchat JF, Mazzei G, Life P, et al. Human CD40 ligand: molecular cloning, cellular distribution and regulation of IgE synthesis. *Res Immunol* 1994;145:240.

203. Graf D, Korthauer U, Mages HW, et al. Cloning of TRAP, a ligand for CD40 on human T cells. *Eur J Immunol* 1992;22:3191.

204. Hollenbaugh D, Grosmaire LS, Kullas CD, et al. The human T cell antigen gp39, a member of the TNF gene family, is a ligand for the CD40 receptor: expression of a soluble form of gp39 with B cell co-stimulatory activity. *EMBO J* 1992;11:4313.

205. Smith CA, Gruss HJ, Davis T, et al. CD30 antigen, a marker for Hodgkin's lymphoma, is a receptor whose ligand defines an emerging family of cytokines with homology to TNF. *Cell* 1993;73:1349.

206. Goodwin RG, Alderson MR, Smith CA, et al. Molecular and biological characterization of a ligand for CD27 defines a new family of cytokines with homology to tumor necrosis factor. *Cell* 1993;73:447.

207. Godfrey WR, Fagnoni FF, Harara MA, et al. Identification of a human OX-40 ligand, a costimulator of CD4+ T cells with homology to tumor necrosis factor. *J Exp Med* 1994;180:757.

208. Goodwin RG, Din WS, Davis ST, et al. Molecular cloning of a ligand for the inducible T cell gene 4-1BB: a member of an emerging family of cytokines with homology to tumor necrosis factor. *Eur J Immunol* 1993;23:2631.

209. Chicheportiche Y, Bourdon PR, Xu H, et al. TWEAK, a new secreted ligand in the tumor necrosis factor family that weakly induces apoptosis. *J Biol Chem* 1997;272:32401.

210. Marsters SA, Sheridan JP, Pitti RM, et al. Identification of a ligand for the death-domain-containing receptor Apo3. *Curr Biol* 1998;8:525.

211. Mauri DN, Ebner R, Montgomery RI, et al. LIGHT, a new member of the TNF superfamily, and lymphotoxin alpha are ligands for herpesvirus entry mediator. *Immunity* 1998;8:21.

212. Lacey DL, Timms E, Tan HL, et al. Osteoprotegerin ligand is a cytokine that regulates osteoclast differentiation and activation. *Cell* 1998;93:165.

213. Yasuda H, Shima N, Nakagawa N, et al. Osteoclast differentiation factor is a ligand for osteoprotegerin/osteoclastogenesis-inhibitory factor and is identical to TRANCE/RANKL. *Proc Natl Acad Sci U S A* 1998;95:3597.

214. Wong BR, Rho J, Arron J, et al. TRANCE is a novel ligand of the tumor necrosis factor receptor family that activates c-Jun N-terminal kinase in T cells. *J Biol Chem* 1997;272:25190.

215. Hahne M, Kataoka T, Schroter M, et al. APRIL, a new ligand of the tumor necrosis factor family, stimulates tumor cell growth. *J Exp Med* 1998;188:1185.

216. Schneider P, MacKay F, Steiner V, et al. BAFF, a novel ligand of the tumor necrosis factor family, stimulates B cell growth. *J Exp Med* 1999;189:1747.

217. Shu HB, Hu WH, Johnson H. TALL-1 is a novel member of the TNF family that is down-regulated by mitogens. *J Leukoc Biol* 1999;65:680.

218. Mukhopadhyay A, Ni J, Zhai Y, et al. Identification and characterization of a novel cytokine, THANK, a TNF homologue that activates apoptosis, nuclear factor-kappaB, and c-Jun NH2-terminal kinase. *J Biol Chem* 1999;274:15978.

219. Harrop JA, McDonnell PC, Brigham BM, et al. Herpesvirus entry mediator ligand (HVEM-L), a novel ligand for HVEM/TR2, stimulates proliferation of T cells and inhibits HT29 cell growth. *J Biol Chem* 1998;273:27548.

220. Cerretti DP, Kozlosky CJ, Mosley B, et al. Molecular cloning of the interleukin-1 beta converting enzyme. *Science* 1992;256:97.

221. Thornberry NA, Bull HG, Calaycay JR, et al. Processing in monocytes. *Nature* 1992;356:768.

222. Kumar S, Kinoshita M, Noda M, et al. Induction of apoptosis by the mouse Nedd2 gene, which encodes a protein similar to the product of the *Caenorhabditis elegans* cell death gene ced-3 and the mammalian IL-1 beta-converting enzyme. *Genes Dev* 1994;8:1613.

223. Wang L, Miura M, Bergeron L, et al. Ich-1, an Ice/ced-3-related gene, encodes both positive and negative regulators of programmed cell death. *Cell* 1994;78:739.

224. Tewari M, Quan LT, O'Rourke K, et al. Yama/CPP32 beta, a mammalian homolog of CED-3, is a CrmA-inhibitable protease that cleaves the death substrate poly(ADP-ribose) polymerase. *Cell* 1995;81:801.

225. Fernandes AT, Litwack G, Alnemri ES. CPP32, a novel human apoptotic protein with homology to *Caenorhabditis elegans* cell death protein Ced-3 and mammalian interleukin-1 beta-converting enzyme. *J Biol Chem* 1994;269:30761.

226. Nicholson DW, Ali A, Thornberry NA, et al. Identification and inhibition of the ICE/CED-3 protease necessary for mammalian apoptosis [see comments]. *Nature* 1995;376:37.

227. Faucheu C, Diu A, Chan AW, et al. A novel human protease similar to the interleukin-1 beta converting enzyme induces apoptosis in transfected cells. *EMBO J* 1995;14:1914.

228. Kamens J, Paskind M, Hugunin M, et al. Identification and characterization of ICH-2, a novel member of the interleukin-1 beta-converting enzyme family of cysteine proteases. *J Biol Chem* 1995;270:15250.

229. Munday NA, Vaillancourt JP, Ali A, et al. Molecular cloning and pro-apoptotic activity of ICErelII and ICErelIII, members of the ICE/CED-3 family of cysteine proteases. *J Biol Chem* 1995;270:15870.

230. Faucheu C, Blanchet AM, Collard D, et al. Identification of a cysteine protease closely related to interleukin-1 beta-converting enzyme. *Eur J Biochem* 1996;236:207.

231. Fernandes AT, Litwack G, Alnemri ES. Mch2, a new member of the apoptotic Ced-3/Ice cysteine protease gene family. *Cancer Res* 1995;55:2737.

232. Fernandes AT, Takahashi A, Armstrong R, et al. Mch3, a novel human apoptotic cysteine protease highly related to CPP32. *Cancer Res* 1995;55:6045.

233. Duan H, Chinnaiyan AM, Hudson PL, et al. ICE-LAP3, a novel mammalian homologue of the *Caenorhabditis elegans* cell death protein Ced-3 is activated during Fas- and tumor necrosis factor-induced apoptosis. *J Biol Chem* 1996;271:1621.

234. Lippke JA, Gu Y, Sarnecki C, et al. Identification and characterization of CPP32/Mch2 homolog 1, a novel cysteine protease similar to CPP32. *J Biol Chem* 1996;271:1825.

235. Fernandes AT, Armstrong RC, Krebs J, et al. In vitro activation of CPP32 and Mch3 by Mch4, a novel human apoptotic cysteine protease containing two FADD-like domains. *Proc Natl Acad Sci U S A* 1996;93:7464.

236. Duan H, Orth K, Chinnaiyan AM, et al. ICE-LAP6, a novel member of the ICE/Ced-3 gene family, is activated by the cytotoxic T cell protease granzyme B. *J Biol Chem* 1996;271:16720.

237. Srinivasula SM, Fernandes AT, Zangrilli J, et al. The Ced-3/interleukin 1beta converting enzyme-like homolog Mch6 and the lamin-cleaving enzyme Mch2alpha are substrates for the apoptotic mediator CPP32. *J Biol Chem* 1996;271:27099.

238. Vincenz C, Dixit VM. Fas-associated death domain protein interleukin-1beta-converting enzyme 2 (FLICE2), an ICE/Ced-3 homologue, is proximally involved in CD95- and p55-mediated death signaling. *J Biol Chem* 1997;272:6578.

239. Wang S, Miura M, Jung Y, et al. Identification and characterization of Ich-3, a member of the interleukin-1beta converting enzyme (ICE)/Ced-3 family and an upstream regulator of ICE. *J Biol Chem* 1996;271:20580.

240. Van-de-Craen M, Vandenabeele P, Declercq W, et al. Characterization of seven murine caspase family members. *FEBS Lett* 1997;403:61.

241. Humke EW, Ni J, Dixit VM. ERICE, a novel FLICE-activatable caspase. *J Biol Chem* 1998;273:15702.

242. Van-de-Craen M, Van-Loo G, Pype S, et al. Identification of a new caspase homologue: caspase-14. *Cell Death Differ* 1998;5:838.

243. Ahmad M, Srinivasula SM, Hegde R, et al. Identification and characterization of murine caspase-14, a new member of the caspase family. *Cancer Res* 1998;58:5201.

244. Rudel T, Bokoch GM. Membrane and morphological changes in apoptotic cells regulated by caspase-mediated activation of PAK2. *Science* 1997;276:1571.

245. Wissing D, Mouritzen H, Egeblad M, et al. Involvement of caspase-dependent activation of cytosolic phospholipase A2 in tumor necrosis factor-induced apoptosis. *Proc Natl Acad Sci U S A* 1997;94:5073.

246. Eichhorst ST, Müller M, Li-Weber M, et al. A novel AP-1 element in the CD95 ligand promoter is required for induction of apoptosis in hepatocellular carcinoma cells upon treatment with anticancer drugs. *Mol Cell Biol* 2000;20:1826.

14

FUNDAMENTALS OF CELLULAR OSMOREGULATION

KEVIN STRANGE

Maintenence of a constant volume in the face of extracellular and intracellular osmotic perturbations is a critical problem faced by all cells. Most cells respond to swelling or shrinkage by activating specific membrane transport and/or metabolic processes that serve to return cell volume to its normal resting state. These processes are essential for normal cell function and survival. This chapter will outline the cellular and molecular events underlying cell volume homeostasis and discuss their relevance to hepatocyte physiology.

FUNDAMENTALS OF CELL VOLUME REGULATION

Water is in thermodynamic equilibrium across the plasma membrane. In other words, the osmotic concentration of cytoplasmic (π_i) and extracellular (π_o) fluids are equal under steady-state conditions. Changes in intracellular or extracellular solute content generate a transmembrane osmotic gradient ($\Delta\pi$). Because cell membranes are freely permeable to water, any such gradient results in the immediate flow of water into or out of the cell until equilibrium is again achieved. Since animal cell membranes are unable

to generate or sustain significant hydrostatic pressure gradients, water flow causes cell swelling or shrinkage.

Cell volume changes are usually grouped into two broad categories, anisosmotic and isosmotic. Anisosmotic volume changes are induced by alterations in extracellular osmolality. Under normal physiological conditions, most mammalian cells, with a few noteworthy exceptions (e.g., cells in the renal medulla and gastrointestinal tract), are protected from anisosmotic volume changes by the kidney's precise regulation of plasma osmolality. However, plasma osmolality can be disrupted by a variety of disease states and their treatments (1,2).

Isosmotic volume changes are brought about by alterations in intracellular solute content. All cells are threatened by possible isosmotic swelling or shrinkage. Under steady-state conditions, intracellular solute levels are held constant by a precise balance between solute influx and efflux across the plasma membrane, and by the metabolic production and removal of osmotically active substances. A variety of physiological and pathophysiological conditions, however, can disrupt this balance. As discussed in more detail below, physiologically relevant isosmotic cell volume disturbances may play an important role in regulating hepatocyte function.

Regulation of Cell Volume

Cells respond to volume perturbations by activating volume regulatory mechanisms. The processes by which swollen and

K. Strange: Anesthesiology Research Division, Laboratories of Cellular and Molecular Physiology, Departments of Anesthesiology and Pharmacology, Vanderbilt University Medical Center, Nashville, Tennessee 37232.

shrunken cells return to a normal volume are collectively termed regulatory volume decrease (RVD) and regulatory volume increase (RVI), respectively (Fig. 14.1). Cell volume can only be regulated by the gain or loss of osmotically active solutes, primarily inorganic ions such as Na^+, K^+, Cl^- or small organic molecules termed organic osmolytes.

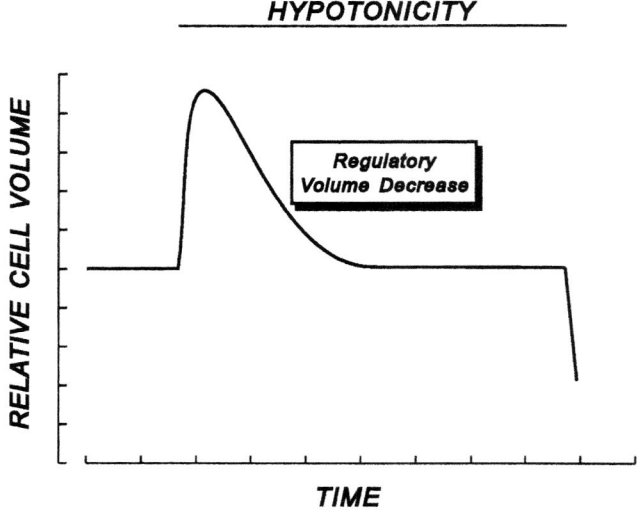

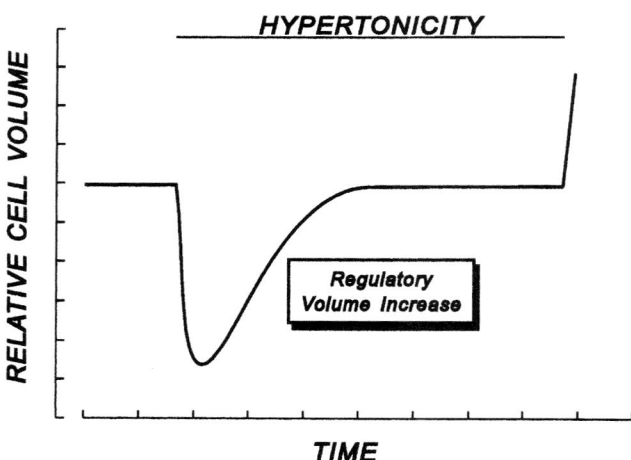

FIGURE 14.1. Cells activate volume regulatory mechanisms in response to volume perturbations,. Volume regulatory solute loss and gain are termed regulatory volume decrease (RVD) and regulatory volume increase (RVI), respectively. The time course of RVD and RVI varies with cell type and experimental conditions. Typically, however, RVI mediated by electrolyte uptake and RVD mediated by electrolyte and organic osmolyte loss occur over a period of minutes. When cells that have undergone RVI or RVD are returned to normotonic conditions they swell above or shrink below their resting volume. This is due to volume regulatory solute accumulation and loss that effectively makes the cytoplasm hypertonic or hypotonic, respectively, compared to normotonic fluid.

Volume regulatory electrolyte loss and gain are mediated exclusively by membrane transport processes (3–5). In most animal cells, RVD occurs through loss of KCl via activation of separate K^+ and Cl^- channels or by activation of the K-Cl cotransporter. In a few cell types, KCl efflux is mediated by activation of K^+/H^+ and Cl^-/HCO_3^- exchangers. Regulatory volume increase occurs by uptake of both KCl and NaCl. Accumulation of these salts is brought about by activation of Na^+/H^+ and Cl^-/HCO_3^- exchangers or the Na-K-2Cl cotransporter.

Figure 14.2 illustrates the ion transport systems commonly involved in cell volume regulation. Activation of these transport pathways is rapid and occurs within seconds after volume perturbation. Rapid stimulation of electrolyte transport is possible because the channels and transporters by which it is mediated reside continuously in the plasma membrane or are stored in submembrane cytoplasmic vesicles. Certain volume-sensitive ion transport systems play multiple roles, participating in volume regulation as well as transepithelial salt and water movement, and intracellular pH control.

Organic osmolytes are found in high (tens to hundreds of millimolar) concentrations in the cytosol of all organisms from bacteria to humans (4,6–8). These solutes play key roles in cell volume homeostasis and may also function as general cytoprotectants. In animal cells, organic osmolytes are grouped into three distinct classes: (a) polyols (e.g., sorbitol, *myo*-inositol), (b) amino acids and their derivatives (e.g., taurine, alanine, proline), and (c) methylamines (e.g., betaine, glycerophosphorylcholine).

Organic osmolytes are "compatible" or "nonperturbing" solutes (6–8). They have unique biophysical and biochemical properties that allow cells to accumulate them to high levels or to withstand large shifts in their concentration without deleterious effects on cellular structure and function. In contrast, so-called "perturbing" solutes such as electrolytes or urea can harm cells or disrupt metabolic processes when they are present at high concentrations or when large shifts in their concentrations occur. For example, elevated electrolyte levels and intracellular ionic strength can denature or precipitate cell macromolecules. Even smaller changes in cellular inorganic ion levels can alter resting membrane potential, the rates of enzymatically catalyzed reactions, and membrane solute transport that is coupled to ion gradients.

Accumulation of organic osmolytes is mediated either by energy-dependent transport from the external medium or by changes in the rates of osmolyte synthesis and degradation (Fig. 14.3) (4,6–8). Volume regulatory organic osmolyte accumulation is typically a slow process relative to electrolyte uptake and requires many hours after initial activation to reach completion. This slow time course is observed because activation of organic osmolyte accumulation pathways usually requires transcription and translation of genes coding for organic osmolyte transporters and synthesis enzymes (Fig. 14.4).

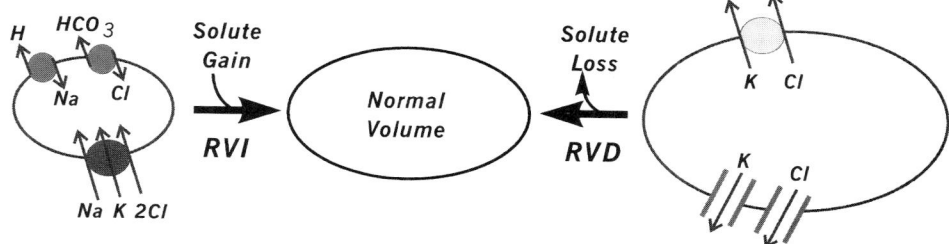

FIGURE 14.2. Volume regulatory electrolyte loss and accumulation is mediated by changes in the activity of membrane carriers and channels. Activation of these transport pathways occurs within seconds after the volume perturbation. This indicates that the channel and carrier proteins are either resident in the cell membrane or are rapidly inserted from a preexisting cytoplasmic pool. *RVD*, regulatory volume decrease; *RVI*, regulatory volume increase.

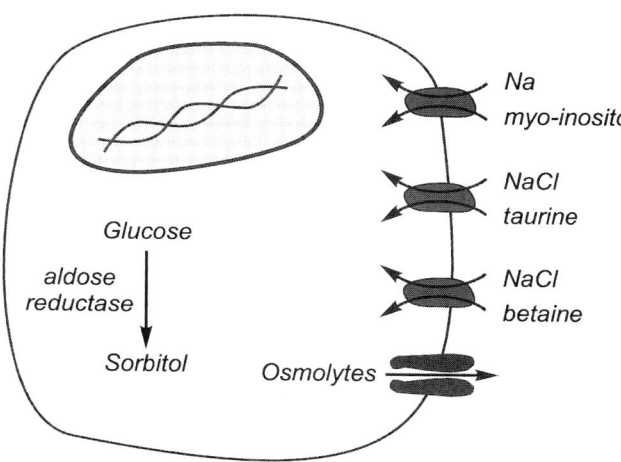

FIGURE 14.3. Mechanisms of organic osmolyte accumulation and loss. Volume regulatory organic osmolyte accumulation in animal cells is mediated largely by changes in the activity of Na^+-coupled membrane transporters and by changes in the rates of synthesis and degradation. Organic osmolyte loss appears to be mediated largely by passive efflux mechanisms.

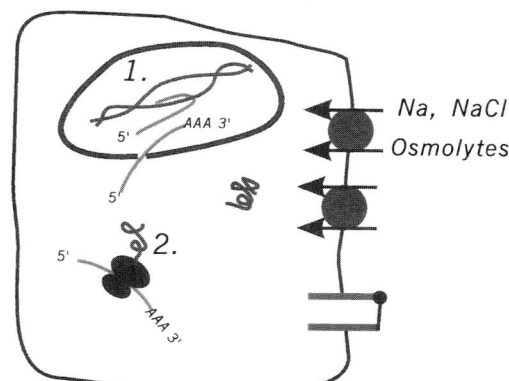

Prolonged exposure
to hypertonicity

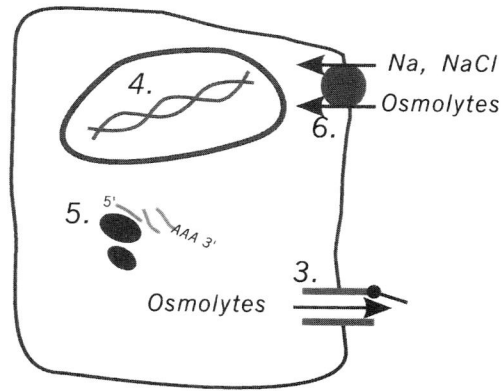

Cell swelling

FIGURE 14.4. Regulation of organic osmolyte transport pathways. Accumulation of organic osmolytes is usually slow (i.e., hours to days) relative to volume regulatory electrolyte uptake and most often involves increased expression of genes coding for organic osmolyte transporters and synthesis enzymes. *1*, Increased gene transcription; *2*, elevated mRNA levels (5'-AAA3') and increased synthesis of transporter and enzyme proteins. Cell swelling induces the loss of organic osmolytes. Downregulation of accumulation pathways is relatively slow. Activation of organic osmolyte efflux is rapid, indicating that organic osmolyte channels preexist in the membrane or a cytoplasmic pool. *3*, Rapid activation of organic osmolyte channels; *4*, inhibition of gene transcription; *5*, reduction of mRNA levels and protein synthesis; *6*, drop in the number of functional transporters and synthesis enzymes.

Loss of organic osmolytes from cells is elicited by swelling and occurs in two distinct steps. First, swelling induces a very rapid (i.e., seconds) increase in passive organic osmolyte efflux (Fig. 14.4). At least one pathway by which organic osmolytes are lost from cells is via a swelling-activated membrane anion channel that also serves as a volume regulatory efflux pathway for Cl^- (3,9,10). Other pathways may exist as well (11).

Downregulation of organic osmolyte synthesis and uptake mechanisms also contribute to the loss of these solutes from the cell. Overall, this process is slow. Cell swelling inhibits transcription of the genes coding for organic osmolyte transporters and synthesis enzymes (6–8). As transcription decreases, mRNA levels drop and the number of functional proteins declines over a period of many hours to days (Fig. 14.4).

How Do Cells Sense Their Size?

Unfortunately, we do not have a good answer to this question. We do know, however, that volume-sensing mechanisms are exquisitely sensitive. For example, studies by Lohr and Grantham (12) on the renal proximal tubule have demonstrated that cells can sense and respond to volume changes of less than 3%.

A number of possible volume signals have been postulated including swelling- and shrinkage-induced changes in membrane tension, cytoskeletal architecture, cellular ion concentrations, and the concentration of cytoplasmic macromolecules (4,5,13). All of these hypotheses have their strengths and weaknesses. At present it appears that no one signaling mechanism can account for the volume sensitivity of the various genes and membrane transport pathways that are activated or inactivated in response to cell volume perturbations. To further complicate the picture, recent evidence suggests that cells can detect more than simple swelling or shrinkage. Cells most likely possess a wide array of volume detector and effector mechanisms that respond selectively to both the magnitude and nature of the volume pertubation (14–16). Such functionally distinct sensor and effector pathways may afford the cell simultaneous control over a variety of parameters (e.g., intracellular pH and ionic composition) in addition to volume.

As with the initial volume signal sensed by the cell, there is little clear-cut understanding of the signaling mechanisms by which cell volume changes are transduced into regulatory responses. Numerous signal transduction pathways have been implicated in the control of volume regulatory transport pathways, including changes in intracellular Ca^{2+} concentration, GTPase activity, serine/threonine and tyrosine phosphorylation/dephosphorylation, and eicosanoid levels (4).

Perhaps the most extensively studied and best understood volume regulatory signaling mechanisms are the phosphorylation/dephosphorylation reactions that regulate swelling- and shrinkage-induced activation of the K-Cl and Na-K-2Cl cotransporters. Swelling-induced activation and shrinkage-induced inactivation of the K-Cl cotransporter are mediated by serine/threonine dephosphorylation and phosphorylation, respectively. The converse is true for the Na-K-2Cl cotransporter; shrinkage-induced activation is mediated by phosphorylation and swelling-induced inactivation is brought by dephosphorylation. Detailed transport studies suggest that both transporters are regulated by a common kinase whose activity is modulated by cell volume changes (13,17,18). The identity of this putative common volume-sensitive kinase is not firmly established. However, recent studies by Klein et al. (19) suggest that c-Jun NH2-terminal kinase (JNK) mediates shrinkage-induced phosphorylation of the Na-K-2Cl cotransporter in endothelial cells. Pharmacological studies suggest that type 1 protein phosphatase mediates protein dephosphorylation (20).

MOLECULAR IDENTIFICATION OF VOLUME REGULATORY MACHINERY

Molecular understanding of how cells sense volume changes requires the cloning of genes and cDNAs coding for volume regulatory transporters, channels, and metabolic enzymes. Significant progress has been made in this area over the past several years.

The genes and cDNAs encoding various organic osmolyte transporters and synthesis enzymes, including the Na^+/*myo*-inositol, Na^+/Cl^-/betaine and Na^+/Cl^-/taurine cotransporters, and aldose reductase (sorbitol synthesis), have been cloned and characterized in detail (6–8). As noted earlier, the activity of the transporters and enzymes themselves does not appear to be osmotically regulated. However, transcription and translation of the genes encoding these proteins are dramatically altered by cellular volume changes. Substantial progress has been made recently in identifying regulatory or so-called "osmotic response elements" (ORE) within the genes that modulate transcription in response to osmotic stress (7,21). It is currently thought that changes in intracellular ionic strength modulate ORE activity (7).

Detailed transport studies on numerous cell types have demonstrated that K-Cl and Na-K-2Cl cotransporters play central roles in RVD and RVI, respectively (4,5). Both transporters belong to the cation–chloride cotransporter (CCC) superfamily. To date, four distinct K-Cl cotransporter (KCC) genes have been identified (22–25). KCC1 is widely expressed and activated by cell swelling, suggesting that it may be a "housekeeping" isoform responsible for cell volume regulation (23). KCC2, which is expressed only in neurons (24), and KCC4 are also activated by swelling (25,26) when heterologously expressed, and may therefore function in volume homeostasis as well.

Two genes encoding Na-K-2Cl cotransporters (NKCC) have been identified (27). NKCC1 is widely expressed and is thought to be responsible for RVI. NKCC2 is found only in the apical membrane of the thick ascending limb of the kidney and most likely mediates apical NaCl and KCl entry and transepithelial salt reabsorption.

The Na^+/H^+ exchanger plays an important role in RVI (4,5). Six Na^+/H^+ exchanger isoforms have been identified to date at the molecular level (28). NHE1 is expressed ubiquitously, is activated by cell shrinkage and likely plays a general housekeeping role in volume homeostasis. NHE2 and NHE4 show a more limited pattern of expression, but are also activated by cell shrinkage when expressed heterologously (28).

Our molecular understanding of volume-sensitive ion channels is limited. To date, no unambiguous molecular candidates for volume regulatory cation channels have been described. However, two mechanosensitive cation channels have been shown to be modulated by cell volume changes. TREK-1 is a two-pore, four-transmembrane domain K^+ channel that is activated by membrane stretch in cell-attached and cell-detached patches (29,30). When expressed in *Xenopus* oocytes, TREK-1 current is inhibited by cell shrinkage (29). Suzuki et al. (31) recently cloned a homologue of the capsaicin receptor that gives rise to stretch-inhibited cation (SIC) channel activity when it is heterologously expressed. Cell shrinkage activates the channel. In addition to these mechanosensitive channels, two K^+ channels, Kv1.3 (32) and mIK1 (33), enhance RVD in cells in which they are heterologously expressed. This enhanced volume regulation is most likely due to complementation of a rate-limiting endogenous K^+ conductance.

ClC-2 is a member of the ClC superfamily of anion channels (34). When heterologously expressed, the channel is activated by cell swelling (35) and participates in RVD (36,37). However, a functional volume regulatory role for native ClC-2 channels or ClC-2-like currents has not been observed (36–40).

Activation of an outwardly rectifying anion current is a ubiquitous response to swelling in mammalian cells, as well as cells of certain lower vertebrates (3). This current is generically termed $I_{Cl,\ swell}$. Molecular identification of the $I_{Cl,\ swell}$ channel has been fraught with controversy and remains uncertain (41). Most recently, it has been suggested that ClC-3, another member of the ClC anion channel superfamily, is responsible for $I_{Cl,\ swell}$ in certain cell types (42,43).

CELL VOLUME HOMEOSTASIS AND HEPATOCYTE FUNCTION

Extensive studies of volume regulation and the effects of volume perturbations on cell function have been performed using hepatocytes (reviewed in refs. 4 and 44). While hepatocytes are not normally exposed to extracellular osmotic perturbations, changes in cell volume can occur under physiologically relevant conditions by alterations in intracellular solute content brought about by hormonal stimulation, uptake of solutes such as amino acids, and oxidative stress (44,45).

Hepatocyte RVD is brought about largely by the loss of K^+, Cl^- and HCO_3^- via swelling-induced activation of K^+ and anion channels. RVI occurs via activation of Na^+/H^+ and Cl^-/HCO_3^- exchangers (44). RVD and RVI are generally not complete in hepatocytes.

In addition to stimulating volume regulatory transport pathways, cell shrinkage or swelling acts as a signal to modify a variety of important liver functions (4,44,45). For example, insulin and glucagon induce cell volume changes by altering the activity of membrane transport pathways. Insulin induces swelling by stimulating the Na^+/H^+ exchanger and the Na-K-2Cl cotransporter. Swelling in turn increases protein and glycogen synthesis. These effects of insulin can be mimicked by anisosmotic cell swelling, and they can be blocked by preventing insulin-induced volume changes. In contrast, glucagon activates K^+ and Cl^- channels resulting in cell shrinkage, which induces breakdown of cellular proteins (Fig. 14.5A).

Figure 14.5B summarizes the effects of hepatocyte volume on proteolysis. The relationship between protein metabolism and cell volume changes induced by a variety of perturbations is linear. Experimental maneuvers that induce swelling inhibit proteolysis, whereas cell shrinkage stimulates protein breakdown. As a general rule, hepatocyte swelling acts as an anabolic signal and shrinkage acts as a catabolic signal (44,45).

CELL VOLUME HOMEOSTASIS AND PATHOPHYSIOLOGY

Disruption of cellular osmoregulatory mechanisms can give rise to a diverse group of disease states and their complications (1). A fundamental understanding of cellular osmoregulation therefore provides insight into patient care on a variety of levels. The following section discusses examples of the relationship between cell volume homeostasis and pathophysiology.

Rapid Regulatory Volume Increase in the Brain: Defeating Osmotherapy

Intravenous injection of hypertonic solutions has been a cornerstone of therapy for cerebral edema and raised intracranial pressure (ICP). Until recently, clinical understanding of intracranial volume has rested on a three-compartment model wherein total intracranial volume is equal to the sum of the volumes of cerebral blood, cerebral spinal fluid (CSF) and brain parenchyma (i.e., $V_{total} = V_{blood} + V_{CSF} + V_{brain}$). In this model, V_{brain} consists of both brain cells and the extracellular fluids or matrix surrounding them. Elevated ICP is commonly treated by decreasing V_{total} through reductions of V_{blood} by measures such as hyperventilation or V_{CSF} by drainage, diversion, or suppression of production.

In urgent situations, raised ICP is most frequently treated by reducing V_{brain} via intravenous injection of hypertonic

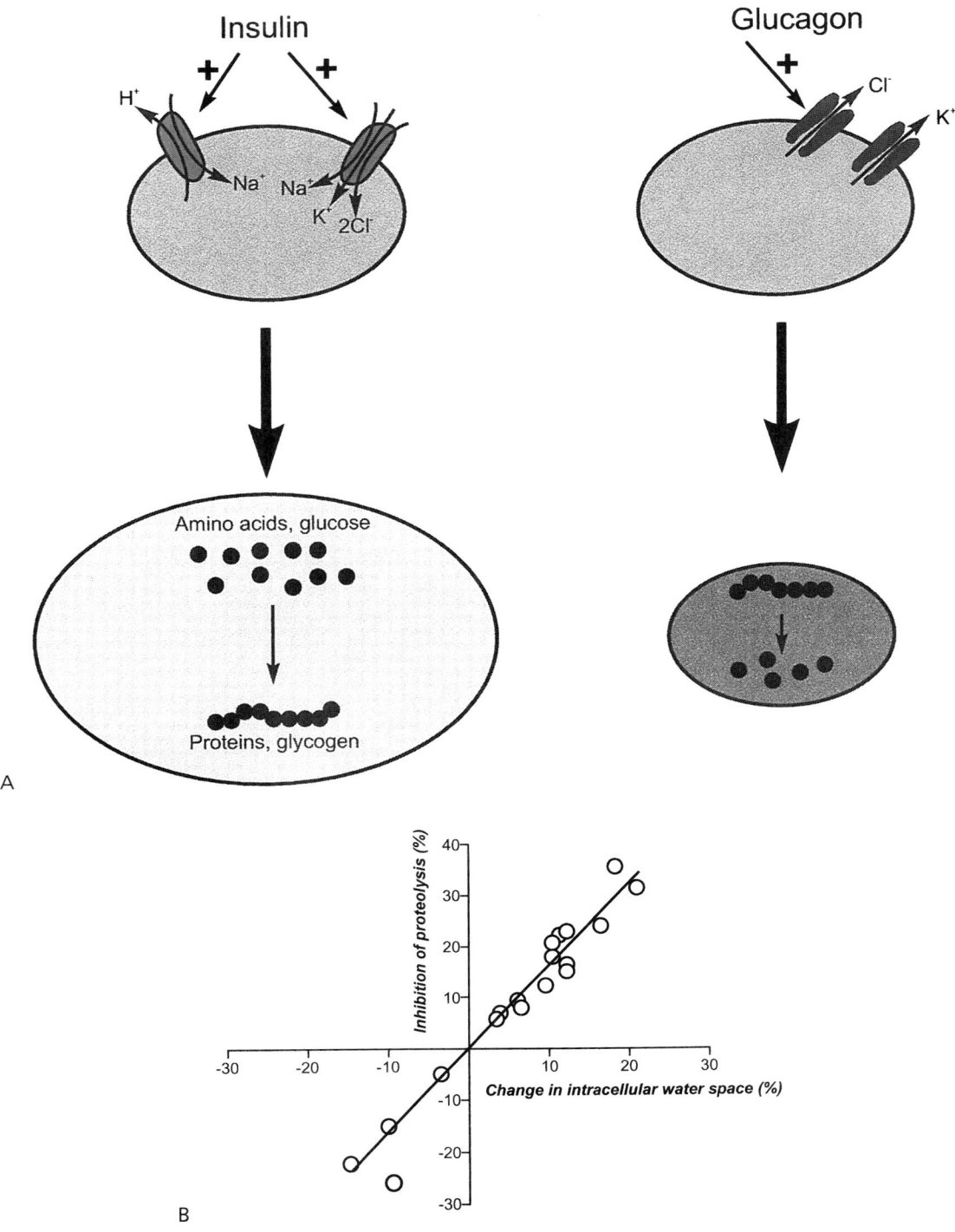

FIGURE 14.5. Effects of cell volume change on liver cell function. **A.** Insulin induces cell swelling by activating Na+/H+ exchange and Na-K-2Cl cotransport. Glucagon activates ion channels and induces cell shrinkage. In general, cell swelling and shrinkage act as anabolic and catabolic signals, respectively. **B.** Relationship between liver cell volume and proteolysis. Cell swelling progressively inhibits protein breakdown. Cell shrinkage increases proteolysis. (From Lang F, Ritter M, Vokl H, et al. The biological significance of cell volume. *Renal Physiology and Biochemistry* 1993;16:48–65, with permission.)

solutions such as mannitol. Mannitol-induced decreases in ICP have traditionally been attributed to osmotic shrinkage of brain cells. It has been observed, however, that changes in brain volume after administration of hypertonic fluids are significantly less than predicted for ideal osmotic behavior. Studies using ion-sensitive microelectrodes have demonstrated that, in fact, intracellular water does not change in the brains of animals injected with hypertonic solutions. Instead, brain cell volume is regulated rapidly by the uptake of Na^+, K^+ and Cl^- (46). This rapid RVI process has also been observed in cultured glial cells and directly opposes any attempts to osmotically reduce cell volume (47). These findings suggest that further progress in the use of osmotherapy for cerebral edema will require investigators to view brain volume in the context of a four-compartment model where $V_{total} = V_{blood} + V_{CSF} + V_{extracellular} + V_{intracellular}$ (47,48).

As discussed above, rapid RVI occurs through electrolyte transport. In a wide range of cell types, RVI may be partially or completely blocked by membrane transport inhibitors such as amiloride or furosemide. Drugs such as furosemide have been used traditionally in combination with plasma hypertonicity to enhance and prolong osmolar effects on ICP. While the synergistic effects of osmotic and loop diuretics in this respect have been attributed to enhanced diuresis, an alternative mechanism involving inhibition of brain cell volume regulatory processes may be at work (47). A four-compartment model, with focus upon the clinical manipulation of $V_{intracellular}$ through membrane transport processes, provides a new avenue for control and treatment of cerebral edema.

Correction of Plasma Hypertonicity: Undermining Nature

A variety of disease states such as diabetes, dehydration, renal failure, and advanced liver disease are associated with significant elevations of plasma osmolality. While correction of acute increases in plasma osmolality is usually well tolerated, correction of chronic plasma hypertonicity can represent a serious clinical challenge. In certain settings, rehydration therapy may be accompanied by brain swelling, herniation, and death.

Clinical differences between acute and chronic osmolar disorders can be understood through consideration of the different mechanisms by which cells in the brain regulate their volume in response to acute and chronic osmotic challenges. As in other cell types, hypertonically stressed brain cells regulate their volume initially by rapid electrolyte uptake (47). With chronic elevation of plasma osmolality, however, most excess electrolytes in the brain are replaced by organic osmolytes. Studies in animal models and cultured cells (reviewed in ref. 49) reveal that idiogenic osmoles are the same organic osmolytes used universally for volume regulation. The most important organic osmolytes in the mammalian brain include *myo*-inositol, taurine, and

certain amino acids. These solutes are accumulated primarily by uptake from the extracellular fluids via activation of Na^+-dependent cotransporters (49).

Cells that have undergone RVI swell above or "overshoot" their resting volume when returned to an isotonic medium (Fig. 14.1). This overshoot is corrected by immediate activation of RVD processes. In cells that have been exposed acutely to hypertonicity, RVD is rapid because accumulated electrolytes are lost rapidly (50). Cells that have accumulated organic osmolytes, however, swell and remain swollen for prolonged periods of time due to slow loss of these solutes. Slow loss of brain organic osmolytes, particularly *myo*-inositol, has been observed in animal models and cultured glial cells (49,50). Lee et al. (51) demonstrated by nuclear magnetic resonance spectroscopy the extremely slow loss of accumulated *myo*-inositol from the brain of a human infant undergoing rehydration therapy.

Why is the loss of *myo*-inositol from brain cells so slow? Strange and coworkers have examined this issue using cultured glial cells (52,53). As discussed earlier, cell swelling activates a broadly selective organic osmolyte efflux channel. *Myo*-inositol is at the upper size limit of solutes that can permeate the channel, however, and efflux is therefore relatively slow. In addition, the Na^+-dependent *myo*-inositol uptake pathway induced by chronic hypertonic stress remains activated for prolonged periods of time. For example, in rat cortical astrocytes, downregulation of the cotransporter does not begin until 16 hours after *abrupt* reduction of extracellular osmolality (54). Downregulation of the cotransporter may be even slower *in vivo* where plasma osmolality is reduced slowly. The net effect of this delayed reduction in cotransporter activity is continued *myo*-inositol accumulation under conditions requiring loss of this solute from the cells.

Sickle Cell Crisis: Blocking Capillaries by Shrinking Cells

Patients with sickle cell disease are homozygous for a gene that codes for the synthesis of an abnormal hemoglobin (HbS). When oxygen tension is low, HbS polymerizes, causing deformation of erythrocytes with production of sickle forms. Sickled cells are poorly compliant and occlude capillaries beds, resulting in microvascular thrombosis, ischemia and pain.

Polymerization of HbS is remarkably sensitive to hemoglobin concentration, with small increases in HbS levels greatly increasing the rate of polymer formation. Sickled erythrocytes are severely dehydrated and have very high mean corpuscular hemoglobin concentrations. Two ion transport pathways, the KCl cotransporter and a K^+ selective channel controlled by cytosolic Ca^{2+} levels (known as the Gardos channel), appear to play major roles in erythrocyte shrinkage (55–57). Both of these K^+ transport pathways are stimulated by deoxygenation, cell swelling and acidosis. The relative contribution of the cotransporter and

Gardos channel to volume decrease in sickled cells is not known. However, an integrated model has been proposed wherein conditions of local tissue acidosis and deoxygenation-induced influx of Ca^{2+} activates the Gardos channel, resulting in K^+ loss and cell shrinkage. A consequence of activation of the Gardos channel is slight cytoplasmic acidification which may, in turn, activate the KCl cotransporter to produce further cell shrinkage. A commonly used antifungal agent, clotrimazole, is a potent blocker of the Gardos channel and cell shrinkage induced by deoxygenation (56,58).

CONCLUSION

An understanding of cellular osmoregulation has provided important insights into basic biological problems such as regulation of gene expression, cellular signal transduction and the molecular basis of transporter protein function. A detailed cellular and molecular understanding of cell volume regulation also provides deeper insight into common pathophysiologic conditions.

ACKNOWLEDGMENTS

This work was supported by National Institutes of Health grants NS30591 and DK45628.

REFERENCES

1. McManus ML, Churchwell KB, Strange K. Regulation of cell volume in health and disease. *N Engl J Med* 1995;333: 1260–1266.
2. McManus ML, Churchwell KB. Clinical significance of cellular osmoregulation. In: Strange K, ed.*Cellular and Molecular Physiology of Cell Volume Regulation*. Boca Raton: CRC Press, 1994; 63–77.
3. Strange K, Emma F, Jackson PS. Cellular and molecular physiology of volume-sensitive anion channels. *Am J Physiol* 1996;270: C711–C730.
4. Lang F, Busch GL, Ritter M, et al. Functional significance of cell volume regulatory mechanisms. *Physiol Rev* 1998;78:247–306.
5. O'Neill WC. Physiological significance of volume-regulatory transporters. *Am J Physiol* 1999;276:C995–C1011.
6. Burg MB. Molecular basis of osmotic regulation. *Am J Physiol* 1995;268:F983–F996.
7. Burg MB, Kwon ED, Kültz D. Regulation of gene expression by hypertonicity. *Annu Rev Physiol* 1997;59:437–455.
8. Yancey PH. Compatible and counteracting solutes. In: Strange K, ed. *Cellular and Molecular Physiology of Cell Volume Regulation*. Boca Raton: CRC Press, 1994;81–109.
9. Kirk K, Strange K. Functional properties and physiological roles of organic solute channels. *Annu Rev Physiol* 1998;60:719–739.
10. Kirk K. Physiological roles and functional properties of swelling-activated organic osmolyte channels. *J Membr Biol* 1997; 158:1–16.
11. Stutzin A, Torres R, Oporto M, et al. Separate taurine and chloride efflux pathways activated during regulatory volume decrease. *Am J Physiol* 1999;277:C392–C402.
12. Lohr JW, Grantham JJ. Isovolumetric regulation of isolated S2 proximal tubules in anisotonic media. *J Clin Invest* 1986;78: 1165–1172.
13. Parker JC. In defense of cell volume? *Am J Physiol* 1993;265: C1191–C1200.
14. Emma F, McManus M, Strange K. Intracellular electrolytes regulate the volume set point of the organic osmolyte/anion channel VSOAC. *Am J Physiol* 1997;272:C1766–C1775.
15. Strange K. Are all cell volume changes the same? *News in Physiological Sciences* 1994;9:223–228.
16. MacLeod RJ, Hamilton JR. Ca^{2+}/Calmodulin kinase II and decreases in intracellular pH are required to activate K^+ channels after substantial swelling in villus epithelial cells. *J Membr Biol* 1999;172:59–66.
17. Jennings ML, al-Rohil N. Kinetics of activation and inactivation of swelling-stimulated K^+/Cl^- transport. The volume-sensitive parameter is the rate constant for inactivation. *J Gen Physiol* 1990;95:1021–1040.
18. Lytle C. A volume-sensitive protein kinase regulates the Na-K-2Cl cotransporter in duck red blood cells. *Am J Physiol* 1998;274: C1002–C1010.
19. Klein JD, Lamitina ST, O'Neill WC. JNK is a volume-sensitive kinase that phosphorylates the Na-K-2Cl cotransporter in vitro. *Am J Physiol* 1999;277:C425–C431.
20. Starke LC, Jennings ML. K-Cl cotransport in rabbit red cells: Further evidence for regulation by protein phosphatase type 1. *Am J Physiol* 1993;264:C118–C124.
21. Ferraris JD, Williams CK, Ohtaka A, et al. Functional consensus for mammalian osmotic response elements. *Am J Physiol* 1999; 276:C667–C673.
22. Hiki K, D'Andrea RJ, Furze J, et al. Cloning, characterization, and chromosomal location of a novel human K^+-Cl^- cotransporter. *J Biol Chem* 1999;274:10661–10667.
23. Gillen CM, Brill S, Payne JA, et al. Molecular cloning and functional expression of the K-Cl cotransporter from rabbit, rat, and human. A new member of the cation-chloride cotransporter family. *J Biol Chem* 1996;271:16237–16244.
24. Payne JA, Stevenson TJ, Donaldson LF. Molecular characterization of a putative K-Cl cotransporter in rat brain. A neuronal-specific isoform. *J Biol Chem* 1996;271:16245–16252.
25. Mount DB, Mercado A, Song L, et al. Cloning and characterization of KCC3 and KCC4, new members of the cation-chloride cotransporter gene family. *J Biol Chem* 1999;274:16355–16362.
26. Singer TD, Delpire E, Morrison R, et al. Molecular and functional characterization of the KCC1 and KCC2 K-Cl cotransporter isoforms. *FASEB J* 1999;13:A712(Abstract)
27. Delpire E, Kaplan MR, Plotkin MD, et al. The Na-(K)-Cl cotransporter family in the mammalian kidney: Molecular identification and function(s). *Nephrol Dial Transplant* 1996;11: 1967–1973.
28. Orlowski J, Grinstein S. Na^+/H^+ exchangers of mammalian cells. *J Biol Chem* 1997;272:22373–22376.
29. Patel AJ, Honore E, Maingret F, et al. A mammalian two pore domain mechano-gated S-like K^+ channel. *EMBO J* 1998;17: 4283–4290.
30. Maingret F, Patel AJ, Lesage F, et al. Mechano- or acid stimulation, two interactive modes of activation of the TREK-1 potassium channel. *J Biol Chem* 1999;274:26691–26696.
31. Suzuki M, Sato J, Kutsuwada K, et al. Cloning of a stretch-inhibitable nonselective cation channel. *J Biol Chem* 1999;274: 6330–6335.
32. Deutsch C, Chen LQ. Heterologous expression of specific K^+ channels in T lymphocytes: functional consequences for volume regulation. *Proc Natl Acad Sci U S A* 1993;90:10036–10040.

33. Vandorpe DH, Shmukler BE, Jiang L, et al. cDNA cloning and functional characterization of the mouse Ca^{2+}-gated K^+ channel, mIK1. Roles in regulatory volume decrease and erythroid differentiation. *J Biol Chem* 1998;273:21542–21553.

34. Jentsch TJ, Günther W. Chloride channels: An emerging molecular picture. *Bioessays* 1997;19:117–126.

35. Grunder S, Thiemann A, Pusch M, et al. Regions involved in the opening of ClC-2 chloride channel by voltage and cell volume. *Nature* 1992;360:759–762.

36. Xiong H, Li C, Garami E, et al. ClC-2 activation modulates regulatory volume decrease. *J Membr Biol* 1999;167:215–221.

37. Furukawa T, Ogura T, Katayama Y, et al. Characteristics of rabbit ClC-2 current expressed in *Xenopus* oocytes and its contribution to volume regulation. *Am J Physiol* 1998;274:C500–C512.

38. Fritsch J, Edelman A. Osmosensitivity of the hyperpolarization-activated chloride current in human intestinal T84 cells. *Am J Physiol* 1997;272:C778–C786.

39. Bond TD, Ambikapathy S, Mohammad S, et al. Osmosensitive C1- currents and their relevance to regulatory volume decrease in human intestinal T84 cells: outwardly vs. inwardly rectifying currents. *J Physiol* 1998;511:45–54.

40. Carew MA, Thorn P. Identification of ClC-2-like chloride currents in pig pancreatic acinar cells. *Pflugers Arch* 1996;433:84–90.

41. Strange K. Molecular identity of the outwardly rectifying, swelling-activated anion channel: time to re-evaluate pICln. *J Gen Physiol* 1998;111:617–622.

42. Duan D, Winter C, Cowley S, et al. Molecular identification of a volume-regulated chloride channel. *Nature* 1997;390:417–421.

43. Duan D, Cowley S, Horowitz B, et al. A serine residue in ClC-3 links phosphorylation-dephosphorylation to chloride channel regulation by cell volume. *J Gen Physiol* 1999;113:57–70.

44. Haussinger D. The role of cellular hydration in the regulation of cell function. *Biochem J* 1996;313:697–710.

45. Haussinger D, Schliess F. Osmotic induction of signaling cascades: role in regulation of cell function. *Biochem Biophys Res Commun* 1999;255:551–555.

46. Cserr HF, DePasquale M, Nicholson C, et al. Extracellular volume decreases while cell volume is maintained by ion uptake in rat brain during acute hypernatremia. *J Physiol* 1991;442:277–295.

47. McManus ML, Strange K. Acute volume regulation of brain cells in response to hypertonic challenge. *Anesthesiology* 1993;78:1132–1137.

48. Cserr HF, Patlak CS. Regulation of brain volume under isosmotic and anisosmotic conditions. In: Gilles R, ed. *Advances in comparative and environmental physiology*. Berlin: Springer-Verlag, 1991;61–80.

49. Strange K. Regulation of solute and water balance and cell volume in the central nervous system. *J Am Soc Nephrol* 1992;3:12–27.

50. Strange K, Morrison R. Volume regulation during recovery from chronic hypertonicity in brain glial cells. *Am J Physiol* 1992;263:C412–9.

51. Lee JH, Arcinue E, Ross BD. Brief report: organic osmolytes in the brain of an infant with hypernatremia. *N Engl J Med* 1994;331:439–442.

52. Strange K, Morrison R, Shrode L, et al. Mechanism and regulation of swelling-activated inositol efflux in brain glial cells. *Am J Physiol* 1993;265:C244–C256.

53. Paredes A, McManus M, Kwon HM, et al. Osmoregulation of Na^+-inositol cotransporter activity and mRNA levels in brain glial cells. *Am J Physiol* 1992;263:C1282–8.

54. Strange K, Emma F, Paredes A, et al. Osmoregulatory changes in *myo*-inositol content and Na^+/*myo*-inositol cotransport in rat cortical astrocytes. *Glia* 1994;12:35–43.

55. Canessa M. Red cell volume-related ion transport systems in hemoglobinopathies. *Hematol Oncol Clin North Am* 1991;5:495–516.

56. Brugnara C, Gee B, Armsby CC, et al. Therapy with oral clotrimazole induces inhibition of the Gardos channel and reduction of erythrocyte dehydration in patients with sickle cell disease. *J Clin Invest* 1996;97:1227–1234.

57. Joiner CH. Cation transport and volume regulation in sickle red blood cells. *Am J Physiol* 1993;264:C251–C270.

58. Brugnara C, De FL, Armsby CC, et al. A new therapeutic approach for sickle cell disease. Blockade of the red cell Ca^{2+}-activated K^+ channel by clotrimazole. *Ann N Y Acad Sci* 1995;763:262–271.

59. Lang F, Ritter M, Vokl H, et al. The biological significance of cell volume. *Ren Physiol Biochem* 1993;16:48–65.

ROLES OF INTRACELLULAR PROTEOLYSIS IN HEPATOCYTE CELL-CYCLE, AGING, AND PROGRAMMED CELL DEATH

J. FRED DICE

The degradation of proteins within hepatocytes and other mammalian cells occurs through several distinct pathways. A major cytosolic and nuclear pathway involves covalent modification of substrate proteins with ubiquitin, followed by their degradation by the 26S proteasome. This pathway of proteolysis also drives the cell cycle by the periodic destruction of cyclins, cyclin-dependent kinase inhibitors, and other critical regulatory proteins. Chaperone-mediated autophagy is one of at least five different lysosomal pathways of protein degradation that are active in hepatocytes. This lysosomal pathway of proteolysis, together with macroautophagy, declines with age and largely accounts for the reduced proteolysis characteristic of aging organisms. This reduced proteolysis may lead to the accumulation of abnormal proteins in aged tissues, including the liver, and probably contributes to other characteristics of aging. Caspases are a family of cytosolic cysteine proteases that cleave after aspartate residues in substrate proteins. A caspase activation cascade commits hepatocytes and other cells to apoptosis or programmed cell death and also plays crucial roles in the execution of apoptosis.

Some pathways of intracellular proteolysis degrade proteins to small peptides or free amino acids, but others hydrolyze proteins in a more limited fashion to activate or inactivate the protein substrates (1–3). Protein degradation is of fundamental importance for cells and organisms. For example, mobilization of amino acids from proteins between meals is essential for survival (1,4,5). Also, degradation of critical signalling proteins provides a more complete inhibition of activity than may be achieved by covalent modifications such as phosphorylation or dephosphorylation (2,6,7). Proteins are also subject to environmental damage by oxidation, nonenzymatic glycosylation, and deamination (8–11). Such posttranslational modifications can be kept to a minimum by continually degrading and resynthesizing proteins.

Eukaryotic cells including hepatocytes have multiple pathways of proteolysis and an abundance of endoproteases and exoproteases (2,3,6,7,12–17). Almost 200 proteases have been reported in hepatocytes (Fig. 15.1, com-

J. F. Dice: Department of Physiology, Tufts University School of Medicine, Boston, Massachusetts 02111.

proteasome subunits (31)
proteasome regulators (36)
ubiquitination (60)
caspases (13)
m-calpains (2)
μ-calpain (2)

tripeptidyl peptidase II
dipeptidyl peptidase III
dipeptidyl peptidase IV
cystinyl aminopeptidase
pyroglutamyl peptidase II
acylaminoacyl peptidase
aspartyl dipeptidase
aminopeptidase B
methionyl aminopeptidase

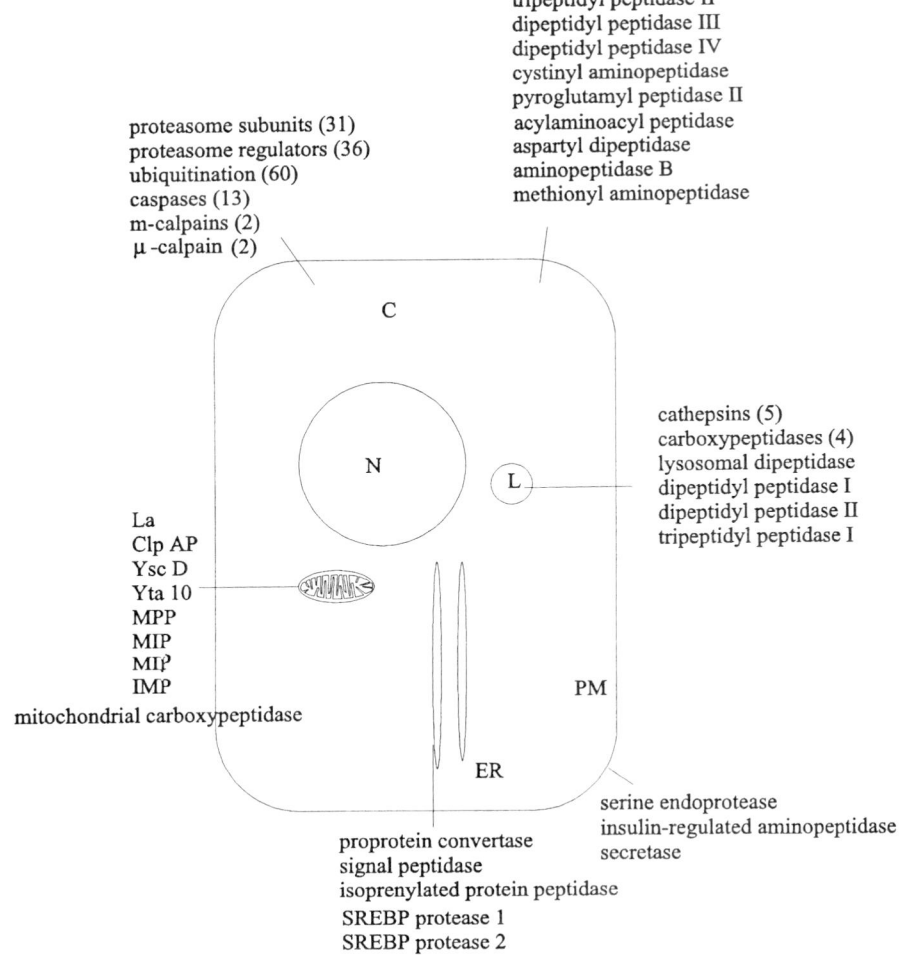

cathepsins (5)
carboxypeptidases (4)
lysosomal dipeptidase
dipeptidyl peptidase I
dipeptidyl peptidase II
tripeptidyl peptidase I

La
Clp AP
Ysc D
Yta 10
MPP
MIP
MIP'
IMP
mitochondrial carboxypeptidase

serine endoprotease
insulin-regulated aminopeptidase
secretase

proprotein convertase
signal peptidase
isoprenylated protein peptidase
SREBP protease 1
SREBP protease 2

FIGURE 15.1. Proteases and peptidases in hepatocytes. Proteases and peptidases and their primary subcellular localization are indicated from infomation gathered from Barrett AJ, Rawlings ND, Woessner JF. *Handbook of proteolytic enzymes.* New York: Academic Press, 1998. Numbers in parentheses indicate numbers of different proteins in that group. For example, cathepsins (5) indicates that there are five different cathepsins in hepatocytes. The cell diagrammed is a hepatocyte. *C*, cytosol; *L*, lysosome; *PM*, plasma membrane; *ER*, endoplasmic reticulum; *SREBP*, sterol regulatory element binding protein.

piled from information in ref. 18), and many of them work in conjuction with other proteins such as molecular chaperones (15,19). The roles of these different proteolytic pathways vary to some extent from tissue to tissue. For example, lysosomal chaperone-mediated autophagy is active in liver, kidney, and certain other tissues in response to prolonged starvation (5,20) but cannot be detected in skeletal muscle (21). Protein breakdown also occurs in muscle in response to starvation, but it is primarily the ubiquitin/proteasome pathway that is activated (22). The ubiquitin/proteasome pathway is also the major proteolytic activity in lymphocytes (23). The evolutionary significance and functional significance of using different

proteolytic pathways to achieve enhanced protein degradation are not known.

THE UBIQUITIN/PROTEASOME SYSTEM AND CELL CYCLE PROGRESSION

Cyclins, cyclin-dependent kinases, and cyclin-dependent kinase inhibitors are critical regulators of cell division in hepatocytes. The ubiquitin/proteasome proteolytic pathway is responsible for the degradation of cyclins, cyclin-dependent kinase inhibitors, and many transcriptional regulators (2,6,7,24–26). If the degradation of these cell cycle regulators is inhibited, the cell cycle arrests at defined points such as G1, G2, or M. Therefore, the ubiquitin/proteasome proteolytic pathway is necessary for cell cycle progression.

The Ubiquitin Conjugation Cycle

The ubiquitin/proteasome system is an important proteolytic pathway in the cytosol and nucleus (2,6,7,27). This pathway involves the covalent ligation of a polyubiquitin chain to a substrate protein (Fig. 15.2). Many details of the conjugation pathway are known and have been extensively reviewed elsewhere (6,7). In brief, ubiquitin is first activated by a ubiquitin-activating enzyme, E1, which activates the ubiquitin C-terminal glycine by forming a thiolester bond in an ATP-dependent manner. A second thiolester bond is formed with one of many ubiquitin-carrier proteins, E2s, and then the E2s alone, or more commonly in association with ubiquitin-conjugating enzymes, E3s, link the C-terminus of ubiquitin to an ε-amino group of lysine in the substrate protein to form an isopeptide bond. In some cases the α-amino group of the N-terminus can be used as a linkage site for the ubiquitin chain (24). The ubiquitin chain is built by sequential coupling of the C-terminus of ubiquitin to an internal lysine of the previous ubiquitin molecule. It is also possible that some ubiquitin chains are preassembled and then linked all at once to the substrate protein. E4 enzymes facilitate the assembly of the ubiquitin chains (28). Coupling to lysine48 (K48) of ubiquitin creates a ubiquitin chain that targets the substrate for degradation by the 26S proteasome. Coupling to other lysines within ubiquitin also occurs *in vivo*, and a K63 linkage may be a signal for endocytosis of plasma membrane receptors and is somehow required for DNA repair (6,7). Ubiquitin chains coupled through K11 and K29 also occur, but their significance is not known. A large family of ubiquitin-specific hydrolases are able to remove ubiquitin from all types of ubiquitin chains as well as from substrate proteins and peptides (6,29,30).

Substrate Specificity

How is a protein selected for ubiquitination? The rate-limiting step appears to be recognition of the substrate protein by one of the E3s (6,7). There are four different families of E3s. Ubr1 or E3α recognizes the amino terminal residue of a protein as well as some internal sequence features (31) and an accessible lysine. E3α also binds to particular E2s to form a complex. Proteins with basic or bulky, hydrophobic amino termini are recognized by E3α, rapidly ubiquitinated, and then rapidly degraded. Substrates for this aspect of ubiquitin-dependent proteolysis termed the N-end rule are listed in Table 15.1. Another family of E3s contain sequences in the hect (*h*omologous to papillomavirus *E6* oncoprotein-associated protein *C-t*erminus; E6-AP) domain family (27).

TABLE 15.1. EXAMPLES OF PROTEIN SUBSTRATES FOR DIFFERENT TYPES OF E3S

Substrates	Role of Protein
E3α (N-end Pathway)	
G protein α subunit	signal transduction
c-Mos	proto-oncoprotein
CUP9	repressor of permeases
Sindbis virus RNA polymerase	viral RNA synthesis
Hect domain E3s	
p53	tumor suppression
RNA polymerase II	transcription
Cdc25 phosphatase	cell cycle progression
c-Jun	transcription
Cyclosome	
mitotic cyclins	cell cycle progression
S-phase cyclins	cell cycle progression
Cut2p	cell cycle progression
Ase1p	cell cycle progression
Cdc6p	cell cycle progression
PULC	
G1 cyclins	cell cycle progression
Sic1p	cell cycle progression
Par1p	cell cycle progression
p27	cell cycle progression
Gcn4p	transcription
NKκB	transcription
IκB	transcription
β-catenin	transcription
E2F-1	transcription
Stat-1	signal transduction
Src	signal transduction

All of these proteins are ubiquitinated and degraded by the 26S proteasome. Citations to original research reports can be found in references 6 and 7.

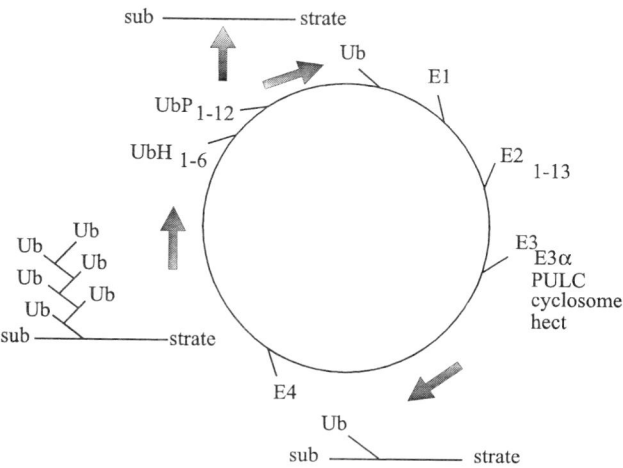

FIGURE 15.2. The protein ubiquitination cycle. The steps and components of this cycle are as described in the text. *Ub*, ubiquitin; *E1*, ubiquitin activating enzyme; *E2*, ubiquitin carrier protein; *E3*, ubiquitin conjugating protein; *E4*, ubiquitin chain-forming enzyme; *PULC*, phosphoprotein–ubiquitin–ligase complexes; *UbH*, ubiquitin hydrolase; *UbP*, ubiquitin protease.

The E6-AP is required for the ubiquitination of p53 and possibly several other proteins (Table 15.1). Other E3s are members of multisubunit complexes. The *phospho-protein–ubiquitin–ligase complexes* (PULCs) act on substrates only after the substrate has been phosphorylated (6). These phosphorylation sites are commonly, but not always, in regions of substrate proteins enriched for the amino acids P, E, S, and T (PEST regions) (25). Sustrates of PULCs include G1 cyclins (Table 15.1). The E3-containing cyclosome (also called the anaphase promoting complex) is a multisubunit structure of 1,500 kd. It ubiquitinates mitotic cyclins and other cell cycle regulatory enzymes (Table 15.1), and the cyclosome activity is dependent on the phosphorylation of cyclosome subunits. The critical region in substrate proteins that is recognized by the cyclosome is the destruction box, nine amino acids with the consensus sequence RxxLxxxxN where x represents any amino acid (6).

Membrane Proteins Can Also Be Ubiquitinated

A growing number of membrane proteins are ubiquitinated and then degraded within lysosomes or the yeast equivalent, the vacuole (Table 15.2) (32–35). However, some membrane proteins and secretory proteins are ubiquitinated and degraded by the 26S proteasome (Table 15.2) (36–39). Such proteins include hepatocye secretory proteins such as apolipoprotein B100 and forms of the α_1-trypsin inhibitor (40). These proteins are ubiquitinated on their cytoplasmic domains and pulled out of the membrane by the binding and proteolytic actions of the 26S proteasome. In the case

of endoplasmic reticulum (ER), the proteins exit through the same translocon complex by which they entered the ER during their synthesis (17,41). Just as molecular chaperones of the 70 kd family are required for efficient entry of proteins into the ER (19,41–43), they are also required for their exit and degradation by the 26S proteasome (17).

The 26S Proteasome

Once the substrate protein has been ubiquitinated, it is either deubiquitinated (Fig. 15.2) or degraded by the 26S proteasome (44–47). The structural and functional properties of the 26S proteasome are shown in Figure 15.3 and are similar in all mammalian cells including hepatocytes. The core 20S proteasome contains two seven-membered rings of α subunits and two seven-membered rings of β subunits arranged into a cylinder. The β subunits contain the proteolytic active sites, while the α subunits bind to unfolded proteins but do not degrade them (6). The 14 α and 14 β subunits are all different gene products in mammalian cells. The 19S regulatory cap forms at one or both ends of the 20S proteasome to produce the 26S proteasome. The regulatory cap can be separated into inner and outer complexes, each of which is made up of eight different subunits (Fig. 15.3). The outer cap contains binding sites for polyubiquitin chains (47), while the inner cap has molecular chaperone activity that presumably acts *in vivo* to unfold proteins (48). The inner cap *in vitro* can also refold proteins in an ATP-dependent manner. Therefore, the model that has emerged for how the 26S proteasome degrades proteins that are conjugated to a polyubiquitin chain is: (a) the polyubiquitin chain

TABLE 15.2. FATES OF MEMBRANE PROTEINS THAT ARE UBIQUITINATED

	Role of Protein
Degraded by the 26S proteasome	
HMGCoA reductase	cholesterol synthesis
Cystic fibrosis transmembrane regulator	calcium channel
T cell receptor subunits	antigen presentation
PDGF receptor	response to PDGF
HGF/SF receptor	response to HGF/SF
Apolipoprotein B100	cholesterol transport
α_1-antitrypsin	trypsin inhibitor
Connexin 43	cell-cell communication
Degraded by lysosomes/vacuoles	
α Factor receptor	mating and signal transduction
Ste6p	transport
Pdr5p	transport
Gal2p	galactose transport
Gap1p	amino acid transport
Fur4	uracil transport
Sodium channel	sodium entry and exit
Growth hormone receptor	response to growth hormone
Kit receptor	signal transduction
Tat2p	tryptophan transport

HMGCoA, hydroxymethylglutaryl coenzyme A; PDGF, platelet-derived growth factor; HGF/SF, hepatocyte growth factor/scatter factor. Citations to original reports can be found in references 6, 7, 32–40.

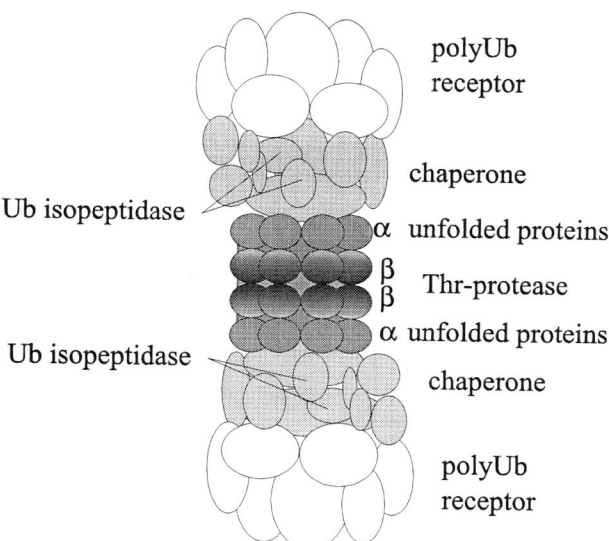

FIGURE 15.3. Structure and activities of the 26S proteasome. The 20S proteasome core consists of 14 α and 14 β subunits arranged in stacked rings. The α subunits bind to unfolded proteins, and the β subunits have threonine protease activities. A regulatory complex binds to both ends of the 20S proteasome to form the 26S proteasome. The outer portion of the regulatory complex binds to ubiquitin chains, and the inner portion acts as a molecular chaperone to unfold proteins. One or two of the proteins in the inner complex is a ubiquitin isopeptidase that removes intact ubiquitin from polypeptides.

is bound by the outer cap, (b) the protein is unfolded by the inner cap, (c) the successfully unfolded protein is bound by the proteasome α subunits, (d) the protein is digested to small peptides in the 8–12 amino acid size range by the proteasome β subunits, and (e) the ubiquitin chains are disassembled from the polypeptide fragments by a ubiquitin hydrolase associated with the outer cap of the proteasome.

A small number of proteins can be degraded by the 26S proteasome even though they are not polyubiquitinated. Such proteins, including ornithine decarboxylase, c-Jun, and IκBα, are probably efficiently unfolded by the inner cap and efficiently bound by α subunits without need for polyubiquitination (6,47).

Other regulatory complexes can also associate with the core 20S proteasome. These regulators activate the peptidase activities of the 20S proteasome but do not permit the degradation of folded proteins. To what extent the 20S proteasome associates with this regulator complex rather than the cap structure *in vivo* is not known (6).

Proteolytic Systems Related to the 26S Proteasome

Other large, multimeric proteases also exist in mammalian cells (16), and their functional relationships with the 26S proteasome are being studied. The tricorn protease was first identified in thermophilic bacteria, but a related larger protease called multicorn exists in mammalian cells including hepatocytes (49). Proteasome inhibitors are usually lethal to cells within a few hours (45), but under particular conditions, cells resistant to proteasome inhibitors can be selected. Many of these cells have increased expression of the multicorn protease, suggesting that the activities of the multicorn at least partially overlap with those of the 26S proteasome.

Ubiquitin-Related Proteins

A variety of ubiquitin-related proteins also exist in hepatocytes and other cell types and are covalently linked to other cellular proteins but do not target them for degradation. For example, the small ubiquitin-like modifier protein, SUMO-1, (50,51) is covalently linked to RanGAP-1, an activator of a Ras-like GTPase required for import of certain proteins into the nucleus. The SUMO-1 modification is required for the activity or localization of the RanGAP-1. Another ubiquitin-like protein, Rub-1, is covalently linked to proteins called cullins and regulates their targeting into multimeric complexes (52). Finally, a protein conjugation system reminiscent of ubiquitination has been identified in both yeast and mammalian cells that is required for the formation of macroautophagic vacuoles as well as later steps of macroautophagy (53–55). More recently, this same protein conjugation system has been shown to be required for microautophagy, at least in its selective mode when peroxisomes are being preferentially degraded (56).

LYSOSOMAL PATHWAYS OF PROTEOLYSIS AND AGING

Hepatocytes have at least five different pathways for the delivery of intracellular proteins to lysosomes for subsequent degradation (Fig. 15.4) (1,13,57–59). Endocytosis in its many forms is responsible for the delivery of extracellular proteins to lysosomes, but membrane proteins can also be delivered to lysosomes by these pathways (60,61). Secreted proteins in the constitutive and regulated pathways can be diverted to lysosomes and degraded when stimuli for their secretion are lacking (14,62–64). This process has been called crinophagy, but may represent several mechanistically distinct pathways. Macroautophagy is a process by which areas of cytoplasm are first sequestered by a double membrane (1,4,13,57,65, 66). These autophagosomes then acidify and fuse to primary lysosomes to form autophagic vacuoles. Microautophagy involves the inward vesiculation of lysosomes with internalized organelles first enclosed in a vesicle within the lysosome (4,13,56,57,66–68). The vesicular membrane is then removed, and the internalized proteins are degraded. Finally, proteins can also be taken into lysosomes in a molecule-by-molecule pathway that we have called chaperone-mediated autophagy (20,57,69).

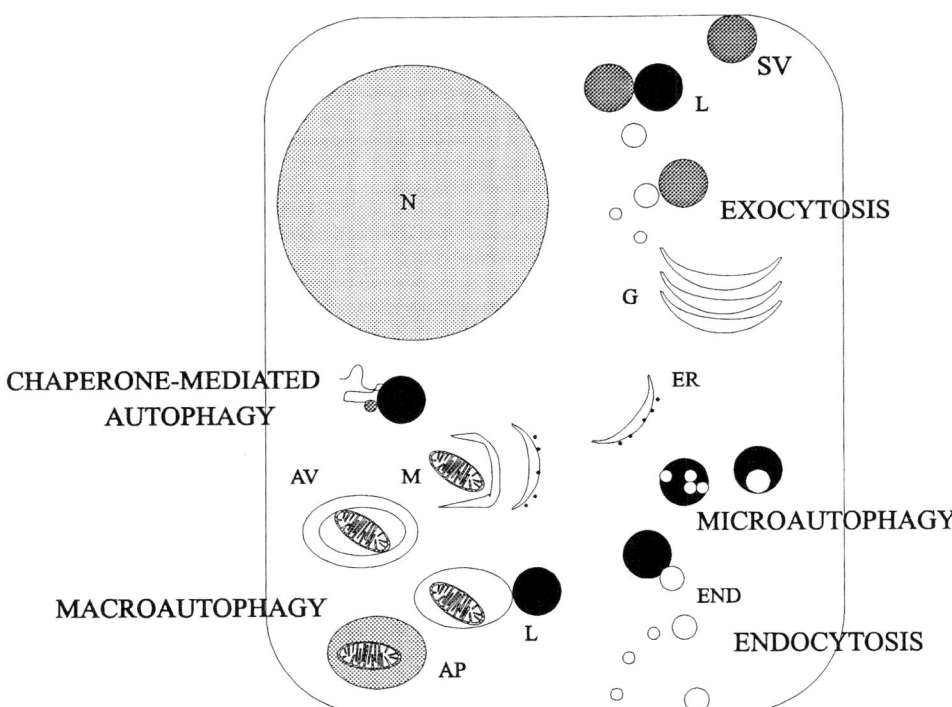

FIGURE 15.4. Lysosomal pathways of intracellular protein degradation. Five different pathways for the delivery of intracellular proteins to lysosomes are shown. Degradation of proteins by endocytosis, exocytosis, macroautophagy, microautophagy, and chaperone-mediated autophagy are described in the text. *SV*, secretory vesicle; *L*, lysosome; *N*, nucleus; *G*, Golgi; *ER*, endoplasmic reticulum; *M*, mitochondrion; *AV*, autophagic vacuole; *AP*, autophagosome; *END*, endosome.

Macroautophagy

Hepatocytes and other cell types can sequester an area of cytoplasm within a double membrane to form an autophagic vacuole (Fig. 15.4). The source of this membrane may be the endoplasmic reticulum (13,65) or it may be formed *de novo* (70). The inner membrane of the autophagic vacuole is lost by unknown mechanisms, and the autophagic vacuole acidifies. Lysosomes then fuse with the autophagic vacuoles to form autophagosomes (1).

Macroautophagy is stimulated in liver, kidney, and other tissues when amino acid concentrations decline (4). Macroautophagy is activated in intact animals by short-term starvation, but a different pathway of lysosomal proteolysis, chaperone-mediated autophagy, is activated during prolonged starvation (5,21). Macroautophagy is largely nonselective in terms of the cytosolic proteins captured (70), and continued operation of such a pathway may not be compatible with survival; long-term starvation may require more selective proteolysis in order for the animal to recover.

Yeasts also stimulate macroautophagy in response to carbon or nitrogen starvation (71). Genetic and biochemical analysis of this process have uncovered signaling components that are required for macroautophagy (72). Recently, these studies revealed a novel protein conjugation system reminiscent of the ubiquitin conjugation pathway (53–55). The pro-

teins that are conjugated have little sequence resemblance to ubiquitin, but enzymes in the conjugation pathway are family members of the ubiquitin activating enzyme, E1. When this protein conjugation system is not functioning, formation of the autophagic vacuoles is deficient (73,74).

Chaperone-Mediated Autophagy

Chaperone-mediated autophagy is mechanistically quite different from macroautophagy (12,20,57,69,75). In this pathway, specific cytosolic proteins are transported to the lysosome through a nonvesicular pathway similar to import pathways into other organelles such as the endoplasmic reticulum, mitochondria, or peroxisomes (Fig. 15.5). Transport of proteins into each of these organelles is stimulated by *h*eat *s*hock *p*roteins of the *70* kd family (hsp70s) especially the constitutively expressed family member (hsc70) (15,19,41,43,76,77) together with cochaperones (78,79). Receptor protein complexes within the organelle membranes (41,77,80) and hsp70s and cochaperones within the organelle (41,77,81–85) are required for protein binding and import, respectively. The receptor in the chaperone-mediated autophagic pathway is the *l*ysosome-*a*ssociated *m*embrane *p*rotein type *2a* (lamp2a) (80), and the hsp70 family member in the lysosomal lumen is a form of hsc70

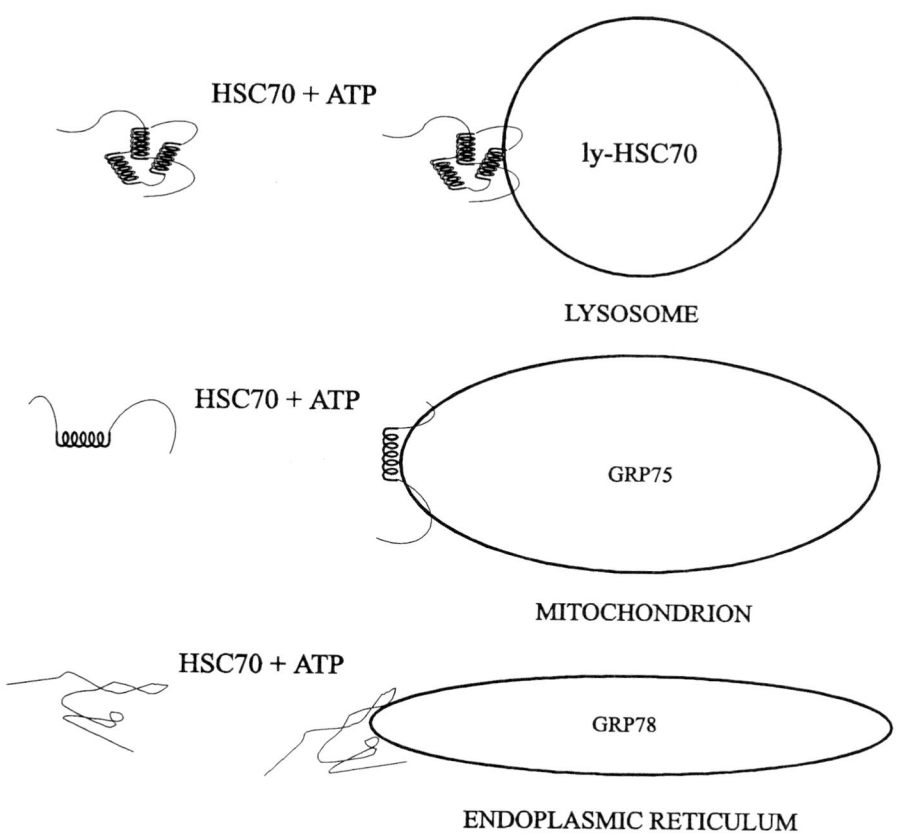

FIGURE 15.5. Requirements for protein import into organelles. Protein import into lysosomes by chaperone-mediated autophagy and import of precursor proteins into mitochondria and endoplasmic reticulum (ER) share common properties. Import is stimulated by the constitutively expressed hsp70, hsc70, together with ATP in the cytosol. Protein substrates bind to receptors at the organelle surface and are pulled across the organelle membrane by an hsp70 family member inside the organelle (ly-hsc70, grp75, and grp78 in lysosomes, mitochondria, and the ER, respectively).

(81). Hsc70/cochaperones, the substrate protein, and lamp2a form a ternary complex at the lysosomal membrane (80). Chaperone-mediated autophagy has recently been reported using isolated vacuoles from yeast (86).

A working model for chaperone-mediated autophagy is shown in Figure 15.6. Substrate proteins in the cytosol interact with hsc70 and cochaperones (step 1). The substrate–hsc70 complex then binds to lamp2a in the lysosomal membrane (step 2). The substrate protein is pulled into the lysosome by the action of a lysosomal hsc70 (step 3). Once the substrate enters the lysosomal matrix, it is rapidly degraded by the lysosomal cathepsins (step 4).

We identified a peptide motif responsible for targeting 30% of cytosolic proteins from hepatocytes or fibroblasts to be degraded by chaperone-mediated autophagy (modified from ref. 12). The targeting peptide can be anywhere within the protein sequence, but its amino acid composition indicates that it will be exposed on the surface of the protein. The motif is related to the pentapeptide, KFERQ, identified experimentally to be the targeting peptide in

microinjected ribonuclease A (87). The concensus peptide motif is: [+,(),−, +/()] QN or QN [+,(),−, +/()], where + = K, R; () = F, I, L, or V; and − = D, E. The parentheses indicate that the order of the amino acids flanking the Q/N is unimportant. We have experimentally confirmed the lack of importance for directionality of the targeting peptide; KFERQ and QREFK were equally effective in tageting a reporter protein for chaperone-mediated autophagy (A. Majeski, A.M. Cuervo, and J.F. Dice, *unpublished data*). This targeting peptide motif is present in 12 proteins that are substrates for chaperone-mediated autophagy and is absent in ten proteins that are not substrates for this pathway of proteolysis. A striking example of the specificity of such targeting peptides comes from analysis of the annexin family (88). Although annexins are 80% identical in sequence, some family members have a KFERQ motif (annexins II and IV) while others do not (annexins V and XI). Annexins II and IV are substrates for chaperone-mediated autophagy, while annexins V and XI are not (88).

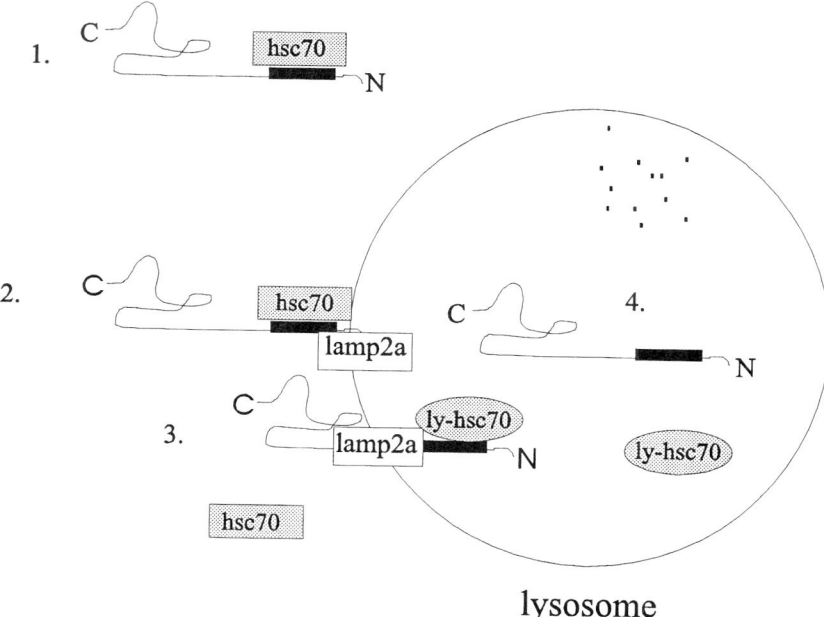

FIGURE 15.6. Steps (*1–4*) in chaperone-mediated autophagy. The constitutively expressed molecular chaperone, hsc70, binds to substrate proteins in the cytosol. The hsc70–substrate complex then binds to lamp2a, a receptor on the lysosomal membrane. A lysosomal hsp70, ly-hsc70, binds to the substrate protein and pulls it into the lysosomal matrix, where the substrate protein is degraded by intralysosomal proteases.

Reduced Proteolysis in Aging

Rates of protein degradation decline with age in many model systems of aging (11,89,90). The ubiquitin/proteasome pathway is not greatly altered in aging (11,91–93) except in certain tissues subjected to oxidative stress (94). The major decline in protein degradation with age is due to reduced macroautophagy and reduced chaperone-mediated autophagy. Macroautophagy declines in liver from aged organisms even though the number of autophagic vacuoles increases (95). The formation of autophagic vacuoles is reduced in aging, but the fusion with lysosomes is delayed even more strikingly (95). The molecular explanations for these deficiencies are not known, but the reduced macroautophagy with age may compromise the normal proteolytic response of the hepatocyte to short-term fasting.

Chaperone-mediated autophagy declines in late-passage human fibroblasts (90) and in liver of aged rats (96). The cause of this decline is a reduced level of lamp2a in both models of aging. The lamp2a in lysosomal membranes of old cells binds to substrates as well as that derived from young cells. Therefore, the lamp2a concentration decreases, and this decline causes the reduced activity of chaperone-mediated autophagy (96). It is not known whether reduced lamp2a also contributes to the age-related decline in macroautophagy.

CASPASES AND PROGRAMMED CELL DEATH

Balanced growth of a multicellular organism requires both cell division and cell death. Mechanisms of cell division

have been studied for at least 150 years, but mechanisms of cell death have been studied only more recently (97–99).

Apoptosis

Apoptosis is a genetically programmed form of cell suicide that can be activated by cytokines, hormones, viruses, and a wide variety of toxic insults including oxidative damage, ethanol, and heat shock (98,99) (see Chapter 13). In hepatocytes, apoptosis is triggered in response to alcohol-induced fatty liver, infections of hepatitis B or C viruses, reperfusion injury, accumulation of intracellular bile acids, and hepatocarcinoma.

Apoptosis requires a family of cysteine asp-cleaving proteases called caspases (3,18,100). The ubiquitin/proteasome system and lysosomal pathways of proteolysis can also be activated in apoptosis, but such activation generally occurs later in the process (6,98). Cells undergoing apoptosis show cytoplasmic shrinkage, blebbing of the plasma membrane, chromatin condensation, and DNA fragmentation (98). Many intracellular proteins are also cleaved, and many of these clips are from the activities of caspases.

Caspases

There are 13 caspases in mammals, and some of them have counterparts in *Candida elegans* and *Drosophila melanogaster* (3,100). They are synthesized as inactive precursors with the general organization shown in Figure 15.7. They are processed into large and small subunits derived from the same precursor. Each active caspase is a tetramer of two large subunits and two small subunits. All caspases cleave

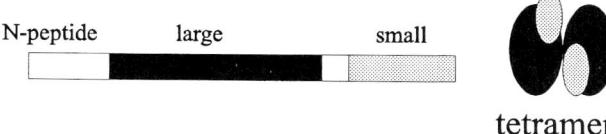

cysteine proteases that cleave after asp

tetramer

cleavage site specificities

caspases 1, 4, 5	W/LEHD
caspases 6, 8, 9, 10	I/V/LEXD
caspases 2, 3, 7	DEXD

FIGURE 15.7. Caspase precursor structure, activated tetramer, and cleavage site specificities. The large and small subunits of caspases are derived from a single precursor polypeptide. The active form of caspases consists of two large and two small subunits. Cleavage site specificities vary for the different caspase family members as indicated.

on the carboxyl side of aspartate residues but have different specificities for amino acids on the amino side of the aspartate (Fig. 15.7).

Some caspases are primarily involved in procytokine activation. For example, caspase 1 clips at a single site in interleukin (IL)-1β and in IL-18. Caspases 1, 4, 5, and 11 are considered to be primarily cytokine activators (3). Other caspase family members are thought to be initiators of apoptosis because they act early after activation of a death receptor such as the Fas receptor (FasR) or tumor necrosis factor receptor (TNFR) (100). These initiator caspases include caspases 2 and 8. Caspase 9 initiates apoptosis following mitochondrial damage and leakage of cytochrome *c* from the mitochondria into the cytoplasm (3,97,101–103). Other caspases act more downstream and may be considered as executioners of apoptosis (caspases 3, 4, 6, and 7) (3). The activation of many of these executioner caspases requires the prior proteolytic activity of the initiator caspases. For example, caspase 8 cleaves procaspases 3, 4, and 7, but these latter caspases are also able to self-activate to some extent.

Caspase 9 Activation

The details of activation of the caspases are complicated, but perhaps can be viewed simply as an explosion of caspase activation (Fig. 15.8). Consider the regulation of caspase 9 activation in hepatocytes as a single example of the complexity of factors that influence caspase activation. Apoptosis in hepatocytes can be triggered by ligand binding to FasR or TNFR. Death signaling complexes then assemble

and lead to the activation of several caspases. The *a*poptotic *p*rotease *a*ctivating *f*actor *1*, Apaf-1, is cytosolic and associates with cytochrome *c* after the cytochrome *c* leaks out of mitochondria (3). The antiapoptotic proteins, Bcl-2 and Bcl-x$_L$, are outer mitochondrial membrane proteins that block the release of cytochrome *c* (101,103). The cytochrome c–Apaf-1 complex then associates with procaspase 9, and in this complex, procaspase 9 cleaves itself into the active species. Caspase 9 is then able to cleave and activate procaspases 3 and 7, and the active caspase 3 can activate procaspase 6. Activated caspase 7, and perhaps other caspases, can enter mitochondria and cleave and inactivate Bcl-2 and Bcl-x$_L$, thereby leading to further cytochrome *c* leakage (103). Several other proteins also affect this apoptotic pathway. For example, the proapoptotic Bcl-2 family member, BID, is cytosolic and is activated by caspase 8-mediated cleavage. The activated BID then associates with the mitochondrial outer membrane and promotes cytochrome *c* release (103).

Caspase Substrates

Substrates of the caspases include a variety of specific proteins that include key components of apoptosis, signal transduction, and cellular architecture. Examples of these substrates, the caspases thought to be responsible for their cleavage, and the effects of the cleavage are listed in Table 15.3. Note that calpastatin, an endogenous inhibitor of the calpains, is a substrate of caspases 1, 3, and 7. The calpastatin is inactivated by the caspase cleavage, so an increase in activity of calpains results. Calpains make limited cleavages in protein substrates, many of which affect cytoskeletal organization.

Effects of Null Mutations in Caspase and Related Genes

Targeted disruptions of caspases 1, 2, 3, 8, 9, and 11 have been carried out in mice (3). Caspase 1 and caspase 11 nulls have similar phenotypes. They are defective in production of cytokines IL-1β, IL-1α, IL-18, and γ-interferon but show no developmental defects. Caspase 2 nulls are developmentally normal, and many cells show normal apoptosis, so the physiological actions of caspase 2 are not known. Caspase 3 nulls die shortly after birth due to defective brain development associated with decreased normal apoptosis of neurons and associated cells. Caspase 8 nulls die as embryos, and the liver and many other tissues derived from such embryos exhibit reduced apoptosis in response to Fas ligand. Caspase 9 nulls show abnormalities in brain development similar to the caspase 3 nulls. Development other organs appears to be normal. Similar results apply Apfa-1 nulls. Finally, BID-deficient mice are significantly delayed in Fas-induced apoptosis in several tissues, especially hepatocytes.

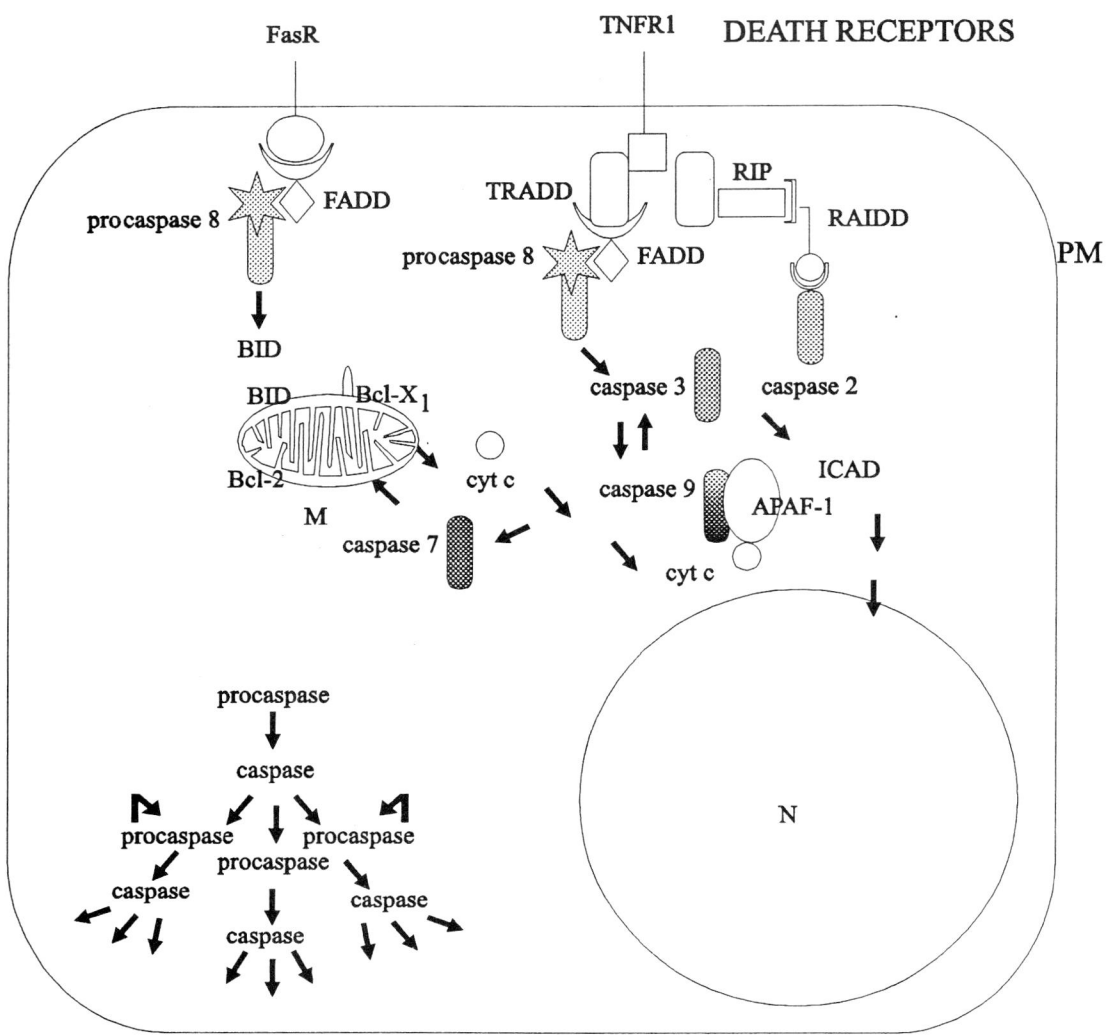

FIGURE 15.8. Interacting proteins and pathways for caspase 9 activation. Apoptosis in hepato-cytes may be initiated by binding of ligands to "death receptors" such as the Fas receptor (*FasR*) or the tumor necrosis factor receptor (*TNFR1*). Binding to FasR recruits the adaptor protein, Fas-associated protein with death domain (*FADD*). Procaspase 8 binds to this death-inducing signal-ing complex, activates itself, and then cleaves several other cellular proteins. These events also take place with the TNFR1 using the adaptor protein, TNF-receptor–associated protein with death domain (*TRADD*). In addition, TNFR interacting protein (*RIP*) recruits TNFR-associated inter-acting protein with death domain (*RAIDD*) and this complex binds to procaspase 2 and leads to its activation. Caspases 2 and 3 degrade an inhibitor of DNase, permitting the degradation of DNA into nucleosome-sized fragments. Caspase 3 is also able to activate procaspase 9, but maxi-mal activation of procaspase 9 requires its interaction with the apoptotic protease-associated fac-tor 1 (*APAF-1*). In addition, cytochrome *c* (cyt *c*) must leak from mitochondria (*M*) and enter this complex for full activation of procaspase 9. Cytochrome *c* will have leaked from the mitochon-dria due to the balance of antiapoptotic (Bcl-2, Bcl-x$_L$) and proapoptotic (*BID*) Bcl-2 family mem-bers that regulate mitochondrial membrane integrity. Activated caspase 9 contributes to the acti-vation of caspase 7 which then associates with mitochondria and leads to further release of cyt *c*. The lower left portion of the cell illustrates the general principal of a caspase explosion in which caspases activate other caspases and even other molecules of their own kind. *N*, nucleus; *PM*, plasma membrane.

TABLE 15.3. EXAMPLES OF SUBSTRATES OF DIFFERENT CASPASES AND THE EFFECT OF CASPASE CLEAVAGE

Protein	Caspase	Effect of Cleavage
caspases	caspases	promotes apoptosis
Bcl-2	?	promotes apoptosis
Bcl-x$_L$	1, 3	promotes apoptosis
BID	8	promotes apoptosis
Inhibitor of DNase	3	DNA fragmentation
Cdc27	3	stabilization of cyclins
Calpastatin	1, 3, 7	activation of calpains
IκB	3	activation of NFκB
Ras GTPase activator protein	3	inhibition of growth
prointerleukin 1β	1	inflammation response
prointerleukin 16	3	T lymphocyte chemotaxis
prointerleukin 18	1	interferon τ synthesis
MEK-kinase1	3	subcellular redistribution
Mst-kinase	3	kinase activation
Focal adhesion kinase	3, 6, 7	kinase inactivation
Protein kinase C	3	kinase activation
Protein kinase N	3	kinase activation
p21-activated kinase	3, 8	kinase activation
Wee1 kinase	3, 7, 8	kinase inactivation
Lamin A	6	nuclear disassembly
Lamin B	3, 6	nuclear disassembly
gelsolin	3	actin disassembly
fodrin	3	plasma membrane blebbing
β-catenin	3	reduction in cell–cell contact

Citations to original reports can be found in reference 3.

CONCLUSION

The importance of intracellular protein degradation in the life and death of eukaryotic cells has become abundantly clear in the last decade. The ubiquitin/proteasome proteolytic pathway controls cell cycle progression (6–8), so division of hepatocytes during liver growth and regeneration is dependent on this proteolytic pathway. Lysosomal proteolytic pathways decline with age and undoubtedly contribute to the accumulation of abnormal proteins in aged tissues (8,11,91,96,104,105). Cells may have mechanisms to detect abnormal proteins and may stop dividing until these abnormal proteins can be repaired or degraded. Finally, programmed cell death requires the activities of several caspases. Protein degradation is as important as protein synthesis in the regulation of hepatocyte life and death.

ACKNOWLEDGMENTS

Research from the author's laboratory was supported by the National Institutes of Health grant AG06116.

REFERENCES

1. Holtzman E. *Lysosomes.* New York and London: Plenum Press, 1989.
2. Kirschner M. Intracellular proteolysis. *Trends Cell Biol* 1999;9:M42–M45.
3. Martins LM, Kaufmann SH. Mammalian caspases: structure, activation, substrates, and functions during apoptosis. *Ann Rev Biochem* 1999;68:383–424.
4. Mortimore G, Pösö A, Lardeux B. Mechanism and regulation of protein degradation in liver. *Diabetes Metab Rev* 1989;5:49–70.
5. Cuervo AM, Knecht E, Terlecky S, et al. Activation of a selective pathway of lysosomal proteolysis in rat liver by prolonged starvation. *Am J Physiol* 1995;269:C1200–C1208.
6. Hershko A, Ciechanover A. The ubiquitin system. *Ann Rev Biochem* 1998;67:425–480.
7. Hochstrasser M. Ubiquitin-dependent protein degradation. *Ann Rev Genet* 1996;30:405–439.
8. Cabiscol E, Levine R. Carbonic anhydrase III. Oxidative modification in vivo and loss of phosphatase activity during aging. *J Biol Chem* 1995;270:14742–14747.
9. Dice JF. Cellular theories of aging as related to the liver. *Hepatology* 1985;5:508–513.
10. Gracy R, Talent J, Zvaigzne A. Molecular wear and tear leads to terminal marking and the unstable isoform of aging. *J Exp Zool* 1998;282:18–27.
11. Dice JF. Cellular and molecular mechanisms of aging. *Physiol Rev* 1993;73:149–159.
12. Dice JF. Peptide sequences that target cytosolic proteins for lysosomal proteolysis. *Trends Biochem Sci* 1990;15:305–309.
13. Dunn WA. Autophagy and related mechanisms of lysosome-mediated protein degradation. *Trends Cell Biol* 1994;4:139–143.
14. Glaumann H. Crinophagy as a means for degrading excess secretory proteins in rat liver. *Revis Biol Celular* 1989;20:97–110.

15. Hayes S, Dice JF. Roles of molecular chaperones in protein degradation. *J Cell Biol* 1996;132:255–258.

16. Lupas A, Flanagan JM, Tamura T, et al. Self-compartmentalizing proteases. *Trends Biochem Sci* 1997;22:399–404.

17. Plemper RK, Wolf DH. Retrograde protein translocation: ERADication of secretory proteins in health and disease. *Trends Biochem Sci* 1999;24:266–270.

18. Barrett AJ, Rawlings ND, Woessner JF. *Handbook of Proteolytic Enzymes.* New York: Academic Press,1998.

19. Hartl F. Molecular chaperones in cellular protein folding. *Nature* 1996;381:571–580.

20. Dice JF, Terlecky SR. Selective degradation of cytosolic proteins by lysosomes. In: A. Ciechanover, A. Schwartz, ed. *Cellular Proteolytic Systems.* New York: Wiley-Liss, 1994; 55–64.

21. Wing SS, Chiang H-L, Goldberg AL, et al. Proteins containing peptide sequences related to Lys-Phe-Glu-Arg-Gln are selectively depleted in liver and heart, but not skeletal muscle, of fasted rats. *Biochem J* 1991;275:165–169.

22. Solomon V, Lecker S, Goldberg AL. The N-end rule pathway catalyzes a major fraction of the protein degradation in skeletal muscle. *J Biol Chem* 1998;273:25216–25222.

23. Rock K, Gramm C, Rothstein M, et al. Inhibitors of the proteasome block the degradation of most cell proteins and the generation of peptides presented on MHC class I molecules. *Cell* 1994;78:761–771.

24. Breitschopf K, Bengal E, Ziv T, et al. A novel site for ubiquitination: the N-terminal residue, and not internal lysines of MyoD, is essential for conjugation and degradation of the protein. *EMBO J* 1998;17:5964–5973.

25. Rechsteiner M, Rogers SW. PEST sequences and regulation by proteolysis. *Trends Cell Biol* 1996;21:267–271.

26. Alkalay I, Yaron A, Hatzubai A, et al. Stimulation-dependent IκBα phosphorylation marks the NFκβ inhibitor for degradation via the ubiquitin–proteasome pathway. *Proc Nat Acad Sci U S A* 1995;92:10599–10603.

27. Scheffner M, Nuber U, Huibregtse JM. Protein ubiquitination involving an E1-E2-E3 enzyme ubiquitin thioester cascade. *Nature* 1995;373:81–83.

28. Koegl M, Hoppe T, Schlenker S, et al. A novel ubiquitination factor, E4, is involved in multiubiquitin chain assembly. *Cell* 1999;96:635–644.

29. D'Andrea A, Pellman D. Deubiquitinating enzymes: A new class of biological regulators. *Crit Rev Biochem Mol Biol* 1998; 33:337–352.

30. Swaminathan S, Amerik AY, Hochstrasser M. The Doa4 deubiquitinating enzyme is required for ubiquitin homoeostasis in yeast. *Mol Biol Cell* 1999;10:2583–2594.

31. Suzuki T, Varshavsky A. Degradation signals in the lysine–asparagine sequence space. *EMBO J* 1999;18: 6017–6026.

32. Hicke L. Gettin' down with ubiquitin: turning off cell-surface receptors, transporters, and channels. *Trends Cell Biol* 1999;9: 107–112.

33. Kölling R, Hollenberg C. The ABC-transporter Ste6p accumulates in the plasma membrane in a ubiquitinated form in endocytosis mutants. *EMBO J* 1994;13:3261–3271.

34. Strous G, van Kerkhof P, Govers R, et al. The ubiquitin conjugation system is required for ligand-induced endocytosis and degradation of the growth hormone receptor. *EMBO J* 1996; 15:3806–3812.

35. Beck B, Schmidt A, Hall MN. Starvation induces vacuolar targeting and degradation of the tryptophan permease in yeast. *J Cell Biol* 1999;146:1227–1237.

36. Ward C, Omura S, Kopito R. Degradation of CFTR by the ubiquitin–proteasome pathway. *Cell* 1995;83:121–127.

37. Mori S, Heldin C, Claesson-Welsh L. Ligand-induced polyubiquitination of the platelet-derived growth factor β-receptor. *J Biol Chem* 1992;267:6429–6434.

38. Plemper R, Böhmler S, Bordallo J, et al. Mutant analysis links the translocon and BIP to retrograde protein transport for ER degradation. *Nature* 1997;388:891–895.

39. Cenciarelli C, Hou D, Hsu K-C, et al. Activation-induced ubiquitination of the T cell antigen receptor. *Science* 1992;257: 795–797.

40. Zhou M, Fisher E, Ginsberg HN. Regulated co-translational ubiquitination of apolipoprotein B100. A new paradigm for proteasomal degradation of a secretory protein. *J Biol Chem* 1998;273:24649–24653.

41. Rapoport T, Jungnickel B, Kutav U. Protein transport across the eukaryotic endoplasmic reticulum and bacterial inner membranes. *Annu Rev Biochem* 1996;65:271–303.

42. Chirico W, Waters M, Blobel G. 70K heat shock related proteins stimulate protein translocation into microsomes. *Nature* 1988;332:805–810.

43. Deshaies R, Koch B, Werner-Washburne M, et al. 70 kD stress protein homologues facilitate translocation of secretory and mitochondrial precursor polypeptides. *Nature* 1988;332: 800–805.

44. Horwich AL, Weber-Ban EU, Finley D. Chaperone rings in protein folding and degradation. *Proc Nat Acad Sci U S A* 1999; 96:11033–11040.

45. Lee DH, Goldberg AL. Proteasome inhibitors: valuable new tools for cell biologists. *Trends Cell Biol* 1998;8:397–403.

46. Voges D, Zwickl P, Baumeister W. The 26S proteasome: a molecular machine designed for controlled proteolysis. *Ann Rev Biochem* 1999;68:1015–1068.

47. Zwickl P, Baumeister W. AAA–ATPases at the crossroads of protein life and death. *Nature Cell Biol* 1999;1:E97–E98.

48. Braun BC, Glickman M, Kraft R, et al. The base of the proteasome regulatory particle exhibits chaperone-like activitiy. *Nature Cell Biol* 1999;1:221–226.

49. Osmulski PA, Gaczynska M. A new large proteolytic complex distinct from the proteasome is present in the cytosol of fission yeast. *Curr Biol* 1998;8:1023–1026.

50. Hodges M, Tissot C, Freemount P. Protein regulation: tag-wrestling with relatives of ubiquitin. *Curr Biol* 1998;8: 749–752.

51. Johnson PR. Hochstrasser M. SUMO-1: ubiquitin gains weight. *Trends Cell Biol* 1997;7:408–413.

52. Hochstrasser M. There's the Rub: a novel ubiquitin-like modification linked to cell cycle regulation. *Genes Dev* 1998;12: 901–907.

53. Kim J, Dalton VM, Eggerton KP, et al. Apg7p/Cvt2p is required for the cytoplasm-to-vacuole targeting, macroautophagy, and peroxisome degradation pathways. *Mol Biol Cell* 1999;10:1337–1351.

54. Mizushima N, Noda T, Yoshimori T, et al. A protein conjugation system essential for autophagy. *Nature* 1998;395:395–398.

55. Mizushima N, Sugita H, Yoshimori T, et al. A new protein conjugation system in humans. The counterpart of the yeast Apg12p conjugation system essential for autophagy. *J Biol Chem* 1998;273:33889–33892.

56. Yuan W, Stromhaug PE, Dunn WA. Glucose-induced autophagy of peroxisomes in *Pichia pastoris* requires a unique E1-like protein. *Mol Biol Cell* 1999;10:1353–1366.

57. Dice JF, *Lysosomal pathways of protein degradation.* Austin: Landes Bioscience, 2000.

58. Chiang HL, Schekman R. Regulated import and degradation of a cytosolic protein in the yeast vacuole. *Nature* 1991;350: 313–318.

59. Klionsky D. Nonclassical protein sorting to the yeast vacuole. *J Biol Chem* 1998;273:10807–10810.

60. Bu G, Schwartz A, Receptor-mediated endocytosis. In: Arias I, ed. *The Liver: Biology and Pathobiology.* 3rd ed: New York: Raven Press, 1994; 259–274.

61. Riezman H, Woodman P, van Meer G, et al. Molecular mechanisms of endocytosis. *Cell* 1997;91:731–738.

62. Lenk S, Fisher D, Dunn WA. Regulation of protein secretion by crinophagy in perfused rat liver. *Eur J Cell Biol* 1991;56: 201–209.

63. Morrissey J, Cohn D. Secretion and degradation of parathormone as a function of intracellular maturation of hormone pools. *J Cell Biol* 1979;83:521–528.

64. Noda T, Farquhar M. A non-autophagic pathway for diversion of ER secretory proteins to lysosomes. *J Cell Biol* 1992;119: 85–97.

65. Dunn WA. Studies on the mechanism of autophagy: Formation of the autophagic vacuole. *J Cell Biol* 1990;110:1923–1933.

66. Tuttle D, Dunn WA. Divergent modes of autophagy in the methylotrophic yeast *Pichia pastoris. J Cell Sci* 1995;108:25–35.

67. Ahlberg J, Glaumann H. Uptake-microautophagy and degradation of exogenous proteins by isolated rat liver lysosomes. Effects of pH, ATP, and inhibitors of proteolysis. *Exp Mol Path* 1985;42:78–88.

68. Sakai Y, Koller A, Rangell L, et al. Peroxisome degradation by microautophagy in *Pichia pastoris.* Identification of specific steps and morphological intermediates. *J Cell Biol* 1998;141: 625–636.

69. Cuervo AM, Dice JF. Lysosomes, a meeting point of proteins, chaperones, and proteases. *J Mol Med* 1998;76:6–12.

70. Seglen P, Gordon P, Holen I. Nonselective autophagy. *Semin Cell Biol* 1990;1:441–448.

71. Tsukada M, Ohsumi Y. Isolation and characterization of autophagy-defective mutants of *Saccharomyces cerevisiae. FEBS Lett* 1993;333:169–174.

72. Noda T, Ohsumi Y. Tor, a phosphatidylinositol kinase homologue, controls autophagy in yeast. *J Biol Chem* 1998;273: 3963–3966.

73. Lenk S, Dunn WA, Trausch J, et al. Ubiquitin-activating enzyme, E1, is associated with maturation of autophagic vacuoles. *J Cell Biol* 1992;118:301–308.

74. Lenk S, Susan P, Hickson I, et al. Ubiquitinated aldolase B accumulates during starvation-induced lysosomal proteolysis. *J Cell Physiol* 1999;178:17–27.

75. Cuervo AM, Terlecky SR, Dice JF, et al. Selective binding and uptake of ribonuclease A and glyceraldehyde-3-phosphate dehydrogenase by rat liver lysosomes. *J Biol Chem* 1994;269: 26374–26380.

76. Chiang H-L, Terlecky S, Plant C, et al. A role for a 70-kilodalton heat shock protein in lysosomal degradation of intracellular proteins. *Science* 1989;246:382–385.

77. Schatz G, Dobberstein B. Common principles of protein translocation across membranes. *Science* 1996;271:1519–1525.

78. Becker J, Walter W, Yan W, et al. Functional interaction of cytosolic hsp70 and a DnaJ-related protein, Ydj1p, in protein translocation in vivo. *Mol Cell Biol* 1996;16:4378–4386.

79. Rassow J, Voos W, Pfanner N. Partner proteins determine multiple functions of hsp70. *Trends Cell Biol* 1995;5:207–212.

80. Cuervo AM, Dice JF. A receptor for the selective uptake and degradation of proteins by lysosomes. *Science* 1996;273: 501–503.

81. Agarraberes F, Terlecky SR, Dice JF. An intralysosomal hsp70 is required for a selective pathway of lysosomal protein degradation. *J Cell Biol* 1997;137:825–834.

82. Cuervo AM, Dice JF, Knecht E. A population of rat liver lysosomes responsible for the selective uptake and degradation of cytosolic proteins. *J Biol Chem* 1997;272:5606–5615.

83. Horst M, Azem A, Schatz G, et al. What is the driving force for protein import into mitochondria? *Biochim Biophys Acta* 1997; 1318:71–78.

84. Kang P, Osterman J, Shilling J, et al. Requirement for hsp70 in the mitochondrial matrix for translocation and folding of precursor proteins. *Nature* 1990;348:137–143.

85. Nicchitta C, Blobel G. Lumenal proteins of the mammalian endoplasmic reticulum are required to complete protein translocation. *Cell* 1993;73:989–998.

86. Horst M, Knecht E, Schu PV. Import into and degradation of cytosolic proteins by isolated yeast vacuoles. *Mol Biol Cell* 1999; 10:2879–2889.

87. Dice JF, Chiang H-L, Spencer E, et al. Regulation of catabolism of microinjected ribonuclease A: Identification of residues 7-11 as the essential pentapeptide. *J Biol Chem* 1986;262:6853–6859.

88. Cuervo AM, Gomes AV, Barnes JA, Dice JF. Selective degradation of annexins by chaperone-mediated autophagy. *J Biol Chem* 2000;275:33329–33335.

89. Makrides S. Protein synthesis and degradation during aging and senescence. *Biol Rev* 1983;83:393–422.

90. Dice JF. Altered degradation of proteins microinjected into senescent human fibroblasts. *J Biol Chem* 1982;257: 14624–14627.

91. Cuervo AM, Dice JF. How do intracellular proteolytic systems change with age? *Front Biosci* 1998;3:25–43.

92. Pan J-X, Short S, Goff S, et al. Ubiquitin pools, ubiquitin mRNA levels, and ubiquitin-mediated proteolysis in aging human fibroblasts. *Exp Gerontol* 1993;28:39–49.

93. Shibatani T, Ward W. Effect of age and food restriction on alkaline protease activity in rat liver. *J Gerontol* 1996;51: B316–B322.

94. Shang F, Gong X, Palmer H, et al. Age-related decline in ubiquitin conjugation in response to oxidative stress in the lens. *Exp Eye Res* 1997;64:21–30.

95. Terman A. The effect of age on formation and elimination of autophagic vacuoles in mouse hepatocytes. *J. Gerontol* 1995;41: 319–325.

96. Cuervo AM, Dice JF. Age-related decline in chaperone-mediated autophagy. *J Biol Chem* 2000; 275:31505–31513.

97. Faubion WA, Gores GJ. Death receptors in liver biology and pathobiology. *Hepatology* 1999;29:1–4.

98. Jacobson MD, Weil M, Raff MC. Programmed cell death in animal development. *Cell* 1997;88:347–354.

99. Pitot HC. Hepatocyte death in hepatocarcinogenesis. *Hepatology* 1998;28:1-5.

100. Nicholson DW, Thornberry NA. Caspases: killer proteases. *Trends Biochem Sci* 1997;22:299–306.

101. Green DR, Martin SJ. The killer and the executioner: how apoptosis controls malignancy. *Curr Opin Immunol* 1995;7:694–703.

102. Green D, Kroemer G. The central executioners of apoptosis: caspases or mitochondria? *Trends Cell Biol* 1998;8:267–271.

103. Porter AG. Protein translocation in apoptosis. *Trends Cell Biol* 1999;9:394–401.

104. Reiss U, Rothstein M. Heat-labile isozymes of isocitrate lyase from aging *Turbatrix aceti. Biochem Biophys Res Commun* 1974; 61:1012–1018.

105. Yuan P, Talent J, Gracy R. Molecular basis for the accumulation of acidic isozymes of triosephosphate isomerase on aging. *Mech Ageing Dev* 1981;17:151–162.

The Liver: Biology and Pathobiology, Fourth Edition, edited by I. M. Arias, J. L. Boyer, F. V. Chisari, N. Fausto, D. Schachter, and D. A. Shafritz.
Lippincott Williams & Wilkins, Philadelphia © 2001.

REGULATION OF HEPATIC CHOLESTEROL HOMEOSTASIS

PHILLIP B. HYLEMON
WILLIAM M. PANDAK
Z. RENO VLAHCEVIC

The liver plays a central role in the regulation of cholesterol homeostasis in the body. Cholesterol is essential for the maintenance of cell membrane integrity, cell growth and differentiation, and is the sole precursor of bile acids and steroid hormones (see Chapter 69 and website chapters W-12, W-22, W-23, and W-24). Interest in cholesterol metabolism has been directed toward defining its role in the pathogenesis of hyperlipidemias, atherosclerosis, and cholesterol gallstones, diseases affecting Western civilization (1). Recent studies have led to better understanding of the role of the multitude of factors which are involved in the maintenance of cholesterol homeostasis. Alterations of cholesterol homeostasis due to genetic defects or environmental factors can lead to hypercholesterolemia and diseases associated with excess cholesterol. Conversely, an understanding of the cellular mechanisms responsible for maintenance of cholesterol homeostasis have also led to interventional therapy aimed at lowering serum cholesterol and reduction of diseases associated with hypercholesterolemia.

Under most physiologic circumstances, several input and output pathways of cholesterol appeared to be coordinately balanced by finely tuned mechanisms with the ultimate aim of preserving cholesterol homeostasis (2,3). Cholesterol *input pathways* in the liver include uptake of lipoprotein cholesterol from chylomicron remnants, low-density lipoproteins (LDL), and high-density lipoproteins (HDL) via separate sinusoidal lipoprotein receptors and *de novo* biosynthesis of cholesterol from acetate (4–6). The liver is a major site for *de novo* biosynthesis of cholesterol, which takes place in a well described cascade of enzymatic reactions of which 3-hydroxy-3-methylglutaryl-CoA reductase (HMG-CoA-reductase) is a rate-determining step. Cholesterol in the liver exists in the form of cholesterol esters (a storage form of cholesterol) and free cholesterol. Free cho-

P. B. Hylemon: Department of Microbiology and Immunology, Medical College of Virginia Campus, Virginia Commonwealth University, Richmond, Virginia 23298.

W. M. Pandak: Division of Gastroenterology, Medical College of Virginia Campus, Virginia Commonwealth University, Richmond, Virginia 23298.

[1]**Z. R. Vlahcevic:** Division of Gastroenterology, Medical College of Virginia Campus, Virginia Commonwealth University, Richmond, Virginia 23298.

[1]Deceased.

lesterol is the sole substrate for conversion to bile acids and for biliary cholesterol secretion. The interchange between these two compartments is facilitated by acyl-CoA:cholesterol acyltransferase (ACAT), a microsomal enzyme which esterifies free cholesterol with long chain fatty acids and neutral cytosolic cholesteryl ester hydrolase (CEH), an enzyme which hydrolyzes cholesterol esters (Fig. 16.1).

Cholesterol output occurs via conversion of cholesterol to primary bile acids and via the canalicular secretion of biliary cholesterol (Fig. 16.1). Approximately 50% of daily cholesterol elimination from the body occurs as a result of its conversion to bile acids, while the remaining 50% occurs in the form of biliary cholesterol secretion. Free cholesterol is a substrate for bile acid biosynthesis which takes place via two pathways; the classic pathway (also called "neutral") and the alternative pathway (also called "acidic"). Daily biosynthesis of cholesterol in humans has been estimated to be 600 to 900 mg/day, while dietary input ranges between 300 and 500 mg; the average total daily input is approximately 1.2 gm/day. Cholesterol output represents a sum of cholesterol converted to bile acids (approximately 500 mg/day), biliary

cholesterol secretion (approximately 600 mg/day), cholesterol loss by sloughing of cells (85 mg/day), and cholesterol used for steroid hormone biosynthesis (50 mg/day). Under physiological circumstances, cholesterol input is equal to output and cholesterol homeostasis is maintained. Another output pathway of cholesterol from the liver is the formation and secretion of very-low-density lipoproteins (VLDL). Hepatic cholesterol incorporated into VLDL circulates through plasma and exchanges with tissue cholesterol but eventually returns to the liver, mostly as LDL cholesterol (Fig. 16.1).

Maintenance of hepatic cholesterol homeostasis is achieved by several integrated feedback and feedforward mechanisms. These include regulation of lipoprotein receptors (LDL and HDL receptors), rate-determining enzymes in the cholesterol and bile acid biosynthetic pathways (HMG-CoA reductase, cholesterol 7α-hydroxylase and sterol 27-hydroxylase), ACAT, CEH, and several transporters involved in biliary lipid secretion (i.e., bile acids, phospholipids, cholesterol). The regulation of these physiological processes in the liver will be described in this review.

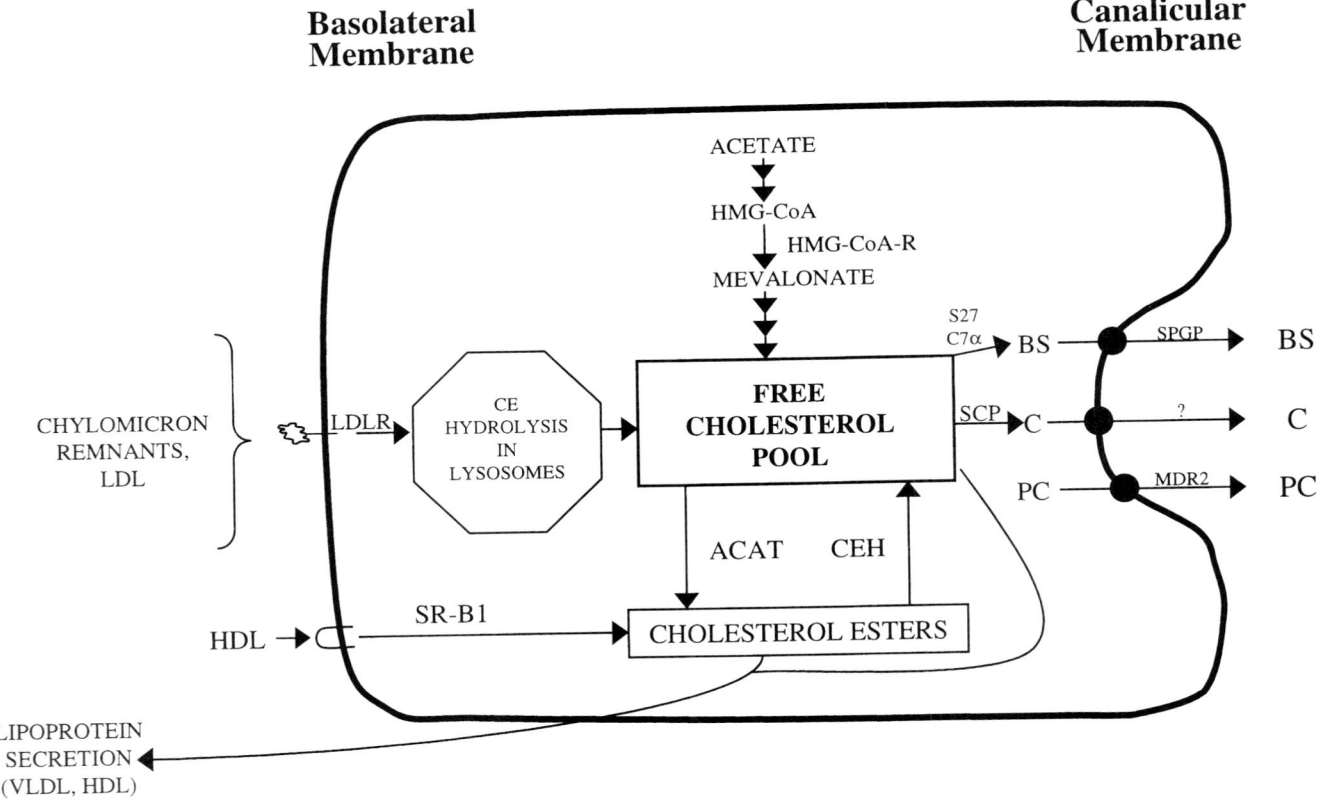

FIGURE 16.1. Cholesterol uptake, metabolism, and secretion in the hepatocyte. Abbreviations are as follows: *LDL*, low-density lipoprotein; *LDLR*, low-density lipoprotein receptor; *HDL*, high-density lipoprotein; *SR-BI*, scavenger receptor class B type I; *VLDL*, very-low-density lipoprotein; *HMG-CoAR*, 3-hydroxy-methylglutaryl coenzyme A reductase; *S27*, sterol 27-hydroxylase; *C7α*, cholesterol 7α-hydroxylase; *BS*, bile salt; *SCP*, sterol carrier protein; *C*, cholesterol; *PC*, phosphotidylcholine; *SPGP*, sister of P-glycoprotein; *mdr2*, multidrug resistance P-glycoprotein.

CHOLESTEROL INPUT PATHWAYS

Low-Density Lipoproteins Receptor–Mediated Endocytosis of Lipoproteins: Its Role in the Maintenance of Cholesterol Homeostasis

The pioneering research of Brown and Goldstein (6) led to the discovery, characterization, and elucidation of the role of the LDL receptor in the regulation of cholesterol homeostasis in the body. The main physiological function of the LDL receptor is to remove apoB100- and apoE-containing lipoproteins from plasma. The liver is solely responsible for removal of cholesterol from the body and contains a large number of LDL receptors per hepatocyte. LDL receptors are found on the surface of hepatic sinusoidal membranes, although virtually all other cells express some LDL receptors. The LDL receptor is a transmembrane glycoprotein containing 893 amino acids (7–9). Site-directed mutagenesis and deletion of individual domains have provided evidence for the relationship between structure and function of various domains of the LDL receptor. The domain includes: (a) the N-terminal ligand binding domain; (b) the region showing amino acid sequence identity with epidermal growth factor receptor; (c) the O-linked oligosaccharide region; (d) the membrane-spanning domain, and (e) the cytogenic domain. LDL binds to a group of Ca^{2+}-dependent, complement-related, cysteine-rich domains at the extracellular N-terminus of the LDL receptor (10–11). Receptor-mediated uptake of LDL occurs in coated pits in the plasma membrane. This complex energy-dependent process involves the recruitment of clathrin from the cytosol to form clathrin-coated vesicles containing LDL receptor and membrane components. Ultimately, the vesicles containing the LDL receptor with bound ligand fuse with lysosomes. The LDL and LDL receptor dissociate due to the lower pH of the lysosome, and the LDL receptor then recycles to the cell surface. LDL is degraded in the lysosomes with release of free cholesterol (9). This process is called "receptor-mediated endocytosis" and differs from HDL cholesterol uptake (see Selective Lipid Uptake via High-Density Lipoprotein Receptor SR-BI, below).

The increased input of cholesterol from lipoproteins plays an important role in the regulation of cholesterol homeostasis in the liver. Cholesterol or "oxysterols" transcriptionally repress the biosynthesis of several key enzymes in the cholesterol biosynthetic pathway, including HMG-CoA reductase, HMG-CoA synthase, and farnesyl diphosphate synthase (Fig. 16.2) (12–13). Excess cholesterol also coordinately represses the biosynthesis of the LDL receptor. Substantial progress has been made in recent years in identifying and characterizing the sterol responsive elements (SREs) in genes regulated by cholesterol, the membrane-bound transcription factors (sterol responsive element-binding proteins), and the cholesterol sensing mechanism (12,14). The coordinate regulation of HMG-CoA reductase activity and the LDL receptor activity and m-RNA has been demonstrated both *in vitro* (15) and *in vivo* (16). Moreover, excess cholesterol also activates ACAT activity (6) and represses CEH (17). Similarly, at least in rats and mice, an increase in cellular cholesterol upregulates the transcriptional activity of the cholesterol 7α-hydroxylase gene by activating LXR, an orphan nuclear receptor (18). The regulation of cholesterol homeostasis is also coordinately regulated with the biosynthesis, secretion, and metabolism of fatty acids and phospholipids.

Selective Lipid Uptake via High-Density Lipoprotein Receptor SR-BI

HDL functions by shuttling cholesterol between cells and other lipoproteins in the body (19). HDL is believed to be important in removing free cholesterol from cells in peripheral tissues. This cholesterol is subsequently esterified in the plasma by lecithin:cholesterol acyl transferase (LCAT) into cholesterol esters. The main target tissue for delivery of cholesterol esters via HDL is the liver. When taken up by the liver, cholesterol esters are hydrolyzed and free cholesterol is secreted into bile, degraded to bile acids, or re-packaged into VLDLs.

The delivery of cholesterol to target tissues from HDL is a fundamentally different cellular process from the LDL receptor-mediated endocytosis. The HDL receptor appears to be involved in the differential uptake of cholesterol esters from HDL, after which the "cholesterol poor" HDL particle is released in the plasma (19). Hepatic and lipoprotein lipases stimulate selective lipid transfer. The HDL-mediated transport of cholesterol from extrahepatic tissues to the liver is also called "reverse cholesterol transport" and appears to be a major pathway for cholesterol elimination from the body. This process plays a critical role in the maintenance of cholesterol homeostasis and has protective effects against atherosclerosis.

Until recently, the receptor responsible for the delivery of HDL cholesterol esters to the liver was unknown. The discovery and cloning of the gene encoding class B, type I scavenger receptor (SR-BI) took place in the laboratory of Krieger and his associates (19–21). They showed that the SR-BI receptor is a cell surface HDL receptor which recognizes apoprotein E. It appears that the SR-BI receptor also binds LDL, but its role in the metabolism of apoprotein B-containing lipoproteins is not well understood. Selective uptake of HDL cholesterol esters is a process by which the core cholesterol ester is taken up without the degradation of the HDL apoprotein. This type of selective transport may be the major route of cholesterol ester delivery into the hepatocytes and steroidogenic tissues (22).

The scavenger receptor SR-BI is a glycoprotein of 509 amino acids and is a member of the CD36 superfamily of proteins (21). Modeling of this receptor has shown that it has a large extracellular loop of about 400 amino acids and

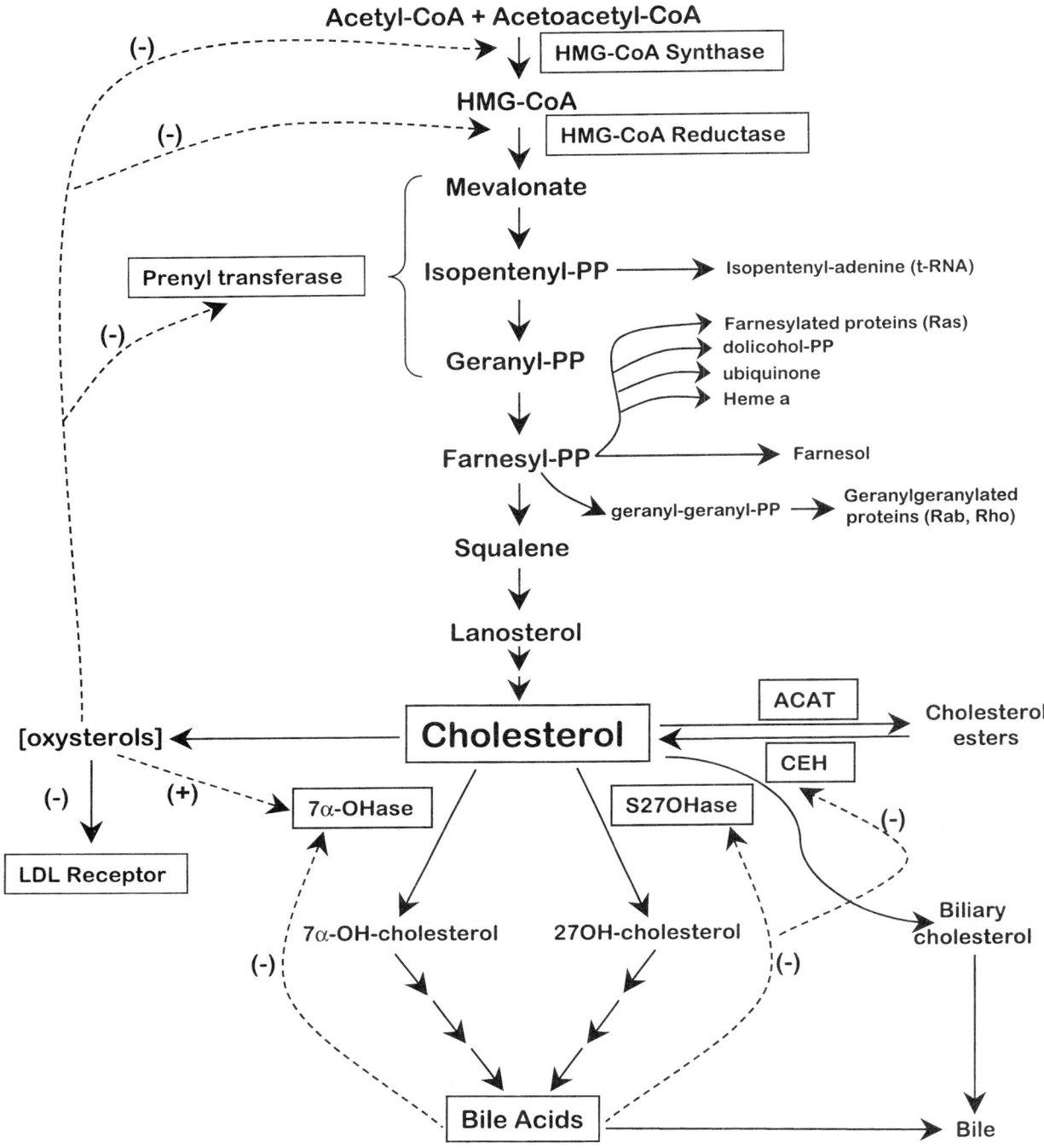

FIGURE 16.2. Cholesterol biosynthesis and metabolism in the liver. Cholesterol homeostasis is maintained by regulation of cholesterol input and output pathways. Key enzymes and pathways that maintain cholesterol homeostasis include: HMG-CoA reductase, the rate-limiting enzyme in the cholesterol biosynthetic pathway; cholesterol 7α-hydroxylase (7α-HOase), the rate-determining enzyme in the neutral pathway of bile acid biosynthesis; sterol 27-hydroxylase (*S27OHase*), the rate-limiting enzyme in the alternative pathway of bile acid biosynthesis; acyl-CoA:cholesterol transferase (*ACAT*), and cholesterol ester hydrolase (*CEH*). Important intermediates in the cholesterol biosynthetic pathway are also indicated. The inhibitory effects (–) and stimulatory (+) effects of bile acids and oxysterols on selected enzymes in the cholesterol and bile acid biosynthetic pathways are indicated by *dashed lines*.

is anchored in the plasma membrane by two membrane-spanning domains, one at the C-terminal and N-terminal domains, respectively. SR-BI recognizes several ligands, including LDL, HDL, and anionic phospholipid vesicles, but its physiologic role in the body is uncertain, except for HDL.

SR-BI expression and hepatic HDL cholesterol ester uptake decrease following ethinyl estradiol treatment or a high cholesterol diet (23). Moreover, hepatic overexpression of SR-BI in mice dramatically reduced plasma HDL and increased biliary cholesterol levels (24). In contrast, SR-BI knockout mice had significantly lower biliary cholesterol levels compared to control mice, suggesting an important role for this receptor in regulating biliary cholesterol secretion (25). The studies in mice are consistent with earlier studies of Schwartz et al. showing that HDL cholesterol is a major source of biliary cholesterol in humans (26,27). If the SR-BI receptor is important in controlling biliary cholesterol secretion in humans, its regulation could play an important role in determining the cholesterol saturation index of bile and the risk of cholesterol gallstone disease.

Role of Dietary Cholesterol Input on Cholesterol Homeostasis

Dietary cholesterol input involves intestinal cholesterol absorption, transport from intestinal cells into plasma as chylomicrons, release of triglycerides from chylomicrons by lipoprotein lipase, and subsequent formation of chylomicron remnants, which are then taken up by the liver via receptor-mediated endocytosis. Cholesterol delivered via chylomicron remnants causes a repression of HMG-CoA reductase activity and a rapid decrease in cholesterol biosynthesis (28–30).

HEPATIC CHOLESTEROL BIOSYNTHESIS

Cholesterol Biosynthetic Pathway

The biosynthesis of cholesterol from acetyl-CoA involves approximately 30 distinct enzymatic steps (31) (Fig. 16.2). The formation of mevalonate from acetyl-CoA occurs in the cytosol and requires three different enzymes. Acetoacetyl-CoA thiolase catalyzes the formation of acetoacetyl-CoA from two acetyl-CoA molecules, and HMG-CoA synthase generates HMG-CoA from acetyl-CoA and acetoacetyl-CoA. HMG-CoA is converted to mevalonate by HMG-CoA reductase, the rate-limiting enzyme in the cholesterol biosynthetic pathway. HMG-CoA reductase is tightly bound to the smooth endoplasmic reticulum (13,32), but the catalytic portion is believed to extend into the cytosol.

Mevalonate is phosphorylated in two steps followed by decarboxylation, yielding isopentenyl pyrophosphate. Isopentenyl pyrophosphate isomerase then catalyzes the conversion of isopentenyl pyrophosphate to dimethylallyl pyrophosphate. The biosynthesis of the C-10 geranyl pyrophosphate from C-5 isopentenyl pyrophosphate and dimethylallyl pyrophosphate is catalyzed by phenyl transferase. The same enzyme adds another isopentenyl group to geranyl pyrophosphate, generating C-15 farnesyl pyrophosphate (31). The biosynthesis of farnesyl pyrophosphate from mevalonate is believed to occur in the cytosol. The biosynthesis of squalene from two molecules of farnesyl pyrophosphate occurs via a two-step process and is catalyzed by squalene synthease, which is located in the endoplasmic reticulum. The formation of squalene is the first committed step in the biosynthesis of sterols. Squalene is next converted to lanosterol by the sequential action of squalene epoxidase and 2,3-oxidosqualene:lanosterol cyclase, respectively. The conversion of lanosterol to cholesterol requires 19 distinct steps that remove three methyl groups, rearrange a double bond at C8–C9 to yield a double bond at C5–C6, and saturate a double bond at C24–25. The enzymes catalyzing these various reactions that convert lansterol to cholesterol are primarily membrane-associated and are not well characterized.

Fate of Isoprenoid Units

The cholesterol biosynthetic pathway yields essential isoprenoid units (Fig. 16.2), which are used in other biosynthetic pathways including those for dolichol, ubiquinone, and heme a (12). Dolicohol is involved in the biosynthesis of glycoproteins and serves as a carrier for oligosaccharides. Ubiquinone is an electron/hydrogen carrier and is essential for the generation of ATP via the electron transport chain in mitochondria. Moreover, polyisoprenoid units (C-15 and C-20) are also utilized in the posttranslational modification of specific membrane-associated proteins. Farnesyl pyrophosphate (C-15) has been shown to be covalently linked to the carboxyl terminus of ras, a membrane-associated GTP/GDP binding protein involved in cell signaling (12,33,34). Geranyl-geranyl pyrophosphate (C-20) has been shown to modify other proteins involved in cell signaling, including Rab, Rho, and the γ subunit of heterotrimeric G proteins (35). Posttranslational modification of these proteins occurs via a carboxy-terminal sequence of Cys-A-A-X where Cys is cysteine, A is an aliphatic amino acid, and X is any amino acid (33–37).

Regulation of 3-Hydroxy-3-Methylglutaryl-CoA Reductase

HMG-CoA reductase is the rate-limiting step in the cholesterol biosynthetic pathway (38,39). The enzyme is a 97-kd glycoprotein located in the smooth endoplasmic reticulum (SER). The N-terminal portion of the enzyme is embedded in the SER membrane by eight putative membrane-spanning regions, while the COOH-terminal portion (approx. 55 kd) contains the active site.

HMG-CoA reductase can be regulated at the transcriptional, translational, and posttranslational levels (12,40,41).

The study of cholesterol biosynthesis in cultured cells by Kandutsch et al. (42) demonstrated that hydroxylated derivatives of cholesterol (oxysterols) are powerful repressors of HMG-CoA reductase. Purification of cholesterol from auto-oxidation products markedly decreased the ability of cholesterol to repress HMG-CoA reductase. Additional studies from several laboratories showed that excess cellular cholesterol transcriptionally repressed a number of genes involved in cellular cholesterol homeostasis, including LDL receptor, HMG-CoA reductase, HMG-CoA synthase, farnesyl diphosphate synthase, and squalene synthase (12,13). Moreover, several genes encoding key enzymes involved in fatty acid (43–46), phospholipid, and triglyceride biosynthesis were subsequently discovered to be regulated by cholesterol/oxysterols (47). Characterization of promoters of genes regulated by cholesterol led to the initial identification of a sterol regulatory element (SRE). Point mutations in the LDL receptor promoter SRE blocked the ability of this gene to be upregulated by cholesterol depletion. These initial data suggested that a positive acting transcription factor was involved in the regulation of this gene by cholesterol/oxysterols (13,14).

Elegant studies by the laboratory of Brown and Goldstein (13,14) led to the purification of sterol responsive element binding proteins (SREBPs). Cloning and characterization of the genes encoding SREBPs showed that there are two SREBP genes (SREBP-1 and SREBP-2). However, these two genes produce three SREBP proteins (SREBP-1a, SREBP-1c, and SREBP-2). SREBP-1a and SREBP-1c are produced from a single gene using different transcriptional initiation sites and different first exons (13,14).

It was discovered that SREBPs are anchored to the endoplasmic reticulum and nuclear membranes by two membrane-spanning domains. The SREBPs contain three functional domains, the N-terminal, central, and COOH-domains. The N-terminal and COOH-terminal domains contain the DNA binding region and regulatory domain, respectively. The central domain contains two transmembrane-spanning regions. The SREBPs are synthesized as approx. 125 kd precursor proteins. In sterol-deleted cells, the precursor protein is released from the membrane as an active transcription factor, in a complex sterol-regulated process that requires two proteolytic cleavage events (47). The initial cleavage of SREBPs requires a Site-1 protease whose activity is regulated by a membrane-bound SREBP cleavage-activating protein (SCAP). SCAP has eight membrane-spanning domains and is thought to bind to SREBPs through protein–protein interactions. Membrane sterol concentrations are hypothesized to be "sensed" by SCAP through the eight membrane-spanning domains (48,49). A second nonsterol-regulated proteolytic cleavage is required for the release of SREBP from the membrane. This is carried out by a Site-2 protease (50). The mature (about 68 kd) SREBP then translocates to the nucleus where it binds and activates promoters containing SRE.

SREs were originally identified in sterol-regulated promoters and contain a direct repeat of 5′-PyCAPy-3′ separated by one nucleotide. Further studies have shown that SREBPs require other transcription factor or coregulatory factors, that is, Sp1, NF-Y, and CREB for activation of sterol responsive genes (51–53).

HMG-CoA reductase can be regulated at the posttranslational level by alteration in protein turnover rates and possibly by phosphorylation (12,13). It was discovered that the protein half-life of HMG-CoA reductase can be rapidly altered by mevalonate-derived metabolites and/or oxysterols in cell culture and in rats (54–57). Additional studies showed that when HMG-CoA reductase activity was inhibited by lovastatin (a competitive inhibitor of HMG-CoA reductase), cholesterol addition did not lead to an enhancement of HMG-CoA reductase degradation unless mevalonate was also added (58–60). These results suggested that a mevalonate-derived product was required for the regulation of HMG-CoA reductase degradation. Subsequent studies showed that farnesol, the C-15 isoprenoid alcohol derived from farnesyl diphosphate (Fig. 16.2), increased the degradation rate of HMG-CoA reductase by an unknown mechanism (61). The transmembrane-spanning domain of HMG-CoA reductase is required for the regulation of enzyme degradation. Finally, the catalytic activity of HMG-CoA reductase can be inhibited *in vitro* by phosphorylation. The phosphorylation of this enzyme can be carried out by three different protein kinases (62). However, the importance of these kinases in the *in vivo* regulation of HMG-CoA reductase activity is unknown.

CHOLESTEROL OUTPUT PATHWAYS

Bile Acid Biosynthetic Pathways

The conversion of cholesterol to primary bile acids (cholic and chenodeoxycholic acid) requires 14 distinct enzymatic steps (63). It has been suggested that in humans there are at least two major bile acid biosynthetic pathways (Fig. 16.3) operating under normal conditions (64). Animal studies (65–68) and studies in primary hepatocytes support this hypothesis (69,70). Cholesterol degradation may be initiated by either a microsomal cholesterol 7α-hydroxylase ("neutral pathway") (Fig.16.3) or by a mitochondrial cholesterol 27-hydroxylase pathway ("acidic or alternative pathway"). In both pathways, the steroid nucleus undergoes a series of modifications including epimerization of the 3β-hydroxyl group, introduction of hydroxyl groups into the 7α and 12α-position (for cholic acid biosynthesis) and saturation of the sterol double bond (Fig. 16.3). The first step in the "neutral" bile acid biosynthetic pathway is the 7α-hydroxylation of cholesterol to form 7α-hydroxycholesterol, which is then converted to 7α-hydroxy-4-cholesten-3-one by an NAD^+-dependent microsomal 3βhydroxy-Δ^5-C_{27}-steroid dehydrogenase/$\Delta^5 \rightarrow \Delta^4$-isomerase. For the biosynthesis of cholic acid, a 12α-hydroxyl group is

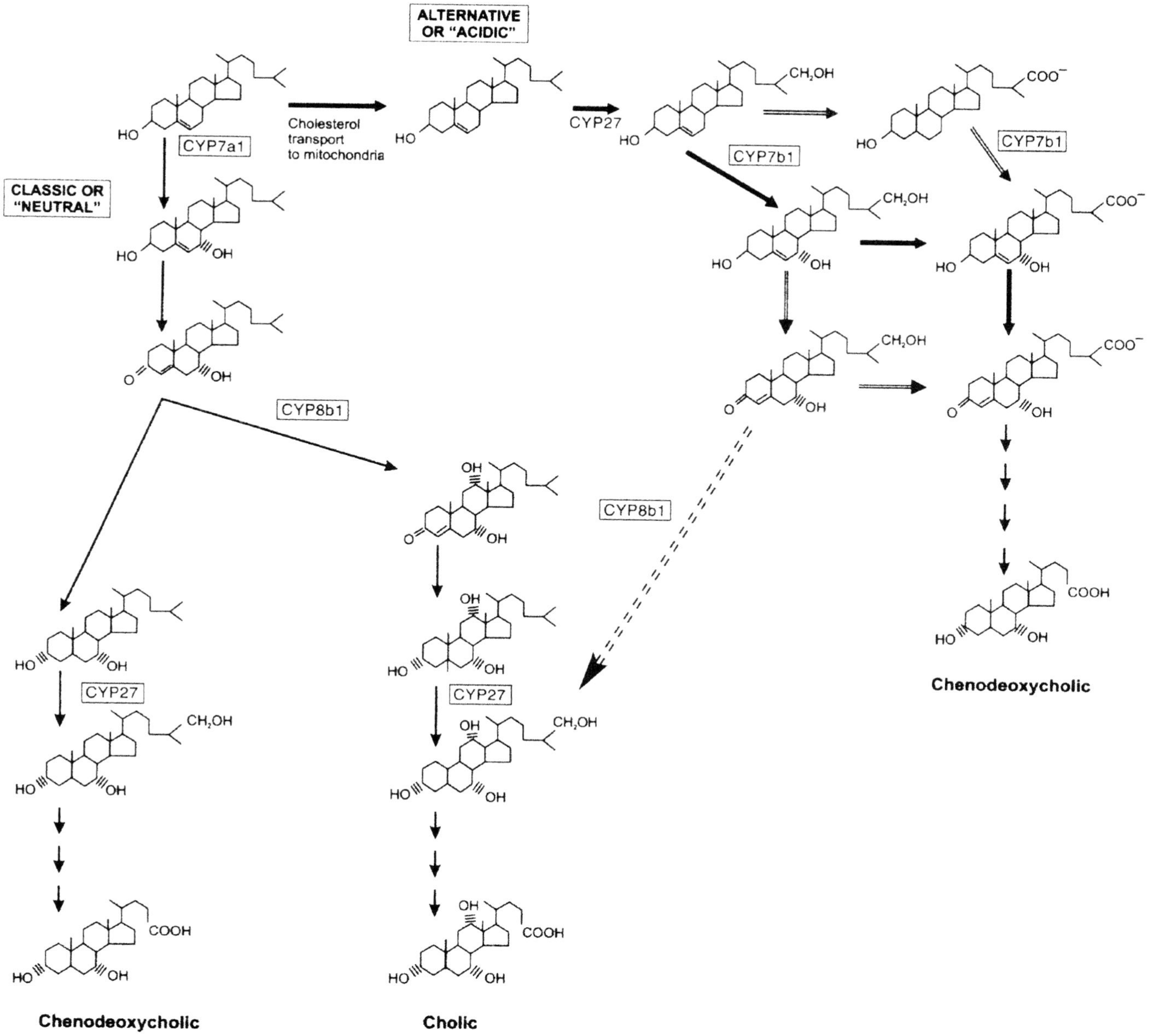

FIGURE 16.3. Neutral and alternative bile acid biosynthetic pathways in the liver. Bile acid biosynthesis can be initiated by either microsomal cholesterol 7α-hydroxylase (*CYP7a1*) or by mitrochondrial sterol 27-hydroxylase (*CYP27*). Oxysterol 7α-hydroxylase (*CYP7b1*) is required for bile acid biosynthesis via the alternative pathway. Sterol 12α-hydroxylase (*CYP8b1*) is crucial for the regulation of the ratio of cholic acid to chenodeoxycholic acid.

inserted by a microsomal sterol 12α-hydroxylase. Cytosolic Δ^4-3-oxosteroid-5β-reductase then reduces the double in the A ring, followed by the reduction of the 3-oxo group to a 3α-hydroxyl group by a soluble 3α-hydroxysteroid dehydrogenase generating 5β-cholestane-3α, 7α, 12α-triol or 5β-cholestane-3α,7α-diol for the biosynthesis of cholic acid or chenodeoxycholic acid, respectively. The cleavage of the side chain of the C_{27}-steroid to form C_{24}-bile acids starts with 27-hydroxylation of cholestane-diol or -triol by mitochondrial

sterol 27-hydroxylase. The 27-hydroxyl group can be oxidized to a COOH group by alcohol and aldehyde dehydrogenases to form 3α,7α-dihydroxy-5β-cholestanoic acids or 3α,7α,12α-trihydroxy-5β-cholestanoic acid (THCA), respectively. However, purified sterol 27-hydroxylase is able to oxidize cholestane triol to THCA (71). Therefore, how the 27-hydroxyl group is oxidized *in vivo* is not clear. A microsomal steroid CoA ligase couples CoA to cholestanoic acid. The terminal steps of side chain cleavage occur in the liver peroxisomes. Most bile acids in humans form glycine or taurine conjugates.

The "acidic" pathway of bile acid biosynthesis is initiated by mitochondrial sterol 27-hydroxylase, which is the same enzyme responsible for the 27-hydroxylation of bile acid biosynthetic intermediates in the "neutral" pathway (72). The second step in the pathway is catalyzed by microsomal oxysterol 7α-hydroxylase (73). The oxysterol 7α-hydroxylase has been shown to recognize side chain hydroxylated derivatives of cholesterol as substrates (74). It is unknown if oxysterol 7α-hydroxylase will recognize COOH metabolites in the "acidic" pathway. However, it is clear that this enzyme is crucial for normal bile acid biosynthesis in humans, as an inborn error in the oxysterol 7α-hydroxylase gene results in severe neonatal liver disease (75). Bile acids biosynthesis initiated by the "acidic" pathway was believed to form primarily chenodeoxycholic acid. However, mice with a disrupted cholesterol 7α-hydroxylase gene continue to synthesize cholic acid. It has been demonstrated that squalestatin, a cholesterol biosynthetic inhibitor, downregulates cholesterol 7α-hydroxylase in rats. Under these conditions the "acidic" pathway becomes the main pathway of bile acid biosynthesis, capable of generating both cholic and chenodeoxycholic acid (67). These results suggest that intermediates in the acidic pathway can be 12α-hydroxylated to yield cholic acid.

Contribution of the Neutral and Acidic Pathways to Total Bile Acid Biosynthesis

The first report on the relative contribution of the classic and alternative pathways to total bile acid biosynthesis was performed in humans with an inserted T-tube. These individuals were injected with [^{3}H] 7α-hydroxycholesterol and [^{3}H] 27-hydroxycholesterol, two intermediates in the classic and alternative pathways, respectively. The results showed that 70% to 95% of [^{3}H] 7α-hydroxycholesterol was promptly and efficiently converted to labeled cholic and chenodeoxycholic acids. In contrast, only about 20% of [^{3}H] 27-hydroxycholesterol was converted to bile acids (predominantly chenodeoxycholic acid) during the same time period. Those authors concluded that the classic pathway of bile acid biosynthesis is the main pathway for elimination of cholesterol from the body and that the alternative pathway plays only a minor role (76). However, in the same series of studies, the alternative pathway was thought to be important in patients with chronic liver disease, since chenodeoxycholic acid was the most abundant bile acid in these patients. Additional information on the role of alternative pathways in liver disease was confirmed with the observation that patients with obstructive jaundice excrete in urine large amounts of 3β-hydroxy-5-cholenoic acid, a known intermediate in the alternative pathway (77). Most convincingly, Axelson et al. (78) have identified intermediates of the alternative pathway in plasma of patients with cir-

rhosis, suggesting that the alternative pathway may be a more important source of bile acid biosynthesis in patients with liver disease.

Our knowledge of the contribution of the alternative pathway to total bile acid biosynthesis was strengthened by the seminal observation by Javitt et al. (79,80), who reported the presence of a significant amount of 27-hydroxycholesterol in human blood. Javitt postulated and subsequently proved that 27-hydroxycholesterol may be formed by sterol 27-hydroxylase in extrahepatic tissues. He suggested that 27-hydroxycholesterol is incorporated into lipoprotein and transported to the liver to be metabolized into bile acids via the alternative pathway. Björkhem et al. (81) postulated that the conversion of cholesterol to more polar 27-hydroxycholesterol should be thought of as a form of reverse cholesterol transport. The physiologic role of 27-hydroxycholesterol, a known powerful repressor of HMG-CoA-reductase *in vitro,* has not been fully established.

In recent years, a significant amount of knowledge has accumulated regarding the relative contribution of the neutral and alternative pathways to total bile acid biosynthesis. Using different experimental designs, two laboratories have reported that in primary rat hepatocytes, the alternative pathway may contribute as much as 50% of total bile acid biosynthesis (82,83). The observation that squalestatin selectively suppresses cholesterol 7α-hydroxylase (classic pathway) but not sterol 27-hydroxylase (alternative pathway) was used in *in vivo* experiments to study bile acid biosynthesis in the absence of contribution from the classic pathway. In rats receiving a 24-hour infusion of squalestatin bile acid, biosynthesis was decreased to 50% of that of controls in the face of undetectable levels of cholesterol 7α-hydroxylase. There was also a marked decrease in the ratio of cholic to chenodeoxycholic acid under these experimental conditions. These latter data suggest that 50% of the remaining bile acid synthesis was derived by pathway(s) other than classic. Infusion of squalestatin for 48 hours showed that bile acid biosynthesis returned to normal in the face of no detectable cholesterol 7α-hydroxylase activity and no induction of sterol 27-hydroxylase. The cholic acid/chenodeoxycholic acid ratio also returned to pre-infusion levels. These latter data suggested that bile acid biosynthesis in rats can proceed without any contribution by the classic pathway (84). This interpretation is consistent with the elegant studies of Ishibashi et al. (85) in cholesterol 7α-hydroxylase knockout (CYP7a1−/−) mice. Although 85% of CYP7a1−/− mice died from fat and fat-soluble vitamin deficiencies in the first three weeks of life, a small fraction (15%) survived with subsequent lifespans which were indistinguishable from those of controls. It became apparent that after two weeks, these surviving mice developed a functioning alternative pathway through which bile acid synthesis continued, albeit at a lower level. Schwarz et al. (86) demonstrated the presence of 7α-hydroxylated intermediates of the acidic pathway in the stool of CYP7−/− mice, suggesting that the alternative pathway is induced between the third and fourth week after birth. Long-term studies did not reveal an expected increase in serum cholesterol in the CYP7a1−/− mice, suggesting continuous cholesterol removal via pathway(s) other than classic. However, these CYP7a1 knockout mice had marked reductions in bile acid biosynthesis and the intestinal bile acid pool, coupled with impaired cholesterol absorption. As expected, cholesterol synthesis increased two-fold. Most interestingly, even though the major pathway for elimination of cholesterol was removed, cholesterol homeostasis was maintained (87).

Regulation of Key Enzymes in the Bile Acid Biosynthetic Pathways

Cholesterol 7α-hydroxylase and sterol 27-hydroxylase are the initial enzymes in the "neutral" and "acidic" bile acid biosynthetic pathways, respectively. Sterol 12α-hydroxylase is the rate-controlling enzyme determining the ratio of cholic acid to chenodeoxycholic acid and metabolites. The genes encoding these enzymes are regulated by hydrophobic bile acids, cholesterol, and specific hormones (summarized in Table 16.1).

Molecular Basis of Regulation of Cholesterol 7-hydroxylase and Sterol 27-hydroxylase

Cholesterol 7α-hydroxylase is regulated at the transcriptional level by hydrophobic bile acids, cholesterol, thyroid hormone, glucocorticoids, insulin, and glucagon (Table 16.1). In recent years, significant progress has been made in elucidating the molecular mechanisms involved in the regulation of the cholesterol 7α-hydroxylase gene by hydrophobic bile acids and cholesterol (oxysterols). Two bile acid responsive elements (BAREs) have been mapped (Fig. 16.4) in the rat cholesterol 7α-hydroxylase promoter by Chiang and co-workers (88,89). Hepatocyte nuclear fac-

tor 4 (HNF-4) and chicken ovalbumin upstream promoter transcription factor II (COUP-TFII) appear to bind to both BARE I and BARE II. In addition, retinoic acid receptor (RAR) and retinoid X receptor (RXR) have been reported to bind to BARE II (90–92). Expression of HNF-4 and COUP-TF-II synergistically activates the rat cholesterol 7α-hydroxylase promoter by approximately 80-fold. In addition, an orphan nuclear receptor (CPF) has been reported to bind and activate the human cholesterol 7α-hydroxylase promoter (93). However, the exact mechanism of regulation by bile acid has not been elucidated. Currently there is evidence for two different modes of transcriptional regulation by bile acids: (a) bile acid activated receptor (94–96) and (b) bile acid signaling through the activation of protein kinase C (PKC) (97–99). Recent results from three independent laboratories reported that hydrophobic bile acids activate the orphan nuclear receptor FXR (94–96). FXR forms a heterodimeric complex with the retinoid X receptor (RXR), and this transcription factor has been shown to repress the gene encoding cholesterol 7α-hydroxylase. The FXR receptor was originally shown to be activated by farnesol, a metabolite derived from the cholesterol biosynthetic pathway (Fig. 16.2) (100). Moreover, the gene encoding the FXR receptor is expressed in the liver, intestines and kidney. Hydrophobic bile acids activated FXR in a concentration range of 10 to 100 µM, which is in the physiological range of bile acids found in portal blood. In this model, bile acids repress the cholesterol 7α-hydroxylase promoter through activation of FXR. However, a binding site for FXR in the CYP7a promoter has not been identified, and the exact mechanism of regulation is uncertain.

Stravitz et al. have reported that bile acids activate protein kinase C (PKC) as a function of their hydrophobicity in a concentration range of 10 to 100 µM (98–99). The addition of phorbol esters (PMA), which activates specific isoforms of PKC, to primary rat hepatocyte cultures down-regulated the cholesterol 7α-hydroxylase gene. Moreover, a

TABLE 16.1. REGULATION OF CHOLESTEROL 7α-HYDROXYLASE, STEROL 27-HYDROXYLASE AND STEROL 12α-HYDROXYLASE ACTIVITY AND MRNA IN THE RAT

Treatment	7αOHase		27OHase		12αOHase	
	Activity	mRNA	Activity	mRNA	Activity	mRNA
Bile acids (hydrophobic)	↓	↓	↓	↓	↓	↓
Cholestyramine	↑	↑	↑	↑	↑	↓
Cholesterol	↑	↑	→	→	↓	↓
Diurnal rhythm						
Dark	↑	↑	↑	↑	?	↑
Light	↓	↓	↓	↓	?	↓
Thyroid hormone	↑	↑	→	→	↓	↓
Glucocorticoids	↑	↑	↑	↑	↑	↑
Insulin	↓	↓	↓	↓	?	?
c-AMP	↓	↓	→	→	?	?

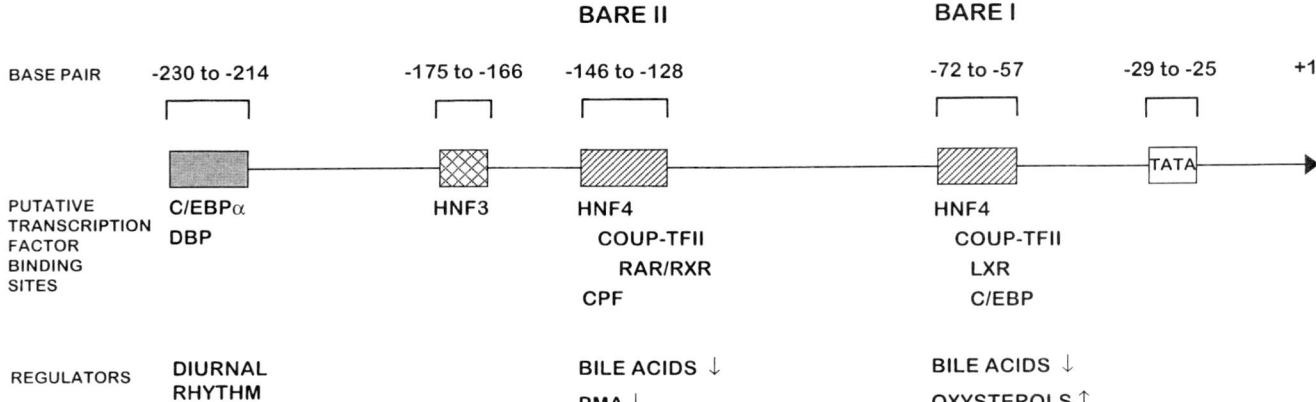

FIGURE 16.4. Proximal 5'-flanking region of the cholesterol 7α-hydroxylase promoter. Shown are the bile acid responsive elements (BAREs), reported transcription factor binding sites, and regulators of gene expression in the rat. Abbreviations: *C/EBP*, CAAT/enhancer binding protein; *DBP*, rat D-element-binding protein; *HNF3*, hepatocyte nuclear factor-3; *HNF4*, hepatocyte nuclear factor-4; *COUP-TFII*, chicken ovalbumin upstream promoter-transcription factor II; *CPF*, CYP7a, promoter binding factor; *BARE*, bile acid responsive element; *RAR*, retinoic acid receptor; *RXR*, retinoid X receptor; *LXR*, nuclear oxysterol receptor; *PMA*, phorbol 12-myristate, 13-acetate.

PMA-responsive element mapped to the BARE II (Fig. 16.4) in the rat cholesterol 7α-hydroxylase promoter (90,101). Finally, inhibitors of PKC blocked the ability of bile acids to downregulate the cholesterol 7α-hydroxylase gene (97). At this point, it is unclear how the activation of FXR and PKC by hydrophobic bile acids might both converge to downregulate the cholesterol 7α-hydroxylase gene or if these are independent mechanisms of regulation. However, it is interesting that both systems respond to hydrophobic bile acids in the same concentration range (10 to 100 μM).

Early studies showed that cholesterol feeding induced the cholesterol 7α-hydroxylase gene in the rat (102). It was demonstrated that the orphan nuclear receptor LXRα is activated by cholesterol metabolites, that is, [24(S),25-epoxycholesterol] and [24(S)-hydroxycholesterol] at physiologic concentrations (103,104). Interestingly, metabolites derived from the cholesterol biosynthetic pathway also appear to be regulators of LXRα (105). For example, geranylgeraniol (Fig. 16.2) has been reported to be an inhibitor of LXRα. A binding site for LXR has been identified (103) in the rat cholesterol 7α-hydroxylase promoter between base pairs −72 and −57 (Fig. 16.4) and has been shown to upregulate this gene. Moreover, mice lacking a functional LXRα gene lose their ability to upregulate cholesterol 7α-hydroxylase when fed a diet high in cholesterol (106). The LXRα-deficient mice accumulated large amounts of cholesterol in the liver on a high-cholesterol diet. These results suggest that LXR plays an important role in the ability of animals to metabolize excess cholesterol via the neutral pathway of bile acid biosynthesis.

Cholesterol 7α-hydroxylase undergoes a circadian rhythm with maximal levels of expression occurring in the dark period of the light cycle (107). Studies by Lavery and Schibler (108) indicate that the liver-enriched transcription factor DBP is responsible for this diurnal variation. DBP was shown to bind and activate the cholesterol 7α-hydroxylase promoter (Fig. 16.4). The levels of DBP in the liver closely parallel the expression of the cholesterol 7α-hydroxylase gene (108).

The gene encoding the sterol 27-hydroxylase gene has been shown to be regulated by hydrophobic bile acids, but not cholesterol or thyroid hormone in the liver (Table 16.1). A single BARE has been mapped in the promoter of the rat sterol 27-hydroxylase gene in primary rat hepatocytes (109). The DNA sequence of this BARE in the sterol 27-hydroxylase promoter is different from the BARE sequences in the rat cholesterol 7α-hydroxylase promoter. The BARE in the rat sterol 27-hydroxylase promoter contains overlapping hepatocyte nuclear factor 1α (HNF1α) and CAAT/enhancer binding protein α (C/EBPα) binding sites. Treatment of primary rat hepatocytes with hydrophobic bile acids resulted in a loss of binding of HNF1α, but not C/EBPα, to this BARE. The mechanism of inhibition of HNF1α binding to the BARE is not clear; however, the amount of nuclear HNF1α protein in bile acid-treated cells does not change. In this case, bile acids appear to downregulate the sterol 27-hydroxylase gene by preventing the binding of a positive-acting transcription factor.

Regulation of Hepatic Sterol 12α-hydroxylase

Sterol 12α-hydroxylase is a key enzyme in the biosynthesis of cholic acid (Fig. 16.3). The levels of this enzyme in the liver are believed to be crucial for maintaining the ratio between cholic acid and chenodeoxycholic acid, and hence, regulating the hydrophobicity of the bile acid pool. The c-

DNA encoding the rabbit sterol 12α-hydroxylase has been cloned and characterized by Eggertsen et al. (110). Interestingly, the gene encoding sterol 12α-hydroxylase was found to lack introns (111). Recent studies show that the specific activity and m-RNA levels of sterol 12α-hydroxylase are downregulated by hydrophobic bile acids, cholesterol feeding, and thyroid hormone in the rat (112,113). The gene encoding this enzyme appears to be very sensitive to the hydrophobicity of the bile acid pool. Feeding cholic acid or deoxycholic acid strongly repressed the m-RNA (93%) and enzyme activity (more than 98%) of sterol 12α-hydroxylase. In contrast, feeding ursodeoxycholic acid, a hydrophilic bile acid, increased sterol 12α-hydroxylase-specific activity (119%) and m-RNA levels (60%)(113). Thyroidectomy of rats caused an increase in both the specific activity and m-RNA levels of sterol 12α-hydroxyalase; in contrast, treatment of intact rats with thyroxine reduced both activity and m-RNA levels of sterol 12α-hydroxylase. However, no apparent thyroid hormone-responsive element was identified in the rat sterol 12α-hydroxylase promoter (–1.9 kb)(112). Therefore, the mechanism of thyroid hormone regulation of the gene encoding sterol 12α-hydroxylase is unclear.

CHOLESTEROL ESTERIFICATION AND HYDROLYSIS

Acyl-CoA:cholesterol acyltransferase (ACAT) and cholesterol ester hydrolase (CEH) play important roles in the regulation of cellular cholesterol homeostasis in the liver (Fig. 16.1) (114). ACAT catalyzes the esterification of cholesterol and certain oxysterols with long chain fatty acids. Cholesterol esters can either be secreted as part of VLDL or hydrolyzed by neutral cholesterol ester hydrolase, yielding free cholesterol and fatty acids. The c-DNA encoding human ACAT-1 was first cloned and characterized from macrophages by T. Y. Chang and co-workers (115). This enzyme is found in the endoplasmic reticulum and contains seven transmembrane domains (116). ACAT-1 has a wide tissue distribution (117) and is catalytically activated by cholesterol and certain oxysterols (118). Gene disruption of ACAT-1 in mice showed reduced ACAT activity and cholesterol ester formation in most tissues except the liver and intestines (119). A c-DNA encoding a second ACAT-2 was cloned and characterized from mouse liver (120,121). This form of ACAT appears to be expressed primarily in the liver and intestines. Enzyme characterization studies showed that ACAT-1 and ACAT-2 differ in their sensitivity to specific inhibitors. Finally, studies by Erickson and Van Zuiden (122) showed that bile salts induce ACAT activity in rat liver, suggesting another physiological link between bile acid and cholesterol metabolism. Steroid hormones also appear to regulate ACAT as progesterone is inhibitory (123) and estrogens are stimulatory (124).

CEH can rapidly mobilize cholesterol and fatty acids by hydrolyzing cholesterol esters found in lipid droplets in the cell cytoplasm. The free cholesterol released can then serve as a substrate for bile acid biosynthesis or biliary cholesterol secretion. The liver contains at least two cholesterol ester hydrolases. Acid cholesterol ester hydrolase is located in lysosomes and hydrolyzes cholesterol esters found in lipoproteins transported into cells by receptor-mediated endocytosis (14). A neutral cholesterol ester hydrolase is located primarily in the cytosol, although some activity is membrane-associated. This enzyme is believed to be responsible for the hydrolysis of cholesterol ester droplets found in the cytoplasm. A c-DNA encoding neutral cholesterol ester hydrolase has been cloned and characterized from rat liver. This c-DNA has a high degree of sequence identity with liver carboxylesterases (125) and encodes a protein of approximately 62 kd. When the c-DNA encoding this enzyme was expressed in COS-7 cells, there was a marked increase in CEH activity. In the rat, hepatic neutral CEH m-RNA and activity is downregulated by hydrophobic bile acids and cholesterol flux (126) (Fig. 16.1). In primary rat hepatocyte cultures, L-thyroxine and glucocorticoids upregulated the gene encoding neutral CEH. Functional sterol responsive elements (SREs) have been identified in the rat CEH promoter (127). The catalytic activity of neutral CEH requires bile salts for maximal activity *in vitro*. Moreover, the *in vitro* activity of this enzyme is increased by phosphorylation by a c-AMP-dependent protein kinase (128). Thus, the level and activity of this enzyme appear to be highly regulated by transcriptional and post-transcriptional mechanisms.

INTRACELLULAR CHOLESTEROL TRANSPORT AND BILIARY CHOLESTEROL SECRETION

Hepatocytes have many unique features and physiological activities that are not shared by other cells. Like other cells, hepatocytes acquire cholesterol by endogenous biosynthesis and via uptake of LDL. In addition, these cells also take up cholesterol and cholesterol esters via chylomicron remnants and HDL. Hepatocytes package cholesterol esters, cholesterol, and triglycerides into VLDLs which are secreted into plasma (Fig. 16.1). Uniquely, the hepatocyte can degrade cholesterol into bile acids or secrete it into bile along with phospholipid (Fig. 16.1). The questions of how hepatocytes coordinately regulate rates of cholesterol biosynthesis, degradation, esterification/hydrolysis, and secretion into both plasma and bile have not been completely elucidated.

It has been estimated that between 65% and 80% of total cellular cholesterol is located in the plasma membrane (reviewed in ref. 129). Lange et al. (130) estimated that the entire plasma membrane cholesterol pool may circulate to the endoplasmic reticulum and back every 40 min. Cholesterol synthesized in the endoplasmic reticulum is rapidly transported to the plasma membrane by an ATP-dependent process (131). Although the exact mechanism(s) of transport is not clear, recent evidence suggests a role for caveolin, a cholesterol-binding protein, and a number of other proteins in this process (132). Plasma membrane cholesterol is continuously transported to the ER in a process requiring an intact intermediate filament network. This process probably occurs via vesicular transport. A fraction (about 30%) of cholesterol entering the hepatocyte via the lysosome-dependent LDL pathway is transported to the endoplasmic reticulum in an energy-dependent process. However, the bulk (about 70%) of LDL cholesterol is believed to be transported to the plasma membrane via a Golgi-dependent pathway (129). In the human disease Niemann–Pick type C, LDL cholesterol enters cells by receptor-mediated endocytosis but is sequestered within lysosomes and does not elicit normal feedback downregulation of HMG-CoA reductase and LDL receptor (reviewed in ref. 133). The human and mouse Niemann–Pick type C (NPC-1) genes have been cloned and characterized (134). The NPC-1 gene encodes a protein of 1,278 amino acids; sequence analyses of this protein suggest that it is a lysosome/endosome membrane-associated protein that is probably involved in the regulation of intracellular cholesterol transport. Although its exact function is unknown, it has been hypothesized that the NPC-1 gene product may help direct the targeting of cholesterol-carrying vesicles derived from lysosomes. Because it appears to have a cholesterol "sensing" domain, it may help to target cholesterol-carrying vesicles to different membranes, depending upon the cholesterol content of the vesicle. There appears to be a second NPC gene that is involved in intracellular cholesterol transport. However, this gene (NPC-2) has not been isolated or characterized.

Tangier disease is a rare autosomal recessive disorder of reverse cholesterol transport characterized by low serum HDL levels, the accumulation of cholesterol esters in various tissues, and defective intracellular lipid trafficking (135). Two pathways have been described to explain the efflux of cholesterol from mammalian cells to HDL: the aqueous diffusion pathway (136) and the apolipoprotein-mediated pathway (137). In the aqueous diffusion model, cholesterol desorbs from the plasma membrane in an energy-independent manner and is accepted by cholesterol-poor HDL. The apolipoprotein-mediated pathway is energy-dependent and requires direct binding of lipid-poor apolipoproteins (apoA-I, apoA-II, apoE) to the cell surface. The low HDL levels in Tangier disease are believed to be due to a markedly reduced rate of lipid transfer from cells to apolipoproteins, resulting in an enhanced degradation of HDL (135).

The molecular basis of Tangier disease and familial HDL deficiency has been elucidated (138–141). It was discovered that patients with Tangier disease and familial HDL deficiency both have mutations in the gene encoding an ATP-binding cassette transporter 1 (ABC-1). The gene encoding ABC-1 is located on human chromosome 9 and consists of 49 exons that range in size from 33 to 249 bp and spans over 70 kb in length. The c-DNA for ABC-1 encodes a protein of 2,201 amino acids. The secondary structure of the ABC-1 transporter is predicted to consist of duplicate six–membrane-spanning domains linked together by a large hydrophobic domain. Two ATP binding motifs are found in this protein, one in the large hydrophobic domain and a second in the carboxyl terminal domain. ABC-1 belongs to a larger gene family of conserved transmembrane proteins that transport a variety of substrates including drugs, lipids, ions, bile acids, vitamins, phospholipids, and peptides across mammalian cell membranes. The levels of the ABC-1 transporter are increased by cholesterol in macrophages (138). Its defect in Tangier disease and familial HDL deficiency shows that it is a key intracellular cholesterol transporter in mammalian cells.

From a clinical point of view, the importance of biliary cholesterol secretion is two-fold: (a) it is responsible for the elimination of 50% of cholesterol from the body each day, and (b) excessive biliary cholesterol secretion is a major factor responsible for supersaturation of bile with cholesterol and subsequently an increased risk for cholesterol gallstone disease (139). It has been known for some time that bile salt transport through the liver is directly coupled to the secretion of biliary phospholipids and cholesterol (140). Bile salts and phospholipid secreted in bile solubilize cholesterol in the form of vesicles and/or mixed micelles.

Only a small part (less than 5%) of cholesterol destined for canalicular excretion is derived from newly synthesized cholesterol. However, recent evidence suggests that selective uptake of HDL cholesterol esters via the SR-B1 receptor is a major source of biliary cholesterol. Overexpression of SR-B1 receptors in mice using adenovirus or transgenic technology resulted in a reduced plasma HDL concentration and increase in biliary cholesterol secretion (19,24). Overexpression of SR-BI in mammalian cells also allows for the more rapid efflux of free cholesterol from cells using either HDL or phospholipid vesicles as cholesterol acceptors (141). However, it is unclear whether the SR-BI receptor plays any direct role in canalicular cholesterol secretion or whether it just provides an expanded pool of cholesterol destined for bile. Moreover, the role of the ABC-1 cholesterol transporter described in Tangiers disease (135–138) is another candidate for a canalicular cholesterol transporter, but data regarding its role in biliary cholesterol secretion are lacking.

The transport of other biliary lipids across the canalicular membrane is more completely understood, with (a) the cloning and characterization of the canalicular bile salt transporter (i.e., sister-P-glycoprotein, SPGP), which mediates ATP-dependent bile salt transport (142) and (b) the discovery that mdr2 p-glycoprotein is a canalicular phospholipid transporter (143).

CONCLUSION

The liver is the major organ for the uptake, biosynthesis, metabolism and secretion of cholesterol from the body. In order to maintain cholesterol homeostasis, the hepatocyte has developed mechanisms for coordinate regulation of the various pathways of cholesterol uptake, biosynthesis, esterification/hydrolysis, degradation to bile acids, intracellular transport, and secretion. Although the cellular mechanisms maintaining cholesterol homeostasis are in place, the system can be overwhelmed as a result of mutations in key genes in this system and/or environmental factors leading to cholesterol-associated diseases. Recent data indicate that there is also coordinate regulation between cholesterol metabolism and the biosynthesis and secretion of other lipids (phospholipids and triglyceride) within the liver.

The last decade has been remarkable for the enormous progress made in our understanding of the molecular mechanisms maintaining cholesterol homeostasis in the liver. The discovery and characterization of SREBPs and the transcription factors involved in transcriptional regulation of LDL and several steps in the cholesterol and fatty acid synthesis pathways have provided a link to our understanding of the coordination of hepatic lipid metabolism. The discovery of SR-B1 receptor as an HDL receptor provided another insight into the relationship of reverse cholesterol transport and cholesterol elimination from the body in the form of biliary cholesterol secretion. Moreover, the importance of bile acid biosynthetic pathways in cholesterol homeostasis is now fully appreciated. The molecular basis of the regulation of genes encoding key enzymes in the bile acid biosynthetic pathways is now being studied. Reports from several laboratories are now identifying key transcription factors, receptors, and second messenger systems which are most likely responsible for the coordinate regulation of these pathways. The general picture emerging is showing an enormous capacity of the liver to provide the ways and means to eliminate excess cholesterol even when the main pathway of bile acid synthesis is eliminated. While the compensatory mechanisms are in place, they are clearly not capable of completely preventing hypercholesterolemia and atherosclerosis in humans and certain other species. However, an in-depth understanding of the mechanisms by which cholesterol homeostasis is maintained provides a rationale for reducing net cholesterol retention, which is a major prerequisite for the prevention of atherosclerosis. One could optimistically predict that in the new millennium, scientific progress leading to a full understanding of factors regulating cholesterol homeostasis may eventually lead to the prevention and eradication of cholesterol-related diseases such as atherosclerosis and cholesterol gallstones.

ACKNOWLEDGMENTS

Supported by the National Institutes of Health Grant PO1 DK38030 and grants by the Department of Veterans Affairs.

REFERENCES

1. Dietschy JM, Turley SD, Spady DK. Role of the liver in the maintenance of cholesterol and low density lipoprotein homeostasis in different animal species including human. *J Lipid Res* 1993;34:1637–1659.
2. Vlhcevic ZR, Pandak WM, Stravitz RT. Regulation of bile acid biosynthesis. In: Cooper A, ed. *Gastroenterology Clinics of North America.* 1999;Vol 28;1:1–25.
3. Javitt NB. Cholesterol homeostasis: Role of the LDL receptor. *FASEB J* 1995;9:1378–1381.
4. Russel DW. Cholesterol biosythesis and metabolism. *Cardiovasc Drugs Ther* 1992;6:103–110.
5. Goldstein L, Brown MS, Anderson RGW, et al. Receptor mediated endocytosis. Concept emerging from the LDL receptor systems. *Annu Rev Cell Biol* 1985;1:1–39.
6. Brown MS, Goldstein JL. A receptor mediated pathway for cholesterol homeostasis. *Science* 1986;323:34–47.
7. Fass D, Blacklos S, Kim PS, et al. Molecular basis of familial hypercholesterolaemia from structure of LDL receptor module. *Nature* 1997;388:691–693.
8. Yamamoto T, Davis CG, Brown MS, et al. The human LDL receptor: a cysteine-rich protein with multiple Alu sequences in its mRNA. *Cell* 1984;39:27–38.
9. Hussain MM, Strickland DK, Bakillah A. The mammalian low-density lipoprotein receptor family. *Annu Rev Nutr* 1999;19:141–172.
10. Bieri S, Atkins AR, Lee HT, et al. Folding, calcium binding, and structural characterization of a concatemer of the first and second ligand-binding modules of the low-density lipoprotein receptor. *Biochemistry* 1998;37:10994–11002.
11. Dirlam-Schatz KA, Attie AD. Calcium induces a conformational change in the ligand domain of the low-density lipoprotein receptor. *J Lipid Res* 1998;39:402–411.
12. Edwards PA, Ericsson J. Sterols and isoprenoids: signaling molecules derived from the cholesterol biosynthetic pathway. *Annu Rev Biochem* 1999;68:157–185.
13. Goldstein JL, Brown MS. Regulation of the mevalonate pathway. *Nature* 1990;343:425–430.
14. Brown MS, Goldstein JL. The SREBP pathway: regulation of cholesterol metabolism by proteolysis of membrane-bound transcription factor. *Cell* 1997;89:331–340.
15. Osborne TG, Gill G, Goldstein JL, et al. Operator constitutive mutation in 3-hydroxy-3-methylglutaryl coenzyme A reductase promoter abolishes protein binding to sterol regulatory element. *J Biol Chem* 1988;263:3380–3387.
16. Rudlin M. Hepatic mRNA levels of the LDL receptor and HMG-CoA reductase show coordinant regulation in vivo. *J Lipid Res* 1992;33:493–501.
17. Ghosh S, Natarajan R, Pandak WM, et al. Regulation of hepatic neutral cholesteryl ester hydrolase by hormones and changes in cholesterol flux. *Am J Physiol* 1998;274:G662–G668.
18. Lehmann JM, Klievwer SA, Moore LB, et al. Activation of the nuclear receptor LXR by oxysterols defines a new hormone response pathway. *J Biol Chem* 1997;272:3137–3140.
19. Krieger M. Charting the fate of the "good cholesterol": Identification and characterization of the high density lipoprotein receptor SR-BI. *Annu Rev Biochem* 1999;68:523–558.
20. Acton SL, Sherer PE, Codish HF, et al. Expression cloning of SR-BI a CD36-related class B scavenger receptor. *J Biol Chem* 1994;269:21003–21009.
21. Acton SL, Rigotti A, Landschulz KT, et al. Identification of scavenger receptor SR-BI as a high density lipoprotein receptor. *Science* 1996;271:518–520.
22. Azhar S, Nomoto A, Leers-Sucheta S, et al. Simultaneous induction of an HDL-receptor protein (SR-BI) and the active

uptake of HDL cholesterol esters in a physiologically relevant steroidogenic cell model. *J Lipid Res* 1996;98:984–995.

23. Fluiter K, van der Westhuijzen DR, van Berkel TJ. In vivo regulation of scavenger receptor BI and the selective uptake of high density lipoprotein cholesteryl esters in rat liver parenchymal and Kupffer cells. *J Biol Chem* 1998;273:8434–8438.

24. Kozarsky KF, Donahee MH, Rigotti A, et al. Overexpression of the HDL receptor SR-BI alters plasma HDL and bile cholesterol levels. *Nature* 1997;387:414–417.

25. Rigotti A, Trigatti BL, Penman M, et al. A targeted mutation in the murine gene encoding the high density lipoprotein (HDL) metabolism. *Proc Natl Acad Sci U S A* 1997;94:12610–12615.

26. Schwartz CC, Halloran LG, Vlahcevic ZR, et al. Preferential utilization of free cholesterol from high-density lipoproteins from biliary cholesterol secretion in man. *Science* 1978;200: 62–64.

27. Schwartz CC, Berman M, Vlahcevic ZR, et al. Multicompartmental analysis of cholesterol metabolism in man. Quantitative kinetic evaluation of precursor sources and turnover of high density lipoprotein cholesterol esters. *J Clin Invest* 1982;70: 863–876.

28. Carrella M, Cooper AD. High affinity binding of chylomicron remnants to rat liver plasma membranes. *Proc Natl Acad Sci U S A* 1979;76:338–345.

29. Havel RJ. Receptor and non-receptor mediated uptake of chylomicron remnants by the liver. *Atherosclerosis* 1998;141:S1–S7.

30. Cooper AD, Ellsworth JL. Lipoprotein metabolism. In: Zakim D, Boyer TD, eds. *Hepatology: A textbook of liver disease.* Philadelphia; WB Saunders Company, 1996;92–130.

31. Rilling HC, Chayet CT. Biosynthesis of cholesterol. In: Danielsson H., Sjövall, J, eds. *Sterols and bile acids.* Amsterdam: Elsevier, 1985;1–39.

32. Olender EH, Simoni RD. The intracellular targeting and membrane topology of 3-hydroxy-3-methylglutaryl-CoA reductase. *J Biol Chem* 1992;267:4223–4235.

33. Hancock JF, Magee AI, Childs JE, et al. All ras proteins are polyisoprenylated but only some are palmitolylated. *Cell* 1989; 57:1167–1177.

34. Casey PJ, Solski PA, Der CJ, et al. p21 ras is modified by a farnesyl isoprenoid. *Proc Natl Acad Sci U S A* 1989;86:8323–8327.

35. Casey PJ. Biochemistry of protein prenylation. *J Lipid Res* 1992; 33:1731–1740.

36. Schafer WR, Kim R, Sterner R, et al. Genetic and pharmacological suppression of oncogenic mutations in RAS genes of yeast and humans. *Science* 1989;245:379–385.

37. Fu HW, Casey PJ. Enzymology and biology of CaaX protein prenylation. *Recent Prog Horm Res* 1999;54:315–342.

38. Rodwell VW, Nordstrom JL, Mitschelen JJ. Regulation of HMG-CoA reductase. *Adv Lipid Res* 1976;14:1–74.

39. Brown MS, Goldstein JL, Dietschy JM. Active and inactive forms of 3-hydroxy-methylglutaryl coenzyme A reductase in the liver of the rat. Comparison with the rate of cholesterol synthesis in different physiological states. *J Biol Chem* 1979;254: 5144–5149.

40. OsborneTF, Goldstein JL, Brown MS. 5′ End of HMG-CoA reductase gene contains sequences responsible for cholesterol-mediated inhibition of transcription. *Cell* 1985;42:203–212.

41. Nakanishi M, Goldstein JL, Brown MS. Multivalent control of 3-hydroxy-3-methylglutaryl coenzyme A reductase. *J Biol Chem* 1988;263:8929–8937.

42. Kandutsch AA, Chen HW, Heiniger HJ. Biological activity of some oxygenated sterols. *Science* 1978;201:498–501.

43. Magana MM, Osborne TF. Two tandem binding sites for sterol regulatory element binding proteins are required for sterol regulation of fatty-acid synthase promoter. *J Biol Chem* 1996;271: 32689–32694.

44. Magana MM, Lin SS, Dooley KA, et al. Sterol regulation of acetyl coenzyme A carboxylase promoter requires two interdependent binding sites for sterol regulatory element binding proteins. *J Lipid Res* 1997;38:1630–1638.

45. Tabor DE, Kim JB, Spiegelman BM., et al. Identification of conserved cis-elements and transcription factors required for sterol-regulated transcription of stearoyl-CoA desaturase 1 and 2. *J Biol Chem* 1999;274:20603–20610.

46. Ericsson J, Jackson SM, Kim JB, et al. Identification of glycerol-3-phosphate acyltransferase as an adipocyte determiantion and differentiation factor 1- and sterol regulatory element-binding protein-responsive gene. *J Biol Chem* 1997;272:7298–7305.

47. Sakai J, Duncan EA, Rawson RB, et al. Sterol-regulated release of SREBP-2 from cell membranes requires two sequential cleavages, one within a transmembrane segment. *Cell* 1996;85: 1037–1046.

48. Nohturfft A, Brown MS, Goldstein JL. Sterols regulate processing of carbohydrate chains of wild-type SREBP cleavage-activating protein (SCAP), but not sterol-resistant mutants Y298C or D443N. *Proc Natl Acad Sci U S A* 1998;95:12848–12853.

49. Nohturfft A, DeBose-Boyd RA, Scheek S, et al. Sterols regulate cycling of SREBP cleavage-activating protein (SCAP) between endoplasmic reticulum and golgi. *Proc Natl Acad Sci U S A* 1999;96:11235–11240.

50. Rawson RB, Zelenski NG, Nijhawan D, et al. Complementation cloning of S2P, a gene encoding a putative metalloprotease required for intramembrane cleavage of SREBPs. *Mol Cell* 1997;1:47–57.

51. Athanikar JN, Sanchez HB, Osborne TF. Promoter selective transcriptional synergy mediated by sterol regulatory element binding protein and Sp1:a critical role for the Btd domain of Sp1. *Mol Cell Biol* 1997;17:5193–5200.

52. Dooley KA, Bennett, MK, Osborne TF. A critical role for cAMP response element-binding protein (CREB) as a Co-activator in sterol-regulated transcription of 3-hydroxy-3-methylglutaryl coenzyme A synthase promoter. *J Biol Chem* 1999;274: 5285–5291.

53. Bennett MK, Ngo TT, Athanikar JN, et al. Co-stimulation of promoter for low density lipoprotein receptor gene by sterol regulatory element-binding protein and Sp1 is specifically disrupted by the yin yang 1 protein. *J Biol Chem* 1999;274: 13025–13032.

54. Edwards PA, Popjak G, Fogelman AM, et al. Control of 3-hydroxy-3-methylglutaryl coenzyme A reductase by endogenously synthesized sterols in vitro and in vivo. *J Biol Chem* 1977;252:1057–1063.

55. Sinensky M, Torget M, Edwards PA. Radioimmune precipitation of 3-hydroxy-3-methylglutaryl coenzyme A reductase in Chinese hamster fibroblasts. Effect of 25-hydroxycholesterol. *J Biol Chem* 1981;256:11774–11779.

56. Liscum L, Luskey KL, Chin DJ, et al. Regulation of 3-hydroxy-3-methylglutaryl coenzyme A reductase and its mRNA in rat liver as studied with a monoclonal antibody and a cDNA probe. *J Biol Chem* 1983;258:8450–8455.

57. Luskey KL, Faust JR, Chin DJ, et al. Amplification of the gene for 3-hydroxy-3-methylglutaryl coenzyme A reductase, but not for the 53-kDa protein, in Ut-1 cells. *J Biol Chem* 1983;258: 8462–8469.

58. Nakanishi M, Goldstein JL, Brown MS. Multivalent control of 3-hydroxy-3-methylglutaryl coenzyme A reductase. Mevalonate-derived product inhibits translation of mRNA and accelerates degradation of enzyme. *J Biol Chem* 1988;263: 8929–8937.

59. Roitelman J, Simoni RD. Distinct sterol and nonsterol signals for the regulated degradation of 3-hydroxy-3-methylglutaryl-CoA reductase. *J Biol Chem* 1992;267:25264–25273.

60. Correll CC, Edwards PA. Mevalonic acid-dependent degradation of 3-hydroxy-3-methylglutaryl-coenzyme A reductase in vivo and in vitro. *J Biol Chem* 1994;269:633–638.

61. Correll CC, Ng L, Edwards PA. Identification of farnesol as the non-sterol derivative of mevalonic acid required for the accelerated degradation of 3-hydroxy-3-methylglutaryl-coenzyme A reductase. *J Biol Chem* 1994;269:17390–17393.

62. Beg ZH, Stonik JA, Brewer HB. Modulation of the enzymatic activity of 3-hydroxy-3-methylglutaryl-CoA reductase by multiple kinase systems involving reversible phosphorylation: a review. *Metabolism* 1987;36:900–917.

63. Russell DW, Setchell KDR. Bile acid biosynthesis. *Biochemistry* 1992;31:4737–4749.

64. Axelson M, Sjövall J. Potential bile acid precursors in plasma-possible indicators of biosynthetic pathways of cholic acid and chenodeoxycholic acid in man. *J Steroid Biochem* 1990;36:631–6.

65. Ishibashi S, Schwarz M, Frykman PK, et al. Disruption of cholesterol 7α-hydroxylase gene in mice. I. Postnatal lethality reversed by bile acid and vitamin supplementation. *J Biol Chem* 1996;271:18017–18023.

66. Schwarz M, Lund EG, Setchell KDR, et al. Disruption of cholesterol 7α-hydroxylase gene in mice. II. Bile acid deficiency is overcome by induction of oxysterol 7α-hydroxylase. *J Biol Chem* 1996;271:18024–18031.

67. Vlahcevic ZR, Stravitz RT, Heuman DM, et al. Quantitative estimations of the contribution of different bile acid pathways to total bile acid synthesis in the rat. *Gasteroenterology* 1997;113:1949–1957.

68. Rosen H, Reshef A, Maeda N, et al. Markedly reduced bile acid synthesis but maintained levels of cholesterol and vitamin D metabolites in mice with disrupted sterol 27-hydroxylase gene. *J Biol Chem* 1998;273:14805–14812.

69. Princen HMG, Meijer P, Wolthers BG, et al. Cyclosporin A blocks bile acid synthesis in cultured hepatocytes by specific inhibition of chenodeoxycholic acid synthesis. *Biochem J* 1991;275:501–505.

70. Stravitz RT, Vlahcevic ZR, Russell TL, et al. Regulation of sterol 27-hydroxylase and an alternative pathway of bile acid biosynthesis in primary cultures of rat hepatocytes. *J Steroid Biochem* 1996;57:337–347.

71. Cole JJ, Russell DW. Characterization of human sterol 27-hydroxylase. A mitrochondrial cytochrome P450 that catalyzes multiple oxidation reactions in bile acid biosynthesis. *J Biol Chem* 1991;266:7774–7778.

72. Okuda KI. Liver mitochondrial P450 involved in cholesterol catabolism and vitamin D activation. *J Lipid Res* 1994;35:361–372.

73. Schwarz M, Lund EG, Lathe R, et al. Identification and characterization of a mouse oxysterol 7-hydroxylase cDNA. *J Biol Chem* 1997;272:23995–24001.

74. Martin KO, Reiss AB, Lathe R, Javitt NB. 7-alpha-hydroxylation of 27-hydroxycholesterol: biologic role in the regulation of cholesterol synthesis. *J Lipid Res* 1997;38:1053–1058.

75. Setchell KD, Schwarz M, O'Connell NC, et al. Identification of a new inborn error in bile acid synthesis mutation of the oxysterol 7-alpha-hydroxylase gene causes severe neonatal liver disease. *J Clin Invest* 1998;102:1690–1703.

76. Swell, L, Gustafsson J, Schwartz CC, et al. An in vivo evaluation of quantitative significance of several potential pathways to cholic and chenodeoxycholic acids from cholesterol in man. *J Lipid Res* 1980;21:455–466.

77. Tazawa Y, Konno T. Urinary monohydroxy bile acids in young infants with obstructive jaundice. *Acta Paediatr Scand* 1982;71:91–95.

78. Axelson M, Mork B, Aly A, et al. Concentration of cholestenoic acid in plasma from patients with liver disease. *J Lipid Res* 1989;30:1877–1882.

79. Javitt NB. 26-hydroxycholesterol: synthesis, metabolism and biologic activities. *J Lipid Res* 1990;31:1527–1533.

80. Javitt NB, Kok E, Burstein S. 26-hydroxycholesterol, identification and quantitation in human serum. *J Biol Chem* 1981;256:12644–12646.

81. Bjorkem I, Andersson O, Diczfalusy U, et al. Atherosclerosis and sterol 27-hydroxylase: Evidence for a role of this enzyme in elimination of cholesterol from human macrophages. *Proc Natl Acad Sci U S A* 1994;91:8592–8596.

82. Princen HMG, Meijer P, Wolthers BG, et al. Cyclosporin A blocks bile acid synthesis in cultured hepatocytes by specific inhibition of chenodeoxycholic acid synthesis. *Biochem J* 1991;275:501–505.

83. Stravitz RT, Vlahcevic ZR, Russell TL, et al. Regulation of sterol 27-hydroxylase and an alternative pathway of bile acid biosynthesis in primary cultures of rat hepatocytes. *J Steroid Biochem Mol Biol* 1996;57:337–347.

84. Vlahcevic ZR, Stravitz RT, Heuman DM, et al. Quantitative estimations of the contribution of different bile acid pathways to total bile acid synthesis in the rat. *Gastroenterology* 1997;113:1949–1957.

85. Ishibashi S, Schwarz M, Frykman PK, et al. Disruption of cholesterol 7α-hydroxylase gene in mice: Postnatal lethality reversed by bile acid and vitamin supplementation. *J Biol Chem* 1996;271:18017–18023.

86. Schwarz M, Lund EG, Setchell KDR, et al. Disruption of cholesterol 7α-hydroxylase gene in mice: II. Bile acid deficiency is overcome by induction of oxysterol 7α-hydroxylase. *J Biol Chem* 1996;271:18024–18031.

87. Schwarz M, Russell DW, Dietschy JM, et al. Marked reduction in bile acid synthesis in cholesterol 7α-hydroxylase deficient mice does not lead to diminished tissue cholesterol turnover or to hypercholesterolemia. *J Lipid Res* 1998;39:1833–43.

88. Chiang JYL, Stroup D. Identification of a putative bile acid-responsive element in cholesterol 7α-hydroxylase gene promoter. *J Biol Chem* 1994;269:17502–17507.

89. Stroup D, Crestani M, Chiang JYL. Identification of a bile acid responsive element in the cholesterol 7α-hydroxylase gene CYP7A. *Am J Physiol* 1997;273:G508–G517.

90. Crestani M, Stroup D, Chiang JYL. Hormonal regulation of the cholesterol 7α-hydroxylase gene (CYP7). *J Lipid Res* 1995;36:2419–2432.

91. Stroup D, Crestani M. Chiang JYL. Orphan receptors chicken ovalbumin upstream promoter transcription factor II (COUP-TFII) and retinoid x receptor (RXR) activate and bind the rat cholesterol 7α-hydroxylase gene (CYP7A). *J Biol Chem* 1997;272:9833–9839.

92. Crestani M, Sadeghpour A, Stroup D, et al. Transcriptional activation of the cholesterol 7-hydroxylase gene (CYP7A) by nuclear hormone receptors. *J Lipid Res* 1998;39:2192–2200.

93. Nitta M, Ku S, Brown C, et al. CPF: an orphan nuclear receptor that regulates liver-specific expression of the human cholesterol 7 alpha-hydroxylase gene. *Proc Natl Acad Sci U S A* 1999;96:6660–6665.

94. Makishima M, Okamoto AY, Repa JJ, et al. Identification of a nuclear receptor for bile acids. *Science* 1999;284:1362–1365.

95. Parks DJ, Blanchard SG, Bledsoe RK, et al. Bile acids: Natural ligands for an orphan nuclear receptor. *Science* 1999:284:1365–1368.

96. Wang H, Chen J, Hollister K, et al. Endogenous bile acids are ligands for the nuclear receptor FXR/BAR. *Mol Cell* 1999;3:543–553.

97. Stravitz RT, Vlahcevic ZR, Gurley EC, et al. Repression of cholesterol 7α-hydroxylase transcription by bile acids is mediated

through protein kinase C in primary cultures of rat hepatocytes. *J Lipid Res* 1995;36:1359–1369.

98. Stravitz RT, Rao YP Vlahcevic ZR, et al. Hepatocellular protein kinase C activation by bile acids: implications for regulation of cholesterol 7α-hydroxylase. *Am J Physiol* 1996:271: G293–G303.

99. Rao YP, Stravitz RT, Vlahcevic ZR, et al. Activation of protein kinase Cα and δ by bile acids: correlation with bile acid structure and diacylglycerol formation. *J Lipid Res* 1997;38: 2446–2454.

100. Forman BM, Goode E. Chen J, et al. Identification of a nuclear receptor that is activated by farnesol metabolites. *Cell* 1995;81: 687–693.

101. Crestani M, Sadeghpour A, Stroup D, et al. The opposing effects of retinoic acid and phorbol esters converge on a common response element in the promoter of the rat cholesterol 7α-hydroxylase gene (CYP7A). *Biochem Biophys Res Commun* 1996;225:585–592.

102. Pandak WM, Li YC, Chiang JYL, et al. Regulation of cholesterol 7α-hydroxylase mRNA and transcriptional activity by bile salts in the chronic bile fistula rat. *J Biol Chem* 1991;266: 3416–3421.

103. Lehmann JM, Kliewer SA, Moore LB, et al. Activation of the nuclear receptor LXR by oxysterols defines a new hormone response pathway. *J Biol Chem* 1997;272:3137–3140.

104. Janowski BA, Grogan MJ, Jones SA, et al. Structural requirements of ligands for the oxysterol liver X receptors LXRalpha and LXRbeta. *Proc Natl Acad Sci U S A* 1999;96:266–271.

105. Forman BM, Ruan B, Chen J, et al. The orphan nuclear receptor LXR is positively and negatively regulated by distinct products of mevalonate metabolism. *Proc Natl Acad Sci U S A* 1997;94:10588–10593.

106. Peet DJ, Turley SD, Ma W, et al. Cholesterol and bile acid metabolism are impaired in mice lacking the nuclear oxysterol receptor LXRα. *Cell* 1998;93:693–704.

107. Mitropoulos KA, Balasubramaniam S, Gibbons GF, et al. Diurnal variation in the activity of cholesterol 7α-hydroxylase in the livers of fed and fasted rats. *FEBS Lett* 1972;27:203–206.

108. Lavery DJ, Schibler U. Circadian transcription of the cholesterol 7α-hydroxylase gene may involve the liver-enriched bZIP protein DBP. *Genes Dev* 1993;7:1871–1884.

109. Rao YP, Vlahcevic ZR, Stravitz RT, et al. Down-regulation of the rat hepatic sterol 27-hydroxylase gene by bile acids in transfected primary hepatocytes: possible role of hepatic nuclear factor 1α. *J Steroid Biochem Mol Biol* 1999;70:1–14.

110. Eggertsen G, Olin M, Andersson U, et al. Molecular cloning and expression of rabbit sterol 12alpha-hydroxylase. *J Biol Chem* 1996;271:32269–32275.

111. Gafvels M, Olin M, Chowdhary BP, et al. Structure and chromosomal assignment of the sterol 12alpha-hydroxylase gene (CYP8b1)in human and mouse: eukaryotic cytochrome P-450 gene devoid of introns. *Genomics* 1999;56:184–196.

112. Andersson U, Yang YZ, Bjorkhem I, et al. Thyroid hormone suppresses hepatic sterol 12alpha-hydroxylase (CYP8b1) activity and messenger ribonucleic acid in rat liver: failure to define known thyroid hormone response elements in the gene. *Biochim Biophys Acta* 1999;1438:167–174.

113. Vlahcevic ZR, Eggertsen G, Bjorkhem I, et al. Regulation of sterol 12α-hydroxylase and cholic acid biosynthesis in the rat. *Gastroenterology* 2000 (*in press*).

114. Chang TY, Chang CC, Cheng D. Acyl-coenzyme A:cholesterol acyltransferase. *Annu Rev Biochem* 1997;66:613–638.

115. Chang CC, Huh HY, Cadigan KM, et al. Molecular cloning and functional expression of human acyl-coenzyme A:cholesterol acyltransferase cDNA in mutant Chinese hamster ovary cells. *J Biol Chem* 1993;268:20747–20755.

116. Lin S, Cheng D, Liu MS, Chen J, et al. Human acyl-CoA:cholesterol acyltransferase-1 in the endoplasmic reticulum contains seven transmembrane domains. *J Biol Chem* 1999;274: 23276–23285.

117. Uelmen PJ, Oka K, Sullivan M, et al. Tissue-specific expression and cholesterol regulation of acycoenzyme A:cholesterol acyltransferase (ACAT) in mice. Molecular cloning of mouse ACAT cDNA, chromosomal localization, and regulation of ACAT in vivo and in vitro. *J Biol Chem* 1995;270:26192–26201.

118. Cheng D, Chang CC, Qu X, et al. Activation of acyl-coenzyme A:cholesterol acyltransferase by cholesterol or by oxysterol in a cell-free system. *J Biol Chem* 1995;270:685–695.

119. Meiner, VL, Cases S, Myers HM, et al. Disruption of the acyl-CoA:cholesterol acyltransferase gene in mice: evidence suggesting multiple cholesterol esterification enzymes in mammals. *Proc Natl Acad Sci U S A* 1996;93:14041–14046.

120. Cases S, Novak S, Zheng YW, et al. ACAT-2, A second mammalian acyl-CoA:cholesterol acyltransferase: its subcloning, expression, and characterization. *J Biol Chem* 1998;273: 26755–26764.

121. Anderson RA, Joyce C, Davis M, et al. Identification of a form of acy-CoA:cholesterol acyltransferase specific to liver and intestine in nonhuman primates. *J Biol Chem* 1998;273; 26747–26754.

122. Erickson SK, Van Zuiden PE. Effects of bile salts on rat hepatic acylCoA:cholesterol acyltransferase. *Lipids* 1995;30:911–915.

123. Del Pozo R, Nervi F, Covarrobias C, et al. Reversal of progesteron-induced biliary cholesterol output by dietary cholesterol and ethynil estradiol. *Biochim Biophys Acta* 1983;753:164–172.

124. Davis RA, Showalter R, Kern F. Reversal by triton WR-1339 of ethynyloestradiol-induced hepatic cholesterol esterification. *Biochem J* 1978;174:45–51.

125. Ghosh S, Mallonee DH, Hylemon PB, et al. Molecular cloning and expression of rat hepatic neutral cholesteryl ester hydrolase. *Biochim Biophys Acta* 1995;1259:305–312.

126. Ghosh S, Natarajan R, Pandak WM, et al. Regulation of hepatic neutral cholesteryl ester hydrolase by hormones and changes in cholesterol flux. *Am J Physiol* 1998;274:G662–G668.

127. Natarajan R, Ghosh S, Grogan WM. Molecular cloning of the promoter for rat hepatic neutral cholesterol ester hydrolase: evidence for transcriptional regulation by sterol. *Biochem Biophys Res Commun* 1998;243;349–355.

128. Martinez MJ, Hernandez ML, Lacort M, et al. Regulation of rat liver microsomal cholesterol ester hydrolase by reversible phosphorylation. *Lipids* 1994;29:7–13.

129. Liscum L, Munn NJ. Intracellular cholesterol transport. *Biochim Biophys Acta* 1999;1438:19–37.

130. Lange Y, Strebel F, Steck TL. Role of the plasma membrane in cholesterol esterification in rat hepatoma cells. *J Biol Chem* 1993;268:13838–13843.

131. DeGrella RF, Simoni RD. Intracellular transport of cholesterol to the plasma membrane. *J Biol Chem* 1982;257:14256–14262.

132. Uittenbogaard A, Ying Y, Smart EJ. Characterization of a cytosolic heat-shock protein-caveolin chaperone complex. Involvement of cholesterol trafficking. *J Biol Chem* 1998;273:6525–6532.

133. Liscum L, Klanse JJ. Niemann-Pick disease type C. *Curr Opin Lipidol* 1998;9:131–135.

134. Carstear ED, Morris JA, Coleman KG, et al. Niemann-Pick C1 disease gene: homology to mediators of cholesterol homeostasis. *Science* 1997;277:228–231.

135. Brooks-Wilson A, Marcil M, Clee SM, et al. Mutations in ABC1 in Tangier disease and familial high-density lipoprotein deficiency. *Nat Genet* 1999;22:336–345.

136. Bodziock M, Orso E, Klucken J, et al. The gene encoding ATP-binding cassette transporter 1 is mutated in Tangier disease. *Nat Genet* 1999;22:347–351.

137. Rust S, Rosier M, Funke H, et al. Tangier disease is caused by mutations in the gene encoding ATP-binding cassette transporter 1. *Nat Genet* 1999;22:352–355.

138. Langmann T. Molecular cloning of the human ATP-binding cassette transporter 1(hABC1): evidence for sterol-dependent regulation in macrophages. *Biochem Biophys Res Commun* 1999; 257:29–33.

139. Apstein MD, Carey MC. Pathogenesis of cholesterol gallstones: a parsimonious hypothesis. *Eur J Clin Invest* 1996;25: 343–352.

140. Mazer NA, Carey MC. Mathematical model of biliary lipid secretion: a quantitative analysis of physiological and biochemical data from man and other species. *J Lipid Res* 1984;25: 932–953.

141. Jian B, de la Llera-Moya M, Ji Y, et al. Scavenger receptor class B type I as a mediator of cellular cholesterol efflux to lipoproteins and phospholipid acceptors. *J Biol Chem* 1999;273:5599–5606.

142. Gerloff T, Steiger B, Hagenbuch B, et al. The sister-P-glycoprotein represents the canalicular bile salt export pump of mammalian liver. *J Biol Chem* 1998;273:10046–10050.

143. Smit JJM, Schinkel AH, Oude Elferink RPJ, et al. Homozygous disruption of the murine mdr2 P-glycoprotein gene leads to complete absence of phospholipid from bile and to liver disease. *Cell* 1993;75:451–462.

The Liver: Biology and Pathobiology, Fourth Edition, edited by I. M. Arias, J. L. Boyer, F. V. Chisari, N. Fausto, D. Schachter, and D. A. Shafritz.
Lippincott Williams & Wilkins, Philadelphia © 2001.

LEPTIN AND THE LIVER

LEE M. KAPLAN

Obesity is a common and increasingly prevalent disorder in the developed and developing world. In the U.S. alone, more than half of the adult population is overweight and nearly a fourth has obesity. Broad-based studies of the U.S. population have shown that the prevalence of obesity, after remaining stable at approximately 12% to 14% from the 1960s to 1980, increased progressively to 23% by 1994 (1–3). The prevalence of both overweight and obesity has increased each year during the 1990s, and it is likely to grow further during the next several decades as the rapidly increasing numbers of overweight and obese children reach maturity. This disorder is not limited to the U.S. and other Western countries. The prevalence of obesity is increasing most rapidly in the developing world, and the World Health Organization estimated that as of 2000, the medical burden of obesity worldwide exceeds that of malnutrition for the first time in human history (1).

Pathophysiologically, obesity is a multisystem disease that results from a failure of normal homeostatic mechanisms regulating food intake, fat storage, and energy utilization. (For presentation of energy metabolism in the liver, see website chapter 🖥 W-11).) At present, approximately 300,000 Americans die each year from the medical complications of obesity, and many more are disabled. These complications can be divided into several groups, including metabolic, anatomic, degenerative, and psychological (1,4). The most common metabolic complications are insulin resistance and type 2 diabetes mellitus, hyperlipidemias, hypertension, platelet dysregulation and atherosclerotic cardiovascular disease, gallstones, and nonalcoholic fatty liver disease (NAFLD). Because of its important roles in lipid and carbohydrate metabolism, the liver appears to play a major role in several of the metabolic complications of obesity. It both contributes to, and is affected by, the insulin resistance that frequently accompanies obesity (5) (see Chapter 36 and website chapter 🖥 W-29). NAFLD in particular appears to result in part from metabolic effects of insulin resistance and hyperinsulinemia (6).

Obesity is likely the outward manifestation of several diseases with complex and varied etiologies, mechanisms, and patterns of complications (4,7,8). In most cases of human obesity, the specific causes are unknown. The regulation of body weight and fat stores is a complex process involving multiple neural, endocrine, and paracrine regulatory pathways (for recent reviews, see refs. 9, 10, and 7). Information about body energy stores and recent food intake is conveyed to several regions of the hypothalamus which integrate these signals and generate a coordinated regulation of energy metabolism. Because weight (and stored energy) is maintained within a narrow range despite changing food sources and availability, tight regulation of energy metabolism is one of the critical homeostatic functions of the hypothalamus. Obesity may result from disturbance of these pathways at any one of several susceptible sites (9,11). Delineation of the mechanisms underlying regulation of weight and energy metabolism is beginning to suggest causes of many forms of human obesity. Understanding of these regulatory pathways has already yielded important clues about the molecular mechanisms by which obesity leads to diabetes, hyperlipidemia, and vascular disease (10,12–14).

LEPTIN AND THE REGULATION OF BODY ENERGY STORES

More than 90% of total body energy is stored in the form of triglycerides, and adipocyte fat comprises nearly all of the fungible energy stores under normal physiological condi-

L. M. Kaplan: Gastrointestinal Unit and MGH Weight Center, Massachusetts General Hospital; and Department of Medicine, Harvard Medical School, Boston, Massachusetts 02114.

tions. Thus, regulation of body weight in adulthood primarily reflects regulation of body fat stores. Until recently, the mechanisms underlying the regulation of body weight have been elusive. A variety of animal studies had revealed an important role for the hypothalamus (7,9,11,15). Surgery or cryoablation of the ventromedial hypothalamus in rats leads to obesity; conversely, damage to the lateral hypothalamus can generate anorexia (15). In addition, several genetic models of obesity in mice and rats were identified and shown to demonstrate Mendelian patterns of inheritance. Most notably, *obese* and *diabetes* mice exhibit autosomal recessive transmission (16).

Investigators had long postulated feedback regulation of body fat stores ("lipostat hypothesis") in which adipose tissue would generate a signal to the hypothalamus, which in turn would regulate food intake and energy expenditure. In now-classical studies, Coleman and colleagues used parabiosis techniques to examine whether circulating factors could account for the differences in phenotype among these different genetic and hypothalamic models of obesity (15,16). In parabiosis studies, the circulations of two animals are linked surgically, with approximately 1% of the blood supply of each animal entering the circulation of the other. Parabiotic linking of an *obese* and a normal mouse leads to correction of the obesity in the mutant animal. Conversely, parabiosis of a *diabetes* and a normal mouse leads to starvation of the normal mouse. Through a wide variety of such studies, these investigators predicted that the *obese* gene encodes a circulating signal that limits body fat deposition and that both the *diabetes* mutation and lesions of the ventromedial hypothalamus interfere with reception of that signal (16). As described below, the circulating factor encoded by the *obese* gene (leptin) fulfills the predictions of the lipostat hypothesis.

Progress in the understanding of the mechanisms of body weight regulation was accelerated by the discovery in 1994 of the hormone leptin. Friedman and colleagues had performed a genome-wide screen for markers linked to the *obese* locus in mice (17). Using positional cloning techniques, they isolated the responsible gene and determined that it encodes a secreted protein that they named after *leptos*, a Greek word meaning "thin." Leptin is a protein produced predominantly, but not exclusively, by adipocytes. It is secreted into the bloodstream and transported into the cerebrospinal fluid (CSF) where it activates receptors on central neurons, predominantly in the arcuate nucleus of the hypothalamus (16). Projections of these leptin-responsive neurons comprise a significant portion of what we now know to be the weight regulatory system of the hypothalamus. Leptin stimulation of neurons in the arcuate nucleus leads to activation of a variety of specific neural pathways that coordinate the regulation of weight and energy metabolism (18). Pathways that appear to be involved in this response include those mediated by neuropeptide Y, melanocortin, agouti gene-related peptide, melanin-concentrating hormone, CART (cocaine and amphetamine-

responsive transcript), orexins A and B, and others (for reviews, see refs. 9 and 14).

In the fasting state, the levels of circulating and CSF leptin are proportional to the amount of body fat. Mobilization of energy (fat) stores in times of decreased food availability leads to decreased leptin levels, activating a coordinated CNS response. As demonstrated by a large number of elegant studies, this response leads to conservation of energy expenditure and stimulation of food-seeking behaviors and food intake (16).

Mutations of the gene encoding leptin, such as seen in the spontaneous *obese* mouse, lead to profound obesity. Lacking the primary signal of body fat stores, the brains of these animals perceive a state of energy depletion. In response, they coordinate an insatiable program of increased food intake and decreased energy utilization that results in a body weight up to five times that of normal animals. A similar phenotype is observed in animals genetically deficient in the leptin receptor, including the *diabetes* mouse and *fatty* (Zucker) rat (19–21). In these animals, the hypothalamus is unable to perceive circulating or CSF leptin, despite the high levels produced by the excess adipose tissue. In normal animals, plasma leptin levels correlate closely with percent body fat, suggesting that leptin is an important signal of fat stores (16,22).

Leptin signaling appears critical for weight regulation in humans as well. Homozygous mutations in the human leptin or leptin receptor (LepR) genes, although extremely rare, are associated with severe, early-onset obesity (23–25). In nearly all cases, however, human obesity is associated with *elevated* leptin levels, suggesting that resistance to the effects of leptin is a major feature, if not the proximal cause, of this disease process.

In normal individuals, an imbalance between energy intake and expenditure leading to increased fat stores is reflected in increased leptin production. The elevated leptin then signals the hypothalamus to decrease food intake and increase energy utilization (16). This simple model, although consistent with the lipostat hypothesis, is inadequate to explain many features of energy homeostasis and leptin action. Circulating leptin levels are not a static reflection of body fat stores. Leptin expression and secretion are affected by many acute physiological influences, including circulating glucose and fatty acids, corticosteroids, and gonadal hormones (9,16,18). Plasma leptin concentrations decrease rapidly with fasting and increase with food intake. They vary with time in a pattern that suggests both pulsatile secretion and circadian rhythmicity. Leptin production and secretion also appear to be altered in response to cytokines and inflammatory mediators. These observations suggest that the physiological roles of this protein extend well beyond the simple signaling of body adipose mass. The inflammatory responses suggest that leptin may contribute to the pathophysiological effects of inflammation, including hepatitis and hepatic fibrosis.

Leptin itself is a member of the cytokine family, most closely related to ciliary neurotrophic factor and leukemia inhibitory factor. It signals through cell surface receptors encoded by the mouse *diabetes* and rat *fatty* genes. By variations in pre-mRNA splicing, the leptin receptor gene encodes several cell-surface receptors and at least one soluble receptor. The receptor subtype with the longest intracellular domain (Ob-R$_L$) is homologous to several other type 1 cytokine receptor subunits, including gp130, the common subunit of several type I cytokine receptors (19,21,22). These proteins contain two intracellular motifs that enable recruitment of members of the Janus kinase (Jak) family of intracellular signaling proteins. Leptin binding leads to receptor homodimerization, and recruitment and activation of several Janus kinases (Jak). Recruited Jak proteins phosphorylate the leptin receptor, leading to recruitment of several cytoplasmic STAT (signal transduction and activators of transcription) proteins. The recruited STAT proteins are subsequently phosphorylated, form bioactive dimers and move to the nucleus, where they promote transcription of selected target genes (22). While activation of the Jak-STAT pathway appears to be the predominant mechanism of leptin signaling in leptin-responsive cells, additional signal transduction pathways appear to be activated in response to leptin, including one that is mediated by phosphatidyl inositol 3-kinase. These additional pathways may also be activated by one or more of the shorter forms of the leptin receptor (Ob-R$_S$) that cannot stimulate Jak-STAT signaling (16). The most common forms of the *diabetes* mutation in mice and *fatty* mutation in rats selectively eliminate the long form of the leptin receptor. Since these animals are obese and insulin-resistant, we can conclude that the Ob-R$_L$ is required for leptin regulation of body weight homeostasis. Ob-R$_L$ receptor is also required for leptin regulation of reproductive function. (Leptin signaling is required for sexual maturation and continued reproductive function at maturity.) The physiological roles of the shorter forms of the leptin receptor are less clear, although at least one form (Ob-R$_a$), expressed heavily in the choroid plexus, is thought to mediate leptin transport into the CSF (19). The shorter forms of the leptin receptor are far more widely distributed than Ob-R$_L$. Demonstration that these shorter forms stimulate intracellular signaling events raises the possibility that they mediate important physiological responses from adipocytes and other cellular sources of leptin (see Leptin and Liver Disease, below).

Although the long form of the leptin receptor is expressed most abundantly in the hypothalamus, it has also been detected in several other tissues, including the pancreatic islets, adipocytes, kidney, and lung (16). In addition, shorter forms of the leptin receptor (Ob-R$_S$) are expressed in many tissues, including the liver and gastrointestinal tract. Their role in these sites is ambiguous. However, as described below, accumulating evidence suggests that leptin can influence metabolic, inflammatory, and fibrogenic responses in the liver.

Obesity in humans and rodents is commonly associated with diabetes mellitus. Animal models of leptin or leptin receptor deficiency (*obese* mice and *diabetes* mice or *fatty* Zucker rats, respectively) exhibit profound insulin resistance and diabetes. Alteration in glucose metabolism does not appear to result exclusively from interruption of the leptin signaling pathway, however. Recent studies show that the genetic background of animals with these mutations exerts a major influence on the degree of insulin resistance. In fact, the rare humans with genetic leptin or leptin receptor deficiency have not had diabetes mellitus and exhibit little or no insulin resistance despite their massive obesity (23–25). The discordance between morbid obesity and diabetes in these individuals is likely due more to the influences of modifying genes than to differences in the role of the leptin pathway in different species. Similarly, diet-induced obesity in both rodents and humans is only variably associated with insulin resistance. In rodents, the proclivity to insulin resistance is strain-dependent. In humans, while the degree of insulin resistance varies dramatically among individuals with similar body fat stores, there appear to be strong genetic influences on this association. Diabetes in one obese member of a family substantially increases the likelihood of diabetes or subclinical insulin resistance in other overweight and obese relatives.

In mice, Hotamisligil and colleagues have demonstrated that tumor necrosis factor α (TNF-α) signaling exerts a permissive role on insulin-resistance in the setting of obesity (13). Obese animals mutated in this cytokine or its receptor are far more insulin-responsive than wild-type mice of the same strain. TNF-α is produced in many tissues, including adipocytes themselves, and it is not yet known which sites of TNF signaling contribute to obesity-associated insulin resistance. Several additional factors likely contribute to the dysregulation of insulin signaling observed in association with obesity.

LEPTIN AND LIVER DISEASE

Fatty liver disease is a common complication of obesity in both animals and humans. As described in Chapter 50, NAFLD encompasses a spectrum of pathological disorders from microvesicular steatosis to steatohepatitis, fibrosis, and frank cirrhosis (26,27). NAFLD, first described in 1980, was initially felt to be a benign process with little medical significance. With longer follow-up times and more careful observation, however, it appears that a small but significant subset of patients with more advanced NAFLD (steatohepatitis) undergo progressive fibrosis and cirrhosis. An increasing number of patients requiring liver transplantation appear to have steatosis-related cirrhosis, without evidence of alcoholic liver disease, toxicity from other drugs, or viral hepatitis. In addition, recent epidemiological studies, conducted since the advent of sensitive serological testing for hepatitis C, have suggested that many if not most cases of cryptogenic cirrhosis represent the last stages of NAFLD. Thus, steatohepatitis has now been recognized as a major cause of progressive liver disease.

The number of patients diagnosed with NAFLD is rising rapidly. Although the increasing diagnosis partly reflects increased physician awareness and screening, the expanding epidemic of obesity is almost certainly causing a dramatic increase in the true prevalence of NAFLD as well. The development of steatohepatitis appears to occur in two discrete steps: steatosis is a necessary precursor to steatohepatitis, but only leads to inflammation in the presence of a second insult, such as enhanced oxidative stress (28).

Epidemiologically, NAFLD is strongly associated with obesity and diabetes (26). Development of NAFLD is most commonly preceded by insulin resistance and hyperinsulinemia, and insulin resistance is a common feature even in lean individuals without diabetes (6). These observations suggest that alteration of insulin-regulated hepatic carbohydrate or fatty acid transport, or of hepatic lipid metabolism, may account for the underlying pathological defect (6,29). In this model, defects in insulin signaling, especially in muscle and liver cells, lead to elevated circulating fatty acid levels. These fatty acids are then transported into hepatocytes, where they are esterified and stored as triglycerides. This model has several shortcomings, most notably the known insulin-responsiveness of fatty acid transport and esterification in the liver. Universal insulin resistance would logically interfere with hepatic steatogenesis, and animals with profound defects in the insulin-response pathways exhibit relatively modest hepatic steatosis despite their profound insulin resistance. It is more likely that tissue- or intracellular signal-specific differences in insulin resistance account for the metabolic derangements leading to hepatocyte fat deposition.

In at least one study, intraperitoneal administration of insulin led to subcapsular hepatic steatosis, suggesting that the steatosis in this case resulted from the action of insulin excess in the local environment (30). Since several types of toxic stimuli lead to fat deposition in hepatocytes, it appears that this process is easily induced and that there may be several distinct pathways of hepatic steatogenesis depending on the model studied. For example, in animal models of lipodystrophy, in which genetic manipulation leads to massive loss of adipose tissue and insulin resistance, hepatic steatosis is thought to represent a secondary pathway of body energy storage. The absence of adipocytes leads to elevated circulating free fatty acids, which are transported into hepatocytes (and to a lesser extent myocytes) for esterification and storage.

Hepatic steatosis is associated with increased delivery of free fatty acids to the liver and elevated intracellular fatty acid levels in hepatocytes. Although the underlying pathophysiology is not fully understood, alterations in insulin signaling and fat metabolism appear to promote the steato-

sis. Liver fat deposition associated with obesity occurs predominantly in the setting of insulin resistance and elevated circulating insulin levels. Impaired insulin responsiveness in adipocytes promotes fat lipolysis and increased delivery of fatty acids to the liver. In the liver, insulin stimulates fatty acid synthesis and inhibits fatty acid oxidation. Impaired insulin signaling should therefore decrease intracellular fatty acid concentrations. However, because of high circulating insulin levels associated with insulin resistance, it is possible that there is a net increase in the insulin signal to hepatocytes in this setting. As noted above, a stimulatory role for insulin signaling in hepatic steatogenesis is further suggested by the observation that intraperitoneal insulin administration in rodents and humans leads to subcapsular fat deposition in the liver (30).

Several studies show that leptin regulates both insulin secretion and tissue responsiveness to this hormone (31–33). Hepatocytes express abundant leptin receptors and respond to leptin administration in cell culture (34). Although the short form of the leptin receptor (Ob-R$_S$) predominates, recent evidence suggests that the long form (Ob-R$_L$) is also expressed. The effects of leptin on insulin response in hepatocytes are complex (35,36) and include direct effects and those mediated through stimulation of central leptin-responsive neurons (37,38). Leptin stimulates glycogenesis, inhibits glycogenolysis and, under most conditions, stimulates gluconeogenesis (39–41). It stimulates glucose transport and turnover, consistent with an insulinotropic effect, and activates intracellular insulin signaling pathways (42). However, it also inhibits insulin-stimulated phosphorylation of other signaling proteins, including IRS-1, suggesting that leptin may help to induce insulin resistance (31,43,44).

The high circulating leptin levels associated with obesity in humans may thus contribute to hepatic steatosis in two ways: (a) by promoting insulin resistance and elevated circulating insulin levels and (b) by altering insulin signaling in hepatocytes so as to promote increased concentrations of intracellular fatty acids and their conversion to triglycerides. Elevated leptin levels may also contribute to fatty liver disease even in the absence of obesity. Tobe et al. (45) observed increased leptin levels in Japanese students with fatty liver, *independent* of body mass index (BMI). In addition, recent studies have demonstrated an elevated leptin/BMI ratio in patients with chronic hepatitis C and steatosis as compared with hepatitis C in the absence of steatosis (46). In this study, individuals with steatohepatitis had the highest circulating leptin/BMI ratio of all.

Leptin may also influence the progression from hepatic steatosis to steatohepatitis. Given the similar intracellular signaling pathways stimulated by leptin and several inflammatory cytokines, it is perhaps not surprising that leptin could regulate inflammatory responses. Loffreda et al. (47) reported that leptin stimulates murine macrophage phagocytic activity *in vitro* and *in vivo*. These effects were dependent on expression of Ob-R$_L$, the long form of the leptin receptor, as macrophages isolated from the *diabetes* mouse were insensitive to these effects of leptin. Moreover, leptin selectively enhanced the secretion of TNF-α, interleukin (IL)-6, and IL-12 from isolated macrophages in response to lipopolysaccharide. Given the known regulatory effects of these cytokines, it thus appears that leptin may help to amplify selected proinflammatory responses (48). Consistent with this hypothesis, recent evidence suggests that leptin facilitates T-lymphocyte-mediated hepatotoxicity by facilitating the activation of TNF-α and IL-18, actions that may contribute to steatosis-associated inflammation (49). Within hepatocytes, leptin appears to regulate the expression and activity of several proteins that mediate oxidative stress, including CYP2E1 and CYP4A (50–52). In obesity, therefore, the increased sensitivity to endotoxic liver injury and steatohepatitis may reflect the observed alterations in leptin expression and signaling.

In a surprising and provocative study, Potter et al. detected leptin expression and protein synthesis in activated hepatic stellate cells grown in cell culture (53). Leptin expression in these cells seems to be dependent on their transdifferentiation into myofibroblast-like cells, similar to the changes that occur after activation *in vivo*. Activation is also associated with release of stored retinoid compounds, which may be essential to regulating differentiation of these cells. Exposure of activated stellate cells in culture to retinoic acid inhibits leptin expression. It remains to be determined whether stellate cells activated *in vivo* express and secrete leptin. Nonetheless, these observations raise the intriguing possibility that locally produced leptin helps mediate the hepatic response to injury. In light of leptin's apparent proinflammatory activities, activation of stellate cells in the setting of steatosis may help to initiate or propagate steatohepatitis, and leptin may contribute to fibrogenesis resulting from stellate cell activation.

Several investigators have found that circulating leptin levels are increased in patients with cirrhosis, independent of changes in circulating TNF-α levels (54,55). In both men and women, observed changes are significant when the reduced body fat mass of cirrhotic patients was taken into account (56). Nonetheless, the physiological significance of this finding is unclear. Do the elevated leptin levels stimulate energy metabolism, decrease appetite, and contribute to the decreased fat stores in these patients? There are numerous other explanations for decreased body fat in cirrhosis, including circulating toxins, inefficient energy utilization, and other inflammatory cytokines. What are the mechanisms underlying increased plasma leptin levels in cirrhosis? Leptin secretion from adipocytes may be enhanced by cytokines released as part of the inflammatory or fibrogenic process. Alternatively, as suggested by some investigators, cirrhotic patients may simply exhibit decreased hepatic clearance of this protein (56). In light of the recent observations by Potter et al., it is intriguing to speculate that

hepatic stellate cells may be a source of additional leptin in these patients (53). Confounding these observations is the finding in one study that leptin levels are *decreased* in adolescents with end-stage liver disease (57). Further studies are necessary to determine the physiological significance of these observations and their applicability to various liver disease states.

A recent study by Lin et al. demonstrated that the fatty liver disease in *obese* (leptin-deficient) mice can be largely reversed by treatment with metformin, an insulin-sensitizing agent used clinically to treat type 2 diabetes mellitus (58). Metformin treatment of the mice was also associated with decreased food intake, increased energy expenditure, decreased adipose tissue mass, and mild inhibition of hepatic TNF-α levels, effects which themselves are predicted to diminish hepatic steatosis and steatohepatitis. Which of these changes are primarily responsible for reversal of fatty liver disease remains unclear (decreased food intake alone was much less effective), but the overall effect of metformin in mice strongly supports the role of insulin resistance in the generation of fatty liver disease. Given our limited understanding of the specific role of insulin signaling in NAFLD, it will be useful to examine the differential effects, if any, of metformin on insulin signaling in various tissues. It will also be important to examine the effects of metformin on NAFLD in humans with and without diabetes mellitus, both for its potential therapeutic benefit as well as to gain increased understanding of the underlying mechanisms in different subgroups of patients.

The specific role of leptin in the pathogenesis of NAFLD is not clear. As noted above, leptin influences both insulin secretion and signaling. Neither clinical leptin resistance nor elevated leptin levels are required for the development of NAFLD, however, as many diabetic patients with normal body mass indices and leptin levels nonetheless develop hepatic steatosis. Whether leptin resistance-mediated insulin signaling defects account for NAFLD in a subset of patients remains to be determined. Loffreda and colleagues have demonstrated elevation of several other cytokines in the serum of patients and animals with hepatic steatosis (47). In particular, they have observed an association of high circulating levels of TNF-α and NAFLD. Interference with TNF-α signaling in leptin-deficient animals appears to prevent hepatic steatosis; however, these animals are more insulin-sensitive than their TNF-α signaling-competent littermates, so the effect of this cytokine may be indirect.

Recent studies have demonstrated that leptin is synthesized and secreted from the stomach as well as adipocytes. Bado et al. (59) detected leptin gene expression and immunoreactive leptin in the rat gastric fundus. Leptin immunoreactivity was localized in the lower half of the fundic glands in the region of the pepsinogen-secreting chief cells (60,61). Unlike leptin expression in adipocytes, gastric leptin content is not affected by fasting. Leptin expression in the stomach appears to be induced by gastric mucosal injury (62), and food ingestion acutely stimulates rapid secretion of gastric leptin stores. This effect is reproduced by cholecystokinin (CCK) administration, leading to increased circulating leptin levels. Because leptin has been shown to enhance the satiety-inducing effect of CCK, CCK-induced leptin secretion may amplify or prolong the intestinal regulation of food ingestion (63). The targets of stomach-derived leptin are currently unknown. In addition to a potential endocrine role, gastric leptin may act locally, exerting paracrine effects within the gastric mucosa or stimulating vagal afferents to signal the central nervous system. Because gastric leptin is likely secreted directly into the portal circulation, leptin may also mediate communication between the stomach and the liver, including information about recent food intake. And because leptin regulates hepatocyte insulin sensitivity, such local leptin signaling pathways would provide a novel mechanism of acutely adjusting the hepatic response to insulin, possibly priming hepatocytes for the increase in insulin levels triggered by postprandial circulating glucose and fatty acid elevations. More detailed studies of the distribution of leptin receptors in the gut, the temporal patterns of leptin secretion in the fundus, and the fate of the secreted leptin will help sort out the physiological roles of gastric leptin and its potential for regulating liver physiology.

CONCLUSION

Leptin is a circulating cytokine discovered through its role in regulating body weight and energy metabolism. Initially thought to be expressed and secreted exclusively by adipocytes, leptin mRNA and/or protein has recently been detected in placenta, gastric mucosa, and hepatic stellate cells. Accumulating evidence suggests that, like other cytokines, leptin has diverse and complex metabolic effects. In the liver, these effects may include a role in the regulation of fat deposition, fibrogenesis, and inflammation. Obesity in humans, like diet-induced obesity in rodents, is associated with elevated circulating leptin levels and hypothalamic insensitivity to this protein. Obesity-associated hepatic steatosis develops primarily in individuals with substantially elevated insulin levels, most commonly as a result of insulin resistance. Because leptin is an important regulator of both insulin secretion and hepatic responsiveness to insulin action, altered leptin signaling in obese individuals may contribute to hepatic steatosis. The recent observations of altered leptin levels in steatohepatitis and cirrhosis, coupled with data suggesting that activated hepatic stellate cells express leptin mRNA, raise the possibility that leptin directly affects the development of hepatic inflammation and fibrosis. In the gastrointestinal tract, leptin is secreted from fundic mucosa in response to food ingestion or CCK, suggesting that it may participate in the gut-derived satiety response. Whether stomach-derived leptin acts locally or systemically and whether it selectively regulates hepatic function after secretion into the portal circulation are unknown. Although considerable work needs to be done to define the nature and magnitude of leptin's activities in the liver, it is becoming increasingly apparent that this protein will take its place among the myriad cytokines that regulate hepatic function in health and disease.

REFERENCES

1. Kopelman P. Obesity as a medical problem. *Nature* 2000;404: 635–643.
2. Bray G. Health hazards of obesity. *Endocrinol Metab Clin North Am* 1996;25:907–919.
3. Van Itallie T. Health implications of overweight and obesity in the United States. *Ann Intern Med* 1985;103:983–988.
4. Hill J, Peters J. Environmental contributions to the obesity epidemic. *Science* 1998;280:1371–1374.
5. Kaplan L. Leptin, obesity and liver disease. *Gastroenterology* 1998;115:997–1001.
6. Marchesini G, et al. Association of nonalcoholic fatty liver disease with insulin resistance. *Am J Med* 1999;107:450–455.
7. Barsh G, Farooqi I, O'Rahilly S. Genetics of body-weight regulation. *Nature* 2000;404:644–651.
8. Comuzzie A, Allison D. The search for human obesity genes. *Science* 1998;280:1374–1377.
9. Schwartz M, et al. Central nervous system control of food intake. *Nature* 2000;404:661–671.
10. Lowell B, Spiegelman B. Towards a molecular understanding of adaptive thermogenesis. *Nature* 2000;404:652–660.
11. Woods S, et al. Signals that regulate food intake and energy homeostasis. *Science* 1998;280:1378–1383.
12. Spiegelman B, Flier J. Adipogenesis and obesity: rounding out the big picture. *Cell* 1996;87:377–389.
13. Uysal K, et al. Protection from obesity-induced insulin resistance in mice lacking TNF-alpha function. *Nature* 1997;389:610–614.
14. Flier J, Maratos-Flier E. Obesity and the hypothalamus: novel peptides for new pathways. *Cell* 1998;92:437–440.
15. Weigle D. Appetite and the regulation of body composition. *FASEB J* 1994;8:302–310.
16. Friedman J, Halaas J. Leptin and the regulation of body weight. *Nature* 1998;395:763–770.
17. Zhang Y, et al. Positional cloning of the mouse obese gene and its human homologue. *Nature* 1994;372:425–432.
18. Elmquist J, Elias C, Saper C. From lesions to leptin: hypothalamic control of food intake and body weight. *Neuron* 1999;22: 221–232.
19. Tartaglia L, et al. Identification and expression cloning of a leptin receptor. *Cell* 1995;83:1263–1271.
20. Chen H, et al. Evidence that the diabetes gene encodes the leptin receptor: identification of a mutation in the leptin receptor gene in db/db mice. *Cell* 1995;84:491–495.
21. Lee G, et al. Abnormal splicing of the leptin receptor in diabetic mice. *Nature* 1996;379:632–635.
22. Tartaglia L. The leptin receptor. *J Biol Chem* 1997;272: 6093–6096.
23. Strobel A, et al. A leptin missense mutation associated with hypogonadism and morbid obesity. *Nat Genet* 1998;18:213–215.
24. Montague C, et al. Congenital leptin deficiency is associated with severe early-onset obesity in humans. *Nature* 1997;387:903–908.
25. Clement K, et al. A mutation in the human leptin receptor gene

causes obesity and pituitary dysfunction. *Nature* 1998;392: 398–401.

26. Matteoni C, et al. Nonalcoholic fatty liver disease: a spectrum of clinical and pathological activity. *Gastroenterology* 1999;116: 1413–1419.

27. Sheth S, Gordon F, Chopra S. Nonalcoholic steatohepatitis. *Ann Intern Med* 1997;126:137–145.

28. Day C, James O. Steatohepatitis: a tale of two "hits"? *Gastroenterology* 1998;114:842–845.

29. Cortez-Pinto H, et al. Non-alcoholic fatty liver: another feature of the metabolic syndrome. *Clin Nutr* 1999;18:353–358.

30. Wanless I, et al. Subcapsular steatonecrosis in response to peritoneal insulin delivery: A clue to the pathogenesis of steatonecrosis in obesity. *Mod Pathol* 1989;2:69–74.

31. Kamohara S, et al. Acute stimulation of glucose metabolism in mice by leptin treatment. *Nature* 1997;389:374–377.

32. Burcelin R, et al. Acute intravenous leptin infusion increases glucose turnover but not skeletal muscle glucose uptake in ob/ob mice. *Diabetes* 1999;48:1264–1269.

33. Ceddia R, et al. Acute effects of leptin on glucose metabolism of in situ rat perfused livers and isolated hepatocytes. *Int J Obes Relat Metab Disord* 1999;23:1207–1212.

34. Wang Y, et al. Leptin receptor action in hepatic cells. *J Biol Chem* 1997;272:16216–16223.

35. Sivitz W, et al. Effects of leptin on insulin sensitivity in normal rats. *Endocrinology* 1997;138:3395–3401.

36. Cohen B, Novick D, Rubinstein M. Modulation of insulin activities by leptin. *Science* 1996;274:1185–1188.

37. Liu L, et al. Intracerebroventricular leptin regulates hepatic but not peripheral glucose fluxes. *J Biol Chem* 1998;273: 31160–31167.

38. Cusin I, et al. Chronic central leptin infusion enhances insulin-stimulated glucose metabolism and favors the expression of uncoupling proteins. *Diabetes* 1998;47:1014–1019.

39. Nemecz M, et al. Acute effect of leptin on hepatic glycogenolysis and gluconeogenesis in perfused rat liver. *Hepatology* 1999;29: 166–172.

40. O'Doherty R, et al. Sparing effect of leptin on liver glycogen stores in rats during the fed-to-fasted transition. *Am J Physiol* 1999;277:E544–E550.

41. Rossetti L, et al. Short term effects of leptin on hepatic gluconeogenesis and in vivo insulin secretion. *J Biol Chem* 1997;272: 27758–27763.

42. Zhao A, et al. Leptin induces insulin-like signaling that antagonizes cAMP elevation by glucagon in hepatocytes. *J Biol Chem* 2000;275:11348–11354.

43. Muller G, et al. Leptin impairs metabolic actions of insulin in isolated rat adipocytes. *J Biol Chem* 1997;272:10585–10593.

44. Szanto I, Kahn C. Selective interaction between leptin and insulin signaling pathways in a hepatic cell line. *Proc Natl Acad Sci U S A* 2000;97:2355–2360.

45. Tobe K, et al. Relationship between serum leptin and fatty liver in Japanese male adolescent university students. *Am J Gastroenterol* 1999;94:3328–3335.

46. Giannini E, et al. Leptin levels in nonalcoholic steatohepatitis and chronic hepatitis C. *Hepatogastroenterology* 1999;46: 2422–2425.

47. Loffreda S, et al. Leptin regulates proinflammatory immune responses. *FASEB J* 1998;12:57–65.

48. Hoppin A, et al. Serum leptin in children and young adults with inflammatory bowel disease. *J Pediatr Gastroenterol Nutr* 1998; 26:500–505.

49. Faggioni R, et al. Leptin-deficient (ob/ob) mice are protected from T cell-mediated hepatotoxicity: role of tumor necrosis factor alpha and IL-18. *Proc Natl Acad Sci U S A* 2000;97: 2367–2372.

50. Watson A, et al. Effect of leptin on cytochrome P-450, conjugation, and antioxidant enzymes in the ob/ob mouse. *Drug Metab Dispos* 1999;27:695–700.

51. Enriquez A, et al. Altered expression of hepatic CYP2E1 and CYP4A in obese, diabetic ob/ob mice, and fa/fa Zucker rats. *Biochem Biophys Res Commun* 1999;255:300–306.

52. Leclercq I, et al. Constitutive and inducible expression of hepatic CYP2E1 in leptin-deficient ob/ob mice. *Biochem Biophys Res Commun* 2000;268:337–344.

53. Potter J, et al. Transdifferentiation of rat hepatic stellate cells results in leptin expression. *Biochem Biophys Res Commun* 1998; 244:178–182.

54. McCullough A, et al. Gender-dependent alterations in serum leptin in alcoholic cirrhosis. *Gastroenterology* 1998;115:947–953.

55. Shimizu H, et al. An increase of circulating leptin in patients with liver cirrhosis. *Int J Obes Relat Metab Disord* 1998;22: 1234–1238.

56. Henriksen J, et al. Increased circulating leptin in alcoholic cirrhosis: relation to release and disposal. *Hepatology* 1999;29: 1818–1824.

57. Roberts G, et al. Serum leptin and insulin in paediatric end-stage liver disease and following successful orthotopic liver transplantation. *Clin Endocrinol (Oxf)* 1998;48:401–406.

58. Lin H, et al. Chronic ethanol consumption induces the production of tumor necrosis factor-alpha and related cytokines in liver and adipose tissue. *Alcohol Clin Exp Res* 1998;22:231S–237S.

59. Bado A, et al. The stomach is a source of leptin. *Nature* 1998; 394:790–793.

60. Cinti S, et al. Secretory granules of endocrine and chief cells of human stomach mucosa contain leptin. *Int J Obes Relat Metab Disord* 2000;24:789–793.

61. Sobhani I, et al. Leptin secretion and leptin receptor in the human stomach. *Gut* 2000;47:178–183.

62. Konturek P, et al. Enhanced expression of leptin following acute gastric injury in rat. *J Physiol Pharmacol* 1999;50:587–595.

63. Barrachina M, et al. Synergistic interaction between leptin and cholecystokinin to reduce short-term food intake in mice. *Proc Natl Acad Sci U S A* 1997;94:10455–10460.

18

HYPOXIC, ISCHEMIC, AND REPERFUSION INJURY TO LIVER

JOHN J. LEMASTERS

J. J. Lemasters: Department of Cell Biology and Anatomy, University of North Carolina–Chapel Hill, Chapel Hill, North Carolina 27599.

HEPATIC OXYGEN METABOLISM (SEE CHAPTER 19 AND WEBSITE CHAPTER 🖳 W-13)

The liver is a highly aerobic organ whose metabolism and viability depend on the availability of oxygen. Oxygen consumption of the liver is 100 to 150 μmol O_2 per hour per gram of wet weight. The hepatic artery and the portal vein together deliver blood to the liver. These vessels furnish about 25% and 75% of blood flow, respectively, although flow rates vary physiologically, particularly in response to digestive activity. Portal blood is better oxygenated than mixed venous blood but is still less oxygenated than arterial blood. Taking oxygenation into account, the portal vein and hepatic artery each provide roughly half of the oxygen supply to the liver. In most circulations, blood flow is regulated primarily by oxygen demand. In the liver, portal blood flow depends on the activity of the digestive organs and increases during active absorption of nutrients. To a considerable extent, hepatic arterial and venous blood flow are reciprocal so as to maintain constant total blood flow through the liver. Because the liver is an important site of first pass clearance of hormones, stable hepatic blood flow prevents fluctuations in hormone levels that would otherwise occur when hepatic blood flow changes.

Portal and arterial blood thoroughly mix inside the hepatic sinusoid. As sinusoidal blood moves through the hepatic lobules, the liver extracts oxygen, nutrients, bile acids, and hormones (Fig. 18.1). At the same time, synthetic products and metabolic wastes are added to the blood. In this way, sinusoidal blood flow and hepatic metabolism create gradients of oxygen, metabolites, and hormones between periportal and pericentral regions of the liver lobule. Tissue responses to these gradients likely contribute to the development of biochemical differences between hepatocytes in different regions of the hepatic lobule, such as the relative enrichment of ureagenesis, gluconeogenesis, and oxidative metabolism in periportal hepatocytes and xenobiotic and glycolytic metabolism in pericentral hepatocytes (1).

Measurements with microlight guides and miniature oxygen electrodes show directly oxygen gradients within the liver lobule with periportal regions more highly oxygenated than pericentral regions. Although still often cited, earlier measurements claiming that intrahepatic oxygen tension is lower than that of the mixed venous drainage are likely the consequence of the decreased sensitivity of Clark-style oxygen electrodes inside solid tissue. When Clark electrodes are calibrated to oxygen inside solid hepatic tissue, intrahepatic oxygen concentrations are in between that of the inflow and outflow blood vessels (2).

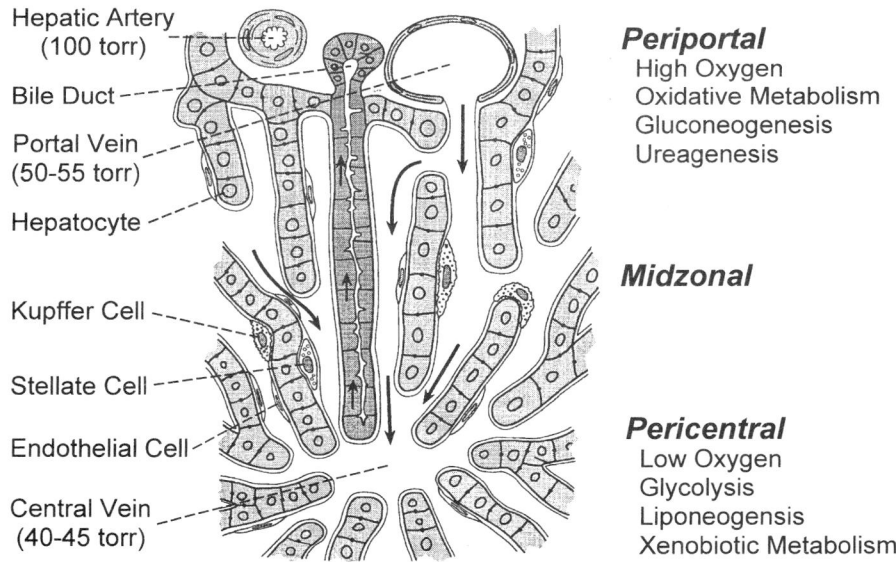

Hepatic Artery (100 torr)
Bile Duct
Portal Vein (50-55 torr)
Hepatocyte
Kupffer Cell
Stellate Cell
Endothelial Cell
Central Vein (40-45 torr)

Periportal
High Oxygen
Oxidative Metabolism
Gluconeogenesis
Ureagenesis

Midzonal

Pericentral
Low Oxygen
Glycolysis
Liponeogensis
Xenobiotic Metabolism

FIGURE 18.1. Oxygen and metabolic gradients within the liver lobule. As blood flows through the liver lobule (*downward arrows*), hepatic tissue extracts oxygen and other blood-borne substances (e.g., hormones, hyaluronic acid, bile acids) while simultaneously adding metabolic wastes and synthetic products. As a consequence, gradients of oxygen and other metabolites form between periportal and pericentral regions. Where blood first enters the lobule, sinusoidal oxygen tension is between that of the hepatic artery and the portal vein. Where blood exits the lobule, oxygen tension is close to that of the central vein (terminal hepatic venule). In low flow and hypoxemic states, pericentral hepatocytes are the first to experience hypoxic stress. Gradients of hepatic enzymes also exist across the liver lobule. Enzymes for oxidative phosphorylation, gluconeogenesis, and ureagenesis are concentrated in periportal regions, whereas enzymes for glycolysis, lipogenesis, and drug metabolism are concentrated in pericentral regions. Bile flow within canaliculi runs countercurrent to blood flow (*upward arrows*).

VULNERABILITY OF LIVER TO HYPOXIC AND ISCHEMIC INJURY

Like the heart and brain, the liver is quite vulnerable to hypoxic injury, but unique features of hepatic vascularization and metabolism afford the liver relative protection against hypoxia. Dual vascularization provides a redundancy of the blood supply, which is the apparent reason why focal ischemic injury secondary to atherosclerosis and related causes is rare in the liver. Livers of well-nourished individuals also contain up to 7% glycogen by weight. This glycogen supports adenosine triphosphate (ATP) generation by anaerobic glycolysis. During anoxia and ischemia, glycolytic ATP formation replaces, in part, ATP lost from oxidative phosphorylation and delays anoxic hepatocellular cell death by hours compared to glycogen-depleted livers.

Even with the protection of a dual blood supply and the anaerobic metabolism of glycogen, hypoxic liver damage is quite common in systemic hypoxemia and cardiogenic, hemorrhagic, and septic shock. Due to the intralobular oxygen gradient, hypoxic injury in low-flow states occurs first in the pericentral region of hepatic lobules (3). Indeed, pericentral and midzonal hepatic necrosis attributable to hypoxic injury is frequently observed at autopsy. If severe enough, pericentral liver hypoxia leads to a syndrome of ischemic hepatitis characterized by a sharp increase in serum transaminase activities in the absence of other causes of hepatic necrosis, such as viral or drug-induced hepatitis (4).

The liver, unlike the heart and brain, has enormous regenerative capacity. Thus, virtually complete restoration of normal liver structure and function can occur after hypoxic injury when normal hepatic perfusion is restored. Repeated cycles of hypoxic injury, however, may lead to chronic liver injury. In alcoholic liver disease, cycles of hypoxic injury are postulated to contribute to hepatic fibrosis and alcoholic cirrhosis (5).

Warm hypoxic liver injury is also of clinical importance in the Budd–Chiari syndrome, veno-occlusive disease, liver surgery, and liver transplantation. The Budd–Chiari syndrome is caused by obstruction of hepatic venous outflow by a thrombus or mass, leading to painful hepatomegaly, microcirculatory stasis, and ascites (6). This outflow obstruction, if untreated by thrombolytic therapy or surgical decompression, leads to progressive hepatic failure requiring liver transplantation. Hepatic veno-occlusive disease, like the Budd–Chiari syndrome, presents clinically as hepatomegaly and ascites most commonly in patients receiving hepatic irradiation and chemotherapy for bone marrow transplantation (7). Veno-occlusive disease is associated with sinusoidal endothelial cell injury and extravasation of red blood cells into the space of Disse. A fibrotic response then leads to obliterative, obstructive lesions of the central veins and smaller hepatic vein branches. Both Budd–Chiari syndrome and veno-occlusive disease cause severe centrilobular congestion and hypoxic hepatocellular necrosis. Ischemia/reperfusion injury is also a concern to the liver surgeon who often needs to occlude branches of the portal vein and hepatic artery temporarily for a blood-free field (Pringle maneuver). Similarly, ischemia/reperfusion injury associated with cold ischemic storage limits liver preservation for transplantation surgery (8).

In animal models, warm ischemia/reperfusion injury to the liver is easily induced by cross-clamping the portal vein and hepatic artery. Clamping the blood supply to specific lobes, such as the median and left lateral lobes, avoids intestinal stasis but still produces ischemia to about 70% of the liver (9). After reflow, hepatic cell death is manifested by release of hepatocellular enzymes (lactate dehydrogenase, transaminases) and uptake of supravital dyes (trypan blue, propidium iodide). Release of enzymes and uptake of normally impermeant dyes signify the breakdown of the plasma membrane permeability barrier, which is the hallmark of onset of necrotic cell death.

CELLULAR CHANGES IN HYPOXIA

One of the earliest hepatocellular changes in hypoxia is the formation of plasma membrane protrusions called blebs (Fig. 18.2) (3,10). Blebs contain cytosol and endoplasmic reticulum but generally exclude larger organelles like mitochondria and lysosomes. Accompanying bleb formation are dilatation of cisternae of endoplasmic reticulum, rounding and moderate swelling of mitochondria, and a 30% to 50% increase of total cellular volume.

These early changes are reversible, and hepatocytes can still recover fully after reoxygenation. Irreversible injury occurs when a plasma membrane bleb literally bursts, causing abrupt failure of the plasma membrane permeability barrier, release of intracellular enzymes and metabolites, and collapse of all electrical and ionic gradients across the plasma membrane (11,12). In hepatocytes, sinusoidal endothelial cells, and other cell types, a metastable state precedes bleb rupture (12). This metastable state begins with mitochondrial permeabilization and lysosomal disruption. Blebs then coalesce and increase in size, low molecular weight anionic fluorophores begin to cross the plasma membrane, and cell swelling accelerates (13). The metastable state culminates in bleb rupture, equilibration of intracellular and extracellular contents, and necrotic cell death.

The cytoprotective amino acid, glycine, inhibits progression into the metastable state after ATP depletion and protects sinusoidal endothelial cells, hepatocytes, and other cell types against the onset of necrotic cell death (14–17). In Madin-Darby canine kidney (MDCK) cells, glycine was reported to block the opening of water-filled pores whose molecular weight exclusion limit increases progressively from about 4,000 d to more than 70,000 d (18). By contrast, in cultured hepatic sinusoidal endothelial cells,

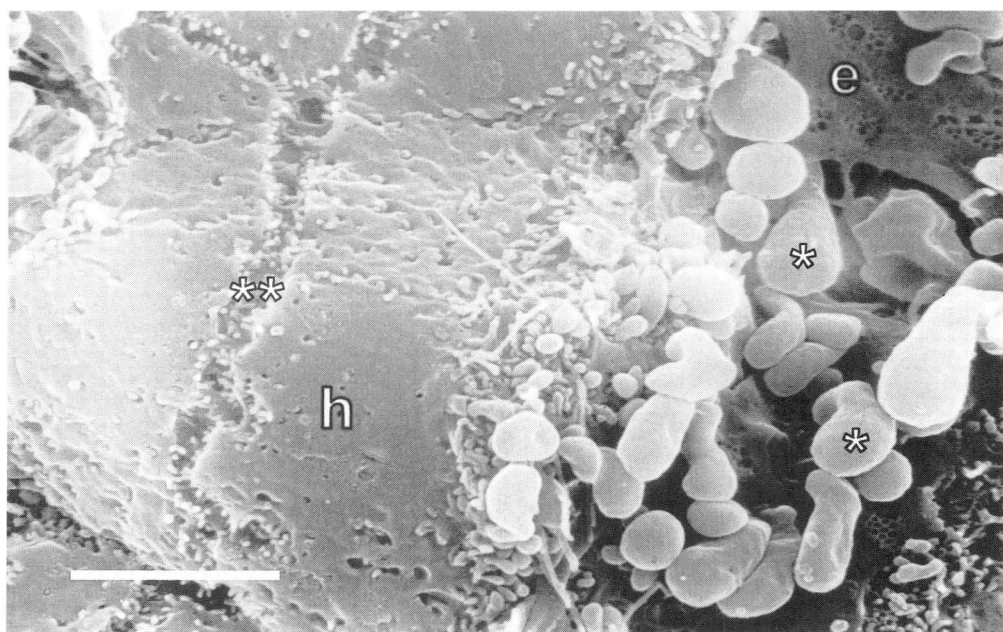

FIGURE 18.2. Scanning electron micrograph of early cell surface bleb formation during hypoxia. Hepatocellular blebs (*single asterisks*) protrude through fenestrations of sinusoidal endothelial cells (*e*) after 15 minutes of low-flow hypoxia in a perfused rat liver. Blebbing occurs on the subsinusoidal surface of the hepatocytes. Intercellular surfaces of the hepatocytes (*h*) are not yet involved, and bile canaliculi (*double asterisks*) are normal. *Bar* is 5 μm. (Adapted from Lemasters JJ, Ji S, Thurman RG. Centrilobular injury following hypoxia in isolated, perfused rat liver. *Science* 1981;213:661–663.)

glycine appeared to inhibit a selective organic anion channel, which is permeable to chloride and polyvalent organic anions up to a molecular size limit of at least 600 d, but not to similarly sized organic cations or larger molecular weight dextrans (17). Opening of the glycine-sensitive organic anion channel leads to the rapid cellular swelling of the metastable state. This swelling likely occurs as Cl⁻ enters through the glycine-sensitive anion channel and Na⁺ enters through monovalent cation channels. The latter channels open earlier in hypoxia (19–21). Colloid osmotic forces drive this swelling, which continues until the plasma membrane bursts. After membrane rupture, cells become permeable to all solutes and further volume growth ceases. Since permeabilization of both mitochondria and lysosomes presage onset of the metastable state (13), a hydrolytic enzyme, such as a protease, or other factor activated by these organelles may be important for opening the glycine gated anion channel.

ADENOSINE TRIPHOSPHATE DEPLETION AND HYPOXIC HEPATOCELLULAR NECROSIS

Failure of aerobic ATP formation by oxidative phosphorylation is the fundamental stress of anoxic and ischemic injury. The importance of ATP depletion in the events leading to necrotic cell death is demonstrated by the ability of glycolytic substrates to rescue hepatocytes and sinusoidal

endothelial cells from lethal cell injury (15,22,23). Glycolytic metabolism partially replaces ATP lost after inhibition of mitochondrial oxidative phosphorylation, and ATP at only 15% to 20% of normal levels is sufficient to prevent onset of necrotic cell death. Glucose, the major glycolytic substrate for most cell types, prevents hypoxic killing of sinusoidal endothelial cells, but glucose does not protect hepatocytes against anoxic injury. Glucose is ineffective in hepatocytes because hepatocytes lack hexokinase. Hexokinase catalyzes the first reaction of glycolysis in most cells and has a high maximum velocity (V_{max}) and a low Michaelis' constant (K_m) for glucose. Hepatocytes have instead glucokinase with a high K_m for glucose and relatively low V_{max}. Glucokinase is metabolically appropriate for hepatocytes, since the liver has the important function of maintaining blood glucose to a concentration of about 5 mM. Even under conditions of anoxia, hepatic consumption of glucose is very low, because rapid hepatic glucose utilization would otherwise lead to systemic hypoglycemia. Instead, fructose protects hepatocytes against hypoxic injury, because hepatocytes contain a highly active fructokinase that feeds fructose into the glycolytic pathway.

In hepatocytes, endogenous glycogen is also an excellent substrate for anaerobic glycolysis. For this reason, hepatocytes of glycogen-rich livers from fed rats are much more resistant to anoxic killing than hepatocytes of glycogen-depleted livers of fasted rats (24). Fructose acts as an alternate glycolytic substrate and prevents anoxic hepatocellular damage in glycogen-depleted livers. Fructose also prevents hepatocellular killing by several toxic chemicals, which implies that mitochondria are important targets of toxic cell killing (25,26). Consistent with these observations in experimental animals, glycogen depletion after fasting predisposes human subjects to acetaminophen-induced liver damage (27).

In aerobic livers, high fructose causes a decrease of ATP and inorganic phosphate (P_i) because of ATP consumed in the fructokinase reaction and the consequent accumulation of sugar phosphate metabolic intermediates. This decline of ATP is often assumed to represent fructose toxicity despite the fact that glucose causes a similar decline of ATP in hexokinase-containing cells. Actually, fructose-treated livers maintain their ATP/adenosine diphosphate (ADP)•P_i ratios, because fructose-induced decreases of ATP are offset by decreases of P_i. The ATP/ADP•P_i ratio is proportional to the free energy of hydrolysis of ATP or phosphorylation potential (ΔG_p). ΔG_p rather than ATP concentration, ATP/ADP ratio, or energy charge is the relevant thermodynamic variable reflecting the energy available from ATP. Furthermore, during anoxia when ATP falls to virtually immeasurable levels, fructose metabolism actually increases ATP substantially. During anoxic and toxic stress, this ATP generation prevents hepatocellular killing (28). Thus, fructose-induced changes of ATP reflect the normal hepatic metabolism of fructose rather than fructose toxicity.

In anoxia, mitochondrial respiration and hence oxidative phosphorylation become fully inhibited. Respiratory inhibitors, such as cyanide and antimycin A, mimic many of the features of hypoxic injury in an experimental model sometimes called "chemical hypoxia" (11). A more severe form of mitochondrial metabolic disruption is uncoupling, which occurs when the mitochondrial inner membrane becomes permeable to hydrogen ions. Uncoupling activates the mitochondrial F_1F_0 adenosine triphosphatase (ATPase). This mitochondrial ATPase normally acts in the reverse direction as the ATP synthase of oxidative phosphorylation. Activation of mitochondrial ATPase by uncoupling causes futile hydrolysis of ATP. As a consequence, glycolytic ATP generation can no longer protect against cell killing. Inhibition of the mitochondrial ATPase with oligomycin prevents mitochondrial hydrolysis of glycolytic ATP after uncoupling and restores the cytoprotection of glycolysis. In the absence of glycolytic substrate, oligomycin actually induces cell killing because it inhibits ATP formation by oxidative phosphorylation. However, in the presence of a glycolytic substrate such as fructose, oligomycin prevents cell killing induced by mitochondrial uncoupling (25,28).

These experimental findings illustrate that mitochondria undergo a progression of injurious changes in response to external stresses (Fig. 18.3). Simple inhibition of mitochondrial respiration with agents such as anoxia or cyanide blocks oxidative phosphorylation. In the absence of glycolysis, respiratory inhibition leads to cellular ATP depletion

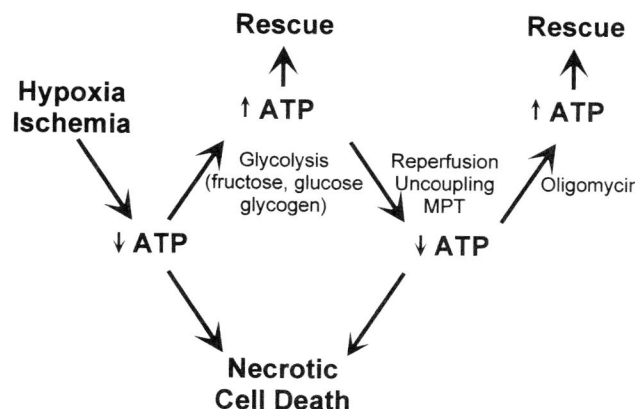

FIGURE 18.3. Progression of mitochondrial injury during hypoxia/ischemia and reperfusion. Oxygen deprivation during ischemia inhibits mitochondrial oxidative phosphorylation, which leads to adenosine triphosphate (*ATP*) depletion and necrotic cell death. Glycolysis restores ATP and prevents anoxic cell killing. Reperfusion induces onset of the mitochondrial permeability transition (*MPT*) and mitochondrial uncoupling, which activates the mitochondrial F_1F_0 adenosine triphosphatase (*ATPase*). This ATPase futilely hydrolyzes ATP made available by glycolysis to overcome the protective effect of glycolytic substrates such as fructose, glucose, and glycogen. Oligomycin inhibits the mitochondrial ATPase, restores glycolytic ATP levels and rescues cells from necrotic cell death. (Adapted from Nieminen AL, Saylor AK, Herman B, et al. ATP depletion rather than mitochondrial depolarization mediates hepatocyte killing after metabolic inhibition. *Am J Physiol* 1994;267:C67–C74.)

and ultimately necrotic cell death. Glycolytic substrates such as fructose in hepatocytes and glucose in sinusoidal endothelial cells partially restore ATP levels and rescue the cells from necrotic killing. However, when mitochondria become uncoupled, then the mitochondrial synthase works in reverse to hydrolyze ATP made available by glycolysis. As a consequence, ATP levels fall profoundly even in the presence of glycolytic substrates, and lethal cell injury ensues. Under these conditions, oligomycin prevents cell killing due to mitochondrial uncoupling by blocking futile uncoupler-induced hydrolysis of glycolytic ATP.

Several toxicants produce cytotoxicity by mitochondrial uncoupling, as shown by cytoprotection with fructose plus oligomycin. These toxicants include the calcium ionophore Br-A23187, often used as a model of Ca^{2+}-dependent cytotoxicity, the monovalent cation ionophore gramicidin D, and the oxidant chemical, *tert*-butylhydroperoxide (25,29). In anoxia/ischemia, free fatty acids accumulate due to activation of phospholipases and inhibition of fatty acid acylation. Free fatty acids are weak mitochondrial uncouplers and may contribute to anoxic and ischemic injury.

PROTECTION BY ACIDOTIC PH AGAINST HYPOXIC KILLING OF LIVER CELLS

Anoxia and *hypoxia* are terms indicating oxygen deprivation that are often used somewhat interchangeably. Anoxia refers to an absolute absence of oxygen, whereas hypoxia refers to relative but not necessarily absolute oxygen deprivation. Ischemia means the loss of blood supply, which can also be relative or absolute. Tissue injury and stress in ischemia begin to occur as tissue oxygen levels approach very low levels. Ischemia produces other tissue changes, particularly a rapid decrease of pH, which can fall by a unit or more (30). This naturally occurring acidosis greatly delays onset of necrotic cell death in hepatocytes and many other cells despite exhaustion of cellular ATP supplies (31–33). Intracellular acidification mediates the protection of acidotic pH. Although anaerobic metabolism contributes to the decline of pH in ischemia, hydrogen ion generation from hydrolysis of high-energy phosphates such as ATP and the release of hydrogen ions from acidic organelles also contribute to cytosolic acidification (32,34). Intracellular acidosis may suppress one or more intracellular enzymes activated by hypoxic stress, such as phospholipase A. ATP depletion activates phospholipase A, phospholipase inhibitors delay hypoxic cell killing, and acidic pH inhibits phospholipase A activity stimulated by hypoxic stress. Phospholipases may in turn activate proteases that further promote cell injury (35).

THE PH PARADOX IN EARLY ISCHEMIA/REPERFUSION INJURY

Although the naturally occurring acidosis of ischemia prevents onset of anoxic cell death, reperfusion after ischemia can paradoxically worsen cell injury and precipitate tissue necrosis within minutes. In experimental models, anoxia at acidotic pH followed by reoxygenation at pH 7.4 simulates oxygen deprivation and acidosis during ischemia and recovery of oxygen and pH after reperfusion. Reperfusion under these conditions leads to loss of cell viability and release of intracellular enzymes such as lactate dehydrogenase (31, 36–40). Restoration of normal pH after reperfusion rather than reoxygenation causes this injury, since reoxygenation at low pH prevents cell killing virtually entirely, whereas return to normal pH without reoxygenation produces the same cell killing as return to normal pH with reoxygenation. This paradoxical injury after recovery of normal pH is called the pH paradox.

Intracellular pH mediates cell injury in the pH paradox. If recovery of intracellular pH is accelerated during reperfusion with an ionophore such as monensin, cell killing occurs more quickly. Conversely, inhibition of the rise of intracellular pH after reperfusion by Na^+/H^+ exchange blockade with dimethylamiloride (in cardiac myocytes) or Na^+-free medium (in hepatocytes) prevents reperfusion-induced necrotic cell killing almost completely. pH-dependent cell killing is independent of extracellular and cytosolic Ca^{2+} and Na^+ and is not linked to pH-dependent secondary changes of cytosolic Na^+ and Ca^{2+} (32,37–39, 41,42).

THE MITOCHONDRIAL PERMEABILITY TRANSITION IN REPERFUSION INJURY

Recent studies in a variety of tissues implicate onset of a phenomenon called the mitochondrial permeability transition in lethal cell injury associated with anoxia, reperfusion, and oxidative stress (reviewed in ref. 43). In the mitochondrial permeability transition, mitochondria become freely permeable to solutes of molecular weight less than about 1500 d (Fig. 18.4) (44). Ca^{2+}, P_i, reactive oxygen species, and numerous oxidant chemicals induce the mitochondrial permeability transition, whereas Mg^{2+}, low pH, and the immunosuppressant drug cyclosporin A block the mitochondrial permeability transition. However, inhibition of the mitochondrial permeability transition by cyclosporin A is unrelated to its immunosuppressive action. At onset of the mitochondrial permeability transition, mitochondria depolarize and undergo large-amplitude swelling. As a consequence, oxidative phosphorylation becomes uncoupled. Patch clamping identifies a highly conductive permeability transition (PT) pore in the mitochondrial inner membrane whose opening causes the mitochondrial permeability transition (45).

The PT pore is likely composed, at least in part, of the adenine nucleotide translocator (ANT) protein in the mitochondrial inner membrane together with cyclophilin D (a cyclosporin A–binding protein) in the mitochondrial matrix, and porin in the outer membrane (Fig. 18.4) (46,47). Translocation of the proapoptotic protein Bax to

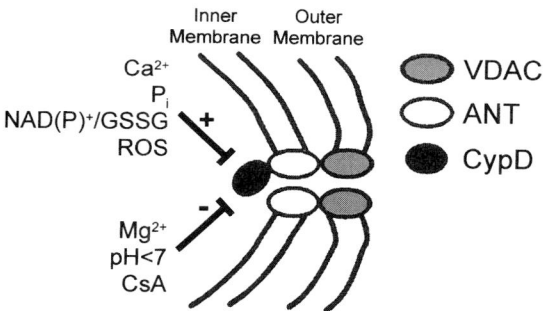

Mitochondrial Permeability Transition

- From opening of a high conductance permeability transition pore conducting solutes up to 1,500 Da.
- Pore formed by adenine nucleotide translocator (ANT), cyclophilin D (CypD) and the voltage dependent anion channel (VDAC).
- Causes mitochondrial depolarization, uncoupling and swelling.
- Promoted by Ca^{2+}, inorganic phosphate (Pi), NAD(P)H/GSH oxidation and reactive oxygen species (ROS).
- Inhibited by Mg^{2+}, low pH, and cyclosporin A (CsA).

FIGURE 18.4. Properties and postulated molecular composition of the permeability transition pore.

the mitochondrial surface also promotes opening of the PT pore (48). This combination of proteins implies that the PT pore spans the inner and outer membrane, presumably at contact sites between the mitochondrial inner and outer membranes. However, our understanding of the exact molecular structure of the PT pore remains incomplete.

pH below 7.0 inhibits the PT pore, and involvement of the mitochondrial permeability transition in pH-dependent reperfusion injury is supported by the observation that cyclosporin A prevents pH-dependent killing of cultured rat hepatocytes after simulated ischemia/reperfusion, even when added only during the reperfusion phase (41). Cyclosporin A also protects heart and brain against anoxia/reoxygenation injury (49,50). Laser scanning confocal microscopy confirms directly a role of the mitochondrial permeability transition in pH-dependent reperfusion injury. When hepatocytes subjected to simulated ischemia are reoxygenated and returned from acidotic pH to normal pH, mitochondria initially begin to repolarize (Fig. 18.5). However, after several minutes the nonspecific permeability of the mitochondrial inner membrane abruptly increases as intracellular pH rises to about 7.0. This is shown by the movement of a normally impermeant fluorophore, calcein, from the cytosol into the mitochondria. Simultaneously, the mitochondria depolarize. Loss of cell viability then occurs after several more minutes (Fig. 18.5). If hepatocytes are reoxygenated at acidic pH or at normal pH in the presence of cyclosporin A, then mitochondrial permeabilization does not occur, and recovery of mitochondrial membrane potential is sustained. Moreover, cell death does not occur. Instead, surface blebs disappear and cellular swelling reverses, indicating restoration of ATP-dependent cellular processes. These findings support the conclusion that the mitochondrial permeability transition is a major causative mechanism in the pathogenesis of reperfusion injury to hepatocytes (41). The mitochondrial permeability transition also plays a causative role in hepatocellular injury due to oxidative stress, various toxicants including Reye's syndrome-related drugs, and cellular calcium overload (43).

pH-dependent reperfusion injury is linked directly to the recovery of intracellular pH from the intracellular acidosis of ischemia. Monensin, a Na^+,H^+-exchanging ionophore that accelerates the recovery of intracellular pH after reperfusion, also accelerates pH-dependent reperfusion injury. Conversely, blockade of plasma membrane Na^+/H^+ exchange by dimethylamiloride (in cardiac myocytes) or a Na^+-free medium (in hepatocytes) delays recovery of intracellular pH after reperfusion and prevents reperfusion-induced loss of cell viability almost completely (38,39,41,42). pH-dependent cell killing occurs independently of levels of cytosolic and extracellular free Ca^{2+}, although a specific increase of mitochondrial free Ca^{2+} precedes onset of mitochondrial permeabilization in both oxidative stress and pH-dependent reperfusion injury (51,52). Intracellular Na^+ increases relatively early during ATP depletion (53). The plasma mem-

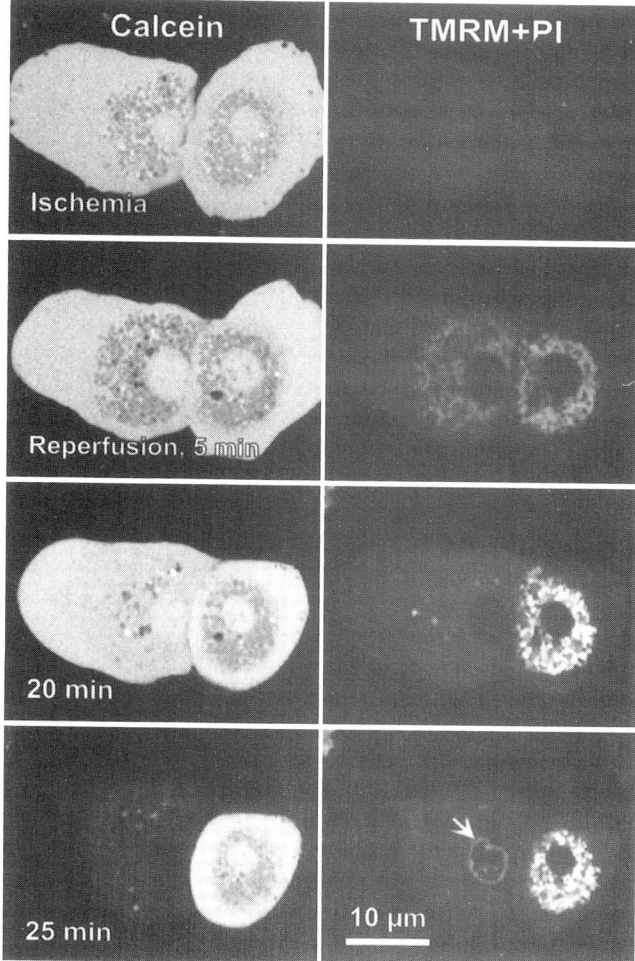

FIGURE 18.5. Induction of the mitochondrial permeability transition by ischemia and reperfusion. Cultured rat hepatocytes were co-loaded with green-fluorescing calcein (**left panels**) and red-fluorescing tetramethylrhodamine methylester (*TMRM*, **right panels**) and subjected to anoxia at pH 6.2, conditions that simulate ischemia. At the end of 4 hours of anoxia, mitochondria were small dark round voids in confocal images of calcein fluorescence, which indicated that the mitochondrial inner membrane remained impermeable to this 623-Da polyanionic fluorophore in the cytosol. At this time, mitochondria were depolarized and did not accumulate TMRM, a membrane potential indicating cationic fluorophore. After rexoxygenation at pH 7.4 to simulate reperfusion, TMRM began to enter the mitochondria of both hepatocytes in the field within 5 minutes. After 20 minutes, one of the hepatocytes then lost TMRM labeling, which indicated mitochondrial depolarization, and its mitochondria filled with calcein, which indicated onset of the mitochondrial permeability transition. The hepatocyte then lost viability after 25 minutes, as indicated by release of cytosolic calcein and nuclear uptake of propidium iodide (PI, *arrow*) included in the incubation medium. The other hepatocyte in the field did not lose viability, and its mitochondria continued to accumulate TMRM and exclude calcein. (Adapted from Qian T, Nieminen AL, Herman B, et al. Mitochondrial permeability transition in pH-dependent reperfusion injury to rat hepatocytes. *Am J Physiol* 1997;273:C1783–C1792.)

brane Na⁺/H⁺ exchanger mediates, in part, this increase. However, prevention of intracellular Na⁺ loading by acidotic pH does not account for cytoprotection by acidotic pH, because acidotic pH protects against cell killing even when intracellular Na⁺ and extracellular Na⁺ are equilibrated with monensin (32).

REACTIVE OXYGEN SPECIES AND REPERFUSION INJURY

Reoxygenation of hypoxic liver also promotes the formation of reactive oxygen species, including hydrogen peroxide (H_2O_2) and superoxide ($O_2^{\bullet-}$). Sources of reactive oxygen species include xanthine oxidase utilizing xanthine and hypoxanthine generated after ATP degradation, reduced nicotinamide adenine dinucleotide phosphate (NADPH) oxidase in Kupffer cells activated by ischemic stress, and the respiratory chain of mitochondria. In the presence of transition metal ions, such as free iron and copper, H_2O_2 and $O_2^{\bullet-}$ react to form the highly reactive and toxic hydroxyl radical (OH•) by the Fenton reaction (Fig. 18.6). In addition, iron catalyzes a lipid peroxidation chain reaction sustained by lipid alkyl and peroxyl radicals. The iron chelator desferal blocks these iron-catalyzed reactions. Superoxide

also reacts nonenzymatically with nitric oxide (NO·) to form peroxynitrite (OONO⁻). Peroxynitrite causes nitrosylation of tyrosyl residues in proteins and also decomposes to a hydroxyl radical-like species. Increasingly, peroxynitrite is recognized as an important toxic intermediate in oxidative tissue injury (54).

Although pH-dependent reperfusion injury occurs in the absence of oxygen and therefore of reactive oxygen species formation, oxidative stress nonetheless also promotes onset of the mitochondrial permeability transition, as shown in hepatocytes treated with *tert*-butylhydroperoxide, a short-chain analogue of the lipid hydroperoxides formed during oxidative stress and ischemia/reperfusion (55). This oxidant chemical initiates a chain of events that culminates in the mitochondrial permeability transition and necrotic cell death. The earliest effect of *tert*-butylhydroperoxide is oxidation of mitochondrial pyridine nucleotides [reduced nicotinamide adenine dinucleotide (NADH) and NADPH] and glutathione, which is followed by an increase of intramitochondrial free Ca^{2+}. Increased mitochondrial Ca^{2+} then stimulates mitochondrial reactive oxygen species formation, which leads to PT pore opening, mitochondrial depolarization, ATP depletion, and cell death (51,56).

In low-flow states, pericentral regions of the liver lobule become anoxic, whereas periportal areas remain normoxic.

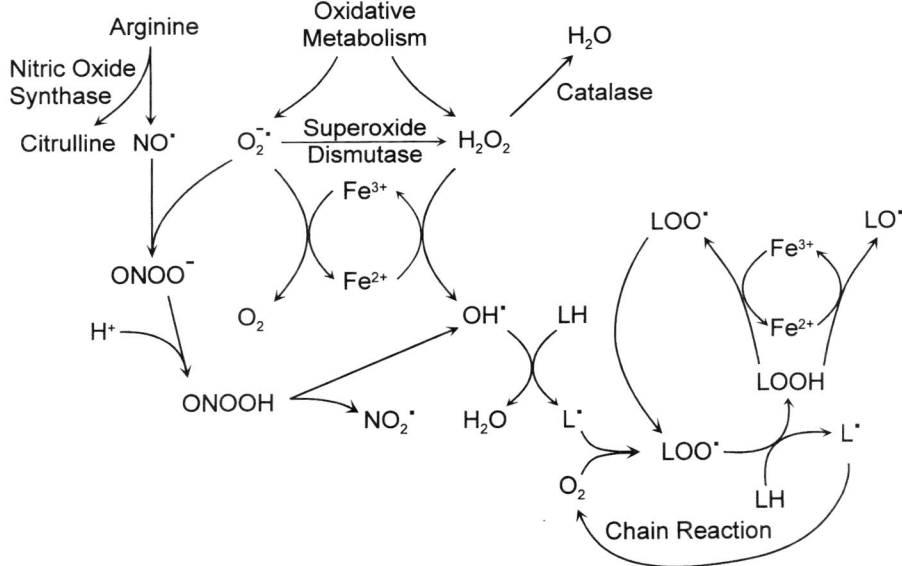

FIGURE 18.6. Iron-catalyzed free radical generation. Oxidative metabolism after reperfusion leads to formation of superoxide ($O_2^{\bullet-}$) and hydrogen peroxide (H_2O_2). Superoxide is detoxified to hydrogen peroxide by superoxide dismutase, and hydrogen peroxide is converted to water by catalase. Iron and other transition metals, including copper, catalyze hydroxyl radical (OH•) formation by the Haber Weiss reaction. Superoxide reduces ferric iron (Fe^{3+}) to ferrous iron (Fe^{2+}), which reacts with hydrogen peroxide to form the highly reactive hydroxyl radical. Hydroxyl radicals react with lipids to form alkyl radicals (L•) that initiate an oxygen-dependent chain reaction generating peroxyl radicals (LOO•) and lipid peroxides (LOOH). Lipid peroxides react with free iron to generate alkoxyl radicals (LO•) and more peroxyl radicals. Nitric oxide synthase catalyzes nitric oxide (NO•) formation from arginine. Nitric oxide reacts nonenzymatically with superoxide to form the unstable peroxynitrite anion (ONOO⁻), which protonates and decomposes to nitrogen dioxide and hydroxyl radical. These toxic radicals also attack proteins and nucleic acids.

The border between normoxic and anoxic tissue is sharp, as reflected by an increase of reduced pyridine nucleotides [nicotinamide adenine dinucleotide (NAD) plus nicotinamide adenine dinucleotide phosphate (NADP)] whose reoxidation is prevented by anoxia (3). Such midzonal border regions are the sites of formation of toxic reactive oxygen species (57). At this border region, the coexistence of hypoxic stress and small amounts of oxygen promotes an accelerated midzonal injury that is blocked by antioxidants. A midzonal pattern of hepatic necrosis is also frequently observed at autopsy after liver hypoperfusion (58).

APOPTOSiS

Apoptosis is another mode of cell death that leads to cell deletion without the inflammation, scarring, and release of cellular contents that characterize necrotic cell death (Table 18.1) (see Chapter 19 and website chapter 💻 W-13). In apoptosis, individual cells shrink and separate from their neighbors. Other characteristic changes of apoptosis include alterations of plasma membrane lipids, condensation of chromatin, internucleosomal DNA degradation, and shedding of membrane-bound cytoplasmic fragments containing ultrastructurally intact organelles and chromatin. Adjacent cells and macrophages take up these apoptotic bodies. In liver pathology, they are Councilman bodies, a characteristic feature of hepatocellular apoptotic cell death (59). Specific physiologic death signals, such as tumor necrosis factor-α (TNF-α) and Fas ligand, trigger apoptosis through a cascade of cysteine-aspartate proteases called caspases.

Apoptosis is also a late sequela of ischemia/reperfusion injury in liver and other tissues and occurs in cells that survive acute onset of necrotic cell death (60,61). Mitochondrial changes, specifically the mitochondrial permeability transition, induced by ischemia reperfusion may play a role in this apoptosis. When purified nuclei and isolated mitochondria are combined in a cell-free system, onset of the mitochondrial permeability transition induces the release of

soluble factors from mitochondria that activate caspases and initiate apoptotic nuclear changes (62). These factors include the loosely bound respiratory protein, cytochrome c, and apoptosis-inducing factor (AIF), which reside in the space between the mitochondrial inner and outer membranes (63,64). Release of cytochrome c occurs when large-amplitude mitochondrial swelling following the mitochondrial permeability transition causes rupture of the outer membrane. Other mechanisms, including the formation of specific cytochrome c release channels in the outer membrane by proapoptotic Bcl2 family members such as Bax, are also proposed to explain the release of cytochrome c and other proapoptotic mitochondrial factors during apoptosis (65,66).

After release from mitochondria, cytochrome c binds to apoptosis-inducing factor-1 (APAF-1) (67). APAF-1 also binds deoxyATP (or dATP) and pro-caspase 9 to form a complex that yields a proteolytically activated caspase 9. Caspase 9, in turn, proteolytically activates pro-caspase 3 to caspase 3, which then initiates the final execution stages of apoptosis, including cell shrinkage, surface blebbing, internucleosomal DNA hydrolysis, chromatin margination, and nuclear lobulation. Other caspases, such as caspase 8, act upstream of mitochondria. For example, binding of TNF-α and Fas ligand to their receptors leads to pro-caspase 8 activation (Fig. 18.7). Caspase 8 then cleaves Bid, another member of the proto-oncogene Bcl2 family of proteins (68), to a truncated form that translocates to mitochondria and induces cytochrome c release. Other pro- and anti-apoptotic members of the Bcl2 family also bind to mitochondria to promote or block, respectively, mitochondrial permeabilization and cytochrome c release. In particular, the protein Bcl2 blocks cytochrome c release and prevents apoptotic signaling through mitochondria (69).

The specific role of the mitochondrial permeability transition in apoptosis is the subject of ongoing controversy. Some studies conclude that release of cytochrome c during apoptosis occurs without mitochondrial depolarization or onset of the mitochondrial permeability transition. In hepa-

TABLE 18.1. FEATURES OF NECROTIC AND APOPTOTIC CELL DEATH

Necrosis	Apoptosis
Accidental cell death	Controlled cell deletion
Contiguous regions of cells	Individual cells separating from their neighbors
Cell swelling	Cell shrinkage
Large plasma membrane blebs without organelles	Zeiotic blebs containing large organelles
Small chromatin aggregates	Condensation of chromatin and nuclear lobulation
Random DNA degradation (smear on gel)	Internucleosomal DNA degradation (ladder on gel)
Cell lysis and release of intracellular contents	Fragmentation into apoptotic bodies
Marked inflammation and scarring	Absence of inflammation and scarring
Mitochondrial swelling and dysfunction	Mitochondrial permeabilization
Phospholipase and protease activation	Caspase activation
ATP depletion and metabolic disruption	ATP and protein synthesis sustained
Cell death precipitated by plasma membrane rupture	Intact plasma membrane

ATP, adenosine triphosphate.

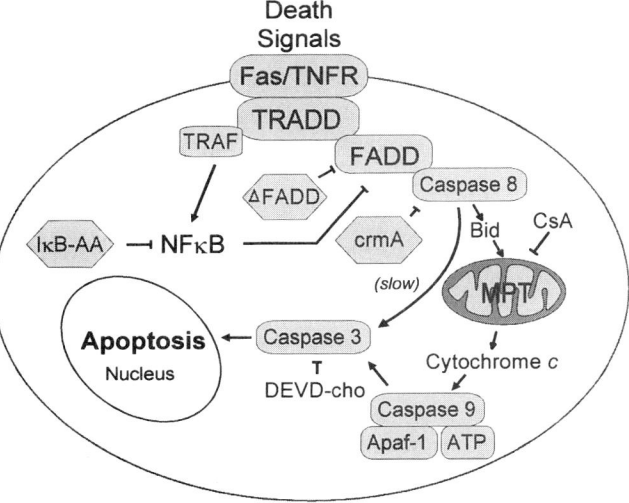

FIGURE 18.7. Scheme of molecular events in death receptor-induced apoptosis. Binding of death signals, such as Fas ligand and tumor necrosis factor-α (TNF-α), to their receptors, Fas or a TNR-α receptor (*TNFR*), activates caspase 8 via the adapter proteins, TNFR-associated death domain (*TRADD*), and Fas-associated death domain (*FADD*). Caspase 8 cleaves the proapoptotic Bcl2 family member, Bid, which then translocates to mitochondria. Subsequently, the mitochondrial permeability transition (*MPT*) occurs, leading to release of cytochrome c. Cyclosporin A (CsA) blocks mitochondrial permeabilization. Cytochrome c binds to apoptosis-inducing factor-1 (Apaf-1) and ATP. This complex activates caspase 9, which in turn proteolytically activates caspase 3. Caspase 3 then initiates the major biochemical and morphologic manifestation of apoptosis. Signaling through another adapter protein, TNF receptor-associated factor (*TRAF*), activates the nuclear transcription factor NFκB. NFκB induces antiapoptotic gene expression acting upstream of mitochondria. Adenoviral expression of an IκB superrepressor, IκB-AA, inhibits the activation of NFκB and is permissive for TNF-α–induced apoptosis to hepatocytes. Adenoviral expression of CrmA, a serpin family protease inhibitor from cowpox virus, inhibits caspase 8 and blocks the mitochondrial permeability transition after TNF-α. Expression of ΔFADD, a truncated dominant-negative FADD, also blocks upstream signaling. Inhibition of downstream caspase 3 with DEVD-cho prevents apoptosis but not mitochondrial permeabilization. Caspase 8 can also activate caspase 3 directly bypassing mitochondria, but this reaction is slow in hepatocytes.

tocytes, however, onset of the mitochondrial permeability transition can be directly visualized after TNF-α treatment and Fas ligation from movement of the normally impermeant green fluorophore calcein into mitochondria from the cytosol (70,71). This mitochondrial permeability transition precedes cytochrome c release, caspase 3 activation, and apoptotic cell death. Cyclosporin A blocks mitochondrial permeabilization induced by TNF-α and Fas ligation in hepatocytes and inhibits cytochrome c release, caspase 3 activation, and apoptosis. Another slower proapoptotic signaling pathway coexists with the mitochondrial pathway. Thus, in the presence of cyclosporin A, apoptosis in hepatocytes may be delayed rather than prevented, in which case apoptosis occurs without mitochondrial permeabilization, depolarization and cytochrome c release (Fig. 18.7). Apoptotic signaling that bypasses mitochondria is the so-called

type 1 pathway and may involve exaggerated activation of caspase 8, whereas apoptotic signaling requiring mitochondrial changes is the type 2 pathway (72).

ADENOSINE TRIPHOSPHATE SWITCH BETWEEN NECROTIC AND APOPTOTIC CELL DEATH

The effect of the mitochondrial permeability transition on ATP is an important factor determining whether apoptosis or necrosis follows onset of the mitochondrial permeability transition. Apoptosis is an ATP-requiring process (73,74), and caspase 9 activation by the cytochrome c/APAF-1 complex requires ATP or dATP (63,67). Necrotic cell death, by contrast, is the consequence of ATP depletion (28). Thus, when the mitochondrial permeability transition develops slowly and heterogeneously within a hepatocyte without fully depleting ATP levels, apoptosis can develop, but when the mitochondrial permeability transition is so rapid and extensive that cellular ATP virtually disappears, then necrotic cell death occurs (Fig. 18.8). A not infrequent event in cells undergoing apoptosis is so-called secondary necrosis, in which necrotic cell killing with breakdown of

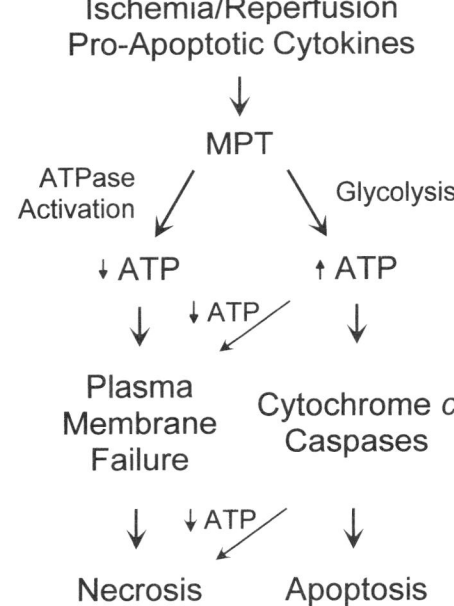

FIGURE 18.8. Role of adenosine triphosphate (*ATP*) in initiating necrosis or apoptosis after the mitochondrial permeability transition. Ischemia/reperfusion and cytokine death signals promote onset of the mitochondrial permeability transition (*MPT*). When mitochondrial permeabilization occurs abruptly, activation of mitochondrial ATPases causes ATP depletion, which leads to plasma membrane failure and necrotic cell death. If mitochondrial permeabilization progresses slowly, glycolysis can maintain ATP levels. In the presence of ATP, cytochrome c release from mitochondria activates cytosolic caspases, causing apoptotic rather than necrotic cell death. At any time, ATP depletion may supervene to induce secondary necrosis.

the plasma membrane permeability barrier occurs as apoptosis is progressing. Secondary necrosis may develop from ATP depletion due to mitochondrial failure (Fig. 18.8).

After ischemia/reperfusion, viral infection, and exposure to toxic chemicals, apoptotic and necrotic features often coexist. For example, massive apoptosis in mouse livers after injection of anti-Fas antibody leads to fulminant hepatic failure, disruption of liver architecture, enzyme release, and liver inflammation, features usually associated with necrosis (75). Moreover, pharmacologic inhibition of apoptosis prevents this liver inflammation (59). Not surprisingly, controversies have developed as to whether cell killing in a particular setting is apoptosis or necrosis (76,77), because conventional distinctions between apoptotic and necrotic cell death often do not hold in pathologic situations. Recently, the term *necrapoptosis* was introduced to emphasize death processes that begin with common signals and stresses, progress through shared pathways, such as mitochondrial permeabilization, and culminate in either cell lysis (necrotic cell death) or programmed cellular resorption (apoptosis) depending on other modifying factors (78). In necrapoptosis, pure apoptosis and pure necrosis are extremes in a continuous spectrum, and the more typical pathophysiologic response is a mixture of features associated with apoptotic and necrotic cell death.

ROLE OF KUPFFER CELLS IN ISCHEMIA/REPERFUSION INJURY

Kupffer cells are the resident macrophages of the liver, which reside in the lining of the hepatic sinusoids directly facing the blood. Ischemia/reperfusion activates Kupffer cells, and this activation also contributes to anoxic, ischemic, and reperfusion injury to liver (see Chapters 19, 30, and 31 and website chapters 🖥 W-13 and W-26). Activated Kupffer cells release cytokines, reactive oxygen species, and other factors that aggravate ischemia/reperfusion injury and promote postischemic neutrophil infiltration and oxidative stress (reviewed in ref. 79). Even prior to reoxygenation, Kupffer cells enhance anoxic killing of hepatocytes in perfused rat livers (80). Kupffer cells also mediate delayed responses occurring up to 24 hours after reperfusion. An intermediate response occurs up to 6 hours after reperfusion and involves release of cytokines, chemokines, reactive oxygen species, and other mediators by Kupffer cells that act to expand the reperfusion injury. A later injury up to 24 hours following reperfusion results from the hepatic infiltration and activation of neutrophils in response to chemoattractants produced by Kupffer cells.

The cytokines produced by activated Kupffer cells include TNF-α and interleukin-1 and -6 (IL-1 and IL-6) (81) (Chapter 40). TNF-α enhances oxidative stress-induced injury and induces apoptosis in hepatocytes, provided that protein synthesis or NFκB-mediated gene expression is sup-

pressed (70,82). Liver-derived TNF-α also induces release of chemokines from the liver, including epithelial neutrophil activating protein (ENA-78), cytokine-induced neutrophil chemoattractant (CINC), macrophage inflammatory protein (MIP-2), monocyte chemoattractant (MCP-1), and others (83–85). These chemokines are strong chemotactic agents for neutrophils. MIP-2 and CINC also increase integrin expression on neutrophils, which further promotes neutrophil margination into the hepatic microvasculature (86).

Like TNF-α, IL-1 increases within minutes of ischemia/reperfusion injury *in vivo* and promotes reactive oxygen species formation (81,87). By contrast, IL-6 release is delayed, and IL-6 treatment protects against warm ischemia/reperfusion injury in rats (88). Kupffer cells are a major source of reactive oxygen species during the intermediate phase of ischemia/reperfusion injury, whereas neutrophils are the major reactive oxygen species source during the late phase of injury (89–92). Oxidative stress is demonstrated by decreased glutathione levels and elevated oxidized glutathione (GSSG) levels (93). Furthermore, treatment with antioxidants, such as superoxide dismutase, *N*-acetylcysteine, desferal, and allopurinol can decrease hepatic ischemia/reperfusion injury and improve survival (57, 94–98). Lipid peroxidation is modest after hepatic ischemia/reperfusion compared to that induced by strong oxidant chemicals. This suggests that reactive oxygen species do not cause cytotoxicity directly, but act as signaling molecules to upregulate nuclear transcription factors like NFκB and subsequent release of TNF-α and IL-1 (99).

Complement (C3a and C5a) generation occurs after ischemia/reperfusion and promotes Kupffer cell oxidant stress (100,101). Platelet activating factor (PAF) also promotes warm reperfusion injury since PAF receptor blockade decreases hepatic damage and improves survival after liver ischemia/reperfusion (102,103). The source of PAF is undefined, but platelets, Kupffer cells, endothelial cells, and neutrophils all can release PAF. PAF increases vascular permeability, and stimulates neutrophils, macrophages, and monocytes to release superoxide, IL-6, IL-8, and TNF-α (102).

MICROCIRCULATORY CHANGES AND THE PROTECTIVE ACTION OF NITRIC OXIDE

Ischemia/reperfusion disturbs the hepatic microcirculation and causes focal narrowing of the sinusoids produced, in part, by obstruction of flow by swollen Kupffer cells (104,105). Endothelin-1 (ET-1), a potent vasoconstrictor released by endothelial cells and stellate cells, also contributes to microcirculatory disturbances (106,107). In addition, neutrophil promote ET-1 formation by releasing proteases that cleave inactive "big ET" to its active form (107,108).

Nitric oxide (NO) generation appears to be a protective response of liver tissue to ischemia/reperfusion. Nitric oxide is a vasodilator that improves hepatic oxygenation and sinusoidal microcirculation. Nitric oxide can be rapidly formed by endothelial cells following shear stress and during hepatic hypoperfusion (109). Inhibition of NO synthase decreases hepatic oxygenation and sinusoidal blood flow, increases adhesion molecule expression, and increases hepatocellular damage after ischemia/reperfusion, whereas L-arginine, an NO precursor, improves blood flow and protects against ischemia/reperfusion injury (107,110–114). NO also scavenges superoxide to form peroxynitrite (112). The resulting decrease of superoxide may be a beneficial effect; however, peroxynitrite is itself a toxic radical. In general, NO production protects against ischemia/reperfusion injury.

HEPATIC NEUTROPHIL INFILTRATION AFTER ISCHEMIC/REPERFUSION INJURY

Chemoattractant molecules produced in large part by Kupffer cells cause hepatic neutrophil infiltration, which mediates the late phase of hepatic ischemia/reperfusion injury. Infiltrating neutrophils perpetuate and amplify injury by releasing many of the same mediators (e.g., reactive oxygen species, cytokines) as Kupffer cells, but often in much larger quantities. Antineutrophil antibodies decrease hepatocellular necrosis 24 hours after hepatic ischemia/reperfusion from 80% to 28% (115).

Neutrophils marginate to the sinusoidal wall and then migrate across the endothelium into the space of Disse. Margination first involves binding of neutrophils to selectin molecules on sinusoidal endothelial cells (116). If endothelial cell damage is severe, transendothelial neutrophil migration occurs easily. Otherwise the interaction of intercellular adhesion molecules (ICAMs) such as ICAM-1 with integrins such as CD11b/CD18 (also called MAC-1) on neutrophils occurs to enhance both adherence and migration through the endothelial lining (see Chapters 32 and 33 and website chapters 🖳 W-27 and W-28). TNF-α, IL-1, and interferon-γ stimulate ICAM-1 expression on hepatocytes and endothelial cells, and anti–ICAM-1 antibodies decrease leukocyte adherence and diminish late hepatic ischemia/reperfusion injury even when added 8 hours after reperfusion (117,118). After warm ischemia/reperfusion, neutrophil CD11b/CD18 expression is upregulated, and antibodies against CD11b attenuate hepatic neutrophil infiltration, superoxide formation, and hepatocellular injury after ischemia/reperfusion (89,119). When neutrophils infiltrate the liver, they worsen hepatic hypoperfusion, exacerbate the effects of ET-1, and may release proteases (cathepsin G, granulocytes elastase) that are toxic to hepatocytes (120,121). Infiltrating neutrophils also produce toxic reactive oxygen species, including superoxide and hydroxyl radicals.

T lymphocytes also play a role in the late phase of hepatic ischemia/reperfusion injury. T-lymphocyte–deficient and CD4+-depleted mice but not CD8+-depleted mice have decreased neutrophil infiltration, liver enzyme release, and hepatocellular necrosis late after hepatic ischemia/reperfusion. CD4+ cells (T-helper cells) infiltrate the liver within an hour after reperfusion and likely provide another signal for neutrophil infiltration (122).

EARLY, INTERMEDIATE, AND LATE PHASES OF REPERFUSION INJURY

Different mechanisms mediate the early, intermediate, and late phases of hepatic ischemia reperfusion injury (Table 18.2). The early phase involves pH-dependent mitochondrial dysfunction and leads to hepatocellular necrosis within minutes of reperfusion and perhaps apoptosis after longer times. Kupffer cell production of free radicals, cytokines, and chemokines principally mediate the intermediate phases of reperfusion injury for up to 6 hours after restoration of blood flow. The late, neutrophil-mediated phase of hepatic ischemia/reperfusion injury involves margination and transendothelial migration of neutrophils in response to Kupffer cell–generated chemoattractants and release of toxic mediators, such as reactive oxygen species and proteases. These three phases of reperfusion injury take on differing importance depending on the length of

TABLE 18.2. PHASES OF HEPATIC ISCHEMIA/REPERFUSION INJURY

Ischemia/anoxia
  Necrotic cell death beginning after 30 min anoxia/ischemia at pH 7.4
  ATP depletion–dependent
  Protection by glycolysis, glycine, and pH <7
  ROS at anoxic/normoxic border
  Phospholipase and protease activation
Reperfusion injury
  Early phase
    Necrotic cell death within 1 h of reperfusion
    Large component of pH-dependent (pH >7), ROS-independent cell killing
    Mitochondrial permeability transition
    Kupffer cell activation and ROS formation
    Microcirculatory disturbances
  Intermediate phase
    Kupffer cell–mediated necrosis and apoptosis after 6 or more h
    Kupffer cell release of ROS, cytokines, and chemokines
    TNF-α–mediated lung injury
    Kupffer cell–initiated neutrophil margination
    T-helper cell infiltration
    Microcirculatory disturbances
  Late phase
    Neutrophil-mediated necrosis and apoptosis after up to 24 h
    Neutrophil transendothelial migration, activation, and release of ROS, cathepsin, and elastase
    Microcirculatory disturbances

ROS, reactive oxygen species; TNF, tumor necrosis factor.

ischemia. After prolonged severe ischemia, the immediate phase predominates. After less severe ischemia, the intermediate and late phases gain more relative importance.

Ischemia/reperfusion injury of the liver can lead to multisystem organ failure. Cytokines and chemokines released by activated Kupffer cells likely promote the pulmonary edema and interstitial infiltration of leukocytes observed after hepatic ischemia/reperfusion. Mononuclear cells in the marginal zones of the spleen also increase, and splenectomy before ischemia/reperfusion decreases neutrophil infiltration into the liver and hepatocellular injury (123). Thus, a systemic inflammatory response involving the spleen also appears to promote liver injury.

ISCHEMIC PRECONDITIONING

Brief periods of myocardial ischemia followed by reperfusion render both human and animal hearts resistant to subsequent prolonged ischemia (124). Such ischemic preconditioning decreases infarct size after subsequent long ischemia and reperfusion. Ischemic preconditioning also protects a variety of other organs, including the liver (125,126). Ischemic preconditioning of the liver decreases hepatocellular enzyme release and mortality after warm ischemia and reperfusion, an effect mediated in part by increased NO formation and heat shock protein synthesis (127,128).

During ischemia, ATP quickly degrades to adenosine. This release is another important mediator of ischemic preconditioning, and in the liver adenosine suppresses TNF-α release from Kupffer cells (129). Adenosine has three types of cellular receptors that differ in their biochemical and pharmacologic responses to adenosine agonists and antagonists (130). Activation of adenosine A_1 and A_3 receptors stimulates inhibitory G proteins that block adenylyl cyclase and decrease $3',5'$-cyclic adenosine monophosphate (cAMP). By contrast, adenosine A_2 receptor activation stimulates adenylyl cyclase and increases cAMP. In the heart, the adenosine A_1 receptor pathway mediates ischemic preconditioning of myocardium, whereas adenosine A_2 receptors mediate ischemic preconditioning of coronary endothelial cells (131,132). In the liver, adenosine A_2 receptors mediate ischemic preconditioning of hepatocytes against warm ischemia/reperfusion by stimulating NO synthesis (133). In the heart, a potential downstream target of adenosine receptor activation is the mitochondrial K_{ATP} channel, and K_{ATP} channel openers such as cromakalin confer protection against ischemic injury (134). The effect of K_{ATP} blockers and openers on hepatic ischemia/reperfusion injury has not yet been studied.

LIVER PRESERVATION FOR TRANSPLANTATION SURGERY

Liver transplantation is the only therapy for children and adults with end-stage liver disease that provides long-term

survival and resumption of a normal life style. Using University of Wisconsin (UW) cold storage solution (Table 18.3), donor livers from brain-dead heart-beating cadaver donors can be preserved successfully by simple cold ischemia for up to 24 hours (135,136). Longer preservation times are limited by a reperfusion injury that occurs predominantly to sinusoidal endothelial and Kupffer cells (Fig. 18.9). A consequence of inadequate preservation is primary graft nonfunction, which still occurs in 5% to 10% of patients (137,138). Metabolic failure of the newly implanted graft, rapidly rising serum transaminases, lack of bile formation, and severe coagulopathy characterize primary nonfunction. Primary nonfunction progresses quickly to hepatic encephalopathy, acute renal failure, disseminated intravascular coagulation, and death unless retransplantation is performed within 3 to 4 days. Since donor livers are in very short supply, every retransplantation due to primary graft nonfunction means another patient on the waiting list dies. For this reason, the continuing need exists to develop new approaches to prevent graft failure from preservation injury and to expand the donor pool to include marginal donor livers, such as fatty livers and livers from non–heart-beating cadavers, which are now considered too risky to use.

Hepatic injury also occurs to grafts that survive and eventually perform well. Serum transaminases typically rise sharply 1 to 3 days postoperatively, which is sometimes followed by a syndrome of primary graft dysfunction or initial poor function characterized by functional cholestasis with sustained high bilirubin, diminished bile flow, and centrilobular hepatocellular ballooning and feathery degeneration (139). Moderate to severe primary graft dysfunction occurs in up to 30% of liver transplant recipients and is associated with two- to fourfold greater overall graft loss, longer intensive care unit and hospital stays, and increased overall mortality (137–140). Nonanastomotic biliary strictures can also develop in transplant patients beginning after

TABLE 18.3. UNIVERSITY OF WISCONSIN (UW) COLD PRESERVATION SOLUTION

Ingredient	Concentration
K-lactobionate	100 mM
Na KH$_2$PO$_4$	25 mM
Adenosine	5 mM
MgSO$_4$	5 mM
Glutathione	3 mM
Raffinose	30 mM
Allopurinol	1 mM
Hydroxyethyl starch	50 g/L
Dexamethasone	8 mg/L
Insulin	100 U/L
Bactrim	0.5 ml/L
Total Na$^+$	30 mM
Total K$^+$	120 mM
pH	7.4
Osmolarity	310–330 mOsm

several weeks (141). The incidence of strictures rises with more prolonged storage times, suggesting a role of preservation injury in their etiology. The clinical incidence of primary graft nonfunction and dysfunction and of ischemic biliary strictures is dependent on time of storage. For example, primary nonfunction and early retransplantation occur nearly four times more often after 20 hours or more of storage than after less than 10 hours. Fatty livers from alcoholic and obese donors tend to do poorly after transplantation (142). In the absence of steatosis, however, metabolic tests and histology of biopsies taken just prior to reperfusion do not discriminate viable grafts from nonviable grafts. Such tests are unable to predict graft performance because the critical injury leading to liver graft failure is a reperfusion injury after storage (143).

ENDOTHELIAL CELL DAMAGE FROM STORAGE/REPERFUSION INJURY

Endothelial cells line the hepatic sinusoids to form a fenestrated sieve plate separating the vascular space from the subsinusoidal surface of the hepatocytes (see Chapters 30 and 31 and website chapters W-26 and W-32). During cold ischemic storage, endothelial cells round up and retract their extended sheet-like cytoplasm (144,145). After shorter periods of storage, these changes are reversible, and the rounded endothelial cells spread out after warm reperfusion. However, after times of cold storage that result in graft failure after transplantation, warm reperfusion leads to the destruction of the sinusoidal lining (Figs. 18.9 and 18.10) (reviewed in ref. 8). Reperfusion initiates a sequence of nuclear membrane vacuolization, mitochondrial swelling

and lysis, ball-like rounding, plasma membrane breaks, cytoplasmic rarefaction, and nuclear condensation. Shredded fragments are all that remain of the sieve plates, and virtually all endothelial cell nuclei label with trypan blue, an indicator of loss of cell viability (Fig. 18.10). Release of the BB isozyme of creatine kinase, an enzyme localized to hepatic nonparenchymal cells, also indicates loss of endothelial cell viability. Similar changes to endothelial cells occur in human livers after storage and reperfusion. Kupffer, stellate (fat-storing or Ito), and bile duct epithelial cells, however, retain viability after cold storage and reperfusion.

Because hepatic sinusoidal endothelial cells are responsible for the clearance of hyaluronic acid from the plasma, levels of serum hyaluronic acid and hepatic clearance of hyaluronic acid provide useful indices of sinusoidal endothelial cell function and viability *in vivo* (146). After cold storage and transplantation of rat livers, decreases of hyaluronic acid clearance and increases of serum hyaluronic acid parallel loss of endothelial cell viability (147,148). Hyaluronic acid content in the initial effluent after reperfusion of stored human livers and measurement of serum hyaluronic acid and hepatic hyaluronic acid clearance are early predictors of liver graft function in clinical transplantation (148,149).

Liver preservation in UW cold storage solution decreases lethal reperfusion injury to endothelial cells after longer periods of cold storage compared to other preservation solutions in current or previous use, including Euro-Collins solution, HTK (*h*istidine–*t*yrptophane–α-*k*etoglutarate solution), and Celsior solution (150,151). The improvement of endothelial cell viability after reperfusion parallels the improvement of graft survival after transplantation. Although hepatic damage after warm anoxic injury is much

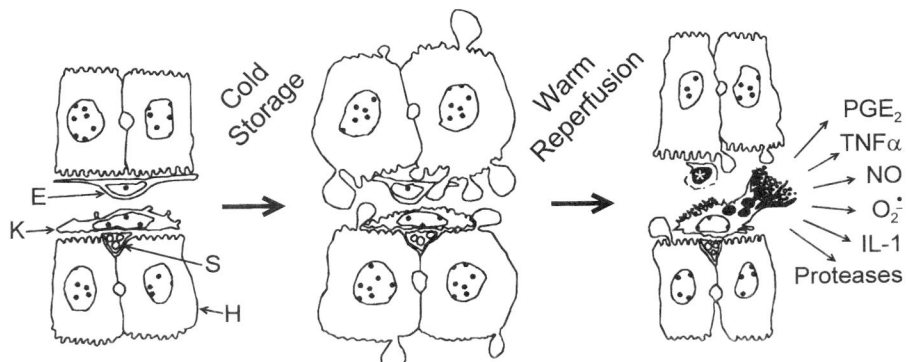

FIGURE 18.9. Reperfusion injury to liver after cold ischemic preservation. During cold ischemic storage, hepatocytes (*H*) swell and form cell surface blebs. Moderate rounding of sinusoidal endothelial cells (*E*) and Kupffer cells (*K*) also occurs. Stellate cells (*S*) change little in structure. After warm reperfusion, endothelial cells lose viability, and their nuclei stain with supravital dyes like trypan blue (*asterisk*). Also after reperfusion, Kupffer cells swell, ruffle, and degranulate. These activated Kupffer cells release inflammatory mediators, including prostaglandin E_2 (PGE$_2$), TNF-α, nitric oxide (*NO•*), superoxide radical (O$_2^{\bullet-}$), interleukin-1 (*IL-1*), and proteases. Hepatocytes recover after reperfusion by resorbing blebs and recovering volume regulation. Stellate cells remain relatively undisturbed. (Adapted from Lemasters JJ, Thurman RG. Reperfusion injury after liver preservation for transplantation. *Annu Rev Pharmacol Toxicol* 1997;37:327–338.)

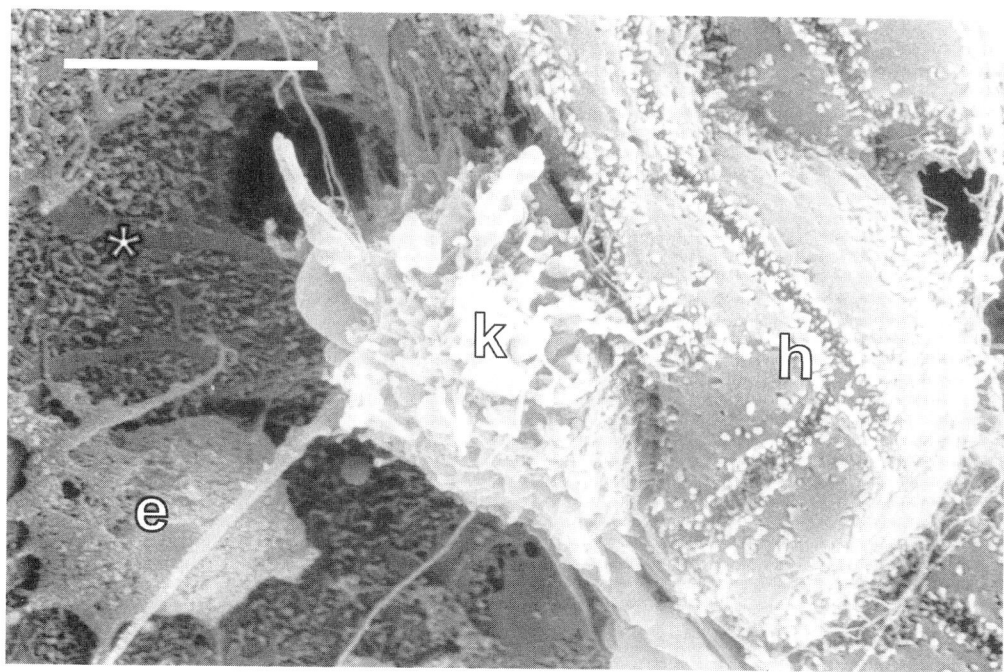

FIGURE 18.10. Scanning electron micrograph of Kupffer cell activation and endothelial cell killing after cold storage and warm reperfusion. A Kupffer cell (*k*) shows swelling, rounding, and ruffling after 24 hours cold storage of a rat liver in Euro-Collins solution and 15 minutes of warm reperfusion. The endothelial lining of the sinusoid is denuded (*asterisk*), and only a remnant of an endothelial cell (*e*) remains. Hepatocytes (*h*) show normal features. *Bar* is 5 μm. (Adapted from Caldwell-Kenkel JC, Currin RT, Tanaka Y, et al. Kupffer cell activation and endothelial cell damage after storage of rat livers: effects of reperfusion. *Hepatology* 1991;13:83–95.)

decreased in livers from fed rats compared to fasted ones because of glycogen accumulation in hepatocytes (24,57), storage/reperfusion injury to endothelial cells is the same in fed and fasted rats (144). However, glycogen superloading of livers appears to decrease endothelial cell injury (152). Protection may be mediated by glucose release from glycogen-loaded hepatocytes, since glucose protects endothelial cells against hypoxic killing (15).

KUPFFER CELL ACTIVATION AFTER COLD STORAGE AND REPERFUSION

During cold ischemic liver storage, relatively minor structural changes occur to Kupffer cells, notably some rounding and blunted ruffling (145). In contrast to these minor changes, warm reperfusion after storage initiates a rapid and marked activation of Kupffer cells (Figs. 18.9 and 18.10) (144,145). Structural changes indicative of activation include vacuolization, cell surface ruffling, formation of wormlike densities, and degranulation within minutes after reperfusion. Cold storage and reperfusion also activate a variety of functional activities in Kupffer cells, including particle phagocytosis, superoxide formation, and hydrolytic enzyme release (145,153,154).

Kupffer cell activation and endothelial cell killing occur in parallel after reperfusion, and both are diminished by storage in UW solution (144,145). These perturbations to nonparenchymal cells are also documented *in vivo* in rat liver grafts that are failing from storage/reperfusion injury (155,156), as well as in human clinical specimens (157,158). Kupffer cells activated by storage/reperfusion injury release TNF-α after liver transplantation, which promotes edema and leukocyte infiltration in the lung (159–162).

REVERSIBLE HEPATOCELLULAR CHANGES DURING LIVER PRESERVATION

During cold ischemic storage, hepatocytes swell and form surface blebs much like those formed during warm hypoxia/ischemia (144,145,163). After longer periods of storage, such blebs literally fill the sinusoids. Hepatocellular swelling and blebbing are less severe after shorter periods of storage, and both occur more slowly during storage in UW solution. Even macroscopically, swelling is much less marked in livers stored in UW solution compared to Euro-Collins solution. Reperfusion after cold storage reverses hepatocellular bleb formation and swelling, and little hepatocellular death and lactate dehydrogenase (LDH) release occur, even after 96 hours of cold storage in Euro-Collins solution, long past the point when liver grafts fail from storage/reperfusion injury (164). Similarly, hepatocellular oxygen consumption and carbohydrate metabolism remain within normal limits (144,164,165). Thus, damage to hepatocytes seems not to underlie liver storage/reperfusion injury.

MICROCIRCULATORY DISTURBANCES AND FREE RADICAL GENERATION AFTER REPERFUSION OF STORED LIVERS

After cold ischemic liver storage, reperfusion with blood leads to microcirculatory disturbances characterized by leukocyte margination, platelet adhesion, fibrin deposition, inflammation, and hemostasis that increases with increasing time of storage (156,166–168). In normal untransplanted livers, leukocyte movement in hepatic sinusoids is rapid and continuous with almost no margination (156,169). In liver grafts failing storage/reperfusion injury, leukocyte velocity decreases substantially, and leukocyte margination increases from virtually 0 to 40% of cells. Kupffer cell phagocytosis is also enhanced. Subsequently, hepatocytes lose viability beginning about 4 hours after transplantation. Even in liver grafts that survive, microcirculatory disturbances occur after reperfusion that are associated with foci of hepatocellular necrosis 24 hours later. Consistent with these experimental findings, platelet trapping in human liver grafts predicts poorer outcomes in clinical liver transplantation (158,170).

Activated Kupffer cells release a variety of inflammatory mediators directly into the blood, including superoxide radicals, NO, proteases, eicosinoids, TNF-α, and other cytokines. These mediators intensify the inflammatory responses and microcirculatory disturbances already created by damage to the sinusoidal endothelium. Spin trapping techniques and nitroblue tetrazolium cytochemistry document free radical formation by Kupffer cells after storage and reperfusion (154,171). Free radicals help stimulate neutrophil margination after reperfusion, since superoxide dismutase decreases neutrophil infiltration into reperfused liver after both warm and cold ischemia (172,173). The systemic release of inflammatory mediators also promotes the adult respiratory distress syndrome and multiple organ failure associated with liver failure (174). Treatments that activate Kupffer cells, such as donor treatment with lipopolysaccharide or physical manipulation of the explanted liver, decrease graft survival dramatically (175–177). Conversely, treatments that suppress Kupffer cell activity, including L-type voltage-sensitive calcium channel blockers, pentoxifylline, adenosine, and prostaglandin E_1, improve graft survival (178–180). Adenosine and prostaglandin E_1 act by cAMP-dependent receptor mechanisms (129), whereas pentoxifylline is a phosphodiesterase inhibitor that blocks cAMP hydrolysis.

Kupffer cell degranulation after cold storage and reperfusion leads to the release of hydrolytic enzymes, including proteases, and the activity of the calcium-dependent protease calpain increases in liver tissue after cold storage and warm reperfusion (181). Free amino acids in the initial reperfusion effluents of stored livers also increase with increasing times of storage (182). Protease inhibition, however, fails to improve long-term graft survival, although some temporary benefit may result (153,183). Thus, protease activation alone does not explain graft failure after storage/reperfusion injury. Rather, a combination of mediators released from Kupffer cells likely promotes graft failure, including reactive oxygen species, proinflammatory cytokines, hydrolytic enzymes such as proteases, and possibly other toxic mediators.

Kupffer cell activation does not cause endothelial cell killing after storage/reperfusion, because Kupffer cell inactivation by pretreatment with $GdCl_3$ fails to decrease endothelial cell killing (184). Similarly, antioxidants, allopurinol, desferal, superoxide dismutase, and catalase, and washout with anoxic buffer have no benefit in preserving endothelial cell viability (154). Thus, oxygen-independent mechanisms mediate lethal storage/reperfusion injury to sinusoidal endothelial cells. Nonetheless, subsequent oxygen-dependent events following endothelial injury involving Kupffer cells contribute to graft failure from storage/reperfusion injury. One consequence is neutrophil infiltration and subsequent neutrophil-mediated hepatic injury by the same mechanisms that occur after warm ischemia/reperfusion injury.

MITOCHONDRIAL CHANGES AND APOPTOSIS FROM STORAGE/REPERFUSION INJURY

Lethal storage/reperfusion injury to sinusoidal endothelial cells is highly pH-dependent, and reperfusion of stored livers with acidotic buffer (pH 6.5 to 6.8) greatly decreases endothelial cell killing (154). The mitochondrial permeability transition may contribute to this pH-dependent injury, since cyclosporin A decreases sinusoidal endothelial cell killing after warm anoxia/reoxygenation (185). Cyclosporin A also decreases reperfusion injury to livers after cold ischemia (186). pH-dependent hypoxic killing of sinusoidal endothelial cells is also associated with mitochondrial depolarization (15). However, cyclosporin A alone does not always prevent the endothelial cell killing associated with warm hypoxia and cold ischemia/reperfusion. Similarly, in isolated mitochondria and hepatocytes, cyclosporin A alone may not be sufficient to prevent the mitochondrial permeability transition after prolonged exposure to strong permeability transition inducers.

Apoptosis to both parenchymal and nonparenchymal cells is also a feature of storage/reperfusion injury and increases with increasing times of cold ischemic storage (187,188). Such apoptosis peaks about 12 hours after transplantation in nonparenchymal cells and after 48 hours for parenchymal cells. A tenfold increase of apoptosis can occur in the absence of primary graft failure and may underlie delayed oxygen-dependent parenchymal cell killing in surviving liver grafts. Activation of caspase 3 and other proteases accompanies apoptosis after storage/reperfusion injury, and the caspase inhibitor IDN-1965 decreases apoptosis by nearly two-thirds (189,190). However, IDN-1965 and other protease inhibitors do not improve long-term graft survival (153,190). Thus, apoptosis may be a consequence rather than a cause of storage/reperfusion injury.

RINSE STRATEGIES TO DECREASE STORAGE/REPERFUSION INJURY

If reperfusion injury is a major contributor to liver graft failure, then modification of the conditions of reperfusion might decrease this injury and improve graft performance and viability. To this end, a new solution was devised at the University of North Carolina to counter potential mechanisms contributing to reperfusion injury (Table 18.4) (191). This solution, named Carolina rinse solution, contains electrolytes similar to Ringer's solution, antioxidants (glutathione, desferal, allopurinol), substrates to regenerate ATP (fructose, glucose, insulin, and adenosine), a calcium channel blocker (nicardipine), colloid osmotic support against interstitial edema (hydroxyethyl starch), a cytopro-

tective amino acid (glycine), and mildly acidic pH (MOPS buffer, pH 6.5). Carolina rinse solution blocks both reperfusion-induced endothelial cell killing after liver storage and the activation of Kupffer cells (192). Carolina rinse solution also improves early bile flow and microvascular perfusion and decreases leukocyte infiltration (192,193). Most significantly, Carolina rinse solution substantially decreases liver graft failure from storage/reperfusion injury when it is flushed into liver explants at the end of storage (194,195). Controversy has existed over whether the injury causing liver graft failure after prolonged cold ischemia in stored livers is a reperfusion injury, or whether irreversible damage occurs during storage prior to reperfusion. The efficacy of Carolina rinse solution used at the end of storage is perhaps the strongest evidence that the injury causing graft failure is a reperfusion-induced event. Two small randomized prospective clinical trials confirm the efficacy of Carolina rinse solution to decrease graft injury after liver transplantation (196,197). However, these pilot studies await confirmation in a large multicenter trial.

Several of the individual components of Carolina rinse solution have been shown to contribute to its efficacy. Adenosine at an optimal concentration of 100 to 200 µM is needed for maximal efficacy, and graft survival decreases when adenosine concentration is either increased or decreased (192,194,195). Antioxidants (glutathione, allopurinol, desferal) and acidic pH (pH 6.5) also are required for efficacy (162). Lastly, the addition of glycine to the other components also improves graft survival after rat liver transplantation (198). The remaining components of Carolina rinse solution, although not specifically demonstrated to contribute to better graft survival, act to counter specific mechanisms contributing to storage/reperfusion injury. The calcium channel blocker (nicardipine) and adenosine suppress lipopolysaccharide-stimulated TNF-α release by cultured Kupffer cells (129,179), and suppression of Kupffer cell activation is one of the likely mechanisms by which Carolina rinse solution improves graft survival after storage/reperfusion injury. Adenine and ribose, the metabolic precursors of adenosine, cannot replace adenosine in Carolina rinse solution (194), supporting the conclusion that adenosine acts via a receptor, possibly adenosine A_2 receptors on both Kupffer cells and endothelial cells. Adenosine also has vasodilatory effects that improve the hepatic microcirculation after reperfusion. As described above, fructose and glucose are substrates for glycolytic ATP formation that protect hepatocytes and sinusoidal endothelial cells, respectively, against hypoxic cell killing.

The efficacy of Carolina rinse solution is also increased when it is used at a warm (30° to 37°C) rather than a cold (1° to 4°C) temperature (195). One benefit of warm temperature is improved microcirculation and decreased vascular resistance to permit more rapid and homogenous reperfusion (159,199). In hepatocytes treated with cyanide to mimic anoxia-induced ATP depletion during organ storage,

TABLE 18.4. CAROLINA RINSE SOLUTION

Ingredient	Concentration
NaCl	115 mM
KCl	5 mM
CaCl$_2$	1.3 mM
KH$_2$PO$_4$	1 mM
MgSO$_4$	1.2 mM
Hydroxyethyl starch	50 g/L
Allopurinol	1 mM
Desferrioxamine	1 mM
Glutathione	3 mM
Fructose	10 mM
Glucose	10 mM
Glycine[a]	5 mM
Adenosine	200 µM
Nicardipine	2 µM
Insulin	100 U/L
3-[N-morpholino]propanesulfonic acid (MOPS)	20 mM
Total Na$^+$	115 mM
Total K$^+$	6 mM
Total Cl$^-$	122
pH	6.5
Osmolarity	290–305 mOsm

[a]Early versions of Carolina rinse solution did not contain glycine.

the rank order of loss of cell viability in various solutions at 0° to 1°C is Ringer's solution > Carolina rinse solution > UW solution (200). However, as temperature increases above 12°C, the rank order of cell killing in different solutions changes to UW solution > Ringer's solution >> Carolina rinse solution. These findings illustrate how UW solution is optimized to be cytoprotective at low temperatures, whereas Carolina rinse solution is optimally effective at warm physiologic temperatures.

ISCHEMIC PRECONDITIONING OF LIVERS PRIOR TO STORAGE

As after warm ischemia, ischemic preconditioning decreases graft injury and improves graft survival after cold ischemic storage of livers. Specifically, ischemic preconditioning prior to storage decreases endothelial cell killing, Kupffer cell activation, and liver graft failure after prolonged cold preservation (201–203). Adenosine mediates this cytoprotection by a cAMP-coupled adenosine A_2 receptor mechanism (184). Similarly, prostaglandin E_2 stimulates Kupffer cells and sinusoidal endothelial cells by cAMP-linked prostaglandin receptors, and donor pretreatment with prostaglandin analogues such as dimethylprostaglandin E_2 decreases endothelial cell killing after cold storage/reperfusion and improves graft success after transplantation (204). These findings in experimental animals hold promise that pretreatment of human donors prior to organ harvest might substantially improve graft function and viability after clinical transplantation.

CONCLUSION

Ischemia/reperfusion involves several different hepatic cell types and involves a variety of mechanisms. During prolonged warm anoxia and ischemia, hepatocellular killing occurs by pH-dependent but oxygen-independent mechanisms. After reperfusion, early hepatocellular killing is also highly pH-dependent and involves a specific injury to mitochondria called the mitochondrial permeability transition. Ischemia/reperfusion also causes Kupffer cell activation, which leads to formation of reactive oxygen species, release of cytokines and chemoattractants, and the recruitment of neutrophils, events that promote liver injury up to 24 hours after reperfusion. Cold ischemia/reperfusion associated with liver preservation for transplantation surgery also involves activation of Kupffer cells, but pH-dependent endothelial cell killing follows reperfusion instead of hepatocyte killing. Studies of hepatic ischemia/reperfusion injury show that multiple mechanisms contribute to hepatic damage. Only by combating these multiple mechanisms of injury can effective strategies be developed to prevent reperfusion injury after warm ischemia and cold ischemic storage.

ACKNOWLEDGMENTS

This work was supported in part by grants DK37034, AG07218, AA09156, and AG13637 from the National Institutes of Health.

REFERENCES

1. Jungermann K, Kietzmann T. Oxygen: modulator of metabolic zonation and disease of the liver. *Hepatology* 2000;31:255–260.
2. Lemasters JJ, Ji S, Thurman RG. New micromethods for studying sublobular structure and function in the isolated, perfused rat liver. In: Thurman RG, Kauffman FC, Jungermann K, eds. *Regulation of hepatic metabolism.* New York: Plenum, 1986:159–184.
3. Lemasters JJ, Ji S, Thurman RG. Centrilobular injury following hypoxia in isolated, perfused rat liver. *Science* 1981;213:661–663.
4. Naschitz JE, Slobodin G, Lewis RJ, et al. Heart diseases affecting the liver and liver diseases affecting the heart. *Am Heart J* 2000;140:111–120.
5. Arteel GE, Iimuro Y, Yin M, et al. Chronic enteral ethanol treatment causes hypoxia in rat liver tissue in vivo. *Hepatology* 1997;25:920–926.
6. Olzinski AT, Sanyal AJ. Treating Budd–Chiari syndrome: making rational choices from a myriad of options. *J Clin Gastroenterol* 2000;30:155–161.
7. Bearman SI. Veno-occlusive disease of the liver. *Curr Opin Oncol* 2000;12:103–109.
8. Lemasters JJ, Bunzendahl H, Thurman RG. Preservation of the liver. In: Maddrey WC, Schiff ER, Sorrell MF, eds. *Transplantation of the liver.* Philadelphia: Lippincott Williams & Wilkins, 2001:251–273.
9. Peng XX, Currin RT, Thurman RG, et al. Protection by pentoxifylline against normothermic liver ischemia/reperfusion in rats. *Transplantation* 1995;59:1537–1541.
10. Lemasters JJ, Stemkowski CJ, Ji S, et al. Cell surface changes and enzyme release during hypoxia and reoxygenation in the isolated, perfused rat liver. *J Cell Biol* 1983;97:778–786.
11. Lemasters JJ, DiGuiseppi J, Nieminen AL, Herman B. Blebbing, free Ca^{2+} and mitochondrial membrane potential preceding cell death in hepatocytes. *Nature* 1987;325:78–81.
12. Nieminen AL, Gores GJ, Wray BE, et al. Calcium dependence of bleb formation and cell death in hepatocytes. *Cell Calcium* 1988;9:237–246.
13. Zahrebelski G, Nieminen AL, al Ghoul K, et al. Progression of subcellular changes during chemical hypoxia to cultured rat hepatocytes: a laser scanning confocal microscopic study. *Hepatology* 1995;21:1361–1372.
14. Dickson RC, Bronk SF, Gores GJ. Glycine cytoprotection during lethal hepatocellular injury from adenosine triphosphate depletion. *Gastroenterology* 1992;102:2098–2107.
15. Nishimura Y, Romer LH, Lemasters JJ. Mitochondrial dysfunction and cytoskeletal disruption during chemical hypoxia to cultured rat hepatic sinusoidal endothelial cells: the pH paradox and cytoprotection by glucose, acidotic pH, and glycine. *Hepatology* 1998;27:1039–1049.
16. Marsh DC, Vreugdenhil PK, Mack VE, et al. Glycine protects hepatocytes from injury caused by anoxia, cold ischemia and mitochondrial inhibitors, but not injury caused by calcium ionophores or oxidative stress. *Hepatology* 1993;17:91–98.
17. Nishimura Y, Lemasters JJ. Glycine blocks opening of a death channel in cultured hepatic sinusoidal endothelial cells during chemical hypoxia. *Cell Death and Differentiation*, in press.

18. Dong Z, Patel Y, Saikumar P, et al. Development of porous defects in plasma membranes of adenosine triphosphate-depleted Madin-Darby canine kidney cells and its inhibition by glycine. *Lab Invest* 1998;78:657–668.

19. Carini R, Bellomo G, Benedetti A, et al. Alteration of Na⁺ homeostasis as a critical step in the development of irreversible hepatocyte injury after adenosine triphosphate depletion. *Hepatology* 1995;21:1089–1098.

20. Ju YK, Saint DA, Gage PW. Hypoxia increases persistent sodium current in rat ventricular myocytes. *J Physiol (Lond)* 1996;497:337–347.

21. Haddad GG, Jiang C. Mechanisms of neuronal survival during hypoxia: ATP-sensitive K⁺ channels. *Biol Neonate* 1994;65:160–165.

22. Nieminen AL, Dawson TL, Gores GJ, et al. Protection by acidotic pH and fructose against lethal injury to rat hepatocytes from mitochondrial inhibitors, ionophores and oxidant chemicals. *Biochem Biophys Res Commun* 1990;167:600–606.

23. Anundi I, King J, Owen DA, et al. Fructose prevents hypoxic cell death in liver. *Am J Physiol* 1987;253:G390–G396.

24. Bradford BU, Marotto M, Lemasters JJ, et al. New, simple models to evaluate zone-specific damage due to hypoxia in the perfused rat liver: time course and effect of nutritional state. *J Pharmacol Exp Ther* 1986;236:263–268.

25. Nieminen AL, Dawson TL, Gores GJ, et al. Protection by acidotic pH and fructose against lethal injury to rat hepatocytes from mitochondrial inhibitors, ionophores and oxidant chemicals. *Biochem Biophys Res Commun* 1990;167:600–606.

26. Wu EY, Smith MT, Bellomo G, et al. Relationships between the mitochondrial transmembrane potential, ATP concentration, and cytotoxicity in isolated rat hepatocytes. *Arch Biochem Biophys* 1990;282:358–362.

27. Whitcomb DC, Block GD. Association of acetaminophen hepatotoxicity with fasting and ethanol use [see comments]. *JAMA* 1994;272:1845–1850.

28. Nieminen AL, Saylor AK, Herman B, et al. ATP depletion rather than mitochondrial depolarization mediates hepatocyte killing after metabolic inhibition. *Am J Physiol* 1994;267:C67–C74.

29. Imberti R, Nieminen AL, Herman B, et al. Mitochondrial and glycolytic dysfunction in lethal injury to hepatocytes by t-butylhydroperoxide: protection by fructose, cyclosporin A and trifluoperazine. *J Pharmacol Exp Ther* 1993;265:392–400.

30. Xia ZF, Horton JW, Zhao PY, et al. Effects of ischemia on intracellular sodium and phosphates in the in vivo rat liver. *J Appl Physiol* 1996;81:1395–1403.

31. Gores GJ, Nieminen AL, Fleishman KE, et al. Extracellular acidosis delays onset of cell death in ATP-depleted hepatocytes. *Am J Physiol* 1988;255:C315–C322.

32. Gores GJ, Nieminen AL, Wray BE, et al. Intracellular pH during "chemical hypoxia" in cultured rat hepatocytes. Protection by intracellular acidosis against the onset of cell death. *J Clin Invest* 1989;83:386–396.

33. Bonventre JV, Cheung JY. Effects of metabolic acidosis on viability of cells exposed to anoxia. *Am J Physiol* 1985;249:C149–C159.

34. Bronk SF, Gores GJ. Efflux of protons from acidic vesicles contributes to cytosolic acidification of hepatocytes during ATP depletion. *Hepatology* 1991;14:626–633.

35. Arora AS, de Groen P, Emori Y, et al. A cascade of degradative hydrolase activity contributes to hepatocyte necrosis during anoxia. *Am J Physiol* 1996;270:G238–G245.

36. Currin RT, Gores GJ, Thurman RG, et al. Protection by acidotic pH against anoxic cell killing in perfused rat liver: evidence for a pH paradox. *FASEB J* 1991;5:207–210.

37. Bond JM, Chacon E, Herman B, et al. Intracellular pH and calcium homeostasis during the pH paradox of reperfusion injury

38. Bond JM, Chacon E, Herman B, et al. Intracellular pH and Ca²⁺ homeostasis in the pH paradox of reperfusion injury to neonatal rat cardiac myocytes. *Am J Physiol* 1993;265:C129–C137.

39. Harper IS, Bond JM, Chacon E, et al. Inhibition of Na⁺/H⁺ exchange preserves viability, restores mechanical function, and prevents the pH paradox in reperfusion injury to rat neonatal myocytes. *Basic Res Cardiol* 1993;88:430–442.

40. Zager RA, Schimpf BA, Gmur DJ. Physiological pH. Effects on posthypoxic proximal tubular injury. *Circ Res* 1993;72:837–846.

41. Qian T, Nieminen AL, Herman B, et al. Mitochondrial permeability transition in pH-dependent reperfusion injury to rat hepatocytes. *Am J Physiol* 1997;273:C1783–C1792.

42. Kaplan SH, Yang H, Gilliam DE, et al. Hypercapnic acidosis and dimethyl amiloride reduce reperfusion induced cell death in ischaemic ventricular myocardium. *Cardiovasc Res* 1995;29:231–238.

43. Lemasters JJ, Nieminen AL, Qian T, et al. The mitochondrial permeability transition in cell death: a common mechanism in necrosis, apoptosis and autophagy. *Biochim Biophys Acta* 1998;1366:177–196.

44. Bernardi P. Mitochondrial transport of cations: channels, exchangers, and permeability transition. *Physiol Rev* 1999;79:1127–1155.

45. Szabo I, Zoratti M. The giant channel of the inner mitochondrial membrane is inhibited by cyclosporin A. *J Biol Chem* 1991;266:3376–3379.

46. Brdiczka D, Beutner G, Ruck A, et al. The molecular structure of mitochondrial contact sites. Their role in regulation of energy metabolism and permeability transition. *Biofactors* 1998;8:235–242.

47. Crompton M, Virji S, Ward JM. Cyclophilin-D binds strongly to complexes of the voltage-dependent anion channel and the adenine nucleotide translocase to form the permeability transition pore. *Eur J Biochem* 1998;258:729–735.

48. Pastorino JG, Tafani M, Rothman RJ, et al. Functional consequences of the sustained or transient activation by Bax of the mitochondrial permeability transition pore. *J Biol Chem* 1999;274:31734–31739.

49. Griffiths EJ, Halestrap AP. Protection by cyclosporin A of ischemia/reperfusion-induced damage to isolated rat hearts. *J Mol Cell Cardiol* 1993;25:1461–1469.

50. Matsumoto S, Friberg H, Ferrand-Drake M, et al. Blockade of the mitochondrial permeability transition pore diminishes infarct size in the rat after transient middle cerebral artery occlusion. *J Cereb Blood Flow Metab* 1999;19:736–741.

51. Byrne AM, Lemasters JJ, Nieminen AL. Contribution of increased mitochondrial free Ca²⁺ to the mitochondrial permeability transition induced by tert-butylhydroperoxide in rat hepatocytes. *Hepatology* 1999;29:1523–1531.

52. Kim J-S, Qian T, Lemasters JJ. Role of mitochondrial Ca²⁺ and reactive oxygen species (ROS) in the mitochondrial permeability transition (MPT) and cell death induced by ischemia/reperfusion in cultured rat hepatocytes. *Hepatology* 2000;32:334A.

53. Carini R, Bellomo G, Benedetti A, et al. Alteration of Na⁺ homeostasis as a critical step in the development of irreversible hepatocyte injury after adenosine triphosphate depletion. *Hepatology* 1995;21:1089–1098.

54. Gutteridge JM, Halliwell B. Free radicals and antioxidants in the year 2000. A historical look to the future. *Ann NY Acad Sci* 2000;899:136–147.

55. Nieminen AL, Saylor AK, Tesfai SA, et al. Contribution of the mitochondrial permeability transition to lethal injury after

exposure of hepatocytes to t-butylhydroperoxide. *Biochem J* 1995;307:99–106.

56. Nieminen AL, Byrne AM, Herman B, et al. Mitochondrial permeability transition in hepatocytes induced by t-BuOOH: NAD(P)H and reactive oxygen species. *Am J Physiol* 1997;272: C1286–C1294.

57. Marotto ME, Thurman RG, Lemasters JJ. Early midzonal cell death during low-flow hypoxia in the isolated, perfused rat liver: protection by allopurinol. *Hepatology* 1988;8:585–590.

58. de la Monte SM, Arcidi JM, Moore GW, et al. Midzonal necrosis as a pattern of hepatocellular injury after shock. *Gastroenterology* 1984;86:627–631.

59. Patel T, Roberts LR, Jones BA, et al. Dysregulation of apoptosis as a mechanism of liver disease: an overview. *Semin Liver Dis* 1998;18:105–114.

60. Sasaki H, Matsuno T, Tanaka N, et al. Activation of apoptosis during the reperfusion phase after rat liver ischemia. *Transplant Proc* 1996;28:1908–1909.

61. Shimizu S, Eguchi Y, Kamiike W, et al. Involvement of ICE family proteases in apoptosis induced by reoxygenation of hypoxic hepatocytes. *Am J Physiol* 1996;271:G949–G958.

62. Zamzami N, Susin SA, Marchetti P, et al. Mitochondrial control of nuclear apoptosis. *J Exp Med* 1996;183:1533–1544.

63. Liu X, Kim CN, Yang J, et al. Induction of apoptotic program in cell-free extracts: requirement for dATP and cytochrome c. *Cell* 1996;86:147–157.

64. Susin SA, Lorenzo HK, Zamzami N, et al. Molecular characterization of mitochondrial apoptosis-inducing factor. *Nature* 1999;397:441–446.

65. Gross A, Pilcher K, Blachly-Dyson E, et al. Biochemical and genetic analysis of the mitochondrial response of yeast to BAX and BCL-X(L). *Mol Cell Biol* 2000;20:3125–3136.

66. Shimizu S, Ide T, Yanagida T, et al. Electrophysiological study of a novel large pore formed by Bax and the voltage-dependent anion channel that is permeable to cytochrome c. *J Biol Chem* 2000;275:12321–12325.

67. Li P, Nijhawan D, Budihardjo I, et al. Cytochrome c and dATP-dependent formation of Apaf-1/caspase-9 complex initiates an apoptotic protease cascade. *Cell* 1997;91:479–489.

68. Li H, Zhu H, Xu CJ, et al. Cleavage of BID by caspase 8 mediates the mitochondrial damage in the Fas pathway of apoptosis. *Cell* 1998;94:491–501.

69. Kroemer G, Reed JC. Mitochondrial control of cell death. *Nat Med* 2000;6:513–519.

70. Bradham CA, Qian T, Streetz K, et al. The mitochondrial permeability transition is required for tumor necrosis factor alpha-mediated apoptosis and cytochrome c release. *Mol Cell Biol* 1998;18:6353–6364.

71. Hatano E, Bradham CA, Stark A, et al. The mitochondrial permeability transition augments Fas-induced apoptosis in mouse hepatocytes. *J Biol Chem* 2000;275:11814–11823.

72. Scaffidi C, Fulda S, Srinivasan A, et al. Two CD95 (APO-1/Fas) signaling pathways. *EMBO J* 1998;17:1675–1687.

73. Nicotera P, Leist M, Ferrando-May E. Intracellular ATP, a switch in the decision between apoptosis and necrosis. *Toxicol Lett* 1998;102–103:139–142.

74. Eguchi Y, Srinivasan A, Tomaselli KJ, et al. ATP-dependent steps in apoptotic signal transduction. *Cancer Res* 1999;59: 2174–2181.

75. Ogasawara J, Watanabe-Fukunaga R, Adachi M, et al. Lethal effect of the anti-Fas antibody in mice [published erratum appears in *Nature* 1993;365:568]. *Nature* 1993;364:806–809.

76. Grasl-Kraupp B, Ruttkay-Nedecky B, Koudelka H, et al. In situ detection of fragmented DNA (TUNEL assay) fails to discriminate among apoptosis, necrosis, and autolytic cell death: a cautionary note. *Hepatology* 1995;21:1465–1468.

77. Ohno M, Takemura G, Ohno A, et al. "Apoptotic" myocytes in infarct area in rabbit hearts may be oncotic myocytes with DNA fragmentation. Analysis by immunogold electron microscopy combined with in situ nick end-labeling. *Circulation* 1998;98: 1422–1430.

78. Lemasters JJ. V. Necrapoptosis and the mitochondrial permeability transition: shared pathways to necrosis and apoptosis. *Am J Physiol* 1999;276:G1–G6.

79. Lichtman SN, Lemasters JJ. Role of cytokines and cytokine-producing cells in reperfusion injury to the liver. *Semin Liver Dis* 1999;19:171–187.

80. Oh K-W, Currin RT, Lemasters JJ. Kupffer cells mediate increased anoxic hepatocellular killing from hyperosmolarity by an oxygen- and prostaglandin-independent mechanism. *Toxicol Lett* 2000;117:95–100.

81. Wanner GA, Ertel W, Muller P, et al. Liver ischemia and reperfusion induces a systemic inflammatory response through Kupffer cell activation. *Shock* 1996;5:34–40.

82. Imanishi H, Scales WE, Campbell DA Jr. Tumor necrosis factor alpha alters the cytotoxic effect of hydrogen peroxide in cultured hepatocytes. *Biochem Biophys Res Commun* 1997;230: 120–124.

83. Hisama N, Yamaguchi Y, Ishiko T, et al. Kupffer cell production of cytokine-induced neutrophil chemoattractant following ischemia/reperfusion injury in rats. *Hepatology* 1996;24: 1193–1198.

84. Yamaguchi Y, Matsumura F, Takeya M, et al. Monocyte chemoattractant protein-1 enhances expression of intercellular adhesion molecule-1 following ischemia-reperfusion of the liver in rats. *Hepatology* 1998;27:727–734.

85. Lentsch AB, Yoshidome H, Cheadle WG, et al. Chemokine involvement in hepatic ischemia/reperfusion injury in mice: roles for macrophage inflammatory protein-2 and Kupffer cells. *Hepatology* 1998;27:507–512.

86. Shanley TP, Schmal H, Warner RL, et al. Requirement for C-X-C chemokines (macrophage inflammatory protein-2 and cytokine-induced neutrophil chemoattractant) in IgG immune complex-induced lung injury. *J Immunol* 1997;158: 3439–3448.

87. Shirasugi N, Wakabayashi G, Shimazu M, et al. Up-regulation of oxygen-derived free radicals by interleukin-1 in hepatic ischemia/reperfusion injury. *Transplantation* 1997;64: 1398–1403.

88. Camargo CA Jr, Madden JF, Gao W, et al. Interleukin-6 protects liver against warm ischemia/reperfusion injury and promotes hepatocyte proliferation in the rodent. *Hepatology* 1997; 26:1513–1520.

89. Jaeschke H, Farhood A. Neutrophil and Kupffer cell-induced oxidant stress and ischemia-reperfusion injury in rat liver. *Am J Physiol* 1991;260:G355–G362.

90. Marubayashi S, Dohi K, Ochi K, et al. Role of free radicals in ischemic rat liver cell injury: prevention of damage by alpha-tocopherol administration. *Surgery* 1986;99:184–192.

91. Jaeschke H, Bautista AP, Spolarics Z, et al. Superoxide generation by Kupffer cells and priming of neutrophils during reperfusion after hepatic ischemia. *Free Radic Res Commun* 1991;15: 277–284.

92. Jaeschke H, Bautista AP, Spolarics Z, et al. Superoxide generation by neutrophils and Kupffer cells during in vivo reperfusion after hepatic ischemia in rats. *J Leukoc Biol* 1992;52:377–382.

93. Sewerynek E, Reiter RJ, Melchiorri D, et al. Oxidative damage in the liver induced by ischemia-reperfusion: protection by melatonin. *Hepatogastroenterology* 1996;43:898–905.

94. Kondo S, Segawa T, Tanaka K, et al. Mannosylated superoxide dismutase inhibits hepatic reperfusion injury in rats. *J Surg Res* 1996;60:36–40.

95. Marzi I. Reduction of leukocyte-endothelial in hepatic sinusoids following cold and warm ischemia by superoxide dismutase. *Cells of the Hepatic Sinusoid* 2000;3:371–375.
96. Fukuzawa K, Emre S, Senyuz O, et al. N-acetylcysteine ameliorates reperfusion injury after warm hepatic ischemia. *Transplantation* 1995;59:6–9.
97. Liu P, Fisher MA, Farhood A, et al. Beneficial effects of extracellular glutathione against endotoxin-induced liver injury during ischemia and reperfusion. *Circ Shock* 1994;43:64–70.
98. Bauer C, Marzi I, Larsen R. Deferoxamine-conjugated hydroxyethyl starch reduces reperfusion injury to the liver following hemorrhagic shock. *Anaesthesist* 1997;46:53–56.
99. Mathews WR, Guido DM, Fisher MA, et al. Lipid peroxidation as molecular mechanism of liver cell injury during reperfusion after ischemia. *Free Radic Biol Med* 1994;16:763–770.
100. Jaeschke H, Farhood A, Bautista AP, et al. Complement activates Kupffer cells and neutrophils during reperfusion after hepatic ischemia. *Am J Physiol* 1993;264:G801–G809.
101. Jaeschke H. Pathophysiology of hepatic ischemia-reperfusion injury: the role of complement activation [editorial;comment]. *Gastroenterology* 1994;107:583–586.
102. Serizawa A, Nakamura S, Suzuki, et al. Involvement of platelet-activating factor in cytokine production and neutrophil activation after hepatic ischemia-reperfusion. *Hepatology* 1996;23:1656–1663.
103. Minor T, Isselhard W, Yamaguchi T. Involvement of platelet activating factor in microcirculatory disturbances after global hepatic ischemia. *J Surg Res* 1995;58:536–540.
104. Clemens MG, Bauer M, Gingalewski C, et al. Hepatic intercellular communication in shock and inflammation [editorial]. *Shock* 1994;2:1–9.
105. McCuskey RS. Morphological mechanisms for regulating blood flow through hepatic sinusoids. *Liver* 2000;20:3–7.
106. Goto M, Takei Y, Kawano S, et al. Endothelin-1 is involved in the pathogenesis of ischemia/reperfusion liver injury by hepatic microcirculatory disturbances. *Hepatology* 1994;19:675–681.
107. Pannen BH, Al Adili F, Bauer M, et al. Role of endothelins and nitric oxide in hepatic reperfusion injury in the rat. *Hepatology* 1998;27:755–764.
108. Ota T, Hirai R, Urakami A, et al. Endothelin-1 levels in portal venous blood in relation to hepatic tissue microcirculation disturbance and hepatic cell injury after ischemia/reperfusion. *Surg Today* 1997;27:313–320.
109. Kelm M, Feelisch M, Deussen A, et al. Release of endothelium derived nitric oxide in relation to pressure and flow. *Cardiovasc Res* 1991;25:831–836.
110. Wang Y, Mathews WR, Guido DM, et al. Inhibition of nitric oxide synthesis aggravates reperfusion injury after hepatic ischemia and endotoxemia. *Shock* 1995;4:282–288.
111. Koeppel TA, Thies JC, Schemmer P, et al. Inhibition of nitric oxide synthesis in ischemia/reperfusion of the rat liver is followed by impairment of hepatic microvascular blood flow. *J Hepatol* 1997;27:163–169.
112. Liu P, Yin K, Nagele R, et al. Inhibition of nitric oxide synthase attenuates peroxynitrite generation, but augments neutrophil accumulation in hepatic ischemia-reperfusion in rats. *J Pharmacol Exp Ther* 1998;284:1139–1146.
113. Shiraishi M, Hiroyasu S, Nagahama M, et al. Role of exogenous L-arginine in hepatic ischemia-reperfusion injury. *J Surg Res* 1997;69:429–434.
114. Jones SM, Thurman RG. L-arginine minimizes reperfusion injury in a low-flow, reflow model of liver perfusion. *Hepatology* 1996;24:163–168.
115. Jaeschke H, Farhood A, Smith CW. Neutrophils contribute to ischemia/reperfusion injury in rat liver in vivo. *FASEB J* 1990;4:3355–3359.
116. Menger MD, Richter S, Yamauchi J, et al. Role of microcirculation in hepatic ischemia/reperfusion injury. *Hepatogastroenterology* 1999;46(suppl 2):1452–1457.
117. Vollmar B, Glasz J, Menger MD, et al. Leukocytes contribute to hepatic ischemia/reperfusion injury via intercellular adhesion molecule-1–mediated venular adherence. *Surgery* 1995;117:195–200.
118. Farhood A, McGuire GM, Manning AM, et al. Intercellular adhesion molecule 1 (ICAM-1) expression and its role in neutrophil-induced ischemia-reperfusion injury in rat liver. *J Leukoc Biol* 1995;57:368–374.
119. Jaeschke H, Farhood A, Bautista AP, et al. Functional inactivation of neutrophils with a Mac-1 (CD11b/CD18) monoclonal antibody protects against ischemia-reperfusion injury in rat liver. *Hepatology* 1993;17:915–923.
120. Ho JS, Buchweitz JP, Roth RA, et al. Identification of factors from rat neutrophils responsible for cytotoxicity to isolated hepatocytes. *J Leukoc Biol* 1996;59:716–724.
121. Kushimoto S, Okajima K, Uchiba M, et al. Role of granulocyte elastase in ischemia/reperfusion injury of rat liver. *Crit Care Med* 1996;24:1908–1912.
122. Zwacka RM, Zhang Y, Halldorson J, et al. CD4(+) T-lymphocytes mediate ischemia/reperfusion-induced inflammatory responses in mouse liver. *J Clin Invest* 1997;100:279–289.
123. Okuaki Y, Miyazaki H, Zeniya M, et al. Splenectomy-reduced hepatic injury induced by ischemia/reperfusion in the rat. *Liver* 1996;16:188–194.
124. Kloner RA, Yellon D. Does ischemic preconditioning occur in patients? *J Am Coll Cardiol* 1994;24:1133–1142.
125. Hotter G, Closa D, Prados M, et al. Intestinal preconditioning is mediated by a transient increase in nitric oxide. *Biochem Biophys Res Commun* 1996;222:27–32.
126. Lloris-Carsi JM, Cejalvo D, Toledo-Pereyra LH, et al. Preconditioning: effect upon lesion modulation in warm liver ischemia. *Transplant Proc* 1993;25:3303–3304.
127. Kume M, Yamamoto Y, Saad S, et al. Ischemic preconditioning of the liver in rats: implications of heat shock protein induction to increase tolerance of ischemia-reperfusion injury. *J Lab Clin Med* 1996;128:251–258.
128. Peralta C, Hotter G, Closa D, et al. Protective effect of preconditioning on the injury associated to hepatic ischemia-reperfusion in the rat: role of nitric oxide and adenosine. *Hepatology* 1997;25:934–937.
129. Reinstein LJ, Lichtman SN, Currin RT, et al. Suppression of lipopolysaccharide-stimulated release of tumor necrosis factor by adenosine: evidence for A2 receptors on rat Kupffer cells. *Hepatology* 1994;19:1445–1452.
130. Ralevic V, Burnstock G. Receptors for purines and pyrimidines. *Pharmacol Rev* 1998;50:413–492.
131. Martin HB, Walter CL. Preconditioning: an endogenous defense against the insult of myocardial ischemia [see comments]. *Anesth Analg* 1996;83:639–645.
132. Schwarz ER, Whyte WS, Kloner RA. Ischemic preconditioning. *Curr Opin Cardiol* 1997;12:475–481.
133. Peralta C, Hotter G, Closa D, et al. The protective role of adenosine in inducing nitric oxide synthesis in rat liver ischemia preconditioning is mediated by activation of adenosine A2 receptors. *Hepatology* 1999;29:126–132.
134. Grover GJ, Garlid KD. ATP-Sensitive potassium channels: a review of their cardioprotective pharmacology. *J Mol Cell Cardiol* 2000;32:677–695.
135. Belzer FO, Southard JH. Principles of solid-organ preservation by cold storage. *Transplantation* 1988;45:673–676.
136. Todo S, Nery J, Yanaga K, et al. Extended preservation of human liver grafts with UW solution. *JAMA* 1989;261:711–714.

137. Porte RJ, Ploeg RJ, Hansen B, et al. Long-term graft survival after liver transplantation in the UW era: late effects of cold ischemia and primary dysfunction. European Multicentre Study Group. *Transplant Int* 1998;11(suppl 1):S164–S167.

138. Rosen HR, Martin P, Goss J, et al. Significance of early amino-transferase elevation after liver transplantation. *Transplantation* 1998;65:68–72.

139. Ploeg RJ, D'Alessandro AM, Knechtle SJ, et al. Risk factors for primary dysfunction after liver transplantation—a multivariate analysis. *Transplantation* 1993;55:807–813.

140. Deschenes M, Belle SH, Krom RA, et al. Early allograft dysfunction after liver transplantation: a definition and predictors of outcome. National Institute of Diabetes and Digestive and Kidney Diseases Liver Transplantation Database. *Transplantation* 1998;66:302–310.

141. Porayko MK, Kondo M, Steers JL. Liver transplantation: late complications of the biliary tract and their management. *Semin Liver Dis* 1995;15:139–155.

142. Laskin DL, Rodriguez del Valle M, Heck DE, et al. Hepatic nitric oxide production following acute endotoxemia in rats is mediated by increased inducible nitric oxide synthase gene expression. *Hepatology* 1995;22:223–234.

143. Gaffey MJ, Boyd JC, Traweek ST, et al. Predictive value of intra-operative biopsies and liver function tests for preservation injury in orthotopic liver transplantation. *Hepatology* 1997;25:184–189.

144. Caldwell-Kenkel JC, Currin RT, Tanaka Y, et al. Reperfusion injury to endothelial cells following cold ischemic storage of rat livers. *Hepatology* 1989;10:292–299.

145. Caldwell-Kenkel JC, Currin RT, Tanaka Y, et al. Kupffer cell activation and endothelial cell damage after storage of rat livers: effects of reperfusion. *Hepatology* 1991;13:83–95.

146. Smedsrod B. Non-invasive means to study the functional status of sinusoidal liver endothelial cells. *J Gastroenterol Hepatol* 1995;10(suppl 1):S81–S83.

147. Reinders ME, van Wagensveld BA, van Gulik TM, et al. Hyaluronic acid uptake in the assessment of sinusoidal endothelial cell damage after cold storage and normothermic reperfusion of rat livers. *Transplant Int* 1996;9:446–453.

148. Suehiro T, Boros P, Emre S, et al. Assessment of liver allograft function by hyaluronic acid and endothelin levels. *J Surg Res* 1997;73:123–128.

149. Rao PN, Bronsther OL, Pinna AD, et al. Hyaluronate levels in donor organ washout effluents: a simple and predictive parameter of graft viability. *Liver* 1996;16:48–54.

150. Peng X-X, Currin RT, Bachmann S, et al. Superiority of UW solution over HTK solution for graft survival and non-parenchymal cell viability after liver preservation for transplantation. *CHS* 1997;6:210–212.

151. Peng XX, Currin RT, Lemasters JJ. Comparison of UW solution and Celsior for storage of rat livers for transplantation surgery. *Hepatology* 2000;32:609A.

152. Morgan GR, Sanabria JR, Clavien PA, et al. Correlation of donor nutritional status with sinusoidal lining cell viability and liver function in the rat. *Transplantation* 1991;51:1176–1183.

153. Takei Y, Marzi I, Kauffman FC, et al. Increase in survival time of liver transplants by protease inhibitors and a calcium channel blocker, nisoldipine. *Transplantation* 1990;50:14–20.

154. Caldwell-Kenkel JC, Currin RT, Coote A, et al. Reperfusion injury to endothelial cells after cold storage of rat livers: protection by mildly acidic pH and lack of protection by antioxidants. *Transplant Int* 1995;8:77–85.

155. Caldwell-Kenkel JC, Currin RT, Gao W, et al. Reperfusion injury to livers stored for transplantation: endothelial cell killing and Kupffer cell activation. *CHS* 1991;3:376–380.

156. Takei Y, Marzi I, Gao W, et al. Leukocyte adhesion and cell death following orthotopic liver transplantation the rat. *Transplantation* 1991;51:959–965.

157. Carles J, Fawaz R, Hamoudi NE, et al. Preservation of human liver grafts in UW solution. Ultrastructural evidence for endothelial and Kupffer cell activation during cold ischemia and after ischemia-reperfusion. *Liver* 1994;14:50–56.

158. Carles J, Fawaz R, Neaud V, et al. Ultrastructure of human liver grafts preserved with UW solution. Comparison between patients with low and high postoperative transaminases levels. *J Submicrosc Cytol Pathol* 1994;26:67–73.

159. Takei Y, Gao W, Hijioka T, et al. Increase in survival of liver grafts after rinsing with warm Ringer's solution due to improvement of hepatic microcirculation. *Transplantation* 1991;52:225–230.

160. Goto M, Takei Y, Kawano S, et al. Tumor necrosis factor and endotoxin in the pathogenesis of liver and pulmonary injuries after orthotopic liver transplantation in the rat. *Hepatology* 1992;16:487–493.

161. Savier E, Shedlofsky SI, Swim AT, et al. The calcium channel blocker nisoldipine minimizes the release of tumor necrosis factor and interleukin-6 following rat liver transplantation. *Transplant Int* 1992;5:S398–S402.

162. Bachmann S, Caldwell-Kenkel JC, Currin RT, et al. Protection by pentoxifylline against graft failure from storage injury after orthotopic rat liver transplantation with arterialization. *Transplant Int* 1992;5(suppl 1):S345–S350.

163. Lemasters JJ, Caldwell-Kenkel JC, Currin RT, et al. Endothelial cell killing and activation of Kupffer cells following reperfusion of rat livers stored in Euro-Collins solution. *Cells of the Hepatic Sinusoid* 1989;2:277–280.

164. Caldwell-Kenkel JC, Thurman RG, Lemasters JJ. Selective loss of nonparenchymal cell viability after cold ischemic storage of rat livers. *Transplantation* 1988;45:834–837.

165. Marzi I, Zhong Z, Lemasters JJ, et al. Evidence that graft survival is not related to parenchymal cell viability in rat liver transplantation: the importance of nonparenchymal cells. *Transplantation* 1989;48:463–468.

166. Clavien PA, Harvey PR, Sanabria JR, et al. Lymphocyte adherence in the reperfused rat liver: mechanisms and effects. *Hepatology* 1993;17:131–142.

167. Arai M, Mochida S, Ohno A, et al. Blood coagulation in the hepatic sinusoids as a contributing factor in liver injury following orthotopic liver transplantation in the rat. *Transplantation* 1996;62:1398–1401.

168. Cywes R, Packham MA, Tietze L, et al. Role of platelets in hepatic allograft preservation injury in the rat. *Hepatology* 1993;18:635–647.

169. Post S, Gonzalez AP, Palma P, et al. Assessment of hepatic phagocytic activity by in vivo microscopy after liver transplantation in the rat. *Hepatology* 1992;16:803–809.

170. Cywes R, Brendan J, Mullen M, et al. Prediction of the outcome of transplantation in man by platelet adherence in donor liver allografts. *Transplantation* 1993;56:316–323.

171. Connor HD, Gao W, Nukina S, et al. Evidence that free radicals are involved in graft failure following orthotopic liver transplantation in the rat—an electron paramagnetic resonance spin trapping study. *Transplantation* 1992;54:199–204.

172. Koo A, Komatsu H, Tao G, et al. Contribution of no-reflow phenomenon to hepatic injury after ischemia-reperfusion: evidence for a role for superoxide anion. *Hepatology* 1992;15:507–514.

173. Marzi I, Knee J, Buhren V, et al. Reduction by superoxide dismutase of leukocyte-endothelial adherence after liver transplantation. *Surgery* 1992;111:90–97.

174. Matuschak GM, Rinaldo JE, Pinsky MR, et al. Effect of end

stage liver failure on the incidence and resolution of adult respiratory distress syndrome. *J Crit Care* 1987;2:162–173.

175. Peng X-X, Currin RT, Muto Y, Musshafen TL, et al. Lipopolysaccharide treatment of donor rats causes graft failure after orthotopic liver transplantation. *Cells of the Hepatic Sinusoid* 1995;5:234–235.

176. Azoulay D, Astarcioglu I, Lemoine A, et al. The effects of donor and recipient endotoxemia on TNF alpha production and mortality in the rat model of syngenic orthotopic liver transplantation. *Transplantation* 1995;59:825–829.

177. Schemmer P, Schoonhoven R, Swenberg JA, et al. Gentle organ manipulation during harvest as a key determinant of survival of fatty livers after transplantation in the rat. *Transplant Int* 1999;12:351–359.

178. Takei Y, Marzi I, Kauffman FC, et al. Increase in survival time of liver transplants by proteases inhibitors and a calcium channel blocker, nisoldipine. *Transplantation* 1990;50:14–20.

179. Currin RT, Reinstein LJ, Lichtman SN, et al. Inhibition of tumor necrosis factor release from cultured rat Kupffer cells by agents that reduce graft failure from storage injury. *Transplant Proc* 1993;25:1631–1632.

180. Tokunaga Y, Wicomb WN, Concepcion W, et al. Successful 20–hour rat liver preservation with chlorpromazine in sodium lactobionate sucrose solution. *Surgery* 1991;110:80–86.

181. Aguilar HI, Steers JL, Wiesner RH, et al. Enhanced liver calpain protease activity is a risk factor for dysfunction of human liver allografts. *Transplantation* 1997;63:612–614.

182. Frankenberg M, Stachlewitz RF, Forman DT, et al. Amino acids in rinse effluents as a predictor of graft function after transplantation of fatty livers in rats. *Transplant Int* 1999;12:168–175.

183. Kohli V, Gao W, Camargo CA Jr, et al. Calpain is a mediator of preservation-reperfusion injury in rat liver transplantation. *Proc Natl Acad Sci USA* 1997;94:9354–9359.

184. Arai M, Thurman RG, Lemasters JJ. Contribution of adenosine A2 receptors and cyclic adenosine monophosphate to protective ischemic preconditioning of sinusoidal endothelial cells against storage/reperfusion injury in rat livers. *Hepatology* 2000;32:297–302.

185. Fujii Y, Johnson ME, Gores GJ. Mitochondrial dysfunction during anoxia/reoxygenation injury of liver sinusoidal endothelial cells. *Hepatology* 1994;20:177–185.

186. Kawano K, Kim YI, Ono M, et al. Evidence that both cyclosporin and azathioprine prevent warm ischemia reperfusion injury to the rat liver. *Transplant Int* 1993;6:330–336.

187. Currin RT, Peng X-X, Arai M, et al. Progression of apoptosis after liver preservation and transplantation. *Hepatology* 1997;26:496A.

188. Gao W, Bentley RC, Madden JF, et al. Apoptosis of sinusoidal endothelial cells is a critical mechanism of preservation injury in rat liver transplantation. *Hepatology* 1998;27:1652–1660.

189. Natori S, Selzner M, Valentino KL, et al. Apoptosis of sinusoidal endothelial cells occurs during liver preservation injury by a caspase-dependent mechanism. *Transplantation* 1999;68:89–96.

190. Sindram D, Kohli V, Madden JF, et al. Calpain inhibition prevents sinusoidal endothelial cell apoptosis in the cold ischemic rat liver. *Transplantation* 1999;68:136–140.

191. Currin RT, Thurman RG, Toole JG, et al. Evidence that Carolina rinse solution protects sinusoidal cells against reperfusion injury after cold ischemic storage of rat liver. *Transplantation* 1990;50:1076–1078.

192. Gao WS, Hijioka T, Lindert KA, et al. Evidence that adenosine is a key component in Carolina rinse responsible for reducing graft failure after orthotopic liver transplantation in the rat. *Transplantation* 1991;52:992–998.

193. Post S, Rentsch M, Gonzalez AP, et al. Effects of Carolina rinse and adenosine rinse on microvascular perfusion and intrahepatic leukocyte-endothelium interaction after liver transplantation in the rat. *Transplantation* 1993;55:972–977.

194. Gao WS, Takei Y, Marzi I, et al. Carolina rinse solution—a new strategy to increase survival time after orthotopic liver transplantation in the rat. *Transplantation* 1991;52:417–424.

195. Bachmann S, Caldwell-Kenkel JC, Oleksy I, et al. Warm Carolina rinse solution prevents graft failure from storage injury after orthotopic rat liver transplantation with arterialization. *Transplant Int* 1992;5:108–114.

196. Sanchez-Urdazpal L, Gores GJ, Lemasters JJ, et al. Carolina rinse solution decreases liver injury during clinical liver transplantation. *Transplant Proc* 1993;25:1574–1575.

197. Haller GW, Langrehr JM, Blumhardt G, et al. Factors relevant to the development of primary dysfunction in liver allografts. *Transplant Proc* 1995;27:1192.

198. Bachmann S, Peng XX, Currin RT, et al. Glycine in Carolina rinse solution reduces reperfusion injury, improves graft function, and increases graft survival after rat liver transplantation. *Transplant Proc* 1995;27:741–742.

199. Rentsch M, Post S, Palma P, et al. Intravital studies on beneficial effects of warm Ringer's lactate rinse in liver transplantation. *Transplant Int* 1996;9:461–467.

200. Currin RT, Thurman RG, Lemasters JJ. Carolina rinse solution protects adenosine triphosphate-depleted hepatocytes against lethal cell injury. *Transplant Proc* 1991;23:645–647.

201. Yin DP, Sankary HN, Chong AS, et al. Protective effect of ischemic preconditioning on liver preservation-reperfusion injury in rats. *Transplantation* 1998;66:152–157.

202. Arai M, Lemasters JJ. Improvement of recipient survival and suppression of Kupffer cell activation by ischemic preconditioning after rat liver transplantation. *Gastroenterology* 1998;114:A1205.

203. Arai M, Thurman RG, Lemasters JJ. Involvement of Kupffer cells and sinusoidal endothelial cells in ischemic preconditioning to rat livers stored for transplantation. *Transplant Proc* 1999;31(1–2):425–427.

204. Arai M, Peng XX, Currin RT, et al. Protection of sinusoidal endothelial cells against storage/reperfusion injury by prostaglandin E2 derived from Kupffer cells. *Transplantation* 1999;68:440–445.

19

PROTECTIVE MECHANISMS AGAINST REACTIVE OXYGEN SPECIES

MASAYASU INOUE

This chapter focuses on mechanisms whereby the liver is protected against reactive oxygen species. Hepatic oxygen metabolism and generation of reactive oxygen species in each cell type in the liver are discussed in website chapter W-13 and in Chapter 18.

METABOLISM OF ANTIOXIDANTS IN THE LIVER

The liver is the major organ for removal of intestinally derived bacteria and toxic compounds, such as endotoxin, oxidants, and pro-oxidants. To detoxify these hazardous compounds, the liver contains high levels of low molecular weight antioxidants and enzymes that degrade reactive oxygen species. Reduced glutathione (GSH), vitamin C, vitamin E, superoxide dismutase (SOD), glutathione peroxidase, and catalase are examples (Table 19.1).

DYNAMIC ASPECTS OF GLUTATHIONE METABOLISM

Glutathione is a naturally occurring major thiol and is synthesized in cytosol in its reduced form. The thiol functions as a multipotential metabolite (1–3). GSH is translocated from cytosol to mitochondria (4) and nucleus (5), and serves as an antioxidant reducer and for detoxifying electrophilic compounds. Since enzymes that hydrolyze GSH, oxidized glutathione (GSSG), and glutathione S-conjugates are localized extracellularly, these tripeptides are translo-

cated out of cells prior to degradation. In rodents, the liver is the major organ that excretes GSH into the circulation and bile (6,7). The liver also excretes GSSG and glutathione S-conjugates preferentially in bile (8). GSH is the major form of glutathione in bile. If fresh bile samples are exposed to air, GSH is oxidized rapidly by a mechanism that is inhibited by ethylenediaminetetraacetic acid (EDTA). GSH is excreted from hepatocytes bidirectionally in plasma and bile. In contrast to bidirectional secretion of GSH, GSSG and glutathione S-conjugates are preferentially excreted in the bile (8,9) (see Chapter 25 and website chapter W-15). However, glutathione S-conjugates formed in erythrocytes and extrahepatic tissues are also excreted into the circulation. Secretory transport of these tripeptides occurs by a carrier-mediated mechanism (10–13).

Studies in hyperbilirubinemic mutant rats [transport defect (TR⁻) or Eisaihyperbilirubinemic rat (EHBR)] revealed that biliary secretion of glutathione is inhibited in these animals. They lack the ability to excrete bilirubin and non–bile acid organic anions into bile (13–16). Biliary secretion of this tripeptide occurs predominantly via an adenosine triphosphate (ATP)-dependent mechanism (see Chapters 24 and 25).

Glutathione and its S-conjugates that are excreted in the bile are degraded to constituent amino acids by γ-glutamyltransferase (GGT) and peptidases localized on the luminal surface of biliary cells (17) (see Chapter 24) and epithelial cells of the pancreas and small intestine. The extent of biliary degradation of the tripeptides differs from one species to another depending on the levels of GGT in biliary cells and pancreatic juice. In the rat, about 50% of biliary glutathione is degraded in bile. In contrast to rodents, hepatic GGT activity is extremely high in humans, rabbits, and sheep. Most of the biliary tripeptide in these species is degraded within the biliary tract. Thus,

M. Inoue: Department of Biochemistry and Molecular Pathology, Osaka City University Medical School, Abeno, Osaka 545-8585, Japan.

TABLE 19.1. ANTIOXIDANTS AND SCAVENGING ENZYMES

Antioxidants	
Glutathione	Major antioxidant in intra- and extracellular compartment (hydrophilic), cellular level: 2–10 mM, levels in arterial plasma: 5–25 μM
Other thiols	Cysteine (significantly lower than GSH)
Vitamin C	Hydrophilic antioxidant in extracellular fluid and cytosol (40–140 μM in plasma) cooperates with vitamin E
Uric acid	Final metabolite of adenosine and xanthine; strong antioxidant (for HO•); 2.6–7.5 mg/dL plasma (0.12–0.45 mM)
Bilirubin	Hydrophobic antioxidant (20 μM); circulates bound to albumin
Vitamin E	Scavenges in hydrophobic compartment; 0.5–1.6 mg/dL plasma (10–40 μM); circulates bound to LDL
β-Carotene	0.055 mg/dL serum
Coenzyme Q10	0.08 mg/dL plasma
Scavenging enzymes	
SOD	Present ubiquitously in all mammalian cells
Cu/Zn-SOD	Cytosol, erythrocytes (2,300 units/g Hb)
Mn-SOD	Mitochondria
Extracellular SOD (EC-SOD)	Plasma and endothelia cell surface, binds to heparin (low specific activity)
Catalase	Peroxisome, RBC (153,000 units/g Hb)
GSH peroxidase	Cytosol (75%), mitochondria (25%), (serenocysteine) RBC (31 units/g Hb) Se-independent (glutathione-S-transferase)
GSSG reductase	NADPH-dependent reduction of GSSG
Thioredoxin system	Redox regulation
Binding Proteins	
Albumin	Strong antioxidant (0.5 mM in plasma); mercapto- and nonmercaptalbumin
Ceruloplasmin	Protection by feroxidase activity; 15–60 mg/dL plasma (1–4 μM)
Transferin	Chelate free iron (200–400 mg/dL, 25–50 μM)
Metalothionein	Chelate heavy metals

[a]Values show the level and activity in humans.
GSH, reduced glutathione; GSSG, oxidized glutathione; HO•, hydroxyl radical; LDL, low-density lipoprotein; RBC, red blood cell; SOD, superoxide dismutase.

cyst(e)ine and other constituent amino acids are the major metabolites in the bile of these animals. In contrast, both glutathione and cyst(e)ine enter the small intestine of rodents. Since GGT is highly enriched in the brush border of intestinal epithelial cells, the remaining glutathione and related peptides are hydrolyzed completely within the lumen. The constituent amino acids are absorbed by active transport systems in the small intestine, transferred to the liver, absorbed by hepatocytes, and used again for GSH synthesis. Thus, the metabolism of biliary glutathione and related metabolites occurs via intrahepatic and enterohepatic cycles (Fig. 19.1).

GSH and its S-conjugates that appear in plasma are degraded in tissues that have GGT. In rodents, the kidney is the major organ that extracts GSH and related peptides in the circulation (18). Since renal GGT is localized on the outer surface of both apical and basolateral membranes of proximal tubule cells, glutathione and related metabolites are degraded both in luminal and contraluminal space of the renal tubules. Since 20% to 30% of low molecular weight compounds in renal arterial plasma is filtered by a single pass through the glomerulus, glutathione and its S-conjugates are degraded by brush border membranes of proximal tubules. The remaining fractions (70% to 80%) are degraded by peritubular transferase activity. Thus, GSH and its metabolites in the circulation are metabolized pre-

dominantly by a hepatorenal cycle (Fig. 19.1). Hepatic GGT activity is less than a few percent of that in the kidney of rodents. In contrast, GGT activity in human liver is as high as in the kidney. Since GGT levels in the liver and other tissues differ from one species to another, the quantitative aspects of GSH cycles may also differ depending on the enzyme activity in tissues. GSH levels in human arterial and hepatic venous plasma are significantly lower (about one-tenth) than those of rodents, which may result from higher activity of hepatic GGT in humans. Hepatic GGT is low in rodents and is localized exclusively on the luminal surface of bile canalicular membranes and biliary cells. However, high activity of rat kidney GGT is localized on the outer surface of both luminal and contraluminal membranes of proximal tubule cells. Although the presence of GGT in bile and on luminal membranes of human liver is well established, direct evidence for absence of the enzyme in sinusoidal plasma membranes is lacking. If hepatic GGT is also localized on the outer surface of contraluminal membranes of hepatocytes, GSH excreted by hepatocytes into the space of Disse may be degraded to constituent amino acids. Since the inferior vena cava in humans contains more circulating glutathione than does the artery, the intestine may possibly be the source for plasma glutathione in humans. Species-specific differences in the interorgan metabolism and transport of GSH exist.

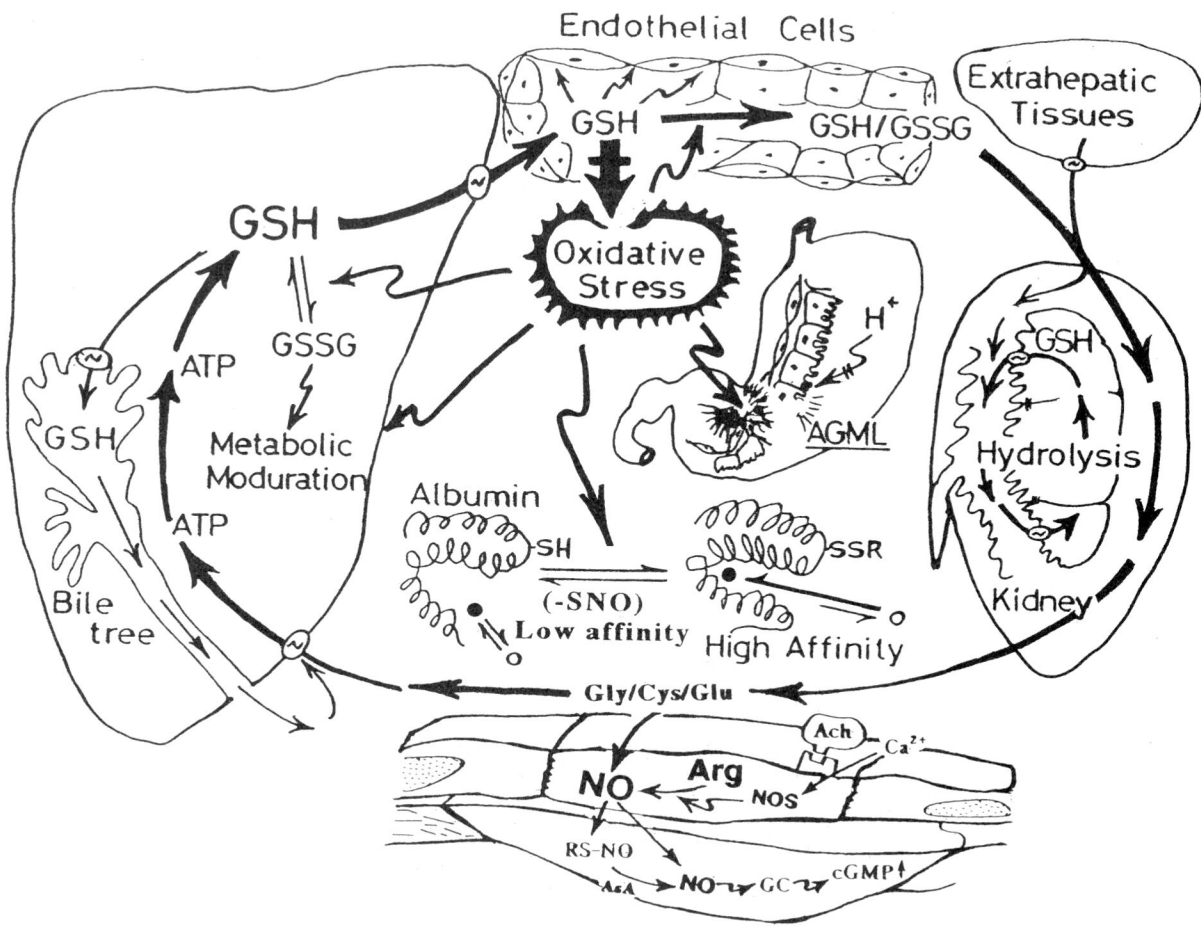

FIGURE 19.1. Interorgan metabolism of reduced glutathione (*GSH*). Glutathione is synthesized exclusively intracellularly in its reduced form (GSH). GSH is secreted by tissues, such as the liver, into the circulation and luminal compartments of epithelial tissues by some adenosine triphosphate (*ATP*)-dependent mechanism. Extracellular GSH and its S-conjugates are hydrolyzed on the outer surface of cells that have γ-glutamyltransferase (*GGT*) activity, such as the kidney and small intestine. The constituent amino acids, such as cysteine, are transported by cells and used for various metabolisms including GSH synthesis. Thus, GSH and its metabolites are handled via inter- and intraorgan cooperation in which liver, kidney, and small intestine play central roles. Both GSH and cysteine function as antioxidants, decrease oxidative stress, and regulate the redox status of various molecules. The ligand-binding activity of albumin is affected by these thiols or by nitric oxide (*NO*) through formation of mixed disulfides or a nitrosothiol at the cys35 residue; nonmercaptalbumin shows higher affinity for hydrophobic anions than does mercaptalbumin (17) while GS-NO shows lowest affinity for the ligands. *AGML*, acute gastric mucosal lesion; *EC*, vascular endothelial cells; *Ach*, acetylcholine; *NOS*, NO synthase; *Arg*, arginine; *RS-NO*, nitrosothiols; *GC*, guanylate cyclase; *AsA*, ascorbic acid.

Other Antioxidants with Low Molecular Weight

In addition to GSH, the liver also contains other antioxidants with low molecular weight such as vitamin C, vitamin E, ubiquinol, carotenoids, and bilirubin. They function in different subcellular compartments depending on their hydrophilic or hydrophobic nature. GSH and vitamin C are potent scavengers of reactive oxygen species, particularly in plasma, cytosol, and other aqueous compartments. In contrast, vitamin E and other hydrophobic antioxidants function predominantly in and around membrane/lipid bilayers.

There is a cooperative mechanism by which free radicals formed in hydrophobic domains are trapped by hydrophilic scavengers in aqueous compartments. For example, vitamin C reacts with vitamin E radicals, thereby regenerating vitamin E. Vitamin C radicals formed in soluble fractions are regenerated to vitamin C by monodehydroascorbate reductase or by spontaneous dismutation. Such synergistic action with lipophilic vitamin E is also seen with other hydrophilic antioxidants, such as cysteine. Thus, in conjunction with vitamin C, cysteine, or other hydrophilic antioxidants, vitamin E effectively scavenges free radicals occurring within lipoproteins and membrane/lipid bilayers of the liver and other tissues (Fig. 19.2). Current topics about vitamin E are described elsewhere (19).

Although the α-form of tocopherol is about ten times more abundant in plants than is its γ-form, only the former is effectively accumulated in the liver. Studies by Arai's group (20) revealed the presence of hepatic-binding protein specific for α-tocopherol. They isolated α-tocopherol transfer protein (α-TTP) from rat liver cytosol, which specifically binds vitamin E and enhances its transfer between membranes. α-TTP also localizes in human liver. The complementary DNA (cDNA) for human α-TTP isolated from a human liver cDNA library predicts 278 amino acids with a molecular mass of 31,749, and the sequence exhibits 94% similarity with rat α-TTP at the amino acid level. The recombinant human α-TTP expressed in *Escherichia coli* exhibits both α-tocopherol transfer activity and cross-reactivity to the anti-(rat α-TTP) monoclonal antibody. Northern blot analysis revealed that human α-TTP is also expressed in the liver. The human and rat α-TTPs show structural similarity with other apparently unrelated lipid-binding/transfer proteins, i.e., retinaldehyde-binding protein present in retina, and yeast SEC14 protein, which possesses phosphatidylinositol-phosphatidylcholine transfer activity. *In situ* hybridization analysis revealed a single α-TTP gene corresponding to the 8q13.1-13.3 region of chromosome 8, which is identical to the locus of a recently described clinical disorder, ataxia with selective vitamin E deficiency.

Patients with isolated vitamin E deficiency have an impaired ability to incorporate α-tocopherol into lipoproteins in the liver and usually have symptoms and signs of spinocerebellar dysfunction before adolescence. The three frame-shift mutations in α-TTP gene were identified. A 744delA mutation accounts for 68% of the mutant alleles

in the 17 families analyzed and appears to have spread in North Africa and Italy. This mutation correlates with a severe phenotype but alters only the C-terminal tenth of the protein. Two other mutations were found in single families. Accumulated evidence suggests that α-TTP is abnormal in these patients. Arai's group (21) studied a patient from an isolated Japanese island who began to have ataxia, dysarthria, and sensory disturbances in the sixth decade of life. The vitamin E concentration in the serum of the patient was low (1.2 mg/mL). Exons of his gene for the α-TTP were analyzed by DNA sequencing. The patient was homozygous for a point mutation that replaces histidine (CAT) with glutamine (CAG) at position 101 of the gene for α-TTP. When expressed in COS-7 cells, the missense mutation produced a functionally defective α-TTP with approximately 11% of the transfer activity of the wild-type protein. Of the 801 island inhabitants examined, 21 were heterozygous for the His101Gln mutation. In all affected subjects, including the patient, this mutation co-segregated with an intron-sequence polymorphism. Heterozygotes were phenotypically normal and had serum vitamin E concentrations that were on average 25% lower than those of normal subjects. Thus, α-TTP is a determinant of serum vitamin E concentrations and an abnormality in this protein causes spinocerebellar dysfunction. The finding of α-TTP gene mutations in the patients substantiates the therapeutic role of vitamin E as a protective agent against neurologic damage in this disease.

Since vitamin C is highly water soluble, this antioxidant functions primarily in cytosol and extracellular fluid. In fact, when plasma was incubated in the presence of radical generating agents, plasma levels of ascorbic acid decreased rapidly (22). Studies using a cytochrome *c* derivative that circulates bound to albumin and, thus, has a prolonged half-life *in vivo*, revealed that significant amounts of ascorbyl radicals are generated in the circulation of normal animals (23,24). These antioxidants function in different subcellular compartments depending on their hydrophilic or hydrophobic nature. There is a cooperative mechanism by which free radicals formed in hydrophobic domains are trapped by hydrophilic scavengers in aqueous compartments (25,26) (Fig. 19.2) (see Chapter 18). The antioxidant activity of bilirubin was initially reported by Bernhard et al. (27). This pigment is as potent as vitamin E in inhibiting the ultraviolet (UV)-induced peroxidation of linoleic acid (28). Bilirubin also inhibits autooxidation of polyunsaturated fatty acids (29). Since hepatocytes have transport systems for bilirubin (see Chapters 20 and 25 and website chapter 🖥 W-16), the circulating bilirubin rapidly undergoes transhepatic transport from plasma to bile. Hence, bilirubin may function as a potent scavenger for reactive oxygen species in plasma, hepatocytes, bile, and the small intestinal lumen. Bernhard et al. suggested that bilirubin may enhance the intestinal absorption of vitamin A and linoleic acid by inhibiting the oxidation of these molecules.

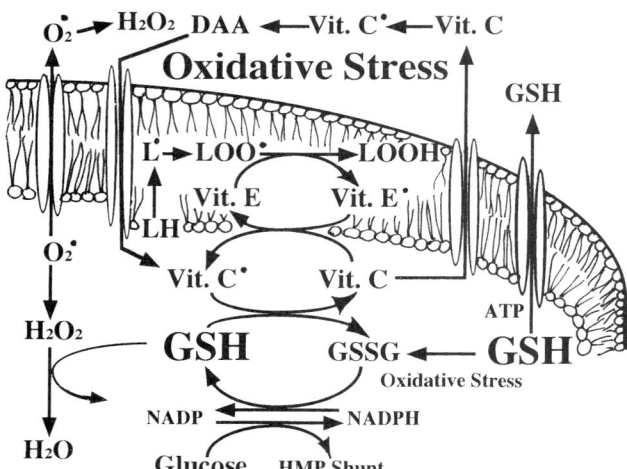

FIGURE 19.2. Radical chain reactions and antioxidant network in membranes and aqueous compartments. *O₂•*, superoxide radical; *LH*, lipids; *L•*, lipid radicals; *LOO•*, peroxy radical; *Vit.E*, vitamin E; *Vit.E•*, vitamin E radical; *Vit.C*, vitamin C; *Vit.C•*, vitamin C radical; *DAA*, dehydroascorbic acid.

When oxidized, bilirubin is converted to stable and water-soluble biliverdin, and excreted in bile without conjugation by glucuronic acid. In the presence of singlet oxygen, bilirubin is degraded to dioxethane and endoperoxide (29). The former is degraded to methylvinylmaleimide and imide dipyrole dialdehyde, whereas the latter is converted to hematinic acid and propentdyopent (30). The rate of bilirubin degradation is enhanced in patients with sepsis or asphyxia. Owing to their relative hydrophobic properties, both conjugated and unconjugated bilirubin circulate, but predominantly the latter bind to albumin. Small amounts of bilirubin also circulate bound to lipoproteins particularly in patients with hypo- and analbuminemia. Thus, plasma bilirubin may function as an antioxidant in the binding sites of albumin and lipoproteins and regions of membrane/lipid bilayers.

Stellate cells (Ito cells or fat-storing cells) contain significantly large amounts of fat and carotenoids; more than 90% of total vitamin A is localized in these cells (see website chapter 🖳 W-20). Although the antioxidant properties of carotenoids have been well documented, the role for stellate cells and retinoids in the metabolism of reactive oxygen species in and around hepatic sinusoids remains to be elucidated.

ANTIOXIDANT ENZYMES

After scavenging reactive oxygen species, some metabolites of low molecular weight antioxidants, such as GSSG and vitamin C and E radicals, are regenerated enzymatically or nonenzymatically, whereas other metabolites of sacrificial scavengers, including bilirubin and uric acid, undergo irreversible degradation. Enzymatic regeneration of the oxidized scavengers may occur principally intracellularly at the expense of GSH, reduced nicotinamide adenine dinucleotide (NADH), or reduced nicotinamide adenine dinucleotide phosphate(NADPH). Under physiologic conditions, the regenerating systems for antioxidants may function sufficiently to maintain their steady-state levels. Since the liver is the main filtering organ for hazardous xenobiotics, high levels of enzymes that metabolize reactive oxygen species (e.g., SOD, catalase, and glutathione peroxidase) are present in the liver (Table 19.1).

Mammalian tissues and cells have three types of SOD isozymes: the first (Cu/Zn-SOD), the homodimer, localizes in cytosol and contains 1 mol of Cu and Zn per mole of monomeric subunit; the second (Mn-SOD), homotetramer, localizes in mitochondrial matrix and contains 1 mol of Mn per subunit; the third (extracellular SOD, EC-SOD), homotetramer, contains 1 mol of Cu and Zn per mole of monomeric subunit and localizes bound to cell surface matrix via its heparin-binding domain. Both Cu/Zn-SOD and Mn-SOD effectively dismutate superoxide radicals and generate hydrogen peroxides by a diffusion-limited

mechanism, whereas the specific activity of EC-SOD is significantly lower than that of other isozymes. The physicochemical properties and catalytic mechanism of Cu/Zn-SOD are well understood (31). Crystallographic analysis of Cu/Zn-SOD suggests that high specific activity of the enzyme (3,000 units/mg) is due, at least in part, to a positively charged lysyl cluster near the active site that drives substrate superoxide anion electrostatically to the Cu-containing catalytic site (32). The specific activity of the enzyme purified from erythrocytes of diabetic patients was significantly lower than that from normal human subjects. Protein chemical analysis suggested that low specific activity of the enzyme from diabetic patients is due to nonenzymatic glycation of lysine residues (Lys^3, Lys^9, Lys^{122}, and Lys^{128}). This observation supports the hypothesis that the positively charged lysyl cluster plays an important role in maintenance of its high catalytic activity. Since mitochondria are highly enriched in Mn-SOD, this enzyme may be the principal one in the dismutation of superoxide radicals within the mitochondrial matrix. Cu/Zn-SOD has been postulated to localize predominantly in cytosol; however, the enzyme also localizes bound to the cytoplasmic surface of mitochondria and peroxisomes. Thus, this isozyme can dismutate superoxide radicals very effectively at the outer surface of these organelles. Such subcellular localization of Cu/Zn-SOD may be important to minimize free radical injury caused by superoxide-dependent reactions in cytosol and nucleus. In this context, mutation of Cu/Zn-SOD has recently been found in patients with familiar amyotrophic lateral sclerosis (32). Interestingly, the affinity of mutant r-SOD to mitochondria and peroxisomes decreased significantly. Thus, changes in subcellular localization of this isozyme may play an important role in the pathogenesis of familiar amyotrophic lateral sclerosis.

Under physiologic conditions, the half-life of the superoxide radical is about 5 seconds. Hence, in compartments with low SOD activity, the superoxide radical is also dismutated nonenzymatically to hydrogen peroxide. Although EC-SOD is localized in plasma and on the vascular endothelial cell surface, total activity of the enzyme in extracellular compartments is low. Thus, nonenzymatic dismutation of superoxide radicals may be important in extracellular compartments with low SOD activity. In fact, some animals, such as rodents, lack this isozyme.

Hydrogen peroxide is relatively stable when compared with other reactive oxygen species, such as superoxide and hydroxyl radicals. Thus, hydrogen peroxide may be more toxic to cultured cells than is superoxide radical (33). However, this need not be the case *in vivo*. Hydrogen peroxide derived from superoxide radicals is further metabolized to water by glutathione peroxidase and catalase. There are two isozymes of glutathione peroxidase inside cells: one is selenium-dependent and the other selenium-independent (34). Both isozymes are highly enriched in human liver. The relative ratio of Se-dependent to -independent enzyme in rat liver is about 2. The Se-independent type of the enzyme is identical with one of the isozyme of glutathione S-transferase (GST 1-1 or YaYa), which catalyzes the conjugation of epoxides and other electrophils with GSH (35). Glutathione S-transferases are a group of isozymes with overlapping specificity whose characteristics have been detailed elsewhere (see website chapters 🖥 W-14 and W-15). The Se-dependent enzyme of the liver is a homotetramer that is synthesized in the cytosol. The amino acid residue at position 45 is catalytically active selenocysteine. Although a major fraction of the enzyme (75%) is localized in the cytoplasmic compartment of hepatocytes, the remainder enters into mitochondria. Hence, conversion of hydrogen peroxide to water occurs in cytosolic and mitochondrial compartments. The substrate is not only hydrogen peroxide but organic peroxides (ROOH) of a lipophylic nature also serve. Selenium deficiency is often associated with cardiomyopathy, liver necrosis, and renal injury. It has been postulated that Se deficiency is the cause of Keshan disease (36). The content of Se in the soil of the Keshan area in China is extremely low, resulting in low Se content in the diet of people living in this area. Patients with Se deficiency show lethal cardiomyopathy. Administration of Se markedly improves the clinical signs of Keshan disease, which suggests that oxidative stress caused by Se-deficiency may underlie the pathogenesis of this disease.

GSH and its redox cycle also play critical roles in catabolizing hydrogen peroxide and other peroxides. In fact, cytotoxicity of hydrogen peroxide increases with low cellular levels of GSH (37). Furthermore, treatment of hepatocytes with L-buthionine sulfoximine, a specific inhibitor of GSH synthase, or 1,3-bis(chloroethyl)-1-nitrosourea, an inhibitor of glutathione reductase, potentiates the cytotoxic effect of hydrogen peroxide.

Since catalase in the liver is localized predominantly in peroxisomes, this enzyme might be the most significant one for degradation of hydrogen peroxide generated in this organelle (see Chapter 18). Hydrogen peroxide is amphipathic and easily penetrates across membrane/lipid bilayers (38). Injury of endothelial cells and hepatocytes caused by hydrogen peroxide was inhibited by erythrocytes, which have high activity of catalase (153,000 units/g Hb). Rao et al. (39) reported that erythrocytes play an important role in preventing cold-storage–induced endothelial cell injury of the liver. Since the protective effect of erythrocytes against hydrogen peroxide-induced cell injury disappeared after treating cells with aminotriazole, an inhibitor of catalase, extracellular hydrogen peroxide can be degraded by intracellular enzyme (40). Hepatic catalase may also function in degrading hydrogen peroxide generated in extraperoxisomal compartments of the liver. The Michaelis' constant (K_m) value of catalase for hydrogen peroxide is much higher than that of glutathione peroxidase. Hence, glutathione peroxidase has been postulated to degrade low levels of hydrogen peroxide physiologically, while catalase might function

when cellular levels of hydrogen peroxide are increased. Consistent with this view are the findings in acatalasemic patients who do not show lethal signs, except for oral gangrene. In Japanese patients with acatalasemia, the defect is inherited as an autosomal-recessive trait (41). Although catalase activity in the heart is only 2% of that in the liver, the enzyme is localized predominantly in peroxisomes and degrades hydrogen peroxide four times more efficiently than does glutathione peroxidase. Cellular levels of catalase and glutathione peroxidase differ from one species to another and show negative correlation; erythrocytes with high glutathione peroxidase activity show low catalase activity, whereas those with low peroxidase activity have high catalase activity. The two enzymes, therefore, appear to compensate for each other in scavenging hydrogen peroxide in intra- and extracellular compartments.

Although reactive oxygen species occur both intracellularly and extracellularly, levels of antioxidants and related enzymes in the former compartments are much higher than those in the latter. Why the metabolism of reactive oxygen species and their scavengers is organized differently in the two compartments is unknown. Oxidative stress, the hepatic circulation, ischemia, and reperfusion-induced liver injury are discussed in website chapter 🖥 W-13 and Chapter 18.

The blood volume circulating through digestive organs comprises about 25% of the cardiac output. Exchange of fluid and solutes between sinusoidal plasma and hepatocytes may be affected by the circulatory status of the liver and metabolic conditions of sinusoidal lining cells. Contraction of sinusoidal endothelial cells and fat-storing Ito cells may decrease the vascular bed in the liver, which could decrease the time and space for interaction of hepatocytes with components in sinusoidal plasma. The hydrostatic pressure of the portal blood is relatively low and, hence, decreases the shear stress for sinusoidal endothelial cells. Presumably because of the circulatory status in the liver, hepatic endothelial cells are able to maintain fenestrae (see Chapter 30 and website chapter 🖥 W-26). Since the size of endothelial fenestrae (about 0.1 um in diameter) is significantly larger than the Stokes' radius of albumin (about 0.014 um) and other plasma proteins, metabolites in sinusoidal plasma interact freely with plasma membranes of hepatocytes. However, sinusoidal endothelial cells and the space of Disse are highly enriched with proteoglycans, such as heparan sulfates. Hence, the functional size of endothelial fenestrae may be considerably smaller than the size observed morphologically. In fact, the concentration of albumin and globulin in hepatic lymph is significantly lower than in sinusoidal plasma, and the ratio of the former to the latter protein in venous plasma (0.7) is lower than in hepatic lymph (0.82). These observations suggest that the transfer of circulating albumin and other plasma proteins to the space of Disse (and to hepatic lymph) may be limited by the sieve plates, particularly when endothelial cells or fenestrae are contracted. Although serotonin induces nitric oxide (NO)-dependent vascular relaxation, it also promotes contraction of endothelial fenestrae (42,43). Serotonin increased portal pressure of an isolated perfused liver of the rat and decreased uptake for albumin-bound cholephilic ligands, such as sulfobromophthalein (44). Thus, endothelial cells and their sieve plates may regulate the extent of interaction of constituents in portal plasma and hepatocytes. In this context, xanthine oxidase induced contraction of fenestrae of cultured hepatic endothelial cells by an SOD-inhibitable mechanism (44). Thus, superoxide or its metabolites could induce contraction of sinusoidal endothelial cells and their fenestrae.

The superoxide radical interacts with NO [endothelium-derived relaxing factor (EDRF)], thereby causing vascular contraction. EDRF is inactivated by superoxide, suggesting that reactive oxygen species may play an important role in regulating the circulatory status of tissues (see website chapter W-32). Although the activities of sinusoidal endothelial cells and Kupffer cells of normal rats to generate reactive oxygen species and NO are relatively low, they increase significantly after treating animals with bacteria (*Propionibacterium acnes*) and endotoxin (45). Thus, such reactive oxygen species as superoxide and NO could also play important roles in the regulation of sinusoidal circulation and hepatic transport across sinusoidal lining cells.

Because NO has high affinity for hemoproteins, it reacts with not only guanylate cyclase but also with other heme proteins, such as mitochondrial electron transfer complexes (see Chapter 39). Thus, the state-3 (ATP-synthesizing state) respiration of mitochondria is inhibited reversibly by NO; cytochrome *c* oxidase (complex IV) is the major site for inhibition (46). The inhibitory effect and EDRF function of NO are enhanced by physiologically low oxygen tensions (47). Thus, cellular production of ATP is regulated pivotally by the coordination of vascular and mitochondrial actions of NO depending on the local concentration of molecular oxygen (48). NO also inhibits ATP synthesis and growth of *E. coli* in an oxygen concentration-dependent manner (49). Thus, a cross-talk of molecular oxygen, superoxide, and NO constitutes a supersystem for the regulation of the circulatory status and energy metabolism and plays a critical role in the defense mechanism against bacterial infection (Fig. 19.3).

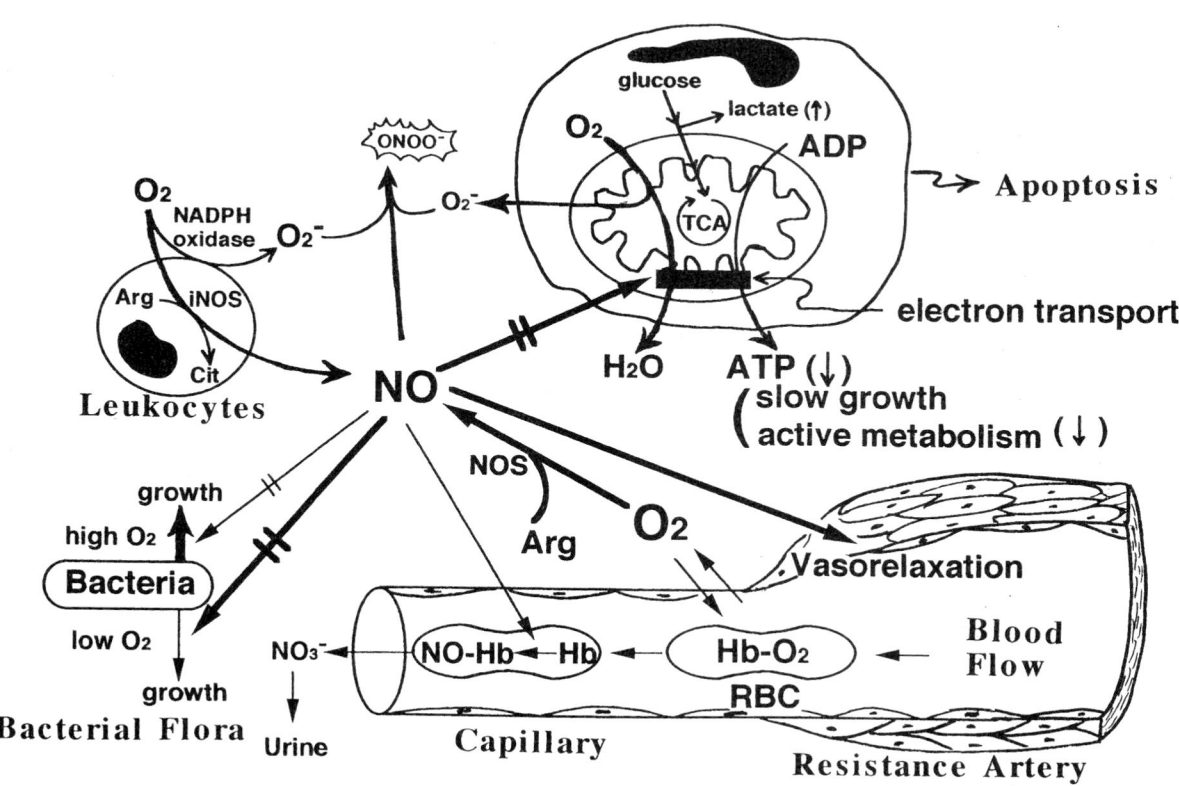

FIGURE 19.3. Supersystem driven by a cross-talk of nitric oxide (*NO*) and oxyradicals regulates circulation, adenosine triphosphate (*ATP*) synthesis, and bacterial growth. NO increases oxygen supply to peripheral tissues by decreasing arterial resistance while it inhibits ATP generation by mitochondria. Biologic activities of NO are enhanced by decreasing local oxygen tensions. Cross-talk of NO, superoxide, and molecular oxygen regulates the circulatory status, mitochondrial ATP generation, and the growth of bacteria. *ADP*, adenosine diphosphate.

ISCHEMIA AND REPERFUSION-INDUCED LIVER INJURY (SEE ALSO CHAPTER 18)

Although liver transplantation is a potential therapy for patients with severe liver injury, a second transplantation of the liver is often required predominantly because of primary nonfunction of a graft. Transient ischemia followed by reperfusion of a tissue also occurs during radical surgical resection. Pathologic metabolites generated during ischemia or reperfusion perturb the circulatory status leading to endothelial cell injury. These changes may underlie the pathogenesis of hepatocellular injury by cold-preservation or postischemic reperfusion of the liver. Kawamoto et al. (50,51) reported that transient occlusion followed by reperfusion of hepatic vessels markedly increased xanthine oxidase activity in plasma of systemic and portal blood. Under such conditions, hepatic circulatory status and transport function for albumin-associated cholephilic ligands were significantly impaired by a mechanism that was inhibited by a long-acting and site-directed SOD derivative that circulates bound to albumin (52,53). Thus, vascular endothelial cells can be impaired by superoxide radicals or related metabolites that are formed during reperfusion (54). Because the mitochondrial electron transport system in ischemic tissues is fully saturated with electrons, molecular oxygen in reperfused blood may undergo one electron reduction by reacting with the released electron to generate superoxide radicals. Since endothelial cells are enriched in xanthine oxidase, the enzyme is also a candidate for generation of superoxide radicals in reperfused liver. Kupffer cells also generate reactive oxygen species particularly when they are primed by endotoxin and various cytokines (see Chapter 30 and 31 and website chapter 🖥 W-26). Thus, cold storage followed by reperfusion of the liver may potentiate the activity of Kupffer cells to generate reactive oxygen species.

Vascular endothelial cells may be injured by reactive oxygen species generated by xanthine oxidase enriched in these cells and/or NADPH-oxidase of leukocytes. Superoxide radicals enhance the adhesion of leukocytes to vascular endothelial cells. Ischemia and reperfusion enhance adhesion of circulating neutrophils to sinusoidal endothelial cells, thereby perturbing the microcirculation in the liver. Hence, activation of leukocytes may also underlie the pathogenesis of reperfusion injury of the liver. Reperfusion injury of the liver and other organs was significantly inhibited by a long-acting and site-directed SOD (50–58). Administration of this SOD derivative markedly inhibited liver injury caused by warm ischemia that followed reperfusion of the graft and improved the survival (59).

Inoue et al. (59–61) developed a fusion gene encoding human Cu/Zn-SOD and a C-terminal heparin-binding domain that has a high affinity for heparan sulfates. When injected intravenously, the fusion SOD binds to heparan sulfates on vascular endothelial cells and hepatic sinusoidal lining cells. The heparin-binding fusion SOD markedly inhibited liver injury caused by ischemia and reperfusion, suggesting that superoxide radicals in and around endothelial cells of hepatic sinusoid play critical roles in its pathogenesis. Thus, site-directed SOD and related enzymes that specifically regulate superoxide metabolism in the region of vascular endothelial cells may have therapeutic potential for decreasing reperfusion injury of the liver and other tissues, and for inhibiting primary nonfunction of a graft. Since reactive oxygen species also underlie the pathogenesis of liver injury, regulation of these hazardous species by site-directed enzymes and antioxidants may also be important.

REFERENCES

1. Arias IM, Jakoby WB, eds. *Glutathione: metabolism and function.* New York: Raven Press, 1976.
2. Sies H, Wendel A, eds. *Functions of glutathione in liver and kidney.* Berlin: Springer–Verlag, 1978.
3. Inoue M. Interorgan metabolism and transport of glutathione and related compounds. In: Kinne R, ed. *Renal biochemistry.* Amsterdam: Elsevier, 1985:225–269.
4. Martensson J, Lai JCK, Meister A. High affinity transport of glutathione is part of a multicomponent system essential for mitochondrial function. *Proc Natl Acad Sci USA* 1990;87:7185–7189.
5. Bellomo G, Vairetti M, Stivala L, et al. Demonstration of nuclear compartmentalization of glutathione in hepatocytes. *Proc Natl Acad Sci USA* 1992;89:4412–4416.
6. Inoue M, Tran T, Kinne R, et al. Rat liver canalicular membrane vesicles: isolation and topological characterization. *J Biol Chem* 1982;258:5183–5188.
7. Bartoli GM, Haeberle D, Sies H. Glutathione efflux from perfused rat liver and its relation to glutathione uptake by the kidney. In: Sies H, Wendel A, eds. *Functions of glutathione in liver and kidney.* Berlin: Springer, 1978:27–31.
8. Sies H, Wahllaender A, Waydhas C. Properties of glutathione disulfide (GSSG) and glutathione S-conjugate release from perfused rat liver. In: Sies H, Wendel A, eds. *Functions of glutathione in liver and kidney.* Berlin: Springer, 1978:120–126.
9. Wahllaender A, Sies H. Glutathione S-conjugate formation from 1-chloro-2,4-dinitrobenzene and biliary S-conjugate excretion in the perfused rat liver. *Eur J Biochem* 1979;96:441–446.
10. Inoue M, Kinne R, Tran T, et al. Glutathione transport across hepatocyte plasma membranes: analysis using isolated rat liver sinusoidal membrane vesicles. *Eur J Biochem* 1984;138:491–495.
11. Inoue M, Kinne R, Tran T, et al. The mechanism of biliary secretion of reduced glutathione: Analysis of transport process in isolated rat-liver canalicular membrane vesicles. *Eur J Biochem* 1983;134:467–471.
12. Inoue M, Akerboom T, Sies H, et al. Biliary transport of glutathione S-conjugate by rat liver canalicular membrane vesicles. *J Biol Chem* 1984;259:4998–5002.
13. Akerboom T, Inoue M, Sies H, et al. Biliary transport of glutathione disulfide studied with isolated rat liver canalicular membrane vesicles. *Eur J Biochem* 1984;141:211–215.
14. Elferink RPJO, Ottenhoff WR, Liefting W, et al. ATP-dependent efflux of GSSG and GS-conjugate from isolated hepatocytes. *Am J Physiol* 1989;258:G699–706.
15. Mikami T, Nozaki Y, Tagaya O. The characters of a new mutant in rats with hyperbilirubinemia syndrome. *Cong Anom* 1986;26:250–251.
16. Nishida T, Hardenbrook C, Gatmaitan Z, et al. ATP-dependent

organic anion transport system in normal and TR⁻ rat liver canalicular membranes. *Am J Physiol* 1992;262:G629–635.

17. Inoue M. Interorgan metabolism of glutathione as the defense mechanism against oxidative stress. In: Sakamoto Y, Higashi T, Taniguchi N, et al., eds. *Glutathione centennial*. New York: Academic Press, 1989:381–394.

18. Hahn R, Wendel A, Floe L. The fate of extracellular glutathione in the rat. *Biochim Biophys Acta* 1978;539:324–337.

19. Packer L, Fuchs J, eds. *Vitamin E in health and disease*. New York: Marcel Dekker, 1993.

20. Arita M, Sato Y, Miyata A, et al. Human alpha-tocopherol transfer protein: cDNA cloning, expression and chromosomal localization. *Biochem J* 1995;306:437–443.

21. Ouahchi K, Arita M, Kayden H, et al. Ataxia with isolated vitamin E deficiency is caused by mutations in the alpha-tocopherol transfer protein. *Nature Genet* 1995;9:141–145.

22. Bendich A, Machlin LJ, Scandurra O, et al. The antioxidant role of vitamin C. *Adv Free Radic Biol Med* 1986;2:419–444.

23. Kunitomo R, Miyauchi Y, Inoue M. Synthesis of a cytochrome C derivative with prolonged in vivo half life and determination of ascorbyl radicals in the circulation of the rat. *J Biol Chem* 1992; 267:8732–8738.

24. Inoue M, Koyama K. In vivo determination of vitamin C radical using long acting cytochrome C- and SOD derivatives. In: Packer L, ed. *Methods of enzymology*, vol. 234. New York: Academic Press, 1993;338–343.

25. Stocker R, Glazer AN, Ames B. Antioxidant activity of albumin-bound bilirubin. *Proc Natl Acad Sci USA* 1979;84:1918–1922.

26. Stocker R, Yamamoto Y, McDonagh AF, et al. Bilirubin is an antioxidant of possible physiological importance. *Science* 1987; 235:1043–1046.

27. Bernhard K, Ritzel G, Steiner KU. Uber eine biologische Bedeutung der Gallenfarbstoffe. Bilirubin und Biliverdin als Antioxidation duer das Vitamin A und die essentiellen Fettsaeuren. *Helv Chim Acta* 1954;37:306–313.

28. Beer H, Bernhard K. Einfluss von Bilirubin und Vitamin E auf die oxidation ungesattigter Fettsaeuren durch UV-Bestrahlung. *Chimia* 1959;13:291–292.

29. Ohnishi S, Yamakawa T, Ogawa J. Photochemical and pathobiological studies on the light-treated newborn infant. In: *XIIIth International Congress of Pediatrics, vol 1. Perinatology*. 1971:373–379.

30. McDonagh AF, Lightner DA. Mechanism of phototherapy of neonatal jaundice. In: Blauer G, Sund H, eds. *Optical properties and structure of tetrapyrroles*. Berlin: Gruyter, 1985:297–310.

31. Steinman HM. Superoxide dismutases: Protein chemistry and structure-function relationships. In: Oberley LW, ed. *Superoxide dismutase*, vol. 1. Boca Raton, FL: CRC Press, 1982:11–68.

32. Rosen DR, Siddique T, Patterson D, et al. Mutations in the cytosolic Cu/Zn-superoxide dismutase gene associated with familial amyotrophic lateral sclerosis. *Nature* 1993;362:59–62.

33. Schraufstatter IU, Hinshaw DB, Hyslop PA, et al. Oxidant injury of cells: DNA strand-breaks activate polyadenosine diphosphate-ribose polymerase and lead to depletion of nicotinamide adenine dinucleotide. *J Clin Invest* 1986;77:1312–1320.

34. Floe L, Guenzler WA, Schock HH. Glutathione peroxidase: a selenoenzyme. *FEBS Lett* 1973;32:132–134.

35. Maruyama H, Inoue M, Arias IM, et al. Ligandins or glutathione S-transferases: a family of multifunctional proteins in the rat. In: Larsson A, Orrenius S, Holmgren A, et al., eds. New York: Raven Press, 1983:89–98.

36. Keshan Disease Research Group. Observations on effect of sodium selenite in prevention of Keshan disease. *Chin Med J* 1979;92:471–476.

37. Suttorp N, Toepfer W, Roka L. Antioxidant defense mechanisms of endothelial cells: Glutathione redox cycle versus catalase. *Am J Physiol* 1986;251:C671–680.

38. Starke PE, Farber JL. Endogenous defense against the cytotoxicity of hydrogen peroxide in cultured hepatocytes. *J Biol Chem* 1985;260:86–92.

39. Rao PN, Walsh TR, Makowka L, et al. Inhibition of free radical generation and improved survival by protection of the hepatic microvascular endothelium by targeted erythrocytes in orthotopic rat liver transplantation. *Transplantation* 1990;49:1055–1059.

40. Inoue M, Watanabe N. Reactive oxygen metabolism and erythrocytes. In: Inoue M, ed. *Pathology of reactive oxygen species: bridging basic science and clinical medicine*. Tokyo: Japan Scientific Society Press, 1992:127–144.

41. Ogata M, Sadamoto M, Takahara S. On the minimal catalytic activity in Japanese acatalasemic blood. *Proc Jpn Acad* 1966;42:828.

42. Oda M, Nakamura M, Watanabe N, et al. Some dynamic aspects of the hepatic microcirculation: demonstration of sinusoidal endothelial fenestrae as a possible regulatory factor. In: Tsuchiya, M, ed. *Intravital observation of organ microcirculation*. Amsterdam: Excerpta Medica, 1987:105–138.

43. Gatmaitan Z, Akamatsu K, Inoue M, et al. Superoxide dismutase prevents hepatic endothelial fenestral contraction and decrease in the Disse's space in response to superoxide anions. *Hepatology* 1989;10:623.

44. Kawamoto S, Inoue M. Changes in the circulatory status and transport function of the liver induced by reactive oxygen species. *Am J Physiol* 1995;268:G47–G53.

45. Kida T, Kuroki T, Kobayashi K, et al. Role of vascular nitric oxide synthase in endotoxin shock of *Propionibacterium acnes*-sensitized rats. *Arch Biochem Biophys* 1994;312:135–141.

46. Nishikawa M, Sato EF, Utsumi K, et al. Oxygen-dependent regulation of energy metabolism in ascites tumor cells by nitric oxide. *Cancer Res* 1996;56:4535–4540.

47. Takehara Y, Kanno T, Yoshioka T, et al. Oxygen-dependent regulation of mitochondrial energy metabolism by nitric oxide. *Arch Biochem Biophys* 1995;323:27–32.

48. Inoue M, Nishikawa M, Sato E, et al. Cross-talk of NO, superoxide and molecular oxygen, a majesty of aerobic life. *Free Radic Res* 1999;31:251–260.

49. Yu H, Sato EF, Nagata K, et al. Oxygen-dependent regulation of the respiration and growth of *E. coli* by nitric oxide. *FEBS Lett* 1997;409:161–165.

50. Kawamoto S, Inoue M, Tashiro S, et al. Inhibition of ischemia and reflow-induced liver injury by an SOD derivative that circulates bound to albumin. *Arch Biochem Biophys* 1990;277:160–165.

51. Kawamoto S, Tashiro S, Miyauchi Y, et al. Mechanism for enterohepatic injury caused by circulatory disturbance of hepatic vessels in the rat. *Proc Soc Exp Biol Med* 1990;198:629–635.

52. Ogino T, Inoue M, Ando Y, et al. Chemical modification of superoxide dismutase: extension of plasma half life of the enzyme through reversible binding to the circulating albumin. *Int J Peptide Protein Res* 1988;32:153–159.

53. Inoue M, Ebashi I, Watanabe N, et al. Synthesis of a SOD derivative that circulates bound to albumin and accumulates in tissues whose pH is decreased. *Biochemistry* 1989;28:6619–6624.

54. Inoue M. Targeting SOD by gene and protein engineering. In: Packer L, ed. *Methods of enzymology*, vol 233. New York: Academic Press, 1993:212–221.

55. Watanabe N, Inoue M, Morino Y. Inhibition of postischemic reperfusion arrhythmias by an SOD derivative that circulated bound to albumin with prolonged in vivo half-life. *Biochem Pharmacol* 1989;38:3477–3483.

56. Hirota M, Inoue M, Ando Y, et al. Inhibition of stress-induced gastric mucosal injury by a long acting superoxide dismutase that circulates bound to albumin. *Arch Biochem Biophys* 1990;280:269–273.

57. Takeda Y, Hashimot H, Kosaka F, et al. Albumin binding superoxide dismutase with prolonged half life reduces reperfusion brain injury. *Am J Physiol* 1993;264:H1708–1716.

58. Hasuoka H, Sakagami K, Takasu S, et al. A new slow delivery type superoxide dismutase improves the survival of swine warm ischemia-damaged transplanted liver. *Transplantation* 1990;50: 164–165.

59. Inoue M, Watanabe N, Sasaki J, et al. Inhibition of oxygen toxicity by targeting superoxide dismutase to endothelial cell surface. *FEBS Lett* 1990;269:89–92.

60. Inoue M, Watanabe N, Sasaki J, et al. Expression of a hybrid Cu,Zn-type superoxide dismutase which has high affinity for heparin-like proteoglycans on vascular endothelial cells. *J Biol Chem* 1991;266:16409–16414.

61. Nakazono K, Watanabe N, Matsuno K, et al. Does superoxide underlie the pathogenesis of hypertension? *Proc Natl Acad Sci USA* 1991;88:10045–10048.

The Liver: Biology and Pathobiology, Fourth Edition, edited by I. M. Arias, J. L. Boyer, F. V. Chisari, N. Fausto, D. Schachter, and D. A. Shafritz. Lippincott Williams & Wilkins, Philadelphia © 2001.

20

DISORDERS OF BILIRUBIN METABOLISM

NAMITA ROY CHOWDHURY
IRWIN M. ARIAS
ALLAN W. WOLKOFF
JAYANTA ROY CHOWDHURY

Bilirubin is the end product of degradation of the heme moiety of hemoproteins. Hemoglobin, derived from senescent erythrocytes, is the major source of bilirubin. Significant fractions are also derived from other hemoproteins of liver and other organs. Historically, hyperbilirubinemia has attracted the attention of clinicians as a marker of liver dys-

N. Roy Chowdhury: Department of Medicine and Molecular Genetics, Albert Einstein College of Medicine, Bronx, New York 10461.

I. M. Arias: Departments of Physiology and Medicine, Tufts University School of Medicine, Boston, Massachusetts 02111.

A. W. Wolkoff: Departments of Medicine and Anatomy and Structural Biology, Albert Einstein College of Medicine, Bronx, New York 10461-1602.

J. Roy Chowdhury: Department of Medicine and Molecular Genetics, Albert Einstein College of Medicine Liver Center; Department of Medicine, Jack D. Weiler Hospital of Albert Einstein College of Medicine, Bronx, New York 10461.

function. Subsequently, the studies of bilirubin chemistry, synthesis, transport, metabolism, distribution, and excretion have provided important insights into the transport, metabolism, and excretion of biologically important organic anions, particularly those with limited aqueous solubility.

Bilirubin is potentially toxic, but is normally rendered harmless by tight binding to albumin, and rapid detoxification and excretion by the liver. Patients with very high levels of unconjugated hyperbilirubinemia are at risk for bilirubin encephalopathy (kernicterus). Kernicterus is found in some cases of severe neonatal jaundice and in inherited disorders associated with severe unconjugated hyperbilirubinemia. This chapter provides a brief review of bilirubin metabolism and its inherited disorders.

FORMATION OF BILIRUBIN

Sources of Bilirubin

The breakdown of hemoglobin, other hemoproteins, and free heme generates 250 to 400 mg of bilirubin daily in humans, approximately 80% of which is derived from the hemoglobin (1). Intravenously administered radiolabeled porphyrin precursors (glycine or δ-aminolevulinic acid) are incorporated into bile pigments in two peaks (2). The "early-labeled" peak appears within 72 hours. The initial component of this peak is derived mainly from hepatic hemoproteins such as cytochromes, catalase, peroxidase, and tryptophan pyrrolase, and a small, rapidly turning over pool of free heme. The slower phase of the early-labeled peak is derived from both erythroid and nonerythroid sources, and is enhanced in conditions associated with "ineffective erythropoiesis," e.g., congenital dyserythropoietic anemias, megaloblastic anemias, iron-deficiency anemia, erythropoietic porphyria and lead poisoning (3), and in accelerated erythropoiesis (4). A "late-labeled" peak appears at approximately 110 days in humans and 50 days in rats, and represents the contribution from the hemoglobin of senescent erythrocytes.

Enzymatic Mechanism of Bilirubin Formation

Heme (ferroprotoporphyrin IX) (Fig. 20.1) is cleaved by selective oxidation of the α-methene bridge, catalyzed by microsomal heme oxygenase. This reaction requires three molecules of O_2 and a reducing agent, such as reduced

nicotinamide adenine dinucleotide phosphate (NADPH), and results in the formation of the linear tetrapyrrole, biliverdin, and 1 mol of CO. The iron molecule is released (5). Three forms of heme oxygenase have been identified (6). Heme oxygenase 1 is ubiquitous and is a major inducible stress-related protein. Heme oxygenase 1 synthesis is upregulated by heme (7). In contrast, heme oxygenase 2 is a constitutive protein, expressed mainly in the brain and the testis. Heme oxygenase 3 has very low catalytic activity and may function mainly as a heme-binding protein. The products of heme oxygenase, biliverdin (which is subsequently reduced to bilirubin), and CO have significant physiologic effects. CO, a potent vasodilator, regulates the vascular tone in the liver and in other organs, such as the heart, under conditions of stress. Biliverdin and bilirubin are potent antioxidants, and may protect tissues under oxidative stress (6,8).

In most mammals, biliverdin is reduced to bilirubin by the action of biliverdin reductases. The physiologic advantage of this process is not clear, because bilirubin requires energy-consuming metabolic modification for excretion in bile. The stronger antioxidant activity of bilirubin may be particularly important during the neonatal period, when concentrations of other antioxidants are low in body fluids. Biliverdin reductases are cytosolic enzymes that require reduced nicotinamide adenine dinucleotide (NADH) or NADPH for activity (9).

Quantification of Bilirubin Production

At a steady-state condition of blood hemoglobin level, the rate of bilirubin production equals the rate of heme synthesis. Therefore, the heme synthesis rate can be estimated from the rate of bilirubin production. In humans, bilirubin production can be quantified from the turnover of intravenously administered radioisotopically labeled bilirubin. Plasma bilirubin clearance (the fraction of plasma from which bilirubin is irreversibly extracted) is proportional to the reciprocal of the area under the radiobilirubin disappearance curve (10). Bilirubin removal is calculated from the product of plasma bilirubin concentration and clearance. When plasma bilirubin concentrations remain constant, removal of bilirubin equals the amount of newly synthesized bilirubin entering the plasma pool. Alternatively, bilirubin formation can also be quantified from carbon monoxide production. Following rebreathing in a closed system, CO production is calculated from the CO concentration in the breathing chamber and/or the increment in blood carboxyhemoglobin saturation (11). CO production exceeds plasma bilirubin turnover by 12% to 18%, because a fraction of bilirubin produced in the liver is excreted into bile without appearing in serum. A small fraction of the CO may be formed by intestinal bacteria (12).

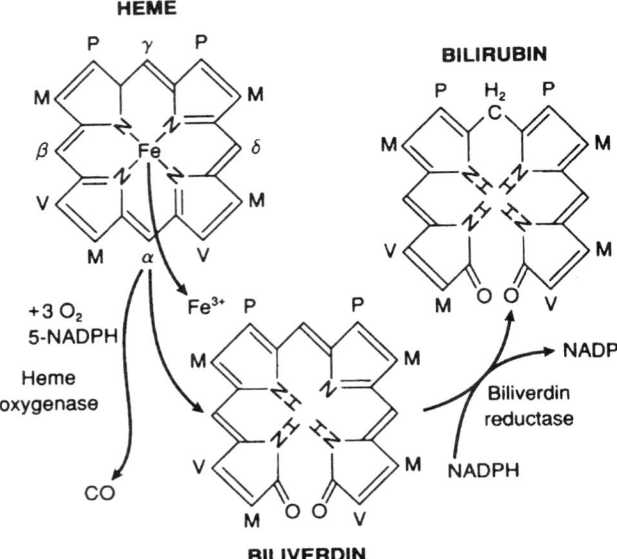

FIGURE 20.1. Mechanism of heme ring opening and subsequent reduction of biliverdin to bilirubin.

Inhibition of Bilirubin Production

Nonmetabolized "dead-end" inhibitors of heme oxygenase, such as tin-protoporphyrin or tin-mesoporphyrin, inhibit heme oxygenase activity (13). Injection of tin-mesoporphyrin in neonates reduces serum bilirubin levels by 76% (14).

CHEMISTRY OF BILIRUBIN

The systemic name of bilirubin IXα is 1,8-dioxo-1,3,6,7-tetramethyl-2,8-divinylbiladiene-a,c-dipropionic acid (15, 16). The linear tetrapyrrole structure of bilirubin was solved by Fischer and Plieninger (17). X-ray diffraction studies of crystalline bilirubin has revealed that the propionic acid side chains of bilirubin are internally hydrogen-bonded to the pyrrolic and lactam sites on the opposite half of the molecule (18). The molecule takes the form of a "ridge tile" in which the two dipyrrolic halves of the molecule lie in two different planes with an interplanar angle of 98 to 100 degrees (Fig. 20.2). The integrity of the hydrogen-bonded structure requires the interpyrrolic bridges at the 5 and 15 position of bilirubin to be in *trans-* or Z configuration. The hydrogen-bonded structure of bilirubin explains many of its physicochemical properties. As both the carboxylic groups, all four NH groups, and the two lactam oxygens are engaged by hydrogen bonding, bilirubin is insoluble in water. The hydrogen bonds "bury" the central methene bridge, so that the molecule reacts very slowly with diazo reagents. *In vivo*, the hydrogen bonds are disrupted by esterification of the propionic acid carboxyl group with glucuronic acid (see below). Because of this disruption, conjugated bilirubin reacts rapidly with diazo reagents ("direct" van den Bergh reaction). Addition of methanol, ethanol, 6 M urea, or dimethyl sulfoxide to plasma disrupts the hydrogen bonds of bilirubin, rendering the molecule water soluble and making the central methene bridge readily accessible, so that both conjugated and unconjugated bilirubin react rapidly with diazo reagents ("total" van den Bergh reaction) (19).

Absorption Spectra and Fluorescence

The main absorption band of unconjugated bilirubin IXα is at 450 to 474 nm in most organic solvents. Although pure bilirubin does not fluoresce, when dissolved in detergents, albumin solution, or alkaline methanol, an intense fluorescence is observed at 510 to 530 nm. Fluorescence determination has been utilized for rapid quantification of blood bilirubin concentrations and the unsaturated bilirubin-binding capacity of albumin (see below).

Effect of Light

The "Z" (trans) configuration of the 5 and/or 15 carbon bridges of bilirubin is changed to the "E" (cis) configuration upon exposure to light. The resulting ZE, EZ, or EE isomers lack internal hydrogen bonds, are more polar than bilirubin IXα-ZZ, and can be excreted in bile without conjugation (20). The vinyl substituent in the endovinyl half of bilirubin IXα-EZ is slowly cyclized with the methyl substituent on the internal pyrrole ring, forming the stable structural isomer, E-cyclobilirubin, which is quantitatively important during phototherapy for neonatal jaundice (21). In the presence of light and oxygen, a fraction of the bilirubin molecules is also converted to colorless fragments (22). A small amount of biliverdin is also formed (22).

QUANTIFICATION OF BILIRUBIN IN BODY FLUIDS

Bile pigments are quantified as native or derivatized tetrapyrroles, or after conversion to azoderivatives. Total bilirubin can also be quantified indirectly by quantification of the intensity of yellow discoloration of the skin. Conversion to azodipyrroles by reaction with diazo reagents is used commonly for determination of serum bilirubin levels for clinical purposes. Electrophilic attack on the central bridge splits bilirubin into two diazotized azodipyrrole molecules.

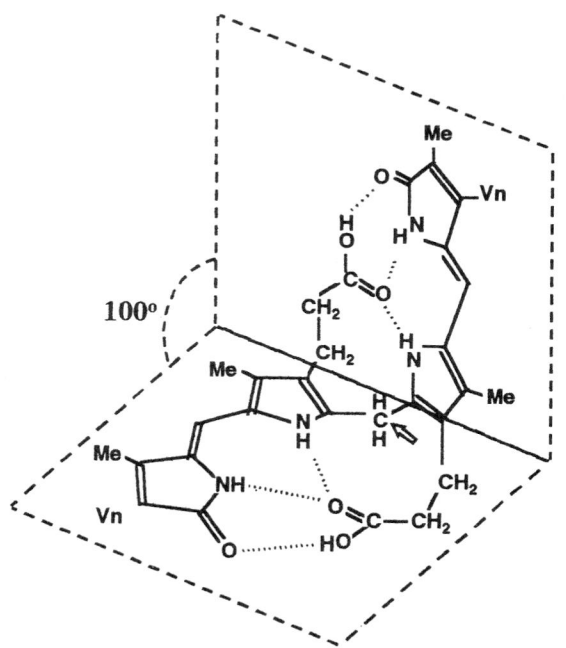

FIGURE 20.2. X-ray crystallographic structure of bilirubin showing a ridge-tile configuration caused by internal hydrogen bonding of the propionic acid carboxyls to the amino groups and the lactam oxygen of the pyrrolenone rings of the opposite half of the molecule. The bonds between the pyrrolenone rings A and B and C and D are in the Z (*trans*) configuration.

As discussed above, conjugated bilirubin reacts rapidly in this system (direct fraction). In the presence of accelerators, both unconjugated and conjugated bilirubin react rapidly (total bilirubin). Unconjugated bilirubin (the "indirect" fraction) is calculated by subtracting the direct fraction from total bilirubin. As 10% to 15% of unconjugated bilirubin may give the direct diazo reaction, this method slightly overestimates conjugated bilirubin. The irreversibly albumin-bound fraction of serum bilirubin, which is formed in the serum of patients with prolonged conjugated hyperbilirubinemia, also exhibits direct diazo reaction (23). For more accurate quantification and for separating the different sugar conjugates, the intact bilirubin tetrapyrroles can be separated by thin-layer or high-performance liquid chromatography (24–26). Bilirubin mono- and diconjugates can be converted to methyl esters by alkaline methanolysis prior to separation (27), but because the sugar groups are cleaved off, this method does not permit identification of specific conjugates.

For repeated bilirubin measurements, particularly in jaundiced infants, special clinical methods have been devised. Measurement of the yellow color of the skin by analysis of reflected light provides a noninvasive approach for estimating serum bilirubin (28), which has been verified in a large study (29). Two slide tests are available for determination of total bilirubin, and the unconjugated, conjugated, and irreversibly protein-bound fractions. Fluorescence characteristics of bilirubin have been utilized for determining total bilirubin, albumin-bound bilirubin, and reserve bilirubin-binding capacity from as little as 0.1 mL of whole blood (30).

About 4% of bilirubin in normal plasma is conjugated, but the clinical diazo-based methods overexpress this fraction (see above). In hemolytic jaundice, there is a proportionate increase of plasma unconjugated and conjugated bilirubin. In contrast, in inherited disorders of bilirubin conjugation, the conjugated bilirubin is absent or reduced in proportion. In biliary obstruction or hepatocellular diseases, both conjugated and unconjugated bilirubin accumulate in plasma. Bilirubin is present in exudates and other albumin containing body fluids and binds to the elastic tissue of skin and sclera. Heme in subcutaneous hematomas is sequentially converted to biliverdin and bilirubin, resulting in a transition from green to yellow discoloration. Because of tight binding to albumin, unconjugated bilirubin is not excreted in urine in the absence of albuminuria, but conjugated bilirubin, which is less strongly bound to albumin, appears in urine. Bilirubin is present in normal human bile predominantly as diglucuronide, with unconjugated bilirubin accounting for only 1% to 4% of the pigments (see below).

TOXICITY OF BILIRUBIN

The toxic effect of bilirubin on the brain of neonates has been known since antiquity. Yellow discoloration of basal ganglia is termed kernicterus. Bilirubin exhibits a wide range of toxic effects in cell culture systems and in cell homogenates. Bilirubin inhibits DNA synthesis in a mouse neuroblastoma cell line (31), and uncouples oxidative phosphorylation and inhibits adenosine triphosphatase (ATPase) activity of brain mitochondria (32). In mutant rats (Gunn strain) with congenital nonhemolytic hyperbilirubinemia (see below), bilirubin inhibited RNA and protein synthesis, and carbohydrate metabolism in brain (33). In a cell-free system, bilirubin inhibited Ca^{2+}-activated, phospholipid-dependent, protein kinase (protein kinase C) activity and $3',5'$-cyclic adenosine monophosphate (cAMP)-dependent protein kinase activity (34), which may be relevant in the mechanism of its toxicity. Albumin binding inhibits toxic effects of bilirubin, both *in vitro* and *in vivo*.

At serum unconjugated bilirubin concentrations over 20 mg/dL, newborn babies are at risk of kernicterus. However, kernicterus can occur at lower concentrations (35). Serum albumin concentrations, pH, and substances that compete for albumin binding are important in the pathogenesis of bilirubin encephalopathy (36). The immaturity of the blood–brain barrier in neonates is often held responsible for increased susceptibility of neonates to kernicterus. Tight junctions between capillary endothelial cells and foot processes of astroglial cells that restrict the exchange of water-soluble substances and proteins between blood and brain are the anatomic constituents of the blood–brain barrier (37). In addition, specific transport processes for ions, water, and nutrients from plasma to brain may provide a functional blood–brain barrier. However, there is little evidence to support the concept of immaturity of the blood–brain barrier in the neonate. The opening of the blood–brain barrier is expected to permit the entrance of albumin-bound bilirubin into the brain, which should not result in increased bilirubin toxicity. The entry of the non–albumin-bound (free) fraction of bilirubin into the brain is independent of the intactness of the blood–brain barrier. Damaged and edematous brain may bind bilirubin avidly, and therefore be unable to clear it rapidly, increasing the susceptibility to bilirubin encephalopathy (38).

DISPOSITION OF BILIRUBIN

Hepatocellular disposition of bilirubin requires several specific physiologic mechanisms, including transport to the hepatocytes from the major sites of production, efficient internalization into the hepatocyte, enzyme-catalyzed conjugation with glucuronic acid, active transport into the bile canaliculus, and degradation in the intestinal tract. These steps are summarized in Fig. 20.3, and briefly discussed below.

Bilirubin Transport in Plasma

Bilirubin is tightly but reversibly bound to plasma albumin. Albumin binding keeps bilirubin in solution and transports the pigment to the liver. Unconjugated bilirubin is bound

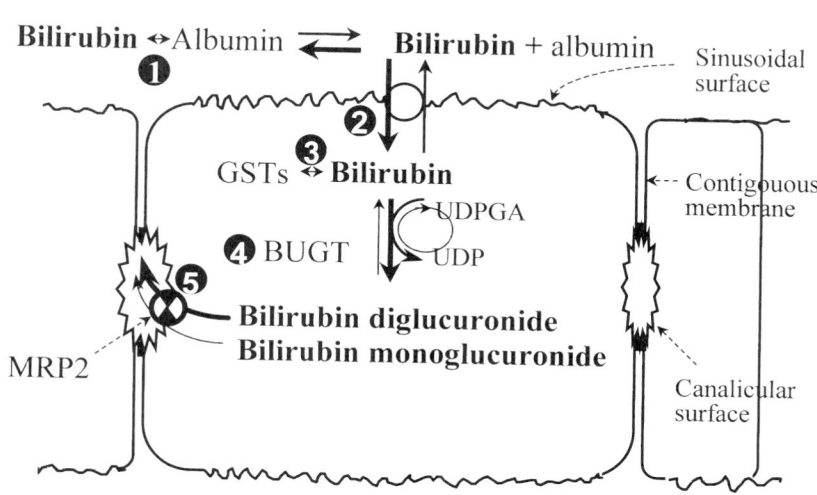

FIGURE 20.3. Summary of hepatic metabolism of bilirubin. Bilirubin is strongly bound to albumin in the circulation (*1*). At the sinusoidal surface of the hepatocyte, this complex dissociates, and bilirubin enters hepatocytes by facilitated diffusion (*2*). This process is non-adenosine triphosphate (ATP)-dependent and bidirectional. Within the hepatocyte, bilirubin binds to a group of cytosolic proteins, mainly to glutathione-S-transferases (*GSTs*) (*3*). GST binding inhibits the efflux of bilirubin from the cell, thereby increasing the net uptake. A specific form of uridine diphosphoglucuronate glucuronosyltransferase (UGT) (*BUGT*, also termed UGT1A1), located in the endoplasmic reticulum, catalyzes the transfer of the glucuronic acid moiety from UDP-glucuronic acid (*UDPGA*) to bilirubin, forming bilirubin diglucuronide and monoglucuronide (*4*). Glucuronidation is necessary for efficient excretion of bilirubin in bile (*5*). Canalicular excretion of bilirubin and other organic anions (except most bile acids) is primarily an energy-dependent process, mediated by the ATP-utilizing transporter multidrug resistance-related protein (*MRP2*), also termed canalicular multispecific organic anion transporter (cMOAT).

tightly to albumin and, therefore, is not excreted in urine, except during albuminuria. Conjugated bilirubin is bound less tightly to albumin, and the unbound fraction is excreted in the urine. During prolonged conjugated hyperbilirubinemia, a fraction of the pigment becomes irreversibly bound to albumin. This fraction, termed deltabilirubin, is not excreted in the bile or urine and disappears slowly, reflecting the long half-life of albumin (23).

Albumin binding protects against the toxic effects of bilirubin. A small unbound fraction of bilirubin is thought to be responsible for its toxicity (39). Normally, the molar concentration of albumin (500 to 700 μmol/L) exceeds that of bilirubin (3 to 17 μmol/L). However, during neonatal jaundice, in patients with Crigler–Najjar syndrome, the molar ratio of unconjugated bilirubin to albumin may exceed 1. Reduction of serum albumin levels during inflammatory states, chronic malnutrition, or liver diseases may accentuate bilirubin toxicity. Sulfonamides, antiinflammatory drugs, and cholecystographic contrast media displace bilirubin competitively from albumin and increase the risk of kernicterus in jaundiced infants (40). Binding of short chain fatty acids to albumin causes conformational changes, decreasing bilirubin binding.

Because of the pathophysiologic importance of the unbound fraction of unconjugated bilirubin, ultrafiltration, ultracentrifugation, gel chromatography, affinity chromatography on albumin agarose polymers, dialysis, and electrophoresis have been used to separate free from bound bilirubin. Unbound bilirubin is rapidly destroyed by treatment with H_2O_2 and horseradish peroxidase, as compared with bound bilirubin. Binding of bilirubin to albumin induces bilirubin fluorescence, and quenches the protein fluorescence. This phenomenon has been utilized for differentiating free from albumin-bound bilirubin.

Bilirubin Uptake by the Hepatocytes

At the sinusoidal surface of the hepatocyte (Fig. 20.3), bilirubin dissociates from albumin and is taken up by the hepatocyte by facilitated diffusion. The transport requires the presence of inorganic anions, such as Cl^-. A family of organic anion transport proteins (oatp) has been identified. One oatp isoform, oatp-1, mediates Na^+-independent taurocholate transport and is associated with HCO_3^- exchange (41). However, the role of oatp family of proteins in bilirubin transport has not been directly established (see Chapter 7).

Hepatocellular Storage of Bilirubin

Within the hepatocyte, bilirubin is kept in solution by binding to cytosolic proteins, which were originally designated Y and Z. The Y group of proteins, which constitute 5% of the liver cytosol, binds various drugs, hormones, organic anions, a cortisol metabolite, and azo-dye carcinogens, and was termed "ligandin" (42). Subsequently, ligandin was found to be a family of proteins, identical to the α class of glutathione-S-transferases (GST) in the rat liver (43). There are corresponding proteins in human hepatocytes as well. Binding to GSTs increases the net uptake of bilirubin by reducing efflux from the hepatocyte (Fig. 20.3). GST binding may inhibit the toxicity of bilirubin by preventing its nonspecific diffusion into specific subcellular compartments. For example, binding to GSTs prevents the inhibition of mitochondrial respiration by bilirubin *in vitro* (44).

Conjugation of Bilirubin

Conversion to bilirubin diglucuronide or monoglucuronide by esterification of both or one of the propionic acid carboxyl groups is critical for efficient excretion of bilirubin across the bile canaliculus (Fig. 20.3). Bilirubin diglucuronide accounts for about 80% of pigments excreted in normal bile (24–26). Bilirubin monoglucuronide constitutes about 10% of the pigments, but in states of partial deficiency of hepatic bilirubin glucuronidation the proportion of bilirubin monoglucuronide increases (see Crigler–Najjar Syndrome Type 2 and Gilbert Syndrome, below). Smaller amounts of glucosyl and xylosyl conjugates are also found.

Bilirubin-Uridine Diphosphoglucuronate Glucuronosyltransferase

Glucuronidation of bilirubin is catalyzed by a specific isoform of uridine diphosphoglucuronate glucuronosyltransferase (UGT). UGTs comprise a family of enzymes that are integral components of the endoplasmic reticulum of various cell types (45). UGTs mediate the conversion of a wide variety of exogenous and endogenous toxic metabolites to less bioreactive, polar compounds that are readily eliminated in bile or urine. Based on the degree of homology of the messenger RNA (mRNA) sequences, UGTs have been categorized into several families and subfamilies (46). Only one of these UGT isoforms, currently termed UGT1A1, contributes significantly to bilirubin glucuronidation (47). The gene that expresses bilirubin-UGT (UGT1A1) is termed *UGT1A* (48). The *UGT1A* locus contains four consecutive exons (exons 2 to 5) at the 3′ end that are used in all mRNAs expressed from this locus, and encode the identical upidine diphospho (UDP)-glucuronic acid-binding carboxy-terminal domain of the UGT isoforms (Fig. 20.4). Upstream to these four common-region exons is a series of unique exons, each preceded by a separate promoter, only one of which is utilized in specific UGT mRNAs. The unique exon encodes the variable aglycone-binding N-terminal domain of individual UGT isoforms. Depending on which promoter is used, transcripts of various lengths are generated. The unique exon, located at the 5′ end of the transcript, is spliced to exon 2, and the intervening sequence is spliced out. Within the *UGT1A* locus, genes encoding individual isoforms are named after the unique exon that is utilized in the specific mRNA. Bilirubin-UGT mRNA, which consists of the first unique region exon of the *UGT1A* locus (plus exons 2 to 5), is named *UGT1A1* according to this terminology.

The presence of a separate promoter upstream to each unique region exon (Fig. 20.4) permits differential expression of individual UGT isoforms during development (49) and enzyme induction (50). UGT1A1 develops after birth (49) and is induced by phenobarbital and clofibrate (51). Treatment of rats with triiodothyronine markedly reduces UGT activity toward bilirubin, whereas the activity toward 4-nitrophenol is increased (50).

Canalicular Excretion of Conjugated Bilirubin (See Chapters 24, 25, and 26)

Conjugated bilirubin is excreted across the bile canaliculus against a concentration gradient, which can be as high as 150-fold. The energy for the uphill transport of bilirubin is provided by an adenosine triphosphate (ATP)-dependent system in the canalicular membranes that is specific for non–bile-acid organic anions, including bilirubin and other glucuronides, and glutathione conjugates (52,53). A canalicular membrane protein, termed canalicular multispecific organic anion transporter (cMOAT) or multidrug resistance-related protein (MRP2) (54), mediates the ATP-dependent canalicular organic anion transport.

Fate of Bilirubin in the Gastrointestinal Tract

Conjugated bilirubin is not substantially absorbed from the gastrointestinal tract. When there is enhanced excretion of unconjugated bilirubin into the intestine, e.g., during phototherapy for neonatal jaundice or Crigler–Najjar syndrome, absorption of unconjugated bilirubin from the intestine may be clinically significant (55). Milk inhibits intestinal absorption of unconjugated bilirubin, but such inhibition is less with human milk than with infant milk formula. Intestinal bacteria degrade bilirubin into a series of urobilinogen and related products (56). Most of the urobilinogen reabsorbed from the intestine is excreted in bile, but a small fraction is excreted in urine. Absence of urobilinogen in stool and urine indicates complete obstruction of the bile duct. In liver disease and states of increased bilirubin production, urinary urobilinogen excretion is increased. Urobilinogen is colorless; its oxidation product, urobilin, contributes to the color of normal urine and stool.

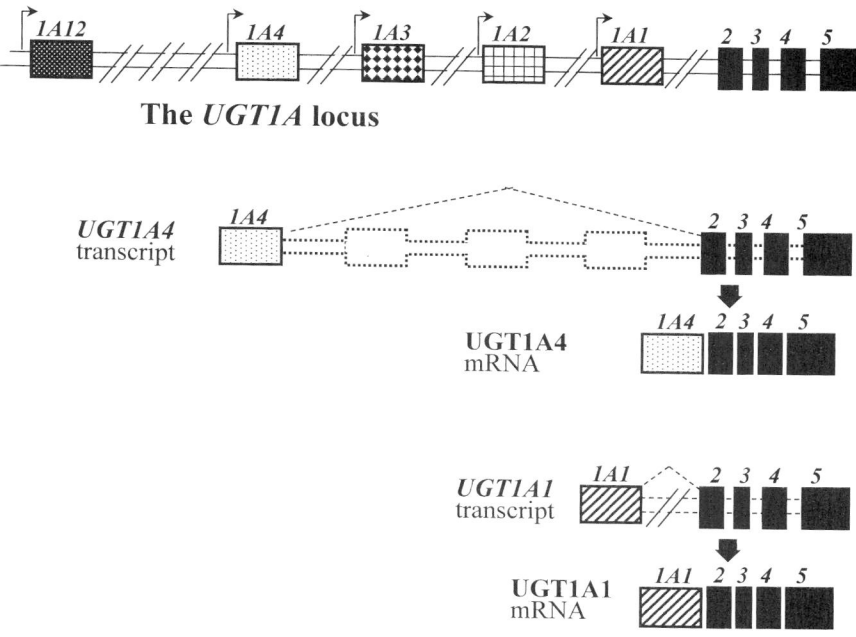

FIGURE 20.4. Schematic representation of the human UGT1A locus, located at 2q37. This locus comprises a number of genes of the UGT1A family that include bilirubin-UGT. Exons 2, 3, 4, and 5, located at the 3′ end of UGT1A, encode the identical carboxyl terminal domains of all UGT1A isoforms expressed from this locus. Upstream to these "common region" exons are a series of "unique exons" (*exons 1A1 through 1A12*), each of which encodes the variable amino terminal domain of a different UGT1A isoform. Each unique region exon is preceded by a separate promoter region (*arrows*), permitting independent regulation of gene expression. Transcription may start from any of the promoters, producing transcripts of varying lengths, two examples of which are shown in the figure. The unique exon located at the 5′ end of the primary transcript is spliced to the 5′ end of exon 2, and other unique region exons present in the transcript (shown in *dotted lines*) are spliced out. Genes belonging to the *UGT1A* locus are named according the unique exon utilized in the processed mRNA. Thus, when the transcription starts at exon 1A4 (**upper** transcript in the figure), the mRNA for UGT1A4 is generated after splicing. This gene, which consists of exon 1A4 plus the common region exons 2 to 5, is termed *UGT1A4*, and the expressed enzyme is termed UGT1A4. Similarly, if the transcription starts at exon 1A1 (**lower** transcript in the figure), an mRNA consisting of exon 1A1 plus exons 2 to 5 is generated. According to the current system of terminology, this gene is named *UGT1A1*, and the expressed isoform is termed UGT1A1. UGT1A1 is the only isoform that contributes significantly to bilirubin glucuronidation in humans. This structure predicts that disorders of bilirubin glucuronidation resulting from genetic lesions within exon 1A1 should affect UGT activity toward bilirubin, but other UGT1A isoforms should be normal. In contrast, mutations of exons 2 to 5 should affect all isoforms of the UGT1A family.

Alternative Routes of Bilirubin Elimination

In the absence of bilirubin glucuronidation, a small fraction of bilirubin is excreted as hydroxylated products. Induction of a specific isoform of microsomal P-450s by administration of 2,3,7,8-tetrachlorodibenzo-p-dioxin (TCDD) in UGT1A1-deficient Gunn rats resulted in a sevenfold increase in the fractional turnover of bilirubin and reduction of the bilirubin pool (57). A mitochondrial bilirubin oxidase in liver (58) and other tissues may catalyze oxidative degradation of bilirubin.

During intrahepatic or extrahepatic cholestasis, the plasma conjugated bilirubin concentrations increase. In total biliary obstruction, renal excretion becomes the major pathway of bilirubin excretion. Renal excretion of conjugated bilirubin depends on glomerular filtration of the non–protein-bound fraction of conjugated bilirubin.

Antioxidant Property of Bilirubin

Although bilirubin has been thought of conventionally as a waste product with little utility, antioxidant activity of bilirubin may serve an important tissue protective role. Both unconjugated (59) and conjugated (60) bilirubin inhibit lipid peroxidation. The tissue cytoprotective role of heme oxygenase in various tissues may be mediated by biliverdin and bilirubin.

DISORDERS OF BILIRUBIN METABOLISM RESULTING IN UNCONJUGATED HYPERBILIRUBINEMIA

Hepatic transport of bilirubin involves four distinct but probably interrelated stages: (a) uptake from the circulation; (b) intracellular binding or storage; (c) conjugation, largely with glucuronic acid; and (d) biliary excretion. Abnormalities in any of these processes may result in hyperbilirubinemia. Complex clinical disorders, such as hepatitis or cirrhosis, may affect multiple processes. In several inherited disorders, the transfer of bilirubin from blood to bile is disrupted at a specific step. Study of these disorders has permitted better understanding of bilirubin metabolism in health and disease. Each disorder is characterized by varied degrees of hyperbilirubinemia of the unconjugated or conjugated type.

Neonatal Jaundice

By adult standards, every newborn baby has increased serum bilirubin levels, and about half of all neonates become clinically jaundiced during the first 5 days of life. Serum bilirubin is predominantly unconjugated. Exaggeration of this "physiologic jaundice" exposes the baby to the risk of kernicterus (see Toxicity of Bilirubin, above). In 16% of newborns, maximal serum bilirubin concentrations equal or exceed 10 mg/dL, and in 5% serum bilirubin levels are above 15 mg/dL. In the normal full-term neonates, serum bilirubin peaks at approximately 72 hours and subsequently declines to normal adult levels in 7 to 10 days. Physiologic jaundice of the newborn results from a combination of increased bilirubin production and immaturity of the bilirubin disposal mechanisms of the liver. Bilirubin production rate is high in newborns, because of the increased early-labeled peak from erythroid and nonerythroid sources, and decreased erythrocyte half-life (61). Net hepatic bilirubin uptake is low in neonates because of low hepatocellular ligandin levels (62). Delayed closure of the ductus venosus may permit the bilirubin-rich portal blood to bypass the liver. Low caloric intake may also reduce hepatic bilirubin clearance. UGT activity toward bilirubin is low in the liver of the newborn and takes about 10 days to mature to adult levels (63). Deficiency of UGT activity may be prolonged and exaggerated in some inherited disorders due to inhibitory factor(s) in maternal milk or serum (see Gilbert syndrome, below). A variant TATAA element within the promoter region of *UGT1A1* has been found to be associated with Gilbert syndrome (64) (see Gilbert syndrome, below). Presence of this variant promoter reduces the expression of bilirubin-UGT (UGT1A1) and may accentuate and prolong neonatal jaundice (65).

Plasma bilirubin concentrations tend to be higher in breast-fed infants than in formula-fed babies. The hyperbilirubinemia resolves on discontinuation of breast-feeding, and kernicterus occurs only rarely (66). Maternal milk jaundice is associated with an inhibitor of UGT activity in maternal milk but not maternal serum (67). Free fatty acids resulting from the digestion of fat by lipase secreted in the milk of some women are thought to inhibit hepatic bilirubin-UGT activity (68). Intestinal absorption of unconjugated bilirubin is high in neonates. Bilirubin absorption may be higher in breast-fed infants than in formula-fed babies.

Inhibitory factors present in the plasma of some mothers may delay the maturation of bilirubin-UGT (69). Peak serum bilirubin concentrations of 8.9 to 65 mg/dL are reached within 7 days. This condition, termed Lucey–Driscoll syndrome, is distinguished from maternal milk jaundice by earlier onset of hyperbilirubinemia, a more severe and protracted course, and occasional kernicterus.

In the great majority of cases, neonatal hyperbilirubinemia is innocuous. But vigilance is needed for the occasional case in which severe neonatal jaundice can expose the newborn to the risk of kernicterus. Although plasma bilirubin levels of 20 mg/dL or higher are considered dangerous, bilirubin encephalopathy may occur at lower concentrations (see Toxicity of Bilirubin, above). Phototherapy is the most common treatment used. In severe cases exchange transfusion is employed to reduce serum bilirubin levels rapidly. Inhibition of heme oxygenase activity by the administration of tin-mesoporphyrin at birth has been shown to prevent the development of significant levels of neonatal jaundice, thereby abrogating the need for phototherapy or exchange transfusion.

Bilirubin Overproduction

Bilirubin overproduction results in unconjugated hyperbilirubinemia, which rarely exceeds 3 to 4 mg/dL in the absence of hepatobiliary dysfunction. Bilirubin overproduction occurs commonly in hemolytic conditions and during resolution of large hematomas. Ineffective erythropoiesis occurs in thalassemia, pernicious anemia, and some rare hereditary anemias, termed congenital dyserythropoietic anemias (70). In addition to unconjugated bilirubin, a small amount of conjugated bilirubin may accumulate in the serum (~4% of total bilirubin), probably because of diffusion out of the hepatocyte. This does not necessarily indicate that the rate of bilirubin production has exceeded the hepatic excretory transport maximum for conjugated bilirubin.

Crigler–Najjar Syndrome Type 1

Crigler–Najjar syndrome type I is a rare disorder, characterized by severe lifelong nonhemolytic unconjugated hyperbilirubinemia (71) (Table 20.1). Hepatic bilirubin-UGT activity is absent or nearly so. Without treatment, the majority of patients used to die of kernicterus during the first 18 months of life. Exceptional patients survived beyond puberty, but succumbed to bilirubin encephalopathy in young adult life (72,73). With the routine use of phototherapy and intermittent plasmapheresis during crises, survival until puberty is usual, but the risk of bilirubin encephalopathy increases at this age (74). Orthotopic or auxiliary liver transplantation cures the disease.

TABLE 20.1. CHARACTERISTICS OF INHERITED UNCONJUGATED HYPERBILIRUBINEMIA

	Crigler–Najjar Syndrome Type 1	Crigler–Najjar Syndrome Type 2	Gilbert Syndrome
Liver function tests other than serum bilirubin and liver histology	Normal	Normal	Normal
Serum bilirubin concentrations	20–50 mg/dL (340–850 μM)	7–20 mg/dL (120–340 μM)	Normal to 5 mg/dL (<85 μM)
Pigments excreted in bile	Small amounts of unconjugated bilirubin and only traces of bilirubin glucuronides	Reduced proportion of bilirubin diglucuronide	Reduced proportion of bilirubin diglucuronide
Hepatic bilirubin-UGT activity	Virtually absent	Markedly reduced but detectable	Reduced to about 30% of normal
Effect of phenobarbital administration	No significant reduction of serum bilirubin levels	Reduction of serum bilirubin levels by >25%	Normalization of serum bilirubin
Inheritance	Autosomal recessive	Autosomal recessive	Autosomal recessive
Molecular basis	Genetic lesions within the coding region or at splice sites of *UGT1A1*	Point mutations within the coding region of *UGT1A1*	Insertion of a TA dinucleotide within the TATAA element of *UGT1A1*[a]
Prevalence	Rare (<1:1,000,000)	Rare (<1:1,000,000)	Phenotype in ~4% of the population; among Caucasians and Africans, ~9% are homozygous for the genotype (less common in Japan)
Prognosis	Kernicterus, unless vigorously treated; currently, liver transplantation is the only curative treatment	Kernicterus is uncommon, but has been reported	No encephalopathy; increased intensity of neonatal jaundice; toxicity of some drugs may be increased
Animal model	Gunn rat	—	Bolivian subpopulation of squirrel monkeys

[a]Some mutations of the coding region of UGT1A1 may be associated with serum bilirubin levels that overlap with the range seen in Gilbert syndrome (Table 20.3).
UGT, uridine-diphosphoglucuronate glucuronosyl-transferase.

Laboratory test results in Crigler–Najjar syndrome type 1 are normal except for the serum bilirubin levels, which are usually 20 to 25 mg/dL, but may increase during intercurrent illness to as high as 50 mg/dL (75). Serum bilirubin is unconjugated and there is no bilirubinuria. There is no evidence of hemolysis. As the canalicular excretion process is normal, oral cholecystography visualizes the gallbladder. There is an increased incidence of pigment gallstones, probably because of increased concentrations of unconjugated bilirubin in bile, resulting from phototherapy. Liver histology is normal except for the presence of "pigment plugs" in bile canaliculi.

As UGT1A1 (bilirubin-UGT1) is the only isoform that contributes significantly to bilirubin metabolism (47), genetic lesions within the coding region of the *UGT1A1* gene can abolish hepatic bilirubin glucuronidation, causing Crigler–Najjar syndrome type 1. Since the initial description of the molecular basis of Crigler–Najjar syndrome in 1992 (48,76) numerous mutations, deletions, and insertions in any of the five exons of UGT1A1 have been shown to cause the disease (77–89) (Table 20.2). In addition to exonic lesions, mutations of the splice donor or splice acceptor sites within the intronic sequences can cause inappropriate splicing of the transcript, resulting in the loss of UGT1A1 activity. These molecular lesions have been

reviewed recently (90). As in all rare recessively inherited disorders, known or unknown consanguinity is common, but not always found (91). Crigler–Najjar syndrome is found in all races. As many different mutations can cause the disease, no single mutation is common in any race. An exception to this is found among the Amish and Mennonite communities of Pennsylvania (92), where the disease is relatively common and all patients have the same mutation, reflecting a strong founder effect. In patients with genetic lesions within the unique exon 1, only UGT1A1 activity is abnormal, but when the mutation affects one of the common region exons (exons 2 to 5), all UGT1A group of isoforms are expected to be abnormal.

The differential diagnosis includes Crigler–Najjar syndrome type 2, with or without coexisting hemolysis. Although serum bilirubin levels are relatively lower in Crigler–Najjar syndrome type 2, the ranges overlap in the two disorders. In most cases of Crigler–Najjar syndrome type 2, the serum bilirubin concentrations are reduced by more than 25% after phenobarbital administration (60 to 120 mg for 14 days), which differentiates it from Crigler–Najjar syndrome type 1 (75). Chromatographic analysis of pigments in bile collected from the duodenum through a perorally placed duodenal catheter or an upper gastrointestinal endoscope provides rapid differentiation of the two conditions. In

TABLE 20.2. GENETIC LESIONS OF *UGT1A1* THAT ABOLISH BILIRUBIN–UGT ACTIVITY (CRIGLER–NAJJAR SYNDROME TYPE 1)

Site of Lesion	Nucleic Acid Alteration	Predicted Mutation of UGT1A1	Activity	Reference
Exon 1	Del C,T at nt 120,121, respectively	Truncated (frameshift)	Inactive	79
Exon 1	Ins 4 bp after codon 80	Truncation (frameshift)	Inactive	80
Exon 1	Ins T after codon 158/del codon 170	Truncated (frameshift)/del of phenylalanine	Inactive/inactive	81
				82
Exon 1	Del of codon 170	Del phenylalanine	Inactive	81–83
Exon 1/exon 2	T529C/del nt 879–892	C177R/truncated (frameshift)	Inactive/inactive	83
Exon 1	G826T	G276R	Inactive	83
Exon 1/exon 3	A835T/C1069T	B279Y/Q357X	ND/inactive	76,83,84
Exon 1	C840A	C280X	Inactive	85
Intron 1	Splice donor, G→C	Truncated	Inactive	86
Exon 2	Skipping of exon 2	Truncated	Inactive	83
Exon 2/exon 4	C872T/A1282G	A291V/K426E	Inactive	84
Exon 2	T880A and del 881–893	Truncated (frameshift)	Inactive	78,83
Exon 2	G923A	G308E	Inactive	84,87
Exon 2	C991T	Q331X	Inactive	77
Exon 3/exon 4	G1005A/G1102A	W335X/A368T	Inactive	84
Exon 3	nt: C1006T	R336W/N	Inactive	88
Exon 3	C1021T	R341X	Inactive	89
Exon 3	C1069T	Q357X	Inactive	76,83,84
Exon 3/exon 4	C1069T/G1201C	Q357X/A401P	Inactive	76,83,84
Exon 3	A1070G	Q357R	Inactive	84
Exon 3/exon 4	C1081T/CC1159,1160GT	Q361X/P387R	Inactive/inactive	79
Intron 3/exon 1	Splice acceptor site, A→G/nt C145T	Truncated protein/Q49X	Inactive	86
Exon 4	C1124T	S376F	Inactive	77,83,87
Exon 4	C1143G	S381R	Inactive	84
Exon 4	CC1159,1160GT	P387R	Inactive	79
Exon 4	G1201C	A401P	Inactive	84
Exon 4/exon 5	G1201C/A1308T	A401P/K437X	Inactive	84

bp, base pair; nt, nucleotide; del, deletion; ins, insertion; N, normal; ND, not determined. Note: A slash separating two mutations indicates that the patient was a compound heterozygote for two different mutations.

Crigler–Najjar syndrome type 1, bilirubin glucuronides are virtually absent in bile, whereas significant amounts of bilirubin conjugates are found in Crigler–Najjar syndrome type 2, although the proportion of bilirubin diglucuronide is reduced (see below). Liver biopsy is not needed for diagnosis, unless a coexisting liver disease is suspected. If a biopsy is performed, UGT activity toward bilirubin is virtually undetectable. The diagnosis can be made also by genetic analysis of DNA extracted from blood, buccal scrapings, or other tissue. The five exons and the flanking intronic sequences are amplified by polymerase chain reaction and the nucleotide sequences are determined (76). If a previously uncharacterized mutation is found, the mutation can be generated in an expression plasmid by site-directed mutagenesis, and its effect can be determined after transfection of the plasmid into COS cells (47). Genetic analysis permits identification of heterozygous carriers and prenatal diagnosis based on chorionic villus sampling or aminocentesis (93).

Animal Model

A mutant strain of Wistar rats, termed Gunn rats (94,95), manifests nonhemolytic unconjugated hyperbilirubinemia due to a lack of bilirubin-UGT activity. The jaundice is inherited as an autosomal trait. The Gunn rat is the only experimental animal that develops kernicterus spontaneously. Much of the knowledge of cellular and biochemical mechanisms of bilirubin encephalopathy has been gained from studies on Gunn rats. The molecular basis of UGT1A1 deficiency in this strain is the deletion of a guanosine base in the common region exon 4. Consequently, in addition to UGT1A1, other enzymes of the UGT1A group are also abnormal.

Treatment

Treatment is aimed at reduction of serum bilirubin levels. Because there is hardly any residual bilirubin-UGT activity, enzyme-inducing agents, such as phenobarbital, are ineffective in Crigler–Najjar syndrome type 1 (75). Phototherapy is the routine treatment. An array of 140-W fluorescent lamps is used for 8 to 12 hours a day with the eyes shielded. After puberty, phototherapy becomes less effective because of skin thickening, pigmentation, and decreased surface area in relation to body mass. Phototherapy converts bilirubin IXα-ZZ into geometric and structural isomers that are excreted in bile without conjugation (see above). A portion of the unconjugated bilirubin excreted in bile is reabsorbed in the small intestine. Oral administration of agar, cholestyramine, or calcium salts inhibits bilirubin reabsorption, thereby slightly enhancing the effect of phototherapy. Plasmapheresis can be used to reduce serum bilirubin concentrations rapidly during crisis, although the effect is short-lived (96). Orthotopic or auxiliary liver transplantation is the only curative therapy available at this time (97). Because of the associated risk of liver transplantation and the need for lifelong immunosuppression, alternative experimental therapies are being explored. Hepatocyte transplantation by infusion into the portal vein through a percutaneously placed portal venous catheter has reduced the serum bilirubin level significantly in one patient (98,99), but the optimum number of cells that should be transplanted for this disease is not known clearly. Immunosuppression is needed for prevention of allograft rejection. Gene therapy methods using recombinant retrovirus, adenovirus, and SV40, as well as nonviral vectors are being explored in studies on Gunn rats. Recently, site-directed gene repair has been used to reduce serum bilirubin levels in Gunn rats. These methods have been reviewed recently (100) and are also described in Chapter 62.

Crigler–Najjar Syndrome Type 2 (Arias Syndrome)

In this variant of Crigler–Najjar syndrome, serum bilirubin concentrations usually range from 7 to 20 mg/dL, the prognosis is much less severe, and serum bilirubin levels are usually reduced by over 25% after administration of bilirubin-

UGT inducing agents, such as phenobarbital (101). Serum bilirubin levels may be as high as 40 mg/dL during fasting (102) or intercurrent illness (103). The bile contains significant amounts of bilirubin glucuronides (Table 20.1). Bilirubin encephalopathy is unusual, but has been reported (102,103). In normal bile, over 90% of the conjugated bilirubin is bilirubin diglucuronide. In Crigler–Najjar syndrome type 2, the major pigment is bilirubin monoglucuronide (103,104). The liver has markedly reduced bilirubin-UGT activity (103).

Crigler–Najjar syndrome type 2 occurs in families (101). There is no sex predilection. The inheritance is autosomal recessive. As in Crigler–Najjar syndrome type I, the disease is caused by mutations of one of the five exons that encode bilirubin-UGT (UGT1A1) (91). However, in Crigler–Najjar syndrome type 2, the genetic lesions are always point mutations that result in the substitution of a single amino acid that markedly reduces, but does not abolish, bilirubin-UGT activity (Table 20.3) (105–115). In Table 20.3, we have classified all published mutations of the *UGT1A1* coding region that result in incomplete deficiency of bilirubin glucuronidating activity as in Crigler–Najjar syndrome type 2. Although in most of these cases serum bilirubin concentrations are clearly consistent with Crigler–Najjar syndrome type 2, some point mutations, described in Japanese individuals, cause serum bilirubin levels that overlap with those seen in Gilbert syndrome (see Gilbert syndrome, below). Based on the serum bilirubin levels, some of the latter cases have been reported in the literature by some Japanese investigators as Gilbert syndrome (106–109,115). Such semantic difficulty in correlating genetic diagnosis with the nomenclature that had been developed before the discovery of molecular

TABLE 20.3. MUTATIONS WITHIN THE CODING REGION OF *UGT1A1* THAT REDUCE, BUT DO NOT ABOLISH BILIRUBIN–UGT ACTIVITY

Site of Mutation	Nucleic Acid Mutation	Predicted Amino Acid Substitution	Activity	Reference
Exon 1	T44G	L15R	Reduced activity	105
Exon 1	G211A[a]	G71R	Reduced activity	106–108
Exon 1	G211A/N	G71R/N	Reduced activity	107,108
Exon 1/exon 5	Double homozygote for G211A and T1456G	G71R and Y486D	Reduced activity[a]	109
Exon 1	T395C	L132P/N	Reduced activity[a]	108
Exon 1	T524A	L175Q	Reduced activity	83
Exon 1/exon 2	T524A/del of nt 973	L175Q/truncated (frameshift)	Reduced activity; truncated—inactive	83
Exon 1	T625C	R209W	Reduced activity	83,111
Exon 1	C686A	P229Q/N	Reduced activity[a]	107
Exon 2	T881C	I294T	Reduced activity	88
Exon 2	A992G	Q331R	Reduced activity	112
Exon 2	C991T	Q331X	Reduced activity[a]	113
Exon 4	C1099G	R367G	Reduced activity[a]	107,108
Exon 5	A1391C	Z464A	Reduced activity	114
Exon 5	T1456G	Y486D	Reduced activity	107,115

[a]These patients had serum bilirubin levels that overlap with the range seen in some patients with Gilbert syndrome, and have been reported in the literature as Gilbert syndrome.
UGT, uridine-diphosphoglucuronate glucuronosyl-transferase.

bases of these conditions is not unexpected. We propose that reduction of UGT1A1 activity, resulting from any structural mutation of *UGT1A1*, should be classified as Crigler–Najjar syndrome type 2, and that due to a promoter abnormality should be classified as Gilbert syndrome (see below).

Gilbert Syndrome

Gilbert syndrome, also known as "constitutional hepatic dysfunction" or "familial nonhemolytic jaundice" (116), is characterized by mild, chronic, and unconjugated hyperbilirubinemia (Table 20.1). Familial occurrence is common, but not always found. The syndrome is often diagnosed in young adults, usually males, who present with mild, predominantly unconjugated hyperbilirubinemia. Serum bilirubin levels may fluctuate from normal to 3 mg/dL, and increase during fasting or intercurrent illness. Occasional patients complain of fatigue and abdominal discomfort, which are probably manifestations of anxiety. Other than icterus, physical examination and routine laboratory tests are normal. Percutaneous liver biopsy, which is not required for diagnosis, when performed, shows normal liver histology, except for a nonspecific accumulation of lipofuscin pigment in the centrilobular zones. Hepatic bilirubin-UGT activity is reduced to approximately 30% of normal. A minority of patients exhibit reduced hepatic uptake of bilirubin and other organic anions (117). Whether such uptake defects are related pathophysiologically to Gilbert syndrome or are merely coincidental is unknown. A 48-hour fast exaggerates the unconjugated hyperbilirubinemia of Gilbert syndrome (118). Serum bilirubin levels also increase in normal individuals and in patients with liver diseases upon fasting. Therefore, the fasting test is of limited diagnostic value. Intravenous injection of nicotinic acid also increases serum bilirubin levels in Gilbert syndrome (119). However, it does not clearly separate patients with Gilbert syndrome from normal subjects or those with hepatobiliary disease. As splenectomy abolishes nicotinic acid-induced hyperbilirubinemia (119), the effect of nicotinic acid may be based on increased erythrocyte fragility and enhanced splenic heme oxygenase activity, leading to increased bilirubin formation.

Molecular Mechanism

The normal TATAA element within the promoter region upstream to exon 1 of *UGT1A1* has the sequence A[TA]$_6$TAA. A variant TATAA box, which contains a longer dinucleotide repeat, A[TA]$_7$TAA, has been found to be associated with Gilbert syndrome (120). Subjects of Caucasian, black, or Asian Indian origin, who have a clinical diagnosis of Gilbert syndrome, have been found to be homozygous for the variant TATAA element, which reduces the expression of the structurally normal UGT1A1. This fits with the definition of autosomal-recessive type of inheritance. However, all subjects with this genotype do not exhibit abnormally high bilirubin levels, which also depend on other contributory factors, including the rate of bilirubin production. For example, Gilbert syndrome is diagnosed clinically much more commonly in males, although the variant promoter is equally distributed in both genders, probably because of a higher daily production of bilirubin in males. Approximately 9% of the general population in Europe and the United States are homozygous for the Gilbert type promoter (gene frequency 0.3). The incidence of this genotype may be lower in Japan. Some mutations in the structural region of *UGT1A1* have been reported to result in levels of hyperbilirubinemia that are consistent with the diagnosis of Gilbert syndrome (106–109,115). These mutations are listed in Table 20.3 (see Crigler–Najjar Syndrome Type 2, above).

Because of the very high incidence of the Gilbert-type promoter, some heterozygous carriers of Crigler–Najjar syndromes type 1 or 2 mutations have the variant TATAA box on the structurally normal allele. The consequent reduction of expression of the only structurally normal allele can reduce the hepatic UGT1A1 activity to a level that may increase serum bilirubin levels to a range compatible with the clinical diagnosis of Crigler–Najjar syndrome type 2. This explains the frequent finding of intermediate levels of hyperbilirubinemia in the family members of patients with Crigler–Najjar syndrome types 1 and 2.

Although Gilbert syndrome is considered innocuous, the diagnosis is important to avoid confusion with other liver diseases and unnecessary investigations. Gilbert syndrome is diagnosed in individuals with mild unconjugated hyperbilirubinemia without evidence of hemolysis or elevation of liver enzymes. Although hemolysis is not a part of the syndrome, coexistent clinical or subclinical hemolysis may increase the bilirubin load, thereby exacerbating the hyperbilirubinemia and bringing the patient to the attention of the physician. When necessary, the diagnosis can be established by analysis of pigments in duodenal juice. The reduced hepatic bilirubin-UGT activity is reflected by a reduction of bilirubin diglucuronide to monoglucuronide ratio in bile (104). Normally, bilirubin monoglucuronide accounts for 10% or less of all forms of bilirubin excreted in bile. In Gilbert syndrome the percentage increases to 14% to 34%. Genetic analysis of DNA extracted from blood leukocytes or any other tissue can aid in the diagnosis.

Animal Model

The Bolivian population of squirrel monkeys (*Saimiri siureus*) has a higher serum unconjugated bilirubin levels and a greater degree of increase upon fasting than does a closely related Brazilian population of the species (121). The Bolivian monkeys have slower plasma clearance of intravenously administered bilirubin, a lower level of hepatic bilirubin-UGT activity, and an increased bilirubin monoglucuronide to diglucuronide ratio in bile. In these respects, the Bolivian squirrel monkeys are a model of human Gilbert syndrome. Fasting hyperbilirubinemia is rapidly reversed by oral or intravenous administration of carbohydrates, but not by lipid administration.

DISORDERS OF BILIRUBIN METABOLISM THAT RESULT IN PREDOMINANTLY CONJUGATED HYPERBILIRUBINEMIA

Conjugated bilirubin may accumulate in plasma because of "leakage" from the liver cells, as in hepatocellular diseases, such as hepatitis, or from disordered canalicular excretion or biliary obstruction. In all such cases, both conjugated and unconjugated bilirubin accumulate in plasma. Rapid advances in molecular genetic studies have revealed the mechanism of several disorders of the hepatocyte that can, directly or indirectly, lead to the accumulation of conjugated bilirubin in plasma. These include Dubin–Johnson syndrome, three types of progressive intrahepatic cholestasis, and benign recurrent intrahepatic cholestasis. Progressive familial intrahepatic cholestasis syndromes have been discussed in Chapter 26. The molecular basis of Rotor syndrome remains unknown. In addition to the hepatocellular excretory abnormalities, developmental anomalies of bile ductules can cause cholestasis. The genetic mechanism of one of these disorders, Alagille syndrome, has been discovered.

Dubin–Johnson Syndrome

Dubin–Johnson syndrome is characterized by conjugated hyperbilirubinemia and black pigmentation of the liver, in the absence of other abnormalities of clinicochemical tests for liver dysfunction, including serum alanine and aspartate aminotransferase, alkaline phosphatase, γ-glutamyltranspeptidase, and albumin levels (122–124) (Table 20.4). Dubin–Johnson syndrome is rare except in Jews of Middle Eastern origin, in whom the incidence is 1 in 1,300 (124). In Middle Eastern Jews, Dubin–Johnson syndrome is associated with clotting factor VII deficiency, but this linkage is not tight. Occasionally, patients complain of vague abdominal discomfort and some have hepatosplenomegaly. In most cases, however, the patients are asymptomatic.

Serum bile acid levels are normal and pruritus is absent (125). Serum bilirubin levels are usually between 2 and 5 mg/dL, but may be normal at times and may be as high as 20 to 25 mg/dL during intercurrent illness, use of oral contraceptives, and pregnancy (125). Fifty percent or more of total serum bilirubin is conjugated and bilirubinuria is frequently found. Continuous retention of bilirubin glucuronides in plasma results in the formation of irreversible adducts of bilirubin with plasma proteins, particularly albumin (δ-bilirubin), which is not excreted in urine or bile and gives a direct van den Bergh reaction.

Organic Anion Excretion

Canalicular excretion of many organic anions, other than bile acids, is defective in Dubin–Johnson syndrome. These anions include bilirubin, bromosulfophthalein (BSP), dibromosulfophthalein (DBSP), indocyanin green (ICG), and ^{125}I-labeled rose Bengal. In most patients, following an intravenous injection of BSP there is normal initial plasma disappearance of the dye, so that the concentration is normal or mildly elevated 45 minutes after the injection. How-

TABLE 20.4. INHERITED DISORDERS CAUSING RETENTION OF BOTH CONJUGATED AND UNCONJUGATED BILIRUBIN

	Dubin–Johnson Syndrome	Rotor Syndrome
Serum bilirubin	Predominantly conjugated, usually 50–85 μM, can be as high as 340 μM	Predominantly conjugated, usually 50–100 μM, occasionally as high as 340 μM
Routine liver function tests	Normal except for hyperbilirubinemia	Normal except for hyperbilirubinemia
Serum bile salt levels	Normal	Normal
Plasma bromsulfophthalein (BSP) retention	Normal at 45 min; secondary rise at 90 min	Elevated; but no secondary rise at 90 min
Plasma BSP clearance	T_{max} is very low; storage is normal	Both T_{max} and storage are reduced
Oral cholecystogram	Usually does not visualize the gallbladder	Usually visualizes the gallbladder
Urinary coproporphyrin excretion pattern	Total—normal; >80% as coproporphyrin I	Total—elevated; ~50–75% coproporphyrin I
Appearance of liver	Grossly black	Normal
Histology of liver	Dark pigments, predominantly in centrilobular areas; otherwise normal	Normal, no increase in pigmentation
Mode of inheritance	Autosomal recessive	Autosomal recessive
Prevalence	Rare (except in Middle Eastern Jews: 1 in 1,300 births)	Rare
Prognosis	Benign	Benign
Animal model	Mutant TR⁻ rats/mutant Corriedale sheep/golden lion Tamarin monkey	None

ever, 90 minutes after the injection, there is a secondary rise because of the reflux of glutathione-conjugated BSP from the liver cell into the circulation prior to excretion by the hepatocytes (126,127). A similar secondary rise has been described following intravenous administration of unconjugated bilirubin. However, such secondary rise can also occur in other cholestatic disorders. Because of the organic anion excretion defect, oral cholecystographic contrast dyes do not visualize the gallbladder even after a double dose.

Hepatic Pigmentation

Macroscopically, the liver is black. Liver histology is normal except for the accumulation of a dense pigment, which is contained within lysosomes (128). Infusion of ^{3}H-epinephrine in the Corriedale sheep (an animal model of Dubin–Johnson syndrome, see below) revealed reduced biliary excretion of radioactivity and incorporation of the isotope into the hepatic pigment, suggesting its relationship with melanin (129). When TR$^-$ rats (another model of Dubin–Johnson syndrome) are fed a diet enriched in aromatic amino acids (phenylalanine, tyrosine, and tryptophan), lysosomal pigmentation develops, probably because of impaired excretion of anionic metabolites of tyrosine, phenylalanine, and tryptophan, with subsequent oxidation, polymerization, and lysosomal accumulation (130). Electron spin resonance spectroscopy suggests that the pigment differs from authentic melanin, but could be composed of polymers of epinephrine metabolites. Computed tomography of the liver shows higher than normal attenuation values in Dubin–Johnson syndrome. Interestingly, the pigment is cleared during acute viral hepatitis and reaccumulates slowly after recovery (131).

Urinary Coproporphyrin Excretion

The total urinary coproporphyrin excretion is normal in Dubin–Johnson syndrome, but the ratio of coproporphyrin I to coproporphyrin III is greater (4:1), than that seen normally (1:3) (132). In obligate heterozygotes (i.e., unaffected parents and children of patients with Dubin–Johnson syndrome), total urinary coproporphyrin excretion is reduced by 40%, because of a 50% reduction in coproporphyrin III excretion (133). In heterozygote carriers, the proportion of coproporphyrin I in urine was intermediate between findings in controls and in patients with Dubin–Johnson syndrome. Based on these data, Dubin–Johnson syndrome is inherited as an autosomal-recessive characteristic. No other hepatobiliary disorder or porphyria has been described in which a combination of normal total urinary coproporphyrin excretion and a great predominance of coproporphyrin I is seen. Thus, in the presence of a consistent history and physical examination, urinary coproporphyrin excretion appears to be diagnostic of this disorder.

Molecular Mechanism

Organic anions, other than bile acids, such as conjugated bilirubin, and other glucuronide or glutathione conjugated substances, are transported across the bile canalicular membrane by an ATP-dependent energy-consuming process, mediated by MRP2 [also known as the canalicular multi-specific organic anion transporter (cMOAT)] (Fig. 20.5) (see Chapters 24 and 25). TR$^-$ rats have a frame-shift mutation in the gene encoding MRP2 (134). The human *MRP2* gene is located on chromosome 10q23-q24. A number of mutations causing Dubin–Johnson syndrome have been identified, a significant proportion of which are in the critical ATP-binding domain (135–139) (Table 20.5). A mutation at an intronic splice donor site that results in abnormal splicing of the transcript has also been identified in a patient with Dubin–Johnson syndrome (139).

Animal Models

A mutant strain of the Corriedale sheep was found to have a metabolic defect similar to that in Dubin–Johnson syndrome. Biliary excretion of conjugated bilirubin, glutathione-conjugated BSP, iopanoic acid, and ICG is decreased in this strain, whereas taurocholate transport is normal. The secretion of unconjugated BSP is unimpaired. As in patients with Dubin–Johnson syndrome, total urinary coproporhyrin excretion is normal with increased proportion of the isomer I. The most extensively studied animal model for Dubin–Johnson syndrome is the TR$^-$ rat (140). The organic anion excretion defect and the pattern of

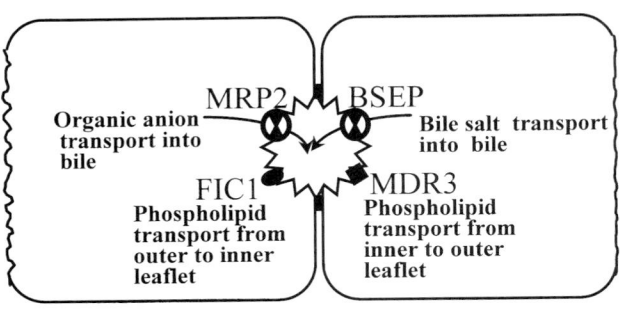

FIGURE 20.5. Four adenosine triphosphate–utilizing transport proteins concentrated in the bile canalicular membrane have been recognized to be important in canalicular transport. Multidrug resistance-related protein (*MRP2*) [also known as canalicular multispecific organic anion transporter (cMOAT)] mediates the transport of most non–bile-acid organic anions, including bilirubin glucuronides. Bile salt export pump (*BSEP*) [also known as sister of p-glycoprotein (SPGP)] is the major bile acid transporter. FIC1 translocates acidic phospholipids (such as phosphatidylserine and phosphatidyl-ethanolamine) from the outer to the inner leaf of the plasma membrane. MDR3 transports phospholipids from the inner to the outer leaflet of the bile canaliculus. Genetic lesions of MRP2 cause Dubin–Johnson syndrome. Inherited abnormalities of the other three genes are associated with various intrahepatic cholestasis syndromes (see text). *FIC*, familial intrahepatic cholestasis; *MDR*, multi drug resistance.

TABLE 20.5. MUTATIONS IDENTIFIED IN PATIENTS WITH DUBIN–JOHNSON SYNDROME TYPE

Site of Mutation	Nucleic Acid Change	Predicted Change of Amino Acid in MRP2	Reference
Exon 13	Del, nt 1669–1815	Truncated protein	138
Intron 15	Splice donor site, T→C	Truncated protein	139
Exon 18	C2302T	R368W	138
Exon 18	Del, nt 2272–2439	Truncated protein	138
Exon 23	C3196T	R1066X—truncated protein	137
Exon 31	Del, nt 4175–4180	Truncated protein	135

MRP, multidrug resistance-related protein.

coproporphyrin excretion in urine are similar to that in Dubin–Johnson syndrome. For organic anions, such as glutathione-conjugated leukotriene (LT)C$_4$, the canalicular secretion defect is nearly complete, whereas for bilirubin glucuronides there is about 10% residual transport activity (141). The TR$^-$ rat and patients with Dubin–Johnson syndrome have normal canalicular excretion of bile salts, except those that have double-negative charges because of conjugation at the 3-OH position (142). The ATP-driven component of bilirubin glucuronide transport by canalicular plasma membrane vesicles is absent in the TR$^-$ rats, but the membrane potential-dependent mechanism provides the residual transport (53). A mutant strain of golden lion tamarins (*Leontopitheous rosalia rosalia*) with Dubin–Johnson-like syndrome has been described (143).

Rotor Syndrome

This disorder is characterized by accumulation of conjugated bilirubin in the plasma in the presence of normal liver function tests (144) (Table 20.4). In contrast to Dubin–Johnson syndrome, there is no increased pigmentation of the liver. Oral cholecystographic agents result in roentgenologic visualization of the gallbladder in Rotor syndrome. Unlike the findings in Dubin–Johnson syndrome, patients with Rotor syndrome exhibit marked retention of BSP at 45 minutes after injection, but biphasic plasma BSP peaks are not found and conjugated BSP does not appear in plasma. There is also marked plasma retention of intravenously administered unconjugated bilirubin and ICG.

Studies using a constant infusion of BSP indicate that while in Dubin–Johnson syndrome the transport maximum (T_{max}) is virtually zero and hepatic storage is normal, in Rotor syndrome the T_{max} is 50% of normal, but the hepatic storage is reduced by 75% to 90%. Thus, Dubin–Johnson syndrome represents a canalicular excretion disorder, whereas Rotor syndrome is a disorder of hepatic storage and may be identical with the so-called familial hepatic storage disease (145).

Urinary Coproporphyrin Excretion

Compared to normal, total urinary coproporphyrin excretion is increased by 250% to 500% and the proportion of coproporphyrin I in urine is approximately 65% of total (146). These results are similar to those seen in many other hepatobiliary disorders and distinguish this disorder from Dubin–Johnson syndrome. Rotor syndrome is inherited as an autosomal-recessive characteristic. Its molecular basis is unknown.

Progressive Familial Intrahepatic Cholestasis Syndromes

In contrast to Dubin–Johnson and Rotor syndromes, progressive familial intrahepatic cholestasis syndromes (PFICs) are autosomal-recessive disorders, associated with various degrees of cholestasis. In most cases PFICs cause progressive liver damage. An exception is benign recurrent intrahepatic cholestasis, which is an episodic and milder disorder. These conditions have been discussed in Chapter 26.

Alagille Syndrome

Several inherited disorders of bile duct development have been described. Of these, the Alagille syndrome was the first to be characterized at the molecular level. Alagille syndrome is characterized by the paucity or absence of small bile ducts, resulting in progressive intrahepatic cholestasis, and abnormalities of the eye, heart, and vertebrae. The disorder is inherited as an autosomal-dominant characteristic. The responsible gene, *JAG1*, has been mapped to chromosome 20p12 (147). *JAG1* encodes an unidentified ligand that binds to the notch receptor, which is crucial for cell plate development in *Drosophila* and mammals. In rare cases, the gene is deleted. In other cases of Alagille syndrome, various point mutations in *JAG1*, each of which abolishes expression of the altered allele, have been described.

ACKNOWLEDGMENTS

The authors thank Dr. Ajit Kadakol for assistance in preparation of this review. This work was supported in part by National Institutes of Health grants DK-46057, DK-39137, DK-41296, DK-23026, DK-35652, and DK-34926.

REFERENCES

1. London IM, West R, Shemin D, et al. On the origin of bile pigment in normal man. *J Biol Chem* 1950;184:351.
2. Schwartz S, Johnson JA, Stephenson BD, et al. Erythropoietic defects in protoporphyria: a study of factors involved in labeling of porphyrins and bile pigments from ALA-3H and glycine-14C. *J Lab Clin Med* 1971;78:411.
3. Robinson SH. Origins of the early-labeled peak. In: Berk PD, Berlin NI, eds. *Bile pigments: chemistry and physiology.* Washington, DC: US Government Printing Office, 1977;175.
4. Come SE, Shohet SB, Robinson SH. Surface remodeling vs. whole-cell hemolysis of reticulocytes produced with erythroid stimulation or iron deficiency anemia. *Blood* 1974;44:817.
5. Tenhunen R, Marver HS, Schmid R. Microsomal heme oxygenase: Characterization of the enzyme. *J Biol Chem* 1969;244:6388.
6. Elbirt KK, Bonkovsky HL. Heme oxygenase: recent advances in understanding its regulation and role. *Proc Assoc Am Physicians* 1999;111:438.
7. Ishizawa S, Yoshida T, Kikuchi G. Induction of heme oxygenase in rat liver. *J Biol Chem* 1983;258:4220.
8. Hayashi S, Takamiya R, Yamaguchi T, et al. Induction of heme oxygenase-1 suppresses venular leukocyte adhesion elicited by oxidative stress: role of bilirubin generated by the enzyme. *Circ Res* 1999;85:663.
9. Tenhunen R, Ross ME, Marver HS, et al. Reduced nicotinamide-adenine dinucleotide phosphate dependent biliverdin reductase: partial purification and characterization. *Biochemistry* 1970;9:298.
10. Jones EA, Bloomer JR, Berk PD, et al. Quantitation of hepatic bilirubin synthesis in man. In: Berk PD, Berlin NI, eds. *Bile pigments: chemistry and physiology.* Washington, DC: US Government Printing Office, 1977;189.
11. Berk PD, Rodkey FL, Blaschke TF, et al. Comparison of plasma bilirubin turnover and carbon monoxide production in man. *J Lab Clin Med* 1974;83:29.
12. Westlake DWS, Roxburgh JM, Talbot G. Microbial production of carbon monoxide from flavinoids. *Nature* 1961;189:510.
13. Kappas A, Drummond GS. Direct comparison of tin-mesoporphyrin, an inhibitor of bilirubin production, and phototherapy in controlling hyperbilirubinemia in term and near-term newborns. *Pediatrics* 1995;95:468.
14. Valaes T, Petmezaki S, Henschke C, et al. Control of jaundice in preterm newborns by an inhibitor of bilirubin production: studies with tin-mesoporphyrin. *Pediatrics* 1994;93:1.
15. Berk PD, Jones EA, Howe RB, et al. Disorders of bilirubin metabolism. In: Bondy PK, Rosenberg LE, ed. *Metabolic control and disease,* 8th ed. Philadelphia: WB Saunders, 1980;1009.
16. Grandchamp B, Bissel DM, Licko V, et al. Formation and disposition of newly synthesized heme in adult rat hepatocytes in primary cultures. *J Biol Chem* 1981;256:11677.
17. Fischer H, Plieninger H. Synthese des biliverdins (uteroverdins) und bilirubins der biliverdine XIII, und III, sowie der Vinulneoxanthosaure. *Hoppe Seyler Z Physiol Chem* 1942;274:231.
18. Bonnet RJ, Davis E, Hursthouse MB. Structure of bilirubin. *Nature* 1976;262:326.
19. Kuenzle CC, Weibel MH, Pelloni RR. The reaction of bilirubin with diazomethane. *Biochem J* 1973;133:357.
20. McDonagh AF, Palma LA, Lightner DA. Phototherapy for neonatal jaundice. Stereospecific and regiospecific photoisomerization of bilirubin bound to human serum albumin and NMR characterization of intramolecularly cyclized photoproducts. *J Am Chem Soc* 1982;104:6867.
21. Itho S, Onishi S. Kinetic study of the photochemical changes of (ZZ)-bilirubin IX bound to human serum albumin. Demonstration of (EZ)-bilirubin IX as an intermediate in photochemical changes from (ZZ)-bilirubin IX to (EZ)-cyclobilirubin IX. *Biochem J* 1985;226:251.
22. McDonagh AF. Thermal and photochemical reactions of bilirubin IX. *Ann NY Acad Sci* 1975;244:553.
23. Lauff JJ, Kasper ME, Ambros RT. Quantitative liquid chromatographic estimation of bilirubin species in pathological serum. *Clin Chem* 1983;29:800.
24. Onishi S, Itho S, Kawade N, et al. An accurate and sensitive analysis by high pressure liquid chromatography of conjugated and unconjugated bilirubin IXα and in various biological fluids. *Biochem J* 1980;185:281.
25. Spivak W, Carey MC. Reverse-phase h.p.l.c. separation, quantification and preparation of bilirubin and its conjugates from native bile. *Biochem J* 1985;225:787.
26. Roy Chowdhury J, Roy Chowdhury N. Quantitation of bilirubin and its conjugates by high pressure liquid chromatography. *Falk Hepatol* 1982;11:1649.
27. Blanckaert N, Kabra PM, Farina FA, et al. Measurement of bilirubin and its mono- and diconjugates in human serum by alkaline methanolysis and high performance liquid chromatography. *J Lab Clin Med* 1980;96:198.
28. Schumacher RE, Thornbery JM, Gutcher GR. Transcutaneous bilirubinometry: a comparison of old and new methods. *Pediatrics* 1985;76:10.
29. Tayba R, Gribetz D, Gribetz I, et al. Non-invasive estimation of serum bilirubin. *Pediatrics* 1998;102:28.
30. Brown AK, Eisinger J, Blumberg WE, et al. A rapid fluorometric method for determining bilirubin levels and binding in the blood of neonates: comparison with other methods. *Pediatrics* 1980;65:767.
31. Schiff D, Chan G, Poznasky MJ. Bilirubin toxicity in neural cell lines N115 and NBR10A. *Pediatr Res* 1985;19:908.
32. Mustafa MG, Cowger ML, Kind TE. Effects of bilirubin on mitochondrial reactions. *J Biol Chem* 1969;244:6403.
33. Catoh R, Kashiwamata S, Niwa F. Studies on cellular toxicity of bilirubin: effect on the carbohydrate metabolism in the young rat brain. *Brain Res* 1975;83:81.
34. Sano K, Nakamura H, Tamotsu M. Mode of inhibitory action of bilirubin on protein kinase C. *Pediatr Res* 1985;19:587.
35. Gourley GR. Bilirubin metabolism and Kernicterus. *Adv Pediatr* 1997;44:173.
36. Odell GB. Influence of binding on the toxicity of bilirubin. *Ann NY Acad Sci* 1973;226:225.
37. Rappaport SI. *Blood-brain barrier in physiology and medicine.* New York: Raven Press, 1976.
38. Lee K-S, Gartner LM. Management of unconjugated hyperbilirubinemia in the newborn. *Semin Liver Dis* 1983;3:52.
39. Bowen WR, Porter E, Waters WF. The protective action of albumin in bilirubin toxicity in new born puppies. *Am J Dis Child* 1959;98:568.
40. Harris RC, Lucey JF, MacLean JR. Kernicterus in premature infants associated with low concentrations of albumin in plasma. *Pediatrics* 1958;21:875.
41. Satlin LM, Amin V, Wolkoff AW. Organic anion transporting polypeptide mediates organic anion/HCO₃- exchange. *J Biol Chem* 1997;272:26340.
42. Fleischner G, Robbins J, Arias IM. Immunological studies of Y protein: a major cytoplasmic organic anion binding protein in rat liver. *J Clin Invest* 1972;51:677.
43. Rowe JD, Nieves E, Listowsky I. Subunit diversity and tissue distribution of human glutathione S-transferases: interpretations based on electrospray ionization-MS and peptide sequence-specific antisera. *Biochem J* 1997;325:481.
44. Kamisaka K, Gatmaitan Z, Moore CL, et al. Ligandin reverses

bilirubin inhibition of liver mitochondrial respiration in vitro. *Pediatr Res* 1975;9:903.

45. Roy Chowdhury J, Novikoff PM, Roy Chowdhury N, et al. Distribution of uridinediphosphoglucuronate glucuronosyl transferase in rat tissues. *Proc Natl Acad Sci USA* 1985;82:2990.

46. Mackenzie PI, Owens IS, Burchell B, et al. The UDP glucosyltransferase gene superfamily: recommended nomenclature update based on evolutionary divergence. *Pharmacogenetics* 1997;7:255.

47. Bosma PJ, Seppen J, Goldhoorn B, et al. Bilirubin UDP-glucuronosyltransferase 1 is the only relevant bilirubin glucuronidating isoform in man. *J Biol Chem* 1994;269:17960.

48. Ritter JK, Chen F, Sheen YY, et al. A novel complex locus UGT1 encodes human bilirubin, phenol and other UDP-glucuronosyltransferase isozymes with identical carboxy termini. *J Biol Chem* 1992;267:3257.

49. Wishart GF. Functional heterogeneity of UDP-glucuronosyl transferase as indicated by its differential development and inducibility by glucocorticoids. *Biochem J* 1978;174:485.

50. Roy Chowdhury J, Roy Chowdhury N, Moscioni AD, et al. Differential regulation by triiodothyronine of substrate-specific uridinediphosphoglucuronate glucuronosyl transferases in rat liver. *Biochim Biophys Acta* 1983;761:58.

51. Lillienblum W, Walli AK, Bock KW. Differential induction of rat liver microsomal UDP-glucuronosyltransferase activities by various inducing agents. *Biochem Pharmacol* 1982;31:907.

52. Ishikaowa T, Muller M, Klunemann C, et al. ATP-dependent primary active transport of cysteinyl leukotrienes transport system for glutathione S-conjugates. *J Biol Chem* 1990;265:19279.

53. Nishida T, Gatmaitan Z, Roy Chowdhury J, et al. Two distinct mechanisms for bilirubin glucuronide transport by rat bile canalicular membrane vesicles. *J Clin Invest* 1992;90:2130.

54. Cole SPC, Bhardwaj G, Gerlach JH, et al. Overexpression of a transporter gene in a multidrug-resistant human lung cancer cell line. *Science* 1992;258:1650.

55. Brodersen R, Herman LS. Intestinal reabsorption of unconjugated bilirubin. A possible contributing factor in neonatal jaundice. *Lancet* 1963;1:1242.

56. Watson CJ. The urobilinoids: milestones in their history and some recent developments. In: Berk PD, Berlin NI, eds. *Bile pigments: chemistry and physiology.* Washington, DC: US Government Printing Office, 1977;469.

57. Kapitulnik J, Ostrow JD. Stimulation of bilirubin catabolism in jaundiced Gunn rats by an inducer of microsomal mixed function mono oxygenases. *Proc Natl Acad Sci USA* 1978;75:682.

58. Cardenas-Vazquez R, Yokosuka O, Billing BH. Enzymic oxidation of unconjugated bilirubin by rat liver. *Biochem J* 1986;236:625.

59. Stocker R, Yamamoto Y, McDonagh AF, et al. Bilirubin is an antioxidant of possible physiological importance. *Science* 1987;235:1043.

60. Stocker R, Peterhans E. Antioxidant properties of conjugated bilirubin and biliverdin; biologically relevant scavanging of hypochlorous acid. *Free Radic Res Commun* 1989;6:57.

61. Vest M, Strebel L, Hauensiein D. The extent of "shunt" bilirubin and erythrocyte survival in the newborn infant measured by the administration of (15N) glycine. *Biochem J* 1965;95:11c.

62. Levi AJ, Gatmaitan Z, Arias IM. Deficiency of hepatic organic anion-binding protein, impaired organic anion uptake by liver and "physiologic" jaundice in newborn monkeys. *N Engl J Med* 1970;283:1136.

63. Brown AK, Zuelzer WW. Studies on the neonatal development of the glucuronide conjugating system. *J Clin Invest* 1958;37:332.

64. Bosma PJ, Roy Chowdhury J, Bakker C, et al. A sequence abnormality in the promoter region results in reduced expression of bilirubin-UDP-glucuronosyltransferase-1 in Gilbert syndrome. *N Engl J Med* 1995;333:1171.

65. Roy Chowdhury N, Deocharan B, Bejjanki HR, et al. The presence of a Gilbert-type promoter abnormality increases the level of neonatal hyperbilirubinemia. *Hepatology* 1997;26:370a.

66. Maisels MJ, Newman TB. Kernicterus in otherwise healthy breast-fed term newborns. *Pediatrics* 1995;96:730.

67. Arias IM, Gartner LM, Seifter S, et al. Prolonged neonatal unconjugated hyperbilirubinemia associated with breast feeding and a steroid, pregnane-3(alpha), 20(beta)-diol, in maternal milk that inhibits glucuronide formation in vitro. *J Clin Invest* 1964;43:2037.

68. Foliot A, Ploussard JP, Housett E, et al. Breast milk jaundice: in vitro inhibition of rat liver bilirubin-uridine diphosphate glucuronyl transferase activity and Z protein-bromosulfophthalein binding by human breast milk. *Pediatr Res* 1976;10:594.

69. Arias IM, Wolfson S, Lucey JF, et al. Transient familial neonatal hyperbilirubinemia. *J Clin Invest* 1965;44:1442.

70. Robinson S, Vanier T, Desforges JF, et al. Jaundice in thalassemia minor: a consequence of ineffective erythropoiesis. *N Engl J Med* 1962;267:512.

71. Crigler JF, Najjar VA. Congenital familial non-hemolytic jaundice with kernicterus. *Pediatrics* 1952;10:169.

72. Childs B, Sidbury JB, Migeon CJ. Glucuronic acid conjugation by patients with familial non-hemolytic jaundice and their relatives. *Pediatrics* 1959;23:903.

73. Berk PD, Martin JF, Blaschke TF, et al. Unconjugated hyperbilirubinemia: physiological evaluation and experimental approaches to therapy. *Ann Intern Med* 1975;82:552.

74. Kapitulnik J, Kaufmann NA, Goitein K, et al. A pigment found in the Crigler-Najjar syndrome and its similarity to an ultra-filterable photo-derivative of bilirubin. *Clin Chim Acta* 1974;57:231.

75. Arias IM, Gartner LM, Cohen M, et al. Chronic nonhemolytic unconjugated hyperbilirubinemia with glucuronosyl transferase deficiency: clinical, biochemical, pharmacologic, and genetic evidence for heterogeneity. *Am J Med* 1969;47:395.

76. Bosma PJ, Roy Chowdhury N, Goldhoorn BG, et al. Sequence of exons and the flanking regions of human bilirubin-UDP-glucuronosyltransferase gene complex and identification of a genetic mutation in a patient with Crigler-Najjar syndrome, type I. *Hepatology* 1992;15:941.

77. Bosma PJ, Roy Chowdhury J, Huang TJ, et al. Mechanism of inherited deficiencies of multiple UDP-glucuronosyltransferase isoforms in two patients with Crigler-Najjar syndrome, type I. *FASEB J* 1992;6:2859.

78. Ritter JK, Yeatman MT, Ferriera P, et al. Identification of a genetic alteration in the code for bilirubin UDP-glucuronosyltransferase in the UGT1 gene complex of a Crigler-Najjar syndrome, type I. *J Clin Invest* 1992;90:150.

79. Ciotti M, Obaray R, Martin M, et al. Genetic disease at the UGT1 locus associated with Crigler-Najjar syndrome type-1 disease, including a prenatal diagnosis. *Am J Med Genet* 1997;68:173.

80. Clarke DJ, Moghrabi N, Monaghan G, et al. Genetic defects of UDP-glucuronosyltransferase-1 (UGT1) gene that cause familial non-hemolytic unconjugated hyperbilirubinemias. *Clin Chem Acta* 1997;266:63.

81. Rosatelli MC, Meloni A, Faa V, et al. Molecular analysis of patients with Sardinian descent with Crigler-Najjar syndrome type 1. *J Med Genet* 1997;34:122.

82. Ritter JK, Yeatman MT, Kaiser C, et al. Phenylalanine codon deletion at the UGT1 gene complex locus of a Crigler-Najjar type I patient generates a pH-sensitive bilirubin UDP-glucuronosyltransferase. *J Biol Chem* 1993;268:23573.

83. Seppen J, Bosma PJ, Goldhoorn BG, et al. Discrimination

between Crigler-Najjar type I and II by expression of mutant bilirubin uridine diphosphate-glucuronosyltransferase. *J Clin Invest* 1994;94:2385.

84. Labrune PH, Myara A, Hadchouel M, et al. Genetic heterogeneity of Crigler-Najjar syndrome type I; a study of 14 cases. *Hum Genet* 1994;94:693.

85. Aono S, Yamada Y, Keino H, et al. A new type of defect in the gene for bilirubin uridine 5′-diphosphate-glucuronosyl-transferase in a patient with Crigler-Najjar syndrome type I. *Pediatr Res* 1994;35:629.

86. Gantla S, Bakker CTM, Deocharan B, et al. Splice site mutations: a novel genetic mechanism of Crigler-Najjar syndrome type 1. *Am J Hum Genet* 1998;62:585.

87. Erps LT, Ritter JK, Hersh JH, et al. Identification of the two single base substitutions in the UGT1 gene locus which abolish bilirubin uridine diphosphate glucuronosyltransferase activity in vitro. *J Clin Invest* 1994;93:564.

88. Ciotti M, Chen F, Rubatelli FF, et al. Coding and a TATA Box mutation at the bilirubin UDP-glucuronosyl transferase gene cause Crigler-Najjar syndrome type 1 disease. *Biochem Biophys Acta* 1998;1407:40.

89. Moghrabi N, Clarke DJ, Burchell B, et al. Cosegregation of intragenic markers with a novel mutation that cause Crigler-Najjar syndrome type I: implication in carrier detection and prenatal diagnosis. *Am J Hum Genet* 1993;53:722.

90. Kadakol A, Ghosh SS, Sappal BS, et al. Genetic lesions of bilirubin uridine-diphosphoglucuronate glucuronosyltransferase (UGT1A1) causing Crigler-Najjar and Gilbert's syndrome: correlation of genotype to phenotype. *Hum Mutat* 2000;16:297.

91. Jansen PLM, Bosma PJ, Roy-Chowdhury J. Molecular biology of bilirubin metabolism. In: Boyer JL, Ockner RK, ed. *Progress liver diseases*, vol 13. Philadelphia: WB Saunders, 1995;125.

92. Deocharan B, Gantla S, Morton DH, et al. Interaction of a Crigler-Najjar syndrome type I mutation and a Gilbert type promoter defect results in two grades of hyperbilirubinemia in members of an Amish and a Mennonite kindred of Lancaster County, Pennsylvania. *Gastroenterology* 1997;112:1255A.

93. Sengupta K, Gantla S, Bommineni VR, et al. Prenatal identification of Crigler-Najjar syndrome type I genotype by analysis of chorionic villus sample DNA. *Hepatology* 1994;20:320A.

94. Gunn CH. Hereditary acholuric jaundice in a new mutant strain of rats. *J Hered* 1938;29:137.

95. Schmid R, Axelrod J, Hammaker L, et al. Congenital jaundice in rats due to a defective glucuronide formation. *J Clin Invest* 1958;37:1123.

96. Blaschke TF, Berk PD, Scharschmidt BF, et al. Crigler-Najjar syndrome. An unusual course with development of neurologic damage at age eighteen. *Pediatr Res* 1974;8:573.

97. van der Veere CN, Sinaasappel M, McDonagh AF, et al. Current therapy for Crigler-Najjar syndrome type 1: report of a world registry. *Hepatology* 1996;24:311.

98. Fox IJ, Roy Chowdhury J, Kaufman SS, et al. Treatment of Crigler-Najjar syndrome type I with hepatocyte transplantation. *N Engl J Med* 1998;338:1422.

99. Roy Chowdhury J, Strom S, Fox IJ. Human hepatocyte transplantation: gene therapy and more? *Pediatrics* 1998;102:647.

100. Ghosh SS, Takahashi M, Thummala NR, et al. Liver-directed gene therapy: promises, problems and prospects at the turn of the century. *J Hepatol* 2000;32:238.

101. Arias IM. Chronic unconjugated hyperbilirubinemia without overt signs of hemolysis in adolescents and adults. *J Clin Invest* 1962;41:2233.

102. Gollan JL, Huang SM, Billing B, et al. Prolonged survival in three brothers with severe type II Crigler-Najjar syndrome. Ultrastructural and metabolic studies. *Gastroenterology* 1975;68:1543.

103. Gordon ER, Shaffer EA, Sass-Kortsak A. Bilirubin secretion and conjugation in the Crigler-Najjar syndrome type II. *Gastroenterology* 1976;70:761.

104. Fevery J, Blanckaert N, Heirwegh KPM, et al. Unconjugated bilirubin and an increased proportion of bilirubin monoconjugates in the bile of patients with Gilbert's syndrome and Crigler-Najjar syndrome. *J Clin Invest* 1977;60:970.

105. Seppen J. Steenken E, Lindhout D, et al. A mutation which disrupts the hydrophobic core of the signal peptide of bilirubin UDP-glucuronosyltransferase, an endoplasmic reticulum membrane protein, causes Crigler-Najjar type II. *FEBS Lett* 1996; 390:294.

106. Soeda Y, Yamamoto K, Adachi Y, et al. Predicted homozygous missense mutation in Gilbert syndrome. *Lancet* 1995;346:1494.

107. Koiwai O, Nishizawa M, Hasada K, et al. Gilbert's syndrome is caused by a heterozygous missense mutation in the gene for bilirubin UDP-glucuronosyltransferase. *Hum Mol Genet* 1995; 4:1183.

108. Aono S, Adachi Y, Uyama E, et al. Analysis of genes for bilirubin UDP-glucuronosyltransferase in Gilbert's syndrome. *Lancet* 1995;345:958.

109. Aono S, Yamada Y, Keino H, et al. Identification of a defect in the gene for bilirubin UDP-glucuronosyltransferase in a patient with Crigler-Najjar syndrome type II. *Biochem Biophys Res Commun* 1993;197:1239.

110. Seppen J, Bosma P, Roy Chowdhury J, et al. Discrimination between Crigler-Najjar syndromes type I and II by expression of mutant bilirubin-UDP-glucuronosyltransferase. *J Clin Invest* 1994;94:2385.

111. Bosma PJ, Golhoorn B, Oude Elferink RP, et al. A mutation in bilirubin uridine 5′-diphosphate glucuronosyltransferase isoforms 1 causing Crigler-Najjar syndrome type II. *Gastroenterology* 1993;105:216.

112. Moghrabi N, Clarke DJ, Boxer M, et al. Identification of an A-to-G missense mutation in exon 2 of the UGT1 gene complex that causes Crigler-Najjar syndrome type 2. *Genomics* 1993;18:171.

113. Koiwai O, Aono S, Adachi Y, et al. Crigler-Najjar syndrome type II is inherited both as a dominant and as a recessive trait. *Hum Mol Genet* 1996;5:645.

114. Chalasani N, Roy Chowdhury N, Roy Chowdhury J, et al. Kernicterus in an adult who is heterozygous for Crigler-Najjar syndrome and homozygous for Gilbert type genetic defect. *Gastroenterology* 1997;112:2099.

115. Maruo Y, Sato H, Yamano T, et al. Gilbert's syndrome caused by homozygous missense mutation (Tyr486Asp) of bilirubin-UDP glucuronosyl transferase. *J Pediatr* 1998;132:1045.

116. Gilbert A, Lereboullet P. La cholamae simple familiale. *Semin Med* 1901;21:241.

117. Berk PD, Bloomer JR, Howe RB, et al. Constitutional hepatic dysfunction (Gilbert's syndrome): a new definition based on kinetic studies with unconjugated radiobilirubin. *Am J Med* 1970;49:296.

118. Felsher BF, Rickard D, Redeker AG. The reciprocal relation between caloric intake and the degree of hyperbilirubinemia in Gilbert's syndrome. *N Engl J Med* 1970;283:170.

119. Fromke VL, Miller D. Constitutional hepatic dysfunction (CHD: Gilbert's disease): a review with special reference to a characteristic increase and prolongation of the hyperbilirubinemia in response to nicotinic acid. *Medicine (Baltimore)* 1972;51:451.

120. Bosma PJ, Roy Chowdhury J, Bakker C, et al. A sequence abnormality in the promoter region results in reduced expression of bilirubin-UDP-glucuronosyltransferase-1 in Gilbert syndrome. *N Engl J Med* 1995;333:1171.

121. Portman OW, Roy Chowdhury J, Roy Chowdhury N, et al. A non-human primate model for Gilbert's syndrome. *Hepatology* 1984;4:175.
122. Dubin IN. Chronic idiopathic jaundice: a review of fifty cases. *Am J Med* 1958;23:268.
123. Sprinz H, Nelson RS. Persistent nonhemolytic hyperbilirubinemia associated with lipochrome-like pigment in liver cells: report of four cases. *Ann Intern Med* 1954;41:952.
124. Shani M, Seligsohn U, Gilon E, et al. Dubin-Johnson syndrome in Israel. I. Clinical, laboratory, and genetic aspects of 101 cases. *West J Med* 1970;39:549.
125. Cohen L, Lewis C, Arias IM. Pregnancy, oral contraceptives, and chronic familial jaundice with predominantly conjugated hyperbilirubinemia (Dubin-Johnson syndrome). *Gastroenterology* 1972;62:1182.
126. Erlinger S, Dhumeaux D, Desjeux JF, et al. Hepatic handling of unconjugated dyes in the Dubin-Johnson syndrome. *Gastroenterology* 1973;64:106.
127. Mandema E, De Fraiture WH, Neiweg HO, et al. Familial chronic idiopathic jaundice (Dubin-Sprinz disease), with a note on bromsulphalein metabolism in this disease. *Am J Med* 1960;28:42.
128. Ehrlick JC, Novikoff AB, Platt R, et al. Hepatocellular lipofuscin and the pigment of chronic idiopathic jaundice. *Bull NY Acad Med* 1960;36:488.
129. Arias IM, Bernstein L, Roffler R, et al. Black liver diseases in Corriedale sheep: metabolism of tritiated epinephrine and incorporation of isotope into the hepatic pigment in vivo. *J Clin Invest* 1965;44:1026.
130. Kitamura T, Alroy J, Gatmaitan Z, et al. Defective biliary excretion of epinephrine metabolites in mutant TR⁻ rats: relation to the pathogenesis of rat liver in Dubin-Johnson syndrome and Corriedale sheep with an analogous excretory defect. *Hepatology* 1992;15:1154.
131. Ware A, Eigenbrodt E, Naftalis J, et al. Dubin-Johnson syndrome and viral hepatitis. *Gastroenterology* 1974;67:560.
132. Koskelo P, Toivonen I, Adlercreutz H. Urinary coproporphyrin isomer distribution in Dubin-Johnson syndrome. *Clin Chem* 1967;13:1006.
133. Wolkoff AW, Cohen LE, Arias IM. Inheritance of the Dubin-Johnson syndrome. *N Engl J Med* 1973;288:113.
134. Paulusma CC, Bosma PJ, Zaman GJR, et al. Congenital jaundice in rats with a mutation in a multidrug resistance-associated protein gene. *Science* 1996;271:1126.
135. Tsujii H, Konig J, Rost D, et al. Exon-intron organization of the human multidrug resistance protein 2 (MRP2) gene mutated in Dubin-Johnson syndrome. *Gastroenterology* 1999;117:653.
136. Toh S, Wada M, Uchuimi T, et al. Genomic structure of the canalicular multispecific organic anion transporter gene (MRP2/cMOAT) and mutations in the ATP-binding cassetted region in Dubin-Johnson syndrome. *Am J Hum Genet* 1999;64:739.
137. Paulusma CC, Kool M, Bosma PJ, et al. A mutation in the human cMOAT gene cause the Dubin-Johnson syndrome. *Hepatology* 1997;25:1539.
138. Wada M, Toh S, Taniguchi K, et al. Mutations in the canalicular multispecific organic anion transporter gene, a novel ABC transporter, in patients with hyperbilirubinemia II/Dubin-Johnson syndrome. *Hum Mol Genet* 1998;7:203.
139. Kajihara S, Hisatomi A, Mizuta T, et al. A splice site mutation in the human canalicular multispecific organic anion transporter (cMOAT) gene causes Dubin-Johnson syndrome. *Biochem Biophys Res Commun* 1998;253:454.
140. Oude Elferink RPJ, Meijer DKF, Kuipers F, et al. Hepatobiliary secretion of organic compounds; molecular mechanisms of membrane transport. *Biochim Biophys Acta* 1995;1241:215.
141. Jansen, PLM, van Klinken JW, van Gelder M, et al. Preserved organic anion transport in mutant TR rats with a hepatobiliary secretion defect. *Am J Physiol* 1993;265:G445.
142. Kobayashi K, Sogame Y, Hayashi K, et al. ATP stimulates the uptake of S-dinitrophenylglutathione by rat liver plasma membrane vesicles. *FEBS Lett* 1988;240:55.
143. Schulman FY, Montali RJ, Bush M, et al. Dubin-Johnson-like syndrome in Golden Lion Tamarins (Leontopithecus rosalia rosalia). *Vet Pathol* 1993;30:491.
144. Rotor AB, Manahan L, Florentin A. Familial nonhemolytic jaundice with direct van den Bergh reaction. *Acta Med Phil* 1948;5:37.
145. Dhumeaux D, Berthelot P. Chronic hyperbilirubinemia associated with hepatic uptake and storage impairment: a new syndrome resembling that of the mutant Southdown sheep. *Gastroenterology* 1975;69:988.
146. Wolkoff AW, Wolpert E, Pascasio FN, et al. Rotor's syndrome. A distinct inheritable pathophysiologic entity. *Am J Med* 1976;60:173.
147. Oda T, Elkaholoun AG, Meltzer PS, et al. Identification and cloning of the human homolog (Jag1) of the rat jagged 1 gene from the Alagille syndrome critical region at 20p12. *Genomics* 1997;43:376.

The Liver: Biology and Pathobiology, Fourth Edition, edited by I. M. Arias, J. L. Boyer, F. V. Chisari, N. Fausto, D. Schachter, and D. A. Shafritz. Lippincott Williams & Wilkins, Philadelphia © 2001.

21

THE PORPHYRIAS

PETER N. MEISSNER
RICHARD J. HIFT
RALPH E. KIRSCH

The porphyrias are a group of metabolic disorders that result from defects of specific enzymes of the heme synthetic pathway (1) (see website chapter 🖳 W-17). Clinically they may be characterized by a propensity to acute neurovisceral crises, photosensitive skin disease, or both. As the pathophysiology, diagnosis, and management of the porphyrias are critically dependent on an understanding of the biochemistry and enzymology of the heme biosynthetic pathway it is necessary to consider this aspect first. Thereafter clinical disorders caused by aberrations in this pathway can be examined in detail.

PORPHYRINS AND HEME

There are a number of excellent reviews on the detailed chemistry and biochemistry of porphyrins (2–6). What fol-

lows is sufficient information to provide a relevant background to this chapter. Porphyrins are tetrapyrrole macrocycles consisting of four weakly aromatic pyrrole rings linked by methene bridges and characterized by their ability to fluoresce a bright red when exposed to ultraviolet light. The porphyrin macrocycle is a rigid planar structure with eight positions where side chains can be attached. The side chain substituents attached to the rings are important in determining the physical characteristics of the porphyrins. Consideration of various arrangements of side chain substituents around the porphyrin ring implies that there are a number of possible different isomeric porphyrin forms. Thus, uroporphyrinogen and coproporphyrinogen can occur in four isomeric forms, but only the I and III forms occur naturally in mammals. All biologically functional tetrapyrroles are derived from uroporphyrinogen-III and the type I isomers of uroporphyrinogen and coproporphyrinogen appear to be biologically useless. As biologic intermediates, the porphyrin tetrapyrroles exist as the partially conjugated, less stable hexahydro-reduced, colorless forms, the porphyrinogens.

An important property of the porphyrin macrocycle is the availability of ligand binding sites within. This attribute gives these compounds the ability to bind metals, particu-

P. N. Meissner, R. J. Hift, and R. E. Kirsch: Medical Research Council/University of Cape Town Liver Research Centre, Department of Medicine, University of Cape Town; and Department of Medicine, Groote Schuur Hospital, Cape Town 7925, South Africa.

larly iron to form heme, magnesium to form chlorophylls, and cobalt to form vitamin B_{12}. Heme is an iron-containing complex of the protoporphyrin-IX molecule that associates with several proteins and is central to virtually all biologic oxidations. Heme, by virtue of its redox-active iron coordinately bound within the tetrapyrrole ring, plays specific roles in oxygen binding, electron transport, reduction of oxygen, and transfer of oxygen for hydroxylation reactions. These roles are in turn determined by the structure of the protein moiety of each specific hemoprotein, their substrates, and the intracellular milieu within which it functions (7).

HEME BIOSYNTHESIS

Heme biosynthesis continues to intrigue medical scientists around the world. The following sections highlight new findings and aspects of heme biosynthesis. Heme is produced by a well-defined pathway in mammals, initiated in the mitochondrial matrix, continuing in the cytosol and ultimately returning to the highly reduced environment of the mitochondrion. All cells are able to produce heme. However, in humans most heme is synthesized in the liver and bone marrow. Estimates of the rate at which hepatic heme is produced in normal humans suggests that in the steady-state situation in which the synthesis of heme is equal to its rate of degradation, heme is produced between 0.7 and 1.6 µmol/kg body weight/day (6).

The key to understanding the conditions referred to as the porphyrias is the fact that each step of heme biosynthesis is catalyzed by an enzyme, or enzymes; deficiency of a particular enzyme (in most instances inherited) may thus lead to a specific pattern of porphyrin accumulation and a characteristic clinical (porphyric) syndrome.

It is thus pertinent to consider the enzymology and molecular biology of each individual enzymatically catalyzed step of heme biosynthesis in detail.

THE ENZYMOLOGY AND MOLECULAR BIOLOGY HEME BIOSYNTHESIS
Formation of the Pyrrole
Biosynthesis of 5-Aminolevulinic Acid

The condensation of succinyl–coenzyme A (CoA) and glycine to form 5-aminolevulinic acid (ALA) is catalyzed by the enzyme ALA synthase (EC 2.3.1.37) (ALAS). Glycine is bound through an essential pyridoxal 5′-phosphate cofactor as a stable Schiff-base carbanion on the enzyme surface, which can react with the electrophilic carbonyl group of succinyl-CoA to produce an α-amino-β-ketoadipic acid with the release of CoA. The carboxyl carbon of glycine is then decarboxylated enzymatically to yield ALA.

Cloning, expression, and detailed characterization of the mouse enzyme have demonstrated a Schiff base linkage between the pyridoxal 5′-phosphate cofactor and a conserved lysine residue [murine ALA synthase (ALAS) Lys-313] in the protein and it is proposed that this lysine residue acts as a general base catalyst (electron "sink") to effect transient quinonoid intermediate formation during catalysis (8). While Lys-313 is thus essential for catalysis, it is not essential for binding the cofactor per se (9) and a conserved tyrosine residue (murine Tyr-121) is now thought to play this role (10). The electron sink function of the pyridoxal 5′-phosphate cofactor may be enhanced by the presence of an aspartate residue (murine ALAS Asp-279) and Arg 439 in the mouse is suggested as playing an essential role in substrate binding (10,11).

Alignment of the predicted amino acid sequences of the mammalian ALA synthases confirms that one should consider two domains. First, the C-terminal two-thirds of the mammalian proteins represents a conserved, ancestral core of the protein, as there is a high degree of homology in this region among ALA synthases. Second, in eukaryotes the N-terminal domain of the newly synthesized protein is not necessary for enzymatic activity and serves as the "presequence," facilitating translocation of the enzyme to the mitochondria. Thus, the human ALA synthase gene encodes a 640 amino acid protein (approximate molecular weight 70,000) in which the N-terminal 56 amino acids constitute the "presequence," which is cleaved on translocation of the protein to the mitochondria.

It is now recognized that there are two separate genes encoding ALA synthase. There is a ubiquitously expressed "housekeeping" (nonerythroid) isoenzyme (ALA-S1; molecular weight 64,600 d) and an erythroid-specific isoenzyme (ALA-S2; molecular weight 59,500 d) (12,13). Although the ALA-S1 and ALA-S2 isoforms share over 50% amino acid identity, they are localized to chromosomes 3p21 and Xp11.21, respectively (14,15). ALA-S1 is the only ALA synthase gene expressed in liver and other nonerythroid tissue and its activity is decreased during differentiation of erythroid cells. During erythropoiesis the gene for ALA-S2 is induced and its gene product is then the dominant form of ALA synthase (16,17).

It is widely accepted that the primary mechanism of regulation of heme synthesis is modulated by ALA synthase. This is therefore considered in some detail in a later section.

Biosynthesis of Porphobilinogen

The condensation of two molecules of ALA to form the monopyrrole PBG is catalyzed by the multisubunit, cytosolic enzyme ALA dehydratase (EC 4.2.1.24) [also referred to as porphobilinogen (PBG) synthase]. The combination of two molecules of ALA to form PBG occurs through a series of stages involving an aldol condensation and formation of a Schiff base.

ALA dehydratase has been purified from a variety of sources and been shown to exist as octamers. The human enzyme is an homo-octamer with subunits of approximately 36,000 d. The holoenzyme contains four catalytic sites and can be viewed as a tetramer of dimers with one active site per dimer. Each active site binds two molecules of ALA at two distinct positions, the A-site and P-site. The ALA molecule contributing the acetate group and the amino-methyl group of PBG binds at the A-site. The ALA contributing the propionate side chain and the pyrrolic nitrogen binds at the P-site. There is an ordered binding in which the keto group of the ALA contributing the propionate side chain forms a transient covalent bond with a conserved lysine (human Lys-252) in the P-site first. Once there is bound substrate at the P-site with an available 5-amino group, binding of the second ALA molecule onto the enzyme at the A-site may occur. The amino-nitrogen then gets incorporated into the pyrrole ring of PBG (18).

Binding of the second substrate at the A-site is dependent on the presence of a divalent metal ion, and removal of these divalent ions prevent binding at the A-site, resulting in loss of activity, but has no effect on ALA binding at the P-site (19). Typically the required metals are Zn^{2+} or Mg^{2+}. Thus in mammalian systems up to a maximum of eight Zn^{2+} ions can bind onto an ALA dehydratase octamer, four being required for catalysis (at the A-site) and four not. Although the binding of the latter four metal ions at the P-site may appear nonessential, they probably play a role in conformational stabilization of the enzyme (20). The two metal binding sites have been specifically identified on the *Escherichia coli* ALA dehydratase and are termed the α and β sites (21).

Cloning technology has allowed several of the genes encoding ALA dehydratases to be sequenced and their cDNAs and protein products characterized. The human gene has been mapped to chromosome 9q34 (22). Furthermore, in humans two tissue-specific forms of ALA dehydratase exist that are encoded by a single gene that contains separate erythroid and housekeeping promoters and can undergo alternative splicing (23,24). It has been proposed that this novel expression of erythroid-specific and housekeeping transcripts evolved to ensure that there is enough supply of heme for high-level tissue-specific hemoglobin production (24).

Cloning has also allowed the development of expression systems for various forms of ALA dehydratase, and ultrapure preparations of the recombinant enzyme have yielded the protein as a crystal, sometimes suitable for x-ray diffraction (25,26). The crystallization and initial x-ray characterization of the ALA dehydratases from *E. coli* and *Saccharomyces cerevisiae* of around 2 Å have been reported (27,28) as well as a more detailed structure down to 1.67 Å for *Pseudomonas aeruginosa* ALA dehydratase (29). In all cases the best crystals were obtained when these proteins were covalently bound to levulinic acid. The x-ray structures have confirmed that ALA dehydratase is a homo-octamer with each of its subunits adopting a "TIM" (*tri*osephosphate *isom*erase) barrel fold with an N-terminal arm of 30 amino acid residues (28). The monomers formed asymmetric dimers with their "arms" wrapped around each other, and four of these dimers interact to form octamers with their active sites located on the surface.

In the *E. coli* enzyme, Lys-247 (equivalent of the essential Lys-252 at the P-site in human ALA dehydratase) formed a Schiff-base link with the bound levulinic acid at the active site. This is also the case in the yeast ALA dehydratase where x-ray analysis shows the formation of a Schiff base with Lys-263 (also equivalent to human Lys-252) (28).

P. aeruginosa ALA dehydratase structural analysis reveals that in each dimer the monomers differed from one another by having a "closed" and an "open" active site pocket. Whereas no metal ions were found in the active site of both monomers, a single well-defined and highly hydrated Mg^{2+} was identified only in the closed form about 14 Å away from the Schiff base forming a nitrogen atom of the active site lysine. Based on this information a structure-based mechanism of action involving Mg^{2+} allosteric binding at the active site and rate enhancement has been proposed (29).

Several ALA dehydratase inhibitors have clinical significance. The enzyme is highly sensitive to lead, which is believed to displace the Zn^{2+} ions. The clinical symptoms of lead poisoning are similar to those described in hereditary ALA dehydratase deficiency (see below), suggesting that ALA dehydratase inhibition is responsible for these effects. Patients with hereditary tyrisonemia also display similar symptoms. In these cases a deficiency in the enzyme 4-fumarylacetoacetate hydrolase causes accumulation of succinylacetone, which is a potent inhibitor of ALA dehydratase.

Assembly of the Tetrapyrrolic (Porphyrinogen) Macrocycle

Biosynthesis of Hydroxymethylbilane

Formation of the basic porphyrinogen tetrapyrrole is initiated in the cytosol by the assembly of four PBG molecules via a stepwise deamination and head-to-tail polymerization into a chemically reactive linear tetrapyrrole, hydroxymethylbilane by the enzyme PBG deaminase (EC 4.3.1.8) (also referred to as uroporphyrinogen-I synthase or hydroxymethylbilane synthase).

PBG deaminase has been purified from many sources, often as a complex together with the next enzyme in the pathway, uroporphyrinogen-III synthase (see next section). PBG deaminase is unique in that it contains a covalently attached dipyrromethane cofactor at the active site that binds substrate molecules during the sequential assembly of the linear tetrapyrrole molecule (30). The structure of the dipyrromethane cofactor and its sites of attachment to the enzyme have been characterized. The PBG deaminase apoenzyme catalyzes the deamination and polymerization of two molecules of PBG at its active site (31). The resultant dipyrrole is covalently linked via a thioether linkage to the enzyme through a conserved cysteine (*E. coli* Cys-242) (32,33). This dipyrrolic cofactor then acts as a primer that gets elongated in a stepwise mechanism, one PBG unit at a time, through enzyme-substrate (ES) intermediate complexes, ES (with one PBG attached); ES_2 (two PBGs attached); ES_3 (three PBGs attached), and finally ES_4 (four PBGs attached) from which the tetrapyrrole product, hydroxymethylbilane, is released by hydrolytic cleavage, regenerating the enzyme-dypyrromethane intact (34). Thus, the two proximal PBGs (i.e., the dipyrromethane cofactor) remain covalently linked to the enzyme and are not turned over. The precise mechanisms by which the enzyme carries out this sequential manipulation of the four substrates and how the tetrapyrrole product is specifically cleaved leaving the intact dipyrromethane cofactor covalently attached to the enzyme have not been fully elucidated.

PBG deaminase was the first of the heme biosynthetic enzymes to benefit from the application of modern recombinant DNA technologic investigation (35). This was primarily driven by investigators attempting to derive diagnostic benefit in the realm of the clinically important diagnosis of acute intermittent porphyria (see below). Consequently, the gene for PBG deaminase has been sequenced and characterized from both prokaryotic and eukaryotic sources.

In mammals there is a single PBG deaminase gene consisting of 15 exons extending over 10 kilobases (kb) of DNA (36). In humans the gene has been mapped to chromosome 11q23, and two different transcripts, differing at their 5′ ends, are produced from the single gene. The first is a ubiquitous, housekeeping messenger RNA (mRNA) transcript produced in all cells in which exon 1 is spliced to exon 3. The second form is specific to erythroid cells and initiates by alternate splicing at exon 2 (37). Activation of transcription of these two forms of PBG deaminase is controlled by two separate, independently regulated promoters.

In addition to the cloning and large-scale expression of recombinant *E. coli* PBG deaminase (38), allowing characterization of the dipyrromethane cofactor, crystallization of the protein was facilitated and the x-ray crystal structure of the *E. coli* PBG deaminase was determined to 1.76 Å resolution (32,39). The high-resolution structure revealed a protein folded into three α/β domains of approximately 100 amino acids each, linked to one another by flexible strands (18,32). Domains 1 and 2, which have similar overall topology, form a cleft at their interface. The dipyrromethane cofactor is bound by extensive contacts, including salt bridges and hydrogen bonds between these two domains in this cleft. Site-directed mutagenesis experiments have demonstrated that several of the salt bridges between arginine and the pyrrole acetates and propionates are important for enzymatic activity (40,41). Domain 3, which is an open-

faced antiparallel sheet of three strands containing the cysteine to which the cofactor is covalently bound, is situated deep within the cleft between domains 1 and 2. Deamination of PBG and formation of the methene bridge occurs here. Thus domain 3 can be considered as containing the single catalytic site. Importantly the crystal structure shows flexible boundaries between the 3 domains, which would allow conformational changes that accommodate each added PBG pyrrole until the tetrapyrrole is synthesized.

Closure of the Tetrapyrrole Ring

The regularly substituted linear tetramer, hydroxymethylbilane, is converted to an asymmetrically substituted cyclic tetramer, uroporphyrinogen-III, by uroporphyrinogen-III synthase (EC 4.2.1.75) (also referred to as uroporphyrinogen cosynthase or hydroxymethylbilane hydrolase), involving intramolecular inversion of the terminal D ring of the substrate. This inversion probably occurs via a chiral spiro intermediate (42).

Uroporphyrinogen-III synthase has been isolated and purified to homogeneity from many sources including human erythrocytes (43). All appear to exist as monomeric subunits with molecular weights around 30,000 d and are extremely thermolabile. Because of this instability, the protein has not been well characterized. Suffice it to say that there is no evidence for a cofactor of any sort. The human enzyme has an isoelectric point of 5.5 and a pH optimum of 7.4, and activity measurements show it to be present in excess over PBG deaminase, favoring the synthesis of the uroporphyrinogen-III over the series I isomeric form (44).

The full-length cDNA for uroporphyrinogen-III synthase has been cloned from a number of sources. The human gene has been isolated, sequenced, and the cDNA expressed in *E. coli* (45). The human uroporphyrinogen-III synthase gene has been mapped to chromosome 10q25.3 (46). In both the human and mouse there are 5′ and 3′ untranslated regions and an open reading frame spanning 10 exons and encoding a polypeptide of 265 amino acids. The mouse gene shares an 80% nucleotide and 78% amino acid identity with that of the human gene (47).

Modification of the Peripheral Side Chains of the Tetrapyrrole

Biosynthesis of Coproporphyrinogen-III

The stepwise decarboxylation of four acetate side chains in the 8-carboxylic (-COOH) uroporphyrinogen-III molecule through formation of 7-, 6-, and 5-COOH intermediates results in the formation of the 4-COOH coproporphyrinogen-III. This reaction takes place in the cytosol and is catalyzed by a single enzyme uroporphyrinogen decarboxylase. At physiologic substrate concentrations this reaction occurs in an orderly manner with the carboxyl groups removed in a clockwise direction starting at ring D and proceeding through A, B, and C before the final formation of copro-porphyrinogen-III. The precise mechanism of achieving this remains elusive especially as it doesn't have a cofactor requirement. The partially decarboxylated intermediates formed in this reaction are relatively stable porphyrinogen species that are detectable *in vivo*. Each intermediate acts as the substrate for further decarboxylation until the requisite coproporphyrinogen is formed. Both the series I and III isomers formed are suitable substrates for this enzyme, but the series III isomer is more rapidly decarboxylated (48). It should be emphasized, however, that only the copro-phyrinogen III isomer can continue in the pathway. The substrate specificity of the enzyme suggests that the active site is flexible, enabling the enzyme "to combine specificity with promiscuity" (49).

This enzyme has been purified from a variety of sources, including human erythrocytes (50). Most forms of the protein have been reported to be monomeric with molecular weights reported from 40,000 to 46,000 d. As with the other heme synthetic enzymes, cloning has followed this earlier protein characterization, and the uroporphyrinogen decarboxylase gene has been studied from a number of sources including human, mouse, and rat (51,52). The interspecies amino acid sequence homology is strong, especially near the N-terminus. The human gene encodes a 367 amino acid residue polypeptide (predicted molecular weight approximately 41 kd), is present as a single copy containing 10 exons within about 3 kb of DNA, and has been mapped to chromosome 1p34. Although two transcriptional start sites separated by six nucleotides have been identified, there is no evidence from either analysis of the gene structure or expression studies in different tissues to suggest tissue-specific promoters or iso-forms of uroporphyrinogen decarboxylase.

Various inhibitor studies suggest that cysteine and histidine residues are important for enzyme activity. However, site-directed mutagenesis experiments indicate that no single cysteine is absolutely critical for the integrity of the catalytic site but one histidine residue (human H339) has been identified as important in imparting isomer specificity (53).

A recombinant human uroporphyrinogen decarboxylase, expressed in *E. coli* and purified has been crystallized and the initial data collected at 3.0-Å resolution (54,55). Subsequently, the crystal structure has been determined at 1.60-Å resolution (56). The 40.8-kd protein is composed of a single domain containing a (β/α) 8-barrel with a deep active site cleft formed by loops at the C-terminal ends of the barrel strands. Many conserved residues cluster at this cleft, including the invariant side chains of human Arg37, Arg41, and His339, which probably function in substrate binding, and human Asp86, Tyr164, and Ser219, which may function in either binding or catalysis. The crystal was dimeric, and assembly of the dimer juxtaposes the active site clefts of the monomers, suggesting a functionally important interaction between the catalytic centers.

Biosynthesis of Protoporphyrinogen-IX

At this point the synthesis of heme reenters the mitochondria, where the enzyme coproporphyrinogen-III oxidase (EC 1.3.3.3) catalyzes the oxidative decarboxylation of coproporphyrinogen-III to form protoporphyrinogen-IX.

The two propionate residues on rings A and B of the tetrapyrrole molecule are converted into vinyl groups in a clockwise fashion, proceeding via a tricarboxylic por-phyrinogen, tripropionate monovinyl porphyrinogen (trivially known as harderoporphyrinogen). It is a stepwise decarboxylation with the decarboxylation of the position-2 proprionate side chain proceeding first and at a faster rate than that of position 4 (57).

Coproporphyrinogen-III oxidase has been purified to homogeneity from a number of sources. The gene encoding coproporphyrinogen-III oxidase has also been cloned from a number of sources, and alignment of the predicted amino acid sequences of a number of oxygen-dependent copro-porphyrinogen-III oxidases indicates a high degree of interspecies conservation (57).

Human coproporphyrinogen-III oxidase has been expressed in *E. coli*, the purified enzyme characterized further, and attempts have been made at crystallization (57–60). Purified human coproporphyrinogen-III oxidase is a nearly globular homodimer (60) composed of subunits of molecular weight approximately 40,000 d. It does not appear to contain any redox reactive metal centers and there was no *in vitro* stimulation by either Fe^{2+} or Cu^{2+} (59,60). This contrasts to other studies that indicate that the mouse enzyme was a metalloprotein associated with Cu^{2+} ions as essential cofactors (61).

The complementary DNA (cDNA) sequence of the human gene encoding coproporphyrinogen-III oxidase has been cloned, sequenced, and characterized (58,59,62,63). In humans there appears to be a single copy of the gene with multiple transcriptional initiation sites. The human gene spans approximately 14 kb, and consists of seven exons and six introns (63). This gene has been mapped to chromosome 3q12 of the human genome. Potential regulatory elements have been identified in the GC-rich promoter region (six Sp1, one CACCC, and four GATA sites) and it is suggested that a single promoter may be differentially regulated in erythroid and nonerythroid tissue (58,62).

It is apparent that newly synthesized coproporphyrinogen-III oxidase has an N-terminal mitochondrial-targeting peptide that is cleaved during transport into the mitochondria. Although the length of this leader sequence was initially proposed to be 31 amino acid residues in length (58), it has more recently been established that it is an unusually long leader sequence of 110 amino acids (62,63).

Oxidation of Protoporphyrinogen-IX and Insertion of Iron

Oxidation of Protoporphyrinogen-IX to Protoporphyrin-IX

While auto-oxidation of protoporphyrinogen-IX to the fully conjugated, planar protoporphyrin-IX can occur in the presence of oxygen, the reducing environment inside cells where this reaction takes place requires catalysis by protoporphyrinogen oxidase (EC 1.3.3.4) (64,65). During this six electron oxidation, the methylene bridges in protoporphyrinogen-IX are converted into methenyl bridges.

There is little direct evidence to suggest a catalytic mechanism for protoporphyrinogen oxidase, but it is possible that diverse mechanisms may exist, especially in prokaryotes that can survive under both aerobic and anaerobic conditions. Three molecules of molecular oxygen, whose ultimate fate is hydrogen peroxide rather than water (66), serves as the final electron acceptor in the aerobic reaction in both eukaryotic and prokaryotic protoporphyrinogen oxidases (66–69). The reaction proceeds via three two-electron oxidations rather than a single six-electron oxidation (H. Dailey, personal communication, 2000).

Partial and, on very rare occasions, homogeneous purification of protoporphyrinogen oxidase from various sources has allowed partial characterization of the enzyme. Most have reported molecular weights within the range of 51,000 to 57,000 d, and it appears that most of these protoporphyrinogen oxidases exist either as monomers or homodimers. Subfractionation studies of rat liver protoporphyrinogen oxidase show it as an intrinsic protein of the inner mitochondrial membrane (67).

Evidence from spectral analysis and gene/protein sequence information shows that protoporphyrinogen oxidases are flavoproteins. Such evidence has come in the form of flavins extracted from various purified protoporphyrinogen oxidases and the identification of the $\beta\alpha\beta$ dinucleotide binding motif (-Gly-x-Gly-x-x-Gly-) near the N-terminal sequences of cloned protoporphyrinogen oxidase genes (68,70,71). Generally the flavin cofactors are noncovalently bound to these proteins and take the form of flavin adenine dinucleotide (FAD) (66).

All protoporphyrinogen oxidases are relatively specific for their natural substrate protoporphyrinogen-IX, although most will also oxidize the nonphysiologic dicarboxylic mesoporphyrinogen-IX.

Of great interest is the inhibition of protoporphyrinogen oxidase by several herbicidal compounds such as the diphenyl ethers. An important feature of these inhibitors is their structural similarity to protoporphyrinogen-IX; while studies on the herbicidal protoporphyrinogen oxidase (PPO) inhibitors showed that a bicyclic structure was the minimum structural requirement for recognition of many molecules by these enzymes (72), it was subsequently shown that some other, but not all, compounds with a tetrapyrrole structure were also effective inhibitors of the enzyme. Thus PPO is effectively inhibited by other compounds such as heme and its metabolic products biliverdin and bilirubin (73). The mode of inhibition is generally competitive.

In recent years several PPO genes have been cloned and sequenced. Initially Hansson and Hederstedt (74) reported an open reading frame in the aerobic bacterium, *Bacillus subtilis*, (*hemY*) which was suggested to be involved in the oxidation of protoporphyrinogen-IX. Following on this Dailey et al. (68) successfully cloned and expressed this *B. subtilis hemY* gene in *E. coli* and showed that it indeed encoded a 53,000 d protein that had oxygen-dependent PPO activity, providing conclusive evidence that this protein was PPO.

Sequence comparisons between various PPO species indicate that most sequence homology is found in the N-terminal sequences containing the dinucleotide binding motif (66,68,75,76).

The cloning, sequencing, and expression of the prokaryotic PPOs from *B. subtilis* (68,69,74) and *E. coli* (77) facilitated the discovery and identification of the mammalian genes encoding mouse (78,79) and human PPOs (80–85). Genomic DNA fragments containing the whole coding sequence for human PPO (1,431 base pairs) have been cloned (85). This gene encodes a 51,000-d (477 amino acid residues) protein that exists as a 100,000-d homodimer (82).

The human PPO gene was mapped by fluorescence *in situ* hybridization to chromosome 1q22-q23 of the human genome (80,85). The human PPO gene has 13 exons spanning approximately 5 kb (85), although some disagreement exists over the lengths of introns 4, 7, and 9 (80,86). Northern blot analysis from a variety of tissues suggests a single mRNA transcript for human PPO of approximately 1.8 kb in length (81,82). These transcripts contain an approximately 300 bp long 5′ untranslated region (UTR) and a short 3′ UTR. Researchers have identified the start and termination codons, as well as a consensus polyadenylation signal and polyadenylation site downstream from the termination site (80,82,86).

The sequence contains no obvious membrane spanning regions and shows no typical mitochondrial targeting signals at the amino terminal (82). Recent data, however, demonstrate that mitochondrial targeting is facilitated by the amino terminal dinucleotide binding motif sequence (H. Dailey, personal communication). Sequence analysis of the protein database suggested that PPOs are members of a protein superfamily that includes plant and animal phytoene desaturases, and animal monoamine oxidases (76). These proteins all share significant homology in a 60 amino acid residue stretch that contains the dinucleotide binding motif. The mouse PPO is similar to the human enzyme in terms of its size, 51,000 d (477 amino acid residues), and homology, as the two proteins share 89% amino acid sequence identity and both lack typical membrane targeting signals despite their localization to the mitochondrial inner membrane (78,80).

Cloning of the various PPO genes and overexpression of this protein in *E. coli* cells have resulted in the establishment of simple rapid purification procedures (87) and enabled researchers to produce large amounts of the protein. Although this has facilitated confirmatory and further characterization of this enzyme from various sources, information on the protein structure, and in particular the understanding of the catalytic mechanism at the enzyme active site, is still lacking.

Insertion of Iron

The terminal step in heme biosynthesis involves the incorporation of Fe^{2+} into the protoporphyrin-IX macrocycle by ferrochelatase (EC 4.99.1.1, protoheme ferrolyase) to form heme or protoheme-IX. Ferrochelatase is located on the matrix side of the inner mitochondrial membrane.

The mechanism of catalysis appears relatively conserved among ferrochelatase species. They have similar substrate specificity with the natural substrates being Fe^{2+} and protoporphyrin-IX (88).

In addition to Fe^{2+}, most ferrochelatases will utilize Co^{2+} and Zn^{2+} as substrates *in vitro*. Several divalent cations including Mn^{2+}, Cd^{2+}, Hg^{2+}, and Pb^{2+} are competitive for all ferrochelatases examined to date (89). Ferrochelatase is thought to use an ordered "bi-bi" reaction mechanism where iron binds prior to porphyrin (90). Following the binding of the metal ion to the enzyme, distortion of the porphyrin to a nonplanar conformation facilitates porphyrin metallation (91,92). This distortion has been demonstrated for the yeast ferrochelatase by Raman resonance to be a simultaneous tilting, or doming, of all four pyrrole rings (92,93). Metallation then occurs with the concomitant removal of the two pyrrolic protons.

Ferrochelatases have been purified and characterized from various sources and exhibit similar properties. The protein is generally encoded as a preprotein of approximately 47,000 d. During importation into the mitochondria the protein is proteolytically processed in an energy-requiring step into a mature protein of approximately 42,000 d (94).

The human ferrochelatase gene has been mapped to chromosome 18q21.3 (95). The characterized gene cDNA sequence consists of 11 exons with an approximate size of 45 kb (96). Both human and mouse ferrochelatase cDNAs contain two polyadenylation signals in the 3′ noncoding regions. A series of elegant experiments reveal that a single ferrochelatase gene is regulated so as to provide for both housekeeping functions and erythroid-specific functions (95,97). The promoter region contains a CpG-rich island, and a Sp1-driven promoter appears to be sufficient for ferrochelatse expression in nonerythroid cell lines. Erythroid

specificity is mediated via GATA-1 and nucleosome transcription factor-E2 (NF-E2) elements. Further studies also suggest a role for chromosomal/chromatin structure and *cis*-acting elements in the regulation of the ferrochelatase mRNA production in erythroid tissue (98,99).

Dailey et al. demonstrated the presence of a labile [2Fe-2S] cluster in purified recombinant human ferrochelatase (100,101), and this feature has now been found in a variety of animal ferrochelatases (102–104). This cluster is readily destroyed by nitric oxide (NO), and its destruction results in the loss of enzyme activity (105). The biophysical properties of this cluster have been described (106), and the four cysteine residues that serve as ligands to the cluster have been identified by site-directed mutagenesis (104,107) and in the crystal structure (H. Dailey, personal communication). The precise function of the [2Fe-2S] cluster, which does not serve to donate iron to the active site, remains to be elucidated, but it does appear to play a role in the stabilization of the ferrochelatase homodimer.

The crystal structure of recombinant *B. subtilis* ferrochelatase, which is a water-soluble monomeric protein that lacks any cofactor or [2Fe-2S] cluster, has been solved to 1.9-Å resolution by Al-Karadaghi et al. (108). More recently the x-ray crystal structure of recombinant human ferrochelatase has been solved at 2.0 Å (H. Dailey, personal communication). The structure reveals that the enzyme is an 86-kd homodimer that contains one [2Fe-2S] cluster per subunit. Each monomer contains 48% α-helix and 14% β-sheet structure and is folded into two similar domains in a fashion that typifies the periplasmic binding protein family. Two differences that exist between the two domains is an additional 50 residues at the amino-terminal end that constitutes a portion of the active site, and a 30-residue addition at the carboxyl-terminus that participates in ligation of the [2Fe-2S] cluster and dimer stabilization. Each monomer contains an active site pocket whose entrance is composed of two hydrophobic lips. In the homodimer, both active sites are present on the same molecular face, and this surface is the largest hydrophobic region of the protein. A proposed function of this region is to serve as the site of membrane attachment. The result of such an organization is that both active sites are within the membrane proper and in position to accept the hydrophobic substrate protoporphyrin from either the hydrophobic milieu of the phospholipid bilayer or directly from the preceding pathway enzyme, protoporphyrinogen oxidase.

The active site pocket contains the majority of highly conserved residues. Key among these may be His263, which has been proposed to be involved in substrate iron donation (109), but most likely participates along with a highly conserved group of carboxylates in proton abstraction and not in iron donation (H. Dailey, personal communication). Substrate iron is proposed to be inserted from the opposite side of the pocket from His263. Residues involved in porphyrin macrocycle distortion remain to be unequivocally identified.

Regulation of Heme Biosynthesis in Nonerythroid and Erythroid Tissue

Heme synthesis is normally an extremely efficient, tightly controlled process in which the amount of heme produced closely matches the needs of the body. This implies that enzymes involved in heme synthesis are normally able to use all of the substrate presented to them, that they can handle an increased flux through the pathway, and that the pathway may be subject to some form of "feedback" control. Indeed, there is much evidence to suggest that, at least in the liver and all nonerythroid tissue, heme itself modulates its own rate of production, principally at the level of ALA synthase, which is considered the rate-determining enzyme of the pathway. This tight regulation of liver cell heme occurs by several mechanisms.

First, heme regulates its own synthesis by controlling the amount of ALA-S1 mRNA. In mammalian systems this occurs primarily at the transcriptional level (110,111), but studies in avian systems suggest the effect may also be on mRNA stability (112,113). The half-life of mammalian ALA-S1 is less than an hour and the half-life of the protein in mitochondria is even shorter. This is an important mechanism as many, but not all, drugs that induce cytochrome P-450 activity also induce transcription of ALA-S1 in mammalian systems and it is suggested that this may be via heme depletion that would accompany the synthesis of P-450 hemoprotein.

Second, heme regulates the translocation of ALA synthase from cytosol to mitochondria (114). This is mediated by two cysteine-containing heme regulatory motifs in the leader sequence (115; H. Dailey, personal communication).

In contrast the mechanisms of controlling erythroid ALA synthase activity are different (116). Transcription of ALA-S2 is controlled primarily by erythroid-specific transcription factors interacting with noncoding regions of the gene (12,117). Interestingly, the same factors are responsible for induction of globin synthesis, but this only occurs following the induction of heme synthesis (118), indicating the importance of heme per se as a regulatory molecule.

Posttranscriptional regulation of ALA-S2 also occurs differently to that of ALA-S1. There is a *cis*-acting regulatory iron element in the 5′ untranslated region (12), similar to the stem-loop structure occurring in the 5′ untranslated region of ferritin mRNAs (119). A protein that binds to the iron regulatory element inhibits translation of the mRNA, but in the presence of iron the protein dissociates and the mRNA binds to ribosomes and is translated (120). In such manner is the translation of ALA-S2 mRNA coupled to the availability of iron.

Although heme does not appear to play a major role in the transcription and translation of ALA-S2, there are identical cysteine-containing heme regulatory motifs to those found in the ALA-S1 gene, in the leader sequence of ALA-S2, and *in vitro* experiments suggest a heme-mediated inhibitory effect (115). Thus translocation of ALA synthase to the mitochondrion may also be a controlled event in erythroid tissue.

CLINICAL DISORDERS ASSOCIATED WITH DEFECTS IN HEME BIOSYNTHESIS

Spectrum of Disorders

Defects in each of the seven heme synthetic enzymes are associated with characteristic clinical disorders. The porphyrias, the associated enzyme defects, and the clinical effects are summarized in Table 21.1. There are two characteristic forms of clinical expression: an acute neurologic syndrome known as the acute attack or porphyric crisis, and skin disease associated with photosensitivity.

The characteristic clinical picture of the acute attack is that it is episodic, may or may not be associated with an obvious precipitating event (such as the administration of porphyrinogenic medication or menstruation), and is marked by a typical constellation of symptoms, notably severe abdominal pain accompanied by few clinical signs and by an absence of peritonism, and features of autonomic neuropathy (121) (particularly hypertension and tachycardia, vomiting, ileus, and constipation). This may proceed to a typical motor neuropathy resembling the Guillain–Barré syndrome; in severe cases, this leads to a severe flaccid quadriparesis and respiratory failure requiring ventilation.

TABLE 21.1. SUMMARY OF THE PORPHYRIAS

Enzyme	Disorder	Inheritance	Clinical Effects
ALA dehydratase	ALA dehydratase deficiency (Doss porphyria)	AR	Acute attacks
PBG deaminase	Acute intermittent porphyria (AIP)	AD	Acute attacks
Uroporphyrinogen cosynthase	Congenital erythropoietic porphyria (CEP)	AR	Photosensitivity
Uroporphyrinogen decarboxylase	Porphyria cutanea tarda (PCT)	Sporadic AD	Photosensitivity
Coproporphyrinogen oxidase	Hereditary coproporphyria (HCP)	AD	Acute attacks, photosensitivity
Protoporphyrinogen oxidase	Variegate porphyria (VP)	AD	Acute attacks, photosensitivity
Ferrochelatase	Erythropoietic protoporphyria (EPP)	AD (AR?)	Photosensitivity

AD, autosomal dominant; AR, autosomal recessive; ALA, 5-aminolevulinic acid; PBG, porphobilinogen.

Pathologically, the neuronal injury is characterized by severe axonal necrosis, though at times there may be a lesser element of demyelination as well (122–126). Once established, the neuropathy is slowly reversible, and typically months to years are required before full function is regained. The clinical features of the acute attack itself are reviewed in detail elsewhere (127–129).

Pathogenesis of the Acute Attack

The pathogenetic mechanisms whereby the acute attack is established are poorly understood. The most likely hypotheses include ALA neurotoxicity and heme deficiency, acting either directly within the neuron or via a deficiency of one or more essential hemoproteins. The subject has recently been concisely and elegantly reviewed by Meyer et al. (128).

5-Aminolevulinic Acid–Induced Neurotoxicity

The invariable observation that the acute attack is always accompanied by an elevation in ALA concentrations has led authorities to suggest that ALA is in itself neurotoxic, though a causal link has not been proven. Many asymptomatic patients, particularly with acute intermittent porphyria (AIP), excrete levels of ALA in excess of those seen in other patients, typically those with hereditary coproporphyria (HCP) and variegate porphyria (VP), who are actively experiencing symptoms (128), and administration of ALA to healthy volunteers, to subjects with AIP (130), and to experimental animals (131,132) does not precipitate the syndrome. Additionally, there is experimental evidence in rodents to suggest that the blood–brain barrier is poorly permeable to ALA (128). In patients with the acute attack, cerebrospinal fluid (CSF) ALA concentrations have been reported to be much lower than those measured simultaneously in blood, representing only 2% to 3% of blood levels (133). However, though this may protect the central nervous system (CNS) against the toxic effects of ALA, the peripheral nervous system would remain exposed to the full blood ALA concentration, a level at which *in vitro* effects on nerve function have been demonstrated (134).

Yet there are lines of evidence to suggest that under certain circumstances ALA *in vivo* is detrimental. Administration into the cerebral ventricle has excitatory effects (135) and reduces seizure latency in rodents (136). There is also evidence that ALA at low concentrations can alter neurophysiologic function, depress spinal reflexes, and induce depolarization of muscle in animals (134), and is neurotoxic in chick embryos (137). Yet ALA at considerably higher concentrations has not proved toxic to human spinal cord neurons in culture (138). The similarity in chemical structure between ALA, the inhibitory neurotransmitter γ-aminobutyric acid (GABA), and the excitatory neurotransmitter L-glutamic acid has suggested a possible effect on

neuronal function, but such an association has not been proven (139,140).

Heme Deficiency

It has been postulated that the acute attack represents the clinical effects of intracellular (and more specifically intraneuronal) heme deficiency (128), since there is experimental evidence in patients with porphyria of a functional heme deficiency in some heme-containing enzymes. Thus, in patients with VP, impaired cytochrome P-450–mediated drug metabolism has been demonstrated (141–143); this function is restored to normal following the administration of exogenous heme. Evidence of direct intraneuronal heme deficiency is lacking (144), and it appears more likely that a deficiency in hemoprotein activity outside the CNS is important. A candidate enzyme is tryptophan dioxygenase, reduced activity of which results in the increased production of serotonin, a known modulator of neuronal function (143,145). It has also been postulated that heme deficiency might lead to deficiencies in cytochrome-dependent energy production in neuronal tissue, leading to axonal degeneration (146), although the evidence is weak.

Treatment of the Acute Attack

This chapter does not describe the clinical management of porphyria in detail. Useful reviews of the general management of the acute attack of porphyria may be found elsewhere (127,147,148). However, the specific therapy of the underlying metabolic defect will be reviewed to throw some light on the physiologic disorders accounting for the porphyria.

The Glucose Effect

The earliest specific therapy advocated for the acute porphyric attack was carbohydrate loading. In early clinical studies, it was suggested that approximately 75% of patients would respond favorably to intravenous or oral glucose administration (149). Additionally, there is experimental evidence that ALAS activity and porphyrin synthesis are repressed when liver cells grown in culture are exposed to porphyrinogenic medication in the presence of high carbohydrate concentrations. Carbohydrate intake also inhibits the induction of hepatic ALAS in experimental porphyria and in human AIP. But no dose-response curve has been shown for the effect of glucose on the induction of hepatic ALAS. Conversely, there is evidence that deficient carbohydrate intake and fasting may precipitate the acute attack of porphyria, and may even increase porphyrin excretion both in healthy subjects and in experimental rats. This, the so-called glucose effect, is demonstrable in AIP, VP, and even in nonacute porphyrias such as erythropoietic protoporphyria (EPP) and porphyria cutanea tarda (PCT). In addition to glucose, fructose and glycerol appear to share this ability to reduce porphyrin synthesis.

Heme Administration

Heme administration in patients with acute attacks of porphyria results in decreased porphyrin production via a repression of ALAS by a process of negative feedback (150), and is clinically highly efficacious. The effect, however, is short-lived (151,152). Since heme is known to induce the enzyme heme oxygenase and thus to mediate its own metabolism, tolerance may result from frequent administration. This has suggested the use of inhibitors of heme oxygenase in clinical practice. A number of substituted metalloporphyrins including tin protoporphyrin, tin mesoporphyrin, and zinc mesoporphyrin will inhibit heme oxygenase. In animal and human experiments, these inhibitors markedly inhibit the induction of hepatic ALAS, the production of ALA and PBG, and the appearance of bilirubin (153,154). There is as yet insufficient experience for their role in the treatment of human porphyria to be defined, but the preliminary evidence suggests that they may be beneficial in unusual patients with severe, recurrent acute attacks (148,155).

THE SPECIFIC SYNDROMES OF PORPHYRIA
5-Aminolevulinic Acid Dehydratase Deficiency

Also known as plumboporphyria or Doss porphyria, this is a rare autosomal-recessive disorder of heme synthesis. Five cases have now been reported since the first description in 1979. The molecular defects have been reported in three of these patients; all have been shown to be compound heterozygotes bearing single base substitutions, unique to each patient, on each allele (118). The patients exhibit a predominately neurologic syndrome similar to the acute attack, with abdominal pain and vomiting progressing to a motor neuropathy and paralysis. One presented in infancy, two in adolescence, and two at an advanced age.

Porphobilinogen Deaminase Deficiency

The clinical syndrome associated with a deficiency of PBG deaminase is acute intermittent porphyria. This is the commonest of the acute porphyrias and is transmitted as an autosomal-dominant trait. Clinical symptoms are restricted to the acute attack, and skin disease is not encountered. This is ascribed to the observation that it is only the precursors ALA and PBG that are elevated in this disorder, rather than the porphyrins. An overall prevalence for Europe of 1 to 2 per 10,000 has been suggested (148), but in Finland, the prevalence is higher, at 2 per 1,000 (156).

Molecular Biology

The human *PBGD* gene has been assigned to chromosome 11q24 (157). The gene contains two distinct promoters; alternative splicing gives rise to two primary transcripts and the production of distinct erythroid and nonerythroid mRNAs, which give rise to two proteins of slightly varying lengths. More than 100 mutations in the *PBGD* gene have been reported in patients with AIP. These have recently been summarized by Grandchamp (158). Most mutations are found in single families. However, the W198X mutation is present in about 50% of AIP families in Sweden (159), and is thought to result from a founder effect for this mutation, and the R116W mutation accounts for a third of AIP cases in the Netherlands (160).

Uroporphyrinogen III Cosynthetase Deficiency

Congenital erythropoietic porphyria (CEP) is the clinical syndrome associated with a deficiency of uroporphyrinogen III cosynthetase (UROS). This is an autosomal-recessive condition and is rare. It is an erythropoietic porphyria that primarily affects heme synthesis in the erythroid compartment, and presents with skin disease alone. Patients are not at risk of developing an acute attack. Severe UROS deficiency results in a failure of production of physiologically relevant series III porphyrin isomers, and series I isomers of uroporphyrin and its decarboxylated derivatives accumulate as a result of spontaneous cyclization and decarboxylation. Characteristic clinical features include hemolysis, mild splenomegaly, anemia, and photomutilation that is usually severe.

Molecular Biology

The molecular basis of CEP has recently been reviewed by Desnick et al. (44). Eighteen mutations have been identified in the UROS gene, comprising deletions, insertions, splice mutations, and single base substitutions. All but one of the known CEP missense mutations occurred in apparently highly conserved UROS peptide sequences. Some patients are homoallelic for a specific mutation, whereas other patients are heteroallelic. CEP is encountered in populations around the world, and several shared mutations have been identified in patients from apparently unrelated families. Particularly striking is the C73R mutation, found in 22 unrelated families and homoallelic in five of the subjects. There is evidence of some genotype–phenotype correlation in CEP. Thus the C73R mutation results in the detection of less than 1% of normal activity when expressed in *E. coli*; human homozygotes for this mutation appear to demonstrate an extremely severe phenotype that may include profound anemia, hydrops fetalis, and transfusion dependency at birth. Patients who carry both C73R and a second mutation that appears to express somewhat more residual activity may demonstrate a moderately severe phenotype, whereas patients who are allelic for mutations with more residual activity have milder forms of CEP (44).

There is considerable interest in gene therapy for CEP, since it is a severe disorder for which therapy is at best largely ineffective. Wild-type UROS cDNA has successfully been introduced into retroviral experiments *in vitro*, which have proved that it is possible to increase greatly UROS activity in hematopoietic progenitor cells and early erythroid cells, as well as in mononuclear cells and fibroblasts from patients with CEP following transfection vectors (161,162).

Uroporphyrinogen Decarboxylase Deficiency

Uroporphyrinogen decarboxylase (UROD) deficiency is associated with PCT, the most common form of porphyria encountered in most countries. The clinical features therefore include blistering, scarring, and pigmentary changes in sun-exposed areas of the skin, and typically a low-grade hepatitis (163). Two forms, clinically indistinguishable, are recognized: familial and sporadic. In both forms hepatic UROD activity is reduced. Additionally, in familial PCT, erythrocyte UROD activity is also reduced, in keeping with a genetic predisposition expressed in all somatic cells, and mutations in the UROPD gene are recognizable. In sporadic PCT, by contrast, the UROD gene is normal (164), reduced UROD activity is restricted to the liver, and, following removal of such precipitating factors as iron overload, may return to normal, suggesting that UROD is subject to the effects of an inhibitor whose effects may be reversed (163). The mechanism for this is not understood, and it is discussed further below.

Molecular Biology

Some 34 UROD gene mutations have been identified in patients with familial PCT. Most are restricted to single families. Where patients are homoallelic for UROD mutation, or are heteroallelic for two such mutations, a severe phenotype referred to as hepatoerythropoietic porphyria may result. This is associated with a severe deficiency in UROD activity in all tissues and is expressed clinically as severe photosensitivity with photomutilation, with onset in childhood (49,51). Familial PCT accounts for approximately 20% of all patients with PCT (165–167), and is inherited as an autosomal-dominant trait but with low clinical penetrance: most clinically expressed cases of familial PCT will be found to have associated risk factors known to produce sporadic PCT, though the average age of onset may be earlier. This suggests that in many cases the presence of a mutant UROD is not of itself sufficient to result in clinical symptoms, but that when exposed to factors thought to inhibit UROD, the threshold for development of symptoms is lower.

Conditions Associated with Sporadic Porphyria Cutanea Tarda

Sporadic PCT is clearly associated with a number of associated, and presumably causally related, factors. These include hepatic iron overload; alcohol consumption; estrogen therapy; viral infection, particularly hepatitis C virus (HCV) and human immunodeficiency virus (HIV); certain hydrocarbon-based toxins such as hexachlorbenzene; and, rarely, some systemic disorders including systemic lupus erythematosus and lymphoma (163,168). In nearly all cases of PCT, at least one of these disorders is present; frequently, several are present in combination.

Iron Loading

In most cases, mild to moderate iron loading of the liver is demonstrable. It has been shown that there is an approximately double allele frequency for the C282Y mutation in the *HFE* gene associated with genetic hemochromatosis in patients of northern European extraction (169–171). This association is not seen in other populations: the H63D mutation may be associated in patients of southern European origin, and suggests that a high transferrin saturation level in a patient with PCT might imply homozygosity for the hemochromatosis gene in European populations (170–172).

Viral Infection

A high prevalence of HCV antibodies in patients with PCT has been demonstrated in several studies from southern Europe with seroprevalences ranging from 62% to over 90% (173). However, studies from northern Europe and South Africa suggest a much weaker association. An association with HIV infection has also been suggested, though it appears that most such patients have other risk factors for the PCT as well (174).

Alcohol, Estrogen, and Other Hepatotoxins

There is a strong association between heavy alcohol ingestion and PCT (168), as well as with the use of natural and synthetic estrogens and toxins such as hexachlorbenzene. Less common factors associated with PCT include some systemic disorders, including systemic lupus erythematosus and lymphoma, and chronic renal failure on hemodialysis.

Pathogenesis

The pathogenesis of PCT has recently been summarized by Elder (163). There is evidence that during the recovery from clinically expressed PCT, in both sporadic and familial forms of the disease, the specific activity of hepatic UROD increases; in sporadic PCT, it may return to normal (175). This suggests that overt disease results from progressive inactivation of a structurally normal enzyme within the liver. The link between factors such as alcohol abuse, iron overload, and viral infection and UROD inhibition is not yet understood. It seems likely that iron serves largely as a powerful oxidant with resultant formation of reactive oxygen species that may bring about the oxidation of uroporphyrinogen to uroporphyrin and of other products that may themselves inhibit UROD (176,177). It is likely that the cytochrome P-450 family is involved. CYP1A is induced by the cyclic hydrocarbons associated with both toxic PCT in humans and its experimental counterpart in animals; in rodents, an isoform of CYP1A catalyzes the microsomal oxidation of uroporphyrinogen to uroporphyrin (178) and reaction is promoted by iron *in vitro*. In a schema suggested by Elder (163), induction of CYP1A results in the oxidation of uroporphyrinogen III to uroporphyrin III (which can therefore participate no further in heme synthesis) and accelerates the production of nonporphyrin oxidation products; these reactions are promoted by the presence of iron-derived reactive oxygen species. These porphyrin products result in the irreversible inhibition of UROD with consequent further accumulation of uroporphyrinogen III, providing further substrate for the oxidation and thus establishing a self-sustaining cycle. Removal of iron may interrupt this cycle, allowing a restoration of normal UROD activity and a reduction in intracellular uroporphyrinogen III. In this schema, iron may be considered a switch controlling the formation of inactivators of UROD.

Treatment

Unlike other forms of porphyria, PCT is treatable. Precipitating factors such as alcohol and estrogen exposure should be removed. Iron removal by venesection is highly effective, and can be shown to result in a restoration of hepatic UROD activity to normal levels in sporadic PCT. Oral administration of chloroquine will also induce remission in most cases by releasing uroporphyrin stored within hepatocyte lysosomes (179), but is not recommended as sole therapy as it will not reduce the potentially deleterious elevation in iron stores.

Coproporphyrinogen Oxidase Deficiency

A deficiency in coproporphyrinogen oxidase is associated with the human disease hereditary coproporphyria and is inherited as an autosomal-dominant trait. Both the acute attack and photosensitive skin disease are encountered. It is a less common condition than other AIP or VP. Frequencies in three different populations have been estimated to range from approximately 1 in 70,000 to 1 in 130,000. It is estimated that only approximately a third of these will be clinically manifest.

Molecular Biology

The gene for coproporphyrinogen oxidase is localized to chromosome 3q12. It has a single promoter region that may be differentially regulated in erythroid and nonerythroid tissues (62,63). In addition to five polymorphisms, at least 19 mutations have been characterized and found to underlie hereditary coproporphyria (180). Homozygous HCP has been seen. A variant coproporphyrinogen oxidase deficiency syndrome has been described and labeled harderoporphyria (181). In this condition, hematologic manifestations predominate and include jaundice, severe hemolytic anemia, hepatosplenomegaly, and skin photosensitivity. The oxidation of coproporphyrinogen is a two-step reaction, proceeding via an intermediate harderoporphyrinogen. In harderoporphyria, it appears that the responsible mutations result in a selective failure of the second step, resulting in accumulation of harderoporphyrin and this unusual syndrome.

Protoporphyrinogen Oxidase Deficiency

Protoporphyrinogen oxidase (PPO) is the penultimate enzyme of the heme synthetic pathway and is responsible for the oxidation of protoporphyrinogen to protoporphyrin IX. Deficiency is clinically associated with variegate porphyria (VP). VP is transmitted as an autosomal-dominant trait and is associated with both acute attacks and photosensitivity. In Britain, VP has been estimated to occur with a prevalence roughly one-third that of AIP, or approximately 0.5 per 100,000 (148). The prevalence is very much higher in South Africa, where it has been estimated to approach 0.6% in the European immigrant population. This is ascribed to a founder effect and has been traced back to a Dutch settler who arrived in the Cape of Good Hope in 1688 (147).

Molecular Biology

The gene for human PPO has been assigned to chromosome 1q22-23 (85). In South Africa a single mutation (R59W) predominates, and has been estimated to account for 95% of the subjects with VP in that country (182); haplotype comparison with the Dutch families with the R59W mutation supports the belief that the mutation was imported from Holland. However, a further nine mutations have been identified in South African families, three of which have been shown heteroallelic to the R59W mutation in compound heterozygotes (183). This suggests a considerable degree of heterogeneity for VP. More than 80 PPO mutations associated with VP have now been reported from around the world. A large study of patients with VP drawn from both England and France has been instructive (184). Most are private mutations, though an R168H mutation appears to have arisen independently on several occasions, as has an L15F mutation.

Kinetic Basis of the Acute Attack

The association between VP and the acute attack is not intuitively obvious, since it is always associated with elevations in the proximal precursors ALA and PBG. In PCT, despite a significant accumulation of intermediate porphyrins, an elevation of ALA and PBG is never encountered and acute attacks are not a feature. Meissner et al. (185,186) demonstrated that in lymphoblasts derived from VP subjects, PBG deaminase activity was decreased by approximately 25% in addition to the expected 50% reduction in PPO activity and was accompanied by an abnormal sigmoidal substrate velocity curve, suggesting allosteric behavior. Furthermore, reduced PBG deaminase activity could be induced *in vitro* in VP-derived lymphoblasts by the addition of protoporphyrinogen IX and coproporphyrinogen III, but not uroporphyrinogen III, and normal kinetic behavior restored by the removal of these porphyrinogens. These findings are in complete agreement with the clinical observation that VP and HCP, the disorders in which coproporphyrinogen and protoporphyrinogen in particular accumulate, may both be associated with acute attack, whereas PCT, associated largely with the accumulation of uroporphyrinogen, is not.

Clinical Expression

In the absence of the ability to make a definitive diagnosis of inheritance of the porphyria at the molecular level, the proportion of patients in whom VP was expressed either clinically or biochemically was unknown. Two previous studies in Cape Town have examined the clinical expression of South African VP. Eales et al. (187) suggested that 17% had experienced only acute attacks, 52% showed evidence of skin disease alone, and 21% had suffered both. A subsequent telephone survey suggested that there had been a change over the period between the two studies, with a decreasing proportion experiencing acute attacks, correspondingly more experiencing skin disease only, and a significant group being clinically silent and only detected as a result of biochemical screening of affected families (147). Recently, using DNA-based testing as the basis of a diagnosis of VP, we have shown in a single large kindred carrying the R59W mutation that only 52% of adult gene carriers demonstrated abnormal stool biochemistry, though abnormal fluorescence peaks were demonstrable in 90%. Only 39% had ever experienced skin symptoms, and 4% had an unequivocal acute attack in addition to skin symptoms; thus 61% were clinically silent. No subject younger than 16 had either biochemical or clinical evidence of VP.

Homozygous Variegate Porphyria

Fourteen subjects with homozygous VP have been reported. The clinical features have been summarized by Hift et al. (188) and include the onset of photosensitivity in infancy, photomutilation, brachydactyly, neurologic features such as nystagmus and seizures, behavioral disorders, a sensory neuropathy, and, in some cases, mental retardation. An unex-

plained observation is that these subjects do not appear to develop acute attacks despite their severely reduced PPO activity. However, we have now identified two sisters, compound heterozygotes, who presented in adolescence, one of whom has experienced acute attacks.

Most of these subjects have now been described genotypically. A minority are true homozygotes; most are compound heterozygotes. Studies of the residual expression of the mutant enzymes support the hypothesis that co-inheritance of two mutations associated with complete loss of PPO kinetic activity is not compatible with life; in every case, a severe mutation was shown to be heteroallelic expressing some residual activity (189). It has not been possible to show a correlation between the phenotypic severity and the activity expressed by the mutant proteins. In all four South African patients with compound heterozygous VP, the common R59W mutation, known to be associated with near-complete loss of kinetic activity, was present on one allele; none of the other mutations were associated with clinically or biochemically expressed VP in the heterozygous state (183), suggesting that they are functionally less damaging: preliminary kinetic data from our laboratory support this. None of the mutations encountered in homozygous and compound heterozygous VP in Europe were associated with clinically expressed VP in heterozygotes, in keeping with the proposition that, in general, these mutations code for mutant enzyme with a variable degree of residual activity sufficient to avoid symptoms except when paired with a second mutant allele (189). Such "mild" mutations are those that appear to preserve 10% to 25% of activity of the wild-type enzyme.

Ferrochelatase Deficiency

This enzyme is responsible for the last step in heme synthesis, that is, the incorporation of ferrous iron into the protoporphyrin line macrocycles. Ferrochelatase deficiency is associated with the human disease EPP. EPP is associated with a characteristic form of cutaneous photosensitivity. In contrast to the skin disease of CEP, PCT, HCP, and VP, which is marked by a vesiculo-erosive pattern of skin injury, skin disease in EPP takes the form of an immediate hypersensitivity. Characteristically, patients who exceed an individual threshold of sun exposure manifest problems of burning, stinging, erythema, and edema in exposed areas, and learn to associate these unpleasant symptoms with sun exposure; they will voluntarily seek to avoid exposure. These features usually begin in childhood rather than postpubertally as in the case with the vesiculo-erosive forms of porphyria. Approximately 10% of clinically expressed cases show evidence of severe protoporphyrin accumulation in the liver, leading to hepatic injury and ultimately to liver failure. Typically liver decompensation occurs late in the illness, but once initiated, progresses rapidly.

Molecular Biology

The gene encoding human ferrochelatase has been mapped to chromosome 18q22 (190). Many mutations have now been identified in the ferrochelatase gene. In most cases, mutations are private and are limited to single families (191). The inheritance of EPP is complex. Though typically described as an autosomal-dominant trait with incomplete penetrance, there is evidence to suggest that, in some families at least, particularly those in whom liver damage occurs, an autosomal-recessive mechanism appears to fit the observed pattern of inheritance more accurately. Most patients with manifest disease have severely reduced ferrochelatase activity, suggesting a disorder carried on both alleles. This has led to the belief that co-inheritance of two defects—one, presumably more severe, from the biochemically abnormal parent and the second, less severe, from an apparently normal parent—is necessary before clinical EPP arises. Since only one parent can be shown biochemically to carry EPP, the disease appears to be dominant, yet its actual inheritance will be recessive (192). In one family a clearly mutated allele was complemented by a poorly expressed ferrochelatase allele associated with markedly reduced mRNA expression (193). It is not known, however, whether a similar mechanism is common to all families with EPP.

Therapy

Recommended therapy includes avoidance of light exposure, the use of topical photoprotectants, and administration of oral β-carotene with or without canthaxanthine. Anecdotally, many patients will report an improvement in light tolerance on β-carotene; this has been described both to be formation of a photoprotectant layer of pigmentation in the skin and to its free radical quenching properties. Yet, in a controlled trial, β-carotene could not be shown to be unequivocally effective (194). A significant intrahepatic circulation of porphyrins has been shown (195), which may be interrupted by the administration of sequestrants such as oral charcoal, cholestyramine, or colestipol (196) with a reduction in protoporphyrin levels. Other theoretically effective measures include the suppression of erythropoiesis by erythrocyte transfusions or the administration of hematin, or by plasmapheresis to reduce free protoporphyrin in the plasma. Liver transplantation has been reported for end-stage protoporphyrin hepatopathy; photosensitivity persists, which proves that the defect in the erythropoietic tissue alone is sufficient to produce symptoms. Furthermore, protoporphyrin-induced liver damage has recurred in the transplanted liver despite the correction of endogenous protoporphyrin production by the transplant. Bone marrow transplantation has not yet been reported in EPP. Of greatest theoretical benefit would be combined liver and bone marrow transplantation (191).

REFERENCES

1. Elder GH. Enzymatic defects in porphyria: an overview. *Semin Liver Dis* 1982;2:87–99.
2. Wyckoff EE, Kushner JP. The porphyrias. In: Arias IM, Boyer JL, Fausto N, et al., eds. *The liver: biology and pathobiology*, 3rd ed. New York: Raven Press, 1994:505–527.
3. Kappas A, Sassa S, Galbraith RA, et al. The porphyrias. In: Wyngaarden CR, Frederickson DS, eds. *The metabolic basis of inherited disease*, 6th ed. New York: McGraw-Hill, 1989:1305.
4. McDonagh AF, Bissell DM. Porphyria and porphyrinology—the past fifteen years. *Semin Liver Dis* 1998;1:3–15.
5. Bissell DM, Schmid R. Hepatic porphyrias. In: Schiff L, Schiff ER, eds. *Diseases of the Liver*, 6th ed. Philadelphia, Toronto: JB Lippincott, 1987:1075–1092.
6. Bloomer JR, Straka JG. Porphyrin metabolism. In: Arias IM, Jakoby WB, Popper H, et al., eds. *The liver: biology and pathobiology*, 2nd ed. New York: Raven Press, 1988:451–466.
7. Bottomley SS, Muller-Eberhard U. Pathophysiology of heme synthesis. *Semin Hematol* 1988;25:282–302.
8. Hunter GA, Ferreira GC. Lysine-313 of 5-aminolevulinate synthase acts as a general base during formation of the quinonoid reaction intermediates. *Biochem* 1999;38:3711–3718.
9. Ferreira GC, Vajapey U, Hafez O, et al. Aminolevulinate synthase: lysine 313 is not essential for binding the pyridoxal phosphate cofactor but is essential for catalysis. *Prot Sci* 1995;4:1001–1006.
10. Tan D, Barber MJ, Ferreira GC. The role of tyrosine 121 in cofactor binding of 5-aminolevulinate synthase. *Prot Sci* 1998;7:1208–1213.
11. Gong J, Hunter GA, Ferreira GC. Aspartate-279 in aminolevulinate synthase affects enzyme catalysis through enhancing the function of the pyridoxal 5′-phosphate cofactor. *Biochemistry* 1998;37:3509–3517.
12. Cox TC, Bawden MJ, Martin A, et al. Human erythroid 5-aminolevulinate synthase: promoter analysis and identification of an iron-responsive element in the mRNA. *EMBO J* 1991;10:1891–1902.
13. Bishop DF. Two different genes encode delta-aminolevulinate synthase in humans: nucleotide sequences of cDNAs for the housekeeping and erythroid genes. *Nucleic Acids Res* 1990;18:7187–7188.
14. Bishop DF, Henderson AS, Astrin KH. Human delta-aminolevulinate synthase: assignment of the housekeeping gene to 3p21 and the erythroid-specific gene to the X chromosome. *Genomics* 1990;7:207–214.
15. Cotter PD, Willard HF, Gorski JL, et al. Assignment of human erythroid delta-aminolevulinate synthase (ALAS2) to a distal subregion of band Xp11.21 by PCR analysis of somatic cell hybrids containing X; autosome translocations. *Genomics* 1992;13:211–212.
16. Riddle RD, Yamamoto M, Engel JD. Expression of delta-aminolevulinate synthase in avian cells: separate genes encode erythroid-specific and nonspecific isozymes. *Proc Natl Acad Sci USA* 1989;86:792–796.
17. Fujita H, Yamamoto M, Yamagami T, et al. Erythroleukemia differentiation. Distinctive responses of the erythroid-specific and the nonspecific delta-aminolevulinate synthase mRNA. *J Biol Chem* 1991;266:17494–17502.
18. Shoolingin-Jordan PM. Structure and mechanism of enzymes involved in the assembly of the tetrapyrrole macrocycle. *Biochem Soc Trans* 1998;26:326–336.
19. Norton E, Sarwar M, Shoolingin-Jordan P. Mechanistic studies on E. coli 5-aminolaevulinic acid dehydratase. *Biochem Soc Trans* 1998;26:S285.
20. Dent AJ, Beyersmann D, Block C, Hasnain SS. Two different

zinc sites in bovine 5-aminolevulinate dehydratase distinguished by extended X-ray absorption fine structure. *Biochemistry* 1990;29:7822–7828.

21. Spencer P, Jordan PM. Characterization of the two 5-aminolaevulinic acid binding sites, the A- and P-sites, of 5-aminolaevulinic acid dehydratase from *Escherichia coli. Biochem J* 1995; 305:151–158.

22. Potluri VR, Astrin KH, Wetmur JG, et al. Human delta-aminolevulinate dehydratase: chromosomal localization to 9q34 by in situ hybridization. *Hum Genet* 1987;76:236–239.

23. Kaya AH, Plewinska M, Wong DM, et al. Human delta-aminolevulinate dehydratase (ALAD) gene: structure and alternative splicing of the erythroid and housekeeping mRNAs. *Genomics* 1994;19:242–248.

24. Bishop TR, Miller MW, Beall J, et al. Genetic regulation of delta-aminolevulinate dehydratase during erythropoiesis. *Nucleic Acids Res* 1996;24:2511–2518.

25. Senior NM, Brocklehurst K, Cooper JB, et al. Comparative studies on the 5-aminolaevulinic acid dehydratases from *Pisum sativum, Escherichia coli* and *Saccharomyces cerevisiae. Biochem J* 1996;320:401–412.

26. Senior NM, Siligardi G, Drake A, et al. Structural studies on 5-aminolaevulinic acid dehydratase from Saccharomyces cerevisiae. *Biochem Soc Trans* 1997;25:78S.

27. Erskine PT, Senior N, Maignan S, et al. Crystallization of 5-aminolaevulinic acid dehydratase from *Escherichia coli* and *Saccharomyces cerevisiae* and preliminary X-ray characterization of the crystals. *Prot Sci* 1997;6:1774–1776.

28. Erskine PT, Senior N, Awan S, et al. X-ray structure of 5-aminolaevulinate dehydratase, a hybrid aldolase. *Nat Struct Biol* 1997;4:1025–1031.

29. Frankenberg N, Erskine PT, Cooper JB, et al. High resolution crystal structure of a Mg2+-dependent porphobilinogen synthase. *J Mol Biol* 1999;289:591–602.

30. Jordan PM, Warren MJ. Evidence for a dipyrromethane cofactor at the catalytic site of *E. coli* porphobilinogen deaminase. *FEBS Lett* 1987;225:87–92.

31. Awan SJ, Siligardi G, Shoolingin-Jordan PM, et al. Reconstitution of the holoenzyme form of *Escherichia coli* porphobilinogen deaminase from apoenzyme with porphobilinogen and preuroporphyrinogen: a study using circular dichroism spectroscopy. *Biochemistry* 1997;36:9273–9282.

32. Louie GV, Brownlie PD, Lambert R, et al. The three-dimensional structure of *Escherichia coli* porphobilinogen deaminase at 1.76-A resolution. *Proteins* 1996;25:48–78.

33. Miller AD, Hart GJ, Packman LC, et al. Evidence that the pyrromethane cofactor of hydroxymethylbilane synthase (porphobilinogen deaminase) is bound to the protein through the sulphur atom of cysteine-242. *Biochem J* 1988;254:915–918.

34. McNeill LA, Shoolingin-Jordan PM. Dipyrromethane cofactor assembly in porphobilinogen deaminase. *Biochem Soc Trans* 1998;26:S286.

35. Grandchamp B, Romeo PH, Dubart A, et al. Molecular cloning of a cDNA sequence complementary to porphobilinogen deaminase mRNA from rat. *Proc Natl Acad Sci USA* 1984;81: 5036–5040.

36. Yoo HW, Warner CA, Chen CH, et al. Hydroxymethylbilane synthase: complete genomic sequence and amplifiable polymorphisms in the human gene. *Genomics* 1993;15:21–29.

37. Grandchamp B, De Verneuil H, Beaumont C, et al. Tissue-specific expression of porphobilinogen deaminase. Two isoenzymes from a single gene. *Eur J Biochem* 1987;162:105–110.

38. Jordan PM, Warren MJ, Mgbeje BI, et al. Crystallization and preliminary X-ray investigation of *Escherichia coli* porphobilinogen deaminase. *J Mol Biol* 1992;224:269–271.

39. Louie GV, Brownlie PD, Lambert R, et al. Structure of porphobilinogen deaminase reveals a flexible multidomain polymerase with a single catalytic site. *Nature* 1992;359:33–39.

40. Jordan PM, Woodcock SC. Mutagenesis of arginine residues in the catalytic cleft of *Escherichia coli* porphobilinogen deaminase that affects dipyrromethane cofactor assembly and tetrapyrrole chain initiation and elongation. *Biochem J* 1991;280:445–449.

41. Lander M, Pitt AR, Alefounder PR, et al. Studies on the mechanism of hydroxymethylbilane synthase concerning the role of arginine residues in substrate binding. *Biochem J* 1991;275:447–452.

42. Spivey AC, Capretta A, Frampton CS, et al. Biosynthesis of porphyrins and related macrocycles. Part 45. Determination by a novel X-ray method of the absolute configuration of the spiro lactam which inhibits uroporphyrinogen III synthase (cosynthase). *J Chem Soc Perkin Trans* 1996;1:2091–2102.

43. Tsai SF, Bishop DF, Desnick RJ. Purification and properties of uroporphyrinogen III synthase from human erythrocytes. *J Biol Chem* 1987;262:1268–1273.

44. Desnick RJ, Glass IA, Xu W, et al. Molecular genetics of congenital erythropoietic porphyria. *Semin Liver Dis* 1998;18:77–84.

45. Tsai SF, Bishop D, Desnick R. Human uroporphyrinogen III synthase: molecular cloning, nucleotide sequence and expression of a full-length cDNA. *Proc Natl Acad Sci USA* 1988;85:7049–7053.

46. Astrin KH, Warner CA, Yoo HW, et al. Regional assignment of the human uroporphyrinogen III synthase (UROS) gene to chromosome 10q25.2-q26.3. *Hum Genet* 1991;87:18–22.

47. Xu W, Kozak CA, Desnick RJ. Uroporphyrinogen III synthase: molecular cloning, nucleotide sequence, expression of a mouse full-length cDNA, and its localization on mouse chromosome 7. *Genomics* 1995;26:556–562.

48. Smith AG, Francis JE. Investigation of rat liver uroporphyrinogen decarboxylase—comparisons of porphyrinogens I and III as substrates and the inhibition by porphyrins. *Biochem J* 1981; 195:241–250.

49. Elder GH, Roberts AG. Uroporphyrinogen decarboxylase. *J Bioenerg Biomembr* 1994;27:207–214.

50. Elder GH, Tovey JA, Sheppard DM. Purification of uroporphyrinogen decarboxylase from human erythrocytes. *Biochem J* 1983;215:45–55.

51. Moran-Jimenez MJ, Ged C, Romana M, et al. Uroporphyrinogen decarboxylase: complete gene sequence and molecular study of three families with hepatoerythropoietic porphyria. *Am J Hum Genet* 1996;58:712–721.

52. Wu C, Xu W, Kozak CA, et al. Mouse uroporphyrinogen decarboxylase: cDNA cloning, expression, and mapping. *Mamm Genom* 1996;7:349–352.

53. Wyckoff EE, Phillips JD, Sowa AM, et al. Mutational analysis of human uroporphyrinogen decarboxylase. *Biochim Biophys Acta* 1996;1298:294–304.

54. Phillips JD, Whitby FG, Kushner JP, et al. Characterization and crystallization of human uroporphyrinogen decarboxylase. *Protein Sci* 1997;6:1343–1346.

55. Laterriere M, d'Estaintot BL, Dautant A, et al. Expression, purification, crystallization and preliminary X-ray diffraction analysis of human uroporphyrinogen decarboxylase. *Acta Crystallogr D Biol Crystallogr* 1998;54:476–478.

56. Whitby FG, Phillips JD, Kushner JP, et al. Crystal structure of human uroporphyrinogen decarboxylase. *EMBO J* 1998;17: 2463–2471.

57. Martásek P. Hereditary coporporphyria. *Semin Liver Dis* 1998; 18:25–32.

58. Taketani S, Kohno H, Furukawa T, et al. Molecular cloning, sequencing and expression of cDNA encoding human coproporphyrinogen oxidase. *Biochem Biophys Acta* 1994;1183(3): 547–549.

59. Medlock AE, Dailey HA. Human coproporphyrinogen oxidase is not a metalloprotein. *J Biol Chem* 1996;271:32507–32510.

60. Martasek P, Camadro J-M, Raman CS, et al. Human coproporphyrinogen oxidase. Biochemical characterization of recombinant normal and R231W mutated enzymes expressed in E. coli as soluble, catalytically active homodimers. *Cell Mol Biol* 1997; 43:47–58.

61. Kohno H, Furukawa T, Tokunaga R, et al. Mouse coproporphyrinogen oxidase is a copper-containing enzyme: expression in *Escherichia coli* and site-directed mutagenesis. *Biochim Biophys Acta* 1996;1292:156–162.

62. Martásek P, Camadro JM, Delfau-Larue MH, et al. Molecular cloning, sequencing, and functional expression of a cDNA encoding human coproporphyrinogen oxidase. *Proc Natl Acad Sci USA* 1994;91:3024–3028.

63. Delfau-Larue MH, Martásek P, Grandchamp B. Coproporphyrinogen oxidase: gene organization and description of a mutation leading to exon 6 skipping. *Hum Mol Genet* 1994;3: 1325–1330.

64. Porra RJ, Falk JE. The enzymic conversion of coproporphyrinogen III into protoporphyrin IX. *Biochem J* 1964;90: 69–75.

65. Meissner PN. Enzyme studies in variegate porphyria. 1990, PhD Thesis, University of Cape Town.

66. Dailey HA, Dailey TA. Protoporphyrinogen oxidase of *Myxococcus xanthus*. Expression, purification, and characterization of the cloned enzyme. *J Biol Chem* 1996a;271:8714–8718.

67. Deybach J-C, Da Silva V, Grandchamp B, et al. The mitochondrial location of protoporphyrinogen oxidase. *Eur J Biochem* 1985;149:435–439.

68. Dailey TA, Meissner P, Dailey HA. Expression of a cloned protoporphyrinogen oxidase. *J Biol Chem* 1994;269:813–815.

69. Hansson M, Hederstedt L. *Bacillus subtilis* hemY is a peripheral membrane protein essential for protoheme IX synthesis which can oxidize coproporphyrinogen III and protoporphyrinogen IX. *J Bacteriol* 1994;176:5962–5970.

70. Camadro J-M, Labbe P. Cloning and characterization of the yeast HEM14 gene coding for protoporphyrinogen oxidase, the molecular target of diphenyl ether-type herbicides. *J Biol Chem* 1996;271:9120–9128.

71. Hansson M, Gustafsson MCU, Kannangara CG, et al. Isolated *Bacillus subtilis* hemY has coproporphyrinogen III to coproporphyrin III oxidase activity. *Biochim et Biophys Acta* 1997;1340: 97–104.

72. Scalla R, Matringe M. Inhibitors of protoporphyrinogen oxidase as herbicides: diphenyl ethers and related photobleaching molecules. *Rev Weed Sci* 1994;6:103–132.

73. Ferreira GC, Dailey HA. Mouse protoporphyrinogen oxidase. Kinetic parameters and demonstration of inhibition by bilirubin. *Biochem J* 1988;250:597–603.

74. Hansson M, Hederstedt L. Cloning and characterization of the *Bacillus subtilis* hemEHY gene cluster, which encodes protoheme IX biosynthetic enzymes. *J Bacteriol* 1992;174: 8081–8093.

75. Corrigall AV, Siziba KB, Maneli MH, et al. Purification of and kinetic studies on a cloned protoporphyrinogen oxidase from the aerobic bacterium Bacillus subtilis. *Arch Biochem Biophys* 1998;358:251–256.

76. Dailey TA, Dailey HA. Identification of an FAD superfamily containing protoporphyrinogen oxidases, monoamine oxidases, and phytoene desaturase. Expression and characterization of phytoene desaturase of *Myxococcus xanthus*. *J Biol Chem* 1998; 273(22):13658–13662.

77. Sasarman A, Nepveu A, Echelard Y, et al. Molecular cloning and sequencing of the hemD gene of *Escherichia coli* K-12 and preliminary data on the *Uro operon*. *J Bacteriol* 1987;169: 4257–4262.

78. Dailey TA, Dailey HA, Meissner PN, et al. Cloning, sequencing, and expression of mouse protoporphyrinogen oxidase. *Arch Biochem Biophys* 1995;324(2):379–384.

79. Taketani S, Yoshinaga T, Furukawa T, et al. Induction of terminal enzymes for heme biosynthesis during differentiation of mouse erythroleukemia cells. *Eur J Biochem* 1995;230: 760–765.

80. Taketani S, Inazawa J, Abe T, et al. The human protoporphyrinogen oxidase gene (PPOX): organization and localization to chromosome 1. *Genomics* 1995;29:698–703.

81. Nishimura K, Taketani S, Inokuchi H. Cloning of a cDNA for protoporphyrinogen oxidase by complementation in vivo of a hemG mutant of *Escherichia coli*. *J Biol Chem* 1995;270: 8076–8080.

82. Dailey TA, Dailey HA. Human protoporphyrinogen oxidase: Expression, purification and characterization of the cloned enzyme. *Prot Sci* 1996;5:98–105.

83. Dailey TA, Dailey HA. Expression, purification and characterization of mammalian protoporphyrinogen oxidase. *Methods Enzymol* 1997;281:340–349.

84. Dailey HA, Dailey TA. Characterization of human protoporphyrinogen oxidase in controls and variegate porphyrias. *Cell Mol Biol* 1997;43:67–73.

85. Roberts AG, Whatley SD, Daniels J, et al. Partial characterization and assignment of the gene for protoporphyrinogen oxidase and variegate porphyria to human chromosome 1q23. *Hum Mol Genet* 1995;4:2387–2390.

86. Puy H, Robreau AM, Rosipal R, et al. Protoporphyrinogen oxidase: complete genomic sequence and polymorphisms in the human gene. *Biochem Biophys Res Commun* 1996;226(1): 226–230.

87. Corrigall AV, Hift RJ, Hancock V, et al. Identification and characterization of a deletion (537 delAT) in the protoporphyrinogen oxidase gene in a South African variegate porphyria family. *Hum Mutat* 1998;12:403–407.

88. Dailey H. Ferrochelatase. In: Eichorn GL, Marzilli LG, Hausinger RP, eds. *Mechanism of metallocenter assembly*. New York: VCH, 1996:77–89.

89. Dailey HA, Dailey TA, Wu CK, et al. Ferrochelatase at the millennium: structures, mechanisms and [2Fe-2S] clusters. *Cell Mol Life Sci* 2000;57:1909–1926.

90. Dailey HA, Fleming JE. Bovine ferrochelatase. Kinetic analysis of inhibition by N-methylprotoporphyrin, manganese, and heme. *J Biol Chem* 1983;258:11453–11459.

91. Lavallee DK. Porphyrin metalation reactions in biochemistry. In: Liebman JF, Greenberg A, eds. *Mechanistic principles of enzyme activity*. New York: VCH, 1988:279–311.

92. Blackwood ME, Rush TS, Medlock A, et al. Resonance spectra of ferrochelatase reveal porphyrin distortion upon metal binding. *J Am Chem Soc* 1997;119:12170–12174.

93. Blackwood ME Jr, Rush TS 3rd, Romesberg F, et al. Alternative modes of substrate distortion in enzyme and antibody catalyzed ferrochelation reactions. *Biochemistry* 1998;37:779–782.

94. Karr SR, Dailey HA. The synthesis of murine ferrochelatase in vitro and in vivo. *Biochem J* 1988;254:799–803.

95. Brenner DA, Didier JM, Frasier F, et al. A molecular defect in human protoporphyria. *Am J Hum Genet* 1992;50:1203–1210.

96. Taketani S, Inazawa J, Nakahashi Y, et al. Structure of the human ferrochelatase gene. Exon/intron gene organization and location of the gene to chromosome 18. *Eur J Biochem* 1992; 205(1):217–222.

97. Brenner DA, Frasier F. Cloning of murine ferrochelatase. *Proc Natl Acad Sci USA* 1991;88(3):849–853.

98. Tugores A, Magness ST, Brenner DA. A single promoter directs both housekeeping and erythroid preferential expression of the human ferrochelatase gene. *J Biol Chem* 1994;269: 30789–30797.

99. Magness ST, Tugores A, Diala ES, et al. Analysis of the human ferrochelatase promoter in transgenic mice. *Blood* 1998;92: 320–328.

100. Dailey HA, Sellers VM, Dailey TA. Mammalian ferrochelatase. Expression and characterization of normal and two human porphyric ferrochelatases. *J Biol Chem* 1994b;269(1):390–395.

101. Dailey HA, Finnegan MG, Johnson MK. Human ferrochelatase is an iron-sulfur protein. *Biochem* 1994;33:403–407.

102. Ferreira GC, Franco R, Lloyd SG, et al. Mammalian ferochelatase, a new addition to the metalloenzyme family. *J Biol Chem* 1994;269:7062–7069.

103. Day AL, Parsons BM, Dailey HA. Cloning and characterization of *Gallus* and *Xenopus* ferrochelatases: Presence of the [2Fe-2S] cluster in nonmammalian ferrochelatase. *Arch Biochem Biophys* 1998;359:160–169.

104. Sellers VM, Wang KF, Johnson MK, et al. Evidence that the fourth ligand to the [2Fe-2S] cluster in animal ferrochelatase is a cysteine. Characterization of the enzyme from *Drosophila melanogaster*. *J Biol Chem* 1998;273:22311–22316.

105. Sellers VM, Johnson MK, Dailey HA. Function of the [2Fe-2S] cluster in mammalian ferrochelatase: a possible role as a nitric oxide sensor. *Biochemistry* 1996;35:2699–2704.

106. Burden AE, Wu CK, Dailey TA, et al. Human ferrochelatase: crystallization, characterization of the [2Fe-2S] cluster and determination that the enzyme is a homodimer. *Biochem Biophys Acta* 1999;1435:191–197.

107. Crouse BR, Sellers VM, Finnegan MG, et al. Site-directed mutagenesis and spectroscopic characterization of human ferrochelatase: identification of residues co-ordinating the [2Fe-2S] cluster. *Biochemistry* 1996;35:16222–16229.

108. Al-Karadaghi S, Hansson M, Nikonov S, et al. Crystal structure of ferrochelatase the terminal enzyme in heme biosynthesis. *Structure* 1997;5:1501–1510.

109. Kohno H, Okuda M, Furukawa T, et al. Site-directed mutagenesis of human ferrochelatase: identification of histidine-263 as a binding site for metal ions. *Biochim Biophys Acta* 1994;1209: 95–100.

110. Srivasata G, Borthwick IA, Macguire DJ, et al. Regulation of 5-aminolevulinate acid synthase mRNA in different rat tissues. *J Biol Chem* 1988;263:5202–5209.

111. Yamamoto M, Kure S, Engel JD. Structure, turnover, and heme-mediated suppression of the level of mRNA encoding rat liver delta-aminolevulinate synthase. *J Biol Chem* 1988;263: 15973–15979.

112. Drew PD, Ades IZ. Regulation of the stability of chicken embryo liver delta-aminolevulinate synthase mRNA by hemin. *Biochem Biophys Res Commun* 1989;162:102–107.

113. Hamilton JW, Bement WJ, Sinclair PR, et al. Heme regulates hepatic 5-aminlevulinate synthase mRNA expression by decreasing mRNA half-life and not by altering its rate of transcription. *Arch Biochem Biophys* 1991;289:387–392.

114. Yamauchi K, Hayashi N, Kikuchi G. Translocation of δ-aminolevulinate synthetase from the cytosol to the mitochondria and its regulation by hemin in the rat liver. *J Biol Chem* 1980;255:1746–1751.

115. Lathrop JT, Timko MP. Regulation by heme of mitochondrial protein transport through a conserved amino acid motif. *Science* 1993;259:522–525.

116. Ponka P. Tissue-specific regulation of iron metabolism and heme synthesis: distinct control mechanisms in erythroid cells. *Blood* 1997;89:1–25.

117. May BK, Dogra SC, Sadlon TJ, et al. Molecular regulation of heme biosynthesis in higher vertebrates. *Prog Nucl Acid Res Mol Biol* 1995;51:1–51.

118. Sassa S. ALAD porphyria. *Semin Liver Dis* 1998;18:95–101.

119. Klausner RD, Rounault TA, Harford, et al. Regulating the fate of mRNA: The control of cellular iron metabolism. *Cell* 1993; 72:19–28.

120. Melefors O, Goossen B, Johansson RS, et al. Translational control of 5-aminolevulinate synthase mRNA by iron-responsive elements in erythroid cells. *J Biol Chem* 1993;268:5974–5978.

121. Blom H, Andersson C, Olofsson BO, et al. Assessment of autonomic nerve function in acute intermittent porphyria: a study based on spectral analysis of heart rate variability. *J Int Med* 1996;240:73–79.

122. Windebank AJ, Bonkovsky HI. Porphyric neuropathy. In: Dyck PJ, Thomas PK, eds. *Peripheral neuropathy*. Philadelphia: WB Saunders, 1992.

123. Cavanagh JB, Mellick RS. On the nature of peripheral nerve lesions associated with acute intermittent porphyria. *J Neurol Neurosurg* 1965;28:320–327.

124. Gibson JB, Goldberg A. The neuropathology of acute porphyria. *J Pathol Bact* 1956;71:495–510.

125. Mustajoki P, Seppäläinen AM. Neuropathy in latent hereditary hepatic porphyria. *Br Med J* 1975;2:310–312.

126. Albers JW, Robertson WC, Daube JR. Electrodiagnostic findings in acute porphyric neuropathy. *Muscle Nerve* 1978;1: 292–296.

127. Kirsch RE, Meissner PN, Hift RJ. Variegate porphyria. *Semin Liver Dis* 1998;18:33–41.

128. Meyer UA, Schuurmans MM, Lindberg RLP. Acute porphyrias: pathogenesis of neurological manifestations. *Semin Liver Dis* 1998;18:43–52.

129. Mustajoki P. Variegate porphyria. *Q J Med* 1980;194:191–203.

130. Shimizu Y, Ida S, Naruto H, et al. Excretion of porphyrins in urine and bile after the administration of delta-aminolevulinic acid. *J Lab Clin Med* 1978;32:795–802.

131. Edwards SR, Shanley BC, Reynoldson JA. Neuropharmacology of delta-aminolaevulinic acid. I. Effect of acute administration in rodents. *Neuropharmacol* 1984;23:477–481.

132. Edwards SR, Shanley BC, Reynoldson JA. Neuropharmacology of delta-aminolaevulinic acid. II. Effect of chronic administration in mice. *Neurosci Lett* 1984;50:169–173.

133. Gorchein A, Webber R. Delta-aminolevulinic acid in plasma, cerebrospinal fluid, saliva and erythrocytes: studies in normal, uraemic and porphyric subjects. *Clin Sci* 1987;72:103–112.

134. Jordan P, Bagust J, Kelly M, et al. A model for acute intermittent porphyria: effects of 5-aminolaevulinic acid on ventral root activity in the hemisected hamster spinal cord. *Mol Asp Med* 1990;11:53–54.

135. Pierach CA, Edwards PS. Neurotoxicity of δ-aminolevulinic acid and porphobilinogen. *Exp Neurol* 1978;62:810–814.

136. Yeung-Lawah AC, Macphee G, Boyle P, et al. Autonomic neuropathy in acute intermittent porphyria. *J Neurol Neurosurg Psychiatry* 1987;48:1025–1030.

137. Percy VA, Lamm MCL, Taljaard JJF. Delta-aminolaevulinic acid uptake, neurotoxicity and effect on [14C] delta-aminobutyric acid uptake into neurons and glia in culture. *J Neurochem* 1981;36:69–76.

138. Gorchein A. δ-aminolaevulinic acid is not directly toxic to human spinal cord neurons in culture. *Biochem Soc Trans* 1989; 17:577–578.

139. Brennan MJW, Cantrill RC. δ-aminolaevulinic acid and amino acid neurotransmitters. *Mol Cell Biochem* 1981;38:49–58.

140. Puy H, Deybach J-C, Bogdan A, et al. Increased δ-aminolevulinic acid and decreased pineal melatonin production. *J Clin Invest* 1996;97:104–110.

141. Mustajoki P, Mustajoki S, Rautio A, et al. Effects of heme arginate on cytochrome P450-mediated metabolism of drugs in patients with variegate porphyria and healthy men. *Clin Pharmacol Ther* 1994;56:9–13.

142. Mustajoki P, Himberg JJ, Tokola O, et al. Rapid normalization

of antipyrine oxidation by heme in variegate porphyria. *Clin Pharmacol Ther* 1992;51:320–324.

143. Bonkovsky HL, Healey JF, Lurie AN, et al. Intravenous heme-albumin in acute intermittent porphyria: evidence for repletion of hepatic hemoproteins and regulatory heme pool. *Am J Gastroenterol* 1991;86:1050–1056.

144. De Matteis F, Ray RE. Studies on cerebellar heme metabolism in the rat in vivo. *J Neurochem* 1982;39:551–556.

145. Puy H, Deybach J-C, Baudry P, et al. Decreased nocturnal plasma melatonin levels in patients with recurrent acute intermittent porphyria attacks. *Life Sci* 1993;53:621–627.

146. Herrick AL, Fisher BM, Moore MR, et al. Elevation of blood lactate and pyruvate levels in acute intermittent porphyria—a reflection of heme deficiency? *Clin Chim Acta* 1990;190:157–162.

147. Hift RJ, Meissner PN, Corrigall AV, et al. Variegate porphyria in South Africa 1688–1996: new developments in an old disease. *S Afr Med J* 1997;87:722–731.

148. Elder GH, Hift RJ, Meissner PN. The acute porphyrias. *Lancet* 1997;349:1613–1617.

149. Doss M, Sixel-Dietrich F, Verspohl F. "Glucose effect" and rate limiting function of uroporphyrinogen synthase on porphyrin metabolism in hepatocyte culture: relationship with human acute porphyrias. *J Clin Chem Clin Biochem* 1985;23:505–513.

150. McColl KEL, Moore MR, Thompson GG, et al. Treatment with hemeatin in acute hepatic porphyria. *Q J Med* 1981;L198:161–174.

151. Mustajoki P. Prevention and treatment of acute porphyric attacks. *Ann Clin Res* 1985;17:289–291.

152. Herrick AL, McColl KE, Moore MR, et al. Controlled trial of heme arginate in acute hepatic porphyria. *Lancet* 1989;1:1295–1297.

153. Galbraith RA, Drummond GS, Kappas A. SN-protoporphyrin suppresses chemically induced experimental hepatic porphyria. Potential clinical implications. *J Clin Invest* 1985;76:2436–2439.

154. Berglund L, Angelin B, Blomstrand R, et al. SN-protoporphyrin lowers serum bilirubin levels, decreases biliary bilirubin output, enhances biliary heme excretion and potently inhibits hepatic heme oxygenase in normal human subjects. *Hepatology* 1988;8:625–631.

155. Dover SB, Moore MR, Fitzsimmons EJ, et al. Tin protoporphyrin prolongs the biochemical remission produced by heme arginate in acute hepatic porphyria. *Gastroenterology* 1993;105:500–506.

156. Mustajoki P, Kauppinen R, Lannfelt L, et al. Frequency of low erythrocyte porphobilinogen deaminase activity in Finland. *J Intern Med* 1992;231:389–395.

157. Namba M, Narahara K, Tsuji K, et al. Assignment of human PBGD to 11q24.1→11q24.2 by in situ hybridization and gene dosage studies. *Cytol Cell Genet* 1991;67:105–108.

158. Grandchamp B. Acute intermittent porphyria. *Semin Liver Dis* 1998;18:17–24.

159. Lee JS, Anvret M. Identification of the most common mutation within the porphobilinogen deaminase gene in Swedish patients with acute intermittent porphyria. *Proc Natl Acad Sci USA* 1991;88:10912–10915.

160. De Rooij FWM, Voortman G, De Baar E, et al. Frequency and distribution of mutations in the gene of porphobilinogen deaminase in Dutch acute intermittent porphyria patients. *Scand J Clin Lab Med* 1995;55(suppl 223):24A.

161. Moreau-Gaudry F, Gedz C, De Verneuil H. Gene therapy for erythropoietic porphyria. *Gene Ther* 1996;3:843–844.

162. Glass IA, Kauppinen R, Atweh G, et al. Toward gene therapy for congenital erythropoietic porphyria. *Am J Hum Genet* 1996;59:A198.

163. Elder GH. Porphyria cutanea tarda. *Semin Liver Dis* 1998;18:67–75.

164. Garey JR, Franklin KF, Brown DA, et al. Analysis of uroporphyrinogen decarboxylase complementary DNAs in sporadic porphyria cutanea tarda. *Gastroenterology* 1993;105:165–169.

165. Elder GH, Roberts AG, De Salamanca RE. Genetics and pathogenesis of human uroporphyrinogen decarboxylase defects. *Clin Biochem* 1989;22:163–168.

166. Held JL, Sassa S, Kappas A, et al. Erythrocyte uroporphyrinogen decarboxylase activity in porphyria cutanea tarda: a study of 40 consecutive patients. *J Invest Dermatol* 1989;93:332–334.

167. Koszo F, Morvay M, Dobozy A, et al. Erythrocyte uroporphyrinogen decarboxylase activity in 80 unrelated patients with porphyria cutanea tarda. *Br J Dermatol* 1992;126:446–449.

168. Hift RJ, Kirsch RE. Porphyria cutanea tarda as a manifestation of alcohol-induced liver disease. In: Hall P, ed. *Alcoholic liver disease*, 2nd ed. London: Edward Arnold, 1995:219–231.

169. Roberts AG, Whatley SD, Morgan RR, et al. Increased frequency of the hemeochromatosis Cys282Tyr mutation in sporadic porphyria cutanea tarda. *Lancet* 1997;349:321–323.

170. Bonkovsky HL, Poh-Fitzpatrick M, Pimstone N, et al. Porphyria cutanea tarda, hepatitis C, and HFE gene mutations in North America. *Hepatology* 1998;27:1661–1669.

171. Stuart KA, Busfield F, Jazwinska EC, et al. The C282Y mutation in the haemochromatosis gene (HFE) and hepatitis C virus infection are independent cofactors for porphyria cutanea tarda in Australian patients. *J Hepatol* 1998;28:404–409.

172. Roberts AG, Whatley SD, Nicklin S, et al. The frequency of hemeochromatosis-associated alleles is increased in British patients with sporadic porphyria cutanea tarda. *Hepatology* 1997;25:159–161.

173. Chuang TY, Brashear R, Lewis C. Porphyria cutanea tarda and hepatitis C virus: a case-control study and meta-analysis of the literature. *J Am Acad Dermatol* 1999;41:31–36.

174. Drobacheff C, Derancourt C, Van Landuyt H, et al. Porphyria cutanea tarda associated with human immunodeficiency virus infection. *Eur J Dermatol* 1998;8:492–496.

175. Elder GH, Urquhart AJ, De Salamanca RE, et al. Immunoreactive uroporphyrinogen decarboxylase in the liver in porphyria cutanea tarda. *Lancet* 1985;2:229–233.

176. De Matteis F. Role of iron in the hydrogen peroxide-dependent oxidation of hexahydroporphyrins (porphyrinogens): a possible mechanism for the exacerbation by iron of hepatic uroporphyria. *Mol Pharmacol* 1988;33:463–469.

177. Francis JE, Smith AG. Polycyclic aromatic hydrocarbons cause hepatic porphyria in iron-loaded CS7 BL/10 mice: comparison of uroporphyrinogen decarboxylase inhibition with induction of alkoxyphenoxazone dealkylations. *Biochem Biophys Res Commun* 1987;146:13–20.

178. Lambrecht RW, Sinclair PR, Gorman N, et al. Uroporphyrinogen oxidation catalyzed by reconstituted cytochrome P450IA2. *Arch Biochem Biophys* 1992;254:504–510.

179. Ashton RE, Hawk JLM, Magnus IA. Low-dose oral chloroquine in the treatment of porphyria cutanea tarda. *Br J Dermatol* 1981;111:609–613.

180. Rosipal R, Lamoril J, Puy H, et al. Systematic analysis of coproporphyrinogen oxidase gene defects in hereditary coproporphyria and mutation update. *Hum Mutat* 1999;13:44–53.

181. Lamoril J, Martasek P, Deybach J-C, et al. A molecular defect in coproporphyrinogen oxidase gene causing harderoporphyria, a variant form of hereditary coproporphyria. *Hum Mol Genet* 1995;4:275–278.

182. Meissner PN, Dailey TA, Hift RJ, et al. A R59W mutation in human protoporphyrinogen oxidase results in decreased

enzyme activity and is prevalent in South Africans with variegate porphyria. *Nat Genet* 1996;13:95–97.

183. Corrigall AV, Hift RJ, Davids LM, et al. Homozygous variegate porphyria in South Africa: Genotypic analysis in two cases. Mol Genet Metabol 2000;69:323–330.
184. Whatley SD, Puy H, Morgan RR, et al. Variegate porphyria in Western Europe: identification of PPOX gene mutations in 104 families, extent of allelic heterogeneity, and absence of correlation between phenotype and type of mutation. *Am J Hum Genet* 1999;65:984–994.
185. Meissner PN, Day RS, Moore MR, et al. Protoporphyrinogen oxidase and porphobilinogen deaminase in variegate porphyria. *Eur J Clin Invest* 1986;16:257–261.
186. Meissner PN, Adams P, Kirsch R. Allosteric inhibition of human lymphoblasts and purified porphobilinogen deaminase by protoporphyrinogen and coproporphyrinogen: a possible mechanism for the acute attack of variegate porphyria. *J Clin Invest* 1993;91:1436–1444.
187. Eales L, Day RS, Blekkenhorst GH. The clinical and biochemical features of variegate porphyria: an analysis of 300 cases studied at Groote Schuur Hospital, Cape Town. *Int J Biochem* 1980;12:837–853.
188. Hift RJ, Meissner PN, Todd G, et al. Homozygous variegate porphyria: an evolving clinical syndrome. *Postgrad Med J* 1993; 69:781–786.

189. Roberts AG, Puy H, Dailey TA, et al. Molecular characterization of homozygous variegate porphyria. *Hum Mol Genet* 1998; 7:1921–1925.
190. Whitcombe DM, Carter NP, Albertson DG, et al. Assignment of the human ferrochelatase gene (FECH) and a locus for protoporphyria to chromosome 18q22. *Genomics* 1991;11: 1152–1154.
191. Cox TM, Alexander GJM, Sarkany RPE. Protoporphyria. *Semin Liver Dis* 1998;18:85–93.
192. Sarkany RPE, Alexander GJM, Cox TM. Recessive inheritance of erythropoietic protoporphyria with liver failure. *Lancet* 1994; 343:1394–1396.
193. Gouya L, Deybach J-C, Lamoril J, et al. Modulation of the phenotype in dominant erythropoietic protoporphyria by a low expression of the normal ferrochelatase allele. *Am J Hum Genet* 1996;58:292–299.
194. Corbett MF, Herxheimer A, Magnus IA, et al. The longterm treatment with beta carotene in erythropoietic protoporphyria: a controlled trial. *Br J Dermatol* 1977;97:655–662.
195. Ibrahim GW, Watson CJ. Enterohepatic circulation and conversion of protoporphyrin to bile pigment in man. *Proc Soc Exp Biol Med* 1968;127:890–895.
196. Davidson DL, Bloomer JR, Klatskin G. Therapy of hepatic disease in erythropoietic protoporphyria. *Gastroenterology* 1973; 65:535.

COPPER METABOLISM AND THE LIVER

IQBAL HAMZA
JONATHAN D. GITLIN

Copper is an essential trace element that plays a critical role in the biochemistry of all aerobic organisms (see website chapter 🖳 W-18). The unique electron structure of this metal permits the facile transfer of electrons, which is exploited by specific enzymes in a select number of critical metabolic pathways (1). In humans, the function of these cuproenzymes is required for neurotransmitter biosynthesis, pigment production, antioxidant defense, peptide amidation, connective tissue processing, iron homeostasis, and cellular respiration (2). The signs and symptoms of copper deficiency are the result of decreased or absent function of these essential cuproproteins. The extraordinary reactivity of copper in biologic systems also accounts for the potential life-threatening toxicity of this metal in circumstances where copper homeostasis is severely impaired. For these reasons, organisms have evolved specific pathways that permit the trafficking and compartmentalization of copper within cells.

The inherited diseases of copper metabolism underscore both the essential need for copper as well as the toxicity of this metal. Elucidation of the molecular genetic basis of these diseases has revealed a remarkable evolutionary conservation of the molecular mechanisms of copper metabolism (3). Wilson disease is an inherited disorder of copper metabolism resulting in hepatic cirrhosis and basal ganglia degeneration. The recognition of a specific genetic disorder resulting in aberrant hepatic copper homeostasis revealed a

central role for the liver in copper metabolism and suggested an intricate specificity to the biochemistry of this metal within hepatocytes that was confirmed with the characterization of the Wilson disease gene (4). In humans, copper balance is entirely maintained by gastrointestinal absorption and biliary excretion, and this process is regulated at the stage of hepatocyte efflux of copper by the transport protein encoded at the Wilson locus.

PHYSIOLOGY

Absorption

The average daily diet in the industrialized world contains approximately 5 mg of copper (Fig. 22.1). About half of this intake of copper is absorbed each day through the gastrointestinal tract, and an equivalent amount is excreted through the biliary tract (5). There is no enterohepatic circulation of copper, and these pathways of absorption and excretion represent the only physiologically relevant mechanisms for maintaining copper balance. Copper can be absorbed through the dermis and mucosa if there is prolonged exposure to the metal such as can occur with jewelry or intrauterine devices, but this is negligible in terms of the total body content. Copper can be excreted from the sweat glands and removed from the plasma by renal filtration, but again these routes are quantitatively irrelevant except in cases of marked copper excess. Gastrointestinal uptake occurs in the duodenum, and although dietary content may influence the efficiency of copper absorption, there is little

I. Hamza and **J. D. Gitlin:** Edward Mallinckrodt Department of Pediatrics, Washington University School of Medicine, St. Louis, Missouri 63110.

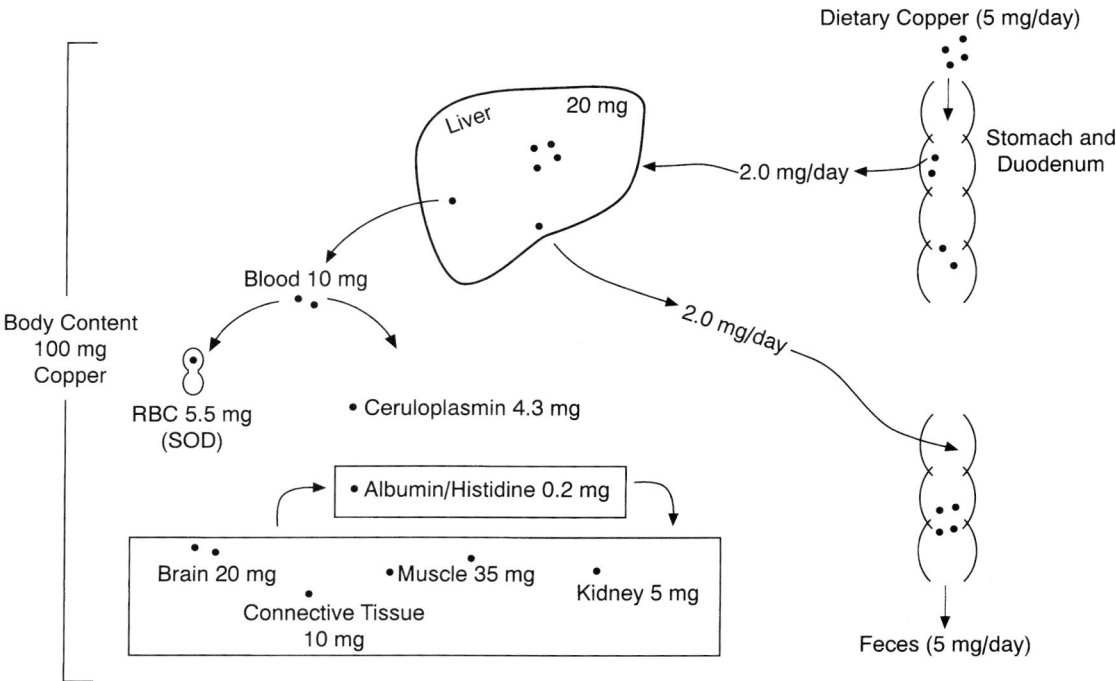

FIGURE 22.1. Pathways of human copper metabolism. Biliary excretion of copper is directly related to the size of the hepatic copper pool and is the only physiologic mechanism determining copper balance. (Modified from Harris ZL, Gitlin JD. Genetic and molecular basis for copper toxicity. *Am J Clin Nutr* 1996;63:8365, with permission.)

variability in total daily uptake among individuals (5). The fractional absorption of copper increases as the total body copper content decreases, but this process of regulation, although mitigating against copper deficiency, is insufficient to maintain balance at very low copper intakes (6).

Recent genetic experiments in *Saccharomyces cerevisiae* have elucidated the mechanisms of copper uptake into mammalian cells. These studies have identified three genes, *CTR1, CTR2,* and *CTR3,* that play an essential role in plasma membrane copper uptake in yeast (7,8). Complementation of a yeast strain deficient in the high-affinity transporter *CTR1* identified a human orthologue, hCTR1, which is expressed in multiple tissues and encodes a protein required for initial copper uptake in mammalian cells (9). Recent cloning of the high-affinity transporter *CTR4* from the fission yeast *Schizosaccharomyces pombe* suggests that hCTR1 is evolutionary derived from a fusion of the yeast *CTR1* and *CTR3* genes, an observation that may provide essential molecular clues for dissecting the mechanisms of mammalian plasma membrane copper uptake (10).

Distribution and Storage

Copper that is absorbed from the gastrointestinal tract appears in the portal circulation bound to histidine and albumin. Radioisotope studies have revealed that a single dose of orally administered ^{64}Cu is rapidly cleared from the plasma by hepatic first-pass kinetics. The liver may play a regulatory role in the distribution of copper to peripheral tissues, but the mechanisms underlying this process have not been elucidated. Nevertheless, within 24 hours following a single administered oral dose of copper, up to 10% will reappear in the plasma in the form of newly synthesized ceruloplasmin. These kinetics reflect only the relative abundance of this cuproenzyme in the plasma, as metabolic and clinical studies reveal no role for ceruloplasmin in copper transport (11,12). Although the precise mechanisms of copper transport and delivery to tissues is unknown, copper is found in plasma complexed to amino acids such as histidine, which may be essential for uptake and utilization of this metal by multiple cell types (2).

Ceruloplasmin is an abundant serum cuproprotein that contains greater than 95% of plasma copper. This protein is synthesized in hepatocytes and secreted into the plasma following incorporation of six atoms of copper per molecule. Copper has no effect on the rate of synthesis or secretion of ceruloplasmin, but impaired incorporation of this metal during synthesis results in an apoprotein that is devoid of enzymatic activity and rapidly catabolized (13,14). The steady-state concentration of ceruloplasmin in the serum represents the sum of the apo and holo forms of the protein, which is determined by hepatocyte copper availability and the half-lives of each moiety. As anticipated from this model, a decrease in copper availability within the hepatocyte as observed in nutritional copper deficiency or Wilson disease results in a decrease in serum ceruloplasmin secondary to the rapid turnover of the secreted apoprotein.

Copper toxicity may result from accidental or intentional ingestion of copper-containing materials, leading to a marked elevation of free serum copper (15). In young children and infants, copper poisoning results in circulatory collapse secondary to copper-induced gastrointestinal hemorrhage. The liver has a considerable capacity to increase biliary copper excretion, and thus chronic copper overload is a rare occurrence in the normal individual. However, in the presence of underlying liver disease where storage capacity is reduced or biliary excretion is impaired, a moderate increase in copper uptake may result in chronic copper toxicosis. Copper can result in free-radical mediated damage once the capacity for storage and sequestration within the hepatocyte has been exceeded, and it is reasonable to presume that this may contribute to hepatic injury in more common disorders such as alcoholic cirrhosis. Evidence of lipid peroxidation and mitochondrial damage in both experimental and clinical copper toxicity supports this concept and suggests the possibility of therapeutic benefit from α-tocopherol or other antioxidants in chronic liver diseases where copper excess may occur (16).

The sites of copper storage within the liver have not been well characterized. Metallothioneins are small intracellular proteins with a multitude of cysteine residues capable of chelating several metal ions including copper. These proteins are found in abundance within the cytoplasm and nuclei of hepatocytes, but transgenic experiments reveal no essential role for metallothioneins in hepatic development or metal metabolism (17). However, experiments in which metallothionein-deficient mice were crossed with Menkes mottled mice reveal a critical role for these proteins in copper sequestration when the homeostasis of this metal is perturbed (18). On the basis of these findings, it seems reasonable to presume that metallothioneins play a similar role in hepatocytes, serving to militate against the effects of copper accumulation in Wilson disease or other situations of hepatic copper excess. What role, if any, these proteins play in the normal process of copper trafficking within cells remains to be elucidated.

Copper deficiency resulting from impaired dietary intake results in hypocupremia, decreased serum ceruloplasmin, decreased hepatic copper stores, neutropenia, anemia, metaphysial dysplasia, osteoporosis, and long-bone fractures (1). Such deficiency is very uncommon but has also been reported in premature infants receiving intravenous nutrition without copper supplementation, in dialysis patients, and in individuals with excess zinc ingestion for therapeutic or megavitamin purposes with resulting interference of copper absorption. The signs and symptoms of copper deficiency are also observed in Menkes disease, an inherited disorder of copper metabolism resulting in impaired copper transport across the placenta, intestine,

and blood–brain barrier due to the absence or dysfunction of a copper-transporting adenosine triphosphatase (ATPase) homologous to the Wilson protein (3).

Excretion

The liver serves as the predominant organ of copper homeostasis, demonstrating considerable capacity for both the storage and excretion of this metal (Fig. 22.1). As noted above, biliary excretion is the sole mechanism determining copper balance, and the amount of copper that is excreted in the bile is directly proportional to the overall size of the hepatic pool of copper (19). The form of copper appearing in the bile is unknown, but radioisotope studies indicate that this exists as an unabsorbable macromolecular complex resulting in no appreciable enterohepatic circulation. Ceruloplasmin is not involved in biliary copper excretion, as clinical and experimental studies of aceruloplasminemia reveal normal hepatic copper metabolism (11,12). All plasma proteins can be detected in small amounts in bile, and the absence of ceruloplasmin in the bile of patients with Wilson disease simply reflects the marked decrease in the serum concentration of this protein in affected patients.

Hepatocytes are the predominant site of copper accumulation within the liver. The intracellular copper concentration of these polarized epithelial cells serves as a set point that reflects the total body copper status. These cells then sense this copper status and regulate copper excretion into bile depending on the intracellular concentration of this metal. The molecular mechanisms of this process have begun to be clarified with elucidation of the molecular genetic defect in patients with Wilson disease. The ATPase encoded at the Wilson locus is abundantly expressed in hepatocytes where it is localized in the *trans*-Golgi network (20–22). When the copper content of the hepatocyte increases, the Wilson ATPase moves to a cytoplasmic vesicular compartment localized near the canalicular membrane (Fig. 22.2). Copper is then accumulated within this compartment by the transport mechanisms of the Wilson ATPase, and the resulting decrease in cytoplasmic copper triggers relocalization of the ATPase to the *trans*-Golgi network. In turn, the copper-containing vesicles move to the canalicular membrane for copper excretion into the bile. This mechanism therefore provides a rapid and efficient posttranslational copper-dependent regulation of the Wilson ATPase essential for maintaining intracellular copper homeostasis. The final steps of copper excretion into the bile have not been clearly elucidated, but immunofluorescent studies reveal the absence of the Wilson ATPase on this membrane during copper excess, suggesting that different transport mechanisms must be involved in this process (21,22).

Development

Clinical and experimental studies indicate that the majority of fetal copper is derived via placental transport. The

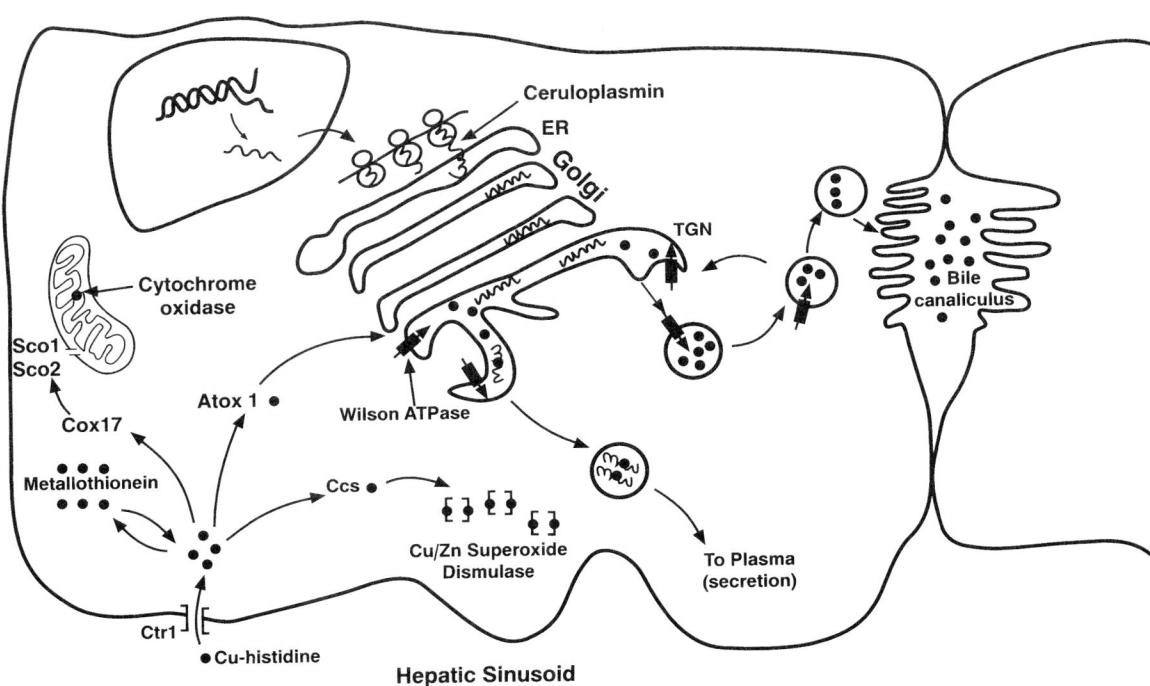

FIGURE 22.2. Cellular biology of copper metabolism. Intracellular trafficking of copper with specific chaperones and target proteins. The copper-dependent recycling of the Wilson adenosine triphosphatase (*ATPase*) is illustrated. *ER*, endoplasmic reticulum; *TGN, trans*-Golgi network. (Modified from Harris ZL, Gitlin JD. Genetic and molecular basis for copper toxicity. *Am J Clin Nutr* 1996;63:8365, with permission.)

Menkes ATPase is essential for this process, as human newborns deficient in this protein are profoundly copper deficient at birth. The Wilson ATPase also plays a role in placental copper transport, as two mouse models of Wilson disease reveal significant copper deficiency at birth, which is exacerbated under circumstances where the mother is also affected and unable to deliver copper from the milk (23,24). In these animal models, hepatic copper is markedly deficient at birth, indicating that the liver plays a critical role in copper metabolism during fetal development, serving as a storage site for maternally derived metal. Experimental and clinical studies reveal a considerable decrease in biliary excretory capacity in the fetus and newborn infant, and as a result copper accumulates in the fetal liver such that the normal concentration at birth greatly exceeds the adult levels. This concentration of hepatic copper does not decrease until several months postpartum due to developmental differences in the handling of copper by the hepatocyte at the level of the secretory pathway (21).

Ceruloplasmin is present in human fetal serum by the fifth week of gestation, and metabolic studies indicate that this is entirely derived from endogenous synthesis without maternal contribution (25). As a result of the differences in copper trafficking within the fetal and newborn liver, the human newborn synthesizes and secretes almost entirely apoceruloplasmin, and the serum concentration of this protein is very low for the first 3 to 6 months postpartum. For

this reason, these developmental differences in hepatic copper metabolism militate against the use of serum ceruloplasmin as a newborn screening test for Wilson disease or aceruloplasminemia. Similarly this normal decrease in ceruloplasmin may result in confusion around the diagnosis of Menkes disease in the neonatal period. The slow rise in serum ceruloplasmin concentration in the first year of life is paralleled by the onset of biliary copper excretion, reflecting a steady increase in the capacity of the hepatocyte for holo-ceruloplasmin biosynthesis.

CELL BIOLOGY

Wilson Adenosine Triphosphatase

Elucidation of the molecular genetic basis of Wilson disease has permitted an initial understanding of the mechanisms of hepatic copper homeostasis. This disease results from the absence or dysfunction of a copper-transporting P-type ATPase that resides in the *trans*-Golgi network of hepatocytes. The Wilson ATPase transports copper into the hepatocyte secretory pathway for incorporation into ceruloplasmin and excretion into the bile, and thus patients with this autosomal-recessive disorder present with signs and symptoms arising from impaired biliary copper excretion. Sequence comparison and hydropathy plot analysis of the derived amino acid sequence of the Wilson protein reveals a polytopic membrane protein predicted to transport copper across a lipid bilayer in an adenosine triphosphate (ATP)-dependent fashion (Fig. 22.3). A homologous ATPase encoded on the X chromosome is defective in the neurodegenerative disorder Menkes disease. The Menkes ATPase resides in the *trans*-Golgi network of specific cells in the placenta, intestine, and blood–brain barrier, functioning to transport copper across these tissues, and thus children with Menkes disease present with signs and symptoms of copper deficiency (2). Homologous copper-transporting P-type ATPases have now been identified in a wide variety of prokaryotic and eukaryotic species (26).

The derived amino acid sequence of the Wilson disease ATPase reveals many features typical of the family of P-type ion transport proteins (Fig. 22.3). The prototypical members of this family of proteins include the Ca^{2+} ATPase in the sarcoplasmic reticulum, the plasma membrane Na$^+$/K$^+$-ATPase, and the H$^+$ ATPase of the gastric mucosa. All P-type ATPases including the Wilson protein contain an invariant aspartate residue within the consensus sequence **D***KTGT*, which is utilized to form a β-aspartyl phosphoryl intermediate essential in the energy-dependent transduction of a specific ion across the membrane. This is accom-

plished utilizing ATP reversibly bound to at a consensus site in the large cytoplasmic loop GDGVND (Fig. 22.3). In all ATPases that have been studied in detail, cation transport is directly coupled to aspartyl phosphorylation with ATP hydrolysis occurring only in the event of ion movement across a membrane. The membrane structure of the Wilson ATPase has not been conclusively determined, but hydropathy analysis and comparison with the known structure of other P-type ATPases as well as site-directed mutagenesis studies suggest the presence of eight transmembrane domains, with the amino and carboxyl terminus on the same side of the membrane within the cytoplasm of the cell. The Wilson ATPase also contains a *CPC* sequence within the sixth transmembrane domain, which is conserved in all P-type ATPases involved in heavy metal transport (27,28). Expression studies have revealed that these amino acids are essential for copper transport by the Wilson ATPase, suggesting a direct role for copper binding by these cysteine residues during transmembrane transport (20,29).

In addition to these common P-type ATPase features noted above, the Wilson protein has two additional domains that are conserved in all known copper-transporting ATPases. The amino terminus contains six highly homologous repeat

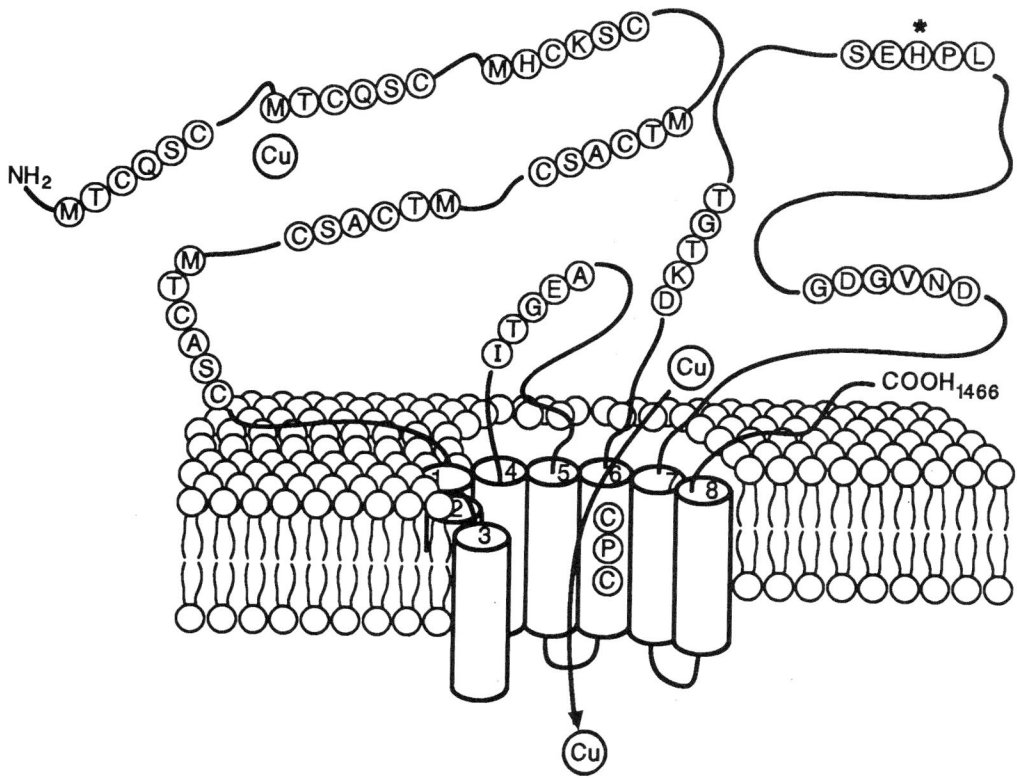

FIGURE 22.3. Topology and motifs of the Wilson adenosine triphosphatase (ATPase). Cytoplasm is viewed at the *top* with amino acids noted for conserved motifs in specific domains. Process of adenosine triphosphate (ATP)-dependent copper transport across the lipid bilayer is shown. (Modified from Payne AS, Gitlin JD. Functional expression of the Menkes disease protein reveals common biochemical mechanisms among the copper-transporting P-type ATPases. *J Biol Chem* 1998;273:3765, with permission.)

domains, each of which is defined by the copper-binding sequence *MXCXXC* (Fig. 22.3). These domains are essential for the copper transport and trafficking functions of the Wilson protein (30,31), and serve as the site of protein-protein interaction with the copper chaperone atox1 (*vide infra*) (32,33). The solution structure of one of these domains from the homologous Menkes copper-transporting ATPase has revealed a novel linear bicoordinate copper-binding environment that is dependent on the cysteine residues of the MXCXXC motif (34). An *SEHPL* sequence is located in the large cytoplasmic loop of the Wilson protein in which the histidine residue is highly conserved in all known copper-transporting P-type ATPases (Fig. 22.3). Although the precise function of this domain is not yet known, this histidine residue is the site of the most common mutation in Wilson disease accounting for up to 40% of the alleles in Northern European populations. This disease mutation (H1069Q) results in impaired folding and trafficking of the Wilson protein, suggesting a role for the *SEHPL* motif in the cellular targeting of the ATPase (35). Although polymerase chain amplification studies have suggested the possibility of multiple splice products of the Wilson ATPase, the only protein isoform identified thus far is a truncated species generated through tissue-specific alternative promoter usage in the retina and pineal gland (36). This isoform exhibits a dramatic 100-fold increase in nocturnal expression under control of the suprachiasmatic nucleus clock, which suggests a potential role for rhythmic copper metabolism in circadian function (36).

Polyclonal antisera generated against the amino-terminus of the Wilson ATPase detects a 165-kd protein that is synthesized as a single polypeptide chain in hepatocytes and localized predominantly to the *trans*-Golgi network (Fig. 22.4). This localization is consistent with the hypothesis that mutations resulting in the absence or dysfunction of this ATPase impair the transport of copper into the secretory pathway, interfering with holoceruloplasmin biosynthesis and biliary copper excretion (Fig. 22.2). In support of

this model, expression of wild-type Wilson protein in a strain of *S. cerevisiae* deficient in the homologous yeast ATPase CCC2 restores copper incorporation into the ceruloplasmin multicopper oxidase homologue Fet3 (20,37). Fet3 is required for high-affinity iron uptake in *S. cerevisiae* (38), and in contrast to the wild-type studies, expression of known Wilson disease mutants in this same *ccc2Δ* yeast is ineffective in restoring holoFet3 biosynthesis or high-affinity iron uptake, providing direct evidence for an essential copper-transport function of the Wilson ATPase (20).

Despite the utility of this yeast system, studies in mammalian cells suggest a greater complexity in Wilson ATPase function, which is essential for maintaining copper homeostasis in health and disease. An elevation of the intracellular copper content of hepatocytes results in the translocation of the Wilson ATPase to a cytoplasmic vesicular compartment (Fig. 22.4). As this increased copper is transported into these vesicles by the ATPase, the copper concentration in the cytoplasm decreases, resulting in translocation of the ATPase back to the *trans*-Golgi network and movement of the vesicles to the canalicular membrane for biliary copper excretion. This process is rapid and independent of new protein synthesis, thus providing a mechanism for the immediate response of the cell to changes in the steady-state intracellular copper concentration (20,21). While the molecular mechanisms involved in this recycling of the Wilson protein have not been fully characterized, site-directed mutagenesis of the Menkes ATPase, which undergoes a similar trafficking pathway, suggest that specific dileucine motifs within the carboxyl terminus provide essential signals for the response of these proteins to intracellular copper (39,40). The vesicular compartment into which copper is transported also remains poorly characterized but experiments utilizing homologous systems in *S. cerevisiae* reveal an essential role for both the H⁺ transporting V-type ATPase (41) and the CLC (chloride channel) Gef1 (42,43). Apparently, these proteins provide an electrogenic shunt for copper and hydrogen transport as well as establish-

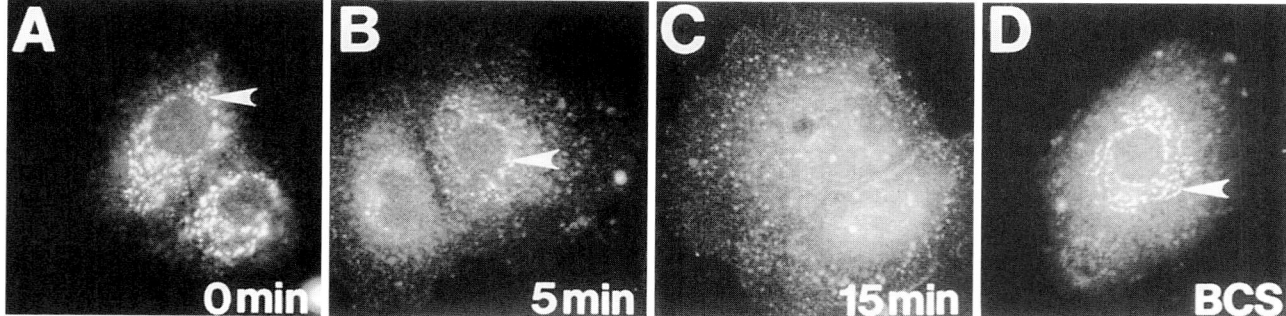

FIGURE 22.4. Effect of copper on the localization of the Wilson adenosine triphosphatase (ATPase). Primary rat hepatocytes were incubated for indicated times (**A–C**) in 50 μM copper or 40 μM bathocuproine disulfonate (*BCS*) after copper incubation (**D**). The Wilson ATPase was detected by immunofluorescence and is indicated in the *trans*-Golgi network with the arrowhead. (From Schaefer M, Hopkins R, Failla M, et al. Hepatocyte-specific localization and copper-dependent trafficking of the Wilson's disease protein in the liver. *Am J Physiol* 1999;276:G639, with permission.)

ing the necessary pH and chloride content within the vesicle to allow for the allosteric assembly of copper into Fet3 (44).

Copper Chaperones

Following the discovery of the copper transporting ATPases, experiments in *S. cerevisiae* revealed that the delivery of copper to specific pathways within the cell is mediated by a group of proteins termed copper chaperones (Fig. 22.2) (45,46). Atx1 and the mammalian homologue atox1 are small cytosolic copper-binding proteins that deliver copper to the transport ATPases for subsequent movement of this metal into the secretory pathway (*vide infra*) (47–50). Similar studies have also revealed the presence of Cox17, a small intracellular protein that is essential for the delivery of copper to cytochrome oxidase in the mitochondria (51). Cox17 contains multiple copper-binding sites and the absence of this protein results in aerobic insufficiency due to impaired respiratory chain assembly (51,52). Genetic studies also reveal that at least two additional proteins, SCO1 and SCO2, are involved in this pathway of copper delivery to cytochrome oxidase, and recent studies reveal that inherited mutations in the human homologue of SCO2 result in profound mitochondrial cardioencephalomyopathy secondary to impaired respiratory chain assembly (53–55). A second copper chaperone termed lys7 has been identified in yeast and shown to be essential for the delivery of copper to cytosolic copper/zinc superoxide dismutase (SOD1) (56). A homologous protein in humans termed the copper chaperone for superoxide dismutase (CCS) can functionally replace lys7 in yeast, and transgenic studies reveal an essential role for CCS in copper incorporation into SOD1 in mammalian cells (56,57).

Understanding why copper chaperones are necessary for copper trafficking within the cell and how these proteins function has permitted a greater understanding of the normal biology of cellular copper homeostasis. Recent experiments reveal that under physiologic circumstances intracellular copper availability is extraordinarily restricted (58). This observation explains why, despite the high affinity of enzymes such as SOD1 for copper, the cell has a need for specific metallochaperones. These proteins provide copper directly to target pathways while protecting this metal from intracellular scavenging. Although the precise cellular mechanisms of determining copper availability and trafficking by these chaperones remains unclear, studies with both the copper transporting ATPases and SOD1 suggest that recognition and directed copper transfer is mediated via interaction of homologous domains between the chaperone and a specific target protein (59–61).

Atox1

Soon after the characterization of the Wilson and Menkes ATPases, experiments in *S. cerevisiae* revealed a small cytosolic protein that functioned as a copper-dependent multicopy suppressor of sod1Δ mutants (47). This protein, termed atx1, was found to be essential in the pathway of copper delivery to the Wilson/Menkes ATPase homologue CCC2 in the yeast secretory pathway, permitting copper incorporation into the multicopper oxidase fet3 required for high-affinity iron uptake (48). The subsequent identification of a homologous protein in humans and mice termed atox1 suggested a similar role for these proteins in mammalian cells and revealed the remarkable evolutionary conservation of this pathway of copper trafficking (49,50). The amino acid sequence of atox1 reveals the presence of a single copy of the *MXCXXC* motif, also found in the amino terminus of the Wilson ATPase, and *in vitro* and *in vivo* studies have demonstrated the essential role of these cysteines in atox1 in copper transport to the secretory pathway (62,63).

Structural analysis of atx1 and atox1 has provided a model of these chaperones that suggests a mechanism for the rapid transfer of copper to the transport ATPases via ligand exchange (Fig. 22.5)(62,64). In such a model, a low activation barrier for transfer between the chaperone and the ATPase, arising from complementary electrostatic forces, is proposed to orient the metal binding loops of these proteins to allow for the formation of copper-bridged intermediates (65). In support of this model, biochemical studies demonstrate direct protein-protein interaction between these chaperones and the ATPases (32,33,59). Taken together these data suggest that copper chaperones overcome the predominant copper scavenging ability of the

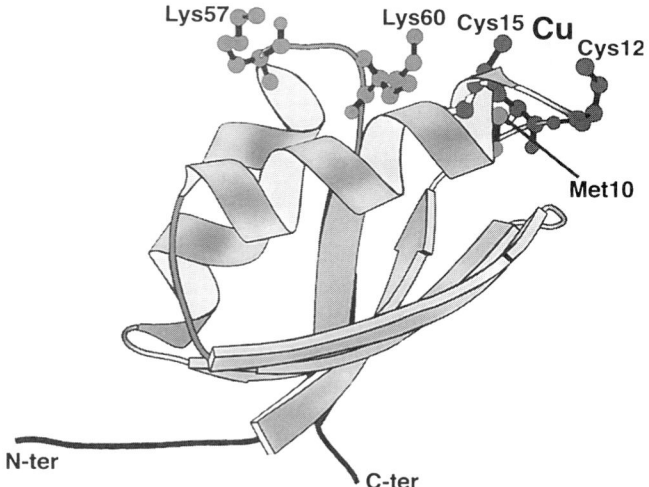

FIGURE 22.5. Solution structure of copper chaperone atox1. Structure reveals α-helices and an opposing antiparallel β-sheet typical of copper binding domains also found in the transport ATPases. The cysteines (*Cys12* and *Cys15*) of the MXCXXC motif are illustrated forming a bicoordinate linear copper ligand at the surface of the protein. (From Hung IH, Casareno RL, Labesse G, et al. HAH1 is a copper-binding protein with distinct amino acid residues mediating copper homeostasis and antioxidant defense. *J Biol Chem* 1998;273:1749, with permission.)

mammalian cytosol by catalyzing the rate of copper transfer between specific targets, tailoring energetic barriers to allow completion of specific reaction pathways (65,66).

WILSON DISEASE

Genetics

Wilson disease is an autosomal-recessive disorder observed in all ethnic groups that occurs worldwide in one in 30,000 individuals with a carrier rate of one in every 90 persons (67). Gene frequency is increased in consanguineous populations, a finding that aided in the establishment of linkage of the Wilson locus to the esterase D gene on chromosome 13 in 1985 (68). In 1993 the Wilson disease gene was cloned and found to encode a novel member of the family of cation transport P-type ATPases (69–71). The Wilson disease gene extends over 21 exons encompassing more than 65 kb on chromosome 13q14.3. DNA analysis from affected individuals has revealed an enormous heterogeneity of mutations consisting of a very small number of common mutations in specific populations and a greater number of rare individual alleles (72–86). A database containing all reported mutations is available through the Department of Medical Genetics at the University of Alberta (http://www.medgen.med.ualberta.ca). Of these reported mutations, about half are missense, the majority of which are located within known consensus motifs or predicted transmembrane domains (Fig. 22.3). The remainder of the mutations consist of small deletions, insertions, splice site errors, and nonsense mutations. As was noted earlier, *H1069Q* accounts for greater than 40% of the alleles identified in populations of Northern European descent. An *A778L* mutation within the fourth transmembrane domain has been identified in 30% of alleles from oriental populations.

The degree of allelic heterogeneity at the Wilson locus indicates that the majority of affected individuals will be compound heterozygotes, thus complicating any phenotype genotype analysis. However, studies in patients and families homozygous for the H1069Q allele have revealed no correlation between this mutation and the age of onset, clinical features, biochemical parameters, or disease activity (81). These data are supported by clinical observations of marked clinical variability among affected siblings and identical twins, supporting the concept that additional genetic and environmental factors significantly influence the outcome of a specific mutation in any given patient (4,67,87). Although to date there are no data regarding the abundance of the Wilson protein in affected patients, the possibility remains that specific mutations such as those resulting in splice site errors may lead to small amounts of functional residual protein resulting in a more predictable and less severe phenotype.

Pathogenesis

Analysis of the cell biology of the Wilson ATPase has allowed for the development of a model illustrating the molecular pathogenesis of Wilson disease (Fig. 22.6). In all cases, this model predicts that aberrant function of the ATPase will result in impaired biliary copper excretion with impaired holoceruloplasmin biosynthesis and eventual cytoplasmic copper accumulation within the hepatocyte. Studies of specific patient mutations support this model and reveal alterations in copper transport (20) as well as subcellular localization and trafficking in response to intracellular copper (35). Expression of the *H1069Q* mutant in a Menkes ATPase–deficient cell line indicates that this mutation results in a temperature-sensitive defect in protein folding leading to mislocalization to the endoplasmic reticulum. Interestingly, studies of this same mutant at a temperature permissive for movement to the *trans*-Golgi network reveal that this histidine residue is also required for copper-induced trafficking, suggesting a role for the SEHPL motif in this cellular process (35).

As noted above, genetic studies in yeast suggest that atox1 plays a role in copper delivery to the transport ATPases in the secretory pathway of the cell. Atox1 directly interacts with the Wilson ATPase in a copper-dependent fashion, and it therefore is reasonable to assume that impairment of this interaction might also lead to a disruption of hepatic copper homeostasis. To directly test this possibility, three disease mutations were identified within the amino-terminal copper-binding domains of the Wilson protein. A marked decrease in atox1 binding was observed with each of these mutants, indicating that impaired copper delivery by atox1 constitutes the molecular basis of Wilson disease in patients harboring these mutations (33). These data provide strong support for the conceptual model of chaperone function and demonstrate another pathway in the cellular pathogenesis of Wilson disease (Fig. 22.6). There are currently three rodent strains available that contain mutations or deletions of the homologous Wilson disease gene, and in all cases the analysis of these animals reveals abnormalities in hepatic copper homeostasis (23,24,88). While these animal models may be useful for therapeutic studies, none develops cirrhosis or neurodegeneration typical of Wilson disease, thus limiting its usefulness in elucidating disease pathogenesis.

Any model of disease pathogenesis must also account for the enormous clinical heterogeneity observed among affected patients. The model illustrated in Fig. 22.6 provides a blueprint for dissecting out additional genetic and environmental factors that may contribute to this heterogeneity. Likely candidates would include vesicular proteins such as homologues of the gef1 chloride channel essential for copper transport in *S. cerevisiae*, which might influence the rates of copper excretion by this pathway in hepatocytes. Although individuals with heterozygosity for muta-

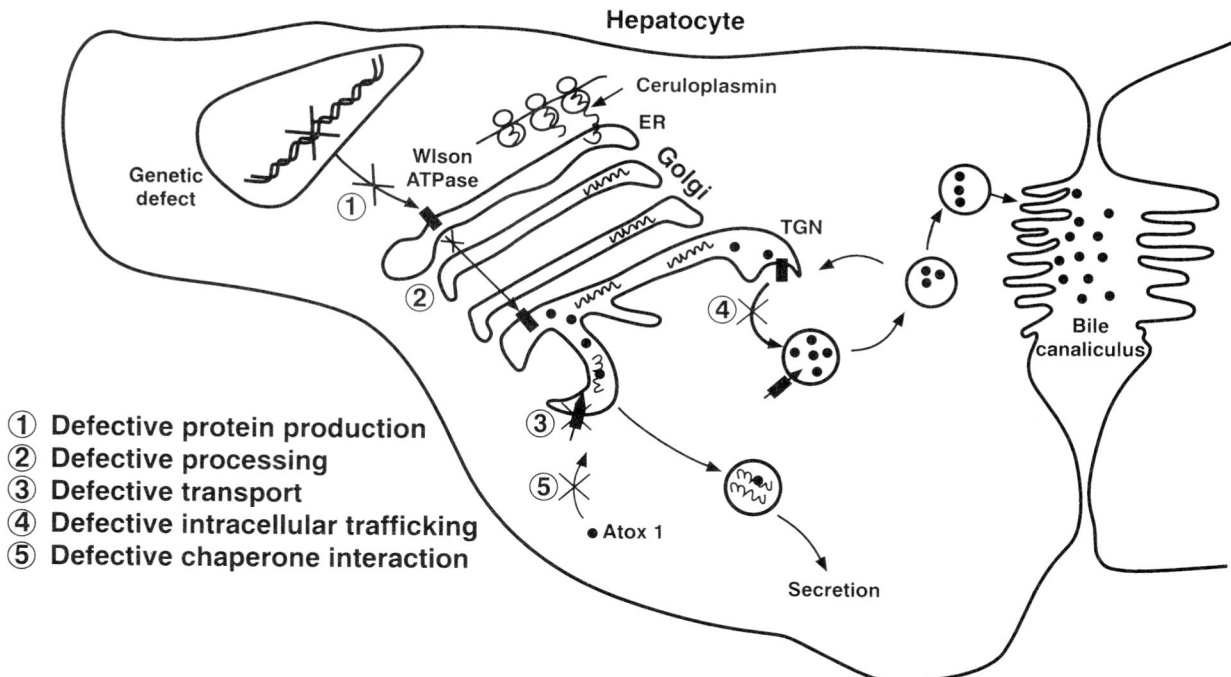

Hepatocyte

① **Defective protein production**
② **Defective processing**
③ **Defective transport**
④ **Defective intracellular trafficking**
⑤ **Defective chaperone interaction**

FIGURE 22.6. Model of the cellular pathogenesis of Wilson disease. The various known pathways of copper transport are shown with molecular mechanisms accounting for impaired copper homeostasis from mutations in the Wilson adenosine triphosphatase (ATPase). ER, endoplasmic reticulum; *TGN, trans*-Golgi network.

tions at the Wilson locus are asymptomatic, the paradigm illustrated above also allows for the intriguing possibility that the presence of such mutant alleles might serve as risk factors promoting copper-associated hepatic toxicity in circumstances of liver dysfunction from more common disorders such as alcoholic cirrhosis (89).

Diagnosis

Although the signs and symptoms of Wilson disease are protean and may arise from copper toxicity in a variety of organ systems, the majority of patients will present with hepatic or neuropsychiatric disease (67,87). Liver dysfunction is the most common presentation in childhood, and the physician should remain alert to the possibility of this diagnosis in any child with unusual symptoms and biochemical evidence of abnormal hepatic function (90). The manifestations of liver disease range from asymptomatic to chronic active hepatitis, and may include acute fulminant hepatic failure. Regardless of presentation, almost all patients will evidence cirrhosis on biopsy resulting from many years of hepatocyte copper accumulation prior to clinical symptoms (91). Eventually, hepatocyte dysfunction results in release of copper into the bloodstream with resultant hemolysis and deposition of this metal in the central nervous system. Neuropsychiatric symptoms are also common at presentation, but generally occur in older individu-

als, most often in the third or fourth decade. Neurologic manifestations may include Parkinsonian movement disorders, diminished facial expressions, dystonia, and choreoathetosis (92). These clinical features reflect neurodegeneration within the basal ganglia resulting from copper accumulation within this region, which may be detected by neuroimaging. The mechanisms resulting in basal ganglia injury with sparing of the motor and sensory cortex despite diffuse brain copper accumulation are unknown. Psychiatric disease may occur in isolation or combined with other neurologic symptoms and includes abnormal behavior, personality changes, depression, impairment in cognition, and schizophrenia (93).

The diagnosis of Wilson disease is based on clinical signs and symptoms that correlate with laboratory studies indicating abnormal copper homeostasis. Diagnostic evaluation should be considered in any individual with isolated elevation in serum transaminases, chronic active hepatitis of undetermined etiology, Kayser–Fleischer rings resulting from copper deposition at the limbus of the cornea, unexplained psychiatric symptoms, or basal ganglia abnormalities on neuroimaging. As noted above, the impairment of copper transfer into the secretory pathway will result in serum ceruloplasmin well below the normal concentration in most cases (94). Urinary copper concentration will be elevated (often >100 μg Cu/24 hours) and is a cost-effective approach to screening. In all cases, where possible, a liver biopsy should be performed to quantitate the hepatic copper content, which will be increased even in presymptomatic individuals. Based on history, physical exam, slit-lamp exam, and these laboratory data, an accurate diagnosis may be made in the majority of cases. While direct molecular diagnosis is precluded in most cases due to the degree of molecular heterogeneity at the Wilson locus, analysis for common mutations in patients of defined ethnic origin may prove of benefit (95,96). Given the low heterozygote frequency and the lack of a reliable biochemical test in the neonatal period, screening is confined to all siblings and first-degree relatives of affected patients. Screening should include the same diagnostic evaluation noted above but in those cases where the proband mutation is identified, direct molecular evaluation can offer a rapid approach to diagnosis. Reproductive and genetic counseling should be made available to any individual identified as a carrier.

Treatment

The goal for treatment in Wilson disease is the restoration of hepatic copper homeostasis by systemic chelation therapy. The first-line drug of choice for this is D-penicillamine, which promotes urinary copper excretion in affected patients and prevents copper accumulation in presymptomatic individuals (67). Most patients will be asymptomatic within 4 months but lifelong therapy is required, and compliance is essential to prevent deterioration from copper mobilization within sequestered tissue sites. Trientine may serve as a second choice in the face of penicillamine toxicity, and in either case the addition of zinc salts to the diet will serve to diminish copper absorption. In the case of progressive liver failure, orthoptic liver transplantation is an efficacious treatment resulting in sustained resolution of hepatic and neurologic disease (97).

COPPER-ASSOCIATED CIRRHOSIS IN CHILDHOOD

Although Wilson disease is the most common disorder resulting in hepatic copper overload, any pathology resulting in impaired biliary outflow has the potential to increase the hepatocyte copper content. Indeed, elevated hepatic copper has been reported in biopsy samples from patients with several forms of cholestatic liver disease (87). The associated signs and symptoms in such cases usually precludes diagnostic confusion with Wilson disease and in all such cases the serum holo-ceruloplasmin is elevated, indicating a defect late in the copper excretory pathway (Fig. 22.2). In contrast to these diseases, a severe form of rapidly progressive cirrhosis has been reported in young children in association with a marked elevation in the hepatic copper content. This disorder was originally described in children from rural, middle-class Hindu families, and was therefore termed Indian childhood cirrhosis (98). Subsequent reports from many other countries of iden-

tical findings in children from families without such ancestry have made it apparent that this rare disease occurs worldwide (99). Affected patients usually present within the first 2 years of life with hepatosplenomegaly and elevation of serum aminotransferases. Liver biopsy often reveals micronodular cirrhosis and hepatic copper content in excess of 2,500 μg/g dry weight. The absence of histologic or biochemical evidence of chronic cholestasis as well as a normal or elevated serum ceruloplasmin concentration in these cases suggests a specific defect in hepatic copper excretion late in the secretory pathway (Fig. 22.2). Interestingly, early treatment with penicillamine has been effective in several cases and hepatic transplantation is curative, suggesting an intrinsic hepatic defect in copper excretion.

The etiology of such cases is unknown, but epidemiologic studies in India and Europe suggest both genetic and environmental influences. Many reports have indicated a marked increase in the copper content of the diet of affected children arising either from the use of copper cooking vessels or acidic water running through copper pipes. However, this increase in dietary copper has not been observed in all cases, and the inability to induce a similar picture of cirrhosis by increasing the copper content of rodent diets has led to the concept of genetic susceptibility in these children. In support of this idea, analysis of a large affected pedigree in Austria has revealed evidence of autosomal-recessive inheritance (99). Much work is still needed to sort out the biochemical and genetic basis of this disorder. Nevertheless, the combined observations do suggest additional as yet undefined steps in the pathway of hepatic copper export, findings that support the concept that the Wilson protein is not the final excretory pathway for copper at the canalicular membrane. Interestingly, a similar form of copper-associated cirrhosis has been observed as an autosomal-recessive disorder in inbred Bedlington terriers. In this case, radioisotope studies have revealed an impairment in biliary copper excretion but not ceruloplasmin copper incorporation, again suggesting a defect late in the pathway of copper excretion. Recent genetic studies in these animals have localized this defect to a region syntenic with human chromosome 2p13-16 (100).

ACKNOWLEDGMENTS

Research from the author's laboratory reported in this chapter was supported in part by National Institutes of Health grants HL41536, DK44464, and DK56783. Jonathan D. Gitlin is the recipient of a Burroughs-Wellcome Scholar Award in Experimental Therapeutics.

REFERENCES

1. Pena M, Lee J, Thiele D. A delicate balance: homeostatic control of copper uptake and distribution. *J Nutr* 1999;129:1251.

2. Camakaris J, Voskoboinik I, Mercer JF. Molecular mechanisms of copper homeostasis. *Biochem Bioph Res Commun* 1999;261: 225.

3. Schaefer M, Gitlin JD. Genetic disorders of membrane transport. IV. Wilson's disease and Menkes disease. *Am J Physiol* 1999;276:G311.

4. Harris ZL, Gitlin JD. Genetic and molecular basis for copper toxicity. *Am J Clin Nutr* 1996;63:8365.

5. Turnlund TR. Human whole-body copper metabolism. *Am J Clin Nutr* 1998;67:9603.

6. Turnlund TR, Jeyes WR, Peiffer GL, et al. Copper absorption, excretion and retention by young men causing low dietary copper determined by using the stable isotope ^{65}cu. *Am J Clin Nutr* 1998;67:1219.

7. Dancis A, Yuan DS, Halle D, et al. Molecular characterization of a copper transport protein in *S. cerevisiae*: an unexpected role for copper in iron transport. *Cell* 1994;76:393.

8. Knight SA, Labbe S, Kwon LF, et al. A widespread transposable element masks expression of a yeast copper transport gene. *Genes Dev* 1996;10:1917.

9. Zhou B, Gitschier J. hCTR1: a human gene for copper uptake identified by complementation in yeast. *Natl Acad Sci* 1997;94: 7481.

10. Labbe S, Pena MM, Fernandes AR, et al. A copper-sensing transcription factor regulates iron uptake genes in *Schizosaccharomyces pombe*. *J Biol Chem* 1999;274:36252.

11. Harris ZL, Takahashi Y, Miyajima H. Aceruloplasminemia: molecular characterization of this disorder of iron metabolism. *Proc Natl Acad Sci USA* 1995;92:2539.

12. Harris ZL, Durley AP, Man TK, et al. Targeted gene disruption reveals an essential role for ceruloplasmin in cellular iron efflux. *Proc Natl Acad Sci USA* 1999;96:10812.

13. Sato M, Gitlin JD. Mechanisms of copper incorporation during the biosynthesis of human ceruloplasmin. *J Biol Chem* 1991; 266:5128.

14. Gitlin JD, Schroeder JJ, Lee-Ambrose LM, et al. Mechanisms of ceruloplasmin biosynthesis in normal and copper-deficient rats. *Biochem J* 1992;282:835.

15. Bremmer I. Manifestation of copper excess. *Am J Clin Nutr* 1998;67:10695.

16. Sokol RJ. Antioxidant defenses in metal-induced liver damage. *Semin Liv Dis* 1996;16:39.

17. Palmiter RD. The elusive function of metallothioneins. *Proc Natl Acad Sci USA* 1998;95:8428.

18. Kelley EJ, Palmiter RJ. A murine model of menkus disease reveals a physiological function of metallothionein. *Nat Genet* 1996;13:219.

19. Arrese M, Ananthananarayanan M, Suchy FJ. Hepatobiliary transport: molecular mechanisms of development and cholestasis. *Pediatr Res* 1998;44:141.

20. Hung IH, Suzuki M, Yamaguchi Y, et al. Biochemical characterization of the Wilson disease protein and functional expression in the yeast *Saccharomyces cerevisiae*. *Biol Chem* 1997;272: 21461.

21. Schaefer M, Hopkins R, Failla M, et al. Hepatocyte-specific localization and copper-dependent trafficking of the Wilson's disease protein in the liver. *Am J Physiol* 1999;276:G639.

22. Schaefer M, Roelofsen H, Wolters H, et al. Localization of the Wilson's disease protein in human liver. *Gastroenterology* 1999; 117:1380.

23. Theophilos MB, Cox DW, Mercer JF. The toxic milk mouse is a murine model of Wilson disease. *Hum Mol Genet* 1996;5:1619.

24. Buiakova OI, Xu J, Lutsenko S, et al. Null mutation of the murine ATP7B (Wilson disease) gene results in intracellular copper accumulation and late-onset hepatic nodular transformation. *Hum Mol Genet* 1999;8:1665.

25. Gitlin D, Biasucci A. Development of gamma G, gamma A, Gamma M, beta 1C, beta 1A, Cl esterase inhibitor, ceruloplasmin, transferrin, hemopexin, haptoglobin, fibrinogen, plasminogen, alpha 1-antritrypsin, orosomucoid, beta-lipoprotein, alpha 2 macroglobulin and prealbumin in the human conceptus. *J Clin Invest* 1969;48:1433.

26. Hamza I, Gitlin JD. Copper-transporting ATPases. In: Creighton TE, ed. *The encyclopedia of molecular medicine*. New York: Wiley, 2000: in press.

27. Lutsenko S, Kaplan JH. Organization of P-type ATPases: significance of structural diversity. *Biochemistry* 1995;34: 15607–15613.

28. Solioz M, Vulpe C. CPx-type ATPases: a class of P-type ATPase that pump heavy metals. *Trends Biochem* 1996;21:237.

29. Payne AS, Gitlin JD. Functional expression of the Menkes disease protein reveals common biochemical mechanisms among the copper-transporting P-type ATPases. *J Biol Chem* 1998; 273:3765.

30. Voskoboinik I, Strausak D, Greenough M, et al. Functional analysis of the N-terminal CXXC metal-binding motifs in the human menkes copper-transporting P-type ATPase expressed in cultured mammalian cells. *J Biol Chem* 1999;274:22008.

31. Forbes J, Hsi G, Cox D. Role of the copper-binding domain in the copper transport function of ATP7B, the P-type ATPase defective in Wilson disease. *J Biol Chem* 1999;274:12408.

32. Larin D, Mekios C, Das K, et al. Characterization of the interaction between the Wilson and Menkes disease proteins and the cytoplasmic copper chaperone, HAH1p. *J Biol Chem* 1999;274: 28497.

33. Hamza I, Schaefer M, Klomp LW, et al. Interaction of the copper chaperone HAH1 with the Wilson disease protein is essential for copper homeostasis. *Proc Natl Acad Sci USA* 1999;96: 13363.

34. Gitschier J, Moffat B, Reilly D, et al. Solution structure of the fourth metal-binding domain from the Menkes copper-transporting ATPase. *Nat Struct Biol* 1998;5:47.

35. Payne AS, Kelly EJ, Gitlin JD. Functional expression of the Wilson disease protein reveals mislocalization and impaired copper-dependent trafficking of the common H1069Q mutation. *Proc Natl Acad Sci USA* 1998;95:10854.

36. Borjigin J, Payne AS, Deng J, et al. A novel pineal night-specific ATPase encoded by the Wilson disease gene. *J Neurosci* 1999; 19:1018.

37. Forbes JR, Cox DW. Functional characterization of missense mutations in ATP7B: Wilson disease mutation or normal variant? *Am J Hum Genet* 1998;63:1663.

38. Askwith C, Eide D, VanHo A, et al. The FET3 gene of *S. cerevisiae* encodes a multicopper oxidase required for ferrous iron uptake. *Cell* 1994;76:403.

39. Francis M, Jones E, Levy E, et al. Identification of a di-leucine motif within the C terminus domain of the menkes disease protein that mediates endocytosis from the plasma membrane. *J Cell Sci* 1999;112:1721.

40. Petris MJ, Mercer JF. The Menkes protein (ATP7A; MNK) cycles via the plasma membrane both in basal and elevated extracellular copper using a C-terminal di-leucine endocytic signal. *Hum Mol Genet* 1999;8:2107.

41. Eide D, Bridgham JT, Zhao Z, et al. The vacuolar H+ ATPase of *Saccharomyces cerevisiae* is required for efficient copper detoxification, melochonidial function and iron metabolism. *Mol Gen Genet* 1993;241:447.

42. Gaxiola RA, Yuan DS, Klausner RD, et al. The yeast CLC chloride channel functions in cation homeostasis. *Proc Natl Acad Sci USA* 1998;95:4046.

43. Schwappach B, Strobrawa S, Hechenberger M, et al. Golgi localization and functionally important domains in the NH_2

and COOH terminus of the yeast CLC putative chloride channel Geflp. *J Biol Chem* 1998;273:15110.

44. Davis-Kaplan SR, Askwith CC, Bengtzen AC, et al. Chloride is an allosteric effector of copper assembly for the yeast multicopper oxidase fet3p: an unexpected role for intracellular chloride channels. *Proc Natl Acad Sci USA* 1998;95:13641.

45. Culotta V, Lin S, Schmidt P, et al. Intracellular pathways of copper trafficking in yeast and humans. *Adv Exp Med Biol* 1999; 448:247.

46. O'Halloran TV, Culotta VC. Metallochaperones, an intracellular shuttle service for metal irons. *J Biol Chem* 2000;275: 25057–25060.

47. Lin SJ, Culotta VC. The ATX1 gene of *Saccharomyces cerevisiae* encodes a small metal homeostasis factor that protects cells against reactive oxygen toxicity. *Proc Natl Acad Sci USA* 1995; 92:3784.

48. Lin SJ, Pufahl RA, Dancis A, et al. A role for the *Saccharomyces cerevisiae* ATX1 gene in copper trafficking and iron transport. *J Biol Chem* 1997;272:9221.

49. Klomp LWJ, Lin SJ, Yuan DS, et al. Identification and functional expression of HAH1, a novel human gene involved in copper homeostasis. *J Biol Chem* 1997;272:9221.

50. Hamza I, Klomp LW, Gaedigk R, et al. Structure, expression, and chromosomal localization of the mouse atox1 gene. *Genomics* 2000;63:294.

51. Glerum DM, Shtanko A, Tzagoloff A. Characterization of COX17, a yeast gene involved in copper metabolism and assembly of cytochrome oxidase. *J Biol Chem* 1996;271:14504.

52. Srinivasan C, Posewitz MC, George GN, et al. Characterization of the copper chaperone Cox 17 of *Saccharomyces cerevisiaeu*. *Biochemistry* 1998;37:7572.

53. Glerum DM, Shtanko A, Tzagoloff A. SCO1 and SCO2 act as high copy suppressors of a mitochondrial copper recruitment defect in *Saccharomyces cerevisiae*. *Biol Chem* 1996;271:20531.

54. Papadopoulou LC, Sue CM, Davidson MM, et al. Fatal infantile cardioencephalomyopathy with cox deficiency and mutations in sco2, a cox assembly gene. *Nat Genet* 1999;23:333.

55. Jaksch M, Ogilvie J, Yao J, et al. Mutations in sco2 are associated with a distinct form of hypertrophic cardiomyopathy and cytochrome c oxidase deficiency. *Hum Mol Genet* 2000;9:795.

56. Culotta VC, Klomp LWJ, Strain J, et al. The copper chaperone for superoxide dismutase. *J Biol Chem* 1997;272:23469.

57. Wong PC, Waggoner D, Subramaniam JR, et al. Copper chaperone for superoxide dismutase is essential to activate mammalian Cu/Zn superoxide dismutase [in process citation]. *Proc Natl Acad Sci USA* 2000;97:2886.

58. Rae T, Schmidt P, Pufahl R, et al. Undetectable intracellular free copper: the requirement of a copper chaperone for superoxide dismutase. *Science* 1999;284:805.

59. Pufahl RA, Singer CP, Peariso KL, et al. Metal ion chaperone function of the soluble Cu(I) receptor, Atx1. *Science* 1997;278: 853.

60. Lamb AL, Wernimont AK, Pufahl RA, et al. Crystal structure of the second domain of the human copper chaperone for superoxide dismutase. *Biochemistry* 2000;39:1589.

61. Schmidt PJ, Rae TD, Pufahl RA, et al. Multiple protein domains contribute to the action of the copper chaperone for superoxide dismutase. *J Biol Chem* 1999;274:23719.

62. Hung IH, Casareno RL, Labesse G, et al. HAH1 is a copper-binding protein with distinct amino acid residues mediating copper homeostasis and antioxidant defense. *J Biol Chem* 1998; 273:1749.

63. Portnoy M, Rosenzweig AR, Huffman TD, et al. Structure-function analyses of the ATX1 metallochaperone. *J Biol Chem* 1999;274:15041.

64. Rosenzweig AC, Huffman DL, Hou MY, et al. Crystal structure

65. Huffman DL, O'Halloran TV. Energetics of copper trafficking between the atx1 metallochaperone and the intracellular copper transporter, Ccc2. *J Biol Chem* 2000;275:18411–18414.

66. Rosenzweig AC, O'Halloran TV. Structure and chemistry of the copper chaperone proteins. *Curr Opin Chem Biol* 2000;4:140.

67. Cuthbert JA. Wilson's disease. Update of a systemic disorder with protean manifestations. *Gastroenterol Clin North Am* 1998; 27:655–681.

68. Frydman M, Bonne-Tamir B, Farrer LA, et al. Assignment of the gene for Wilson disease to chromosome 13:linkage to the esterase D locus. *Proc Natl Acad Sci USA* 1985;82:1819.

69. Bull PC, Thomas GR, Rommens JM, et al. The Wilson disease gene is a putative copper transporting P-type ATPase similar to the Menkes gene. *Nat Genet* 1999;5:327.

70. Tanzi RE, Petrukhin K, Chernov I, et al. The Wilson disease gene is a copper transporting ATPase with homology to the Menkes disease gene. *Nat Genet* 1993;5:344.

71. Yamaguchi Y, Heiny ME, Gitlin JD. Isolation and characterization of a human liver cDNA as a candidate gene for Wilson disease. *Biochem Biophys Res Commun* 1993;197:271.

72. Curtis D, Durkie M, Balac P, et al. A study of Wilson disease mutations in Britain. *Hum Mutat* 1999;14:304.

73. Haas R, Gutierrez-Rivero B, Knoche J, et al. Mutation analysis in patients with Wilson disease: identification of 4 novel mutations. Online. *Hum Mutat* 1999;14:88.

74. Kalinsky H, Funes A, Zeldin A, et al. Novel ATP7B mutations causing Wilson disease in several Israeli ethnic groups. *Hum Mutat* 1998;11:145.

75. Kim EK, Yoo OJ, Song KY, et al. Identification of three novel mutations and a high frequency of the Arg778Leu mutation in Korean patients with Wilson disease. *Hum Mutat* 1998;11:275.

76. Petrukhin K, Lutsenko S, Chernov L, et al. Characterization of the Wilson disease gene encoding a P-type copper transporting ATPase: genomic organization, alternative splicing, and structure/function predicting. *Hum Mol Genet* 1994;3:1647.

77. Loudianos G, Dessi V, Angius A, et al. Wilson disease mutations associated with uncommon haplotypes in Mediterranean patients. *Hum Genet* 1996;98:640.

78. Loudianos G, Dessi V, Lovicu M, et al. Haplotype and mutation analysis in Greek patients with Wilson disease. *Eur J Hum Genet* 1998;6:487.

79. Loudianos G, Dessi V, Lovicu M, et al. Further delineation of the molecular pathology of Wilson disease in the Mediterranean population. *Hum Mutat* 1998;12:89.

80. Nanji MS, Nguyen VT, Kawasoe JH, et al. Haplotype and mutation analysis in Japanese patients with Wilson disease. *Am J Hum Genet* 1997;60:1423.

81. Shah AB, Chernov I, Zhang HT, et al. Identification and analysis of mutations in the Wilson disease gene (ATP7B): population frequencies, genotype-phenotype correlation, and functional analyses. *Am J Hum Genet* 1997;61:317.

82. Shimizu N, Kawase C, Nakazono H, et al. A novel RNA splicing mutation in Japanese patients with Wilson disease. *Biochem Biophys Res Commun* 1995;217:16.

83. Thomas GR, Forbes JR, Roberts EA, et al. The Wilson disease gene: spectrum of mutations and their consequences. *Nat Genet* 1995;9:210.

84. Tsai CH, Tsai FJ, Wu JY, et al. Mutation analysis of Wilson disease in Taiwan and description of six new mutations. *Hum Mutat* 1998;12:370.

85. Waldenstrom E, Lagerkvist A, Dahlman T, et al. Efficient detection of mutations in Wilson disease by manifold sequencing. *Genomics* 1996;37:303.

86. Loudianos G, Dessi V, Lovicu M, et al. Mutation analysis in

patients of Mediterranean descent with Wilson disease: identification of 19 novel mutations. *J Med Genet* 1999;36:833.

87. Schilsky ML. Wilson disease: genetic basis of copper toxicity and natural history. *Semin Liver Dis* 1996;16:83.

88. Li Y, Togashi Y, Sato S, et al. Spontaneous hepatic copper accumulation in Long-Evans Cinnamon rats with hereditary hepatitis. A model of Wilson's disease. *J Clin Invest* 1991;87:1858.

89. Pyeritz RE. Genetic heterogeneity in Wilson disease: lessons from rare alleles. *Ann Intern Med* 1997;127:70.

90. Walshe JM. Wilson's disease presenting with features of hepatic dysfunction: a clinical analysis of eighty-seven patients. *Q J Med* 1989;70:253.

91. Davies SE, Williams R, Portmann B. Hepatic morphology and histochemistry of Wilson's disease presenting as fulminant hepatic failure: a study of 11 cases. *Histopathology* 1989;15:385.

92. Oder W, Grimm G, Kollegger H, et al. Neurological and neuropsychiatric spectrum of Wilson's disease: a prospective study of 45 cases. *J Neurol* 1991;238:281.

93. Dening TR, Berrios GE. Wilson's disease: psychiatric symptoms in 195 cases. *Arch Gen Psychiatry* 1989;46:1126.

94. Schilsky ML, Sternlieb I. Overcoming obstacles to the diagnosis of Wilson's disease. *Gastroenterology* 1997;113:350.

95. Maier-Dobersberger T, Ferenci P, Polli C, et al. Detection of the His1069Gln mutation in Wilson disease by rapid polymerase chain reaction. *Ann Intern Med* 1997;127:21.

96. Cox DW. Molecular advances in Wilson disease. *Prog Liver Dis* 1996;14:245.

97. Schilsky ML, Scheinberg IH, Sternlieb I. Liver transplantation for Wilson's disease: indications and outcome. *Hepatology* 1994;19:583.

98. Pandit A, Bhave S. Present interpretation of the role of copper in Indian childhood cirrhosis. *Am J Clin Nutr* 1996;63:830S.

99. Muller T, Feichtinger H, Berger H, et al. Endemic Tyrolean infantile cirrhosis: an ecogenetic disorder. *Lancet* 1996;347:877.

100. van de Sluis BJ, Breen M, Nanji M, et al. Genetic mapping of the copper toxicosis locus in Bedlington terriers to dog chromosome 10, in a region syntenic to human chromosome region 2p13-p16. *Hum Mol Genet* 1999;8:501.

23

THE LIVER AND IRON

MARK D. FLEMING
NANCY C. ANDREWS

ROLE OF THE LIVER IN IRON METABOLISM (SEE WEBSITE CHAPTER 🖳 W-19)

Iron is essential in a wide variety of biochemical reactions, and therefore extremely well conserved in humans. Average daily losses are normally limited to 1 mg (about 0.02% of total body iron) in normal adult men. Average losses are about twice as high in menstruating women. Loss of iron is almost precisely compensated by absorption of iron from the gut to maintain a near-zero balance of the metal. While the erythron is the major site for iron utilization, the liver plays an essential, dual role in iron recycling and storage. The Kupffer cell, as part of the reticuloendothelial system, is involved in the recovery and remobilization of iron from senescent and damaged erythrocytes. It thus helps maintain a steady-state supply of iron for the biosynthesis of hemo-globin and other iron proteins and enzymes. In addition, the hepatocyte stores iron to provide an expandable reserve to deal with iron deficiency and iron excess. In this way, the body can assure its supply of this essential metal, yet avoid potential toxicity (see website chapter 🖳 W-18).

THE BODY'S IRON ECONOMY

Normal adults have approximately 3 to 5 g of total body iron. There is no physiologic mechanism for iron excretion through the liver or kidneys; rather, iron balance is primarily controlled at the level of intestinal absorption. The past few years have seen major advances in our understanding of this process (reviewed in ref. 1). Iron is absorbed in the proximal portion of the small intestine, where it must pass through two membranes to traverse the epithelium. Nonheme iron uptake through the apical membrane is carried out by a transport process that is distinct from transfer through the basolateral membrane to the plasma. Divalent metal transporter 1 (DMT1, formerly known as Nramp2 or DCT1) brings dietary nonheme iron into duodenal villus enterocytes through the apical membrane (2–4). At least

M. D. Fleming: Department of Pathology, Children's Hospital and Harvard Medical School, Boston, Massachusetts 02115.
N. C. Andrews: Department of Pediatrics, Harvard Medical School; Division of Hematology/Oncology, Howard Hughes Medical Institute, Children's Hospital, Boston, Massachusetts 02115.

two proteins are important for basolateral transfer of enterocyte iron to the plasma. Ferroportin (also known as Ireg1, MTP1), transports iron across the basolateral membrane (5–7). It likely acts in concert with a multicopper ferroxidase, hephaestin (8), but the role of the ferroxidase and its functional relationship to ferroportin are not well understood. Both DMT1 and ferroportin are widely expressed, and probably have iron transport roles in other tissues as well. Dietary heme iron, primarily from meat sources, is taken up through a separate process that has not yet been elucidated. The control of intestinal iron absorption is also not yet understood, though genetic iron overload diseases typically result from perturbation of normal regulatory mechanisms (see below).

CELLULAR ASPECTS OF HEPATIC IRON METABOLISM

Storage of Iron

Hepatocytes

About 0.4 g (10%) of the total body content of iron is present in hepatic stores in adult men, primarily in the form of ferritin. Although the mechanisms of iron uptake into and release from hepatocytes are not fully understood at the molecular level, several factors are known to affect hepatocyte iron balance. Uptake is regulated in response to cellular iron stores, serum iron concentration, iron saturation of circulating transferrin, and the number of transferrin receptors per cell. Release of iron depends in part on the availability of iron-sequestering agents to capture iron exiting the cell, thereby preventing its reuptake.

Uptake of Iron from Transferrin by Cells

Plasma transferrin serves three purposes. First, it solubilizes ferric ions, preventing them from precipitating out of solution at neutral pH. Second, it attenuates the reactivity of iron, eliminating its toxicity. Third, it delivers iron to cell-surface transferrin receptors. Our current understanding of the transferrin cycle for iron uptake is shown in Fig. 23.1. The initial event in the cellular acquisition of transferrin-bound iron is the association of iron-bearing transferrin with transferrin receptors on the plasma membrane. At neutral extracellular pH the receptor effectively recognizes only iron-bearing transferrin. Thus, an abundance of apo-transferrin in the circulation, which may exceed 90% of total transferrin in iron deficiency, does not interfere with binding of iron-transferrin to cell-surface receptors. The complex of transferrin and its receptor is then internalized by invagination of clathrin-coated pits. Specialized endosomes form, and become acidified through the action of a proton pump. This leads to protein conformational changes that allow release of iron from transferrin. The released iron is reduced to the ferrous state by an endosomal ferric reductase activity (9). Ferrous iron then traverses the endosomal membrane through the action of DMT1, the same transmembrane iron transporter that functions in apical iron uptake in the intestine (10). Cytoplasmic iron enters a low molecular weight cytosolic transit pool available for re-release to the plasma, incorporation into iron enzymes, or storage in ferritin. Meanwhile, iron-depleted transferrin, still bound to its receptor, is returned to the cell surface. There, encountering a neutral pH environment, transferrin is freed for another cycle of iron transport.

Since the concentration of iron-bearing transferrin in the circulation usually exceeds the availability of cellular transferrin receptors, the transferrin receptor is the ultimate gatekeeper, controlling uptake of transferrin-bound iron for most cells. Proliferating cells and erythroid precursors have increased iron needs, and consequently express high levels of transferrin receptor. Most differentiated cells, however, express little transferrin receptor. Hepatocytes are an exception to this generalization; even with their low rate of turnover, they express substantial numbers of transferrin receptors, reflecting the special role of these cells in iron storage. The normal rat hepatocyte has about 40,000 receptors for transferrin that bind the iron-saturated protein with dissociation constant (K_d) of 60 nM. Kupffer cells also express transferrin receptors.

Other Sources of Liver Iron

In chronic iron overload, much of the body's excess iron is found in the liver. Although transferrin is normally the major source of iron for the liver, hepatocytes can utilize iron derived from the uptake of heme-hemopexin, hemoglobin-haptoglobin, methemalbumin, free plasma hemoglobin, lactoferrin, ferritin, and low molecular weight ferrous iron. In iron overload disorders and acute iron poisoning, the plasma concentration of non–transferrin-bound iron becomes significant, and the liver is often a primary target of damage. Severe iron overload, as in thalassemia and hereditary hemochromatosis, leads to complete saturation of serum transferrin and appearance of low molecular weight forms of iron in the circulation (non–transferrin-bound iron). This iron also is cleared by the hepatocyte. The capacity of the liver for uptake of non–transferrin-bound iron is dramatically demonstrated by patients with genetic atransferrinemia (11). As described later in this chapter, they develop tissue iron overload, particularly in the liver. The molecular basis of non–transferrin-bound iron uptake by hepatocytes has not been determined, though the biochemical features of the transport process have been characterized in cell culture systems (12,13). In contrast to non–transferrin-bound iron uptake by absorptive enterocytes of the intestine (2,3), non–trans-

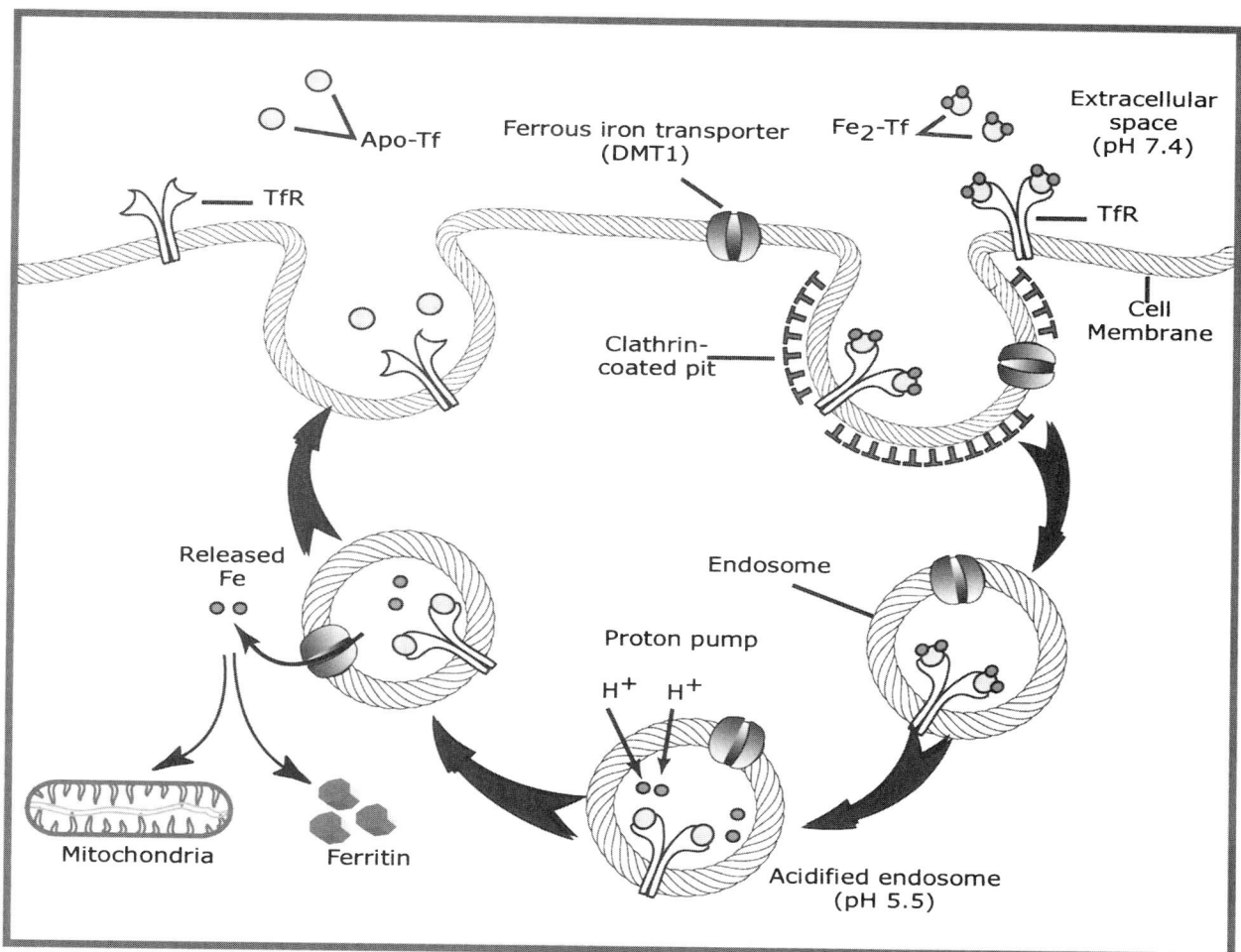

FIGURE 23.1. The transferrin cycle. Our current understanding of the transferrin cycle is depicted in this cartoon. Diferric transferrin (*Fe₂*-Tf) binds to cell surface transferrin receptors (TfRs) to initiate receptor-mediated endocytosis. Clathrin-coated pits invaginate to form specialized endosomes, which contain both TfR and the ferrous iron transporter, divalent metal transporter 1 (DMT1), in their membrane. The endosomes become acidified through the action of a proton pump. At low pH iron is released from transferrin. It leaves the endosome through DMT1, to go to sites of utilization (mitochondria) and storage (ferritin) in the cytoplasm. Meanwhile, apo-Tf and TfR are recycled to the cell surface for further rounds of iron uptake.

ferrin-bound iron uptake by hepatocytes does not appear to involve DMT1 (Hiromi Gunshin and Nancy Andrews, unpublished observations, 2000).

Kupffer Cells

Reticuloendothelial macrophages, including Kupffer cells, serve as the major clearinghouse for iron in the body. The molecular details of this process, however, are unknown. At one time it was thought that cells of the reticuloendothelial system were the principal sites of long-term storage of iron. It now appears that hepatocytes probably carry the major burden of this function. Little ferritin or nonheme iron is found in Kupffer cells in normal rats, but stainable iron may be observed in hypertransfused or otherwise iron over-

loaded animals. Injection of iron dextran or hemoglobin in large doses increases the nonheme iron in these cells. About 85% of the iron of heat-damaged erythrocytes can be captured by the human reticuloendothelial system and returned to circulating erythrocytes within 12 days, the remainder presumably exchanging with parenchymal iron stores and other non–hemoglobin iron-containing compartments. Recycling is delayed by iron overload and enhanced by iron depletion, in concert with the physiologic needs of the organism. Kupffer cells are also capable of taking up iron from transferrin. This uptake is much slower than uptake into hepatocytes or erythroid precursor cells, perhaps explaining why ferrokinetic studies in humans show only insignificant removal of iron bound to transferrin by reticuloendothelial cells.

Mobilization of Iron

Hepatocytes

Release of iron from hepatocytes to apotransferrin has been demonstrated in the perfused rat liver and in suspensions of isolated hepatocytes. In neither system can release of iron be increased above basal level by increasing the apotransferrin concentration, suggesting that the rate of release is predominantly modulated by intracellular factors, possibly involving ferroportin. A variable fraction of released iron is also found as ferritin; the importance of this fraction in iron turnover by hepatocytes is not known.

Kupffer Cells

The intracellular degradation of erythrocytes engulfed by phagocytes initially entails digestion of cells in secondary lysosomes to release heme from hemoglobin. Iron is then liberated from heme by the microsomal heme oxygenase. Much of the iron freed from senescent red blood cells is immediately returned to the plasma, but some may be retained by Kupffer cells and be incorporated into ferritin or hemosiderin. Iron released by macrophages is in a form that is readily available for binding by vacant sites of transferrin

The mechanism of iron release from Kupffer cells is poorly understood. Iron must be exported from the cell,

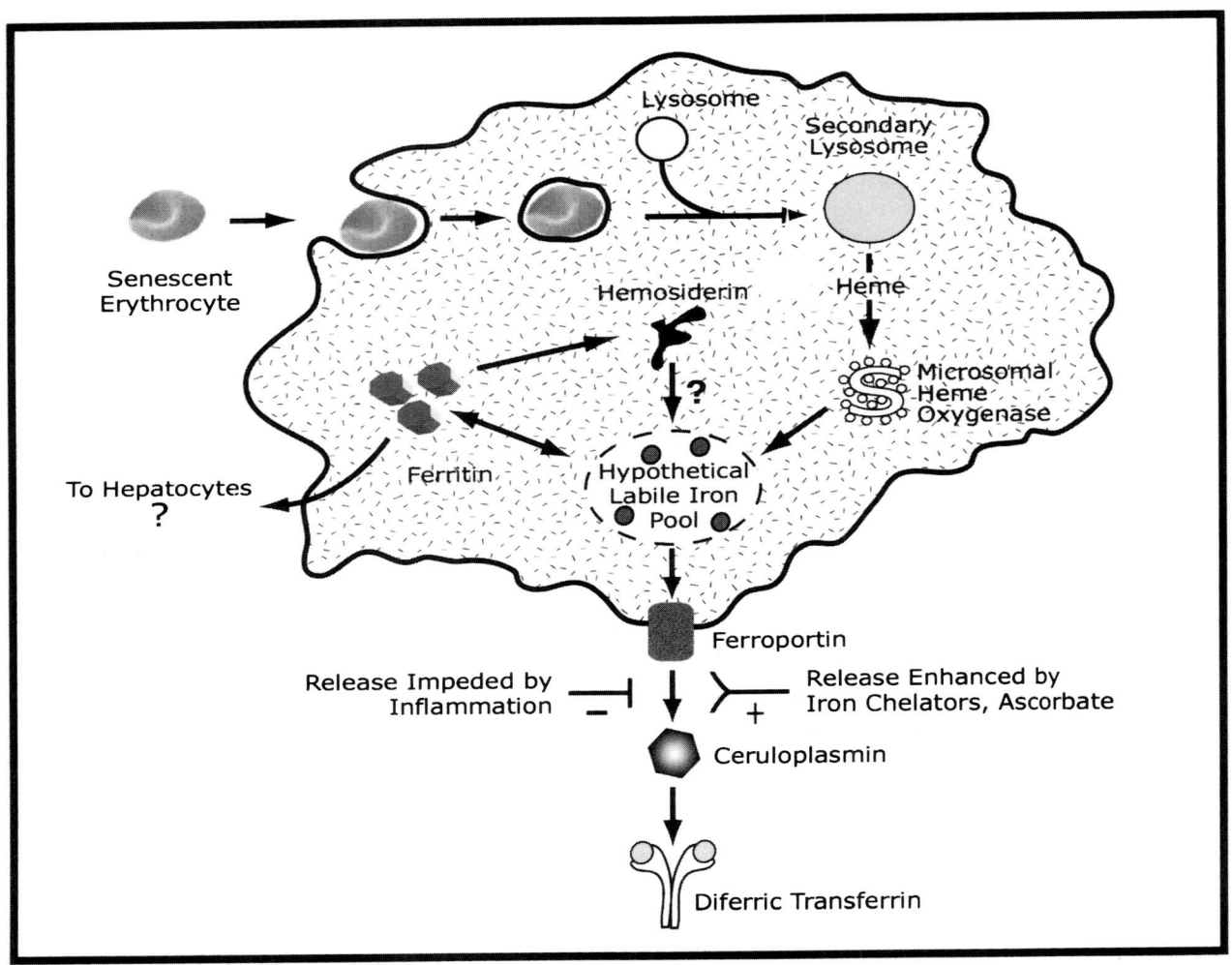

FIGURE 23.2. Iron recycling by reticuloendothelial macrophages. Kupffer cells and other reticuloendothelial macrophages recycle iron from effete erythrocytes by engulfing them and degrading hemoglobin. This diagram shows a model for how that process may occur. Aging erythrocytes are phagocytosed, and lysed in a lysosomal compartment. Heme is released, and degraded with the aid of heme oxygenase. Liberated iron probably enters a labile iron pool, from which it can be incorporated into ferritin, or exported to reload apotransferrin. We speculate that the iron exporter, ferroportin, may be involved in transfer of iron across the cellular membrane. Ceruloplasmin is involved in iron release, but its precise role has not yet been determined. Iron release is impeded by inflammation, probably as a result of inflammatory cytokines that act upon the macrophages. External iron chelators and ascorbate enhance iron release. Ultimately, recycled iron ends up on plasma transferrin.

and loaded onto transferrin for reuse. The recent identification of a transmembrane iron exporter, ferroportin (also known as Ireg1, MTP1) may help elucidate this process (5–7). Studies of animals lacking the plasma protein ceruloplasmin further suggest that ceruloplasmin plays a role in assisting either macrophage iron export or transferrin loading (14). A model incorporating our current understanding of iron recycling is shown in Fig. 23.2.

PROTEINS OF IRON METABOLISM

Ferritin

Widely distributed throughout nature, ferritin has been identified in microorganisms and plants as well as higher organisms. The protein molecule consists of a roughly spherical, hollow shell, within which iron is stored in a microcrystalline core of magnetic, polymeric, ferric oxyhydroxide phosphate. The average iron content of rat liver ferritin molecules is about 2,500 to 3,000 atoms, but as many as 4,500 atoms can be included in the 70 Å cavity. In this fully loaded state, iron represents almost 30% of the dry molecular mass. The protein shell has a molecular weight of about 450,000 and consists of 24 subunits of two apparent size classes designated L [molecular weight (MW) 19 kd] and H (MW 21 kd) for their relative sizes (light and heavy) or the tissues in which they predominate (liver and heart).

With entry of iron into the cell, ferritin messenger RNA (mRNA) is recruited from an inactive, stored pool to polysomes where active translation takes place. In keeping with the role of the protein in iron storage, the rate of ferritin synthesis is sensitive to the presence of iron. Iron stimulates ferritin synthesis primarily at the level of translation. Translational control of ferritin expression by iron is due to a highly conserved 28-nucleotide sequence in the 5′ untranslated region of the mRNA, which forms an iron regulatory element (IRE). The structure and function of IREs are discussed in detail below. Newly synthesized ferritin subunits probably assemble first into apoferritin, which then progressively incorporates iron. Oxidation of ferrous iron, the form most efficiently taken up by ferritin *in vitro*, is a function localized to a ferroxidase site in the H-chain of human ferritin. No corresponding site has been identified in the human L-chain. Once polymerization of ferric iron in the core has commenced, the growing polymer itself facilitates oxidation of the iron. In addition, oxidation may continue at the ferroxidase sites with the resulting Fe^{3+} then translocated to the core.

Effective mobilization of iron from ferritin requires reduction of iron from the ferric to the ferrous state. This may account for the well-known ability of ascorbate to assist in the mobilization and excretion of iron from subjects with chronic iron overload. However, reduction itself is not sufficient to release iron from ferritin. An acceptor of

Fe^{2+} must be present to provide sufficient thermodynamic driving force for release to proceed. Some reductants—thioglycollate, ascorbate, or dihydrolipoate, for example—may bind Fe^{2+} sufficiently tightly to effect release in the absence of other ferrous iron chelators. However, it is not known whether reductive release actually occurs *in vivo*; degradation of ferritin may be necessary to secure its iron for cellular metabolic needs or for export.

Transferrin

The transferrin molecule consists of a single polypeptide chain arranged in two lobes with greater than 40% amino acid identity between them. Each lobe is formed of two domains surrounding a cleft bearing a specific iron-binding site. The two sites are similar, but not identical, in structure and physicochemical properties. However, they differ in their occupancies in the circulation and hence in their physiologic functions. The crystal structures of human serum transferrin (15), human lactoferrin, and rabbit serum are very similar. At each iron-binding site, the protein provides one histidyl, one aspartyl, and two tyrosal ligands. A carbonate anion completes the coordination requirement of ferric iron by serving as a bridging ligand between protein and metal, thereby locking the metal ion in place. Each lobe of the transferrin molecule may exist in two conformations, open and closed (16). The open conformation of a lobe is assumed in solution when the lobe is devoid of metal; binding of iron drives the protein to the closed conformation. Release of iron occurs readily from the open conformation, but is impeded by the closed conformation that normally predominates at pH 7.4. In monoferric transferrin, open and closed conformations may coexist.

The gene encoding transferrin is found on human chromosome 3, at 3q21. The human transferrin gene is organized into 17 exons, the first of which specifies the cleavable 19-residue leader sequence of the preprotein and the last containing the 3′ untranslated sequence. The gene can be divided into two halves, which show close sequence homology reminiscent of the internal homologies in the N-terminal and C-terminal halves of the transferrin molecule. This reinforces the hypothesis that the modern transferrin gene arose by the contiguous duplication and recombination of sequences in an ancestral gene specifying a single-sited "half-transferrin."

In mammals, many cells are capable of transferrin synthesis, but the hepatocyte is by far the most important source of circulating transferrin. Hepatic synthesis of transferrin is sensitive to iron status, so that iron deficiency is often associated with a modest rise in plasma transferrin, reflecting an increase in transferrin synthesis, while iron overload may be accompanied by a slight decline in transferrin levels. Transferrin expression appears to be controlled primarily at the level of transcription.

Transferrin Receptor

The transferrin receptor is a homodimer of 90-kd subunits, each capable of binding a transferrin molecule for an overall 2:2 stoichiometry. It is a type II membrane protein, with the amino terminus in the cytoplasm, and a single membrane-spanning domain. Its subunits are joined by disulfide bonds and anchored in the cell membrane by hydrophobic interactions assisted by a fatty acid covalently bound to each receptor subunit. The transferrin receptor is glycosylated at asparaginyl *N*- and threonyl *O*-sites. Loss of glycosylation sites results in impaired function of the receptor. Most of the receptor, including its carbohydrate moieties, lies extracellularly; a 70-kd fragment bearing the transferrin recognition site can be cleaved from the receptor by trypsin or by an endogenous protease (17) to release a soluble form of the protein that circulates in plasma. The molecular function of the soluble form is unknown, but its levels tend to reflect body iron status and erythropoietic iron needs (18). Soluble transferrin receptor is increased in patients with iron deficiency anemia and disorders characterized by ineffective erythropoiesis, such as thalassemia and sideroblastic anemia. The crystal structure of the transferrin receptor ectodomain was recently determined (19). However, neither the receptor recognition site of the transferrin molecule nor the transferrin-binding site of the receptor has been identified.

Like transferrin, the gene encoding the transferrin receptor is also found on human chromosome 3, at 3q29. It contains 18 exons. Synthesis of the transferrin receptor is highly regulated by iron, much more so than synthesis of transferrin. An increase in cellular iron or heme causes decreased receptor synthesis and downregulation of the number of receptors in the cell. Depletion of cellular iron by desferrioxamine has a converse effect, promoting receptor synthesis and upregulation of receptor number. At least part of the iron-dependent regulation is mediated by IREs in the 3′ untranslated region of transferrin receptor mRNA (see below). Receptors are also upregulated when hepatocytes are driven to proliferate by partial hepatectomy.

Transferrin Receptor-2

Direct sequencing of the human genome recently revealed the presence of a gene encoding a transferrin receptor homologue, transferrin receptor-2, mapping to chromosome 7q22 (20). It is 45% identical and 66% similar to transferrin receptor in its extracellular domain. Transferrin receptor-2 mRNA is expressed at extremely high levels in the liver and at much lower levels in several other tissues. Transferrin receptor-2 can mediate uptake of diferric transferrin by cells (20), but with a lower affinity for the ligand (21). Unlike transferrin receptor, its mRNA is not regulated in response to iron deficiency or iron overload; levels of transferrin receptor-2 expression do not change with iron

status (22). Its role in iron metabolism is not yet established, though a subclass of patients with an inherited form of hemochromatosis has been shown to have a nonsense mutation disrupting the transferrin receptor-2 gene (23) (see below).

Divalent Metal Transporter 1

The DMT1 protein has 12 transmembrane domains. Both amino- and carboxyl-termini are predicted to be within the cytoplasm. There is a substantial extracellular loop between transmembrane domains 7 and 8 with probable asparagine-linked glycosylation sites. Mutations in transmembrane domain 4 have been shown to interfere with DMT1 protein function (2,10). The expression of DMT1 is regulated in response to iron status (3,4).

The gene encoding DMT1 is located on chromosome 12, at 12q13. It consists of 17 exons spread over more than 36 kilobases (kb). There are at least two different splice forms, encoding alternative carboxyl-termini and alternative 3′ untranslated regions (10). One of the 3′ untranslated regions contains an IRE (3), suggesting that DMT1 protein expression may be controlled posttranslationally by intracellular iron concentration, but that hypothesis has not yet been validated experimentally.

Ferroportin

The gene encoding ferroportin is located on human chromosome 2 (Adriana Donovan, unpublished results). It encodes a protein with ten predicted transmembrane domains with iron exporter activity in cultured cells (5–7). Immunohistochemical studies show that the protein is expressed at high levels on the basolateral surface of duodenal enterocytes and placental syncytiotrophoblasts as well as in Kupffer cells (5,7), consistent with a physiologic role in iron export. There is a perfectly conserved IRE element in the 5′ untranslated region of the mRNA (see below), but because it is only recently discovered, little is known about regulation of ferroportin protein expression or its involvement in disease.

Iron Regulatory Proteins and Posttranscriptional Control of Gene Expression

IREs are RNA hairpin structures to which either of two iron regulatory proteins (IRPs) specifically bind when cellular iron is depleted (reviewed in ref. 24). Binding of IRPs to IREs upstream of coding sequences inhibits translation by preventing the recruitment of the small ribosomal subunit to the mRNA (25). When the intracellular iron level rises, the repressor protein is discharged, and mRNA molecules are available for translation. IRE stem-loop motifs occur in the 5′ untranslated regions of mRNAs encoding ferritin subunits and ferroportin (Ireg1, MTP1) (5–7) and the first enzyme in heme biosynthesis, erythroid aminolevulinate synthase.

IREs are also found in the 3′ untranslated regions of mRNAs encoding the transferrin receptor and DMT1 (3). In this position they also confer posttranscriptional regulation, but through a very different mechanism. Five IRE stem-loop structures are found in the 3′ untranslated region of the transferrin receptor message, each capable of interacting with IRPs. Mutagenesis of the transferrin receptor IREs prevents binding of IRPs and destabilizes the mRNA. Thus, occupancy of the IRE of the transferrin receptor mRNA by IRPs stabilizes the message, thereby enhancing expression of the receptor. This is opposite to the effect of 5′ IREs in ferritin mRNAs; when they are occupied translation is impeded.

The two known IRPs are related proteins of approximately 90 to 100 kd (26,27). IRP1 is 30% identical to mitochondrial aconitase, and similarly contains an iron sulfur (4Fe·4S) cluster. The 18 active site residues of mitochondrial aconitase are identical to those in IRP1, and purified IRP1 has been shown to have aconitase activity. Very likely, therefore, cytoplasmic aconitase, a protein of hitherto unclear identity, is IRP1. Manipulations that alter the iron-sulfur cluster of IRP1 reciprocally alter its RNA-binding and aconitase activities. Under iron-loaded conditions, the iron-sulfur cluster is fully formed, and the protein functions exclusively as an aconitase. In contrast, when cellular iron stores are depleted, the iron-sulfur cluster is not assembled, and IRP1 functions as an RNA binding protein. Consequently, the posttranslational regulation of IRP1 centers on the iron-sulfur cluster, which responds to the availability of intracellular iron, and this, in turn, regulates its RNA-binding activity. Modulation of IRP1 activity by chelatable iron is thus reversible, and thus does not involve permanent alterations of the integrity of the protein.

IRP2, though similar in amino acid sequence to IRP1 (27), is regulated by a different mechanism (28). IRP2 does not contain an iron-sulfur cluster. Instead, it contains a polypeptide insertion that confers susceptibility to proteosome-mediated proteolysis in an iron-enriched environment (29). When cellular iron is depleted, however, IRP2 is stabilized, and binds to RNA in a fashion similar to that of IRP1. Both IRP1 and IRP2 proteins are widely expressed. If they function differentially as translational regulators, differences are most likely determined by the precise structure of the IREs. Accordingly, it has been shown that the preferred binding sites for IRP1 and IRP2 differ significantly (30,31).

In addition to iron, nitric oxide and oxidative stress have also been shown to modulate IRP function (reviewed in ref. 32). In this way, protection of the cell against iron excess and potentially oxidative damage is enhanced by coordinate changes that increase the rate of synthesis of ferritin protein and reduce the synthesis of proteins important for accepting iron into the cell.

MECHANISMS OF IRON TOXICITY

Because of the liver's singular role in iron storage, it is particularly vulnerable to the effects of systemic iron overload. It not only provides a freely available reservoir of iron for distribution to other tissues, but also serves to protect tissues from the toxic effects of the free metal. When its capacity is exceeded, toxicity supervenes. The precise mechanisms underlying the noxious effects of iron are still a matter of debate. However, it is generally accepted that the ability of iron to catalyze the production of reactive oxygen species and other free radicals underlies the pathogenesis of iron toxicity. Iron may react with reducing agents and oxygen to form the superoxide radical anion $O_2^-\bullet$, leading in turn to generation of the highly reactive hydroxyl radical, OH•. The actual oxidants responsible for cell damage by iron may be adducts or analogues of the hydroxyl radical such as the ferryl ion, FeO^{2+}.

Circulating low molecular weight iron complexes associated with supersaturation of serum transferrin have been reported to stimulate lipid peroxidation and promote formation of the hydroxyl radical. For example, iron-mediated peroxidation of unsaturated fatty acids occurs in the presence of ascorbic acid and probably occurs via a free radical intermediate. Nucleotide complexes of iron are also potent initiators of lipid peroxidation. Red blood cells in patients with β-thalassemia and sickle cell disease are particularly susceptible to membrane lipid peroxidation perhaps because precipitated hemoglobin also catalyzes the peroxidation reaction. Hepatic lipid peroxidation occurs in iron-overloaded rats and may be a fundamental event in liver disease consequent to iron overload. Damage to nucleic acids caused by free radicals induced by iron overload has been postulated to be a factor in carcinogenesis.

IRON OVERLOAD DISORDERS

The liver is susceptible to iron overload; iron deficiency has little clinical consequence on the liver. Iron overload disorders can be broadly segregated into those that are a result of a primary inherited defect in iron metabolism and those that are secondary to another genetic or acquired condition (Table 23.1). While relatively little progress has been made in the field of secondary iron overload disorders, the past decade has seen an explosion in the clinical and molecular definition of genetic causes of primary iron overload. Whereas the term *hereditary hemochromatosis* once encompassed all patients with an inherited clinical phenotype of primary hepatic iron overload, we now recognize multiple distinct, primary iron overload disorders. The discussion in this chapter focuses primarily on the features of the primary inherited iron overload disorders.

TABLE 23.1. IRON OVERLOAD DISORDERS

Primary
  Molecular/biochemical cause defined
    Hereditary hemochromatosis (HLA-linked or *HFE*-related
      hemochromatosis)
    Transferrin receptor-2–related hemochromatosis
    Aceruloplasminemia
    Atransferrinemia or hypotransferrinemia
  Molecular/biochemical cause undefined
    Non–*HFE*-related hemochromatosis
    African iron overload (Bantu siderosis)
    Melanesian iron overload
    Neonatal hemochromatosis (idiopathic neonatal iron
      storage disease)
    Finnish lethal metabolic syndrome
Secondary
  Ineffective erythropoiesis/hemolytic anemia
    Thalassemia syndromes
    Sideroblastic anemias
    Congenital dyserythropoietic anemias
    Pyruvate kinase deficiency
  Excessive iron intake
    Transfusional siderosis
    Excessive dietary iron supplements
    Excessive parenteral iron therapy
  Other liver diseases
    Alcoholic liver disease
    Porphyria cutanea tarda
    Viral hepatitis
    Nonalcoholic steatohepatitis
    Portacaval shunt
  Other systemic diseases
    Chronic renal failure
    Chronic inflammatory diseases

HLA, human leukocyte antigen.

Hereditary Hemochromatosis

The term *hereditary hemochromatosis* (HH) has evolved to refer only to the most common inherited form of iron overload, a human leukocyte antigen (HLA)-linked disease associated with mutations in the *HFE* gene (see below). To clearly distinguish this genetic iron overload disorder from other primary causes, some prefer to add the qualifying term "HLA-linked" or "*HFE*-related." HH is prevalent in individuals of Northern European ancestry. Consequently, the mid-19th century description by Trousseau of the clinical triad of hepatic cirrhosis, hyperpigmentation of the skin, and glycosuria almost certainly described patients with HH. von Recklinghausen was the first to attribute the clinical findings to iron overload and coined the term "hemochromatosis." The inherited nature of the disorder was recognized by Sheldon, who further described the clinical features of the disease. As awareness of HH has grown, a greater number of patients are diagnosed prior to the onset of clinically significant end-organ damage; patients are now often recognized with early symptoms such as fatigue and arthralgias, frequently as the result of investigation of family members of an affected individual (reviewed in ref. 33).

Conventional laboratory diagnosis of HH relies upon finding an elevated transferrin saturation, over 50% in women and over 60% in men, and an increased serum ferritin (34). The hepatic iron index [(μmol Fe/g liver tissue)/patient age] determined from a liver biopsy has been considered the "gold-standard" diagnostic test. A hepatic iron index of 1.9 or more is typical of patients with HH (35), but in certain populations, including younger women and patients with established cirrhosis, these tests may be misleading.

Pathologically, HH is characterized by iron accumulation in parenchymal cells of the liver, pancreas, heart, pituitary, and other tissues. The liver is most severely affected by excess iron deposition. Early in the disease, the metal accumulates in hepatocytes surrounding the portal tracts, creating a gradient of iron deposition between the portal tract and central vein. Iron is incorporated into ferritin and hemosiderin granules that are characteristically aligned with the canalicular surfaces of the cells. Liver Kupffer cells, like other reticuloendothelial cells in the bone marrow and spleen, are relatively spared of iron deposition, particularly early in the course of the disease. While not unique to HH, this pattern of iron deposition is distinct from that seen in African iron overload and transfusional siderosis, in which reticuloendothelial cell iron deposition is an early feature (36). If HH is not treated by phlebotomy, iron deposition extends throughout the hepatic lobule and gradually also involves Kupffer cells as the cumulative iron burden grows. Ultimately, hepatic fibrosis ensues, leading to cirrhosis. Cirrhosis resulting from HH may not be distinguishable from other etiologies of cirrhosis on histologic grounds alone, as conspicuous iron deposition, particularly in stromal cells and histiocytes, may be seen in end-stage liver disease resulting from many causes (37). When venesection therapy is instituted in the precirrhotic, prediabetic stage of hemochromatosis, life expectancy may be restored to normal.

Although the functional consequences of iron overload in HH are most pronounced in the liver, the fundamental metabolic defect in HH appears to be one of dysregulated intestinal iron absorption. This is graphically, but anecdotally, illustrated by cases of inadvertent transplantation of hemochromatotic livers into patients who do not have hemochromatosis, and transplantation of normal livers into HH patients (38); further iron loading of the transplanted liver correlates with the genotype of the recipient, and not with the genotype of the liver.

In normal individuals, absorption of iron varies inversely with body iron stores, decreasing as iron accumulates and increasing as stores diminish. In patients with HH, this regulatory mechanism appears grossly intact, but, for any given amount of storage iron, HH patients absorb proportionately more iron from the intestine than normal individuals (39,40). Aberrant mucosal uptake of iron and excessive transfer of iron into the circulation have both been investigated as possible mechanisms important to the pathogenesis of HH. Those studies that have directly investigated HH patients, rather than relying on inferences from normal or iron deficient individuals, suggest that mucosal transfer of intestinal epithelial iron is enhanced in HH (40).

The discovery by Marcel Simon in 1976 that HH was associated with homozygosity for HLA-A3 definitively established the recessive mode of inheritance of HH and provided the first piece of information that would ultimately lead to cloning the HH gene. Linkage to the HLA-A locus on human chromosome 6p focused future cloning efforts. The high degree of association with the HLA-A3 allele strongly indicated a founder effect. It suggested that most patients are descended from a single individual and would share a common mutation. Many groups had failed to identify the disease gene using conventional positional cloning techniques, because the very property of the HLA locus that preserved the association of HLA-A3 with the disease causing mutation, a relatively low frequency of meiotic recombination over the genetic interval, hindered a family-based genetic recombination approach. By assuming a strong founder effect and treating all HH patients as part of a single extended family, however, Mercator Genetics succeeded where others had failed (41). After pursuing this approach, a single plausible candidate gene, *HFE*, encoding an atypical HLA class I molecule, was identified. Most patients with HH had a missense mutation at position 282 that converts a structurally important cysteine to a tyrosine (C282Y).

The C282Y mutation is strongly associated with hemochromatosis, with a reported incidence of homozygosity for the allele range from 60% to 100% in European, North American, and Australian populations (reviewed in ref. 42). Most people homozygous for this mutation have evidence of iron overload; however, there is a great variation in clinical severity of the disease (43,44). Several other polymorphisms in the *HFE* gene have been described. An aspartate substitution for histidine at position 63 (H63D) is a prevalent polymorphism, particularly in HH patients from Southern Europe; however, its association with iron overload is inconsistent (45). Another polymorphism, a cysteine for serine substitution at position 65 (S65C), appears to be associated with a mild phenotype (46). Other point mutations, as well as a single mutation that alters *HFE* mRNA splicing, have been associated with clinical disease (47,48).

Targeted disruption of the *Hfe* gene in mice (*Hfe*$^{-/-}$) leads to a hepatic iron overload phenotype (49–51). Nonheme iron is deposited in the liver, in a pattern similar to HH in humans. Interestingly, hepatic iron overload begins prior to complete saturation of serum transferrin, suggesting that non–transferrin-bound iron is not a significant factor in the pathogenesis of iron overload early in the disease. Radioiron absorption studies have confirmed excessive iron absorption in knockout animals maintained on iron-replete, iron-deficient, or iron-excessive diets (49). Not surprisingly, *β2m* knockout mice also accumulate iron in a fashion similar to

Hfe knockout mice, confirming the idea that the Hfe functions as a heterodimer with β2m (52,53).

Introduction of the equivalent of the human C282Y mutation into the murine *Hfe* gene results in a milder phenotype than the null allele, indicating that the C282Y mutation is not a complete loss of function mutation (50). Heterozygosity for either a null or C282Y allele confers slight, but significantly increased, hepatic iron stores (50). The murine *Hfe*$^{-/-}$ and *Hfe*$^{C282Y/C282Y}$ phenotypes can be modified by abnormalities in other proteins involved in iron metabolism, including DMT1, β2m, transferrin receptor, and hephaestin (54). Most notably, crossing *Hfe*$^{-/-}$ animals with microcytic anemia (*mk*) mice, which have a severe loss of function mutation in DMT1 (2), results in complete abrogation of the *Hfe*$^{-/-}$ phenotype, indicating that DMT1 mediates iron uptake in HH (54). Similar variant forms of the human homologues of these and other iron-related genes may account for the clinical variability seen in human patients with identical *HFE* genotypes.

HFE is expressed in most tissues at low levels, and is present at the highest levels in liver and small intestine. It is not immediately apparent how an atypical major histocompatibility complex (MHC) class I protein can influence iron absorption. There is, however, an important clue from the fact that the HFE/β2m heterodimer interacts with the transferrin receptor to form a high-affinity complex (55–58). Affinity measurements performed with purified proteins show that the interaction of HFE with transferrin receptor decreases its affinity for transferrin (57). It is not yet known, however, in which tissues this association between HFE and transferrin receptor is important, or how exactly it influences iron metabolism.

Transferrin Receptor-2-Related Hemochromatosis

Coincident with the description of transferrin receptor-2, two Sicilian families were described with an autosomal-recessive form of hemochromatosis not linked to *HFE* (59). The clinical features seen in two affected individuals in one of the two families are remarkable only for a high estimated total body iron at a young age. Mapping showed linkage to 7q22 in one family known to be consanguineous, and demonstrated that affected individuals in both families share homozygosity for a common haplotype over a region that included the transferrin receptor-2 locus. Each patient was homozygous for a nonsense mutation in the transferrin receptor-2 gene at codon 250 (Y250X) (23). At present, it is unclear how a loss of function mutation in transferrin receptor-2 results in iron overload.

Juvenile Hemochromatosis

Juvenile hemochromatosis (JH) is a rare, autosomal-recessive form of inherited iron overload typically presenting in the second or third decade of life (60,61). The histopathologic patterns of iron distribution and tissue injury are similar to HH. However, JH patients typically present with complications of extrahepatic iron overload, particularly hypogonadotrophic hypogonadism and cardiac dysfunction, even though they have liver iron burdens that are comparable to patients with symptomatic HH. It is not clear why extrahepatic manifestations of iron overload predominate in JH. It may be related to the fact that iron overload is present at the time of puberty; the rapidly growing heart and developing neuroendocrine axis may be particularly susceptible to iron toxicity. Alternatively, it may be due to the rate at which iron loading occurs. JH is not linked to the *HFE* locus, and patients are not homozygous for the C282Y mutation (60,61). Similar to other rare autosomal-recessive disorders, JH is more common in inbred pedigrees. This has facilitated mapping of the disorder to the ~4cM interval on human chromosome 1q (62).

Non–*HFE*-Related Hemochromatosis

There are a number of other well-documented pedigrees with inherited iron overload with clinical and pathologic features similar to HH, whose disease is not linked to the HLA locus and is not associated with *HFE* mutations (59,63–65). These patients have been broadly categorized as having "non–HFE-related" hemochromatosis (42). Their existence indicates that mutations in other genes can be responsible for a hereditary hemochromatosis-like phenotype. Given the iron overload seen in β2m-deficient mice, β2m has been considered as a candidate gene for these orphan inherited iron overload syndromes; however, no mutations have been found in the patients examined (65).

African Iron Overload

A distinctive hepatic iron overload syndrome is prevalent in sub-Saharan Africa, affecting 10% or more of the population in some rural areas of Zimbabwe (66). Historically, the disorder was called "Bantu siderosis" and was attributed to the consumption of an iron-rich diet that included traditional beer brewed in nongalvanized steel drums. It is now evident that while dietary intake may contribute to iron overload, many affected individuals have not consumed significant amounts of iron-rich food or beverages, implicating other factors (67). More recent studies have indicated an interaction between dietary and genetic factors in the development of African iron overload (AIO) (68). Based on pedigree analysis, it is suggested that individuals heterozygous for a putative mutation in an unknown gene are predisposed to iron overload, while homozygotes for this mutation may be more severely affected (68). The putative gene is not linked to the HLA locus, and the *HFE* C282Y mutation has not been identified in any patient (68,69). A limited number of cases of primary iron overload have been reported in African Americans (70,71). *HFE* mutations are distinctly uncommon in this ethnic group (72). Although ancestral relationships would suggest that these individuals might be affected by AIO, it is uncertain if it is indeed the same process.

In addition to the ethnic background of AIO patients, the disorder is unique in the tissue pattern of iron deposition (36,73). In contrast to HH, iron is typically present within Kupffer cells early in the course of the disease and there is typically no gradient of iron deposition between the portal tracts and central vein (66). Iron deposition is also a prominent feature in the bone marrow and spleen, which are relatively spared in HH (36,69). Serum transferrin saturations may also be normal or only modestly elevated in the setting of significant iron overload (66). Overall, these pathologic and laboratory features suggest an abnormality in reticuloendothelial iron recycling; however, physiologic measurements of cellular iron efflux have not been performed.

Melanesian Iron Overload

A single large Melanesian kindred with familial hepatic iron overload with an apparent autosomal-dominant pattern of inheritance has been described (74). As early as their early teenage years, both male and female members of this pedigree develop hepatic iron overload largely restricted to the hepatocytes. Hepatomegaly and liver failure are the most common clinical signs of disease; clinical diabetes, hypogonadism, and cardiomyopathy were not observed. Linkage analysis in a subgroup of the pedigree excluded linkage to the HLA locus.

Aceruloplasminemia

Individuals deficient in the serum multicopper oxidase ceruloplasmin suffer from a progressive neurodegenerative disorder associated with diabetes and systemic hemosiderosis (reviewed in refs. 75 and 76). Loss of ceruloplasmin, which is thought to facilitate iron efflux from cells, results in iron accumulation in hepatocytes, reticuloendothelial macrophages, pancreatic acinar and islet cells, and neurons of the basal ganglia, among other cell types (77). Although hepatic iron deposition is a characteristic feature of this disorder, clinically important signs and symptoms are primarily related to neuronal damage. The clinical findings, molecular genetics, and pathophysiology of aceruloplasminemia are discussed in greater detail in Chapter 22 and website chapter 🖳 W-18.

Congenital Atransferrinemia or Hypotransferrinemia

Seven families with a severe deficiency or absence of serum transferrin have been reported (reviewed in ref. 11). Patients typically present as children, ranging in age from infancy to 7 years, with hypochromic, microcytic anemia, accompanied by a low serum iron level and a very low total iron-binding capacity, commonly in the range of 3 to 15 μmol/L. Transferrin may be present in trace amounts or undetectable. In one family, a transferrin variant with an abnormal isoelectric focusing pattern was identified (78). Compound heterozygosity for a complex deletion/insertion mutation and a missense mutation in the transferrin gene has been described in one patient (119). Treatment with plasma or purified transferrin, even in small amounts, restores hemoglobin production. Hepatic iron deposition is a common feature. When reported, excess hepatic iron is detected in both parenchymal and Kupffer cells.

The pathophysiology of iron overload in congenital atransferrinemia has been studied extensively in a murine model, the hypotransferrinemic (*hpx*) mouse. These animals have less than 1% of normal serum transferrin levels. Similar to the human disorder, homozygous *hpx* mice have a profound hypochromic, microcytic anemia associated with hepatic, pancreatic, and cardiac hemosiderosis (79,80). Heavy iron deposition is present in both hepatocytes and Kupffer cells. The underlying genetic defect is a mutation in a splice donor site in the last intron of the gene that results in inefficient and aberrant splicing of the mRNA (81,82). The small amount of transferrin made by these animals contains an internal deletion of 9 amino acids near the carboxyl terminus (82). Intestinal iron absorption is greatly increased in untreated animals, and approximately three to five times normal in *hpx* homozygotes given a maintenance dose of transferrin (83,84). Expression of DMT1, the apical intestinal iron transporter, is significantly upregulated in these animals (120). Transfusion of red blood cells to correct the anemia partially reverses the increase in iron absorption, indicating that anemia, and not transferrin deficiency per se, is the inciting stimulus for some of the increase in intestinal iron uptake (84,85). Whereas in wild-type animals most iron is used for hematopoiesis, in *hpx/hpx* animals the majority of iron is deposited in the liver (86,87). This illustrates the dependence of the erythron on transferrin-bound iron, and the relative avidity of the liver for non–transferrin-bound iron species (88).

Neonatal Hemochromatosis

Neonatal hemochromatosis is a clinicopathologic syndrome in which infants typically present *in utero* or at birth with liver failure associated with diffuse hepatic fibrosis, pseudoacinar and giant cell transformation of hepatocytes, hepatic iron deposition, and siderosis of extrahepatic tissues, which tends to spare the reticuloendothelial system (89). Minor salivary gland biopsies may reveal hemosiderosis, and facilitate the diagnosis when liver biopsy is impractical. Most infants develop progressive hepatic failure

requiring hepatic transplantation for survival; however, in a small subset, full recovery without adverse sequelae has been reported (90). Treatment with deferoxamine or antioxidants has been attempted in several reported cases, with modest effects (91).

It is clear that the NH phenotype can be associated with a number of acquired conditions, including congenital infections, immune and nonimmune fetal hydrops, and maternal Sjögren's syndrome. Numerous other sporadic cases with or without other congenital anomalies and no identifiable inciting factor have been reported. Features of NH may be seen in infants with trisomy 21. In a number of cases, including those with syndromic and nonsyndromic features, there are multiple affected siblings and no attributable extrinsic cause. In most families, inheritance is presumed to be autosomal recessive (92), but several pedigrees are consistent with maternal or codominant inheritance (93). Recently, two unique polymorphisms in mitochondrial DNA encoding subunits of the electron transport apparatus have been reported to be associated with NH (94).

Because NH can result from a variety of causes, a common pathophysiologic mechanism of disease is unlikely. In some cases excessive iron transport across the placenta has been postulated. In other cases, intrinsic hepatocellular defects have been cited. Most notably, a bile acid synthesis defect, Δ^4-3-oxosteroid 5β-reductase deficiency, has been reported to be associated with some cases (95,96). However, it is uncertain if this is a cause or a consequence of the hepatic dysfunction, as this finding can be in seen in patients with severe liver disease from other causes (97).

Finnish Lethal Neonatal Metabolic Syndrome

An autosomal-recessive inherited, uniformly fatal, metabolic syndrome consisting of fetal growth retardation, lactic acidosis, aminoaciduria, and mild to moderate hemosiderosis of the liver has been described in Finland (98). Stainable iron was not seen in organs other than the liver. In patients surviving beyond 1 month of age, progression of portal fibrosis was noted, despite the fact that iron was relatively decreased in hepatocytes (98). The pathophysiology of the disorder remains undefined, but the genetic locus lies on chromosome 2q33-37 (99).

Liver Iron in Other Diseases

Secondary iron overload may be seen in a great number of clinical situations (Table 23.1). Of these, secondary cases of hepatic siderosis, alcoholic liver disease, hepatitis C infection, porphyria cutanea tarda, and iron-loading anemias with or without transfusion are the most commonly encountered disease processes.

Alcoholic Liver Disease

Mild to moderate hepatic iron overload is frequently encountered in alcoholic cirrhosis; however, a hepatic iron index of greater than 1.9 is unusual (see Chapter 50 and website chapter 🖳 W-41). Very likely, many cases of severe iron overload in alcoholics actually represent underlying hereditary hemochromatosis. Mechanisms driving hepatic accumulation of iron in alcoholic cirrhosis are not well understood. Subjects with alcoholic cirrhosis often display increased absorption of iron derived from ferrous sulfate or hemoglobin, but nonanemic and abstaining alcoholic subjects may exhibit normal or even decreased absorption of iron. Acute and chronic hemolysis in alcoholics may also dispose toward increased absorption of iron.

Porphyria Cutanea Tarda

Iron is one of several factors that may contribute to the pathogenesis of porphyria cutanea tarda (PCT) (see Chapter 21 and website chapter 🖳 W-17). Hepatic siderosis is present in most patients with PCT, and phlebotomy therapy often ameliorates the symptoms (100). Until recently, it was uncertain if the hepatic iron overload was a cause or a consequence of PCT. However, with the advent of linkage analysis for HH and molecular determination of *HFE* gene mutations, it is clear that abnormal HFE alleles are over-represented in both familial and sporadic cases of PCT (101–105). In one large American study, homozygosity or compound heterozygosity for the C282Y and/or H63D mutations was present in approximately one-third of PCT patients (102). In this study, heterozygosity for the C282Y mutation alone did not appear to confer susceptibility to PCT. The pathogenesis of iron overload in patients without two mutated *HFE* alleles may be related to other conditions. For example, hepatitis C virus infection is associated with abnormalities in hepatic iron metabolism and also prevalent in patients with PCT. In experimental models, iron potentiates the effects of porphyrogenic agents (106,107). How it does so is uncertain, but it may be that the ferrous iron enhances porphyrin synthesis or further exacerbates the enzymatic deficiency.

Viral Hepatitis

An increased serum iron concentration and transferrin saturation associated with mildly elevated liver iron concentrations is a common finding in patients with chronic hepatitis C virus (HCV) (108). Studies have shown that HCV patients responding to interferon-α therapy have significantly lower hepatic iron concentrations (reviewed in ref. 109). A poor response to therapy has been correlated with increased iron in Kupffer cells (reviewed in ref. 110). High iron concentrations may impair the immune response to the virus. Early studies suggest that phlebotomy therapy may have a beneficial role in the patients treated with interferon-α for hepatitis C infection (111,112).

Iron Overload Associated with Inherited or Acquired Anemias

In the absence of transfusion, patients with inherited anemias such as thalassemia syndromes, X-linked sideroblastic anemia, and congenital dyserythropoietic anemias are susceptible to hepatic iron overload (reviewed in ref. 113). Each of these anemias is characterized by lysis of a fraction of erythroid precursors prior to their complete maturation and release as reticulocytes—a process referred to as ineffective erythropoiesis. Intramedullary lysis of red cell precursors leads to increased plasma iron turnover and accelerated intestinal iron absorption. Treatment with regular transfusions suppresses the erythropoietic drive, but contributes significantly to the iron burden, as each milliliter of packed red blood cells contains approximately 1 mg of iron. In those anemias in which red cell life span is near normal, iron deposition tends to be hepatocellular. However, in certain anemias, such as β-thalassemia, in which there is a significant hemolytic component, or those treated with transfusion, there is prominent reticuloendothelial iron deposition. Congenital hemolytic anemias, including hereditary spherocytosis, which do not have significant ineffective erythropoiesis, are not typically associated with iron overload (114), except when they are present in association with HLA-A3, often linked to a mutated HH allele (115,116). HLA-A3 or mutations in *HFE* may also be associated with an increased iron burden in patients with β-thalassemia or β-thalassemia trait (117,118).

ACKNOWLEDGMENTS

We appreciate the careful work that S. P. Young and P. Aisen put into writing the earlier version of this chapter. We thank Karyn Giarla for preparing Figs. 23.1 and 23.2. Due to space limitations, many older references, particularly those cited in previous editions of this book, have been omitted from the text. Our iron research has been supported by the Howard Hughes Medical Institute (N.C.A.), the March of Dimes Foundation (N.C.A.), the National Institutes of Health (N.C.A. and M.D.F.), the American Society of Hematology (M.D.F.), and the American Liver Foundation (M.D.F.).

REFERENCES

1. Andrews NC. Medical progress: disorders of iron metabolism. *N Engl J Med* 1999;341:1986–1995.
2. Fleming MD, Trenor CCI, Su MA, et al. Microcytic anemia mice have a mutation in Nramp2, a candidate iron transporter gene. *Nature Genet* 1997;16:383–386.
3. Gunshin H, Mackenzie B, Berger UV, et al. Cloning and characterization of a mammalian proton-coupled metal-ion transporter. *Nature* 1997;388:482–488.
4. Canonne-Hergaux F, Gruenheid S, Ponka P, et al. Cellular and

subcellular localization of the Nramp2 iron transporter in the intestinal brush border and regulation by dietary iron. *Blood* 1999;93:4406–4417.

5. Donovan A, Brownlie A, Zhou Y, et al. Positional cloning of zebrafish ferroportin1 identifies a conserved vertebrate iron exporter. *Nature* 2000;403:776–781.

6. McKie AT, Marciani P, Rolfs A, et al. A novel duodenal iron-regulated transporter, IREG1, implicated in the basolateral transfer of iron to the circulation. *Mol Cell* 2000;5:299–309.

7. Abboud S, Haile DJ. A novel mammalian iron-regulated protein involved in intracellular iron metabolism. *J Biol Chem* 2000;275:19906–19912.

8. Vulpe CD, Kuo YM, Murphy TL, et al. Hephaestin, a ceruloplasmin homologue implicated in intestinal iron transport, is defective in the sla mouse. *Nature Genet* 1999;21:195–199.

9. Watkins JA, Altazan JD, Elder P, et al. Kinetic characterization of reductant dependent processes of iron mobilization from endocytic vesicles. *Biochemistry* 1992;31:5820–5830.

10. Fleming MD, Romano MA, Su MA, et al. Nramp2 is mutated in the anemic Belgrade (b) rat: evidence of a role for Nramp2 in endosomal iron transport. *Proc Natl Acad Sci USA* 1998;95:1148–1153.

11. Hamill RL, Woods JC, Cook BA. Congenital atransferrinemia: a case report and review of the literature. *Am J Clin Pathol* 1991;96:215–218.

12. Barisani D, Berg CL, Wessling-Resnick M, et al. Evidence for a low Km transporter for non-transferrin-bound iron in isolated rat hepatocytes. *Am J Physiol* 1995;269:G570–576.

13. Parkes JG, Randell EW, Olivieri NF, et al. Modulation by iron loading and chelation of the uptake of non-transferrin-bound iron by human liver cells. *Biochim Biophys Acta* 1995;1243:373–380.

14. Harris ZL, Durley AP, Man TK, et al. Targeted gene disruption reveals an essential role for ceruloplasmin in cellular iron efflux. *Proc Natl Acad Sci USA* 1999;96:10812–10817.

15. MacGillivray RT, Moore SA, Chen J, et al. Two high-resolution crystal structures of the recombinant N-lobe of human transferrin reveal a structural change implicated in iron release. *Biochemistry* 1998;37:7919–7928.

16. Grossmann JG, Neu M, Pantos E, et al. X-ray solution scattering reveals conformational changes upon iron uptake in lactoferrin, serum and ovo-transferrins. *J Mol Biol* 1992;225:811–819.

17. Baynes RD, Shih YJ, Hudson BG, et al. Production of the serum form of the transferrin receptor by a cell membrane-associated serine protease. *Proc Soc Exp Biol Med* 1993;204:65–69.

18. Cook JD. The measurement of serum transferrin receptor. *Am J Med Sci* 1999;318:269–276.

19. Lawrence CM, Ray S, Babyonyshev M, et al. Crystal structure of the ectodomain of human transferrin receptor. *Science* 1999;286:779–782.

20. Kawabata H, Yang R, Hirama T, et al. Molecular cloning of transferrin receptor 2. A new member of the transferrin receptor-like family. *J Biol Chem* 1999;274:20826–20832.

21. Kawabata H, Germain RS, Vuong PT, et al. Transferrin receptor 2-alpha supports cell growth both in iron-chelated cultured cells and in vivo. *J Biol Chem* 2000;275:16618–16625.

22. Fleming RE, Migas MC, Holden CC, et al. Transferrin receptor 2: continued expression in mouse liver in the face of iron overload and in hereditary hemochromatosis. *Proc Natl Acad Sci USA* 2000;97:2214–2219.

23. Camaschella C, Roetto A, Cali A, et al. The gene TFR2 is mutated in a new type of haemochromatosis mapping to 7q22. *Nat Genet* 2000;25:14–15.

24. Rouault T, Klausner R. Regulation of iron metabolism in eukaryotes. *Curr Top Cell Regul* 1997;35:1–19.

25. Muckenthaler M, Gray NK, Hentze MW. IRP-1 binding to ferritin mRNA prevents the recruitment of the small ribosomal subunit by the cap-binding complex eIF4F. *Mol Cell* 1998;2:383–388.

26. Rouault TA, Tang CK, Kaptain S, et al. Cloning of the cDNA encoding an RNA regulatory protein—the human iron-responsive element-binding protein. *Proc Natl Acad Sci USA* 1990;87:7958–7962.

27. Samaniego F, Chin J, Iwai K, et al. Molecular characterization of a second iron-responsive element binding protein, iron regulatory protein 2. Structure, function, and post-translational regulation. *J Biol Chem* 1994;269:30904–30910.

28. Henderson BR, Kuhn LC. Differential modulation of the RNA-binding proteins IRP-1 and IRP-2 in response to iron. IRP-2 inactivation requires translation of another protein. *J Biol Chem* 1995;270:20509–20515.

29. Guo B, Phillips JD, Yu Y, et al. Iron regulates the intracellular degradation of iron regulatory protein 2 by the proteasome. *J Biol Chem* 1995;270:21645–21651.

30. Henderson BR, Menotti E, Kuhn LC. Iron regulatory proteins 1 and 2 bind distinct sets of RNA target sequences. *J Biol Chem* 1996;271:4900–4908.

31. Butt J, Kim HY, Basilion JP, et al. Differences in the RNA binding sites of iron regulatory proteins and potential target diversity. *Proc Natl Acad Sci USA* 1996;93:4345–4349.

32. Hentze MW, Kuhn LC. Molecular control of vertebrate iron metabolism: mRNA-based regulatory circuits operated by iron, nitric oxide, and oxidative stress. *Proc Natl Acad Sci USA* 1996;93:8175–8182.

33. Bacon BR, Sadiq SA. Hereditary hemochromatosis: presentation and diagnosis in the 1990s. *Am J Gastroenterol* 1997;92:784–789.

34. Edwards CQ, Kushner JP. Screening for hemochromatosis. *N Engl J Med* 1993;328:1616–1620.

35. Bassett ML, Halliday JW, Powell LW. Value of hepatic iron measurements in early hemochromatosis and determination of the critical iron level associated with fibrosis. *Hepatology* 1986;6:24–29.

36. Brink B, Disler P, Lynch S, et al. Patterns of iron storage in dietary iron overload in idiopathic hemochromatosis. *J Lab Clin Med* 1976;88:725–731.

37. Ludwig J, Hashimoto E, Porayko MK, et al. Hemosiderosis in cirrhosis: a study of 447 native livers. *Gastroenterology* 1997;112:882–888.

38. Koskinas J, Portmann B, Lombard M, et al. Persistent iron overload 4 years after inadvertent transplantation of a haemochromatotic liver in a patient with primary biliary cirrhosis. *J Hepatol* 1992;16:351–354.

39. Lynch SR, Skikne BS, Cook JD. Food iron absorption in idiopathic hemochromatosis. *Blood* 1989;74:2187–2193.

40. McLaren GD, Nathanson MH, Jacobs A, et al. Regulation of intestinal iron absorption and mucosal iron kinetics in hereditary hemochromatosis. *J Lab Clin Med* 1991;117:390–401.

41. Feder JN, Gnirke A, Thomas W, et al. A novel MHC class I-like gene is mutated in patients with hereditary haemochromatosis. *Nature Genet* 1996;13:399–408.

42. Bacon BR, Powell LW, Adams PC, et al. Molecular medicine and hemochromatosis: at the crossroads. *Gastroenterology* 1999;116:193–207.

43. Adams PC, Chakrabarti S. Genotypic/phenotypic correlations in genetic hemochromatosis: evolution of diagnostic criteria. *Gastroenterology* 1998;114:319–323.

44. Olynyk JK, Cullen DJ, Aquilia S, et al. A population-based study of the clinical expression of the hemochromatosis gene. *N Engl J Med* 1999;341:718–724.

45. Rochette J, Pointon JJ, Fisher CA, et al. Multicentric origin of

hemochromatosis gene (HFE) mutations. *Am J Hum Genet* 1999;64:1056–1062.

46. Mura C, Raguenes O, Ferec C. HFE mutations analysis in 711 hemochromatosis probands: evidence for S65C implication in mild form of hemochromatosis. *Blood* 1999;93:2502–2505.

47. Barton JC, Sawada-Hirai R, Rothenberg BE, et al. Two novel missense mutations of the HFE gene (I105T and G93R) and identification of the S65C mutation in Alabama hemochromatosis probands. *Blood Cells Mol Dis* 1999;25:147–155.

48. Wallace DF, Dooley JS, Walker AP. A novel mutation of HFE explains the classical phenotype of genetic hemochromatosis in a C282Y heterozygote. *Gastroenterology* 1999;116:1409–1412.

49. Bahram S, Gilfillan S, Kuhn LC, et al. Experimental hemochromatosis due to MHC class I HFE deficiency: immune status and iron metabolism. *Proc Natl Acad Sci USA* 1999;96:13312–13317.

50. Levy JE, Montross LK, Cohen DE, et al. The C282Y mutation causing hereditary hemochromatosis does not produce a null allele. *Blood* 1999;94:9–11.

51. Zhou XY, Tomatsu S, Fleming RE, et al. HFE gene knockout produces mouse model of hereditary hemochromatosis. *Proc Natl Acad Sci USA* 1998;95:2492–2497.

52. de Sousa M, Reimao R, Lacerda R, et al. Iron overload in beta 2-microglobulin-deficient mice. *Immunol Lett* 1994;39:105–111.

53. Santos M, Schilham MW, Rademakers LHPM, et al. Defective iron homeostasis in beta2-microglobulin knockout mice recapitulates hereditary hemochromatosis in man. *J Exp Med* 1996;184:1975–1985.

54. Levy JE, Montross LK, Andrews NC. Genes that modify the hemochromatosis phenotype in mice. *J Clin Invest* 2000;105:1209–1216.

55. Parkkila S, Waheed A, Britton RS, et al. Association of the transferrin receptor in human placenta with HFE, the protein defective in hereditary hemochromatosis. *Proc Natl Acad Sci USA* 1997;94:13198–13202.

56. Feder JN, Penny DM, Irrinki A, et al. The hemochromatosis gene product complexes with the transferrin receptor and lowers its affinity for ligand binding. *Proc Natl Acad Sci USA* 1998;95:1472–1477.

57. Lebron JA, Bennett MJ, Vaughn DE, et al. Crystal structure of the hemochromatosis protein HFE and characterization of its interaction with transferrin receptor. *Cell* 1998;93:111–123.

58. Bennett MJ, Lebron JA, Bjorkman PJ. Crystal structure of the hereditary haemochromatosis protein HFE complexed with transferrin receptor. *Nature* 2000;403:46–53.

59. Camaschella C, Fargion S, Sampietro M, et al. Inherited HFE-unrelated hemochromatosis in Italian families. *Hepatology* 1999;29:1563–1564.

60. Camaschella C, Roetto A, Cicilano M, et al. Juvenile and adult hemochromatosis are distinct genetic disorders. *Eur J Hum Genet* 1997;5:371–375.

61. Camaschella C. Juvenile haemochromatosis. *Baillieres Clin Gastroenterol* 1998;12:227–235.

62. Roetto A, Totaro A, Cazzola M, et al. Juvenile hemochromatosis locus maps to chromosome 1q. *Am J Hum Genet* 1999;64:1388–1393.

63. Pietrangelo A, Montosi G, Totaro A, et al. Hereditary hemochromatosis in adults without pathogenic mutations in the hemochromatosis gene. *N Engl J Med* 1999;341:725–732.

64. Walker EM Jr, Wolfe MD, Norton ML, et al. Hereditary hemochromatosis. *Ann Clin Lab Sci* 1998;28:300–312.

65. Walker AP, Wallace DF, Partridge J, et al. Atypical haemochromatosis: phenotypic spectrum and beta2-microglobulin candidate gene analysis. *J Med Genet* 1999;36:537–541.

66. Gordeuk V, Mukiibi J, Hasstedt SJ, et al. Iron overload in Africa. Interaction between a gene and dietary iron content. *N Engl J Med* 1992;326:95–100.

67. Moyo VM, Gangaidzo IT, Gomo ZA, et al. Traditional beer consumption and the iron status of spouse pairs from a rural community in Zimbabwe. *Blood* 1997;89:2159–2166.

68. Moyo VM, Mandishona E, Hasstedt SJ, et al. Evidence of genetic transmission in African iron overload. *Blood* 1998;91:1076–1082.

69. Gangaidzo IT, Moyo VM, Saungweme T, et al. Iron overload in urban Africans in the 1990s. *Gut* 1999;45:278–283.

70. Barton JC, Edwards CQ, Bertoli LF, et al. Iron overload in African Americans. *Am J Med* 1995;99:616–623.

71. Wurapa RK, Gordeuk VR, Brittenham GM, et al. Primary iron overload in African Americans. *Am J Med* 1996;101:9–18.

72. Monaghan KG, Rybicki BA, Shurafa M, et al. Mutation analysis of the HFE gene associated with hereditary hemochromatosis in African Americans. *Am J Hematol* 1998;58:213–217.

73. Bothwell TH, Bradlow BA. Siderosis in the Bantu: a combined histopathological and chemical study. *Arch Pathol* 1960;70:279–292.

74. Eason RJ, Adams PC, Aston CE, et al. Familial iron overload with possible autosomal dominant inheritance. *Aust NZ J Med* 1990;20:226–230.

75. Gitlin JD. Aceruloplasminemia. *Pediatr Res* 1998;44:271–276.

76. Harris ZL, Klomp LW, Gitlin JD. Aceruloplasminemia: an inherited neurodegenerative disease with impairment of iron homeostasis. *Am J Clin Nutr* 1998;67:972S–977S.

77. Morita H, Ikeda S, Yamamoto K, et al. Hereditary ceruloplasmin deficiency with hemosiderosis: a clinicopathological study of a Japanese family. *Ann Neurol* 1995;37:646–656.

78. Hayashi A, Wada Y, Suzuki T, et al. Studies on familial hypotransferrinemia: unique clinical course and molecular pathology. *Am J Hum Genet* 1993;53:201–213.

79. Simpson RJ, Konijn AM, Lombard M, et al. Tissue iron loading and histopathological changes in hypotransferrinaemic mice. *J Pathol* 1993;171:237–244.

80. Simpson RJ, Deenmamode J, McKie AT, et al. Time-course of iron overload and biochemical, histopathological and ultrastructural evidence of pancreatic damage in hypotransferrinaemic mice. *Clin Sci (Colch)* 1997;93:453–462.

81. Huggenvik JI, Craven CM, Idzerda RL, et al. A splicing defect in the mouse transferrin gene leads to congenital atransferrinemia. *Blood* 1989;74:482–486.

82. Trenor CC, Campagna DR, Sellers VM, et al. The molecular defect in hypotransferrinemic mice. *Blood*, 2000;96:1113–1118.

83. Raja KB, Simpson RJ, Peters TJ. Intestinal iron absorption studies in mouse models of iron overload. *Br J Hematol* 1994;86:156–162.

84. Raja KB, Pountney DJ, Simpson RJ, et al. Importance of anemia and transferrin levels in the regulation of intestinal iron absorption in hypotransferrinemic mice. *Blood* 1999;94:3185–3192.

85. Buys SS, Martin CB, Eldridge M, et al. Iron absorption in hypotransferrinemic mice. *Blood* 1991;78:3288–3290.

86. Dickinson TK, Devenyi AG, Connor JR. Distribution of injected iron 59 and manganese 54 in hypotransferrinemic mice. *J Lab Clin Med* 1996;128:270–278.

87. Raja KB, Simpson RJ, Peters TJ. Plasma clearance of transferrin in control and hypotransferrinaemic mice: implications for regulation of transferrin turnover. *Br J Haematol* 1995;89:177–180.

88. Simpson RJ, Cooper CE, Raja KB, et al. Non-transferrin-bound iron species in the serum of hypotransferrinaemic mice. *Biochim Biophys Acta* 1992;1156:19–26.

89. Knisely AS. Neonatal hemochromatosis. *Adv Pediatr* 1992;39:383–403.

90. Colletti RB, Clemmons JJ. Familial neonatal hemochromatosis with survival. *J Pediatr Gastroenterol Nutr* 1988;7:39–45.

91. Sigurdsson L, Reyes J, Kocoshis SA, et al. Neonatal hemochromatosis: outcomes of pharmacologic and surgical therapies. *J Pediatr Gastroenterol Nutr* 1998;26:85–89.

92. Ferrell L, Schmidt K, Sheffield V, et al. Neonatal hemochromatosis: genetic counseling based on retrospective pathologic diagnosis. *Am J Med Genet* 1992;44:429–433.

93. Verloes A, Temple IK, Hubert AF, et al. Recurrence of neonatal haemochromatosis in half sibs born of unaffected mothers. *J Med Genet* 1996;33:444–449.

94. Brown MD, Chitayat D, Allen J, et al. Mitochondrial DNA mutations associated with neonatal hemochromatosis. *Am J Hum Genet* 1999;45:A45(abst).

95. Shneider BL, Setchell KD, Whitington PF, et al. Delta 4-3-oxosteroid 5 beta-reductase deficiency causing neonatal liver failure and hemochromatosis. *J Pediatr* 1994;124:234–238.

96. Siafakas CG, Jonas MM, Perez-Atayde AR. Abnormal bile acid metabolism and neonatal hemochromatosis: a subset with poor prognosis. *J Pediatr Gastroenterol Nutr* 1997;25:321–326.

97. Clayton PT. Delta 4-3-oxosteroid 5 beta-reductase deficiency and neonatal hemochromatosis. *J Pediatr* 1994;125:845–846.

98. Fellman V, Rapola J, Pihko H, et al. Iron-overload disease in infants involving fetal growth retardation, lactic acidosis, liver haemosiderosis, and aminoaciduria. *Lancet* 1998;351:490–493.

99. Visapaa I, Fellman V, Varilo T, et al. Assignment of the locus for a new lethal neonatal metabolic syndrome to 2q33-37. *Am J Hum Genet* 1998;63:1396–1403.

100. Rocchi E, Cassanelli M, Borghi A, et al. Liver iron overload and desferrioxamine treatment of porphyria cutanea tarda. *Dermatologica* 1991;182:27–31.

101. Bonkovsky HL, Poh-Fitzpatrick M, Pimstone N, et al. Porphyria cutanea tarda, hepatitis C, and HFE gene mutations in North America. *Hepatology* 1998;27:1661–1669.

102. Bulaj ZJ, Phillips JD, Ajioka RS, et al. Hemochromatosis genes and other factors contributing to the pathogenesis of porphyria cutanea tarda. *Blood* 2000;95:1565–1571.

103. Roberts AG, Whatley SD, Morgan RR, et al. Increased frequency of the haemochromatosis Cys282Tyr mutation in sporadic porphyria cutanea tarda. *Lancet* 1997;349:321–323.

104. Roberts AG, Whatley SD, Nicklin S, et al. The frequency of hemochromatosis-associated alleles is increased in British patients with sporadic porphyria cutanea tarda. *Hepatology* 1997;25:159–161.

105. Sampietro M, Piperno A, Lupica L, et al. High prevalence of the His63Asp HFE mutation in Italian patients with porphyria cutanea tarda. *Hepatology* 1998;27:181–184.

106. Sinclair PR, Gorman N, Dalton T, et al. Uroporphyria produced in mice by iron and 5-aminolaevulinic acid does not occur in Cyp1a2(−/−) null mutant mice. *Biochem J* 1998;330:149–153.

107. Smith AG, Carthew P, Francis JE, et al. Influence of iron on the induction of hepatic tumors and porphyria by octachlorostyrene in C57BL/10ScSn mice. *Cancer Lett* 1994;81:145–150.

108. Di Bisceglie AM, Axiotis CA, Hoofnagle JH, et al. Measurements of iron status in patients with chronic hepatitis. *Gastroenterology* 1992;102:2108–2113.

109. Bonkovsky HL, Banner BF, Lambrecht RW, et al. Iron in liver diseases other than hemochromatosis. *Semin Liver Dis* 1996;16:65–82.

110. Banner BF, Barton AL, Cable EE, et al. A detailed analysis of the Knodell score and other histologic parameters as predictors of response to interferon therapy in chronic hepatitis C. *Mod Pathol* 1995;8:232–238.

111. Fong TL, Han SH, Tsai NC, et al. A pilot randomized, controlled trial of the effect of iron depletion on long-term response to alpha-interferon in patients with chronic hepatitis C. *J Hepatol* 1998;28:369–374.

112. Fontana RJ, Israel J, LeClair P, et al. Iron reduction before and during interferon therapy of chronic hepatitis C: results of a multicenter, randomized, controlled trial. *Hepatology* 2000;31:730–736.

113. Bottomley SS. Secondary iron overload disorders. *Semin Hematol* 1998;35:77–86.

114. Pootrakul P, Kitcharoen K, Yansukon P, et al. The effect of erythroid hyperplasia on iron balance. *Blood* 1988;71:1124–1129.

115. Fargion S, Cappellini MD, Piperno A, et al. Association of hereditary spherocytosis and idiopathic hemochromatosis. A synergistic effect in determining iron overload. *Am J Clin Pathol* 1986;86:645–649.

116. Mohler DN, Wheby MS. Hemochromatosis heterozygotes may have significant iron overload when they also have hereditary spherocytosis. *Am J Med Sci* 1986;292:320–324.

117. Fargion S, Piperno A, Panaiotopoulos N, et al. Iron overload in subjects with beta-thalassaemia trait: role of idiopathic haemochromatosis gene. *Br J Haematol* 1985;61:487–490.

118. Longo F, Zecchina G, Sbaiz L, et al. The influence of hemochromatosis mutations on iron overload of thalassemia major. *Haematologica* 1999;84:799–803.

119. Beutler E, Gelbart T, Lee P, et al. Molecular characterization of a case of atransferrinemia. *Blood* 2000;96:4071–4074.

120. Cannone-Hergaux F, Levy JE, Fleming MD, et al. Expression of DMT1 (NRAMP2/DCT1) iron transporter in mice with genetic iron overload disorders. *Blood* 2001;97:1138–1140.

24

THE BIOLOGY OF THE BILE CANALICULUS

PETER UJHÁZY
HELMUT KIPP
SUNITI MISRA
YOSHIYUKI WAKABAYASHI
IRWIN M. ARIAS

Apical membranes of hepatocytes form the bile canaliculus, which is a distinct structural and functional unit (see chapters 7 and 8, website chapters 🖥 W-1, W-2, and W-5). Although only 10% to 15% of the entire hepatocyte surface is devoted to the canalicular membrane, which is the most proximal channel of the biliary tree, it is an important checkpoint for biliary secretion and enterohepatic circulation.

Research on bile canalicular structure and function followed several stages. Study of structure relied mostly on established light, electron, and confocal microscopic methods, and immunofluorescence and biochemical analysis. Functional studies underwent a more radical development. Due to the relative inaccessibility of the bile canaliculus, information on bile secretion was initially based on indirect methods using animal models and collection of common duct bile. These methods, particularly isolated liver perfusion, served well to evaluate the kinetics of secretion and allowed testing of modifying agents. Later studies involved secretion of fluorescent organic molecules by hepatocyte doublets (i.e., two or more hepatocytes that retain an apical domain in the form of a closed cyst-like structure). However, because these preparations contain portions of canalicular domains that remain after removal of adjacent hepatocytes, they are of limited use in studying secretion and intracellular trafficking. A more stable variation was developed in WIFB9 cells, an immortalized chimera between a human fibroblast (WI38) and rat hepatoma line (Fao) (1,2). WIFB9 cells form canalicular structures and proved to be valuable in the study of intracellular trafficking and biliary secretion. Transfection technologies, confocal microscopy, and image analysis make this model especially attractive and versatile in studies of the genes and their products that are involved in bile formation. Advances in purification of canalicular membrane vesicles with right-side out and inside-out orientation (3) prompted experimental designs to evaluate substrate transport through the canalicular membrane in either direction. More recently, time lapse video-imaging permitted functional studies of bile canaliculus and exchange of its components with intracellular compartments (4). These molecular, cell, physiologic, and biochemical approaches have resulted in significant understanding of bile canalicular biology.

P. Ujházy, H. Kipp, S. Misra, Y. Wakabayashi, and **I. M. Arias:** Department of Physiology, Tufts University School of Medicine, Boston, Massachusetts 02111.

STRUCTURE OF THE BILE CANALICULUS

Scanning electron microscopic images depict bile canaliculi as half-tubules carved out of the hepatocytes' surface (see website chapters 🖥 W-1 and W-8). Channels created by two or more adjacent hepatocytes are 0.75 μm in diameter and may bifurcate so that several branches appear on the same face of a cell. Some canaliculi show lateral sacculations corresponding to short intracellular branches. Often bile canaliculi are in a close proximity (0.1 μm) to the Disse space, which may explain the regurgitation of bile components into sinusoidal blood. The biliary canalicular membrane has several pits and/or small holes, which may be related to secretory processes (5). Numerous actin-containing microvilli can be seen along each channel. Canaliculi are delimited from the basolateral part of the hepatocyte membrane by tight junctions, which are supported by adherens junctions and which prevent free tangential exchange of ions, proteins, and lipids between the apical and sinusoidal membranes (see Chapter 8 and website chapter 🖥 W-5). Quantitative differences in lipid composition distinguish each domain of the plasma membrane; the canalicular is characterized by higher total lipid, cholesterol, and sphingomyelin content per milligram protein and increased molar ratios of cholesterol/phospholipid and sphingomyelin/phosphatidylcholine.

The canalicular structure is supported by a complex cytoskeleton (see Chapter 3 and website chapters 🖥 W-1 and W-2). Canalicular microvilli contain arrays of actin filaments that extend from the plasma membrane to the canalicular space. Filaments are accompanied by actin-binding proteins such as myosin II, tropomyosin, vinculin, α-actin, villin, as well as non–actin-related proteins α-tubulins and cytokeratin. Three actin filaments regions were identified: microvillous core filaments, a membrane-associated microfilamentous network, and circumferential pericanalicular actin filament band associated with the zonula adherens junction. Intermediate keratin filaments insert into desmosomes. The cytoskeletal support of the bile canaliculus is essential for its contractile movement, which facilitates the distal movement of bile.

CONTRACTION OF THE BILE CANALICULUS

Contraction of canaliculi is a normal and spontaneous phenomenon that promotes the movement of bile through the canalicular network (6,7). Canalicular contractility is dependent on Ca^{2+}, actin-myosin adenosine triphosphatase (ATPase) activity, and myosin light chain kinase (8) and is inhibited by cytochalasins B and D, which disrupt actin polymerization and aggregate microfilaments around the bile canaliculus. Despite these effects, secretion of bile substrates remains unimpaired (9). Another pathway for contraction

inhibition involves nitric oxide, which, by stimulation of 3′,5′-cyclic guanosine monophosphate (cGMP) production, decreases inositol triphosphate-dependent Ca^{2+} release from internal stores (10). Nitric oxide and cGMP also stimulate bile secretion in isolated rat hepatocyte douplets but not in isolated bile duct units (11) (see Chapters 29 and 39 and website chapter 🖥 W-25). A similar effect on canalicular contraction was observed by using carbon monoxide (12).

Disruption of microtubules and intermediate keratin filaments has no impact on canalicular motility; however, it results in complete inhibition of secretory function (13). These results suggest that actin filaments are necessary for canalicular contractility and that microtubules and keratin filaments are required for delivery of transporters and/or their substrates toward the apical pole of the hepatocyte.

PROTEINS OF THE CANALICULAR MEMBRANE

The search for protein components of the canalicular membrane occurred in two directions. Some molecules were found by virtue of their activity (i.e., several ATPases); others (i.e., cCAM105), although structurally characterized, still require functional elucidation. Canalicular ATPase activity was detected by enzyme histochemistry over 40 years ago and was postulated to participate in transport. Most canalicular ATPase activity results from ectoenzymes (see website chapters 🖥 W-4 and W-5), although adenosine triphosphate (ATP) fuels several transporters, at least four of which have been well defined (Fig. 24.1).

The canalicular membrane contains numerous ectoenzymes, which have substrate-binding sites that face the canalicular lumen. Most of these enzymes either have single transmembrane domains or are linked to the plasma membrane by phosphoinositol-glycan linkages (see Chapter 8). The ectoenzymes include γ-glutamyl transpeptidase (GGTP), dipeptidylpeptidase (DPPIV), leucinaminopeptidase (LAP), COOH-terminal peptidase, NH_2-peptidase, phospholipid methyltransferase, canalicular cell adhesion molecule (cCAM), Ca^{2+}/Mg^{2+} ATPase, ecto-5′-nucleotidase (5′-NT), and ATP diphosphohydrolase (ATPDase). The first two degrade extracellular glutathione into cysteine, glutamic acid, and glycine; the last three serve in detoxification and/or salvage pathway for extracellular nucleotides (14) (see Chapter 28). Other enzymatic activities in the canalicular membrane include alkaline phosphatase and alkaline phosphodiesterase. High concentrations of small G proteins, 3′,5′-cyclic adenosine monophosphate (cAMP) (15), and several isoforms of phosphoinositide 3 (PI3)-kinase occur in the canalicular membrane and suggest the presence of signaling pathways that originate in the apical pole of the hepatocyte (see Chapters 34 and 35).

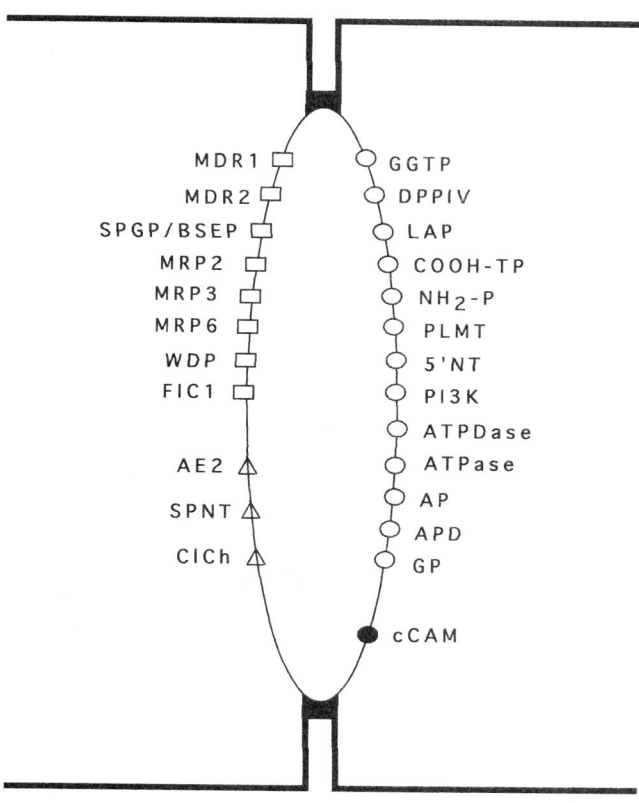

□ Transporters (ATP-dependent)
△ Channels
○ Enzymes
● Adhesion molecule

FIGURE 24.1. Membrane proteins of the bile canaliculus. *5'NT*, ecto-5'-nucleotidase; *AE2*, chloride bicarbonate anion exchanger isoform 2; *AP*, alkaline phosphatase; *APD*, alkaline phosphodiesterase; *ATPase*, Ca^{2+}/Mg^{2+} ATPase; *ATPDase*, ATP diphosphohydrolase; *cCAM*, canalicular cell adhesion molecule; *ClCh*, chloride channel; *COOH-TP*, COOH-terminal peptidase; *DPPIV*, dipeptidylpeptidase; *FIC1*, familial intrahepatic cholestasis type 1 protein; *GGTP*, γ-glutamyl transpeptidase; *GP*, small G proteins; *LAP*, leucinaminopeptidase; *MDR1*, multidrug resistance protein 1/P-glycoprotein 170; *MDR3*, multidrug resistance protein 3; *MRP2*, multidrug resistance associated protein 2/canalicular multiorganic anion transporter; *MRP3*, multidrug resistance associated protein 2; *MRP6*, multidrug resistance associated protein 6; *NH₂-P*, NH_2-peptidase; *PI3K*, phosphoinositide 3-kinase; *PLMT*, phospholipid methyltransferase; *SPGP/BSEP*, sister of P-glycoprotein/bile salt export pump; *SPNT*, sodium-dependent purine-specific nucleoside cotransporter; *WDP*, Wilson's disease protein. (From Gatmaitan ZC, Nies AT, Arias IM. Regulation and translocation of ATP-dependent apical membrane proteins in rat liver. *Am J Physiol* 1997;272:G1041–G1049, with permission.)

CANALICULAR TRANSPORTERS

An increasing number of canalicular proteins have been shown to be transporters, which are directly or indirectly connected with bile formation. Non–ATP-dependent

transporters include the chloride bicarbonate anion exchanger isoform 2, which secretes bicarbonate into bile, controls volume, and stimulates bile flow independently of bile acids (see Chapter 14 and website chapters 🖥 W-22, W-23, and W-24); the chloride channel, the putative glutathione transporter, and the sodium-dependent purine-specific nucleoside cotransporter, which conserves nucleosides and amino acids, respectively.

The existence of ATP-dependent transporters for large hydrophobic metabolites of many endogenous compounds was predicted when it became clear that the physiologic intracellular negative membrane potential (35 mV) in hepatocytes could not account for the 100-fold concentration difference between intracellular and biliary content of secreted substrates, such as bile salts and other organic anions. To date, four ATP-dependent pumps have been well characterized (16,17). They utilize the hydrolysis of ATP to drive transport of organic cations, xenobiotics, phospholipids, and cytokines [multidrug resistance protein 1 (MDR1) and P-glycoprotein 170)] (17,18); phosphatidylcholine from the inner to the outer leaflet of the membrane bilayer (MDR3) (19,20); multispecific organic anions including glutathione conjugates and bilirubin diglucuronide [multidrug resistance-associated protein 2 (MRP2) and canalicular multiorganic anion transporter (cMOAT)] (see Chapters 25 and 26); and bile salts [sister of P-glycoprotein (SPGP) and bile salt export pump (BSEP)] (21) (see Chapter 26). All four transporters are members of the large ATP-binding cassette (ABC) membrane transporter family (see Chapters 25 and 26) (16,22).

Another ABC transporter, MRP3, has also been identified in this location; however, it has also been localized to the basolateral membrane (23,24) (see Chapter 7). MRP3 transports various organic anions, including glycocholate and taurocholate (25). Mrp6, a member of this family, mediates ATP-dependent transport of the anionic cyclopentapeptide BQ-123, estradiol 17-D-glucuronide, and S-(2,4-dinitrophenyl)-glutathione, and is localized in the lateral and canalicular borders of normal rat hepatocytes.

Wilson's disease is an autosomal-recessive disorder of copper metabolism that results from the absence or dysfunction of a copper-transporting P-type ATPase, which leads to impaired biliary copper excretion and disturbed holoceruloplasmin synthesis (see Chapter 22 and website chapter 🖥 W-18). Another member of the P-type ATPase family, the newly discovered *FIC1* gene product (26), is a putative aminophospholipid translocase. Mutations in *FIC1* occur in progressive familiar intrahepatic cholestasis 1 (PFIC1), Byler disease, and benign recurrent intrahepatic cholestasis (BRIC) (see Chapter 26). *FIC1* was detected in the canalicular membrane of rat hepatocytes (27). The normal function of *FIC1* and the mechanism whereby its mutations lead to two phenotypically different forms of cholestasis are presently unknown (see Chapter 26).

MULTIDRUG RESISTANCE PROTEIN TRANSPORTER FAMILY

The MDR family of transporters was originally discovered in an effort to delineate molecules responsible for multidrug resistance in cancer. The first protein characterized in this regard was P-glycoprotein 170, also known as multidrug resistance protein 1 (MDR1) (28). Rodents have two forms of this gene: *mdr1a* and *mdr1b*. MDR1 pumps many hydrophobic cytostatic agents across the membrane in an ATP-dependent way, which prevents high intracellular cytotoxic concentrations of these drugs (29).

In search of the physiologic function of MDR1, the protein was localized in the apical membrane of several polarized epithelial cells (e.g., hepatocytes, intestinal cells, kidney epithelium, and adrenal cells), and it was proposed to serve as an effective mechanism for the extrusion of many xenobiotic cationic compounds (see website chapter 🖳 W-14) (30). So far, the only plausible candidates for its endogenous substrates are membrane lipids (phosphatidylcholine, phosphatidylethanolamine, and sphingomyelin), which are translocated from the inner to the outer leaflets of the membrane (31). According to the "hydrophobic vacuum cleaner" hypothesis, MDR1 translocates substrates bound in the inner membrane leaflet, as opposed to the "channel" hypothesis, in which substrates are translocated from the cytosol to the extracellular environment. The vacuum cleaner mechanism is supported by recent structural studies, which reveal that substrates are translocated along the groove on one side of the channel, which is created by the 12 α-helical transmembrane domains. MDR1 has two nucleotide-binding sites, glycosylation sites on the first N-terminus extracellular loop, and several phosphorylation sites, and the whole sequence has extensive homology between different MDR gene family members and across species. Mouse knockouts for the *mdr1a* gene display an impairment of the blood–brain barrier (32), and *mdr1a/b* double knockouts developed colitis similar to the human inflammatory bowel disease (33).

MDR1 is expressed in the bile canaliculus at low levels. Another member of this family, MDR3 (rodents have a homologue named mdr2), accounts for approximately 80% of all MDR family members in canalicular plasma membrane (34). MDR3 transports phosphatidylcholine from the inner to the outer leaflet of the canalicular membrane. Phosphatidylcholine-containing vesicles that encapsulate bile salts are constantly released from the canalicular membrane to bile, and protect hepatocytes and small bile duct cells against the detergent effect of high concentrations of bile salts. Homozygous disruption of the murine *mdr2* gene causes complete absence of phospholipid from bile and liver disease (35). Homology between MDR1 and MDR2 led to studies of exchangeability of their domains. The N-terminal halves of MDR1 and MDR2 were exchangeable except for a few residues in TM6. This degree of exchangeability was not found in the C-terminal half of MDR1 and MDR2 (36).

Promoters for both MDR1 and MDR3 (mdr2) genes were isolated and studied for functional motifs. Binding sites for several transcription factors (AP-1, Sp-1, and AP-2) and nuclear factors (NF-1, NF-IL6) were found. Exposure to chemotherapeutic drugs, carcinogens, heat shock, and ultraviolet (UV) light increases transcriptional activity of the mdr promoter *in vivo* and *in vitro*.

THE BILE SALT TRANSPORTER SISTER OF P-GLYCOPROTEIN/BILE SALT EXPORT PUMP

A long-standing effort to discover the predicted ATP-dependent bile salt export pump was finally rewarded in 1997 when Gerloff and colleagues discovered that the sister of P-glycoprotein I [relative molecular mass (M_r) = 160 kd] is the major, if not exclusive, bile transporter in bile canaliculus (21). The sister of P-glycoprotein was described in Victor Ling's laboratory in 1995 as a canalicular member of the MDR1 family (37). At that time no function was assigned to this molecule. The full-length gene was isolated from rat liver, and function was demonstrated in transfected *Xenopus laevis* oocytes and Sf9 cells. The ATP-dependent transport activity of various bile salts was inhibitable by vanadate and exhibited saturability [Michaelis' constant (K_m) = 5 μM for taurocholate]. The specificity for bile salts mirrored that found in rat plasma membrane vesicles: taurochenodeoxycholate > tauroursodeoxycholate = taurocholate > glycocholate = cholate. SPGP was found predominantly in liver, where it was localized to the canalicular microvilli and subcanalicular vesicles. Cloning of the murine spgp/bsep followed (34), and the sequence is 94% similar to rat and 89% similar to human bsep. The discovery of the bile salt export pump has important implications for understanding of bile formation, since bile salts are the driving force in bile secretion. Mutation in SPGP results in progressive familial intrahepatic cholestasis type 2 (see Chapter 23).

MRPs, the second major class of ABC transporters are reviewed in Chapter 25.

REGULATION OF CANALICULAR TRANSPORTERS

Canalicular ABC transporters play a key role in bile formation in mammalian liver. Insufficient amounts or malfunctioning of these transporters in the canalicular membrane may be anticipated to impair bile secretion, resulting in cholestasis. Therefore, it is critical to understand their molecular and cellular regulation.

The amount of each ABC transporter in the canalicular membrane is regulated by the physiologic demand to secrete bile acids. Intravenous administration to rats of taurocholate or dibutyryl-cAMP rapidly and selectively increased the functional activity and amount of each ABC transporter in the canalicular membrane. This effect was inhibited by prior administration of colchicine, which disrupts microtubules (38), and Wortmannin, which inhibits PI3-kinase (39). These observations indicate that an intracellular microtubule dependent transport mechanism, which is sensitive to active PI3-kinase, is required to traffic ABC transporters to the canalicular membrane. In addition, the specific 3′-phosphoinositides regulate the ATP-dependent substrate transport activity of spgp and mrp2 in the canalicular membrane (40). Taurocholate and cAMP increase the amount of ABC transporters in the bile canalicular membrane.

Taurocholate (TC) stimulates biliary secretion of phospholipids (41), cholesterol (42), and canalicular membrane and lysosomal enzymes (43,44). The mechanisms responsible for transcellular transport of these compounds are unclear. *In vitro*, taurocholate stimulates microtubule function and vesicle fusion, and directly affects properties of membrane vesicles (45). cAMP increases biliary secretion of bile acids by increasing the microtubule-dependent intracellular vesicle transport system (46) and regulating intracellular Ca^{2+} levels and/or phosphorylation of microtubule associated proteins by cAMP kinases (47–49). In rats, simultaneous infusion of dibutyryl-cAMP (DBcAMP) and taurocholate summate in their effects on secretion of phospholipids and bile acids (46). Whether the TC and DBcAMP effects are due to changes in the affinity, capacity, or number of individual transporters was not known until recently.

Gatmaitan et al. (38) used canalicular membrane vesicles (CMVs) prepared from rats that were treated with TC and/or DBcAMP, and quantified changes in the relative amount of ABC transporters and other canalicular proteins. Intravenous administration of TC or DBcAMP increased (1.5- to 3-fold) the amount of the two ABC transporters, mdr1 and mdr2, and of the canalicular cell adhesion molecule, cCAM105, in canalicular membranes. Prior administration of colchicine abolished the TC-induced increase in membrane proteins and, to a lesser extent, the effect of DBcAMP. Changes in the relative amount of canalicular ABC transporters after treatment with TC or cAMP were paralleled by altered ATP-dependent transport in CMV for TC, a substrate for spgp; daunomycin (DAU), a substrate for mdr1; dinitrophenyl-glutathione (GS-DNP), a substrate for mrp2; and nucleoside binding domain (NBD) hatidylcholine (NBD-PC), a substrate for mdr2 (Fig. 24.2). CMV from rats simultaneously injected with both TC and DBcAMP exhibited greater uptake of ABC transporter substrates when compared to results in CMV from rats that were treated with only one effector. The effects of TC and DBcAMP were additive rather than alternative.

This study demonstrated for the first time that enhancement of bile secretion caused by TC or DBcAMP resulted

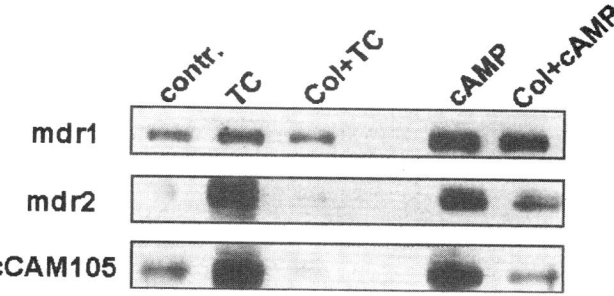

FIGURE 24.2. Protein levels (Western blots) of canalicular proteins in a canalicular membrane vesicle (CMV) prepared from rats receiving various combinations of intravenous pretreatment with taurocholate (*TC*), colchicine (*Col*), and 3′,5′-cyclic adenosine monophosphate (*cAMP*). CMV (equal amounts of protein) were separated by sodium dodecyl sulfate–polyacrylamide gel electrophoresis (SDS-PAGE), transferred onto nitrocellulose, and probed with antibodies against mdr1, mdr2, and cCAM105. (From Gatmaitan ZC, Nies AT, Arias IM. Regulation and translocation of ATP-dependent apical membrane proteins in rat liver. *Am J Physiol* 1997;272:G1041–G1049, with permission.)

from an increase in the specific amount of ABC transporters in the bile canalicular membrane. Where do these additional ABC transporters originate from and how do they traffic to the bile canaliculus? Since the observed responses to TC and DBcAMP occurred within minutes, enhanced transcription on translation appears unlikely as the source of the additional bile canalicular ABC transporters. More likely is recruitment of preexisting transporters from intracellular pool(s). The finding that TC and DBcAMP effects are additive suggests the possibility of two different intracellular pools from which transporters are recruited to the canalicular membrane in response to stimulation with TC or DBcAMP. Since colchicine abolished the effect of TC and to a lesser extent, the effect of DBcAMP, an intracellular vesicular pathway that is dependent on intact microtubules was proposed to be required for the trafficking of ABC transporters from intracellular pools to the bile canalicular membrane. PI3-kinases regulate intrahepatic trafficking and activity of bile canalicular ABC transporters.

PI3-kinase (PI3K) was discovered in Cantley's laboratory over 10 years ago; major interest initially focused on its role in growth factor and oncogene tyrosine kinase-mediated signal transduction (see Chapters 34 and 35). Subsequent studies revealed that PI3Ks are ubiquitous lipid kinases that function as signal transducers downstream of cell surface receptors and are essential for cell proliferation, adhesion, survival, and cytoskeletal rearrangement (49,50). The products of PI3K-catalyzed reactions are $PtdIns(3,4,5)P_3$, $PtdIns(3,4)P_2$, and $PtdIns(3)P$, which serve as second messengers in many signal transduction pathways. Serendipitous observation following characterization of yeast proteins that were involved in intracellular trafficking resulted in many studies that demonstrate that PI3K is required for vesicle trafficking in plant, yeast, and animal cells (51).

Studies of the function of PI3K were greatly facilitated by discovery that, at low nanomolar concentration, Wortmannin, which is a fungal component, specifically inhibits PI3K (52,53). Other PI3K inhibitors of the LY series were subsequently synthesized. When used at the proper concentrations, these inhibitors have high specificity for PI3K in isolated systems and in cells.

Folli and colleagues (52) were among the first to demonstrate that Wortmannin administration in perfused rat liver resulted in intracellular vacuolation, intracellular and canalicular membrane disruption, and impaired transcytosis. Misra and co-workers (39) investigated the effect of Wortmannin on TC-stimulated bile secretion in isolated perfused rat liver. Different schedules of TC and Wortmannin administration in perfused liver and comparison with ABC transporter protein levels in CMV revealed two unexpected effects of Wortmannin on TC-induced bile secretion. When compared to a control experiment, TC perfusion increased bile secretion that resulted from an increased amount of canalicular ABC transporters. Administration of Wortmannin before TC prevented increased bile secretion and simultaneously prevented increase in the amount of canalicular ABC transporters. These observations indicate that active PI3K is required for recruitment and vesicular trafficking of additional ABC transporters from intracellular pools to the bile canalicular membrane after stimulation by TC. When Wortmannin was administered following TC administration, the levels of canalicular ABC transporters remained elevated; however, bile secretion rapidly decreased by 50% following addition of Wortmannin to the perfusion. In these experiments, the amount of canalicular ABC transporters remained elevated; however, transport activity and bile secretion were impaired, which suggests that active PI3K is not only required for TC induced vesicular trafficking, but also may play a role in regulation of ABC transporter activity in the canalicular membrane.

In studies in which the transport of [3H]-TC into CMV was measured, preincubation of CMV with Wortmannin (50 nM) for 5 minutes inhibited ATP-dependent [3H]-TC transport by more than 50%, whereas ATP-independent uptake remained unaltered (40). The concentration that inhibits 50% (IC_{50}) for Wortmannin was 25 nM. The same inhibitory effect was observed with a different PI3K inhibitor, LY294002 (IC_{50} 20 μM). CMV as well as SMV contain substantial amounts of active PI3K. Preincubation for 5 minutes with Wortmannin and LY294002 was necessary in order to inhibit [3H]-TC transport into CMV. These observations suggest that PI3K products, which facilitate ABC TRANS-transporter activity, undergo rapid turnover in the bile canalicular membrane.

That PI3K lipid products are sufficient to enhance ATP-dependent transport activity of canalicular ABC transporters was proven by adding the lipid products to CMVs that were prepared from rats that received various pretreatments, and ATP-dependent [3H]-TC and [3H]-GS-NDP

transport were measured. ATP-dependent transport of [3H]-TC into CMV was enhanced by prior treatment of rats with TC and inhibited by addition of Wortmannin. Addition of PI3K lipid product $PtdIns(3,4)P_2$ to CMV not only rescued Wortmannin inhibition, but restored ATP-dependent [3H]-TC transport above the level induced following TC administration. A similar effect was observed on addition of PI3K lipid products $PtdIns(3,4,5)P_3$ and $PtdIns(3)P$, but not for the structurally related $PtdIns(4,5)P_2$, which lacks 3-hydroxyl phosphorylation. These studies reveal the specificity of PI3K lipid products on ABC transporter activation. Further evidence of the involvement of PI3K lipid products in maximal ABC transporter function was gained by investigation of the effect of a synthetic peptide, which specifically activates PI3K. A rhodamine-linked decapeptide selectively increases $PtdIns(3,4)P_2$ and $PtdIns(3,4,5)P_3$. Addition of the peptide to CMV doubled ATP-dependent [3H]-TC transport into CMV in a dose-dependent and saturable manner. Studies of the kinetics at ATP-dependent transport of TC by spgp and DNP-GSH by mrp2 in CMV were previously performed at saturating levels of all substrates, and kinetic constants, K_m and maximum velocity (V_{max}), were determined. Addition of the PI3K-stimulating peptide increased ATP-dependent transport of TC and DNP-GSH 1.5- to 3-fold. The mechanism responsible for this unexpected result is uncertain; however, we speculate that an active PI3K signal transduction system within the canalicular membrane resulted in lipid kinase products that alter and may physiologically regulate transporter activity and overall bile secretion.

These studies indicate not only that active PI3K is required for intracellular vesicular trafficking of ABC transporters in rat liver, but also that the lipid products of PI3K are necessary for maximal ATP-dependent transport of canalicular ABC transporters in the canalicular membrane. The mechanism by which PI3K regulates ATP-dependent transporters is not known; however, a direct interaction with phospholipids has been proposed for the multidrug resistance protein (mdr1). Trafficking of newly synthesized canalicular proteins has been demonstrated in rat hepatocytes *in vivo*.

Membrane targeting of the newly synthesized canalicular ectoenzymes dipeptidylpeptidase IV, aminopeptidase N and 5′-nucleotidase, and the canalicular cell adhesion molecule cCAM105 (also known as HA4) has been studied in rat liver by *in vivo* metabolic pulse chase labeling. After biosynthesis, these canalicular proteins are transferred from the Golgi network to the basolateral membrane and subsequently reach the bile canaliculus only by transcytosis (Janmey PA, Cunningham CC, Stossel TP, et al. U.S. Patent 5,846,743). Based on these results, it was proposed that all newly synthesized canalicular proteins, including canalicular ABC transporters, are targeted via this indirect route.

An important observation from previous studies was that the canalicular cell adhesion molecule cCAM105, but not canalicular ABC transporters, were readily detected in SMV using Western blots. The presence of cCAM105 in SMV can be explained by the fact that cCAM105 is initially transferred to the basolateral membrane after biosynthesis and subsequently reaches the apical pole by transcytosis. This scenario is in good accordance with detectable steady-state levels of cCAM105 in SMV. These observations also suggest that canalicular ABC transporters may not undergo transcytosis after biosynthesis. The hypothesis of direct apical targeting of canalicular ABC transporters in rat hepatocytes was subsequently tested using metabolic pulse chase labeling (54).

Rats were injected with ^{35}S-methionine, and labeling of newly synthesized proteins was terminated 15 minutes later by injection of an excess of unlabeled methionine. Liver from individual rats was excised after a chase time of 15 minutes, 30 minutes, and 1, 2, and 3 hours from which CMV, SMV, and Golgi membranes were prepared. Each fraction was immunoprecipitated with anti-cCAM105, C219 (mdr1 and mdr2), and anti-spgp antibodies, immunoprecipitates were separated by sodium dodecyl sulfate–polyacrylamide gel electrophoresis (SDS-PAGE), and radioactive bands were detected and quantified with a phosphorimager (Fig. 24.3).

Radiolabeled mdr1, mdr2, and spgp peaked in Golgi membranes after a chase time of 30 minutes and were virtually absent from the Golgi membrane at later time points, indicating that processing and passage through the Golgi of these ABC transporters is complete after 30 to 60 minutes. This is also supported by the observation that immature forms of spgp disappeared from homogenates at chase times greater than 30 minutes. The rate of trafficking of ABC transporters to the canalicular membrane was considerably faster than that of cCAM105. In Golgi membranes, cCAM105 was detected up to 2 hours in parallel with the presence of immature forms of the protein in the homogenate during this time period.

Besides passage through Golgi, major differences were also observed between the canalicular membrane proteins with regard to their membrane targeting. After a chase time of 15 minutes, newly synthesized cCAM105 appeared exclusively in SMV, increased to peak at 1 hour, and progressively declined thereafter. In CMV, cCAM105 was first detected after 1 hour and subsequently increased for 3 hours. These observations are in good accordance with transcytotic targeting of cCAM105 and confirm results of earlier studies (Janmey PA, Cunningham CC, Stossel TP, et al. U.S. Patent 5,846,743). In contrast, after a chase time of 30 minutes, mdr1 and mdr2 appeared exclusively in CMV and increased thereafter for the remaining time investigated. At no time were mdr1 or mdr2 detected in SMV. The absence of mdr1 and mdr2 from SMV at all time points and the time course of their appearance in CMV strongly suggest direct targeting from Golgi to the canalicular membrane. A transcytotic pathway can also be

excluded for the plasma membrane targeting of spgp. At no time was spgp detected in SMV, but when compared to mdr1 and mdr2, it appeared in CMV, but only after 2 hours. Particularly interesting are results after 1-hour labeling: the homogenate contained only mature spgp, indicating that spgp had already trafficked through Golgi but had not reached the cell surface. The most likely explanation for retarded spgp trafficking is that spgp is transiently sequestered in an intracellular pool(s) before being delivered to the canalicular membrane.

The membrane targeting of bile canalicular proteins found in these recent studies (37) is summarized in Fig. 24.4. Electronmicroscopic immunogold detection of spgp in rat hepatocytes revealed that the distribution of spgp in rat hepatocyte is not restricted to the bile canaliculus; labeling of spgp was also detected in electron translucent vacuoles close to the apical membrane, but not in the basolateral membrane (21). Pericanalicular distribution of spgp was also demonstrated by immunofluorescent staining of isolated rat hepatocyte couplets. These subapical structures, which contain spgp, may represent the intracellular pool in which newly synthesized spgp is transiently sequestered prior to its targeting to the bile canaliculus.

In addition to results of *in vivo* labeling studies and the absence of steady-state levels of canalicular ABC transporters in SMV, there is additional evidence for a direct Golgi to bile canaliculus pathway after biosynthesis of ABC transporters. Disturbance of transhepatic trafficking by colchicine, which disrupts microtubules, or Wortmannin, which inhibits PI3K, resulted in accumulation of the transcytosing molecule cCAM105 in the basolateral membrane, but did not result in detectable levels of ABC transporters in the basolateral membrane (39). These results further support nontranscytotic trafficking of canalicular ABC transporters. Moreover, direct targeting from Golgi to the bile canalicular domain of an ABC transporter has recently been visualized in polarized WIFB cells, which were stably transfected with a mdr1-green fluorescent protein chimera gene (55).

WIFB cells are a hybrid of rat hepatoma cells and human fibroblasts, have functional bile canaliculi, and serve as a useful model for hepatocytes (1,2). Functional features of hepatocytes are also observed in WIFB cells: e.g., basolateral to apical membrane transcytosis of canalicular ectoenzymes (51); secretion of fluorescent bile acids and substrates for mdr1 and mrp2; inhibition of the secretion of fluorescent substrates by the PI3K inhibitor, Wortmannin (55); and enhancement of the secretion of fluorescent substrates by TC and PI3K activating synthetic peptide (55).

Intracellular distribution and trafficking of mdr1-green fluorescent protein (GFP) was recently studied in stably transfected WIFB cells (55). Fluorescence of the mdr1-GFP chimera was exclusively detected in Golgi and bile canalicular membranes; no labeling of basolateral plasma membranes was observed. To visualize movement of mdr1-GFP chimeric

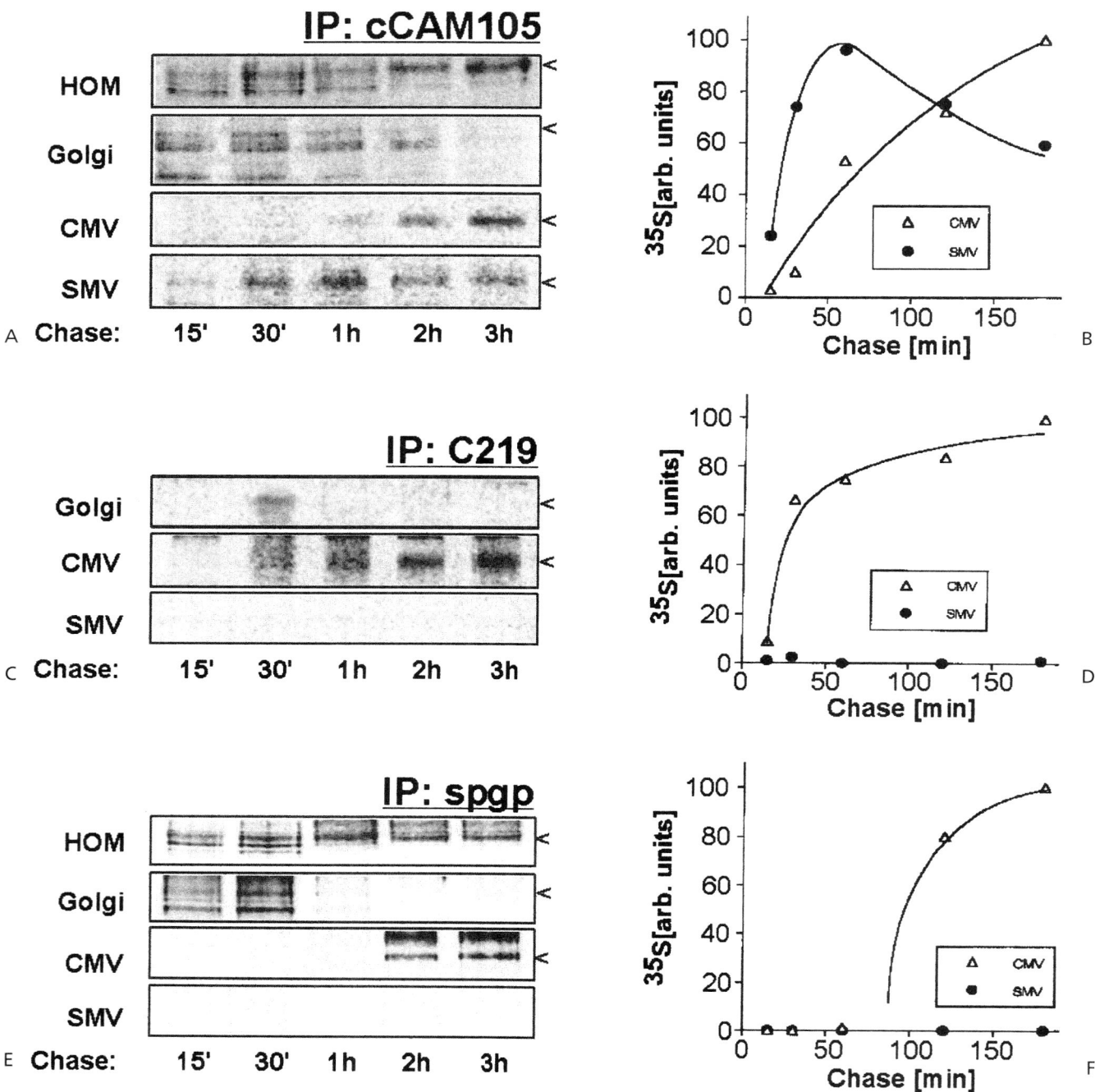

FIGURE 24.3. Metabolic pulse-chase labeling. Rats were pulse labeled for 15 minutes with ^{35}S-methionine and then chased with unlabeled methionine for 15 minutes, 30 minutes, and 1, 2, and 3 hours. cCAM105 (**A**), mdr1, mdr2 (**C**) and spgp (**E**) were then immunoprecipitated from liver homogenates (*HOM*), Golgi membranes, canalicular membrane vesicles (*CMV*), and sinusoid membrane vesicles (*SMV*). ^{35}S in immunoprecipitates from CMV and SMV were quantified with a phosphorimager and plotted versus the chase time to illustrate the membrane targeting of each membrane protein (panels **B, D, F**). *Arrowheads* indicate the positions of mature antigens.

protein between Golgi and bile canaliculi, fluorescent images of stably transfected WIFB cells were serially examined by confocal microscopy. Digital fluorescent images were collected for 20 minutes and converted into a QuickTime movie (see complete movie at http://www.healthsci.tufts.edu/ LABS/IMArias/SaiF9.htm); selected sequences from the movie are depicted in Fig. 24.5. The upper six panels show a time sequence over 2 to 6 minutes, in which mdr1-GFP moved rapidly from the Golgi (G), directly along straight or curvilinear paths, and merged with the bile canaliculus (BC).

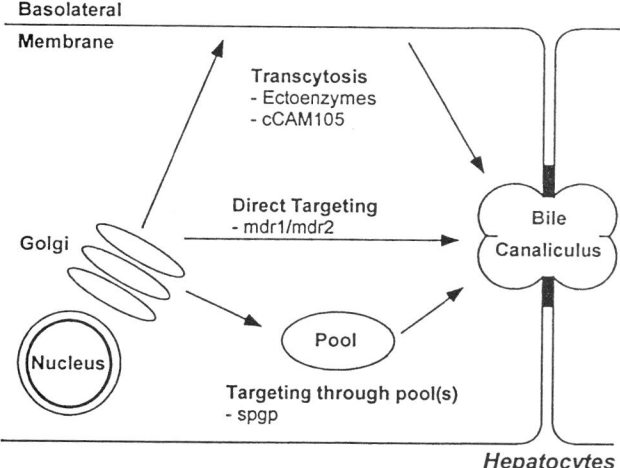

FIGURE 24.4. Membrane targeting of newly synthesized canalicular proteins in rat hepatocytes.

In the middle right nine panels, tubulovesicular movement of mdr1-GFP was also observed between the bile canaliculus and pericanalicular region (arrows). Single long tubules shrank, formed vesicles, and subsequently fused with the canalicular membrane. Other tubular structures extended from the canalicular membrane into the subapical region and retracted to the canalicular membrane (arrowhead in Fig. 24.5A, left middle panel). Figure 24.5B shows a series of confocal images with tubular structures reaching directly from Golgi to the bile canaliculus (arrows). Movement of mdr1-GFP was not synchronous. Individual tubulovesicular structures frequently changed shape during translocation. Frequently there was a brief delay following which tubular vesicles fused with the canalicular membrane. This event appeared distinct from movements of tubules in other directions (i.e., those presumably not fusing). Multiple confocal examinations of many cells indicated that the tubule is not moving in and out of focus but fuses with the canalicular membrane.

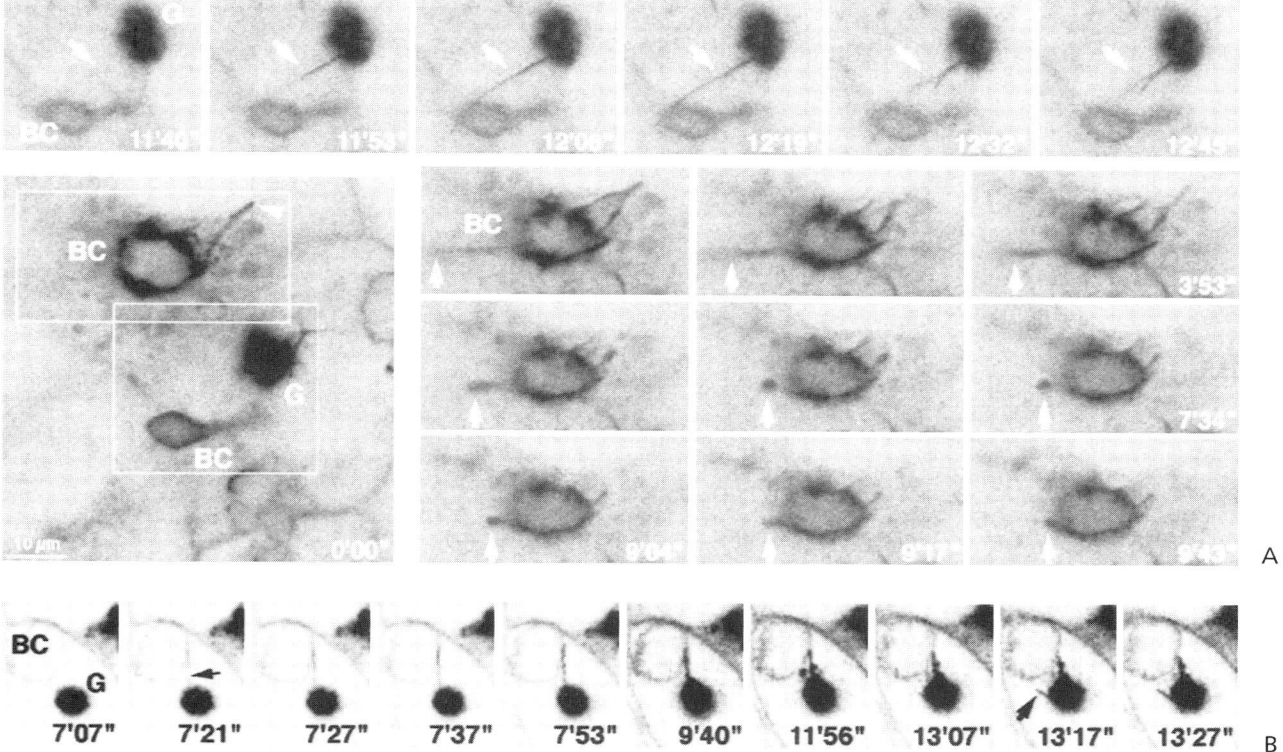

FIGURE 24.5. Visualization of intracellular movement of mdr1-GFP protein between the Golgi and canalicular membranes in stably transfected WIFB9 cells. WIFB9 cells stably transfected with mdr1-GFP were grown on glass cover slips, mounted on the microstage and maintained at 37°C. **A** and **B** represent independent experiments using independent cell cultures. The cells that express mdr1-GFP both in canaliculi and perinuclear Golgi region were identified under the phase and epifluorescence microscope. Digital images were collected using confocal microscope at 3.24-second intervals for about 20 minutes. Every four images were averaged to reduce background noise. See QuickTime movie at http://www.healthsci.tufts.edu/LABS/IMArias/Sa_F9.htm. Smaller panels on **top** and **right** were time sequences of clipped images (actual time in observation was indicated) from *white rectangles* in the **large middle-left panel**. G, Golgi compartment; BC, canalicular membranes. See text for explanation.

In addition, incubation of mdr1-FGP stably transfected WIFB9 cells at 15°C for 20 hours revealed only colocalization of mdr1-FGP with Golgi markers. Following increase in incubation temperature to 37°C, mdr1-FGP progressively moved to the canalicular plasma membrane within 30 to 60 minutes; this process was accelerated on incubation of cells with TC, and the entire process including release from Golgi was prevented by preincubation with Wortmannin. At no time was basolateral membrane localization of mdr1-GFP observed. This model provides further opportunity to examine the role of specific candidate participants in intracellular trafficking and membrane localization.

The observed direct Golgi to bile canalicular trafficking of mdr1-FGP in WIF-B9 cells is consistent with the membrane targeting detected using C219 antibody in rat metabolic labeling studies *in vivo*. Furthermore, the movement of mdr1-GFP from Golgi to the canalicular membrane was tubulovesicular in appearance and intermittent (occurring every 5 to 20 minutes). A speed of 0.02 to 0.6 μm/second was slightly lower than values obtained from other studies, which were up to 1 μm/second (see Chapter 9 and website chapter 🖳 W-6). The process closely resembles the movement of vesicular stomatitis virus-GFP (VSV-G) protein from ER to Golgi in nonpolarized cells (see Chapter 9 and website chapter 🖳 W-6) and previously described Golgi to plasma membrane trafficking involving large tubular–vesicular structures rather than discrete vesicles, which has been the conventional postulate.

CONCLUSION

The mechanism of formation of the tubular vesicles and factors that control their movement to the canalicular membrane are unknown. Based on other studies of vesicular transport in other polarized cells, the process probably requires ATP, Ca^{2+}, dynein and other motors, PI3K lipids, many specific guanosine triphosphatases (GTPases) including dynamin and rab family members, and other factors yet to be identified (see Chapter 10). The recent manufacture of green, yellow, blue, and red fluorescent proteins now permits simultaneous monitoring of different dynamic processes including apical and basolateral sorting of proteins in living cells, and should elucidate further the mechanisms and regulation of these processes. In their brilliant review entitled "The Road Taken: Past and Future Foundations of Membrane Traffic," Mellman and Warren (56) make the following prescient comment: "What is needed is the development of instruments and methods that are familiar to Star Trek fans, namely tools that will allow real-time visualization of events occurring *in vitro* as well as within cells at the molecular level." Current attention is directed toward optical methods that utilize fluorescent probes, such as GFP chimeric proteins. The future holds the promise of greater on-line molecular analysis based on atomic force microscopy, video electron microscopy, and, perhaps, eventual video x-ray or nuclear magnetic resonance (NMR) microscopy.

These studies prompt revision of current hypotheses regarding the trafficking of canalicular membrane proteins from Golgi. Present investigations are directed toward understanding (a) the sequential participation of lipids and proteins that direct ABC transporters to the canalicular domain; (b) identification of kinetics and rate-limiting steps in recruitment and trafficking of canalicular ABC transporters under physiologic conditions; (c) how canalicular membrane lipids, particularly 3′-phosphoinositides, lecithin, and aminophospholipids, regulate the activity of ABC transporters in the membrane; (d) identification of specific targeting motifs, such as PDZ domains, for targeting of apical membrane proteins; (e) the mechanisms whereby cAMP regulates ABC transporter traffic and activity in canalicular membranes; and (f) the relation of each of these studies to liver function in health and disease.

Since the discovery and cloning of several canalicular ABC transporters, inheritable defects in the transporters have been demonstrated to be the molecular basis for at least three forms of familial inheritable cholestasis (see Chapters 25 and 26). Inasmuch as bile acid secretion is essential for optimal bile secretion, defects in the formation, trafficking, membrane insertion, and regulation of spgp (and other canalicular ABC transporters) are likely to be critical in the pathogenesis of acquired intrahepatic cholestasis. We propose that acquired cholestasis associated with hepatocellular effects of viruses, drugs, metals, and other factors may result from impaired regulation of one or more participants in normal canalicular transporter biology. According to this scenario, the common feature of intrahepatic cholestasis is an "intracellular traffic jam," which results in defective function and regulation of canalicular ABC transporters, particularly spgp. This concept also offers novel possibilities of new targets for pharmacotherapy of cholestasis.

REFERENCES

1. Cassio D, Harmon-Benais C, Guerin M, et al. Hybrid cell lines constitute a potential reservoir of polarized cells: isolation and study of highly differentiated hepatoma-derived hybrid cells able to form functional bile canaliculi in vitro. *J Cell Biol* 1993;115: 1397–1408.
2. Ihrke G, Neufeld EB, Meads T, et al. WIF-B cells: an *in vitro* model for studies of hepatocyte polarity. *J Cell Biol* 1993;123: 1761–1775.
3. Inoue M, Kinne R, Tran T, et al. Rat liver canalicular membrane vesicles. Isolation and topological characterization. *J Biol Chem* 1983;258:5183–5188.
4. Sai Y, Nies AT, Arias IM. Bile acid secretion and direct targeting of mdr1-green fluorescent protein from Golgi to the canalicular membrane in polarized WIF-B cells. *J Cell Sci* 1999;112: 4535–4545.

5. Motta P, Fumagalli G. Structure of rat bile canaliculi as revealed by scanning electron microscopy. *Anat Rec* 1975;182:499–513.
6. Tsukada N, Phillips MJ. Bile canalicular contraction is coincident with reorganization of pericanalicular filaments and co-localization of actin and myosin-II. *J Histochem Cytochem* 1993;41:353–363.
7. Watanabe N, Tsukada N, Smith CR, et al. Motility of bile canaliculi in the living animal: implications for bile flow. *J Cell Biol* 1991;113:1069–1080.
8. Kitamura T, Brauneis U, Gatmaitan Z, et al. Extracellular ATP, intracellular calcium and canalicular contraction in rat hepatocyte doublets. *Hepatology* 1991;14:640–647.
9. St-Pierre MV, Dufour JF, Arias IM. Disruption of actin organization by cytochalasin D does not impair biliary secretion of organic anions in the rat. *Hepatology* 1997;25:970–975.
10. Dufour JF, Turner TJ, Arias IM. Nitric oxide blocks bile canalicular contraction by inhibiting inositol trisphosphate-dependent calcium mobilization. *Gastroenterology* 1995;108:841–849.
11. Trauner M, Mennone A, Gigliozzi A, et al. Nitric oxide and guanosine 3′,5′-cyclic monophosphate stimulate bile secretion in isolated rat hepatocyte couplets, but not in isolated bile duct units. *Hepatology* 1998;28:1621–1628.
12. Shinoda Y, Suematsu M, Wakabayashi Y, et al. Carbon monoxide as a regulator of bile canalicular contractility in cultured rat hepatocytes. *Hepatology* 1998;28:286–295.
13. Kawahara H, French SW. Role of cytoskeleton in canalicular contraction in cultured differentiated hepatocytes. *Am J Pathol* 1990;136:521–532.
14. Che M, Ortiz DF, Arias IM. Primary structure and functional expression of a cDNA encoding the bile canalicular, purine-specific Na(+)-nucleoside cotransporter. *J Biol Chem* 1995;270:13596–13599.
15. Ali N, Milligan G, Evans WH. Distribution of G-proteins in rat liver plasma-membrane domains and endocytic pathways. *Biochem J* 1989;261:905–912.
16. Gatmaitan ZC, Arias IM. ATP-dependent transport systems in the canalicular membrane of the hepatocyte. *Physiol Rev* 1995;75:261–275.
17. Higgins CF. ABC transporters: from microorganisms to man. *Annu Rev Cell Biol* 1992;8:67–113.
18. Kamimoto Y, Gatmaitan Z, Hsu J, et al. The function of Gp170, the multidrug resistance gene product, in rat liver canalicular membrane vesicles. *J Biol Chem* 1989;264:11693–11698.
19. Ruetz S, Gros P. Phosphatidylcholine translocase: a physiological role for the mdr2 gene. *Cell* 1994;77:1071–1081.
20. Nies AT, Gatmaitan Z, Arias IM. ATP-dependent phosphatidyl-choline translocation in rat liver canalicular plasma membrane vesicles. *J Lipid Res* 1996;37:1125–1136.
21. Gerloff T, Stieger B, Hagenbuch B, et al. The sister of P-glycoprotein represents the canalicular bile salt export pump of mammalian liver. *J Biol Chem* 1998;273:10046–10050.
22. Muller M, Jansen PL. Molecular aspects of hepatobiliary transport. *Am J Physiol* 1997;272:G1285–1303.
23. Ortiz DF, Li S, Iyer R, et al. MRP3, a new ATP-binding cassette protein localized to the canalicular domain of the hepatocyte. *Am J Physiol* 1999;276:G1493–1500.
24. Konig J, Rost D, Cui Y, et al. Characterization of the human multidrug resistance protein isoform MRP3 localized to the basolateral hepatocyte membrane. *Hepatology* 1999;29:1156–1163.
25. Hirohashi T, Suzuki H, Takikawa H, et al. ATP-dependent transport of bile salts by rat multidrug resistance-associated protein 3 (Mrp3). *J Biol Chem* 2000;275:2905–2910.
26. Bull LN, van Eijk MJ, Pawlikowska L, et al. A gene encoding a P-type ATPase mutated in two forms of hereditary cholestasis. *Nat Genet* 1998;18:219–224.
27. Ujhazy P, Ortiz DF, Misra S, et al. ATP-dependent aminophos-

pholipid translocase activity in rat canalicular membrane vesicles and its relationship to FIC1. *Hepatology* 1999;30:1208.
28. Riordan JR, Ling V. Purification of P-glycoprotein from plasma membrane vesicles of Chinese hamster ovary cell mutants with reduced colchicine permeability. *J Biol Chem* 1979;254:12701–12705.
29. Shustik C, Dalton W, Gros P. P-glycoprotein-mediated multidrug resistance in tumor cells: biochemistry, clinical relevance and modulation. *Mol Aspects Med* 1995;16:1–78.
30. Higgins CF, Callaghan R, Linton KJ, et al. Structure of the multidrug resistance P-glycoprotein. *Semin Cancer Biol* 1997;8:135–142.
31. van Helvoort A, Smith AJ, Sprong H, et al. MDR1 P-glycoprotein is a lipid translocase of broad specificity, while MDR3 P-glycoprotein specifically translocates phosphatidylcholine. *Cell* 1996;87;507–517.
32. Schinkel AH, Smit JJ, van Tellingen O, et al. Disruption of the mouse mdr1a P-glycoprotein gene leads to a deficiency in the blood-brain barrier and to increased sensitivity to drugs. *Cell* 1994;77:491–502.
33. Panwala CM, Jones JC, Viney JL. A novel model of inflammatory bowel disease: mice deficient for the multiple drug resistance gene, mdr1a, spontaneously develop colitis. *J Immunol* 1998;161:5733–5744.
34. Buschman E, Arceci RJ, Croop JM, et al. mdr2 encodes P-glycoprotein expressed in the bile canalicular membrane as determined by isoform-specific antibodies. *J Biol Chem* 1992;267;18093–18099.
35. Smit JJM, Schinkel AH, Oude-Elferink RPJ, et al. Homozygous disruption of the murine mdr2 P-glycoprotein gene leads to a complete absence of phospholipid from bile and to liver disease. *Cell* 1993;75:451–462.
36. Zhou Y, Gottesman MM, Pastan I. Domain exchangeability between the multidrug transporter (MDR1) and phosphatidyl-choline flippase (MDR2). *Mol Pharmacol* 1999;56:997–1004.
37. Childs S, Yeh RL, Georges E, et al. Identification of a sister gene to P-glycoprotein. *Cancer Res* 1995;55:2029–2034.
38. Gatmaitan ZC, Nies AT, Arias IM. Regulation and translocation of ATP-dependent apical membrane proteins in rat liver. *Am J Physiol* 1997;272:G1041–G1049.
39. Misra S, Ujhazy P, Gatmaitan Z, et al. The role of phosphoinositide 3-kinase in taurocholate-induced trafficking of ATP-dependent canalicular transporters in rat liver. *J Biol Chem* 1998;273:26638–26644.
40. Misra S, Ujhazy P, Varticovski L, et al. Phosphoinositide 3-kinase lipid products regulate ATP-dependent transport by sister of P-glycoprotein and multidrug resistance associated protein 2 in bile canalicular membrane vesicles. *Proc Natl Acad Sci USA* 1999;96:5814–5819.
41. Paumgartner G, Herz R, Sauter K, et al. Taurocholate exertion and bile formation in the isolated perfused rat liver. An in vitro–in vivo comparison. *Naunyn Schmeidebergs Arch Pharmacol* 1974;285:165–174.
42. Lowe PJ, Barnwell SG, Coleman R. Rapid kinetic analysis of the bile-salt-dependent secretion of phospholipid, cholesterol and a plasma-membrane enzyme into bile. *Biochem J* 1984;222:631–637.
43. Barnwell SG, Godfrey PP, Lowe PJ, et al. Biliary protein output by isolated perfused rat livers. Effects of bile salts. *Biochem J* 1983;210:549–557.
44. LeSage GD, Robertson WE, Baumgart MA. Bile acid-dependent vesicular transport of lysosomal enzymes into bile in the rat. *Gastroenterology* 1993;105:889–900.
45. Crawford JM, Berken CA, Gollan JL. Role of the hepatocyte microtubular system in the excretion of bile salts and biliary lipid: implications for intracellular vesicular transport. *J Lipid Res* 1988;29:144–156.

46. Hayakawa T, Bruck R, Ng OC, et al. DBcAMP stimulates vesicle transport and HRP excretion in isolated perfused rat liver. *Am J Physiol* 1990;259:G727–G735.

47. Davidson HW, McGovan CH, Balch WE. Evidence for the regulation of exocytic transport by protein phosphorylation. *J Cell Biol* 1992;116:1343–1355.

48. Richter-Landsberg C, Jastorff B. In vitro phosphorylation of microtubule-associated protein 2: differential effects of cyclic AMP analogues. *J Neurochem* 1985;45:1218–1222.

49. Toker A, Cantley LC. Signalling through the lipid products of phosphoinositide-3–OH kinase. *Nature* 1997;387:673–676.

50. Fruman DA, Meyers RE, Cantley LC. Phosphoinositide kinases. *Annu Rev Biochem* 1998;67:481–507.

51. Sai Y, Nies AT, Arias IM. Bile acid secretion and direct targeting of mdr1-green fluorescent protein from golgi to the canalicular membrane in polarized WIF-B cells. *J Cell Sci* 1999;112:4535–4545.

52. Folli F, Alvaro D, Gigliozzi A et al. Regulation of endocytic-transcytotic pathways and bile secretion by phosphatidylinositol 3-kinase in rats. *Gastroenterology* 1997;113:954–965.

53. Arcaro A, Wymann MP. Wortmannin is a potent phosphatidylinositol 3-kinase inhibitor: the role of phosphatidylinositol 3,4,5-trisphosphate in neutrophil responses. *Biochem J* 1993;296:297–301.

54. Bartles JR, Feracci HM, Stieger B, Hubbard AL. Biogenesis of the rat hepatocyte plasma membrane in vivo: comparison of the pathways taken by apical and basolateral proteins using subcellular fractionation. *J Cell Biol* 1987;105:1241–1251.

55. Kipp H, Arias IM. Newly synthesized canalicular ABC Transporters are directly targeted from Golgi to the hepatocyte apical domain in rat liver. *J Biol Chem* 2001;276:7218–7224.

56. Mellman I, Warren G. The road taken: past and future foundations of membrane traffic. *Cell* 2000;100:99–112.

25

CONJUGATE EXPORT PUMPS OF THE MULTIDRUG RESISTANCE PROTEIN (MRP) FAMILY IN LIVER

DIETRICH KEPPLER
JÖRG KÖNIG
ANNE T. NIES

The conjugation of many endogenous and exogenous lipophilic substances with glucuronate, glutathione, sulfate, or other negatively charged groups precedes their transport across the plasma membrane into the extracellular space (see website chapters ⌨ W-14 and W-15 and Chapter 24). Hepatocytes are particularly active in the formation of such conjugates, as exemplified by the glucuronidation of bilirubin. The transport of conjugates across the hepatocyte canalicular membrane has been characterized as a unidirectional, primary-active adenosine triphosphate (ATP)-dependent process (1–5). The molecular identification and cloning of this canalicular conjugate export pump, also known as canalicular multispecific organic anion transporter (cMOAT) and now termed multidrug resistance protein 2 (MRP2) (6–10), was a consequence of the discovery that the multidrug resistance protein 1 (MRP1) functions as an ATP-dependent export pump for glutathione S-conjugates and glucuronides (11–13). The members of the MRP family belong to the superfamily of ATP-binding cassette (ABC) transporters, subfamily C; the symbols for MRP1 to MRP6 are thus ABCC1 to ABCC6. The substrate specificity of the conjugate export pumps MRP1 and MRP2 is similar, although differences in their kinetic properties and in their domain-specific localization have been recognized (9,10,14). Mutant rat strains deficient in the hepatobiliary secretion of conjugates and additional organic anions (15–17) were

shown to lack the MRP2 protein in their hepatocyte canalicular membrane (7,8) because of point mutations introducing premature termination codons in the *MRP2* gene (8,18). Studies in these mutant rats support the conclusion that anionic conjugates of many lipophilic substances cannot exit across the plasma membrane into bile in the absence of the MRP2 pump (Fig. 25.1). The lack of MRP2 prevents the secretion into bile of substances such as the glutathione S-conjugate leukotriene C_4 and N-acetyl leukotriene E_4 (16,19), which are both high-affinity substrates for MRP2 (3,10). These studies have indicated that there is no alternative transport protein in the canalicular membrane for the secretion of these conjugates into bile. On the other hand, conjugates formed in hepatocytes can be transported into the sinusoidal blood, particularly under conditions of cholestasis and impaired function of MRP2 (20,21). The recent localization (21,22) and functional characterization of MRP3 as a conjugate export pump (23–25) provides a molecular explanation for the release of conjugates across the basolateral hepatocyte membrane. The cloning (26) and functional characterization of MRP1 (11–13) and additional human MRP family members (14,27) prompted subsequent identification of orthologous ATP-dependent conjugate export pumps in many organisms including yeast, plants, and nematodes (reviewed in refs. 14 and 28). Moreover, the identification of mutations in the human *MRP2* gene (29–31) and in the *MRP6* gene (32,33) has contributed to the molecular understanding of Dubin–Johnson syndrome and of pseudoxanthoma elasticum, respectively.

D. Keppler, J. König, and **A. T. Nies:** Division of Tumor Biochemistry, German Cancer Research Center, D-69120 Heidelberg, Germany.

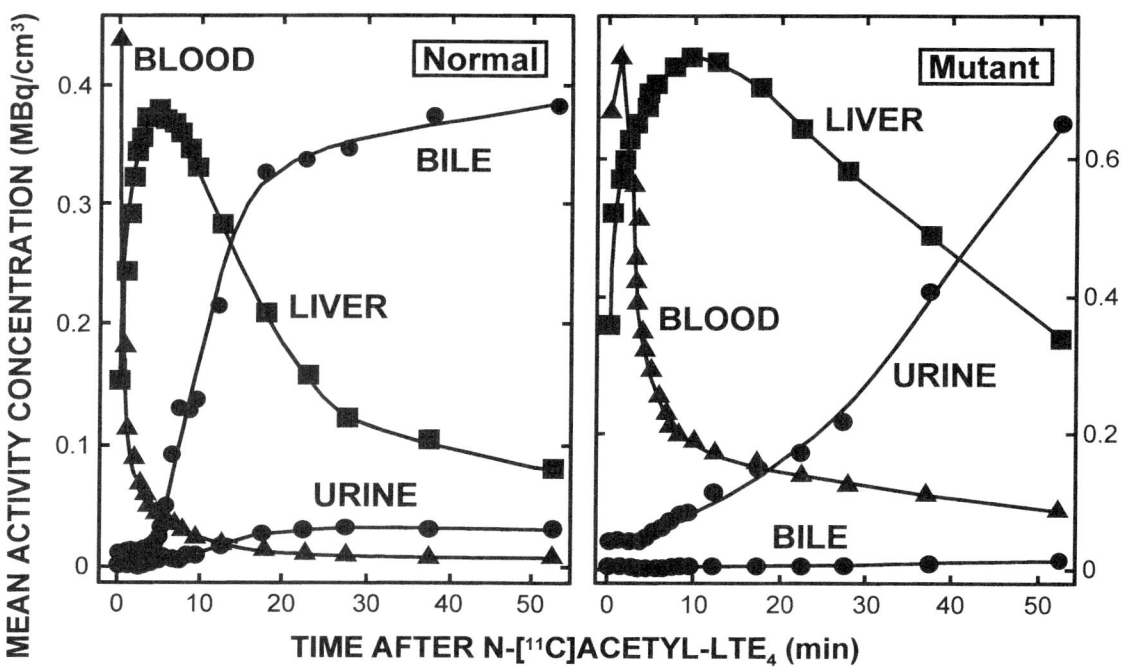

FIGURE 25.1. Hepatobiliary elimination of the lipophilic anionic conjugate *N*-acetyl leukotriene E4 in normal and MRP2-deficient mutant rats. The endogenous cysteinyl leukotriene, *N*-acetyl-LTE4, was labeled in its acetyl moiety with the positron-emitting short-lived carbon isotope ^{11}C to analyze noninvasively its uptake into the liver and its excretion into bile by positron-emission tomography (19). Rapid elimination from blood is due to the selective uptake of the tracer into hepatocytes, where the maximal concentration is already reached after 4 minutes. MRP2-mediated canalicular secretion of *N*-acetyl-LTE4 (3,16,19) leads to the appearance of this conjugate in bile after a mean transit time through the liver in normal rats of 17 minutes (**left panel**). In MRP2-deficient mutant rats the mean transit time is 54 minutes and secretion into bile is below detectability (**right panel**). In the mutant rat, *N*-acetyl-LTE4 is in part metabolized in hepatocytes, secreted back into blood, and excreted via the kidneys into urine (19). This experiment demonstrates that the selective absence of the adenosine triphosphate (ATP)-dependent conjugate export pump MRP2 from hepatocytes (7) precludes transport of this anionic conjugate across the canalicular membrane into bile. The same conclusion holds true for the transport of many other mercapturate, glutathione, and glucuronate conjugates.

THE MULTIDRUG RESISTANCE PROTEIN FAMILY OF CONJUGATE EXPORT PUMPS

The first member of the MRP family was identified in 1992 by the cloning of human MRP1 (previously termed multidrug resistance-associated protein, MRP). MRP1 (symbol ABCC1) was cloned from a doxorubicin-selected multidrug resistant human small cell lung cancer cell line (H69AR) (26) that had no increased level of the known multidrug resistance P-glycoprotein (MDR1 P-gp). The analysis of the amino acid sequence of MRP1 (26) followed by the elucidation of its function (11,12) suggested the presence of related transporters in other tissues. The comparison of MRP1-mediated substrate transport (11–13) with the transport properties of hepatocyte canalicular membrane vesicles from normal and GY/TR⁻ or EHBR mutant rats led to the characterization and cloning of the first MRP1-related partial complementary DNA (cDNA) sequence (6). The protein encoded by the full-length cDNA is now

termed MRP2 [symbol ABCC2; formerly known as canalicular MRP (cMRP) or canalicular multispecific organic anion transporter (cMOAT)] and is localized to the canalicular membrane of hepatocytes (7,8), in addition to several other apical membrane domains including the luminal membrane of kidney proximal tubules (34,35) and the luminal membrane of small intestine (36). The identification of the additional MRP family members, MRP3, MRP4, MRP5, and MRP6, was mainly based on database analyses. MRP6 was first identified by analyzing a genomic clone, MRP3, MRP4, and MRP5 by analyses of expressed sequence tag (EST) databases (37) followed by the cloning of partial cDNA sequences (38). The six currently identified MRP family members are encoded by different genes located on different chromosomes, except for *MRP1* and *MRP6*, which are both located on chromosome 16 in close vicinity (Table 25.1). The *MRP1* gene, located on chromosome 16, contains 31 exons and a high proportion of class 0 introns (39). It spans approximately 150 kilobases (kb)

TABLE 25.1. CHARACTERISTICS OF HUMAN MRP FAMILY MEMBERS

Protein	Symbol	Chromosome	Amino Acids	Identity %	Substrates	Localization (Hepatocyte)	Disorder
MRP1	ABCC1	16p13.1	1531	48	LTC$_4$, E$_2$17βG, GSH, GSSG		
MRP2	ABCC2	10q24	1545	100	MGB, BGB, LTC$_4$, E$_2$17βG, GSH, GSSG	Apical	Dubin–Johnson syndrome
MRP3	ABCC3	17q21.3	1527	46	MGB, BGB, glycocholate	Basolateral	
MRP4	ABCC4	13q32	1325	36	nucleotide analogs		
MRP5	ABCC5	3q27	1437	36	cGMP, cAMP	Basolateral	
MRP6	ABCC6	16p13.1	1503	38		Basolateral	Pseudoxanthoma elasticum

LTC$_4$, leukotriene C$_4$; E$_2$17βG, estradiol 17β-glucuronide; MGB, monoglucuronosyl bilirubin; BGB, bisglucuronosyl bilirubin; MRP, multidrug resistance protein; cAMP, 3′,5′-cyclic adenosine monophosphate; cGMP, 3′,5′-cyclic guanosine monophosphate; GSH, reduced glutathione; GSSG, oxidized glutathione.
Amino acid identities are given in relation to human MRP2 (in box). Only prototypic substrates and disorders caused by mutations in the respective gene are mentioned.

and is thus larger than the *MRP2* gene that spans around 69 kb. The latter is located on chromosome 10 (40) and contains 32 exons (31,41). The *MRP2* gene has a high proportion of class 0 introns (31). The comparison of the genomic organization of *MRP1* and *MRP2* displays some remarkable similarities as indicated by the number and size of exons, by the high proportion of class 0 introns, and by 21 identical splice junction sites when the exon-intron organization is transferred to the amino acid sequence alignment (31). The genomic organization of *MRP3* was analyzed by means of a cosmid clone containing the entire *MRP3* gene. A comparison of the *MRP3* gene structure with the two experimentally analyzed gene structures of *MRP1* and *MRP2* again revealed remarkable similarities. The *MRP3* gene contains 31 exons, as does the *MRP1* gene (25), and a high proportion of class 0 introns. A gene structure alignment of these three genes transferred to the amino acid alignment of the three proteins indicates 21 splice junction sites at the same position (25). The similar gene structure of *MRP1*, *MRP2*, and *MRP3* demonstrates the close evolutionary relationship of these three transporters.

The topology of the transport proteins of the MRP family is characterized by two types of structural domains shared with other members of the superfamily of the ABC transporters: the hydrophobic, polytopic membrane-spanning domains, and the hydrophilic, cytosolic ATP-binding domains. Within the MRP family, the topology is most similar between MRP1, MRP2, MRP3, and MRP6, which share three membrane-spanning domains and two ATP-binding domains (7,14,27,42). Direct evidence has been obtained for an extracellularly located amino terminus of MRP1 (42) and MRP2 (10). This structural feature is not predicted for the topology of MRP4 and MRP5, which are shorter in length (Table 25.1) and lack the amino-terminal extension of the first membrane-spanning domain of the other currently known members of the MRP family (27,43). MRP4 and MRP5 are predicted to have a total of

12 transmembrane segments arranged in a similar fashion as in MDR1 P-glycoprotein (27,44). The number of transmembrane segments between the first and the second ATP-binding domain is predicted to be four for MRP2 (5,7,14) and it may be six or four in MRP1 (44). The amino-terminal membrane-spanning domain is predicted to contain five transmembrane segments, followed by six transmembrane segments for the second membrane-spanning domain. Accordingly, the total number of transmembrane segments in MRP1, MRP2, MRP3, and MRP6 should be 15 or 17.

The members of the MRP family (Table 25.1) differ by their cell-type–specific expression (38), by their domain-specific localization in polarized cells (14,27), and by their substrate specificity (10,14,45) and kinetic properties (10,14,46). While all currently known members may be expressed at different levels in the liver, only some are expressed in membrane domains of the hepatocyte (Table 25.1).

SUBSTRATES FOR HEPATOCELLULAR MULTIDRUG RESISTANCE PROTEIN ISOFORMS

Based on RNA expression data, the following members of the MRP family have been detected in liver (27): *MRP2*, *MRP3*, *MRP5*, and *MRP6*. Immunolocalization in human hepatocytes has demonstrated MRP2 in the canalicular membrane (20,29,31) and MRP3 in the basolateral membrane (21,22). Moreover, MRP5 (27) and MRP6 (Fig. 25.2) are localized to the basolateral domain. The substrate specificity of the recombinant MRP proteins examined in inside-out membrane vesicles has been established for MRP2 (10,14,47,48), MRP3 (23–25), and MRP5 (45). Indirect information on the substrate specificity of rat MRP2 has been obtained from comparative transport studies with canalicular membrane vesicles from normal and

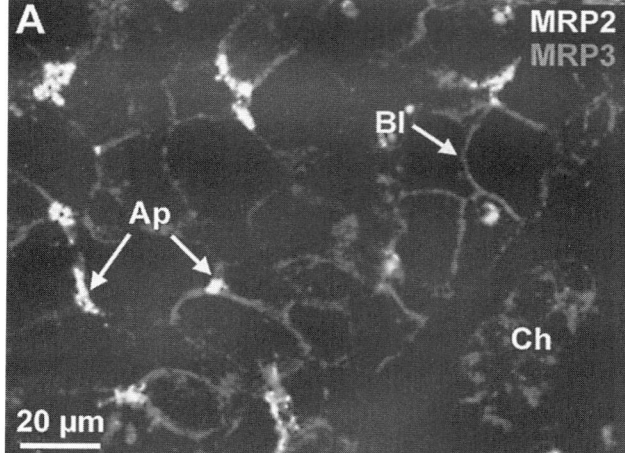

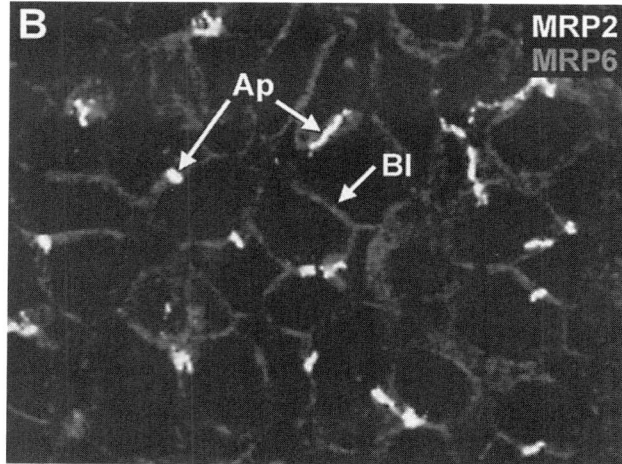

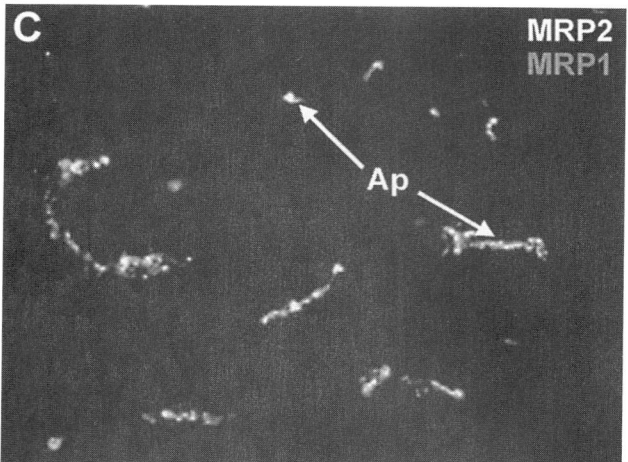

FIGURE 25.2. Localization of multidrug resistance protein 2 (*MRP2*), *MRP3*, and *MRP6* with isoform-specific antibodies in human liver. Double-label immunofluorescence microscopy of frozen liver sections (5 μm) was performed as described (21). Pictures of an optical thickness of 1.5 μm were taken on a confocal laser scanning microscope. *Ap*, apical (canalicular) membrane of hepatocytes; *Bl*, basolateral membrane of hepatocytes; *Ch*, cholangiocytes. The apical isoform MRP2 (*red fluorescence* in **A–C** of color plate 10 and *white* here) is restricted to the canalicular membrane domain of hepatocytes as detected either with the monoclonal antibody M₂ III-6 (29) in **A** and **B**, or with the polyclonal antiserum EAG5 in **C** (10,34). The isoforms MRP3 (*green fluorescence* in **A**, using the antiserum FDS (21) and MRP6 (*green* fluorescence in **B**, using the antiserum AQL (21) are localized to the basolateral membrane of human hepatocytes and are excluded from the bile canalicular domain. In addition to its expression in hepatocytes, MRP3 is expressed in cholangiocytes (**A**). MRP1 was not detected in hepatocytes using the MRP1-specific antibody QCRL-1 (**C**) (64). *Bar* in **A**, 20 μm; same magnification for all panels. See Color Plate 10.

MRP2-deficient mutant rats (summarized in refs. 14 and 49). Prototypic endogenous substrates for ATP-dependent transport by human MRP2 include monoglucuronosyl bilirubin, bisglucuronosyl bilirubin, the glutathione S-conjugate leukotriene C₄, and 17β-glucuronosyl estradiol with Michaelis' constant (K_m) values of 0.7, 0.9, 1.0, and 7.2 μM, respectively (10,48). Many other glutathione and glucuronate conjugates of lipophilic endogenous substances have been recognized as substrates for MRP2 (14). In addition, several xenobiotics and chemotherapeutic agents are exported from cells by MRP2, indicating the importance of this ABC transporter in drug resistance (9,10,50). Although several prototypic high-affinity substrates for MRP2 are anionic conjugates, nonconjugated organic anions are substrates as well, as indicated by the ATP-dependent transport of fluo-3 (14,51), methotrexate (52), ochratoxin, and *para*-aminohippurate (53). Glutathione complexes with various substances may also function as substrates for MRP2. This was first indicated by the cotransport of reduced glutathione with vincristine mediated by MRP1 (54). Relatively unstable complexes of glutathione with arsenic were recently identified as MRP2 substrates (55). The detection of arsenic triglutathione and methylarsenic diglutathione in bile of normal rats but not of MRP2-deficient mutant rats indicates an important role of MRP2 in detoxification of arsenic (55).

Both oxidized glutathione (GSSG) (4) and reduced glutathione (GSH) (47,50) are transported by MRP2. This is in line with the severely impaired excretion of GSSG and GSH into bile of MRP2-deficient mutant rats (47). MRP2-mediated transport of GSH proceeds with low affinity; however, since hepatocellular GSH concentrations are high (5 to 10 mM), this may be adequate for the controlled release of GSH into bile (47). Furthermore, MRP2-mediated cotransport of GSH with drugs (50) and yet unidentified endogenous substances may contribute to GSH secretion.

MRP3-mediated transport has been most extensively characterized for the recombinant rat orthologue (23,24). Substrates include glucuronides, such as 17-glucuronosyl estradiol (23) and several bile salts, such as sulfatolithocholyl taurine and sulfatochenodeoxycholyl taurine (24).

Cholyl taurine and cholyl glycine are substrates with a lower affinity for rat MRP3 when compared with the sulfated bile salts (24). It should be noted that glutathione conjugates, such as leukotriene C_4, are poor substrates for MRP3 (23,24). Glucuronosyl conjugates of bilirubin were shown to be substrates for human recombinant MRP3 (25). The localization of human MRP3 to the basolateral membrane of human cholangiocytes (22) suggests that MRP3 may play a role in the cholehepatic circulation of bile salts and glucuronides (24). Moreover, because of the basolateral localization of MRP3 in human hepatocytes (21,22), this member of the MRP family can mediate the export of bile salts and glucuronides from hepatocytes into the sinusoidal blood during cholestasis (also see Chapters 24 and 46).

The physiologic transport function of MRP5 has only recently been elucidated (45). Recombinant human MRP5 mediates the ATP-dependent transport of the cyclic nucleotides 3′,5′-cyclic guanosine monophosphate (cGMP), with a K_m value of 2.1 μM, and 3′,5′-cyclic adenosine monophosphate (cAMP), with a K_m value of 379 μM (45). This finding indicates that cellular levels of cyclic nucleotides are controlled not only by the activity of cyclases and phosphodiesterases but also by the ATP-dependent export by MRP5 (45). cGMP and cAMP are the first substrates for a MRP family member where a phosphate residue represents the negatively charged moiety of the anionic conjugate.

The physiologic substrates for MRP6 are unknown at present. Identification of the transport function of MRP6 may contribute to the molecular understanding of pseudoxanthoma elasticum, which is associated with mutations in the *MRP6* gene (32,33).

LOCALIZATION OF HEPATIC MULTIDRUG RESISTANCE PROTEIN ISOFORMS

Antibodies of high affinity and specificity are required for the detection of individual MRP isoforms in different cell types of the liver and for the localization of distinct MRP isoforms to different membrane domains of the hepatocyte (Fig. 25.2). MRP2 is the only apical isoform detected so far (Table 25.1). With the use of immunofluorescence microscopy, MRP2 was localized to the canalicular membrane of rat and human hepatocytes (7,20,29,56) and to the apical vacuole membrane of rat (51) and human (57) hepatoma cells. In normal rat liver, MRP2 is homogeneously distributed throughout the entire liver lobule; however, in cholestasis induced by bile duct ligation, MRP2 expression is concentrated to the central (perivenous) areas of the liver lobules (58). On the subcellular level, as an early event in intrahepatic or obstructive cholestasis in rats, selective retrieval of MRP2 from the canalicular membrane to pericanalicular vesicles was observed by immunofluorescence (56,59–61) and quantitative immunogold electron microscopy (61). MRP2 was also detected in the apical

membrane of extrahepatic tissues including the proximal tubule epithelia of rat and human kidney (34,35), and the epithelial cells of rat (62) and rabbit (36) small intestine. Transfection of rat (10) and human (9,10) *MRP2* cDNA resulted in an apical localization of the recombinant protein in polarized Madin–Darby canine kidney (MDCK) cells.

In addition to the expression of MRP2 in the canalicular membrane domain, hepatocytes express distinct MRP isoforms in their basolateral membrane domain (6,20). RNA transcripts of *MRP1*, the first cloned member of the MRP family (26), were not detected in human liver in significant amounts (26,63). With the use of isoform-specific antibodies, MRP1 was localized to the plasma membrane of many different cell types (64–66) and to the basolateral membrane of polarized epithelia in lung (67,68). However, MRP1 was not detected in hepatocytes when using a MRP1-specific antibody (64) for immunofluorescence microscopy (Fig. 25.2). The isoform MRP3 was recently cloned by several groups from rat (69,70) and human liver (21,22) and localized to the basolateral membrane of human hepatocytes (21,22) and human cholangiocytes (22) (Fig. 25.2). Extrahepatic tissues in which *MRP3* messenger RNA (mRNA) was detected include colon, small intestine, pancreas, prostate, and kidney (21,71,72). After transfection, recombinant human MRP3 was localized to the lateral membrane of polarized MDCK cells (14,22). A more recently identified member of the MRP family, the MRP6 isoform, is highly expressed in rat (69,73) and human liver (74), and in human kidney (74). MRP6 was localized to the basolateral membrane of human hepatocytes (Fig. 25.2).

MULTIDRUG RESISTANCE PROTEIN ISOFORMS IN CHOLESTASIS

The formation and subsequent biliary excretion of anionic conjugates of endogenous and xenobiotic substances is of vital importance in detoxification and cellular homeostasis. When the canalicular conjugate secretion via MRP2 is impaired in intrahepatic cholestasis or in biliary obstruction, alternative pathways are required for conjugate export, and basolateral MRP isoforms may then mediate the release of conjugates from the hepatocyte into sinusoidal blood (20) (see Chapters 24 and 46). The recent localization (21,22) and functional characterization (23,24) of MRP3 indicates that this member of the MRP family has the properties to compensate for the impaired biliary conjugate secretion in cholestasis. MRP3 has been recognized as an inducible transporter upregulated in the liver of rats after bile duct ligation and in hereditary MRP2 deficiency as indicated by Northern blotting (23,24,69,70). In human liver, both the absence of MRP2 in Dubin–Johnson syndrome and cholestatic liver disease in primary biliary cholangitis were associated with a strong expression of the MRP3 protein in basolateral hepatocyte membranes when compared with normal liver (21). The basal expression of MRP3 in hepatocytes is low, and the mechanisms underlying its induction in intrahepatic and extrahepatic cholestasis are incompletely understood (75). Characterization of the 5′-flanking region of human MRP3 indicated that it is under the control of a TATA-less promoter. The basal promoter activity of human MRP3 is only 4% of that determined under the same conditions for MRP2 (76). Human MRP3 promoter activity, mRNA, and protein are strongly increased after disruption of microtubules by nocodazole and after administration of the genotoxic acetylaminofluorene (76). However, none of the endogenous substances known to accumulate in hepatocytes during cholestasis has been shown to induce human MRP3 expression. The apical isoform MRP2 is often inversely regulated in comparison to MRP3 (76). In extrahepatic and in intrahepatic cholestasis, MRP2 is downregulated, as studied extensively in rats after bile duct ligation, in endotoxin-induced cholestasis, and after treatment with the cholestatic steroid ethinylestradiol (56,59). Interestingly, endocytic retrieval of MRP2 precedes the reduction of MRP2 protein and mRNA in rats treated with endotoxin (59). The hereditary deficiency of MRP2 in mutant rats is associated with a reduction of bile flow to about 50% of normal (77). This suggests that MRP2 significantly contributes to bile flow by uphill transport into bile of substrates including reduced glutathione, glutathione S-conjugates, and glucuronides. The present knowledge on the regulation of other MRP isoforms, particularly MRP5 and MRP6, does not suggest major changes of these basolateral export pumps in cholestasis.

HEREDITARY DEFICIENCY OF MULTIDRUG RESISTANCE PROTEIN 2 IN DUBIN–JOHNSON SYNDROME

An increasing number of mutations in the *MRP2* gene has been identified (Fig. 25.3) since the initial demonstration that the MRP2 protein is absent from the hepatocyte canalicular membrane in Dubin–Johnson syndrome (20,78). The Dubin–Johnson syndrome is an autosomal-recessive inherited disorder characterized by conjugated hyperbilirubinemia and deposition of a dark pigment in hepatocytes (79–81). The impaired transport of conjugated bilirubin and other anionic conjugates across the canalicular membrane into bile is caused by the absence of functionally active MRP2 from the apical membrane (20,29,31,78). Up to now, mutations in the *MRP2* gene leading to a functionally deficient protein still inserted into the apical membrane have not been identified. Furthermore, we have detected neither truncated MRP2 protein in hepatocytes from a Dubin–Johnson syndrome patient with a premature termination codon in exon 23 of the *MRP2* gene nor a mutated protein in a patient with a 6-nucleotide deletion in exon 30 (31). The latter mutation leads to a loss of two amino acids, arginine 1392 and methionine 1393, in the second ATP-binding domain. Transfection and expression of this mutated *MRP2* cDNA demonstrated that the mutated protein is recognized by the cellular quality control machinery, retained in the endoplasmic reticulum, and subsequently degraded by proteasomes (82). The currently known mutations in the coding sequence and in splice sites

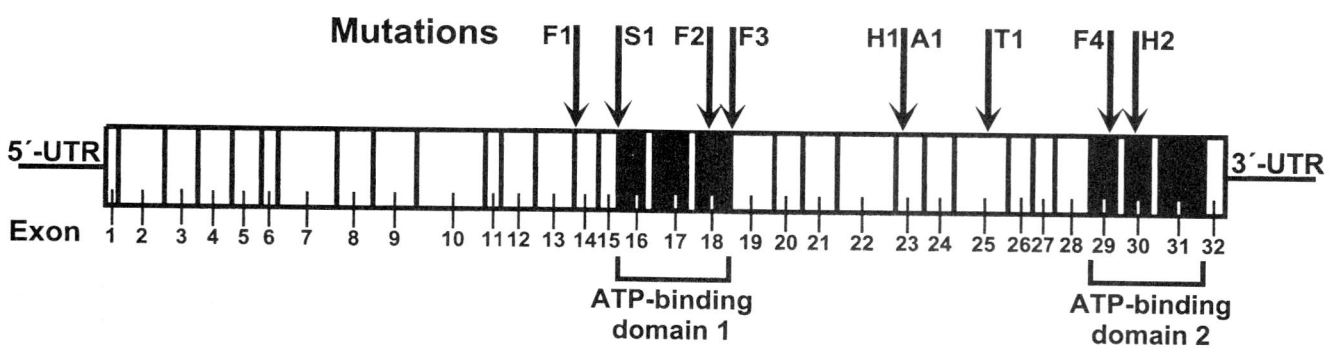

FIGURE 25.3. Mutations in the multidrug resistance protein (*MRP2*) gene leading to Dubin–Johnson syndrome. Exon numbers are indicated and exon boundaries are represented by vertical lines. Both adenosine triphosphate (*ATP*)-binding domains are marked by *black boxes*. *Arrows* indicate sites of currently known mutations:

Designation (Reference)	Nucleotide Change	Predicted Consequence or Amino Acid Change
F1 (41)	1815+2T>A	Splice donor, loss of exon 13
S1 (83)	1967+2T>C	Splice donor, loss of exon 15
F2 (41)	2302C>T	R768W
F3 (41)	2439+2T>C	Splice donor, loss of exon 18
H1/A1 (31,29)	3196C>T	R1066X
T1 (84)	3517A>T	I1173F
F4 (41)	4145A>G	Q1382R
H2 (31)	4175–4180delGGATGA	R1392+M1393del

of the *MRP2* gene leading to Dubin–Johnson syndrome together with the exon-intron organization of the gene are depicted in Fig. 25.3. These mutations are mostly found in the 3′-proximal half of the mRNA and particularly in the exons encoding both ATP-binding domains. Of special interest is the mutation in exon 25 causing an exchange of isoleucin 1173 to phenylalanine in the large group of Dubin–Johnson syndrome patients of Iranian–Jewish origin (84). In addition to the mutations identified in the human *MRP2* gene, two distinct mutations have been described in two well-characterized hyperbilirubinemic rat strains, the GY/TR⁻ mutant rat (8,15) and the EHBR mutant (17,18). These mutations introduce premature termination at codon 401 and 805 in GY/TR⁻ and EHBR mutant rats, respectively (8,18). In both mutant rat livers, however, no truncated MRP2 protein was detectable (7), and the mRNA was below detectability when analyzed by Northern blotting (7,8,18). These premature termination codons may cause the enhanced rate of mRNA degradation by a mechanism termed nonsense-mediated decay (85). Thus, some mutations in Dubin–Johnson syndrome may lead to a rapid degradation of the mutated mRNA, while others, such as the H2 mutation in exon 30 (Fig. 25.3), cause a defective maturation of the MRP2 protein (82). Moreover, certain mutations in the *MRP2* gene may affect the interaction of MRP2 with chaperone proteins required for the correct trafficking of MRP2 to the apical membrane.

CONCLUSION AND PROSPECTS

The membrane glycoproteins mediating the ATP-dependent transport of many lipophilic substances conjugated to anionic residues have been identified as members of the multidrug resistance protein (MRP) family. Human hepatocytes express several members of these ABC transporters of the subfamily C, including the apical isoform MRP2 (ABCC2), and the basolateral isoforms MRP3 (ABCC3) (Fig. 25.4), MRP5 (ABCC5), and MRP6 (ABCC6). Transporters of the MRP family differ markedly in sequence and substrate specificity from the members of the smaller MDR P-glycoprotein (ABCB) family. The conjugate export pumps within the MRP family differ by their domain-specific localization in polarized cells, by their substrate specificity, and by their regulation under pathophysiologic conditions such as cholestasis. Prototypic substrates for MRP2 and MRP3 include glucuronosyl bilirubin conjugates. Several mutations in the *MRP2* gene lead to Dubin–Johnson syndrome, which is caused by a lack of functionally active MRP2 protein in the canalicular membrane and is associated with conjugated hyperbilirubinemia. Hereditary deficiency of MRP2 or its downregulation in cholestasis are compensated for in part by an upregulation of MRP3 in the basolateral membrane. The secretion of glutathione and glucuronate conjugates of toxic substances into bile illustrates the essential role of MRP2 in hepatic detoxification.

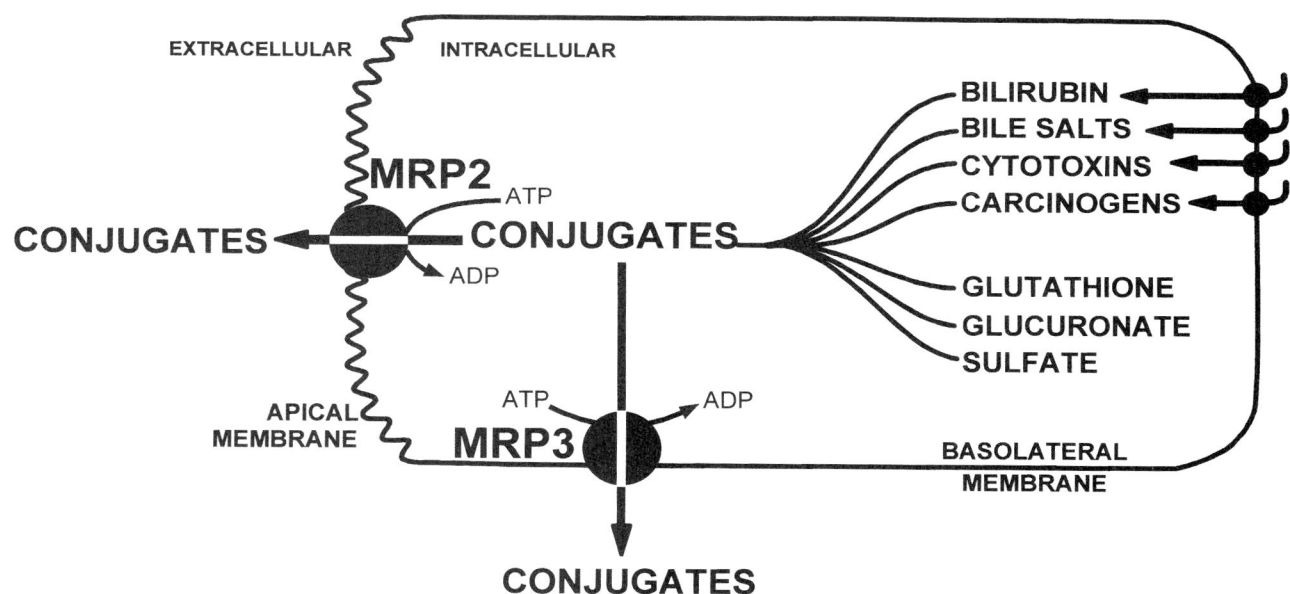

FIGURE 25.4. Localization and function of apical and basolateral multidrug resistance proteins (*MRP*) isoforms. Many endogenous substances, xenobiotics, and drugs are transported into hepatocytes across the basolateral membrane, some of them oxidized in phase-1 reactions, and subsequently conjugated with glutathione, glucuronate, or sulfate. Adenosine triphosphate (*ATP*)-dependent export of these conjugates across the apical membrane into bile or, for instance in cholestasis, across the basolateral membrane into sinusoidal blood depends on the presence of MRP isoforms in the respective plasma membrane domain. *ADP*, adenosine diphosphate.

Overexpression of several members of the MRP family, including MRP2, confers multidrug resistance. In most cells and organisms the export pumps of the MRP family are indispensable for the release of many organic anions into the extracellular space.

ACKNOWLEDGMENTS

We thank our colleagues Jürgen Kartenbeck, Yunhai Cui, Gabriele Jedlitschky, and Inka Leier for their contributions to our work on multidrug resistance proteins in liver. Our studies were supported by the Deutsches Krebsforschungszentrum and by grants SFB601 and SFB352 from the Deutsche Forschungsgemeinschaft.

REFERENCES

1. Kobayashi K, Sogame Y, Hayashi K, et al. ATP stimulates the uptake of S-dinitrophenylglutathione by rat liver plasma membrane vesicles. *FEBS Lett* 1988;240:55–58.
2. Kitamura T, Jansen P, Hardenbrook C, et al. Defective ATP-dependent bile canalicular transport of organic anions in mutant (TR⁻) rats with conjugated hyperbilirubinemia. *Proc Natl Acad Sci USA* 1990;87:3557–3561.
3. Ishikawa T, Müller M, Klünemann C, et al. ATP-dependent primary active transport of cysteinyl leukotrienes across liver canalicular membrane. Role of the ATP-dependent transport system for glutathione S-conjugates. *J Biol Chem* 1990;265:19279–19286.
4. Fernandez-Checa JC, Takikawa H, Horie T, et al. Canalicular transport of reduced glutathione in normal and mutant Eisai hyperbilirubinemic rats. *J Biol Chem* 1992;267:1667–1673.
5. Keppler D, König J. Hepatic canalicular membrane 5: expression and localization of the conjugate export pump encoded by the *MRP2 (cMRP/cMOAT)* gene in liver. *FASEB J* 1997;11:509–516.
6. Mayer R, Kartenbeck J, Büchler M, et al. Expression of the MRP gene-encoded conjugate export pump in liver and its selective absence from the canalicular membrane in transport-deficient mutant hepatocytes. *J Cell Biol* 1995;131:137–150.
7. Büchler M, König J, Brom M, et al. cDNA cloning of the hepatocyte canalicular isoform of the multidrug resistance protein, cMRP, reveals a novel conjugate export pump deficient in hyperbilirubinemic mutant rats. *J Biol Chem* 1996;271:15091–15098.
8. Paulusma CC, Bosma PJ, Zaman GJ, et al. Congenital jaundice in rats with a mutation in a multidrug resistance-associated protein gene. *Science* 1996;271:1126–1128.
9. Evers R, Kool M, van Deemter L, et al. Drug export activity of the human canalicular multispecific organic anion transporter in polarized kidney MDCK cells expressing *cMOAT (MRP2)* cDNA. *J Clin Invest* 1998;101:1310–1319.
10. Cui Y, König J, Buchholz U, et al. Drug resistance and ATP-dependent conjugate transport mediated by the apical multidrug resistance protein, MRP2, permanently expressed in human and canine cells. *Mol Pharmacol* 1999;55:929–937.
11. Jedlitschky G, Leier I, Buchholz U, et al. ATP-dependent transport of glutathione S-conjugates by the multidrug resistance-associated protein. *Cancer Res* 1994;54:4833–4836.
12. Leier I, Jedlitschky G, Buchholz U, et al. The MRP gene encodes an ATP-dependent export pump for leukotriene C₄ and structurally related conjugates. *J Biol Chem* 1994;269:27807–27810.
13. Jedlitschky G, Leier I, Buchholz U, et al. Transport of glutathione, glucuronate, and sulfate conjugates by the MRP gene-encoded conjugate export pump. *Cancer Res* 1996;56:988–994.
14. König J, Nies AT, Cui Y, et al. Conjugate export pumps of the multidrug resistance protein (MRP) family: localization, substrate specificity, and MRP2-mediated drug resistance. *Biochim Biophys Acta* 1999;1461:377–394.
15. Jansen PL, Peters WH, Lamers WH. Hereditary chronic conjugated hyperbilirubinemia in mutant rats caused by defective hepatic anion transport. *Hepatology* 1985;5:573–579.
16. Huber M, Guhlmann A, Jansen PL, et al. Hereditary defect of hepatobiliary cysteinyl leukotriene elimination in mutant rats with defective hepatic anion excretion. *Hepatology* 1987;7:224–228.
17. Takikawa H, Sano N, Narita T, et al. Biliary excretion of bile acid conjugates in a hyperbilirubinemic mutant Sprague-Dawley rat. *Hepatology* 1991;14:352–360.
18. Ito K, Suzuki H, Hirohashi T, et al. Molecular cloning of canalicular multispecific organic anion transporter defective in EHBR. *Am J Physiol* 1997;272:G16–G22.
19. Guhlmann A, Krauss K, Oberdorfer F, et al. Noninvasive assessment of hepatobiliary and renal elimination of cysteinyl leukotrienes by positron emission tomography. *Hepatology* 1995;21:1568–1575.
20. Keppler D, Kartenbeck J. The canalicular conjugate export pump encoded by the cmrp/cmoat gene. *Prog Liver Dis* 1996;14:55–67.
21. König J, Rost D, Cui Y, et al. Characterization of the human multidrug resistance protein isoform MRP3 localized to the basolateral hepatocyte membrane. *Hepatology* 1999;29:1156–1163.
22. Kool M, van der Linden M, de Haas M, et al. MRP3, an organic anion transporter able to transport anti-cancer drugs. *Proc Natl Acad Sci USA* 1999;96:6914–6919.
23. Hirohashi T, Suzuki H, Sugiyama Y. Characterization of the transport properties of cloned rat multidrug resistance-associated protein 3 (MRP3). *J Biol Chem* 1999;274:15181–15185.
24. Hirohashi T, Suzuki H, Takikawa H, et al. ATP-dependent transport of bile salts by rat multidrug resistance-associated protein 3 (Mrp3). *J Biol Chem* 2000;275:2905–2910.
25. Keppler D, Kamisako T, Leier I, et al. Localization, substrate specificity, and drug resistance conferred by conjugate export pumps of the MRP family. *Adv Enzyme Regul* 2000;40:339–349.
26. Cole SP, Bhardwaj G, Gerlach JH, et al. Overexpression of a transporter gene in a multidrug-resistant human lung cancer cell line. *Science* 1992;258:1650–1654.
27. Borst P, Evers R, Kool M, et al. The multidrug resistance protein family. *Biochim Biophys Acta* 1999;1461:347–357.
28. Rea PA, Li Z, Lu Y, et al. From vacuolar GS-X pumps to multispecific ABC transporters. *Annu Rev Plant Physiol Plant Mol Biol* 1998;49:727–760.
29. Paulusma CC, Kool M, Bosma PJ, et al. A mutation in the human canalicular multispecific organic anion transporter gene causes the Dubin-Johnson syndrome. *Hepatology* 1997;25:1539–1542.
30. Wada M, Toh S, Taniguchi K, et al. Mutations in the canalicular multispecific organic anion transporter (cMOAT) gene, a novel ABC transporter, in patients with hyperbilirubinemia II/Dubin-Johnson syndrome. *Hum Mol Genet* 1998;7:203–207.
31. Tsujii H, König J, Rost D, et al. Exon-intron organization of the human multidrug resistance protein 2 (MRP2) gene mutated in Dubin-Johnson syndrome. *Gastroenterology* 1999;117:653–660.
32. Le Saux O, Urban Z, Tschuch C, et al. Mutations in a gene encoding an ABC transporter cause pseudoxanthoma elasticum. *Nature Genet* 2000;25:223–227.
33. Ringpfeil F, Lebwohl MG, Christiano AM, et al. Pseudoxanthoma elasticum: mutations in the MRP6 gene encoding a trans-

membrane ATP-binding cassette (ABC) transporter. *Proc Natl Acad Sci USA* 2000;97:6001–6006.

34. Schaub TP, Kartenbeck J, König J, et al. Expression of the MRP2 gene-encoded conjugate export pump in human kidney proximal tubules and in renal cell carcinoma. *J Am Soc Nephrol* 1999;10:1159–1169.

35. Schaub TP, Kartenbeck J, König J, et al. Expression of the conjugate export pump encoded by the mrp2 gene in the apical membrane of kidney proximal tubules. *J Am Soc Nephrol* 1997;8:1213–1221.

36. van Aubel RA, Hartog A, Bindels RJ, et al. Expression and immunolocalization of multidrug resistance protein 2 in rabbit small intestine. *Eur J Pharmacol* 2000;400:195–198.

37. Allikmets R, Gerrard B, Hutchinson A, et al. Characterization of the human ABC superfamily: isolation and mapping of 21 new genes using the expressed sequence tags database. *Hum Mol Genet* 1996;5:1649–1655.

38. Kool M, de Haas M, Scheffer GL, et al. Analysis of expression of cMOAT (MRP2), MRP3, MRP4, and MRP5, homologues of the multidrug resistance-associated protein gene (MRP1), in human cancer cell lines. *Cancer Res* 1997;57:3537–3547.

39. Grant CE, Kurz EU, Cole SP, et al. Analysis of the intron-exon organization of the human multidrug-resistance protein gene (MRP) and alternative splicing of its mRNA. *Genomics* 1997;45:368–378.

40. Taniguchi K, Wada M, Kohno K, et al. A human canalicular multispecific organic anion transporter (cMOAT) gene is overexpressed in cisplatin-resistant human cancer cell lines with decreased drug accumulation. *Cancer Res* 1996;56:4124–4129.

41. Toh S, Wada M, Uchiumi T, et al. Genomic structure of the canalicular multispecific organic anion-transporter gene (MRP2/cMOAT) and mutations in the ATP-binding-cassette region in Dubin-Johnson syndrome. *Am J Hum Genet* 1999;64:739–746.

42. Hipfner DR, Almquist KC, Leslie EM, et al. Membrane topology of the multidrug resistance protein (MRP). A study of glycosylation-site mutants reveals an extracytosolic NH_2 terminus. *J Biol Chem* 1997;272:23623–23630.

43. Tusnady GE, Bakos E, Varadi A, et al. Membrane topology distinguishes a subfamily of the ATP-binding cassette (ABC) transporters. *FEBS Lett* 1997;402:1–3.

44. Hipfner DR, Deeley RG, Cole SP. Structural, mechanistic and clinical aspects of MRP1. *Biochim Biophys Acta* 1999;1461:359–376.

45. Jedlitschky G, Burchell B, Keppler D. The multidrug resistance protein 5 (MRP5) functions as an ATP-dependent export pump for cyclic nucleotides. *J Biol Chem* 2000;275:30069–30074.

46. Leier I, Jedlitschky G, Buchholz U, et al. ATP-dependent glutathione disulphide transport mediated by the MRP gene-encoded conjugate export pump. *Biochem J* 1996;314:433–437.

47. Paulusma CC, van Geer MA, Evers R, et al. Canalicular multispecific organic anion transporter/multidrug resistance protein 2 mediates low-affinity transport of reduced glutathione. *Biochem J* 1999;338:393–401.

48. Kamisako T, Leier I, Cui Y, et al. Transport of monoglucuronosyl and bisglucuronosyl bilirubin by recombinant human and rat multidrug resistance protein 2. *Hepatology* 1999;30:485–490.

49. Oude Elferink RP, Meijer DK, Kuipers F, et al. Hepatobiliary secretion of organic compounds; molecular mechanisms of membrane transport. *Biochim Biophys Acta* 1995;1241:215–268.

50. Evers R, de Haas M, Sparidans R, et al. Vinblastine and sulfinpyrazone export by the multidrug resistance protein MRP2 is associated with glutathione export. *Br J Cancer* 2000;83:375–383.

51. Nies AT, Cantz T, Brom M, et al. Expression of the apical conjugate export pump, Mrp2, in the polarized hepatoma cell line, WIF-B. *Hepatology* 1998;28:1332–1340.

52. Hooijberg JH, Broxterman HJ, Kool M, et al. Antifolate resis-

tance mediated by the multidrug resistance proteins MRP1 and MRP2. *Cancer Res* 1999;59:2532–2535.

53. Leier I, Hummel-Eisenbeiss J, Cui Y, et al. ATP-dependent para-aminohippurate transport by apical multidrug resistance protein MRP2. *Kidney Int* 2000;57:1636–1642.

54. Loe DW, Deeley RG, Cole SP. Characterization of vincristine transport by the M(r) 190,000 multidrug resistance protein (MRP): evidence for cotransport with reduced glutathione. *Cancer Res* 1998;58:5130–5136.

55. Kala SV, Neely MW, Kala G, et al. The MRP2/cMOAT transporter and arsenic-glutathione complex formation are required for biliary excretion of arsenic. *J Biol Chem* 2000;275:33404–33408.

56. Trauner M, Arrese M, Soroka CJ, et al. The rat canalicular conjugate export pump (Mrp2) is down-regulated in intrahepatic and obstructive cholestasis. *Gastroenterology* 1997;113:255–264.

57. Cantz T, Nies AT, Brom M, et al. MRP2, a human conjugate export pump, is present and transports fluo 3 into apical vacuoles of Hep G2 cells. *Am J Physiol* 2000;278:G522–G531.

58. Paulusma CC, Kothe MJ, Bakker CT, et al. Zonal down-regulation and redistribution of the multidrug resistance protein 2 during bile duct ligation in rat liver. *Hepatology* 2000;31:684–693.

59. Kubitz R, Wettstein M, Warskulat U, et al. Regulation of the multidrug resistance protein 2 in the rat liver by lipopolysaccharide and dexamethasone. *Gastroenterology* 1999;116:401–410.

60. Rost D, Kartenbeck J, Keppler D. Changes in the localization of the rat canalicular conjugate export pump Mrp2 in phalloidin-induced cholestasis. *Hepatology* 1999;29:814–821.

61. Dombrowski F, Kubitz R, Chittattu A, et al. Electron-microscopic demonstration of multidrug resistance protein 2 (Mrp2) retrieval from the canalicular membrane in response to hyperosmolarity and lipopolysaccharide. *Biochem J* 2000;348:183–188.

62. Mottino AD, Hoffman T, Jennes L, et al. Expression and localization of multidrug resistant protein mrp2 in rat small intestine. *J Pharmacol Exp Ther* 2000;293:717–723.

63. Zaman GJ, Versantvoort CH, Smit JJ, et al. Analysis of the expression of MRP, the gene for a new putative transmembrane drug transporter, in human multidrug resistant lung cancer cell lines. *Cancer Res* 1993;53:1747–1750.

64. Hipfner DR, Gauldie SD, Deeley RG, et al. Detection of the M(r) 190,000 multidrug resistance protein, MRP, with monoclonal antibodies. *Cancer Res* 1994;54:5788–5792.

65. Flens MJ, Izquierdo MA, Scheffer GL, et al. Immunochemical detection of the multidrug resistance-associated protein MRP in human multidrug-resistant tumor cells by monoclonal antibodies. *Cancer Res* 1994;54:4557–4563.

66. Flens MJ, Zaman GJ, van der Valk P, et al. Tissue distribution of the multidrug resistance protein. *Am J Pathol* 1996;148:1237–1247.

67. Brechot JM, Hurbain I, Fajac A, et al. Different pattern of MRP localization in ciliated and basal cells from human bronchial epithelium. *J Histochem Cytochem* 1998;46:513–517.

68. Wright SR, Boag AH, Valdimarsson G, et al. Immunohistochemical detection of multidrug resistance protein in human lung cancer and normal lung. *Clin Cancer Res* 1998;4:2279–2289.

69. Hirohashi T, Suzuki H, Ito K, et al. Hepatic expression of multidrug resistance-associated protein-like proteins maintained in Eisai hyperbilirubinemic rats. *Mol Pharmacol* 1998;53:1068–1075.

70. Ortiz DF, Li S, Iyer R, et al. MRP3, a new ATP-binding cassette protein localized to the canalicular domain of the hepatocyte. *Am J Physiol* 1999;276:G1493–G1500.

71. Kiuchi Y, Suzuki H, Hirohashi T, et al. cDNA cloning and inducible expression of human multidrug resistance associated protein 3 (MRP3). *FEBS Lett* 1998;433:149–152.

72. Uchiumi T, Hinoshita E, Haga S, et al. Isolation of a novel human canalicular multispecific organic anion transporter, cMOAT2/MRP3, and its expression in cisplatin-resistant cancer

cells with decreased ATP-dependent drug transport. *Biochem Biophys Res Commun* 1998;252:103–110.

73. Madon J, Hagenbuch B, Landmann L, et al. Transport function and hepatocellular localization of mrp6 in rat liver. *Mol Pharmacol* 2000;57:634–641.

74. Kool M, van der Linden M, de Haas M, et al. Expression of human *MRP6*, a homologue of the multidrug resistance protein gene *MRP1*, in tissues and cancer cells. *Cancer Res* 1999;59:175–182.

75. Ogawa K, Suzuki H, Hirohashi T, et al. Characterization of inducible nature of MRP3 in rat liver. *Am J Physiol* 2000;278:G438–G446.

76. Stöckel B, König J, Nies AT, et al. Characterization of the 5′-flanking region of the human multidrug resistance protein 2 (MRP2) gene and its regulation in comparison with the multidrug resistance protein 3 (MRP3) gene. *Eur J Biochem* 2000;267:1347–1358.

77. Böhme M, Müller M, Leier I, et al. Cholestasis caused by inhibition of the adenosine triphosphate-dependent bile salt transport in rat liver. *Gastroenterology* 1994;107:255–265.

78. Kartenbeck J, Leuschner U, Mayer R, et al. Absence of the canalicular isoform of the MRP gene-encoded conjugate export pump from the hepatocytes in Dubin-Johnson syndrome. *Hepatology* 1996;23:1061–1066.

79. Sprinz H, Nelson RS. Persistent nonhemolytic hyperbilirubine-mia associated with lipochrome-like pigment in liver cells; report of four cases. *Ann Intern Med* 1954;41:952–962.

80. Dubin IN, Johnson FB. Chronic idiopathic jaundice with unidentified pigment in liver cells; a new clinicopathologic entity with report of 12 cases. *Medicine* 1954;33:155–179.

81. Roy Chowdhury J, Roy Chowdhury N, Wolkoff AW, et al. Heme and bile pigment metabolism. In: Arias IM, Boyer JL, Fausto N, et al., eds. *The liver: biology and pathology.* New York: Raven Press, 1994:471–504.

82. Keitel V, Kartenbeck J, Nies AT, et al. Impaired protein maturation of the conjugate export pump multidrug resistance protein 2 as a consequence of a deletion mutation in Dubin-Johnson syndrome. *Hepatology* 2000;32:1317–1328.

83. Kajihara S, Hisatomi A, Mizuta T, et al. A splice mutation in the human canalicular multispecific organic anion transporter gene causes Dubin-Johnson syndrome. *Biochem Biophys Res Commun* 1998;253:454–457.

84. Mor-Cohen R, Zivelin A, Rosenberg N, et al. Identification of a common Ile1173Phe mutation in the canalicular multispecific organic anion transporter gene in patients with Dubin-Johnson syndrome of Iranian-Jewish origin. *Am J Hum Genet* 1999;65 (suppl):581.

85. Thermann R, Neu-Yilik G, Deters A, et al. Binary specification of nonsense codons by splicing and cytoplasmic translation. *EMBO J* 1998;17:3484–3494.

The Liver: Biology and Pathobiology, Fourth Edition, edited by I. M. Arias, J. L. Boyer, F. V. Chisari, N. Fausto, D. Schachter, and D. A. Shafritz.
Lippincott Williams & Wilkins, Philadelphia © 2001.

GENETIC DEFECTS OF CANALICULAR TRANSPORT

RICHARD J. THOMPSON
SANDRA S. STRAUTNIEKS

The conditions described in this chapter represent inheritable defects in hepatocyte-derived bile acid–dependent and –independent bile secretion. The phenotypic differences between the different conditions reflect the underlying defects. However, normal bile secretion requires contributions from all components, which are interdependent and not isolated. The consequence is that cholestasis caused by different specific defects often results in a similar clinical phenotype, particularly late in the disease process. These diseases have helped unravel the physiology. Now that their basis is understood, it is hoped that better treatments will follow.

The diseases discussed in this chapter are defects in specific mechanisms of bile formation. Normal bile formation and secretion and various mechanisms of cholestasis are discussed in website chapters 🖳 W-22 through W-24 and Chapters 24 and 27. Whereas clinical and histologic features may vary between conditions in the early stages, even the most selective of defects often results in secondary liver damage, which gradually becomes less specific.

In 1930 Arnold Rice Rich predicted that most causes of jaundice result from a reduced secretory capacity of the liver. Although this remains correct, the reduction in secretory capacity is usually secondary to quite distinct pathology, for instance bile duct damage. However, molecular mechanisms of hepatocellular excretory transport have been discovered in the last few years. A significant portion of this progress resulted from identification of patients with specific defects in hepatocyte secretory function. The general classification that has come to be applied to these patients is progressive familial intrahepatic cholestasis (PFIC) (1,2), which is currently being replaced by specific terminology based on the underlying defect. PFIC is a descriptive term; however, the name does embrace important information. It recognizes that many, if not all, cases have a genetic cause. Because the defect is genetic, the disease is progressive and not transient.

DEFECTS IN BILE ACID SECRETION

Normal bile production depends on the active transport of many constituents into the biliary space. The largest contribution to bile flow is made by bile acids. A defect in canalicular bile acid transport would be expected to cause severe liver disease because bile acids are highly toxic. They are powerful detergents and also have significant functions in the regulation of gene transcription. As a consequence of one or both of these properties, they are potent apoptotic agents. A failure of bile acid export from hepatocytes, therefore, would be anticipated to cause fat malabsorption as well as hepatocellular dysfunction and progressive liver damage secondary to the retained bile acids. Early in the disease, the biochemical findings in patients with such defects are characteristic (3). Biochemical markers are low biliary bile acids and high serum levels of bile acids in the absence of a defect in bile acid synthesis. In practice, few patients have biliary bile acid mea-

R. J. Thompson: Paediatric Liver Service, Department of Child Health, Guy's, King's, and St. Thomas' School of Medicine, King's College Hospital, London SE5 9RS, United Kingdom.

S. S. Strautnieks: Department of Child Health, Guy's, King's, and St. Thomas' School of Medicine, King's College Hospital, London SE5 9RS, United Kingdom.

surements. Fortuitously, there is good correlation between low biliary bile acids and normal serum levels of γ-glutamyl transpeptidase (GGT) (4,5). In the liver, GGT is normally bound to the canalicular membrane and to (cholangiocyte) biliary epithelium. In cholestasis, it is presumed that the detergent action of bile acids liberates GGT from the plasma membrane. When this is combined with poor bile flow, GGT leaks back into the circulation and elevated plasma levels result. In the absence of bile acids in bile, even in the presence of poor bile flow, GGT is not released and serum levels remain normal. Therefore, in cholestasis, normal serum GGT levels correlate well with low biliary bile acid levels. The original patients described with this phenotype were among the old order Amish (1). One of the original families was named Byler, and this condition has become widely known as Byler disease.

BILE SALT EXPORT PUMP DEFICIENCY

Many, but not all, patients with low-GGT PFIC have been shown to have a specific defect in bile acid transport. The gene encoding the human bile salt export pump was identified and subsequently shown to be mutated in these patients. An expressed sequence tag (EST) from this gene was first identified from a porcine complementary DNA (cDNA) library (6). The full-length rat cDNA was cloned, expressed *in vitro* (7), and demonstrated to represent competent, adenosine triphosphate (ATP)-dependent bile acid transporter. The human orthologue was mapped to the long arm of chromosome 2 (8), in the same region to which a locus for PFIC had previously been mapped using Middle Eastern families (9). The predicted protein sequence represents an ATP-binding cassette (ABC) transporter. The nearest human homologues are MDR1 or P-glycoprotein (encoded by *ABCB1*) and MDR3 (encoded by *ABCB4*), which is discussed below. Mutations in this gene have subsequently been identified in patients from a wide range of ethnic and geographic origins (5,10). The human gene was originally termed *SPGP* (sister of P-glycoprotein), and then *BSEP*, and officially redesignated as *ABCB11*. The protein it encodes is termed the bile salt export pump (BSEP). These patients mostly present in the first few months with a neonatal hepatitis. However, the disease progresses and pruritus usually becomes a prominent problem toward the end of the first year. The rate of progression is variable, resulting in end-stage liver disease at 2 to 10 years of age or older. No treatment short of transplantation has shown to be of benefit. These patients appear to be incapable of excreting ursodeoxycholic acid (UDCA) (5). However, treatment with modest doses of UDCA may have a beneficial effect by further suppressing endogenous bile acid production. Because expression of the gene appears to be limited to the liver, liver transplantation has proved successful in correcting the phenotype.

FIC1 DEFICIENCY

Other patients with low-GGT PFIC, including members of the original Byler family, have a disease that does not map to chromosome 2 but rather to chromosome 18 (11). The locus coincides with that which had previously been identified using patients with the similar, but much milder, phenotype of benign recurrent intrahepatic cholestasis (BRIC) (12). The gene responsible has been cloned and is predicted to encode a P-type adenosine triphosphatase (ATPase) (13). The gene is termed *FIC1* and the protein is FIC1. Mutations have been found in both BRIC and PFIC patients, with some phenotype-genotype correlation; however, several significant questions arise from this finding. First, the gene is widely expressed and there is relatively low-level expression in the liver, which correlates with the finding that some patients with FIC1 disease also have extrahepatic manifestations. This is in contrast to patients with BSEP-related disease where the phenotype and the expression of the gene are restricted to the liver. Expression of *FIC1* is particularly high in the small intestine and pancreas. FIC1-related PFIC patients have been described with pancreatitis and many have malabsorption, which is not improved by liver transplantation. Anecdotally, in a few cases, liver transplantation has made the gastrointestinal disease worse. Genetically proven FIC1 deficiency has been identified in many populations (13). Greenland cholestasis (14), which had previously shown possible mapping to chromosome 18 (15), has recently been mapped to the same locus (16).

The function of the FIC1 protein remains unclear. Based on sequence homology, it may serve as an aminophospholipid translocase (17). There is need for such a protein to maintain enrichment of the inner leaflet of the plasma membrane with aminophospholipids, such as phosphatidylserine. Such a function has been demonstrated in normal canalicular membrane vesicles, and FIC1 is present in hepatocyte canalicular membrane (18). What is not clear is how the loss of this function would lead to manifestation of this disease. FIC1-deficient patients do not have neonatal hepatitis and manifest mild cholestasis, which suggests that there is not the same intracellular accumulation of bile acids, as in BSEP-deficient disease. The other hepatic feature that may distinguish between FIC1 deficiency and BSEP deficiency is the appearance of canalicular bile at electron microscopy. In BSEP-deficient disease, the bile has an amorphous appearance. However, in FIC1 deficiency, the bile is coarsely granular, which is termed Byler bile (4). It is not known what is different about the composition of the canalicular bile. However, the coarse granules may represent disrupted microvilli, which, due to their altered lipid composition, have a different appearance in FIC1-deficient patients. The mature bile in both groups of patients has remarkably low bile acid levels. In FIC1-associated disease, chenodeoxycholate conjugates appear to be more depleted than are cholate conjugates. However, very few samples have been obtained early in the disease, and some of the effects may be secondary. FIC1-deficient patients do have particularly low serum levels of GGT, which suggests that biliary bile acid secretion is severely impaired from an early stage.

These findings may be explained in several ways. Abnormal lipid composition in the canalicular membrane may result in failure of correct targeting of BSEP protein to the canalicular membrane. Failure of insertion alone would be expected to result in a BSEP-deficiency–like picture. However, a small proportion of BSEP in the basolateral membrane may ameliorate intracellular bile acid accumulation and change the phenotype. Alternatively, bile acids might be exported normally, but the abnormal lipid composition in the outer leaflet of the membrane and biliary space may not permit normal formation of mixed micelles, resulting in precipitation of lipids (Byler bile). The nonmicellar monomeric bile acids must then be reabsorbed because they are not present in mature bile. This process may be the function of the apical sodium-dependent bile acid transporter (ASBT), which is expressed in cholangiocytes. It would be reasonable that excess monomeric bile acids are reabsorbed under normal circumstances because they may be harmful to the biliary tree. It is difficult to understand why GGT is low under these circumstances, if free monomeric bile acids are present in the canaliculi. Failure of canalicular targeting is currently our favored mechanism, which may also be responsible for the extrahepatic manifestations of FIC1 deficiency.

MDR3 DEFICIENCY

There is another disease that has some similarities with PFIC and BSEP and that has helped to elucidate mechanisms of normal bile formation and secretion. Phospholipid in the form of phosphatidylcholine (PC) is the major lipid in mammalian bile and combines with bile acids, cholesterol, and small amounts of other lipids, to form mixed micelles. A defect in PC secretion would be predicted to result in the production of highly detergent bile, which would be expected to cause considerable damage. This is the phenotype in a condition called high-GGT PFIC (19). Mice in which mdr2 has been "knocked out" by homologous recombination show a similar phenotype and mechanism (20). Patients with high-GGT PFIC and mdr2 homozygous knockout mice have high bile acid to phospholipid ratios in bile. The human orthologue of *mdr2* is generally known as *MDR3* and the new gene symbol is *ABCB4*. This gene is mutated in patients with this phenotype (21). The conclusion must be that the gene product (MDR3) plays a critical role in PC secretion. The critical step is enrichment of the outer leaflet of the plasma membrane with PC (see Chapter 24). It is still a matter of debate as to how the lipid constituents get from the membrane into bile. In the absence of phospholipid, the detergent action of bile acids is unopposed by micelle formation. Thus high concentrations of bile acid in the canalicular lumen gain access to small bile duct epithelial cells and damage them. The disease is further characterized by marked portal inflammation and bile duct proliferation. Some patients, particularly those with residual MDR3 function, clinically respond to ursodeoxycholic acid, which would be expected to reduce the hydrophobicity of the bile. Preliminary data from the murine model reveal that transplanted hepatocytes are capable of largely ameliorating the phenotype and, due to their built-in survival advantage, manifest proliferation. This work provides good evidence to support the concept that such transport defects in humans are good candidates for hepatocyte transplantation or gene therapy.

Some mothers of patients with MDR3 deficiency, themselves carrying heterozygous mutations, have suffered from intrahepatic cholestasis of pregnancy (ICP) (21). More recently, cases of ICP occurring in families with no history of PFIC have been associated with MDR3 mutations (22,23). However, in these cases, serum GGT increased during cholestatic episodes. An alternative explanation is needed regarding the majority of ICP cases in which GGT is not elevated.

DUBIN–JOHNSON SYNDROME

The fourth genetic defect of hepatocanalicular transport that has emerged recently involves canalicular transport of non-bile acid organic anions, including reduced glutathione (GSH) and glucuronide adducts of various drugs and metabolites.. Accumulation of conjugated bilirubin (and other nonbile acid organic anions) within cells is not particularly harmful, and bilirubin conjugates, although contributing to bile flow, have a relatively minor role in bile formation. Bilirubin glucuronides are transported across the canalicular membrane by a multispecific organic anion transporter (cMOAT) (see Chapters 24 and 25). Mutations in the gene encoding this protein have been demonstrated in the relative benign condition, Dubin–Johnson syndrome (24). The gene encoding cMOAT has been variously termed CMOAT and *MRP2*, but has now been designated as ABCC2. A potentially important spin-off from this disease is the observation that a related gene product is overexpressed in the basolateral membrane in this syndrome (25). MRP3 (26), encoded *ABCC3*, may serve as a basolateral "escape" mechanism. MRP3 has a broad substrate specificity and may act as an alternative basolateral transporter when canalicular secretion is impaired in cholestasis (27).

OTHER POTENTIAL TRANSPORT DEFECTS

Not all autosomal-recessive cholestatic liver diseases can be accounted for by the genes described above. There may be other transporters in the canalicular membrane, or indeed transporter associated proteins that when mutated lead to cholestasis. Furthermore cholangiocyte membrane transporters are already known to be responsible for other cholestatic liver diseases. The best example is the cystic fibrosis transmembrane conductance regulator. However other "biliary" cholestases may be due to similar defects. Examples include neonatal sclerosing cholangitis and North American Indian childhood cirrhosis (NAICC), the latter having been recently mapped to chromosome 16 (28), though the gene has yet to be cloned.

FUTURE DIAGNOSIS AND TREATMENT OF PROGRESSIVE FAMILIAL INTRAHEPATIC CHOLESTASIS

The majority of patients with PFIC have, until recently, probably never been diagnosed. We now realize, however, that many patients with FIC1 deficiency, a few with MDR3 deficiency, and a majority of patients with BSEP deficiency are compound heterozygotes. That is to say that parental consanguinity is not an issue and, in most cases, there is no family history. These patients have largely been labeled as having cryptogenic cirrhosis. Current treatments for these conditions are not dependent on precise diagnosis. Unfortunately, the best treatments available are essentially supportive, until liver function is sufficiently poor that transplantation is required. Having said that, a definitive diagnosis is always preferable, and treatments are going to change, once we can reliably distinguish between different groups of patients.

BSEP, FIC1, and MDR3 deficiencies are currently genetic diagnoses. Clinically they are either low- or high-GGT PFIC. It is important to realize that not all PFIC is caused by one of these genetic defects. In addition to BSEP and FIC1 deficiency, there is at least one other cause of low-GGT PFIC, and in addition to MDR3 deficiency and

NAICC, there is at least one other cause of high-GGT PFIC. The underlying defects in these other groups remain to be identified.

In MDR3 deficiency, bile has a high bile acid/phospholipid ratio (29). Immunohistochemical staining for the MDR3 protein shows a fairly good correlation with identification of mutations (21,29).

In low-GGT PFIC, the morphologic differences between BSEP and FIC1 deficiencies have been described (4), notably the presence of a giant-cell hepatitis in BSEP-related disease, but only bland cholestasis in FIC1 disease. The presence or absence of "Byler" bile on electron microscopy may also help. Immunohistochemical staining for BSEP reveals good correlation with genetic defects (5). Staining for FIC1 has not yet been systematically examined. Immunohistochemical staining for any of these proteins is not yet available as a routine clinical tool. No laboratory currently provides routine genetic diagnostic service.

Only limited data have been published on the precise mutations found in these patients. In *ABCB4* (MDR3), 22 different mutations have been found in 17 families with PFIC (21,29,30) (Table 26.1). There is retention of immunostaining in some missense mutations, which, in some cases, correlates with secretion of phospholipid in bile. Nine mutations have been described in *FIC1* (13,31,32). In addition to those in Table 26.2, one large deletion has been described (13). The protein truncating mutations are all associated with PFIC rather than BRIC. As would be anticipated, one mutation accounts for all the FIC1-related disease in the Amish (G308V). I661T was found to be homozygous in nearly all European patients with BRIC.

Some 42 different mutant *BSEP* alleles have been detected in patients with PFIC (5,6,32,33). All those detected in more than one family are listed in Table 26.3. E297G and D482G have been found in 25 and 16 European families, respectively. These mutations are not at pre-

TABLE 26.1. MDR3 (*ABCB4*) MUTATIONS IN PFIC PATIENTS (29)

Amino Acid	Base Change	Predicted Consequence	MDR3 Immunostaining	Phospholipid in Bile	Patients
26	A to G	Disrupts splice site	−		2 homozygotes
132	7-bp deletion	Truncation	−		1 homozygote
138	T to C	W to R		6%	1 homozygote
346	G to T	S to I	+/−	1%	1 homozygote
424	A to G	T to A	+/−	7%	1 heterozygote
425	G to A	V to M	+++		1 heterozygote
541	A to T	I to F	−		1 homozygote
556	T to G	L to R			1 heterozygote
571	1-bp del	Truncation			1 homozygote
636	C to T	Stop	−		2 homozygotes
652	A to G	R to G			1 homozygote
					4 heterozygotes
957	C to T	Stop	−		1 homozygote

MDR, multi-drug resistance protein; PFIC, progressive familial intrahepatic cholestasis.

TABLE 26.2. FIC1 (*FIC1*) MUTATIONS IN PFIC AND BRIC PATIENTS (13,31,32)

Amino Acid	Base Change	Predicted Consequence	Patient	Disease	Origin
288	T to C	L to S	1 homozygote	PFIC	Poland
308	G to T	G to V	9 homozygotes	PFIC	Amish
412	G to C	R to P	1 homozygote	PFIC	Japan
554	G to A	D to R	12 homozygotes	PFIC	Greenland
661	T to C	I to T	Many	BRIC	Europe
699 (+2)	T to C	Disrupts splice site	1 heterozygote	PFIC	
795	9 bp deletion	Deletes GNR	1 homozygote	BRIC	Netherlands
892	G to A	G to R	1 homozygote	PFIC	Europe

BRIC, benign recurrent intrahepatic cholestasis.

dicted mutation "hot spots," and from geographic and haplotype data, they appear to be due to founder effects. One of these two mutations is present in 30% of European patients (33). The other mutations listed are all at cytosine-guanine (CpG) dinucleotides, which are known mutation hot spots. Therefore, these probably represent different mutational events in each family. In addition to those listed, a further two missense and two nonsense mutations have been found at CpG sites, but only in single families. Some 25 other sporadic mutations have been found in individual families; 11 are missense mutations, at conserved residues; one is a nonsense mutation; three disrupt splice sites; eight are small insertions and deletions; and two are large intragenic rearrangements. A further six alleles represent major deletions, detected by hemizygosity for intragenic polymorphisms and mutations. One such patient also has cleft palate and coloboma. These features have previously been described in patients with chromosome 2 deletions (34). Patients with low-GGT cholestasis and craniofacial abnormalities should be investigated for chromosome 2q24-31 deletions.

Our increased understanding of the molecular basis of PFIC has not yet translated into improved treatment. There is already limited evidence that reduction of the cytotoxic-

ity of bile is of value in some patients with MDR3 deficiency in particular (29). Real advances can now be envisaged in both cell and gene therapy (see Chapters 61–63). In MDR3 deficiency, the lack of phospholipid in bile makes it cytotoxic to all cells. Cells expressing wild-type protein would be expected to protect not only themselves, but also adjacent hepatocytes and downstream cholangiocytes. Such cells could be introduced by gene therapy or hepatocyte transplantation. The potential for this approach has been demonstrated in the murine model of MDR3 deficiency (35). In the case of BSEP deficiency, the effect should be even greater, as the cells expressing wild-type proteins that are therefore capable of exporting bile acids would have greater selective advantage over mutant cells. Allogeneic hepatocytes could be used for this purpose, but require immunosuppression. However, autologous hepatocytes could be used in combination with *ex vivo* gene therapy. More exciting still is the prospect of gene repair using RNA/DNA oligonucleotides (36,37). Widespread application of this technique may be limited by the relatively low level of correction achieved; however, in diseases such as PFIC, where there is significant selective advantage to the corrected cells, this approach may be clinically applicable in the near future.

TABLE 26.3. BSEP (*ABCB11*) MUTATIONS IN PFIC PATIENTS (5,10,32,33)

Amino Acid	Base Change	Predicted Consequence	BSEP Immunostaining	Patients	Origin
297	A to G	E to G	–	10 homozygotes	European and Caucasian
				15 heterozygotes	
482	A to G	D to G		3 homozygotes	Poland and Slovakia
				13 heterozygotes	
575	C to T	R to X	–	4 heterozygotes	CpG site
948	C to T	R to C		3 heterozygotes	CpG site
982	G to A	G to R	–	1 homozygote	CpG site
				2 heterozygotes	
1,057	C to T	R to X	–	2 heterozygotes	CpG site
1,153	C to T	R to C		2 homozygotes	CpG site
	G to A	R to H		3 heterozygotes	

BSEP, bile salt export pump; PFIC, progressive familial intrahepatic cholestasis.

REFERENCES

1. Clayton RJ, Iber FL, Ruebner BH, et al. Byler disease. Fatal familial intrahepatic cholestasis in an Amish kindred. *Am J Dis Child* 1969;117:112–124.
2. Whitington PF, Freese DK, Alonso, et al. Clinical and biochemical findings in progressive familial intrahepatic cholestasis. *J Pediatr Gastroenterol Nutr* 1994;18:134–141.
3. Jacquemin E, Dumont M., Bernard O, et al. Evidence for defective primary bile acid secretion in children with progressive familial intrahepatic cholestasis (Byler disease). *Eur J Pediatr* 1994;153:424–428.
4. Bull LN, Carlton VE, Stricker VL, et al. Genetic and morphological findings in progressive familial intrahepatic cholestasis (Byler disease (PFIC-1) and Byler syndrome): evidence for heterogeneity. *Hepatology* 1997;26:155–164.
5. Jansen PL, Strautnieks SS, Jacquemin E, et al. Hepatocanalicular bile salt export pump deficiency in patients with progressive familial intrahepatic cholestasis. *Gastroenterology* 1999;117:1370–1379.
6. Childs S, Yeh RL, Georges E, et al. Identification of a sister gene to P-glycoprotein. *Cancer Res* 1995;55:2029–2034.
7. Gerloff T, Steiger B, Hagenbuch B, et al. The sister of P-glycoprotein represents the canalicular bile salt export pump of mammalian liver. *J Biol Chem* 1998;273:10046–10050.
8. Childs S, Yeh RL, Hui D, et al. Taxol resistance mediated by transfection of the liver-specific sister gene of P-glycoprotein. *Cancer Res* 1998;58:4160–4167.
9. Strautnieks SS, Kagalwalla AF, Tanner MS, et al. Identification of a locus for progressive familial intrahepatic cholestasis PFIC2 on chromosome 2q24. *Am J Hum Genet* 1997;61:630–633.
10. Strautnieks SS, Bull LN, Knisely AS, et al. A gene encoding a liver-specific ABC transporter is mutated in progressive familial intrahepatic cholestasis. *Nat Genet* 1998;20:233–238.
11. Carlton VE, Knisely AS, Freimer NB. Mapping of a locus for progressive familial intrahepatic cholestasis (Byler disease) to 18q21-q22, the benign recurrent intrahepatic cholestasis region. *Hum Mol Genet* 1995;4:1049–1053.
12. Houwen RH, Baharloo S, Blankenship K, et al. Genome screening by searching for shared segments: mapping a gene for benign recurrent intrahepatic cholestasis. *Nat Genet* 1994;8:380–386.
13. Bull LN, van Eijk MJ, Pawlikowska L, et al. A gene encoding a P-type ATPase mutated in two forms of hereditary cholestasis. *Nat Genet* 1998;18:219–224.
14. Ornvold K, Nielsen IM, Poulsen H. Fatal familial cholestatic syndrome in Greenland Eskimo children. A histomorphological analysis of 16 cases. *Virchows Arch [A]* 1989;415:275–281.
15. Eiberg H, Nielsen IM. Linkage studies of cholestasis familiaris groenlandica/Byler-like disease with polymorphic protein and blood group markers. *Hum Hered* 1993;43:250–256.
16. Eiberg H, Nielsen IM. Linkage of cholestasis familiaris Groenlandica/Byler-like disease to chromosome 18. *Int J Circumpolar Health* 2000;59:57–62.
17. Tang X, Helleck MS, Schlegel RA, et al. A subfamily of P-type ATPases with aminophospholipid transporting activity. *Science* 1996;272:1495–1497.
18. Ujhazy P, Ortiz DF, Misra S, et al. ATP-dependent aminophospholipid translocase activity in rat canalicular membrane vesicles and its relationship to FIC1. *Hepatology* 1999;30:462A.
19. Deleuze JF, Jacquemin E, Sturm E, et al. Defect of multidrug-resistance 3 gene expression in a subtype of progressive familial intrahepatic cholestasis. *Hepatology* 1996;2:904–908.
20. Smit JJ, et al. Homozygous disruption of the murine mdr2 P-glycoprotein gene leads to a complete absence of phospholipid from bile and to liver disease. *Cell* 1993;75:451–462.
21. de Vree JM, Jacquemin E, Sturm E, et al. Mutations in the MDR3 gene cause progressive familial intrahepatic cholestasis. *Proc Natl Acad Sci USA* 1998;95:282–287.
22. Jacquemin E, Cresteil D, Manouvrier S, et al. Heterozygous nonsense mutation of the MDR3 gene in familial intrahepatic cholestasis of pregnancy. *Lancet* 1999;353:210–211.
23. Dixon PH, Weerasekera N, Linton KJ, et al. Heterozygous MDR3 missense mutation associated with intrahepatic cholestasis of pregnancy: evidence for a defect in protein trafficking. *Hum Mol Genet* 2000;9:1209–1217.
24. Paulusma CC, Kool M, Bosma PJ, et al. A mutation in the human canalicular multispecific organic anion transporter gene causes the Dubin-Johnson syndrome. *Hepatology* 1997;25:1539–1542.
25. Konig J, et al. Characterization of the human multidrug resistance protein isoform MRP3 localized to the basolateral hepatocyte membrane. *Hepatology* 1999;29:1156–1163.
26. Kiuchi Y, Suzuki H, Hirohashi T, et al. cDNA cloning and inducible expression of human multidrug resistance associated protein 3 (MRP3). *FEBS Lett* 1998;433:149–152.
27. Hirohashi T, Suzuki H, Takikawa H, et al. ATP-dependent transport of bile salts by rat multidrug resistance-associated protein 3 (Mrp3). *J Biol Chem* 2000;275:2905–2910.
28. Bétard C, Rasquin-Weber A, Brewer C, et al. Localization of a recessive gene for North American Indian childhood cirrhosis to chromosome region 16q22 and identification of a shared haplotype. *Am J Hum Genet* 2000;67:222–228.
29. de Vree JM. *Defects in hepatobiliary lipid transport.* Amsterdam: University of Amsterdam, Department of Gastroenterology and Hepatology, 1999.
30. Jacquemin E, de Vree M, Cresteil D, et al. MDR3 deficiency in patients with progressive familial intrahepatic cholestasis with high serum gamma-glutamyl transferase (ggt) activity (PFIC3). *J Pediatr Gastroenterol Nutr* 2000;31:S207.
31. Klomp LW, Bull LN, Knisely AS, et al. A missense mutation in FIC1 is associated with greenland familial cholestasis. *Hepatology* 2000;32:1337–1341.
32. Sumazaki R, Hasegawa M, Matsui A. FIC1 and BSEP analysis in Japanese patients with chronic intrahepatic cholestasis. *J Pediatr Gastroenterol Nutr* 2000;31:S122.
33. Strautnieks S, Bryne J, Knisely A, et al. Clinical and genetic analysis of progressive familial intrahepatic cholestasis. *J Pediatr Gastroenterol Nutr* 2000;31:S207.
34. Slavotinek A, Schwartz C, Getty JF, et al. Two cases with interstitial deletions of chromosome 2 and sex reversal in one. *Am J Med Genet* 1999;86:75–81.
35. De Vree JM, Ottenhoff R, Bosma PI, et al. Correction of liver disease by hepatocyte transplantation in a mouse model of progressive familial intrahepatic cholestasis. *Gastroenterology* 2000;119:1720–1730.
36. Kren BT, et al. Correction of the UDP-glucuronosyltransferase gene defect in the gunn rat model of Crigler-Najjar syndrome type I with a chimeric oligonucleotide. *Proc Natl Acad Sci USA* 1999;96:10349–10354.
37. Yoon K, Cole-Strauss A, Kmiec EB. Targeted gene correction of episomal DNA in mammalian cells mediated by a chimeric RNA.DNA oligonucleotide. *Proc Natl Acad Sci USA* 1996;93:2071–2076.

27

HORMONAL REGULATION OF BILE SECRETION

FRANCIS R. SIMON

Hormones transported to the liver by the portal and systemic circulation regulate many hepatic functions. The mechanisms by which these hormones regulate gene expression and protein functions have been under intensive investigation in recent years. It is clear that hepatic metabolic responses to steroid and peptide hormones are generally similar to those for other hormone-sensitive tissues. Thus, liver is increasingly recognized as a target tissue for actions of many hormones of endogenous as well as exogenous origin. In addition, liver also participates in clearance and metabolism of many hormones from the circulation. This chapter summarizes some of the interrelationships between hormones and bile secretion.

BILE FORMATION

Components of bile formation are localized to hepatocytes and bile ductular cells. A simplified model of hepatic bile formation is shown in Figure 27.1 (Chapters 24–29 and website chapters 🖳 W-22 through W-24). In hepatocytes, bile generation involves diffusion of water and electrolytes into canaliculi along osmotic gradients that are generated by secretion of organic and inorganic solutes (1–10). Bile salts, which undergo a dynamic enterohepatic circula-

tion, are the primary driving force for bile secretion. Following intestinal absorption, bile salts are transported to the liver, where the majority is efficiently cleared by the proximal lobular hepatocytes by transport proteins localized to the sinusoidal domain (11,12). This enterohepatic circulation is integral to the metabolism of cholesterol to bile acids

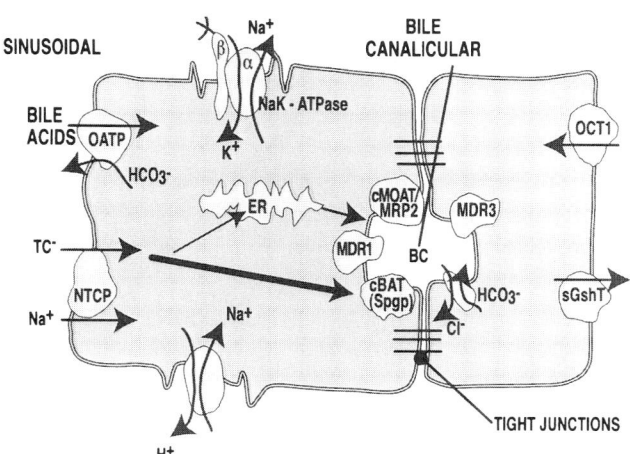

FIGURE 27.1. Hepatic transporters involved in bile formation. *NTCP*, sodium/dependent taurocholate transporter; *OATP*, sodium/independent organic anion transporter proteins; *OCT1*, organic cation transporter; *sGshT*, glutathione transporter; *cMOAT/MRP2*, multidrug resistance-associated protein 2; *MDR1*, multidrug resistance transporter; *MDR3*, phosphatidylcholine flippase; *cBAT/Spgp*, bile salt export protein/sister of P-glycoprotein.

F. R. **Simon:** Department of Medicine, University of Colorado Health Sciences Center; and Department of Medicine, Denver Veterans Affairs Medical Center, Denver, Colorado 80262

and the generation of bile flow (Chapters 16 and 69). After uptake into hepatocytes, bile salts are translocated to the canalicular membrane and excreted by ABC-transporters, in particular the bile salt export protein (Bsep) (13). This is the so-called bile salt–dependent fraction of bile flow (BSDBF). In addition, a bile salt–independent fraction of bile secretion has been characterized (BSIBF) (14,15). This component of hepatic bile flow is due in part to secretion of glutathione (GSH) and the Cl/HCO$_3$ exchanger (16,17). Although the specific glutathione transporters are still controversial, evidence suggests that the ABC-transporter known as multidrug resistance protein (Mrp2) may be involved in the low-affinity secretion of GSH (18–21). Bile ductular secretion and absorption of electrolytes including chloride and bicarbonate modify the primary bile.

Hepatocytes, like other epithelial cells, are polarized for efficient vectorial transport of organic compounds, electrolytes and lipids (22–27) (Chapters 7, 8, and 24 and website chapter 🖳 W-5). The surface membrane is organized into sinusoidal and bile canalicular domains which are structurally and functionally asymmetric. Polarized distribution of specific transport proteins is responsible for vectorial translocation of biliary constituents (22). Osmotically active compounds secreted by hepatocytes include bile salts, GSH, and glucuronide- and GSH-conjugated compounds and inorganic anions such as bicarbonate and chloride. Bile salts, the major cholephilic compound in bile, are very efficiently cleared during a single pass through the liver. Clearance involves both sodium-dependent and -independent mechanisms (28). Sodium-dependent taurocholate cotransporter (Ntcp) is the principal transporter involved, while sodium-independent uptake of bile salts is mediated largely by the organic anion transport proteins (oatp1, 2, and 3). These transporters are promiscuous and also transport many endo- and xenobiotics (29,30) that in turn may also behave as osmotic components of bile. Bile salts are translocated across the hepatocyte cytoplasm probably bound in part to intracellular proteins (2), whereas the role of vesicular transport in the intracellular movement of biliary solutes is unclear. The vesicular process has been suggested to be involved in sequestration of detergent-like molecules during high bile salt loads. In addition, increasing evidence indicates that both sinusoidal and bile canalicular transporters may exist in intracellular vesicles (31,32).

Canalicular transport is generally considered to be rate-limiting in the overall hepatocellular transport of organic anions into bile (Chapter 24). However, several studies using steady-state kinetics and physiological bile salt concentrations indicate that taurocholate uptake may become rate-limiting in bile secretion (Table 27.1) (33–35) (Chapter 7 and website chapter 🖳 W-5). Secretion of bile acids into the canalicular space takes place against a high osmotic and chemical gradient, indicating that an active transport system is required. At least five primary-active ATP-dependent export carriers have been identified in the hepatocyte canalicular

TABLE 27.1. MICHAELIS–MENTEN PARAMETERS FOR HEPATIC TAUROCHOLATE UPTAKE AND EXCRETION IN RATS USING STEADY-STATE MODELING

Parameters	Uptake	Excretion
Km (µM)	68 ± 35	504 ± 266
Vmax (mmol/min/g liver)	343 ± 64	394 ± 89

From Deroubaix X, Coche T, Depiereux E, et al. Saturation of hepatic transport of taurocholate in rats *in vivo*. Am J Physiol 1991;260:G189–196, with permission.

membrane (36) (Chapters 8 and 24–26). Three of these primary active export pumps comprise the multidrug resistance family (7,36–43). Multidrug resistance transporter (Mdr1) is primarily responsible for export of hydrophobic, mostly cationic compounds, while the Mdr2/3 (rat/human) gene product acts as a phospholipid filppase (7). Recently bile salt export protein/sister of P glycoprotein (Bsep/Spgp) was shown to mediate ATP-dependent bile acid transport (13). The cystic fibrosis transmembrane regulator, which is also an ABC-transporter, is not located in hepatocytes, but rather has been identified in the bile ductular cells.

HORMONAL REGULATION OF HEPATIC TRANSPORT

A number of studies in animals and especially in rats have addressed the effect of hormones on bile flow (website chapters 🖳 W-22 through W-24). Fewer studies have confirmed these effects in humans. Particularly striking has been the demonstration of the sexual dimorphic differences in hepatic transport processes and xenobiotic metabolism demonstrated in rats (44–53). However, little evidence exists to support similar differences in humans (54). Mechanisms for hormonal action on the liver and other tissues can be divided into two broad categories: (1) hormones whose effects are mediated by the steroid nuclear receptor family, and (2) peptide hormones whose intracellular actions are mediated by surface membrane receptors.

EFFECTS OF STEROID HORMONES ON THE LIVER

Steroid hormones are produced in the adrenal gland or gonads, then transformed in other tissues such as liver and excreted in urine or undergo a enterohepatic circulation. Considerable progress has been achieved in understanding the mechanisms involved in the action of these hormones in liver and other tissues. In particular, many of the intracellular hormone (and xenobiotic) binding factors have been identified and cloned. This remarkable progress has opened up new understanding of the regulation of hepatic genes.

The nuclear hormone receptors are transcriptional regulators that activate gene expression upon binding of their respective ligands. These receptors are ligand-inducible transcription factors that are involved in a number of physiological and cellular events (Table 27.2). Together, they form a superfamily which includes the classic steroid receptors (estrogen, androgen, glucocorticoid, mineralocorticoid, and progesterone receptors); the thyroid, vitamin D, and retinoid receptors, and many others (called orphan receptors) that have been characterized (55–65). For example LXR, PXR, and CAR mediate bile acid and cholesterol synthesis and have xenobiotic effects on metabolism and excretion (62).

Unlike water-soluble peptide hormones and growth factors, which bind to cell surface receptors, the fat-soluble steroid hormones pass through the lipid bilayer of cell membranes and interact with their cognate receptors. It has been more than 15 years since the initial cloning of the glucocorticoid and estrogen receptors. The cloning of these receptors demonstrated that chemically distinct ligands interact with structurally related receptors. The discovery that the vitamin A metabolite retinoic acid bound to similar receptors (66) demonstrated the existence of a nuclear receptor superfamily. Discovery of retinoid X receptors advanced our understanding of receptor heterodimerization as well as homodimerization in the mediation of hormone action (67).

A central DNA-binding domain (DBD) that targets the receptor to specific DNA sequences known as hormone response elements (HRE) characterizes nuclear receptors. The DBD is composed of two highly conserved zinc fingers (68). The carboxy-terminal half of the receptor encompasses the ligand-binding domain (LBD), which possesses the essential property of hormone recognition. More than 150 different members of this family have been identified including the so-called orphan receptors. The superfamily is further divided into the steroid receptor family and the thyroid/retinoid/vitamin D (or nonsteroid) receptor family. The steroid hormone receptors function as ligand-induced homodimers and bind to DNA half-sites organized as inverted repeats. In contrast, thyroid hormone, retinoic acid and peroxisome proliferator-activated receptors heterodimerize with RXR and typically bind to direct repeats. In addition, there is now compelling evidence that many of the orphan receptors are steroid receptors and are capable of mediating signaling pathways for bile acids, oxysterols and xenobiotics (62,69).

Bile formation has been demonstrated to be influenced by ligands which bind to each of these categories of receptors, including steroids (glucocorticoids, sex steroid hormones), thyroid hormone, and orphan receptors (xenobiotics and bile acids).

Steroid Hormone Receptors

Estrogens

The major endogenous estrogens are estradiol, estrone, and estriol, which are produced in the ovaries, testes and placenta through conversion of androgens by enzymatic aromatization of the steroid A ring (70,71). Estradiol and estrone in plasma are interconvertible. Estrone is also derived from androstenedione, an androgen produced by the adrenal cortex and in women by the ovaries. Estradiol and its major metabolites are excreted primarily in urine as conjugates, mostly as glucuronides and sulfates. However, as much as half of the circulating estrogens are secreted in bile after conjugation in liver. Eighty percent of this fraction is reabsorbed after hydrolysis in the intestine.

Clinical and research work over a more than three-decade span has established an association of estrogens with bile flow (72–77). Initially in humans and subsequently in experimental animals it was demonstrated that estrogen administration is associated with cholestasis. In numerous animal studies, estrogens decreased bile flow and organic anion excretion in a time-dependent and reversible manner (78–80). Morphological studies do not demonstrate classical changes in bile canalicular surface by light, transmission

TABLE 27.2. NUCLEAR RECEPTORS: ENDOGENOUS AND XENOBIOTIC LIGANDS AND REPRESENTATIVE RESPONSE GENES

Nuclear Receptor	Representative Ligands	Prototypic Responsive Liver Genes
Homodimers		
Estrogen	17β-Estradiol	Ceruloplasmin
Androgen	5α-dihydrotestosterone	Estrogen 2-hydroxylase
Glucocorticoid	Corticosterone/Dexamethasone	Tyrosine
		Aminotransferase/Mrp2
Heterodimers		
Thyroid	Thyroid hormone	NaK-ATPase/Malic enzyme
Retinoid	9-*cis*-retinoic acid	Liver fatty acid binding protein
PPARs	Linoleic acid/Clofibrates	CYP4A
LXR	25-hydroxycholesterol	CYP7A
FXR	Chenodeoxycholic acid	CYP7A/IBAT
CAR	Androstanol/PB	CYP2B1
PXR	Pregnenolone/PCN	CYP3A/MRP2

PB, phenobarbital; PCN, pregnenolone-16a-carbonitrile.

or scanning microscopy (81,82). In addition, serum markers of cholestasis, except for elevated bile acids, are normal (83). Thus, ethinyl estradiol induces subclinical cholestasis, which could be called "bland cholestasis."

Studies in animals were stimulated by the observations that cholestasis develops in some women after administration of oral contraceptive steroids containing synthetic estrogens and during the last trimester of pregnancy where bromosulfophthalein (BSP) maximum excretory transport (Tm) was decreased (77,84). Kreek et al. (77) first observed that estrogen administration to rats decreased bile flow. Forker (85) and later Gumucio et al. demonstrated that decreased bile salt-independent bile flow was the major defect. In addition, other studies found that estrogen administration decreased the maximum capacity for excretion of bile acids, BSP, and bilirubin (86–89). Reyes and Kern (90) showed that pregnancy in hamsters was associated with decreased bile acid-dependent bile flow, decreased NaK-ATPase and cholic acid secretion, similar to changes reported for estrogen administration in hamsters and rats.

Estrogen-mediated changes in hepatic organic anion transport are generalized since both sinusoidal and bile canalicular membrane domain functions are altered (79,83,91). Furthermore, the alterations are selective, since organic anion transport is decreased, while alanine transport is increased (83). With the use of cDNA probes and antibodies specific to transporters, it has been shown that ethinyl estradiol markedly decreased sodium-taurocholate cotransporter and the organic anion transporter at the sinusoidal surface, indicating pre-translational changes (78). Alterations at the bile canalicular domain are varied (Table 27.3). Mrp2 and Mdr2 protein content was markedly reduced, while Bsep was only modestly decreased at 5 days (and not significantly altered after 10 days of treatment) (92,93). Furthermore, there is a poor correlation between changes in protein content and mRNA levels. Probably also contributing to the development of cholestasis is decreased sinusoidal membrane fluidity, which results in abnormal activity of the sodium pump, the major driving force for the uptake of conjugated bile acids (79).

TABLE 27.3. EXPRESSION OF CANALICULAR AND SINUSOIDAL TRANSPORTERS IN ESTROGEN-INDUCED CHOLESTASIS

Transporter	Protein Content	mRNA level
Bsep/Spgp	↓	NC
Mrp2	↓↓↓	NC
Pgp/Mdr1	↑↑	ND
Mdr2	↓↓	NC
EctoATPase/cCAM	↑	NC
Ntcp	↓↓↓	↓↓
Oatp1	↓↓↓	↓↓

Data derived from references 78, 92, 93 and unpublished data. ↓, decreased; ↑, increased; NC, no change; ND, not determined.

A number of hypotheses have been proposed to explain the pathogenesis of estrogen-induced cholestasis. However, recently reported observations indicate that biochemical alterations in hepatocytes are primarily involved in the pathogenesis of decreased bile secretion. Initially it was suggested that increased biliary permeability permitting the back-diffusion of water, electrolytes, and organic anions was the major defect (85). However, later studies found that permeability changes followed the development of cholestasis (94,95), and freeze-fracture examination of tight junctions showed only minor abnormalities in the arrangement of strands (96). A second hypothesis suggested that decreased transport of organic anions and electrolytes was attributable to alteration in transport function secondary to decreased liver plasma membrane lipid fluidity (97,98). However, decreased fluidity was later localized to the sinusoidal domain and not the bile canalicular surface (79). Although NaK-ATPase activity was reported to be decreased without changes in the protein content of its subunits (78), other investigators reported that decreased fluidity was associated with increased bile flow (99) or that correction of bile flow was not associated with correction of fluidity (100).

Estrogen receptors are present in liver, but at low levels compared to target tissues (101,102). Although it has been assumed that estrogens act directly on liver (73), this has not been directly shown for most sex steroid-regulated genes. For example, increased hepatic low-density lipoprotein receptor (LDL-R) with estrogen administration is dependent on an intact pituitary, and more specifically it requires GH secretion (103–105). Since estrogens alter the secretion of growth hormone (GH), it is probable that ethinyl estradiol also indirectly alters hepatic transport protein expression by changing the GH secretory pattern, as discussed later in this chapter (Fig. 27.7 on page 402) (44,48). In support of this hypothesis, which is schematically shown in Figure 27.2, hepatic taurocholate uptake, protein and mRNA demonstrated sexually dimorphic expression (106) (Fig. 27.3). The mechanism(s) will be discussed below in the Growth Hormone section.

Another mechanism for inhibition of apical bile acid transport has been shown for estrogen metabolites, in particular estradiol-17-O-glucuronide (107). Estradiol-17-O-glucuronide is a potent and rapid inhibitor of bile flow (108). In contrast to ethinyl estradiol, which takes hours to exert its effects, bile flow is decreased immediately after exposure to the estrogen-glucuronide in a dose-dependent fashion (109). This estrogen metabolite is transported into bile by Mrp2, and produces trans-inhibition of Bsep leading to cholestasis (110).

Estrogens, Pregnancy, and Intrahepatic Cholestasis of Pregnancy (ICP)

The effects of natural and synthetic estrogens on liver excretory function in humans have been studied more

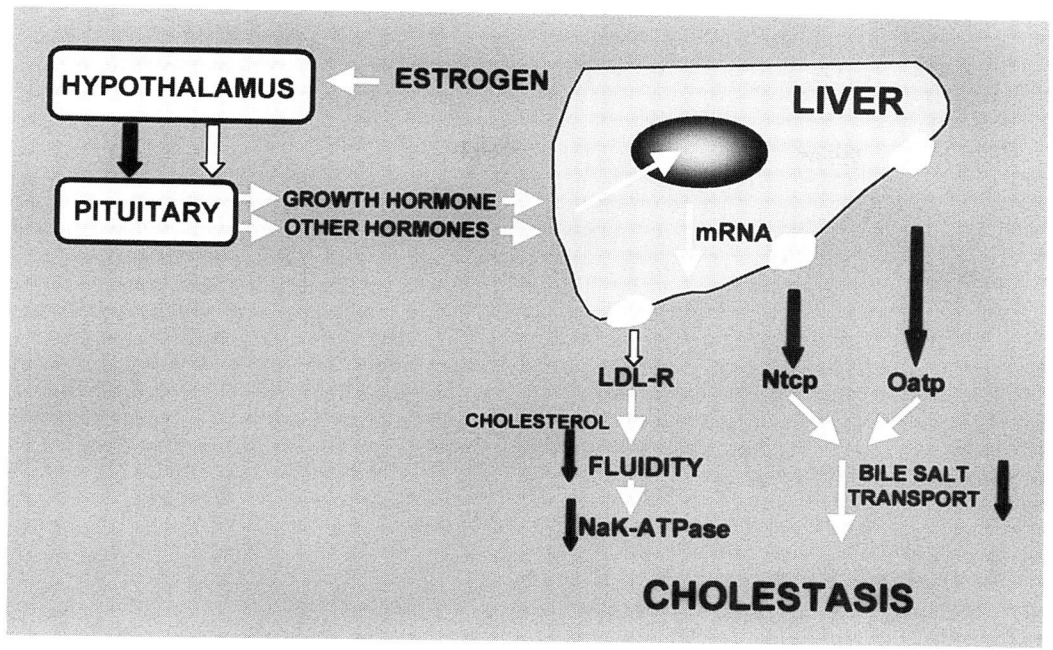

FIGURE 27.2. Hypothesis for alterations in sinusoidal membrane lipids and transporters: Pathogenesis of estrogen-induced cholestasis. Estrogen administration to male rats alters secretion of growth hormone leading to increased low-density lipoprotein receptors (*LDL-R*). Increased LDL-receptors cause hepatic accumulation of cholesterol and decreased sinusoidal membrane fluidity. In addition, altered growth hormone secretion decreased levels of sinusoidal bile acid transport proteins, sodium-dependent taurocholate cotransporter (*Ntcp*), and organic anion transport proteins (*Oatp*). (From Simon FR, Fortune J, Iwahashi M, et al. Ethinyl estradiol cholestasis involves alterations in expression of liver sinusoidal transporters. *Am J Physiol* 1996,271:G1043–1052, with permission).

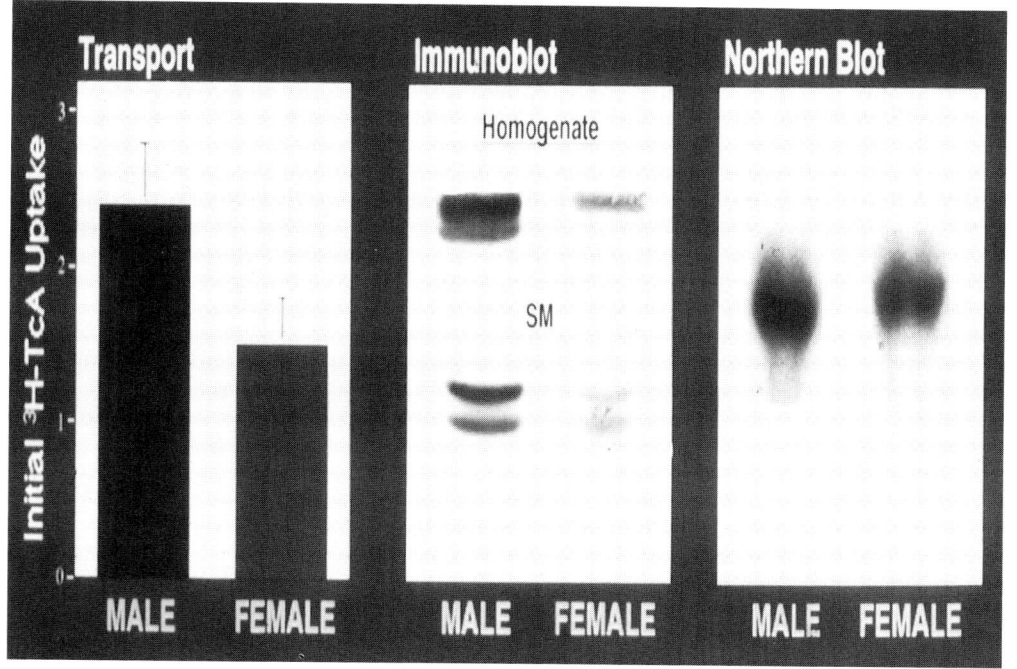

FIGURE 27.3. Sexual dimorphic expression of the sodium/dependent taurocholate transporter. Maximum transport uptake rate, protein content in liver homogenates and sinusoidal membrane (*SM*) fractions, and mRNA levels were measured in male and female rat livers.

extensively than those of other hormones. It is generally assumed that the mechanisms by which estrogens alter bile formation and organic anion excretion in animals are related to the changes in hepatic function that occur during pregnancy and with the use of oral contraceptives containing estrogen.

Retention of BSP (an organic anion predominately cleared from plasma by oatp1 and excreted into bile by Mrp2) was shown to be abnormal in humans treated with natural estrogens, as early as 1964 (111). The effect was seen within one day and was reversible when the estrogen was discontinued. Subsequent studies using the Wheeler BSP infusion technique showed that estrogens consistently depressed hepatic secretory transport maximum (Tm) for the dye (112–114). BSP Tm was decreased during the latter half of pregnancy to 77% of control, and with oral contraceptive steroid administration to 60% (113,114). Since Preisig et al. (115) had shown that BSP Tm is similar in male and female subjects, these studies established that "high" levels of estrogens are associated with dye retention. Pregnancy and oral contraceptives may also increase serum bilirubin in previously anicteric individuals with the Dubin–Johnson syndrome, intrahepatic cholestasis of pregnancy (ICP) or underlying chronic liver disease (72,116,117).

ICP is a well-characterized liver disorder usually manifested in the last trimester of pregnancy and disappears spontaneously after delivery. ICP is diagnosed when skin pruritus appears during the second half of a previously uneventful pregnancy. These symptoms are associated with increased serum bile salts (30-fold), a mild or moderate increase in aminotransferases and occasionally mild hyperbilirubinemia (less than 5mg/dL). Values for alkaline phosphatase and γ-glutamyltranspeptidase are usually in the range detectable during normal pregnancy (118). Symptoms and laboratory values usually return to normal less than one month postpartum.

The cause of ICP is unknown. A number of clinical observations relate its pathogenesis to hepatic metabolism of female sex hormones (72,119). The temporal pattern of ICP is similar to that for estrogen synthesis, which attains its highest levels during the last trimester of pregnancy (120). Also, the prevalence of ICP is five times greater in twin compared to single pregnancies; the synthesis of estrogens and progesterone is higher than during single pregnancy (121). Other possibilities include production of an abnormal estrogen metabolite or an increase in the hepatic susceptibility to cholestatic effects of normal estrogen metabolites. Impairment in sulfation, which is an important metabolic pathway in the detoxification of estrogens, has been reported in patients with ICP and in women taking contraceptive pills (122). The imbalance of sulfation and glucuronidation associated with high levels of estrogens might also play a role. In most studies, serum levels and urinary excretion of estrogens and metabolites have not been found to be different during ICP as compared to in normal pregnancies (120,123). Thus, direct evidence supporting the role of estrogens and their metabolites is lacking.

An alternative hypothesis proposes that the formation of large amounts of sulfated progesterone metabolites might predispose susceptible women to an inhibition of hepatic transport of organic anions (124). Elevated levels of serum sulfated metabolites of progesterone have been reported (124), and other studies have found that a majority of patients with ICP in France had taken oral, natural progesterone for risk of premature delivery (125). Further controlled studies demonstrated that administration of progesterone increased serum bile acid levels during the third trimester of pregnancy (126,127). However, the mechanisms involved in progesterone-induced cholestasis are unclear, since progestins have not been shown to decrease hepatic clearance of BSP (76).

Because ICP occurs in families and is particularly prevalent in certain countries (Chile and Scandinavia), both genetic and environmental factors have been evoked. It is possible that the susceptibility trait is related to an abnormal hepatic metabolic response to physiologic increases in estrogens during pregnancy or following their administration. In support of this hypothesis, Reyes et al. (128) demonstrated an exaggerated abnormal BSP clearance following low-dose estrogen administration in women with a history of ICP, and most importantly a similar exaggerated response was observed in nulligestant women and even men whose sisters or mothers had ICP. Furthermore, there is a higher prevalence of the disorder in mothers and sisters of patients with ICP, and pedigree studies have documented a familial clustering of ICP (129). Further support for the hypothesis was recently reported where a number of individuals in a large pedigree had a heterozygous nonsense mutation in the MDR3 gene associated with ICP (130). However, other preliminary studies have found defects in the bile salt export transporter and the FIC1 gene regions. Thus, ICP may present with similar phenotypic features due to different underlying genetic abnormalities in organic anion transport.

Epidemiological studies have supported a familial association. However, although Scandinavian countries and Chile showed very high incidences of ICP in early studies, more recent reports have demonstrated a markedly lower incidence, suggesting that environmental factors may also contribute (119). It is not known what exogenous factors may participate to make ICP apparent. For instance, ICP recurs in only 65% of the pregnancies, the clinical and biochemical severity fluctuates during an affected pregnancy, and there is a seasonal variability to its occurrence (131).

Androgens

Treatment of patients with anabolic steroids has been associated with hepatic complications including peliosis hepatitis, liver tumors and cholestasis (132). In humans, methyl testosterone and norethandrolone, but not physiological androgens, impair BSP transport (133,134). Addition of "cholestatic" androgens to isolated rat hepatocytes also impairs bile salt uptake (135,136). However, little is known about the mechanisms involved in the pathogenesis of androgen-induced impairment of transport function, since animal models have not been reported.

Androgen receptors are reported to be present in human and rat liver (137). Similar to other steroid nuclear receptors, androgen receptors mediate physiological actions of androgens, primarily testosterone and 5 α-dihydrotestosterone. Ligand binding induces receptor homodimerization, resulting in binding to a glucocorticoid-like DNA hormone response element (138). To date, none of the genes involved in bile flow have been demonstrated to be altered by androgens. It is possible that androgens inhibit function by competing for a glucocorticoid or other hormone response element. Other possibilities include polymorphism in androgen metabolism, and norethandrolone alteration of microfilaments (139).

Glucocorticoids

The naturally occurring adrenal glucocorticoid corticosterone, 11-deoxycorticosterone, cortisone and cortisol regulate a variety of metabolic pathways in liver including carbohydrate, protein and lipid metabolism. Many of these effects are due to the direct effect of glucocorticoids on liver gene expression. Indeed, liver proteins have been model genes to study glucocorticoid regulation of gene expression. Studies have demonstrated that glucocorticoids may influence gene expression through the glucocorticoid receptor, the PXR receptor (at high doses) and by interacting with other transcription factors (140).

Glucocorticoids increase bile flow in dogs and rats (141–145). Most studies used pharmacological doses of glucocorticoids, and few studies have been directed at mechanism(s). At pharmacological doses, PXR rather than the glucocorticoid receptor may mediate the molecular process (146). Miner et al. (141) examined the effect of adrenalectomy and cortisone replacement on bile salt-independent bile flow (BSIBF), bile salt excretion and BSP Tm. Adrenalectomy decreased BSIBF, but did not change bile salt excretion or the maximal capacity to transport BSP. They further demonstrated that adrenalectomy reduced and glucocorticoid replacement increased NaK-ATPase activity and protein content. Together these studies demonstrated that glucocorticoids increase bile secretion, but the mechanism was unclear since glucocorticoids might modulate other transporters or alter the membrane lipid environment.

In rats deficient in the canalicular cMOAT/Mrp2 gene, BSIBF and glutathione secretion are reduced, suggesting this transporter contributes at least in part to the generation of this component of bile flow (147,148). Both rat and human Mrp2 genes have been cloned, and DNA elements in the promoter region have been identified which potentially recognize glucocorticoids (149,150). Although physiological doses of glucocorticoids have not been reported, dexamethasone, a potent glucocorticoid, increased Mrp2 (151,152) and protected against downregulation following administration of lipopolysaccharide (153). In addition, Simon et al. described induction of Mrp2 in intact rats and isolated hepatocytes at both physiological and pharmacological concentrations of dexamethasone (154). Thus, these studies suggest that physiological as well as pharmacological administrations of glucocorticoids increase bile flow, possibly by involving induction of both the sodium pump and Mrp2.

Glucocorticoids mediate changes in gene expression classically by binding to cytosolic glucocorticoid receptors which homodimerize and bind to hormone response elements (55,58). Glucocorticoids bind to other transcription factors such as PXR, which induces CYP3A (146). In addition, glucocorticoid receptors may interact with AP1 elements through binding to the fos/jun heterodimer (58). Studies to define the molecular regulation of transporters by glucocorticoids have not been reported, but are of importance since these drugs are frequently used to treat patients with liver disease.

Nonsteroid Nuclear Receptors

This family of receptors is characterized by heterodimerization of one partner with the retinoid X receptor (RXR) (59). Potentially important ligands and/or receptors that may be involved in regulation of bile secretion include thyroid hormone (TR), so-called orphan receptors for bile acids (FXR) and oxysterols (LXR), xenobiotics including phenobarbital (CAR), and the antisteroid pregnenolone-16a-carbonitrile (PCN) (PXR) (Chapter 69).

Thyroid Hormone

Two different modes of action have been described for thyroid hormone: (a) nongenomic or plasma membrane and mitochondrial effects, and (b) genomic or nuclear effects. Genomic effects are mediated only by T_3 and require at least several hours to detect changes in rates of gene transcription.

The liver removes circulating thyroxine and T_3, where T_4 is converted to its active form T_3 by 5'-deiodinase. T_3 passes into the nucleus and binds to the thyroid receptor (TR). TRs can bind to thyroid response element (TREs) with or without ligand. T_3-bound TR may dimerize with itself or form a homodimer or with the 9-*cis*-retinoic acid receptor (RXR) to form a heterodimer. In addition, coactivators and corepressors interact with the DNA-bound TR to induce positive or negative transcriptional regulation (65,155,156).

Hyperthyroidism and hypothyroidism are associated with changes in liver function such as BSP retention, and transaminase and alkaline phosphatase elevation (157). Minor histological changes such as steatosis may be seen on liver biopsy. Thyroid hormone is an important modulator of intermediary metabolism. Its actions include stimulation of both lipogenesis and lipolysis and protein synthesis. Hypothyroidism is associated with altered lipoprotein metabolism, including decreased LDL receptors, hepatic lipase activity, and sterol and bile acid turnover (158). Thyroid status in the rat influences bile secretion and composition. Thyroid administration increases the bile salt pool size due to increased synthesis (159,160). Increased bile flow is due to alterations in the bile salt-independent fraction as well as the bile salt-dependent bile flow, but changes in the bile salt-independent flow are more prominent (161).

Several studies have demonstrated that hyperthyroidism and hypothyroidism modulate the BSIBF (98,161,162). These changes in BSIBF correlate with lipid composition, membrane fluidity and NaK-ATPase activity in hepatic plasma membranes (98). However, the effect of thyroid status on other transporters involved in the generation of bile flow has not been examined. Preliminary studies suggest that thyroid hormone may also regulate levels of Ntcp and especially Mrp2 (163,164). Since hepatic bilirubin transport is also decreased in thyroidectomized as well as hypophysectomized rats (162), this indicates that thyroid hormone may be a critical factor in regulating bilirubin transport as well as BSIBF, both functions associated with Mrp2 activity.

Orphan Nuclear Receptor Ligands

The term "orphan receptor" was coined over ten years ago to describe gene products that appeared to belong to the nuclear receptor family on the basis of sequence identity, but that lacked identified hormones. Discovery of these gene products has lead to the development of the field of "reverse endocrinology" (60). A number of these receptors have helped in the understanding of drug and lipid metabolism, and this very likely is the beginning of unraveling molecular mechanisms underlying hormonal and drug effects on bile secretion as well. At least four families of orphan receptors may participate in the regulation of bile secretion. Two receptors are involved in the control of cholesterol and bile acid metabolism: farnesol X receptor (FXR) and liver X receptor (LXR) (69). In addition, the pregnane X receptor (PXR) and the androstane receptor (CAR) mediate xenobiotics which are known to induce cytochrome P450s as well as increase bile flow (Chapter 69).

Bile acids are the major driving force for bile secretion. Chenodeoxycholate was shown to interact with the nuclear hormone receptor, FXR, to suppress transcription of cholesterol 7α-hydroxylase and to induce the ileal bile

acid binding protein (165–167). In contrast, LXR, the oxysterol receptor, activates cholesterol 7α-hydroxylase (168–170). Other tissue-specific factors are undoubtedly involved in regulation of this critical step in bile acid synthesis. Recent studies have also shown that Ntcp and Mrp2 may be downregulated by RAR/RXR heterodimers following stimulation by interleukin-1β (171). Together these observations have suggested a model for regulation of cholesterol and bile acid metabolism where FXR is involved in feedforward regulation whereas LXR participates in feedback regulation (69).

PXR was discovered to be involved in the regulation of CYP3A, the cytochrome that metabolizes a majority of xenobiotics (146). PXR, which is selectively expressed in liver and intestine, is activated by an array of compounds and binds as a heterodimer with RXR to a xenobiotic response element. Pregnanes such as PCN are the most potent compounds, but corticosteroids and estrogens also activate PXR (60,62). Xenobiotic response elements have also been identified in Mrp2, UDP-gluconyltransferase and other cytochromes (62). Thus, in addition to being a potential steroid hormone "sensor," PXR may be involved in a coordinated process of drug metabolism and biliary excretion.

The fourth class of orphan receptors that may be involved in bile secretion is constitutive androstane receptor (CAR). Phenobarbital (PB) is well established to increase bile flow and has been shown to increase Mrp2 mRNA and protein content (89,172,173). A major advance in our understanding of the mechanism of PB induction was provided by the recent discovery of Negishi and coworkers that the liver-enriched orphan nuclear receptor CAR is the factor that interacts with the PB-response element (174,175). CAR binds as a heterodimer with RXR. Recent evidence suggests that CAR is a constitutive androstane receptor and that PB derepresses the androstane inhibition of CAR binding leading to gene induction (176). PB also binds to PXR, and thus its effects may also be mediated by this receptor. Thus, PB like PCN utilizes endogenous steroid nuclear receptors to induce genes which may be involved in the generation of bile flow.

EFFECTS OF PEPTIDE HORMONES ON LIVER

Nonpituitary Hormones

Peptide hormones such as vasopressin, glucagon and insulin bind to specific receptors on the liver sinusoidal surface. Intracellular signals are mediated by a number of mechanisms including receptor phosphorylation (insulin), synthesis of cAMP through activation of adenylate cyclase, and guanosine (GTP)-binding protein (177). Hormonal binding to the GTP-binding protein leads to activation of a specific phospholipase, resulting in hydrolysis of phosphatidylinositol 4,5 bisphosphate and 1,2 diacylglycerol. Diacylglycerol as well as intracellular calcium activates protein kinase C (PKC), which involves the translocation of PKC from the cytosol to the cell membrane, where it phosphorylates serine/threonine sites on proteins. In addition to being integral in many cellular regulatory processes, PKC has also been implicated in the regulation of bile acid synthesis and bile secretion. It was shown to modulate 7α-hydroxylase in cultured rat hepatocytes (178) and to inhibit bile secretion in the perfused rat liver (179). In contrast, hormones such as glucagon and vasoactive intestinal peptide as well as β-adrenergic agonists promote hepatocellular cAMP synthesis from ATP through activation of adenylate cyclase, mediated by a stimulatory GTP-binding protein. Through cAMP synthesis and cAMP-dependent protein kinase activation, these hormones play an important role in hepatic regulation of glycogenolysis and gluconeogenesis as well as DNA synthesis (177). They also regulate bile acid synthesis and bile secretion (180–182). Glucagon and secretin, through the generation of cAMP, have choleretic effects involving both biliary bile acid excretion and bile flow (183–186).

cAMP stimulates both bile salt uptake and excretion. Increased uptake may be related in part to hyperpolarized sinusoidal membrane, which in turn would stimulate sodium-dependent uptake of taurocholate (187). A recent series of studies demonstrated that Ntcp is phosphorylated, and this is associated with increased translocation of the transporter from an endosomal location to the sinusoidal domain (32,188,189). Bile acid efflux is also stimulated by cAMP. Other studies have identified that cAMP increases the translocation of ABC-transporters involved in bile secretion from an intracellular pool to the bile canalicular domain through a mechanism involving microtubule-dependent transcytotic vesicular translocation (31,180,181,190–192). These effects support a coordinated mechanism for rapidly adjusting bile acid efflux as a function of bile acid concentrations and intracellular signaling processes.

Insulin, in addition to promotion of protein synthesis and control of carbohydrate metabolism, produces choleresis in dogs (193,194). Diabetes alters the composition of bile as a result of changes in cholesterol and bile acid metabolism (195,196). Diabetes also increases ileal taurocholate uptake, which may contribute to a markedly enlarged bile salt pool size (196,197). In addition to stimulation of bile flow rates, diabetes also alters biliary excretion of several organic anions (198). Since diabetes increases bile salts and not BSP Tm, selective regulation of bile salt Tm probably is due to increased bile salt bile size, rather than a direct effect of insulin on Bsep function (199). On the other hand, other investigators have shown that diabetes induces cholestasis (200,201). These latter studies suggested that hyperglycemia as well as hypoinsulinemia decreased BSIBF, but the specific mechanisms were not determined.

Pituitary Hormones

Studies in rats, dogs, and humans have indicated that pituitary hormones also participate in the regulation of hepatic transport of organic anions and generation of bile flow. Following hypophysectomy, bile acid synthesis, bile flow, and biliary excretion of bile acids, bilirubin and BSP are reduced (160,162,202). As discussed above, glucocorticoids and thyroid hormone make important contributions to the regulation of bile flow and organic anion transport. However, a number of studies also indicate that GH and prolactin contribute significantly to bile acid transport and bile flow. Another class of intracellular signaling molecules mediates the cellular action of these hormones. Growth hormone and prolactin receptors do not contain tyrosine kinase activity, but rather rely on the so-called JAK/STAT pathway for signal transduction (203–215). In addition to their recognized role in the determination of sexual dimorphic metabolism of xenobiotic and endogenous steroid compounds, these hormones are important regulators of both sinusoidal and bile canalicular transporters.

Growth Hormone

Growth hormone (GH) belongs to a family of hormones that includes prolactin (Prl) and somatomammotropin/placental lactogen (216,217). The role of GH in maintaining growth and its influence on the intermediary metabolism of glucose, lipids and protein are well known. However, its roles in drug metabolism and bile flow are not as well appreciated. Many of the functional effects of GH are mediated by insulin-like growth factors (IGF-1 and IGF-II) which are produced primarily in liver (218). One important experimental task is to determine which GH-associated effects are caused indirectly through IGF actions and which are due to GH. In addition, GH secretion is partially regulated by other steroid hormones, especially estrogens and androgens (48,219–223). Thus it is also important to separate the direct sex steroid effects on liver from those mediated by GH.

Growth Hormone Secretion and Cellular Signaling

GH secretion by the pituitary in rats is pulsatile, with the frequency of pulsations being sex-dependent and under the influence of gonadal steroid hormones (221–228). In adult female rats, a high pulse frequency results in the continuous presence of GH in the circulation (10 to 20 ng/ml). In contrast, in adult male rats GH is intermittently present in plasma, with regular peaks (100 or 200 ng/ml) detected each 3 or 4 hours followed by trough periods of no detectable GH. This pattern of pituitary GH secretion is ultimately regulated by sex steroids, primarily at the level of the hypothalamus, affecting the balance between the secretion of GHRH and somatostatin. In addition, peripheral hormones including thyroid hormone, glucocorticoids and IGF-I, as well as GH, regulate GH secretion (47). Thus, it is difficult to interpret whether sex steroid hormones administered to intact animals act directly or indirectly on the liver.

The sexually differentiated plasma GH profiles regulate the expression of a number of liver proteins, including many cytochrome P450s, receptors, and secretory proteins (Table 27.4). For example, the continuous plasma GH pattern positively regulates the female-specific CYP2C12 gene, while the expression of the male-specific CYP 2C11 is stimulated by the male pattern of intermittent GH pulsation (229–230). In addition, GH may require other pituitary hormones to initiate its regulation (231,232). Steroid 5α-reductase, which is also a female-expressed gene, is dependent on the interaction of the steady plasma level of GH with T$_4$ to upregulate its expression in females (232). In contrast, intermittent GH secretion plus thyroid hormone is important in the downregulation of alcohol dehydrogenase gene expression found in male rats (233).

The effects of GH on liver gene expression involves a direct action of the hormone on hepatocytes (234,235), through specific receptors which are expressed prominently in the liver in approximately equal density in male and female rats (Fig. 27.4) (236). The GH receptor is structurally related to members of the cytokine/hematopoietin superfamily of receptors, with the highest degree of homology to the prolactin receptor (237). One molecule of GH binds to the receptor at the cell surface, inducing homodimerization and activation of intracellular signaling events. Dimerization of receptors results in a conformational change in the intracellular domain, allowing association and activation of JAK2 (192). This leads to tyrosine phosphorylation of the receptor, recruitment of SH2-containing

molecules to the complex and subsequently tyrosine phosphorylation of STAT molecules (STATs 1, 3, and 5) (203–205). Phosphorylation permits dimerization of STAT5 with movement to the nucleus and binding to specific gamma activated sequences (GAS). Specific phosphatases within the cell presumably terminate transcriptional enhancement (204). It has been shown that the male pattern of GH secretion increases the content of phosphorylated STAT5 (especially 5b), whereas the female pattern downregulates its nuclear content (208–212). In STAT5b knockout mice, their intrinsic response to the male GH secretory pattern is lost (204). GH also elicits intracellular signaling through the activation of the mitogen-activated protein (MAP) kinase transduction pathway, phosphorylation of IRS-1 and activation of PI$_3$ kinase, and enhanced formation of diacylglycerol by phospholipase C with subsequent activation of PKC (203,238,239). Thus, multiple and interacting pathways converge within the cell to mediate the cellular responses to GH. Most likely the combinatorial interplay of these transcription pathways is important in the sexual dimorphic expression of hepatic genes.

GH, like other polypeptide hormones, is secreted in a pulsatile fashion in humans and animals. However, differences in the secretion patterns exist among rats, mice, and humans. In male mice and rats, serum GH peaks occur in a regular pattern. The two rodent species differ, however, in that GH profiles of mice do not demonstrate a sex difference in either the peak height or baseline level (240). In humans, the mean GH levels are higher in females than males (241,242). In addition, during pregnancy serum GH levels are markedly elevated, due to placental lactogen secretion (223).

Human studies have shown that GH status alters BSP Tm. The results are summarized in Figure 27.5. Preisig et al. studied 11 patients with acromegaly, using the Wheeler BSP infusion technique (115). Liver size was greater in the acromegalic patients compared to controls. Their BSP storage capacity was within normal limits, but BSP Tm was markedly increased and on average was double the normal values (115). Similar changes were measured in dogs with chronic administration of GH (243). On the other hand, a study of patients with hypopituitarism revealed normal BSP storage capacity, but BSP Tm was decreased by 40% (244). Importantly, in one patient with selective GH deficiency, BSP Tm was also decreased (244). Cholestasis and jaundice is also a common finding (30%) in neonatal hypopituitarism (245). In rats, hypophysectomy in addition to resulting in reductions in bile acid synthesis and bile flow also decreased bilirubin and BSP maximum transport (162,202). Although thyroid hormone was important for the correction of bile flow and bilirubin transport, GH had a major role in restoration of normal function. These results are consistent with the molecular interaction of GH and thyroid hormone in the regulation of Mrp2 (164), the canalicular transporter principally responsible for both bilirubin and BSP excretion.

TABLE 27.4. PROTEINS REGULATED BY GROWTH HORMONE IN THE RAT

Liver Proteins	Relative Expression Levels	
	Male	Female
Secretory Proteins		
IGF-1	++++	++++
Serine protease inhibitor	+++	+++
α$_1$-antitrypsin	+++	+++
Mouse urinary protein	++++	+
α$_2$-microglobulin	++++	+
Lipoprotein lipase	+++	+++
Enzymes		
CYP2E1	++	++++
CYP2C11	++++	+
CYP2C12	+	++++
CYP3A2	+++	+
Steroid 5α-reductase	+	++++
Alcohol dehydrogenase	++	++++
Receptors		
GH-R	+++	+++
Prl-R	+	+++
LDL-R	++	+++

GH-R, growth hormone receptor; IGF, insulin-like growth factors; LDL-R, low-density lipoprotein receptor; Prl-R, prolactin receptor.

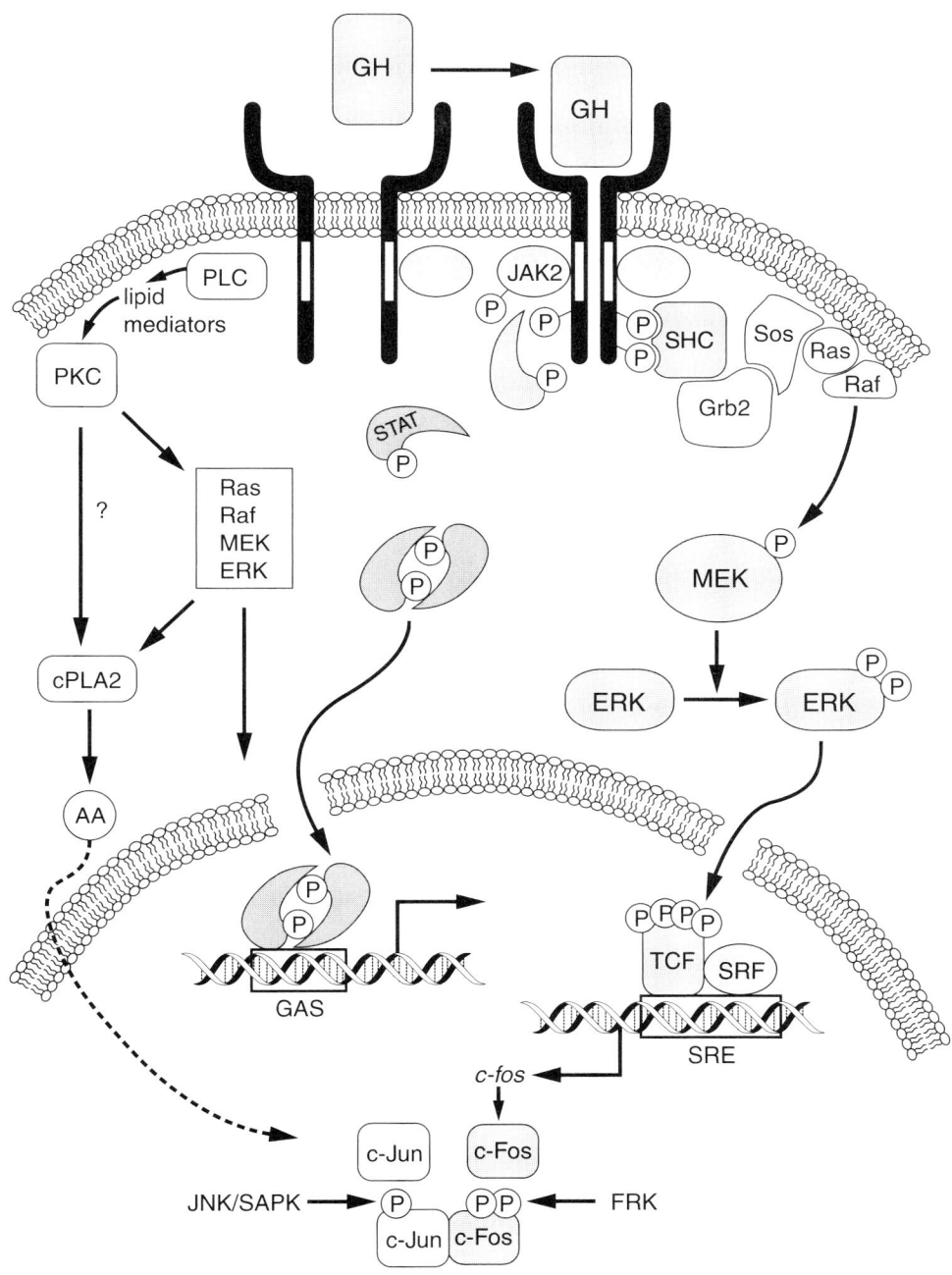

FIGURE 27.4. Signal transduction pathways for growth hormone action. Three major pathways are shown: the JAK/STAT pathway, the Ras-ERK pathway and the DAG-PKC pathway, for gene regulation. *GAS*, gamma activated sequences; *GH*, growth hormone; *PKC*, protein kinase C. See text for details. Adapted from Mode A (Ph.D. thesis, unpublished).

Sexual Dimorphic Expression of Hepatic Function

It has become clear that the liver is a sexually differentiated tissue (44,48,50,52). This phenomenon has been demonstrated best in rodents and is measured as sex differences in the level of many hepatic proteins ranging from receptors and secretory proteins to enzymes (Table 4). The most extensively studied enzymes exhibiting dimorphic levels are members of the cytochrome (CYP) P450 family (45–47). These enzymes catalyze the oxidation of a vast array of drugs, xenobiotics and steroids (246). Although most CYP P450-catalyzed reactions are more efficient in male than in female liver, a prominent exception is CYP2C12, which is

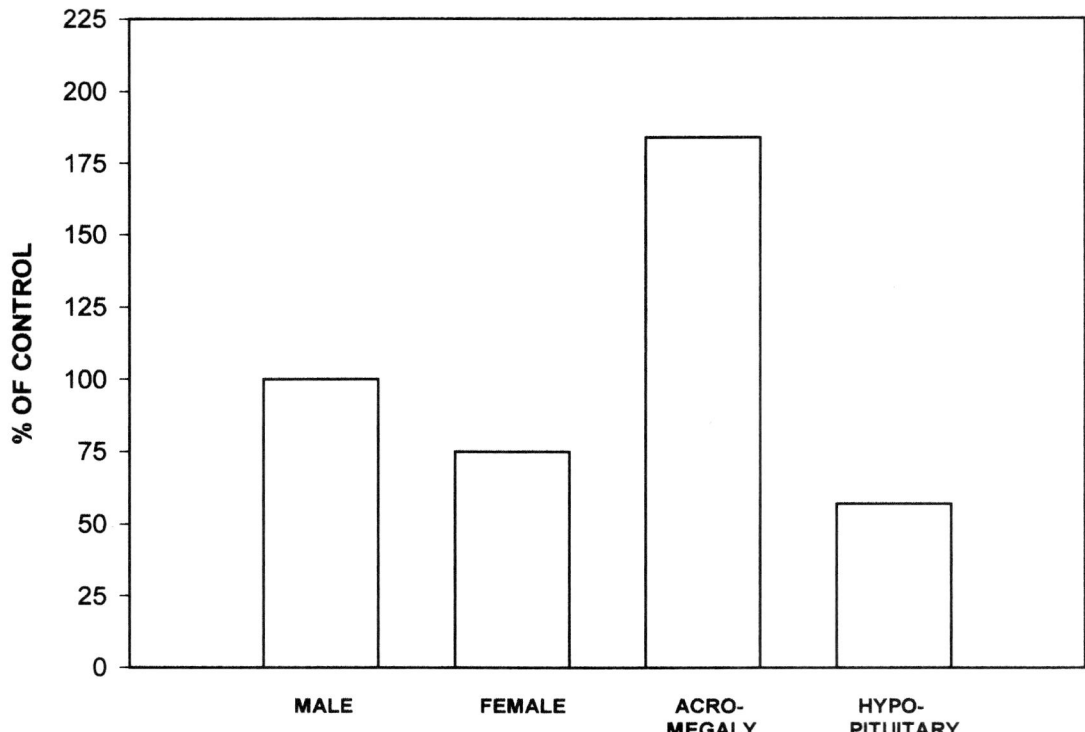

FIGURE 27.5. Effect of gender, acromegaly, and hypopituitarism on BSP Tm in humans compared to controls. The graph is derived from data in Preisig R, Morris TQ, Shaver JC, et al. Volumetric, hemodynamic, and excretory characteristics of the liver in acromegaly. *J Clin Invest* 1966; 45:1379–1387 and Schmidt ML, Gartner LM, Arias IM. Studies of hepatic excretory function. 3. Effect of hypopituitarism on the hepatic excretion of sulfobromophthalein sodium in man. *Gastroenterology* 1967;52:998–1002, with permission.

expressed dominantly in female rat liver (50). The physiological significance of sex differences in the liver is largely unknown, especially in humans, but these differences may be important in maintaining appropriate endocrine balance and metabolism of drugs (247). In addition, several diseases occur in a sex-dependent manner, including development of hepatoma, cholestasis and susceptibility to drug toxicity.

CYP2C11 and CYP2C12 are steroid hydroxylases that are differentially expressed in livers from male and female rats (50). In hypophysectomized rats, devoid of GH, there is no sex difference in mRNA levels for these cytochromes (230). The importance of the GH pattern is shown by the administration of a continuous infusion of GH (mimicking the female pattern of GH secretion), where CYP2C12 is increased and CYP2C11 is further decreased (248,249). In contrast, the administration of GH intermittently in the male pattern selectively increased CYP2C11 (230,249, 250). These effects are the direct effect of GH on hepatocytes and not due to release of IGF-1 (244). Although GH is the major regulator of hepatic GH-responsive genes, as with other hormone-regulated genes, glucocorticoids, insulin and especially thyroid hormone contribute to their regulation (231,232). The promoter regions of CYP2C11

and 12 were cloned years ago; however, despite intensive investigation, the GH-responsive region for CYP2C12 had not been definitively identified until recently, when a STAT binding site far upstream was uncovered (251).

Studies utilizing STAT knockout mice and cell lines expressing GH receptors have provided strong evidence for the role of STAT5b and its differential phosphorylation in the regulation of sexual dimorphic expression of hepatic GH-responsive genes (52,210,211,213–215). Waxman and associates demonstrated that STAT5b is tyrosine phosphorylated in male but not female rats in response to GH pulses. Intermittent plasma GH pulses initiate rapid tyrosine phosphorylation and nuclear translocation of liver STAT5b, while the continuous pattern of GH secretion downregulates STAT5b signaling. Furthermore, in mice, STAT5b gene disruption leads to loss of sexually differentiated responses including the sexually dimorphic pattern of liver genes, and male-characteristic body growth rates (213). However, other studies show that STAT5a and STAT5b are both required for constitutive expression in female liver of female predominate cytochromes (215).

In addition to drug metabolism, gender differences have been described for hepatic transport for organic anions including taurocholate, bilirubin, BSP, indocyanine green, fatty acids and some steroid hormones (106,252–258). Although some studies indicate that gender differences in drug excretion may exist, sex differences in bile flow have not been shown (259). Brock and Vore first demonstrated that taurocholate uptake was two-fold greater in males compared to females (252). Simon et al. (106) confirmed these results and further demonstrated that the difference in taurocholate uptake was due to increased content of the sodium-dependent taurocholate cotransporter, which was transcriptionally determined. The mechanism for transport differences in other organic anions has not been reported. Figure 27.6 demonstrates mRNA levels for several bile canalicular transporters and proteins present at the bile canalicular domain. Bile salt export protein and MDR2/3 were not sexually differentiated. However, Mrp2 mRNA level was four-fold greater in females. This differential expression was determined by the GH secretory pattern (164). At the present time it is not clear that similar gender differences are present in humans, but GH is an important factor in the control of BSP transport (115,244).

Sexual dimorphic expression of hepatic genes is determined for the most part by the secretory pattern of GH and only rarely by a direct effect of sex steroids on the liver (44,48). Although hepatic drug metabolism and uptake of organic anions is established to be differentially expressed in male and female rats, sexual dimorphic biliary excretion of organic anions and bile flow has not been extensively examined (259). Thus the effect of estrogen administration on the hepatic transport, at least at the sinusoidal level, may be determined in large part by the effect of estrogens on GH secretion, as shown in the schematic model in Figure 27.7. Although it is not clear that GH secretion in humans has as marked a differential secretory pattern as the rat, studies in humans as well as animals implicate GH and possibly thyroid hormone in the regulation of biliary transport processes.

Prolactin

Prolactin (Prl) is a 23kd peptide hormone secreted by the anterior pituitary (260). Secretion of Prl is markedly stimulated by suckling and by estrogen (260). Prl actions are mediated by binding to its receptor, which belongs to the GH/cytokine receptor family (237). The Prl receptor is expressed predominately in female liver with only low levels in male (263,264). In contrast to the GH receptor, the Prl receptor exists as a long form in the breast and liver, but in liver the short or inactive form of the receptor is present at greater levels (262,263). Prl receptor levels are also regulated by the GH secretory pattern and greatly reduced in hypophysectomized rats (264). Intracellular signaling mechanisms for Prl in the breast are similar to GH in that both involve the JAK/STAT pathway (265). However, in breast one sees an increase in STAT5a, while Choi and Waxman were unable to demonstrate a similar response in liver (266).

At supraphysiological levels, Prl stimulates both sodium-dependent taurocholate uptake (267,268) and ATP-dependent taurocholate transport (269). In addition, in postpartum female rats, taurocholate transport, Ntcp mRNA and protein were increased compared to controls (267,268). It was proposed that Prl stimulated STAT phosphorylation and binding to putative STAT (GAS) sites in the Ntcp promoter (270). However, suckling also stimulates GH release, which may lead to similar signaling processes.

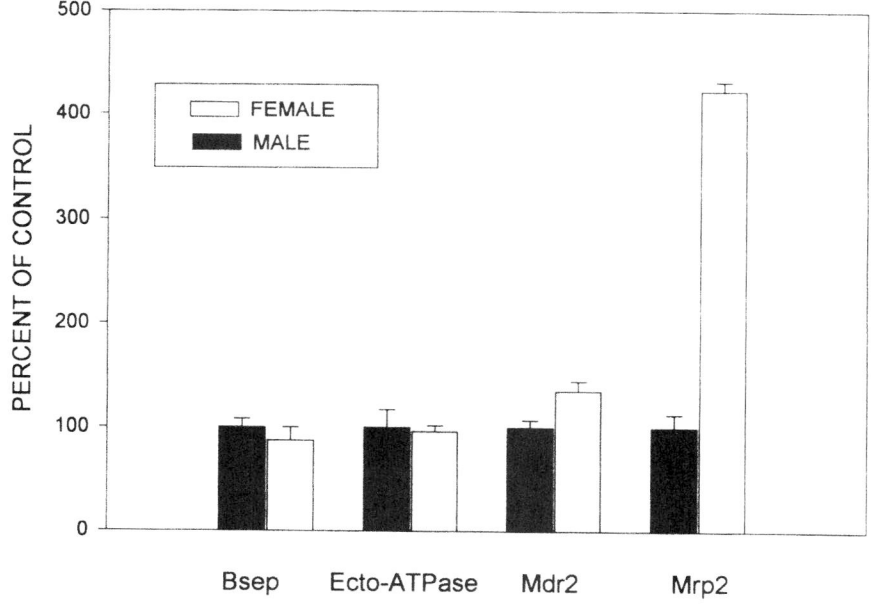

FIGURE 27.6. Steady-state mRNA levels of bile canalicular transporters in male and female rats. Levels are relative to male values. Mrp2 mRNA levels were expressed in a sexually dimorphic pattern.

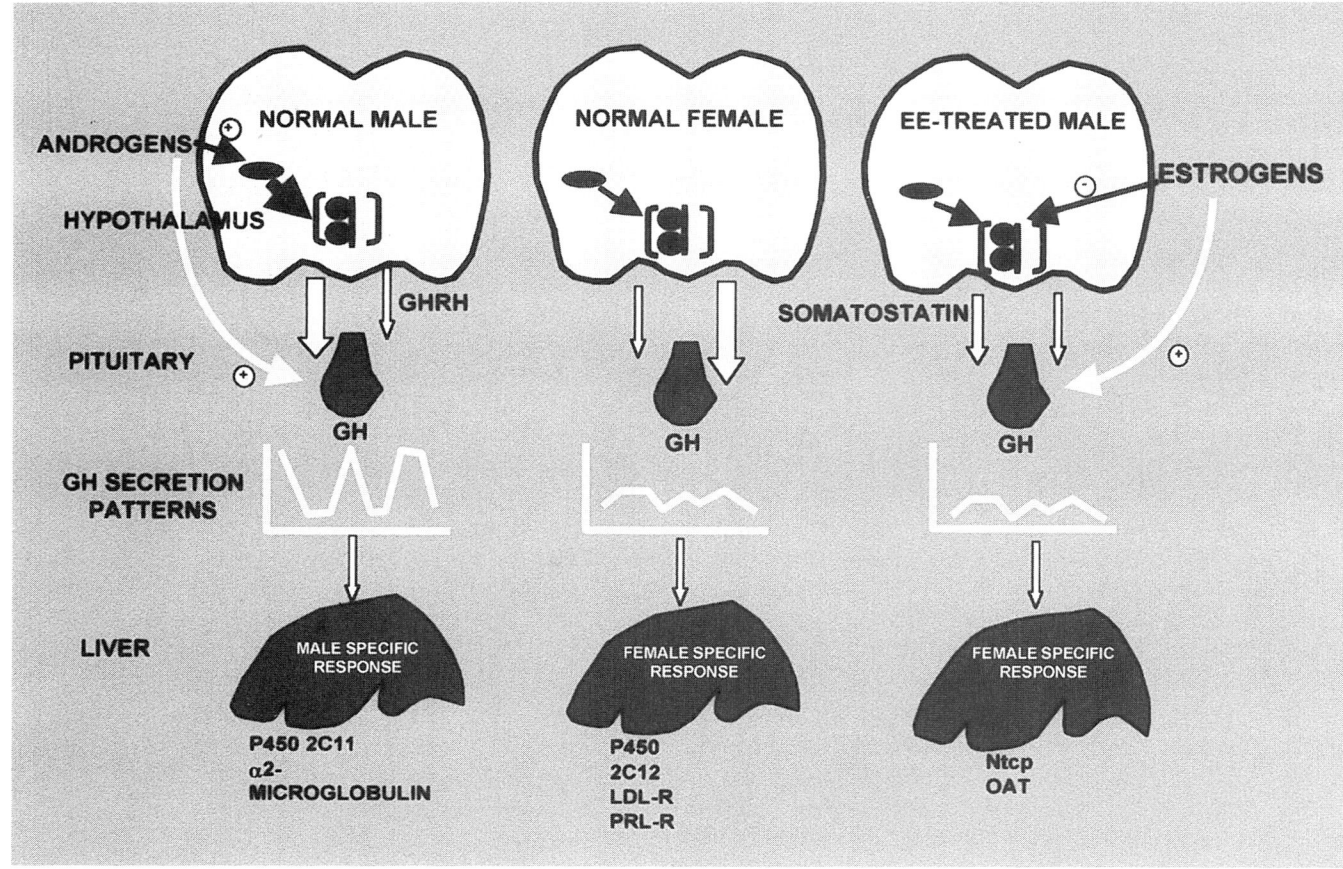

FIGURE 27.7. Model of the hypothalamic–pituitary–liver axis and sex steroid regulation of the sexual dimorphic pattern of growth hormone secretion in the rat. Growth hormone (*GH*) secretory patterns regulate the differential expression of specific genes in liver. Estrogen administration to male rats converts the intermittent male growth hormone pattern to a constant female pattern. This change in GH secretion alters the expression of hepatic GH-responsive genes. *LDL-R*, low-density lipoprotein receptor; *Ntcp*, sodium-dependent taurocholate cotransporter; OAT, organic anion transporter protein. (From Gustafsson J-A: The hypothalamic-pituitary-liver axis. Growth hormone controls liver sex. In: Arias IM, Boyer JL, Fausto N, Jakoby WB, Schachter DA, Shafritz DA, eds. *The Liver: Biology and Pathobiology*, 3rd Edition. New York: Raven Press, 1994: 1209–1214, with permission.)

CONCLUSION

There have been remarkable advances in our knowledge of both the bile secretory pathway and intracellular signaling mechanisms involved in regulating hormone actions in the liver. The merging of disciplines should provide a better understanding of the mechanisms involved in the pathogenesis of cholestasis, and may lead to pharmacological insights toward the development of therapeutic tools to treat some forms of cholestasis.

ACKNOWLEDGMENTS

The work was supported by National Institutes of Health Grant RO1 DK-15851 and Veterans Affairs Merit Review grants. Appreciation is also extended to J.-A. Gustafsson and A. Mode, who provided many of the ideas for this review during discussions with the author during his sabbatical leave at the Department of Medical Nutrition, NOVUM, Karolinska Institute. The author is also grateful to his longtime associates Mieko Iwahashi and Eileen Sutherland, who have contributed many extra hours to the successful generation of experimental data.

REFERENCES

1. Trauner M, Meier PJ, Boyer JL. Molecular pathogenesis of cholestasis. *N Engl J Med* 1998;339:1217–1227.
2. Bahar RJ, Stolz A. Bile acid transport. *Gastroenterol Clin North Am* 1999;28:27–58.
3. Oude Elferink RP, Meijer DK, Kuipers F, et al. Hepatobiliary secretion of organic compounds; molecular mechanisms of membrane transport. *Biochim Biophys Acta* 1995;1241:215–268.

4. Stieger B, Meier PJ. Bile acid and xenobiotic transporters in liver. *Curr Opin Cell Biol* 1998;4:462–467.

5. Hagenbuch B, Meier PJ. Sinusoidal (basolateral) bile salt uptake systems of hepatocytes. *Semin Liver Dis* 1996;16:129–136.

6. Meier PJ. Molecular mechanisms of hepatic bile salt transport from sinusoidal blood into bile. *Am J Physiol* 1995;269: G801–812.

7. Gatmaitan ZC, Arias IM. ATP-dependent transport systems in the canalicular membrane of the hepatocyte. *Physiol Rev* 1995; 75:261–275.

8. Muller M, Jansen PL. Molecular aspects of hepatobiliary transport. *Am J Physiol* 1997;272:G1285–1303.

9. Simon FR. Drug-induced cholestasis: pathobiology and clinical features. *Clinics in Liver Disease* 1998;2:483–499.

10. Arrese M, Ananthananarayanan M, Suchy FJ. Hepatobiliary transport: molecular mechanisms of development and cholestasis. *Pediatr Res* 1998, 44:141–147.

11. Groothuis GMM, Hardonk MJ, Keulemans KPT, et al. Autoradiographic and kinetic demonstration of acinar heterogeneity of taurocholate transport. *Am J Physiol* 1982;243:G455–462.

12. Ananthanarayanan M, Ng OC, Boyer JL, et al. Characterization of cloned rat liver Na(+)-bile acid cotransporter using peptide and fusion protein antibodies. *Am J Physiol* 1994;267:G637–643.

13. Gerloff T, Stieger B, Hagenbuch B, et al. The sister of P-glycoprotein represents the canalicular bile salt export pump of mammalian liver. *J Biol Chem* 1998;273:10046–10050.

14. Erlinger S, Dhumeaux D. Mechanisms and control of secretion of bile water and electrolytes. *Gastroenterology* 1974;66:281–304.

15. Boyer JL, Klatskin G. Canalicular bile flow and bile secretory pressure. Evidence for a non-bile salt dependent fraction in the isolated perfused rat liver. *Gastroenterology* 1971;59:853–859.

16. Ballatori N, Truong AT. Glutathione as a primary osmotic driving force in hepatic bile formation. *Am J Physiol* 1992;263: G617–624.

17. Benedetti A, Strazzabosco M, Ng OC, et al. Regulation of activity and apical targeting of the Cl–/HCO3– exchanger in rat hepatocytes. *Proc Natl Acad Sci U S A* 1994;91:792–796.

18. Ballatori N, Rebbeor JF. Roles of MRP2 and oatp1 in hepatocellular export of reduced glutathione. *Semin Liver Dis* 1998;18:377–387.

19. Lee TK, Li L, Ballatori N. Hepatic glutathione and glutathione S-conjugate-transport mechanisms. *Yale J Biol Med* 1997;70: 287–300.

20. Ballatori N, Dutczak WJ. Identification and characterization of high and low affinity transport systems for reduced glutathione in liver cell canalicular membranes. *J Biol Chem* 1994;269: 19731–19737.

21. Elferink RP, Ottenhoff R, Liefting W, et al. Hepatobiliary transport of glutathione and glutathione conjugate in rats with hereditary hyperbilirubinemia. *J Clin Invest* 1989;84:476–483.

22. Simon FR. The role of membrane lipids and fluidity in hepatic plasma membrane transport processes. In: Tavoloni N, Berk PD, eds. *Hepatic Anion Transport and Bile Secretion: Physiology and Pathophysiology.* New York: Marcel Dekker, 1992.

23. Ihrke G, Hubbard AL. Control of vesicle traffic in hepatocytes. *Prog Liver Dis* 1995;3:63–99.

24. Maurice M, Schell MJ, Lardeux B, et al. Biosynthesis and intracellular transport of a bile canalicular plasma membrane protein: studies in vivo and in the perfused rat liver. *Hepatology* 1994;19:648–655.

25. Hubbard AL, Stieger B, Bartles JR. Biogenesis of endogenous plasma membrane proteins in epithelial cells. *Annu Rev Physiol* 1989;51:755–770.

26. Bartles JR, Hubbard AL. Plasma membrane protein sorting in epithelial cells: do secretory pathways hold the key? *Trends Biochem Sci* 1988;13:181–184.

27. Bartles JR, Feracci HM, Stieger B, et al. Biogenesis of the rat hepatocyte plasma membrane in vivo: comparison of the pathways taken by apical and basolateral proteins using subcellular fractionation. *J Cell Biol* 1987;105:1241–1251.

28. Hagenbuch B, Meier PJ. Sinusoidal (basolateral) bile salt uptake systems of hepatocytes. *Semin Liver Dis* 1996;16:129–136.

29. van Montfoort JE, Hagenbuch B, Fattinger KE, et al. Polyspecific organic anion transporting polypeptides mediate hepatic uptake of amphipathic type II organic cations. *J Pharmacol Exp Ther* 1999;291:147–152.

30. Eckhardt U, Schroeder A, Stieger B, et al. Polyspecific substrate uptake by the hepatic organic anion transporter Oatp1 in stably transfected CHO cells. *Am J Physiol* 1999;276:G1037–1042.

31. Kipp H, Arias IM. Newly synthesized canalicular ABC transporters are directly targeted from the Golgi to the hepatocyte apical domain in rat liver. *J Biol Chem* 2000;275:15917–15925.

32. Muklopadhyay S, Ananthanarayanan M, Stieger B, et al. cAMP increases liver Na+-taurocholate cotransport by translocating transporter to plasma membranes. *Am J Physiol* 1997;273: G842–848.

33. Coche T, Deroubaix X, Depiereux E, et al. Compartmental analysis of steady-state taurocholate transport kinetics by isolated rat hepatocytes. *Hepatology* 1991;13:1203–1214.

34. Deroubaix X, Coche T, Depiereux E, et al. Saturation of hepatic transport of taurocholate in rats in vivo. *Am J Physiol* 1991;260: G189–196.

35. Deroubaix X, Coche T, Depiereux E, et al. Compartmental modeling of the hepatic transport of taurocholate in the rat in vivo. *Am J Physiol* 1989;257:G210–220.

36. Keppler D, Arias IM. Hepatic canalicular membrane. Introduction: transport across the hepatocyte canalicular membrane. *FASEB J* 1997;11:15–18.

37. Leveille-Webster CR, Arias IM. The biology of the P-glycoproteins. *J Membr Biol* 1995;143:89–102.

38. Silverman JA, Thorgeirsson SS. Regulation and function of the multidrug resistance genes in liver. *Prog Liver Dis* 1995;13: 101–123.

39. Silverman JA, Schrenk D. Hepatic canalicular membrane 4: expression of the multidrug resistance genes in the liver. *FASEB J* 1997;11:308–313.

40. Germann UA. P-glycoprotein—a mediator of multidrug resistance in tumour cells. *Eur J Cancer* 1996;32A,927–944.

41. Cole SP, Deeley RG. Multidrug resistance mediated by the ATP-binding cassette transporter protein MRP. *Bioessays* 1998; 20:931–940.

42. Deeley RG, Cole SP. Function, evolution and structure of multidrug resistance protein (MRP). *Semin Cancer Biol* 1997;8: 193–204.

43. Loe DW, Deeley RG, Cole SP. Biology of the multidrug resistance-associated protein, MRP. *Eur J Cancer* 1996;32A: 945–957.

44. Roy AK, Chatterjee B. Sexual dimorphism in the liver. *Annu Rev Physiol* 1983;45:37–50.

45. Shapiro BH, Agrawal AK, Pampori NA. Gender differences in drug metabolism regulated by growth hormone. *Int J Biochem Cell Biol* 1995,27:9–20.

46. Kobliakov V, Popova N, Rossi L. Regulation of the expression of the sex-specific isoforms of cytochrome P-450 in rat liver. *Eur J Biochem* 1991;195:585–591.

47. Gustafsson JA, Mode A, Norstedt G, et al. Growth hormone: a regulator of the sexually differentiated steroid metabolism in rat liver. *Prog Clin Biol Res* 1983;135:37–59.

48. Gustafsson J-A, Mode A, Norstedt G, et al. Sex steroid induced changes in hepatic enzymes. *Annu Rev Physiol* 1983;45:51–60.

49. Legraverend C, Mode A, Wells T, et al. Hepatic steroid hydroxylating enzymes are controlled by the sexually dimorphic pat-

tern of growth hormone secretion in normal and dwarf rats. *FASEB J* 1992;6:711–718.

50. Zaphiropoulos PG, Mode A, Norstedt G, et al. Regulation of sexual differentiation in drug and steroid metabolism. *Trends Pharmacol Sci* 1989;10:149–153.

51. Mode A. Sexually differentiated expression of genes encoding the P4502C cytochromes in rat liver—a model system for studying the action of growth hormone. *J Reprod Fertil Suppl* 1993;46:77–86.

52. Davey HW, Wilkens RJ, Waxman DJ. STAT5 signaling in sexually dimorphic gene expression and growth patterns. *Am J Hum Genet* 1999;65:959–965.

53. Mode A, Ahlgren R, Lahuna O, et al. Gender differences in rat hepatic CYPZC gene expression-regulation by growth hormone. *Growth Horm IGF Res* 1998;Suppl B:61–67.

54. Schmucker DL, Woodhouse KW, Wang RK. et al. Effects of age and gender on in vitro properties of human liver microsomal monooxygenase. *Clin Pharmacol Ther* 1991;48:365–374.

55. Beato M. Gene regulation by steroid hormones. *Cell* 1989;6:335–344.

56. Manelsdorf DJ, Thummel C, Beato M, et al. The nuclear receptor superfamily: The second decade. *Cell* 1995;83:835–839.

57. Mangelsdorf DJ, Evans R. The RXR heterodimers and orphan receptors. *Cell* 1995;83:841–850.

58. Beato M, Herrlich P, Schutz G. Steroid hormone receptors: Many actors in search of a plot. *Cell* 1995;83:851–857.

59. Ribeiro RCJ, Kushner PJ, Baxter JD. The nuclear hormone receptor gene superfamily. *Annu Rev Med* 1995;46:443–453.

60. Kliewer SA, Lehmann JM, Willson TM. Orphan nuclear receptors: Shifting endocrinology into reverse. *Science* 1999;284:757–760.

61. Giguere V. Orphan nuclear receptors: From gene to function. *Endocr Rev* 1999;20:689–725.

62. Waxman, DJ. P450 induction by structurally diverse xenochemicals: Central role of nuclear receptors CAR, PXR, and PPAR. *Arch Biochem Biophys* 1999;369:11–23.

63. Desvergne B, Wahli W. Peroxisome proliferator-activated receptors: Nuclear control of metabolism. *Endocr Rev* 1999;20:649–688.

64. MeKenna NJ, Lanz RB, O'Malley BW. Nuclear receptor coregulators: Cellular and molecular biology. *Endocr Rev* 1999;20:321–344.

65. Glass CK. Some new twists in the regulation of gene expression by thyroid hormone and retinoic acid receptors. *J Endocrinology* 1996;150:349–357.

66. Giguere V, Ong ES, Segui P, et al. Identification of a receptor for the morphogen retinoic acid. *Nature* 1987;330:624–629.

67. Mangelsdorf DJ, Ong ES, Dyck JA, et al. Nuclear receptor that identifies a novel retinoic acid response pathway. *Nature* 1990;345:224–229.

68. Beg JM. DNA binding specificity of steroid receptors. *Cell* 1989;57:1065–1068.

69. Russell DW. Nuclear orphan receptors control cholesterol catabolism. *Cell* 1999;97:539–542.

70. Aldecreutz H. Hepatic metabolism of estrogens in health and disease. *N Engl J Med* 1974;290:1081–1083.

71. Bolt HM. Metabolism of estrogens—natural and synthetic. *Pharmacol Ther* 1979;4:155–181.

72. Reyes H, Simon FR. Intrahepatic cholestasis of pregnancy: an estrogen-related disease. *Semin Liver Dis* 1993;13:289–301.

73. Vore M. Estrogen cholestasis. Membranes, metabolites or receptors? *Gastroenterology* 1987;93:643–649.

74. Svanborg A. A study of recurrent jaundice in pregnancy. *Acta Obstet Gynecol Scand* 1954;33:434–444.

75. Kreek MJ, Sleisenger MH, Jeffries GH. Recurrent cholestatic jaundice of pregnancy with demonstrated estrogen sensitivity. *Am J Med* 1967;43:795–803.

76. Kreek MJ. Female sex steroids and cholestasis. *Semin Liver Dis* 1987;7:8–23.

77. Kreek MJ, Peterson RE, Sleisenger MH, et al. Effects of ethinyl estradiol induced cholestasis on bile flow and biliary excretion of estradiol and estradiol glucuronide by the rat. *Proc Soc Exp Biol Med* 1969;131:646–650.

78. Simon FR, Fortune J, Iwahashi M, et al. Ethinyl estradiol cholestasis involves alterations in expression of liver sinusoidal transporters. *Am J Physiol* 1996;271:G1043–1052.

79. Rosario J, Sutherland E, Zaccaro L, et al. Ethinylestradiol administration selectively alters liver sinusoidal membrane lipid fluidity and protein composition. *Biochemistry* 1988;27:3939–3946.

80. Tritapepe R, DiPadova C, Rovagnati P. Spontaneous reversal of ethinyl estradiol-induced cholestasis in the rat. *Experientia* 1980;36:580–581.

81. Vial JD, Simon FR, Mackinnon AM. Scanning electron microscopic studies of hepatocytes under different experimental conditions. In: Leavy CM, ed. *Diseases of Liver and Biliary Tract*, Basel: S. Karger AG, 1975:42–47.

82. Layden TJ, Schwarz, Boyer JL. Scanning electron microscopy of the rat liver. Studies of the effect of taurolithocholate and other models of cholestasis. *Gastroenterology* 1975;69:724–738.

83. Bossard R, Stieger B, O'Neill B, et al. Ethinylestradiol treatment induces multiple canalicular membrane transport alterations in rat liver. *J Clin Invest* 1993;91:2714–2720.

84. Combes B, Shibata H, Adams R, et al. Alterations in sulphobromophthalein sodium removal mechanisms from blood during normal pregnancy. *J Clin Invest* 1963;42:1431–1442.

85. Forker EL. The effect of estrogen on bile formation in the rat. *J Clin Invest* 1969;48:654–663.

86. Gumucio J, Valdivieso V. Studies on the mechanisms of ethinyl estradiol impairment of bile flow and bile salt excretion in the rat. *Gastroenterology* 1971;61:339–344.

87. Heikel TAJ, Lathe GH. The effect of oral contraceptive steroids on bile secretion and bilirubin Tm in rats. *Br J Pharmacol* 1970;38:593–601.

88. Simon FR, Gonzalez M, Sutherland E, et al. Reversal of ethinyl estradiol induced bile secretory failure with Triton WR-1339. *J Clin Invest* 1980;65:851–860.

89. Gumucio J, Accatino L. Macho AM, et al. Effect of phenobarbital on the ethinyl estradiol induced cholestasis in the rat. *Gastroenterology* 1973;65:651–657.

90. Reyes H, Kern F. Effect of pregnancy on bile flow and biliary lipids in the hamster. *Gastroenterology* 1979;76:144–150.

91. Berr F, Simon FR, Reichen J. Ethinylestradiol impairs bile salt uptake and Na,K pump function of rat hepatocytes. *Amer J Physiol* 1984;247:G437–443.

92. Trauner M, Arrese M, Soroka CJ, et al. The rat canalicular conjugate export pump (Mrp2) is down-regulated in intrahepatic and obstructive cholestasis. *Gastroenterology* 1997;113:255–264.

93. Lee, JM, Trauner M, Soroka, CJ, et al. Expression of the bile salt export pump is maintained after chronic cholestasis in the rat.*Gastroenterology* 2000;118:163–172.

94. Jaeschke H, Trummer E, Krell H. Increase in biliary permeability susequent to intrahepatic cholestasis by estradiol valerate in rats. *Gastroenterolgy* 1987;93:533–538.

95. Jaeschke H, Krell H, Pfaff E. No increase of biliary permeability in ethinyl estradiol-treated rats. *Gastroenterolgy* 1983;85:808–814.

96. Robenek H, Rassat J, Grosser V, et al. Ultrastructural study of cholestasis induced by long-term treatment with estradiol valerate. Tight junction analysis and tracer experiments. *Virchows Arch B Cell Pathol* 1982;40:201–215.

97. Davis R, Kern F, Showalter R, et al. Alterations of hepatic (Na+K)ATPase and bile flow by estrogen: Effects on liver surface membrane lipid structure and function. *Proc Natl Acad Sci U S A* 1978;75:4130–4134.

98. Keefee EB, Scharschmidt BF, Blankenship NM, et al. Studies of relationships among bile flow, liver membrane NaK-ATPas, and membrane microviscosity in the rat. *J Clin Invest* 1979;64: 1590–1598.

99. Smith DJ, Gordon ER. Role of liver plasma membrane fluidity in the pathogenesis of estrogen-induced cholestasis. *J Lab Clin Med* 1988;112:679–685.

100. Miccio M, Orzes N, Lunazzi GC, et al. Reversal of ethinyl estradiol induced cholestasis by epomediol in rat. The role of liver plasma-membrane fluidity. *Biochem Pharmacol* 1989;38: 3559–3563.

101. Eisenfeld AJ, Alen R, Weinberger M, et al. Estrogen receptor in the mammalian liver. *Science* 1976;191:862–865.

102. Porter LE, Elm MS, Van Thiel DH, et al. Characterization and quantitation of human hepatic estrogen receptor. *Gastroenterology* 1983;84:704–712.

103. Kovanen PT, Brown MS, Goldstein JL. Increased binding LDL to liver membranes from rats treated with 17-ethinyl estradiol. *J Biol Chem* 1979;254:11367–11373.

104. Patrick T, Ma S, Yamamoto T, et al. Increased mRNA for low density lipoprotein receptor in livers of rabbits treated with 17α-ethinyl estradiol. *Proc Natl Acad Sci U S A* 1986;83:792–796.

105. Rudling M, Norstedt G, Olivecrona H, et al. Importance of growth hormone for the induction of hepatic low density lipoprotein receptors. *Proc Natl Acad Sci U S A* 1992;89: 6983–6987.

106. Simon FR, Fortune J, Iwahashi M, et al. Characterization of the mechanisms involved in the gender differences in hepatic taurocholate uptake. *Am J Physiol* 1999;276:G556–565.

107. Vore M, Slikker W. Steroid D-ring glucuronides: a new class of cholestatic agents. *Trends Pharmacol Sci* 1985;6:256–259.

108. Meyers M. Slikker W, Pascoe G, et al. Characterization of cholestasis induced by estradiol-17b-D-glucuronide in the rat. *J Pharmacol Exp Ther* 1980;214:87–93.

109. Meyers M. Slikker W, Vore M. Steroid D-ring glucuronides: Characterization of a new class of cholestatic agents in the rat. *J Pharmacol Exp Ther* 1981;218:6–73.

110. Stieger B. Fattinger L. Madon J, et al. Drug- and estrogen-induced cholestasis through inhibition of the hepatocellular bile salt export pump (Bsep) of rat liver. *Gastroenterology* 2000;118: 422–430.

111. Mueller MN, Kappas A. Estrogen pharmacology I. The influence of estradiol and estriol on hepatic disposal of sulfobromophthallein (BSP) in man. *J Clin Invest* 1964;43:1905–1909.

112. Wheeler HO, Meltzer JL, Bradley S, et al. Biliary transfer and hepatic storage of sulfobrompthalein in the unanesthetized dog, in normal man and in patients with hepatic disease. *J Clin Invest* 1960;39:1131–1144.

113. Combes B, Shibata H, Adams R, et al. Alterations in sulphobromophthalein sodium removal mechanisms from blood during normal pregnancy. *J Clin Invest* 1963;42:1431–1442.

114. Kleiner GJ, Kresch L, Arias IM. Studies of hepatic excretory function II. The effect of norethynodrel and mestranol on bromsulfalein sodium metabolism in women of childbearing age. *N Engl J Med* 1965;273:420–423.

115. Preisig R, Morris TQ, Shaver JC, et al. Volumetric, hemodynamic, and excretory characteristics of the liver in acromegaly. *J Clin Invest* 1966;45:1379–1387.

116. Cohen L, Lewis C, Arias IM. Pregnancy, oral contraceptives, and chronic familial jaundice with predominantly conjugated hyperbilirubinemia (Dubin–Johnson syndrome). *Gastroenterology* 1972;62:1182–1190.

117. Boake WC, Schade SG, Morrissey JF, et al. Intrahepatic cholestatic jaundice of pregnancy followed by Enovid-induced cholestatic jaundice. Report of a case. *Ann Intern Med* 1965;63: 302–308.

118. Bacq Y, Zarka O, Brechot J-F, et al. Liver function tests in normal pregnancy: A prospective study of 103 pregnant women and 103 matched controls. *Hepatology* 1996;23:1030–1034.

119. Bacq Y. Intrahepatic cholestasis of pregnancy. *Clinics Liver Disease* 1999;3:1–13.

120. Leslie KK, Reznikov L, Simon FR, et al. Estrogens in intrahepatic cholestasis of pregnancy. *Obstet Gynecol* 2000;95:372–376.

121. Gonzalez MC, Reyes H, Arrese M, et al. Intrahepatic cholestasis of pregnancy in twin pregnancies. *J Hepatol* 1989;9:84–90.

122. Davies MH, Ngong JM, Yucesoy M, et al. The adverse influence of pregnancy upon sulfation: A clue to the pathogenesis of intrahepatic cholestasis of pregnancy? *J Hepatol* 1994;21: 1127–1133.

123. Adlercreutz H, Tikkanen MJ, Wichman K, et al. Recurrent jaundice in pregnancy. IV. Quantitative determination of urinary and biliary estrogens, including studies in pruritis gravidarum. *J Clin Endocrinol Metab* 1974;38:51–57.

124. Meng LJ, Reyes H, Axelson M, et al. Progesterone metabolites and bile acids in serum of patients with intrahepatic cholestasis of pregnancy. Effect of ursodeoxycholic acid therapy. *Hepatology* 1997;26:1573–1582.

125. Bacq Y, Sapey T, Bechot MC, et al. Intrahepatic cholestasis of pregnancy: A French prospective study. *Hepatology* 1997;26: 358–365.

126. Noblot G, Audra P, Dargent D, et al. The use of micronized progesterone in the treatment of menace of preterm delivery. *Eur J Obstet Gynaecol Reprod Biol* 1991;40:203–209.

127. Erny R, Pigne A, Prouvost C, et al. The effects of oral administration of progesterone for premature labor. *Am J Obstet Gynecol* 1986;154:525–529.

128. Reyes H, Ribalta J, Gonzalez MC, et al. Sulfobromophthalein clearance tests before and after ethinyl estradiol administration in women and men with familial history of intrahepatic cholestasis of pregnancy. *Gastroenterology* 1981;81:226–231.

129. Reyes H, Ribaltra J, Gonzalez MC. Idiopathic cholestasis of pregnancy in a large kindred. *Gut* 1976;17:709–713.

130. Jacquemin E, Cresteil D, Manouvrier S, et al. Heterozygous non-sense mutation of the MDR3 gene in familial intrahepatic cholestasis of pregnancy. *Lancet* 1999;353:210–211.

131. Reyes H. The enigma of intrahepatic cholestasis of pregnancy: Lessons from Chile. *Hepatology* 1982;2:87–96.

132. Zimmerman HJ. *Hepatotoxicity, The Adverse Effects of Drugs and Other Chemicals on the Liver,* New York: Appleton-Century-Crofts, 1978.

133. Scherb J, Kirschner M, Arias IM. Studies of hepatic excretory function. The effect of 17a-ethyl-19-nortestosterone on sulfobromophthalein sodium metabolism in man. *J Clin Invest* 1963;42:404–408.

134. DeLorimier AA, Gordon GS, Lowe RC, et al. Methyltestosterone, related steroids, and liver function. *Arch Intern Med* 1965;116:289–294.

135. Roberts RJ, Shriver SL, Plaa GL. Effect of norethandrolone on the biliary excretion of bilrubin in the mouse and rat. *Biochem Pharmacol* 1969;17:1261–1268.

136. Schwarz LR, Schwenk M, Pfaff E, et al. Cholestatic steroid hormones inhibit taurocholate uptake into isolated rat hepatocytes. *Biochem Pharmacol* 1977;26:2433–2437.

137. Eagon PK, Elm MS, Stafford EA, et al. Androgen receptor in human liver: characterization and quantitation in normal and diseased liver. *Hepatology* 1994;19:92–100.

138. Brinkmann AO, Blok LJ, deRuiter PE, et al. Mechanisms of androgen receptor activation and function. *J Steroid Biochem Mol Biol* 1999;69:307–313.

139. Phillips MJ, Oda M. Fumatsu K. Evidence for microfilament involvement in norethandrolone-induced intrahepatic cholestasis. *Am J Pathol* 1978;93:729–739.

140. Glass CK. Differential recognition of target genes by nuclear receptor monomers, dimers and heterodimers. *Endocr Rev* 1994; 15:391–407.

141. Miner Jr PB, Sutherland E, Simon FR. Regulation of hepatic sodium plus potassium-activated adenosine triphosphatase activity by glucocorticoids in the rat. *Gastroenterology* 1980; 79:212–221.

142. Zsigmond G, Solymoss B. Increased canalicular bile production induced by pregnenolone-16alpha-carbonitrile, spironolactone and cortisol in rats. *Proc Soc Exp Biol Med* 1974;145:631–635.

143. Solymoss B, Zsigmond G. Effect of various steroids on the hepatic glucuronidation and biliary excretion of bilirubin. *Can J Physiol Pharmacol* 1973;51:319–323.

144. Zsigmond G, Solymoss B. Effect of spironolactone, pregnenolone-16-carbonitrile and cortisol on the metabolism and biliary excretion of sulfobromophthalein and phenol-3,6-dibromophthalein disulfonate in rats. *J Pharmacol Exp Ther* 1972; 183:499–507.

145. Macarol V, Morris TQ, Baker KJ, et al. Hydrocortisone choleresis in the dog. *J Clin Invest* 1970;49:1714–1723.

146. Kliewer SA, Moore JT, Wade L, et al. An orphan nuclear receptor activated by pregnanes defines a novel steroid signaling pathway. *Cell* 1998;9:92:73–82.

147. lferink RP, Ottenhoff R, Liefting W, et al. Hepatobiliary transport of glutathione and glutathione conjugate in rats with hereditary hyperbilirubinemia. *J Clin Invest* 1989;84:476–483.

148. Paulusma CC, Oude Elferink RP. The canalicular multispecific organic anion transporter and conjugated hyperbilirubinemia in rat and man. *J Mol Med* 1997;75:420–428.

149. Kauffmann HM, Schrenk D. Sequence analysis and functional characterization of the 5′-flanking region of the rat multidrug resistance protein 2 (mrp2) gene. *Biochem Biophys Res Commun* 1998;245:325–331.

150. Tanaka T, Uchiumi T, Hinoshita E, et al. The human multidrug resistance protein 2 gene: Functional characterization of the 5′-flanking region and expression in hepatic cells. *Hepatology* 1999;30:1507–1512.

151. Demeule M, Jodoin J, Beaulieu E, et al. Dexamethasone modulation of multidrug transporters in normal rats. *FEBS Lett* 1999;442:208–214.

152. Kubitz R, Warskulat U, Schmitt M, et al. Dexamethasone- and osmolarity-dependent expression of the multidrug-resistance protein 2 in cultured rat hepatocytes. *Biochem J* 1999;340:585–591.

153. Kubitz R, Wettstein M, Warskulat U, et al. Regulation of the multidrug resistance protein 2 in the rat liver by lipopolysaccharide and dexamethasone. *Gastroenterology* 1999;116:401–410.

154. Simon FR, Sutherland E, Iwahashi M, et al. Hormonal and xenobiotic regulation of rat nultidrug resistance protein2 (cMOAT/Mrp2): sexual dimorphic expression and regulation by pregnane X receptors (PXR). *Hepatology 2000 (in press)*.

155. Motomura K, Brent GA. Mechanisms of thyroid hormone action. Implications for the clinical manifestation of thyrotoxicosis. *Endocrinol Metab Clin North Am* 1998;27:1–23.

156. Brent GA. Mechanisms of disease: the molecular basis of thyroid hormone action. *New Engl J Med* 1994;331:847–853.

157. Ashkar FS. Liver disease in hyperthyroidism. *South Med J* 1971;64:462–467.

158. Ness GC, Chambers CM. Feedback and hormonal regulation of hepatic 3-hydroxy-3-methylglutaryl coenzyme A reductase: the concept of cholesterol buffering capacity. *Proc Soc Exp Biol Med* 2000;224:8–19.

159. Eriksson S. Influence of thyroid activity on excretion of bile acids and cholesterol in the rat. *Proc Soc Exp Biol Med* 1957;94: 582–589.

160. Beher WT, Beher ME, Semenuk G. The effect of pituitary and

161. Layden TJ, Boyer JL. The effect of thyroid hormone on bile salt-independent bile flow and Na+, K+-ATPase activity in liver plasma membranes enriched in bile canaliculi. *J Clin Invest* 1976;57:1009–1018.

162. Gartner LM, Arias IM. Hormonal control of hepatic bilirubin transport and conjugation. *Am J Physiol* 1972;222:1091–1099.

163. Bowman SB, Fortune J, Sutherland E, et al. Sex differences and hormonal regulation of hepatic organic anion transporters. *Hepatology* 1995;22:312A.

164. Simon FR, Hu L-J, Arias IM, et al. Thyroid hormone is necessary for growth hormone regulated sexually dimorphic expression of hepatic multidrug resistance associated protein 2. *Mol Biol Cell* 1999;10:79a.

165. Parks DJ, Blanchard SG, Bledsoe RK, et al. Bile acids: natural ligands for an orphan nuclear receptor. *Science* 1999;284: 1365–1368.

166. Makishima M, Okamoto AY, Repa JJ, et al. Identification of a nuclear receptor for bile acids. *Science* 1999;284:1362–1365.

167. Grober J, Zaghini I, Fujii H, et al. Identification of a bile acid-responsive element in the human ileal bile acid-binding protein gene. Involvement of the farnesoid X receptor/9-cis-retinoic acid receptor heterodimer. *J Biol Chem* 1999;274:29749–29754.

168. Peet DJ, Turley SD, Ma W, et al. Cholesterol and bile acid metabolism are impaired in mice lacking the nuclear oxysterol receptor LXRα. *Cell* 1998;93:693–704.

169. Janowski BA, Willy PJ, Devi TR, et al. An oxysterol signaling pathway mediated by the nuclear receptor LXR alpha. *Nature* 1996;383:728–731.

170. Lehmann JM, Kiewer SA, Moore LB, et al. Activation of the nuclear receptor LXR by oxysterols defines a new hormone response pathway. *J Biol Chem* 1997;272:3137–3140.

171. Denson LA, Auld KL, Schiek DS, et al. Interleukin-1β suppresses retinoid transactivation of two hepatic trasporter genes involved in bile formation. *J Biol Chem* 2000;275:8835–8843.

172. Berthelot P, Erlinger S, Dhumeaux D, et al. Mechanism of phenobarbitol-induced hypercholeresis in the rat. *Am J Physiol* 1970;221:809–813.

173. Simon FR, Sutherland E, Accatino L. Stimulation of hepatic (Na+-K+)ATPase activity by phenobarbital: Its possible role in regulation of bile flow. *J Clin Invest* 1977;59:849–861.

174. Honkakoski P, Negishi M. Regulation of cytochrome P450 (CYP) genes by nuclear receptors. *Biochem J* 2000;347: 321–337.

175. Honkakoski P, Zelko I, Sueyoshi T, et al. The nuclear orphan receptor CAR-retinoid X receptor heterodimer activates the phenobarbital-responsive enhancer module of the CYP2B gene. *Mol Cell Biol* 1998;18:5652–5658.

176. Sueyoshi T, Kawamoto T, Zelko I, et al. The repressed nuclear receptor CAR responds to phenobarbital in activating the human CYP2B6 gene. *J Biol Chem* 1999;274:6043–6046.

177. Bouscarel B, Kroll SD, Fromm H. Signal transduction and hepatocellular bile acid transport: cross talk between bile acids and second messengers. *Gastroenterolgy* 1999;117:433–452.

178. Stravitz RT, Rao Y-P, Vlahcevic ZR, et al. Hepatocellular protein kinase C activation by bile acids: implications for regulation of cholesterol 7a-hydroxylase. *Am J Physiol* 1996;271: G293–G303.

179. Corasanti JG, Smith ND, Gordon ER, et al. Protein kinase C agonists inhibit bile secretion independently of effects on the microcirculation in the isolated perfused rat liver. *Hepatology* 1989;10:8–13.

180. Boyer JL, Soroka CJ. Vesicle targeting to the apical domain regulates bile excretory function in isolated rat hepatocyte couplets. *Gastroenterolgy* 1995;109:1600–1611.

181. Gatmaitan ZC, Nies AT, Arias IM. Regulation and translocation of ATP-dependent apical membrane proteins in rat liver. *Am J Physiol* 1997;272:G1041–G1049.
182. Botham KM, Suckling KE, Boyd GS. The effect of glucagon-adenosine 3′,5′-monophosphate concentrations on bile acid synthesis in isolated rat liver cells. *FEBS Lett* 1984;168:317–320.
183. Kaminski DL, Deshpande Y, Beinfeld MC. Role of glucagon in cholecystokinin-stimulated bile flow in dogs. *Am J Physiol* 1988;254:G864–G869.
184. Lenzen R, Hruby VJ, Tavaloni N. Mechanism of glucagon-induced choleresis in guinea pigs. *Am J Physiol* 1990;259:G736–G744.
185. Branum GD, Bowers BA, Watters CR, et al. Biliary response to glucagon in humans. *Ann Surg* 1991;213:335–340.
186. Thomsen OO, Larsen JA. The effect of glucagon, dibutyrylic cyclic AMP and insulin on bile production in the intact rat and the perfused rat liver. *Acta Physiol Scand* 1981;111:23–30.
187. Edmondson JW, Miller BA, Lumeng L. Effect of glucagon on hepatic taurocholate uptake: relationship to membrane potential. *Am J Physiol* 1985;249:G427–G433.
188. Mukhopadhyay S, Ananthanarayanan M, Stieger B, et al. Sodium taurocholate cotransporting polypeptide is a serine, threonine phosphoprotein and is dephosphorylated by cyclic adenosine monophosphate. *Hepatology* 1998;28:1629–1636.
189. Mukhopadhyay S, Webster CR, Anwer MS. Role of protein phosphatases in cyclic AMP-mediated stimulation of hepatic Na+/taurocholate cotransport. *J Biol Chem* 1998;273:30039–30045.
190. Roelofsen H, Soroka CJ, Keppler D, et al. Cyclic AMP stimulates sorting of the canalicular organic anion transporter (Mrp2/cMoat) to the apical domain in hepatocyte couplets. *J Cell Sci* 1998;111:1137–1145.
191. Misra S, Ujhazy P, Varticovski L, et al. Phosphoinositide 3-kinase lipid products regulate ATP-dependent transport by sister of P-glycoprotein and multidrug resistance associated protein 2 in bile canalicular membrane vesicles. *Proc Natl Acad Sci U S A* 1999;96:5814–5819.
192. Misra S, Ujhazy P, Gatmaitan Z, et al. The role of phosphoinositide 3-kinase in taurocholate-induced trafficking of ATP-dependent canalicular transporters in rat liver. *J Biol Chem* 1998;273:26638–26644.
193. Jefferson LS. Role of insulin in the regulation of protein synthesis. *Diabetes* 1980;29:487–496.
194. Jones RS. Effect of insulin on canalicular bile formation. *Am J Physiol* 1976;231:40–43.
195. Uchida K, Takase H, Kadowaki M, et al. Altered bile acid metabolism in alloxan diabetic rats. *Jpn J Pharmacol* 1979;29:553–562.
196. Nervi F, Severin CH, Valdivieso VD. Bile acid pool changes and regulation of cholate synthesis in experimental diabetes. *Biochem Biophys Acta* 1978;529:212–223.
197. Caspary WF. Increase of active transport of conjugated bile salts in streptozotocin-diabetic rat small intestine. *Gut* 1973;14:949–955.
198. Watkins JB, Noda H. Biliary excretion of organic anions in diabetic rats. *J Pharmacol Exp Ther* 1986;239:467–473.
199. Icarte MA, Pizarro M, Accatino L. Adaptive regulation of hepatic bile salt transport: effects of alloxan diabetes in the rat. *Hepatology* 1991;14:671–678.
200. Carnovale CE, Marinelli RA, Garay EAR. Bile flow decrease and altered bile composition in streptozotocin-treated rats. *Biochem Pharmacol* 1986;35:2625–2628.
201. Garcoa KK, Voamieva GR, Esteller A. Diabetes-induced cholestasis in the rat: possible role of hyperglycemia and hypoinsulinemia. *Hepatology* 1988;8:332–340.
202. Cersonsky C, Simon FR. Selective alterations of organic anion transport capacity in rats following hypophysectomy and thyroidectomy. *Clin Res* 1977;108A.
203. Carter-Su C, Schwartz J, Smit LS. Molecular mechanism of growth hormone action. *Annu Rev Physiol* 1996;58:187–207.
204. Davey HW, Wilkins RJ, Waxman DJ. STAT5 signaling in sexually dimorphic gene expression and growth patterns. *Am J Hum Genet* 1999;65:959–965.
205. Darnell JE. STATs and gene regulation. *Science* 1997;277:1630–1635.
206. Waxman DJ, Ram PA, Park S-H, et al. Intermittent plasma growth hormone triggers tyrosine phosphorylation and nuclear translocation of a liver-expressed, Stat 5-related DNA binding protein. *J Biol Chem* 1995;270:13262–13270.
207. Ram PA, Park SH, Choi HK, et al. Growth hormone activation of Stat 1, Stat 3, and Stat 5 in rat liver. Differential kinetics of hormone desensitization and growth hormone stimulation of both tyrosine phosphorylation and serine/threonine phosphorylation. *J Biol Chem* 1996;271:5929–5940.
208. Gebert CA, Park S-H, Waxman DJ. Regulation of STAT 5b activation by the temporal pattern of growth hormone stimulation. *Mol Endocrinol* 1997;11:400–414.
209. Park SH, Liu X, Hennighausen L, et al. Distinctive roles of STAT5a and STAT5b in sexual dimorphism of hepatic P450 gene expression. Impact of STAT5a gene disruption. *J Biol Chem* 1999;274:7421–7430.
210. Gebert CA, Park SH, Waxman DJ. Down-regulation of liver JAK2-STAT5b signaling by the female plasma pattern of continuous growth hormone stimulation. *Mol Endocrinol* 1999;13:213–227.
211. Gebert CA, Park SH, Waxman DJ. Termination of growth hormone pulse-induced STAT5b signaling. *Mol Endocrinol* 1999;13:38–56.
212. Subramanian A, Wang J, Gil G. STAT 5 and NF-Y are involved in expression and growth hormone-mediated sexually dimorphic regulation of cytochrome P450 3A10/lithocholic acid 6β-hydroxylase. *Nucleic Acids Res* 1998;26:2173–2178.
213. Udy GB, Towers RP, Snell RG, et al. Requirement of STAT5b for sexual dimorphism of body growth rates and liver gene expression. *Proc Natl Acad Sci U S A* 1997;94:7239–7244.
214. Teglund S, McKay C, Schuetz E, et al. Stat5a and Stat5b proteins have essential and nonessential, or redundant, roles in cytokine responses. *Cell* 1998;93:841–850.
215. Park SH, Liu X, Hennighausen L, et al. Distinctive roles of STAT5a and STAT5b in sexual dimorphism of hepatic P450 gene expression. Impact of STAT5a gene disruption. *J Biol Chem* 1999;274:7421–7430.
216. Moutoussamy S, Kelly PA, Finidori J. Growth-hormone-receptor and cytokine-receptor-family signaling. *Eur J Biochem* 1998;255:1–11.
217. Horseman ND, Yu-Lee LY. Transcriptional regulation by the helix bundle peptide hormones: growth hormone, prolactin and hematopoeitic cytokines. *Endocr Rev* 1994;15:627–649.
218. Daughaday WH, Rotwein P. Insulin-like growth factors I and II. Peptide, messenger ribonucleic acid and gene structures, serum, and tissue concentrations. *Endocr Rev* 1989;10:68–91.
219. Russell WE. Growth hormone, somatomedins, and the liver. *Semin in Liver Dis* 1985;5:46–58.
220. Painson JC, Thorner MO, Krieg RJ, et al. Short-term adult exposure to estradiol feminizes the male pattern of spontaneous and growth hormone-releasing factor-stimulated growth hormone secretion in the rat. *Endocrinol* 1992;130:511–519.
221. Zachmann M. Interrelations between growth hormone and sex hormones: physiology and therapeutic consequences. *Horm Res (Suppl)* 1992;38 1:1–8.
222. Mode A, Norstedt G. Effects of gonadal steroid hormones on the hypothalamo-pituitary-liver axis in the control of sex differences in hepatic steroid metabolism in the rat. *J Endocrinol* 1982;95:181–187.

223. Jansson JO, Ekberg S, Isaksson OG, et al. Influence of gonadal steroids on age- and sex-related secretory patterns of growth hormone in the rat. *Endocrinol* 1984;114:1287–1294.

224. Waxman DJ, Pampori NA, Ram PA, et al. Interpulse interval in circulating growth hormone patterns regulates sexually dimorphic expression of hepatic cytochrome P450. *Proc Natl Acad Sci U S A* 1991;88:6868–6872.

225. Norstedt G, Palmiter R. Secretory rhythm of growth hormone regulates sexual differentiation of mouse liver. *Cell* 1984;36:805–812.

226. Mode A, Norstedt G, Simic B, et al. Continuous infusion of growth hormone feminizes hepatic steroid metabolism in the rat. *Endocrinol* 1981;108:2103–2108.

227. Tollet P, Mode A, Gustafsson J-A. The hypothalamic-pituitary-liver axis: growth hormone controls liver sex. In: HB Reyes, U Leuschner, IM Arias, eds. *Pregnancy, Sex Hormones and the Liver. Falk Symposium 89.* 1995:16–48.

228. Gustafsson J-A: The hypothalamic-pituitary-liver axis. Growth hormone controls liver sex. In: IM Arias, JL Boyer, N Fausto, WB Jakoby DA Schachter and DA Shafritz, eds. *The Liver: Biology and Pathobiology*, 3rd Edition. New York:Raven Press, 1994:1209–1214.

229. Liddle C, Mode A, Gustafsson J-A. Constitutive expression and hormonal regulation of male sexually differentiated cytochromes P450 in primary cultured rat hepatocytes. *Arch Biochem Biophys* 1992;298:159–166.

230. Legraverend C, Mode A, Westin S, et al. Transcriptional regulation of rat P-450 2C gene subfamily members by the sexually dimorphic pattern of growth hormone secretion. *Mol Endocrin* 1992;6:259–266.

231. Tollet P, Legraverend C, Gustafsson JA, et al. Growth hormone (GH) regulation of cytochrome P-450IIC12, insulin-like growth factor-I (IGF-I), and GH receptor messenger RNA expression in primary rat hepatocytes: A hormonal interplay with insulin, IGF-I, and thyroid hormone. *Mol Endocrin* 1990;4:1934–1942.

232. Ram PA, Waxman DJ. Pretranslational control by thyroid hormone of rat liver steroid 5 α-reductase and comparison to the thyroid dependence of two growth hormone-regulated CYP2C mRNAs. *J Biol Chem* 1990;265:19223–19229.

233. Simon FR, Fortune, J, Iwahashi M, et al. Gender differences in alcohol dehydrogenase are regulated by growth hormone secretory patterns. *Gastroenterology* 1996;110:A1327.

234. Kempe KC, Isom HC, Greene FE. Responsiveness of an SV40-immortalized hepatocyte cell line to growth hormone. *Biochem Pharmacol* 1995;49:1091–1098.

235. Guzelian PS, Li D, Schuetz EG, et al. Sex changes in cytochrome P450 phenotype by growth hormone treatment of adult rat hepatocytes maintained in a new culture system on matrigel. *Proc Natl Acad Sci U S A* 1988;85:9783–9787.

236. Mathews LS, Enberg B, Norstedt G. Regulation of rat growth hormone receptor gene expression. *J Biol Chem* 1986;264:9905–9910.

237. Kelly PA, Dijiane J, Postel-Vinay M-C, et al. The prolactin/growth hormone receptor family. *Endocr Rev* 1991;12:235–251.

238. Kopchick JJ, Bellush LL, Coschigano KT. Transgenic models of growth hormone action. *Annu Rev Nutr* 1999;19:437–461.

239. Tollet P, Hamberg M, Gustafsson JA, et al. Growth hormone signaling. *J Biol Chem* 1995;270:12569–12577.

240. Gevers E, Pincus SM, Robinson IC, et al. Differential orderliness of the GH release process in castrated male and female rats. *Am J Physiol* 1998;274:R437–R444.

241. Veldhuis JD, Metzger DL, Martha Jr PM, et al. Estrogen and testosterone, but not a nonaromatizable androgen, direct network integration of the hypothalamo-somatotrope (growth hor-

mone)-insulin-like growth factor I axis in the human: evidence from pubertal pathophysiology and sex-steroid hormone replacement. *J Clin Endocrinol Metab* 1997;82:3414–3420.

242. Winer LM, Shaw MA, Baumann G. Basal plasma growth hormone levels in man: new evidence for rhythimicity of growth hormone secretion. *J Clin Endocrinol Metab* 1990;70:1678–1686.

243. Morris TQ, Preisig R, Shaver JC, et al. Effects of growth hormone administration on hepatic excretion of bromsulfalein (BSP). *Proc Soc Exp Biol Med* 1969;130:1183–1188.

244. Schmidt ML, Gartner LM, Arias IM. Studies of hepatic excretory function. 3. Effect of hypopituitarism on the hepatic excretion of sulfobromophthalein sodium in man. *Gastroenterology* 1967;52:998–1002.

245. Krahe J, Hauffa BP, Wollmann HA, et al. Transient elevation of urinary catecholamine excretion and cholestatic liver disease in a neonate with hypopituitarism. *J Pediatr Gastroenterol Nutr* 1992;14:153–159.

246. Nelson DR. Cytochrome P450 and the individuality of species. *Arch Biochem Biophys* 1999;369:1–10.

247. Cheung NW, Liddle C, Coverdale S, et al. Growth hormone treatment increases cytochrome P450-mediated antipyrine clearance in man. *J Clin Endocrinol Metab* 1996;81:1999–2001.

248. Pampori NA, Shapiro BH. Gender differences in the responsiveness of the sex-dependent isoforms of hepatic P450 to the feminine plasma growth hormone profile. *Endocrinology* 1999;140:1245–1254.

249. Mode A, Wiersma-Larsson E, Strom A, et al. A dual role of growth hormone as a feminizing and masculinizing factor in the control of sex-specific cytochrome P-450 isozymes in rat liver. *J Endocrinol* 1988;120:311–317.

250. Liddle C, Mode A, Gustafsson J-A. Constitutive expression and hormonal regulation of male sexually differentiated cytochromes P450 in primary cultured rat hepatocytes. *Arch Biochem Biophysics* 1992;298:159–166.

251. Sasaki Y, Takahashi Y, Nakayama K, et al. Cooperative regulation of CYP2C12 gene expression by STAT5 and liver-specific factors in female rats. *J Biol Chem* 1999,274:37117–37124.

252. Brock WJ, Vore M. Characterization of uptake of steroid glucuronides into isolated male and female rat hepatocytes. *J Pharmacol Exp Ther* 1984;229:175–181.

253. Martin JF, Mikulecky M, Blaschke TF, et al. Differences between the plasma indocyanine green disappearance rates of normal men and women. *Proc Soc Exp Biol Med* 1975;150:612–617.

254. Orzes N, Bellentani S, Aldini R, et al. Sex differences in the hepatic uptake of sulphobromophthalein in the rat. *Clin Sci* 1985;69:587–593.

255. Muraca J, DeGroote J, Fevery J. Sex differences of hepatic conjugation of bilirubin determine its maximal biliary excretion in non-anaesthetized male and female rats. *Clin Sci* 1983;64:85–90.

256. Sorrentino D, Licko V, Weisiger RA. Sex differences in sulfobromophthalein-glutathione transport by perfused rat liver. *Biochem Pharmacol* 1988;37:3119–3126.

257. Weisiger RA, Fitz JG. Sex differences in membrane potential in the intact perfused rat liver. *Am J Physiol* 1988;255:G8222–G825.

258. Luxon BA, Holly DC, Milliano MT, et al. Sex differences in multiple steps in hepatic transport of palmitate support a balanced uptake mechanism. *Am J Physiol* 1998;274:G52–G61.

259. Klaassen CD, Strom SC. Comparison of biliary excretory function and bile composition in male, female, and lactating female rats. *Drug Metab Dispos* 1978;6:120–124.

260. Ben-Johnson N, Arbogast LA, Hyde JF. Neuroendocrine regulation of prolactin release. *Prog Neurobiol* 1989;333:399–447.

261. Kelly PA, Posner BI, Tsushima T, et al. Studies of insulin, growth hormone and prolactin binding: ontogenesis, effect of sex and pregnancy. *Endocrinology* 1974;95:532–539.

262. Robertson JA, Haldosen LA, Wood TJ, et al. Growth hormone pretranslationally regulates the sexually dimorphic expression of the prolactin receptor gene in rat liver. *Mol Endocrin* 1990;4:1235–1239.

263. Jahn GA, Daniel N, Jolivet G, et al. In vivo study of prolactin (PRL) intracellular signalling during lactogenesis in the rat: JAK/STAT pathway is activated by PRL in the mammary gland but not in the liver. *Biol Reprod* 1997;57:894–900.

264. Barash I, Cromlish W, Posner BI. Prolactin (PRL) receptor induction in cultured rat hepatocytes: Dual regulation by PRL and growth hormone. *Endocrinol* 1988;122:1151–1158.

265. Wakao H, Gouilleux F, Groner B. Mammary gland factor (MGF) is a novel member of the cytokine regulated transcription factor gene family and confers the prolactin response. *EMBO J* 1994;13:2182–2191.

266. Choi HK, Waxman DJ. Growth hormone, but not prolactin, maintains low-level activation of STAT5a and STAT5b in female rat liver. *Endocrinol* 1999;140:5135–5185.

267. Ganguly TC, Liu Y, Hyde JF, et al. Prolactin increases hepatic Na+/taurocholate co-transport activity and messenger RNA postpartum. *Biochem J* 1994;303:33–36.

268. Ganguly T, Hyde JF, Vore M. Prolactin increases Na+/taurocholate cotransport in isolated hepatocytes from postpartum rats and ovariectomized rats. *J Pharmacol Exp Ther* 1993;267:82–87.

269. Liu Y, Suchy FJ, Silverman JA, et al. Prolactin increases ATP-dependent taurocholate transport in canalicular plasma membrane from rat liver. *Am J Physiol* 1997;272:G46–G53.

270. Ganguly TC, O'Brien ML, Karpen SJ, et al. Regulation of the rat liver sodium-dependent bile acid cotransporter gene by prolactin. Mediation of transcriptional activation by Stat5. *J Clin Invest* 1997;99:2906–2914.

NUCLEOTIDE TRANSPORT AND REGULATION OF BILE FORMATION

RICHARD M. ROMAN
J. GREGORY FITZ

The formation of bile by the liver depends upon functional interactions between hepatocytes and cholangiocytes, two distinct cell types that together form the bile secretory unit. Recent studies indicate that adenosine triphosphate (ATP) may serve as a signaling molecule that is released by hepatocytes and targets cholangiocytes, suggesting a role for ATP in local autocrine/paracrine regulation of bile formation. Consequently, the purpose of this chapter is to (a) review the evidence supporting a role for ATP in the regulation of cholangiocyte Cl^- secretion, (b) assess the potential sources of ATP in bile, and (c) describe the cellular mechanisms thought to contribute to the regulation of ATP release. Based on the recent identification of multiple ATP-responsive receptors in liver cells, it is attractive to speculate that pharmacological modulation of ATP release and purinergic receptors might provide novel strategies for the management of cholestasis and other disorders characterized by impaired cholangiocyte function.

R. M. Roman and J. G. Fitz: Department of Medicine, University of Colorado Health Sciences Center, Denver, Colorado 80262.

HEPATOBILIARY COUPLING — HOW DO HEPATOCYTES TALK TO CHOLANGIOCYTES?

Traditional models emphasize that the final volume and composition of bile depends upon separate contributions from bile salt-dependent secretion (hepatocytes), bile salt-independent secretion (hepatocytes), and intrahepatic ductular secretion (cholangiocytes). Transport of bile salts, glutathione and other solutes into the canalicular space between hepatocytes generates an osmotic gradient favoring influx of water. Subsequently, this primary product is alkalinized and diluted as it flows through the extensive network of intrahepatic ducts as a result of cholangiocyte Cl^- and HCO_3^- secretion (7). There has been rapid progress in the molecular identification of the transporters involved, and the results have underscored the important contribution of each pathway. Importantly, the cellular mechanisms involved in solute transport are quite different, with ATP-dependent transport of bile salts (bsep) and glutathione (mrp2) across the canalicular membrane of hepatocytes, and channel-mediated secretion of Cl^- (cftr) and Cl^-/HCO_3^- exchange (AE) across the apical membrane of cholangiocytes (Fig. 28.1). Curiously, bile salt transport by hepatocytes also appears to increase biliary Cl^- secretion. For example, a 1962 study by Wheeler et al. using intact liver showed that bile salt infusion not only increased bile

Hepatocytes:
organic and inorganic solute secretion

Cholangiocytes:
Cl⁻ and HCO₃⁻ secretion

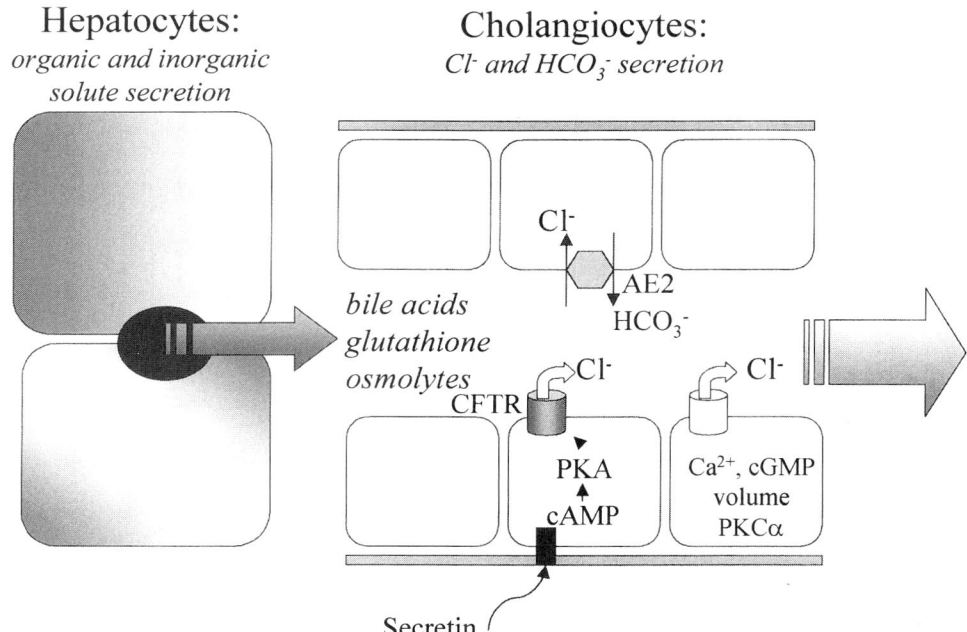

FIGURE 28.1. Cellular mechanisms of bile formation. Bile formation is initiated by transport of bile acids, glutathione and other organic solutes into the canalicular space between hepatocytes. Subsequently, the volume and composition of bile is altered as it flows through the lumen of intrahepatic bile ducts. The mechanisms of secretion by the cholangiocytes which line these ducts is thought to involve Cl^- efflux through cftr and other Cl^- channels as well as Cl^-/HCO_3^- mediated by AE2 in the apical membrane.

volume, but also increased biliary Cl^- and HCO_3 excretion (23). This observation raises the intriguing possibility that there are factors released into bile by hepatocytes that are capable of stimulating cholangiocyte anion secretion.

THE CASE FOR ADENOSINE TRIPHOSPHATE—PURINERGIC SIGNALING PATHWAYS

ATP has recently been recognized to be a versatile autocrine and paracrine-signaling molecule targeting many different cell types. ATP is found inside cells in relatively high concentrations of 3 to 6 mM. In response to specific physiologic signals, most cells are capable of releasing ATP [and uridine triphosphate (UTP)], leading to the appearance of low concentrations of nucleotides in blood, bile, and interstitial fluids under normal conditions (Fig. 28.2). The amount of ATP released is small, representing less than 1% of total cellular stores. However, the amount of extracellular ATP required for signaling is in the nanomolar range, concentrations 10,000-fold below that found within cells.

The biological effects of extracellular nucleotides are mediated by binding to specific purinergic receptors in the plasma membrane (27). The molecular identification of these receptors has proceeded at a rapid pace, with the cloning and expression of complementary DNAs encoding

four adenosine-preferring (P1) and at least eighteen ATP and/or UTP-preferring (P2) receptors. In general, the adenosine-preferring P1 receptors are positively or negatively coupled to adenylyl cyclase and modulate cellular cAMP levels. The proposed structure is characteristic of other G-protein coupled receptors, with seven α-helical transmembrane domains, an extracellular amino terminus, and an intracellular carboxy terminus. Sequences within the intracellular domains are thought to interact with GTP-binding proteins, and agonist binding increases GTPase activity and liberates α and βγ subunits that interact with ion channels, kinases, and other effector mechanisms.

The *nucleotide-preferring P2 receptors* are molecularly distinct from the P1 family and can be divided into two groups (Fig. 28.3). Receptors in the *P2X* category have intrinsic cation channel properties, and receptors in the *P2Y* category belong to the G protein-coupled receptor superfamily. While P2X receptors are expressed in liver, information regarding their function is just beginning to emerge. In contrast, P2Y receptors have been identified in all of the different cell types within liver, and their pharmacologic and signaling properties have been reviewed by Harden, Boyer and Nicholas (10). When expressed in heterologous models, most P2Y receptors stimulate phospholipase C, and mobilize intracellular Ca^{2+}. Other signaling pathways may be targeted as well, depending on the cell type under investigation. Classically, P2Y receptors have an

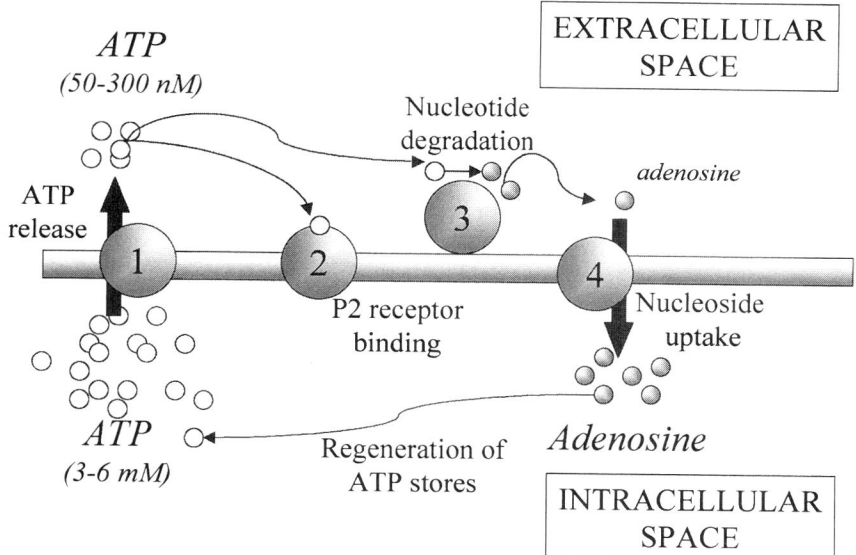

FIGURE 28.2. Purinergic signaling pathways. Autocrine/paracrine signaling involves (*1*) release of adenosine triphosphate (*ATP*) or uridine triphosphate (UTP) from the cell interior, probably through a specific channel, (*2*) binding to one or purinergic receptors in the plasma membrane, (*3*) nucleotide degradation through cell surface-associated ecto-nucleotidases, and (*4*) reuptake of adenosine and uridine through specific transport proteins. This signaling scheme offers several potential sites for regulation of purinergic signaling.

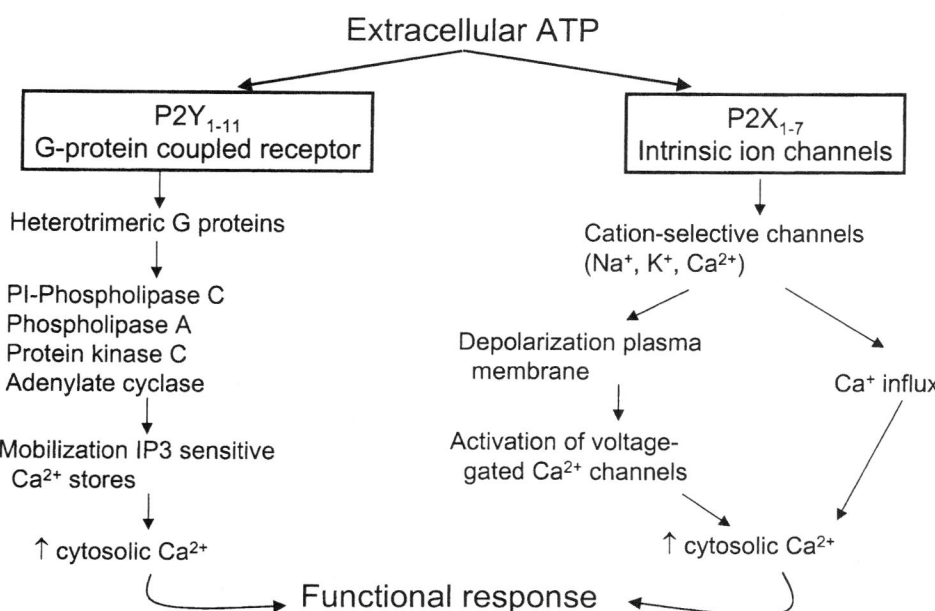

FIGURE 28.3. P2 receptor categorization. The functional response to adenosine triphosphate (*ATP*) depends in large part on the cellular repertoire of P2 receptors. Broadly, these include P2Y receptors which are generally coupled through G proteins to phospholipase C and other pathways; and P2x receptors which have intrinsic cation channel properties and permit the influx of Na^+ and Ca^{2+} ions.

agonist potency order for ATP > ADP > AMP >> adenosine, with half-maximal responses to ATP at concentrations of 300 to 500 nM. However, ADP and the pyrimidine nucleotides UTP and UDP are the preferred agonists for certain P2Y receptor subtypes (27). With the rapid progress in this area, the web sites maintained by the Molecular Recognition Section of the National Institutes of Health (http://mgddk1.niddk.nih.gov:8000/nomenclature.html) are a valuable guide to current information regarding receptor structure and function.

Small concentrations of nucleotides can exert potent regulatory effects on liver cells. However, the response can be complex based on the types of nucleotides and nucleosides available at the cell surface, the repertoire of receptors expressed by target cells, and the subcellular localization of the receptors. While much remains to be learned, this model suggests several potential sites for regulation of purinergic signaling including (a) modulation of *nucleotide release* through opening of channels or other pathways, (b) modulation of *nucleotide degradation* by extracellular nucleotidases, which dephosphorylate ATP and generate other active metabolites, and (c) expression of more than one type of receptor to transduce specific signals to the cell interior. In the following sections, the potential role of these mechanisms in the regulation of bile formation is explored.

P2Y2 RECEPTORS ARE PRESENT IN THE APICAL MEMBRANE OF CULTURED CHOLANGIOCYTES

See Chapter 29 and website chapter 🖳 W-25. In cholangiocytes, exposure to ATP and/or UTP stimulates phospholipase C and increases intracellular $[Ca^{2+}]$ with equal potency (half-maximal effects at approximately 300 nM), consistent with the expression of receptors in the P2Y2 (also known as P2u) subclass. Interestingly, ATP is present in bile in concentrations sufficient to activate these receptors (2). Consequently, if P2Y2 (or other) receptors are present in the apical membrane of cholangiocytes, then ATP in bile could function as a signaling molecule regulating ductular secretion. Several observations support this concept (31). First, in normal rat cholangiocytes (NRCs) in monolayer culture, selective exposure of the apical membrane to ATP causes an increase in short-circuit current (ΔI_{sc}), the electrophysiologic signature of apical Cl^- secretion (Fig. 28.4). Second, the pharmacologic properties of the response, including equal agonist potency for ATP, UTP and the non-hydrolyzable analog ATPγS, are consistent with that anticipated for P2Y2 receptors. There is no significant apical response to ADP, AMP or adenosine. Third, a cDNA encoding P2Y2 receptors has been cloned from a rat liver cDNA library, and encodes a protein of 374 amino acids, highly homologous to other rat P2Y2 receptors. When expressed in *Xenopus laevis* oocytes, the pharmacologic properties are analogous to the apical response of NRC cells.

Normal Rat Cholangiocyte monolayer: Cl⁻ secretory response to apical ATP

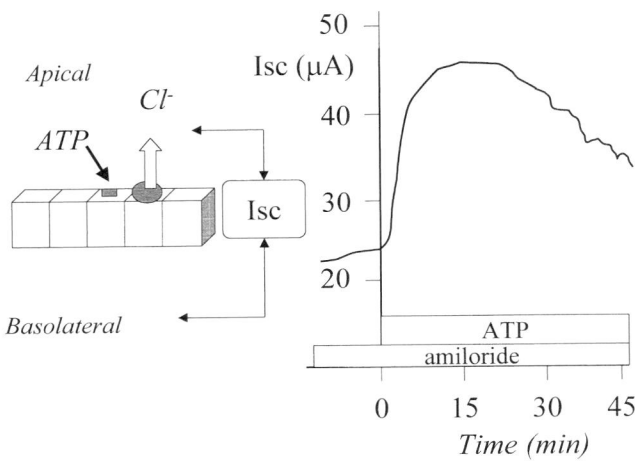

FIGURE 28.4. Adenosine triphosphate (*ATP*) stimulates transepithelial secretion across cholangiocyte monolayers. In polarized cell monolayers, transepithelial movement of Cl^- ions from the basolateral to apical space is measured as short circuit current (I_{sc}). In the preence of miloride to block Na+ absorption, exposure to ATP activates P2Y₂ receptors (P2R) in the apical membrane, and elicits a brisk Cl^- secretory response.

Finally, P2Y2 mRNA as assessed by Northern analysis is detectable as a 33 kb band in NRC cells (31). Collectively, these molecular and functional findings are consistent with a role for nucleotides as regulatory factors modulating biliary secretion through activation of P2Y2 receptors in the apical membrane of cholangiocytes. It is notable that there are also P2Y2 (and other) receptors in the basolateral membrane of cholangiocytes (19), and that purinergic agonists modulate other transport pathways as well.

THE CELLULAR ORIGIN OF BILIARY NUCLEOTIDES

Outside of the central nervous system where ATP serves as a neurotransmitter, the mechanisms responsible for nucleotide release are not well defined. Nonetheless, there are many examples where, in the absence of cell injury or necrosis, ATP is released in response to mechanical stress, changes in cell volume, increased intracellular Ca^{2+}, increased cAMP and membrane receptor stimulation, as reviewed recently (27). While the molecular basis of ATP release remains controversial, an electrophysiologic approach using whole-cell patch clamp techniques is capable of detecting transmembrane currents carried by the movement of ionized ATP molecules across the membrane. This observation suggests that ATP release is electrogenic and is mediated through the opening of membrane pores or channels. Initial studies suggested that the Cl^- channel proteins encoded by cftr and the multidrug resistance P-glycoprotein encoded by mdr1 were each capable of functioning as ATP channels under defined conditions. Native expression, upregulation and heterologous expression of these proteins are associated with enhanced ATP permeability and ATP channel activity in some but not all model systems (1,29,33). However, more recent studies indicate that cftr and mdr are more likely to serve as ATP channel regulators, increasing the amount of ATP released through an as yet unidentified mechanism (22). This relationship between cftr, mdr1 and ATP release remains controversial, and it is clear that many cells exhibit regulated ATP release in the absence of apparent cftr or mdr1 expression. It seems likely that multiple ATP transport pathways will be defined in the future, and mechanisms of regulation are likely to be cell type-specific in order to respond to different physiologic demands.

There is convincing evidence that hepatocytes and cholangiocytes each exhibit regulated ATP release. In intact liver, ATP is present in venous effluent and in bile (2,20). In cells in culture, low levels of ATP in the nanomolar range are always detectable in the supernatant fluid due to constitutive release of ATP from the cell interior. In addition, the rate of release can be increased ten-fold or more by increases in cell volume or other stimuli. In the example of human hepatocytes in culture shown in Figure 28.5, extracellular ATP concentrations were measured using a sensitive luciferin–luciferase assay (4). Mechanical stimulation caused by addition of isotonic buffer (Iso) caused a small increase in release, but cell volume increases caused by addition of hypotonic buffer (hypo, 20% or 40% decrease in NaCl) caused a much larger increase in ATP release (4). The response occurs rapidly, peaking within one minute, and then gradually decreases toward basal levels. Other studies indicate that the response is decreased by chelation of intracellular Ca^{2+} with BAPTA-AM; and Gd^{3+} appears to be a potent and reversible inhibitor of the ATP pore in many cell types, uncoupling changes in ATP release from cell volume (25).

A limitation of the hepatocyte studies to date is that there has been no clear localization of the cellular sites of ATP release. If ATP signals to cells further down the bile secretory unit, then an apical/canalicular orientation of release into the bile lumen would be anticipated. At present, there is no direct evidence in support of this due to the difficulty in sampling from the small (less than 1μ) canalicular space between cells. However, ATP is present in bile and there is considerable evidence for a heavy cellular investment in the enzymes and transporters involved in local canalicular ATP availability. For example, the ATP channel regulator mdr1 is present in the apical/canalicular membrane, and ATP released into the canalicular lumen is subject to degradation by resident ecto-ATPase (apyrase) and 5′ nucleotidase activity (3). Due to the anatomical relationship between the canalicular space and the lumen of intra-

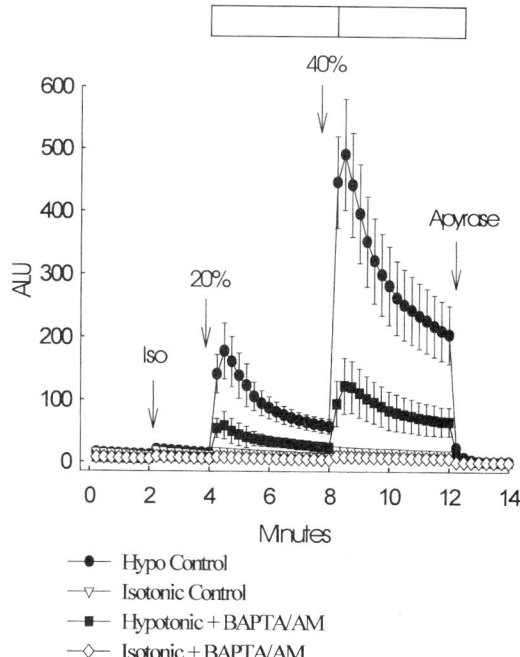

FIGURE 28.5. Adenosine triphosphate (ATP) release was measured from human hepatocytes in culture using a luciferin–luciferase assay. Using this assay, the concentration of ATP in the extracellular space is proportional to the Arbitrary Light Units (*ALUs*). A small ATP signal was detectable under basal conditions, and mechanical stimulation caused by media addition (*Iso*) increased this slightly but significantly. In contrast, increases in cell volume caused by exposure to hypotonic (*hypo*) media caused a large increase in ATP release. The response was inhibited by preincubation in BAPTA-AM to inhibit increases in cytosolic [Ca2+]. (From Feranchak AP, Fitz JG, Roman RM. Volume-sensitive purinergic signaling in human hepatocytes. *J Hepatol* 2000;33:174–182, with permission.)

hepatic bile ducts, any ATP that escapes local degradation within the canaliculus would have direct access to the apical membrane P2Y2 receptors in cholangiocytes.

More recently, the luciferase–luciferin assay has been utilized to demonstrate that cholangiocytes are also capable of releasing ATP into bile. These studies also demonstrate that there are significant differences in nucleotide trafficking in the apical versus basolateral compartments (30). In NRCs in monolayer culture, the apical and basolateral compartments are isolated by high resistance junctions (greater than 1,000 ohm cm²) between cells, so the different compartments can be studied in isolation. Interestingly, both membrane domains exhibit constitutive ATP efflux and express P2 receptors. However, ATP release is polarized, with concentrations in the apical (lumenal) chamber of about 250 nM, about five-fold greater than concentrations of approximately 50 nM in the basolateral chamber. Interestingly, these values are very close to those required for half-maximal stimulation of ΔI_{sc}. Second, the cellular signals that stimulate ATP release are different, although increases in cell volume are the most dramatic. Finally, there are differences in the kinetics of ATP degradation. In the apical compartment, the time course of nucleotide degradation can be described by a single exponential, resulting in the clearance of 13% of ATP in the first minute. In the basolateral compartment, the time course for clearance is faster and more complex, suggesting the presence of more than one degradation pathway. This degradation is likely due to the presence of biliary cell ecto-ATPases (30).

Taken together, these findings indicate that the majority of ATP in bile is likely to be derived from release across the apical membranes of both hepatocytes and cholangiocytes. At present, the relative contribution of the two cell types is unknown due to the inability to make measurements within the lumen of the canalicular space. Maintenance of local ATP concentrations within the lumen is likely to be complex due to changes in bile flow, changes in the rates of ATP release, and potent mechanisms for nucleotide degradation (3). However, even small changes in ATP availability would be expected to effect cholangiocyte Cl^- secretion, since the best evidence suggests that local concentrations are within the range required for receptor binding (31).

CELLULAR SIGNALS REGULATING NUCLEOTIDE RELEASE

In liver epithelia, cell volume is not a static parameter. Rather, there are regulated changes of ±10% that occur in response to hormonal signals and changes in solute transport (11). Interestingly, volume-sensitive changes in ATP release are not limited to liver cells, but have been demonstrated in many unrelated cell types (14,17,18,33). Consequently, considerable attention has been focused on the cellular mechanisms that sense these changes in cell volume and stimulate ATP release.

Both intracellular $[Ca^{2+}]$ and protein kinase $C\alpha$ modulate liver cell responses to cell volume increases, mediating adaptive opening of K^+ and Cl^- channels, solute efflux, and restoration of cell volume toward basal values (24,28). These effects may be mediated in part through calcium-dependent modulation of ATP release (Fig. 28.5). For example, in human hepatocytes, chelation of intracellular $[Ca^{2+}]$ by exposure to BAPTA-AM inhibits constitutive and volume-sensitive ATP release by approximately 60% and approximately 90%, respectively, and prevents Cl^- channel activation and recovery from cell swelling (4). Similarly, BAPTA-AM and the protein kinase C inhibitor calphostin C (500 nM) inhibit ATP release from biliary cells (30). In contrast, neither increases in cAMP levels nor inhibition of cAMP-dependent signaling has any effect on ATP release. It is notable that increases in cell volume have only small effects on intracellular $[Ca^{2+}]$ in these cells (unpublished observations), and that increases

in intracellular $[Ca^{2+}]$ caused by exposure to ionomycin (2 μM) or thapsigargin (1 μM) stimulate ATP release but to a much smaller extent (30). Thus, intracellular $[Ca^{2+}]$ appears to be necessary for ATP release, but may not be the primary signaling pathway involved.

More recently, increases in cell volume have been shown to cause parallel activation of a number of kinases, including phosphoinositide 3-kinase (PI 3-kinase) (12) (see Chapters 34 and 35). Upon activation, PI 3-kinase phosphorylates phosphatidylinositol, producing phosphatidylinositol 3-phosphate (PtdIns 3-P), phosphatidylinositol 3,4-biphosphate (PtdIns-3,4 P_2), and phosphatidylinositol 3,4,5-trisphosphate (PtdIns-3,4,5 P_3). In liver cells, there is increasing evidence that these phospholipids play a major role in vesicular trafficking, movement of bile acid transporters to the canalicular membrane and bile formation (8,15,16) (see Chapter 24 and website chapters 🖳 W-22 through W-24).

Several observations indicate that PI 3-kinase also plays a central role in the regulation of hepatic ATP release (5,6). Since volume-sensitive ATP release leads to receptor binding and activation of Cl^- channels in liver and biliary cells, measurement of volume-sensitive Cl^- currents provides a convenient bioassay for ATP available at the cell surface (34). First, exposure to the PI 3-kinase inhibitors wortmannin and LY294002 sharply decreases cellular ATP release and prevents volume-sensitive activation of Cl^- currents. Second, the same inhibitors also prevent recovery from swelling in isolated cells and ΔI_{sc} in NRC monolayers (5,6). Each effect is attributable to impaired delivery of ATP to the cell surface, since the Cl^- secretory response to exogenous ATP is retained. Finally, intracellular dialysis with the synthetic products of PI 3-kinase leads to activation of Cl^- currents even in the absence of cell volume changes (5). Using whole-cell recording techniques, this experimental approach, illustrated in Fig. 28.6, takes advantage of the low resistance access to the cell interior provided by the patch pipette. When synthetic PtdIns-3,4-P_2 and/or PtdIns-3,4,5-P_3 in concentrations of 10 μM is delivered to the cell interior, there is a gradual activation of Cl^- currents. In contrast, neither PIP2 nor PtdIns-3-P has any effect, suggesting that only the bis- or trisphosphate products of PI 3-kinase serve in this signaling capacity. Since the current response is blocked by removal of extracellular ATP with apyrase, the results are most consistent with a model wherein the lipid products of PI 3-kinase directly modulate membrane ATP permeability (5). This represents an attractive mechanism for site-specific regulation of membrane ATP permeability by a membrane-derived phospholipid. Based on the established role of PI 3-kinase in the regulation of vesicular trafficking, including other transporters involved in bile formation (15,16), it is possible that PI 3-kinase signaling leads to insertion of new ATP channels or to opening of preexisting ATP channels. However, the molecular basis of ATP release has not been defined, so the specific site of action of these lipids is not known.

Basal

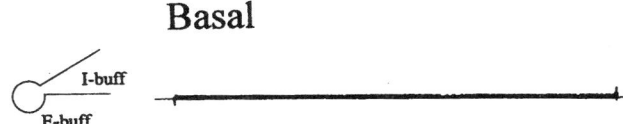

Hypotonic Exposure

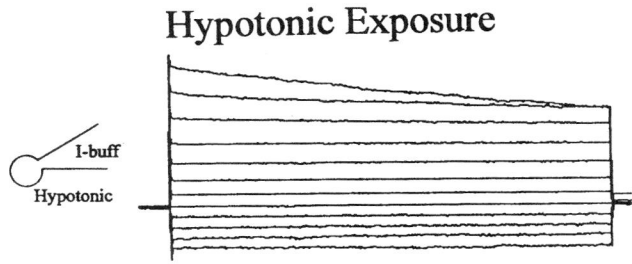

PI 3-kinase Lipid Products

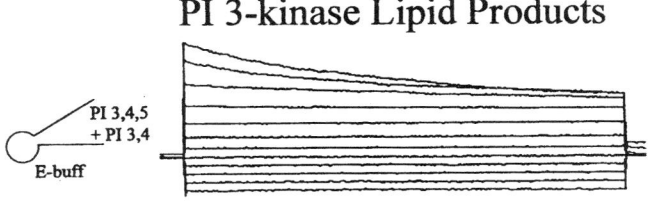

Control Lipid

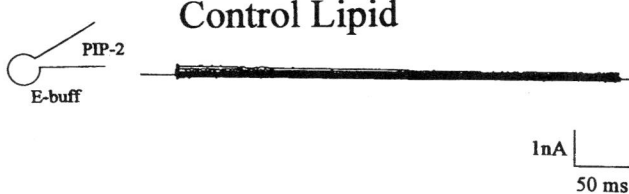

1nA ⌐
     └
     50 ms

FIGURE 28.6. The lipid products of PI 3-kinase activate Cl⁻ currents. In human cholangiocarcinoma cells, whole cell patch clamp techniques were utilized to measure membrane Cl⁻ currents, a bioassay for adenosine triphosphate (ATP) release (5). This approach permits intracellular delivery of lipids by their inclusion in the patch pipette. Under basal conditions in the absence of lipids, currents are small (**top**). Exposure to hypotonic media activates large Cl⁻ currents (**second tracing**). Interestingly, exposure to phosphoinositide 3-kinase (*PI 3-kinase*) lipid products by inclusion of PtdIns-3,4-P$_2$ and PtdIns-3,4,5-P$_3$ in the patch pipette has similar effects (**third tracing**). The effect appears to be specific since PIP-2 has no effects. These findings suggest that PI 3-kinase may contribute to regulation of ATP release. (From Feranchak AP, Roman RM, Schwiebert EM, et al. Phosphatidyl inositol 3-kinase represents a novel signal regulating cell volume through effects on ATP release. *J Biol Chem* 1998;273:14906–14911, with permission.)

TESTING THE ROLE OF ENDOGENOUS ADENOSINE TRIPHOSPHATE RELEASE IN THE REGULATION OF DUCTULAR SECRETION

It is difficult to estimate the overall contribution of purinergic signaling to the regulation of bile formation. In humans, secretin acts on cholangiocytes to increase bile flow from 0.67 to 1.54 mL/min⁻¹, indicating that ductular secretion contributes importantly to the volume and composition of bile (13). In NRC cells in culture, the amplitude of the ΔI_{sc} response to apical ATP exceeds that of secretin (unpublished observations). While there are obvious limitations that preclude extrapolation of these observations *in vitro* to intact liver, the robust responses observed in isolated cells are sufficient to suggest that ATP represents a good candidate for local regulation of constitutive and volume-stimulated cholangiocyte Cl⁻ secretion.

To test this hypothesis more directly, the role of endogenous ATP release as a mediator of the secretory response in cells in culture has recently been assessed (26). In isolated Mz-ChA-1 cholangiocarcinoma cells, there is significant ATP release detectable under basal conditions. This constitutive ATP release appears to be physiologically significant, since removal of extracellular ATP leads to a gradual increase in cell volume and prevents volume-dependent activation of Cl⁻ channels and recovery from swelling (Fig. 28.7). Moreover, in intact monolayers, increases in cell volume stimulate changes in ΔI_{sc} due to apical Cl⁻ secretion, and the response is dependent on ATP release and apical P2Y2 receptor stimulation (26). In the examples shown in Figure 28.8, I_{sc} was measured under control conditions and during exposure to hypotonic (30% decrease in NaCl) buffer to increase cell volume and stimulate ATP release. Hypotonic exposure caused a rapid increase in ΔI_{sc} of 41% to 69%. This response appears to be mediated by ATP release and P2 receptor binding, since it is inhibited by apyrase to degrade extracellular ATP and suramin to block P2 receptors (26). Taken together, these findings suggest that volume-sensitive ATP release across the apical membrane of cholangiocytes acts in an autocrine/paracrine manner to bind P2Y2 receptors on adjacent cells and stimulate Cl⁻ secretion.

POTENTIAL IMPLICATIONS FOR BILE FORMATION

These findings suggest that ATP in bile derived from both hepatocytes and cholangiocytes regulates cholangiocyte secretion through activation of P2Y2 receptors in the apical membrane (Fig. 28.9). If these findings are relevant to cholangiocyte secretion *in vivo*, several general points merit further investigation. First, it is notable that the ATP effects emphasized here focus on events taking place at the apical

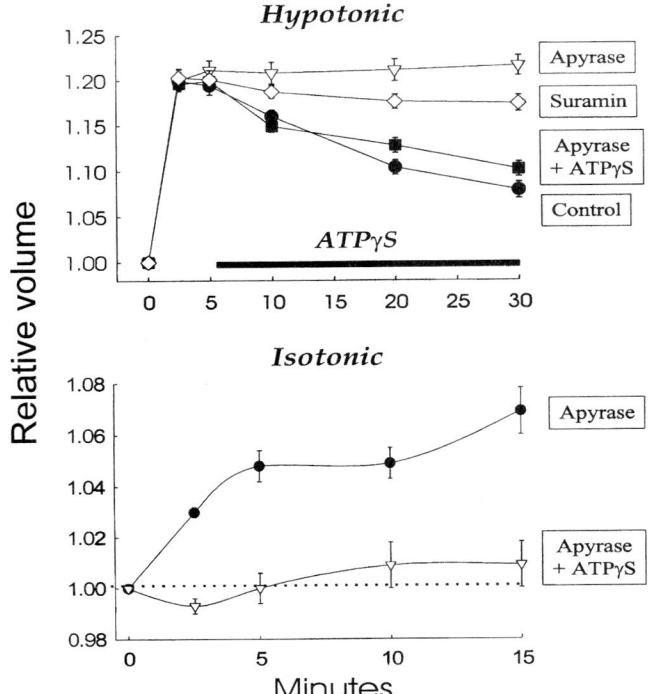

FIGURE 28.7. Extracellular adenosine triphosphate (*ATP*) regulates biliary cell volume. The volume of Mz-ChA-1 cholangiocarcinoma cells was measured using a Coulter multisizer, and data are presented as relative cell volume by normalization to basal values in isotonic buffer. **Top:** Exposure to hypotonic buffer caused a rapid initial increase in cell volume, followed by gradual recovery mediated in part by opening of Cl⁻ channels (Control). Interruption of purinergic signaling by addition of the ATP scavenger apyrase or the P2 receptor blocker suramin inhibited cell volume recovery. **Bottom:** Exposure of cells suspended in isotonic buffer to apyrase to remove extracellular ATP led to an increase in cell volume. The effects were reversed by the presence of the non-hydrolyzable P2 receptor analog ATPγS. These findings suggest that endogenous release of ATP contributes to cell volume homeostasis through regulation of P2 receptors. (From Roman RM, Feranchak AP, Salter KD, et al. Endogenous ATP regulates Cl⁻ secretion in cultured human and rat biliary epithelial cells. *Am J Physiol* 1999;276:G1391–G1400, with permission.)

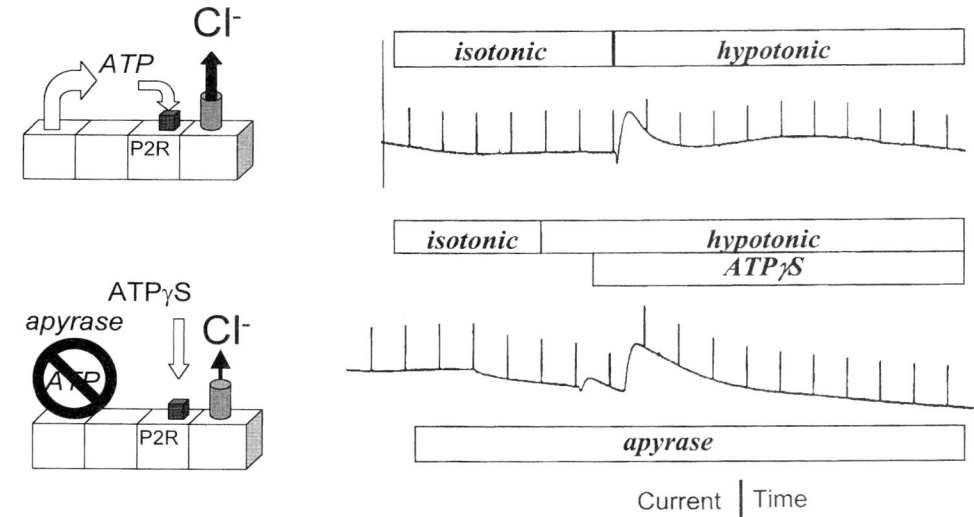

FIGURE 28.8. Endogenous adenosine triphosphate (*ATP*) release regulates transepithelial Cl⁻ secretion. In biliary cell monolayers, I_{sc} was measured as a guide to transepithelial Cl⁻ secretion. Exposure to hypotonic buffer to stimulate ATP release increases I_{sc} (**top tracing**). In the presence of apyrase to eliminate extracellular ATP, this response is minimized. However, exposure to exogenous ATPγS still elicits a response. These findings indicate that the swelling-activated secretory current is related to apical ATP release and P2 receptor stimulation. (From Roman RM, Feranchak AP, Salter KD, et al. Endogenous ATP regulates Cl⁻ secretion in cultured human and rat biliary epithelial cells. *Am J Physiol* 1999;276:G1391–G1400, with permission.)

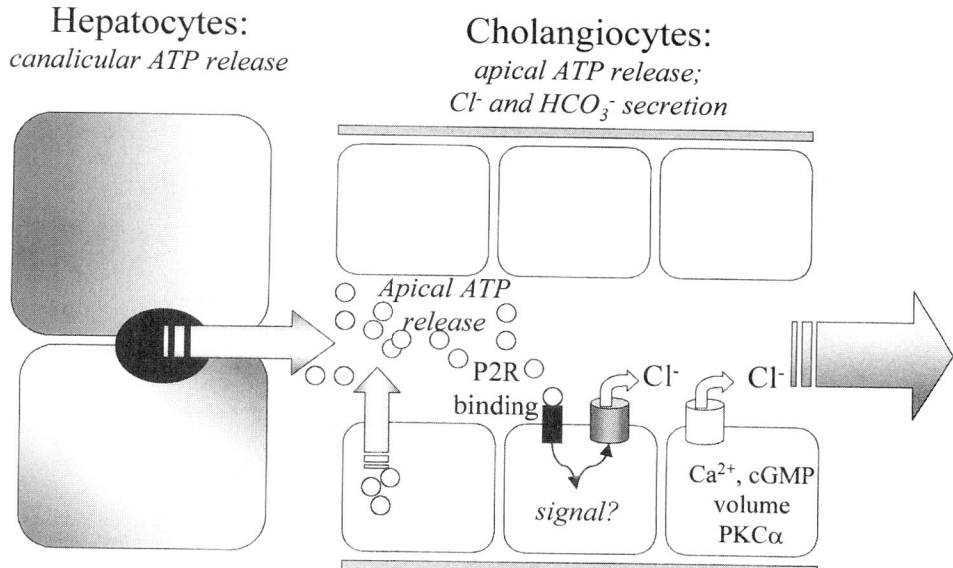

FIGURE 28.9. Proposed model for purinergic modulation of biliary secretion. *ATP*, adenosine triphosphate. (From Roman RM, Feranchak AP, Salter KD, et al. Endogenous ATP regulates Cl⁻ secretion in cultured human and rat biliary epithelial cells. *Am J Physiol* 1999;276:G1391–G1400, with permission.)

membrane. This represents an anatomic orientation that is well suited for hepatocyte-to-cholangiocyte or cholangiocyte-to-cholangiocyte signaling by release of ATP into bile. This orientation differs from secretin and other hormones which are delivered to the basolateral membrane through the bloodstream. However, it should be emphasized that purinergic receptors are also present in the basolateral domains of these cells. These pathways are presumably designed to respond to different stimuli that may be unrelated to bile formation (32). For example, in rat liver epithelial cells (WB-F344), mechanically-induced Ca^{2+} wave propagation appears to depend not only on intercellular gap junctions, but requires ATP release and paracrine P2 receptor stimulation as well (9).

A second issue is that there are substantial cell-to-cell differences in the Cl⁻ channels responsible for apical efflux, and the intracellular signals that couple P2 receptor binding to ion channel opening are not fully defined. This represents an issue of particular importance due to the recognition that CFTR functions as a cAMP-regulated Cl⁻ channel in many gastrointestinal secretory cells. Interestingly, in cells with the cystic fibrosis phenotype, activation of P2 receptors still elicits potent secretory responses. Thus, P2 receptors appear capable of stimulating secretion through opening of anion channels unrelated to CFTR. Accordingly, there is great interest in exploring options for use of P2 receptor agonists to bypass the Cl⁻ secretory defect associated with cystic fibrosis (21).

Finally, identification of the molecular basis of ATP permeability and the cellular signals controlling ATP release represent very high priorities. The best evidence suggests

that transport occurs through an electrogenic pathway consistent with a channel or pore. If so, opening of an ATP permeable channel would lead to rapid efflux of ATP^{4-} or $MgATP^{2-}$ from the high (mM) concentrations in the cell interior to the low (nM) concentrations near the cell surface.

The recent progress in identification in liver of the many contributors to purinergic signaling, including ATP channels, P-glycoproteins, nucleotidases, and purinergic receptors suggests that nucleotides in bile are likely to play a physiologic role in hepatobiliary coupling and paracrine regulation of bile formation. Moreover, these pathways offer new options for the development of pharmacologic strategies to increase bile flow and biliary pH based on increasing the concentration of ATP in bile and stimulation of P2Y2 receptors in the apical membrane of cholangiocytes.

REFERENCES

1. Bosch I., Jackson G, Croop JM, et al. Expression of *Drosophilia melanogaster* P-glycoproteins is associated with ATP channel activity. *Am J Physiol* 1996;271:C1527–C1538.
2. Chari RS, Schutz SM, Haebig JA, et al. Adenosine nucleotides in bile. *Am J Physiol* 1996;270:G246–G252.
3. Che M, Gatmaitan Z, Arias IM. Ectonucleotidases, purine nucleoside transporter, and function of the bile canalicular plasma membrane of the hepatocyte. *FASEB J* 1997;11:101–108.
4. Feranchak AP, Fitz JG, Roman RM. Volume-sensitive purinergic signaling in human hepatocytes. *J Hepatol* 2000;33:174–182.
5. Feranchak AP, Roman RM, Doctor RB, et al. The lipid products of phosphoinositide 3-kinase contribute to regulation of cholangiocyte ATP and chloride transport. *J Biol Chem* 1999;274:30979–30986.
6. Feranchak AP, Roman RM, Schwiebert EM, et al. Phosphatidyl inositol 3-kinase represents a novel signal regulating cell volume

through effects on ATP release. *J Biol Chem* 1998;273: 14906–14911.

7. Fitz JG. Cellular mechanisms of bile secretion. In: Zakim D, Boyer TD, eds. *Hepatology*. Philadelphia: WB Saunders, 1996: 362–376.

8. Folli F, Alvaro D, Gigliozzi A, et al. Regulation of endocytic-transcytotic pathways and bile secretion by phosphatidylinositol 3-kinase in rats. *Gastroenterology* 1997;113:954–965.

9. Frame MK, de Feijter AW. Propagation of mechanically induced intercellular calcium waves via gap junctions and ATP receptors in rat liver epithelial cells. *Exp Cell Res* 1997;230:197–207.

10. Harden TK, Boyer JL, Nicholas RA. P$_2$-purinergic receptors: subtype-associated signaling responses and structure. *Annu Rev Pharmacol Toxicol* 1997;35:541–579.

11. Haussinger D. Regulation and functional significance of liver cell volume. In: Boyer JL, Ockner RK, eds. *Progress in liver disease*. Philadelphia: WB Saunders, 1996:29–53.

12. Krause U, Rider MH, Hue L. Protein kinase signalling pathway triggered by cell swelling and involved in the activation of glycogen synthase and acetyl-CoA carboxylase in isolated rat hepatocytes. *J Biol Chem* 1996;271:16668–16673.

13. Lenzen R, Elster J, Behrend C, et al. Bile acid-independent bile flow is differentially regulated by glucagon and secretin in humans after orthotopic liver transplantation. *Hepatology* 1997; 26:1272–1281.

14. Light DB, Capes TL, Gronau RT, et al. Extracellular ATP stimulates volume decrease in Necturus red blood cells. *Am J Physiol* 1999;277:C480–C491.

15. Misra S, Ujhazy P, Gatmaitan Z, et al. The role of phosphoinositide 3-kinase in taurocholate-induced trafficking of ATP-dependent canalicular transporters in rat liver. *J Biol Chem* 1998; 273:26638–26644.

16. Misra S, Ujhazy P, Varticovski L, et al. Phosphoinositide 3-kinase lipid products regulate ATP-dependent transport by sister of P-glycoprotein and multidrug resistance associated protein 2 in bile canalicular membrane vesicles. *Proc Natl Acad Sci U S A* 1999; 96:5814–5819.

17. Mitchell CH, Carre DA, McGlinn MA, et al. A release mechanism for stored ATP in ocular ciliary epithelial cells. *Proc Natl Acad Sci U S A* 1998;95:7174–7178.

18. Musante L, Zegarra-Moran O, Montaldo PG, et al. Autocrine regulation of volume-sensitive anion channels in airway epithelial cells by adenosine. *J Biol Chem* 1999;274:11701–11707.

19. Nathanson M. Burgstahler H, Mennone AD. Characterization of cytosolic Ca2+ signalling in rat bile duct epithelia. *Am J Physiol* 1996;271:G86–G96.

20. Nukina S, Fusaoka T, Thurman RG. Gylcogenolytic effect of adenosine involves ATP from hepatocytes and eicosanoids from Kupffer cells. *Am J Physiol* 1994;266:G99–G105.

21. Parr CE, Sullivan DM, Paradiso AM, et al. Cloning and expression of a human P2u nucleotide receptor, a target for cystic fibrosis pharmacotherapy. *Proc Natl Acad Sci U S A* 1994;91:3275–3279.

22. Pasyk EA, Foskett JK. Cystic fibrosis transmembrane conductance regulator-associated ATP and adenosine 3'-phosphate 5'-phosphosulfate channels in endoplasmic reticulum and plasma membranes. *J Biol Chem* 1997;272:7746–7751.

23. Preisig R, Cooper HL, Wheeler HO. The relationship between taurocholate secretion rate and bile production in the unanesthetized dog during cholinergic blockade and during secretin administration. *J Clin Invest* 1962;41:1152–1162.

24. Roman RM, Bodily K, Wang Y, et al. Activation of protein kinase C alpha couples cell volume to membrane Cl$^-$ permeability in HTC hepatoma and Mz-ChA-1 cholangiocarcinoma cells. *Hepatology* 1998;28:1073–1080.

25. Roman RM, Feranchak AP, Davison AK, et al. Evidence for Gd^{3+} inhibition of membrane ATP permeability and purinergic signaling. *Am J Physiol* 1999;277:G1222–G1230.

26. Roman RM, Feranchak AP, Salter KD, et al. Endogenous ATP regulates Cl$^-$ secretion in cultured human and rat biliary epithelial cells. *Am J Physiol* 1999;276:G1391–G1400.

27. Roman RM, Fitz JG. Emerging roles of purinergic signaling in gastrointestinal epithelial secretion and hepatobiliary function. *Gastroenterology* 1999;116:964–979.

28. Roman RM, Wang Y, Fitz JG. Regulation of cell volume in a human biliary cell line: Calcium-dependent activation of K+ and Cl− currents. *Am J Physiol* 1996;271:G239–G248.

29. Roman RM, Wang Y, Lidofsky SD, et al. Hepatocellular ATP-binding cassette protein expression enhances ATP release and autocrine regulation of cell volume. *J Biol Chem* 1997;272:21970–21976.

30. *Salter KD, Fitz JG, Roman RM. Domain-specific purinergic signaling in polarized rat cholangiocytes.* Am J Physiol 2000;278: G492–G500.

31. Schlenker TJ. Romac MJ, Sharara A, et al. Regulation of biliary secretion through apical purinergic receptors in cultured rat cholangiocytes. *Am J Physiol* 1997;273:G1108–G1117.

32. Schlosser SF, Burgstahler AD, Nathanson MH. Isolated rat hepatocytes can signal to other hepatocytes and bile duct cells by release of nucleotides. *Proc Natl Acad Sci U S A* 1996;93:9948–9953.

33. Taylor AL, Kudlow BA, Marrs KL, et al. Bioluminescence detection of ATP release mechanisms in epithelia. *Am J Physiol* 1998; 275:C1391–C1406.

34. Wang Y, Roman RM, Lidofsky SD, et al. Autocrine signaling through ATP release represents a novel mechanism for cell volume regulation. *Proc Natl Acad Sci U S A* 1996;93:12020–12025.

The Liver: Biology and Pathobiology, Fourth Edition, edited by I. M. Arias, J. L. Boyer, F. V. Chisari, N. Fausto, D. Schachter, and D. A. Shafritz.
Lippincott Williams & Wilkins, Philadelphia © 2001.

29

THE PATHOBIOLOGY OF BILIARY EPITHELIA

GIANFRANCO ALPINI
RICHARD T. PRALL
NICHOLAS F. LARUSSO

The liver is composed of two types of epithelial cells: (a) hepatocytes representing approximately 60% of the endogenous liver cell population in the rodent liver, and (b) intrahepatic bile duct epithelial cells (i.e., cholangiocytes), which account for 3% to 5% of the nucleated liver cell population. Major progress has recently been made in our understanding of the pathobiology of cholangiocytes, primarily due to the development of techniques to isolate and culture normal, hyperplastic and neoplastic cholangiocytes from rodents and humans. In recognition of the physiological and pathophysiological importance of cholangiocytes and of the recent advances in our understanding of the pathobiology of these cells, it is timely to summarize current knowledge of cholangiocyte biology since the previous edition.

G. Alpini: Department of Internal Medicine and Medical Physiology, Scott & White Hospital, The Texas A&M University System Health Science Center, College of Medicine and Central Texas Veterans Health Care System, Temple, Texas 76504.
R. Prall: Center for Basic Research in Digestive Diseases, Division of Gastroenterology and Hepatology, and the Departments of Medicine and Biochemistry and Molecular Biology, Mayo Medical School, Clinic, and Foundation, Rochester, Minnesota, 55905.
N. F. LaRusso: Center for Basic Research in Digestive Diseases, Division of Gastroenterology and Hepatology, and the Departments of Medicine and Biochemistry & Molecular Biology, Mayo Medical School, Clinic, and Foundation, Rochester, Minnesota, 55905.

ANATOMY

Nerves

This chapter thus emphasizes recent findings regarding the pathobiology of biliary epithelia. (For background, see website chapter W-25.)

Parasympathetic nerves regulate cholangiocyte growth (1) and secretion (1–3). Acetylcholine (ACh) elicits both Ca^{2+} increases and oscillations in isolated intrahepatic bile duct units (IBDU) and cholangiocytes due to both influx of extracellular Ca^{2+} and mobilization of thapsigargin-sensitive Ca^{2+} stores (3). Furthermore, other studies (2) have demonstrated that ACh, by interaction with M3 ACh receptor subtypes on cholangiocytes, stimulates secretin-induced ductal secretory activity by a Ca^{2+}-calcineurin PKA-dependent modulation of adenyl cyclase.

Recent studies (1) have shown that interruption of the cholinergic innervation by vagotomy in bile duct–ligated (BDL) rats inhibits cholangiocyte proliferation and increases cholangiocyte apoptosis (Fig. 29.1) through downregulation of intracellular adenyl cyclase. Restoration of cholangiocyte cAMP levels, by *in vivo* chronic forskolin administration, maintained cholangiocyte proliferation and decreased cholangiocyte apoptosis (Fig. 29.1) due to vagotomy in BDL rats (1).

Morphologic Heterogeneity

Electron microscopic analysis of liver sections and IBDU from normal rats shows that cholangiocytes are heterogeneous with regard to distribution of some cellular organelles (4). For example, rough endoplasmic reticulum is inconspicuous in small ducts but abundant in the largest ducts (4). In support of ultrastructural differences between ducts of different sizes, the nucleus to cytoplasmic ratio is much greater in small ducts compared to large bile ducts (4).

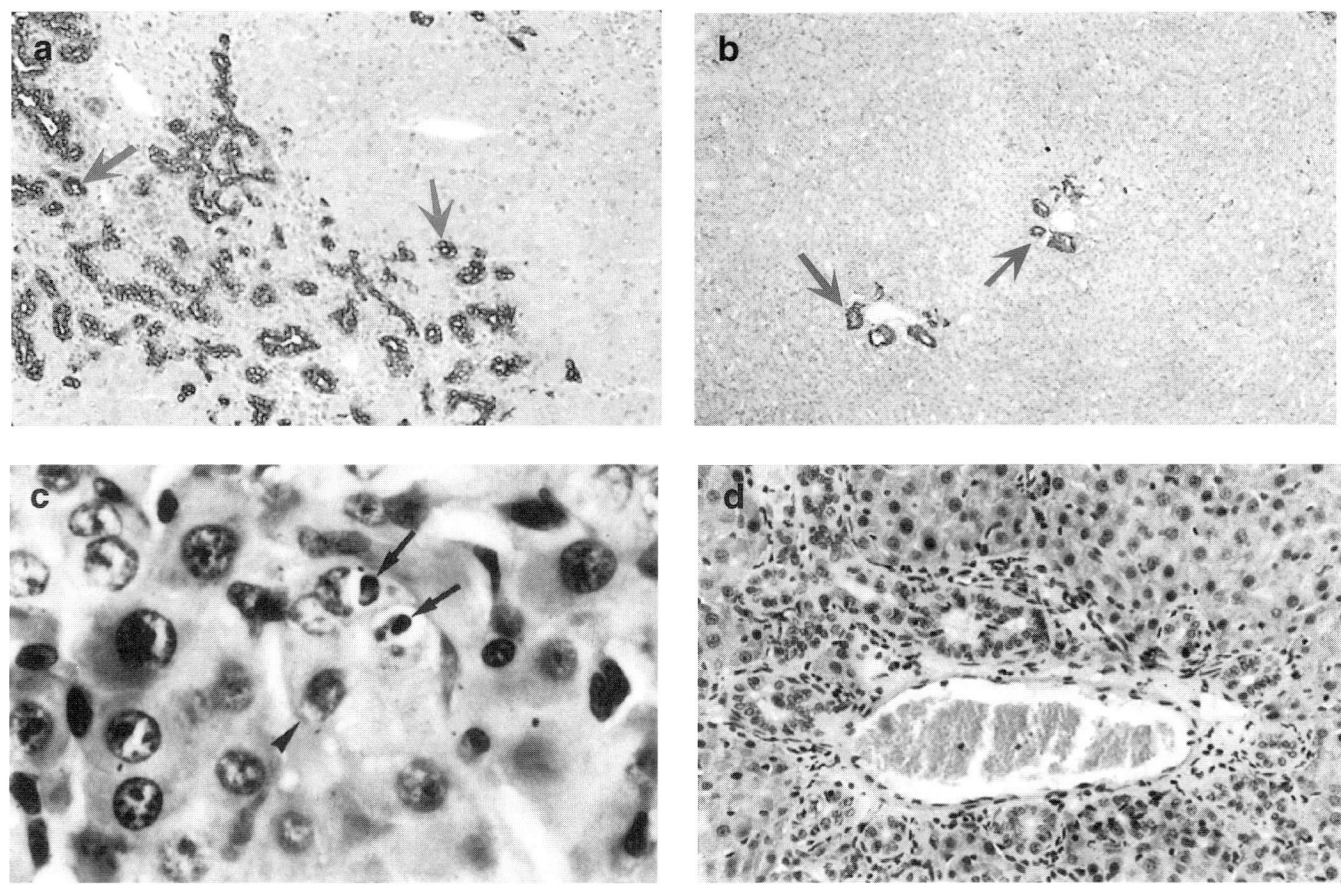

FIGURE 29.1. Immunohistochemistry for CK-19 in frozen liver sections from bile duct–ligated (BDL) **(A)** and BDL+vagotomy **(B)** rats. Vagotomy induced a decrease in the number of ducts as compared with BDL control rats. Original magnification x125. Evaluation of apoptosis in liver sections (stained with hematoxylin and eosin) from BDL **(C)** and BDL+vagotomy **(D)** rats. **C:** Liver section from a BDL+vagotomy rat. Two apoptotic bodies (*arrows*) appear in the epithelium of a bile duct (*arrowhead*) which is surrounded by hepatocytes and located in the proximity of an enlarged portal space (representative section of six examined). **D:** Rat liver section seven days after BDL + vagotomy + forskolin treatment showing proliferating bile ducts without any evidence of apoptosis. Original magnification x100. (From LeSage G, Alvaro D, Benedetti A, et al. Cholinergic system undulates growth, apoptosis, and secretion in cholangiocytes from bile duct–ligated rats. *Gastroenterology* 1994;117:191–199, with permission.) (See Color Plate 11.)

PHENOTYPIC CHARACTERISTICS

Specific Proteins

Endothelin 1 (ET-1) (a) is secreted by human gallbladder epithelial cells in primary culture, and (b) inhibits, via a Gi protein-coupled receptor, cAMP-dependent electrolyte secretion in the human gallbladder epithelium (5). Rat cholangiocytes express both endothelin (ET) ET_A and ET_B receptors, and ET-1 inhibits secretin-stimulated ductal bile secretion by interaction with ET_A but not ET_B receptors (5a).

A functional Na^+-dependent apical bile acid transporter (ABAT) was identified in freshly isolated cholangiocytes (6) and confluent polarized monolayers of normal rat cholangiocytes (NRC) (7). This bile acid transporter plays an important role in the modulation of ductal secretion in normal states and cholangiocyte growth in cholestasis by regulating cholangiocyte uptake of conjugated bile acids from the duct lumen (6–9). An alternatively spliced, truncated form of apical sodium-dependent bile acid transporter (ASBT) transports bile acids in a Na^+-independent manner and was localized to the basolateral domain of cholangiocytes where it serves as an efflux protein for bile acids (10).

Functional receptors for CCK-B/gastrin and M3 Ach are expressed by cholangiocytes and regulate proliferative and secretory activities of the intrahepatic biliary epithelia (2,11–13). The Na^+-dependent glucose transporter (SGLT1) is present on the apical domain of cholangiocytes, which, together with GLUT1 (a facilitative glucose transporter) on the basolateral domain, is responsible for glucose absorption from bile (14).

Aquaporin-1 (AQP1) water channels in the apical and basolateral plasma membrane domains of cholangiocytes (Fig. 29.2) have proposed that hormone-regulated cholangiocyte transport of bile water is critically dependent on cholangiocyte expression of this and other water-channel proteins (15,16). Purinergic receptors have been identified in the apical membrane of rat (17) and human (17,18) cholangiocytes, and are thought to regulate ductal secretion through exposure to biliary ATP (17,18).

Cholangiocytes in the normal human liver express the message for laminin (19). In the fibrotic liver, the expression of laminin RNA is markedly increased in proliferating cholangiocytes, a finding supporting the concept that cholangiocytes may contribute to the development of liver fibrosis (19). Cholangiocytes from cholestatic BDL rats synthesize the message for platelet-derived growth factor-B (PDGF-B) chain (19a), which is a major fibrogenic factor in chronic liver disease (20). *In situ* hybridization of liver sections from patients with chronic liver diseases has shown that the messages for both the transforming growth factor (TGF) β-1 and PDGF-A were expressed by proliferating cholangiocytes (20). The expression of TGF β-1 and PDGF-A in proliferating human cholangiocytes (20) further support the concept that these cells are involved in the development of liver fibrosis.

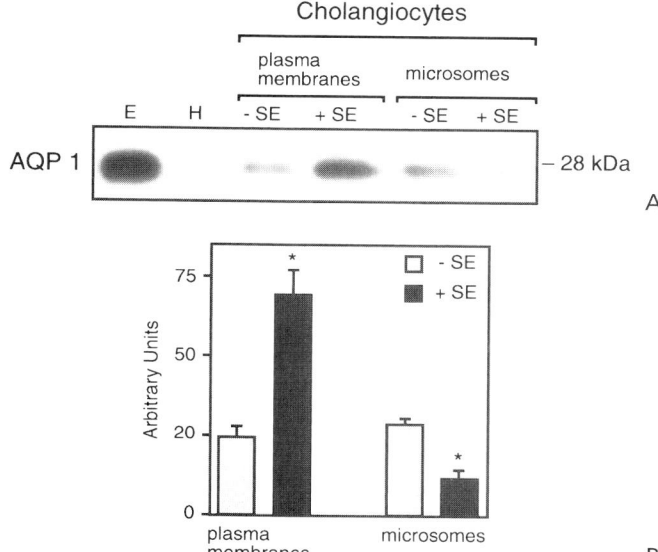

FIGURE 29.2. Effect of secretin (*SE*) on the amount of AQP1 protein in cholangiocyte membranes. **A:** Representative immunoblot for AQP1 on plasma and microsomal membrane fractions. Cells were incubated in the absence (–) or presence (+) of 10^{-7} M secretin, and cholangiocyte membrane fractions were prepared. *E,* erythrocyte plasma membranes (positive control); *H,* hepatocyte plasma membranes (negative control). Each lane was loaded with 10 μg of protein for cholangiocyte membrane fractions and hepatocyte plasma membranes and 1 μg for erythrocyte plasma membranes. **B:** Densitometric analysis of four separate experiments expressed in arbitrary units as mean ± SE *, p < 0.01 for secretin effect as compared with basal value (Student's t test). (From Marinelli RA, Pham L, Agre P, et al. Secretin promotes osmotic water transport in rat cholangiocytes by increasing aquaporin-1 water chanel in plasma membrane. Evidence for a secretin-induced vesicular translocation of aquaporin-1. *J Biol Chem* 1997;272:12984–12988, with permission.)

Functional Heterogeneity

Protein Expression

The intrahepatic biliary epithelia are heterogeneous regarding morphological characteristics (Fig. 29.3), secretory processes and response to liver injury and/or toxins.

Hyperplastic cholangiocytes are heterogeneous regarding the expression of selected enzymes including leucine aminopeptidase, BD.1 antigen, and alkaline phosphatase (21). In normal mouse liver, annexin-V is expressed only by small intrahepatic bile ducts, which suggests that this protein may be a unique marker for small intrahepatic bile ducts (22). Since annexin-V is involved in membrane-cytoskeletal interactions during vesicular transport and apoptosis (22), we propose the possible involvement of small bile ducts in transport processes and their resistance to agents/drugs inducing cell apoptosis, a concept supported by other studies (13). In support of the concept that small cholangiocytes are more resistant than large cholangiocytes to toxins/injury, the antiapoptotic protein bcl-2 was found only in cholangiocytes lining ductules and small bile ducts

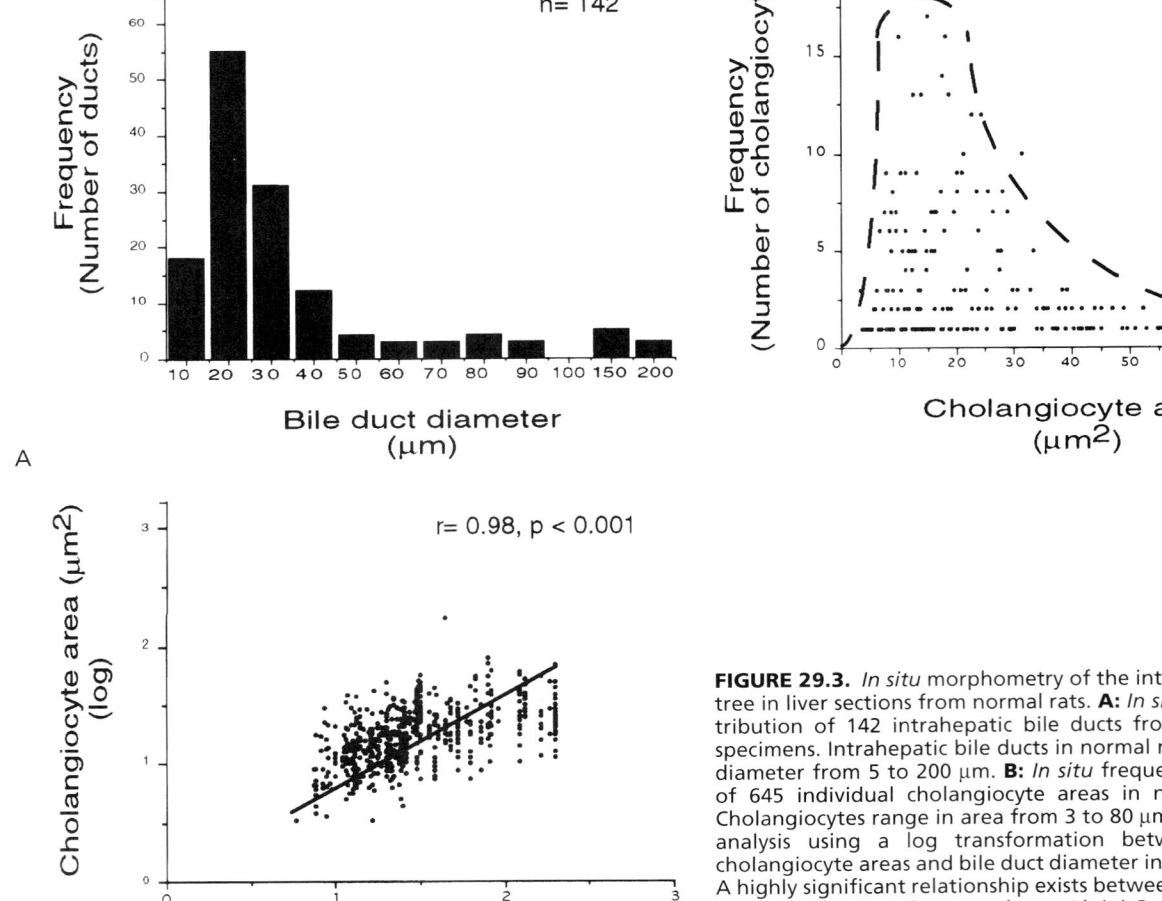

FIGURE 29.3. *In situ* morphometry of the intrahepatic biliary tree in liver sections from normal rats. **A:** *In situ* diameter distribution of 142 intrahepatic bile ducts from two rat liver specimens. Intrahepatic bile ducts in normal rat liver range in diameter from 5 to 200 μm. **B:** *In situ* frequency distribution of 645 individual cholangiocyte areas in normal rat liver. Cholangiocytes range in area from 3 to 80 μm². **C:** Regression analysis using a log transformation between individual cholangiocyte areas and bile duct diameter in normal rat liver. A highly significant relationship exists between cholangiocyte area and bile duct diameter. (From Alpini G, Roberts S, Kuntz S, et al. Morphological, molecular and functional heterogeneity of cholangiocytes from normal rat liver. *Gastroenterology* 1996;110:1636–1643, with permission.)

in normal human liver and human liver with cirrhosis and focal nodular hyperplasia (23). Moreover, the cytochrome P4502E1 (the enzyme that initiates CCl_4 (carbon tetrachloride) hepatotoxicity) (24) is present in large but not small cholangiocytes (13). The absence of cytochrome P4502E1 in small cholangiocytes (13) may explain the resistance of these cells to CCl_4.

Secretory Response

The isolation of distinct subpopulations of small (about 8 μm in size) and large (about 13 μm in size) cholangiocytes (5a,6,13,25–27) and small (less than 15 μm in diameter) and large (greater than 15 μm in diameter) IBDU (28) from different portions of the rat biliary tree has enabled the demonstration that large (but not small) cholangiocytes and large-diameter IBDU express: (a) the secretin (5a,13,25–28) and somatostatin ($SSTR_2$) (27) receptors,

the Cl^-/HCO_3^- exchanger (25,28) and the Cl^- channel, cystic fibrosis transmembrane regulator (CFTR) (26); and (b) respond to secretin (Fig. 29.4) and somatostatin with changes in ductal secretory activity (5a,13,25–28). Large human bile ducts express the Cl^-/HCO_3^- exchanger (29) that regulates the secretion of HCO_3^- in the duct lumen (2,25,30). In addition, endothelin 1 (ET-1) receptors (i.e., ET_A and ET_B) are expressed by both small and large cholangiocytes, and ET-1 decreases the secretin-induced secretion from large cholangiocytes by selectively interacting with ET_A receptors (5a). Since ET_A receptors are expressed in small cholangiocytes (5a), and since ET-1 regulates cell function in other epithelia through the second messengers IP_3 and Ca^{2+} (32), we suggest the possible role of small cholangiocytes in the regulation of ductal bile secretion through Ca^{2+}- and IP_3-dependent mechanisms different from that shown for secretin (1,2,5a,6,12, 13, 25–28,30,33–36).

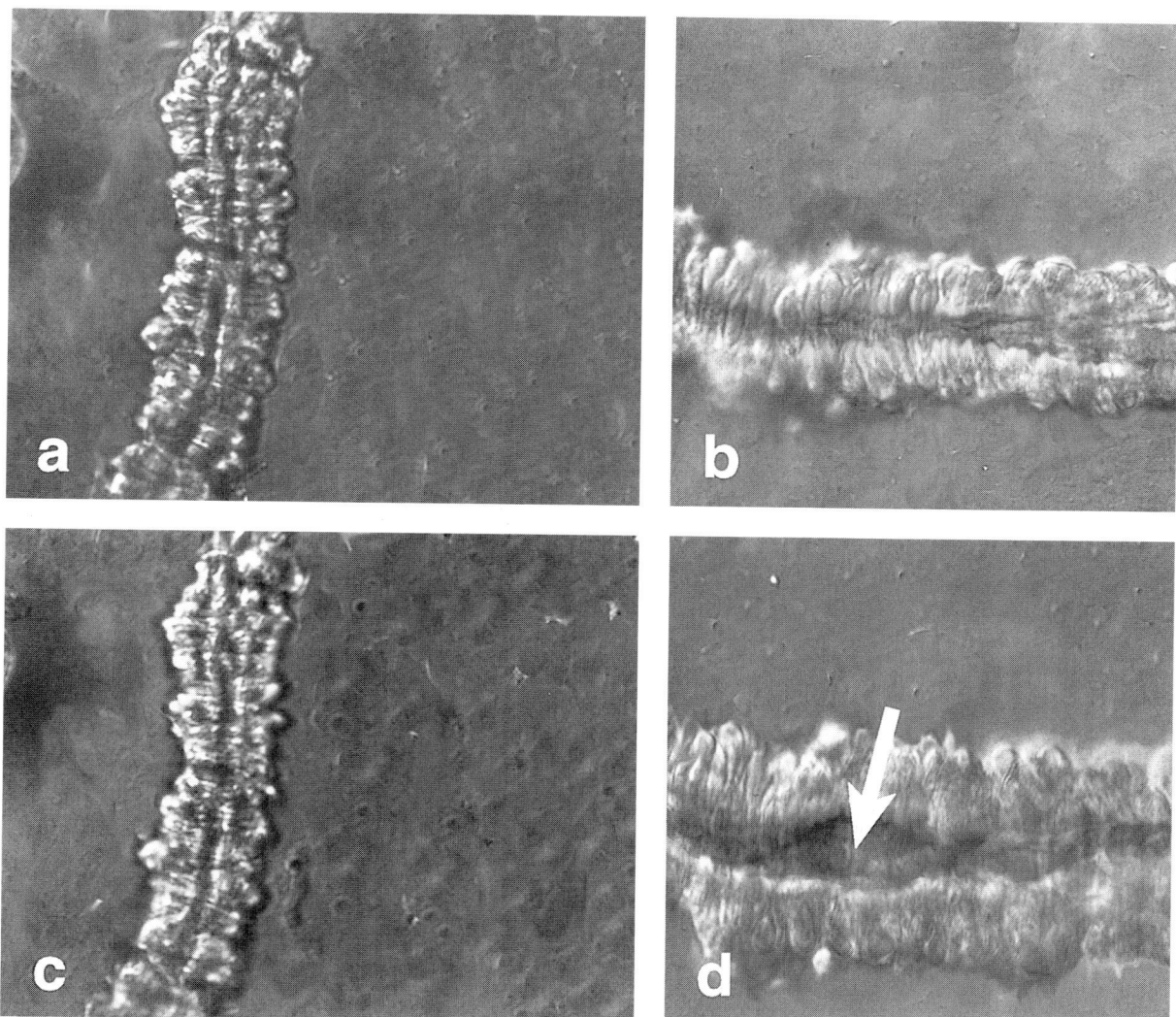

FIGURE 29.4. Ductal secretion in small and large intrahephatic bile duct unit (*IBDU*) following the addition of secretin (10^{-7} M). Small (**a**, **c**) or large (**b**, **d**) IBDU were mounted in a perfusion chamber of a light microscope, and the lumen size was measured before (**upper panel**) or 10 minutes after (**lower panel**) the addition of secretin. In response to secretin, lumen (*arrow*) expanded in large but not small IBDU, indicating the presence of hormone-induced ductal secretion in large but not small IBDU. (From Alpini G, Glaser S, Robertson W, et al. Large but not small intrahepatic bile duct units are involved in secretin-regulated ductal bile secretion in normal rat liver. *Am J Physiol* 1997;272:G1064–G1074. with permission.)

Response to Injury and/or Toxins

In the intrahepatic biliary tree, there are specific proliferative compartments that differentially respond to injury and/or toxins (e.g., BDL, partial hepatectomy, or acute CCl$_4$ administration) with proliferation/loss of certain sized bile ducts (13,27,37) accompanied by up- or downregulation of secretory processes (13,27,37). Following BDL, for example, mitosis and increased secretory activity are restricted to large intrahepatic bile ducts (26,27). Large cholangiocytes are damaged *in vivo* (with loss of proliferative and secretory activities) by a single dose of CCl$_4$, whereas small cholangiocytes, resistant to CCl$_4$-induced

damage, transiently proliferate and secrete, thus compensating for the loss of the proliferative and secretory capacity of large cholangiocytes (13). Moreover, following partial hepatectomy, both small and large bile ducts participate in the regrowth of the biliary tree through increases in cholangiocyte growth and secretion (37).

Typical Proliferation

Selected bile acids [i.e., taurocholate (TCH) and taurolithocholate (TLCH)] stimulate the proliferative capacity of cholangiocytes *in vitro* (8). In addition, accumulation of bile acids in serum (due to chronic feeding of TCH and TLCH to normal rats (9)) induces a hyperplastic duct reaction confined to portal areas that resembles that of the BDL rat model (13,27,33). Other bile acids [e.g., ursodeoxycholate (UDCA) and tauroursodeoxycholate (TUDCA)] have been shown to inhibit cholangiocyte proliferative capacity (38,39).

A number of intracellular [e.g., adenosine 3′,5′-monophosphate (cAMP) and protein kinase C (PKC) system] (1,11,13) and extracellular components (e.g., gastrointestinal hormones, growth factors and parasympathetic and sympathetic innervation) (1,11,40) have been shown to regulate "typical" cholangiocyte growth.

The cholinergic system plays a role in sustaining cholangiocyte growth following BDL, since interruption of the parasympathetic innervation by vagotomy inhibits cholangiocyte mitosis induced by BDL (1). The intracellular cAMP system also regulates the growth of cholangiocytes in rats with BDL and partial hepatectomy (1,13,30).

The gastrointestinal hormone somatostatin inhibits the cholangiocyte hyperplastic reaction in response to BDL (27) by selectively interacting with $SSTR_2$ somatostatin receptors and through a decrease in intracellular cAMP levels (27,36). Similarly, a recent study (11) indicates that gastrin inhibits cholangiocyte growth by interacting with CCK-B/gastrin receptors through membrane translocation of the Ca^{2+}-dependent PKC isoform, PKC-α.

The functional expression of the secretin receptor (SR) in cholangiocytes may play an important role in the regulation of ductal hyperplasia (1,9,12,13,26,27,30,34). In support of this concept, downregulation of SR gene expression and secretin-induced cAMP levels occurs when cholangiocyte mitosis is reduced in BDL rats by vagotomy (1) or depletion of the endogenous bile acid pool (41). The functional expression of the SR is upregulated in most animal models of ductal hyperplasia (1,9,12,13,26,27,30,34), which suggests that the SR may play an important role in the regulation of cholangiocyte proliferation.

Cholangiocyte Apoptosis

Several studies have explored the mechanisms by which cholangiocytes die in liver diseases and the role of apoptosis in this process (42–46). The first requirement was to develop and characterize rodent models of cholangiocyte apoptosis. The first model (46) demonstrated that beauvericin, a K^+ ionophore, induces apoptosis of rat cholangiocytes by a Ca^{2+}-dependent, CPP-32 protease-sensitive pathway. A single gavage dose of the toxin CCl_4 to normal or BDL rats induces damage (by apoptosis) of large hormone-responsive ducts, whereas small ducts resistant to apoptosis compensate by *de novo* proliferation (13). Resistance of cholangiocytes to injury and/or toxins may be due to over-expression of B-cell lymphoma/leukemia 2 (Bcl-2) family members (47). The expression of Bcl-2 in cholangiocytes is regulated by the antioxidant glutathione (GSH), since GSH

depletion is associated with decreased Bcl-2 expression and increased apoptosis in immortalized human cholangiocytes (43). Cholangiocarcinomas escape immune surveillance either by disabling FasR signaling through the expression of Fas-associated death domain–like IL-1 converting enzyme (I-FLICE) and/or increased FasL expression, thus causing apoptosis of T cells (45). Reduction of I-FLICE expression in cholangiocarcinoma cells restores Fas-mediated apoptosis (45). These important studies suggest that maneuvers to inhibit the expression of I-FLICE may be a new therapeutic window in the treatment of cholangiocarcinoma.

FUNCTIONAL PARAMETERS

Regulation of Secretion

Secretin stimulates cholangiocyte secretory activity by interaction with specific receptors expressed only by cholangiocytes in rat liver (34), which causes an increase in intracellular cAMP levels (1,5a,12,13,25–27,30,). Increased cAMP levels lead to opening, by phosphorylation, of the CFTR Cl^- channels (48), and activation of the apically located Cl^-/HCO_3^- exchanger (2,25), which stimulates bicarbonate secretion in ductal bile (2,12,25,33). Furthermore, secretin stimulates exocytosis via a cAMP-dependent, but cGMP-, IP_3- and Ca^{2+}-independent mechanism (35), further supporting the concept that secretin stimulates transport of water and electrolytes in the intrahepatic biliary tree.

Protein kinase A (PKA) but not PKC regulates secretin-stimulated bicarbonate-enriched cholangiocyte secretion (49). Specifically, Sp-adenosine 3′,5′-cyclic monophosphothiolate (Sp-cAMPs), a PKA-specific agonist, stimulates cholangiocyte bicarbonate secretion whereas Rp-cAMPs, a specific PKA inhibitor, decreased secretin-stimulated ductal bicarbonate secretion (49). Once CFTR is activated by cAMP-PKA-dependent phosphorylation, secretin-induced cholangiocyte secretion is regulated by a dephosphorylation step driven by endogenous protein serine/threonine protein phosphatases 1 and 2A (49). These phosphatases, by dephosphorylating the regulatory domain of CFTR, promote conformational changes opposite to those caused by PKA, changes that lead to occlusion of the Cl^- conductance pathway, thus restoring the basal quiescent state (49). The findings suggest that secretin-stimulated ductal bile secretion is regulated, at the level of CFTR, by a balance between the activities of kinases (inducing activation) and phosphatases (causing inactivation) (49). Alkaline phosphatase may play an important role in this regulatory balance between kinases and phosphatases (50).

Somatostatin inhibits both basal and secretin-stimulated ductal secretory activity, perhaps by interfering with exocytosis through interactions with a subtype (i.e., $SSTR_2$) of somatostatin receptors (27,36).

Cholangiocytes express the CCK-B/gastrin receptor and gastrin inhibits secretin-induced ductal secretory activity of hyperplastic cholangiocytes from BDL through activation of Ca^{2+}-dependent PKC-α (11).

Intrahepatic biliary epithelium express both ET_A and ET_B, and ET-1 inhibits secretin-stimulated ductal bile secretion by selectively interacting with ET_A receptors through IP_3- and Ca^{2+}-dependent inhibition of intracellular adenylyl cyclase (5a). Intrahepatic bile ducts express (both at the message and protein levels) the insulin receptor, and insulin inhibits the stimulatory effects of secretin on cholangiocyte secretion by interacting with its own receptor (51). Bombesin stimulates the activity of Cl^-/HCO_3^- exchanger in cholangiocytes, presumably with specific receptors (sensitivity to the bombesin receptor inhibitor [Tyr4, D-Phe12]-bombesin) (52). Stimulation of Cl^-/HCO_3^- exchanger activity by bombesin is independent of the increase in the second messengers cAMP, cGMP or intracellular Ca^{2+} (52). Vasoactive intestinal peptide (VIP) stimulates ductal bile secretion by the activation of the Cl^-/HCO_3^- exchanger (53).

Drug Metabolism

Phase I and phase II drug-metabolizing enzymes are differentially expressed by the intrahepatic biliary epithelia (13,54,55), which may explain the heterogeneous susceptibility/response of cholangiocytes to drugs, toxins (e.g., CCl_4), injury (e.g., BDL) virus, and carcinogens (13,56). While phase I or mixed-function oxygenase enzymes (e.g., microsomal cytochrome P-450, aminopyrine-N-demethylases, G_{-6}-PO_4, and NADPH cytochrome C reductase) possess oxidative metabolic activities (55), phase II or glutathione (GSH) redox cycle enzymes (e.g., GSH-peroxidase, UDP-glucuronosyltransferase, and glutathione-S-transferase) possess conjugating properties (55). Cholangiocytes have been shown to contain both phase I and phase II enzymes (13,54). A recent study (13) showed that cytochrome P4502E1, the enzyme that initiates CCl_4 hepatotoxicity (24), is present in large but not small cholangiocytes. The presence of cytochrome P4502E1 in large cholangiocytes may explain in part the loss of large bile duct function in response to CCl_4 (13). Conversely, small bile ducts are resistant to CCl_4-induced damage due to absence of CCl_4 metabolism by cytochrome P4502E1 in small cholangiocytes (13).

Membrane Channel Activity

Activation of purinergic P_{2u} receptors on the apical membranes of cholangiocytes stimulates Cl^- efflux (18) (see Chapter 28). Physiologic concentrations of ATP in bile activate P_{2u} receptors, which mobilize intracellular Ca^{2+} stores and activate Ca^{2+}-dependent apical membrane Cl^- channels (18). These findings suggest that ATP secreted into bile by hepatocytes regulates Ca^{2+}-dependent Cl^- channels and cholangiocyte secretion through activation of purinergic P_{2u} receptors. A recent study (17) in polarized NRC showed that transepithelial Cl^- secretion is also regulated by changes in the osmolality of the extracellular environment. For example, ATP release from NRC increased rapidly during cell swelling induced by hypotonic exposure, which stimulates Cl^- efflux through interaction with purinergic receptors. Other studies have also shown that ATP activates chloride permeability in human biliary epithelial cell lines (48) through Ca^{2+}- and calmodulin-dependent protein kinase II mechanisms (57). cGMP-dependent Cl^- channels have also been identified in human cholangiocarcinoma cell lines (58). Specifically, natriuretic peptide stimulates cGMP production in human biliary epithelial cells, which in turn stimulates ductal secretion through the opening of Cl^- channels (58). Moreover, phosphoinositide (PI) 3-kinase dependent Cl^- channels, which were localized in human cholangiocarcinoma cell lines, stimulate lipid products of PI 3-kinase, thus triggering ATP release, Cl^- efflux and subsequently cholangiocyte secretion (59).

The cholangiocarcinoma cell line Mz-ChA-1 expresses functional K^+ channels and demonstrated that biliary K^+ efflux helps to minimize cell injury (during ATP depletion) through Ca^{2+} and PKC α-dependent mechanisms (60). The data suggest that K^+ channel efflux may inhibit cholangiocyte injury during the ischemia and metabolic stress that accompany liver preservation (61).

K^+ and Cl^- channels are also important in the regulation of cell volume of the biliary epithelia during osmotic stress. Exposure to hypotonic buffer (40% less NaCl) rapidly increases the relative cell volume of cholangiocarcinoma cell lines by activation of separate K^+ and Cl^- conductance through a mechanism that depends in part on Ca^{2+}-sensitive signaling pathways (62). Moreover, PKC-dependent opening of membrane Cl^- channels has been shown to play an important role in the regulation of cell volume homeostasis in the cholangiocarcinoma cell line Mz-ChA-1 (63).

Regulation of Absorption

Water

Evidence that the intrahepatic biliary epithelia play a key role in water transport comes from recent studies showing that both human and rat cholangiocytes express functional water channels (i.e., aquaporins (AQP) such as AQP1) (15,16), which regulate biliary water transport (15,16). Cholangiocyte water transport (through AQP1) is regulated by secretin (15,16) via microtubule-dependent (sensitivity to colchicine) exocytic insertion of AQP1 into the apical domain of cholangiocytes (15), a process that plays a fundamental role in ductal bile secretion.

The sulfonylurea glybenclamide stimulates bile secretion and bicarbonate excretion in the isolated perfused rat liver (IPRL) by direct interaction with cholangiocytes rather than hepatocytes (64). The stimulatory effect of glybenclamide on ductal bile secretion is associated with activation of the Na^+-K^+-$2Cl^-$ cotransport.

Carbohydrates

The demonstration of carbohydrate transport by bile ducts comes from a study (14) that evaluated the uptake and transcellular transport of a nonmetabolizable monosaccharide, methyl α-D-glucopyranoside, in polarized NRC. Both the Na $(^+)$-glucose cotransporter (SGLT1) and the facilitative glucose transporter (GLUT1) were identified in the apical and basolateral domain, respectively, of cholangiocytes (14). The data indicate that SGLT1 (on the apical domain), in conjunction with GLUT1 (on the basolateral domain) regulates ductal glucose absorption from bile (14).

Bile Acids

Evidence of a role for bile acids in the regulation of biliary functions comes from recent studies showing that a Na^+-dependent ABAT is present in the apical domain of cholangiocytes and that ABAT mediates bile acid uptake from the duct lumen, resulting in modification of canalicular bile secretion and modulation of cholangiocyte secretion and growth (6–9). A bile acid transporter was functionally identified in the basolateral membrane of rat cholangiocytes that facilitates carrier-mediated transport of conjugated bile acids across the basolateral membrane of the intrahepatic biliary epithelia (65). More recently, a truncated form of ASBT derived by alternate splicing has been identified, shown to be located in the basolateral domain of cholangiocytes, and to function as a Na^+-independent efflux carrier from bile acids (10).

Ursodeoxycholate (UDCA) increases cytosolic calcium concentration and activates Cl^- currents in a biliary cell line (66). Both UDCA and tauroursodeoxycholate (TUDCA) *in vivo* and *in vitro* inhibit cholangiocyte growth and decrease secretin-stimulated ductal bile secretion (38,39). In contrast, UDCA does not affect the secretory activity of human cholangiocarcinoma cell lines (67). In support of the role of UDCA in inhibiting cholangiocyte proliferation, the human cholangiocyte cell line H69 possesses a functional bile acid transporter, and glycoursodeoxycholic acid (GUDC) decreases beauvericin-induced apoptosis and inhibits the activity of caspase 3 protease by blocking cytochrome *c* release from mitochondria (44). The data suggest that the beneficial effect of UDCA on liver diseases may involve decreased apoptosis after GUDC uptake by cholangiocytes (44).

Endocytosis, Exocytosis, and Membrane Recycling

As mentioned above, the intrahepatic biliary tree participates in secretin-regulated water transport through the apical insertion of aquaporin-1 water channels in rat cholangiocytes (15,16). Moreover, other studies have observed exocytosis in short-term cultures of normal rat cholangiocytes by a novel fluorescence unquenching assay and demonstrated that secretin, a choleretic hormone, stimulates exocytosis through an increase in cAMP levels (35). In contrast, somatostatin, which is cholestatic, decreases both secretin-induced exocytosis and secretin-induced increases in cAMP levels in rat cholangiocytes (36).

On the basis of these findings, and cognizant of the roles of endocytosis and exocytosis in water and electrolyte transport in other epithelia, a membrane microdomain recycling system in cholangiocytes has been postulated, which involves exocytic insertion into the apical plasma membrane of ion or water channels sequestered on intracellular vesicles (15,16,35). In contrast, somatostatin-induced cholestasis occurs by endocytic retrieval of transporters and ion and water channels from the apical plasma membrane through a decrease in intracellular levels of cAMP (36).

Regulation of Intralumenal and Intracellular pH

The apically located Cl^-/HCO_3^- exchanger regulates bicarbonate secretion into bile (2,25,30,67). The Cl^-/HCO_3^- exchanger is regulated by hormones with stimulation by secretin (25,30,33), bombesin (52), and VIP (53), and inhibition by somatostatin (36), gastrin (12), ET-1 (5a), and insulin (51). Stimulation of the Cl^-/HCO_3^- exchanger by secretin requires activation, by phosphorylation, of cAMP-dependent Cl^- channels (48). The dependence of the Cl^-/HCO_3^- exchanger activity on Cl^- channel opening is presumably due to the requirement for lumenal-directed Cl^- secretion to replenish Cl^- internalized into cholangiocytes by the Cl^-/HCO_3^- exchanger (48). Other studies have shown that the depolarization induced by Cl^- channel opening leads to increased HCO_3^- internalization by the Na^+-HCO_3^- symporter (68). The increase in intracellular HCO_3^- and pH directly activates the apically located Cl^-/HCO_3^- exchanger. Insertion of CFTR or Cl^-/HCO_3^- exchanger to the apical domain of cholangiocytes from intracellular cytoplasmic stores activates their activity (69). According to these studies (69), secretin-induced choleresis is due to the activation of a Na^+/H^+ exchanger by secretin, which causes intracellular alkalinization in cholangiocytes. The Cl^-/HCO_3^- exchanger is subsequently stimulated by high intracellular pH due to the presence of a pH-dependent domain on the exchanger (69).

Purinergic receptors regulate the intracellular pH of cholangiocytes. Parallel with the role for biliary ATP in paracrine and autocrine control of cholangiocyte Cl^- secretion (17,18), extracellular ATP also stimulates cholangiocyte basolateral Na^+-H^+ exchange (NHE) activity through purinergic receptors located on the apical cell membrane of cholangiocytes (18).

Regulation of Growth

Growth Factors

The expression of the oncogene c-erb-B2 markedly increased after BDL in rats (40), thus suggesting a potential role for c-erb-B2 in the regulation of cholangiocyte growth. Hepatocyte growth factor stimulates DNA synthesis of cultured human cholangiocytes (70). The interleukin-6 (IL-6)/gp-80 ligand/receptor system stimulates *in vitro* cholangiocyte proliferative capacity (71). Periductal hematolymphoid and stromal cells secrete putative cholangiocyte growth factors (HGF/met and IL-6/gp-80 systems), and receptors for these factors are upregulated following BDL (71). The data suggest that complex, coordinate interactions between inflammatory and stromal elements and cholangiocytes result in a dysmorphogenic repair response leading to hyperplasia. Furthermore, the stem cell factor/c-kit system, TGF-α, and TGF-β regulate cholangiocyte proliferation of young rats with BDL (72).

Inflammation

The intrahepatic biliary epithelium is exposed to mediators of inflammation such as bacterial endotoxin or lipopolysaccharide (LPS) in a variety of inflammatory conditions (73). These conditions are also characterized by cholangiocyte proliferation and a predisposition to malignancy (74). Cholangiocytes secrete IL-6 in response to inflammatory stimuli such as LPS, tumor necrosis factor-α (TNF-α) and IL-1β. IL-6 is mitogenic for normal as well as malignant cholangiocytes (74). Cholangiocytes possess the IL-6 receptor complex subunits and intact signaling mechanisms leading to activation of STAT transcription factors as well as mitogen-activated protein kinase (MAPK) signaling pathways (74). Although both p38 and p44/p42 MAP kinases are constitutively present and active in cholangiocytes, IL-6 increases p44/p42 and not p38 MAPK activity in normal, nonmalignant cholangiocytes (74). This proliferative response is blocked by selective inhibition of the p44/p42 MAPK pathway (74). Thus the proliferative response of cholangiocytes to inflammatory mediators such as LPS involves IL-6-mediated activation of the p44/p42 MAPK pathway.

Malignant cholangiocytes secrete IL-6 constitutively, and proliferate in response to IL-6 via a receptor-mediated signaling mechanism involving MAPK activation (74). Thus, IL-6 can contribute to the autocrine and/or paracrine growth stimulation of malignant cholangiocytes (74). In contrast to nonmalignant cholangiocytes, mitogen stimulation increases activity of both p38 and p44/p42 MAP kinases in cholangiocarcinoma cells (74). Selective inhibition of either the p44/p42 MAPK pathway by PD098059 or the p38 MAPK pathway by SB203580 blocks proliferation in response to IL-6. Thus, recruitment of p38 MAPK signaling pathways may contribute to aberrant growth of malignant cholangiocytes (74).

Activation of inducible nitric oxide synthase (iNOS) and excess production of nitric oxide (NO) in response to inflammatory cytokines cause DNA damage and inhibit DNA repair proteins (75) (see Chapter 39). NO inactivation of DNA repair enzymes may provide a link between inflammation and the initiation, promotion, and/or progression of malignant cholangiocyte growth (e.g., cholangiocarcinoma) (75).

PATHOLOGY

The biliary epithelium is the target of both acquired and inherited disease processes collectively termed the cholangiopathies. Research into the molecular etiopathogenesis of these entities has progressed over the past few years. Space limitations preclude a thorough discussion of the spectrum of biliary pathology, and therefore, where appropriate, the reader is referred to additional sources. The following synopsis puts forth our current level of insight into the pathogenic mechanisms of biliary disease, highlighting recent advances in research.

Immune-Mediated Cholangiopathies

Primary biliary cirrhosis (PBC) and primary sclerosing cholangitis (PSC), while relatively rare, are the two most common biliary diseases seen by hepatologists and are frequent indications for liver transplantation. Immune mechanisms are postulated in the pathogenesis of both PBC and PSC, and are thought to be intimately involved in allograft rejection and graft-versus-host disease after transplantation.

Primary Biliary Cirrhosis

PBC is an autoimmune disease of unknown etiology primarily affecting middle-aged women, characterized by segmental, chronic, nonsuppurative, destructive cholangitis involving the small septal and interlobular bile ducts of the intrahepatic biliary tree. Continued damage leads to cholestasis and portal fibrosis, and eventually, biliary cirrhosis. Histologically, lymphocytes and plasma cells infiltrate portal areas and bile ducts, causing focal ruptures. Periportal lymphoid follicles and granulomas are distinguishing features (76). Apoptosis of cholangiocytes may be responsible for bile duct loss (42). Although the clinical course is variable, most symptomatic patients left untreated progress to cirrhosis and liver failure an average of eight years after diagnosis (77).

Patients with PBC frequently exhibit concomitant autoimmune diseases. This association, along with a long list of humoral and cellular immune abnormalities, strongly implicates an autoimmune etiology. Ninety-five percent of PBC patients exhibit antibodies against mitochondrial antigens (AMA), antibodies directed against metabolic enzymes found on the inner membrane of mitochondria. Nine types of AMA, termed M1-M9, have been determined, but only the M2 subtype is specific for PBC (78). The dominant immunogenic epitopes have been mapped to residues 128–221 of the inner lipoyl domain of the E2 subunit of the pyruvate dehydrogenase complex (79). Antibodies against other mitochondrial antigens, although less specific for PBC, may provide prognostic information (80). The absolute titer of AMA does not correlate with prognosis. Despite the high sensitivity of AMA positivity as a diagnostic test for PBC, 5% of patients with PBC of do not exhibit these characteristic antibodies but have indistinguishable disease. These patients have an increased incidence of antibodies to nuclear antigens such as proteins associated with nuclear pore complexes, the nuclear envelope, and nuclear matrix proteins. These antibodies also appear to be specific for PBC, but their significance is not currently known (81).

Abnormalities of cellular immunity have also been characterized. Increased numbers of T lymphocytes are found in periportal infiltrates in patients with PBC, but studies have differed as to whether CD4-positive helper cells or CD8-positive cytotoxic T cells are the predominant subset (82). Recent studies utilizing cloned liver-derived lymphocytes from patients with PBC show a predominance of the T helper 1 (Th1)-type cytokines IFN-γ and IL-2, whereas in a separate study, the T helper 2 (Th2) cytokine IL-4 was not detected, suggesting a Th1-type immune response, a profile associated with organ-specific autoimmunity (83). In addition, studies with peripheral blood lymphocytes and liver-derived clones indicate that T cell recognition of the E2 components of the pyruvate dehydrogenase complex (PDC-E2) is increased in patients with PBC (84). T cell recognition of cholangiocytes may be aided by the appearance of MHC II (major histocompatibility complex class II) and ICAM-1 (intercellular adhesion molecule type I) on cholangiocytes. MHC II and ICAM-1 are not found in normal liver but are inducible with cytokine stimulation. However, these molecules are present constitutively on cholangiocytes in PBC. This is most likely not causative but an epiphenomenon common to cholestatic liver disease (85,86). Taken as a whole, this combination of findings does imply an increased cellular immune response in PBC, but whether this is a primary causative factor or secondary response remains to be determined.

What factors are responsible for initiating this response? Autoreactivity against cholangiocytes could be generated if cholangiocytes were capable of presenting antigen in association with MHC II complexes; however, this does not seem to be conducted efficiently by human cholangiocytes. This is in contrast to what has been observed with rat cholangiocytes, which express costimulatory molecules not found on human cholangiocytes thought necessary for efficient lymphocyte activation (86). What has been demonstrated is that cholangiocytes aberrantly express PDC-E2 on the outer surface of the plasma membrane in PBC but not normal liver, and that antibodies recognizing these antigens are not simply cross-reacting (87). In addition, luminal expression of PDC-E2

occurs early in PBC, preceding MHC II expression (88). Together, these findings could explain why antimitochondrial antibodies, not alone pathogenic, can cause disease in PBC, and why antibody to an antigen found sequestered in all cells causes disease focused on the biliary tract. The trigger initiating this cascade remains to be identified.

What role genetic factors may play is still being elucidated. There is evidence of increased genetic susceptibility in some patients, as indicated by 100-fold increased relative risk of acquiring PBC in siblings and positive associations with HLA DR8 haplotypes (89). Polymorphisms in the gene encoding TNF-α have been suggested to be important in the development and severity of other autoimmune diseases, but this remains controversial for PBC and PSC (90). The immunogenetics of PBC are reviewed elsewhere (89).

Primary Sclerosing Cholangitis

PSC is an idiopathic cholestatic liver disease strongly associated with ulcerative colitis, characterized by fibrosing inflammation and destruction of the extra- and intrahepatic bile ducts (76). The disease primarily afflicts young to middle-aged men, with a median survival from time of diagnosis of approximately 12 years (91). There are no proven medical therapies, and liver transplantation remains the only effective treatment. The lack of medical therapies reflects our lack of understanding into the pathogenesis of this disease. Given the strong association with ulcerative colitis, portal bacteremia and increased permeability of the diseased colon to bacterial toxins and/or toxic bile acids released into the enterohepatic circulation have been implicated in disease pathogenesis. However, the fact that PSC can occur without any colonic involvement and years after colectomy indicates that these factors are not necessary for PSC to occur. Ischemia and injection with floxuridine (presumed to cause toxic and ischemic effects) can cause changes mimicking PSC, but no primary role for ischemia causing PSC has been proven (92). Similarly, cross-antigenicity or antigenic mimicry of cholangiocyte cell surface proteins by a virus or bacterium has been proposed as an etiologic agent, but none has been identified. PSC is generally regarded to be an immune-mediated disease, which is triggered by an unknown event in a genetically susceptible person.

Like PBC, there are numerous abnormalities of humoral and cellular immunity in patients with PSC, which have led many to invoke an autoimmune etiology. Past studies have reported frequent associations with other autoimmune syndromes, hypergammaglobulinemia, increased levels of circulating immune complexes, activation of the complement system, and the presence of anti-smooth muscle, anti-nuclear, and perinuclear anti-neutrophil cytoplasmic antibodies. While present with high frequency, the significance of these antibodies remains unclear, as they are neither specific nor lend prognostic information. Antibodies to a shared epitope between colonic and biliary epithelium may provide an etiologic connection between PSC and ulcerative colitis (93). Cellular abnormalities, including decreased total numbers of circulating T cells with a disproportionate decrease in the CD8 fraction, leading to an increased CD4 to CD8 ratio, and increased numbers of $\gamma\delta$ T cells in the liver and peripherally have been described (94). Cytokine mRNA expression studies have demonstrated the presence of both T-helper 1 and 2 (Th1 and Th2) lymphocytes, although reports differ as to whether there is a shift towards the Th1 profile (95). In addition, serum levels of markers of an inflammatory Th1 response in PSC patients have been found to be normal, whereas serum levels of the Th2 cytokine IL-10 have been elevated (96). At present, although seemingly logical, there is no good evidence to support a primary role for a Th1 shift in the pathogenesis of PSC. Higher levels of TNF-α in response to lipopolysaccharide or as the result of a genetic polymorphism may be shown to be important in disease severity, and remain to be fully explored (90).

As with PBC, recent work has focused on the role of cholangiocytes in immune recognition and targeting of the biliary epithelium. Again, as with PBC, there is increased expression of MHC II antigens and ICAM-1 on cholangiocytes. These changes are not specific to PSC or PBC, occur also in extrahepatic biliary obstruction, and likely represent an epiphenomenon (85). A role for other unidentified adhesion molecules or costimulatory molecules allowing increased immune recognition and activation of lymphocytes cannot be excluded.

The increased frequency of PSC among family members suggests an immunogenetic basis for susceptibility to PSC. HLA haplotype associations have been extensively examined. PSC occurs more frequently in persons of HLA haplotypes B8, DR3, DR2, and DRw52a, whereas reports differ as to whether the DRw52a and the DR4 allele are associated with a more severe course (97). The elucidation of the complex interplay of polygenic factors initiating autoimmune diseases remains one of the great challenges in biomedical research, hopefully to be aided considerably by the sequencing of the human genome.

Liver Allograft Rejection and Graft-Versus-Host Disease

Liver allograft rejection and graft-versus-host disease (GVHD) are problematic liver diseases occurring after orthotopic liver transplantation and bone marrow transplantation (BMT), respectively. Both are characterized by damage and destruction of the small intrahepatic bile ducts and are clearly immune-mediated, although the precise antigenic targets leading to bile duct loss are not known. Acute rejection is characterized histopathologically by a predominantly mononuclear portal inflammation, endotheliitis, and bile duct inflammation and injury. Chronic rejection typically does not occur for at least two months posttransplant, and is characterized by bile duct loss and obliterative arteriopathy.

GVHD commonly affects the skin, gastrointestinal tract, and liver, occurring acutely within the first month post-BMT and also chronically in 30% to 50% of patients. In acute GVHD, endotheliitis and injury to the small bile ducts with a predominantly mononuclear, portal infiltrate are also seen but are typically less severe than seen in acute rejection. With chronicity, endotheliitis subsides but the portal inflammation may drastically worsen, in contrast to chronic rejection, presumably occurring with immune reconstitution. Bile duct injury worsens, eventually leading to bile duct destruction. Both rejection and GVHD are characterized by mononuclear portal inflammation, endotheliitis, and small bile duct injury and loss. The obliterative arteriopathy distinguishes allograft rejection from GVHD and suggests either different antigenic targets or immune effector mechanisms in the pathogenesis of these disorders. This subject has recently been reviewed in depth elsewhere (98).

Genetic Cholangiopathies

To date, there are a small number of diseases in which an identifiable genetic mutation is responsible for biliary disease. Mutations responsible for the syndromic paucity of intrahepatic bile ducts observed in neonatal patients with Alagille syndrome have recently been mapped to the Jagged1 gene (99). Mutations in the cystic fibrosis transmembrane conductance regulator (CFTR) are the first recognized mutations responsible for causing human biliary disease due to defective transport by cholangiocytes. Liver disease occurs in approximately 17% of patients with cystic fibrosis (CF) and is increasingly recognized as patients live longer due to improvements in treatments for the pulmonary complications of CF. It is presumed that defective chloride transport and chloride-mediated secretion by cholangiocytes are responsible for the reduced fluidity and alkalinity of bile, leading to bile duct damage. Specific mutations in CFTR responsible for the development of liver disease have not yet been defined. Our knowledge of the natural history and best treatments for CF-associated liver disease is continuing to evolve (100).

Infectious Cholangiopathies

The human biliary tree is typically a sterile environment. When the normal architecture is disrupted, such as occurs with stricture, stones, obstruction, or congenital malformation, the biliary tree is subject to infections with enteric pathogens such as *Escherichia coli* and *Salmonella typhimurium*. A detailed review of how these cells cause cholangitis is beyond the scope of this chapter, but an interesting paper demonstrates that *S. typhimurium* can invade intestinal epithelial cells via CFTR (101). This may represent a novel means for entry by bacteria into cholangiocytes as well.

Immunocompromised patients have a unique set of opportunistic biliary infections. In particular, AIDS patients can develop a unique cholangiopathy characterized by variable cholangiographic patterns and combinations of papillary stenosis and extra- and intrahepatic sclerosing cholangitis (102). When carefully sought after, infectious agents are usually identified, and include *Cryptosporidium, Microsporidium, Cytomegalovirus, Mycobacterium avium* complex, and *Cyclospora* (103). Animal models using immunodeficient mice and targeted knockouts infected with *Cryptosporidium parvum* suggest that T cell cytokines are required for the bile duct inflammation and sclerosis induced in these animals by the parasite (104). Studies into the cytopathic mechanisms of *C. parvum* on cholangiocytes indicate that widespread cell death occurs via an apoptotic mechanism in an *in vitro* model of biliary cryptosporidiosis using human biliary epithelial cells (105). Further studies are underway to elucidate the mechanisms of entry by the parasite and the intracellular apoptotic pathways activated by infection with *C. parvum*.

Neoplastic Cholangiopathies

Neoplastic transformation of cholangiocytes can result in the formation of both benign (adenomas and cystadenomas) or malignant tumors (cholangiocarcinoma and cystadenocarcinoma). Cholangiocarcinoma is of greatest concern due to its greater frequency and grave prognosis. PSC, chronic infection with parasitic liver flukes, and congenital dilatation of the bile ducts are conditions associated with a high risk of developing this malignancy (106). Chronic inflammation and toxic bile acids have been imputed as possible factors leading to tumor formation, but to date the molecular biological mechanisms have remained elusive. Recent *in vitro* work utilizing human cholangiocarcinoma cell lines have demonstrated genotoxic effects of nitric oxide, both by directly damaging DNA and inactivating DNA repair enzymes via nitrosylation (75). This suggests that induction of nitric oxide synthase and hence nitric oxide production that occurs during chronic inflammatory states may be a mechanistic link between inflammation and cancer in the biliary tree. Alterations in apoptotic thresholds resulting from a chronic inflammatory state may also be important in cholangiocarcinoma development. Cholangiocytes are inherently resistant to apoptosis, but are observed to undergo programmed cell death in PBC and PSC, leading to bile duct loss (42). In PSC, the inflammatory milieu may lead to a further dysregulation of apoptosis, allowing genetically damaged cells to proliferate and perhaps escape immune recognition, ultimately leading to the dreadful 10% to 20% incidence of bile duct malignancy observed in this condition.

SUMMARY: CURRENT STATUS AND FUTURE PERSPECTIVES

Recent information is presented concerning the pathobiology of biliary epithelia, a rapidly evolving field receiving increasing attention from investigators with interests ranging from epithelial cell biology to clinical hepatology.

The principal reasons for this flurry of investigative activity include: (a) the development of new experimental models and techniques that allow specific hypotheses related to cholangiocyte biology to be directly addressed; (b) the recognition that biliary epithelia are important to the normal functions of the liver, especially transport; and (c) the growing appreciation that cholangiocytes represent the major target in a variety of debilitating, life-threatening diseases, cholangiopathies. While our grasp of the embryology and anatomy of the biliary system is generally adequate, we know much less about functional aspects of the biliary tree, under either normal or pathological conditions. In our judgment, the most important advances in this field have been: (a) the development of distinct subpopulations of small and large cholangiocytes from different portions of the biliary tree, which permits demonstration of secretory, proliferative, and apoptotic activities; and (b) the role of bile salts and aquaporins in the regulation of ductal secretory activity. The concept that cholangiopathies may develop from pathogenic mechanisms as diverse as altered immunity infections with cholangiotrophic microbes, direct toxicity from chemicals or genetic abnormalities makes the cholangiocyte a cell of great interest to experimental hepatologists. It thus seems likely that the pathobiology of biliary epithelia will continue to grow as a focus of increasing attention and importance.

ACKNOWLEDGMENTS

This work was supported by Grants DK24031 and DK07198 from the National Institutes of Health and by the Mayo Foundation (N.F.L.) and Scott & White Hospital and Texas A&M University Health Science Center, College of Medicine, by Grant DK54208 and a Veterans Administration Merit Review Grant (G.A.).

REFERENCES

1. LeSage G, Alvaro D, Benedetti A, et al. Cholinergic system modulates growth, apoptosis and secretion of cholangiocytes from bile duct ligated rats. *Gastroenterology* 1999;117:191–199.
2. Alvaro D, Alpini G, Jezequel AM, et al. Role and mechanisms of acetylcholine in the regulation of cholangiocyte secretory functions. *J Clin Invest* 1997;100:1349–1362.
3. Nathanson MH, Burgstahler AD, Mennone A, et al. Characterization of cytosolic Ca²⁺ signaling in rat bile duct epithelia. *Am J Physiol* 1996;271:G86–G96.
4. Benedetti A, Bassotti C, Rapino K, et al. A morphometric study of the epithelium lining the rat intrahepatic biliary tree. *J Hepatol* 1996;24:335–342.
5. Fouassier L, Chinet T, Robert B, et al. Endothelin-1 is synthesized and inhibits cyclic adenosine monophosphate-dependent anion secretion by an autocrine/paracrine mechanism in gallbladder epithelial cells. *J Clin Invest* 1998;101:2881–2888.
5a. Caligiuri A, Glaser S, Rodgers R, et al. Endothelin 1 inhibits

secretin-stimulated ductal secretion by interacting with ET$_A$ receptors on large cholangiocytes. *Am J Physiol* 1998;275: G835–G846.

6. Alpini G, Glaser SS, Rodgers R, et al. Functional expression of the apical Na$^+$-dependent bile acid transporter in large but not small rat cholangiocytes. *Gastroenterology* 1997;113:1734–1740.

7. Lazaridis KN, Pham L, Tietz P, et al. Rat cholangiocytes absorb bile acids at their apical domain via the ileal sodium-dependent bile acid transporter. *J Clin Invest* 1997;100:2714–2721.

8. Alpini G, Glaser S, Robertson W, et al. Bile acids stimulate proliferative and secretory events in large but not small cholangiocytes. *Am J Physiol* 1997;273:G518–G529.

9. Alpini G, Glaser S, Ueno Y, et al. Bile acid feeding induces cholangiocyte proliferation and secretion: evidence for bile acid-regulated ductal secretion. *Gastroenterology* 1999;116:179–186.

10. Lazaridis KN, Tietz PS, Wu T, et al. Alternative splicing of the rat sodium/bile acid transporter changes its cellular localization and transport properties. *Proc Natl Acad Sci U S A* 2000;97: 11092–11097.

11. Glaser S, Benedetti A, Marucci L, et al. Gastrin inhibits cholangiocyte growth in bile duct ligated rats by interaction with CCK-B/gastrin receptors via IP$_3$-, Ca^{2+}-, and PKCα-dependent mechanisms. *Hepatology* 2000;32:17–25.

12. Glaser SS, Rodgers R, Phinizy JL, et al. Gastrin inhibits secretin-induced ductal secretion by interaction with specific receptors on rat cholangiocytes. *Am J Physiol* 1997;273:G1061–G1070.

13. LeSage G, Glaser S, Marucci L, et al. Acute carbon tetrachloride feeding induces damage of large but not small cholangiocytes from bile duct ligated rat liver. *Am J Physiol* 1999;276:G1289–G1301.

14. Lazaridis KN, Pham L, Vroman B, et al. Kinetic and molecular identification of sodium-dependent glucose transporter in normal rat cholangiocytes. *Am J Physiol* 1997;272:G1168–G1174.

15. Marinelli RA, Pham L, Agre P, et al. Secretin promotes osmotic water transport in rat cholangiocytes by increasing aquaporin-1 water channels in plasma membrane. Evidence for a secretin-induced vesicular translocation of aquaporin-1. *J Biol Chem* 1997;272:12984–12988.

16. Marinelli RA, Tietz PS, Pham LD, et al. Secretin induces the apical insertion of aquaporin-1 water channels in rat cholangiocytes. *Am J Physiol* 1999;276:G280–G286.

17. Roman RM, Feranchak AP, Salter KD, et al. Endogenous ATP release regulates Cl$^-$ secretion in cultured human and rat biliary epithelial cells. *Am J Physiol* 1999;276:G1391–G1400.

18. Zsembery A, Spirli C, Granato A, et al. Purinergic regulation of acid/base transport in human and rat biliary epithelial cell lines. *Hepatology* 1998;28:914–920.

19. Milani S, Herbst H, Schuppan D, et al. Cellular localization of laminin gene transcripts in normal and fibrotic human liver. *Am J Pathol* 1989;134:1175–1182.

19a. Grappone C, Pinzani M, Parola M, et al. Expression of platelet-derived growth factor in newly formed cholangiocytes during experimental biliary fibrosis in rats. *J Hepatol* 1999;31:100–109.

20. Malizia G, Brunt EM, Peters MG, et al. Growth factor and procollagen type I gene expression in human liver disease. *Gastroenterology* 1995;108:145–156.

21. Mathis GA, Wyss PA, Schuetz EG, et al. Expression of multiple proteins structurally related to gamma-glutamyl transpeptidase in non-neoplastic adult rat hepatocytes in vivo and in culture. *J Cell Physiol* 1991;146:234–241.

22. Katayanagi K, Van de Water J, Kenny T, et al. Generation of monoclonal antibodies to murine bile duct epithelial cells: identification of annexin V as a new marker of small intrahepatic bile ducts. *Hepatology* 1999;29:1019–1025.

23. Charlotte F, L'Hermine A, Martin N, et al. Immunohistochem-

ical detection of bcl-2 protein in normal and pathological human liver. *Am J Pathol* 1994;144:460–465.

24. Handler JA, Goldstein RS. Xenobiotic metabolism and toxic responses of intrahepatic biliary epithelium. In: Sirica AE, Longnecker DS, eds. *Biliary and pancreatic ductal epithelia pathobiology and pathophysiology.* New York: Raven Press, 1996; 181–199.

25. Alpini G, Roberts SK, Kuntz SM, et al. Morphological, molecular and functional heterogeneity of cholangiocytes from normal rat liver. *Gastroenterology* 1996;110:1636–1643.

26. Alpini G, Ulrich C, Roberts S, et al. Molecular and functional heterogeneity of cholangiocytes from rat liver after bile duct ligation. *Am J Physiol* 1997;272:G289–G297.

27. Alpini G, Glaser SS, Ueno Y, et al. Heterogeneity of the proliferative capacity of rat cholangiocytes after bile duct ligation. *Am J Physiol* 1998;274:G767–G775.

28. Alpini G, Glaser S, Robertson W, et al. Large but not small intrahepatic bile duct units are involved in secretin-regulated ductal bile secretion in normal rat liver. *Am J Physiol* 1997;272: G1064–G1074.

29. Martinez-Anso E, Castillo JE, Diez, et al. Immunohistochemical detection of chloride/bicarbonate anion exchangers in human liver. *Hepatology* 1994;19:1400–1406.

30. LeSage G, Glaser S, Gubba S, et al. Regrowth of the rat biliary tree after 70% partial hepatectomy is coupled to increased secretin-induced ductal bile secretion. *Gastroenterology* 1996; 111:1633–1644.

31. Reference deleted.

32. Pinzani M, Milani S, De Franco R, et al. Endothelin 1 is overexpressed in human cirrhotic liver and exerts multiple effects on activated hepatic stellate cells. *Gastroenterology* 1996;110:534–548.

33. Alpini G, Lenzi R, Sarkozi L, et al. Biliary physiology in rats with bile ductular cell hyperplasia. Evidence for a secretory function of proliferated bile ductules. *J Clin Invest* 1988;81: 569–578.

34. Alpini G, Ulrich C II, Phillips J, et al. Upregulation of secretin receptor gene expression in rat cholangiocytes after bile duct ligation. *Am J Physiol* 1994;266:G922–G928.

35. Kato A, Gores GJ, LaRusso NF, et al. Secretin stimulates exocytosis in isolated bile duct epithelial cells by a cyclic AMP–mediated mechanism. *J Biol Chem* 1992;267:15523–15529.

36. Tietz P, Alpini G, Pham LD, et al. Somatostatin inhibits secretin-induced ductal choleresis in vivo and exocytosis by cholangiocytes. *Am J Physiol* 1995;269:G110–G118.

37. LeSage G, Glaser S, Robertson W, et al. Partial hepatectomy induces proliferative and secretory events in small cholangiocytes. *Gastroenterology* 1996;110:A1250.

38. Alpini G, Glaser S, Caligiuri A, et al. Ursodeoxycholic acid feeding inhibits secretin-induced cholangiocyte secretory processes in bile duct ligated rats. *Gastroenterology* 1998;114: AL0016.

39. Baiocchi L, Alpini G, Glaser S, et al. The inhibitory effect of ursodeoxycholate (UDCA) on cholangiocyte growth and secretion in bile duct ligated (BDL) rats is not affected by its conjugation with taurine. *Gastroenterology* 1999;116:AL0033.

40. Polimeno L, Azzarone A, Zeng QH, et al. Cell proliferation and oncogene expression after bile duct ligation in the rat: evidence of a specific growth effect on bile duct cells. *Hepatology* 1995; 21:1070–1088.

41. Alpini G, Glaser S, Phinizy JL, et al. Bile acid depletion decreases cholangiocyte proliferative capacity and secretin-stimulated ductal bile secretion in bile duct ligated (BDL) rats. *Gastroenterology* 1997;112:A1210.

42. Celli A, Que FG. Dysregulation of apoptosis in the cholangiopathies and cholangiocarcinoma. *Semin Liver Dis* 1998;18: 177–185.

43. Grubman SA, Perrone RD, Lee DW, et al. Regulation of intracellular pH by immortalized human intrahepatic biliary epithelial cell lines. *Am J Physiol* 1994;266:G1060–G1070.
44. Que FG, Phan VA, Phan VH, et al. GUDC inhibits cytochrome c release from human cholangiocyte mitochondria. *J Surg Res* 1999;83:100–105.
45. Que FG, Phan VA, Phan VH, et al. Cholangiocarcinomas express Fas ligand and disable the Fas receptor. *Hepatology* 1999;30:1398–1404.
46. Que FG, Gores GJ, LaRusso NF. Development and initial application of an in vitro model of apoptosis in rodent cholangiocytes. *Am J Physiol* 1997;272:G106–G115.
47. Harnois DM, Que FG, Celli A, et al. Bcl-2 is overexpressed and alters the threshold for apoptosis in a cholangiocarcinoma cell line. *Hepatology* 1997;26:884–890.
48. McGill JM, Basavappa S, Gettys TW, et al. Secretin activates Cl⁻ channels in bile duct epithelial cells through a cAMP-dependent mechanism. *Am J Physiol* 1994;266:G731–G736.
49. Alvaro D, Mennone A, Boyer JL. Role of kinases and phosphatases in the regulation of fluid secretion and Cl⁻/HCO₃⁻ exchange in cholangiocytes. *Am J Physiol* 1997;273:G303–G313.
50. Alvaro D, Benedetti A, Marucci L, et al. The function of alkaline phosphatase in the liver: regulation of intrahepatic biliary epithelium secretory activities in the rat. *Hepatology* 2000;32:174–184.
51. LeSage G, Glaser S, Caligiuri A, et al. Insulin inhibits secretin-stimulated ductal bile secretion in bile duct ligated (BDL) rats by interaction with insulin receptors on cholangiocytes. *Gastroenterology* 1998;114:L0367.
52. Cho WK, Mennone A, Ryderg SA, et al. Bombesin stimulates bicarbonate secretion from rat cholangiocytes: implications for neural regulation of bile secretion. *Gastroenterology* 1995;113:311–321.
53. Cho WK, Boyer JL. Vasoactive intestinal polypeptide is a potent regulator of bile secretion from rat cholangiocytes. *Gastroenterology* 1999;117:420–428.
54. Lakehal F, Wendum D, Barbu V, et al. Phase I and phase II drug-metabolizing enzymes are expressed and heterogeneously distributed in the biliary epithelium. *Hepatology* 1999;30:1498–1506.
55. Roomi MW, Ho RK, Sarma DS, et al. A common biochemical pattern in preneoplastic hepatocyte nodules generated in four different models in the rat. *Cancer Res* 1985;45:564–571.
56. Reference deleted.
57. Kwiatkowski AP, McGill JM. Human biliary epithelial cell line Mz-ChA-1 expresses new isoforms of calmodulin-dependent protein kinase II. *Gastroenterology* 1995;109:1316–1323.
58. St. Pierre MV, Schlenker T, Dufour JF, et al. Stimulation of cyclic guanosine monophosphate production by natriuretic peptide in human biliary cells. *Gastroenterology* 1998;114:782–790.
59. Feranchak AP, Roman RM, Doctor RB, et al. The lipid products of phosphoinositide 3-kinase contribute to regulation of cholangiocyte ATP and chloride transport. *J Biol Chem* 1999;274:30979–30986.
60. Wang Y, Roman R, Schlenker T, et al. Cytosolic Ca²⁺ and protein kinase Calpha couple cellular metabolism to membrane K⁺ permeability in a human biliary cell line. *J Clin Invest* 1997;12:2890–2897.
61. Tian Y, Fukuda C, Schilling MK. Interstitial accumulation of Na⁺ and K⁺ during flush-out and cold storage of rat livers: implications for graft survival. *Hepatology* 1998;28:1327–1331.
62. Roman RM, Wang Y, Fitz JG. Regulation of cell volume in a human biliary cell line: activation of K⁺ and Cl⁻ currents. *Am J Physiol* 1996;271:G239–G248.
63. Roman RM, Bodily KO, Wang Y, et al. Activation of protein kinase Calpha couples cell volume to membrane Cl⁻ permeability in HTC hepatoma and Mz-ChA-1 cholangiocarcinoma cells. *Hepatology* 1998;28:1073–1080.
64. Nathanson MH, Burgstahler AD, Mennone A, et al. Stimulation of bile duct epithelial secretion by glybenclamide in normal and cholestatic rat liver. *J Clin Invest* 1998;101:2665–2676.
65. Benedetti A, Di Sario A, Marucci L, et al. Carrier-mediated transport of conjugated bile acids across the basolateral membrane of biliary epithelial cells. *Am J Physiol* 1997;272:G1416–G1424.
66. Shimokura GH, McGill JM, Schlenker T, et al. Ursodeoxycholate increases cytosolic calcium concentration and activates Cl⁻ currents in a biliary cell line. *Gastroenterology* 1995;109:965–972.
67. Strazzabosco M, Poci C, Spirli C, et al. Effect of ursodeoxycholic acid on intracellular pH in a bile duct epithelium-like cell line. *Hepatology* 1994;19:145–154.
68. Strazzabosco M, Boyer JL. Regulation of intracellular pH in the hepatocyte. Mechanisms and physiological implications. *J Hepatol* 1996;24:631–644.
69. Strazzabosco M, Mennone A, Boyer JL. Intracellular pH regulation in isolated rat bile duct epithelial cells. *J Clin Invest* 1991;87:1503–1512.
70. Sawma JT, Isseroff H, Reino D. Proline in fascioliasis. Induction of bile duct hyperplasia. *Comp Biochem Physiol* 1978;61A:239–243.
71. Liu Z, Sakamoto T, Ezure T, et al. Interleukin-6, hepatocyte growth factor, and their receptors in biliary epithelial cells during a type I ductular reaction in mice: interactions between the periductal inflammatory and stromal cells and the biliary epithelium. *Hepatology* 1998;28:1260–1268.
72. Omori M, Evarts RP, Omori N, et al. Expression of alpha-fetoprotein and stem cell factor/c-kit system in bile duct ligated young rats. *Hepatology* 1997;25:1115–1122.
73. Hoffmann R, Grewe M, Estler HC, et al. Regulation of tumor necrosis factor-alpha-mRNA synthesis and distribution of tumor necrosis factor-alpha-mRNA synthesizing cells in rat liver during experimental endotoxemia. *J Hepatol* 1994;20:122–128.
74. Park J, Gores GJ, Patel T. Lipopolysaccharide induces cholangiocyte proliferation via an interleukin-6-mediated activation of p44/p42 mitogen-activated protein kinase. *Hepatology* 1999;29:1037–1043.
75. Jaiswal M, LaRusso N, Burgart L, et al. Inflammatory cytokines induce DNA damage and inhibit DNA repair in cholangiocarcinoma cells by a nitric oxide-dependent mechanism. *Cancer Res* 2000;60:184–190.
76. Portmann B, MacSween R. Diseases of the intrahepatic bile ducts. In: MacSween R, Anthony P, Scheuer P, eds. *Pathology of the Liver*. Edinburgh: Churchill Livingstone, 1994.
77. Dickson ER, Grambsch PM, Fleming TR, et al. Prognosis in primary biliary cirrhosis: model for decision making [see comments]. *Hepatology* 1989;10:1–7.
78. Coppel RL, McNeilage LJ, Surh CD, et al. Primary structure of the human M2 mitochondrial autoantigen of primary biliary cirrhosis: dihydrolipoamide acetyltransferase. *Proc Natl Acad Sci U S A* 1988;85:7317–7321.
79. Surh CD, Coppel R, Gershwin ME. Structural requirement for autoreactivity on human pyruvate dehydrogenase-E2, the major autoantigen of primary biliary cirrhosis. Implication for a conformational autoepitope. *J Immunol* 1990;144:3367–3374.
80. Klein R, Pointner H, Zilly W, et al. Antimitochondrial antibody profiles in primary biliary cirrhosis distinguish at early stages between a benign and a progressive course: a prospective study on 200 patients followed for 10 years. *Liver* 1997;17:119–128.
81. Joplin RE, Neuberger JM. Immunopathology of primary biliary cirrhosis. *Eur J Gastroenterol Hepatol* 1999;11:587–593.

82. Hoffmann RM, Pape GR, Spengler U, et al. Clonal analysis of liver-derived T cells of patients with primary biliary cirrhosis. *Clin Exp Immunol* 1989;76:210–215.

83. Harada K, Sudo Y, Kono N, et al. In situ nucleic acid detection of PDC-E2, BCOADC-E2, OGDC-E2, PDC-E1alpha, BCOADC-E1alpha, OGDC-E1, and the E3 binding protein (protein X) in primary biliary cirrhosis. *Hepatology* 1999;30: 36–45.

84. Jones DE, Palmer JM, James OF, et al. T-cell responses to the components of pyruvate dehydrogenase complex in primary biliary cirrhosis. *Hepatology* 1995;21:995–1002.

85. Adams DH, Hubscher SG, Shaw J, et al. Increased expression of intercellular adhesion molecule 1 on bile ducts in primary biliary cirrhosis and primary sclerosing cholangitis. *Hepatology* 1991;14:426–431.

86. Leon MP, Bassendine MF, Gibbs P, et al. Immunogenicity of biliary epithelium: study of the adhesive interaction with lymphocytes. *Gastroenterology* 1997;112:968–977.

87. Joplin RE, Wallace LL, Lindsay JG, et al. The human biliary epithelial cell plasma membrane antigen in primary biliary cirrhosis: pyruvate dehydrogenase X? *Gastroenterology* 1997;113: 1727–1733.

88. Tsuneyama K, Van De Water J, Van Thiel D, et al. Abnormal expression of PDC-E2 on the apical surface of biliary epithelial cells in patients with antimitochondrial antibody-negative primary biliary cirrhosis. *Hepatology* 1995;22:1440–1446.

89. Agarwal K, Jones DE, Bassendine MF. Genetic susceptibility to primary biliary cirrhosis. *Eur J Gastroenterol Hepatol* 1999;11: 603–606.

90. Bernal W, Moloney M, Underhill J, et al. Association of tumor necrosis factor polymorphism with primary sclerosing cholangitis. *J Hepatol* 1999;30:237–241.

91. Wiesner RH, Grambsch PM, Dickson ER, et al. Primary sclerosing cholangitis: natural history, prognostic factors and survival analysis. *Hepatology* 1989;10:430–436.

92. Ludwig J, Kim CH, Wiesner RH, et al. Floxuridine-induced sclerosing cholangitis: an ischemic cholangiopathy? *Hepatology* 1989;9:215–218.

93. Mandal A, Dasgupta A, Jeffers L, et al. Autoantibodies in scle-rosing cholangitis against a shared peptide in biliary and colon epithelium. *Gastroenterology* 1994;106:185–192.

94. Martins EB, Graham AK, Chapman RW, et al. Elevation of gamma delta T lymphocytes in peripheral blood and livers of patients with primary sclerosing cholangitis and other autoimmune liver diseases. *Hepatology* 1996;23:988–993.

95. Dienes HP, Lohse AW, Gerken G, et al. Bile duct epithelia as target cells in primary biliary cirrhosis and primary sclerosing cholangitis. *Virchows Arch* 1997;431:119–124.

96. Bansal AS, Thomson A, Steadman C, et al. Serum levels of interleukins 8 and 10, interferon gamma, granulocyte-macrophage colony stimulating factor and soluble CD23 in patients with primary sclerosing cholangitis. *Autoimmunity* 1997;26:223–229.

97. Farrant JM, Doherty DG, Donaldson PT, et al. Amino acid substitutions at position 38 of the DR beta polypeptide confer susceptibility to and protection from primary sclerosing cholangitis. *Hepatology* 1992;2:390–395.

98. Demetris AJ. Immune cholangitis: liver allograft rejection and graft-versus-host disease. *Mayo Clin Proc* 1998;73:367–379.

99. Li L, Krantz ID, Deng Y, et al. Alagille syndrome is caused by mutations in human Jagged1, which encodes a ligand for Notch1 [see comments]. *Nat Genet* 1997;16:243–251.

100. Colombo C, Battezzati PM, Strazzabosco M, et al. Liver and biliary problems in cystic fibrosis. *Sem Liver Dis* 1998;18:227–35.

101. Pier GB, Grout M, Zaidi T, et al. Salmonella typhi uses CFTR to enter intestinal epithelial cells. *Nature* 1998;393:79–82.

102. Cello JP. Acquired immunodeficiency syndrome cholangiopathy: spectrum of disease. *Am J Med* 1989;86:539–546.

103. Cello JP. AIDS-Related biliary tract disease. *Gastrointest Endosc Clin N Am* 1998;8:963.

104. Stephens J, Cosyns M, Jones M, Hayward A. Liver and bile duct pathology following Cryptosporidium parvum infection of immunodeficient mice. *Hepatology* 1999;30:27–35.

105. Chen XM, Levine SA, Tietz P, et al. Cryptosporidium parvum is cytopathic for cultured human biliary epithelia via an apoptotic mechanism. *Hepatology* 1998;28:959–960.

106. Chapman RW. Risk factors for biliary tract carcinogenesis. *Ann Oncol* 1999;10:308–311.

The Liver: Biology and Pathobiology, Fourth Edition, edited by I. M. Arias, J. L. Boyer, F. V. Chisari, N. Fausto, D. Schachter, and D. A. Shafritz.
Lippincott Williams & Wilkins, Philadelphia © 2001.

30

ENDOTHELIAL AND PIT CELLS

FILIP BRAET
DIANZHONG LUO
ILAN SPECTOR
DAVID VERMIJLEN
EDDIE WISSE

LIVER SINUSOIDAL ENDOTHELIAL CELLS

Liver sinusoidal endothelial cells (LSECs) constitute the sinusoidal wall, also called the endothelium, or endothelial lining (see website chapter ⌨ W-26). The liver sinusoids can be regarded as unique capillaries which differ from other capillaries in the body, because of the presence of fenestrae lacking a diaphragm and a basal lamina underneath the endothelium. The first electron microscopic observation of LSEC fenestrae was accomplished in 1970 by Wisse (1), who applied perfusion fixation to the rat liver and demonstrated groups of fenestrae arranged in sieve plates. In subsequent reports, Widmann (2) and Ogawa (3) confirmed the existence of fenestrae in LSECs by using transmission electron microscopy (TEM). In general, endothelial fenestrae measure 150 to 175 nm in TEM, occur at a frequency of 9 to 13 per μm^2, and occupy 6% to 8% of the

F. Braet: Laboratory for Cell Biology and Histology, Free University of Brussels, 1090 Brussels, Belgium.

D. Luo: Laboratory for Cell Biology and Histology, Free University of Brussels, 1090 Brussels, Belgium; and Department of Pathology, First Affiliated Hospital, Guangxi Medical University, Nanning 530021, Guangxi, China.

I. Spector: Department of Physiology and Biophysics, Health Science Center, State University of New York at Stony Brook, New York.

D. Vermijlen: Laboratory for Cell Biology and Histology, Free University of Brussels, 1090 Brussels, Belgium.

E. Wisse: Laboratory for Cell Biology and Histology, Free University of Brussels, 1090 Brussels, Belgium.

endothelial surface in scanning electron microscopy (SEM) (4). In addition, differences in fenestrae diameter and frequency in periportal and centrilobular zones were demonstrated; in SEM the diameter decreases slightly from 110.7 ± 0.2 nm to 104.8 ± 0.2 nm, whereas the frequency increases from 9 to 13 per μm^2, resulting in an increase in porosity from 6% to 8% from periportal to centrilobular (5). Recent atomic force microscopic observations on glutaraldehyde-fixed and living LSECs in culture revealed that the fenestrae diameter is about 240 to 280 nm (6,7).

Other ultrastructural characteristics of LSECs are the presence of numerous bristle-coated micropinocytotic vesicles and many lysosome-like vacuoles in the perikaryon, indicating a well developed endocytotic activity. The nucleus sometimes contains a peculiar body, the sphaeridium (8).

On the basis of morphological and physiological evidence, it was reported that the grouped fenestrae act as a dynamic filter (4,9). Fenestrae filter fluids, solutes and particles that are exchanged between the sinusoidal lumen and the space of Disse, allowing only particles smaller than the fenestrae to reach the parenchymal cells or to leave the space of Disse (Fig. 30.1). At present, it has become clear that alteration of the endothelial filter affects the bidirectional macromolecular exchange, and therefore may determine the balance between health and disease. Although the majority of the research has been descriptive, the role of the liver sieve has been demonstrated in various diseases such as hyperlipoproteinemia, cirrhosis and cancer (Reviewed in ref. 10). Another functional

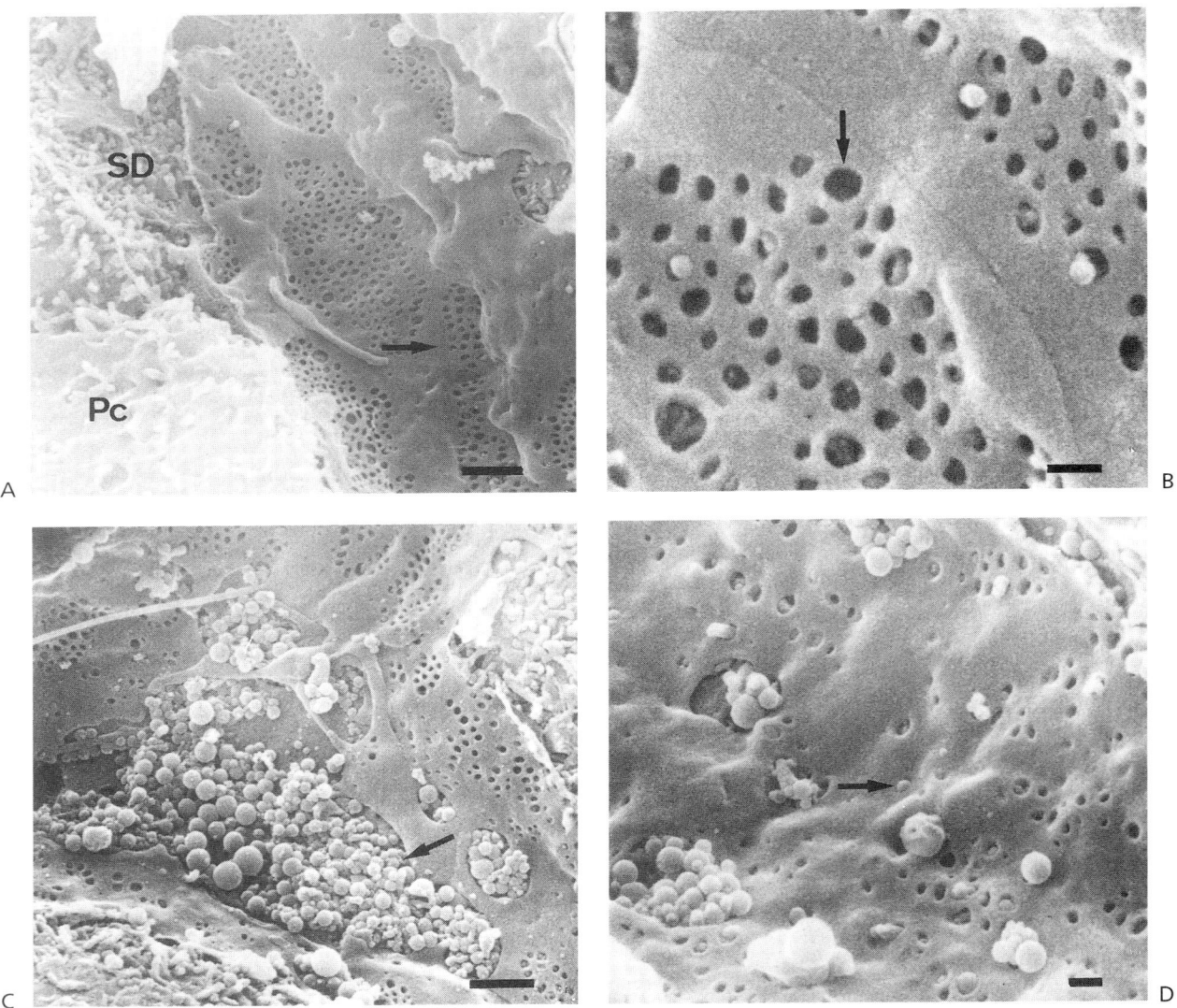

FIGURE 30.1. Scanning electron micrographs of the sinusoidal endothelium from rat liver. **A:** Low magnification showing the fenestrated wall, the space of Disse (*SD*) and the bordering parenchymal cells (*Pc*). Notice also the clustering of fenestrae in sieve plates (*arrow*). *Scale bar*, 1 µm. **B:** Higher-power micrograph depicting fenestrae (*arrow*). *Scale bar*, 250 nm. **C:** Low magnification showing the sinusoidal endothelium of a corn oil-fed rat. After administration of a dose of corn oil, chylomicrons (*arrow*) with diameters in the range of 250 to 600 nm were present in the liver sinusoids. *Scale bar*, 1 µm. **D:** Higher magnification shows lipid particles passing the fenestrae (*arrow*), illustrating the sieving effect of fenestrae. *Scale bar*, 250 nm. (Courtesy of Dr. R. De Zanger.)

characteristic of LSECs is their high endocytotic capacity. This function is reflected by the presence of numerous endocytotic vesicles and by the effective uptake of a wide variety of substances from the blood by receptor-mediated endocytosis [(11), reviewed in ref. 12]. This endocytotic capacity, together with the presence of fenestrae and the absence of a regular basal lamina, makes these cells different and unique from any other type of endothelial cell in the body (13).

Preparation of Endothelial Cells

LSECs seem to be vulnerable cells, a fact that becomes obvious during the isolation, purification and cultivation proce-

dures for *in vitro* studies. LSEC suspensions from rats and mice can be obtained through a variety of isolation and purification techniques, all including perfusion of the liver with one or more tissue-dissociating enzymes. Specific methods can be chosen to satisfy particular requirements in terms of cell yield, purity, intact morphology, responsiveness, and ability to survive in culture (Reviewed in ref. 14).

We found that the use of a low-rate nonrecirculating perfusion of rat liver with collagenase plus fetal calf serum, followed by purification using isopycnic sedimentation in a two-step Percoll gradient and removal of contaminating cells by selective adherence, gave a vital and morphologic intact LSEC population of high purity, enabling the study

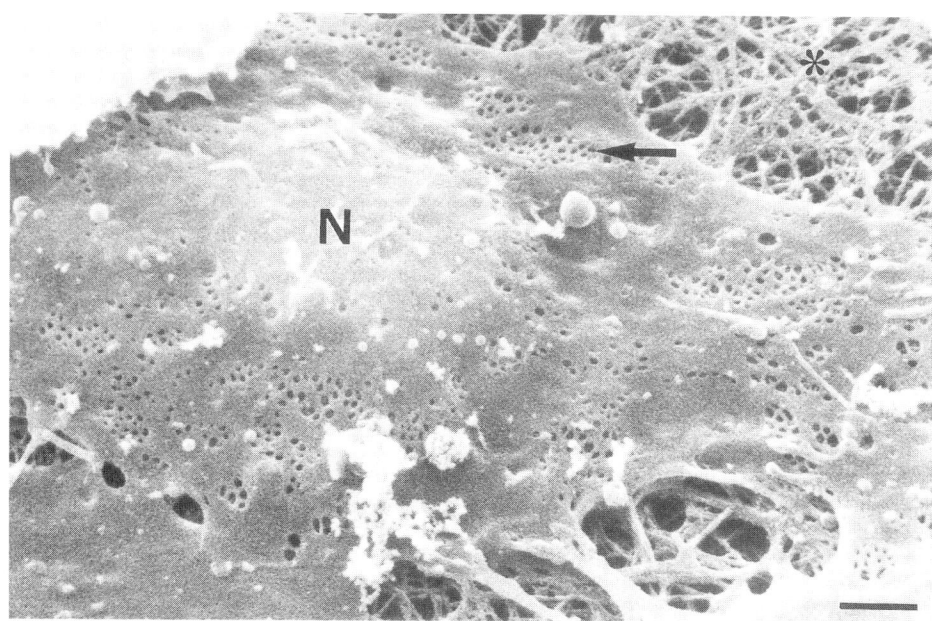

FIGURE 30.2. Scanning electron micrograph of a spread liver sinusoid endothelial cells after 8-hour culture on a collagen-matrix (*asterisk*). Nucleus (*N*); Sieve plate (*arrow*). *Scale bar*, 2 μm.

of structure and function of these cells *in vitro* (Fig. 30.2) (15). Comparable isolation and purification methods have been described to obtain LSEC cultures from pig (16) and humans as well (17).

Identification of Endothelial Cells

To discriminate LSECs from other liver cells (pit cells, stellate cells, Kupffer cells (KC), parenchymal cells, and bile duct cells), immunocytochemical, receptor ligand, and ultrastructural studies can be used. RECA-1 and SE-1 have been reported as suitable antibodies to stain rat LSECs *in vitro* and *in situ* (18,19). However, RECA-1 antibodies do in fact label other microvascular endothelia as well (18). A commercial LSEC-specific human monoclonal antibody named HM 15/3 (BMA Biomedical AG, Switzerland) is available as well. Staining with von Willebrand factor or factor VIII-related antigen is commonly used as a cytochemical marker for vascular endothelium and has been used in attempts to identify LSECs (16,20–21). However, this marker should be used with caution, because the presence of von Willebrand factor in LSECs is controversial. Variations in activity and presence among various species make it inadvisable to use this marker. Until this controversy has been settled, markers other than von Willebrand should be used to identify LSECs.

LSECs possess cell membrane receptors, which enable them to clear rapidly from the blood specific substances such as hyaluran and other extracellular matrix components, which can be used to specifically label LSECs (12).

Besides hyaluronan, Smedsrød et al. (22) conjugated fluorescein isothiocyanate to chondroitin sulphate proteoglycan, collagen alpha chains, and N-terminal propeptide of procollagen type I. All these substances are endocytosed exclusively and with a remarkable efficiency by LSECs. Therefore, in systems with viable cells, this way of distinguishing LSECs from other types of cells is probably the most reliable and specific method available at present.

LSECs in culture display their normal morphologic and functional characteristics, such as fenestrae and pinocytotic vesicles (1), and can also be identified easily from other liver cells by their ultrastructural morphology (Fig. 30.2) (13,15).

Biology of Endothelial Cells

At present, studies are focused on the molecular biology and the clinical aspects of this intriguing class of cells (23–24). LSECs can be regarded as outlined earlier: (a) as a "selective sieve" for substances passing from the blood to parenchymal and stellate cells, and *vice versa* (10), and (b) as a "scavenger system" which clears the blood from many different macromolecular waste products, which originate from turnover processes in different tissues (22). In addition, LSECs have (c) a variety of adhesion molecules (25–26), (d) a capacity to secrete cytokines (26–27), and (e) an important role in various diseases such as liver cancer (28), posttransplantation rejection (29), alcoholic liver disease (30), lipoprotein metabolism (31), fibrosis (32), and viral infection (23).

Interactions between leukocytes or cancer cells and LSECs have been known to be involved in the pathogenesis of liver injury (26). In these cell-to-cell interactions, a wide spectrum of adhesion molecules play a key role, and their expression is mainly regulated by inflammatory cytokines such as interleukin-1, tumor necrosis factor-α and interferon-γ (27). LSECs in normal liver express intercellular adhesion molecule-1, intercellular adhesion molecule-2, leukocyte function-associated-3, very late antigen-5, and CD44. In patients with acute or chronic liver disease, intercellular adhesion molecule-1 and vascular cell adhesion molecule-1 expression are markedly enhanced in the inflamed liver tissue (27,33–34). Selectins are not present in normal conditions, but are induced after lipopolysaccharide administration (35).

Colorectal tumors often metastasize in the liver. In general, it has been supposed that single tumor cells get stuck in the sinusoids when entering the liver, because their size largely exceeds the diameter of a sinusoid. After plugging, their adhesion molecules might react with the surface molecules of the LSECs, enabling them to extravasate and enter the liver parenchyma. Therefore, the adherence of tumor cells to LSECs is a crucial step in early stages of hepatic metastasis [(36), reviewed in ref. 37].

The success of liver transplantation depends at least partially on the functioning of LSECs in the transplanted liver. Preparing the liver for transplantation includes perfusion of preserving fluid, lowering the temperature, stagnant flow during preservation, and reperfusion with warm oxygenated blood when connecting the liver to the donor circulation (29). Many studies point to the LSECs as being very sensitive in this procedure, possibly leading to essential and lethal deficiency during the posttransplantation period (23,38).

Experimental data have accumulated suggesting that alcohol-induced pathological changes of LSECs precede the pathological changes of the hepatocytes. Moreover, due to its strategic position in the liver sinusoid, LSEC dysfunction and structural alterations have far-reaching repercussions for the whole liver (39). There is evidence suggesting that alcohol-induced LSEC alterations are mostly due to KC activation induced by alcohol rather than to a direct action of alcohol on LSEC. In alcoholemia, the activated KC secrete a spectrum of mediators that affect both the structure and function of LSECs. Alcohol-induced LSEC dysfunction comprises a dramatic decrease in hyaluronan uptake by the scavenger receptors of LSECs, a decreased porosity of the liver sieve, and an increment in the secretion of the vasoconstrictor endothelin-1 (40).

LSECs also have important functions in the handling of lipoproteins and the regulation of lipoprotein metabolism (31). They possess several cell membrane receptors for the various types of apoproteins. Moreover, these scavenger receptors have been implicated in adhesion, clearance of dying cells, and host defense against foreign organisms [(41), reviewed in ref. 42].

The role of LSECs in liver fibrosis seems to be quite passive; that is, the cells might become involved in the process of capillarization, but active participation in the synthesis of extracellular matrix products seems to be the task of activated stellate cells (reviewed in ref. 32). However, in cirrhotic liver, compared to normal liver, LSECs exhibit as much as five times the collagen type I mRNA, whereas mRNA for type IV collagen and laminin is decreased by up to 50% (43). Moreover, transforming growth factor-β1 stimulates the synthesis of basement membrane proteins laminin, collagen type IV and entactin in rat LSEC cultures (44).

LSECs are permissive for mouse hepatitis virus 3, at the same time showing a decrease in the number of fenestrae *in vivo* and *in vitro* (45). Therefore, it has been hypothesized that viral infection of LSECs may cause hyperlipoproteinemia. However, feline immunodeficiency virus, as a model for human immunodeficiency virus type 1, did not change the number of fenestrae upon infection. Moreover, the infection of LSECs with the feline immunodeficiency virus contributed to the progression of the infection (46). When human LSECs were infected with human immunodeficiency virus type 1 *in vitro*, they showed the budding of new viral particles, indicating the production of new viruses. This infection was probably facilitated by CD4 surface antigens on LSECs, as were shown to be present by immunogold-EM (47). Therefore, it is concluded that LSECs might be a target and a reservoir for human immunodeficiency viruses.

Biology of Fenestrae

To date, one of the widely accepted hypotheses maintains that drugs which dilate fenestrae, such as pantethine, acetylcholine and ethanol improve the extraction of dietary cholesterol from the circulation while drugs such as nicotine, long-term ethanol abuse, adrenalin, noradrenalin and serotonin, which decrease the endothelial porosity, play a role in the development of drug- and stress-related atherogenesis (48). As a consequence, alterations in the number or diameter of fenestrae by drugs, hormones, toxins, and diseases can produce serious perturbations in liver function (10).

Current interest focuses on the role of the actin cytoskeleton in regulating the diameter and number of fenestrae. Immunoelectron microscopic studies of LSECs in the early 1980s revealed the first information regarding the structural basis of the contraction and dilatation machinery of fenestrae. Oda et al. (49) described in 1983 the presence of actin filaments in the neighborhood of fenestrae, indicating that the cytoskeleton of LSECs plays an important role in the modulation of fenestrae. At present, it is widely accepted that contractile bundles of actin and myosin around fenestrae regulate fenestrae diameter under the control of intracellular calcium levels (Fig. 30.3) (50–53).

In 1986, Steffan et al. (54–55) provided the first evidence that LSEC fenestrae are inducible structures. Treatment of LSECs *in situ* and *in vitro* with the microfilament-

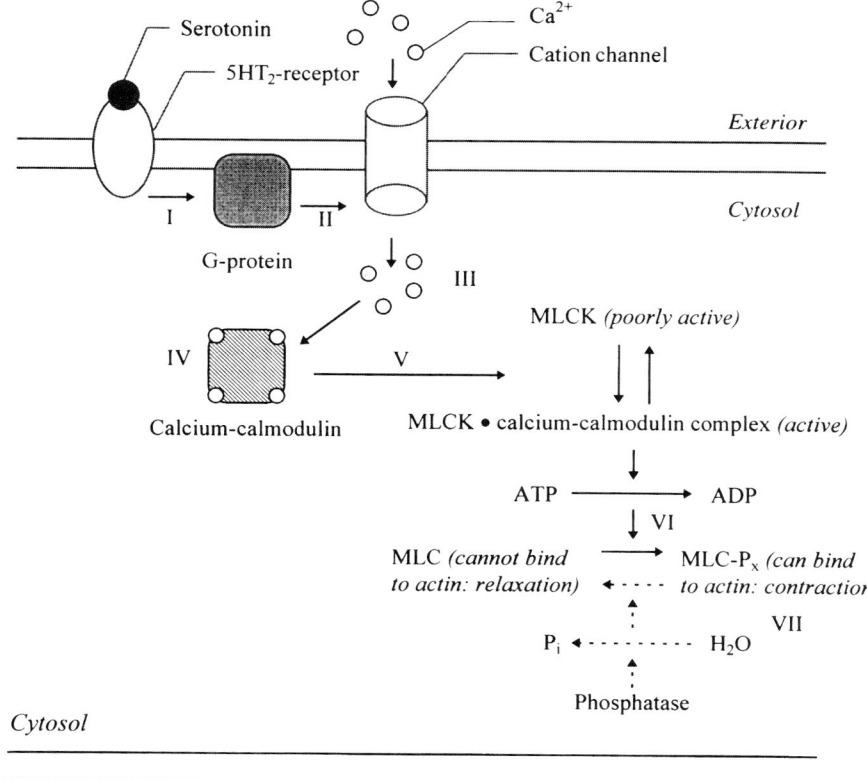

FIGURE 30.3. Scheme of the serotonin signal pathway showing the steps in fenestral contraction and relaxation, as postulated by Arias and co-workers (50–53): (*I*) serotonin binds to a ketanserin-inhibitable receptor, coupled to a pertussis-toxin sensitive G-protein; (*II*) a calcium channel opens, causing an influx of calcium ions; (*III*) the intracellular calcium level increases rapidly, and (*IV*) calcium binds to calmodulin, (*V*) the calcium-calmodulin complex activates myosin light chain kinase, and (*VI*) as a result phosphorylation of the 20-kd light chain of myosin occurs, resulting in (*VII*) an increased actin-activated myosin ATPase activity, which finally initiates contraction of fenestrae. The mechanism for the relaxation of liver sinoidal endothelial cell fenestrae is presently unclear and probably involves dephosphorylation of myosin light chains (*MLC*) as represented by *dashed lines*: a decrease in the cytosolic free calcium concentration leads to dissociation of calcium and calmodulin from the kinase, thereby inactivating myosin light chain kinase (*MLCK*); under these conditions myosin light chain phosphatase, which is not dependent on calcium for activity, dephosphorylates myosin light chain and finally causes relaxation of fenestrae. *ADP*, adenosine diphosphate; *ATP*, adenosine triphosphate.

inhibiting drug cytochalasin B resulted in an increased number of fenestrae. SEM observations of detergent-extracted LSECs revealed that the increase in the number of fenestrae was related to an alteration of the cytoskeleton. Moreover, the effect of cytochalasin B on the number of fenestrae and cytoskeleton could be reversed after removal of the drug. However, when LSECs were treated with various microtubule-altering drugs, there was no effect on the number of fenestrae, thereby demonstrating that microtubules are not involved in the formation of the endothelial pores (55–56). These observations indicate that fenestrae are dynamic structures which may undergo changes in number in response to local external stimuli and that the actin-cytoskeleton has a major role in this process. Later, Bingen et al. (57) noted, in freeze-fracture replicas of cytochalasin B-treated LSECs, areas which were more or less devoid of intramembrane particles having the size of fenestrae. Those authors proposed that fenestrae are formed by fusion between opposite sheets of plasma membrane which are depleted of intramembrane particles. In addition, Taira (58) elaborated the study of Bingen et al. (57) and found some new evidence about the formation of sieve plates or clustered fenestrae. The study of the luminal cell membrane of freeze-fractured LSECs revealed the presence of trabecular meshworks which were attached to the E- and P-face of the cell membrane of both the cell body and the attenuated cell processes. The author demon-

strated that these meshworks give rise to a stepwise formation of sieve plates by ballooning, fusion and flattening of the cell membrane and cytosol among these plasmalemmal invaginations.

The recent availability of a battery of new actin binding drugs that affect the polymerization of actin by different mechanisms greatly enhances the precision with which the dynamics and functions of the actin cytoskeleton in various cell types can be dissected (59). The study of the numerical dynamics of LSEC fenestrae is an example of such a cellular process, in which the use of several microfilament-disrupting drugs was necessary to identify one that could selectively reveal the process of fenestrae formation. In the past we demonstrated that treatment of LSECs with cytochalasin B, latrunculin A, swinholide A, misakinolide A or jasplakinolide induce an increased number of fenestrae (59–61). However, only by treating LSECs with misakinolide were we able to visualize the process of fenestrae formation and to identify a new structure involved in the process of fenestrae formation, as we describe below (61).

Actin filament staining of untreated LSECs displays intense circular bundles lining the cell periphery and few straight bundles oriented parallel to the long axis of the cell (Fig. 30.4A). The maximal effect of misakinolide on F-actin was obtained as soon as 10 to 15 minutes after treatment and caused loss of F-actin bundles. Further incubation did

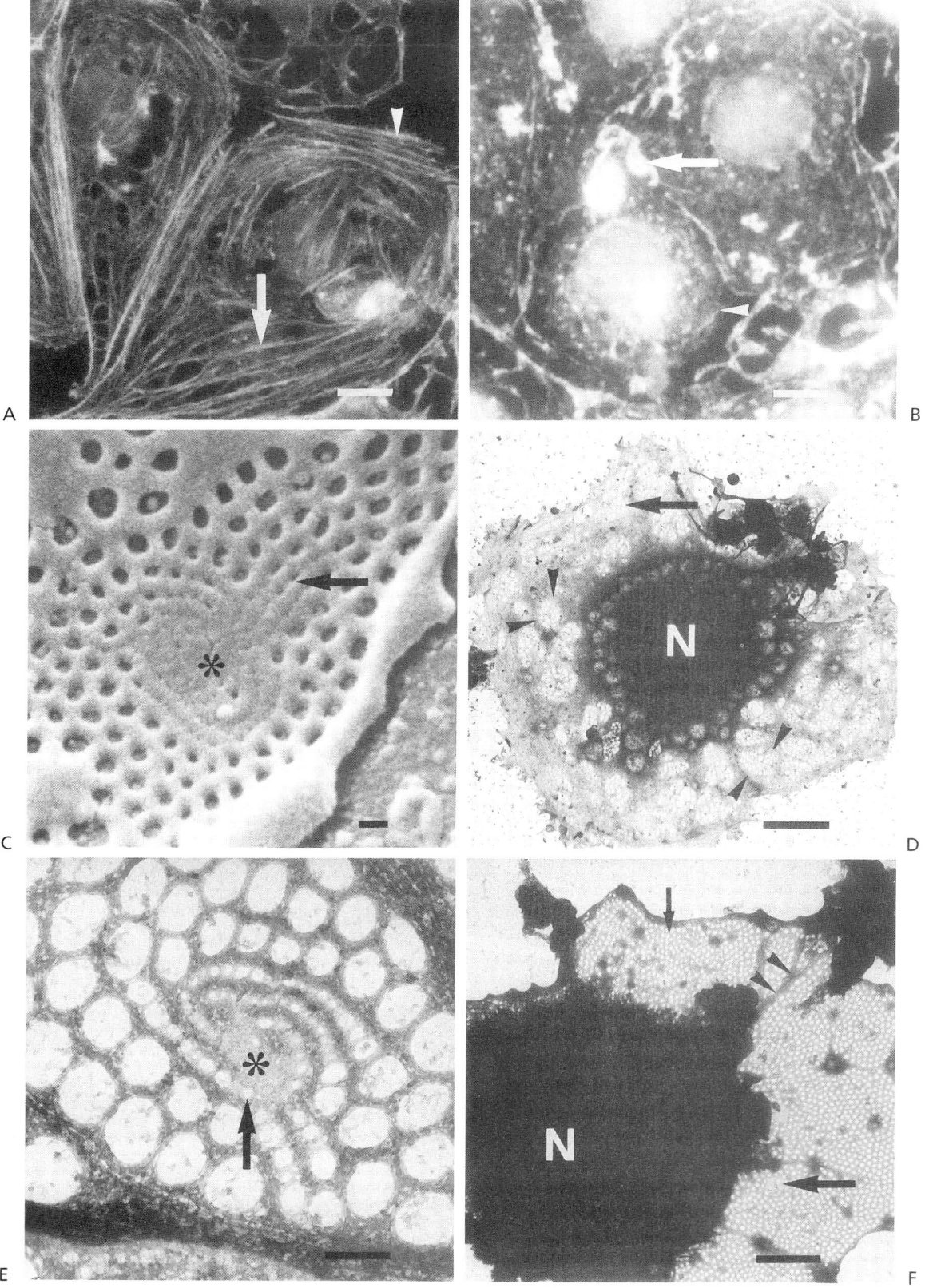

not result in additional alterations in actin organization or in adverse effects on cell shape and viability (Fig. 30.4B). Remarkably, within one hour of misakinolide treatment, we could observe with the aid of SEM small cytoplasmic unfenestrated areas, surrounded by rows of very small fenestrae within the area of fenestrated cytoplasm (Fig. 30.4C). To study these areas in more detail we applied whole-mount TEM to LSECs cultured on collagen-coated grids, after slight prefixation and extraction with detergent, as this technique allows the visualization of the cytoskeleton with minimal disruption of the cells (62) (Fig. 30.4D-F). Examination of control LSECs at low magnification showed the existence of an extensive network of cytoskeletal elements that fills and structurally organizes the cytoplasm (Fig. 30.4D). Treatment with misakinolide for 10 to 30 minutes resulted in the disappearance of microfilaments, and in the appearance of small cytoplasmic unfenestrated areas of intermediate electron density (gray centers) within the cytoplasm of all treated cells. In several of these unfenestrated areas, a singular structure could be observed, consisting of rows of fenestrae with increasing diameter, emanating from the gray centers and fanning out into the surrounding cytoplasm (Fig. 30.4E). These structures are suggestive of *de novo* fenestrae formation, and we therefore named them "fenestrae-forming center" (FFC). By two hours of treatment, the burst of fenestrae formation has subsided and the small unfenestrated areas (gray centers) did not show the presence of rows of fenestrae (Fig. 30.4F). Thorough investigation of swinholide A-, jasplakinolide-, cytochalasin B-, and latrunculin A-treated LSECs revealed only small unfenestrated areas, but no sign of connected fenestrae rows. The disassembly of actin filaments in LSECs by these compounds, together with the increase in the number of fenestrae and the presence of inactive FFCs, suggests nevertheless a common mechanism of fenestrae formation for all actin binding agents. Appar-

ently, specific alterations in actin organization at particular locations and at particular times are required to bring to light nascent fenestrae emerging from the FFCs.

When the short period of time necessary to form new fenestrae is taken into account, it is most likely that this process does not involve *de novo* protein synthesis. We have performed experiments with cycloheximide, an inhibitor of protein synthesis, to check this hypothesis. In this set-up, the use of cycloheximide in combination with misakinolide resulted also in the appearance of active FFCs and in an increment in the number of fenestrae. Therefore, it is obvious that the process of fenestrae formation is not driven via protein synthesis. Instead, we consider a reorganization of preexisting FFCs. By using dry-cleaving of LSECs, we recently observed a sponge-like framework of three-dimensional organized fenestrae grouped along the nucleus, as early as 5 minutes after microfilament-disruption (59). We suppose therefore that FFCs are normally anchored to the actin cytoskeleton in the perinuclear area of LSECs, where they cannot be resolved in whole-mount TEM or TEM sections due to the mass thickness and/or the complex three-dimensional organization of the cytoskeletal proteins in this area (59). Disruption of the actin cytoskeleton can, therefore, free the preexisting FFCs from their anchor in the perinuclear region, resulting in their translocation into the 300- to 400-nm–thick peripheral cytoplasm, thereby giving rise to flattened FFCs as depicted in Figure 30.4E.

The fusion of two opposing cell membranes to form fenestrae in LSECs requires the presence of unique compositional membrane microdomains (57,63) and a cell membrane-associated cytoskeletal structure (61). Several theories have been used to model the possible mechanisms of membrane fusion and pore formation. In general, the process leading to membrane fusion is subdivided into the following: adhesion-dehydration; disappearance of the hydration bar-

FIGURE 30.4. A: Actin distribution in control liver sinusoidal endothelial cells (LSECs) showing the presence of stress fibers (*arrow*), mainly oriented parallel to the long axis of the cells, and peripheral bands (*arrowhead*) of actin bundles that line the cell margin. *Scale bar*, 5 μm. **B:** LSECs treated with 25 nM misakinolide A for 10 minutes show a loss of actin bundles and the appearance of curly actin aggregates (*arrow*). Peripheral actin bands (*arrowhead*) are less dense and interrupted. *Scale bar*, 5 μm. **C:** High-power scanning electron micrograph of the fenestrated cytoplasm obtained after 1 hour of exposure to 25 nM misakinolide. Note a typical cytoplasmic unfenestrated area (*asterisk*), surrounded by rows of very small fenestrae (*arrow*). *Scale bar*, 250 nm. **D–F:** Transmission electron micrographs of whole-mount, formaldehyde-prefixed, cytoskeleton buffer-extracted LSEC of control (**D**) and misakinolide-treated LSECs. (**E–F**) **D:** Low magnification showing the cell nucleus (*N*) and extracted cytoplasm. Note that the sieve plates are well defined by a dark border (*arrowheads*). Inside the sieve plates, fenestrae can be observed (*arrow*). *Scale bar*, 2 μm. **E:** Treatment with 25 nM misakinolide A for 30 to 60 minutes resulted in the appearance of small cytoplasmatic unfenestrated areas of intermediate density (*asterisk*) within the fenestrated cytoplasm and showing the initial step of fenestrae formation (*arrow*). *Scale bar*, 200 nm. **F:** Low magnification showing the cell nucleus (*N*) and the highly fenestrated cytoplasm (*small arrow*) after 120 minutes of 25 nM misakinolide treatment. Compare with Fig. 4D for the difference from control. Note the thin cytoplasmic arms (*arrowheads*) which run from the nucleus into the cytoplasm. In the cytoplasm, inactive FFCs (*large arrow*) can be observed. *Scale bar*, 5 μm.

rier; contact between phospholipid bilayers, and molecular rearrangement, resulting in pore formation (64–66). As for LSECs, the first step corresponds to the formation of intramembrane protein-free zones (57), while the appearance of peristomal rings of sterols around fenestrae probably corresponds to the final step (63). It seems reasonable to consider that these events take place in the rim of FFCs. However, although nothing realistic can be said about the molecular composition of FFCs, we speculate that the presence of fusion proteins (64), which pull the bilayers of the cell membranes together on the rim of FFCs, may contribute as well to the fusion-fission process. In addition, based on our gallery of electron micrographs taken from misakinolide-treated LSECs, it became clear that the nascent fenestrae emanating from an FFC are already decorated with the earlier described fenestrae-associated cytoskeleton ring (FACR) (Fig. 30.4E) (62). This probably indicates that FFCs already contain the necessary cytoskeletal proteins for assembling the FACR.

In conclusion, despite the multidisciplinary approach taken to study the structure, origin, dynamics and formation of fenestrae, there are still important gaps in information. Our knowledge needs considerable consolidation and expansion at the structural and biochemical level to reveal how the different proteins form a contractile unit, and which signal transduction pathways are involved in fenestral dilatation and relaxation. Moreover, further investigation is needed to determine the molecular composition of the FACR, the FFC, and the exact mechanism of fenestrae formation in the FFCs.

For the near future, we expect that forthcoming research will focus on therapeutic strategies by altering the sieve's porosity. For example, the discovery of new drugs that increase the porosity of the liver sieve may be of great benefit. Such agents may not only improve the extraction of atherogenic lipoproteins from the circulation; they could also be used for enhancing the efficiency of liposome-mediated gene or drug delivery to parenchymal cells.

PIT CELLS, THE LIVER-SPECIFIC NATURAL KILLER CELLS

Natural killer (NK) cells are functionally defined by their ability to kill certain tumor cells and virus-infected cells without prior sensitization (67). NK cells comprise about 10% to 15% of lymphocytes in the peripheral blood, and most of these cells in human and rat have the morphology of large granular lymphocytes (LGL) (68). However, it has been demonstrated that small agranular lymphocytes, lacking CD3 expression, have cytolytic activity comparable to that of NK cells (69). These variations may be related to the stage of NK cell differentiation or heterogeneity (70). Moreover, some cytotoxic T lymphocytes (CTL) also display LGL characteristics (70). Besides NK cells in peripheral blood, NK cells are also found in tissue compartments

such as the spleen, lung, intestine, lymph nodes, bone marrow and liver (70). NK cells in the liver, also called pit cells (71), constitute a unique resident population in the liver sinusoids. Their immunophenotypical, morphological and functional characteristics differ from those of blood NK cells (72). Morphologic and cytotoxic differences between pit cells of different species have been observed (73).

Identification, Structure, and Tissue Distribution of Pit Cells

Pit cells were first described in 1976 by Wisse (71). The name pit cell was introduced because of the characteristic cytoplasmic granules, which in Dutch language are called pit, resembling the pits in a grape (71). The hypothesis that pit cells might possess NK activity was formulated by Kaneda et al. (74), and was based on their morphologic resemblance to LGL. The isolation and purification of pit cells from rat liver and the evidence of spontaneous cytotoxicity against YAC-1 cells confirmed these cells to be hepatic NK cells (75–76).

Pit cells inhabit the liver sinusoids and often adhere to LSECs, although they incidentally contact KCs (Fig. 30.5).

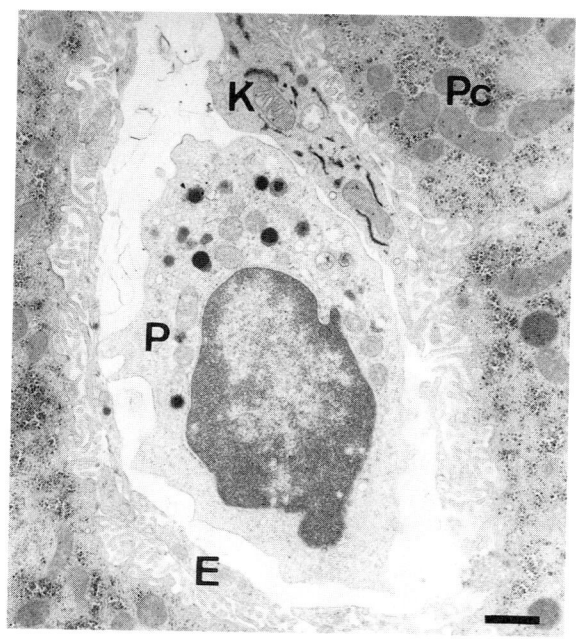

FIGURE 30.5. Transmission electron micrograph of a pit cell in a rat hepatic sinusoidal lumen. The pit cell (*P*) shows a polarity with an eccentric nucleus. The cytoplasm is abundant and contains characteristic electron-dense granules and other organelles lying mainly on one side of the nucleus. The cell contacts an endothelial cell (*E*) and a portion of a Kupffer cell (*K*) with a positive peroxidase reaction product in the rough endoplasmic reticulum. Note the relation with parenchymal cells (*Pc*). *Scale bar*, 1μm. (From Bouwens L, Wisse E. Tissue localization and kinetics of pit cells or large granular lymphocytes in the liver of rats treated with biological response modifiers. *Hepatology* 1988;8: 46–52, with permission.)

They face the blood directly. Pseudopodia of pit cells can penetrate the fenestrae of the LSECs and enter the space of Disse, and can directly contact the microvilli of hepatocytes (4,71). Their appearance in the space of Disse is not a common feature (77). By morphological investigation, the frequency of pit cells in rat liver tissue was found to be about an average of 1 pit cell per 10 KCs. The number of pit cells, in untreated rats, is therefore estimated to be 1.4 to 2×10^6 cells per gram liver weight (75). By immunohistochemistry, using mAb 3.2.3 against NKR-P1A (a specific marker of NK cells), the number of pit cells in frozen sections of rat liver was counted as 13.7 per mm^2 (78). After intravenous injection of biological response modifiers (BRM), the number of pit cells increases 4- to 6-fold in rat liver treated with zymosan (79), and 43-fold with interleukin-2 (IL-2) (80). The surplus of pit cells is considered to originate from local proliferation and from the bone marrow (79–80). Pit cells were found to be more numerous in the periportal than in the pericentral region of the liver lobule (74,78).

Pit cells have essentially the same morphology as NK cells from blood and other organs, that is, LGL morphology (Fig. 30.5). The cells are characterized by a relatively large size compared to other lymphocytes, the presence of granules in the cytoplasm, a pronounced asymmetry of the cell and an indented or kidney-shaped nucleus of high density (81). Pit cells in the rat are about 7 μm in diameter and vary in shape, possessing well-developed pseudopodia. They show a pronounced polarity with an eccentric nucleus and most organelles lying at one side of the nucleus.

The most conspicuous organelles are the electron-dense granules. These granules have several characteristics. They are azurophilic and can be seen after Giemsa staining of a cell smear or cytospin preparation with light microscopic examination. As measured by electron microscopy, the granules differ in size between different pit cell subpopulations [low-density (LD) and high-density (HD) pit cells], but within one cell type the granules are rather homogeneous with respect to size, shape and electron density (82). The granules are membrane-bound and range in size between 0.2 μm in LD pit cells and 0.5 μm in lymphokine-activated killer (LAK) cells. The granules contain lysosomal enzymes, such as acid phosphatase (75,83). Although perforin and granzymes, which have been isolated from NK cell granules (84–85), have not yet been identified in pit cell granules, it is believed by analogy that these molecules are present in the granules of pit cells.

Rod-cored vesicles are small inclusions, ranging in diameter from 0.17 to 0.2 μm, and are exclusively found in LGL (74,83). They contain a straight rod structure that is 30 to 50 nm in length, which bridges the entire diameter of the vesicle (74,83). Rod-cored vesicles derive from and distribute preferentially around the Golgi apparatus. Possibly rod-cored vesicles may also contain cytotoxic factors functioning in natural cytotoxicity (77).

Pit cells also exist in human and mouse liver, but their identification is difficult because they contain a low number of small granules and only a very few rod-cored vesicles (86–88). On the other hand, 5% to 25% of human pit cells contain "parallel tubular arrays" (PTA), which were also reported in human blood NK cells and are considered as a characteristic of these cells (72,87).

Surface Phenotype of Pit Cells

Most surface antigens found on rat pit cells are similar to those found on spleen or blood NK cells (Table 30.1) (76,78,89,90). Pit cells were found to express NKR-P1 (78) (Fig. 30.6). NKR-P1 was first identified in the rat (91) and has now been shown to be expressed by mouse and human

TABLE 30.1. CHARACTERISTICS OF RESTING NK CELLS, LD, HD PIT CELLS, AND IL-2-ACTIVATED-NK CELLS

	Resting NK Cells	HD Pit Cells	LD Pit Cells	IL-2-Activated-NK Cells
Morphology				
Size of the cell (øin μm)	6–7	6–7	6–7	8–13
Number of rod-cord vesicles per cell	0.5	0.8	1.0	n.d.[a]
Size of specific granules (øin μm)	Large (0.3–0.5)	Intermediate (±0.2)	Small (±0.17)	Very Large (0.5–0.9)
Number of granules per cell	Low (n = 10)	Intermediate (n = 20)	High (n = 50)	n.d.
Surface antigens[b]				
CD2	80	80	80	100
CD8	40	100	100	n.d.
CD11a	54	90	90	90–100
CD18	90	90	90	90–100
CD54	35	35	35	97
Asialo-GM1	100	70	36	n.d.
NKR-PI	94	95	95	95
Cytotoxicity				
NK activity	+	++	+++	++++
P815 cell killing	−	−	+	+

Data summarized from references 68, 76, 78, 82, 83, 89, and 91; [a]n.d., no data; [b]Approximate percentage of cells that express antigen.

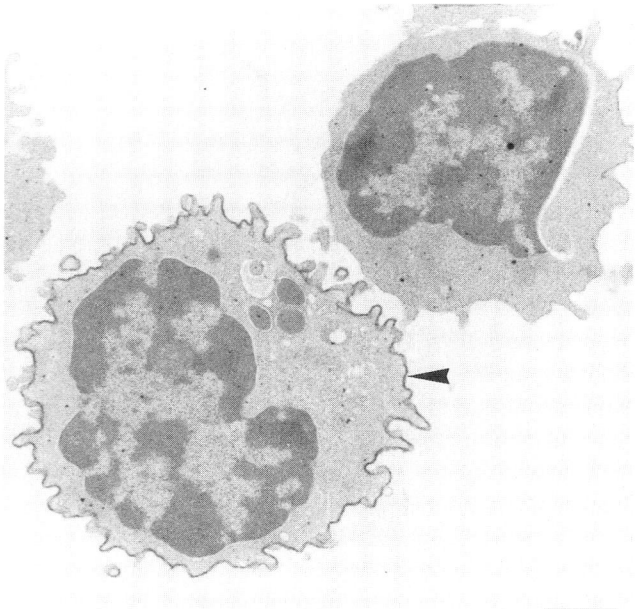

FIGURE 30.6. Immunotransmission electron micrograph showing a 3.2.3-positive LGL (pit cell) (*arrowhead*) and a 3.2.3-negative agranular cell. The 3.2.3⁺ pit cell shows characteristic electron-dense granules in the cytoplasm and immunoperoxidase reaction product on the surface. *Scale bar*, 1μm. (From Luo D, Vanderkerken K, Bouwens L, et al. The number and distribution of hepatic natural killer cells (pit cells) in normal rat liver: an immunohistochemical study. *Hepatology* 1995;21:1690–1694, with permission.)

NK cells (92–93). NKR-P1 is present on 94% of rat LGL and serves as a molecule triggering cytotoxic action (91). The anti-NKR-P1 monoclonal antibody (mAb) 3.2.3 is considered to be useful for NK cell identification (91). However, a subset of T lymphocytes and polymorphonuclear leukocytes (PMN) also expresses NKR-P1 (91,93). CD11a is present on 90% of rat pit cells, which is different from rat peripheral blood NK cells (54%) (89). Approximately 90% of rat pit cells express CD18, 35% express CD54 and 80% express CD2 (89). Asialo-GM1, which is expressed by all rat blood NK cells (82), is present on 36% of LD pit cells and 70% of HD pit cells (82). CD8, a marker of NK cells and cytotoxic T lymphocytes (68), is present on all rat pit cells (76). However, the composition of CD8 in NK cells and T lymphocytes is different. Most CD8⁺ NK cells express CD8α/CD8α homodimers rather than the CD8α/CD8β heterodimers prevalent on cytotoxic T cells (94). In addition, rat pit cells do not express T cell receptor and CD5 antigen (a pan T cell marker) (76–77).

Isolation and Purification of Pit Cells

The isolation method for rat pit cells is based on a nonenzymatic, high-pressure washout technique (75) followed by purification, based on the magnetic negative selection of cells using mAbs against surface antigens found on T and B cells (72,95). Since pit cells are apparently not heavily anchored in the liver sinusoids, the cells can be washed out by a nonenzymatic, high-pressure (50 cm water) perfusion of the liver via the portal vein with phosphate-buffered saline supplemented with 0.1% EDTA (75). The washout is collected from the vena cava. The erythrocytes, granulocytes and cell debris in the washout are removed by Ficoll-Paque gradient centrifugation. The mononuclear cells recovered from the interface of Ficoll-Paque gradient are composed of T cells, pit cells, B cells, monocytes, and a few LSECs. Adherent monocytes and B cells in this population can be selectively removed in a nylon wool column (75). Pit cells are further purified by magnetic cell sorting (95). With this system, a highly purified population of pit cells can be obtained by negative selection, that is, by elimination of remaining monocytes, T and B cells using specific antibodies and immunomagnetic beads. By this method, pit cells with a purity of more than 90% and a viability of more than 95% can be obtained (Fig. 30.7). Moreover, this nonenzymatic method does not destroy cell surface molecules.

Heterogeneity and Origin of Pit Cells

A considerable set of data indicates that rat pit cells constitute a heterogeneous population. Based on the cell density, pit cells can be separated into LD and HD cells by apply-

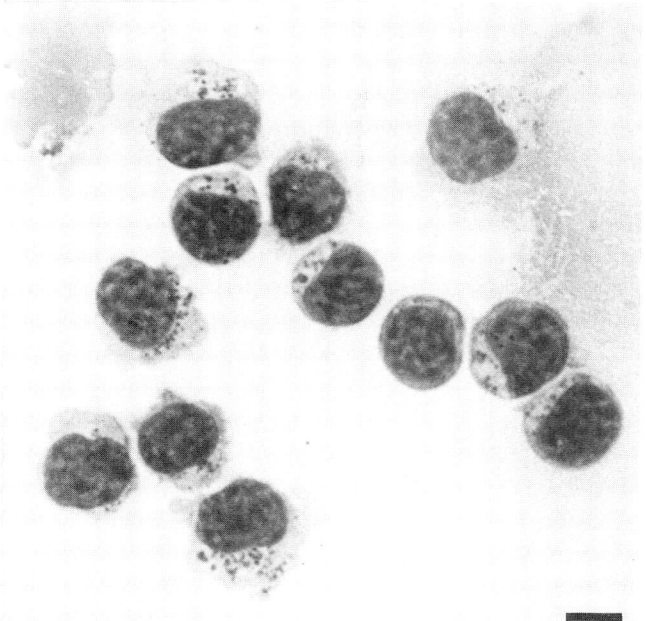

FIGURE 30.7. Light micrograph of an isolated and purified pit cell population in a May-Grünwald-stained cytospin. The cells contain cytoplasmic granules, which can be used to recognize and count the number of pit cells in freshly isolated liver-associated lymphocyte population. *Scale bar*, 5 μm.

ing 45% iso-osmotic Percoll gradient centrifugation (82). These two cell populations have been shown to differ immunophenotypically, morphologically and functionally from each other and from blood LGL (Table 30.1)

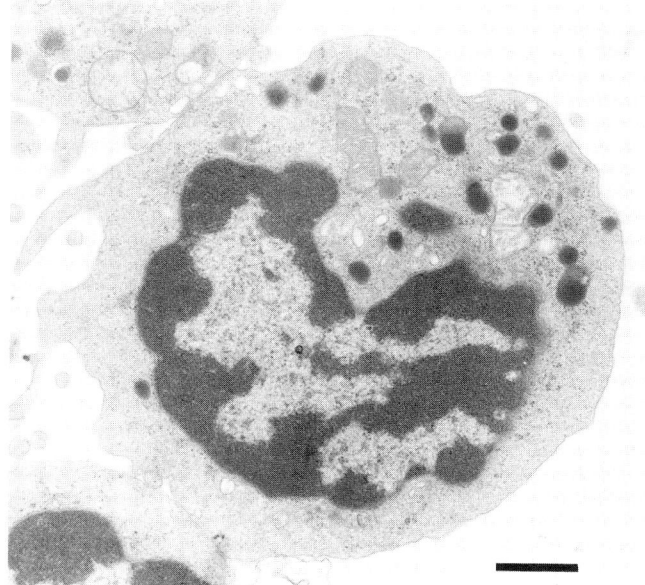

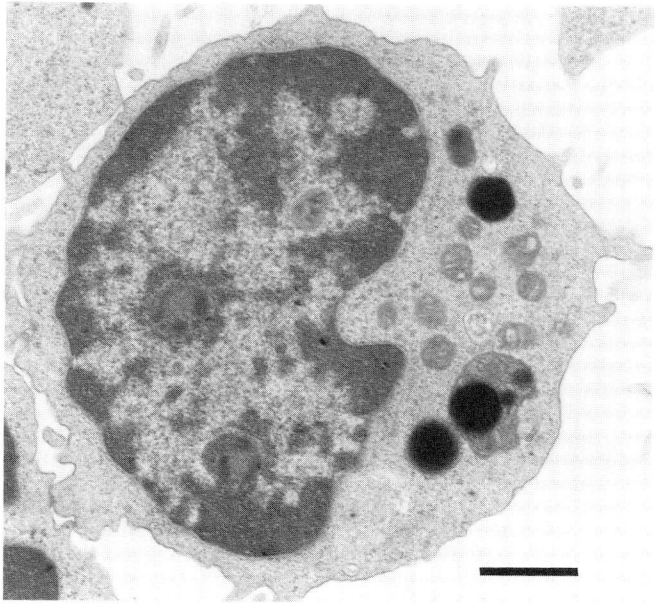

FIGURE 30.8. Transmission electron micrograph of a typical low-density (LD) pit cell (**A**) and a blood NK cell (**B**). **A:** The main morphological characteristics of LD pit cells, compared to high-density (HD) cells and blood NK cells, is the presence of numerous small cytoplasmic granules. **B:** Note the few, but large granules in blood NK cell. *Scale bar*, 1 μm. (From Vanderkerken K, Bouwens L, Wisse E. Characterization of a phenotypically and functionally distinct subset of large granular lymphocytes (pit cells) in rat liver sinusoids. *Hepatology*, 1990,12:70–75, with permission.)

(82,89,90,96). LD pit cells (Fig. 30.8A) contain more rod-cored vesicles and more but smaller granules than blood NK cells (Fig. 30.8B) (82). The number of rod-cored vesicles and granule composition (number and size) of HD pit cells are intermediate between LD pit cells and blood NK cells (82). Immunophenotypically, almost all blood NK cells are asialo-GM1 positive, and 70% of HD pit cells are strongly positive, whereas only 36% of LD pit cells are weakly positive (82). Furthermore, functional differences have been observed among these three populations. The LD pit cells are more cytotoxic against YAC-1 cells and colon carcinoma (CC531s) cells than blood NK cells (96). The HD pit cells have intermediate cytotoxic activity between LD pit cells and blood NK cells (96). In addition, LD pit cells are able to lyse LAK-sensitive P815 mastocytoma targets, which are resistant to normal blood NK cells and hepatic HD pit cells (96).

Pit cells are considered to originate from blood NK cells (97). Several types of evidence support the concept that blood NK cells immigrate into the hepatic sinusoids to become HD pit cells, which further differentiate into LD pit cells. Importantly, the characteristics and functions of HD pit cells are intermediate between blood NK cells and LD pit cells (97). Kinetic experiments with sublethal total body irradiation (700 cGy) showed that blood NK cells and HD pit cells were depleted about one week after irradiation, whereas LD pit cells had totally disappeared at two weeks after irradiation. Shielding of the liver gave similar results, and splenectomy did not affect pit cell number (97). With the use of intravenous anti-asialo-GM1 antiserum injection, blood NK and HD pit cells totally disappeared within one week of treatment, whereas LD pit cells disappeared from the liver one week later (97). The direct evidence for LD pit cells originating from asialo-GM1-positive precursors (blood NK and HD pit cells) was given by the adoptive transfer of fluorescent-labeled HD pit cells into syngeneic rats. After three days, 5% of labeled cells were recovered in the LD fraction, and these cells displayed typical LD pit cell morphology (97). These observations also indicate that the lifespan of pit cells in the liver is about two weeks (72,97).

The mechanism behind the migration of blood NK cells to the liver sinusoids is not fully understood. Several adhesion molecules were found to be involved in the process (89). Rat blood NK and pit cells express LFA-1 (CD11a/CD18) and CD2 (LFA-2) adhesion molecules (89). Their ligands, CD54 (ICAM-1) and CD58 (LFA-3) were found to be present on liver LSECs (98). After intravenous injection of antibodies against CD2, CD11a and CD18 into rats, the number of pit cells in the liver decreased significantly, indicating that the interactions of LFA-1/CD54 and CD2/CD58 are involved in the recruitment of pit cells in the liver (89).

Once marginated in the liver sinusoids, blood NK precursors first differentiate into HD pit cells, then into LD pit cells. The microenvironment of the liver sinusoid is believed to be responsible for this differentiation process (99). Van-

derkerken et al. (99) found that KCs were selectively eliminated three days after intravenous injection of liposomes
containing the cytotoxic drug dichloromethylene diphos-
phonate. This treatment kills the KCs, whereas other cells
remain unharmed. The number of HD pit cells declined
three days after the injection. At that time, the LD pit cell
population showed no change, but a decline of about 80%
was seen seven days after the injection (99). These data
indicate that pit cells are KC-dependent, and therefore it is
supposed that KCs play a role in the differentiation of pit
cells in the liver. However, it remains unclear what factor(s)
derived from KC are responsible for this differentiation. In
addition, LSECs may work synergically with KCs and may
contribute to pit cell differentiation, since co-culture of HD
pit cells with KCs failed to induce the full differentiation of
HD into LD pit cells (99).

Functions of Pit Cells

As a member of the NK cell family, pit cells have demonstrated cytotoxic activity against various tumor cells. The
production of cytokines and participation in the resistance
to microbial pathogens is less well known (67). Rat pit cells
have a high spontaneous cytotoxic activity against various
tumor cell lines, such as YAC-1, P815, CC531s, DHD-
K12, L929, 3LL, and 3LL-R (81). Compared with blood
NK cells, pit cells are four to eight times more cytotoxic
against YAC-1 and CC531s cells, and are able to kill the
NK-resistant but LAK-sensitive P815 cells (82,96,100).
This evidence supports the fact that pit cells become activated by the hepatic microenvironment. Furthermore, NK
activity in the liver could be augmented by BRM (79,88).
Interestingly, an increase in function seems to coincide with
a large increase in the number of LGL (79,88).

Mechanisms in Pit Cell-Mediated Cytotoxicity

It is believed that, like NK cells (101), pit cell-mediated target killing is a multistep process, including recognition of
target cells, binding of effector to target cells (conjugation),
activation of effector cells, delivery of the lethal signal to
target cells, and effector cell detachment and recycling
(68,70,101).

The prerequisite of pit cell killing is the binding of one
or more effector cells to a target cell (72). Adhesion molecules are considered to be responsible for this process. It has
been found that the interaction between β2 integrins
(CD11a-c/CD18) and ICAMs (intercellular adhesion molecules) is the most important mechanism of binding of NK
cells to their targets (102–103). In addition, LFA-1
(CD11a/CD18) also participates in the signal transduction
in NK cells required for NK cell activation (104). Cross-
linking of LFA-1 on NK cells with its antibody is known to
induce a calcium influx, phosphoinositide turnover, and

tumor necrosis factor-α (TNF-α) production (104), and to
inhibit the target cell killing by NK cells (105). LFA-1 was
also found to be involved in pit cell-mediated cytotoxicity.
The antibody against LFA-1 inhibits not only the binding
of pit cells to target cells, but also the killing of target cells
by pit cells (106). Taken together, this information suggests
that LFA-1 on effector cells may have a dual function of
binding to target cells and triggering cytolysis.

CD2 is an adhesion molecule involved in T cell (107)
and NK cell cytotoxicity (108–109). Approximately 80%
of rat pit cells express CD2 (89). Anti-CD2 mAb had no
effect on the binding of pit cells to CC531s, or on the cytotoxicity against CC531s cells (106). However, the anti-
CD2 mAb enhanced the cytolytic activity of rat pit cells
against FcγR+ P815 target cells (106).

NKR-P1 is a well-known triggering receptor on NK cells
(102,110). mAbs against mouse and rat NKR-P1 were
found to trigger NK cell-mediated lysis of FcγR+ target
cells, termed re-directed antibody-dependent cellular cytotoxicity (ADCC) (91). This action also involves a rise in
intracellular Ca++ levels (111) and cytokine production
(112). Furthermore, mAbs to NKR-P1 stimulate phosphoinositide turnover (111), arachidonic acid generation (113)
and granule exocytosis (91). NKR-P1 has been found to be
involved in pit cell-mediated cytotoxicity against FcγR+
P815 target, but not in FcγR− CC531s target killing (114).
These data indicate that NKR-P1 and CD2 depend on subclass specificity of target cell IgG-FcR (109), and may serve
as activation structures on pit cells.

NK cytotoxicity was originally thought to be spontaneous and major histocompatibility complex (MHC) class
I-unrestricted. However, increasing evidence indicates that
NK cells preferentially kill cells lacking MHC class I
(115–119). Masking of MHC class I by an mAb enhances
pit cell-mediated cytotoxicity against CC531s cells, indicating that MHC class I on CC531s cells protects these cells
from being killed by rat pit cells (114). An explanation of
this observation is that the cytotoxic activity of NK cells is
regulated by positive and negative signals from triggering
and inhibitory membrane receptors. The final outcome,
that is, triggering of cytotoxic activity or inhibition of cytotoxicity, appears to depend on the balance between the positive and negative signals (102,120). Inhibitory receptors on
effector cells recognize MHC class I, and this recognition
generally inhibits the lysis of MHC class I+ cells
(110,120–123). However, inhibitory receptors like Ly49
have not been directly identified on pit cells yet.

Studies have demonstrated that NK cell-mediated cytotoxicity can mainly be implemented by two pathways, the
perforin/granzyme (granule exocytosis) pathway and the
Fas/FasL pathway (124,125). The perforin/granzyme pathway is a Ca++-dependent pathway and is mediated by the
pore-forming protein perforin and granzymes, especially
granzyme B, both of which are stored in NK cell granules
(125), of which pit cells have plenty (82). After contact

between effector and target cells, perforin and granzymes are released in a directed manner into the intercellular space between these cells. Perforin alone induces lysis without inducing apoptosis, that is, fragmentation of target cell DNA. Granzymes play a critical role in the rapid induction of DNA fragmentation by CTLs, NK cells and pit cells (126,127). It has been shown that pit cells induce apoptosis in CC531s tumor cells (Fig. 30.9) by the perforin/granzyme pathway (126).

The Fas pathway of apoptosis is mediated by the interaction of Fas ligand (FasL, CD95L) with the apoptosis-inducer Fas (CD95/APO-1) molecule expressed on target cells (124,128,129). Fas is widely expressed on lymphoid and nonlymphoid cells, and some tumor cells (126,129). FasL is expressed by activated T cells, NK cells and pit cells (126,129). It has been demonstrated that Fas/FasL plays an important role in the killing of virus-infected cells and tumor cells by CTLs and NK cells (130). Although Fas is expressed on CC531s cells and FasL is expressed on rat pit cells, pit cell-mediated CC531s apoptosis was found to be exclusively implemented by the perforin/granzyme exocytosis pathway (126).

In conclusion, there is growing evidence that pit cells are highly active, liver-specific NK cells. Pit cells are located in the liver sinusoids and can be separated into LD

and HD fractions by 45% iso-osmotic Percoll gradient centrifugation. These two subpopulations differ morphologically, phenotypically and functionally from each other and from blood NK cells. LD pit cells contain a higher number of small granules, have a higher expression of LFA-1, are more cytotoxic against several tumor cell lines as compared to blood NK cells, and are able to kill NK-resistant but LAK-sensitive P815 cells. The characteristics of HD cells are intermediate between those of LD pit cells and blood NK cells. Pit cells most probably originate from blood NK cells, and the recruitment of pit cells in the liver is mediated by adhesion molecules. A major challenge is to achieve a better understanding of the mechanisms of pit cell cytotoxicity and the cooperation between pit cells and other cells in the liver (i.e., KCs, LSECs, T-, and NK-T cells). Moreover, since pit cells are located in a strategic position in the hepatic sinusoids, they represent a first line of cellular defense against metastasizing colon cancer cells. The role of pit cells in a number of liver pathologies, such as viral hepatitis, deserves more attention.

ACKNOWLEDGMENTS

The authors thank Chris Derom, Marijke Baekeland, Carine Seynaeve, and Ann De Dobbeleer for their photographic, technical, and administrative support. F.B. is a postdoctoral fellow of the Fund for Scientific Research — Flanders.

REFERENCES

1. Wisse E. An electron microscopic study of the fenestrated endothelial lining of rat liver sinusoids. *J Ultrastruct Res* 1970; 31:125–150.
2. Widmann JJ, Cotran RS, Fahimi HD. Mononuclear phagocytes (Kupffer cells) and endothelial cells in regenerating rat liver. *J Cell Biol* 1972;52:159–170.
3. Ogawa K, Minase T, Enomoto K, et al. Ultrastructure of fenestrated cells in the sinusoidal wall of rat liver after perfusion fixation. *Tohoku J Exp Med* 1973;110:89–101.
4. Wisse E, De Zanger RB, Charels K, et al. The liver sieve: Considerations concerning the structure and function of endothelial fenestrae, the sinusoidal wall and the space of Disse. *Hepatology* 1985;5:683–692.
5. Wisse E, De Zanger RB, Jacobs R, et al. Scanning electron microscope observations on the structure of portal veins, sinusoids and central veins in rat liver. *Scanning Microsc* 1983;3: 1441–1452.
6. Braet F, Kalle WHJ, De Zanger RB, et al. Comparative atomic force and scanning electron microscopy; an investigation on fenestrated endothelial cells in vitro. *J Microsc* 1996;181:10–17.
7. Braet F, Rotsch C, Wisse E, et al. Comparison of fixed and living liver endothelial cells by atomic force microscopy. *Appl Phys A* 1998:66;S575–S578.
8. Wisse E. An ultrastructural characterization of the endothelial cell in the rat liver sinusoid under normal and various experimental conditions, as a contribution to the distinction between endothelial and Kupffer cells. *J Ultrastruct Res* 1972;38:528–562.
9. Fraser R, Bosanquet AG, Day WA. Filtration of chylomicrons

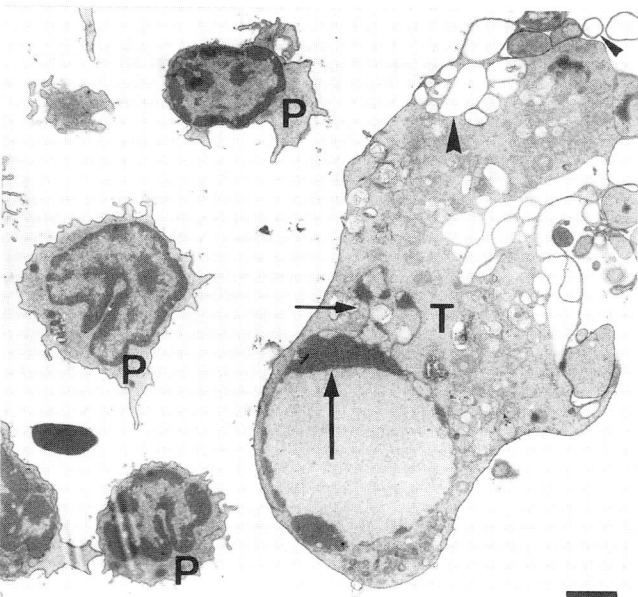

FIGURE 30.9. Transmission electron micrograph of an apoptotic CC531s cell (*T*) coincubated with pit cells (*P*) for 3 hours. The apoptotic CC531s cell (*T*) shows vacuolization (*large arrowhead*), blebbing of the cell surface (*small arrowhead*), chromatin condensation (*large arrow*), and fragmentation of the nucleus (*small arrow*). *Scale bar*, 2 μm. (From Vermijlen D, Luo D, Robaye B, et al. Pit cells (hepatic natural killer cells) of the rat induce apoptosis in colon carcinoma cells by the perforin/granzyme pathway. *Hepatology* 1999;29:51–56, with permission.)

by the liver may influence cholesterol metabolism and atherosclerosis. *Atherosclerosis* 1978;29:113–123.

10. Fraser R, Dobbs BR, Rogers GWT. Lipoproteins and the liver sieve: the role of the fenestrated sinusoidal endothelium in lipoprotein metabolism, atherosclerosis, and cirrhosis. *Hepatology* 1995;21:863–874.

11. Smedsrød B, Melkko J, Araki N, et al. Advanced glycation end products are eliminated by scavenger-receptor-mediated endocytosis in hepatic sinusoidal Kupffer and endothelial cells. *Biochem J* 1997;322:567–573.

12. Smedsrød B, De Bleser PJ, Braet F, et al. Cell biology of liver endothelial and Kupffer cells. *Gut* 1994;35:1509–1516.

13. De Leeuw AM, Brouwer A, Knook DL. Sinusoidal endothelial cells of the liver: fine structure and function in relation to age. *J Electron Microsc Tech* 1990;14:218–236.

14. Alpini G, Philips JO, Vroman B, et al. Recent advances in the isolation of liver cells. *Hepatology* 1994;20:494–514.

15. Braet F, De Zanger R, Sasaoki T, et al. Assessment of a method of isolation, purification and cultivation of rat liver sinusoidal endothelial cells. *Lab Invest* 1994;70:944–952.

16. Cattan P, Zhang B, Braet F, et al. Comparison between aortic and sinusoidal liver endothelial cells as targets of hyperacute xenogeneic rejection in the pig to human combination. *Transplantation* 1996:62;803–810.

17. Daneker GW, Lund SA, Caughman W, et al. Culture and characterization of sinusoidal endothelial cells isolated from human liver. *In Vitro Cell Dev Biol - Anim* 1998:34;370–377.

18. Duijvestijn AM, Van Goor H, Klatter F, et al. Antibodies defining rat endothelial cells: RECA-1, a pan-endothelial cell-specific monoclonal antibody. *Lab Invest* 1992;66:459–466.

19. Ohna A, Mochida S, Aria M, et al. The novel monoclonal antibody against rat sinusoidal endothelial (SE-1): usefulness in characterization of the cells in diseased rat livers. *Hepatology* 1994;20:212.

20. Harrison RL, Boudreau R. Human hepatic sinusoidal endothelium cells in culture produce von Willebrand factor and contain Weibel-Palade bodies. *Liver* 1989;9:242–249.

21. Petrovic L, Burroughs A, Scheuer PJ. Hepatic sinusoidal endothelium: Ulex lectin binding. *Histopathology* 1989;14:233–243.

22. Smedsrød B. Non-invasive means to study the functional status of sinusoidal liver endothelial cells. *J Gastroenterol Hepatol* 1995;10:S81–S83.

23. Le Bail B, Bioulac-Sage P, Senuita R, et al. Fine structure of hepatic sinusoids and sinusoidal cells in disease. *J Electron Microsc Tech* 1990;14:257–282.

24. Wisse E, Braet F, Dianzhong L, et al. Endothelial cells of the hepatic sinusoids: a review. In: Tanikawa K, Ueno T, eds. *Liver diseases and hepatic sinusoidal cells*. Tokyo: Springer-Verlag, 1999:17–55.

25. Scoazec JY, Feldmann G. The cell adhesion molecules of hepatic sinusoidal endothelial cells. *J Hepatol* 1994;20:296–300.

26. Ohira H, Ueno T, Tanikawa K, et al. Changes in adhesion molecules of sinusoidal endothelial cells in liver injury. In: Tanikawa K, Ueno T, eds. *Liver diseases and hepatic sinusoidal cells*. Tokyo: Springer-Verlag, 1999:91–100.

27. Rieder H, zum Buschenfelde M, Ramadori G. Functional spectrum of sinusoidal endothelial liver cells — Filtration, endocytosis, synthetic capacities and intercellular communication. *J Hepatol* 1992;15:237–250.

28. Vidal-Vanaclocha F, Rocha MA, Asumendi A, et al. Role of periportal and perivenous sinusoidal endothelial cells in hepatic homing of blood and metastatic cancer cells. *Semin Liver Dis* 1993;13:60–71.

29. Lemasters JJ, Thurman RG. Reperfusion injury after liver preservation for transplantation. *Annu Rev Pharmacol Toxicol* 1997;37:327–338.

30. Sarphie TG, Deaciuc IV, Spitzer JJ, et al. Liver sinusoid during chronic alcohol consumption in the rat: an electron mirsocpic study. *Alcohol Clin Exp Res* 1995;19:291–298.

31. Kuiper J, Brouwer A, Knook DL, et al. Kupffer and sinusoidal endothelial cells. In: Arias I, Boyer JL, Fausto N, et al., eds. *The liver: biology and pathobiology*, 3rd ed. New York: Raven Press, 1994:791–818.

32. Geerts A, De Bleser P, Hautekeete M, et al. Fat-storing (Ito) cell biology. In: Arias I, Boyer JL, Fausto N, et al., eds. *The liver: bology and pathobiology.* 3rd ed. New York: Raven Press, 1994: 819–838.

33. Volpes R, van den Oord JJ, Desmet VJ. Vascular adhesion molecules in acute and chronic liver inflammation. *Hepatology* 1992;15:269–275.

34. Steinhoff G, Behrend M, Schrader B, et al. Expression patterns of leucocyte adhesion ligand molecules on human liver endothelial — lack of ELAM-1 and CD62 inducibility on sinusoidal endothelia and distinct distribution of VCAM-1, ICAM-1, ICAM-2 and LFA-3. *Am J Pathol* 1993;142:481–488.

35. Essani NA, McGuire GM, Manning AM, et al. Differential induction of mRNA for ICAM-1 and selectins in hepatocytes, Kupffer cells and endothelial cells during endotoxemia. *Biochem Biophys Res Commun* 1995;211:74–82.

36. Wisse E, Braet F, Luo D, et al. Sinusoidal liver cells. In: Bircher J, Benhamou JP, McIntyre N, et al., eds. *Oxford textbook of clinical hepatology*. New York: Oxford University Press, 1999; 33–49.

37. Wisse E, Luo D, Vermijlen D, et al. On the function of pit cells, the liver-specific natural killer cells. *Semin Liver Dis* 1997:17; 265–286.

38. Gao W, Bentley RC, Madden JF, et al. Apoptosis of sinusoidal endothelial cells is a critical mechanism of preservation injury in rat liver transplantation. *Hepatology* 1998;27:1652–1660.

39. Deaciuc IV, Spitzer JJ. Hepatic sinusoidal endothelial cells in alcoholemia and endotoxemia. *Alcohol Clin Exp Res* 1996;20: 607–614.

40. Deaciuc IV, Spitzer JJ, Shellito JE, et al. Acute alcohol administration to mice induces hepatic sinusoidal cell dysfunction. *Int Hepatol Commun* 1994;2:81–85.

41. Dini L, Lentini A, Diez GD, et al. Phagocytosis of apoptotic bodies by liver endothelial cells. *J Cell Sci* 1995;108:967–973.

42. Terpstra V, van Amersfoort ES, van Velzen AG, et al. Hepatic and extrahepatic scavenger receptors: function in relation to disease. *Arterioscler Thromb Vasc Biol* 2000;20:1860–1872.

43. Mather JJ, McGuire RF. Extracellular matrix gene expression increases preferentially in rat lipocytes and sinusoidal endothelial cells during hepatic fibrosis in vivo. *J Clin Invest* 1990;86: 1641–1648.

44. Neubauer K, Krüger M, Quondamatteo F, et al. Transforming growth factor-β1 stimulates the synthesis of basement membrane proteins laminin, collagen type IV and entactin in rat liver sinusoidal endothelial cells. *J Hepatol* 1999;31:692–702.

45. Steffan AM, Pereira CA, Bingen A, et al. Mouse hepatitis virus type 3 infection provokes a decrease in the number of sinusoidal endothelial cell fenestrae both in vivo and in vitro. *Hepatology* 1995;22:395–401.

46. Steffan AM, Lafon ME, Gendrault JL, et al. Productive infection of primary cultures of endothelial cells from cat liver sinusoid with the feline immunodeficiency virus. *Hepatology* 1996; 23:964–970.

47. Steffan AM, Lafon ME, Gendrault JL, et al. Primary cultures of endothelial cells from the human liver sinusoid are permissive for human immunodeficiency virus type-1. *Proc Natl Acad Sci U S A* 1992;89:1582–1586.

48. Oda M, Azuma T, Watamabe N, et al. Regulatory mechanism of hepatic microcirculation: Involvement of the contraction and

dilatation of sinusoids and sinusoidal endothelial fenestrae. In: Messemer K, Hammersen F, eds.*Gastrointestinal microcirculation, Progress in applied microcirculation.* Basel: Karger, 1990:103–128.

49. Oda M, Nakamura M, Watanabe N, et al. Some dynamic aspects of the hepatic microcirculation — demonstration of sinusoidal endothelial fenestrae as a possible regulatory factor. In: Tsuchiya M, Wayland H, Oda M, et al., eds. *Intravital observation of organ microcirculation.* Amsterdam: Excerpta Medica, 1983:105–138.

50. Arias IM. The biology of hepatic endothelial cell fenestrae. In: Schaffer F, Popper H, eds. *Progress in liver disease.* Philadelphia: WB Saunders, 1990:11–26.

51. Brauneis U, Gatmaitan Z, Arias IM. Serotonin stimulates a Ca^{2+} permeant nonspecific cation channel in hepatic endothelial cells. *Biochem Biophys Res Commun* 1992;186:1560–1566.

52. Gatmaitan Z, Arias IM. Hepatic endothelial cell fenestrae. In: Knook DL, Wisse E, eds. *Cells of the hepatic sinusoid 4.* Leiden: Kupffer Cell Foundation, 1993:3–7.

53. Gatmaitan Z, Varticovski L, Ling L, et al. Studies on fenestral contraction in rat liver endothelial cells in culture. *Am J Pathol* 1996;148:2027–2041.

54. Steffan AM, Gendrault JL, McCuskey RS, et al. Phagocytosis, an unrecognized property of murine endothelial liver cells. *Hepatology* 1986;6:830–836.

55. Steffan AM, Gendrault JL, Kirn A. Increase in the number of fenestrae in mouse endothelial liver cells by altering the cytoskeleton with cytochalasin B. *Hepatology* 1987;7:1230–1238.

56. Braet F, De Zanger R, Kalle WHJ, et al. Comparative scanning, transmission and atomic force microscopy of the microtubular cytoskeleton in fenestrated endothelial cells. *Scanning Microsc* 1996;10;225–236.

57. Bingen A, Gendrault JL, Kirn A. Cryofracture study of fenestrae formation in mouse liver endothelial cells treated with cytochalasin B. In: Wisse E, Knook DL, Decker K, eds.*Cells of the hepatic sinusoid 2.* Leiden: Kupffer Cell Foundation, 1989:466–470.

58. Taira K. Trabecular meshworks in the sinusoidal endothelial cells of the golden hamster liver: a freeze-fracture study. *J Submicrosc Cytol Pathol* 1994;26:271–277.

59. Spector I, Braet F, Shochet NR, et al. New anti-actin drugs in the study of the organization and function of the actin cytoskeleton. *Microsc Res Tech* 1999;47;18–37.

60. Braet F, De Zanger R, Jans D, et al. Microfilament disrupting agent latrunculin A induces an increased number of fenestrae in rat liver sinusoidal endothelial cells: comparison with cytochalasin B. *Hepatology* 1996;24:627–635.

61. Braet F, Spector I, De Zanger R, et al. A novel structure involved in the formation of liver endothelial cell fenestrae revealed using the actin inhibitor misakinolide. *Proc Natl Acad Sci U S A* 1998;95;13635–13640.

62. Braet F, De Zanger R, Baekeland M, et al. Structure and dynamics of the fenestrae-associated cytoskeleton of rat liver sinusoidal endothelial cells. *Hepatology* 1995;21:180–189.

63. Simionescu N, Lupu F, Simionescu M. Rings of membrane sterols surround the openings of vesicles and fenestrae, in capillary endothelium. *J Cell Biol* 1983;97:1592–1600.

64. Lindau M, Almers W. Structure and function of fusion pores in exocytosis and exoplasmic membrane fusion. *Curr Opin Cell Biol* 1995;7:509–517.

65. Monck JR, Fernandez JM. The fusion pore and mechanisms of biological membrane fusion. *Curr Opin Cell Biol* 1996;8: 524–533.

66. White JM. Membrane fusion. *Science* 1992;258:917–923.

67. Trinchieri G. Biology of natural killer cells. *Adv Immunol* 1989;47:187–376.

68. Robertson MJ, Ritz J. Biology and clinical relevance of human natural killer cells. *Blood* 1990;76:2421–2438.

69. Inveraldi L, Witson JC, Fuad SA, et al. CD3 negative "small agranular lymphocytes" are natural killer cells. *J Immunol* 1991;146:4048–4052.

70. Lotzova E. Definition and functions of natural killer cells. *Nat Immun* 1993;12:169–176.

71. Wisse E, van't Noordende JM, van der Meulen J, et al. The pit cell: description of a new type of cell occurring in rat liver sinusoids and peripheral blood. *Cell Tissue Res* 1976;173:423–435.

72. Wisse E, Luo D, Vermijlen D, et al. On the function of pit cells, the liver-specific natural killer cells. *Sem Liver Dis* 1997;17: 265–286.

73. Wright PFA, Stacey NH. A species/strain comparison of hepatic natural lymphocytotoxic activities in rats and mice. *Carcinogenesis* 1991;12:1365–1370.

74. Kaneda K, Wake K. Distribution and morphological characteristics of the pit cells in the liver of the rat. *Cell Tissue Res* 1983;233:485–505.

75. Bouwens L, Remels L, Baekeland M, et al. Large granular lymphocytes or "pit cells" from rat liver: isolation, ultrastructural characterization and natural killer activity. *Eur J Immunol* 1987; 17:37–42.

76. Bouwens L, Wisse E. Immuno-electron microscopic characterization of large granular lymphocytes (natural killer cells) from rat liver. *Eur J Immunol* 1987;17:1423–1428.

77. Bouwens L, Wisse E. Pit cells in the liver. *Liver* 1992;12:3–9.

78. Luo D, Vanderkerken K, Bouwens L, et al. The number and distribution of hepatic natural killer cells (pit cells) in normal rat liver: an immunohistochemical study. *Hepatology* 1995;21: 1690–1694.

79. Bouwens L, Wisse E. Tissue localization and kinetics of pit cells or large granular lymphocytes in the liver of rats treated with biological response modifiers. *Hepatology* 1988;8:46–52.

80. Bouwens L, Marinelli A, Kuppen PJK, et al. Electron microscopic observations on the accumulation of large granular lymphocytes (pit cells) and Kupffer cells in the liver of rats treated with continuous infusion of interleukin-2. *Hepatology* 1990;12:1365–1370.

81. Bouwens L. Isolation and characteristics of hepatic NK cells. In: Bouwens L, ed. *NK cells in the liver.* Springer-Verlag, New York, 1995:1–19.

82. Vanderkerken K, Bouwens L, Wisse E. Characterization of a phenotypically and functionally distinct subset of large granular lymphocytes (pit cells) in rat liver sinusoids. *Hepatology* 1990; 12:70–75.

83. Kaneda K. Nagamuta M, Kataoka M, et al. Ultrastructural characteristics of lymphokine-activated killer cells of the rat in comparison with natural killer cells. *Arch Histol Cytol* 1991; 54:119–132.

84. Liu CC, Perussia B, Cohn ZA, et al. Identification and characterization of a pore-forming protein of human peripheral blood natural killer cells. *J Exp Med* 1986;164:2061–2076.

85. Kamada MM, Michon J, Ritz J, et al. Identification of carboxypeptidase and tryptic esterase activities that are complexed to proteoglycans in the secretory granules of human cloned natural killer cells. *J Immunol* 1989;142:609–615.

86. Hata K, Zhang XR, Iwatsuki S, et al. Isolation, phenotyping, and functional analysis of lymphocytes from human liver. *Clin Immunol Immunopathol* 1990;56:401–419.

87. Bouwens L, Brouwer A, Wisse E. Ultrastructure of human hepatic pit cells. In: Wisse E, Knook DL, Decker K, eds. *Cells of the hepatic sinusoid.* The Kupper Cell Foundation: Rijwijk, The Netherlands, 1989:471–476.

88. Wiltrout RH, Mathieson BJ, Talmadge JE, et al. Augmentation of organ-associated natural killer activity by biological response modifiers. Isolation and characterization of large granular lymphocytes from the liver. *J Exp Med* 1984;160:1431–1449.

89. Luo D, Vanderkerken K, Bouwens L, et al. The role of adhesion molecules in the recruitment of hepatic natural killer cells (pit cells) in rat liver. *Hepatology* 1996;4:1475–1480.

90. Luo D, Vermijlen D, Ahishali B, et al. On the cell biology of pit cells, the liver-specific NK cells. *World J Gastroenterol* 2000;6: 1–11.

91. Chambers WH, Vujanovic NL, DeLeo AB, et al. Monoclonal antibody to a triggering structure expressed on rat natural killer cells and adherent lymphokine-activated killer cells. *J Exp Med* 1989;169:1373–1389.

92. Giorda R, Trucco M. Mouse NKR-P1: a family of genes selectively coexpressed in adherent lymphokine-activated killer cells. *J Immunol* 1991;147:1701–1708.

93. Lanier LL, Chang C, Philips JH. Human NKR-P1A: a disulfide-linked homodimer of the C-type lectin superfamily expressed by a subset of NK and T lymphocytes. *J Immunol* 1994;153:2417–2428.

94. Baume DM, Caligiuri MA, Manley TJ, et al. Differential expression of CD8α and CD8β associated with MHC-restricted and non-MHC restricted cytolytic effector cells. *Cell Immunol* 1990;131:352–365.

95. Kanellopoulou C, Seynaeve C, Crabbé E, et al. Isolation of pure pit cells with a magnetic cell sorter and effect of contaminating T cells on their cytolytic capability against CC531. In: Wisse E, Knook DL, Balabaud C, eds. *Cells of the hepatic sinusoid.* The Kupffer Cell Foundation: Leiden, The Netherlands. 1997: 471–473.

96. Vanderkerken K, Bouwens L, Wisse E. Heterogeneity and differentiation of pit cells or large granular lymphocytes of the rat. In: Wisse E, Knook DL, Decker K, eds. *Cells of the hepatic sinusoid.* The Kupffer Cell Foundation: Rijswijk, The Netherlands, 1989:456–461.

97. Vanderkerken K, Bouwens L, De Neve W, et al. Origin and differentiation of hepatic natural killer cells (pit cells). *Hepatology* 1993;18:919–925.

98. Lukomska B, Garcia-Barcina M, Gawron W, et al. Adhesion molecules on liver associated lymphocytes and sinusoidal lining cells of human livers. In: Wisse E, Knook DL, Wake K, eds. *Cells of the hepatic sinusoid.* The Kupffer Cell Foundation: Leiden, The Netherlands. 1995:99–102.

99. Vanderkerken K, Bouwens L, Van Rooijen N, et al. The role of Kupffer cells in the differentiation process of hepatic natural killer cells. *Hepatology* 1995;22:283–290.

100. Bouwens L, Wisse E. Hepatic pit cells have natural cytotoxic (NC) activity against solid tumor-derived target cells. In: Wisse E, Knook DL, Decker K, eds. *Cells of the hepatic sinusoid.* The Kupffer Cell Foundation: Rijwijk, The Netherlands, 1989: 215–221.

101. Berke G. The binding and lysis of target cells by cytotoxic lymphocytes: Molecular and cellular aspects. *Annu Rev Immunol* 1994;12:735–773.

102. Timonen T, Helander TS. Natural killer cell-target cell interactions. *Curr Opin Cell Biol* 1997;9:667–673.

103. Robertson MJ, Caligiuri MA, Manley TJ, et al. Human natural killer cell adhesion molecules: Differential expression after activation and participation in cytolysis. *J Immunol* 1990;145: 3194–3201.

104. Melero I, Balboa M, Alonso JL, et al. Signaling through the LFA-1 leucocyte integrin actively regulates intercellular adhesion and tumor necrosis factor-α production in natural killer cells. *Eur J Immunol* 1993;23:1859–1865.

105. Smits KM, Kuppen PJK, Eggermont AMM, et al. Rat interleukin-2-activated natural killer (A-NK) cell-mediated lysis is determined by the presence of CD18 on A-NK cells and the absence of major histocompatibility complex class I on target cells. *Eur J Immunol* 1994;24:171–175.

106. Luo D, Vermijlen D, Vanderkerken K, et al. Involvement of LFA-1 in hepatic NK cell (pit cell)-mediated cytolysis and apoptosis of colon carcinoma cells. *J Hepatol* 1999;31:110–116.

107. Springer TA. Adhesion receptors of the immune system. *Nature* 1990;346:425–434.

108. Anasetti C, Martin PJ, June CH, et al. Induction of calcium flux and enhancement of cytolytic activity in natural killer cells by cross-linking of the sheep erythrocyte binding protein (CD2) and the Fc-receptor (CD16). *J Immunol* 1987;139: 1772–1779.

109. Van De Griend RJ, Bolhuis RLH, Stoter G, et al. Regulation of cytolytic activity in CD3− and CD3+ killer cell clones by monoclonal antibodies (anti-CD16, anti-CD2, anti-CD3) depends on subclass specificity of target cell IgG-FcR. *J Immunol* 1987; 138:3137–3144.

110. Lanier LL. NK cell receptors. *Annu Rev Immunol* 1998;16: 359–393.

111. Ryan JC, Niemi EC, Goldfien RD, et al. NKR-P1, an activating molecule on rat natural killer cells, stimulates phosphoinositide turnover and a rise in intracellular calcium. *J Immunol* 1991;147:3244–3250.

112. Arase H, Arase N, Saito T. Interferon γ production by natural killer (NK) cells and NK1.1+ T cells upon NKR-P1 cross-linking. *J Exp Med* 1996;183:2391–2396.

113. Cifone MG, Roncaioli P, Cironi L, et al. NKR-P1A stimulation of arachidonate-generating enzymes in rat NK cells is associated with granule release and cytotoxic activity. *J Immunol* 1997; 159:309–317.

114. Luo D, Vermijlen D, Vanderkerken K, et al. Participation of CD45 on pit cells and MHC class I on target cells in rat hepatic NK cell (pit cell)-mediated cytotoxicity against colon carcinoma cells. In: Wisse E, Knook DL, eds. *Cells of the hepatic sinusoid.* The Kupffer Cell Foundation: Leiden, The Netherlands, 1999: 287–291.

115. Giezeman-Smits KM, Kuppen PJK, Ensink NG, et al. The role of MHC class I expression in rat NK cell-mediated lysis of syngeneic tumor cells and virus-infected cells. *Immunobiology* 1996;195:286–299.

116. Carlow DA, Payne U, Hozumi N, et al. Class I (H-2Kb) gene transfection reduces susceptibility of YAC-1 lymphoma targets to natural killer cells. *Eur J Immunol* 1990;20:841–846.

117. Piontek GE, Taniguchi K, Ljunggren HG, et al. YAC-1 MHC class I variants reveal an association between decreased NK sensitivity and increased H-2 expression after interferon treatment or in vivo passage. *J Immunol* 1985;135:4281–4288.

118. Kraus E, Lambracht D, Wonigeit K, et al. Negative regulation of rat natural killer cell activity by major histocompatibility complex class I recognition. *Eur J Immunol* 1996;26: 2582–2586.

119. Storkus WJ, Howell DN, Salter RD, et al. NK susceptibility varies inversely with target cell class l HLA antigen expression. *J Immunol* 1987;138:1657–1659.

120. Burshtyn DN, Long EO. Regulation through inhibitory receptors: lessons from natural killer cells. *Trends Cell Biol* 1997;7: 473–479.

121. Lanier LL. Follow the leader: NK cell receptors for classical and nonclassical MHC class I. *Cell* 1998;92:705–707.

122. Yokoyama WM. Natural killer cell receptors. *Curr Opin Immunol* 1995;7:110–120.

123. Trinchieri G. Recognition of major histocompatibility complex class I antigens by natural killer cells. *J Exp Med* 1994;180: 417–421.

124. Moretta A. Molecular mechanisms in cell-mediated cytotoxicity. *Cell* 1997;90:13–18.

125. Kagi D, Ledermann B, Burki K, et al. Molecular mechanisms of lymphocyte-mediated cytotoxicity and their role in immuno-

logical protection and pathogenesis in vivo. *Annu Rev Immunol* 1996;14:207–232.

126. Vermijlen D, Luo D, Robaye B, et al. Pit cells (hepatic natural killer cells) of the rat induce apoptosis in colon carcinoma cells by the perforin/granzyme pathway. *Hepatology* 1999;29:51–56.

127. Shresta S, MacIvor DM, Heusel JW, et al. Natural killer and lymphokine-activated killer cells require granzyme B for the rapid induction of apoptosis in susceptible target cells. *Proc Natl Acad Sci U S A* 1995;92:5679–5683.

128. Berke G. The CTL's kiss of death. *Cell* 1995;81:9–12.

129. Nagata S, Golstein P. The Fas death factor. *Science* 1995;267:1449–1456.

130. Ashkenazi A, Dixit VM. Death receptors: signaling and modulation. *Science* 1998;281:1305–1308.

The Liver: Biology and Pathobiology, Fourth Edition, edited by I. M. Arias, J. L. Boyer, F. V. Chisari, N. Fausto, D. Schachter, and D. A. Shafritz. Lippincott Williams & Wilkins, Philadelphia © 2001.

HEPATIC STELLATE CELLS: MORPHOLOGY, FUNCTION, AND REGULATION

DAN LI
SCOTT L. FRIEDMAN

Hepatic stellate cells (previously known as lipocytes, Ito cells, fat-storing cells or perisinusoidal cells) are a major regulator of normal liver homeostasis and play a central role in the response to liver injury. These insights have resulted from progress in several areas: (a) the use of immunocytochemical markers to identify hepatic stellate cells *in situ*, since this cell type is not readily visible on routine hematoxylin and eosin staining; (b) the development of techniques to isolate and purify stellate cells from rodent and human liver; (c) the application of molecular techniques to characterize the cellular phenotype of the stellate cell and its profiles of gene expression and protein secretion, and (d) advances in cytokine biology and signaling pathways that provide insights into cell–matrix and cell–cell interactions which are essential for stellate cell function. These advances paint a more comprehensive picture of how this cell type contributes to normal liver function and to fibrosis following injury.

D. Li: Division of Liver Diseases, Department of Medicine, Mount Sinai School of Medicine, New York, New York 10029

S. L. Friedman: Division of Liver Diseases, Department of Medicine, Mount Sinai School of Medicine; and Division of Liver Diseases, Mount Sinai Hospital, New York, New York 10029

HISTORICAL ASPECTS OF STELLATE CELL BIOLOGY AND NOMENCLATURE

The first description of the hepatic stellate cell was made by von Kupffer in 1876. Using a gold chloride method that specifically identifies vitamin A-containing droplets, he named these cells "*sternzellen*," or "star cells" (1). Other investigators used different staining methods to characterize perisinusoidal stellate cells. Among these were the "hepatic pericytes" described by Zimmermann using the Golgi silver method, "fat-storing cells" by Ito using a fat staining method (2), and Suzuki's "interstitial cells" using a silver impregnation method. Bronfenmajer proposed the name "lipocytes" to reflect their role in fat (vitamin A) uptake and pointed out their resemblance to fibroblasts "when their fat content is small" (3). Using von Kupffer's original gold chloride method, Wake provided the definitive description of stellate cells *in situ*, and concluded that the "perisinusoidal cells" were the same cells as von Kupffer's *sternzellen* (4,5) (Fig. 31.1).

Stellate cells began to attract increasing attention when Kent demonstrated their intimate association with collagen fibers in injured liver (6). Further studies established the importance of stellate cells in hepatic injury and fibro-

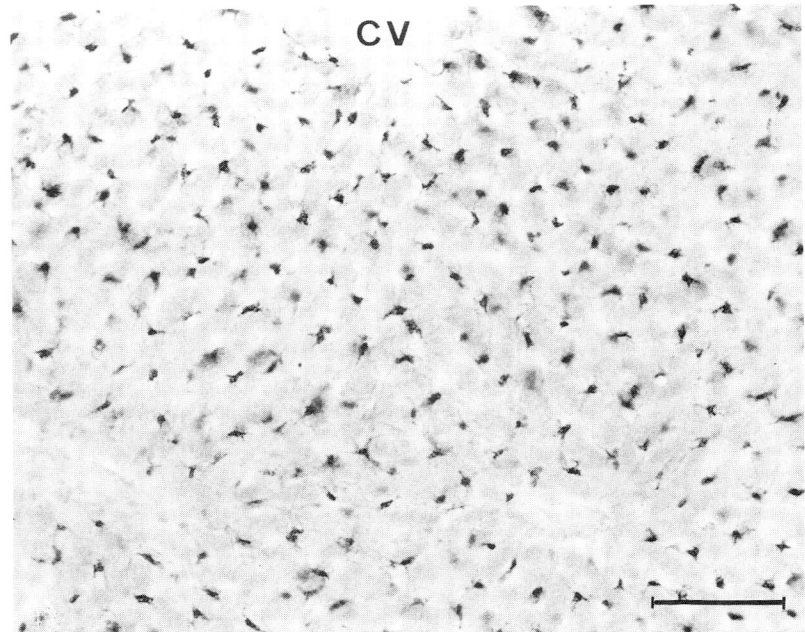

FIGURE 31.1. Human hepatic stellate cells stained by Kupffer's gold chloride method. Star-shaped cells are distributed throughout the liver lobule. *CV*, central vein. *Bar*, 100 μm. Original magnification: ×200. (Courtesy of Professor K. Wake.)

sis, and stimulated efforts to isolate and characterize this cell type from rodent and human liver (7–9). In recent years, knowledge of this cell type expanded dramatically, and the term hepatic stellate cell was widely adopted by investigators.

MORPHOLOGY

Anatomy and Ultrastructure

Hepatic stellate cells are located in the subendothelial space, between the basolateral surface of hepatocytes and the ablumenal side of sinusoidal endothelial cells. They comprise approximately one-third of the nonparenchymal cell population, or about 15% of the total number of resident cells in normal liver (10). In some studies, a slight pericentral predominance has been described.

Stellate cells have spindle-shaped cell bodies with oval or elongated nuclei. Their perikaryons are usually found in recesses between neighboring parenchymal cells. Ultrastructurally, they have moderately developed rough endoplasmic reticulum (rER), juxtanuclear small Golgi complex, and prominent dendritic cytoplasmic processes. These subendothelial processes extend beneath endothelial cells and wrap around sinusoids (Fig. 31.2). On each of these processes are numerous thorny microprojections (spines). A single stellate cell usually surrounds more than two nearby sinusoids (11). On the lumenal side, multiple processes extend across the space of Disse to make contact with hepatocytes. This intimate contact between stellate cells and neighboring cell types may facilitate intercellular transport of soluble mediators and cytokines. In addition, stellate cells have direct connections with nerve endings (12),

which may be important for neurally mediated vasoregulation.

The most characteristic feature of stellate cells in normal liver is cytoplasmic droplets which contain vitamin A, primarily in the form of retinyl esters (Fig. 31.3). In unfixed tissue or isolated cells, the vitamin A droplets exhibit a striking, rapidly fading greenish autofluorescence when excited

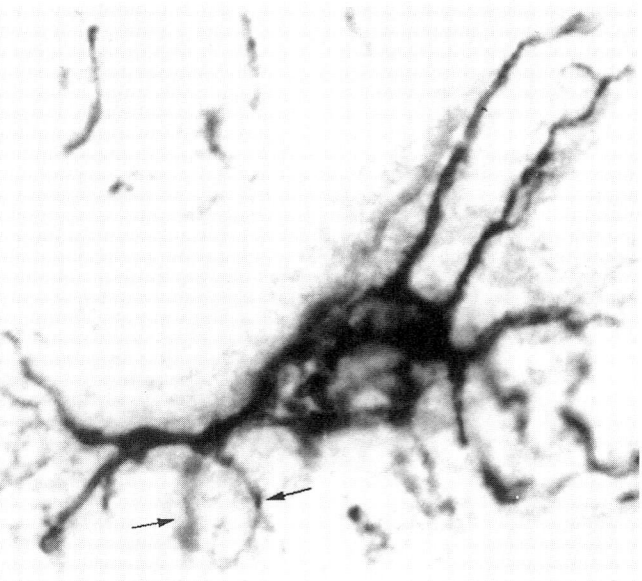

FIGURE 31.2. Indirect immunoperoxidase staining of GFAP in a rat hepatic stellate cell *in situ*. Fine cytoplasmic processes are evident, two of which encircle a sinusoid (*arrows*). Peroxidase was visualized using DAB/H$_2$O$_2$/Ni^{2+}/Co^{3+} substrate solution. (Courtesy of Professor A. Geerts.)

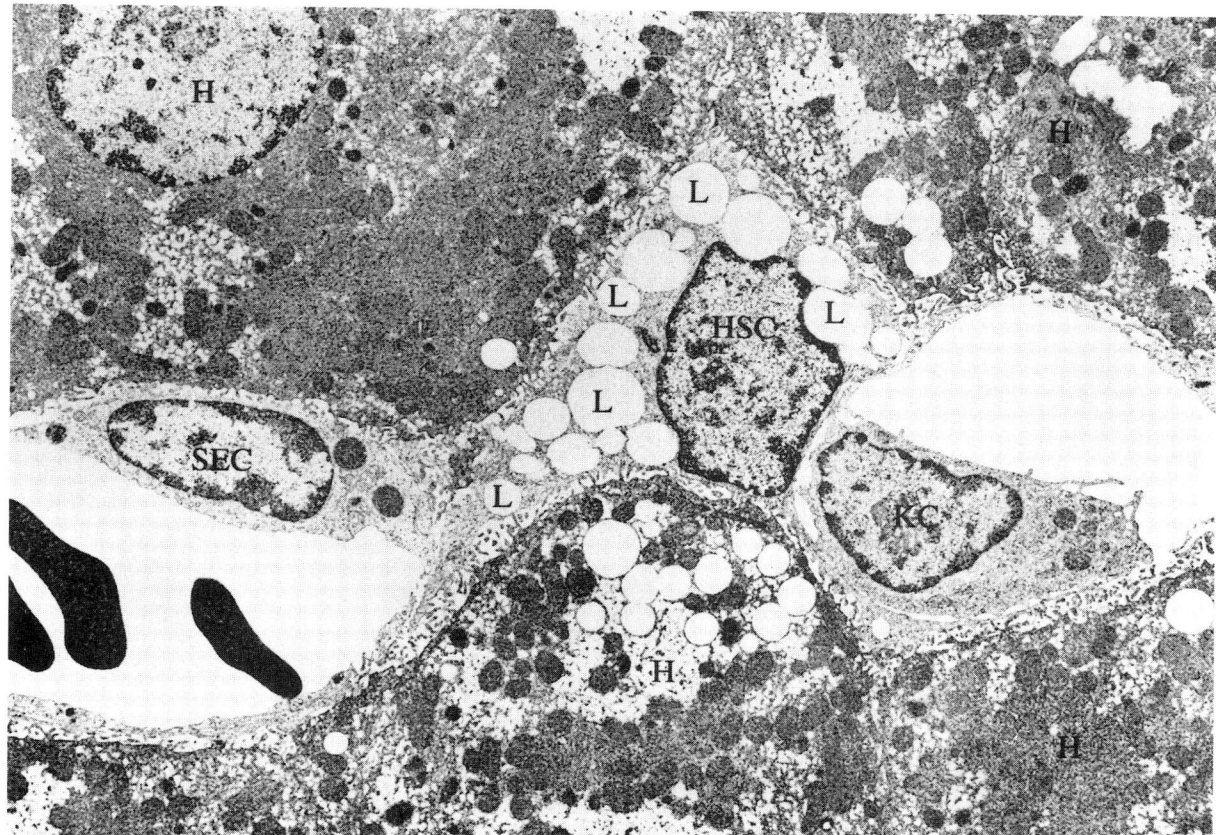

FIGURE 31.3. Quiescent rat hepatic stellate cell in normal liver. The stellate cell (*HSC*) lies outside the hepatic sinusoids in the recess between neighboring parenchymal cells. Abundant lipid (vitamin A) droplets (*L*) in its cytoplasm are a prominent feature of this cell type. *H*, hepatocyte; *SEC*, sinusoidal endothelial cell; *KC*, Kupffer cell. Original magnification: ×5,000. (Courtesy of Professors H. Senoo and K. Imai.)

with the light of 328 nm. The number of droplets varies according to species and abundance of vitamin A stores of the organism. The pattern of vitamin A storage among stellate cells is heterogeneous. The volume of vitamin A droplets differs depending on the intralobular position of the cells. Vitamin A fluorescence is more concentrated in periportal than pericentral regions.

During liver injury, the fine structure of stellate cells changes considerably. They lose their characteristic droplets and become "activated." The rER becomes enlarged, accompanied by a well-developed Golgi apparatus, suggesting active protein synthesis (13) (Fig. 31.4). Bundles of numerous microfilaments appear beneath the cell membrane. The cells then transdifferentiate into myofibroblast-like cells (see below) surrounded by newly formed collagen fibrils.

Cytoskeletal Phenotype of Stellate Cells

Embryologically, stellate cells have traditionally been ascribed to mesenchymal cells of the septum transversum; however, this view has been challenged by the expression of

several neural markers (see below). Their distinct location in the subendothelial space suggests that they are tissue-specific pericytes (14); other members of this group include interstitial cells in lung and mesangial cells in kidney. During liver injury, pericytes display characteristic features of myofibroblasts which are important in wound healing and scar contraction in most adult tissues.

The development of antibodies to a number of cytoskeletal proteins has made it possible to classify the phenotypes of mesenchymal cells. Analysis of stellate cells reveals a heterogeneous pattern of cytoskeletal markers depending on lobular location, species, and whether the tissue is normal or injured. In 1984, Yokoi detected desmin in stellate cells, an intermediate filament typical of contractile cells. This finding suggested similarity between stellate cells and myogenic cell types. Desmin has been widely used as a "gold standard" for identifying stellate cells in rodent liver. In human liver, however, its expression is inconsistent (15). A significant proportion of vitamin A-storing cells may be desmin-negative, but still may contain vitamin A droplets, vimentin, laminin, and tenascin. They are concentrated in the peri-

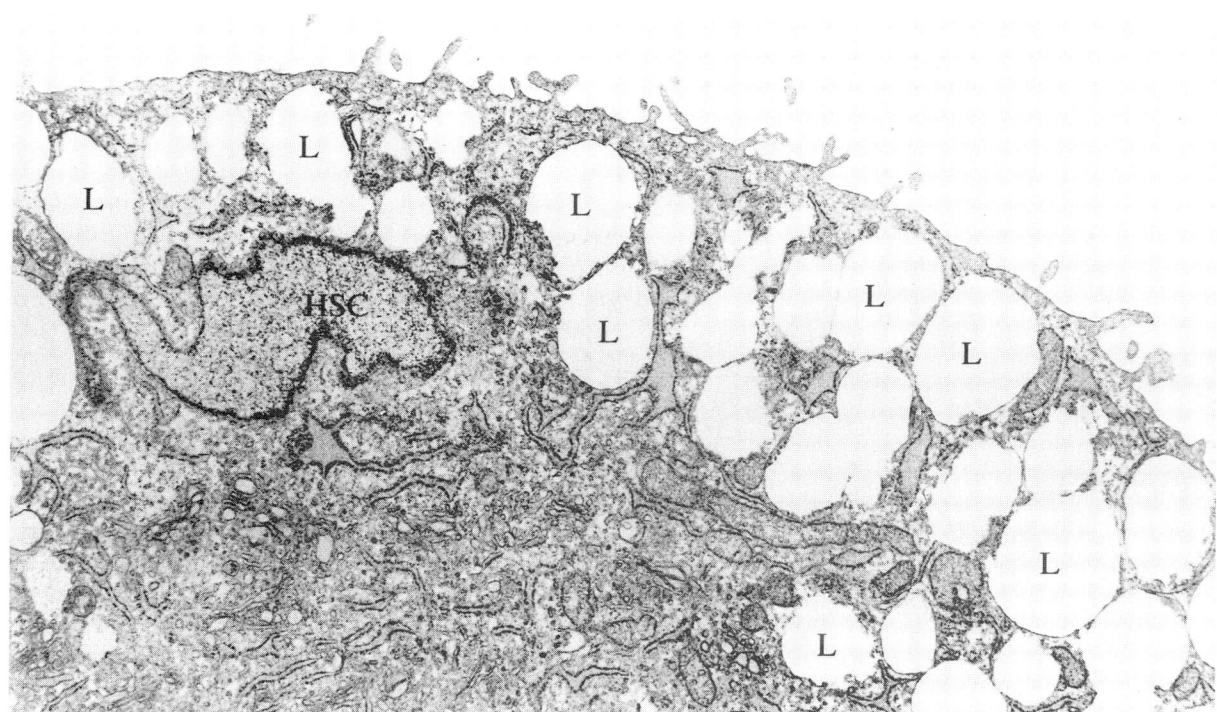

FIGURE 31.4. Rat hepatic stellate cell (*HSC*) in culture. This cell is undergoing transition from a quiescent state to an activated state. Although lipid (vitamin A) droplets (*L*) are still present, rough endoplasmic reticulum is well developed and dilated. Original magnification: ×12,000. (Courtesy of Professors H. Senoo and K. Imai.)

central zone, where they represent up to 50% of stellate cells, whereas periportal stellate cells are typically desmin-positive. It is unclear whether a functional difference exists between desmin-positive and -negative stellate cells.

Vimentin, a mesenchymal intermediate filament, is consistently found in rat and human stellate cells (16). However, because it is widely expressed in most mesenchymal cells, it is not useful in distinguishing stellate cells from other mesenchymal cell types in liver. Stellate cells also express laminin and tenascin, which are two matrix glycoproteins.

Alpha smooth muscle actin (α-SMA) is a functionally important marker of stellate cells, especially during experimental liver injury. α-SMA is one of the six actin isoforms in mammalian tissues and is considered to be typical for vascular smooth muscle cells (17,18). It is the most reliable marker of myofibroblast cells (19). In acute liver injury due to CCl$_4$ or biliary obstruction, the appearance of α-SMA indicates the conversion of stellate cells to myofibroblast-like cells. This marker is absent from other resident liver cells in normal or injured liver, except in smooth muscle cells surrounding large vessels. In human and rat liver, α-SMA is greatly increased during liver injury and is localized in microfilament bundles within cells (15).

The expression by stellate cells of desmin and α-SMA links them closely to cells of myogenic origins; however, neural-associated markers have also been identified in this cell type. Rat hepatic stellate cells express glial fibrillary acidic protein (GFAP) (Fig. 2), the major intermediate filament of astrocytes (20). Another neural-related intermediate filament, nestin, has also been identified in rat stellate cells (21). Nestin is expressed in a variety of cells including neural precursor cells (22) and reactive astrocytes (23), both of which are of neural crest origin. These findings suggest cytoskeletal similarity between hepatic stellate cells and astrocytes, the central effectors of "gliosis"—the wound healing process in the central nervous system. In addition, stellate cells express neural cell adhesion molecule (N-CAM) (24), as well as a neuron-specific guanosine triphosphate-binding protein, RhoN (25). The appearance of neural crest markers in stellate cells raises new questions about their embryonic origin.

The Heterogeneity of Stellate Cells

As reviewed above, "hepatic stellate cells" are a heterogeneous cell population. Although this cell type was originally identified by retinoid droplets, the vitamin A storage capacity differs considerably across the lobule. Cells in pericentral regions are devoid of vitamin A. The variable expression of desmin further underscores its heterogeneity. As noted above, a vitamin A-poor and desmin-negative subpopulation of stellate cells has been described, which has the similar capacity to transform into myofibroblasts and become indistinguishable from vitamin A-rich, desmin-positive stellate cells (26).

Several studies have examined the behavior of fibroblast-like cells in the periportal region and around the central veins, whose relationship to "classical" stellate cells is uncertain (27). The term "second-layer cells" describes the cells in the second layer of the walls of central veins that have a fibroblast-like appearance, but rarely contain lipid droplets. These cells are also vimentin- and desmin-positive and have fibrogenic potential. Whether they are of an origin similar to that of typical vitamin A-rich stellate cells is unclear. Another study explored stellate cell heterogeneity (28) using an isolation method that destroys vitamin A-rich stellate cells. A population of myofibroblast-like cells was obtained from rat liver which has distinct patterns of cytoskeletal markers and expresses the matrix protein fibulin-2; the functional relevance of these patterns to normal and diseased liver remains uncertain.

In summary, the data to date suggest that the pattern of vitamin A storage and cytoskeletal filament is a continuum among stellate cells within liver lobules, indicating that efforts to classify stellate cells into subpopulations based on cytoskeletal phenotype may have limited relevance *in vivo*. It is possible that different subpopulations of stellate cells are derived from similar embryonic origins, and acquire different phenotypes as they adapt to specialized local microenvironments within the liver lobule. If subpopulations of stellate cells differ in their fibrogenic capability or propensity for apoptosis, this information may be important for targeting antifibrotic therapies (29).

FUNCTIONS OF STELLATE CELLS

Retinoid Storage and Metabolism

Vitamin A Storage and Transport (also see website chapter 🖥 W-20)

In normal liver, stellate cells play a key role in the storage and transport of retinoids (vitamin A compounds). Under physiologic conditions, about 50% to 80% of total retinoid of the body is stored in the liver, of which 80% to 90% is in stellate cells. Most vitamin A is stored as cytoplasmic droplets in the form of retinyl esters, predominantly retinyl palmitate (30). The composition of these droplets is affected by dietary intake. They also contain small amounts of triglycerides, phospholipids, cholesterol and free fatty acids (30).

In the intestinal epithelium, dietary retinol is esterified with long-chain fatty acids and packaged into chylomicrons for transport to the systemic circulation through mesenteric lymphatics. These retinol-containing chylomicrons are taken up by hepatocytes and transferred to stellate cells for storage; a small amount remains in hepato-

cytes. Retinyl esters are hydrolyzed to free retinol before their transfer to stellate cells. This process is mediated by retinol-binding protein (RBP). In addition, stellate cells take up RBP-bound retinoids directly from blood. A direct release of RBP-bound retinol from stellate cells into plasma may also occur. The storage and transport of retinoids are influenced by the vitamin A status of the animal. In vitamin A-deficient conditions, dietary retinoids transported to the liver are rapidly bound to RBP in hepatocytes and exported to the circulation without transfer to stellate cells.

Several retinoid-related proteins have been identified in stellate cells, including cellular retinol-binding protein (CRBP), retinol palmitate hydrolase, cellular retinoic acid-binding protein (CRABP), bile salt-dependent and -independent retinol ester hydrolase, and acyl coenzyme A:retinal acyltransferase (31). Whether stellate cells produce RBP is controversial.

Stellate cells also express nuclear retinoid receptors, including retinoic acid receptors (RAR) α, β, and γ, retinoid X receptors (RXR) α and β, but not γ (32), and peroxisome proliferator-activated receptors (PPARs). These receptors are members of the nuclear hormone receptor superfamily (33). The role of nuclear hormone receptors and their specific ligands in stellate cells is not fully defined, although RARα may mediate activation of transforming growth factor β (TGFβ) by retinoic acid metabolites (see next section, below).

Biologic Effects of Retinoids on Stellate Cells

The biological role of retinoids in regulating stellate cell activation remains a puzzle. Although loss of retinoid is a prominent feature accompanying stellate cell activation *in vivo* and in culture (34), it is unknown whether this process is a prerequisite for activation. Reports describing effects of retinoids on stellate cells and fibrogenesis are contradictory (35–38). In culture, both retinol and retinoic acid suppress the proliferation of stellate cells, with retinoic acid 1000 times more potent than retinol. In rats, 9-*cis*-RA and 9,13-di-*cis*-RA, two metabolites of retinoic acid, promote porcine serum-induced liver fibrosis. Both 9-*cis*-RA and 9,13-di-*cis*-RA promote fibrosis by upregulating plasminogen activator, which increases the production and activation of TGFβ. This process is mediated by RARα. However, in another study using a rat fibrosis model induced by bile duct ligation, the increase in TGFβ production was attributed to diminished RA signaling in stellate cells. These reports suggest that retinoic acid affects stellate cell fibrogenesis through more than one pathway, depending on the mechanism of liver injury.

Synthesis of Apolipoproteins and Prostaglandins

Stellate cells secrete apolipoprotein E (39,40), a feature characteristic of smooth muscle cells. In one study, they reportedly express apo A-I and apo A-IV (40), whereas other investigators did not detect mRNAs for apo A-I and A-IV by polymerase chain reaction (39). The functional importance of apolipoprotein production in stellate cells is not clearly defined.

Prostaglandins are also secreted by stellate cells. Prostaglandins play important roles in hepatic metabolism, inflammation, and neural-mediated vasoregulation. In early primary culture, rat stellate cells rapidly release prostaglandin (PG)F2α and D2 when incubated with the neurotransmitter noradrenaline or adenosine triphosphate (ATP) (41). This finding has special relevance *in vivo* because of the close proximity of stellate cells to nerve endings in the normal liver. Activated rat stellate cells also produce PGI2 and PGE2 in response to ethanol, which is mediated by acetaldehyde. Leukotriene C4 and B4 production has also been reported.

The roles of prostaglandins in stellate cell activation and fibrogenesis are not yet clear.

Production of Cytokines and Expression of Membrane Receptors

Stellate cells are an important source of cytokines in the liver. Signal-transduction mediated by the binding of cytokines to their membrane receptors comprises the main mode of cell–cell interaction in normal and injured liver (42) (Table 31.1).

Stellate cells secrete transforming growth factor α (TGFα) and epidermal growth factor (EGF), two potent epithelial growth factors which are important in hepatocyte proliferation during liver regeneration (see Chapter 42 and website chapter ⌨ W-31). TGFα and EGF also stimulate

TABLE 31.1. PRODUCTS AND COMPONENTS OF HEPATIC STELLATE CELLS

Vitamin A-related components and lipids

Retinoids	Retinol, retinyl esters, retroretinoids
Binding proteins	CRBP, CRABP, RBP (controversial)
Enzymes	Retinyl palmitate hydrolase, acetylcoenzyme A: retinyl acyltransferase
Nuclear retinoid receptors	RARα, RARγ, RXRα, RXRβ, PPARs (controversial)
Apolipoproteins	Apo E, apo A-I and A-IV (controversial)

Cytoskeletal markers
Vimentin, desmin, α-SMA, GFAP, nestin

Extracellular matrix

Collagens	Types I, III, IV, V, VI, XIV
Proteoglycans	Heparan, dermatan and chondroitin sulfates, perlecan, syndecan-1, biglycan, decorin
Glycoproteins	Cellular fibronectin, laminin, merosin, tenascin, nidogen/entactin, undulin, hyaluronic acid

Proteases and inhibitors

Matrix proteases	MMP-2, stromelysin-1 (transin), MMP-1, MT-MMP
Protease inhibitors	TIMP-1, TIMP-2, PAI-1

Cytokines, growth factors and inflammatory mediators

Prostanoids	Prostaglandin (PG) F2α, PGD2, PGI2, PGE2; LTC4, LTB4
Leukocyte mediators	M-CSF, MCP-1, PAF
Acute phase components	α2-macroglobulin, IL-6
Mitogens	HGF, EGF, PDGF, SCF, IGF I and II, αFGF
Adhesion molecules	I-CAM-1, V-CAM-1, N-CAM
Vasoactive mediators	ET-1, NO
Fibrogenic compounds	TGFβ1, TGFβ2, TGFβ3, CTGF,
Others	IL-10, CINC

Receptors

Cytokine receptors	PDGF-R, TGFβ-R types I, II and III, ET-R, EGF-R, VEGF-R
Others	Integrin, DDR, thrombin-R, mannose 6 phosphate-R, uPA-R

Signaling molecules and transcription factors

Signaling components	Raf; raf and MAP kinase
Transcription factors	Sp1, NFκB, c-myb, Zf9

CINC, cytokine-induced neutrophil chemoattractant; CRABP, cellular retinoic acid-binding protein; CRBP, cellular retinol-binding protein; CTGF, connective-tissue growth factor; DDR, discoidin domain receptor; EGF, epidermal growth factor; ET, endothelin; FGF, fibroblast growth factor; GF, growth factor; HGF, hepatocyte GF; I-CAM-1, intercellular adhesion molecule 1: IGF, insulin-like GF; IL, interleukin; MAP kinase, mitogen-activated protein kinase; M-CSF, macrophage colony-stimulating factor; MCP-1, monocyte chemotactic peptide 1; MMP, matrix-metalloproteinase; N-CAM, neural cell adhesion molecule; PAF, platelet-activating factor; PPARs, peroxisome proliferator-activated receptors; PDGF, platelet-derived GF; RAR, retinoic acid receptors; RBP, retinol-binding protein; RXR, retinoid X receptor; TGF, transforming GF; TIMP, tissue inhibitor of metalloproteinase; VEGF, vascular endothelial GF.

mitosis in stellate cells (43), thereby creating an autocrine loop for cellular proliferation. Hepatocyte growth factor (HGF) (see Chapter 45) is produced by stellate cells, whose production diminishes during acute liver injury (44). Insulin-like growth factors I and II (IGF-I and -II) and their receptors are also products of stellate cells (45).

Platelet-derived growth factor (PDGF) is the most potent stellate cell mitogen described to date (46,47). PDGF-A chain mRNA has been detected in activated human stellate cells. During liver injury, stellate cells produce more PDGF and upregulate PDGF receptors (48). Following ligand binding, PDGF receptor recruits Ras, followed by activation of the ERK/MAP kinase pathway (see Chapter 35). In addition, phosphoinositol 3 kinase (PI3K) and STAT-1 may mediate PDGF signaling in stellate cells (see Chapters 34 and 35).

Acidic fibroblast growth factor (aFGF), another mitogenic cytokine, has been identified in stellate cells *in situ* during liver injury, late hepatic development, and hepatic regeneration. Stellate cells also create an autocrine loop for basic FGF (bFGF), which is mitogenic towards culture-activated rodent and human stellate cells (49,50).

Stellate cells produce macrophage colony-stimulating factor (M-CSF) and monocyte chemotactic peptide 1 (MCP-1) (51), which regulate macrophage accumulation and growth. MCP-1 production is stimulated by thrombin, interleukin-$l\alpha$, interferon γ and tissue necrosis factor α (TNFα) (52). It is blocked by H-7, an inhibitor of protein kinase C (PKC), suggesting the involvement of PKC in the signaling pathway leading to MCP production. M-CSF synthesis is stimulated by PDGF and bFGF (47). Secretion by stellate cells of these macrophage growth factors may amplify inflammatory and fibrogenic responses during liver injury.

The neutrophil inflammatory response in injured liver is also amplified by stellate cells through the production of platelet-activating factor (PAF). PAF promotes chemotaxis of neutrophils and stimulates their activation. Its production is increased by thrombin, lipopolysaccharide, and calcium ionophores. Rat stellate cells also produce cytokine-induced neutrophil chemoattractant (CINC), a rat form of human interleukin-8 (53). Upregulation of CINC expression accompanies stellate cell activation *in vivo* and in culture.

Stellate cells secrete interleukin-6 (IL-6), thereby contributing to the acute phase response (54) (see Chapter 40). Interleukin-10 (IL-10), an antiinflammatory cytokine, is also produced by stellate cells and is upregulated in early stellate cell activation (55). IL-10 has prominent antifibrogenic activity by downregulating collagen type I expression while upregulating interstitial collagenase. IL-10 knockout mice develop more severe hepatic fibrosis following CCl$_4$ administration than do wild-type mice (56). It is uncertain whether the antifibrotic effect of IL-10 is direct or is mediated through immune downregulation. Clinical trials are currently evaluating IL-10's efficacy in chronic liver fibrosis (57).

Stellate cells also express several adhesion molecules (see Chapter 33 and website chapter 🖳 W-28), including intercellular adhesion molecule 1 (I-CAM-1), vascular cell adhesion molecule 1 (V-CAM-1) and neural cell adhesion molecule (N-CAM) (58). Expression of I-CAM-1 increases following stellate cell activation and may regulate lymphocyte adherence to activated stellate cells. *In situ*, both I-CAM-1 and V-CAM-1 are upregulated following CCl$_4$-induced liver injury (58). Peak immunoreactivity of these molecules coincides with maximal cell infiltration, and the inflammatory cytokine TNFα increases the transcripts of both CAMs. Therefore, it is likely that I-CAM and V-CAM are involved in modulating recruitment of inflammatory cells during liver injury. Stellate cells which express N-CAM lie in close proximity to nerve endings in the liver.

Transforming growth factor β (TGFβ) is one of the most important stimulators of hepatic fibrosis (see Chapte 49). In response to injury, stellate cells secrete latent TGFβ1, which, after activation, exerts potent fibrogenic effects in both autocrine and paracrine patterns. Of these two sources, autocrine activity is most important (59). TGFβ1 expression is increased in experimental and human hepatic fibrosis. Upregulation of TGFβ1 in activated stellate cells occurs through multiple mechanisms. Factors including Sp1 and Zf9/KLF6 transactivate the TGFβ1 promoter through interactions with multiple 'GC box' motifs (60,61). Several mechanisms mediate the activation of latent TGFβ1, including cell surface activation following binding to cell-surface mannose-6-phosphate/IGF-II receptor, and binding to several proteins secreted by stellate cells, including α2-macroglobulin, decorin, and biglycan, and local plasminogen activator (PA)/plasmin. The signaling of TGFβ1 in rat stellate cells involves the activation of Ras, Raf-1, MEK and MAP kinase. A family of signaling molecules, known as SMAD proteins, is also involved in TGFβ signaling (62,63), and their role in stellate cells is under study (64).

Connective tissue growth factor (CTGF) promotes fibrogenesis in skin, lung and kidney and is strongly expressed in stellate cells during hepatic fibrosis (65). Regulation of its expression in stellate cells is not defined, although it is a downstream target of TGFβ in other cellular systems.

Endothelin-1 (ET-1) was originally identified as a potent vasoconstrictor produced mainly by endothelial cells (66). More recent studies identified stellate cells as both a major source and a target of this cytokine during liver injury (67). Interestingly, stellate cells also produce nitric oxide (NO) (see Chapter 39), a physiological antagonist to ET-1 (68).

Expression of Membrane Receptors

Several cytokines regulate stellate cell behavior through specific, high-affinity binding to their cognate membrane receptors.

PDGF receptor was the first receptor identified in stellate cells. It is composed of α or β subunits as either homodimers or heterodimers. In rat stellate cells, the β subunit is the predominant isoform, whereas in human stellate cells both α and β subunits are detectable.

All three forms of TGFβ receptors, types I, II and III (betaglycan), are expressed in rat stellate cells. TGFβ1 binding and responsiveness are enhanced during activation *in vivo* and *in vitro*.

The effects of ET-1 are mediated through two G-protein coupled receptors. Receptor types A and B have been identified in quiescent and activated stellate cells (69). The relative prevalence of ETA and ETB receptors changes during the activation of stellate cells. The ETB receptor is the predominant mediator of stellate cell contraction and growth inhibition. In contrast, the proliferative effect of ET-1 in quiescent stellate cells is mediated through the ETA receptor.

Induction of receptors for vascular endothelial growth factor (VEGF) (see Chapter 65) occurs during stellate cell activation *in vivo* and in culture (70). VEGF receptor upregulation is associated with enhanced mitogenesis in response to VEGF, which is further synergized by bFGF. Because VEGF plays a critical role in angiogenesis, this finding suggests that stellate cells may be involved in typical "angiogenic" responses, thereby broadening their potential role in both wound healing and tumor formation.

Stellate cells express the receptor for thrombin, a serine protease derived from prothrombin. The binding of thrombin to its receptor leads to cellular proliferation and increased production of MCP-1.

In addition to receptors for cytokines, membrane receptors for matrix molecules have been characterized in stellate cells (see Chapter 32 and website chapter 🖥 W-27). Several integrins and their downstream effectors have been identified in stellate cells, including α1β1, α2β1, αvβ1 and α6β4 (71–73). In particular, integrin ligands contain an arginine (Arg) – glycine (Gly) – aspartate (Asp) tripeptide sequence. The common presence of Arg-Gly-Asp (RGD) within many integrin ligands has raised the possibility of using competitive RGD antagonists to block integrin-mediated pathways in fibrogenesis.

A special family of tyrosine kinase receptors called "discoidin domain receptors" (DDR) has ligands which are fibrillar collagens rather than growth factors (74). Identification of DDR mRNA in activated stellate cells (70) raises the possibility that this receptor mediates interactions between stellate cells and the surrounding interstitial matrix during progressive liver injury.

Synthesis of Extracellular Matrix and Involvement in Matrix Degradation

The extracellular matrix (ECM) (see Chapter 32 and website chapters 🖥 W-27 and W-28) of the liver consists of collagens, glycoproteins and proteoglycans. In normal liver, the subendothelial space of Disse contains a basement membrane-like matrix, which is composed of non–fibril forming collagens including types IV, VI and XIV, glycoproteins, and proteoglycans. In contrast, the so-called interstitial ECM is largely confined to the capsule, around large vessels and in the portal areas. The main components are fibril-forming collagens (e.g., types I and III), cellular fibronectin, undulin (collagen XIV) and other glycoconjugates.

Hepatic stellate cells are the major cellular source of ECM in normal and injured liver (75,76). Stellate cells produce a wide array of ECM components, including collagens I, III, IV, V, VI, and XIV; proteoglycans: heparan, dermatan and chondroitin sulfate, perlecan, syndecan-1, biglycan and decorin; glycoproteins: cellular fibronectin, laminin, tenascin, undulin, and hyaluronic acid. The list of matrix products of stellate cells is still expanding and includes virtually every ECM component of normal and injured liver.

During chronic liver injury, the matrix phenotype of stellate cells changes qualitatively and quantitatively. Overall, its ECM production increases remarkably, accompanied by a shift in the type of ECM in subendothelial space from the normal low-density basement membrane-like matrix to the interstitial type.

The accumulation of ECM, especially collagen, is a dynamic process reflecting the imbalance between the matrix accumulation and degradation (see Chapter 33 and website chapters 🖥 W-27 and W-28). Hepatic stellate cells, the main producer of ECM, are also the major participant in its degradation. The repertoire of factors responsible for ECM remodeling is continually being identified (77). These include a family of zinc-dependent enzymes named matrix-metalloproteinases (MMPs), their inhibitors (tissue inhibitor of metalloproteinases, TIMPs) and several converting enzymes (MT1-MMP and stromelysin, for example). Although cellular sources of matrix proteases and their regulators in liver have not been fully elucidated, stellate cells are a key source of MMP-2 and stromelysin (78). They also express TIMP-1 and -2 mRNA, and produce TIMP-1 and MT1-MMP. MMP-9, which is a type IV collagenase, is locally secreted by Kupffer cells (79). The hepatic source of MMP-1 (interstitial collagenase, collagenase I), which plays a crucial role in degrading the excess interstitial matrix in advanced liver disease, is still uncertain, although it is known that upregulation of plasmin and stromelysin-1 can activate latent MMP1.

In human liver diseases, there is a downregulation of MMP1 and upregulation of MMP2 (gelatinase A) and MMP9 (gelatinase B). Because these enzymes have different substrate specificities, the result is increased degradation of basement membrane collagen and decreased degradation of interstitial type collagen (see Chapter 33 and website chapter 🖥 W-28).

Contractility

Because of their unique location in the subendothelial space encircling hepatic sinusoids, stellate cells have long been proposed as tissue-specific pericytes, which regulate blood flow through their perivascular contractility (80). Human and rat stellate cells contract in response to several vasoconstrictors, including thrombin and angiotensin II, thromboxane A2 and prostaglandin F2α (81,82). Only activated stellate cells are fully contractile, whereas quiescent stellate cells are less so (83). Contractility of stellate cells appears concomitantly with expression of α-smooth muscle actin, but it is unclear whether this protein is required for the cell to contract, or alternatively is simply a nonfunctional marker of a contractile phenotype.

It is uncertain whether quiescent stellate cells are contractile in normal liver. Freshly isolated stellate cells from normal rat liver do not contract in collagen gel contraction assays (83). However, based on *in vivo* microscopy, stellate cell-associated fluorescence colocalizes with sinusoidal contraction in response to endothelin-1 (ET-1) (84). Considering the strategic position of stellate cells, the abundance of endothelin receptors on their surface, and close proximity to nerve endings containing vasoactive neurotransmitters, stellate cells may play a role in regulating hepatic microcirculation under physiological as well as pathological conditions.

Among many factors that induce stellate cell contraction, ET-1 is the most potent agonist. Accompanying endothelin-1-mediated contraction is an increase in cytoplasmic calcium (81). Activated stellate cells express prepro-ET-1 mRNA (85) and release ET-1 in the supernatant, indicating an autocrine activity of this cytokine, in addition to the paracrine action provided by endothelial cells. In cirrhotic liver, expression of ET-1 is markedly increased in endothelial cells and stellate cells (85). The ET-1 antagonist, bosentan, reduces portal pressure when perfused into the cirrhotic rat liver with portal hypertension (86). These studies suggest that activated stellate cells regulate sinusoidal blood flow during liver injury, possibly via the action of ET-1. In cirrhotic liver, contractility of stellate cells could lead to sinusoidal constriction and organ contraction, resulting in portal hypertension.

The vasoconstrictive effects of endothelin-1 may be counteracted by locally produced vasodilators. Prominent among these is nitric oxide (NO) (see Chapter 39), which is produced from L-arginine by different forms of NO synthase (NOS) (87). When stimulated with interferon γ, TNFα and lipopolysaccharide, stellate cells rapidly produce NO (88), largely as the product of the inducible form of NO synthase. The endogenously produced NO strongly opposes contractility induced by ET-1 during liver injury, especially within regions of inflammation. In addition to NO, carbon monoxide, a product of heme cleavage, also mediates sinusoidal relaxation *in vivo* through its effects on stellate cells (89).

REGULATION OF STELLATE CELLS: "ACTIVATION" IN LIVER INJURY

The past two decades have witnessed rapid elucidation of the role of stellate cells in liver injury and fibrosis. In nor-

mal liver, stellate cells are quiescent perisinusoidal vitamin A-storing cells in the subendothelial space of Disse. During injury, they undergo a gradient of phenotypic changes collectively called *activation* (sometimes referred to as *"trans-differentiation"*), through which they transform into proliferative, fibrogenic and contractile myofibroblasts (90,91). The regulation of their different phenotypes in normal and injured liver is the result of interactions with neighboring cells through paracrine and autocrine pathways, as well as interactions between stellate cells and the extracellular matrix (Fig. 31.5).

The detailed pathways responsible for maintaining the quiescent phenotype of stellate cells in normal liver are unclear. Nonetheless, culture studies have demonstrated the importance of the basement membrane-like ECM in this process. When cultured on Engelbreth–Holm–Swarm (EHS) murine tumor-derived ECM, a gel matrix mimicking basement membrane-type ECM, stellate cells maintain the quiescent phenotype (92), in contrast to the activated phenotype when cultured on uncoated plastic. Individual components of the matrix (laminin, type IV collagen, and heparan sulfate proteoglycan) do not replicate the activity of the complete gel matrix, suggesting the requirement for complex matrix assembly in mediating this effect (92). When stellate cells are cultured on type I collagen, TGFβ stimulates the synthesis of collagen type I and III, whereas TGFβ has no such stimulating effects when cells are grown on type IV collagen (93).

The role of stellate cells in human liver disease has been greatly clarified. Features of stellate cell activation have been observed in viral hepatitis (94,95), massive hepatic necrosis (94) and alcohol-induced liver disease (96). In some diseases such as those associated with iron overload, lipid peroxides stimulate stellate cell activation, leading to increased collagen production and liver fibrosis (97,98). Activated stellate cells participate in tumor stroma accumulation in hepatocellular carcinoma (99). Stellate cell activation has also been implicated in a number of other human liver diseases, including biliary obstruction (15), hematologic malignancy (15), vascular disease (15), mucopolysaccharidosis (100), acetaminophen overdose (101), leishmaniasis (102), and in drug abusers (103).

A Model of Stellate Cell Activation

Stellate cell activation can be conceptually viewed as a two-stage process, initiation and perpetuation (90,91). Initiation refers to early changes in gene expression and phenotype that render the cells responsive to other cytokines and stimuli, while perpetuation results from the effects of these stimuli on maintaining the activated phenotype and generating fibrosis. Initiation is largely due to paracrine stimulation, whereas perpetuation involves autocrine as well as paracrine loops (Fig. 31.6).

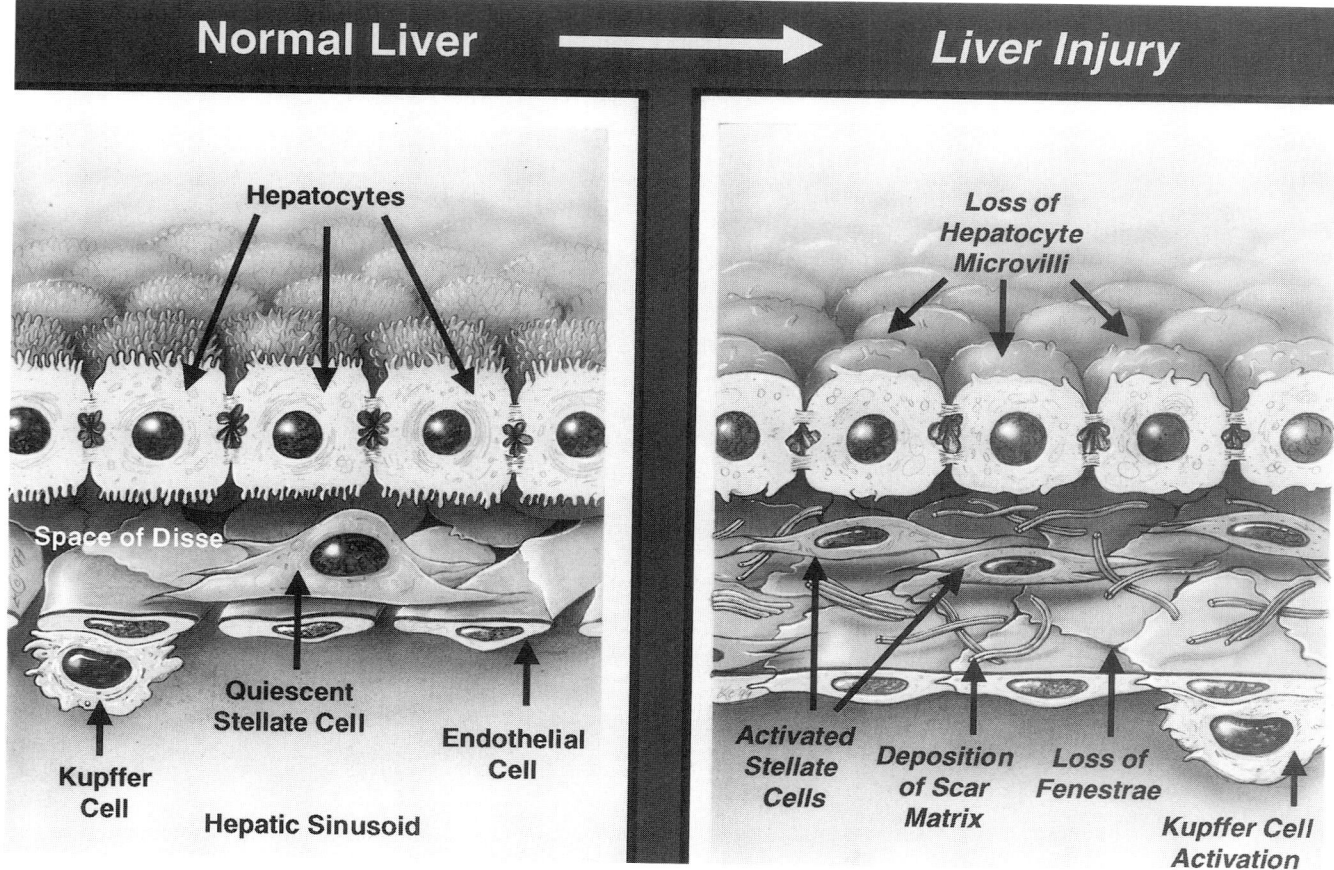

FIGURE 31.5. Sinusoidal events during fibrosing liver injury. Stellate cell activation leads to accumulation of scar (fibril-forming) matrix, which in turn contributes to the loss of hepatocyte microvilli and sinusoidal endothelial fenestrae. Kupffer cell (macrophage) activation accompanies liver injury and contributes to paracrine activation of stellate cells. (From Friedman SL. Molecular regulation of hepatic fibrosis, an integrated cellular response to tissue injury. *J Biol Chem* 2000; 275:2247–2250, with permission.)

Initiation

Stellate cell activation is initiated by paracrine stimuli from injured neighboring cells, including hepatocytes, endothelial and Kupffer cells, and platelets, as well as infiltrating tumor cells in primary and metastatic cancer (92). Among the most well studied paracrine stimuli are fibronectin (71), lipid peroxides (104), and cytokines including platelet-derived growth factor (PDGF), transforming growth factor beta 1 (TGFβ1) and epidermal growth factor (EGF). In recent years, increasing interest has been focused on transcription factors involved in stellate cell activation, including Sp1, c-myb, NFκB, c-jun/AP1, and STAT-1 and Zf9/KLF6.

Perpetuation

After initiation, activated stellate cells undergo a series of phenotypic changes which collectively lead to the accumulation of extracellular matrix. These changes include: (a) *proliferation:* this is partly due to local proliferation in response to

paracrine and autocrine mediators (105), including PDGF, ET-1, thrombin, FGF, IGF (106), and TGFβ1(107), among others (107). (b) *contractility:* contraction by stellate cells may be a major determinant of early and late increases in portal resistance during liver fibrosis and cirrhosis. A key contractile stimulus towards stellate cells is ET-1 (108). Other contractile agonists include arginine vasopressin, adrenomedullin, and eicosanoids. (c) *fibrogenesis:* A large number of fibrogenic factors have been identified, including interleukin-1β, tumor necrosis factor, lipid peroxides and acetaldehyde, but none is as potent as TGFβ1 (109). (d) *chemotaxis:* the accumulation of stellate cells during liver injury may be the result of both proliferation and directed migration into regions of injury. PDGF and the chemoattractant monocyte chemotactic peptide-1 (MCP-1) have been identified as stellate cell chemoattractants. (e) *matrix degradation:* quantitative and qualitative changes in the activity of MMPs and their inhibitors play a vital role in ECM remodeling in liver fibrogenesis. The net effect is the conversion of the low-density subendothelial matrix to one rich in interstitial collagens. (f) *retinoid loss:*

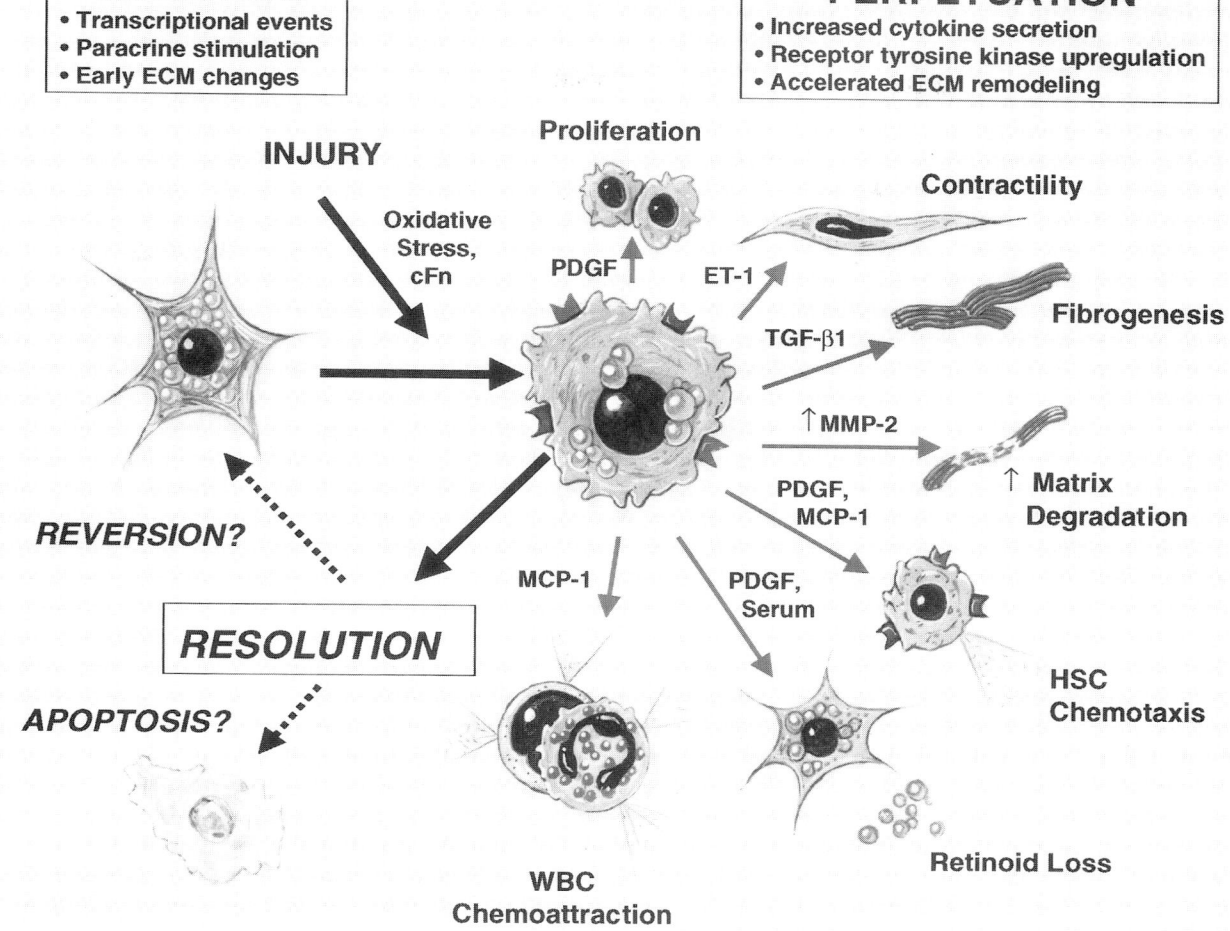

FIGURE 31.6. Features of hepatic stellate cell activation during liver injury and resolution. Following liver injury, hepatic stellate cells undergo "activation," a transition from quiescent vitamin A-rich cells into proliferative, fibrogenic and contractile myofibroblasts. The major phenotypic changes after activation include proliferation, contractility, fibrogenesis, matrix degradation, chemotaxis, retinoid loss, and white blood cell (*WBC*) chemoattraction. Key mediators underlying these effects are shown. The fate of activated stellate cells during resolution of liver injury is uncertain, but may include reversion to a quiescent phenotype and/or selective clearance by apoptosis. *ECM*, extracellular matrix; *ET-1*, endothelin-1; *MCP-1*, monocyte chemotactic peptide 1; *MMP*, matrix-metalloproteinase; *PDGF*, platelet-derived growth factor; TGF-β1, transforming growth factor-β1. (From Friedman SL. Molecular regulation of hepatic fibrosis, an integrated cellular response to tissue injury. *J Biol Chem* 2000;275:2247–2250, with permission.)

activation of stellate cells is accompanied by the loss of their characteristic perinuclear retinoid droplets. It is still unknown whether retinoid loss is a requirement for stellate cell activation. (g) *cytokine release:* increased production of cytokines may be critical for the perpetuation of stellate cell activation. These cytokines include TGFβ1, PDGF, FGF, HGF, PAF, ET-1, MCP-1 and cytokine-induced neutrophil chemoattractant (CINC).

The Fate of Activated Stellate Cells

The fate of activated stellate cells as liver injury resolves is unclear. It is not certain whether activated stellate cells can

revert to the quiescent state or are selectively cleared by apoptosis. Increasing evidence implicates apoptosis *in vivo*. During the resolution of liver injury, the percentage of stellate cells undergoing apoptosis is increased (110). Interestingly, these cells express high levels of TIMP (110). Therefore, their selective clearance may remove a key molecule that prevents the degradation of fibrotic scar by interstitial collagenase, unleashing the liver's capacity to resorb excess ECM. Activated stellate cells also display increased susceptibility to apoptotic signals (such as soluble Fas ligand) and decreased expression of the antiapoptotic protein bcl-2 (111). These findings are consistent with wound healing in other tissues such as kidney and vascular wall.

The signals in the hepatic microenvironment responsible for modulating stellate cell apoptosis are not yet clarified. The ECM may play a role in regulating apoptosis by providing permissive or inhibitory signals (112). Interruption of integrin-mediated interaction between stellate cells and ECM induces apoptosis (113) and similar effects occur in the kidney. Interestingly, TGFβ and TNFα inhibit apoptosis of activated stellate cells, suggesting that fibrogenic cytokines may promote the survival of activated, fibrogenic stellate cells (114).

FUTURE PROSPECTS

The dramatic advance in our understanding of stellate cells during the past two decades has provided a well-delineated picture of this cell type. However, several key questions still remain, including: (a) What are the key genes that initiate stellate cell activation? (b) Are there any stellate cell-specific genes, and how are they involved in liver fibrogenesis? (c) What is the fate of activated stellate cells during resolution of liver injury? Can they revert to a quiescent state? What factors determine the reversibility of liver fibrosis? (d) What is the relation, if any, between the loss of vitamin A and stellate cell activation? The elucidation of these questions may ultimately translate into effective therapies for chronic liver disease and fibrosis.

REFERENCES

1. Aterman K. The parasinusoidal cells of the liver: a historical account. *Histochem J* 1986;18:279–305.
2. Ito T. Cytological studies on stellate cells of Kupffer and fat storing cells in the capillary wall of human liver. *Acta Anat Nippon* 1951;26:2.
3. Bronfenmajer S, Schaffner F, Popper H. Fat-storing cells (lipocytes) in human liver. *Arch Pathol* 1966;82:447–453.
4. Wake K. Perisinusoidal stellate cells (Fat-storing cells, interstitial cells, lipocytes), their related structure in and around liver sinusoids, and vitamin A storing cells in extrahepatic organs. *Int Rev Cytol* 1980;66:303–353.
5. Wake K. Liver perivascular cells revealed by gold and silver impregnation methods and electron microscopy. In: Motta PM, ed. *Biopathology of the liver, an ulrastructural approach.* Dordrecht: Kluwer, 1988:23–36.
6. Kent G, Gay S, Inouye T, et al. Vitamin A containing lipocytes and formation of type III collagen in liver injury. *Proc Natl Acad Sci U S A* 1976; 73:3719–3722.
7. Knook DS, Seffelaar AM; de Leeuw AM. Fat-storing cells of the rat liver. Their isolation and purification. *Exp Cell Res* 1982;139:468–471.
8. Friedman SL, Roll FJ. Isolation and culture of hepatic lipocytes, Kupffer cells, and sinusoidal endothelial cells by density gradient centrifugation with Stractan. *Anal Biochem* 1987;161:207–218.
9. Friedman SL, Rockey DC, McGuire RF, et al. Isolated hepatic lipocytes and Kupffer cells from normal human liver: morphological and functional characteristics in primary culture. *Hepatology* 1992;15:234–243.
10. Jezequel AM, Novelli G, Venturini C, et al. Quantitative analysis of the perisinusoidal cells in human liver; the lipocytes. *Front Gastrointest Res* 1984; 8:85–90.
11. Wake K. Structure of the sinusoidal wall in the liver. In: Wisse

E, Knook DL, Wake K, eds. *Cells of the hepatic sinusoid.* Leiden: The Kupffer Cell Foundation, 1995:241–246.
12. Bioulac-Sage P, Lafon ME, Saric J, et al. Nerves and perisinusoidal cells in human liver. *J Hepatol* 1990;10:105–112.
13. Brouwer A, Wisse E, Knook DL. Sinusoidal endothelial cells and perisinusoidal fat-storing cells. In: Arias IM, Jakoby WB, eds. *The liver: biology and pathobiology.* 2nd ed. New York: Raven Press, 1988:665–682.
14. Sims DE. The pericyte—a review. *Tissue Cell* 1986;18:153–174.
15. Schmitt-Graff A, Kruger S, Bochard F, et al. Modulation of alpha smooth muscle actin and desmin expression in perisinusoidal cells of normal and diseased human livers. *Am J Pathol* 1991;138:1233–1242.
16. Rockey DC, Friedman SL. Cytoskeleton of liver perisinusoidal cells (lipocytes) in normal and pathological conditions. *Cell Motil Cytoskeleton* 1992;22:227–234.
17. Skalli O, Ropraz P, Trzeciak A, et al. A monoclonal antibody against alpha-smooth muscle actin: a new probe for smooth muscle differentiation. *J Cell Biol* 1986;103:2787–2796.
18. Gabbiani G, Schmid E, Winter S, et al. Vascular smooth muscle cells differ from other smooth muscle cells: predominance of vimentin filaments and a specific alpha-type actin. *Proc Natl Acad Sci U S A* 1981;78:298–302.
19. Serini G, Gabbiani G. Mechanisms of myofibroblast activity and phenotypic modulation. *Exp Cell Res* 1999;250:273–283.
20. Niki T, De Bleser PJ, Xu G, et al. Comparison of glial fibrillary acidic protein and desmin staining in normal and CCl₄-induced fibrotic rat livers. *Hepatology* 1996;23:1538–1545.
21. Niki T, Pekny M, Hellemans K, et al. Class VI intermediate filament protein nestin is induced during activation of rat hepatic stellate cells. *Hepatology* 1999;29:520–527.
22. Lendahl U, Zimmerman LB, McKay RD. CNS stem cells express a new class of intermediate filament protein. *Cell* 1990; 60:585–595.
23. Frisen J, Johansson CB, Torok C, et al. Rapid, widespread, and long-lasting induction of nestin contributes to the generation of glial scar tissue after CNS injury. *J Cell Biol* 1995;131:453–464.
24. Nakatani K, Seki S, Kawada N, et al. Expression of neural cell adhesion molecule (N-CAM) in perisinusoidal stellate cells of the human liver. *Cell Tissue Res* 1996;283:159–165.
25. Nishi M, Takeshima H, Houtani T, et al. RhoN, a novel small GTP-binding protein expressed predominantly in neurons and hepatic stellate cells. *Brain Res Mol Brain Res* 1999;67:74–81.
26. Ramm GA, Britton RS, O'Neill R, et al. Vitamin A-poor lipocytes: a novel desmin-negative lipocyte subpopulation, which can be activated to myofibroblasts. *Am J Physiol* 1995; 269:G532–G541.
27. Bhunchet E, Wake K. Role of mesenchymal cell populations in porcine serum-induced rat liver fibrosis. *Hepatology* 1992;16:1452–1473.
28. Knittel T, Kobold D, Saile B, et al. Rat liver myofibroblasts and hepatic stellate cells: different cell populations of the fibroblast lineage with fibrogenic potential. *Gastroenterology* 1999;117:1205–1221.
29. Friedman SL. The virtuosity of hepatic stellate cells. *Gastroenterology* 1999;117:1244–1246.
30. Moriwaki H, Blaner WS, Piantedosi R, et al. Effects of dietary retinoid and triglyceride on the lipid composition of rat liver stellate cells and stellate cell lipid droplets. *J Lipid Res* 1988;29:1523–1534.
31. Friedman SL, Wei S, Blaner WS. Retinol release by activated rat hepatic lipocytes: regulation by Kupffer cell-conditioned medium and PDGF. *Am J Physiol* 1993;264:G947–G952.
32. Ulven SM, Natarajan V, Holven KB, et al. Expression of retinoic acid receptor and retinoid X receptor subtypes in rat liver cells: implications for retinoid signalling in parenchymal, endothelial, Kupffer and stellate cells. *Eur J Cell Biol* 1998;77:111–116.

33. Mangelsdorf DJ, Thummel C, Beato M, et al. The nuclear receptor superfamily: the second decade. *Cell* 1995;83:835–839.

34. Bachem MG, Meyer D, Melchior R, et al. Activation of rat liver perisinusoidal lipocytes by transforming growth factors derived from myofibroblastlike cells. A potential mechanism of self perpetuation in liver fibrogenesis. *J Clin Invest* 1992;89:19–27.

35. Seifert WF, Bosma A, Brouwer A, et al. Vitamin A deficiency potentiates carbon tetrachloride-induced liver fibrosis in rats. *Hepatology* 1994;19:193–201.

36. Senoo H, Wake K. Suppression of experimental hepatic fibrosis by administration of vitamin A. *Lab Invest* 1985;52:182–194.

37. Seifert WF, Bosma A, Hendriks HFJ, et al. Dual role of vitamin A in experimentally induced liver fibrosis. In: Wisse E, Knook DL, Decker K, eds. *Cells of the hepatic sinusoid.* Rijswijk: The Kupffer Cell Foundation, 1989;43–48.

38. Leo MA, Lieber CS. Hepatic fibrosis after long-term administration of ethanol and moderate vitamin A supplementation in the rat. *Hepatology* 1983;3:1–11.

39. Friedman G, Liu LM, Friedman SL, et al. Apolipoprotein E is secreted by cultured lipocytes of the rat liver. *J Lipid Res* 1991;32:107–114.

40. Ramadori G, Rieder H, Theiss F, et al. Fat-storing (Ito) cells of rat liver synthesize and secrete apolipoproteins: comparison with hepatocytes. *Gastroenterology* 1989;97:163–172.

41. Athari A, Hanecke K, Jungermann K. Prostaglandin F2 alpha and D2 release from primary Ito cell cultures after stimulation with noradrenaline and ATP but not adenosine. *Hepatology* 1994;20:142–148.

42. Friedman SL. Cytokines and fibrogenesis. *Semin Liver Dis* 1999;19:129–140.

43. Win KM, Charlotte F, Mallat A, et al. Mitogenic effect of transforming growth factor-β 1 on human Ito cells in culture: evidence for mediation by endogenous platelet-derived growth factor. *Hepatology* 1993;18:137–145.

44. Maher JJ. Cell-specific expression of hepatocyte growth factor in liver. Upregulation in sinusoidal endothelial cells after carbon tetrachloride. *J Clin Invest* 1993;91:2244–2252.

45. Pinzani M, Abboud HE, Aron DC. Secretion of insulin-like growth factor-I and binding proteins by rat liver fat-storing cells: regulatory role of platelet-derived growth factor. *Endocrinology* 1990;127:2343–2349.

46. Pinzani M, Knauss TC, Pierce GF, et al. Mitogenic signals for platelet-derived growth factor isoforms in liver fat-storing cells. *Am J Physiol* 1991;260:C485–C491.

47. Pinzani M, Abboud HE, Gesualdo L, et al. Regulation of macrophage colony-stimulating factor in liver fat-storing cells by peptide growth factors. *Am J Physiol* 1992;262:C876–C881.

48. Pinzani M, Milani S, Grappone C, et al. Expression of platelet-derived growth factor in a model of acute liver injury. *Hepatology* 1994;19:701–707.

49. Rosenbaum J, Blazejewski S, Preaux AM, et al. Fibroblast growth factor 2 and transforming growth factor β1 interactions in human liver myofibroblasts. *Gastroenterology* 1995;109:1986–1996.

50. Marsden ER, Hu Z, Fujio K, et al. Expression of acidic fibroblast growth factor in regenerating liver and during hepatic differentiation. *Lab Invest* 1992;67:427–433.

51. Czaja MJ, Geerts A, Xu J, et al. Monocyte chemoattractant protein 1 (MCP-1) expression occurs in toxic rat liver injury and human liver disease. *J Leukoc Biol* 1994;55:120–126.

52. Marra F, Valente AJ, Pinzani M, et al. Cultured human liver fat-storing cells produce monocyte chemotactic protein-1. Regulation by proinflammatory cytokines. *J Clin Invest* 1993; 92:1674–1680.

53. Maher JJ, Lozier JS, Scott MK. Rat hepatic stellate cells produce cytokine-induced neutrophil chemoattractant in culture and in vivo. *Am J Physiol* 1998;275:G847–G853.

54. Tiggelman AM, Boers W, Linthorst C, et al. Interleukin-6 production by human liver (myo)fibroblasts in culture. Evidence for a regulatory role of LPS, IL-1β and TNFα. *J Hepatol* 1995; 23:295–306.

55. Wang SC, Tsukamoto H, Rippe RA, et al. Expression of interleukin-10 by in vitro and in vivo activated hepatic stellate cells. *J Biol Chem* 1998;273:302–308.

56. Thompson K, Maltby J, Fallowfield J, et al. Interleukin-10 expression and function in experimental murine liver inflammation and fibrosis. *Hepatology* 1998;28:1597–1606.

57. Nelson DR, Lauwers GY, Lau JY, et al. Interleukin 10 treatment reduces fibrosis in patients with chronic hepatitis C: a pilot trial of interferon nonresponders. *Gastroenterology* 2000;118:655–660.

58. Knittel T, Dinter C, Kobold D, et al. Expression and regulation of cell adhesion molecules by hepatic stellate cells (HSC) of rat liver: involvement of HSC in recruitment of inflammatory cells during hepatic tissue repair. *Am J Pathol* 1999;154:153–167.

59. Bissell DM, Wang SS, Jarnagin WR, et al. Cell-specific expression of transforming growth factor-β in rat liver. Evidence for autocrine regulation of hepatocyte proliferation. *J Clin Invest* 1995;96:447–455.

60. Ji C, Casinghino S, McCarthy TL, et al. Multiple and essential Sp1 binding sites in the promoter for transforming growth factor-β type I receptor. *J Biol Chem* 1997;272:21260–21267.

61. Kim Y, Ratziu V, Choi SG, et al. Transcriptional activation of transforming growth factor β1 and its receptors by the Kruppel-like factor Zf9/core promoter-binding protein and Sp1. Potential mechanisms for autocrine fibrogenesis in response to injury. *J Biol Chem* 1998;273:33750–33758.

62. Attisano L, Wrana JL. Mads and Smads in TGFβ signaling. *Curr Opin Cell Biol* 1998;10:188–194.

63. Heldin CH, Miyazono K, ten Dijke P. TGF-β signaling from cell membrane to nucleus through SMAD proteins. *Nature* 1997;390:465–471.

64. Dooley S, Delvoux B, Lahme B, et al. Modulation of transforming growth factor β response and signaling during transdifferentiation of rat hepatic stellate cells to myofibroblasts. *Hepatology* 2000;31:1094–1106.

65. Paradis V, Dargere D, Vidaud M, et al. Expression of connective tissue growth factor in experimental rat and human liver fibrosis. *Hepatology* 1999;30:968–976.

66. Yanagisawa M, Kurihara H, Kimura S, et al. A novel potent vasoconstrictor peptide produced by vascular endothelial cells [see comments]. *Nature* 1988;332:411–415.

67. Rockey DC, Fouassier L, Chung JJ, et al. Cellular localization of endothelin-1 and increased production in liver injury in the rat: potential for autocrine and paracrine effects on stellate cells. *Hepatology* 1998;27:472–480.

68. Rockey DC, Chung JJ. Inducible nitric oxide synthase in rat hepatic lipocytes and the effect of nitric oxide on lipocyte contractility. *J Clin Invest* 1995;95:1199–1206.

69. Housset C, Rockey DC, Bissell DM. Endothelin receptors in rat liver: lipocytes as a contractile target for endothelin 1. *Proc Natl Acad Sci U S A* 1993;90:9266–9270.

70. Ankoma-Sey V, Matli M, Chang KB, et al. Coordinated induction of VEGF receptors in mesenchymal cell types during rat hepatic wound healing. *Oncogene* 1998;17:115–121.

71. Jarnagin WR, Rockey DC, Koteliansky VE, et al. Expression of variant fibronectins in wound healing: cellular source and biological activity of the EIIIA segment in rat hepatic fibrogenesis. *J Cell Biol* 1994;127:2037–2048.

72. Carloni V, Romanelli RG, Pinzani M, et al. Focal adhesion kinase and phospholipase C γ involvement in adhesion and migration of human hepatic stellate cells. *Gastroenterology* 1997;112:522–531.

73. Racine-Samson L, Rockey DC, Bissell DM. The role of α1β1 integrin in wound contraction. A quantitative analysis of liver myofibroblasts in vivo and in primary culture. *J Biol Chem* 1997;272:30911–30917.

74. Shrivastava A, Radziejewski C, Campbell E, et al. An orphan

receptor tyrosine kinase family whose members serve as nonintegrin collagen receptors. *Mol Cell* 1997;1:25–34.

75. Friedman SL, Roll FJ, Boyles J, et al. Hepatic lipocytes: the principal collagen-producing cells of normal rat liver. *Proc Natl Acad Sci U S A* 1985;82:8681–8685.

76. Kawase T, Shiratori Y, Sugimoto T. Collagen production by rat liver fat-storing cells in primary culture. *Exp Cell Biol* 1986;54:183–192.

77. Arthur MJ. Fibrosis and altered matrix degradation. *Digestion* 1998;59:376–380.

78. Vyas SK, Leyland H, Gentry J, et al. Rat hepatic lipocytes synthesize and secrete transin (stromelysin) in early primary culture. *Gastroenterology* 1995;109:889–898.

79. Winwood PJ, Schuppan D, Iredale JP, et al. Kupffer cell-derived 95-kd type IV collagenase/gelatinase B: characterization and expression in cultured cells. *Hepatology* 1995;22:304–315.

80. Wake K, Kishiye T, Yamamoto H, et al. Sinusoidal cell function life under the microscope. In: Gressner AM, Ramadori G, eds. *Molecular and cell biology of liver fibrogenesis*. Dordrecht: Kluwer Academic Publishers, 1992:45–51.

81. Pinzani M, Failli P, Ruocco C, et al. Fat-storing cells as liver-specific pericytes. Spatial dynamics of agonist-stimulated intracellular calcium transients. *J Clin Invest* 1992;90:642–646.

82. Kawada N, Tran TT, Klein H, et al. The contraction of hepatic stellate (Ito) cells stimulated with vasoactive substances. Possible involvement of endothelin 1 and nitric oxide in the regulation of the sinusoidal tonus. *Eur J Biochem* 1993;213:815–823.

83. Rockey DC, Housset CN, Friedman SL. Activation-dependent contractility of rat hepatic lipocytes in culture and in vivo. *J Clin Invest* 1993;92:1795–1804.

84. Zhang JX, Pegoli W, Jr., Clemens MG. Endothelin-1 induces direct constriction of hepatic sinusoids. *Am J Physiol* 1994;266: G624–G632.

85. Pinzani M, Milani S, De Franco R, et al. Endothelin 1 is overexpressed in human cirrhotic liver and exerts multiple effects on activated hepatic stellate cells. *Gastroenterology* 1996;110:534–548.

86. Rockey DC, Weisiger RA. Endothelin induced contractility of stellate cells from normal and cirrhotic rat liver: implications for regulation of portal pressure and resistance. *Hepatology* 1996; 24:233–240.

87. Moncada S, Higgs A. The L-arginine-nitric oxide pathway. *N Engl J Med* 1993;329:2002–2012.

88. Helyar L, Bundschuh DS, Laskin JD, et al. Induction of hepatic Ito cell nitric oxide production after acute endotoxemia. *Hepatology* 1994;20:1509–1515.

89. Suematsu M, Goda N, Sana T, et al. Carbon monoxide: an endogenous mediator of sinusoidal tone in the perfused liver. *J Clin Invest* 1995;96:2431–2437.

90. Friedman SL. Seminars in medicine of the Beth Israel Hospital, Boston. The cellular basis of hepatic fibrosis. Mechanisms and treatment strategies. *N Engl J Med* 1993;328:1828–1835.

91. Friedman SL. Molecular regulation of hepatic fibrosis, an integrated cellular response to tissue injury. *J Biol Chem* 2000;275: 2247–2250.

92. Friedman SL, Roll FJ, Boyles J, et al. Maintenance of differentiated phenotype of cultured rat hepatic lipocytes by basement membrane matrix. *J Biol Chem* 1989;264:10756–10762.

93. Davis BH. Transforming growth factor β responsiveness is modulated by the extracellular collagen matrix during hepatic Ito cell culture. *J Cell Physiol* 1988;136:547–553.

94. Enzan H, Himeno H, Iwamura S, et al. Sequential changes in human Ito cells and their relation to postnecrotic liver fibrosis in massive and submassive hepatic necrosis. *Virchows Archiv* 1995;426:95–101.

95. Inuzuka S, Ueno T, Torimura T, et al. Immunohistochemistry of the hepatic extracellular matrix in acute viral hepatitis. *Hepatology* 1990;12:249–256.

96. Schmitt-Graff A, Chakroun G, Gabbiani G. Modulation of perisinusoidal cell cytoskeletal features during experimental hepatic fibrosis. *Virchows Arch A Pathol Anat Histopathol* 1993; 422:99–107.

97. Bedossa P, Houglum K, Trautwein C, et al. Stimulation of collagen α 1(I) gene expression is associated with lipid peroxidation in hepatocellular injury: a link to tissue fibrosis? *Hepatology* 1994;19:1262–1271.

98. Houglum K, Bedossa P, Chojkier M. TGF-β and collagen-α 1 (I) gene expression are increased in hepatic acinar zone 1 of rats with iron overload. *Am J Physiol* 1994;267:G908–G913.

99. Enzan H, Himeno H, Iwamura S, et al. Alpha-smooth muscle actin-positive perisinusoidal stromal cells in human hepatocellular carcinoma. *Hepatology* 1994;19:895–903.

100. Resnick JM, Whitley CB, Leonard AS, et al. Light and electron microscopic features of the liver in mucopolysaccharidosis. *Hum Pathol* 1994;25:276–286.

101. Mathew J, Hines JE, James OF, et al. Non-parenchymal cell responses in paracetamol (acetaminophen)-induced liver injury. *J Hepatol* 1994;20:537–541.

102. el Hag IA, Hashim FA, el Toum IA, et al. Liver morphology and function in visceral leishmaniasis (Kala-azar). *J Clin Pathol* 1994;47:547–551.

103. Trigueiro de Araujo MS, Gerard F, Chossegros P, et al. Cellular and matrix changes in drug abuser liver sinusoids: a semiquantitative and morphometric ultrastructural study. *Virchows Archiv A* 1993;422:145–152.

104. Paradis V, Kollinger M, Fabre M, et al. In situ detection of lipid peroxidation by-products in chronic liver diseases. *Hepatology* 1997;26:135–142.

105. Friedman SL. Hepatic stellate cells. *Prog Liver Dis* 1996;14: 101–130.

106. Skrtic S, Wallenius V, Ekberg S, et al. Insulin-like growth factors stimulate expression of hepatocyte growth factor but not transforming growth factor β1 in cultured hepatic stellate cells. *Endocrinology* 1997;138:4683–4689.

107. Pinzani M, Marra F, Carloni V. Signal transduction in hepatic stellate cells. *Liver* 1998;18:2–13.

108. Rockey DC. The cellular pathogenesis of portal hypertension: stellate cell contractility, endothelin, and nitric oxide. *Hepatology* 1997;25:2–5.

109. Pietrangelo A. Metals, oxidative stress, and hepatic fibrogenesis. *Semin Liver Dis* 1996;16:13–30.

110. Iredale JP, Benyon RC, Pickering J, et al. Mechanisms of spontaneous resolution of rat liver fibrosis. Hepatic stellate cell apoptosis and reduced hepatic expression of metalloproteinase inhibitors. *J Clin Invest* 1998;102:538–549.

111. Gong W, Pecci A, Roth S, et al. Transformation-dependent susceptibility of rat hepatic stellate cells to apoptosis induced by soluble Fas ligand. *Hepatology* 1998;28:492–502.

112. Shi YB, Li Q, Damjanovski S, et al. Regulation of apoptosis during development: Input from the extracellular matrix (Review). *Int J Mol Med* 1998;2:273–282.

113. Iwamoto H, Sakai H, Tada S, et al. Induction of apoptosis in rat hepatic stellate cells by disruption of integrin-mediated cell adhesion. *J Lab Clin Med* 1999;134:83–89.

114. Saile B, Matthes N, Knittel T, et al. Transforming growth factor-β and tumor necrosis factor-α inhibit both apoptosis and proliferation of activated rat hepatic stellate cells. *Hepatology* 1999;30:196–202.

32

THE EXTRACELLULAR MATRIX OF THE LIVER

PATRICIA GREENWEL
MARCOS ROJKIND

With the advent of molecular biology, new macromolecules belonging to the various classes of extracellular matrix (ECM) components have been cloned. Although in some instances their tissue distribution and cellular sources have been established, in others, neither their function nor the molecular events involved in their regulation have been fully elucidated. Nonetheless, over the past few decades, the ECM has gained "respectability" because in addition to its traditional function as an inert support, multiple and very exciting functions for some of its components have been discovered. These include, among others, its role in development, cell differentiation, storage of cytokines and growth factors and in keeping cells informed of critical events occurring in their microenvironment. These latter signals provide cells with key information which allows them to regulate the expression of sets of genes required to maintain and/or restore homeostasis (reviewed in refs. 1–5).

Early studies to determine the role of laminin in cell attachment and function revealed that multiple cytokines and growth factors are retained in the purified matrix and that they could thus directly influence the behavior of cells (6). Therefore, in this regard, the ECM acts as a reservoir for cytokines and growth factors or, alternatively, prevents their biological activity by sequestering them (see website

chapter 🖳 W-36). Since these initial observations, multiple publications have demonstrated that different ECM components bind cytokines and/or growth factors, and that these interactions are important in regulating their biological activity (2,5,7–15). These findings are important because active cytokines and growth factors that are trapped in the ECM can be released upon tissue injury. Thus, they represent the earliest response to injury and play a key role in activating the inflammatory and wound healing cascades. In addition, because different ECM components have multiple domains whose biological activity is only manifested upon their limited proteolytic digestion, they also contribute to this very early response by releasing peptides with multiple biological activities. These include, among others, peptides with cell-binding and epidermal-like growth factor domains, chemoattractants for inflammatory cells and fibroblasts, modulators of vascular permeability, and inducers of proteolytic cascades, including the production and activation of matrix metalloproteinases. Because of the cryptic nature of these domains, these peptides have been named "matricryptins" (5).

The overall composition of the ECM as well as the actual concentration and distribution of its components varies from tissue to tissue. This is due in part to the nature and quantity of ECM components produced by each cell type within a given tissue, and also to the production and/or elimination of components whose expression is modulated by cell–cell and cell–matrix interactions. For each tissue, and irrespective of the nature and/or actual concentration

P. Greenwel: Department of Biochemistry and Molecular Biology, Mount Sinai School of Medicine, New York, New York 10029.

M. Rojkind: Departments of Medicine and Pathology, Albert Einstein College of Medicine, Bronx, New York 10461.

of its ECM components, the amount of these proteins is maintained constant by an active process of synthesis and degradation. However, during physiological and pathological processes, production and deposition of ECM components may be altered. For example, during liver regeneration occurring post-hepatectomy, changes in ECM production and/or deposition are transient, there is active remodeling, and upon completion of the regenerative process, homeostasis is restored and the overall composition and distribution of ECM return to normal values. In contrast, during pathological conditions such as those occurring after chronic liver injury, abnormalities in matrix deposition result in excess deposition of fibrous scar tissue. These changes are in many instances permanent and irreversible (see Chapter 33 and website chapter 💻 W-28).

The multiple macromolecules that compose the ECM of the liver have been previously reviewed (see website chapter 💻 W-27). In this chapter we will summarize information pertaining to recently described ECM components whose presence in the liver has been demonstrated.

COLLAGENS

During the past few years the collagen family has grown significantly. At least 19 types, the product of 33 genes, have been described (16). Types I, II, III, V and XI constitute the fibrillar collagens, whereas type IV, types VI to X and types XII to XIX represent the structurally diverse nonfibrillar members (see website chapter 💻 W-27). Of all collagens, the most abundant ones in the liver are types I, III, IV and V and VI. Their general features and localization in the liver have been reviewed (see website chapter 💻 W-27). Recent work from several laboratories has demonstrated that the liver also contains several "minor" collagens, including types IX, XI, XIV, XV, XVIII and XIX. Although the exact role of each of these proteins remains unknown, they are likely to confer critical biomechanical properties to the liver and play important roles in maintaining tissue homeostasis. In the next section, we will briefly describe some general features of these collagens, as well as their location in the liver, when known.

Type IX Collagen

Type IX collagen is a heterotrimer composed of three genetically distinct chains. This 270 kd protein belongs to the *fibril-associated collagens with interrupted triple helices* (FACIT) subgroup of collagens (see website chapter 💻 W-27). Each chain contains four noncollagenous domains separated by three triple helical collagenous domains. Interestingly, this protein is also a proteoglycan, because a glycosaminoglycan side chain is covalently attached to the α2(IX) chain. Type IX collagen is located primarily on the surface of fibrillar collagens. Its major function is to regulate

the size of collagen fibrils, and to act as a macromolecular bridge between fibrils and other ECM components (17). During mouse development, this protein (a high molecular weight splice variant) is present in low, but significant levels in the liver (18). However, its exact location and cellular source are not known.

Type XI Collagen

Type XI collagen is a component of fibrils in both cartilage and a wide variety of noncartilaginous tissues, including liver. Interestingly, in noncartilaginous tissues, collagen XI has been found to coassemble with chains of the highly homologous type V collagen. This protein belongs to the fibrillar subgroup of collagens, and is a heterotrimeric molecule consisting of three different chains. The α3(XI) chain is an overglycosylated form of the α1(II) collagen chain, whereas the α1(XI) and α2(XI) chains are distinct gene products. In noncartilaginous tissues, type XI collagen is found within the major fibrils of type I collagen, and its major role in these tissues is to regulate collagen types I and V fibrillogenesis (16,19). This protein is present in low levels during human liver development (20). Unfortunately, its exact location and cellular source remain unknown.

Type XIV Collagen

Type XIV collagen is a member of the FACIT subgroup of collagens (see website chapter 💻 W-27). It has an approximate molecular weight of 220 kd, and consists of two short collagenous and three noncollagenous domains. It is a modular protein with fibronectin type III repeats and von Willebrand factor A domains which mediate interactions with cellular receptors and other extracellular matrix proteins. Type XIV collagen associates with the surface of collagen fibrils, where it contributes to the maintenance of the organization and stability of the extracellular matrix (16). During chick embryogenesis, this protein is expressed in low levels in liver stroma (21). Undulin, an alternatively spliced variant of type XIV collagen, has been well studied in normal and cirrhotic liver (see website chapter 💻 W-27).

Type XV Collagen

Type XV collagen is a nonfibrillar collagen which, together with type XVIII collagen, form the multiplexins subgroup of collagens (*multiple* triple-helix domains with *in*terruptions) (22). This 225 to 250 kd protein has a widespread distribution in tissues, and is also a chondroitin sulfate proteoglycan. The complete primary structure of the human α1(XV) chain consists of 1,388 residues, with the following domains: a 25-residue putative signal peptide, a 530-residue N-terminal noncollagenous domain, a 577-residue collagenous sequence consisting of nine collagenous domains separated by eight noncollagenous domains, and a 256-residue

C-terminal noncollagenous domain (16). In the liver, this protein is found in basement membrane zones surrounding vascular and ductular structures, as well as in the portal interstitium (23).

Type XVIII Collagen

Type XVIII collagen is a nonfibrillar collagen that belongs to the multiplexins subgroup of collagens (22). It has an approximate molecular weight of 180 to 200 kd and contains a central interrupted triple helical domain flanked at the N- and C-termini by larger globular structures. Several variant forms exist that differ with respect to the length of the N-terminal region (16). The liver is the major source of type XVIII collagen production, as well as of endostatin, a 20 kd fragment derived from its C-terminal domain (24–27). This fragment, generated via proteolysis, is a powerful inhibitor of endothelial cell proliferation *in vitro*, and of angiogenesis and tumor growth *in vivo*. During development, type XVIII collagen is expressed along the developing sinusoidal structures between hepatocytes and around portal areas and in the basement membrane zones under the endothelium in the blood vessels. In adult liver, this protein is present along the sinusoids, the walls of the arteries of the portal tracts, capillaries in the portal areas, and in basement membrane zones under the epithelium of the bile ducts. Hepatocytes, and to a lesser degree endothelial and epithelial cells, are the major producers of type XVIII collagen in the liver. During cirrhosis, production of this protein increases, particularly in hepatic stellate cells (HSCs) (see Chapter 31).

Type XIX Collagen

Type XIX collagen is a member of the FACIT subgroup of collagens (see website chapter W-27). It has an approximate molecular weight of 150 kd and consists of five collagenous domains interspersed and flanked with six noncollagenous domains. Several splice variants exist. This protein may act as a crossbridge between collagen fibrils and other ECM molecules (16). In the liver, it is localized to the basement membrane zones of the ductal and vascular structures. In addition, it is observed in low levels in the hepatic sinusoids (23).

NONCOLLAGENOUS PROTEINS

The major noncollagenous proteins of the hepatic ECM have been described previously (see website chapter W-27). Excellent reviews have been published (28–40). In the following section we summarize the current knowledge regarding novel noncollagenous proteins whose expression has been detected in liver.

Fibulin-2

This microfibril-associated protein belongs to a family of proteins containing at least five members (41–43). It binds several ECM proteins including fibronectin, nidogen, collagen types IV and VI, and fibrillin. Its major role is to stabilize interactions between structural elements of the ECM and during developmental processes. Fibulin-2 is a 175 kd disulfide-linked homodimer. Structurally, it contains three consecutive anaphylatoxin-related segments and a central region followed by 10 tandem arrays of calcium-binding epidermal growth factor-like motifs. The N-terminal region consists of two separate subdomains, a cysteine-rich segment, and a cysteine-free segment, and is unique to fibulin-2, not showing any sequence homology to other known proteins (41). Fibulin-2 is expressed in liver myofibroblasts, but not HSC; thus, it has been suggested that fibulin-2 can be used as a marker to discriminate the phenotypical and functional characteristics of these two cell populations (44,45).

FLRT3

FLRT3 is a poorly characterized member of a novel gene family. It was isolated in a screen for laminin-binding proteins expressed in muscle. The FLRT3 gene encodes for a putative type I transmembrane protein, containing ten leucine-rich repeats flanked by N-terminal and C-terminal cysteine-rich regions, a fibronectin/collagen-like domain, and an intracellular tail. Based on these features, it has been suggested that this protein may play a role in cell adhesion and/or cell signaling. FLRT3 mRNA (4.4 kb) is expressed in several tissues, including liver (46). Unfortunately, its localization and cellular source are unknown.

Ladinin

Ladinin is a 528 amino acid polypeptide with an approximate molecular mass of 59 kd. This protein is located in basement membrane zones in association with anchoring filaments. Ladinin mRNA is predominantly expressed in kidney and lung. It is also present, albeit in smaller amounts, in liver, brain and spleen. Its function is still unknown, although it has been proposed that it may play a role in contributing to the stability of the association of epithelial layers with the underlying mesenchyme (47).

Nectinepsin

This is a 54 kd protein abundant during embryonic development. It contains an RGD cell binding motif of integrin ligands, and shares homology with vitronectin. It is present in the liver, but its exact location and cellular source have not been determined (48).

Osteopontin

Osteopontin is a negatively charged glycosylated phospho-protein with an approximate molecular weight of 32 kd. It is a secreted protein which binds calcium and binds covalently to fibronectin via transglutaminase-catalyzed crosslinking. Osteopontin production is modulated by cytokines such as transforming growth factor-β, epidermal growth factor and platelet-derived growth factor. This protein is chemotactic for several cell types including smooth muscle cells and macrophages, and induces cell migration. It can bind to integrins and serve as attachment substrate to several cell types. Moreover, it acts as a signaling ligand for cells, inducing a transient increase in intracellular calcium and activating the calcium ATPase pump. This protein is produced and secreted in response to injury and may play a major role in the injury/repair cascade (49). In the liver, production of this protein increases after carbon tetrachloride-induced acute damage in Kupffer cells and HSC (50).

ACKNOWLEDGMENTS

Part of this work was supported with Grants RO1 AA09231 and RO1 AA10541 (M.R.), RO1 AA12196 (P.G.) and grants from the Alcohol Medical Beverage Research Foundation to M.R. and P.G.

REFERENCES

1. Bork P. The modular architecture of vertebrate collagens. *FEBS Lett* 1992;307:49–54.
2. Taipale J, Keski-Oja J Growth factors in the extracellular matrix. *FASEB J* 1997;11:51–59.
3. Streuli C. Extracellular matrix remodelling and cellular differentiation. *Curr Opin Cell Biol* 1999;11:634–640.
4. Boudreau NJ, Jones PL. Extracellular matrix and integrin signalling: the shape of things to come. *Biochem J* 1999;339:481–488.
5. Davis GE, Bayless KJ, Davis MJ, et al. Regulation of tissue injury response by the exposure of matricryptic sites within extracellular matrix molecules. *Am J Pathol* 2000;156:1489–1498.
6. Vukicevic S, Kleinman HK, Luyten FP, et al. Identification of multiple active growth factors in basement membrane Matrigel suggests caution in interpretation of cellular activity related to extracellular matrix components. *Exp Cell Res* 1992;202:1–8.
7. Khachigian LM, Chesterman CN. Structural basis for the extracellular retention of PDGF A-chain using a synthetic peptide corresponding to exon 6. *Peptides* 1994;15:133–137.
8. Somasundaram R, Schuppan D. Type I, II, III, IV, V, and VI collagens serve as extracellular ligands for the isoforms of platelet-derived growth factor (AA, BB, and AB). *J Biol Chem* 1996;271: 26884–26891.
9. Schuppan D, Schmid M, Somasundaram R, et al. Collagens in the liver extracellular matrix bind hepatocyte growth factor. *Gastroenterology* 1998;114:139–152.
10. Ortega N, L'Faqihi FE, Plouet J. Control of vascular endothelial growth factor angiogenic activity by the extracellular matrix. *Biol Cell* 1998;90:381–390.
11. Pedrozo HA, Schwartz Z, Mokeyev T, et al. Vitamin D3 metabolites regulate LTBP1 and latent TGF-beta1 expression and latent TGF-beta1 incorporation in the extracellular matrix of chondrocytes. *J Cell Biochem* 1999;72:151–165.
12. Somasundaram R, Ruehl M, Tiling N, et al. Collagens serve as an extracellular store of bioactive interleukin 2. *J Biol Chem* 2000; 275:38170–38175.
13. Ortega N, Hutchings H, Plouet J. Signal relays in the VEGF system. *Front Biosci* 1999;4:D141–D152.
14. Verderio E, Gaudry C, Gross S, et al. Regulation of cell surface tissue transglutaminase: effects on matrix storage of latent transforming growth factor-beta binding protein-1. *J Histochem Cytochem* 1999;47:1417–1432.
15. Palka J, Banikowski E, Jaworski S. An accumulation of IGF-I and IGF-binding proteins in human umbilical cord. *Mol Cell Biochem* 2000;206:133–139.
16. Brown JC, Timpl R. The collagen superfamily. *Int Arch Allergy Immunol* 1995:107:484–490.
17. Olsen BR. Collagen IX. *Int J Biochem Cell Biol* 1997;29:555–558.
18. Liu CY, Olsen BR, Kao WW. Developmental patterns of two alpha 1(IX) collagen mRNA isoforms in mouse. *Dev Dyn* 1993; 198:150–157.
19. van der Rest M, Garrone R. Collagen family of proteins. *FASEB J* 1991;5:2814–2823.
20. Sandberg MM, Hirvonen HE, Elima KJ, et al. Co-expression of collagens II and XI and alternative splicing of exon 2 of collagen II in several developing human tissues. *Biochem J* 1993;294:595–602.
21. Castagnola P, Tavella S, Gerecke DR, et al. Tissue-specific expression of type XIV collagen—a member of the FACIT class of collagens. *Eur J Cell Biol* 1992;59:340–347.
22. Oh SP, Kamagata Y, Muragaki Y, et al. Isolation and sequencing of cDNAs for proteins with multiple domains of Gly-Xaa-Yaa repeats identify a distinct family of collagenous proteins. *Proc Natl Acad Sci U S A* 1994;91:4229–4233.
23. Myers JC, Li D, Bageris A, et al. Biochemical and immunohistochemical characterization of human type XIX defines a novel class of basement membrane zone collagens. *Am J Pathol* 1997; 151:1729–1740.
24. Rehn M, Pihlajaniemi T. Alpha 1(XVIII), a collagen chain with frequent interruptions in the collagenous sequence, a distinct tissue distribution, and homology with type XV collagen. *Proc Natl Acad Sci U S A* 1994;91:4234–4238.
25. Schuppan D, Cramer T, Bauer M, et al. Hepatocytes as a source of collagen type XVIII endostatin. *Lancet* 1998;352:879–880.
26. Saarela J, Rehn M, Oikarinen A, et al. The short and long forms of type XVIII collagen show clear tissue specificities in their expression and location in basement membrane zones in humans. *Am J Pathol* 1998;153:611–626.
27. Musso O, Rehn M, Saarela J, et al. Collagen XVIII is localized in sinusoids and basement membrane zones and expressed by hepatocytes and activated stellate cells in fibrotic human liver. *Hepatology* 1998;28:98–107.
28. Kosmehl H, Berndt A, Katenkamp D. Molecular variants of fibronectin and laminin: structure, physiological occurrence and histopathological aspects. *Virchows Arch* 1996;429:311–322.
29. Romberger DJ. Fibronectin. *Int J Biochem Cell Biol* 1997;29: 939–943.
30. Miyamoto S, Katz BZ, Lafrenie RM, Yamada KM. Fibronectin and integrins in cell adhesion, signaling, and morphogenesis. *Ann N Y Acad Sci* 1998;857:119–129.
31. Ekblom M, Falk M, Salmivirta K, et al. Laminin isoforms and epithelial development. *Ann N Y Acad Sci* 1998;857:194–211.
32. Colognato H, Yurchenco PD. Form and function: The laminin family of heterotrimers. *Dev Dyn* 2000;218:213–234.
33. Scheetz Jones F, Lloyd Jones P. The tenascin family of ECM glycoproteins: Structure, function and regulation during embryonic development and tissue remodeling. *Dev Dyn* 2000;218: 235–259.

34. Iozzo RV, Danielson KG. Transcriptional and posttranscriptional regulation of proteoglycan gene expression. *Prog Nucleic Acid Res Mol Biol* 1999;62:19–53.
35. Adams JC. Thrombospondin-1. *Int J Biochem Cell Biol* 1997;29:861–865.
36. Motamed K. SPARC (osteonectin/BM-40). *Int J Biochem Cell Biol* 1999;31:1363–1366.
37. Rapraeger AC. Syndecan-regulated receptor signaling. *J Cell Biol* 2000;149:995–998.
38. Sadler JE. Thrombomodulin structure and function. *Thromb Haemost* 1997;78:392–395.
39. Lebaron RG. Versican. *Perspect Dev Neurobiol* 1996;3:261–271.
40. Olsen BR. Life without perlecan has its problems. *J Cell Biol* 1999;147:909–912.
41. Grassel S, Sicot FX, Gotta S, et al. Mouse fibulin-2 gene. Complete exon-intron organization and promoter characterization. *Eur J Biochem* 1999;263:471–477.
42. Giltay R, Timpl R, Kostka G. Sequence, recombinant expression and tissue localization of two novel extracellular matrix proteins, fibulin-3 and fibulin-4. *Matrix Biol* 1999;18:469–480.
43. Kowal RC, Jolsin JM, Olson EN, et al. Assignment of fibulin-5 (FBLN5) to human chromosome 14q31 by in situ hybridization and radiation hybrid mapping. *Cytogenet Cell Genet* 1999;87:2–3.
44. Knittel T, Kobold D, Saile B, et al. Rat liver myofibroblasts and hepatic stellate cells: different cell populations of the fibroblast lineage with fibrogenic potential. *Gastroenterology* 1999;117:1205–1221.
45. Knittel T, Kobold D, Piscaglia F, et al. Localization of liver myofibroblasts and hepatic stellate cells in normal and diseased rat livers: distinct roles of (myo-)fibroblast subpopulations in hepatic tissue repair. *Histochem Cell Biol* 1999;112:387–401.
46. Lacey SE, Bonnemann CG, Buzney EA, et al. Identification of FLRT1, FLRT2 and FLRT3: a novel family of transmembrane leucine-rich repeat proteins. *Genomics* 1999;62:417–426.
47. Motoki K, Megahed M, LaForgia S, et al. Cloning and chromosomal mapping of mouse ladinin, a novel basement membrane zone component. *Genomics* 1997;39:323–330.
48. Blancher C, Omri B, Bidou L, et al. Nectinepsin: a new extracellular matrix protein of the pexin family. Characterization of a novel cDNA encoding a protein with an RGD cell binding motif. *J Biol Chem* 1996;271:26220–26226.
49. Rodan GA. Osteopontin overview. *Ann N Y Acad Sci* 1995;760:1–5.
50. Kawashima R, Mochida S, Matsui A, et al. Expression of osteopontin in Kupffer cells and hepatic macrophages and stellate cells in rat liver after carbon tetrachloride intoxication: a possible factor for macrophage migration into hepatic necrotic areas. *Biochem Biophys Res Commun* 1999;256:527–531.

INTEGRINS

LUCIA R. LANGUINO
REBECCA G. WELLS

Integrins have emerged as modulators of a variety of cellular functions (1). They have been implicated in organ and tissue development, normal and aberrant cellular growth, and modulation of intracellular signal transduction mechanisms (2–5). In this chapter, the structural and functional characteristics of integrins, their ability to control cell functions and signaling, and their expression and potential role in liver development and disease will be discussed.

THE INTEGRIN FAMILY OF ADHESION RECEPTORS

Adhesive contacts between cells and extracellular matrix (ECM) components play a crucial role in organ development, abnormal tissue growth, and tumor progression (see Chapter 32 and website chapters 🖥 W-27 and W-28. These interactions are mediated by *integrins*, the most widely distributed gene superfamily of adhesion receptors, expressed by all mammalian cells (3). Integrins can also mediate cell–cell interactions, although the ability to mediate cell–cell contact is restricted to a few members of the family [$\alpha_L\beta_2$, $\alpha_M\beta_2$, $\alpha_X\beta_2$, $\alpha_D\beta_2$, $\alpha_4\beta_1$, and $\alpha_4\beta_7$(3)].

α and β Subunits

Based on immunochemical and molecular evidence, integrins are structurally organized into heterodimeric transmembrane complexes, variously assembled through the noncovalent association between an α and a β subunit (6). So far, 18 α subunits, 8 β subunits, and 22 complexes have been identified and their expression and function characterized in various cell types. The integrin family is divided into subfamilies that share the β subunit (7). Each β subunit associates with one to eight α subunits and each α can associate with more than one β subunit. Functional specificity is determined by the specific associated subunits and by the cell type that expresses the heterodimeric complex (Table 33.1).

Integrins are expressed as constitutively active or inactive receptors for ECM ligands. Their functional state is cell type-dependent as well as ligand-dependent (8,9). These different functional states might be crucial in modulating integrin-mediated functions *in vivo*.

Integrin Cytoplasmic Domains

Recent experimental evidence obtained with recombinant deletion mutants and chimeric forms of integrin α and β cytoplasmic domains has demonstrated that cytoplasmic tails modulate receptor distribution, receptor surface expression, ligand binding affinity of the extracellular domain, cell adhesion, and cell spreading (6,10). Therefore, structural differences in the primary sequences of the integrin intracellular domains are predicted to determine the

L. R. Languino: Department of Pathology, Yale University School of Medicine, New Haven, Connecticut 06520.

R. G. Wells: Departments of Medicine and Pathology, Yale University School of Medicine; Department of Medicine, Yale New Haven Hospital, New Haven, Connecticut 06520.

TABLE 33.1. THE INTEGRIN FAMILY

Subunit		Ligand
$\beta_{1(A)}$	α_1	laminin, collagen
	α_2	laminin, collagen
	α_{3A}, α_{3B}	laminin, collagen, fibronectin entactin
	α_4	fibronectin, VCAM1
	α_5	fibronectin, L1
	α_{6A}, α_{6B}, α_{6X1}, α_{6X2}	laminin
	α_{7A}, α_{7B}, α_{7X1}, α_{7X1X2}	laminin
	α_8	fibronectin, tenascin, vitronectin, osteopontin
	α_9	tenascin
	α_v	fibronectin, osteopontin
β_{1B}, β_{1C}, β_{1D}		
β_2	α_L	ICAM1, ICAM2, ICAM3, ICAM4
	α_M	iC3B, fibrinogen, Factor X, ICAM1, ICAM2, ICAM4
	α_X	iC3b, fibrinogen
	α_D	ICAM3
β_{3A}	α_{IIb}, α_{IIbalt}	fibrinogen, fibronectin, von Willebrand factor, vitronectin, thrombospondin, disintegrin, osteopontin
	α_v	vitronectin, fibrinogen, fibronectin, von Willebrand factor, thrombospondin, disintegrin, L1, MMP2, osteopontin
$\beta_{3B,3C}$		
β_{4A}	α_{6A}, α_{6B}	laminin-5
β_{4B}, β_{4C}, β_{4D}		
β_{5A}	α_v	vitronectin, osteopontin
β_{5B}		
β_6	α_v	fibronectin, tenascin
β_7	α_4	fibronectin, VCAM, MAdCAM1
	α_{IEL}	
β_8	α_v	vitronectin, fibronectin, laminin

specificity of a variety of integrin-mediated events. In support of this hypothesis, mutations and deletions in the integrin cytoplasmic domain have been found in the β_3 and β_4 integrin subgroups in, respectively, Glanzmann's thrombasthenia (11) and junctional epidermolysis bullosa (12), thus pointing to the cytoplasmic domain as a key player in determining crucial cellular responses *in vivo*.

Alternatively spliced forms of the α (α_3, α_6, α_7) and β (β_1, β_3, β_4) integrin cytoplasmic domains have been identified (reviewed in refs. 6,10), thus adding further complexity to the regulatory pathways mediated by integrins. It is well established that the cytoplasmic domain of the β_1 subunit is required for integrins to modulate many cellular functions as well as to trigger signaling events which result in protein phosphorylation and interactions with intracellular proteins (10). Four different β_1 isoforms containing alternatively spliced cytoplasmic domains have been identified (β_{1A}, β_{1B}, β_{1C}, and β_{1D}) that differentially affect receptor localization, cell proliferation, cell adhesion and migration, interactions with intracellular proteins and, ultimately, phosphorylation and activation of signaling molecules (10).

The expression of integrin variants is tissue- and cell type-specific (10). Selective expression has been shown for the β_{1C} integrin subunit, an inhibitor of cell proliferation (10), in hematopoietic cells, platelets, activated endothelial cells and epithelial cells of liver, kidney, lung and prostate. The β_{1B} isoform is restricted to skin and liver, while the β_{1D} subunit was detected in striated muscle, where it replaces the common β_{1A} isoform. Similar to β_1 variants, a differential distribution of the variant forms β_{3A}, β_{3B}, α_{3A}, α_{3B}, α_{6A}, α_{6B}, α_{7A}, and α_{7B} in relationship to their wild-type counterparts has been described using protein and mRNA analysis (10). The functional differences described for these variants suggest that modulation of splicing patterns of β_1 mRNA may provide an accessory mechanism to regulate signaling pathways initiated by integrins (13).

INTEGRIN MODULATION OF CELL PROLIFERATION

By interacting with the ECM and, inside the cell, with the cytoskeleton, integrins transfer signals from the extracellular environment to intracellular compartments and control many cellular functions, such as proliferation, migration, differentiation, and gene expression (14–16). These signals are initiated after integrin engagement with natural ligands or surrogate antibody ligands and include increases in cytosolic free [Ca2+]i, tyrosine phosphorylation, elevation of intracellular pH, and stimulated transcription and translation of immediate and early inflammatory genes (16). Integrins can act synergistically with growth factors in modulating cellular functions (16).

The ability of integrins to modulate cell proliferation has been extensively characterized (14). Several studies reveal that cell adhesion to the ECM is required for cell cycle progression and proliferation in different cell types (14). Cell adhesion and spreading on fibronectin, vitronectin, and collagen activates mitogen-activated protein (MAP) kinase (17,18). Ras-independent and -dependent pathways have been implicated in MAP kinase activation by integrins (13,19,20). Cell adhesion mediated by integrins modulates the cell cycle, whereas detachment from the matrix induces apoptosis and cell cycle arrest (21). Cyclin A expression and cyclin E-dependent kinase activity are induced by cell attachment to the matrix, adding to the evidence that complex pathways of growth control are mediated by integrins and their ligands (14).

Loss of cell anchorage to the ECM upregulates the expression of the cyclin-dependent kinase inhibitors p27[kip1] and p21[cip1/waf1], while decreasing the levels of cyclin A (14). Changes in p27[kip1] occur in response to integrin expression (22). Overall, these studies show that modulation of cell cycle regulators is mediated by adhesion- and spreading-dependent events as well as by integrin expression.

Integrin ligation contributes to the abnormal proliferation of transformed cells (23) and, in the absence of their ligands, integrins block cell proliferation and downregulate *c-fos* and c-jun early genes. The mechanisms of signaling that occur proximal to the membrane are poorly known; integrin clustering or association with members of the transmembrane 4 superfamily may trigger proliferation signals and, consequently, regulate tumor growth (24).

SIGNALING PATHWAYS ACTIVATED BY INTEGRINS

Integrin engagement and consequent cell adhesion and spreading activate a cascade of intracellular signaling events. The best characterized pathways activated by integrins are Focal Adhesion Kinase (FAK), Phosphoinositide 3 (PI 3)-kinase and Ras/MAP kinase pathways (see Chapters 34–36).

Focal Adhesion Kinase Pathway

Integrins activate the tyrosine kinase FAK, which is a substrate for src (reviewed in refs. 25, 26). FAK is a nonreceptor protein tyrosine kinase that colocalizes with integrins at focal contact sites; FAK becomes tyrosine phosphorylated in response to integrin engagement and prevents apoptosis (26). FAK activation is accompanied by anchorage-independent growth and significant tumorigenic potential (15). FAK binds to paxillin, p130cas, phosphatidylinositol-3 kinase, c-src and Grb2; Grb2 forms complexes with SOS that ultimately activate ras (26). FAK is also activated by mitogens such as platelet-derived growth factor, suggesting a role in mediating the synergistic effects of integrins and growth factors (16). Further investigations are necessary to determine whether integrin-ligand interactions act synergistically or independently from growth factor activity.

Phosphoinositide 3-Kinase Pathway

In addition to stimulating FAK, integrins also activate the phosphoinositide 3 (PI 3)-kinase pathway (27) (see Chapter 35). PI 3-kinases are a family of lipid kinases activated by a wide variety of extracellular stimuli. The lipid products of PI 3-kinases, specifically phosphatidylinositol(3,4)biphosphate $[PI(3,4)P_2]$ and (3,4,5)triphosphate $[PI(3,4,5)P_3]$, affect cell proliferation, survival, differentiation, and migration by targeting specific signaling molecules such as the serine/threonine protein kinase B, also known as AKT, and protein kinase C. Integrin-mediated adhesion to the ECM stimulates the production of $PI(3,4)P_2$ and $PI(3,4,5)P_3$, the association of the p85 PI 3-kinase subunit with FAK (27), and AKT activation (28). AKT plays an important role in transducing survival signals in response to several growth factors and integrin engagement (28).

Ras/Mitogen-Activated Protein Kinase Pathway

The small GTPase Ras is a critical component of signaling pathways that control cell proliferation, differentiation and survival. The Ras/extracellular signal-regulated kinase 1 and 2 (ERK1 and 2) MAP kinase pathway plays a pivotal role in modulating gene expression and cell cycle progression in response to mitogens (29). Integrin clustering stimulates Ras GTP-loading and activates specific effectors of the Ras/MAP kinase signaling cascade such as Raf-1 and the MAP kinase, MEK (30).

INTEGRINS AND THE LIVER

The regulated expression of integrins in the liver during development and in healthy and diseased adult liver reflects the functions and cell–cell interactions of the different types of liver cells, and may have an important role in tissue remodeling and disease pathogenesis. Integrin expression in the liver has been well described (see Chapter 32 and website chapters W-27 and W-28); future research will focus on functional correlates, combining general knowledge of integrins with an increasing appreciation of the role of the ECM in the liver.

Integrin Expression in the Developing and Adult Liver

The microenvironment of the liver sinusoid is unique, with a matrix unlike that surrounding any other vascular structure in the body. The two major epithelial cell populations in the adult liver, hepatocytes and biliary epithelial cells, have distinctive integrin profiles reflecting the composition of their basement membranes (Fig. 33.1). The biliary epithelium, which has a standard basement membrane composed of laminin, entactin, perlecan, and type IV collagen, expresses a variety of integrins including the $\beta 1$ integrins α_2, α_3, α_5, α_6, and α_v, as well as α_6/β_4 (31–33). Hepatocytes lack an orga-

nized basement membrane, and their integrin profile, unique among epithelial cells, reflects an adaptation to the special microenvironment of the sinusoid (see Chapters 30 and 31 and website chapter ⌨ W-26). The perisinusoidal matrix includes large amounts of tenascin, but no laminin and entactin; hepatocytes lack the laminin receptors $\alpha_3\beta_1$, $\alpha_6\beta_1$, and $\alpha_6\beta_4$, but express the tenascin receptor $\alpha_9\beta_1$ (31). Hepatocytes also express fibronectin on all surfaces, with corresponding expression of the fibronectin receptor $\alpha_5\beta_1$, and they express $\alpha_1\beta_1$, correlating with their unusual expression (for an epithelial cell) of type I collagen (31,32).

The two epithelial cell populations of the liver diverge from a common precursor cell (Fig. 33.1) (see Chapter 2)

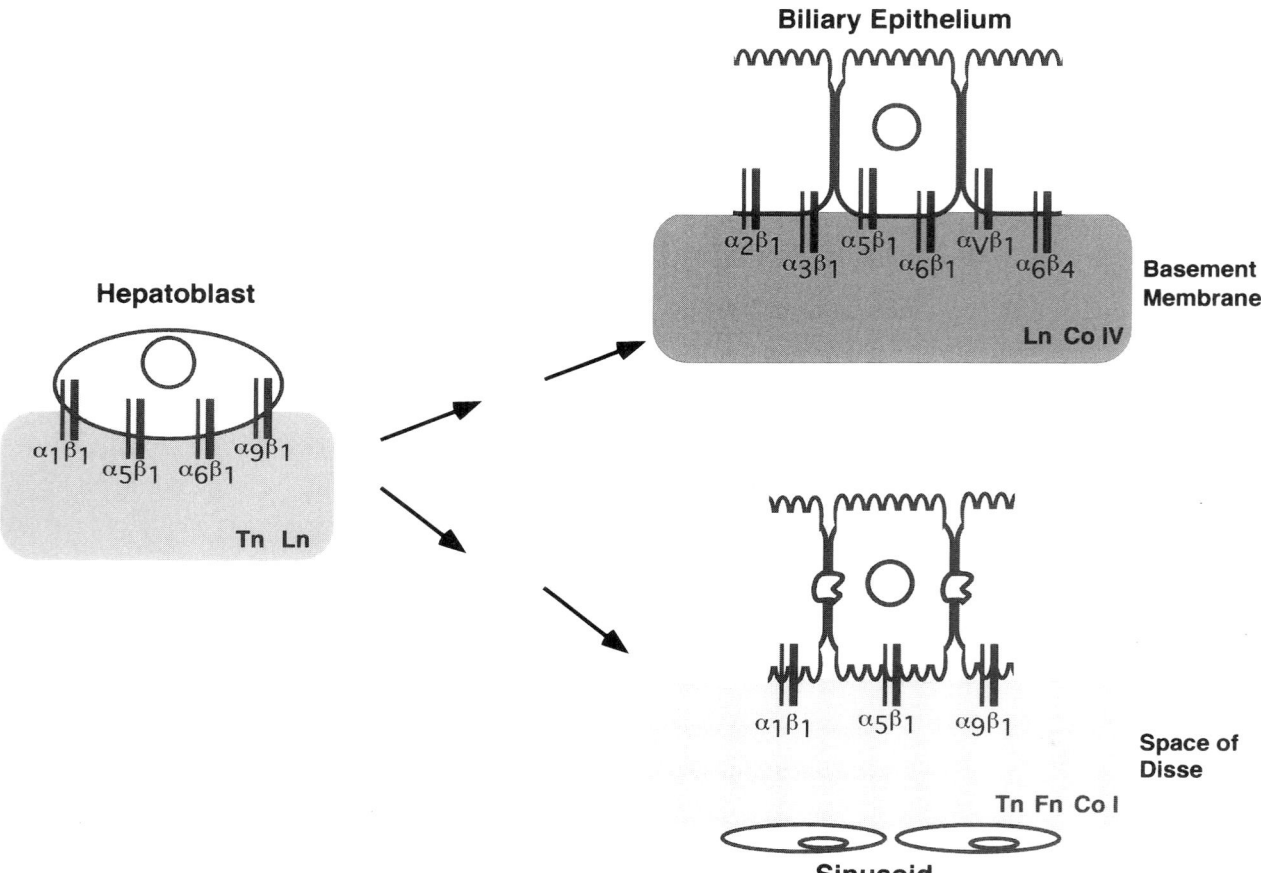

FIGURE 33.1. Integrin expression in the fetal and adult liver. Schematic of a precursor hepatoblast in the 5- to 7-week human liver developing into mature biliary epithelial cells (**top right**) and hepatocytes (**bottom right**) From Couvelard A, Bringuier AF, Dauge MC, et al. Expression of integrins during liver organogenesis in humans. *Hepatology* 1998;27:839–847 and Volpes R, van den Oord JJ, Desmet VJ. Distribution of the VLA family of integrins in normal and pathological human liver tissue. *Gastroenterology* 1991;101:200–206, with permission. Shaded areas represent the basement membrane (biliary epithelium) or its equivalent (perisinusoidal matrix for hepatoblasts and Space of Disse for hepatocytes). The major integrins expressed by the three cell types are shown, as are some of the major matrix components (*Tn*, tenascin; *Ln*, laminin; *Co IV*, type IV collagen; *Co I*, type I collagen; *Fn*, fibronectin). Sinusoidal endothelial cells, shown opposing the hepatocytes, have an integrin expression profile similar to that of hepatocytes. For the sake of clarity, only matrix components that vary among the cell types and are relevant to integrin expression are shown; additionally, details are shown for only one of the hepatocyte sinusoidal surfaces.

early in liver organogenesis (7 to 9 weeks). At the same time, integrin expression on the increasingly distinct cells changes, paralleling changes in the composition of the surrounding ECM (31). Precursor hepatoblasts in the 5 to 7 week human fetal liver express only the β_1 integrins α_1, α_5, α_6, and α_9, similar except for $\alpha_6\beta_1$ to adult hepatocytes. The perisinusoidal matrix, in which the hepatocytes will reside, expresses laminin at 5 to 7 weeks, but has lost it completely by 10 weeks; tenascin increases progressively to reach adult levels by 15 weeks. Primitive hepatocytes, which differentiate from the primitive hepatoblasts between 8 and 30 weeks, gradually lose expression of α_6, consistent with the disappearance of surrounding laminin. By 30 weeks, fetal hepatocytes demonstrate a pattern of integrin expression similar to adult hepatocytes (31).

The biliary epithelium undergoes a marked change in integrin expression beginning at eight weeks, when ductal plate differentiation begins; there is increased α_2, α_3, α_6 and β_4, and decreased α_1, consistent with ECM expression of the developing portal tracts (see Chapter 32 and website chapters 🖥 W-27 and W-28). Laminin and collagen IV expression begins at eight weeks at the point of contact with the ductal plate, and there is a progressive decrease in tenascin expression. The changes in the biliary epithelium are progressive, and there are transitional cells during development that express both $\alpha_1\beta_1$, characteristic of the hepatoblast, and $\alpha_6\beta_1$, characteristic of the mature cells (31). By 12 weeks, the biliary epithelial cells demonstrate a mature pattern of integrin expression. The expression of $\alpha_6\beta_1$ in association with the deposition of laminin on the ductal plate is crucial for bile duct morphogenesis, as these interactions are critical for morphogenesis in other organs. The importance of β_1 integrin subunits in liver development is supported by the finding that mice chimeric for β_1-null cells failed to show colonization of the liver by the knockout cells (34).

Similar interactions may be important in liver regeneration (see Chapter 42 and website chapter 🖥 W-31). After partial hepatectomy, there is rapid and transient upregulation of integrin β_1 and α_V subunits associated with rapid reorganization of other ECM components, suggesting that integrin-mediated processes are important in ECM reorganization and proliferation involved in regeneration (35).

Sinusoidal endothelial cells, which reside in the unique environment of the sinusoid with hepatocytes, have an integrin expression profile similar to hepatocytes, but different from that of most microvascular endothelial cells, including those lining the capillaries of the portal system. Specifically, sinusoidal endothelial cells express high levels of integrins $\alpha_1\beta_1$ and $\alpha_5\beta_1$, consistent with the high levels of collagen and fibronectin in the perisinusoidal space, and $\alpha_9\beta_1$ (32,33,36). They express little or no β_3, β_4, α_2, α_3, or α_6, consistent with the lack of laminin in the perisinusoidal space and with the lack of β_3 ligands such as von Willebrand factor, thrombospondin, and vitronectin.

Integrins in Diseased Liver

The relationship between matrix components and integrin expression persists in inflammatory and cholestatic liver disease, and raises questions about the causal nature and functional relevance of changes in integrin expression. In inflammatory liver diseases, there is an increase in laminin expression, and a corresponding increase in the expression of the laminin receptors $\alpha_3\beta_1$ and $\alpha_6\beta_1$, which are potentially important in liver repair and rearrangement (32). In cholestatic liver disease, hepatocytes can undergo a biliary metaplastic reaction to become more phenotypically similar to biliary epithelial cells, and express increased α_2, α_3, and α_6 (32). Intraductal bipotent stem cells have been described in the human liver (37) and reside within the canals of Hering. Although the integrin expression of these cells has not been reported, the role of integrins in their differentiation is an interesting question for future research.

Integrins in Hepatocellular Carcinoma and Metastases

Tumor cells in hepatocellular carcinoma (HCC) have a markedly different surrounding matrix compared to normal hepatocytes, and a correspondingly different integrin profile that may be functionally relevant. Detailed immunohistologic studies of integrins in normal and cirrhotic liver and in high-grade dysplastic nodules (also referred to as "macroregenerative nodules" and "atypical adenomatous hyperplasia") and HCC demonstrate localization of laminin in the sinusoids of all these except normal liver, with evidence that the laminin is produced by hepatocytes, endothelial cells, and stellate cells (38). There is a corresponding increase in expression of the laminin receptors $\alpha_1\beta_1$ and $\alpha_6\beta_1$. Of these, $\alpha_6\beta_1$, which is not expressed by normal adult hepatocytes, is induced *de novo* during carcinogenesis and correlates best with laminin localization in HCC (38,39). High-grade dysplastic nodules and small HCC have common laminin and $\alpha6$ subunit expression, lending support to the hypothesis that dysplastic nodules progress to HCC (39). Attachment of various HCC lines to laminin *in vitro* is blocked by antibodies against α_6 and β_1 or by knockouts of $\alpha_6\beta_1$ expression, highlighting the importance of the $\alpha_6\beta_1$ integrin in HCC/laminin attachment (40–42). In these experiments, migration, invasion of basement membrane type matrix, and anchorage-independent growth were also decreased, suggesting that $\alpha_6\beta_1$ has an additional role in maintaining the transformed phenotype of at least some HCC. There is also a focal decrease in the fibronectin receptor subunit α_5 in high-grade dysplastic nodules and HCC, and it has been postulated that this integrin has a role in HCC invasion due to loss of cell–cell and cell–matrix contacts (39). Intrahepatic invasion of human HCC in SCID mice was blocked by antibodies against β_1 and α_5 integrins, supporting this hypothesis (43).

Integrin expression mediates *in vivo* metastasis establishment and growth in the liver and other organs (7). Cell invasion mediated by integrins, a crucial step in *in vivo* metastasis establishment and growth, is supported *in vitro* by signaling molecules FAK, PI 3-kinase, and members of the MAP kinase family. Thus, it is predicted that study of these signaling pathways will contribute to understanding of mechanisms that support metastasis growth *in vivo* in liver and other organs.

Integrins in the Fibrotic Liver

Fibrosis is marked by changes in the integrin expression of hepatocytes and sinusoidal endothelial cells which mimic those seen in HCC, and which reflect alterations in the composition of the perisinusoidal ECM (36). The major change is expression of laminin in the sinusoidal space, where it is normally absent. Correspondingly, laminin receptors on hepatocytes and sinusoidal endothelial cells are upregulated. In hepatocytes, the laminin receptors $\alpha_1\beta_1$, $\alpha_3\beta_1$, and $\alpha_6\beta_1$ are increased, as well as receptors for collagen and fibronectin ($\alpha_2\beta_1$ and $\alpha_5\beta_1$, respectively). Sinusoidal endothelial cells demonstrate similar increases in these integrins, but also broadly upregulate other integrins including those for $\alpha_3\beta_1$ and $\alpha_4\beta_1$. Of note, these changes occur very early in fibrosis, before the onset of cirrhosis, and may not only represent adaptation to changes in the ECM but also play a causal role in the initiation of fibrosis (36).

Hepatic stellate cells (HSC) and myofibroblasts are the primary matrix-producing cells in the diseased liver, although little is known about their expression of integrins or its relevance to fibrosis (see Chapter 31). In particular, details of stellate cell activation to the fibrogenic phenotype are not known; it is likely that matrix interactions play a major role in initiating this activation.

Stellate cells express integrins $\alpha_1\beta_1$, $\alpha_v\beta_1$, $\alpha_8\beta_1$, and $\alpha_6\beta_4$, consistent with their binding of collagens, fibronectin, and laminin (44,45). $\alpha_2\beta_1$ expression, which occurs in cells *in vitro*, is likely to be an artifact of culture (46). HSC in culture activate if grown on uncoated plastic, but remain quiescent if grown on the basement membrane-like substrate Matrigel; growth on laminin, type IV collagen, and heparan sulfate proteoglycans does not have the same result (47). Interestingly, growing culture-activated cells on Matrigel results in their reversion to the nonfibrogenic, quiescent state (48), suggesting that matrix interactions not only play a role in initiating activation, but also play a role in maintaining the activated state. It may be relevant that integrins are upregulated by the cytokine transforming growth factor (TGF)-β, which is produced in autocrine fashion by activated HSC and is the most potent fibrogenic cytokine in these cells (49). Additionally, TGF-β induces production of the (EIIIA) splice variant of fibronectin by sinusoidal endothelial cells, which contributes to HSC activation (50).

Integrins are also likely to be important in other aspects of HSC function. Integrin $\alpha_1\beta_1$ mediates adhesion to collagen, and may regulate contractility of HSC, potentially related to the development of portal hypertension in cirrhosis (see Chapter 47). Antibodies to this integrin inhibit HSC contraction, although it is expressed constitutively, not just in activated and contractile cells, and there are likely to be other important factors (46). There is a dramatic increase in fibronectin production in the diseased liver; soluble RGD peptides result in decreased production of type I collagen by HSC in culture (by increasing MMP-1 activity) and result overall in decreased activation of these cells through the inhibition of FAK tyrosine phosphorylation, implicating FAK in the cytoskeletal reorganization of HSC as they activate (51,52). Integrins may also be involved in initiation and perpetuation of the inflammatory phase of liver injury: activation of β_1 integrins, by plating on β_1 substrates or by plating on anti-β_1 subunit antibodies, results in increased secretion of monocyte chemotactic protein-1 by HSC (53).

CONCLUSION

Integrins are cell surface receptors for ECM proteins which mediate a variety of functions related to cell proliferation, differentiation, and survival. Although the specific functions of integrins and their ligands in the liver are not well understood, recent publications outlining their expression pave the way for investigations describing integrin isoforms and signaling pathways involved in liver development, malignancy, fibrosis, and differentiation.

ACKNOWLEDGMENTS

We thank Neil Theise for reviewing parts of the manuscript. This work was supported by grants to L.R.L. from the National Institutes of Health (CA-71870) and the PCRP (DAMD17-98-1-8506) and to R.G.W. from the Yale Liver Center (DK-34989). We thank Ms. N. Bennett for expert assistance in preparing the manuscript.

REFERENCES

1. Ruoslahti E, Reed JC. Anchorage dependence, integrins and apoptosis. *Cell* 1994;77:477–478.
2. Damsky CH, Werb Z. Signal transduction by integrin receptors for extracellular matrix: cooperative processing of extracellular information. *Curr Opin Cell Biol* 1992;4:772–781.
3. Hynes RO. Cell adhesion: old and new questions. *Trends Cell Biol* 1999;9:M33–37.
4. Juliano R. Cooperation between soluble factors and integrin-mediated cell anchorage in the control of cell growth and differentiation. *BioEssays* 1996;18:911–917.

5. Haas TL, Madri JA. Extracellular matrix-driven matrix metallo-proteinase production in endothelial cells: Implications for angiogenesis. *Trends Cardiovasc Med* 1999;9:70–77.

6. Hemler ME, Weitzman JB, Pasqualini R, et al. Structure, biochemical properties, and biological functions of integrin cytoplasmic domains. In: Takada Y, ed. *Integrins: the biological problems.* Boca Raton: CRC Press, 1995:1–35.

7. Ruoslahti E. Integrins as signaling molecules and targets for tumor therapy. *Kidney Int* 1997;51:1413–1417.

8. Byzova TV, Rabbani R, D'Souza SE, et al. Role of integrin $\alpha_V\beta_3$ in vascular biology. *Thromb Haemost* 1998;80:726–734.

9. Zheng DQ, Woodard AS, Tallini G, et al. Substrate specificity of $\alpha_V\beta_3$ integrin-mediated cell migration and PI 3-kinase/AKT pathway activation. *J Biol Chem* 2000;275:24565–24574.

10. Fornaro M, Languino LR. Alternatively spliced variants: a new view of the integrin cytoplasmic domain. *Matrix Biol* 1997;16:185–193.

11. Williams MJ, Hughes PE, O'Toole TE, et al. The inner world of cell adhesion: integrin cytoplasmic domains. *Trends Cell Biol* 1994;4:109–112.

12. Vidal F, Aberdam D, Miquel C, et al. Integrin $\beta4$ mutations associated with junctional epidermolysis bullosa with pyloric atresia. *Nat Genet* 1995;10:229–234.

13. Fornaro M, Steger CA, Bennett AM, et al. Differential role of β_{1C} and β_{1A} integrin cytoplasmic variants in modulating focal adhesion kinase, protein kinase B/AKT, and Ras/Mitogen-activated protein kinase pathways. *Mol Biol Cell* 2000;11:2235–2249.

14. Bottazzi ME, Assoian RK. The extracellular matrix and mitogenic growth factors control G1 phase cyclins and cyclin-dependent kinase inhibitors. *Trends Cell Biol* 1997;7:348–352.

15. Frisch SM, Ruoslahti E. Integrins and anoikis. *Curr Opin Cell Biol* 1997;9:701–706.

16. Schwartz MA, Schaller MD, Ginsberg MH. Integrins: emerging paradigms of signal transduction. *Annu Rev Cell Dev Bio* 1995;11:549–599.

17. Chen Q, Kinch M, Lin T, et al. Integrin-mediated cell adhesion activates mitogen-activated protein kinases. *J Biol Chem* 1994;269:26602–26605.

18. Zhu X, Assoian RK. Integrin-dependent activation of MAP kinase: a link to shape-dependent cell proliferation. *Mol Biol Cell* 1995;6:273–282.

19. Chen H-C, Appeddu PA, Isoda H, et al. Phosphorylation of tyrosine 397 in focal adhesion kinase is required for binding phosphatidylinositol 3-kinase. *J Biol Chem* 1996;271:26329–26334.

20. Clark E, Hynes R. Ras activation is necessary for integrin-mediated activation of extracellular signal-regulated kinase 2 and cytosolic phospholipase A_2 but not for cytoskeletal organization. *J Biol Chem* 1996;271:14814–14818.

21. Fang F, Orend G, Watanabe N, et al. Dependence of cyclin E-CDK2 kinase activity on cell anchorage. *Science* 1996;271:499–502.

22. Fornaro M, Tallini G, Zheng DQ, et al. p27kip1 acts as a downstream effector of and is coexpressed with the β_{1C} integrin in prostatic adenocarcinoma. *J Clin Invest* 1999;103:321–329.

23. Varner JA, Emerson DA, Juliano RL. Integrin $\alpha_5\beta_1$ expression negatively regulates cell growth: reversal by attachment to fibronectin. *Mol Biol Cell* 1995;6:725–740.

24. Hemler M, Mannion B, Berditchevski F. Association of TM4SF proteins with integrins: relevance to cancer. *Biochim Biophys Acta* 1996;1287:67–71.

25. Malik RK, Parsons JT. Integrin-mediated signaling in normal and malignant cells: a role of protein-tyrosine kinases (review). *Biochim Biophys Acta* 1996;1287:73–76.

26. Schlaepfer DD, Hunter T. Integrin signalling and tyrosine phosphorylation: just the FAKs? *Trends Cell Biol* 1998;8:151–157.

27. Keely P, Parise L, Juliano R. Integrins and GTPases in tumor cell growth, motility and invasion. *Trends Cell Biol* 1998;8:101–106.

28. Rameh LE, Cantley LC. The role of phosphoinositide 3-kinase lipid products in cell function. *J Biol Chem* 1999;274:8347–8350.

29. Campbell SL, Khosravi-Far R, Rossman KL, et al. Increasing complexity of Ras signaling. *Oncogene* 1998;17:1395–1413.

30. Howe A, Aplin AE, Alahari SK, et al. Integrin signaling and cell growth control. *Curr Opin Cell Biol* 1998;10:220–231.

31. Couvelard A, Bringuier AF, Dauge MC, et al. Expression of integrins during liver organogenesis in humans. *Hepatology* 1998;27:839–847.

32. Volpes R, van den Oord JJ, Desmet VJ. Distribution of the VLA family of integrins in normal and pathological human liver tissue. *Gastroenterology* 1991;101:200–206.

33. Fornaro M, Manzotti M, Tallini G, et al. β_{1C} integrin in epithelial cells correlates with a nonproliferative phenotype: forced expression of β_{1C} inhibits prostate epithelial cell proliferation. *Am J Pathol* 1998;153:1079–1087.

34. Fassler R, Meyer M. Consequences of lack of β_1 integrin gene expression in mice. *Genes Dev* 1995;9:1896–1908.

35. Kim TH, Mars WM, Stolz DB, et al. Extracellular matrix remodeling at the early stages of liver regeneration in the rat. *Hepatology* 1997;26:896–904.

36. Scoazec JY. Expression of cell-matrix adhesion molecules in the liver and their modulation during fibrosis. *J Hepatol* 1995;22:20–27.

37. Theise ND, Saxena R, Portmann BC, et al. The canals of Hering and hepatic stem cells in humans. *Hepatology* 1999;30:1425–1433.

38. Torimura T, Ueno T, Kin M, et al. Coordinated expression of integrin $\alpha_6\beta_1$ and laminin in hepatocellular carcinoma. *Hum Pathol* 1997;28:1131–1138.

39. Le Bail B, Faouzi S, Boussarie L, et al. Extracellular matrix composition and integrin expression in early hepatocarcinogenesis in human cirrhotic liver. *J Pathol* 1997;181:330–337.

40. Carloni V, Romanelli RG, Mercurio AM, et al. Knockout of $\alpha_6\beta_1$-integrin expression reverses the transformed phenotype of hepatocarcinoma cells. *Gastroenterology* 1998;115:433–442.

41. Nejjari M, Hafdi Z, Dumortier J, et al. $\alpha_6\beta_1$ integrin expression in hepatocarcinoma cells: regulation and role in cell adhesion and migration. *Int J Cancer* 1999;83:518–525.

42. Torimura T, Ueno T, Kin M, et al. Integrin $\alpha_6\beta_1$ plays a significant role in the attachment of hepatoma cells to laminin. *J Hepatol* 1999;31:734–740.

43. Genda T, Sakamoto M, Ichida T, et al. Loss of cell–cell contact is induced by integrin-mediated cell–substratum adhesion in highly-motile and highly-metastatic hepatocellular carcinoma cells. *Lab Invest* 2000;80:387–394.

44. Carloni V, Romanelli RG, Pinzani M, et al. Expression and function of integrin receptors for collagen and laminin in cultured human hepatic stellate cells. *Gastroenterology* 1996;110:1127–1136.

45. Levine D, Rockey DC, Milner TA, et al. Expression of the integrin $\alpha_8\beta_1$ during pulmonary and hepatic fibrosis. *Am J Pathol* 2000;156:1927–1935.

46. Racine-Samson L, Rockey DC, Bissell DM. The role of $\alpha_1\beta_1$ integrin in wound contraction. A quantitative analysis of liver myofibroblasts *in vivo* and in primary culture. *J Biol Chem* 1997;272:30911–30917.

47. Friedman SL, Roll FJ, Boyles J, et al. Maintenance of differentiated phenotype of cultured rat hepatic lipocytes by basement membrane matrix. *J Biol Chem* 1989;264:10756–10762.

48. Gaca MDA, Kiriella KB, Issa R, et al. Hepatic stellate cell phenotype is regulated by extracellular matrix: implications for liver fibrogenesis. *Mol Biol Cell* 1999;10:62a.

49. Heino J, Ignotz RA, Hemler ME, et al. Regulation of cell adhe-

sion receptors by transforming growth factor-β. Concomitant regulation of integrins that share a common β₁ subunit. *J Biol Chem* 1989;264:380–388.

50. Jarnagin WR, Rockey DC, Koteliansky VE, et al. Expression of variant fibronectins in wound healing: cellular source and biological activity of the EIIIA segment in rat hepatic fibrogenesis. *J Cell Biol* 1994;127:2037–2048.

51. Iwamoto H, Sakai H, Kotoh K, et al. Soluble Arg-Gly-Asp pep-tides reduce collagen accumulation in cultured rat hepatic stellate cells. *Dig Dis Sci* 1999;44:1038–1045.

52. Iwamoto H, Sakai H, Nawata H. Inhibition of integrin signaling with Arg-Gly-Asp motifs in rat hepatic stellate cells. *J Hepatol* 1998;29:752–759.

53. Marra F, Pastacaldi S, Romanelli RG, et al. Integrin-mediated stimulation of monocyte chemotactic protein-1 expression. *FEBS Lett* 1997;414:221–225.

The Liver: Biology and Pathobiology, Fourth Edition, edited by I. M. Arias, J. L. Boyer, F. V. Chisari, N. Fausto, D. Schachter, and D. A. Shafritz.
Lippincott Williams & Wilkins, Philadelphia © 2001.

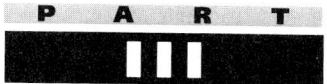

INTERRELATED CELL FUNCTIONS

34

ROLE OF INOSITOL TRISPHOSPHATE AND DIACYLGLYCEROL IN THE REGULATION OF LIVER FUNCTION

JOHN H. EXTON

Many hormones and neurotransmitters exert their biological actions by stimulating the breakdown of a specific phospholipid (phosphatidylinositol 4,5-bisphosphate) in the plasma membrane of their target cells (Chapter 35). This breakdown yields inositol 1,4,5-trisphosphate, which enters the cytosol, and 1,2-diacylglycerol, which remains in the membrane. Inositol trisphosphate has a second messenger role in that it rapidly releases Ca^{2+} ions from components of the endoplasmic reticulum, and the resulting rise in cytosolic Ca^{2+} causes many of the physiological responses observed, through the mediation of calmodulin and other Ca^{2+}-binding proteins. A major mechanism is the phosphorylation of specific proteins by isozymes of Ca^{2+}-calmodulin-dependent protein kinase. Diacylglycerol is also a second messenger because it activates most isozymes of the Ca^{2+}-phospholipid-dependent protein kinase, termed protein kinase C. This leads to the phosphorylation of a number of cellular proteins contributing to the observed responses.

Liver cells respond to many agonists that promote the breakdown of phosphatidylinositol bisphosphate, namely, epinephrine and norepinephrine (acting through α_1-adrenergic receptors), vasopressin (acting through V_1-vasopressin receptors), adenosine triphosphate (ATP) and adenosine diphosphate (ADP) (acting through P_{2y}-purinergic receptors), angiotensin II (acting through AT_{1A} receptors) leu-enkephalin, and epidermal growth factor. These agents increase inositol trisphosphate, cytosolic Ca^{2+}, and diacylglycerol in isolated hepatocytes. The α_1-adrenergic responses to epinephrine and norepinephrine play an important role in the control of liver function by the sympathetic nervous system, but the physiological significance of the hepatic actions of angiotensin II, leu-enkephalin, epidermal growth factor, vasopressin, and the adenine nucleotides is presently unclear. Since ATP is released concurrently with norepinephrine during activation of the sympathetic nervous system, it may contribute to the responses seen in this situation. Hepatic processes regulated by Ca^{2+}-mobilizing hormones include glycogen breakdown and synthesis, gluconeogenesis, ureogenesis, fatty acid oxidation and synthesis, amino acid transport, bile secretion, respiration, ion fluxes and membrane polarization, regeneration, and DNA synthesis.

PHOSPHOINOSITIDE METABOLISM (CHAPTER 35)

Phosphatidylinositol 4,5-bisphosphate is a minor phospholipid that is derived from phosphatidylinositol and is present mainly in the inner leaflet of the plasma membrane (1). Phosphatidylinositol represents 7% of the total liver phospholipids and 7% of the plasma membrane lipids. Of the total inositol phospholipids, phosphatidylinositol 4,5-bisphosphate represents approximately 1% of those in the cell or approximately 10% of those in the plasma membrane. The synthesis of phosphatidylinositol 4,5-bisphosphate is shown schematically in Figure 34.1. Phosphatidylinositol (PI) is sequentially converted to phosphatidylinositol 4-

J. H. Exton: Department of Molecular Physiology and Biophysics, Vanderbilt University School of Medicine, Nashville, Tennessee 37232.

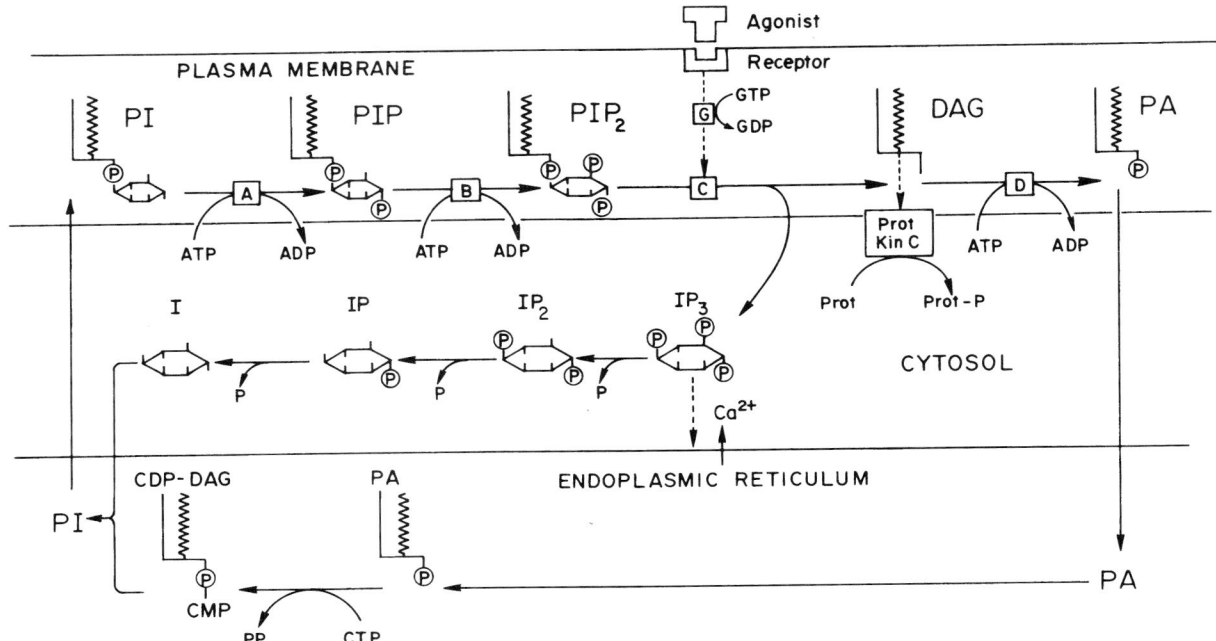

FIGURE 34.1. Phosphoinositide metabolism and its regulation by Ca²⁺-mobilizing agonists. *ADP*, adenosine diphosphate; *ATP*, adenosine triphosphate; *DAG*, 1,2-diacylglyerol; *PA*, phosphatidic acid; *I*, *myo*-inositol; *IP*, inositol 4-phosphate; *IP₂*, inositol 1,4-bisphosphate; *A*, phosphatidylinositol 4-kinase; *B*, phosphatidylinositol 4-P 5-kinase; *C*, phospholipase C; *D*, diacylglycerol kinase; *G*, G protein.

phosphate (PI 4-P) and phosphatidylinositol 4,5-bisphosphate (PI 4,5-P₂) by ATP-requiring kinases (1). Phosphomonoesterases that reverse these reactions are also present in the plasma membrane.

In addition to PI 4-P and PI 4,5-P₂, cells contain PI 3-P, PI 3,4-P₂ and PI 3,4,5-P₃, especially after stimulation with growth factors and certain other agonists. These 3-phosphorylated inositol phospholipids are present at low concentrations relative to PI 4-P and PI 4,5-P₂ and are formed by the action of phosphatidylinositol 3-kinase, which is activated by many growth factors (2). The formation and physiological functions of these lipids are described in detail in Chapter 35.

PI 4,5-P₂ is hydrolyzed by specific phospholipase C isozymes to yield inositol 1,4,5-trisphosphate (IP₃) and 1,2-diacylglycerol (DAG). As will be described below, these isozymes are regulated by hormones and neurotransmitters via guanine nucleotide binding proteins or by growth factors through their receptor tyrosine kinases, and the products of the reaction act as intracellular signals (3,4).

As expected for a signaling molecule, IP₃ is rapidly metabolized after release. This occurs by two pathways. The first is sequential dephosphorylation to inositol 1,4-bisphosphate, inositol 4-phosphate, and *myo*-inositol (5) (Fig. 34.1). The second is by phosphorylation to inositol 1,3,4,5-tetrakisphosphate by an ATP-dependent 3-kinase (5). The tetrakisphosphate is subsequently broken down by phosphomono-

esterases to inositol 1,3,4-trisphosphate, inositol 3,4-bisphosphate, inositol 3-phosphate, and *myo*-inositol. The inositol bis- and monophosphates appear to be biologically inert. There is continuing controversy about whether inositol 1,3,4,5-tetrakisphosphate acts as an intracellular messenger and regulates Ca²⁺ entry (6). The various inositol phosphates can be further converted by kinases and phosphomonoesterases to a large number of additional compounds (5), but their physiological functions, if any, are unknown.

The metabolic fate of the DAG released by PIP₂ breakdown is not well defined. The current view is that it remains in the plasma membrane and is mainly phosphorylated to phosphatidic acid (PA) by 1,2-diacylglycerol kinase (7) (Fig. 34.1). An alternative fate is hydrolysis by lipases to monoacylglycerol, glycerol, and fatty acids. It is believed that much of the phosphatidic acid generated by phospholipid breakdown in the plasma membrane is transferred to the endoplasmic reticulum (ER) by carrier proteins. There it is utilized for the synthesis of PI or phosphatidylglycerol by reaction with CTP to form CDP-diacylglycerol (CDP-DAG) under the action of CDP-diacylglycerol synthetase (7,8) (Fig. 34.1). Alternative fates are its hydrolysis by phosphatidate phosphohydrolase to DAG for utilization in the synthesis of triacylglycerol, phosphatidylcholine, or phosphatidylethanolamine.

Myo-inositol formed from the breakdown of inositol phospholipids, transported into the cell or synthesized from glucose, is incorporated into PI by two reactions (7,8). The first is the reaction with CDP-DAG to form PI and CMP, which is catalyzed by CDP-diacylglycerol:inositol transferase (Fig. 34.1). The second is the exchange reaction with other phospholipids to form PI with release of the corresponding head group. PI formed in the ER is transferred to the plasma membrane by a carrier protein.

The inositol phospholipids are enriched in stearic and arachidonic acids in the sn 1 and sn 2 positions of glycerol, respectively (8). This is the result of remodeling by acyl exchange that occurs following synthesis (8). Such exchange occurs by deacylation-reacylation reactions catalyzed by phospholipases A_2 and A_1 and acylCoA:lysophospholipid acyltransferases, including 1-acyl-*sn*-glycero-3-phosphorylinositol acyltransferase, which has a high preference for arachidonic acid in liver (8).

HORMONAL CONTROL OF PHOSPHATIDYLINOSITOL BISPHOSPHATE BREAKDOWN

Several agonists stimulate PIP_2 breakdown in hepatic parenchymal cells, leading to an elevation of cytosolic Ca^{2+}. This elevation results in a diversity of physiological responses (9) (Fig. 34.1). Each agonist interacts with its specific receptor subtype located on the external surface of the cell. Many of the receptor subtypes have been cloned and expressed, including the epidermal growth factor receptor (10) and the α1B-adrenergic (11), V_1-vasopressin (12), and AT_{1A}-angiotensin II (13,14) receptors. The latter three receptors have an extracellular N-terminal domain, seven transmembrane segments, three cytoplasmic and extracellular loops, and a C-terminal cytoplasmic tail of variable length (15). Activating ligands interact with certain of the extracellular or transmembrane domains, and this leads to conformational changes in the cytoplasmic domains which promote their interaction with and activation of specific guanine nucleotide-binding regulatory proteins (G proteins), namely members of the G_q family of G proteins, which includes G_q, G_{11}, G_{14}, G_{15}, and G_{16} (16–18). Activation of the G proteins is due to the release of GDP from the guanine nucleotide-binding site of their α-subunits and its replacement by GTP (19,20). This results in dissociation of the $\beta\gamma$ complex from the α-subunits. The GTP-liganded α-subunits then interact with β-isozymes of PIP_2 phospholipase C, causing a large increase in their activity (16). Due to the intrinsic GTPase activity of the α-subunits, which is activated by the phospholipase, the bound GTP is hydrolyzed to GDP and the α-subunits become inactive (19,20). They then recombine with the $\beta\gamma$ subunits to form inactive G protein heterotrimers. In the continued presence of agonist and with active (nondesensitized) receptors, the G proteins undergo further cycles of activation-inactivation. There is maintenance of a fraction of the α-subunits

in the GTP-liganded, active state and continued activation of the phospholipase.

Unlike the G proteins involved in the regulation of adenylate cyclase (G_s and G_i), the activity of the Gq family of G proteins is not modified by either cholera toxin or pertussis toxin (10,18). However, PIP_2 breakdown induced by some agonists in neutrophils, mesangial cells, and mast cells is inhibited by pertussis toxin (10), implying the involvement of a member(s) of the G_i family. In these cases, the activating subunit is the G protein $\beta\gamma$ complex which stimulates the β_2- and β_3-isozymes of phospholipase C. The phosphoinositide-specific phospholipase C isozymes that are mostly potently activated by the G_q family of G proteins are the β_1- and β_3-isozymes (16,20,21). Other isozymes of the β class, for example, β_2 and β_4, are activated by these G proteins, but the response of the β_2-isozyme is much less (20) and the β_4-isozyme is confined to the retina and brain.

In contrast to the phospholipase C isozymes that are the target of agonists that activate G proteins, the isozymes that are activated by growth factor receptors, the T cell antigen receptor, the IgE and IgG receptors, and the receptors for certain cytokines are of the γ_1 and γ_2 types (21). Occupancy of growth factor receptors by their ligands leads to oligomerization and activation of the intrinsic tyrosine kinase activity of the receptors. As a result, tyrosine-containing domains in the cytoplasmic tail of the receptors are phosphorylated (autophosphorylation) (22). Certain cytoplasmic proteins, including phosphoinositide phospholipase Cγ_1, p21*ras*-GAP, Shc, Grb2, Nck, protein tyrosine phosphatase 1D, and phosphatidylinositol 3-kinase then associate with specific P-tyrosine domains through their SH2 (*src*-homology) domains (21–23). Upon association with the cytoplasmic tail of the receptor, phospholipase Cγ_1 becomes activated and phosphorylated on tyrosine (21). The T-cell receptor, the IgE and IgG receptors, and the receptors for some cytokines do not possess intrinsic tyrosine kinase activity. However, they activate a variety of soluble tyrosine kinases which phosphorylate and activate phospholipase Cγ isozymes (21). The physiological significance of PIP_2 hydrolysis induced by epidermal growth factor (EGF) in liver and by growth factors in general is unclear, but, in combination with other signals, it appears to control cell growth. Deletion of phospholipase Cγ_1 causes embryonic lethality in mice. The activation of phospholipase Cγ_1 by EGF in liver is unusual in that it is inhibited by pertussis toxin, implying the involvement of a G protein of the G_i family (24,25).

Since the plasma membrane pool of PIP_2 is very small, continuous stimulation of its breakdown would rapidly lead to its depletion unless resynthesis occurred. There is evidence that increased flux through PI kinase and PI 4-P 5-kinase accompanies PIP_2 hydrolysis in some cells, and this is presumed to also occur in liver. A possible explanation for the increased flux from PI to PIP_2 is simple mass action, but other mechanisms may be involved. Transfer of phosphatidylinositol from its site of synthesis in the ER to the plasma membrane by phosphatidylinositol transfer proteins is essential for continued production of inositol trisphosphate in stimulated cells.

Glucagon increases cytosolic Ca^{2+} in hepatocytes (26,27), but there is some uncertainty regarding the mechanisms involved and also the physiological importance of the effect. The increase in Ca^{2+} is due to both intracellular Ca^{2+} mobilization and influx of extracellular Ca^{2+}. There is a small increase in IP_3 which probably contributes to the release of internal Ca^{2+} (27), but in addition, there is evidence that activation of cAMP-dependent protein kinase sensitizes the intracellular Ca^{2+} release mechanism to IP_3 (28). Glucagon also potentiates the effects of Ca^{2+}-mobilizing agonists (norepinephrine, vasopressin, and angiotensin II) on IP_3 formation and Ca^{2+} mobilization and influx (29–32). Since all the effects of glucagon on liver Ca^{2+} are mimicked by cAMP analogues and by other agents that elevate cAMP (27–32), it appears that they are secondary to the increase in the nucleotide.

In remains unclear which, if any, of the physiological responses to glucagon are due to the increase in Ca^{2+} *per se*. Since the ability of the hormone to activate phosphorylase is unaffected by Ca^{2+} depletion of liver cells, it appears that Ca^{2+} mobilization is not required for activation of hepatic glycogenolysis. A role for the increase in Ca^{2+} in other glucagon effects, especially the stimulation of gluconeogenesis, is possible.

INOSITOL TRISPHOSPHATE AND CALCIUM RELEASE (SEE CHAPTERS 35 AND 38)

The generation of IP_3 in response to agonists in hepatocytes is sufficiently rapid to account for the mobilization of intracellular Ca^{2+} (Fig. 34.2), although there is amplification in the system in that a submaximal rise in IP_3 can maximally elevate cytosolic Ca^{2+} (33). The response of permeabilized hepatocytes to exogenous IP_3 is very rapid and is observed with IP_3 concentrations within the probable intracellular range, that is, 0.1 to 1 µM (3,28,34).

The initial increase in IP_3 in response to agonists is not sustained (Fig. 34.2), since it is rapidly metabolized in hepatocytes and other tissues (5). The concentration of IP_3 does not, however, decline to the basal level for several minutes in the continuing presence of agonists, and it is assumed that its level is sufficiently high to prevent reuptake of cytosolic Ca^{2+} by the ER. The gradual decline in the IP_3 level following its initial rapid rise is due to a decrease in its production. This has been attributed to deactivation of certain components of the transmembrane signaling system due to their phosphorylation by protein kinase C (21). However, the specific targets of the kinase, for example, receptors, G protein subunits, phospholipase C, and IP_3 receptor, are unclear.

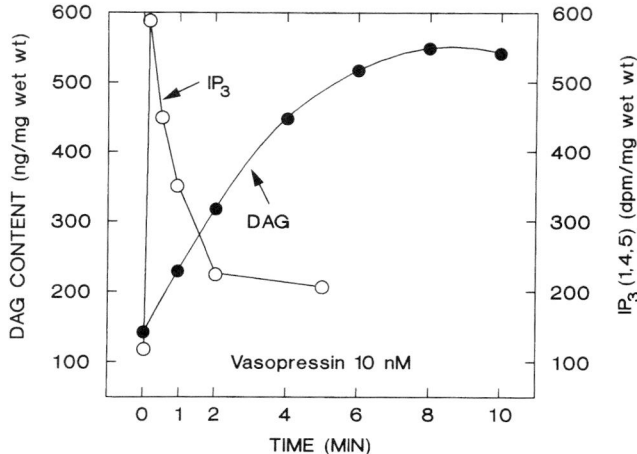

FIGURE 34.2. Time course of IP_3 and 1,2-diacylglycerol (*DAG*) formation in hepatocytes treated with vasopressin. Cells were labeled to isotopic equilibrium with [³H]*myo*-inositol and [³H]IP_3 and unlabeled DAG were measured by high performance liquid chromatography.

The intracellular target of IP_3 is the IP_3 receptor, which exists in three subtypes and is localized to subcomponents of the smooth and rough ER (35). The receptors subtypes share 60% to 70% amino acid identity and can form homo- and heterotetrameric assemblies. They have been shown, by expression, to mediate Ca^{2+} release in an IP_3-sensitive manner. They contain an IP_3-binding domain at the amino terminus, a coupling domain with sites for phosphorylation and ATP binding, and a transmembrane domain with eight membrane-spanning segments (35). The last four transmembrane segments show high homology with the ryanodine receptor, which mobilizes Ca^{2+} from the sarcoplasmic reticulum in skeletal muscle. Because of this, these segments are believed to form the Ca^{2+}-permeable pore of the receptor. Incorporation of the purified IP_3 receptor in lipid vesicles provides an electrophysiologically detectable Ca^{2+} channel that is activated by IP_3, proving that the receptor itself can form the channel. The physiological function of the ATP binding sites is unclear, but it has been observed that the nucleotide cooperatively enhances the ability of IP_3 to stimulate Ca^{2+} flux. The receptor can be phosphorylated by cAMP-dependent protein kinase, protein kinase C and Ca^{2+}-calmodulin-dependent protein kinase (35), but the specific functions of these phosphorylations remain conjectural.

Cytosolic Ca^{2+} rises very rapidly following the release of IP_3 induced by vasopressin in hepatocytes, and the resulting physiological responses, for example, phosphorylase activation, occur within seconds (10). A similar rapidity is seen with other Ca^{2+}-mobilizing agonists (10,33). In contrast, the increase in cyclic AMP and resulting rise in phosphorylase α induced by glucagon or β-adrenergic agonists are significantly slower. These data illustrate the general finding that Ca^{2+}-mobilizing agonists induce their physiological responses more rapidly than cyclic AMP-dependent agonists.

Since the intracellular Ca^{2+} stores mobilized by IP_3 are limited in magnitude, increased Ca^{2+} entry is necessary in order for agonists to produce a sustained elevation of cytosolic Ca^{2+} and hence sustained responses. In excitable cells such as neurons and muscle cells, neurotransmitters open ion channel(s) in the plasma membrane that allow the influx of extracellular Ca^{2+} (36). However, in nonexcitable cells such as hepatocytes, the depletion of intracellular Ca^{2+} stores leads to the opening of plasma membrane Ca^{2+} channels that are termed store-operated Ca^{2+} channels (36,37). However, the signaling mechanisms involved in controlling these channels remain obscure (37).

CALCIUM AND CALCIUM-REGULATED PROTEINS

The release of Ca^{2+} from the ER and the influx of Ca^{2+} through plasma membrane ion channels induced by agonists in hepatocytes result in an abrupt increase in the cytosolic Ca^{2+} concentration. In the absence of extracellular Ca^{2+}, the concentration declines rapidly to reach basal levels after several minutes, whereas in the presence of physiological extracellular Ca^{2+} concentrations, the elevation persists (9).

When the Ca^{2+} responses to agonists are measured in single hepatocytes, it is seen that the cytosolic Ca^{2+} concentration undergoes oscillations (38,39). The form of the Ca^{2+} wave shows differences depending on the specific agonist for reasons that are not clear. With increasing agonist concentration, the frequency of the oscillations increases, but the amplitude is unchanged (38,39). The waves begin at a specific focus adjacent to the plasma membrane and spread across the cell (39). Several hypotheses have been proposed to explain the oscillations (40), including the proposal that Ca^{2+} released from the IP_3-sensitive stores causes an efflux of Ca^{2+} from surrounding Ca^{2+} stores (calcium-induced calcium release). This, in turn, causes a propagated wave of Ca^{2+} release through the cell (40).

Ca^{2+} exerts effects on cellular processes by interacting with various Ca^{2+}-binding proteins. A major target is calmodulin, which is a ubiquitous 17 kd protein that has four nonidentical Ca^{2+}-binding domains of high affinity (41). The binding of Ca^{2+} to calmodulin results in a conformational change in the protein that increases its reversible interaction with certain enzymes and other proteins, thereby altering their activities (Fig. 34.3). Some of the common targets of the Ca^{2+}-calmodulin complex are isozymes of Ca^{2+}-calmodulin-dependent protein kinase, certain isozymes of cyclic nucleotide phosphodiesterase, and a specific phosphoprotein phosphatase termed 2B or calcineurin (10,41). In addition, Ca^{2+} interacts directly with liver phosphorylase *b* kinase through its calmodulin (δ) subunit (10). It can also activate this enzyme in other tissues via the Ca^{2+}-calmodulin complex. These interactions are undoubtedly responsible for the rapid breakdown of

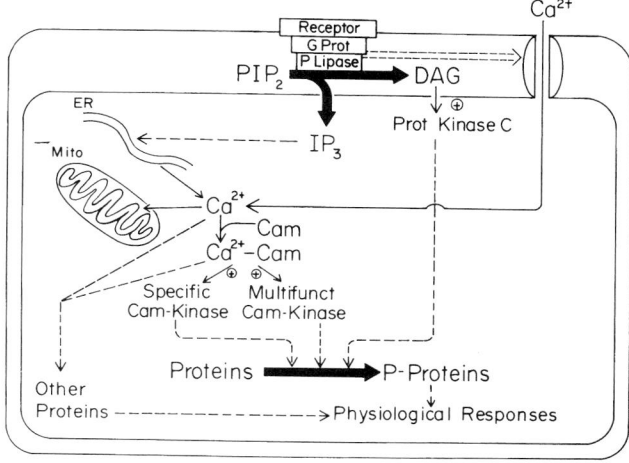

FIGURE 34.3. Mechanisms involved in physiological responses to Ca^{2+}-mobilizing agonists. *Cam*, calmodulin. *DAG*, 1,2-diacylglycerol; *ER*, endoplasmic reticulum; *mito*, mitochondria.

glycogen induced by Ca^{2+}-mobilizing agonists in liver and other tissues. The Ca^{2+}-calmodulin complex interacts with a variety of other proteins in other cells (myosin light chain kinase, types I and III adenylate cyclase, tubulin, a plasma membrane Ca^{2+}-ATPase), but some of these proteins do not seem to be targets in liver cells (9,41).

A major physiological target of Ca^{2+}-calmodulin in liver and other cells is the multifunctional type II calmodulin-dependent protein kinase (42) (Fig. 34.3) (Chapter 38). This phosphorylates and inactivates glycogen synthase, pyruvate kinase, acetyl-CoA carboxylase, ATP-citrate lyase, and phenylalanine hydroxylase, and these phosphorylations probably account for the inhibition of glycogen synthesis, glycolysis, and lipogenesis, and certain other effects seen with Ca^{2+}-mobilizing agonists in liver (9). The enzyme has additional substrates in other tissues (42). EGF produces many metabolic changes in liver that are similar to those exerted by other Ca^{2+}-mobilizing agonists, but some that are different, for example, stimulation of glycogen synthesis and glycolysis. These differences are due to the tyrosine phosphorylation of other proteins in addition to phospholipase C.

Some of the Ca^{2+} released from the ER and entering the cell during agonist stimulation of hepatocytes is taken up by mitochondria, leading to an increase in the Ca^{2+} concentration of the matrix (43,44). This leads to an activation of pyruvate dehydrogenase (45), since the phosphatase which dephosphorylates and activates the enzyme is stimulated half-maximally by approximately 1 μM Ca^{2+} (43,44). The resting free Ca^{2+} concentration in liver mitochondria *in vivo* is estimated at 0.3 μM (43), and the calcium content of these organelles can increase two-fold within a few minutes of exposure to hormones (45).

Another Ca^{2+}-sensitive intramitochondrial enzyme that is activated by Ca^{2+}-mobilizing agonists in liver is α-oxyglutarate dehydrogenase (43–45). NAD$^+$-isocitrate dehydrogenase also responds to increases in matrix Ca^{2+} *in vitro* (43,44), and there is evidence that it is activated by agonists in intact liver also. The activation of these dehydrogenases probably accounts for the reduction of $NAD(P)^+$ and the stimulation of the citrate cycle and of respiration observed in hepatocytes exposed to Ca^{2+}-mobilizing agonists. The stimulation of the cycle would also account for the increased oxidation of fatty acids to CO_2 and decreased ketogenesis seen under these conditions (9).

The roles of Ca^{2+}-binding proteins other than calmodulin in the hepatic actions of Ca^{2+}-mobilizing agonists have not been defined, although they are well documented in other tissues. For example, in some of these tissues, Ca^{2+} can interact with troponin C, gelsolin, and related proteins to influence cell contraction or movement.

DIACYLGLYCEROL AND PROTEIN KINASE C

The breakdown of PIP_2 induced by agonists releases DAG in addition to IP_3. In liver, the accumulation of DAG induced by agonists develops more slowly than IP_3 and persists at a very high level for a longer duration (46) (Fig. 34.2). This is due to the fact that the DAG is derived from another lipid besides PIP_2, namely phosphatidylcholine (PC) (47).

DAG has signaling properties, since it can activate most isozymes of protein kinase C (4,48,49)(Fig. 34.3). The α, β and γ isozymes of this kinase require Ca^{2+} and a phospholipid for activity, with phosphatidylserine being the most effective. The activity of these isozymes is low at cytosolic concentrations of Ca^{2+}, but is markedly increased by the addition of *sn*-1,2-DAG (4,48). DAG not only increases the activity of these enzymes at maximum Ca^{2+}, but, importantly, decreases the concentration of Ca^{2+} for half-maximal activity down to the submicromolar range found in the cytosol (4). The addition of arachidonic or other unsaturated long-chain fatty acids further enhances the effects of DAG on some isozymes.

The δ, ε, and ζ isozymes of protein kinase C are unaffected by Ca^{2+} since they lack the C2 (Ca^{2+}-binding) domain found in the α, β, and γ isozymes (4,48,49). The δ and ε isozymes respond to DAG, but the ζ and ι/λ isozymes do not, since they lack one of the cysteine-rich, Zn^{2+}-binding fingers of the C1 domain. The ε and ζ isozymes are stimulated by unsaturated fatty acids, but the δ isozyme is not. Additional protein kinase C isozymes (η and θ) have been identified, but their regulation is unknown.

Tumor-promoting phorbol esters such as phorbol myristate acetate have some structural similarity to DAG and produce similar changes in the activity of protein kinase C (48). This enzyme probably represents the major cellular target for these compounds *in vivo*, although other "receptors" have not been excluded. The protein kinase C isozymes are present mainly in the cytosol, and when DAG is elevated with or without Ca^{2+}, all except the ζ and ι isozymes are translocated to the plasma membrane.

Fatty acid and molecular species analyses of the DAG generated in liver in response to agonists indicate that it is initially derived from inositol phospholipids, whereas it arises later from other phospholipids, especially PC, which is the major phospholipid of cell membranes (46,49,50). Almost all the agonists that activate PIP_2 hydrolysis in cells also promote the hydrolysis of PC (47,49–52; Fig. 34.4). In general, the later phase of DAG production from PC is of slower onset but is much more prolonged than is the initial phase, which is due to PIP_2 hydrolysis (Fig. 34.2). The principal PC hydrolyzing enzyme that is activated is phospholipase D, which yields choline and PA (47,51). A large fraction of the PA derived from PC is converted to DAG by phosphatidate phosphohydrolase, accounting for the second phase of DAG formation (47,49,51).

The mechanisms by which phospholipase D is activated by agonists remain unclear. The principal mechanism appears to involve protein kinase C (47,51,52) (Fig. 34.4). Thus, the initial activation of protein kinase C, due to PIP_2 hydrolysis, leads secondarily to activation of phospholipase D (47,51,52). However, it is not known whether phospholipase D is activated by a protein–protein interaction with protein kinase C, or if phosphorylation of the enzyme or another protein is involved (51,52). Since the activation of phospholipase D yields PA, which is then converted to DAG, there is continuing production of DAG, which maintains the activation of protein kinase C and hence

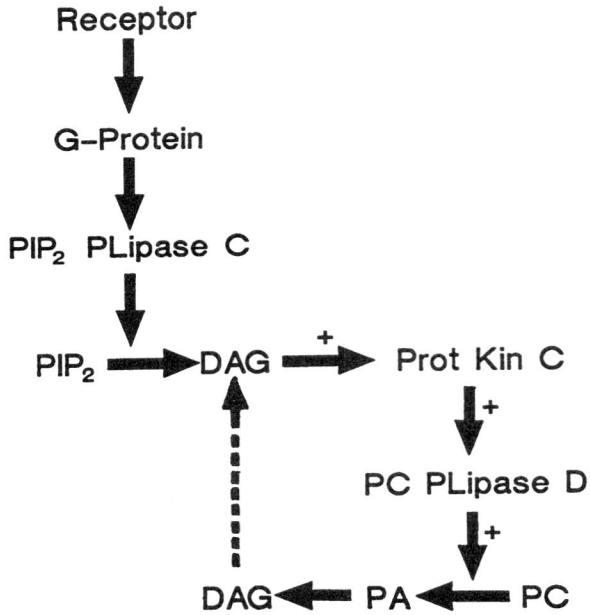

FIGURE 34.4. Role of protein kinase C (*Prot Kin C*) in the activation of phosphatidylcholine (*PC*) hydrolysis by Ca^{2+}-mobilizing agonists. *DAG*, 1,2-diacylglycerol; *PA*, phosphatidic acid.

phospholipase D. In other words, the system exhibits positive feedback. Phospholipase D can be activated directly by small G proteins of the ARF and Rho families, and there is evidence that these proteins are also involved in regulation of the enzyme by agonists (51,52). Lipids such as PIP_2 and unsaturated fatty acids may also play a role. There is evidence of a role for Ca^{2+} in the activation of phospholipase D in some cells (51,52), but this ion has little effect on the enzyme in liver.

Agonist-induced PC hydrolysis and PIP_2 hydrolysis cause differential translocation of the α, β and ϵ isozymes of protein kinase C in many cells (53–56). The situation with respect to the other isozymes is unclear, except for the ζ isozyme, which is not affected by DAG (57,58). These findings indicate that the molecular species of DAG derived from PC and PIP_2 activate different protein kinase C isozymes. The functional consequences of this differential activation are presently unclear, but it may result in the phosphorylation of different cellular substrates.

The physiological roles of the PA produced by phospholipase D action remain to be defined (47,51). There is evidence that PA stimulates protein phosphorylation, and the enzymes involved may be protein kinase Cζ (58) and another undefined protein kinase (59). A role for PA in the activation of the NADPH oxidase that generates O_2^- in polymorphonuclear leukocytes has been postulated (59,60), and there are reports that it activates Raf-1 kinase and acts as a mitogen (51). It has been speculated that it is involved in agonist-induced changes in actin polymerization (51).

As noted above, a major metabolic fate of PA in cells is conversion to DAG, but it can also be acted on by a phospholipase A_2 to form lysoPA (61). This lipid interacts with surface receptors encoded by certain edg genes (62). These receptors are coupled to G proteins, leading to the activation of many signaling enzymes including phospholipase C, phospholipase A_2, and phospholipase D (61,62). Stimulation of these enzymes leads to Ca^{2+} mobilization, release of arachidonic acid, and PA formation. As a result of the increase in cytosolic Ca^{2+}, other changes can occur, including an increase in Cl^- current and changes in cell morphology and secretory activity (61). The activation of phospholipase C is mediated by members of the G_q or G_i families, but the mechanisms of activation of the other phospholipases are unclear (61,62). In several cell types, lysoPA inhibits cAMP accumulation and activates the Raf1/MAP kinase cascade. These effects are mediated by G_i, since they are inhibited by pertussis toxin (61).

Although protein kinase C phosphorylates many proteins *in vitro*, the *in vivo* substrates in liver and most tissues remain to be defined. It is likely that many of them are located in the plasma membrane, since this is where the kinase is activated. Examples include the receptors for epidermal growth factor and α_1-adrenergic agonists (63). The phosphorylation of these receptors by protein kinase C probably accounts in part for their desensitization following agonist stimulation or

phorbol ester administration. Other receptors, for example, those for insulin, insulin-like growth factor 1, and transferrin, may be targets for protein kinase C, but the physiological consequences of their phosphorylation are presently unknown (63). There is evidence that the Na^+ pump and the Na^+/H^+ antiporter are controlled by DAG and protein kinase C (63), and this may involve phosphorylation of these entities. Ca^{2+}-mobilizing agonists cause a transient uptake of K^+ by the liver and an associated hyperpolarization. In some species, this is due to the activation of the Na^+, K^+ ATPase by protein kinase C, whereas in other species, there is evidence that a K^+ channel is controlled by Ca^{2+}. In many cells, the plasma membrane exhibits high Na^+/H^+ exchange activity, and this is regulated by Ca^{2+}-mobilizing agonists through protein kinase C, and by growth factors through their receptor tyrosine kinases (64). Regulation of ion fluxes by this system appears to be minor in liver.

With respect to other physiological substrates of protein kinase C in liver, glycogen synthase is inactivated by agents that activate protein kinase C in this tissue, but it is not clear that this involves direct phosphorylation of the enzyme (63). Several other cytoplasmic substrates have been identified as probable targets of the kinase in liver, platelets, brain, and pituitary (63,65). A prominent substrate in most tissues is a myristoylated, alanine-rich protein called MARCKS (64). This protein binds Ca^{2+}-calmodulin, but not when it is phosphorylated. It also binds actin filaments and crosslinks them, but this activity is inhibited by Ca^{2+}-calmodulin or by phosphorylation, apparently because one of the actin-binding sites is inactivated or there is dissociation of the MARCKS dimer (66). Phosphorylation of MARCKS by protein kinase C in cells is thought to promote its release from the plasma membrane and inhibition of its crosslinking action, whereas dephosphorylation allows MARCKS to provide a crossbridge between actin and the plasma membrane. In this way, it is proposed that MARCKS regulates the actin cytoskeleton (66).

Although the IP_3/Ca^{2+} and DAG/protein kinase C limbs of the PIP_2 signaling system have been shown to interact synergistically in platelets and other cell types (64), this has not been observed in liver and many other tissues. In fact, phorbol esters are usually inhibitory because they induce desensitization to Ca^{2+}-mobilizing agonists at the level of the receptor and beyond (67), presumably because of the phosphorylation of certain signaling components.

CONCLUSION

The actions of epinephrine, norepinephrine, vasopressin, angiotensin II, leu-enkephalin, ATP, and ADP on liver cells are mediated wholly or partly by an oscillating increase in cytosolic Ca^{2+}. These agonists interact with specific receptors on the cell surface to cause the activation of the β_1- and β_3-isozymes of phospholipase C, which catalyze the hydrolysis of phosphatidylinositol 4,5-bisphosphate in the inner leaflet of the plasma membrane. The coupling of the receptors to these phospholipase C isozymes involves G proteins of the G_q family. Epidermal growth factor also raises cytosolic Ca^{2+} in hepatocytes through activation and autophosphorylation of its receptor. The association of the γ_1-isozyme of phospholipase C with phosphorylated tyrosine residues in the cytoplasmic tail of the receptor leads to its activation. The hydrolysis of phosphatidylinositol 4,5-bisphosphate releases inositol l,4,5-trisphosphate and 1,2-diacylglycerol. The inositol trisphosphate enters the cytosol and binds to receptors on certain components of the ER. This causes the release of Ca^{2+} through the opening of a channel that is part of the receptor. This release initiates the propagation of a Ca^{2+} wave through the cell. The diacylglycerol remains in the plasma membrane, where it causes the translocation and activation of major isozymes of the Ca^{2+}-phospholipid-dependent protein kinase, protein kinase C.

Calcium ions released from the ER bind to several proteins, in particular the calcium-binding regulatory protein, calmodulin. The Ca^{2+}-calmodulin complex in turn interacts with a variety of enzymes and other proteins, thereby changing their activities. Major targets in liver are phosphorylase b kinase, which has calmodulin as its δ subunit, and the multisubstrate type II calmodulin-dependent protein kinase. The former enzyme phosphorylates and activates phosphorylase, leading to the breakdown of glycogen and release of glucose, whereas the latter enzyme phosphorylates and inactivates glycogen synthase and pyruvate kinase, resulting in inhibition of glycogen synthesis and glycolysis. The calmodulin-dependent protein kinase can also phosphorylate acetyl-CoA carboxylase, ATP-citrate lyase, and phenylalanine hydroxylase *in vitro*.

The increase in cytosolic Ca^{2+} induced by Ca^{2+}-mobilizing agonists in liver and other cells involves an influx of Ca^{2+} across the plasma membrane in addition to release from the ER. This results in prolongation of the Ca^{2+} increase beyond the point when the intracellular Ca^{2+} stores are depleted. Influx of Ca^{2+} occurs because depletion of Ca^{2+} in the ER activates Ca^{2+} channels in the plasma membrane. The mechanisms involved remain obscure.

The elevation of Ca^{2+} in the cytosol that is caused by Ca^{2+}-mobilizing agonists in liver and other tissues is associated with activation of certain mitochondrial enzymes, due to a rise in free Ca^{2+} in the mitochondrial matrix. These enzymes are pyruvate dehydrogenase, α-oxoglutarate dehydrogenase, and NAD^+-isocitrate dehydrogenase. The former dehydrogenase is activated because of the stimulatory effect of Ca^{2+} on pyruvate dehydrogenase phosphatase, whereas the latter dehydrogenases are directly activated by Ca^{2+}. The activation of these dehydrogenases is partly responsible for the increases in respiration, citrate cycle activity, and reduction state of $NAD(P)^+$ induced by Ca^{2+}-mobilizing agonists in liver.

The diacylglycerol released by the breakdown of phosphatidylinositol bisphosphate accumulates in the plasma membrane, where it causes the translocation and activation of certain protein kinase C isozymes, by lowering their requirement for Ca^{2+} to the cytosolic range. Tumor-promoting phorbol esters produce a similar activation and translocation of the enzyme from the cytosol to the membrane. The physiological substrates for protein kinase C have not been defined for most tissues. Probable targets in liver plasma membranes are the receptors for epidermal growth factor and α_1-adrenergic agonists, and perhaps some components of the pathways for regulating adenylate cyclase and phospholipase C. Phosphorylation of these substrates probably accounts for the desensitization caused by phorbol esters or prolonged exposure to Ca^{2+}-mobilizing agonists.

REFERENCES

1. Michell RH. Inositol phospholipids and cell surface receptor function. *Biochim Biophys Acta* 1975;415:81–147.
2. Stephens LR, Jackson TR, Hawkins PT. Agonist-stimulated synthesis of phosphatidylinositol (3,4,5)-trisphosphate: a new intracellular signaling system? *Biochim Biophys Acta* 1993;1179:27–75.
3. Berridge MJ. Inositol trisphosphate and calcium signaling. *Nature* 1993;361:315–325.
4. Nishizuka Y. The molecular heterogeneity of protein kinase C and its implications for cellular regulation. *Nature* 1988;334:661–665.
5. Shears SB. Metabolism of inositol phosphates. In: Putney JW Jr., ed. *Advances in second messenger and phosphoprotein research.* New York: Raven Press, 1992:63–92.
6. Irvine RF. Inositol phosphates and Ca^{2+} entry: toward a proliferation or a simplification? *FASEB J* 1992;6:3085–3091.
7. Thompson GA. *The regulation of membrane lipid metabolism.* Boca Raton: CRC Press, 1980.
8. Holub BJ, Kuksis A. Metabolism of molecular species of diacylglycerophospholipids. *Adv Lipid Res* 1978;16:1–125.
9. Exton JH. Mechanisms involved in calcium mobilizing agonist responses. *Adv Cyclic Nucleotide Protein Phosphorylation Res* 1986;20:211–262.
10. Ullrich A, Coussens L, Hayflock JS, et al. Human epidermal growth factor receptor cDNA sequence and aberrant expression of the amplified gene in A431 epidermoid carcinoma cells. *Nature* 1984;309:418–425.
11. Schwinn DA, Lomasney JW, Lorenz W, et al. Molecular cloning and expression of the cDNA for a novel α_1-adrenergic receptor subtype. *J Biol Chem* 1990;265:8183–8189.
12. Morel A, O'Carroll AM, Brownstein MJ, et al. Molecular cloning and expression of a rat Vla arginine vasopressin receptor. *Nature* 1992;356:523–526.
13. Sasaki K, Yamano Y, Bardhan S, et al. Cloning and expression of a complementary DNA encoding a bovine adrenal angiotensin II type-1 receptor. *Nature* 1991;351:230–232.
14. Murphy TJ, Alexander RW, Griendling KK, et al. Isolation of a cDNA encoding the vascular type-1 angiotensin II receptor. *Nature* 1991;351:233–236.
15. Savarese TM, Fraser CM. *In vitro* mutagenesis and the search for structure–function relationships among G protein-coupled receptors. *Biochem J* 1992;283:1–19.
16. Taylor SJ, Chae HZ, Rhee SG, et al. Activation of the $\beta1$ isozyme of phospholipase C by α subunits of the G_q class of G proteins. *Nature* 1991;350:516–518.

17. Smrcka AV, Hepler JR, Brown KO, et al. Regulation of polyphosphoinositide-specific phospholipase C activity by purified G_q. *Science* 1991;251:804–807.

18. Simon MI, Strathmann MP, Gautam N. Diversity of G proteins in signal transduction. *Science* 1991;252:802–808.

19. Bourne HR, Sanders DA, McCormick F. The GTPase superfamily: a conserved switch for diverse cell functions. *Nature* 1990; 348:125–132.

20. Hepler JR, Gilman AG. G Proteins. *TIBS* 1992;17:383–387.

21. Lee SB, Rhee SG. Significance of PIP_2 hydrolysis and regulation of phospholipase C isozymes. *Curr Biol* 1995;7:183–189.

22. Cadena DL, Gill GN. Receptor tyrosine kinases. *FASEB J* 1992; 6:2332–2337.

23. Koch CA, Anderson D, Moran MF, et al. SH2 and SH3 domains: elements that control interactions of cytoplasmic signaling proteins. *Science* 1991;252:668–674.

24. Johnson RM, Garrison JC. Epidermal growth factor and angiotensin II stimulate formation of inositol l,4,5- and inositol l,3,4-trisphosphate in hepatocytes. Differential inhibition by pertussis toxin and phorbol 12-myristate 13-Acetate. *J Biol Chem* 1987;262:17285–17293.

25. Yang L, Baffy G, Rhee SG, et al. Pertussis toxin-sensitive G_i protein involvement in epidermal growth factor-induced activation of phospholipase C-γ in rat hepatocytes. *J Biol Chem* 1991;266: 22451–22458.

26. Sistare FD, Picking RA, Haynes RC Jr. Sensitivity of the response of cytosolic calcium in quin-2-loaded rat hepatocytes to glucagon, adenine nucleosides, and adenine nucleotides. *J Biol Chem* 1985;260:12744–12747.

27. Blackmore PF, Exton JH. Studies on the hepatic calcium-mobilizing activity of aluminum fluoride and glucagon. Modulation by cAMP and phorbol myristate acetate. *J Biol Chem* 1986;261: 11056–11063.

28. Burgess GM, Bird GJ, Obie JF, et al. The mechanism for synergism between phospholipase C- and adenylylcyclase-linked hormones in liver. Cyclic AMP-dependent kinase augments inositol trisphosphate-mediated Ca^{2+} mobilization without increasing the cellular levels of inositol polyphosphates. *J Biol Chem* 1991;266:4772–4781.

29. Morgan NG, Charest R, Blackmore P, et al. Potentiation of $α_1$-adrenergic responses in rat liver by a cAMP-dependent mechanism. *Proc Natl Acad Sci U S A* 1984;81:4208–4212.

30. Mauger JP, Poggioli J, Claret M. Synergistic stimulation of the Ca^{2+} influx in rat hepatocytes by glucagon and the Ca^{2+}-linked hormones vasopressin and angiotensin II. *J Biol Chem* 1985;260: 11635–11642.

31. Mauger JP, Claret M. Mobilization of intracellular calcium by glucagon and cyclic AMP analogues in isolated rat hepatocytes. *FEBS Lett* 1986;195:106–108.

32. Pittner RA, Fain JN. Exposure of cultured hepatocytes to cyclic AMP enhances the vasopressin-mediated stimulation of inositol phosphate production. *Biochem J* 1989;257:455–460.

33. Lynch CJ, Blackmore PF, Charest R, et al. The relationships between receptor-binding capacity for norepinephrine, angiotensin II, and vasopressin and release of inositol trisphosphate, Ca^{2+} mobilization, and phosphorylase activation in rat liver. *Mol Pharmacol* 1985;28:93–99.

34. Joseph SK, Williamson JR. Characteristics of inositol trisphosphate-mediated Ca^{2+} release from permeabilized hepatocytes. *J Biol Chem* 1986;261:14658–14664.

35. Taylor CW. Inositol trisphosphate receptors: Ca^{2+}-modulated intracellular Ca^{2+} channels. *Biochim Biophys Acta* 1998;1436:19–33.

36. Berridge MJ, Bootman MD, Lipp P. Calcium — a life and death signal. *Nature* 1998;395:645–648.

37. Barritt GJ. Receptor-activated Ca^{2+} inflow in animal cells: a variety of pathways tailored to meet different intracellular Ca^{2+} signaling requirements. *Biochem J* 1999;337:153–169.

38. Cobbold PH, Sanchez-Bueno A, Dixon CJ. The hepatocyte calcium oscillator. *Cell Calcium* 1991;12:87–95.

39. Thomas AP, Renard DC, Rooney TA. Spatial and temporal organization of calcium signaling in hepatocytes. *Cell Calcium* 1991;12:111–126.

40. Berridge MJ. Calcium oscillations. *J Biol Chem* 1990;265: 9583–9586.

41. Klee CB, Vanaman TC. Calmodulin. In: Anfinsen CB, Edsall JT, Richards FM, eds. *Advances in Protein Chemistry*. New York: Academic Press, 1982:213–321.

42. Colbran RJ, Schworer CM, Hashimoto Y, et al. Calcium/ calmodulin-dependent protein kinase II. *Biochem J* 1989;258: 313–325.

43. Denton RM, McCormack JG. Ca^{2+} transport by mammalian mitochondria and its role in hormone action. *J Physiol* 1985; 249:E545–E554.

44. Hansford RG. Relation between mitochondrial calcium transport and control of energy metabolism. *Rev Physiol Biochem Pharmacol* 1985;102:1–72.

45. Assimacopoulos-Neannet F, McCormack JG, Jeanrenaud B. Vasopressin and/or glucagon rapidly increases mitochondrial calcium and oxidative enzyme activities in the perfused rat liver. *J Biol Chem* 1986;261:8799–8804.

46. Bocckino SB, Blackmore PF, Exton JH. Stimulation of 1,2-diacylglycerol accumulation in hepatocytes by vasopressin, epinephrine, and angiotensin II. *J Biol Chem* 1985;260:14201–14207.

47. Exton JH. Signaling through phosphatidylcholine breakdown. *J Biol Chem* 1990;265:1–4.

48. Bell RM, Burns DJ. Lipid activation of protein kinase C. *J Biol Chem* 1991;266:4661–4664.

49. Asaoka Y, Nakamura S, Yoshida K, et al. Protein kinase C, calcium, and phospholipid degradation. *TIBS* 1991;17:414–417.

50. Augert G, Bocckino SB, Blackmore PF, et al. Hormonal stimulation of diacylglycerol formation in hepatocytes. Evidence for phosphatidylcholine breakdown. *J Biol Chem* 1989;264:21689–21698.

51. Exton JH. Phospholipase D: Enzymology, mechanisms of regulation, and function. *Physiol Rev* 1997;77:303–320.

52. Exton JH. Regulation of phospholipase D. *Biochim Biophys Acta* 1999;1439:121–133.

53. Pfeffer LM, Eisenkraft BL, Reich NC, et al. Transmembrane signaling by interferon α involves diacylglycerol production and activation of the ε isoform of protein kinase C in Daudi cells. *Proc Natl Acad Sci U S A* 1991;88:7988–7992.

54. Kiley SC, Parker PJ, Fabbro D, et al. Differential regulation of protein kinase C isozymes by thyrotropin-releasing hormone in GH_4C_1 cells. *J Biol Chem* 1991;266:23761–23768.

55. Leach, KL, Ruff VA, Wright TM, et al. Dissociation of protein kinase C activation and *sn* -1,2-diacylglycerol formation. Comparison of phosphatidylinositol- and phosphatidylcholine-derived diglycerides in α-thrombin-stimulated fibroblasts. *J Biol Chem* 1991;266:3215–3221.

56. Baldassare JJ, Henderson PA, Burns D. Translocation of protein kinase C isozymes in thrombin-stimulated human platelets. Correlation with 1,2-diacylglycerol levels. *J Biol Chem* 1992;267: 15585–15590.

57. Ways DK, Cook PP, Webster C, et al. Effect of phorbol esters on protein kinase C-ζ. *J Biol Chem* 1992;267:4799–4805.

58. Nakanishi H, Exton JH. Purification and characterization of the ζ isoform of protein kinase C from bovine kidney. *J Biol Chem* 1992;267:16347–16354.

59. Waite KA, Wallin R, Qualliotine-Mann D, et al. Phosphatidic acid-mediated phosphorylation of the NADPH oxidase component p47-*phox*. *J Biol Chem* 1997;272:15569–15578.

60. Agwu DE, McPhail LC, Sozzani S, et al. Phosphatidic acid as a second messenger in human polymorphonuclear leukocytes. Effects on activation of NADPH oxidase. *J Clin Invest* 1991;88: 531–539.

61. Moolenaar WH. Lysophosphatidic acid, a multifunctional phospholipid messenger. *J Biol Chem* 1995;270:12949–12952.

62. Goetzl EJ, An S. Diversity of cellular receptors and functions for the lysophospholipid growth factors lysophosphatidic acid and sphingosine 1-phosphate. *FASEB J* 1998;12:1589–1598.

63. Exton JH. Mechanisms of α_1-adrenergic responses. Roles of calcium, phosphoinositides, guanine nucleotides, diacylglycerol, calmodulin, and changes in protein phosphorylation. In: Elson EL, Frazier WA, Glaser L, eds. *Methods and Reviews*, New York: Plenum, 1988:113–182.

64. Seifter JL, Aronson PS. Properties and physiological roles of the plasma membrane sodium–hydrogen exchanger. *J Clin Invest* 1986;78:859–864.

65. Nishizuka Y. The role of protein kinase C in cell surface signal transduction and tumour promotion. *Nature* 1984;308:693–698.

66. Aderem A. Signal transduction and the action cytoskeleton: the roles of MARCKS and profilin. *TIBS* 1992;17:438–443.

67. Nishizuka Y. The molecular heterogeneity of protein kinase C and its implications for cellular regulation. *Nature* 1988;334:661–665.

SYNTHESIS OF AND SIGNALING THROUGH D-3 PHOSPHOINOSITIDES

RIAL A. CHRISTENSEN
ISABEL DE AÓS SCHERPENSEEL
LYUBA VARTICOVSKI

Inositol-containing lipids were recognized as early as 1930 as components of biological membranes in mycobacteria, plants, and mammalian cells (reviewed in ref. 1). Over the next 20 years, the structure of these lipids as phosphorylated derivatives of phosphatidylinositol (PI) was elucidated (2). PI is the simplest component of this family and has an inositol ring attached by its D-1-OH group to phosphatidic acid. In cells, the free hydroxyl groups of inositol ring, except those at the D-2 and D-6 positions, can be phosphorylated in different combinations, which gives each carbon atom its unique identity and creates the diversity among the inositol-containing phospholipids. Eight different PI species have been identified in eukaryotic cells to date. The function of these lipids began to be clarified in the early 1950s. However, their participation in intracellular signal transduction was not recognized until the early 1980s, and the nature of the protein–phospholipid interactions has only been appreciated in the last few years. In this chapter, we focus on the enzymes that generate polyphosphoinositides phosphorylated in the D-3 position and their role in signal transduction.

Regarding the liver, PI 3-kinase has been increasingly demonstrated to play a critical role in apoptosis (Chapter 34), differentiation (Chapter 2), regeneration (Chapter 42 and website chapter 🖥 W-3), malignant transformation (Chapter 68), intracellular trafficking (Chapter 24), and membrane transport (Chapter 10). PI 3-kinase participates in these and other functions in hepatocytes (Chapter 36), endothelial cells (Chapter 30), Kupffer cells (website chapter 🖥 W-26), stellate cells (Chapter 31), and biliary epithelial cells (Chapter 29). These rapid developments are remarkable because, until recent years, PI 3-kinase had been associated only with activity of tyrosine kinase growth factors and oncogenes. In addition, the mechanisms whereby the 3' phosphoinositide products of the enzyme affect these processes were unknown.

SUBSTRATES FOR THE SYNTHESIS OF D-3 PHOSPHOINOSITIDES

Phospholipids constitute approximately 3% of the total cell weight of mammalian cells (3). The inositol-containing phospholipids represent less than 20% of total cellular phospholipids (reviewed in ref. 4). The majority (up to 80%) of the inositol-containing lipids are present as PI (132). PI 4-phosphate (PI 4-P) and PI 4,5-bisphosphate (PI 4,5-P_2) share the remaining fraction of the inositol-containing lipids in nonstimulated mammalian cells. The 3' phosphorylated polyphosphoinositide, PI 3-P, constitutes a

R. A. Christensen and I. De Aós Scherpenseel: Department of Medicine, Center for Biomedical Research, St. Elizabeth's Medical Center, Tufts University School of Medicine, Boston, Massachusetts 02135.

L. Varticovski: Departments of Medicine and Physiology, Tufts University School of Medicine, Boston, Massachusetts 02115; Department of Medicine, St. Elizabeth's Medical Center, Boston, Massachusetts 02135.

small fraction (less than 0.25%) of total inositol-containing phospholipids, and even smaller fractions are detected as PI $3,4-P_2$ and PI $3,4,5-P_3$ in transformed or growth factor-stimulated cells. These polyphosphoinositides are not substrates for the PI-specific phospholipases C (PLC) (6,7), enzymes that cleave inositol phospholipids into membrane-bound diacylglycerol and soluble inositol phosphates. Thus, this separates PI 3-kinase signaling from the PLC/PI $4,5-P_2$ pathway, a pathway that leads to Ca^{2+} release and activation of protein kinase C (PKC). Instead, phosphoinositides phosphorylated in the D-3 position are substrates for lipid kinases and phosphatases that act on the inositol ring.

THE PI 3-KINASE FAMILY

PI 3-kinase was initially recognized as a novel enzymatic activity associated with the virally encoded protein-tyrosine kinases, v-*src*, and v-*ros* (8,9). Subsequently, this activity was found in association with other receptor and nonreceptor protein-tyrosine kinases, such as platelet-derived growth factor receptor (PDGFR) and the polyoma middle T/pp 60^{c-src} complex (10–15). This PI kinase activity was shown to be different from the previously characterized PI 4-kinase based on its sensitivity to detergents and adenosine (16,17). Further studies identified a distinct activity that phospho-

rylated the D-3 position of the inositol ring of purified PI, PI 4-P and PI $4,5-P_2$ (18). This discovery led to the purification of PI 3-kinase from rat liver and brain (19,20). Nine mammalian genes have been cloned to date, and their protein products are part of the PI 3-kinase family that has been grouped into three classes (I–III) (21) based on their structure, *in vitro* substrate specificity and probable mechanism of regulation (Table 35.1).

Class I PI 3-Kinases

Structure of Class I PI 3-Kinases

Class I PI 3-kinases are heterodimeric complexes that consist of a catalytic subunit and an adaptor/regulatory subunit. Class I enzymes are further subdivided into Class I_A PI 3-kinases and Class I_B PI 3-kinases, based on association with different regulatory subunits (Table 35.1). The mammalian Class I_A catalytic subunits include three isoforms: p110α, p110β, and p110δ. The catalytic subunits, p110α and p110β are found in most mammalian tissues, whereas p110δ is expressed in leukocytes (22). There are five adaptor/regulatory subunits for mammalian Class I_A PI 3-kinases. These arise from three different genes: p85α, p85β, and p55PIK/p55γ with two additional protein products (p55α and p50α) that result from the alternate splicing of p85α (reviewed in ref. 23). p85α is ubiquitously distrib-

TABLE 35.1. CLASSIFICATION OF THE MAMMALIAN MEMBERS OF THE PI 3-KINASE FAMILY: STRUCTURAL AND DOMAIN ORGANIZATION OF THE SUBUNITS, LIPID SUBSTRATES OF THE ENZYMES, AND MECHANISMS OF REGULATION

Enzyme	Subunits Catalytic	Subunits Adaptor	Structural Features		Lipid Substrates *in vitro*	Lipid Substrates *in vivo*	Regulation
Class I A	p110α p110β p110δ			p110 α,β,δ	PI PI 4-P PI $4,5-P_2$	PI $4,5-P_2$	p85 Ras Heterotrimeric G-proteins
		p85α		p85α			
		p85β		p85β			Tyrosine Kinases SH3 domains PIP_3
		p55α,γ		p55α,γ			
		p50α		p50α			
B				p110γ			Ras Heterotrimeric G-proteins
	p110γ	p101		p101			
Class II	PI3K-C2α PI3K-C2β PI3K-C2γ			PI3K-C2	PI PI 4-P PI $4,5-P_2$	?	Unknown ? Tyrosine Kinases or Heterotrimeric G-proteins. Not Ras
Class III	VpS34p homologue (PI 3-K III)	VpS15p homologue (p150)		PI 3-K III VpS34p			
				p150 VpS15p	PI	PI	Constitutive

Kinase domain   ● p85 binding domain   ⌒ SH2 domain   ▯ proline-rich domain   ⊙ C2 domain

⊠ Ras domain   □ PIK domain   ● SH3 domain   Rho-GAP domain   △ PX domain

uted, whereas p85β is expressed primarily in bovine brain and lymphoid tissues (24). Although there are no reports of preferential interactions between the regulatory and catalytic subunits, differential tissue distribution may be responsible for some differences in function.

The p110 subunits contain a C-terminal catalytic domain that is also found in related protein and lipid kinases, a PIK domain that is found in all lipid kinases to which no known function has been assigned, and a region for association with p21^{ras} (25). The Class I$_A$ PI 3-kinases also have an N-terminal region that is required for interaction with the regulatory subunits. In addition to lipid kinase activity, the catalytic subunit has an intrinsic serine/threonine (Ser/Thr) protein kinase activity and phosphorylates the inter-SH2 domain of p85 (19,26), and autophosphorylates p110δ (27), which results in downregulation of the lipid kinase activity. The p110δ PI 3-kinase has one proline-rich region and a leucine-zipper-like domain whose functions have not been fully characterized (27).

The p85α and β regulatory subunits contain two *src* homology-2 (SH2) domains and one N-terminal *src* homology-3 (SH3) domain. The region between the two SH2 domains (inter-SH2 domain) interacts with the Class I$_A$ catalytic subunits (26,28). Two proline rich regions (P1 and P2) of p85 associate with SH3 domains of *c-abl*, p56^{lck}, p59^{fyn}, and p60^{v-src}. The SH3 domain of the p85 subunit can also self-associate through the proline-rich regions and bind to proline-rich regions in other proteins (29). p85 also has a domain which is homologous to the C-terminal region of the breakpoint cluster region gene product (BH domain). The BH domain of p85 contains a GTPase-activating protein domain (GAP domain) which provides binding sites for the Rho family proteins, Cdc42 and Rac1, although p85 itself does not have GTPase activity (30).

Alternative splicing of p85α mRNA gives rise to proteins that migrate at 50 and 55 kd in sodium dodecyl sulfate polyacrylamide gels (31,32). These proteins contain only the second proline-rich region and lack the SH3 and GAP domains. The N-terminal region of p55α contains a 34-amino-acid (aa) fragment which is not found in p85. The other splice form, p50α, contains a 6-aa extension (32). The third gene, p55PIK/p55γ, encodes for a protein with similar overall structure to p55α (33). Thus, there is a multitude of mechanisms by which the regulatory subunits could modulate the constitutive and signal-mediated interactions of PI 3-kinase with other intracellular proteins.

The only Class I$_B$ PI 3-kinase identified to date is p110γ, which is found only in mammals and is expressed highly in white blood cells (34). The structure of p110γ is similar to other Class I enzymes except for the lack of the N-terminal p85-binding sequence. The p110γ isoform binds to a 101-kd regulatory protein which has no sequence homology to any other known protein (35). Although the binding sites have not been mapped, p101 is required for activation of p110γ by heterotrimeric G proteins (35–37).

Activity and Regulation of Class IA PI 3-Kinases

The *in vitro* substrates for all Class I PI 3-kinases include PI, PI 4-P, and PI 4,5-P$_2$, whereas their preferred substrate *in vivo* is PI 4,5-P$_2$ (38). The delayed generation of PI 3,4-P$_2$ in response to some growth factors is likely due to dephosphorylation of PI 3,4,5-P$_3$ by a 5′-inositol phosphatase rather than a direct effect of the Class I PI 3-kinases (39,40). PI 3,4-P$_2$ or PI 3,4,5-P$_3$ are not detectable in quiescent cells, and transient accumulation of these products is only observed in response to growth factors (18,41). Class I$_A$ PI 3-kinases can also phosphorylate PI 5-P *in vitro* (38), although there is no evidence for accumulation of PI 3,5-P$_2$ in response to Class I$_A$ PI 3-kinase agonists (reviewed in ref. 42).

Activation of Class I$_A$ PI 3-kinases is tightly controlled by growth factor receptors that have intrinsic protein tyrosine kinase activity, as well as by receptors coupled to *src*-like protein tyrosine kinases, p21^{ras} or heterotrimeric G proteins. Receptor-mediated PI 3-kinase activation, which have been well characterized, include: platelet-derived growth factor (PDGF), insulin, insulin-like growth factor 1 (IGF-1) (see Chapter 36), nerve growth factor (NGF), stem cell growth factor (SCF), epidermal growth factor (EGF), and hepatocyte growth factor (HGF) (see Chapter 43) (reviewed in refs. 23,42). Translocation of PI 3-kinase to the plasma membrane brings the catalytic subunit in proximity to its substrates, which is required for accumulation of PI 3-kinase lipid products in adherent cells (43,44), but not in hematopoietic cells (44). Activation of PI 3-kinase based on translocation to the plasma membrane has been verified by myristoylated or C-terminal isoprenylated PI 3-kinase mutants (45). The adaptor subunits are recruited to the membrane by an interaction of their SH2 domains with specific tyrosine-phosphorylated motifs, pTyr-X1-X2-Met (YXXM) on the intracellular domain of the receptor or other adaptor proteins (46). The mechanism whereby p85 increases the lipid kinase activity in the catalytic subunit is still unclear. However, association of phosphotyrosine-containing synthetic peptides with the SH2 domain of p85 increases the catalytic activity of the p110 subunit *in vitro* (47,48). The downregulation of PI 3-kinase activity could be mediated by the highly phosphorylated product, PI 3,4,5-P$_3$, which competes with pYXXM motifs for p85 SH2 docking sites and could result in dissociation of PI 3-kinase from the plasma membrane (49). The versatility of the regulatory subunits to interact with multiple signaling molecules and the ability to form direct complexes with the receptors allows tight regulation of intracellular PI 3-kinase.

PI 3-kinase may also be recruited by interaction with the p85 SH3 domain. Two proline-rich consensus motifs with higher affinity for the p85 SH3 domain have been identified, RXLPPRPXX and XXXPPXPXX, where X could be any amino acid except cysteine (50). A constitutive interaction of the p85 SH3 domain with widely expressed adaptor proteins, such as *c-cbl*, *in vitro* and *in vivo* has been identified (51,52). The SH3 domain of p85, expressed as a GST-fusion protein, binds to the microtubule-associated protein, dynamin (53) (see Chapter 10), and this interaction occurs *in vivo* (231).

The p85α SH3 domain also binds to each of the proline-rich regions, P1 and P2, within p85 itself (29). The P1 and P2 domains of p85 can also associate with SH3 domains of Src family kinase members, *src, lck, lyn, fyn,* and *abl* (29,54–57). The binding of p85 to *lyn* and *fyn* increases the lipid kinase activity (58). The N-terminal proline-rich region, preferentially binds to the SH3 domain of *c-src* (58). The p50α, p55α, and p55γ subunits have only one proline-rich motif, and lack the N-terminal proline-rich region that preferentially binds *c-src*. The p85β possesses a distinct C-terminal proline-rich motif. Thus, a different subset of SH3-containing proteins could associate *in vivo* with each of the regulatory subunits.

The catalytic subunits also have intrinsic protein Ser/Thr kinase activity (26,27,59). The substrates of this activity are serine residues within the catalytic and the regulatory subunits. The p85α regulatory subunit has been shown to be phosphorylated by p110α on Ser 608, which reduces the lipid kinase activity several-fold (26,59). p110δ autophosphorylation also downregulates the lipid kinase activity (27). In contrast, p110γ autophosphorylation does not seem to affect its enzymatic activity (60). Several investigators have reported that p85 subunits become tyrosine-phosphorylated in response to growth factors (11,61–65). No change in lipid kinase activity has been attributed to this modification (66,67).

Class I$_A$ and I$_B$ enzymes are activated by the interaction of p110 subunits with GTP-loaded p21^{ras}, which signals through a number of downstream effectors. When GTP-loaded Ras is bound to p110α, the lipid kinase activity increases two- to three-fold *in vitro* and *in vivo* (25,68). Immunoprecipitation with anti-Ras antibodies provided evidence for the physical association of p21^{ras} and the p85/p110α heterodimer (69). Amino acid residues 133–314 within p110α are necessary for binding to GTP-Ras (68,70). Transient transfection of constitutively active Ras (V12Ras) leads to an accumulation of PI 3,4-P$_2$ and PI 3,4,5-P$_3$ lipid products, while dominant negative Ras (N17Ras) abrogates growth factor-mediated activation of PI 3-kinase (25). These data provided evidence for Ras as an upstream regulator of PI 3-kinase, whereas other studies using a PDGFR mutant that lacks the PI 3-kinase docking site fail to activate Ras (71), which suggests that Ras could be a downstream target of PI 3-kinase.

In addition, βγ subunits of G-protein coupled receptors stimulate p85 immunoprecipitable PI 3-kinase activity (72,73), and insulin-activated PI 3-kinase is synergistically activated by a pertussis toxin-sensitive G-protein (72). The βγ subunits specifically activate p85-associated p110β but not p110α isoforms *in vitro*, and Gβγ-sensitive PI 3-kinase partially purified from rat liver is activated synergistically by phosphotyrosyl peptides (72–75). Thus, the p110β isoform

can function as a cross-talk between protein–tyrosine kinases and G-protein-mediated signaling.

Other proposed models for activation of Class I$_A$ PI 3-kinase have been reported, but their significance in intracellular signaling is controversial. The phosphatidylinositol transfer protein (PITP) (76), profilin and gelsolin have also been shown to increase PI 3-kinase activity in an Src-dependent manner (reviewed in ref. 77). A membrane-permeable peptide generated from the PI 4,5-P$_2$-binding site of gelsolin is a potent activator of PI 3-kinase in intact cells (78,79,230). It has been proposed that calmodulin could activate PI 3-kinase by binding to p85 SH2 domains (80). The binding of the p85 BH domain to the Rho family GTPases, Rac and Cdc42, also increases PI 3-kinase activity (30,81), although other studies failed detect this interaction *in vivo* (25).

The use of knockout and transgenic mice has been useful in establishing the function of Class I$_A$ PI 3-kinases. Deletion or expression of catalytically inactive PI 3-kinase subunits p110α or p110β result in embryonic lethality between E9.5 and E10.5 (82). The results for the p110α knockout were not surprising due to the broad tissue distribution, whereas the similar phenotype observed for the p110β mutant was less expected. The study of Class I PI 3-kinases in the nematode *C. elegans* has also revealed interesting results. Deletion of Class I$_A$ PI 3-kinase results in the entry into the arrested dauer stage and prolongs the lifespan of the nematode (83), which suggests a role for PI 3-kinase as a regulator of longevity.

Most mice which lack p85α and its splice variants, p50α and p55α, do not survive to birth, and those that do have impaired B cell development with normal T cell lineages (84). Gene targeting of the first exon of p85α, which leads to deletion of p85α without affecting the expression of p50α and p55α isoforms, results in mice that are viable but develop B cell immunodeficiency that is reminiscent of Btk$^{-/-}$ mice. These mice also have increased sensitivity to insulin by producing elevated PI 3,4,5-P$_3$ levels, which suggests that p50α participates in insulin-mediated signaling (85,86). Mice which lack p85α invariably manifest extensive hepatic necrosis of unknown pathogenesis. The p85β knockout mice are also viable, which is consistent with the restricted expression of this subunit (87). The p85α is over-expressed in p110β$^{-/-}$ animals, whereas expression of catalytic subunits is reduced in p85α$^{-/-}$ mice (84), which indicates that the expression of PI 3-kinase subunits is interdependent.

Activity and Regulation of Class I$_B$ PI 3-Kinase

The p110γ catalytic subunit is the only member of this group and differs from the Class I$_A$ PI 3-kinases in that it lacks an N-terminal p85-binding domain. Class I$_B$ PI 3-kinase is activated directly by the βγ subunits of heterotrimeric G proteins (30,90–92). Some groups have also reported that p110γ can be activated by G-protein associated α subunits (90,93). In addition, a modest activation of p110γ is mediated by p21^{ras} (94). The interaction of Ras with p110γ occurs through the N-terminal region homologous to the Ras-binding site of Class I$_A$ isoforms (94). Interestingly, the Ras/p110γ interaction prevents Ras from GTPase activity, suggesting a reciprocal modulation (95).

Receptors coupled to heterotrimeric G proteins (GPCR) are one of the largest known families of integral membrane receptors. Binding of ligands to growth factor receptors or activation of odor and taste receptors coupled to heptahelical GPCR triggers the exchange of GDP for GTP in the α subunit. This leads to dissociation of βγ subunits. This process is amplified in a way that activation of one GPCR leads to activation of multiple G proteins, leading GTP-bound α and free βγ subunits to participate, independently, in regulation of other pathways. G-protein-mediated activation of PI 3-kinase *in vivo* was reported prior to cloning and characterization of the catalytic subunits (96). The precise mechanism of regulation of p110γ is not well understood. However, recent identification of an adaptor protein, p101 (35), which is required for activation of p110γ by Gβγ (36), provides a plausible mechanism.

Ligands that activate heterotrimeric G-proteins have also been reported to stimulate Class I$_A$ PI 3-kinase activity as discussed in the section that describes the activity and regulation of Class I$_A$ PI 3-kinases. This activity is most likely mediated by p110β. The activation of p85-associated PI 3-kinase isoforms and p110γ are probably interdependent and may explain the synergy between responses initiated by protein–tyrosine kinase receptors and heterotrimeric G-protein receptors.

The functional role of p110γ has been difficult to study because of the crossover effects between the Class I PI 3-kinase isoforms. Recent studies involving mice which lack p110γ identified a link to a chemotactic response provided by G-type receptors, interleukin-8 (IL-8), C5a and the formylated peptide, fMLP (97,98). Neutrophils from these mice have defective homing with increased accumulation in the peripheral blood, impaired chemoattractant-induced migration and activation of Akt but no apparent changes in responses generated by receptor protein–tyrosine kinases. These results complement studies which suggest that activation of chemotactic GPCRs is required for migration of neutrophils in response to chemoattractants (99,100).

Mice which lack p110γ have impaired thymocyte development (101), in contrast to p85 knockout mice that showed a defect in B-cell development (84). Thus, type I PI 3-kinase-mediated activation of Akt is required for survival of lymphoid cells in both lymphoid lineages at specific stages of differentiation. In addition, p110γ$^{-/-}$ mice are defective in T cell-mediated secretion of IL-2 (101) despite normal phosphotyrosine-mediated binding of PI 3-kinase to the T cell receptor. Therefore, T cell receptor-mediated secretion of IL-2 requires functional p110γ, which suggests that p110γ participates in vesicular trafficking and secretion.

Class II PI 3-Kinases

Structure of Class II PI 3-Kinases

Class II PI 3-kinase catalytic subunits are larger proteins (170 to 220 kd) that contain a C2 domain, a PX domain, a PIK domain and a catalytic domain which shares 40% to 50% sequence homology with Class I enzymes. Three different isoforms of Class II PI 3-kinases are encoded by separate genes: PI 3-K-C2α, β, and γ. PI 3-K-C2α and β have a PX domain identified in other signaling molecules, phox-40 and phox-70, whose function is unclear (reviewed in ref. 42). PI 3-K-C2α and β are found ubiquitously in mammals, whereas PI 3-kinase-C2γ is found primarily in the liver (102,103).

The defining feature of this class of PI 3-kinases is the C-terminal C2 domain (104–106). C2 domains have been implicated in the Ca^{2+}-dependent binding of proteins to lipid vesicles. However, Class II PI 3-kinases lack a critical Asp residue that is required for Ca^{2+}-sensitive phospholipid binding. In contrast to the cytosolic distribution of Class I enzymes, Class II enzymes are associated with the membrane fraction (104).

Activity and Regulation of Class II PI 3-Kinases

In vitro, Class II PI 3-kinases phosphorylate only PI and PI 4-P, although PI 3-K-C2α also phosphorylates PI 4,5-P$_2$ in the presence of phosphatidylserine (106). Regulation may be provided by weak acidic phospholipid binding to the C2 domain in a Ca^{2+}-independent fashion (105). Class II PI 3-kinases are activated by insulin, EGF, PDGF, integrins, and a chemokine, MCP-1, and are sensitive to nanomolar concentrations of wortmannin (107–109). No adaptor proteins have been identified, and the mechanisms of control for these PI 3-kinases is still unknown. The *Drosophila* Class II PI 3-kinase, PI3K-68D/cpk, has been found in association with 90 kd and 190 kd tyrosine-phosphorylated proteins, implying that they could participate in the activation of Class II PI 3-kinases (110).

Class III PI 3-Kinases

Structure of Class III PI 3-Kinases

The first Class III PI 3-kinase was identified in yeast (Vps34p). This enzyme exists as a complex with Vps15p, whereas in mammalian cells the homologue of Vps34p, PI 3-K III, associates with a p150 regulatory subunit (111–114). The catalytic subunit of PI 3-K III has a kinase domain, a PIK domain, and a Vps15p/p150 binding motif (114). The mammalian regulatory subunit, p150, has 30% identity with its yeast counterpart (115). Vps15p and p150 are N-terminally myristoylated Ser/Thr kinases. Myristoylation of these proteins recruits them to the plasma membrane, thus providing a constitutive interaction of PI 3-kinase with its substrates. In addition to having a Ser/Thr domain, the p150 adaptor subunit has a series of HEAT repeats (116) and C-terminal WD motifs (117) which may regulate interactions with other proteins.

Activity and Regulation of Class III PI 3-Kinases

Vps34p and its homologues in *Dictyostelium, Drosophila* and humans use only PI as their substrate and will not phosphorylate PI 4-P or PI 4,5-P$_2$ *in vitro* (114). PI 3-P is the only 3' phosphorylated phosphoinositide detected in yeast and is constitutively present in all mammalian cells (114,118). Although PI 3-P levels do not change in response to activation of receptor–tyrosine kinases, large increases in PI 3-P are observed only in platelets in response to agonists (119). Mutational analysis of the yeast Vps34p demonstrated that this lipid kinase is essential for accurate vesicle-mediated transport, osmoregulation, and endocytosis (120).

PI 3-KINASE INHIBITORS

There are two extensively studied cell-permeable inhibitors of PI 3-kinases, wortmannin and LY294002 (121–123). They are not structurally related and block the enzymatic activity by different mechanisms. Wortmannin binds covalently to the PI 3-kinase catalytic subunits (124), whereas LY294002 is a competitive inhibitor of ATP binding (123). Formation of a Schiff-base between p110α and wortmannin involves a conserved Lys[802] residue which is also required for ATP hydrolysis (124). *In vitro,* Class I PI 3-kinases are blocked by 1 nM wortmannin or by 1μM LY294002. Treatment of cells with 25 to 50 nM wortman-

nin or by 10 to 20μM LY294002 blocks PI 3-kinase-dependent biological responses. At higher concentrations, these compounds lose specificity. Class II PI 3-kinases are less sensitive to these agents, and the ubiquitously expressed PI 3-K-C2α isoform is ten-fold more resistant to wortmannin (106,125). The mammalian Class III PI 3-kinase are also sensitive to wortmannin (114), whereas their *S. cerevisiae* and *S. pombe* counterpart, Vps34, is resistant (126,127).

ALTERNATE PATHWAYS FOR GENERATING D-3 POLYPHOSPHOINOSITIDES

Until recently, PI 4-P was the only PIP product detected in cells. Although PI 4-P is the most abundant monophosphoinositide, PI 3-P and PI 5-P also occur physiologically. A number of kinases and phosphatases that generate PI 3,4-P$_2$ or PI 3,5-P$_2$ from PIPs have recently been identified.

In the early 1990s, two types of PIP kinases were isolated from human erythrocytes based on their ability to phosphorylate PI 4-P in vitro (128). These were subsequently designated as type I (68 kd) and type II (53 kd) PIP kinases based on their biochemical properties (Table 35.2). In addition, a 90 kd PIP kinase was isolated from rat brain which was immunologically similar to type I PIP kinase and was, therefore, designated type Ib (129). Biochemical characterization of these enzymes indicated that both type Ia and type Ib, but not the type II isoform, were stimulated in vitro by phosphatidic acid (PA) (129).

TABLE 35.2. CLASSIFICATION OF THE PIP 4-KINASES AND PIP 5-KINASES: STRUCTURAL FEATURES OF THE ENZYMES, THEIR LIPID SUBSTRATES, AND MECHANISMS OF REGULATION

| Enzyme | Subunits | | Structural Features | Lipid Substrates | | Regulation |
	Catalytic	Adaptor		*in vitro*	*in vivo*	
PIP 4-K	*Human* PIP 4-K IIα (47 kd) IIβ (47 kd) *Rat* PIP 4-K IIγ (47 kd)	TNFR	⊐▯⫽▯⊏ PIP 4-KII (α, β, γ)	PI 5-P PI 3-P	PI 5-P PI 3-P	Integrin-mediated pathway TNFα stimulates PIP 4-KIIβ Inhibited by: PI 4,5-P$_2$ Heparin
PIP 5-K	*Human* PIP 5-K Iα (61 kd) Iβ (68 kd) (90 kd) (110 kd) *Mouse* PIP 5-K Iα (68 kd) Iβ (68 kd) Iγ (90 kd)		⊢⫽⊣ PIP 5-KI (α, β)	PI 4-P PI 3-P PI 3,4-P$_2$ PI 3,5-P$_2$	PI 4-P PI 3-P PI 3,4-P$_2$ PI 3,5-P$_2$	Regulated by: Heterotrimeric G proteins Small g proteins Rac I and Rho A Activated by: Phosphatidic acid Heparin Spermine Inhibited by: PI 4,5-P$_2$

⫽⫽⫽ catalytic domain ▯ proline-rich domain

Structure of PIP Kinase Family

The type II PIP kinase (type IIα) was the first enzyme in this family to be cloned (130,131). Since then, two other type II PIP kinases (β and γ) have been cloned and characterized (reviewed in ref. 132). The structure and distribution of the type II PIP kinases are similar to those of the type I PIP kinases and are discussed in the next section.

Three distinct type I PIP 5-kinases have been cloned in the mouse. The type Iα and β isoforms migrate at 68 kd, whereas the third, type Iγ, migrates at 87 to 90 kd (133). There are several different isoforms for each of the type I PIP 5-kinases which result from alternate splicing. Human homologues of the murine type Iα and β isoforms have also been cloned (reviewed in ref. 132). The human type Iα is closer to the mouse type Iβ (134). Two PIP kinases have also been identified in *S. cerevisiae*; Mss4, which is biochemically similar to mammalian type I PIP 5-kinase (135,136), and FAB1. FAB1 is unique in that it converts PI 3-P to PI 3,5-P_2 and does not utilize other types of phosphoinositides (137). Therefore, this enzyme could be considered as a type III PIP kinase.

PIP 4-kinases and PIP 5-kinases are about 35% identical in their putative catalytic core domain, but are different in their N- and C-terminal regions, and neither share homology with other lipid or protein kinases (reviewed in refs. 42,132). The PIP 4- but not 5-kinases contain two proline-rich domains within their catalytic core which could provide binding sites for SH3 domain-containing proteins.

Although at least one of the isoforms of types I and II PIP kinases is found in mammalian tissues, the expression level varies considerably for each isoform (reviewed in ref. 132). With the exception of the type IIα PIP kinase, both types I and II PIP kinases are found at very low levels in the liver (132).

Activity and Regulation of PIP Kinases

Despite homology in the DNA sequence, PIP kinases phosphorylate the inositol ring at different positions. Type II PIP kinase phosphorylates the D-4- position of PI 3-P and PI 5-P *in vitro* (138,139) and *in vivo* (140,141), and could be considered a 4-OH kinase. Type I PIP kinase phosphorylates PI 4-P on the D-5-position of the inositol ring and thus can be considered a 5-OH kinase as suggested previously (138,139) and could provide an alternative pathway for the synthesis of PI 3,4-P_2. PI is not a substrate for PIP 4-kinases (139). The activity of PIP 4-kinases is inhibited by its product, PI 4,5-P_2, and by heparin. Indirect evidence suggests that PIP 4-kinases associate with the p55 subunit of the tumor necrosis factor (TNF) receptor. Binding of TNFα to its receptor leads to an increase in PIP 4-kinase IIβ activity (142). In platelets, the generation of PI 3,4-P_2 from PI 3-P in integrin-dependent signaling involves PIP 4-kinase (143).

In addition, Iα and β isoforms of PIP 5-kinase generate PI 3,5-P_2 from PI 3-P and PI 3,4,5-P_3 from PI 3,4-P_2 *in vitro*, although at a lower rate than PI 3-kinases (139,144,145). Recombinant purified PIP 5-kinase generates significant amounts of PI 3,4,5-P_3 from PI 3,4-P_2 (139). It is unclear whether PI 3-P is preferentially phosphorylated to PI 3,4-P_2 or PI 3,5-P_2 (139) and whether these intermediates can be further phosphorylated to PI 3,4,5-P_3 (reviewed in ref. 42).

The activity of PIP 5-kinases is stimulated by heparin and spermine (138) and, as much as 50-fold, by phosphatidic acid (129,146). PIP 5-kinase activity is inhibited by its product, PI 4,5-P_2. *In vivo*, PIP 5-kinase activity may be influenced by small G proteins. The nonhydrolyzable GTP analog GTPγS increases PIP 5-kinase activity in several cell types (147). PIP 5-kinase has also been found to associate with Rac1 (30) and RhoA (148) and, in intact cells, the addition of rac-GTP or RhoA results in the accumulation of PI 4,5-P_2 (79,148,149). Furthermore, PIP 5-kinase activity is regulated by a cholera toxin-sensitive heterotrimeric G protein in rat liver membranes (150). It is clear that the number of enzymes belonging to these two families will continue to grow.

Phosphatases

Phosphatases can be divided into three groups based on the specificity for the phosphate on the inositol ring to use PI 3-P, PI 3,4-P_2 or PI 3,5-P_2. It has been proposed that a phosphatase that hydrolyzes the phosphate on the D-3 position could play a role in tumor suppression. A tumor suppressor gene located on human chromosome 10q23, PTEN (phosphatase and tensin homologue deleted on chromosome ten) or MMAC1 (mutated in multiple advanced cancers), was identified by several groups (151,152). PTEN is deleted or mutated in a wide variety of tumors (reviewed in ref. 153). The DNA sequence of PTEN suggested that it is a dual-specificity phosphatase, and PTEN can dephosphorylate some Ser/The phosphorylated proteins, although it prefers highly acidic substrates, such as poly(Glu-pTyr) (154). In contrast to a weak protein phosphatase activity, PTEN is a potent phosphatase for PI 3,4,5-P_3 *in vivo* and *in vitro* (155). Subsequent studies established that PTEN hydrolyzes PI 3,4-P_2, PI 3,4,5-P_3 and, to a lesser extent, PI 3-P (154). In addition to its catalytic domain, PTEN has a C-terminal potential binding site for PDZ domain-containing proteins and a region which overlaps the catalytic domain that is similar to the cytoskeletal proteins tensin and auxilin. The function of these domains is still unclear, but other PDZ proteins have been shown to direct the assembly of multiprotein complexes, often at the membrane/cytoskeletal interface, whereas the "tensin domain" may constitute a binding site for the phosphoinositides. PTEN affects several signal transduction pathways including PI 3-kinase-dependent activation of Akt (156) and dephosphorylation of focal adhesion kinase (FAK) (157). The lipid phosphatase activity of PTEN is required for its tumor suppressor activity and for its role in normal development (reviewed in ref. 153).

A group of magnesium-independent phosphatases that remove the phosphate from the D-4 position of the inositol ring also participate in the turnover of PI 3-kinase lipid products. The D-4-phosphatases are encoded for by two genes (types I and II) which are alternately spliced and contain a phosphatase consensus sequence (CKSAKDRT) within the catalytic domain (158). Both types catalyze the hydrolysis of PI 3,4-P$_2$ and, to a lesser extent, inositol 3,4-bisphosphate (158,159). The alternately spliced isoforms contain a C-terminal putative transmembrane domain (158). Type I phosphatase can be inactivated by proteolytic cleavage from the transmembrane domain by calcium-dependent protease, calpain, which may be responsible for the calcium-dependent accumulation of PI 3,4-P$_2$ in platelets (158).

Several 5′-phosphatases have been cloned and characterized, and there are others for which the sequence has not been identified (40,160). All identified 5′-phosphatases are magnesium-dependent phosphomonoesterases (160). Members of this family share a conserved domain of about 300 amino acids in the central portion of the molecule and are defined by two signature motifs: (F/I)WXGDXN(F/Y)R and (R/N)XP(S/A)(W/Y)(C/T)DR(I/V)(L/I) and are subdivided based on their substrate specificity (reviewed in ref. 160). Type I 5′-phosphatases hydrolyze only inositol polyphosphates. Type II enzymes specifically remove D-5-phosphate from soluble inositols and phosphatidylinositol polyphosphates. Type II enzymes are further subdivided based on their sequences and subcellular localization (40). Human and mouse platelet 5′-phosphatase (INPP5P) have a C-terminal prenylation site that targets this enzyme to mitochondria and plasma membranes, in addition to an N-terminal domain which is also thought to be important for association with cellular membranes (75). Another member of this group, OCRL-1, is not modified by a lipid moiety but is found on the surface of lysosomes (161). INPP5P and OCRL-1 may have overlapping functions in mice, although this is probably not the case in humans (162). Cell lines derived from the proximal tubules of the kidney from a patient with Lowe syndrome were shown to lack OCRL-1 and have missorting of lysosomal enzymes and accumulation of PI 4,5-P$_2$ and PI 3,4,5-P$_3$ (162). Two other members of this family isolated from nerve terminals are synaptojanin 1 and 2. These proteins are related to synaptic vesicle trafficking proteins and have PI 4,5-P$_2$ 5′-phosphatase activity (163). Synaptojanins play a role in osmoregulation and vacuole morphology in yeast (164) and form complexes with dynamin and amphiphysin and thus may participate in vesicular trafficking.

The SH2 domain-containing 5′-inositol phosphatases (SHIP1 and SHIP2) constitute the type III enzymes and hydrolyze specifically the 5′-phosphate from PI 3-kinase lipid products (reviewed in ref. 160). In addition to the N-terminal SH2 domain, both enzymes contain a C-terminal proline-rich region which interacts with SH3-containing proteins (165,166). SHIP1 contains two phosphotyrosine-binding (PTB) domains within the proline-rich region, whereas SHIP2 contains only one. The SH3 and PTB domains of SHIP1 and SHIP2 are probably responsible for their association with Shc and Grb2-Sos1 complexes, which link these phosphatases to signal transduction initiated by protein–tyrosine kinases (167,168). SHIP1 is expressed almost exclusively in cells of hematopoietic origin, but it is also found in lung and testis (168), whereas SHIP2 is expressed ubiquitously. SHIP1 and SHIP2 have been implicated in the downregulation of cellular responses to cytokines and growth factors, specifically insulin (169).

A different enzymatic activity has recently been isolated from platelets and placed in a separate group (type IV). This enzyme is found in a complex with PI 3-kinase and specifically hydrolyzes PI 3,4,5-P$_3$ (170).

LIPID PRODUCTS AS MEDIATORS OF PI 3-KINASE DOWNSTREAM SIGNALING

The ability of PI 3-kinase to initiate intracellular signals is derived from the direct interaction of the catalytic and regulatory subunits with other proteins and from protein–lipid interactions provided by lipid-binding domains in target proteins (Fig. 35.1). Two lipid-binding domains have been identified that specifically recognize inositol-containing phospholipids: the FYVE and PH domains. A novel method for the identification of protein-lipid interactions has recently been described (171). This technology is based on screening peptide libraries with biotinylated analogs of the lipids and may uncover novel mechanisms for interaction with lipid moieties.

FYVE Domains

The FYVE domain was named after the first four proteins known to contain the conserved protein sequence: *F* ab1p, *Y* OTB, *V* ac1p, and *E* EA1. It selectively binds to PI 3-P (172–174). To date, over 40 FYVE domain-containing proteins have been described in mammals, and most of them have been implicated in intracellular trafficking. The discovery of the FYVE domain as a target of PI 3-P opened a new level of understanding for the role of PI 3-P in vesicular trafficking (reviewed in ref. 175). The 60–80 amino acid residue FYVE domain is a special RING zinc finger structure with eight conserved cysteines forming two separate zinc coordination centers (173,176). Many FYVE domain-containing proteins are involved in secretion, vacuolar targeting, receptor recycling and multivesicular endosome formation (reviewed in ref. 175). The FYVE domain of EEA1, a protein that regulates fusion of endocytic membranes (177), is necessary for Rab-5-directed vesicular trafficking (178,179). The crystal structure of

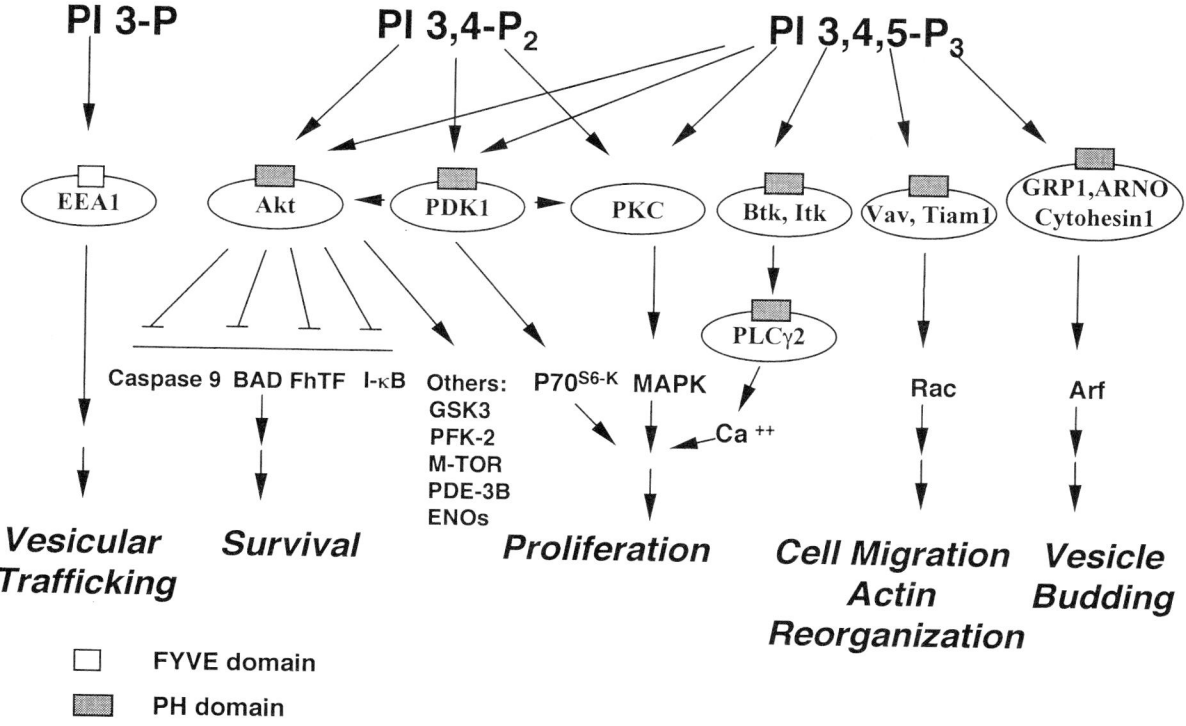

FIGURE 35.1. Downstream signaling through PI 3-kinase lipid products. The targets of lipid products are indicated, as are their roles in cellular responses. The PH and FYVE protein domains that bind phospholipids are highlighted.

VPS27p protein suggests that PI 3-P but not other lipids, including PI 5-P, can be accommodated in the binding site, and mutation of the zinc coordinating cysteines or removal of zinc reduces the affinity for PI 3-P (180). The crystal structure of a homodimer of FYVE domains derived from *Drosophila* Hrs (HGF-regulated tyrosine kinase substrate) has a parallel rather than perpendicular orientation to the membrane (181). Hrs is involved in targeting the endosome to the lysosome and is required for normal mouse development. Dimerization of the Hrs FYVE domain creates two identical pockets, resulting in higher affinity for PI 3-P.

Pleckstrin Homology Domains

The pleckstrin homology (PH) domain contains 90–110 amino acids and was initially found in pleckstrin, the major protein kinase C substrate in platelets. PH domains are found in more than 100 proteins with a wide range of cellular functions, including kinases, phospholipases, nucleotide-exchange factors, and adaptor proteins and proteins which mediate protein–phospholipid and protein–protein interactions (182). The inositol head group binding site in the PH domain is formed by two β-sheets capped by an α-helix. Divergent basic residues in the PH domain core structure determine the binding affinity (reviewed in ref. 175). Most

PH domains bind inositol-containing phospholipids but only some bind with high affinity. There are no PH domains that bind PI 3-P, a role that seems to be assigned to FYVE domains. Some PH domains preferentially bind to PI 3,4-P$_2$, whereas others specifically bind PI 3,4,5-P$_3$ (138,183). In addition, PH domains have been used as probes for the visualization of subcellular compartments that transiently accumulate polyphosphoinositides in response to specific stimuli (184), and led to the identification of novel signaling cascades in membrane ruffling, adhesion, and chemotaxis (reviewed in ref. 175).

The PH domain of Akt, also referred to as PKB, preferentially binds to PI 3,4-P$_2$ and PI 3,4,5-P$_3$ over other phosphoinositides. The mechanism of activation of Akt is not fully understood, but the interaction of PH domain with phosphoinositides leads to a three- to five-fold stimulation of its activity *in vitro* (185–187). *In vivo*, Akt activation requires PI 3-kinase and phosphorylation of Thr[308] and Ser[473] (188). Thr[308] is phosphorylated by PDK1, a constitutively active Ser/Thr kinase that also contains a PH domain with high affinity for PI 3,4,5-P$_3$ and, to a lesser degree, PI 3,4-P$_2$ (189–192). Phosphorylation of Akt on Thr[308] is enhanced over one thousand-fold in the presence of lipid micelles containing PI 3,4-P$_2$ or PI 3,4,5-P$_3$. An enzymatic activity named PDK2 phosphorylates Ser[473]. Embryonic stem cells, which lack PDK1, fail to phosphorylate Thr[308] in response to IGF-1 but have phosphorylation on Ser [473], which suggests that PDK2 is functional in these cells (193).

PI 3-kinase-dependent activation of Akt is required for its role in cell survival. Akt participates in counteracting the apoptotic pathway on several levels, and its effect on cell survival may depend on the specific apoptotic pathway affected in different cell types. Akt phosphorylates BAD, a protein that in a dephosphorylated state promotes apoptosis by binding to Bcl-x$_L$, a cell survival factor. Phosphorylation of BAD disrupts the BAD/Bcl-x$_L$ complex and allows Bcl-x$_L$ to homodimerize and thereby protect mitochondria from apoptosis. Caspase 9, a protease necessary for the initiation of the apoptotic cascade, is also phosphorylated and inhibited by Akt (194,195). Two additional targets that interfere with the apoptotic pathway have recently been identified. Akt phosphorylates forkhead transcription factor, which leads to its accumulation in the cytosol, thus preventing expression of proapoptotic molecules such as Fas (196–199). Akt also associates with and activates I-κB kinases (200–202). This leads to degradation of I-B, which allows NF-κB-dependent transcription of antiapoptotic proteins (203). In the liver, PI 3-kinase-dependent activation of Akt also protects hepatocytes from apoptosis (204,205).

In addition to cell survival, activation of Akt affects other cellular responses, including regulation of enzymes involved in glycogen turnover in response to insulin. These include glycogen synthase kinase 3 (GSK3) (206), the cardiac isoform of 6-phosphofructo-2-kinase (207), phosphodiesterase-3B (208) which is involved in the regulation of intracellular levels of cAMP, and mTOR (209), which regulates protein translation. Akt also participates in the generation of nitric oxide (NO) in endothelial cells by activation of endothelial NO synthase (210–212).

PDK1 is a constitutively active protein Ser/Thr kinase that is recruited to the plasma membrane by the interaction of its PH domain with PI 3,4-P$_2$ and PI 3,4,5-P$_3$. PDK1 has targets other than Akt. PDK1 phosphorylates and activates p70 S6 kinase (213,214) and several members of the PKC family, PKCε, and PKCζ (215). These PKC isoforms also contain PH domains and can be independently activated by PI 3,4-P$_2$ or PI 3,4,5-P$_3$ (216,217). Additional targets for PDK1 may be activated independently of PI 3-kinase signaling.

Another large group of proteins which contain PH domains are GTP/GDP exchange factors (GEFs) and GTPase-activating proteins (GAPs), proteins which regulate the GTPase activity of small G proteins. The presence of PH domains in Rho family GTPases and ARF-GTPases supports the experimental evidence that these small G proteins are regulated by 3′-polyphosphoinositides (218). Two GEFs for Rac, Vav and Tiam1, specifically bind to PI 3,4,5-P$_3$, which results in activation of Rac (182,219). PI 3-kinase-dependent activation of Rac may be responsible for growth factor-mediated membrane ruffling, actin reorganization and chemotaxis (220,221). Other examples include

GAP1^m and GAP1^{IP4BP}, which are Ras-GAPs; their PH domains also bind PI 3,4,5-P$_3$. Although the role of this binding is unclear because it does not lead to increased Ras-GAP activity, it may facilitate the recruitment of PI 3-kinase to the plasma membrane and Ras-dependent activation of PI 3-kinase, as discussed in the earlier section entitled Activity and Regulation of Class I$_A$ PI 3-kinase.

Three ARF-GEFs which participate in vesicular membrane trafficking are known to be regulated by PI 3-kinase lipid products: GRP1, ARNO, and cytohesin-1 (reviewed in refs. 222,223). Their PH domains preferentially bind to PI 3,4,5-P$_3$ and have relatively low affinity for PI-3-P and PI 3,4-P$_2$. This leads to translocation of these proteins from the cytosol to the plasma membrane, where they regulate vesicle coating and budding. In addition, centaurins, which are ARF-GAPs, specifically bind to PI 3,4,5-P$_3$ or the soluble Ins(1,3,4,5)-P$_4$ *in vitro*. The role of PI 3-kinase in vesicular trafficking is further supported by studies of PDGF-dependent trafficking of the PDGF receptor to lysosomes and for the insulin-dependent trafficking of the glucose transporter, GLUT4, to the plasma membrane (224,225).

Other proteins that contain PH domains are Tec nonreceptor tyrosine kinases. Tec family members include Bruton's tyrosine kinase (Btk) and the inducible T-cell kinase (Itk). Btk is critical for B cell development and function. Mutation in the Btk PH domain that affects binding to PI 3,4,5-P$_3$ results in X-linked immunodeficiency in mice (226). The mechanism of Btk activation resembles the activation of Akt by PDK1. The PH domain of Btk mediate its translocation to the plasma membrane where it can be further activated by phosphorylation on Tyr and Ser by Src family kinases (reviewed in ref. 23). Btk regulates tyrosine phosphorylation of PLCγ2, which also has a PI 3,4,5-P$_3$-specific PH domain (227). Thus, the recruitment to the plasma membrane and activation of PLCγ2 provides a role for PI 3-kinase lipid products in hematopoietic cells.

Other Targets for D-3 Phosphoinositides

As described in the earlier section entitled Activity and Regulation of Class I$_A$ PI 3-kinases, PI 3,4,5-P$_3$ binds to p85 SH2 domains and may compete for its interaction with phosphotyrosine-containing sequences. This binding could terminate the PI 3-kinase cascade by inducing dissociation of PI 3-kinase from the lipid substrates. In contrast, binding of PI 3,4,5-P$_3$ to the SH2 domain of PLCγ enhances its phospholipase activity (49,228,229). Other targets for PI 3-kinase lipid products are continuously identified.

REFERENCES

1. Balla T. Phosphatidylinositol 4-kinases. *Biochim Biophys Acta* 1998;1436:69–85.
2. Divecha N, Irvine RF. Phospholipid signaling. *Cell* 1995;80: 269–278.

3. Alberts B, Bray D, Lewis J, et al. Macromolecules: structure, shape, and information. In: *Molecular biology of the cell.* New York: Garland Publishing, 1989:88–134.

4. Varticovski L, Harrison-Findik D, Keeler ML, et al. Role of PI 3-kinase in mitogenesis. *Biochim Biophys Acta* 1994;1226:1–11.

5. Monaco ME, Greshengton MC. Subcellular organization of receptor-mediated phosphoinositide turnover. *Endocr Rev* 1992; 13:707–718.

6. Serunian LA, Haber MT, Fukui T, et al. Phosphoinositides produced by phosphatidylinositol 3-kinase are poor substrates for phospholipases C from rat liver and bovine brain. *J Cell Biol* 1989;264:17809–17815.

7. Lips DL, Majerus PW, Gorga FR, et al. Phosphatidylinositol 3-phosphate is present in normal and transformed fibroblasts and is resistant to hydrolysis by bovine brain phospholipase C II. *J Biol Chem* 1989;264:8759–8763.

8. Sugimoto Y, Whitman M, Cantley LC, et al. Evidence that the Rous sarcoma virus transforming gene product phosphorylates phosphatidylinositol and diacylglycerol. *Proc Natl Acad Sci U S A* 1984;81:2117–2121.

9. Macara IG, Marinetti GV, Balduzzi PC. Transforming protein of avian sarcoma virus UR2 is associated with phosphatidylinositol kinase activity: possible role in tumorigenesis. *Proc Natl Acad Sci U S A* 1984;81:2728–2732.

10. Whitman M, Kaplan DR, Schaffhausen B, et al. Association of phosphatidylinositol kinase activity with polyoma middle-T component for transformation. *Nature* 1985;315:239–242.

11. Kaplan DR, Whitman M, Schaffhausen BS, et al. Common elements in growth factor stimulation and oncogenic transformation: 85 kd protein and phosphatidylinositol kinase activity. *Cell* 1987;50:1021–1029.

12. Escobedo JA, Kaplan DR, Kavanaugh M, et al. A phosphatidylinositol-3 kinase binds to platelet-derived growth factor receptor through a specific receptor sequence containing phosphotyrosine. *Mol Cell Biol* 1991;11:1125–1132.

13. Escobedo JA, Navankasattussa S, Kavanaugh WM, et al. cDNA cloning of a novel 85 kd protein that has SH2 domains and regulates binding of PI3-kinase to the PDGF β-receptor. *Cell* 1991;65:75–82.

14. Skolnik EY, Margolis B, Mohammadi M, et al. Cloning of PI 3-kinase-associated p85 utilizing a novel method for expression/cloning of target proteins for receptor tyrosine kinases. *Cell* 1991;65:83–90.

15. Otsu M, Hiles I, Gout I, et al. Characterization of two 85 kd proteins that associate with receptor tyrosine kinases, middle-T/pp60c-src complexes, and PI 3-kinase. *Cell* 1991;65:91–104.

16. Whitman M, Kaplan DR, Roberts TM, et al. Evidence for two distinct phosphatidylinositol kinases in fibroblasts: Implications for cellular regulation. *Biochem J* 1987;247:165–174.

17. Whitman M, Downes CP, Keeler M, et al. Type I phosphatidylinositol kinase makes a novel inositol phospholipid, phosphatidylinositol 3-phosphate. *Nature* 1988;332:644–646.

18. Auger KR, Serunian LA, Soltoff SP, et al. PDGF-dependent tyrosine phosphorylation stimulates production of novel polyphosphoinositides in intact cells. *Cell* 1989;57:167–175.

19. Carpenter CL, Duckworth BC, Auger KR, et al. Purification and characterization of phosphoinositide 3-kinase from rat liver. *J Biol Chem* 1990;265:19704–19711.

20. Morgan SJ, Smith AD, Parker PJ. Purification of bovine brain type I phosphatidylinositol kinase. *Eur J Biochem* 1990;191:761–767.

21. Domin J, Waterfield MD. Using structure to define the function of phosphoinositide 3-kinase family members. *FEBS Letters* 1997;410:91–95.

22. Vanhaesebroeck B, Welham MJ, Kotani K, et al. P110δ, a novel

phosphoinositide 3-kinase in leukocytes. *Proc Natl Acad Sci U S A* 1997;94:4330–4335.

23. Vanhaesebroeck B, Waterfield MD. Signaling by distinct classes of phosphoinositide 3-kinases. *Exp Cell Res* 1999;253:239–254.

24. Volinia S, Patracchini P, Otsu M, et al. Chromosomal localization of human p85α, a subunit of phosphatidylinositol 3 kinase, and its homologue, p85β. *Oncogene* 1991;7:789–793.

25. Rodriguez-Viciana P, Warne PH, Dhand R, et al. Phosphatidylinositol-3-OH kinase as a direct target of Ras. *Nature* 1994;370:527–532.

26. Dhand R, Hiles I, Panayotou G, et al. PI 3-kinase is a dual specificity enzyme: Autoregulation by an intrinsic protein-serine kinase activity. *EMBO J* 1994;13:522–533.

27. Vanhaesebroeck B, Higashi K, Raven K, et al. Autophosphorylation of p110δ phosphoinositide 3-kinase: a new paradigm for the regulation of lipid kinases *in vitro* and *in vivo. EMBO J* 1999;18:1292–1302.

28. Klippel A, Escobedo JA, Hu Q, et al. A region of the 85-kilodalton (kd) subunit of phosphatidylinositol 3-kinase binds the 110-kd catalytic subunit *in vivo. Mol Cell Biol* 1993;13:5560–5566.

29. Kapeller R, Prasad KVS, Janssen O, et al. Identification of two SH3-binding motifs in the regulatory subunit of phosphatidylinositol 3-kinase. *J Biol Chem* 1994;269:1927–1933.

30. Tolias KF, Cantley LC, Carpenter CL. Rho family GTPases bind to phosphoinositide kinases. *J Biol Chem* 1995;270:17656–17659.

31. Antonetti DA, Algenstaedt P, Kahn CR. Insulin receptor substrate 1 binds two novel splice variants of the regulatory subunit of phosphatidylinositol 3-kinase in muscle and brain. *Mol Cell Biol* 1996;16:2195–2203.

32. Inukai K, Funaki M, Ogihara T, et al. p85α gene generates three isoforms of regulatory subunit for phosphatidylinositol 3-kinase (PI 3-kinase), p50α, p55α, and p85α, with different PI 3-kinase activity elevating responses to insulin. *J Biol Chem* 1997;272:7873–7882.

33. Pons S, Asano T, Glasheen E, et al. The structure and function of p55PIK reveal a new regulatory subunit for phosphatidylinositol 3-kinase. *Mol Cell Biol* 1995;15:4453–4465.

34. Stephens L, Smrcka A, Cooke FT, et al. A novel phosphoinositide 3 kinase activity in myeloid-derived cells is activated by G protein βγ subunits. *Cell* 1994;77:83–93.

35. Stephens LR, Eguinoa A, Erdjument-Bromage H, et al. The G βγ sensitivity of a PI3K is dependent upon a tightly associated adaptor, p101. *Cell* 1997;89:105–114.

36. Krugmann S, Hawkins PT, Pryer N, et al. Characterizing the interactions between the two subunits of the p101/p110γ phosphoinositide 3-kinase and their role in the activation of this enzyme by Gβγ subunits. *J Biol Chem* 1999;274:17152–17158.

37. Metjian A, Roll RL, Ma AD, et al. Agonists cause nuclear translocation of phosphatidylinositol 3-kinase γ. A Gβγ-dependent pathway that requires the p110gamma amino terminus. *J Biol Chem* 1999;274:27943–27947.

38. Stephens LR, Hughes KT, Irvine RF. Pathway of phosphatidylinositol (3,4,5)-trisphosphate synthesis in neutrophils. *Nature* 1991;351:33–39.

39. Woscholski R, Parker PJ. Inositol lipid 5-phosphatases—traffic signals and signal traffic. *Trends Biochem Sci* 1997;22:427–431.

40. Erneux C, Govaerts C, Communi D, et al. The diversity and possible functions of the inositol polyphosphate 5-phosphatases. *Biochim Biophys Acta* 1998;1436:185–199.

41. Varticovski L, Druker B, Morrison D, et al. The CSF-1 receptor associates with and activates PI 3-kinase. *Nature* 1989;342:699–702.

42. Fruman DA, Meyers RE, Cantley LC. Phosphoinositide kinases. *Annu Rev Biochem* 1998;67:481–507.

43. Ling LE, Drucker BJ, Cantley LC, et al. Transformation-defec-

tive mutants of polyoma middle T antigen associate with phosphatidylinositol 3-kinase (PI 3-kinase) but are unable to maintain wild-type levels of PI 3-kinase products in intact cells. *J Virol* 1992;66:1702–1708.

44. Varticovski L, Daley GQ, Jackson P, et al. Activation of phosphatidylinositol 3-kinase in cells expressing abl oncogene variants. *Mol Cell Biol* 1991;11:1107–1113.

45. Klippel A, Reinhard C, Kavanaugh WM, et al. Membrane localization of phosphatidylinositol 3-kinase is sufficient to activate multiple signal-transducing kinase pathways. *Mol Cell Biol* 1996;16:4117–4127.

46. Songyang Z, Shoelson SE, Chaudhuri M, et al. SH2 domains recognize specific phosphopeptide sequences. *Cell* 1993;72:767–778.

47. Backer JM, Myers MGJ, Shoelson SE, et al. Phosphatidylinositol 3′-kinase is activated by association with IRS-1 during insulin stimulation. *EMBO J* 1992;11:3469–3479.

48. Carpenter CL, Auger KR, Chanudhuri M, et al. Phosphatidylinositol 3-kinase is activated by phosphopeptides that bind to the SH2 domains of the p85 kD subunit. *J Biol Chem* 1993;268:9478–9483.

49. Rameh LE, Chen C-S, Cantley LC. Phosphatidylinositol (3,4,5)P3 interacts with SH2 domains and modulates PI 3-kinase association with tyrosine-phosphorylated proteins. *Cell* 1995;83:1–20.

50. Yu H, Chen JK, Feng S, et al. Structural basis for the binding of proline-rich peptides to the SH3 domains. *Cell* 1994;76:933–945.

51. Jain SK, Langdon WY, Varticovski L. Tyrosine phosphorylation of p120cbl in BCR/abl transformed hematopoietic cells mediates enhanced association with phosphatidylinositol 3-kinase. *Oncogene* 1997;14:2217–2228.

52. Harrison-Findik D, Misra S, Jain SK, et al. Dynamin inhibits phosphatidylinositol 3-kinase in hematopoietic cells. *Biochem Biophys Acta* 2001;1538:10–19.

53. Gout I, Dhland R, Hiles I, et al. The GTPase dynamin binds and is activated by a subset of SH3 domains. *Cell* 1993;75:25–36.

54. Liu X, Marengere LM, Koch CA, et al. The v-src SH3 domain binds phosphatidylinositol 3-kinase. *Mol Cell Biol* 1993;13:5225–5232.

55. Prasad KVS, Jannsen O, Kapeller R, et al. Src-homology 3 domain of protein kinase p59fyn mediates binding to phosphatidylinositol 3-kinase in T cells. *Proc Natl Acad Sci U S A* 1993;90:7366–7370.

56. Pleiman CM, Clark MR, Timson Gauen LK, et al. Mapping of sites on the Src family protein tyrosine kinases p55blk, p59fyn, and p56lyn which interact with the effector molecules phospholipase C-γ2, microtubule-associated protein kinase, GTPase-activating protein, and phosphatidylinositol 3-kinase. *Mol Cell Biol* 1993;13:5877–5887.

57. Jain SK, Susa-Spring M, Carlesso N, et al. PI 3-kinase activation in BCR/abl-transformed hematopoietic cells does not require interaction of p85 SH2 domains with p210 BCR/abl. *Blood* 1996;88:1542–1550.

58. Pleiman CM, Hertz WM, Cambier JC. Activation of phosphatidylinositol-3′ kinase by Src-family kinase SH3 binding to the p85 subunit. *Science* 1994;263:1609–1612.

59. Carpenter CL, Auger KR, Duckworth BC, et al. A tightly associated serine/threonine protein kinase regulates phosphoinositol 3-kinase activity. *Mol Cell Biol* 1993;13:1657–1665.

60. Stoyanova S, Bulgarelli-Leva G, Kirsch C, et al. Lipid kinase and protein kinase activities of G-protein-coupled phosphoinositide 3-kinase γ: structure-activity analysis and interactions with wortmannin. *Biochem J* 1997;324:489–495.

61. Auger KR, Carpenter CL, Shoelsen SE, et al. Polyoma virus middle T antigen-pp60c-src complex associates with purified phosphatidylinositol 3-kinase *in vitro*. *J Biol Chem* 1992;267:5408–5415.

62. Gout I, Dhland R, Panayotou G, et al. Expression and characterization of the p85 subunit of the PI 3-kinase complex and related p85 protein using the baculovirus expression system. *Biochem J* 1992;288:395–405.

63. Hayashi Y, Nakazawa S. [Clinical features of childhood Ph1 positive acute leukemia]. *Rinsho Ketsueki* 1991;32:338–344.

64. De Aós I, Metzger M, Exley M, et al. Tyrosine phosphorylation of the CD3-ε subunit of the T cell receptor mediates enhanced association with phosphoinositol 3-kinase in Jurkat T cells. *J Biol Chem* 1997;272:26638–26644.

65. Soltoff SP, Rabin SL, Cantley LC, et al. Nerve growth factor promotes the activation of phosphatidylinositol 3-kinase and its association with the trk tyrosine kinase. *J Biol Chem* 1992;267:17472–17477.

66. Reif K, Gout I, Waterfield MD, et al. Divergent regulation of phosphatidylinositol 3-kinase P85α and P85β isoforms upon T cell activation. *J Biol Chem* 1993;268:10780–10788.

67. Cantrell D, Izquierdo-Pastor M, Reif K, et al. Signal transduction by the T-cell antigen receptor: Regulation and function of p21ras and PtdIns-3 kinase. *Chem Immunol* 1994;59:115–127.

68. Rodriguez-Viciana P, Warne PH, Vanhaesebroeck B, et al. Activation of phosphoinositide 3-kinase by interaction with Ras and by point mutation. *EMBO J* 1996;15:2442–2451.

69. Sjolander A, Yamamoto K. Association of p21ras with phosphatidylinositol 3-kinase. *Proc Natl Acad Sci U S A* 1991;88:7908–7912.

70. Kodaki T, Woscholski R, Hallberg B, et al. The activation of phosphatidylinositol 3-kinase by Ras. *Curr Biol* 1994;4:798–806.

71. Satoh T, Fantl WJ, Escobedo JA, et al. Platelet-derived growth factor receptor mediates activation of ras through different signaling pathways in different cell types. *Mol Cell Biol* 1993;13:3706–3713.

72. Okada T, Hazeki O, Ui M, et al. Synergystic activation of PtdIns 3-kinase by tyrosine-phosphorylated peptide and by βγ-subunits of GTP-binding proteins. *Biochem J* 1996;317:475–480.

73. Thomason PA, James SR, Casey PJ, et al. A G-protein βγ-subunit-responsive phosphoinositide 3-kinase activity in human platelets. *J Biol Chem* 1994;269:16525–16528.

74. Kurosu H, Maehama T, Okada T, et al. Heterodimeric phosphoinositide 3-kinase consisting of p85 and p110b is synergistically activated by the bg subunits of G proteins and phosphotyrosyl peptide. *J Biol Chem* 1997;272:24252–24256.

75. Speed CJ, Little PJ, Hayman JA, et al. Underexpression of the 43 kd inositol polyphosphate 5-phosphatase is associated with cellular transformation. *EMBO J* 1996;15:4852–4861.

76. Kular G, Loubtchenkov M, Swigart P, et al. Co-operation of phosphatidylinositol transfer protein with phosphoinositide 3-kinase γ in the formylmethionyl-leucylphenylalanine-dependent production of phosphatidylinositol 3,4,5-trisphosphate in human neutrophils. *Biochem J* 1997;325:299–301.

77. Toker A. The synthesis and cellular roles of phosphatidylinositol 4,5-bisphosphate. *Curr Opin Cell Biol* 1998;10:254–261.

78. Misra S, Ujhazy P, Varticovski L, et al. Phosphoinositide 3-kinase lipid products regulate ATP-dependent transport by sister-P-glycoprotein and multidrug resistance associated protein 2 in bile canalicular membrane vesicles. *Proc Natl Acad Sci U S A* 1999;96:5814–5819.

79. Hartwig JH, Bockoch GM, Carpenter CL, et al. Thrombin receptor ligation and activated Rac uncap actin filament barbed ends through phosphoinositide synthesis in permeabilized human platelets. *Cell* 1995;82:643–653.

80. Joyal JL, Burks DJ, Pons S, et al. Calmodulin activates phosphatidylinositol 3-kinase. *J Biol Chem* 1997;272:28183–28186.

81. Zheng Y, Bagrodia S, Cerione RA. Activation of phosphoinositide 3-kinase activity by Cdc42Hs binding to p85. *J Biol Chem* 1994;269:18727–18730.

82. Bi L, Okabe I, Bernard DJ, et al. Proliferative defect and embryonic lethality in mice homozygous for a deletion in the p110α subunit of phosphoinositide 3-kinase. *J Biol Chem* 1999;274:10963–10968.

83. Morris JZ, Tissenbaum HA, Ruvkun G. A phosphatidylinositol-3-OH kinase family member regulating longevity and diapause in *caenorhabditis elegans*. *Nature* 1996;382:536–539.

84. Fruman D, Snapper SB, Yballe CM, et al. Impaired B cell development and proliferation in absence of phosphoinositide 3-kinase p85α. *Science* 1999;283:393–397.

85. Terauchi Y, Tsuji Y, Satoh S, et al. Increased insulin sensitivity and hypoglycaemia in mice lacking the p85α subunit of phosphoinositide 3-kinase. *Nat Genet* 1999;21:230–235.

86. Suzuki H, Terauchi Y, Fujiwara M, et al. Xid-like immunodeficiency in mice with disruption of the p85α subunit of phosphoinositide 3-kinase. *Science* 1999;283:390–392.

87. Cantley LC, Yballe C. *personal communication* 1999.

88. Fujikawa K, de Aós I, Jain SK, et al. Role of PI 3-kinase in angiopoietin-1-mediated migration and attachment-dependent survival of endothelial cells. *Exp Cell Res* 1999;253:663–672.

89. Gerber H-P, McMurtrey A, Kowalski J, et al. Vascular endothelial growth factor regulates endothelial cell survival through the phosphatidylinositol 3′-kinase/Akt signal transduction pathway. *J Biol Chem* 1998;273:30336–30343.

90. Stoyanov B, Volinia S, Hanck T, et al. Cloning and characterization of a G protein-activated human phosphoinositide 3-kinase. *Science* 1995;269:690–693.

91. Lopez-Ilasaca M, Crespo P, Pellici PG, et al. Linkage of G protein-coupled receptors to the MAPK signaling pathway through PI 3-kinase γ. *Science* 1997;275:394–397.

92. Maier U, Babich A, Nurnberg B. Roles of noncatalytic subunits in Gβγ-induced activation of class I phosphoinositide 3-kinase isoforms β and γ. *J Biol Chem* 1999;274:29311–29317.

93. Murga C, Laguinge L, Wetzker R, et al. Activation of Akt/protein kinase B by G protein-coupled receptors. A role for α and β γsubunits of heterotrimeric G proteins acting through phosphatidylinositol-3-OH kinase γ. *J Biol Chem* 1998;273:19080–19085.

94. Rubio I, Rodriguez-Viciana P, Downward J, et al. Interaction of Ras with phosphoinositide 3-kinase γ. *Biochem J* 1997;326:891–895.

95. Rubio I, Wittig U, Meyer C, et al. Farnesylation of Ras is important for the interaction with phosphoinositide 3-kinase γ. *Eur J Biochem* 1999;266:70–82.

96. Okada T, Sakuma L, Fukui Y, et al. Blockage of chemotactic peptide-induced stimulation of neutrophils by wortmannin as a result of selective inhibition of phosphatidylinositol 3-kinase. *J Biol Chem* 1994;269:3563–3567.

97. Li Z, Jiang H, Xie W, et al. Roles of PLC-β2 and -β3 and PI3Kγ in chemoattractant-mediated signal transduction. *Science* 2000;287:1046–1049.

98. Hirsch E, Katanaev VL, Garlanda C, et al. Central role of phosphoinositide 3-kinase γ in inflammation. *Science* 2000;287:1049–1053.

99. Servant G, Weiner OD, Herzmark P, et al. Polarization of chemoattractant receptor signaling during neutrophil chemotaxis. *Science* 2000;287:1037–1040.

100. Jin T, Zang N, Long Y, et al. Localization of the G-protein βγ complex in living cells during chemotaxis. *Science* 2000;287:1034–1036.

101. Sasaki T, Sasaki JI, Jones RG, et al. Function of PI3Kγ in thymocyte development, T cell activation, and neutrophil migration. *Science* 2000;287:1040–1046.

102. Misawa H, Ohtsubo M, Copeland NG, et al. Cloning and characterization of a novel class II phosphoinositide 3-kinase containing C2 domain. *Biochem Biophys Res Commun* 1998;244:531–539.

103. Ono F, Nakagawa T, Saito S, et al. A novel class II phosphoinositide 3-kinase predominantly expressed in the liver and its enhanced expression during liver regeneration. *J Biol Chem* 1998;273:7731–7736.

104. Arcaro A, Volinia S, Zvelebil MJ, et al. Human phosphoinositide 3-kinase C2β, the role of calcium and the C2 domain in enzyme activity. *J Biol Chem* 1998;273:33082–33090.

105. MacDougall LK, Domin J, Waterfield MD. A family of phosphoinositide 3-kinases in *Drosophila* identifies a new mediator of signal transduction. *Curr Biol* 1995;5:1404–1415.

106. Domin J, Pages F, Volinia S, et al. Cloning of a human phosphoinositide 3-kinase with a C2 domain that displays reduced sensitivity to the inhibitor wortmannin. *Biochem J* 1997;15:139–147.

107. Brown RA, Domin J, Arcaro A, et al. Insulin activates the α isoform of class II phosphoinositide 3-kinase. *J Biol Chem* 1999;274:14529–14532.

108. Zhang J, Banfic H, Straforini F, et al. A type II phosphoinositide 3-kinase is stimulated via activated integrin in platelets. A source of phosphatidylinositol 3-phosphate. *J Biol Chem* 1998;273:14081–14084.

109. Turner SJ, Domin J, Waterfield MD, et al. The CC chemokine monocyte chemotactic peptide-1 activates both the class I p85/p110 phosphoinositol 3-kinase and the class II PI3K-C2α. *J Biol Chem* 1998;273:25987–25995.

110. Molz L, Chen YW, Hirano M, et al. Cpk is a novel class of *Drosophila* PtdIns 3-kinase containing a C2 domain. *J Biol Chem* 1996;271:13892–13899.

111. Herman PK, Stack JH, DeModena JA, et al. A novel protein kinase homolog essential for protein sorting to the yeast lysosomal-like vacuole. *Cell* 1991;64:425–437.

112. Herman PK, Emr SD. Characterization of VPS34, a gene required for vacuolar protein sorting and vacuolar segregation in *Saccharomyces cerevisiae*. *Mol Cell Biol* 1990;10:6742–6754.

113. Schu PV, Takegawa K, Fry MJ, et al. Phosphatidylinositol 3-kinase encoded by yeast VPS34 gene is essential for protein sorting. *Science* 1993;260:88–91.

114. Volinia S, Dhand R, Vanhaesebroeck B, et al. A human phosphatidylinositol 3-kinase complex related to the yeast Vps34p-Vps15p protein sorting system. *EMBO J* 1995;14:3339–3348.

115. Panaretou C, Domin J, Cockcroft S, et al. Characterization of p150, an adaptor protein for the human phosphatidylinositol (PtdIns) 3-kinase. Substrate presentation by phosphatidylinositol transfer protein to the p150 Ptdins 3-kinase complex. *J Biol Chem* 1997;271:2477–2485.

116. Andrade MA, Bork P. HEAT repeats in the Huntington's disease protein. *Nat Genet* 1995;11:115–116.

117. Neer EJ, Schmidt CJ, Nambudripad R, et al. The ancient regulatory protein family of WD-repeat proteins. *Nature* 1994;371:297–300.

118. Auger KR, Serunian LA, Cantley LC, et al. Phosphatidylinositol 3-kinase and its novel product, phosphatidylinositol 3-phosphate, are present in *Saccharomyces cerevisiae*. *J Biol Chem* 1989;264:20181–20184.

119. Toker A, Bachelot C, Chen C-S, et al. Phosphorylation of the platelet p47 phosphoprotein is mediated by the lipid products of phosphoinositide 3-kinase. *J Biol Chem* 1995;270:1–7.

120. Stack JH, DeWald DB, Takegawa K, et al. Vesicle-mediated protein transport: Regulatory interactions between the Vps15 protein kinase and the Vps34 PtdIns 3-kinase essential for protein sorting to the vacuole in yeast. *J Cell Biol* 1995;129:321–334.

121. Arcaro A, Wymann MP. Wortmannin is a potent phosphatidylinositol 3-kinase inhibitor: The role of phosphatidyli-

nositol 3,4,5-trisphosphate in neutrophil responses. *Biochem J* 1993;296:297–301.

122. Yano H, Nakanishi S, Kimura K, et al. Inhibition of histamine secretion by wortmannin through the blockade of phosphatidylinositol 3-kinase in RBL-2H3 cells. *J Biol Chem* 1993;268:25846–25856.

123. Vlahos CJ, Matter WF, Hui KY, et al. A specific inhibitor of phosphatidylinositol 3-kinase, 2-(4-morpholinyl)-8-phenyl-4H-1-benzopyran-4-one (LY294002). *J Biol Chem* 1994;269:5241–5248.

124. Wymann MP, Bulgarelli-Leva G, Zvelebil MJ, et al. Wortmannin inactivates phosphoinositide 3-kinase by covalent modification of Lys-802, a residue involved in the phosphate transfer reaction. *Mol Cell Biol* 1996;16:1722–1733.

125. Virbasius JV, Guilherme A, Czech MP. Mouse p170 is a novel phosphatidylinositol 3-kinase containing a C2 domain. *J Biol Chem* 1996;271:13304–13307.

126. Stack JH, Emr SD. Vps34p required for yeast vacuolar protein sorting is a multiple specificity kinase that exhibits both protein kinase and phosphatidylinositol-specific PI 3-kinase activities. *J Biol Chem* 1994;269:31552–31562.

127. Takegawa K, DeWald DB, Emr SD. *Schizosaccharomyces pombe* Vps34p, a phosphatidylinositol-specific PI 3-kinase essential for normal cell growth and vacuole morphology. *J Cell Sci* 1995; 108:3745–3756.

128. Bazenet CE, Ruano AR, Brockman JL, et al. The human erythrocyte contains two forms of phosphatidylinositol-4-phosphate 5-kinase which are differentially active toward membranes. *J Biol Chem* 1990;265:18012–18022.

129. Jenkins GH, Fisette PL, Anderson RA. Type I phosphatidylinositol 4-phosphate 5-kinase isoforms are specifically stimulated by phosphatidic acid. *J Biol Chem* 1994;269:11547–11554.

130. Boronenkov IV, Anderson RA. The sequence of phosphatidylinositol-4-phosphate 5-kinase defines a novel family of lipid kinases. *J Biol Chem* 1995;270:2881–2884.

131. Divecha N, Truong O, Hsuan JJ, et al. The cloning and sequence of the C isoform of PtdIns4P 5-kinase. *Biochem J* 1995;309:715–719.

132. Hinchliffe KA, Ciruela A, Irvine RF. PIPkins, their substrates and their products: New functions for old enzymes. *Biochim Biophys Acta* 1998;1436:87–104.

133. Ishihara H, Shibasaki Y, Kizuki N, et al. Type I phosphatidylinositol-4-phosphate 5-kinases. Cloning of the third isoform and deletion/substitution analysis of members of this novel lipid kinase family. *J Biol Chem* 1998;273:8741–8748.

134. Loijens JC, Anderson RA. Type I phosphatidylinositol-4-phosphate 5-kinases are distinct members of this novel lipid kinase family. *J Biol Chem* 1996;271:32937–32943.

135. Homma K, Terui S, Minemura M, et al. Phosphatidylinositol-4-phosphate 5-kinase localized on the plasma membrane is essential for yeast cell morphogenesis. *J Biol Chem* 1998;25: 15779–15786.

136. Desrivieres S, Cooke FT, Parker PJ, et al. MSS4, a phosphatidylinositol-4-phosphate 5-kinase required for organization of the actin cytoskeleton in *Saccharomyces cerevisiae*. *J Biol Chem* 1998;273:15787–15793.

137. Cooke FT, Dove SK, McEwen RK, et al. The stress-activated phosphatidylinositol 3-phosphate 5-kinase Fab1p is essential for vacuole function in *Saccharomyces cerevisiae*. *Curr Biol* 1998;8: 1219–1222.

138. Rameh LE, Tolias KF, Duckworth BC, et al. A new pathway for synthesis of phosphatidylinositol-4,5-bisphosphate. *Nature* 1997;390:192–196.

139. Zhang X, Loijens JC, Boronenkov IV, et al. Phosphatidylinositol-4-phosphate 5-kinase isozymes catalyze the synthesis of 3-phosphate-containing phosphatidylinositol signaling molecules. *J Biol Chem* 1997;272:17756–17761.

140. Yamamoto K, Graziani A, Carpenter CL, et al. A novel pathway for the formation of phosphatidylinositol(3,4)bisphosphate: Phosphorylation of phosphatidylinositol(3)monophosphate by phosphatidylinositol(3)monophosphate 4-kinase. *J Biol Chem* 1990;265:22086–22089.

141. Graziani A, Ling LE, Endemann G, et al. Purification and characterization of human erythrocyte phosphatidylinositol 4-kinase. Phosphatidylinositol 4-kinase and phosphatidylinositol 3-monophosphate 4-kinase are distinct enzymes. *Biochem J* 1992;284:39–45.

142. Castellino AM, Parker GJ, Boronenkov IV, et al. A novel interaction between the juxtamembrane region of the p55 tumor necrosis factor receptor and phosphatidylinositol-4-phosphate 5-kinase. *J Biol Chem* 1997;272:5861–5870.

143. Banfic H, Tang X-W, Batty IH, et al. A novel integrin-activated pathway forms PKB/Akt-stimulatory phosphatidylinositol 3,4-bisphosphate via phosphatidylinositol 3-phosphate in platelets. *J Biol Chem* 1998;273:13–16.

144. Whiteford CC, Brearley CA, Ulug ET. Phosphatidylinositol 3,5-bisphosphate defines a novel PI 3-kinase pathway in resting mouse fibroblasts. *Biochem J* 1997;323:597–601.

145. Dove SK, Cooke FT, Douglas MR, et al. Osmotic stress activates phosphatidylinositol-3,5-bisphosphate synthesis. *Nature* 1997;390:187–192.

146. Moritz A, De Graan PN, Gispen WH, et al. Phosphatidic acid is a specific activator of phosphatidylinositol-4-phosphate kinase. *J Biol Chem* 1992;267:7207–7210.

147. Loijens JC, Boronenkov IV, Parker GJ, et al. The phosphatidylinositol 4-phosphate 5-kinase family. *Adv Enzyme Regul* 1996;36:115–140.

148. Chong LD, Traynor-Kaplan A, Bokoch GM, et al. The small GTP-binding protein regulates a phosphatidylinositol 4-phosphate 5-kinase in mammalian cells. *Cell* 1994;79:507–513.

149. Zigmond SH, Joyce M, Borleis J, et al. Regulation of actin polymerization in cell-free systems by GTPγS and Cdc42. *J Cell Biol* 1997;138:363–374.

150. Urumow T, Wieland OH. Evidence for a cholera-toxin-sensitive G-protein involved in the regulation of phosphatidylinositol 4-phosphate kinase of rat liver membranes. *Biochim Biophys Acta* 1988;972:232–238.

151. Li J, Yen C, Liaw D, et al. PTEN, A putative protein tyrosine phosphatase gene mutated in human brain, breast, and prostate cancer. *Science* 1997;275:1943–1947.

152. Steck PA, Pershouse MA, Jasser SA, et al. Identification of a candidate tumor suppressor gene, MMAC1, at chromosome 10q23.3 that is mutated in multiple advanced cancers. *Nat Genet* 1997;15:356–362.

153. Cantley LC, Neel BG. New insights into tumor suppression: PTEN suppresses tumor formation by restraining the phosphoinositide 3-kinase/akt pathway. *Proc Natl Acad Sci U S A* 1999;96:4240–4245.

154. Myers MP, Pass I, Batty IH, et al. The lipid phosphatase activity of PTEN is critical for its tumor suppressor function. *Proc Natl Acad Sci U S A* 1998;95:13513–13518.

155. Maehama T, Dixon JE. The tumor suppressor, PTEN/MMAC1, dephosphorylates the lipid second messenger, phosphatidylinositol 3,4,5-triphosphate. *J Biol Chem* 1998;273: 13375–13378.

156. Li J, Takahashi M, Miliaresis C, et al. The PTEN/MMAC1 tumor suppressor induces cell death that is rescued by the AKT/protein kinase B oncogene. *Cancer Res* 1998;58:5667–5672.

157. Tamura M, Gu J, Matsumoto K, et al. Inhibition of cell migration, spreading, and focal adhesions by tumor suppressor PTEN. *Science* 1998;280:1614–1617.

158. Norris FA, Atkins RC, Majerus PW. The cDNA cloning and characterization of inositol polyphosphate 4-phosphatase type

II. Evidence for conserved alternative splicing in the 4-phosphatase family. *J Biol Chem* 1997;272:23859–23864.

159. Norris FA, Majerus PW. Hydrolysis of phosphatidylinositol 3,4-bisphosphate by inositol polyphosphate 4-phosphatase isolated by affinity elution chromatography. *J Biol Chem* 1994; 269:8716–8720.

160. Majerus PW, Kisseleva MV, Anderson Norris F. The role of phosphatases in inositol signaling reactions. *J Biol Chem* 1999; 274:10669–10672.

161. Zhang X, Hartz PA, Philip E, et al. Cell lines from kidney proximal tubules of a patient with Lowe Syndrome lack OCRL inositol polyphosphate 5-phosphatase and accumulate phosphatidylinositol 4,5-bisphosphate. *J Biol Chem* 1998;273: 1574–1582.

162. Janne PA, Suchy SF, Bernard D, et al. Functional overlap between murine INPP5B and OCRL1 may explain why deficiency of the murine ortholog for OCRL1 does not cause Lowe Syndrome in mice. *J Clin Invest* 1998;101:2042–2053.

163. Srinivasan S, Seaman M, Nemoto Y, et al. Disruption of three phosphatidylinositol-polyphosphate 5-phosphatase genes from *Saccharomyces cerevisiae* results in pleiotropic abnormalities of vacuole morphology, cell shape, and osmohomeostasis. *Eur J Cell Biol* 1997;74:350–360.

164. Sha B, Phillips SE, Bankaitis VA, et al. Crystal structure of the *Saccharomyces cerevisiae* phosphatidylinositol-transfer protein. *Nature* 1998;391:506–510.

165. Damen JE, Liu L, Rosten P, et al. The 145-kd protein induced to associate with Shc by multiple cytokines is an inositol tetraphosphate and phosphatidylinositol 3,4,5-triphosphate 5-phosphatase. *Proc Natl Acad Sci U S A* 1996;93:1689–1693.

166. Kavanaugh WM, Pot DA, Chin SM, et al. Multiple forms of an inositol polyphosphate 5-phosphatase form signaling complexes with Shc and Grb2. *Curr Biol* 1996;6:438–445.

167. Lioubin MN, Algate PA, Tsai S, et al. p150Ship, a signal transduction molecule with inositol polyphosphate-5-phosphatase activity. *Genes Dev* 1996;10:1084–1095.

168. Liu Q, Shalaby F, Jones J, et al. The SH2-containing inositol polyphosphate 5-phosphatase, Ship, is expressed during hematopoiesis and spermatogenesis. *Blood* 1998;91:2753–2759.

169. Habib T, Hejna JA, Moses RE, et al. Growth factors and insulin stimulate tyrosine phosphorylation of the 51C/SHIP2 protein. *J Biol Chem* 1998;273:18605–18609.

170. Jackson SP, Schoenwaelder SM, Matzaris M, et al. Phosphatidylinositol 3,4,5-triphosphate is a substrate for the 75 kd inositol polyphosphate 5-phosphatase and a novel 5-phosphatase which forms a complex with the p85/p110 form of phosphoinositide 3-kinase. *EMBO J* 1995;14:4490–4500.

171. Rao VR, Corradetti MN, Chen J, et al. Expression cloning of protein targets for 3-phosphorylated phosphoinositides. *J Biol Chem* 1999;274:37893–37900.

172. Patki V, Lawe DC, Corverra S, et al. A functional PtdIns(3)P-binding motif. *Nature* 1998;394:433–434.

173. Burd CG, Emr SD. Phosphatidylinositol(3)-phosphate signaling mediated by specific binding to RING FYVE domains. *Mol Cell* 1998;2:157–162.

174. Kutateladze TG, Ogburn KD, Watson WT, et al. Phosphatidylinositol 3-phosphate recognition by the FYVE domain. *Mol Cell* 1999;3:805–811.

175. Fruman DA, Rameh LE, Cantley LC. Phosphoinositide binding domains: Embracing 3-phosphate. *Cell* 1999;97:817–820.

176. Gaullier J-M, Simonsen A, D'Arrigo A, et al. FYVE fingers bind PtdIns(3)P. *Nature* 1998;394:432–433.

177. Mills IG, Jones AT, Clague MJ. Involvement of the endosomal autoantigen EEA1 in homotypic fusion of early endosomes. *Curr Biol* 1998;8:881–884.

178. Simonsen A, Lippé R, Christoforidis S, et al. EEA1 links PI(3)K

179. Christoforidis S, Miaczynska M, Ashman K, et al. Phosphatidylinositol-3-OH kinases are Rab5 effectors. *Nat Cell Biol* 1999;1:249–252.

180. Misra S, Hurley JH. Crystal structure of a phosphatidylinositol 3-phosphate-specific membrane-targeting motif, the FYVE domain of Vps27p. *Cell* 1999;97:657–666.

181. Mao Y, Nickitenco A, Duan X, et al. Crystal structure of the VHS and FYVE tandem domains of Hrs, a protein involved in membrane trafficking and signal transduction. *Cell* 2000;100: 447–456.

182. Rameh LE, Cantley LC. The role of phosphoinositide 3-kinase lipid products in cell function. *J Biol Chem* 1999;274: 8347–8350.

183. Isakoff SJ, Cardozo T, Andreev J, et al. Identification and analysis of PH domain-containing targets of phosphatidylinositol 3-kinase using a novel in vivo assay in yeast. *EMBO J* 1998;17:5374–5387.

184. Honda A, Nogami M, Yokozeki T, et al. Phosphatidylinositol 4-phosphate 5-kinase α is a downstream effector of the small G protein ARF6 in membrane ruffle formation. *Cell* 1999;99: 521–532.

185. Franke TF, Kaplan DR, Cantley LC, et al. Direct regulation of the Akt proto-oncogene product by phosphatidylinositol-3,4-bisphosphate. *Science* 1997;275:665–668.

186. Klippel A, Kavanaugh WM, Pot D, et al. A specific product of phosphatidylinositol 3-kinase directly activates the protein kinase Akt through its pleckstrin homology domain. *Mol Cell Biol* 1997;1997:338–344.

187. Andjelkovic M, Alessi DR, Meier R, et al. Role of translocation in the activation and function of protein kinase B. *J Biol Chem* 1997;272:31515–31524.

188. Alessi DR, Andjelkovic M, Caudwell B, et al. Mechanism of activation of protein kinase B by insulin and IGF-1. *EMBO J* 1996;15:6541–6551.

189. Alessi DR, Deak M, Casamayor A, et al. 3-Phosphoinositide-dependent protein kinase-1 (PDK1): structural and functional homology with the *Drosophila* DSTPK61 kinase. *Curr Biol* 1997;7:776–789.

190. Alessi DR, James SR, Downes CP, et al. Characterization of a 3-phosphoinositide-dependent protein kinase which phosphorylates and activates protein kinase Bα. *Curr Biol* 1997; 7:261–269.

191. Stephens L, Anderson K, Stokoe D, et al. Protein kinase B kinases that mediate phosphatidylinositol 3,4,5-trisphosphate-dependent activation of protein kinase B. *Science* 1998; 279:710–714.

192. Stokoe D, Stephens LR, Copeland T, et al. Dual role of phosphatidylinositol-3,4,5-trisphosphate in the activation of protein kinase B. *Science* 1997;277:567–570.

193. Williams MR, Simon J, Arthur C, et al. The 3-phosphoinositide-dependent protein kinase 1 mediates the activation of AGC kinases in embryonic stem cells. *Curr Biol* 2000;10:439–448.

194. Cardone MH, Roy N, Stennicke HR, et al. Regulation of cell death protease-9 by phosphorylation. *Science* 1998;282: 1318–1321.

195. Alnemri ES. Hidden powers of the mitochondria. *Nat Cell Biol* 1999;1:E40–E42.

196. Brunet A, Bonni A, Zigmond M, et al. Akt promotes cell survival by phosphorylating and inhibiting a forkhead transcription factor. *Cell* 1999;96:857–868.

197. Rena G, Guo S, Cichy SC, et al. Phosphorylation of the transcription factor forkhead family member FKHR by protein kinase B. *J Biol Chem* 1999;274:17179–17183.

198. Kops GJ, de Ruiter ND, De Vries-Smits AM, et al. Direct con-

trol of the forkhead transcription factor AFX by protein kinase B. *Nature* 1999;398:630–634.

199. Biggs WHR, Meisenhelder J, Hunter T, et al. Protein kinase B/Akt-mediated phosphorylation promotes nuclear exclusion of the winged helix transcription factor FKHR1. *Proc Natl Acad Sci U S A* 1999;96:7421–7426.

200. Romashkova JA, Makarov SS. NF-kappaB is a target of AKT in antiapoptotic PDGF signaling. *Nature* 1999;401:86–90.

201. Ozes ON, Mayo LD, Gustin JA, et al. NF-kappaB activation by tumour necrosis factor requires the Akt serine-threonine kinase. *Nature* 1999;401:82–85.

202. Kane LP, Shapiro VS, Stokoe D, et al. Induction of NF-kappaB by the Akt/PKB kinase. *Curr Biol* 1999;9:601–604.

203. Khwaja A. Akt is more than just a Bad kinase. *Nature* 1999; 401:33–34.

204. Rust C, Karnitz LM, Paya CV, et al. The bile acid taurochenodeoxycholate activates a phosphatidylinositol 3-kinase-dependent survival signaling cascade. *J Biol Chem* 2000 (*in press*).

205. Webster C, Anwer M. Cyclic adenosine monophosphate-mediated protection against bile acid-induced apoptosis in cultured rat hepatocytes. *Hepatology* 1998;27:1324–1331.

206. Cross DA, Alessi DR, Cohen P, et al. Inhibition of glycogen synthase kinase-3 by insulin mediated by protein kinase B. *Nature* 1995;378:785–789.

207. Deprez J, Vertommen D, Alessi DR, et al. Phosphorylation and activation of heart 6-phosphofructo-2-kinase by protein kinase B and other protein kinases of the insulin signaling cascades. *J Biol Chem* 1997;272:17269–17275.

208. Kitamura T, Kitamura Y, Kuroda S, et al. Insulin-induced phosphorylation and activation of cyclic nucleotide phosphodiesterase 3B by the serine-threonine kinase Akt. *Mol Cell Biol* 1999;19:6286–6296.

209. Nave BT, Ouwens M, Withers DJ, et al. Mammalian target of rapamycin is a direct target for protein kinase B: Identification of a convergence point for opposing effects of insulin and amino acid deficiency on protein translation. *Biochem J* 1999;344:427–431.

210. Dimmeler S, Fleming I, Fisslthaler B, et al. Activation of nitric oxide synthase in endothelial cells by Akt-dependent phosphorylation. *Nature* 1999;399:601–605.

211. Fulton D, Gratton JP, McCabe TJ, et al. Regulation of endothelium-derived nitric oxide production by the protein kinase Akt. *Nature* 1999;399:597–601.

212. Fujio Y, Walsh K. Akt mediates cytoprotection of endothelial cells by vascular endothelial growth factor in an anchorage-dependent manner. *J Biol Chem* 1999;274:16349–16354.

213. Jensen CJ, Buch MB, Krag TO, et al. 90-kd ribosomal S6 kinase is phosphorylated and activated by 3-phosphoinositide-dependent protein kinase-1. *J Biol Chem* 1999;274: 27168–27176.

214. Pullen N, Dennis PB, Andjelkovic A, et al. Phosphorylation and activation of p70s6k by PDK1. *Science* 1998;279:707–710.

215. Le Good JA, Ziegler WH, Parekh DB, et al. Protein kinase C isotypes controlled by phosphoinositide 3-kinase through the protein kinase PDK1. *Science* 1998;281:2042–2045.

216. Toker A, Meyer M, Reddy KK, et al. Activation of protein kinase C family members by the novel polyphosphoinositides PtdIns-3,4-P$_2$ and PtdIns-3,4-P$_3$. *J Biol Chem* 1994;269: 32358–32367.

217. Nakanishi H, Brewer KA, Exton JH. Activation of the ζ isomer of protein kinase C by phosphatidylinositol 3,4,5-trisphosphate. *J Biol Chem* 1993;268:13–16.

218. Musacchio A, Gibson T, Rice P, et al. The PH domain: A common piece in the structural patchwork of signaling proteins. *Trends Biochem Sci* 1993;18:343–348.

219. Han J, Luby-Phelps K, Das B, et al. Role of substrates and products of PI 3-kinase in regulating activation of Rac-related guanosine triphosphatases by Vav. *Science* 1998;279: 558–560.

220. Lockyer PJ, Wennstrom S, Kupzig S, et al. Identification of the ras GTPase-activating protein GAP1(m) as a phosphatidylinositol-3,4,5-trisphosphate-binding protein in vivo. *Curr Biol* 1999;9:265–268.

221. Venkateswarlu K, Oatey PB, Tavare JM, et al. Identification of centaurin-α1 as a potential in vivo phosphatidylinositol 3,4,5-trisphosphate-binding protein that is functionally homologous to the yeast ADP-ribosylation factor (ARF) GTPase-activating protein, Gcs1. *Biochem J* 1999;340:359–363.

222. Roth MG. Inheriting the golgi. *Cell* 1999;99:559–562.

223. Leevers SJ, Vanhaesebroeck B, Waterfield MD. Signaling through phosphoinositide 3-kinases: The lipids take centre stage. *Curr Opin Cell Biol* 1999;11:219–225.

224. Haruta T, Morris AJ, Rose DW, et al. Insulin-stimulated GLUT4 translocation is mediated by a divergent intracellular signaling pathway. *J Biol Chem* 1995;270:27991–27994.

225. Cheatham B, Vlahos CJ, Cheatham L, et al. Phosphatidylinositol 3-kinase activation is required for insulin stimulation of pp70 S6 kinase, DNA synthesis, and glucose transporter translocation. *Mol Cell Biol* 1994;14:4902–4911.

226. Baraldi E, Carugo KD, Hyvonen M, et al. Structure of the PH domain from Bruton's tyrosine kinase in complex with inositol 1,3,4,5-tetrakisphosphate. *Structure* 1999;7:449–460.

227. Falasca M, Logan SK, Lehto VP, et al. Activation of phospholipase C γ by PI 3-kinase-induced PH domain-mediated membrane targeting. *EMBO J* 1998;17:414–422.

228. Rameh LE, Rhee SG, Spokes K, et al. Phosphoinositide 3-kinase regulates phospholipase Cγ-mediated calcium signaling. *J Biol Chem* 1998;273:23750–23757.

229. Bae YS, Cantley LG, Chen CS, et al. Activation of phospholipase C-γ by phosphatidylinositol 3,4,5-trisphosphate. *J Biol Chem* 1998;273:4465–4469.

221. Gatmaitan ZC, Nies AT, Arias IM. Regulation and translocation of ATP-dependent apical membrane proteins in rat liver. *Am J Physiol* 1997;272:G1041–G1049.

231. Harrison-Findik D, Misra S, Jain SK, et al. Dynamin inhibits phosphatidylinositol 3-kinase in hematopoietic cells. *Biochem Acta* 2001;1538:10–19.

INSULIN AND OTHER GROWTH FACTORS

M. DODSON MICHAEL
NEIL B. RUDERMAN

The liver is the central organ in energy metabolism, and insulin is the primary anabolic hormone promoting the storage of energy in the fed state (1–3) (see website chapter 🖳 W-11). In response to nutrient secretagogues, insulin is secreted from the pancreatic β-cells directly into the portal circulation. The resulting high portal insulin levels prime the liver for rapid alterations in hepatic carbohydrate and lipid homeostasis, such as stimulation of glycogen synthesis, lipogenesis, and lipoprotein synthesis and suppression of gluconeogenesis/glycogenolysis and VLDL formation (4–6) (see website chapter 🖳 W-12). Many of these effects are mediated by the regulation of gene expression, with insulin having positive effects on genes encoding glycolytic and lipogenic enzymes and negative effects on genes encoding gluconeogenic enzymes (7). In addition, insulin affects the messenger RNA stability of specific transcripts, promotes translation by activation of p70 S6 kinase, stimulates phosphorylation and dephosphorylation of many metabolic enzymes, and is required for hepatic growth and regeneration.

The effects of insulin on metabolism are mediated by high-affinity cell surface receptors. Insulin binding activates the intrinsic tyrosine kinase activity of the receptor's intracellular domain, leading to autophosphorylation of the receptor as well as phosphorylation of a family of insulin receptor substrate (IRS) proteins (Fig. 36.1). The phosphorylated IRS proteins serve as docking sites for the binding and activation of intracellular effector molecules that contain Src homology 2 (SH2) domains including the regulatory subunit of phosphatidylinositol 3'-kinase (PI 3-kinase), the tyrosine phosphatase SHP-2, and the adapter molecule Grb2. Subsequently, these effector molecules propagate specific signals that elicit the biological effects of insulin on protein, lipid, and carbohydrate metabolism. This chapter reviews the molecular mechanisms by which insulin and the related insulin-like growth factors exert their biological effects, and how aberrant signaling contributes to pathophysiological states.

M. D. Michael: Endocrine Research, Eli Lilly and Company, Indianapolis, Indiana 46285.
N. B. Ruderman: Departments of Medicine and Physiology, Boston University School of Medicine; Diabetes Unit, Department of Medicine, Section of Endocrinology, Boston Medical Center, Boston, Massachusetts 02118.

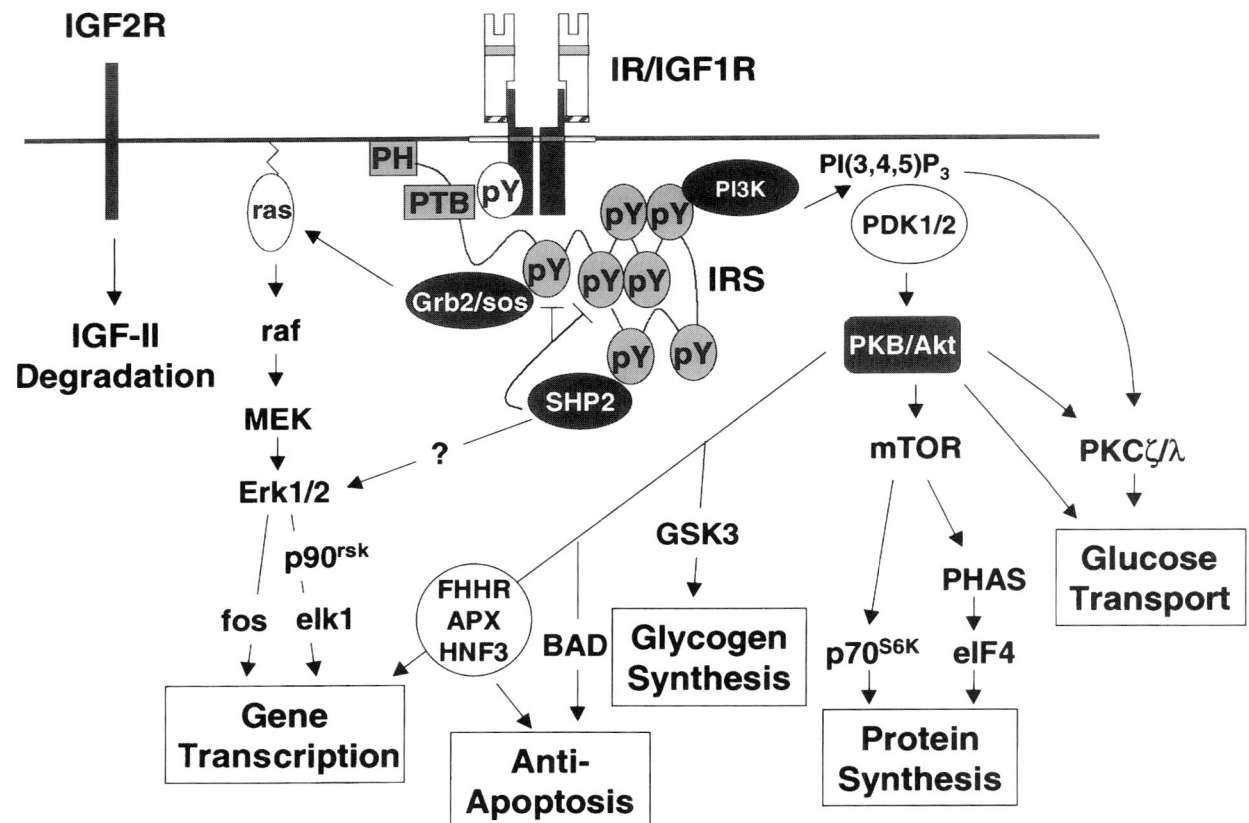

FIGURE 36.1. The insulin/insulin-like growth factor (IGF) signaling cascade. Insulin and IGFs bind to three different transmembrane receptors: the insulin receptor (*IR*), the type 1 IGF receptor (*IFG1R*) and the type 2 IGF receptor (*IGF2R*). Whereas the IGF2R targets IGF-II for intracellular degradation, the IR and IGF1R initiate an intracellular signaling cascade. Binding of ligand to its cognate receptor induces autophosphorylation of the receptor on tyrosine residues of the intracellular domain. These phosphotyrosines serve as docking sites for a family of insulin receptor substrate (*IRS*) proteins, which serve as multi-site docking proteins for downstream effector molecules such as PI 3-kinase (*PI3K*), Grb2, and SHP2. PI 3-kinase activation results in the production of PI(3, 4, 5)P$_3$ in the membrane, ultimately leading to the activation of PKB/Akt. PKB/Akt has been implicated in mediating the action of insulin to stimulate glucose transport, protein synthesis, and glycogen synthesis, to inhibit apoptosis, and to affect gene transcription. Activation of Grb2 couples the insulin signaling pathway to the ras/MAP kinase pathway for the stimulation of mitogenesis and gene expression. Activation of the tyrosine phosphatase, SHP2, is thought to attenuate insulin signaling by dephosphorylating the IRS proteins, and it may also have effects on MAP kinases. *PH*, pleckstrin homology; *PTB*, phosphotyrosine binding domain.

FUEL HOMEOSTASIS

The Role of the Liver in Glucose Homeostasis

The liver has a critical role as an integrator of whole-body fuel homeostasis in great measure by closely regulating the concentration of glucose in the blood (see website chapter 🖥 W-11) (2,3). Glucose occupies a unique position in fuel homeostasis, since it serves as the only fuel source for the brain, except in conditions of prolonged fasting. The liver is a major depot for glucose uptake and storage, and may account for disposal up to one-third of an oral glucose load. The major postprandial stimuli for the storage of glucose as glycogen in the liver are insulin, glucose, and parasympathetic nerve stimulation (6). The expression of glucokinase, which catalyzes the rate-limiting step in glycogen synthesis, is dependent on insulin. Insulin stimulation directly activates glycogen synthase by inactivating the negative regulatory protein glycogen synthase kinase-3 (GSK-3), and by increasing the activity of protein phosphatase 1, although the precise role of these enzymes remains controversial (8). In addition, insulin stimulates the intracellular accumulation of Na$^+$, K$^+$, and Cl$^-$ ions, resulting in an increase in cell volume, which also activates glycogen synthase. Insulin not only activates glycogen synthesis but also inhibits the breakdown of endogenous glycogen stores by inhibiting the cAMP-dependent activation of glycogen phosphorylase. While most extracellular signals control glycogen metabolism by transmembrane receptors, glucose activates glycogen synthesis by binding directly to glycogen phosphorylase. Glucose binding to the active site of the active form of glycogen phosphorylase, phosphorylase *a*, not only acts as a competitive inhibitor of phosphorylase enzymatic activity but also induces a conformational change that makes phosphorylase *a* more susceptible to inactivation by dephosphorylation. The decrease in phosphorylase *a* further releases the glycogen-associated Ser/Thr protein phosphatase PP1G from an allosteric inhibitor, thus allowing dephosphorylation and activation of glycogen synthase. This mechanism prevents the simultaneous synthesis and degradation of glycogen.

When blood glucose concentrations and insulin levels decline in the postabsorptive state, the liver is the major organ capable of releasing physiologically significant amounts of glucose into the circulation (see website chapter 🖥 W-11). The glucose released by the liver is produced by the synthesis of glucose from amino acids, lactate, pyruvate, and glycerol via the gluconeogenic pathway or glycogenolysis. Increased hepatic glucose production is stimulated by glucagon, catecholamines, and/or eicosanoids and decreased levels of insulin. This adaptive mechanism whereby the liver maintains blood glucose concentrations in the normal range is possible because hepatocytes express the enzyme glucose-6-phosphatase, which hydrolyzes the phosphate from glucose-6-phosphate allowing free glucose to exit the cell. Muscle and other tissues synthesize and degrade glycogen for their own energy needs, but because they do not express glucose-6-phosphatase, these organs do not release significant amounts of glucose into the circulation for use by other tissues. The only exception is the kidney, which serves a significant role in amino acid-derived gluconeogenesis in states of prolonged fasting and possibly other situations (9).

Metabolic Adaptations to Fasting and Starvation

Liver glycogen is a short-lived but readily mobilized source of glucose, whereas gluconeogenesis is a more long-lived but less flexible source of glucose (1–3). The first few hours after a meal, glucose in the blood originates predominately from gastrointestinal tract absorption. The absorbed glucose that is in excess of the immediate needs of the brain and other glucose-dependent tissues is used to rebuild fuel reservoirs. During this time period, plasma glucose and insulin levels are high, plasma glucagon levels are low, and glycogen synthesis is favored in liver and muscle. After an overnight fast (about 12 hours), 35% to 60% of the circulating glucose is derived from hepatic glycogenolysis and the remainder from gluconeogenesis. After 24 to 36 hours of starvation, gluconeogenesis is the sole source of glucose

entering the circulation. The principal gluconeogenic precursors are amino acids (primarily alanine), which originate from the degradation of protein in muscle and other tissues; lactate, which arises from the anaerobic glycolysis of glucose, and glycerol, derived principally from the hydrolysis of triglycerides in adipose stores. Release of these metabolites is enhanced by the catabolic effect of low plasma insulin and elevated plasma glucagon levels. Concomitant with hepatic gluconeogenesis, these hormones also stimulate the hepatic production of ketone bodies (acetoacetate and β-hydroxybutyrate) from fatty acids derived from the hydrolysis of adipose triglycerides. Upon even more prolonged fasting, the ketone body concentration in cerebrospinal fluid increases, and ketone metabolism by brain displaces glucose utilization, thus sparing crucial proteins from muscle and other tissues from further degradation. Moreover, the decreased alanine release from muscle results in decreased gluconeogenic precursors for extraction by the liver and therefore decreased hepatic glucose production. In the starved state, the kidney assumes a primary role in amino acid-derived gluconeogenesis (primarily from glutamine), accounting for as much as 20% to 25% of whole-body glucose turnover (9,10).

INSULIN ACTION

Insulin Synthesis and Structure

Insulin is synthesized and secreted from the β-cells of the islets of Langerhans. Because of its critical role in regulating metabolism, the insulin protein and the gene encoding preproinsulin have been extensively studied (see website chapter 🖥 W-29). The human preproinsulin gene, located on human chromosome 11p15.5, is 1,355 base pairs in length and contains three exons. Translation of the preproinsulin mRNA yields an 11.5-kd preproinsulin peptide that is rapidly translocated into the lumen of the rough endoplasmic reticulum (ER), where the ER-targeting "pre" signal sequence is cleaved. This results in the formation of proinsulin, a 9-kd peptide containing A and B domains, which are processed to form a molecule composed of the A and B chains of insulin, linked by a 33-amino-acid connecting peptide (C-peptide). One major function of the C-peptide is to align the cysteine residues in the A and B domains for appropriate disulfide bridge formation, but whether C-peptide independently has a physiological role is not clear. Following transport to the Golgi, proinsulin is packaged into secretory granules, and processed to insulin by the sequential action of two endopeptidases, prohormone convertase (PC)-3 and -2. In normal subjects, less than 5% of proinsulin remains unprocessed and is secreted in that form. The mature insulin molecule consists of a 21-amino-acid A-chain with an intrachain disulfide bond linking residues 6 and 11 linked to a 30-amino-acid B-chain by two disulfide bridges between A7-B7 and A20-B19. The high insulin concentration together with the low pH of the secretory granule promotes the precipitation of insulin with Zn^{2+} to form a 2 Zn^{2+}-insulin hexamer composed of three identical insulin dimers associated in a three-fold symmetrical pattern. Insulin and C-peptide remain stored together in the secretory granule, and upon stimulation, are secreted together in equimolar amounts. If the number of stored insulin granules exceeds the requirements for secretion, the cargo of the secretory granules is destroyed by granule fusion with lysosomes in a process called crinophagy.

Insulin Secretion and Clearance

The major physiological determinant of insulin secretion from the pancreatic β-cells is the concentration of glucose in the blood, although other metabolites, hormones, and neural signals are involved in this process as well. As depicted in Figure 36.2, glucose enters the β-cell via the Glut2 glucose transporter and is phosphorylated by glucokinase, which acts as a sensitive glucose sensor that ultimately couples insulin secretion to the prevailing glucose level. Insulin secretion requires the active metabolism of glucose, which results in an increase in the adenosine triphosphate (ATP)/adenosine diphosphate (ADP) ratio and subsequent closure of the ATP-sensitive K^+ channels in the β-cell membrane. Blockage of the efflux of K^+ ions from the β-cell causes depolarization of the plasma membrane,

which in turn opens voltage-gated Ca^{2+} channels. The increase in cytosolic calcium initiates an acute phase of insulin granule exocytosis from a primed releasable pool of insulin secretory granules. This first phase of insulin release is followed by a second phase of sustained release of secretory vesicles that undergo priming as the result of cellular metabolism. Wollheim and colleagues (11) have proposed that the Ca^{2+}-dependent production of glutamate by the β-cell mitochondria is involved in priming the pool of secondary insulin secretory granules for release. The massive dilution that occurs following insulin secretion causes the dissociation of the 2 Zn^{2+}-insulin hexamer to the monomer form, which predominates in the circulation.

The amino acids leucine and arginine are also potent stimulators of insulin secretion in the absence of glucose. Metabolism of leucine within the β-cell generates ATP, which in turn promotes insulin secretion in a manner analogous to glucose. Arginine, on the other hand, has been proposed to depolarize the β-cell membrane upon entry into the cell, causing a Ca^{2+} influx. In addition to insulin and amino acids, free fatty acids have been shown to be important insulin secretagogues; indeed, they appear to be necessary to maintain the low but finite rate of insulin secretion during starvation (12). In addition to fuels and amino acids, a wide variety of hormones and neuropeptides may enhance insulin secretion. Glucagon, gastric inhibitory peptide, and glucagon-like peptide augment insulin secre-

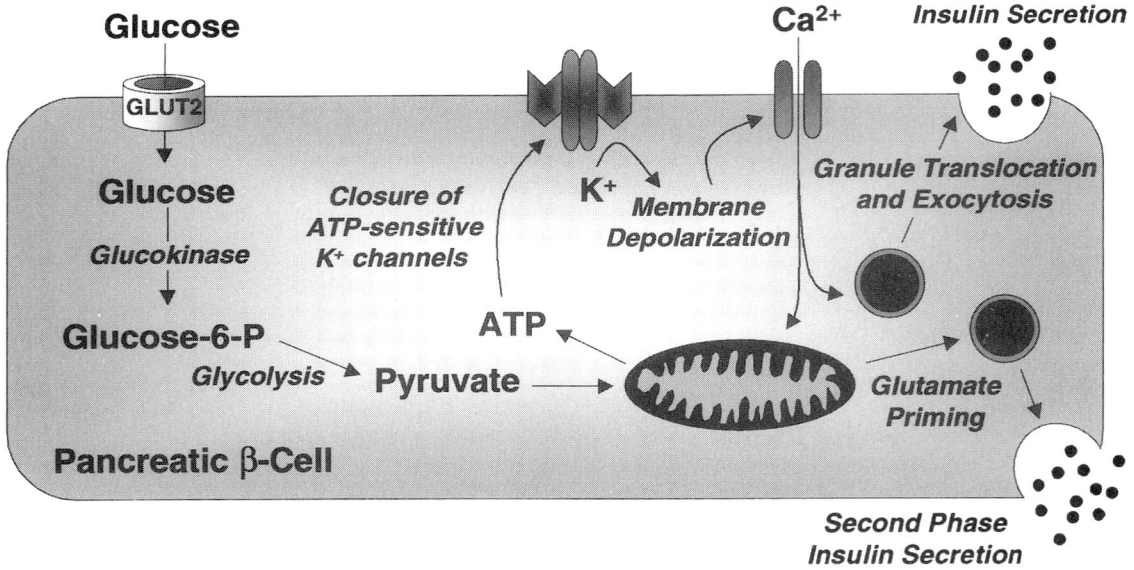

FIGURE 36.2. Glucose-stimulated insulin secretion from the pancreatic β-cell. Glucose enters the β-cell via the GLUT-2 facilitative transporter, and is subsequently metabolized to produce adenosine triphosphate (*ATP*). Increased levels of ATP close ATP-sensitive potassium channels in the β-cell membrane, leading to membrane depolarization and opening of voltage-gated calcium channels. The influx of calcium initiates an acute phase of insulin granule exocytosis from a primed pool of granules, and further stimulates glutamate production from the mitochondria. Glutamate plays a role in priming a secondary pool of insulin granules for a second, more prolonged phase of insulin secretion.

tion by increasing intracellular cAMP, whereas acetylcholine, cholecystokinin, vasoactive intestinal peptide, and gastrin-releasing peptide as well as insulin itself stimulate insulin secretion by promoting the release of Ca^{2+} from intracellular stores. Other hormones and neuropeptides that decrease intracellular cAMP and Ca^{2+} levels inhibit insulin secretion.

Due to the rapid effects of insulin to regulate cellular metabolism and maintain blood glucose within the normal range, the process of rapid, efficient insulin clearance from the circulation is just as important as tightly regulated insulin secretion. The liver is the primary site of insulin clearance, with as much as 50% of insulin being removed by a receptor-mediated process during the first pass through the portal circulation. Upon binding the hepatocyte insulin receptor, insulin is internalized into endosomal vesicles, where the insulin-degrading enzyme (IDE) initiates insulin degradation. As much as 50% of internalized insulin is degraded in endosomes with the remaining degradation occurring in lysosomes, the cytosol, and possibly the nucleus. At least some portion of the internalized insulin escapes endosomal degradation and is returned to the cell surface with the recycled receptor. Since insulin clearance by the liver is a receptor-mediated process, disease states that affect receptor number, such as obesity, type 2 diabetes mellitus, and liver disease, can decrease insulin clearance, thereby increasing the residence time of insulin in the circulation. The kidney plays a secondary role in insulin clearance, which occurs by both glomerular filtration and proximal tubule reabsorption and degradation. In addition, glomerular filtration by the kidney serves as the major clearance mechanism for both proinsulin and C-peptide.

The Insulin Receptor

The insulin receptor is a ubiquitously expressed, transmembrane glycoprotein consisting of two 135 kd α-subunits and two 95 kd β-subunits linked by disulfide bonds to form an $\alpha_2\beta_2$ heterotetramer (Fig. 36.3). The α and β subunits are derived by proteolytic processing of a prorecptor polypeptide that is encoded by a single gene located on human chromosome 19p13.2. Alternative splicing of exon 11 results in two insulin receptor isoforms that are called −exon 11 or the A-form and +exon 11 or the B-form. The abundance of the +exon 11 isoform shows a marked predominance in liver, whereas the −exon 11 isoform is predominant in leukocytes. The two receptor isoforms have slightly different affinities for insulin; however, there is no definitive evidence that expression of either isoform is altered in insulin-resistant states.

The extracellular α-subunits are responsible for insulin binding, and in the absence of ligand inhibit the activity of the intracellular tyrosine kinase domain located in the β-subunits. Binding of insulin leads to a conformational change in the receptor that is propagated through the membrane by the β-subunits to the intracellular domain. This in turn relieves the inhibition of the tyrosine kinase domain, resulting in autophosphorylation of the β-subunit on at least six residues. Phosphotyrosine 960, which is located in the juxtamembrane region, resides in an NPXpY motif that is recognized by the phosphotyrosine binding (PTB) domains of IRS proteins. This NPXpY motif also serves a second function as a ligand-dependent receptor internalization motif. Three of the autophosphorylated tyrosine residues, that is, Tyr1146, Tyr1150, and Tyr1151, reside in an activation domain of the receptor. When phosphorylated, these tyrosines promote enhanced tyrosine kinase activity towards nonreceptor substrates.

Attenuation of Insulin Receptor Signaling

Several mechanisms have evolved to attenuate insulin signaling and prevent sustained signaling from the occupied and unoccupied receptor. Insulin receptors on the cell surface have a half-life of about 12 to 18 hours, but insulin stimulation accelerates receptor internalization and degradation, reducing the half-life to only 2 to 3 hours. Thus, ligand-mediated endocytosis and degradation of the receptor play a major role in acutely diminishing insulin signaling as well as preventing chronic hyperstimulation.

A second mechanism for signal attenuation is inactivation of the tyrosine kinase activity of the receptor by dephosphorylation. Two protein tyrosine phosphatases (PTPases), that is, the receptor-type PTPase LAR and the cytosolic PTP-1B, have been implicated in the dephosphorylation of the insulin receptor *in vitro*. Studies using gene knockout mice have directly tested the *in vivo* significance of these two PTPases in regulating insulin signaling. Targeted mutagenesis of LAR demonstrated impaired mammary gland development with no apparent effect on carbohydrate metabolism or insulin signaling (13). However, Ren and colleagues (14) demonstrated lower plasma insulin and glucose levels, as well as reduced hepatic glucose production, in LAR knockout mice created by insertional mutagenesis. The discrepancy between these two models of LAR deficiency is not understood. In contrast to the inconclusive involvement of LAR in insulin signaling, studies with PTP-1B knockout mice strongly implicate this tyrosine phosphatase in modulating both insulin sensitivity and fuel metabolism. PTP-1B knockout mice showed decreased blood glucose and insulin concentrations, with enhanced insulin sensitivity evident in both glucose and insulin tolerance tests. Furthermore, PTP-1B knockout mice showed increased tyrosine phosphorylation of the insulin receptor in liver and muscle tissue in response to insulin (15).

Insulin Receptor Substrates and the Insulin Signaling Cascade

Phosphorylation of cytosolic IRS proteins allows propagation of the signal from the activated tyrosine kinase domain of the

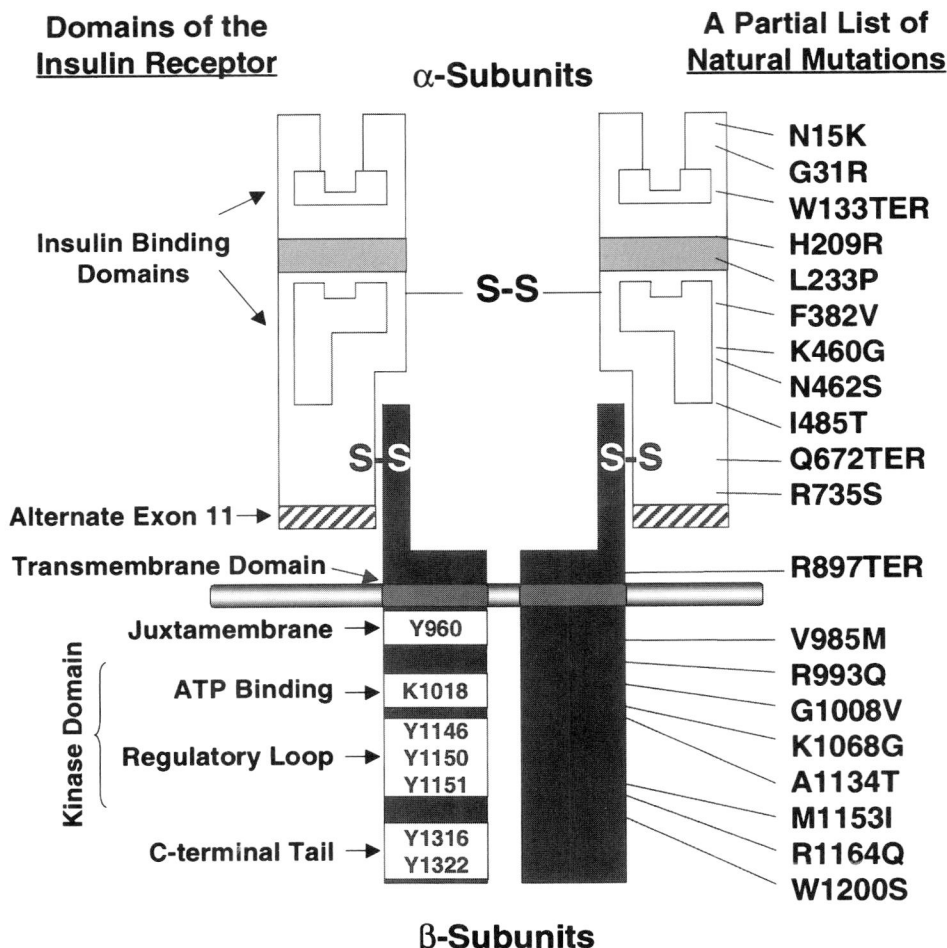

FIGURE 36.3. Structural domains of the insulin receptor with a partial list of naturally occurring mutations in humans. The insulin receptor is an $\alpha_2\beta_2$ heterotetramer that is held together by three disulfide bridges. Two distinct insulin binding domains are found in the α-subunits. The alternative exon 11 is located at the carboxy-terminus of the α-subunits. The β-subunits contain a 23-amino-acid transmembrane domain and the intracellular tyrosine kinase domains. Several tyrosine residues of the β-subunits that are critical for signaling are shown. Naturally occurring mutations that are associated with insulin resistance are shown on the right half of the heterotetramer. *ATP*, adenosine triphosphate.

insulin receptor (Fig. 36.1). At least nine members of a family of IRS proteins have been identified. These include IRS-1, -2, -3, and -4, which are regarded as the most specific substrates for insulin signaling, as well as the three isoforms of Shc, Gab-1, and p62^{dok}. IRS-1 and IRS-2 are both expressed in many tissues at varying levels, with IRS-1 and -2 predominating in liver. Shc, which couples the insulin receptor to the Ras/MAP kinase pathway through interaction with Grb-2, is phosphorylated by insulin, but the in vivo significance of Shc to regulate insulin-dependent growth and metabolism has not been studied in detail. Very little data exist to support a role for IRS-3, IRS-4, Gab-1 or p62^{dok} in insulin signaling in liver.

IRS proteins possess several discrete structural domains. Near the amino-terminus is a pleckstrin homology (PH) domain that targets IRS proteins to specific membrane domains that contain certain phospholipids. This is followed by a PTB domain, which is critical in facilitating the interaction of IRS proteins with the insulin receptor. The PH domain is found in all substrates of the insulin receptor tyrosine kinase except Shc, which has a unique PTB domain that allows interaction with the receptor. Gab-1 is the only substrate that lacks a PTB domain. The carboxy-terminal tail of these substrates contains most of the tyrosine phosphorylation sites, which vary in number from only one in Shc to as many as 22 in IRS-1. Once phosphorylated, these tyrosines in the context of the surrounding residues become specific binding sites for proteins containing SH2 interaction motifs.

Three types of intracellular signaling partners couple with IRS proteins to propagate the insulin signal: SH2 adaptor proteins, SH2 enzymes, and other non-SH2 proteins that act by unknown mechanisms. The SH2 domains of IRS protein signaling partners consist of about 100 amino acids, including a highly conserved phosphotyrosine-binding pocket that promotes specific, high-affinity interactions. Some of these SH2 proteins also contain SH3 domains, which bind to proline-rich sequences and thereby provide a link between the SH2 protein and an associated catalytic subunit or downstream target. The most important SH2 adaptor proteins involved in insulin signaling are the regulatory subunits of PI 3-kinase and Grb-2. The physiological roles of Crk and Nck in insulin signaling are less well understood. The SH2 enzymes that bind tyrosine-phosphorylated IRS proteins include the protein kinases Fyn, Cbl, and Csk as well as the phosphatases SHIP and SHP-2.

Phosphatidylinositol 3′-Kinase Regulatory Subunits

PI 3-kinase is a lipid kinase and a key element in the pathway leading to most of the metabolic effects of insulin. Inhibition of PI 3-kinase activity by dominant negative mutants or by pharmacological inhibitors such as wortmannin or LY294002 abolishes many of the metabolic effects of insulin, including stimulation of glucose uptake and activation of fatty acid, glycogen, protein, and DNA synthesis (see website chapter 💻 W-29).

Grb-2

Grb-2 is a 27-kd molecule with an SH2-SH3-SH2 structure that links the insulin signaling cascade to the Ras/MAP kinase pathway. Grb-2 constitutively associates with the mammalian homolog of the *Drosophila* protein son-of-sevenless (mSOS), the guanine nucleotide exchange factor for the small G-protein, Ras. The binding of Grb-2 to either the insulin receptor-associated IRS proteins or receptor-associated Shc brings mSOS in proximity to the membrane-bound Ras, thereby facilitating GTP loading and activation of Ras. Activated Ras then sets in motion a cascade of serine/threonine kinases including Raf-1, MEK, the MAP kinases ERK1 and ERK2, and p90rsk. Activation of the Ras/MAP kinase pathway is believed to mediate some of the stimulatory effects of insulin on gene transcription, mitogenesis, and cell survival.

Fyn/Cbl Complex

Fyn is a cytoplasmic protein tyrosine kinase that can be activated by association with other phosphotyrosine proteins through its SH2 domain or by dephosphorylation of its carboxy-terminal tyrosine. Fyn is not activated directly by the insulin receptor, but rather by its association with IRS proteins and the insulin receptor substrate, c-Cbl (16,17). c-

Cbl contains a PTB domain and binds to the SH2 adaptor proteins Grb-2, Crk, and the p85 regulatory subunit of PI 3-kinase (18). Once it is tyrosine phosphorylated by the activated insulin receptor kinase, c-Cbl binds to Fyn, and the bound partners are translocated to small invaginations of the plasma membrane, called caveolae (17). Fyn has been demonstrated to phosphorylate two isoforms of the caveolae-specific protein, caveolin (17); however, the biological significance of this modification of caveolin with respect to insulin action has not been elucidated.

Csk

The carboxy-terminal Src kinase (Csk) is a cytoplasmic tyrosine kinase that inactivates Src-type kinases by tyrosine phosphorylation. Csk associates with IRS-1 through its SH2 domain and promotes a decrease in the phosphorylation of focal adhesion kinase (FAK) in an insulin-dependent manner. FAK is one of the key kinases in regulating cell–cell interactions and cell–extracellular matrix interaction in the integrin and other growth factor signaling pathways. This action of Csk, which may be mediated by its inhibition of Src kinases, may promote the insulin-induced rearrangement of cytoskeletal components.

SHIP

Insulin stimulation of PI 3-kinase produces both $PI(3,4,5)P_3$ and $PI(3,4)P_2$. The SH2-containing phosphatase, SHIP, has been identified as a 5′-phosphate phosphatase with specificity for inositol 1,3,4,5-tetraphosphate, and $PI(3,4,5)P_3$, converting the latter to $PI(3,4)P_2$ (19). Overexpression of SHIP specifically decreases the amount of $PI(3,4,5)P_3$ produced following insulin stimulation (20); therefore it appears that SHIP is involved in attenuation of insulin signaling events.

SHP-2

SHP-2 (also called SH-PTP2, PTP1D, and Syp) is a phosphotyrosine phosphatase that is activated upon binding the carboxy-terminal phosphotyrosines of IRS-1. The physiological substrates of SHP-2 are not known, but overexpression of SHP-2 modulates cell adhesion and migration as well as insulin activation of both the Ras/MAP kinase pathway and c-Jun NH_2-terminal kinases (JNKs) (21–24).

ALTERATIONS OF INSULIN SIGNALING IN DISEASE STATES

Insulin receptors and IRS proteins are essential to insulin action. Alterations in receptor and postreceptor function occur in disease states such as type 2 diabetes mellitus and obesity. Insulin resistance exists whenever normal concentrations of insulin produce a less than normal biological response. In most cases, insulin resistance is accompanied by increased insulin secretion from the pancreas in an effort to compensate for the resistance. When compensatory insulin secretion cannot override the insulin resistance in target tissues, disease states develop.

Obesity

The most common pathophysiological state of insulin resistance is obesity, especially in people adapted to Western diets. Insulin action on metabolism is impaired in obese subjects, as demonstrated by decreased insulin-stimulated glucose uptake and phosphorylation and decreased glycogen synthesis. In both humans and rodents, obesity is typically associated with elevated fasting plasma insulin levels, which correlate directly with the level of insulin resistance and inversely with insulin receptor number and kinase activity in muscle. As described in detail above, insulin receptor content is regulated by rates of synthesis, internalization, and degradation, whereas receptor tyrosine kinase activity is activated by tyrosine phosphorylation and inhibited by serine/threonine phosphorylation. Two potential mechanisms, that is, activation of PTPases and serine kinases, have recently been suggested to be involved in modulating receptor kinase activity in obese states. Increased PTPase activity in the skeletal muscle of obese subjects is associated with increased expression of the PTPases, LAR, and PTP-1B (25).

Despite the presence of abnormalities in insulin receptor number and tyrosine kinase activity, it is unlikely that decreased receptor function is responsible for the insulin resistance associated with obesity. In animals and in humans, insulin receptor expression and tyrosine kinase activity as well as whole-body insulin sensitivity are restored by weight reduction, streptozotocin treatment or diazoxide therapy, all of which cause a lowering of plasma insulin levels. These data support the concept that the reduction of insulin receptor number and tyrosine kinase activity is a secondary effect to the hyperinsulinemia associated with obesity and not the primary defect underlying insulin resistance.

A potential link between increased adiposity and insulin resistance has come from the discovery that adipocytes themselves produce and secrete hormones and cytokines that negatively affect metabolism and insulin sensitivity. The first recognized of these was the cytokine, tumor necrosis factor-α (TNFα), which not only diminishes insulin-stimulated tyrosine phosphorylation and increases inhibitory serine/threonine phosphorylation of IRS proteins in some cells but also decreases the activity of the insulin receptor tyrosine kinase (26). Neutralization of TNFα with antibodies in obese rats (27) and gene knockout of both TNFα receptor isoforms in diet-induced obese mice (28,29) are associated with improved insulin sensitivity; however, anti-TNFα treatment of obese humans does not improve insulin sensitivity. Adipocytes also produce the hormone leptin, which affects appetite regulation and insulin sensitivity (see Chapter 17). Leptin is the product of the *obese* gene that was identified by positional cloning of the defective gene in the obese, hyperinsulinemic *ob/ob* mouse (30). Since circulating leptin concentrations in humans closely correlate with the percentage of body fat (31), obese humans seem to be leptin-resistant rather than leptin-deficient.

Type 2 Diabetes Mellitus

Type 2 diabetes mellitus is among the most common metabolic disorders worldwide, and is characterized by at least two distinct defects: (a) insulin resistance, that is, a decrease in the ability of insulin to stimulate glucose disposal and inhibit hepatic glucose production, and (b) a relative insulin deficiency, that is, an inability of the pancreatic β-cells to compensate for this insulin resistance by appropriate increases in insulin secretion. The exact site of the insulin resistance leading to decreased glucose disposal remains a matter of debate. In the earliest phases of human type 2 diabetes, insulin resistance appears to be greatest in skeletal muscle; however, mice with severe insulin resistance in skeletal muscle due to a muscle-specific insulin receptor knockout have surprisingly normal whole-body glucose homeostasis (32). Insulin resistance in the liver has been suggested to be a later factor in the development of hyperglycemia, with increased hepatic glucose production tightly correlated with fasting hyperglycemia in type 2 diabetic individuals (33).

Polymorphisms and Mutations of the Insulin Receptor Gene

Over 50 mutations in the insulin receptor gene have been described (Fig. 36.3). Taylor has classified these mutations into five distinct classes: Class 1 mutations prevent receptor synthesis; Class 2 mutations impair receptor transport and/or posttranslational processing; Class 3 mutations decrease insulin binding; Class 4 mutations directly decrease tyrosine kinase activity; and Class 5 mutations increase receptor degradation (34). The phenotypes associated with these mutations are wide-ranging and include: the severe insulin resistance, acanthosis nigricans, and growth retardation associated with leprechaunism and Rabson–Mendenhall syndrome; glucose intolerance, insulin resistance, acanthosis nigricans, and hyperandrogenism of the type A syndrome of insulin resistance; and mild insulin resistance or even no apparent clinical phenotype. Although there are many reports in the literature describing polymorphisms in the insulin receptor gene in patients with type 2 diabetes, genomic analysis of large populations indicates that mutations in the insulin receptor are not significant contributors to the insulin resistance associated with typical type 2 diabetes or obesity.

Polymorphisms and Mutations of the Insulin Receptor Substrate Protein Genes

The originally described IRS protein, IRS-1, serves as a substrate for the insulin receptor and the related insulin-like growth factor (IGF)-1 receptor as well as for other tyrosine kinase receptors of the cytokine receptor family. The IRS-1 gene, which is an intronless gene located on human chromosome 2q36, contains many naturally occurring polymorphisms. The most extensively studied of these mutations, G972R, is found in white populations, with a higher prevalence in type 2 diabetic patients (10.7%) compared to healthy control patients (5.8%) (35). IRS-2 shares many similarities with IRS-1 including sequence similarities in the PH and PTB domains and many tyrosine phosphorylation sites that are recognized by similar effector molecules. Three polymorphisms of IRS-2 have recently been identified (36,37). One of these, L647V, has a rare association with type 2 diabetes (37); however, linkage analysis in two different populations of patients with type 2 diabetes failed to reveal a significant association of IRS-2 with this disease (36,38).

INSULIN-LIKE GROWTH FACTORS

In 1957, Salmon and Daughaday proposed that the effects of growth hormone on cartilage sulfation are mediated not directly by growth hormone itself, but rather by the production of growth hormone-stimulated mediators, originally called somatomedins. The somatomedin most regulated by growth hormone was identified as somatomedin C, now referred to as IGF-I. A second somatomedin, IGF-II (somatomedin A), is similar in primary sequence and three-dimensional structure to IGF-I, but it is less regulated by growth hormone. In addition to their effects to stimulate growth and metabolism, the IGFs stimulate differentiation of myoblasts and osteoblasts, increase the differentiation, migration, and clonal expansion of T lymphocytes, enhance gonadal steroidogenesis, and induce mitogenesis in a wide variety of cell types. These polypeptide hormones, which are made by the liver and by most, if not all, peripheral tissues, bind to two classes of receptors: the insulin receptor/type 1 IGF receptor (IGF1R) class and the type 2 IGF receptor (IGF2R), which is analogous to the cation-independent mannose-6-phosphate receptor. Binding of IGFs to the insulin receptor/IGF1R class mediates all known signaling events, whereas the IGF2R serves a role in clearance of IGF-II from the circulation. In addition to the cell surface IGF binding proteins (i.e., receptors), a large family of IGF binding proteins (IGFBPs) present in biological fluids and the extracellular matrix serve to modulate IGF action.

Insulin-Like Growth Factor Biosynthesis

IGF-I and IGF-II are small (approximately 70 amino-acid), secreted peptides that are homologous to insulin in both primary amino acid sequence and in three-dimensional structure. The structural similarity of the IGFs with insulin explains, at least in part, the ability of both of these hormones to bind the insulin receptor and exert insulin-like effects. The IGFs are synthesized as preprohormones with amino-terminal sequences that target the peptides to a constitutive secretion pathway. Like insulin, the IGFs have A and B domains; however, the connecting C-peptide is not cleaved from the IGFs, thereby giving them a molecular weight greater than that of insulin.

Despite an exceptional degree of amino acid sequence homology between the IGFs and insulin, the genes that encode both IGF-I and IGF-II are remarkably more complex. The IGF-I gene, located on human chromosome 12q22-q24.1, spans more than 100 kb and has multiple 5'- and 3'-untranslated regions, which may regulate mRNA translation and/or stability. Transcription of the IGF-I gene is influenced by many factors and nutritional states. Growth hormone is a primary regulator of IGF-I gene expression in both the liver and the periphery. Conversely, when its synthesis and secretion are increased, the resultant increase in plasma IGF-I negatively feeds back on the pituitary to decrease growth hormone secretion. Insulin also stimulates IGF-I gene expression, and humans with poorly controlled type 1 diabetes mellitus have decreased IGF-1 secretion that can be restored following insulin therapy. In extrahepatic tissues, IGF-I expression is increased by estrogen (in endometrium), ACTH, angiotensin II, and FGF (in adrenal) and gonadotropic hormones (in gonads). Other hormones including thyroid hormone and glucocorticoids have stimulatory effects on hepatic IGF-I expression, whereas somatostatin inhibits IGF-I expression in liver. IGF-I gene expression is also dramatically inhibited in states of undernutrition, such as protein- or protein-calorie-restricted diets, uncontrolled diabetes mellitus, chronic liver disease, and cirrhosis.

The IGF-II gene, which is located near the insulin gene on human chromosome 11p15.5, is similarly complex, consisting of nine exons spread over more that 80 kb. There are four distinct transcriptional promoters, three of which regulate IGF-II expression in the fetus and one that drives IGF-II expression after birth. Like the IGF-I gene, the IGF-II gene has multiple 3'-untranslated regions that control IGF-II mRNA translation and stability. Although the factors that regulate IGF-II gene expression are not well characterized, it is known that in rodents, (a) IGF-II expression is high in the fetus, in which it plays a major role in growth and development, and (b) its expression subsequently declines in the perinatal period. In humans, however, IGF-II gene expression and hormone secretion persist into adulthood (31). The physiological role of IGF-II in adults is not clear.

Insulin-Like Growth Factor Receptors

The type 1 IGF receptor is highly related to the insulin receptor in both structure and function. The IGF1R is expressed in all tissues except the liver, where it is expressed very little or not at all, from a single copy gene on human chromosome 15q25-q26. The subsequent cascade of intracellular signaling events that is initiated by IGF1R activation is similar to the insulin signaling cascade described previously in this chapter; however, some differences do exist (40). IGF-I, IGF-II, and insulin can interact with the IGF1R and the insulin receptor albeit with different affinities (IGF1R: IGF-I>IGF-II>>insulin; insulin receptor: insulin>IGF-II>IGF-I). The IGF2R is important in the uptake and intracellular trafficking of mannose-6-phosphate-containing lysosomal enzymes, and it serves as a scavenger receptor that facilitates the internalization and degradation of IGF-II from the circulation (41,42). This receptor is unrelated to the IGF1R and insulin receptor both structurally and functionally. It remains questionable whether the IGF2R has a signaling function.

Insulin-Like Growth Factor Binding Proteins

The IGFs exist in the circulation bound to a superfamily of IGFBPs that are differentially expressed in a wide variety of tissues. To date there have been six homologous IGFBPs (IGFBP-1 through -6) identified that bind IGFs, but not insulin. The general structure of the IGFBPs is a conserved amino-terminal domain that contains 10 to 12 cysteine residues, a variable middle domain, and a conserved carboxy-terminal domain that contains six cysteine residues. The large number of cysteines allows the IGFBPs to form highly ordered structures that are stabilized by disulfide bridges. In addition to the conventional IGFBPs, a family of at least nine low-affinity IGFBP-related proteins (IGFBP-rP) has been identified that shares homology in the cysteine-rich amino-terminal domain (43). The exact biological role of this family of proteins remains to be elucidated.

Insulin-Like Growth Factors in Disease and Disease Prevention

Growth Disorders

Growth deficiencies may result from both a lack of adequate growth hormone production from the pituitary due to either hypothalamic or pituitary abnormalities or to growth hormone insensitivity [as in Laron-type dwarfism (44)]. The former is characterized by low growth hormone and IGF-I levels, whereas patients with the latter condition have normal to high growth hormone levels and low IGF-I and IGFBP-3.

Diabetes Mellitus

Patients with both type 1 and type 2 diabetes mellitus have abnormalities in the growth hormone–IGF–I axis. Hepatic resistance to growth hormone in type 1 diabetics affects IGF-I production, thereby decreasing the linear growth during puberty (45).

Cancer

The role of the IGF system has been studied in a number of human malignancies including liver, breast, colon, brain, and others (46–52). IGF-I, IGF-II, IGF1R, and IGFBPs are variably expressed in many human cancers, and experimental therapies such as antisense techniques and receptor antagonists have been shown to inhibit proliferation and/or induce apoptosis (53–55).

LESSONS FROM GENE KNOCKOUT MICE

One approach to determine the role of the multiple insulin and IGF signaling proteins has been the disruption of genes that encode these proteins (see Chapter 63). Because a large number of transgenic and gene knockout mice have been generated, only a sampling will be presented here.

Insulin and Insulin Receptor Knockout Mice

Rodents possess two genes for insulin, and mice in which both genes were disrupted by homologous recombination display intrauterine growth retardation of 20% (56). After suckling, glycosuria, hepatomegaly with steatosis, and high serum triglycerides and ketone bodies followed by early neonatal lethality were observed in the mutant mice. The insulin-deficient mice showed normal pancreas development with enlarged islets, suggesting either that insulin exerts negative influences on islet growth or that a circulating hormone or metabolite that is increased in the insulin-deficient state promotes islet hypertrophy. Similar to the insulin knockout mice, mice with a whole-body knockout of the insulin receptor gene die within a few days of birth from severe ketoacidosis and metabolic abnormalities (57,58). Unlike humans with null insulin receptor alleles who show intrauterine growth retardation, the insulin receptor knockout mice are normal in size at birth, suggesting that there are species differences in the role of insulin and IGF receptors in intrauterine growth. These findings further suggest that insulin mediates most if not all of its metabolic effects via the insulin receptor, but taken together with the results from the insulin knockout mice, insulin's effects on intrauterine growth is likely mediated by another receptor. Heterozygous insulin receptor knockout mice, which have a 50% reduction in receptor number, have only mild insulin resistance that is compensated by slight hyper-insulinemia (57,58).

To directly assess the role of insulin signaling in the liver on whole-body fuel homeostasis, Kahn and colleagues (60) used Cre/*lox*P-mediated gene targeting to generate mice with a *liver-specific insulin receptor gene knockout* (LIRKO) (59). LIRKO mice were viable, but suffered from glucose intolerance, insulin resistance, and severe hyperglycemia in the fed state. In addition, insulin levels in LIRKO mice were elevated 15- to 20-fold due to both increased insulin secretion and decreased insulin clearance. Insulin failed to suppress hepatic glucose production, and genes that control gluconeogenesis were highly overexpressed in the LIRKO liver. Serum lipids were suppressed in LIRKO mice likely due to both decreased delivery of substrates for lipid synthesis and decreased expression of lipogenic enzymes. In addition, alterations in the growth hormone-IGF axis were noted, including overexpression of liver-derived IGFBP-1 and -2. Taken together, these data provide *in vivo* genetic evidence that insulin action in the liver is critical for the control of many aspects of fuel metabolism.

Insulin-Like Growth Factor (IGF)-I, IGF-II, IGF1R, and IGF2R Knockout Mice

Several null mutation experiments in mice over the past ten years have substantially clarified the roles of IGF-I and -II and the IGF receptors in growth and development. Mice lacking IGF-I expression in all tissues exhibit growth retardation at birth (60% of normal birthweight) (61). Depending on the genetic background of the mice, some IGF-I null mice die shortly after birth while others survive to adulthood. Those that survive show further exacerbation of their dwarfism with body weights reaching only 30% of normal in adulthood (62). Likewise, mice lacking IGF-II show a similar decrease in birthweight as the IGF-I null mice, yet these animals grow normally in the postnatal period, indicating that IGF-II is important for intrauterine growth but is dispensable for growth after birth (63).

In contrast to the milder phenotypes observed in the IGF ligand knockouts, IGF1R knockout mice die invariably at birth due to respiratory failure (61). The IGF1R knockout mice are more severely growth retarded (45% of normal birthweight) than either of the IGF ligand knockouts alone. In addition to generalized organ hypoplasia, the IGF1R null mice also had defects in ossification, skin development and central nervous system morphology. Interestingly, IGF2R knockout mice have high serum and tissue levels of IGF-II and exhibit intrauterine overgrowth (135% of normal birthweight) with generalized organomegaly, postaxial polydactyly, heart abnormalities, kinky tail, and edema (64). Most IGF2R mice die in the perinatal period; some survive and are fertile. Consistent with the hypothesis that the phenotype of the IGF2R mouse is caused by defective clearance of IGF-II and subsequent overstimulation of

IGF1R, the IGF2R knockout phenotype is completely rescued by a second mutation eliminating either IGF-II or IGF1R (64). Furthermore, IGF1R/IGF2R double knockout mice develop normally *in utero* due to the ability of excessive IGF-II to stimulate growth through binding the insulin receptor, but they fail to exhibit normal postnatal growth (64). On the other hand, IGF-I/IGF-II double knockout mice are severely growth retarded (30% of normal birth weight), showing a phenotype that is indistinguishable from IGF1R/insulin receptor and IGF1R/IGF-II double knockouts (65). These results provide strong genetic evidence that both IGF-I and -II regulate fetal growth by binding the IGF1R and the insulin receptor, that IGF2R is critical for IGF-II clearance, and that postnatal growth is dependent on IGF-I stimulation of IGF1R.

The classical somatomedin hypothesis states that growth hormone stimulates body growth by stimulating the production of somatomedins (i.e., IGFs) by the liver. IGFs act in an endocrine manner to stimulate bone growth and increase body mass. To directly test this hypothesis, two groups used Cre/*lox*P-mediated gene targeting to disrupt the expression of hepatic IGF-I (66,67). Circulating IGF-1 levels were reduced by more than 75% in the hepatic IGF-I knockout mice, yet surprisingly the loss of hepatically derived IGF-I did not affect postnatal linear growth in any way. Although growth hormone levels were generally elevated in these mice, the level of IGF-I mRNA in peripheral target tissues was not increased. These results call for a revision of the classical somatomedin hypothesis to indicate that autocrine/paracrine IGF-I is the critical regulator of postnatal growth.

Insulin Receptor Substrate-1 Knockout Mice

Inactivation of IRS-1 by insertional mutagenesis results in a 50% retardation in embryonic and postnatal growth, and pronounced resistance to the blood glucose-lowering effects of exogenously administered insulin, IGF-I, and IGF-II (68,69). Restoration of IRS-1 expression in liver by recombinant adenovirus-mediated gene transfer results in almost complete recovery from the whole-body insulin resistance, even though disturbance of insulin signaling in the skeletal muscle of IRS-1-deficient mice seems to be more severe than that in the liver (70). Together, these data suggest that IRS-1 is a major signaling intermediate in the insulin-mediated activation of glycogen metabolism and suppression of glucose production in liver and in the stimulation of glucose transport, protein synthesis, and IGF-I-mediated proliferation in muscle.

Insulin Receptor Substrate-2 Knockout Mice

In contrast to the IRS-1 knockout mice, mice with disruption of the IRS-2 gene (71) display hyperglycemia and hyperinsulinemia as early as 3 days after birth and subsequently develop severe glucose intolerance and insulin resistance by 6 to 10 weeks of age. At 12 to 16 weeks of age, IRS-2 knockout mice have fasting blood glucose levels in excess of 400 mg/dl, develop polydypsia and polyuria without ketosis, and ultimately die from dehydration and hyperosmolar coma. The nature of the profound insulin resistance in IRS-2 knockout mice is failure to suppress hepatic glucose production and peripheral insulin resistance that is secondary to hyperglycemia. In addition, IRS-2 knockout mice fail to produce a compensatory increase in pancreatic β-cell mass in the presence of hyperglycemia and insulin resistance.

REFERENCES

1. Cahill GF. Starvation in man. *New Engl J Med* 1970;282: 668–675.
2. Shulman GI, Barrett E, Sherwin RS. Integrated fuel metabolism. In: Porte D, Sherwin RS, eds. *Diabetes mellitus*, 5th ed. Stamford: Appleton & Lange, 1996;1–18.
3. Ruderman NB, Tornheim K, Goodman MN. Fuel homeostasis and intermediary metabolism of carbohydrate, fat and protein. In: Becker K, ed. *Principles and practice of endocrinology and metabolism,* 3rd ed. Philadelphia: Lippincott, 2001:1257–1272.
4. Cryer PE, Polonsky KS. Glucose homeostasis and hypoglycemia. In: Wilson JD, Foster DW, Kronenberg HM, et al., eds. *Williams textbook of endocrinology,* 9th ed. Philadelphia: WB Saunders, 1998:939–972.
5. Mahley RW, Weisgraber KH, Farese RVJ. Disorders of lipid metabolism. In: Wilson JD, Foster DW, Kronenberg HM, et al., eds. *Williams textbook of endocrinology,* 9th ed. Philadelphia: WB Saunders, 1998:1099–1154.
6. Cherrington AD. Banting Lecture 1997. Control of glucose uptake and release by the liver in vivo. *Diabetes* 1999;48: 1198–1214.
7. O'Brien RM, Granner DK. Regulation of gene expression by insulin. *Physiol Rev* 1996;76:1109–1161.
8. Lawrence JC, Roach PJ. New insights into the role and mechanism of glycogen synthase activation by insulin. *Diabetes* 1997; 46:541–547.
9. Stumvoll M, Meyer C, Perriello G, et al. Human kidney and liver gluconeogenesis: evidence for organ substrate selectivity. *Am J Physiol* 1998;274:E817–E826.
10. Ekberg K, Landau BR, Wajngot A, et al. Contributions by kidney and liver to glucose production in the postabsorptive state and after 60 h of fasting. *Diabetes* 1999;48:292–298.
11. Maechler P, Wollheim CB. Mitochondrial glutamate acts as a messenger in glucose-induced insulin exocytosis. *Nature* 1999; 402:685–689.
12. Dobbins RL, Chester MW, Daniels MB, et al. Circulating fatty acids are essential for efficient glucose-stimulated insulin secretion after prolonged fasting in humans. *Diabetes* 1998;47: 1613–1618.
13. Schaapveld RQ, Schepens JT, Robinson GW, et al. Impaired mammary gland development and function in mice lacking LAR receptor-like tyrosine phosphatase activity. *Dev Biol* 1997;188: 134–146.
14. Ren JM, Li PM, Zhang WR, et al. Transgenic mice deficient in the LAR protein-tyrosine phosphatase exhibit profound defects in glucose homeostasis. *Diabetes* 1998;47:493–497.
15. Elchebly M, Payette P, Michaliszyn E, et al. Increased insulin sensitivity and obesity resistance in mice lacking the protein tyrosine phosphatase-1B gene. *Science* 1999;283:1544–1548.
16. Sun XJ, Pons S, Asano T, et al. The Fyn tyrosine kinase binds IRS-1 and forms a distinct signaling complex during insulin stimulation. *J Biol Chem* 1996;271:10583–10587.
17. Mastick CC, Saltiel AR. Insulin-stimulated tyrosine phosphorylation of caveolin is specific for the differentiated adipocyte phenotype in 3T3-L1 cells. *J Biol Chem* 1997;272:20706–20714.
18. Liu YC, Altman A. Cbl: complex formation and functional implications. *Cell Signal* 1998;10:377–385.
19. Erneux C, Govaerts C, Communi D, et al. The diversity and possible functions of the inositol polyphosphate 5-phosphatases. *Biochim Biophys Acta* 1998;1436:185–199.
20. Vollenweider P, Clodi M, Martin SS, et al. An SH2 domain-containing 5′ inositolphosphatase inhibits insulin-induced GLUT4 translocation and growth factor-induced actin filament rearrangement. *Mol Cell Biol* 1999;19:1081–1091.
21. Xiao S, Rose DW, Sasaoka T, et al. Syp (SH-PTP2) is a positive mediator of growth factor-stimulated mitogenic signal transduction. *J Biol Chem* 1994;269:21244–21248.
22. Noguchi T, Matozaki T, Horita K, et al. Role of SH-PTP2, a protein-tyrosine phosphatase with Src homology 2 domains, in insulin-stimulated Ras activation. *Mol Cell Biol* 1994;14: 6674–6682.
23. Fukunaga K, Noguchi T, Takeda H, et al. Requirement for protein-tyrosine phosphatase SHP-2 in insulin-induced activation of c-Jun NH(2)-terminal kinase. *J Biol Chem* 2000;275: 5208–5213.
24. Inagaki K, Noguchi T, Matozaki T, et al. Roles for the protein tyrosine phosphatase SHP-2 in cytoskeletal organization, cell adhesion and cell migration revealed by overexpression of a dominant negative mutant. *Oncogene* 2000;19:75–84.
25. Ahmad F, Azevedo JL, Cortright R, et al. Alterations in skeletal muscle protein-tyrosine phosphatase activity and expression in insulin-resistant human obesity and diabetes. *J Clin Invest* 1997; 100:449–458.
26. Paz K, Hemi R, LeRoith D, et al. A molecular basis for insulin resistance. Elevated serine/threonine phosphorylation of IRS-1 and IRS-2 inhibits their binding to the juxtamembrane region of the insulin receptor and impairs their ability to undergo insulin-induced tyrosine phosphorylation. *J Biol Chem* 1997;272: 29911–29918.
27. Hotamisligil GS, Shargill NS, Spiegelman BM. Adipose expression of tumor necrosis factor-alpha: direct role in obesity-linked insulin resistance. *Science* 1993;259:87–91.
28. Uysal KT, Wiesbrock SM, Hotamisligil GS. Functional analysis of tumor necrosis factor (TNF) receptors in TNF-α-mediated insulin resistance in genetic obesity. *Endocrinology* 1998;139: 4832–4838.
29. Uysal KT, Wiesbrock SM, Marino MW, et al. Protection from obesity-induced insulin resistance in mice lacking TNF-α function. *Nature* 1997;389:610–614.
30. Zhang Y, Proenca R, Maffei M, et al. Positional cloning of the mouse obese gene and its human homologue. *Nature* 1994;372: 425–432.
31. Considine RV, Sinha MK, Heiman ML, et al. Serum immunoreactive-leptin concentrations in normal-weight and obese humans. *N Engl J Med* 1996;334:292–295.
32. Brüning JC, Michael MD, Winnay JN, et al. A muscle-specific insulin receptor knockout exhibits features of the metabolic syndrome of NIDDM without altering glucose tolerance. *Mol Cell* 1998;2:559–569.
33. DeFronzo RA. Pathogenesis of type 2 diabetes: metabolic and molecular implications for identifying diabetes genes. *Diabetes Rev* 1997;5:177–269.

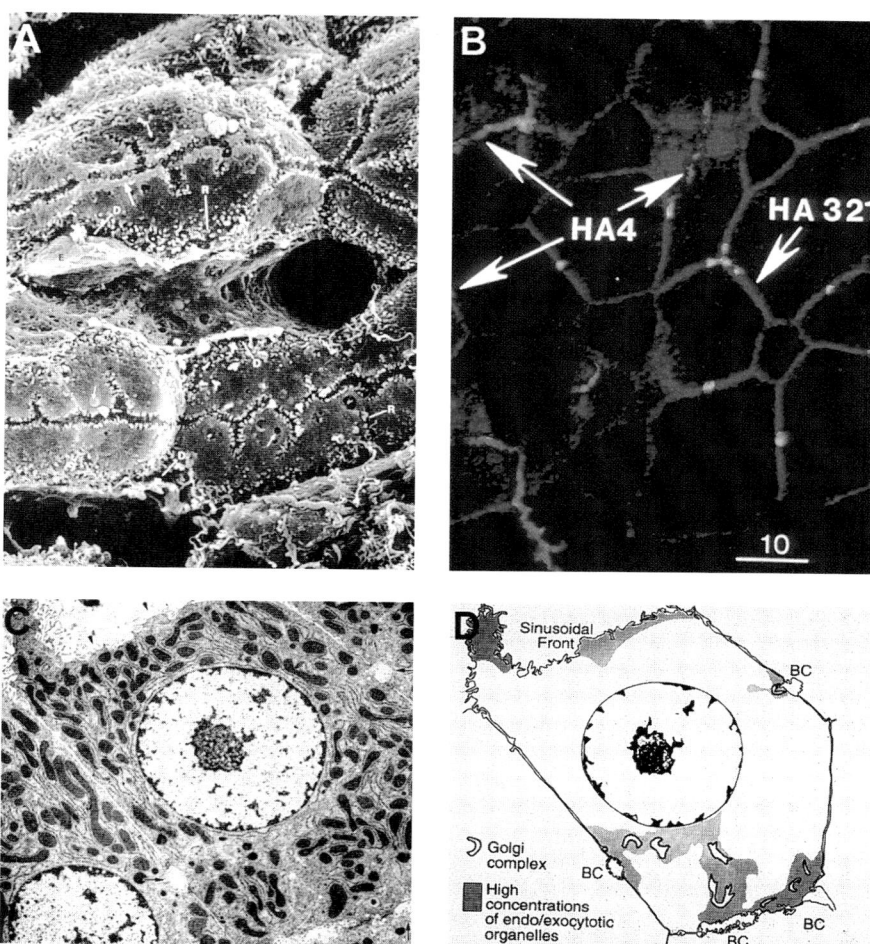

COLOR PLATE 1. The architecture of the liver is unique. **A:** A scanning electron micrograph of a portion of a liver lobule. A continuous network of bile canaliculi (*BC*) runs along the exposed cell surfaces of the liver plate. **B:** The two distinct plasma membrane (PM) domains are visualized by immunofluorescence detection of the basolateral PM protein, HA321/BEN (*red*) and the apical PM protein, HA4/cell-CAM105/ecto-adenosine triphosphatase (ATPase) (*blue*). An electron micrograph of a hepatocyte (**C**) and a corresponding schematic drawing (**D**) highlight the "active zones" in vesicular trafficking. The major sorting organelles [*trans*-Golgi network (TGN) and endosomes] and transport vesicles are concentrated in small "clear" zones that are probably the most active in vesicle traffic. These zones are located between the Golgi and the apical PM and near the basolateral PM (the *shaded regions* in **D**). See Figure 8.1 on page 98.

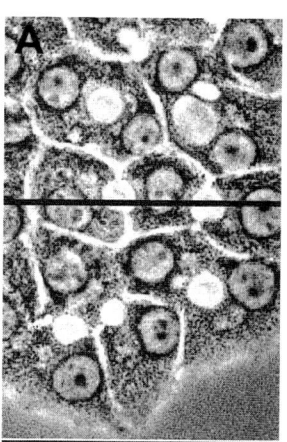

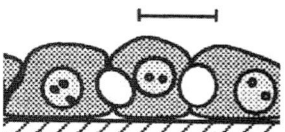

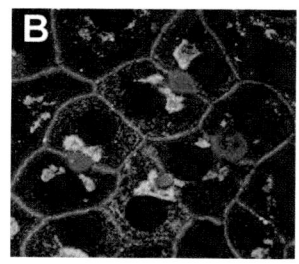

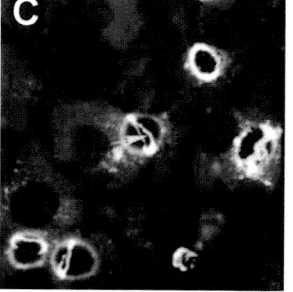

COLOR PLATE 2. WIF-B cells are an *in vitro* model of polarized hepatocytes. **A:** The phase contrast morphology of living WIF-B cells is shown (**top**). The phase-lucent "blisters" between neighboring cells correspond to the "bile canalicular" or apical space. A cross-sectional "reconstruction" of the cell monolayer (**bottom panel**) taken along the line indicated in the **upper panel** shows that the bile canalicular spaces (BCs) are closed off from both the substrate and overlying medium. **B:** Triple immunofluorescence labeling of apical (*blue*), basolateral (*red*), and Golgi (*green*) proteins is shown in fully polarized WIF-B cells. The apical protein, HA4/ cell-CAM105/ecto–adenosine triphosphatase (ATPase), is localized to the membrane lining the dilated spaces, HA321/BEN is found along the basolateral surface, and albumin is concentrated at the Golgi. **C:** The tight junction protein, ZO-1 (*yellow*) marks the borders between the apical and basolateral domains. HA4/ cell-CAM105/ecto-ATPase is also labeled (*blue*) to mark the apical surface. See Figure 8.2 on page 100.

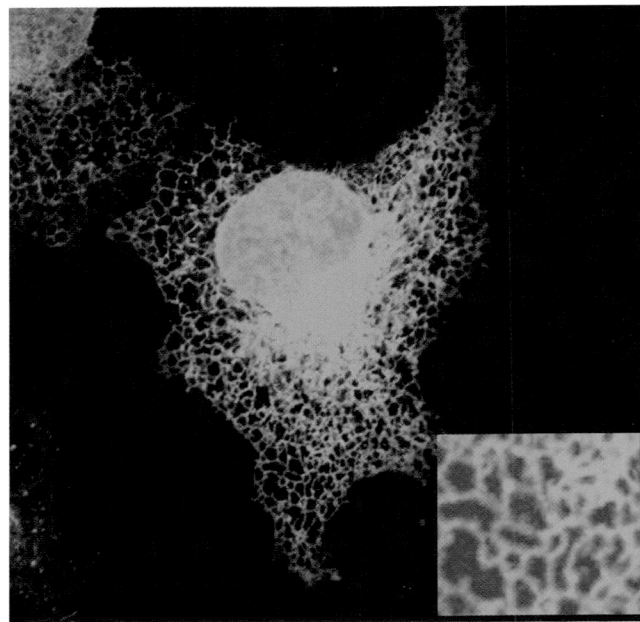

COLOR PLATE 3. Morphology of the endoplasmic reticulum (ER) labeled with the cargo protein vesicular stomatitis virus tagged with green fluorescent protein (VSVG-GFP) retained in the ER at its restrictive temperature of 40°C. See Figure 9.2 on page 120.

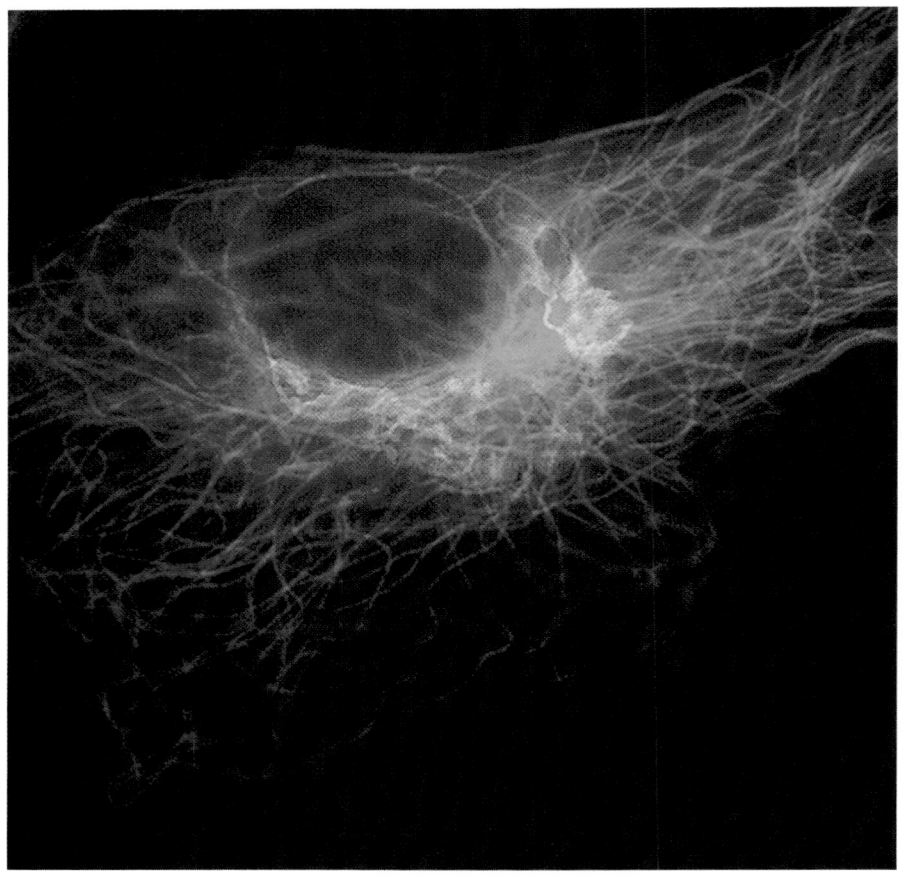

COLOR PLATE 4. Localization of the Golgi complex in mammalian cell. *Green* is antibody labeling of tubulin, and *yellow* is antibody staining to the Golgi enzyme mannosidase II. See Figure 9.5B on page 125.

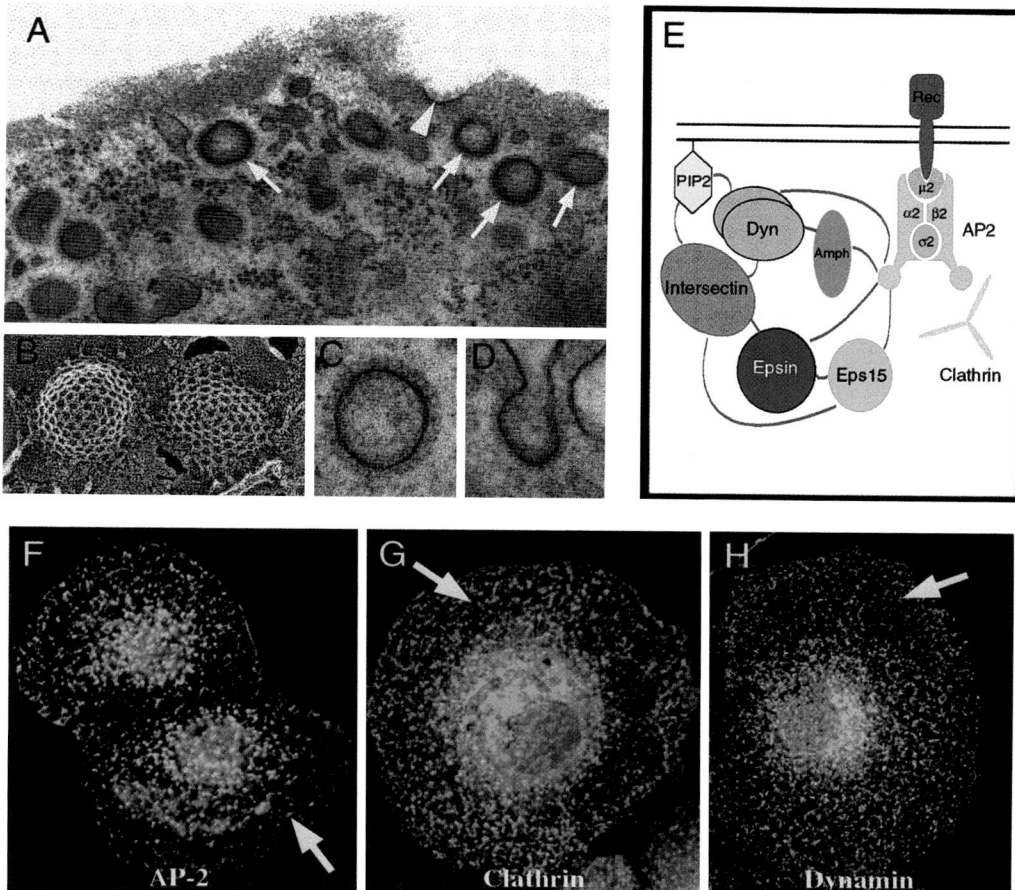

COLOR PLATE 5. Clathrin-coated vesicle formation at the plasma membrane. **A:** Thin-section electron micrograph of a rat hepatocyte taken from original collections of Dr. Keith Porter. Numerous electron-dense bristle coats are found to line the cytosolic side of cell surface invaginations (*arrowhead*) and small internalized vesicles (*arrows*). **B:** Electron micrographs showing an intracellular view of clathrin-coated pits in fibroblasts. Clathrin lattices are clearly visualized in these replicas. (From Heuser J. Effects of cytoplasmic acidification on clathrin lattice morphology. *J Cell Biol* 1989;108:401–411, with permission.) **C and D:** Clathrin-coated vesicle and clathrin-coated pit in rat liver hepatocyte micrographs from Dr. Keith Porter. **E:** Clathrin-coated vesicle formation involves clathrin and a number of accessory proteins that are known to interact with each other via specific protein:protein interaction domains (see text) and in this way effect a regulatory role on coated vesicle biogenesis. **F–H:** Immunofluorescence images of plasma membrane adaptor complex, adaptor protein 2 (*AP2*), clathrin, and the molecular pinchase dynamin in clone 9 cultured rat hepatocytes reveal a punctate pattern of labeling at the cell surface (*arrows*). In double-labeling experiments, these three clathrin-coated pit components are found to colocalize. (Images from Dr. Hong Cao, Mayo Clinic.). See Figure 10.2 on page 135.

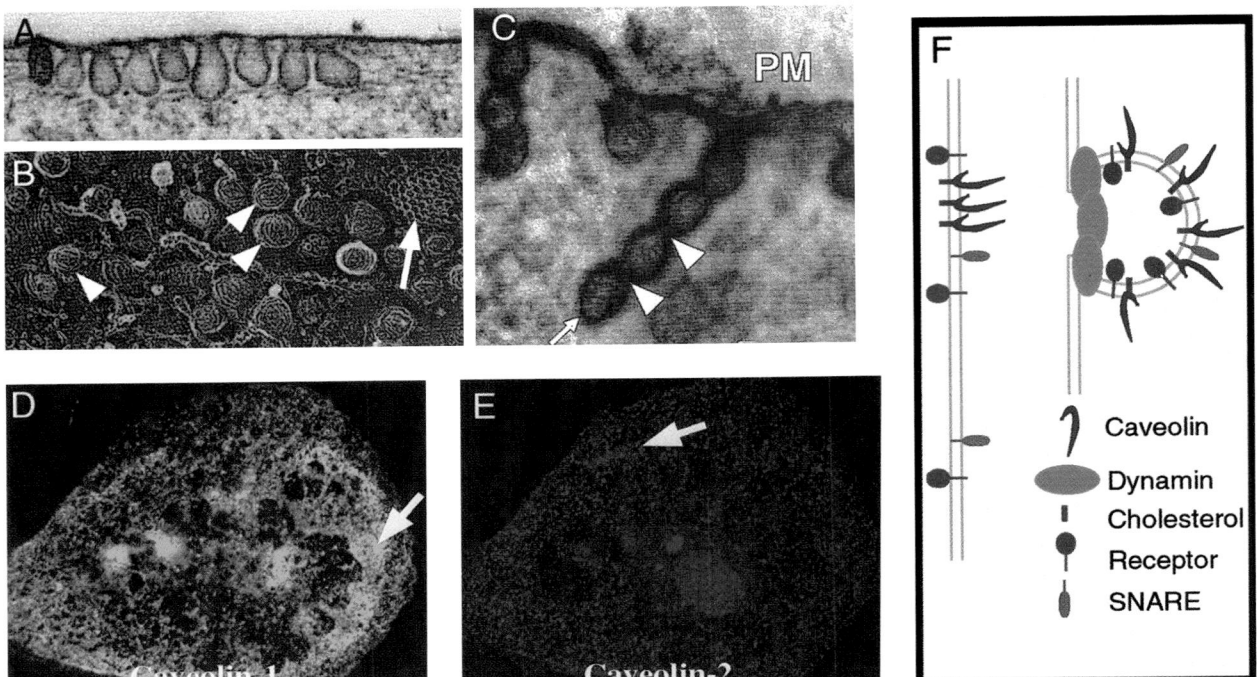

COLOR PLATE 6. Caveolae and flask-shaped structures at the plasma membrane (*PM*). **A:** Thin-section electron micrograph showing homogenous small flask-shaped invaginations, caveolae, at the cell surface of human fibroblasts. (From Rothberg KG, Heuser JE, Donzell WC, et al. Caveolin, a protein component of caveolae membrane coats. *Cell* 1992;68:673–682, with permission.) **B:** Deep-etch intracellular view of caveolae (*arrowheads*) clearly showing the characteristic spiral coat distinct from the organized lattice coat structure of a clathrin coated pit (*arrow*). (From Rothberg KG, et al., as above.) **C:** Cultured hepatocytes microinjected with inhibitory dynamin antibodies exhibit accumulated chains of caveolae separated by constrictions still attached to the PM. This shows the key role of dynamin in caveolae scission (From Henley JR, Krueger EW, Oswald BJ, et al. Dynamin-mediated internalization of caveolae. *J Cell Biol* 1998;141:85–99, with permission.) **D and E:** Immunofluorescence images of caveolin-1 (as revealed by a GFP-tagged caveolin-1) and caveolin-2 demonstrate a patchy versus punctate cell surface distribution for these caveolin isoforms, respectively (Images from Dr. Hong Cao, Mayo Clinic.) **F:** Caveolae vesicle formation is known to involve the presence of caveolin-1, cholesterol, and dynamin. SNAREs are known to also be present in caveolae and are involved in addressing caveolae to their correct target membrane. See Figure 10.3 on page 142.

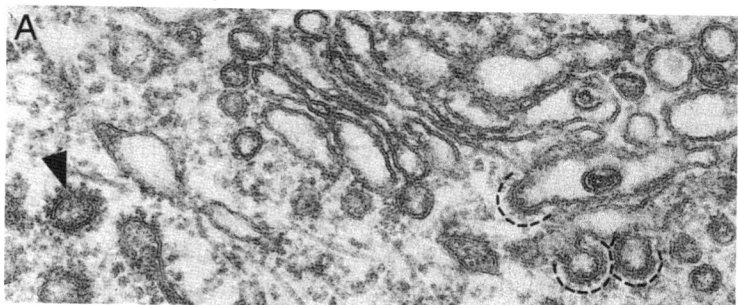

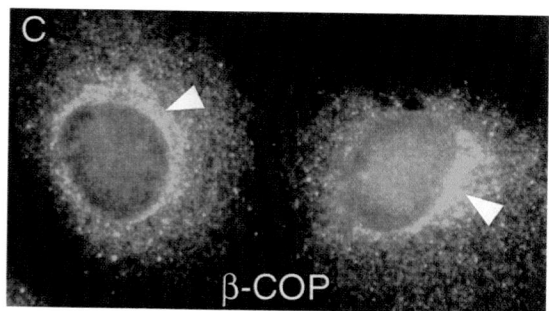

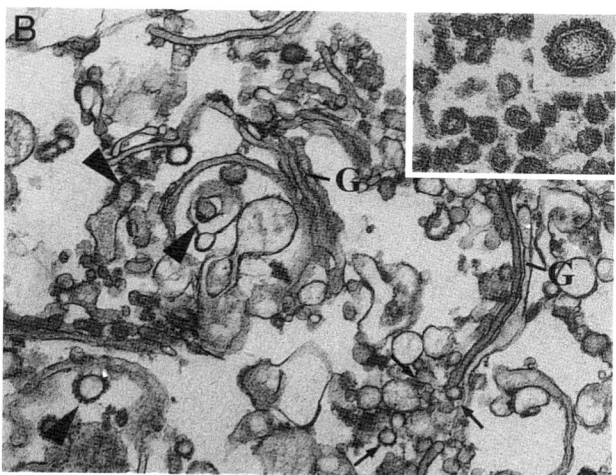

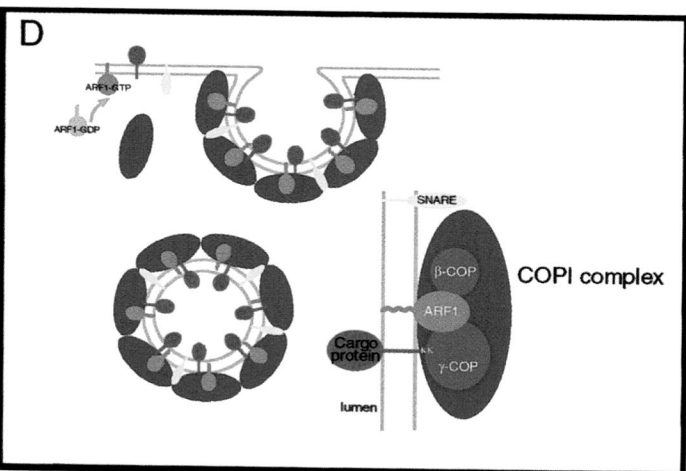

COLOR PLATE 7. COPI-coated vesicles in protein trafficking through the secretory pathway. **A:** *COPI-coated buds* (dotted lines) on Golgi cisternae from Chinese Hamster Ovary (CHO) cells are distinct from the spiny coats of clathrin-coated vesicles (*arrowhead*) (From Orci L, Glick BS, Rothman JE. A new type of coated vesicular carrier that appears not to contain clathrin; its possible role in protein transport within the Golgi stack. *Cell* 1986;46:171–184, with permission.) **B:** An isolated rat liver Golgi fraction shows Golgi stacks of 2–3 flattened cisternae (*G*) and scores of vesicular and budding profiles. The bristle coat of clathrin on some of these profiles (*arrowheads*) is visibly different from the thin electron-dense coat of COPI buds and vesicles (*arrows*). (Images from Dr. John Bergeron, McGill University, Montreal, Canada.) **Inset:** Purified yeast COPI vesicles. (From Schekman R, Orci L. Coat proteins and vesicle budding. *Science* 1996;271:1526–1533, with permission.) **C:** Immunofluorescence labeling with antibodies against a COPI component, β-COP, reveals prominent perinuclear staining of cultured clone 9 rat hepatocytes. (Image from Dr. Yisang Yoon, Mayo Clinic.) **D:** COPI-coated vesicle formation is known to involve the COPI coatomer complex consisting of 7 subunit proteins. Two of these, β-COP and γ-COP, are known to mediate important interactions with the small GTP binding protein ARF1 and the cytosolic tails (specifically dilysine, or KK, motifs) of transmembrane proteins (such as p24 family members, see text). ARF–GDP/GTP exchange is one of the initial steps in the recruitment of the coatomer complex for COPI vesicle biogenesis. See Figure 10.4 on page 146.

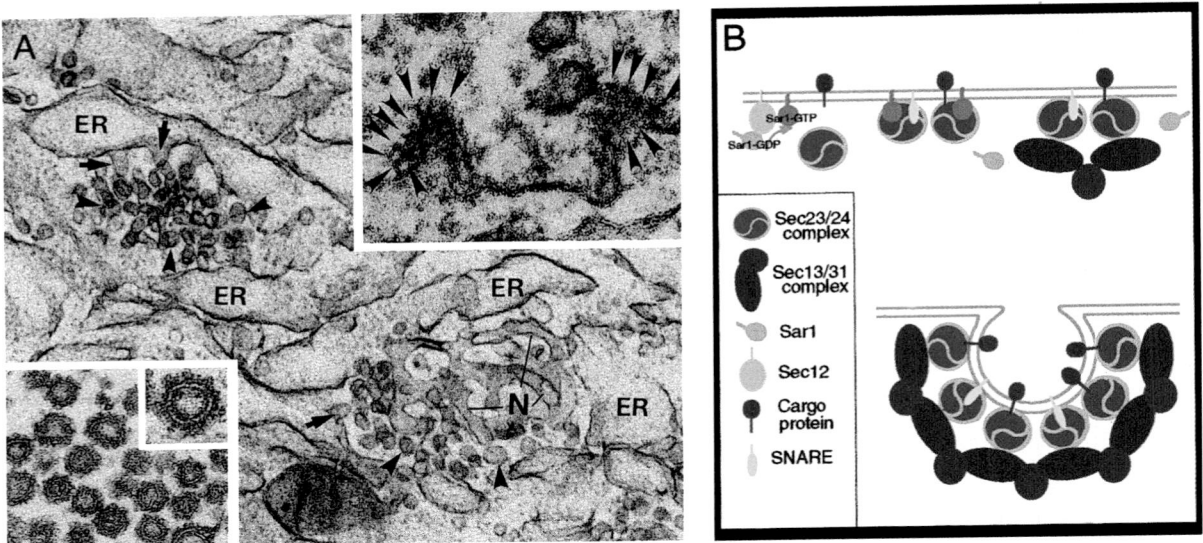

COLOR PLATE 8. COPII-coated vesicles in endoplasmic reticulum (*ER*)-to-Golgi protein trafficking. **A:** Clusters of small vesicular profiles, likely representing COPII vesicles (*arrowheads*), can be seen to be closely surrounded by ER cisternae and budlike projections (*arrows*) in this electron micrograph of principal cells of the epididymal initial segment (From Hermo L, Green H, Clermont Y. Golgi apparatus of epithelial principal cells of the epididymal initial segment of the rat: structure, relationship with endoplasmic reticulum, and role in the formation of secretory vesicles. *Anat Rec* 1991;229:159–176, with permission.) **Top inset:** Honeycombed appearance of the coat (*arrowheads*) of COPII vesicles in rat basophilic leukemia cells (From Bannykh SI, Rowe T, Balch WE. The organization of endoplasmic reticulum export complexes. *J Cell Biol* 1996;135:19–35, with permission.) **Bottom inset:** Purified yeast COPII vesicles (From Schekman R, Orci L. Coat proteins and vesicle budding. *Science* 1996;271:1526–1533, with permission.) **B:** COPII-coated vesicle formation, like COPI, involves several protein complexes, and a small GTP-binding protein, Sar1, which is known to be one of the initiating factors in the generation of COPII vesicles. Membrane association of Sar1 is regulated by Sec12, GTPase-activating protein for Sar1. *N*, anastomosing network of tubules. See Figure 10.5 on page 148.

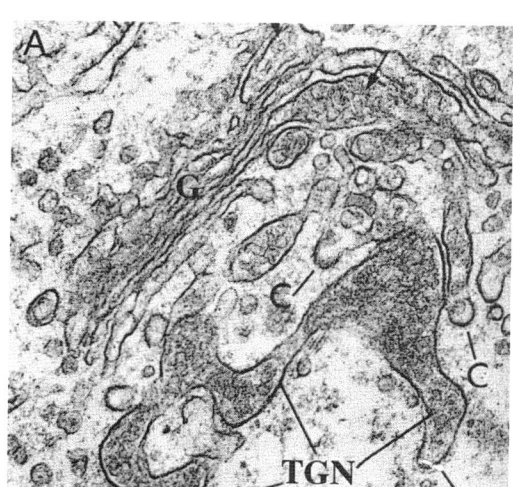
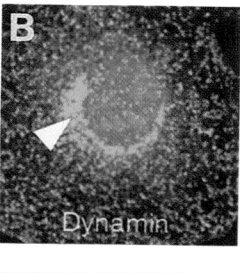
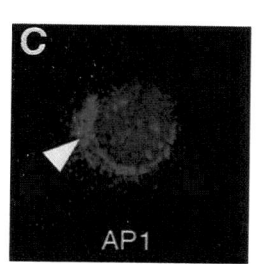
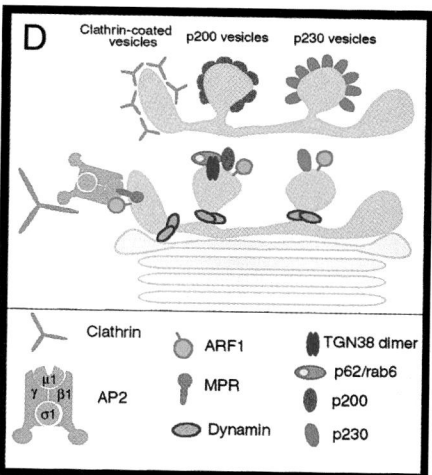

COLOR PLATE 9. Secretory vesicles derived from the *trans*-Golgi network (*TGN*). **A:** Electron micrograph of a Golgi apparatus from a rat liver hepatocyte. The tubular network of the TGN is clearly visible in this micrograph as are uncoated and coated buds (*C*) (From Novikoff PM, Yam A. Sites of lipoprotein particles in normal rat hepatocytes. *J. Cell Biol.* 1978;76:1–11, with permission.) **B–C:** Immunofluorescence images of clone 9 cultured rat hepatocytes labeled for dynamin and AP1. These two accessory proteins involved in TGN-derived clathrin-coated vesicle formation are colocalized in a perinuclear location. (Images from Dr. Hong Cao, Mayo Clinic). **D:** Several vesicle types are known to arise from the TGN. Formation of clathrin-coated vesicles is known to involve membrane receptors [such as the mannose-6-phosphate receptor (*MPR*)], the Golgi adaptor protein complex, AP1, ARF1, which mediates AP1 membrane association, and the molecular pinchase dynamin. p200 vesicles are known to involve p62/rab6/TGN38. Notably, a lacelike coated vesicle population identified in normal rat kidney cells have been suggested to be coated by p200 (196). p230 vesicles are known to have a distinct coat from p200. Formation of non–clathrin-coated vesicles is known to require ARF1 and dynamin for vesicle release. See Figure 10.6 on page 150.

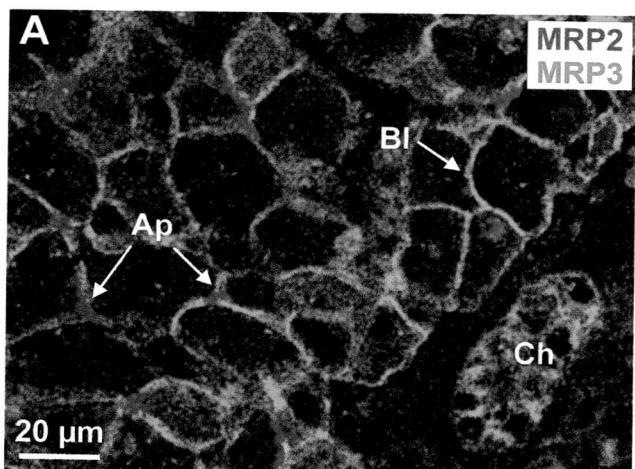
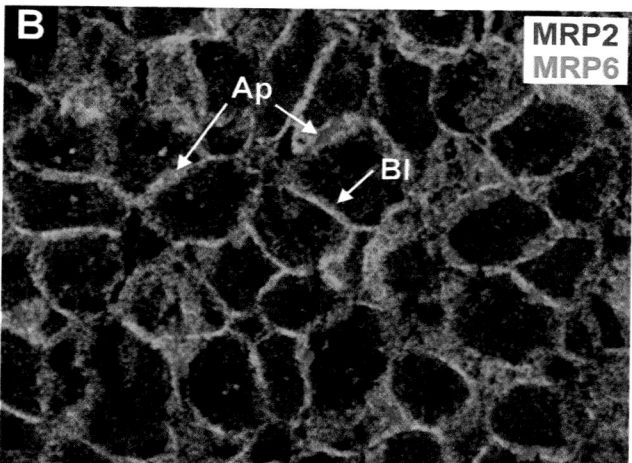
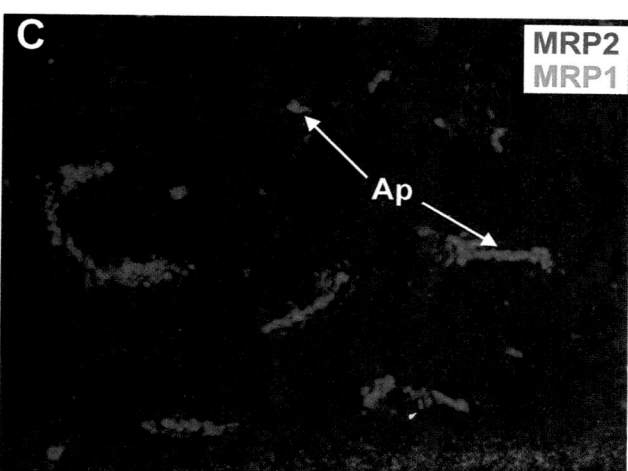

COLOR PLATE 10. Localization of multidrug resistance protein 2 (*MRP2*), *MRP3*, and *MRP6* with isoform-specific antibodies in human liver. Double-label immunofluorescence microscopy of frozen liver sections (5 μm) was performed as described (21). Pictures of an optical thickness of 1.5 μm were taken on a confocal laser scanning microscope. *Ap*, apical (canalicular) membrane of hepatocytes; *Bl*, basolateral membrane of hepatocytes; *Ch*, cholangiocytes. The apical isoform MRP2 (*red fluorescence* in **A–C**) is restricted to the canalicular membrane domain of hepatocytes as detected either with the monoclonal antibody M₂ III-6 (29) in **A** and **B**, or with the polyclonal antiserum EAG5 in **C** (10,34). The isoforms MRP3 (*green fluorescence* in **A**, using the antiserum FDS (21) and MRP6 (*green fluorescence* in **B**, using the antiserum AQL (21) are localized to the basolateral membrane of human hepatocytes and are excluded from the bile canalicular domain. In addition to its expression in hepatocytes, MRP3 is expressed in cholangiocytes (**A**). MRP1 was not detected in hepatocytes using the MRP1-specific antibody QCRL-1 (**C**) (64). *Bar* in **A**, 20 μm; same magnification for all panels. See Figure 25.2 on page 376.

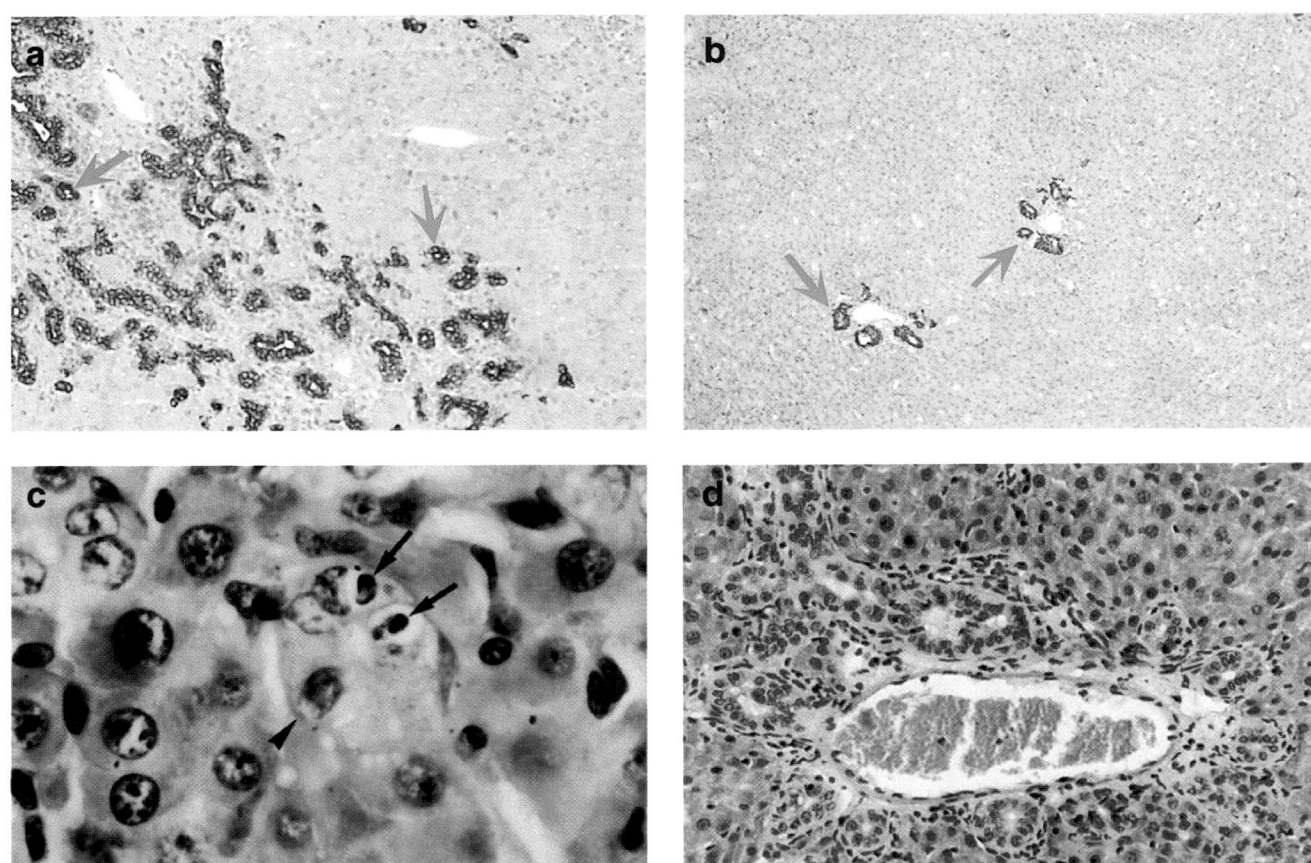

COLOR PLATE 11. Immunohistochemistry for CK-19 in frozen liver sections from bile duct–ligated (BDL) (**A**) and BDL+vagotomy (**B**) rats. Vagotomy induced a decrease in the number of ducts as compared with BDL control rats. Original magnification x125. Evaluation of apoptosis in liver sections (stained with hematoxylin and eosin) from BDL (**C**) and BDL+vagotomy (**D**) rats. **C:** Liver section from a BDL+vagotomy rat. Two apoptotic bodies (*arrows*) appear in the epithelium of a bile duct (*arrowhead*) which is surrounded by hepatocytes and located in the proximity of an enlarged portal space (representative section of six examined). **D:** Rat liver section seven days after BDL + vagotomy + forskolin treatment showing proliferating bile ducts without any evidence of apoptosis. Original magnification x100. (From LeSage G. Alvaro D, Benedetti A, et al. Cholinergic system modulates growth, apoptosis, and secretion of cholangiocytes from bile duct–ligated rats. *Gastroenterology* 1999;117:191–199, with permission.) See Figure 29.1 on page 422.

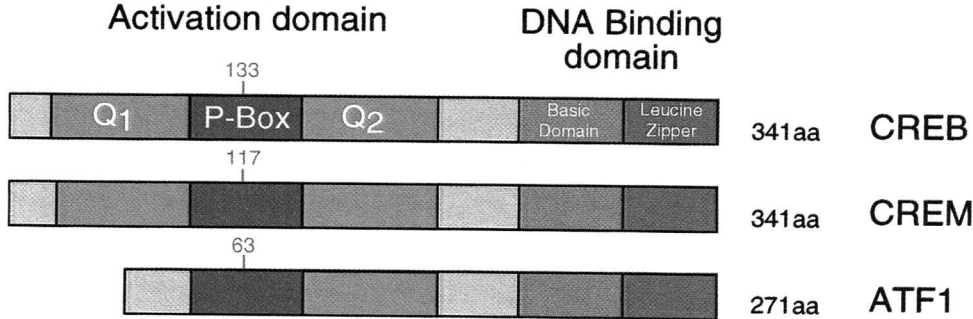

AESEDSQESVDSVTDSQKRREILSRRPSYRKILNDLSSDAPGVPRIEEEKSEEETSA   **CREB**

AETDDSADS..EVIDSHKRREILSRRPSYRKILNELSSDVPGIPKIEEEKSEEEGTP   **CREM**

SESEESQDSSDSIGSSQKAHGILARRPSYRKILKDLSSEDTRGRKGDGENSGVSAAV   **ATF1**

COLOR PLATE 12. Structure of cyclic AMP-responsive element (CRE)–binding proteins (*CREB*), CRE modulators (*CREM*), and activating transcription factor-1 (*ATF1*): (a) The glutamine-rich domains (*Q1* and *Q2*), the DNA-binding region (basic domain and leucine zipper) and the P-box are shown. The position of the serine residue phosphorylated by the cAMP-dependent protein kinase (PKA) and other kinases (see Fig. 37.3) is also indicated; and (b) Sequence alignment of the P-box domain from these proteins. The serine corresponding to the PKA-phosphoacceptor site is shown in blue. (From De Cesare D, Fimia GM, Sassone-Corsi P. Signaling routes to CREM and CREB: plasticity in transcriptional activation. *Trends Biochem Sci* 1999;24:281–285, with permission.) See Figure 37.2 on page 528.

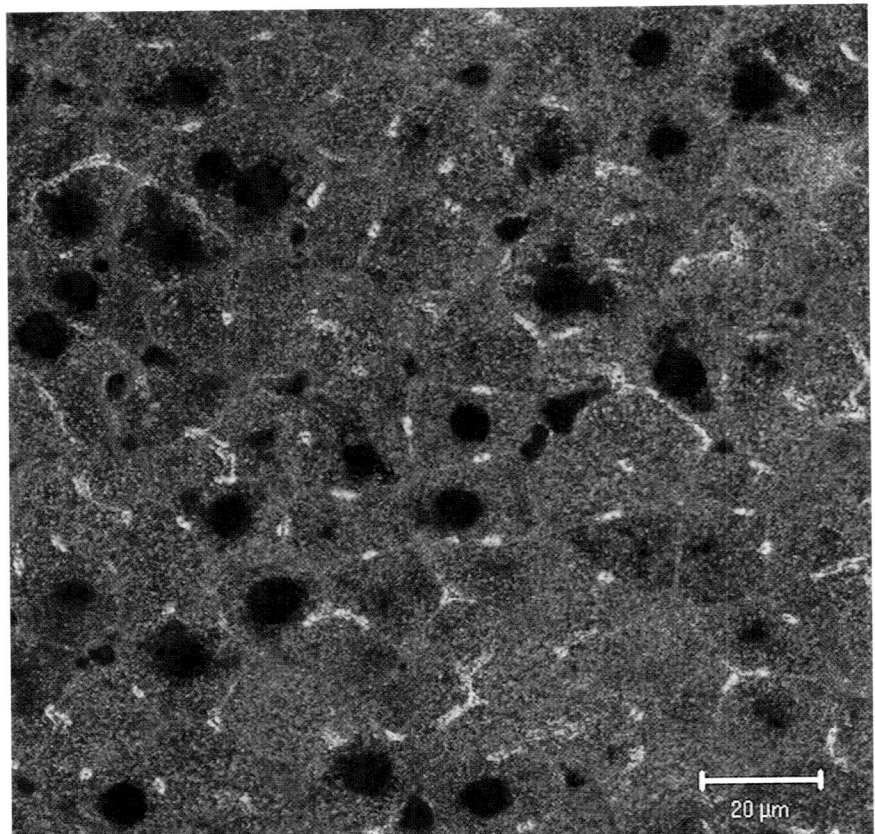

COLOR PLATE 13. Distribution of the InsP3 receptor (InsP3R) in the liver. A confocal immunofluorescence image of rat liver shows the distribution of the InsP3R (*green*). The specimen also is labeled with rhodamine phalloidin (*red*) to identify canaliculi. The InsP3R is most concentrated in the pericanalicular regions, with lesser staining elsewhere in the cytosol. See Figure 38.2 on page 540.

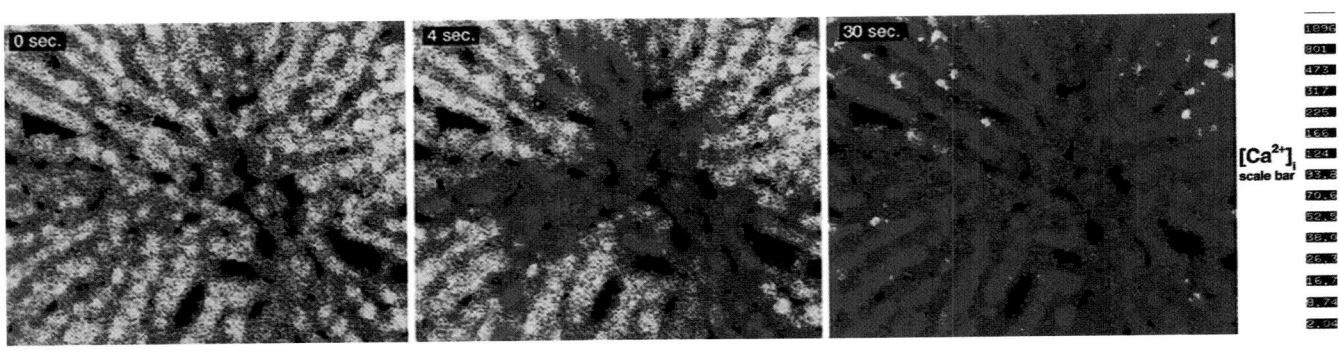

COLOR PLATE 14. Organization of Ca^{2+} signals in the intact liver. Serial confocal images of a vasopressin-induced Ca^{2+} wave in the isolated perfused rat liver demonstrates that the increase in Ca^{2+} begins in the pericentral region, then spreads as a wave toward the periportal regions. Images were obtained at baseline and after 4 and 30 seconds of stimulation with vasopressin (20 nM). (From Motoyama K, Karl IE, Flye MW, et al. Effect of Ca2+ agonists in the perfused liver: determination via laser scanning confocal microscopy. *Am J Physiol Regul Integr Comp Physiol* 1999;276:R575–R585, with permission.) See Figure 38.5A on page 544.

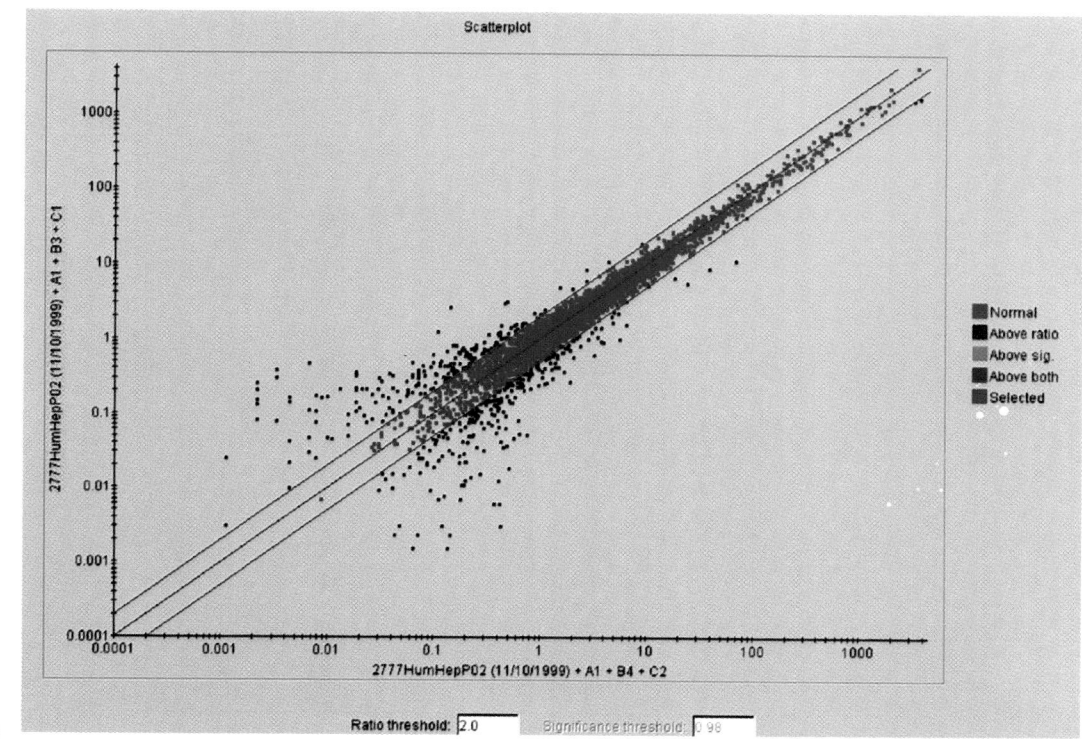

A

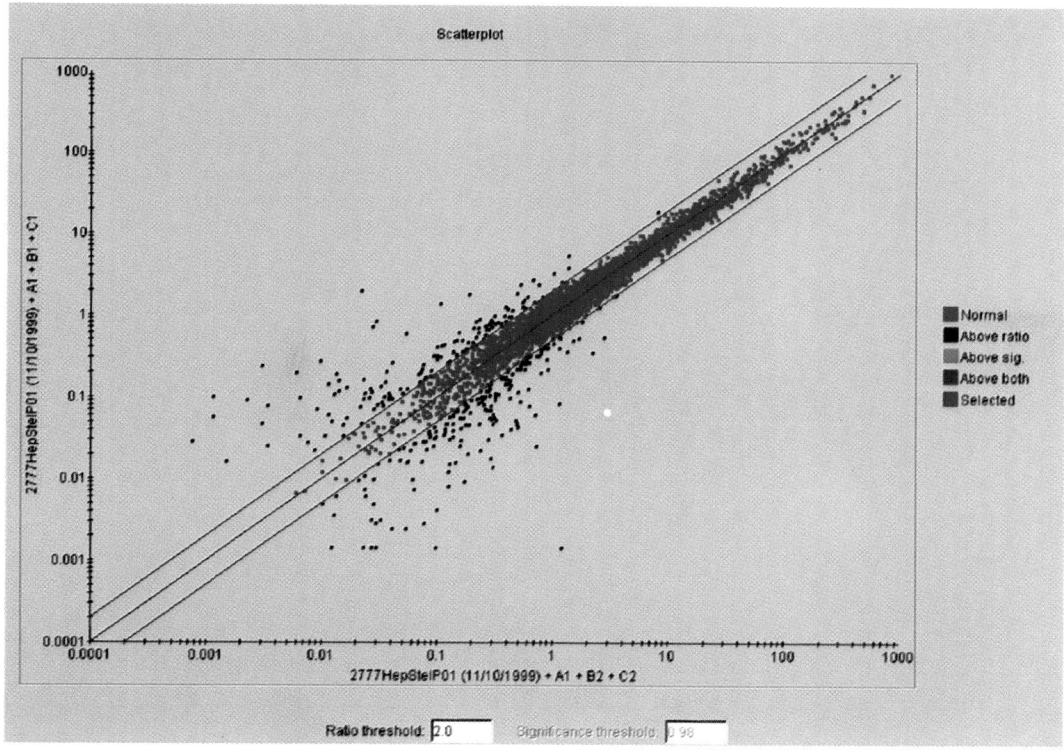

B

COLOR PLATE 15. Scatterplots corresponding to filters hybridized with human hepatocyte RNA (**A**) or human activated stellate cell RNA (**B**). *Spots within the two blue parallel lines* represent those for which the absolute values did not differ more than two-fold in the duplicate filters. Genes with low expression levels (left-lower corner) tend to present a higher degree of variation, as expected. See Figure 59.1 on page 913.

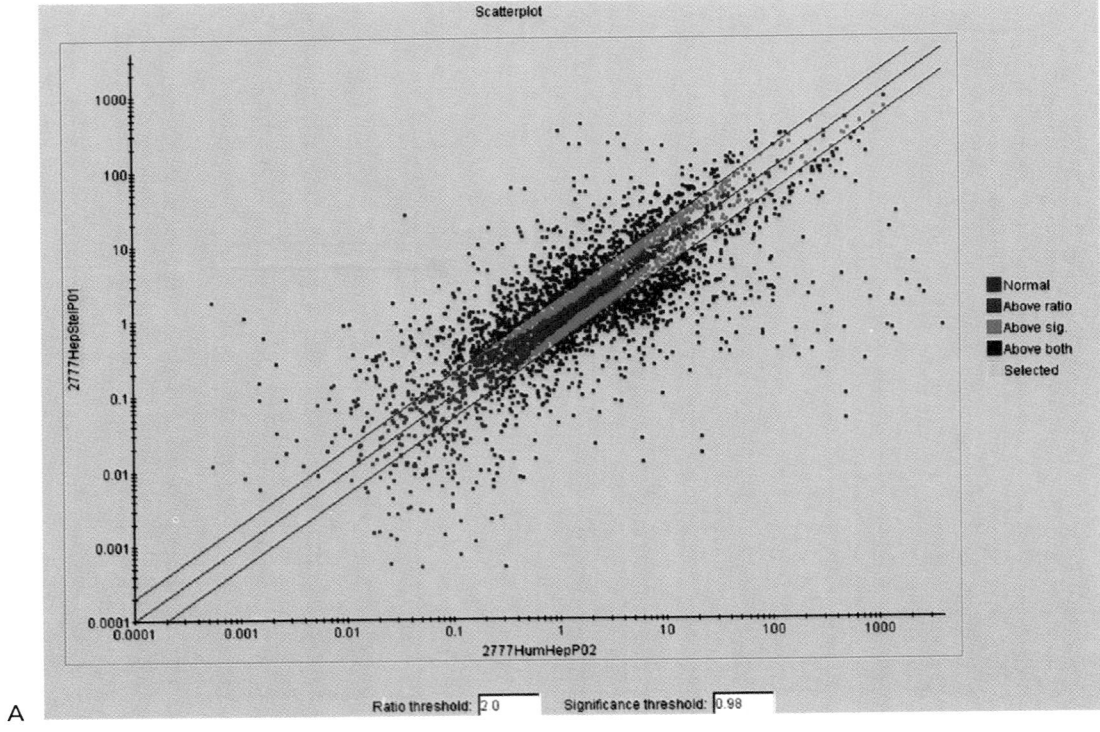

A

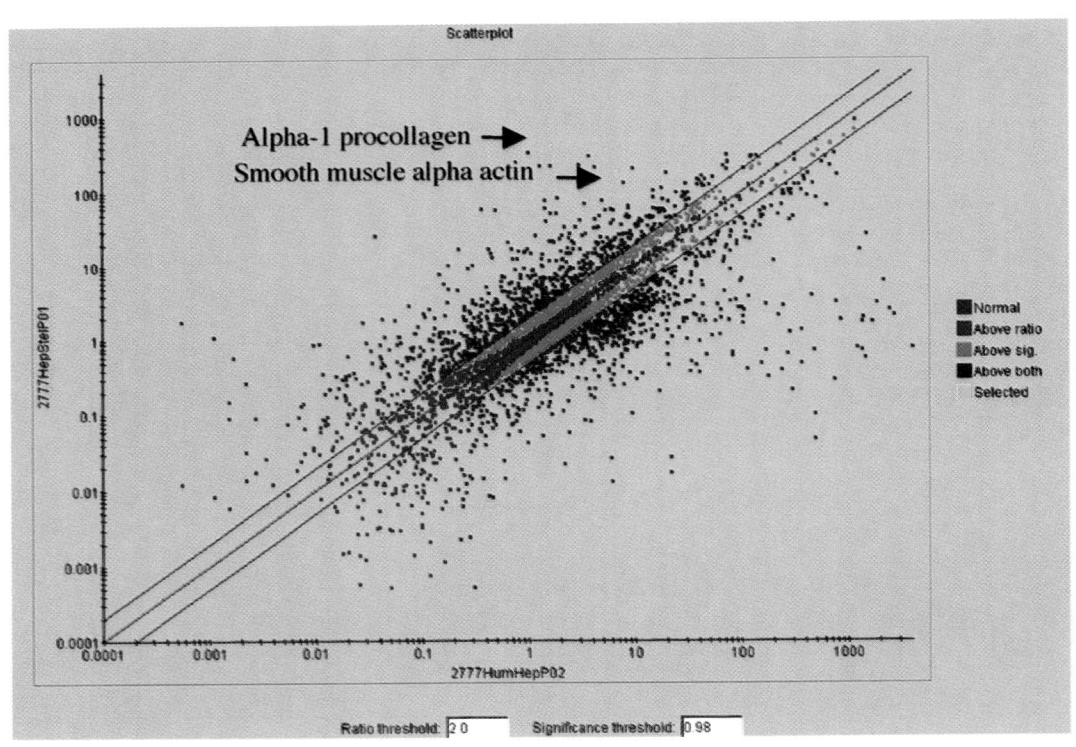

B

COLOR PLATE 16. Scatterplots comparing activated hepatic stellate cells (aHSCs) with hepatocyte expression. **A:** *Spots to the left of the upper blue line* represent genes whose expression levels in aHSC compared to hepatocytes are higher than two-fold. *Spots to the right of the lower blue line* represent genes whose expression levels in hepatocytes compared to aHSC are higher than two-fold. **B:** Two representative marker genes, procollagen and smooth muscle α-actin, are indicated. See Figure 59.2 on page 914.

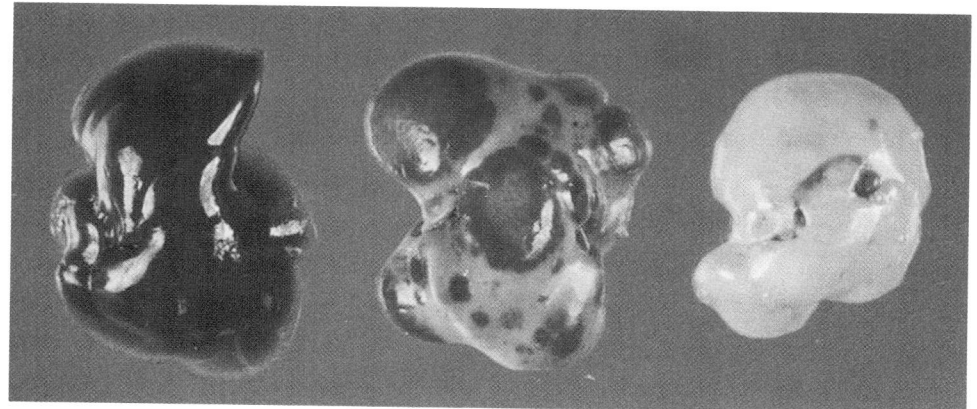

COLOR PLATE 17. Spontaneous liver repopulation of urokinase plasminogen activator (uPA) transgenic mouse liver by endogenous hepatocytes that have deleted the uPA transgene. **Left,** liver from a 5-week-old nontransgenic mouse; **center,** liver from a hemizygous uPA transgenic mouse; **right,** liver from a homozygous uPA transgenic mouse. (From Sandgren EP, Palmiter RD, Heckel JL, et al. Complete hepatic regeneration after somatic deletion of an albumin-plasminogen activator transgene. *Cell* 1991;66:245–256, with permission.) See Figure 61.1 on page 929.

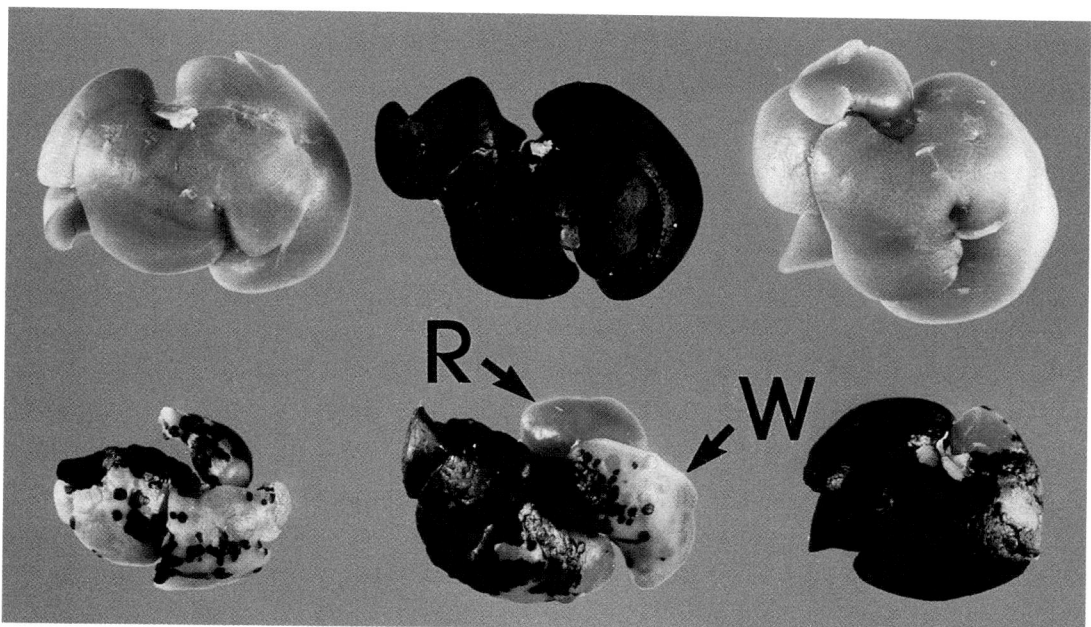

COLOR PLATE 18. Repopulation of uPA transgenic mouse liver with transplanted normal mouse hepatocytes containing a lacZ marker transgene. Livers from a nontransgenic control (**top, left**), a lacZ-positive control (**top, center**), a control mouse lacking the Alb-uPA transgene and transplanted with lacZ cells (**top, right**), and three livers from Alb-uPA transgenic mice receiving lacZ cells (**bottom**). All tissues were stained with X-gal, which produces a blue color in lacZ-positive cells. Red areas (*R*) represent endogenous cells that have lost uPA transgene expression, and white areas (*W*) represent residual endogenous liver still expressing the uPA transgene. (From Rhim JA, Sandgren EP, Degen JL, et al. Replacement of disease mouse liver by hepatic cell transplantation. *Science* 1994;263,1149–1152, with permission.) See Figure 61.3 on page 930.

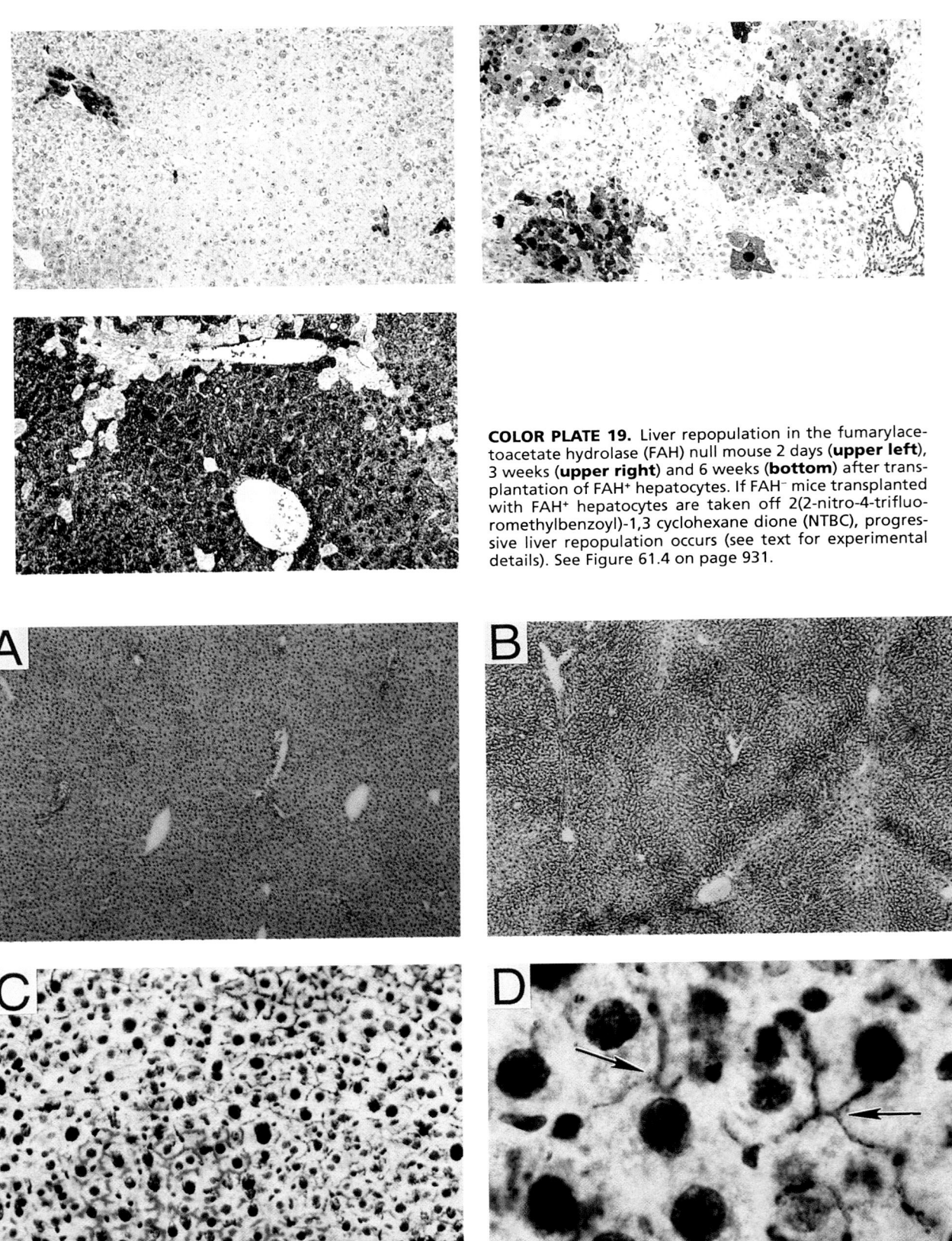

COLOR PLATE 19. Liver repopulation in the fumarylace-toacetate hydrolase (FAH) null mouse 2 days (**upper left**), 3 weeks (**upper right**) and 6 weeks (**bottom**) after transplantation of FAH+ hepatocytes. If FAH− mice transplanted with FAH+ hepatocytes are taken off 2(2-nitro-4-trifluoromethylbenzoyl)-1,3 cyclohexane dione (NTBC), progressive liver repopulation occurs (see text for experimental details). See Figure 61.4 on page 931.

COLOR PLATE 20. Liver repopulation by dipeptidyl peptidase IV (DPPIV)+hepatocytes in DPPIV− mutant Fischer 344 rats in the retrorsine/partial hepatectomy model. **A:** Liver from DPPIV− rat before hepatocyte transplantation. **B:** Liver from same DPPIV− rat 9 months after transplantation of DPPIV+ hepatocytes. **C:** Expanding clusters of DPPIV+ hepatocytes in DPPIV− rat liver two months after transplantation of DPPIV+ hepatocytes. **D:** Higher magnification of region from panel C showing formation of hybrid bile canaliculi between endogenous (DPPIV−) and transplanted (DPPIV+) hepatocytes as denoted by *arrows*. (From Laconi E, Oren R, Mukhopadhyay DK, et al. Long-term, near-total liver replacement by transplantation of isolated hepatocytes in rats treated with retrorsine. *Am J Pathol* 1998;153:319–329, with permission.) See Figure 61.6 on page 934.

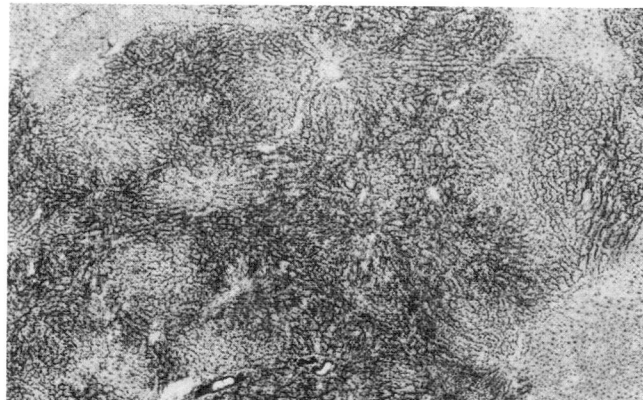

COLOR PLATE 21. Repopulation of dipeptidyl peptidase IV (DPPIV)⁻ mutant rat liver by transplanted DPPIV⁺ day E13 fetal liver cells, showing completely new liver lobules containing DPPIV⁺ hepatocyte cords and DPPIV⁺ bile ducts. See Figure 61.7 on page 936.

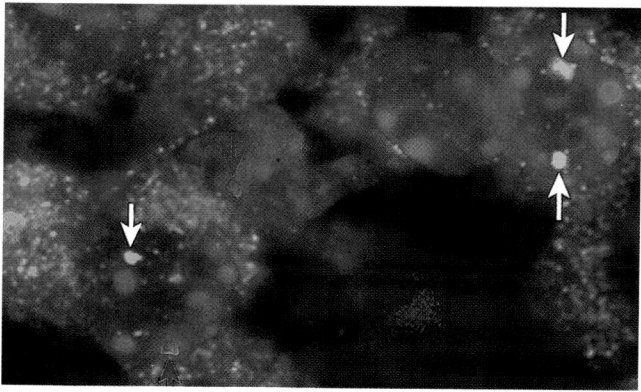

COLOR PLATE 22. Detection of Y chromosome-positive hepatocytes in the liver of a female mouse after transplantation of bone marrow cells from a male donor. *Bright green dots* in blue-stained nuclei of hepatocyte (highlighted by *white arrows*) indicate transcription centers for albumin mRNA. The finely stippled, bright green staining surrounding the nuclei is cytoplasmic albumin mRNA. One hepatocyte also contains a red-labeled Y chromosome (*red arrows*), indicating that it is of male origin and derived from the transplanted bone marrow. A second cell of undetermined phenotype also contains a red-labeled Y chromosome, indicating that it also is of male bone marrow origin. See Figure 61.8 on page 937.

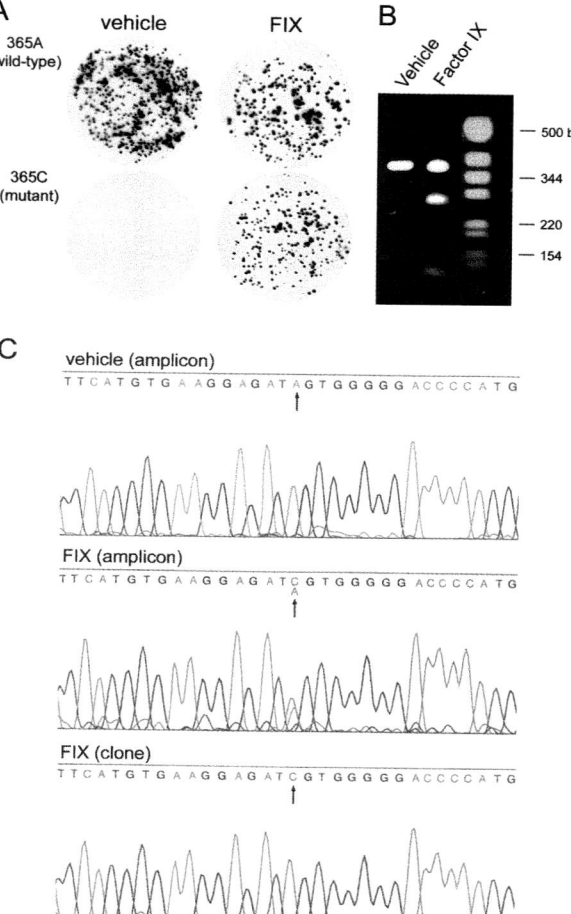

COLOR PAGE 23. Filter lift hybridizations, restriction fragment length polymorphism and sequence analyses of DNA isolated from the liver. **A:** Hybridization patterns of duplicate filter lifts of the cloned polymerase chain reaction (PCR) products from liver DNA of rats 18 months postinjection with vehicle (left) or factor IX (*FIX*) chimeraplasts (**right**). **B**: PCR amplicons were subjected to *Sau*3AI restriction enzyme digestion and analyzed by agarose gel electrophoresis and ethidium bromide staining. The site-specific A to C conversion creates a new restriction site, resulting in the partial cleavage of the amplicons from the factor IX-treated animals, but not from vehicle-treated controls. **C:** Direct DNA sequencing of the PCR-amplified *factor IX* gene surrounding the targeted C insertion site at Ser³⁶⁵ (*arrows*) is shown for wild-type/vehicle (**top**), factor IX amplicon (**middle**), and factor IX clone (**bottom**). See Figure 62.7 on page 955.

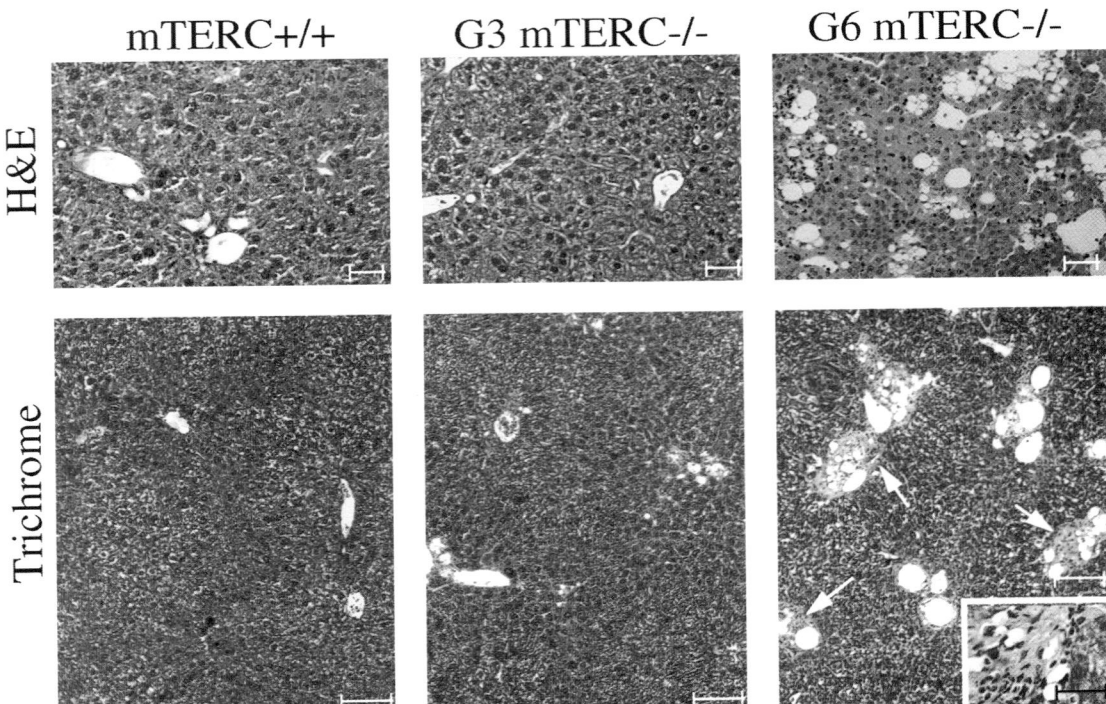

COLOR PLATE 24. Telomere shortening in the essential telomerase RNA component (*mTERC–/–*) mice correlates with accelerated induction of liver cirrhosis by repeated CCl₄ injections. mTERC+/+ (telomerase activity, long telomeres), G3 mTERC–/– (no telomerase activity, intermediate telomere length), and G6 mTERC–/– mice (no telomerase activity, short telomeres) were treated with six intraperitoneal injections of CCl₄. No obvious liver damage was present in mice with long telomeres, but increased centrilobular fibrosis (*blue areas* in Trichrome stain, *bar: 100 μm.* **Inset:** *bar:* 50 μm) and steatosis [Hematoxilin–Eosin-stain (*H&E*), *bar:* 50 μm] were present in liver sections of mice with short telomeres. In addition, serum bilirubin levels were increased and serum albumin levels were decreased in mice with short telomeres. These features of accelerated cirrhosis were rescued in G6 mTERC–/– mice, which were pretreated with a telomerase-expressing adenovirus. (From Rudolph KL, Chang S, Millard M, et al. Inhibition of experimental liver cirrhosis in mice by telomerase gene delivery. *Science* 2000;287:1253–1258, with permission.) See Figure 67.2 on page 1006.

34. Taylor SI. Lilly Lecture: Molecular mechanisms of insulin resistance. Lessons from patients with mutations in the insulin-receptor gene. *Diabetes* 1992;41:1473–1490.

35. Hitman GA, Hawrami K, McCarthy MI, et al. Insulin receptor substrate-1 gene mutations in NIDDM; implications for the study of polygenic disease. *Diabetologia* 1995;38:481–486.

36. Kalidas K, Wasson J, Glaser B, et al. Mapping of the human insulin receptor substrate-2 gene, identification of a linked polymorphic marker and linkage analysis in families with Type II diabetes: no evidence for a major susceptibility role. *Diabetologia* 1998;41:1389–1391.

37. Almind K, Frederiksen SK, Bernal D, et al. Search for variants of the gene-promoter and the potential phosphotyrosine encoding sequence of the insulin receptor substrate-2 gene: evaluation of their relation with alterations in insulin secretion and insulin sensitivity. *Diabetologia* 1999;42:1244–1249.

38. Bektas A, Warram JH, White MF, et al. Exclusion of insulin receptor substrate 2 (IRS-2) as a major locus for early-onset autosomal dominant type 2 diabetes. *Diabetes* 1999;48:640–642.

39. Engstrom W, Shokrai A, Otte K, et al. Transcriptional regulation and biological significance of the insulin like growth factor II gene. *Cell Prolif* 1998;31:173–189.

40. Butler AA, Yakar S, Gewolb IH, et al. Insulin-like growth factor-I receptor signal transduction: at the interface between physiology and cell biology. *Comp Biochem Physiol B Biochem Mol Biol* 1998;121:19–26.

41. Morgan DO, Edman JC, Standring DN, et al. Insulin-like growth factor II receptor as a multifunctional binding protein. *Nature* 1987;329:301–307.

42. Tong PY, Tollefsen SE, Kornfeld S. The cation-independent mannose 6-phosphate receptor binds insulin-like growth factor II. *J Biol Chem* 1988;263:2585–2588.

43. Hwa V, Oh Y, Rosenfeld RG. The insulin-like growth factor-binding protein (IGFBP) superfamily. *Endocr Rev* 1999;20:761–787.

44. Laron Z. Disorders of growth hormone resistance in childhood. *Curr Opin Pediatr* 1993;5:474–480.

45. Connors MH. Growth in the diabetic child. *Pediatr Clin North Am* 1997;44:301–306.

46. Cullen KJ, Yee D, Sly WS, et al. Insulin-like growth factor receptor expression and function in human breast cancer. *Cancer Res* 1990;50:48–53.

47. Gammeltoft S, Ballotti R, Kowalski A, et al. Expression of two types of receptor for insulin-like growth factors in human malignant glioma. *Cancer Res* 1988;48:1233–1237.

48. Harris TM, Rogler LE, Rogler CE. Reactivation of the maternally imprinted IGF2 allele in TGFa induced hepatocellular carcinomas in mice. *Oncogene* 1998;16:203–209.

49. Hakam A, Yeatman TJ, Lu L, et al. Expression of insulin-like growth factor-1 receptor in human colorectal cancer. *Hum Pathol* 1999;30:1128–1133.

50. Long L, Rubin R, Brodt P. Enhanced invasion and liver colonization by lung carcinoma cells overexpressing the type 1 insulin-like growth factor receptor. *Exp Cell Res* 1998;238:116–121.

51. Macaulay VM, Everard MJ, Teale JD, et al. Autocrine function for insulin-like growth factor I in human small cell lung cancer cell lines and fresh tumor cells. *Cancer Res* 1990;50:2511–2517.

52. Minuto F, Del Monte P, Barreca A, et al. Evidence for an increased somatomedin-C/insulin-like growth factor I content in primary human lung tumors. *Cancer Res* 1986;46:985–988.

53. Pietrzkowski Z, Mulholland G, Gomella L, et al. Inhibition of growth of prostatic cancer cell lines by peptide analogues of insulin-like growth factor 1. *Cancer Res* 1993;53:1102–1106.

54. Upegui-Gonzalez LC, Duc HT, Buisson Y, et al. Use of the IGF-I antisense strategy in the treatment of the hepatocarcinoma. *Adv Exp Med Biol* 1998;451:35–42.

55. Ellouk-Achard S, Djenabi S, De Oliveira GA, et al. Induction of apoptosis in rat hepatocarcinoma cells by expression of IGF-I antisense cDNA. *J Hepatol* 1998;29:807–818.

56. Duvillie B, Cordonnier N, Deltour L, et al. Phenotypic alterations in insulin-deficient mutant mice. *Proc Natl Acad Sci U S A* 1997;94:5137–5140.

57. Accili D, Drago J, Lee EJ, et al. Early neonatal death in mice homozygous for a null allele of the insulin receptor gene. *Nat Genet* 1996;12:106–109.

58. Joshi RL, Lamothe B, Cordonnier N, et al. Targeted disruption of the insulin receptor gene in the mouse results in neonatal lethality. *Embo J* 1996;15:1542–1547.

59. Michael MD, Kulkarni RN, Postic C, et al. Loss of insulin signaling in hepatocytes leads to severe insulin resistance and progressive hepatic dysfunction. *Mol Cell* 2000;6:87-97.

60. Michael MD, Kahn CR. Circulating levels of insulin-like growth factor binding proteins are altered in liver-specific insulin receptor knockout mice. *Proc Endo Soc* 2000;221(abst).

61. Liu JP, Baker J, Perkins AS, et al. Mice carrying null mutations of the genes encoding insulin-like growth factor I (Igf-1) and type 1 IGF receptor (Igf1r). *Cell* 1993;75:59–72.

62. Baker J, Liu JP, Robertson EJ, et al. Role of insulin-like growth factors in embryonic and postnatal growth. *Cell* 1993;75:73–82.

63. DeChiara TM, Efstratiadis A, Robertson EJ. A growth-deficiency phenotype in heterozygous mice carrying an insulin-like growth factor II gene disrupted by targeting. *Nature* 1990;345:78–80.

64. Ludwig T, Eggenschwiler J, Fisher P, et al. Mouse mutants lacking the type 2 IGF receptor (IGF2R) are rescued from perinatal lethality in Igf2 and Igf1r null backgrounds. *Dev Biol* 1996;177:517–535.

65. Louvi A, Accili D, Efstratiadis A. Growth-promoting interaction of IGF-II with the insulin receptor during mouse embryonic development. *Dev Biol* 1997;189:33–48.

66. Yakar S, Liu JL, Stannard B, et al. Normal growth and development in the absence of hepatic insulin-like growth factor I. *Proc Natl Acad Sci U S A* 1999;96:7324–7329.

67. Sjogren K, Liu JL, Blad K, et al. Liver-derived insulin-like growth factor I (IGF-I) is the principal source of IGF-I in blood but is not required for postnatal body growth in mice. *Proc Natl Acad Sci U S A* 1999;96:7088–7092.

68. Araki E, Lipes MA, Patti ME, et al. Alternative pathway of insulin signalling in mice with targeted disruption of the IRS-1 gene. *Nature* 1994;372:186–190.

69. Tamemoto H, Kadowaki T, Tobe K, et al. Insulin resistance and growth retardation in mice lacking insulin receptor substrate-1. *Nature* 1994;372:182–186.

70. Ueki K, Yamauchi T, Tamemoto H, et al. Restored insulin-sensitivity in IRS-1-deficient mice treated by adenovirus-mediated gene therapy. *J Clin Invest* 2000;105:1437–1445.

71. Withers DJ, Gutierrez JS, Towery H, et al. Disruption of IRS-2 causes type 2 diabetes in mice. *Nature* 1998;391:900–904.

CYCLIC AMP SIGNALING IN THE LIVER: COUPLING TRANSCRIPTION TO PHYSIOLOGY AND PROLIFERATION

GIUSEPPE SERVILLO
MARIA AGNESE DELLA FAZIA
PAOLO SASSONE-CORSI

Control of gene expression involves a panoply of nuclear proteins governing transcription, RNA processing, and chromatin remodeling (1–4). A major outcome of studies conducted during the past two decades is that a large number of these proteins are under direct control of intracellular responses to external signals (5). In particular, the function of many transcription factors has been found to be modulated by a number of signal transduction pathways activated by selected second messengers (6,7). One of the best examples of a transcription factor being controlled by transduction pathways is AP-1, which is composed of the Fos and Jun oncoproteins, products of the early response genes *fos* and *jun* (8). AP-1 activity may be increased by inducing c-*fos* gene transcription, a process mediated by the ERK-1 and ERK-2 mitogen-activated protein (MAP) kinases, which directly phosphorylate the transcription factor Elk1/TCF, responsible for stimulation of c-*fos* expression through a serum response element within the promoter. Alternatively, AP-1 activity may be enhanced by direct phosphorylation of Jun by a different type of MAPK, the stress-activated protein kinases (JNK/SAPK) (9). Importantly, both *fos* and *jun* genes are known to be activated rapidly and transiently in the liver upon partial hepatectomy (10).

The cyclic AMP (cAMP)-dependent signaling pathway governs a number of essential liver functions (11). In particular, hormones acting on liver physiology (e.g., glucagon, adrenaline, noradrenaline) bind to specific receptors and via G proteins regulate the intracellular concentration of this second messenger (12). Thus, the understanding of the signaling routes and the molecular events leading to regulated gene expression by cAMP is central to the deciphering of liver physiological responses.

THE CYCLIC AMP TRANSDUCTION ROUTE

Cyclic AMP, identified in 1959 in prokaryotic and eukaryotic cells as a mediator of hormonal action, is chemically derived from a molecule of adenosine triphosphate (ATP) by action of the enzyme adenylate cyclase (AC). AC is a plasma membrane-bound enzyme comprised of two clusters of six transmembrane segments spanning two intracellular catalytic domains (13–15). AC is composed of a multigene family of at least nine components. Different

P. Sassone-Corsi: Institute of Genetics and of Molecular and Cellular Biology, Louis Pasteur University, 67404 Illkirch-Strasbourg, France.

G. Servillo and **M.A. Della Fazia:** Department of Biochemical Science and Cellular and Molecular Biotechnology, Department of Physiopathology, Policlinico Monteluce, 06100 Perugia, Italy.

external stimuli, which act on specific receptors coupled to trimeric G proteins, change AC activity (G proteins are constituted by three chains, α, β, and γ) (16,17) (Fig. 37.1).

Regulation of the intracellular concentration of cAMP relies on what type of receptor is activated; indeed, depending on the coupling of receptors to G proteins, these will elicit either activation or inhibition of AC function (18,19). Specif-

ically, receptors can couple two different forms of G protein α-subunits: the activating form, called stimulatory G protein (Gs) (i.e., coupled to the β-adrenergic receptor), or the inhibitory form, known as inhibitory G protein (Gi) (i.e., coupled to the α2-adrenergic receptor). Gs is constituted by a α^s chain which hydrolyzes a molecule of GTP in GDP, and a complex of β and γ chains which anchors the G protein to the

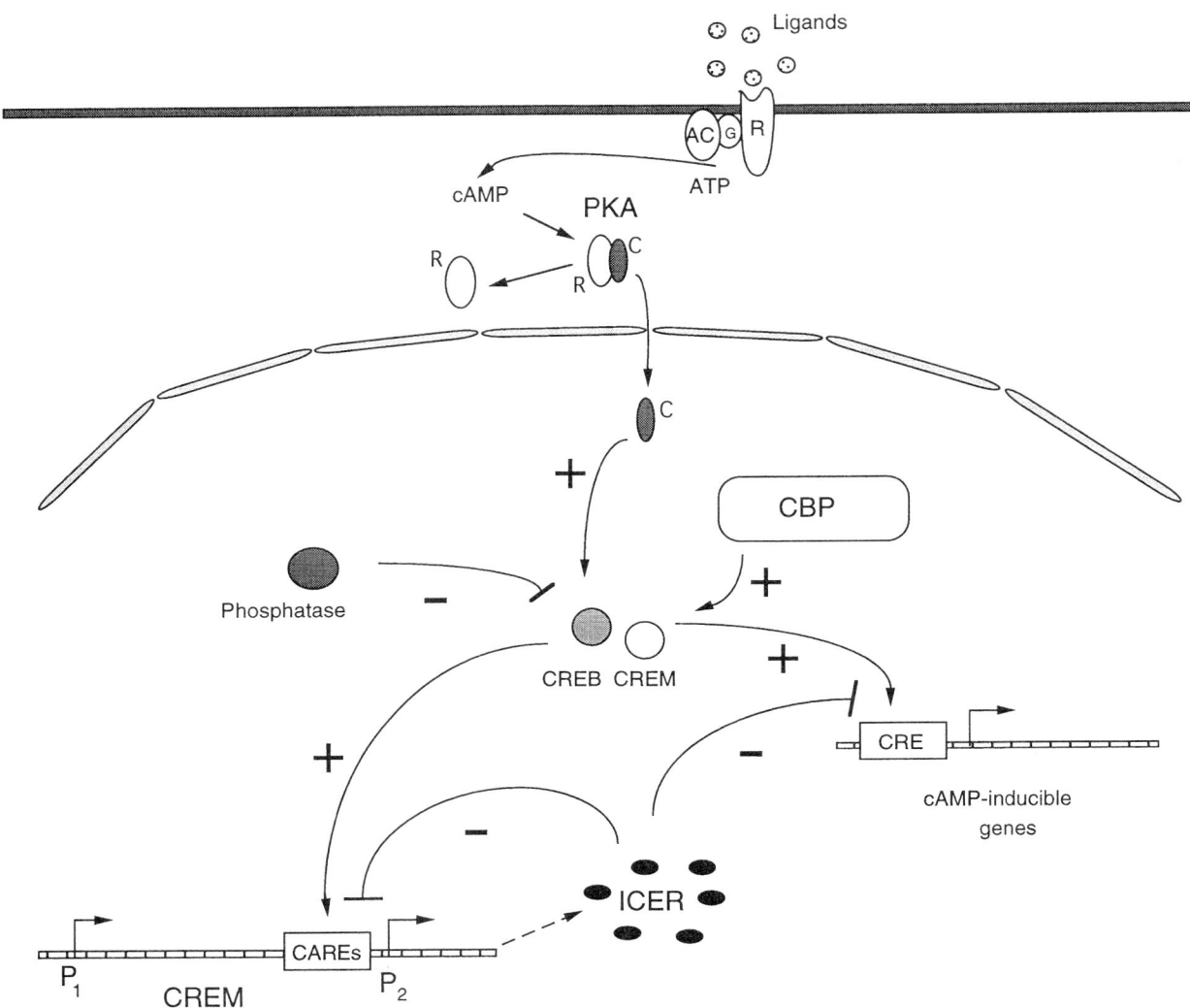

FIGURE 37.1. Schematic representation of the cyclic AMP (*cAMP*) signal transduction pathway and its nuclear effectors controlling gene expression. Ligands binding to specific membrane receptors activate coupled G proteins (*G*), which in turn stimulate the activity of the membrane-associated adenylyl cyclase (*AC*), which converts adenosine triphosphate (*ATP*) to cAMP. Increased intracellular levels of cAMP cause the dissociation of the inactive tetrameric protein kinase A (*PKA*) complex into the active catalytic subunits (*C*) and the regulatory subunits (*R*). Catalytic subunits migrate into the nucleus where they phosphorylate (*P*) and induce transcriptional activators such as cAMP-responsive element (*CRE*)–binding proteins (*CREB*) and CRE modulators (*CREM*). Phosphorylation allows the recruiting of CREB-binding protein (*CBP*), a large coactivator. DNA binding to CRE found in promoters of cAMP-responsive genes is a key step in transcriptional activation. Products of cAMP-inducible genes are involved in the hormonal response, differentiation and proliferation. An intronic, cAMP-inducible promoter (*P2*) of the CREM gene directs the synthesis of inducible cAMP early repressor (*ICER*), which downregulates the expression of CRE-containing promoters, including P2, generating a negative autoregulatory transcriptional loop. *CARES*, cAMP autoregulatory elements; *P1*, promoter 1.

membrane by a prenyl group. After stimulation, the α^s of Gs releases the GDP molecule bound to the trimeric complex and binds GTP. This change permits the dissociation of the complex and the binding of α^s to AC, thereby resulting in an increase in cAMP intracellular levels. An inhibitory stimulus acts on the α^i subunit and permits the binding of GTP and the release of the complex in α^i and $\beta\gamma$. These molecules in turn inhibit the activity of AC (16,20,21). A number of G protein subunit isoforms exist, some displaying differential tissue distribution, particularly in the liver (22).

The increased level of cAMP elicited by AC activation triggers the cAMP-dependent protein kinase A (PKA). In the absence of cAMP, PKA is a tetrameric holoenzyme composed of two regulatory and two catalytic subunits (R and C subunits) (23–25). Binding of cAMP on the two regulatory subunits (RI and RII) results in the dissociation of the protein complex. The activated catalytic subunits are released from cytoplasmic and Golgi complex anchoring sites and become able to phosphorylate a number of cytoplasmic and nuclear substrates on serine sites within the canonical peptidic setting X-Arg-Arg-X-*Ser*-X (where X is any amino acid) (19,26,27). RI subunits contain binding sites for MgATP. Binding of MgATP stabilizes the holoenzyme by raising the threshold of cAMP concentration required to cause activation and enhancing holoenzyme reassociation. RII subunits do not bind MgATP, but are targets of autophosphorylation, which destabilizes and activates the holoenzyme. Multiple isoforms of both R and C subunits have been identified, namely, RIα, RIβ, RIIα RIIβ, Cα, Cβ, and Cγ (28–33). Each subunit isoform has a characteristic pattern of tissue-specific expression (33). In particular, the Cα-subunit is expressed in brain, heart, adrenal gland, testis, lung, kidney, spleen, and liver, whereas the Cβ-subunit is expressed in the brain and adrenal gland and in much lesser amounts in other tissues. The differential distribution of the various C subunit isoforms suggests that individual subunits are involved in specialized functions (34).

COUPLING CYCLIC AMP TO LIVER GENE TRANSCRIPTION

A primary checkpoint in the control of transcription is provided by the specific arrangement of regulatory sequences within the promoter region. DNA sequences responsible for determining the exact initiation site and the levels of mRNA are now well known for a large number of transcription factors. The analysis of promoter sequences of several cAMP-responsive genes allowed the identification of a promoter element that could mediate transcriptional activation in response to increased levels of intracellular cAMP. The CRE (*cAMP responsive element*) (27,35) is composed of a consensus palindromic sequence of eight base pairs (bp) (TGACGTCA, Table 37.1) with higher conservation in the 5′ half of the palindrome with respect to the 3′ sequence (27).

CRE sites have been identified in a number of promoters (36–38), among which many display a neuroendocrine-specific expression. Mutation of these elements causes a significant decline not only in cAMP-inducibility, but also in the basal transcriptional activity (39). CRE consensus sequences have also been found in promoters where they appear to confer transcriptional properties of tissue-specificity (40), of nonendocrine expression (41,42) and in viral transcription units (43,44).

A number of genes essential for liver physiology are under control of the cAMP signaling pathway (Table 37.1). Genes involved in gluconeogenesis such as *tyrosine-aminotransferase* (TAT), *phosphoenolpyruvate carboxykinase* (PEPCK), *serine dehydratase* (SDH), and *glucose-6-phosphatase* (G-6-P) contain CREs in their promoter and present cAMP-inducible expression (44–48). TAT and PEPCK share common features and constitute two useful models to study cAMP-responsive transcription in the liver. Both are gluconeogenetic enzymes localized in periportal hepatocytes; their expression increases upon fasting and decreases

TABLE 37.1. EXPRESSION PROFILES OF SOME LIVER GENES AND LOCATION OF CREs IN THEIR PROMOTERS

Gene	CRE Location	Fetal Life	Normal Liver	Induction Upon Liver Regeneration (h after PH)
TAT	−3651/−3644	−	+	2–10
PEPCK	−90/−83	−	+	1–4
SDH	−1129/−1122	−	+	2–5
G-6-Pase	−136/−129	+	+	30 min to 24
	−161/−152			
CREM (ICER)	−105/−98	?	+	2–5
	−116/109			
	−136/−129			
	−148/140			
c-*fos*	−66/−59	?	−	30 min to 2 h
Cyclin A	−80/−73	?	−	38–72

TAT, tyrosine aminotransferase; PEPCK, phosphoenolpyruvate carboxykinase; SDH, serine dehydratase; G-6-Pase, glucose-6-phosphatase; CREM, cyclic AMP-responsive element modulator; ICER, inducible cyclic AMP early repressor; PH, partial hepatectomy.

during diets rich in glucose. Glucagon stimulates the expression of both genes by acting through the cAMP pathway (49–51).

TAT is a rate-limiting enzyme for tyrosine catabolism. It is synthesized exclusively in hepatocytes and is involved in gluconeogenesis (50). The enzyme synthesis is absent during the fetal life and rises within the first hours after birth. Administration of glucagon starting from the 17th day of rat fetal life results in the transient induction of TAT synthesis (52). In addition, TAT is highly expressed during liver regeneration following partial hepatectomy (53). The TAT promoter contains a functional CRE 3.6 kb upstream of the transcription start site (45).

PEPCK catalyses the synthesis of phosphoenol-pyruvate from oxaloacetate; its expression is high in the liver, kidney, and adipose tissue and low in skeletal muscle, heart, mammary gland, ovary, and lung (54). A peculiar feature of the PEPCK promoter is that distinct segments confer differential activity in different tissues. For example, sequences between positions −2088 and −888 are essential for expression in fat, heart, ovary, and muscle tissues, while for expression in kidney sequences located between −460 and −355 appear crucial. In the liver, PEPCK expression is controlled by sequences located between −460 and +73 (55). Interestingly, this region contains two CREs, named CRE-1 and CRE-2, CRE-1 more active than CRE-2 (55). Yet, it has been shown that CRE-1 exerts its full activity only if the integrity of other flanking elements is preserved (56). Indeed, in addition to the CREs, the promoter contains multiple critical binding sites for liver-enriched nuclear proteins within the region which directs liver-specific expression. In support of this observation, cooperative actions of various transcription factors on this essential region of the PEPCK promoter have been shown (see Role of Cyclic AMP-Responsive Element Modulators in Liver Regeneration, below).

NUCLEAR EFFECTORS OF CYLIC AMP SIGNALING: THE CYCLIC AMP-RESPONSIVE ELEMENT–BINDING PROTEIN FAMILY

The search for nuclear factors binding specifically to CRE sites revealed a class of proteins bearing common structural and functional characteristics (57,58). The identification and the cloning of the first CRE-binding factor (58,59), CRE-binding protein (CREB), opened the way for the

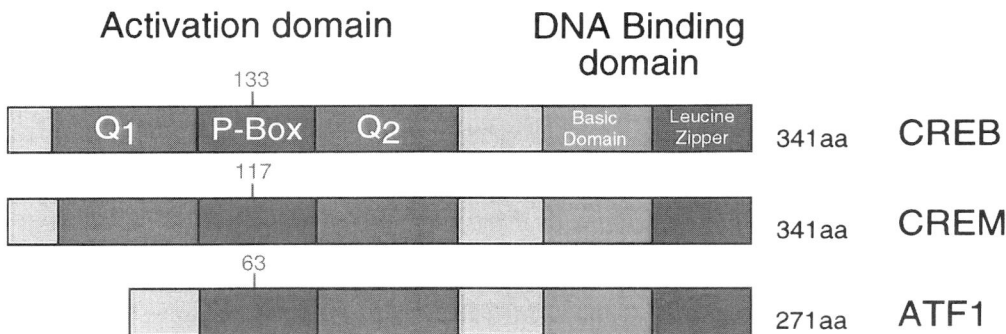

FIGURE 37.2. Structure of cyclic AMP-responsive element (CRE)–binding proteins (*CREB*), CRE modulators (*CREM*), and activating transcription factor-1 (*ATF1*): (a) The glutamine-rich domains (*Q1* and *Q2*), the DNA-binding region (basic domain and leucine zipper) and the P-box are shown. The position of the serine residue phosphorylated by the cAMP-dependent protein kinase (PKA) and other kinases (see Fig. 37.3) is also indicated; and (b) Sequence alignment of the P-box domain from these proteins. The serine corresponding to the PKA-phosphoacceptor site is shown in blue. (From De Cesare D, Fimia GM, Sassone-Corsi P. Signaling routes to CREM and CREB: plasticity in transcriptional activation. *Trends Biochem Sci* 1999;24:281–285, with permission.) See Color Plate 12.

identification of a large number of cDNA-encoding-related but distinct CREBs.

All the members of CREB family share common characteristics: they all belong to the bZip (basic domain-leucine zipper) transcription factor class. A basic domain about 50% rich in lysine and arginine residues and needed for direct contact with DNA is located near a leucine zipper, an α-helical-coiled-coil structure which is needed for parallel dimerization. The number of leucines in the zipper heptad repeat varies from four to six (27).

Outside the bZip region, the CREB family members share little similarity at the level of primary amino acid sequence. However, CREB, activating transcription factor-1 (ATF-1) and CRE modulator (CREM) show similar domains in their structural organization (60–62) (Fig. 37.2). The members of this subfamily are able to heterodimerize with each other, but only in certain combinations following a specific "dimerization code."

The genes encoding these transcription factors share the common feature of alternative splicing. For example, two CREB isoforms, CREB341 and CREB327, are encoded by the CREB gene (63). In CREM, alternative splicing is extensive since more than ten isoforms are generated. In addition, CREM displays alternative polyadenylation, alternative use of two promoters, and alternative translation, all determining different functional transcripts (57,62,64).

Alternative isoforms of CREB may act as transcriptional activators (CREMτ, CREB, and ATF1) (62,65,66) or repressors (CREMα, β, γ, and CREB-2) (64,67,68). A notable repressor is ICER (*i*nducible *c*AMP *e*arly *r*epressor), the only inducible repressor of the class, which is generated by an alternative promoter within CREM gene (57,69,70; see also Mechanisms of Repression, below).

MECHANISMS OF ACTIVATION

Regulated Phosphorylation

Two independent, well-conserved regions mediate the transcriptional activation by CREB family activator proteins (Fig. 37.2). The first, termed *k*inase *i*nducibile *d*omain (KID) or phosphorylation box (P-box), contains a serine residue within a consensus phosphorylation site for PKA at position 133 in CREB and 117 in CREM (27,65,71–73). The second region is composed of two glutamine-rich domains, termed Q1 and Q2, which flank the P-box (27,57). The phosphorylation event is a prerequisite for turning these transcription factors into powerful activators. The central serine within the P-box constitutes the direct link between cAMP signaling and activation of gene expression. Importantly, this same serine was also found to be phosphorylated by other kinases, thus representing a convergence site of various signaling pathways (57,74–77) (Fig. 37.3). For example, in Hep-G2 and 3T3-L1 cells, insulin induces CREB phosphorylation and stimulates transcriptional activity (78).

An important example of signaling crosstalk in the nucleus involves the pathway coupled to the nerve growth factor (NGF) receptor, Trk, which results in the activation of several kinases. Trk is a receptor tyrosine kinase which, once activated, stimulates the activity of the small GTP-binding protein Ras (79). Activation of Ras triggers the MAPK pathway, which includes the MAP kinase kinase (MEK) and the ribosomal S6 kinase pp90^{rsk} (80). Interestingly, constitutively-activated expression of MAPK and MEK is sufficient to induce neurite outgrowth in PC12 cells (81,82), indicating a direct role of this pathway in eliciting the changes in gene expression required for the neuronal differentiation program. Although MAPK and MEK have not been shown to directly phosphorylate CREB, the use of cells expressing a dominant-interfering Ras mutant has revealed the involvement of this pathway for CREB phosphorylation upon NGF-induction (76). Indeed, the involvement of a CREB-kinase with characteristics similar to pp90^{rsk} has been proposed. pp90^{rsk} is likely to be responsible for CREB phosphorylation in human melanocytes (83), while a different member of the RSK family, p70^{s6k}, also possesses CREB phosphorylation activity (84). We used cells from patients with Coffin–Lowry syndrome which carry mutations in the gene encoding the RSK-2 protein, one of the four isoforms of pp90^{rsk} (85). We have demonstrated that RSK-2 is responsible for CREB phosphorylation in response to epidermal growth factor (EGF) and for the consequent transcriptional induction of c-*fos* (77). Finally, CREB has been shown to be phosphorylated upon activation of the stress pathway involving the p38/MAPKAP-2 kinases (86). Thus, various signaling pathways may converge to modulate gene expression via the same transcriptional regulator, CREB. The complexity of the signaling pathways controlling transcription factors is a demonstration of the pleiotropic functions performed by these molecules in the regulation of physiology and metabolism.

Modularity of the Activation Domain

The two domains rich in glutamine, Q1 and Q2, are crucial for activation function. In other transcription factors, such as AP-2 and SP-1, Q-rich regions also exist (87,88). These domains are believed to mediate the interaction of activators with other components of the transcriptional machinery to elicit efficient initiation. The contribution of Q2 to the activation function seems more significant than that of Q1 (57). The demonstration of the role of the Q2-rich domain is offered by a splicing form of CREM and by ATF-1 (89,90), both of which lack a counterpart of Q1 yet are still able to activate transcription (66). Thus, the P-box region and Q2 are sufficient for induction.

The identification of the CREB-binding protein (CBP), a 265-kd protein that interacts selectively with the phosphorylated form of CREB, increased the understanding of the mechanism by which the cAMP pathway controls tran-

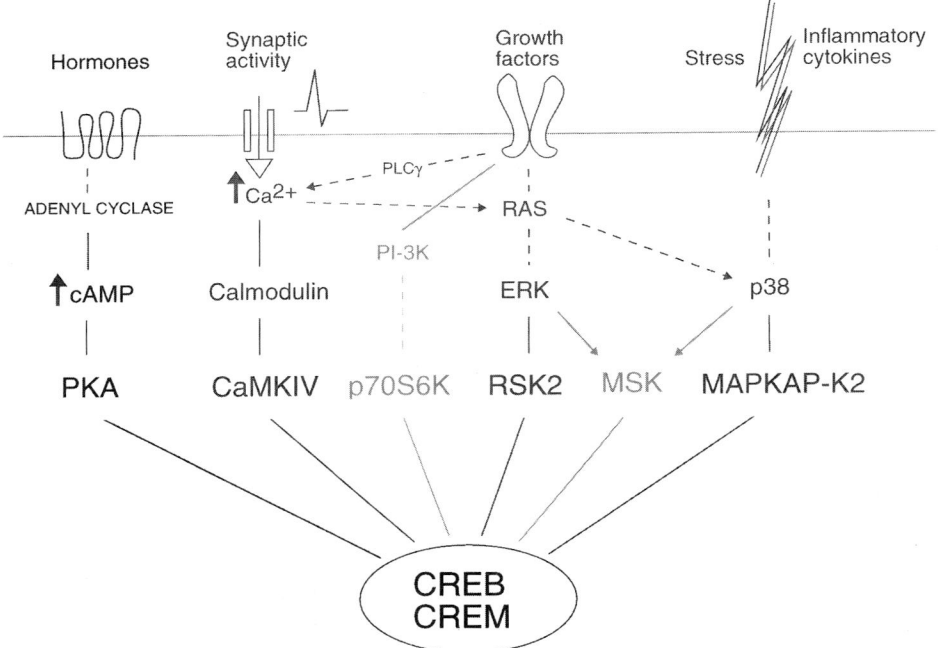

FIGURE 37.3. Signal transduction pathways that lead to phosphorylation of the activators cyclic AMP (*cAMP*)-responsive element (CRE) modulators (*CREM*) and CRE-binding proteins (*CREB*). Various signaling cascades are color-coded according to the external stimulus by which they are activated. Crosstalk between pathways is indicated by *arrows*. *Dashed lines* indicate the presence of intermediate kinases not shown. *CaMKIV*, Ca2+-calmodulin-dependent kinase IV; *ERK*, extracellular-regulated kinase; *MAPKAP-K2*, MAP-kinase-activated protein kinase 2; *MSK*, mitogen- and stress-activated kinase; *p70S6K*, p70 S6 kinase; *PI-3K*, phosphoinositide-3 kinase; *PKA*, cyclic AMP-dependent protein kinase; *PLCγ*, phospholipase C; *RSK2*, ribosomal S6 kinase 2. (From De Cesare D, Fimia GM, Sassone-Corsi P. Signaling routes to CREM and CREB: plasticity in transcriptional activation. *Trends Biochem Sci* 1999;24:281–285, with permission.)

scription (91). CBP presents two zinc finger domains, a glutamine-rich domain and PKA consensus sites. Upon phosphorylation, CREB binds to CBP, an interaction that facilitates the binding of CBP to TFIIB, a factor directly linked to RNA polymerase II (92). Another protein similar to CBP, p300 (93,94), shares similar regulatory functions in differentiation (95), cell growth (96), apoptosis, and DNA repair (97). Both p300 and CBP interact with the basal transcription factors, including TFIIB, TBP, and an RNA helicase. In addition, they have an intrinsic or associated histone acetyltransferase (HAT) activity, establishing a direct link with chromatin remodeling (92,98–101). Moreover, CBP and p300 interact with several other transcription factors (e.g., Jun, Fos, MyoD, p53, NF-κB) and nuclear receptors (102).

Additional Routes to Activation

A coactivator factor has recently been isolated in testis that is able to interact with and modulate the CREM transcriptional activity. This protein, named *a*ctivator of *CR*EM in *t*estis (ACT), presents four complete LIM domains and one amino-terminal half-LIM motif. ACT is a tissue-specific coactivator that shares a high degree of homology with a family of proteins expressed in heart and skeletal muscle. ACT is able to perform its function independently of CREM phosphorylation at Ser-117, and thus independently of the interaction with CBP. This suggests a new way to elicit activation by the transcription factors of the CREB class, possibly bypassing classical signaling pathways (103). As it is likely that ACT defines a novel class of tissue-specific coactivators, it would be of great interest to determine whether proteins of this type exist in the liver.

MECHANISMS OF REPRESSION

Dephosphorylation of Cyclic AMP-Responsive Element–Binding Protein

One of the mechanisms involved in the negative regulation of CREB is represented by dephosphorylation. After the well-studied rapid phosphorylation of CREB in response to various stimuli (57,58), protein phosphatases, presumably PP-1 and PP-2a, are likely to be involved in the dephosphorylation of CREB. Some *in vitro* results appear to support this possibility (104). However, the signals required to trigger phosphatase activity and their regulation remain obscure.

Thus, the role played by phosphatases in the *in vivo* regulation of CREB function remains to be determined.

Cyclic AMP-Responsive Element–Binding Repressors

The dynamic and versatile CREM expression, combined with its tissue- and developmental-specific expression pattern, opened a new dimension in the study of the transcriptional response to cAMP (64). These characteristics contrast with those of the remaining members of the CRE-binding factor family, whose expression seems to be constant and ubiquitous (61,105).

Several studies have demonstrated that differential transcript processing plays a central role in the regulation of CREM expression (57,64). Three isoforms (CREMα, -β, -γ,) generated from the GC-rich housekeeping promoter (P1) lack the activation domain and thereby act as antagonists of cAMP-responsive transcription by either competing for binding to CREs or by blocking CREB by heterodimerizing with it (57).

A particularly noteworthy repressor is the CREM isoform ICER. This is a small protein of 120 aa consisting only of the bZip domain whose synthesis is directed by an alternative P2 promoter lying within an intron near the 3' end of the CREM gene (Fig. 37.1). ICER is one of the smallest transcription factors ever isolated and functions as a powerful repressor of cAMP-induced transcription (69,70). An essential feature of ICER is its inducibility. The P2 promoter is strongly inducible by cAMP, since it contains two pairs of closely spaced CREs (69). Thus, following cAMP treatment there is a rapid and transient increase of ICER expression characteristic of the early response gene class (69). ICER then turns off its own expression by repressing the activity of the P2 promoter, establishing a negative autoregulatory loop.

ROLE OF CYCLIC AMP-RESPONSIVE ELEMENT MODULATORS IN LIVER REGENERATION

Partial hepatectomy is well-known for inducing a finely-tuned program of gene expression leading to the regeneration of the tissue (see Chapter 42 and website chapter 🖳 W-31). A look at the temporal kinetics of transcriptional activation after hepatectomy reveals a pattern of early induction for several genes (Fig. 37.4). A central role for cAMP signaling in

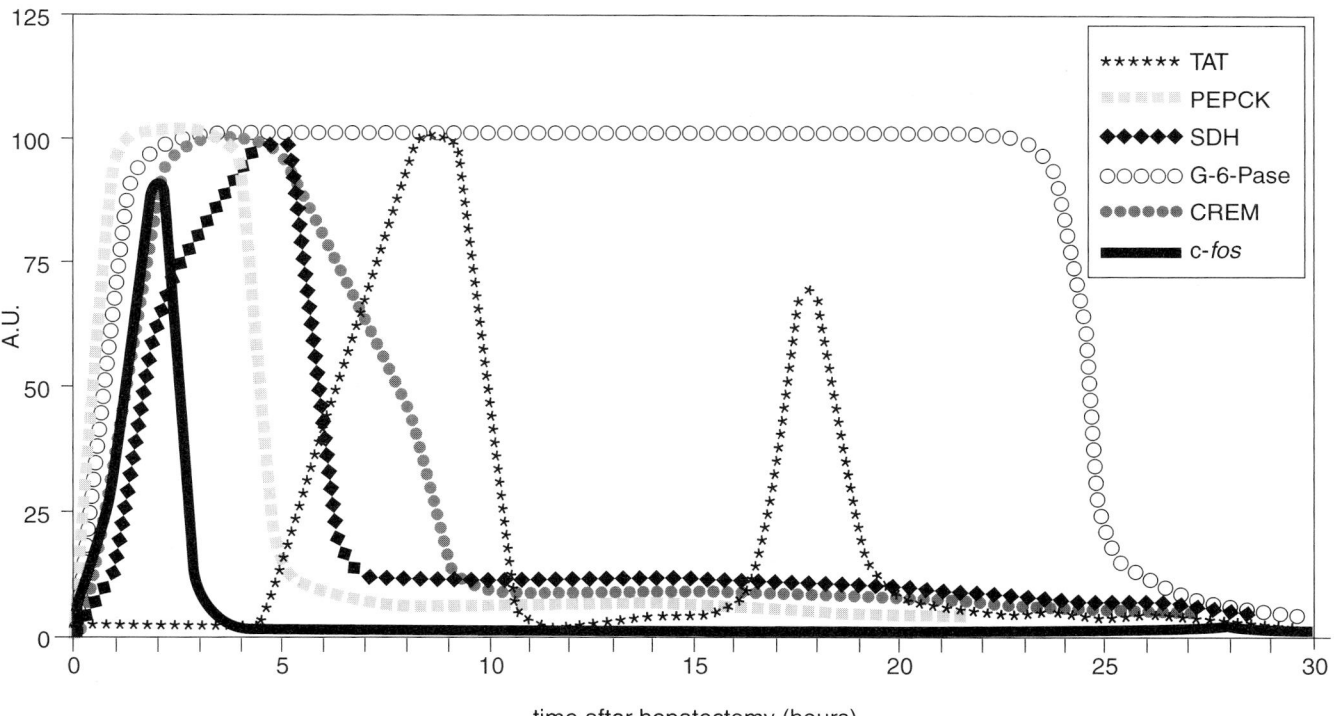

FIGURE 37.4. Expression profiles of genes bearing at least one cyclic AMP-responsive element (CRE) site in their promoter regulatory region at different times after partial hepatectomy. This representation reveals the various kinetics of gene expression in response to the proliferative stimulus. The relative levels of expression of the various genes are not respected, and data are expressed in arbitrary units (*A.U.*). *TAT*, tyrosine aminotransferase; *PEPCK*, phosphoenolpyruvate carboxykinase; *SDH*, serine dehydratase; *G-6-Pase*, glucose-6-phosphatase; *CREM*, CRE modulator.

the early phases of the regeneration has been invoked. In particular, increased levels of cAMP in hepatocytes lead to CREB phosphorylation and activation of TAT synthesis by virtue of the CRE present in the promoter (106). CREB also binds to the CRE-1 in the promoter of the PEPCK gene, playing a role in both basal and cAMP-stimulated expression (107). Other transcription factors, such as C/EBPα, C/EBPβ, and DBP bind to the PEPCK promoter and are thought to synergize with CREB (108,109). Thus, one important issue concerns the interplay that cAMP-responsive transcription factors have with other proteins regulating liver-specific promoters. This issue has not yet been satisfactorily explored, but it is likely that future experiments will reveal functional interactions with liver-specific transcription factors.

Because cAMP has a central role in the regulation of hepatocyte function, the way cAMP-responsive nuclear proteins are regulated in these cells is of interest. When hepatocytes in culture are induced to proliferate, there is a remarkable induction in CREB phosphorylation and a subsequent induction of ICER expression (110). Importantly, the same pattern is observed *in vivo* by treating rats with an intraperitoneal injection of cAMP. In these animals, ICER expression is powerfully induced at 2, 4, and 8 hours following treatment with cAMP. These observations suggest that CREM may play a role in the control of the hepatocyte response to cAMP (110).

The role of cAMP signaling in proliferation has been debated for a long time. In certain cell types, cAMP appears to act as a promoting factor, while in other cells it appears to suppress proliferation. High concentrations of cAMP in primary hepatocyte cultures result in inhibition of DNA synthesis, a notion in apparent contrast to the increased levels of cAMP that are normally observed in animals at birth and during liver regeneration. During liver regeneration, there are two peaks of intracellular concentration of cAMP in residual hepatocytes. The second peak precedes the first round of mitosis and has been associated with hepatocyte proliferation (111). Pharmacological inhibition of the second peak of cAMP correlates with a delay in DNA synthesis (112). In the first hours following partial hepatectomy, ICER expression was shown to be rapidly and transiently induced, suggesting a role for this transcriptional repressor in the regulation of the early proliferation phases (110). Indeed, subsequent studies postulated a role for CREM in the proliferation of hepatocytes and other cells (113,114) (Fig. 37.5).

The role of CREM was established with the use of mutant mice in which the CREM gene was targeted by homologous recombination (113). In CREM-deficient mice, there is a significant delay in the first round of mitosis following partial hepatectomy. Expression of the genes encoding cyclins A, B, D1, E, and cdc2 undergoes a switch, confirming a delay in mitosis. In addition, the expression of the liver-specific markers TAT and PEPCK is affected, as well as the immediate early gene c-*fos* (113). Since the protein product of the c-*jun* gene combines with the Fos protein to constitute the transcription factor AP-1, which has been involved in various proliferative processes, the pattern of AP-1 expression upon partial hepatectomy in the CREM-deficient mice was also worth being analyzed. Intriguingly, no differences with respect to normal mice have been observed (*our unpublished data*), indicating that alteration of one of the AP-1 components is sufficient to cause a delay in hepatocyte proliferation. This observation is also interesting in light of results obtained with c-*jun* liver-specific conditional mutant mice, which display a phenotype highly reminiscent of the CREM-deficient mice (E. Wagner, *personal communication,* 2000). The role of CREM as a cAMP-responsive factor in liver physiology is thus quite attractive. It is noteworthy that the promoter regulatory regions of several genes whose expression is altered in the CREM-deficient mice, that is, cyclin A, cyclin D1, TAT, PEPCK, and c-*fos*, contain CRE sequences (55,104,115, 116), establishing a direct link with the regulatory function of the CREM products. These results provide clear evidence that CREM has an important function in regulating hepatocyte proliferation.

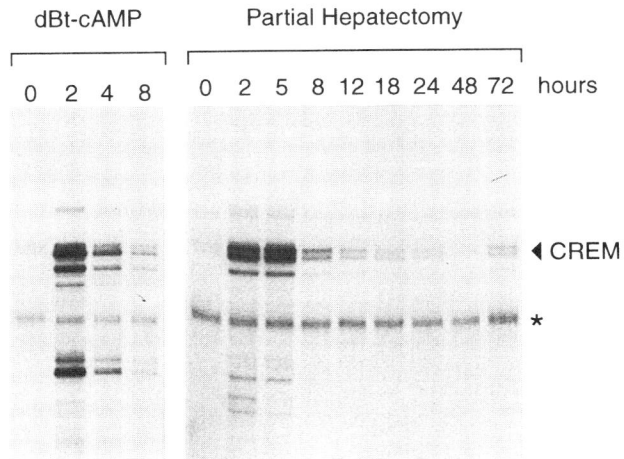

FIGURE 37.5. Cyclic AMP-responsive element modulator (*CREM*) gene induction in the liver. Expression of inducible cAMP early repressor (*ICER*) in rat liver was analyzed after dBtcAMP intraperitoneal injection (*lanes 2 through 4*) (*lane 1*, saline injection) and in the regenerating liver at different times after partial hepatectomy (*lane 5*, nonoperated control). The *arrowhead* corresponds to the ICER-specific transcript generated from the CREM P2 promoter. (From Servillo G, Della Fazia MA, Sassone-Corsi P. Transcription factor CREM coordinates the timing of hepatocyte proliferation in the regenerating liver. *Genes Dev* 1998;12:3639–3643,with permission.)

CONCLUSION

The complex process of liver regeneration is governed by a highly specialized program of gene expression. Signals to transcription factors are utilized to integrate the information required to direct synchronized waves of hepatocyte proliferation. A central role for the cAMP-signaling transduction cascade in this process has long been considered, and evidence involving cAMP-responsive transcription factors is now present. Although some clear links with cell proliferation are provided by, for example, the direct control that CREM appears to exert on cyclin gene expression, many questions remain: what are the target genes of cAMP-responsive transcription factors? What role is played by crosstalk among signaling pathways? In what way does cAMP influence the cell cycle of proliferating hepatocytes? Various experimental approaches will be needed to further elucidate the molecular mechanisms governing normal and pathological liver physiology. The available technology of targeted disruption of specific genes in the mouse by homologous recombination, especially if coupled to tissue-specific and conditional mutagenesis, will very likely provide a great deal of novel, essential information.

ACKNOWLEDGMENTS

We thank all the members of the Sassone-Corsi laboratory for their help and discussions. We also acknowledge G.M. Fimia, M.P. Viola-Magni, and E. Borrelli for insights. G. Servillo was supported by a fellowship from the Fondation de la Recherche Médicale, and M.A. Della Fazia was supported by the Institut National de la Santé et de la Recherche Médicale. Work in Sassone-Corsi's laboratory is supported by grants from the Centre National de la Recherche Scientifique, the Institut National de la Santé et de la Recherche Médicale, the Centre Hospitalier Universitaire Régional, the Fondation de la Recherche Médicale, the Université Louis Pasteur, the Association pour la Recherche sur le Cancer, and the Human Frontiers Scientific Programme.

REFERENCES

1. Strahl BD, Allis CD. The language of covalent histone modifications. *Nature* 2000;403:41-45.
2. Lamond AI, Earnshaw WC. Structure and function in the nucleus. *Science* 1998;280:547–553.
3. Cheung P, Allis CD, Sassone-Corsi P. Signaling to chromatin through histone modifications. *Cell* 2000;103:263–271.
4. Hirose Y, Manley JL. RNA polymerase II and the integration of nuclear events. *Genes Dev* 2000;14:1415–1429.
5. Hunter T. Signaling 2000 and beyond. *Cell* 2000;100:113–127.
6. Pawson T, Saxton TM. Signaling networks: do all roads lead to the same genes? *Cell* 1999;97:675–678.
7. De Cesare D, Fimia GM, Sassone-Corsi P. Signaling routes to CREM and CREB: plasticity in transcriptional activation. *Trends Biochem Sci* 1999;24:281–285.
8. Vogt PK, Bos TJ. The oncogene *jun* and nuclear signaling. *Trends Biochem Sci* 1989;14:172–175.
9. Davis RJ. MAPKs: new JNK expands the group. *Trends Biochem Sci* 1994;19:470–473.
10. Morello D, Lavenu A, Babinet C. Differential regulation and

11. Diehl AM, Rai RM Liver regeneration 3: regulation of signal transduction during liver regeneration. *FASEB J* 1996;10: 215–227.
12. Freissmuth M, Casey PJ, Gilman AG. G-proteins control diverse pathways of transmembrane signaling. *FASEB J* 1989;3: 2125–2131.
13. Schramm M, Selinger Z. Message transmission: receptor-controlled adenylate cyclase system. *Science* 1984;225:1350–1356.
14. Tang WJ, Gilman AG. Adenylyl cyclases. *Cell* 1992;70:869–872.
15. Houslay MD, Milligan G. Tailoring cAMP-signaling responses through isoform multiplicity. *Trends Biochem Sci* 1997;22: 217–224.
16. Gilman AG. G-proteins: transducers of receptor generated signals. *Ann Rev Biochem* 1987;56:615–649.
17. Sunahara RK, Dessauer CW, Gilman AG. Complexity and diversity of mammalian adenylyl cyclases. *Annu Rev Pharmacol Toxicol* 1996;36:461–480.
18. Choi EJ, Xia Z, Villacres EC, et al. The regulatory diversity of the mammalian adenylyl cyclases. *Curr Opin Cell Biol* 1993;5: 269–273.
19. McKnight GS, Clegg CH, Uhler MD, et al. Analysis of the cAMP-dependent protein kinase system using molecular genetic approaches. *Recent Prog Horm Res* 1988;44:307–335.
20. Iniguez-Lluhi J, Kleuss C, Gilman AG. The importance of G-protein βγ subunits. *Trends Cell Biol* 1993;3:230–235.
21. Kaziro Y, Itoh H, Kozasa T, et al. Structure and function of signal-transducing GTP-binding proteins. *Annu Rev Biochem* 1991;60:349–400.
22. Manning DR, Woolkalis MJ. G protein function and diversity. In: Arias IM, Boyer JL Fausto N, Jakoby WB, Schachter DA, Shafritz D, eds. *The liver: biology and pathobiology,* 3rd ed. New York: Raven Press, 1994:919–931.
23. Taylor SS, Buechler JA, Yonemoto W. cAMP-dependent protein kinase: framework for a diverse family of regulatory enzymes. *Annu Rev Biochem* 1990;59:971–1005.
24. Francis SH, Corbin JD. Structure and function of cyclic nucleotide-dependent protein kinases. *Annu Rev Physiol* 1994; 56:237–272.
25. Beebe SJ. The cAMP-dependent protein kinases and cAMP signal transduction. *Semin Cancer Biol* 1994;5:285–294.
26. Roesler WJ, Vanderbark GR, Hanson RW. Cyclic AMP and the induction of eukaryotic gene expression. *J Biol Chem* 1988;263: 9063–9066.
27. Lalli E, Sassone-Corsi P. Signal transduction and gene regulation: the nuclear response to cAMP. *J Biol Chem* 1994;269: 17359–17362.
28. Lee DC, Carmichael DF, Krebs EG, et al. Isolation of a cDNA clone for the type I regulatory subunit of bovine cAMP-dependent protein kinase. *Proc Natl Acad Sci U S A* 1983;80: 3608–3612.
29. Clegg CH, Cadd GG, McKnight GS. Genetic characterization of a brain-specific form of the type I regulatory subunit of cAMP-dependent protein kinase. *Proc Natl Acad Sci U S A* 1988;85:3703–3707.
30. Scott JD, Glaccum MB, Zoller MJ, et al. The molecular cloning of a type II regulatory subunit of the cAMP-dependent protein kinase from rat skeletal muscle and mouse brain. *Proc Natl Acad Sci U S A* 1987;84:5192–5196.
31. Jahnsen T, Hedin L, Kidd VJ, et al. Molecular cloning, cDNA structure, and regulation of the regulatory subunit of type II cAMP-dependent protein kinase from rat ovarian granulosa cells. *J Biol Chem* 1986;261:12352–12361.
32. Adavani SR, Schwarz M, Showers MO, et al. 1990 multiple

expression of *jun*, c-*fos* and c-*myc* proto-oncogenes during mouse liver regeneration and after inhibition of protein synthesis. *Oncogene* 1990;5:1511–1519.

mRNA species code for the catalytic subunit of the cAMP-dependent protein kinase from LLC-PK1 cells. Evidence for two forms of the catalytic subunit. *Eur J Biochem* 1987;167: 221–226.

33. Beebe SJ, Oyen O, Sandberg M, et al. Molecular cloning of a tissue-specific protein kinase (C γ) from human testis representing a third isoform for the catalytic subunit of cAMP-dependent protein kinase. *Mol Endocrinol* 1990;4:465–475.

34. Shuntoh H, Sakamoto N, Matsuyama S, et al. Molecular structure of the C β catalytic subunit of rat cAMP-dependent protein kinase and differential expression of C α and C β isoforms in rat tissues and cultured cells. *Biochim Biophys Acta* 1992; 1131:175–180.

35. Ziff EB. Transcription factors: a new family gathers at the cAMP response site. *Trends Genet* 1990;6:69–72.

36. Ishiguro H, Kim KT, Joh TH, et al. Neuron-specific expression of the human dopamine β-hydroxylase gene requires both the cAMP-response element and a silencer region. *J Biol Chem* 1993;268:17987–17994.

37. Steger DJ, Hecht JH, Mellon PL. GATA-binding proteins regulate the human gonadotropin α-subunit gene in the placenta and pituitary gland. *Mol Cell Biol* 1994;14:5592–5602.

38. Horiuchi M, Nakamura N, Tang SS, et al. Molecular mechanism of tissue-specific regulation of mouse renin gene expression by cAMP. Identification of an inhibitory protein that binds nuclear transcriptional factor. *J Biol Chem* 1991;266: 16247–16254.

39. Robertson LM, Kerppola TK, Vendrell M, et al. Regulation of c-*fos* expression in transgenic mice requires multiple interdependent transcription control elements. *Neuron* 1995;14:241–252.

40. Wu H, Mahata SK, Mahata M, et al. A functional cyclic AMP response element plays a crucial role in neuroendocrine cell type-specific expression of the secretory granule protein chromogranin A. *J Clin Invest* 1995;96:568–578.

41. Dean DC, McQuillan JJ, Weintraub S. Serum stimulation of fibronectin gene expression appears to result from rapid serum-induced binding of nuclear proteins to a cAMP response element. *J Biol Chem* 1990;265:3522–3527.

42. Liou HC, Boothby MR, Glimcher LH. Distinct cloned class II MHC DNA-binding proteins recognize the X-box transcription element. *Science* 1988;242:69–71.

43. Wagner S, Green MR. DNA-binding domains: targets for viral and cellular regulators. *Curr Opin Cell Biol* 1994;6:410–414.

44. Sassone-Corsi P. Cyclic AMP induction of early adenovirus promoters involves sequences required for E1A transactivation. *Proc Natl Acad Sci U S A* 1988;85:7192–7196.

45. Boshart M, Weih F, Schmidt A, et al. A cyclic AMP response element mediates repression of tyrosine aminotransferase gene transcription by the tissue-specific extinguisher locus Tse-1. *Cell* 1990;61:905–916.

46. Liu JS, Park EA, Gurney AL, et al. Cyclic AMP induction of phosphoenolpyruvate carboxykinase (GTP) gene transcription is mediated by multiple promoter elements. *J Biol Chem* 1991;266:19095–19102.

47. Su Y, Pitot HC. Identification of regions in the rat serine dehydratase gene responsible for regulation by cyclic AMP alone and in the presence of glucocorticoids. *Mol Cell Endocrinol* 1992;90: 141–146.

48. Lin B, Morris DW, Chou JY. The role of HNF1α, HNF3γ, and cyclic AMP in glucose-6-phosphatase gene activation. *Biochemistry* 1997;36:14096–14106.

49. Hanson RW, Reshef L. Regulation of phosphoenolpyruvate carboxykinase (GTP) gene expression. *Annu Rev Biochem* 1997; 66:581–611.

50. Granner DK, Hargrove JL. Regulation of the synthesis of tyro-sine aminotransferase: the relationship to mRNATAT. *Mol Cell Biochem* 1983;54:113–128.

51. Montoliu L, Blendy JA, Cole TJ, et al. Analysis of the cAMP response on liver-specific gene expression in transgenic mice. *Fundam Clin Pharmacol* 1994;8:138–146.

52. Greengard O. The developmental formation of enzyme in rat liver. In: Litwack IG, ed. *Mechanism of hormone action.* New York: Academic Press, 1970:53–85.

53. Della Fazia MA, Servillo G, Viola-Magni M. Different expression of tyrosine aminotransferase and serine deydratase in rat livers after partial hepatectomy. *Biochem Biophys Res Commun* 1992;182:753–759.

54. Lemaigre FP, Rousseau GG. Transcriptional control of genes that regulate glycolysis and gluconeogenesis in adult liver. *Biochem J* 1994;303:1–14.

55. Roesler WJ, Vandenbark GR, Hanson RW. Identification of multiple protein-binding domains in the promoter–regulatory region of the phosphoenolpyruvate carboxykinase (GTP) gene. *J Biol Chem* 1989;264:9657–9664.

56. Roesler WJ, Graham JG, Kolen R, et al. The cAMP response element-binding protein synergizes with other transcription factors to mediate cAMP responsiveness. *J Biol Chem* 1995;270: 8225–8232.

57. Sassone-Corsi P. Transcription factors responsive to cAMP. *Annu Rev Cell Dev Biol* 1995;11:355–377.

58. Montminy M. Transcriptional regulation by cyclic AMP. *Annu Rev Biochem* 1997;66:807–822.

59. Hoffler JP, Meyer TE, Yun Y, et al. Cyclic AMP-responsive DNA-binding protein: structure based on a cloned placental cDNA. *Science* 1988;242:1430–1433.

60. Shaywitz AJ, Greenberg ME. CREB: a stimulus-induced transcription factor activated by a diverse array of extracellular signals. *Annu Rev Biochem* 1999;68:821–861.

61. Hai TY, Liu F, Coukos WJ, et al. Transcription factor ATF cDNA clones: an extensive family of leucine zipper proteins able to selectively form DNA-binding heterodimers. *Genes Dev* 1989;3:2083–2090.

62. Foulkes NS, Sassone-Corsi P. More is better: activators and repressors from the same gene. *Cell* 1992;68:411–414.

63. Yamamoto KK, Gonzalez GA, Menzel P, et al. Characterization of a bipartite activator domain in transcription factor CREB. *Cell* 1990;60:611–617.

64. Foulkes NS, Borrelli E, Sassone-Corsi P. CREM gene: Use of alternative DNA-binding domains generates multiple antagonists of cAMP-induced transcription. *Cell* 1991;64: 739–749.

65. Gonzalez GA, Montminy MR. Cyclic AMP stimulates somatostatin gene transcription by phosphorylation of CREB at Ser 133. *Cell* 1989;59:675–680.

66. Rehfuss RP, Walton KM, Loriaux MM, et al. The cAMP-regulated enhancer-binding protein ATF-1 activates transcription in response to cAMP-dependent protein kinase A. *J Biol Chem* 1991;266:18431–18434.

67. Cowell IG, Skinner A, Hurst HC. Transcriptional repression by a novel member of the bZip of transcription factors. *Mol Cell Biol* 1992;12:3070–3076.

68. Karpinski BA, Morle GD, Huggenvik J, et al. Molecular cloning of human CREB-2: an ATF/CREB transcription factor that can negatively regulate transcription from the cAMP response. *Proc Natl Acad Sci U S A* 1992;89:4820–4824.

69. Molina CA, Foulkes NS, Lalli E, et al. Inducibility and negative autoregulation of CREM: An alternative promoter directs the expression of ICER, an early response repressor. *Cell* 1993; 75:875–886.

70. Stehle JH, Foulkes NS, Molina CA, et al. Adrenergic signals

70. direct rhythmic expression of transcriptional repressor CREM in the pineal gland. *Nature* 1993;365:314–320.

71. Lee CQ, Yun Y, Hoeffler JP. Cyclic AMP-responsive transcriptional activation involves interdependent phosphorylated subdomains. *EMBO J* 1990;9:4455–4465.

72. de Groot RP, den Hertog J, Vandenheede JR, et al. Multiple and cooperative phosphorylation events regulate the CREM activator function. *EMBO J* 1993a;12:3903–3911.

73. de Groot RP, Derua R, Goris J, et al. Phosphorylation and negative regulation of the transcriptional activator CREM by p34cdc2. *Mol Endocrinol* 1993b;7:1495–1501.

74. Sheng M, McFadden G, Greenberg ME. Membrane depolarization and calcium induce c-*fos* transcription via phosphorylation of transcription factor CREB. *Neuron* 1990;4:571–582.

75. Dash PK, Karl KA, Colicos MA, et al. cAMP response element-binding protein is activated by Ca2+/calmodulin- as well as cAMP-dependent protein kinase. *Proc Natl Acad Sci U S A* 1991;88:5061–5065.

76. Ginty DD, Bonni A, Greenberg ME. Nerve growth factor activates a Ras-dependent protein kinase that stimulates c-*fos* transcription via phosphorylation of CREB. *Cell* 1994;77:713–725.

77. De Cesare D, Jacquot S, Hanauer A, et al. Rsk-2 activity is necessary for epidermal growth factor-induced phosphorylation of CREB protein and transcription of c-*fos* gene. *Proc Natl Acad Sci U S A* 1998;95:12202–12207.

78. Klemm DJ, Roesler WJ, Boras T, et al. Insulin stimulates cAMP-response element-binding protein activity in HepG2 and 3T3-L1 cell lines. *J Biol Chem* 1998;273:917–923.

79. Gomez N, Cohen P. Dissection of the protein kinase cascade by which nerve growth factor activates MAP kinases. *Nature* 1991;353:170–173.

80. Cobb MH, Goldsmith EJ. How MAP kinases are regulated. *J Biol Chem* 1995;270:14843–14846.

81. Cowley S, Paterson H, Kemp P, et al. Activation of MAP kinase kinase is necessary and sufficient for PC12 differentiation and for transformation of NIH 3T3 cells. *Cell* 1994;77:841–852.

82. Fukuda M, Gotoh Y, Tachibana T, et al. Induction of neurite outgrowth by MAP kinase in PC12 cells. *Oncogene* 1995;11:239–244.

83. Böhm M, Moellmann G, Cheng E, et al. Identification of p90RSK as the probable CREB-Ser133 kinase in human melanocytes. *Cell Growth Differ* 1995;6:291–302.

84. de Groot RP, Ballou LM, Sassone-Corsi P. Positive regulation of the cAMP-responsive activator CREM by the p70 S6 kinase: an alternative route to mitogen-induced gene expression. *Cell* 1994;79:81–91.

85. Trivier E, De Cesare D, Jacquot S, et al. Mutations in the kinase Rsk-2 associated with Coffin–Lowry syndrome. *Nature* 1996;384:567–570.

86. Tan Y, Rouse J, Zhang A, et al. FGF and stress regulate CREB and ATF-1 via a pathway involving p38 MAP kinase and MAP-KAP kinase-2. *EMBO J* 1996;15:4629–4642.

87. Williams T, Admon A, Luscher B, et al. Cloning and expression of AP-2, a cell-type-specific transcription factor that activates inducible enhancer elements. *Genes Dev* 1988;2:1557–1569.

88. Courey AJ, Tjian R. Analysis of Sp1 *in vivo* reveals multiple transcriptional domains, including a novel glutamine activation motif. *Cell* 1989;55:887–898.

89. Laoide BM, Foulkes NS, Schlotter F, et al. The functional versatility of CREM is determined by its modular structure. *EMBO J* 1993;12:1179–1191.

90. Brindle P, Linke S, Montminy M. Protein-kinase-A-dependent activator in transcription factor CREB reveals a new role for CREM repressors. *Nature* 1993;364:821–824.

91. Chrivia JC, Kwok RPS, Lamb N, et al. Phosphorylated CREB binds specifically to the nuclear protein CBP. *Nature* 1993;365:855–859.

92. Kwok RP, Lundblad JR, Crivia JC, et al. Nuclear protein CBP is a coactivator for the transcription factor CREB. *Nature* 1994;370:223–226.

93. Eckner R, Ewen ME, Newsome D, et al. Molecular cloning and functional analysis of the adenovirus E1A-associated 300-kd protein (p300) reveals a protein with properties of a transcriptional adaptor. *Genes Dev* 1994;8:869–884.

94. Arany Z, Sellers WR, Livingston DM, et al. E1A-associated p300 and CREB-associated CBP belong to a conserved family of coactivators. *Cell* 1994;77:799–800.

95. Eckner R, Yao TP, Oldread E, et al. Interaction and functional collaboration of p300/CBP and bHLH proteins in muscle and B-cell differentiation. *Genes Dev* 1996a;10:2478–2490.

96. Eckner R. p300 and CBP as transcriptional regulators and targets of oncogenic events. *J Biol Chem* 1996b;377:685–688.

97. Giordano A, Avantaggiati ML. p300 and CBP: partners for life and death. *J Cell Physiol* 1999;181:218–230.

98. Nakajima T, Uchida C, Anderson SF, et al. RNA helicase A mediates association of CBP with RNA polymerase II. *Cell* 1997;90:1107–1112.

99. Bannister AJ, Kouzarides T. The CBP coactivator is a histone acetyltransferase. *Nature* 1996;384:641–643.

100. Korzus E, Torchia J, Rose DW, et al. Transcription factor-specific requirements for coactivators and their acetyltransferase functions. *Science* 1998;279:703–707.

101. Goldman PS, Tran VK, Goodman RH. The multifunctional role of the coactivator CBP in transcriptional regulation. *Recent Prog Horm Res* 1997;52:103–120.

102. Janknecht R, Hunter T. Transcription. A growing coactivator network. *Nature* 1996;383:22–23.

103. Fimia GM, De Cesare D, Sassone-Corsi P. CBP-independent activation of CREM and CREB by the LIM-only protein ACT. *Nature* 1999;398:165–169.

104. Nichols M, Weih F, Schmid W, et al. Phosphorylation of CREB affects its binding to high- and low-affinity sites: implications for cAMP-induced gene transcription. *EMBO J* 1992;11:3337–3346.

105. Sassone-Corsi P. Goals for signal transduction pathways: linking up with transcriptional regulation. *EMBO J* 1994;13:4717–4728.

106. Weih F, Stewart AF, Boshart M, et al. *In vivo* monitoring of a cAMP-stimulated DNA-binding activity. *Genes Dev* 1990;4:1437–1449.

107. Quinn PG, Wong TW, Magnuson MA, et al. Identification of basal and cyclic AMP regulatory elements in the promoter of the phosphoenolpyruvate carboxykinase gene. *Mol Cell Biol* 1988;8:3467–3475.

108. Park EA, Gurney AL, Nizielski SE, et al. Relative roles of CCAAT/enhancer-binding protein β and cAMP regulatory element-binding protein in controlling transcription of the gene for phosphoenolpyruvate carboxykinase (GTP). *J Biol Chem* 1993;268:613–619.

109. Roesler WJ, McFie PJ, Puttick DM. Evidence for the involvement of at least two distinct transcription factors, one of which is liver-enriched, for the activation of the phosphoenolpyruvate carboxykinase gene promoter by cAMP. *J Biol Chem* 1993;268:3791–3796.

110. Servillo G, Penna L, Foulkes NS, et al. Cyclic AMP-signaling pathway and cellular proliferation: induction of CREM during liver regeneration. *Oncogene* 1997;14:1601–1606.

111. Diehl AM, Yang SQ, Wolfgang D, et al. Differential expression of

guanine nucleotide-binding proteins enhances cAMP synthesis in regenerating rat liver. *J Clin Invest* 1992;89:1706–1712.

112. Mac Manus JP, Franks DJ, Youdale T, et al. Increases in rat liver cyclic AMP concentrations prior to the initiation of DNA synthesis following partial hepatectomy or hormone infusion. *Biochem Biophys Res Commun* 1972;49:1201–1207.

113. Servillo G, Della Fazia MA, Sassone-Corsi P. Transcription factor CREM coordinates the timing of hepatocyte proliferation in the regenerating liver. *Genes Dev* 1998;12:3639–3643.

114. Uyttersprot N, Costagliola S, Dumont JE, et al. Requirement for cAMP-response element (CRE)-binding protein/CRE modulator transcription factors in thyrotropin-induced proliferation of dog thyroid cells in primary culture. *Eur J Biochem* 1999;259:370–378.

115. Desdouets C, Matesic G, Molina CA, et al. Cell cycle regulation of cyclin A gene expression by the cyclic AMP-responsive transcription factors CREB and CREM. *Mol Cell Biol* 1995;15:3301–3309.

116. Lamas M, Molina C, Foulkes NS, et al. Ectopic ICER expression in pituitary corticotroph AtT20 cells: effects on morphology, cell cycle, and hormonal production. *Mol Endocrinol* 1997;11:1425–1434.

38

Ca²⁺ SIGNALING IN THE LIVER

MARIA DE FATIMA LEITE
MICHAEL H. NATHANSON

Cytosolic Ca^{2+} (Ca_i^{2+}) is a ubiquitous second messenger that regulates a range of functions in virtually every type of tissue (1,2). Mechanisms and effects of Ca_i^{2+} signaling have been studied extensively in the liver in particular (3,4). Ca_i^{2+} signaling in hepatocytes is mediated by inositol 1,4,5-trisphosphate (InsP3), and this mechanism is highly conserved from primitive marine organisms to mammals (1,5). Functions that are mediated by Ca_i^{2+} in the liver include bile secretion, glucose metabolism, mitochondrial activity, cell volume regulation, cell motion, and cell growth and death (4). A major advance in our understanding of Ca_i^{2+} signaling has come with the appreciation that this second messenger can regulate multiple activities simultaneously. This occurs by careful modulation of Ca_i^{2+} signals, not only over time, but in different subcellular regions and from cell to cell as well (2,6). This chapter examines the basis for regulation of liver function by Ca_i^{2+}. Mechanisms of Ca_i^{2+} signaling are described, and are the basis for understanding the Ca_i^{2+} signaling patterns that are observed in the liver. This chapter also provides illustrative examples of how Ca_i^{2+} regulates distinct functions in the hepatocyte.

M. de Fatima Leite: Department of Physiology and Biophysics, Federal University of Minas Gerais, Belo Horizonte, Brazil.

M.H. Nathanson: Department of Internal Medicine, Yale University School of Medicine, New Haven, Connecticut 06520-8019; Department of Internal Medicine, Yale–New Haven Hospital–Yale University School of Medicine, New Haven, Connecticut 06511.

MECHANISMS OF Ca²⁺ SIGNALING

Hormone Receptors and Initiation of Ca²⁺ Signals

Hormones, neurotransmitters, and growth factors initiate Ca_i^{2+} signaling through a variety of mechanisms (1). Hydrophobic substances such as corticosteroids and nitric oxide rapidly penetrate the plasma membrane to stimulate intracellular receptors. Hydrophilic substances such as peptide hormones, nucleotides, and bioactive amines bind to and stimulate specific surface membrane receptors, which in turn initiate intracellular signal transduction pathways. Of these various mechanisms for initiating Ca_i^{2+} signals, the role of plasma membrane receptors has been studied in the most detail.

There are several types of plasma membrane receptors. The largest family is the G-protein–coupled receptors, which are associated with guanosine triphosphate (GTP)-binding regulatory proteins, or G proteins (1,7). These receptors have seven hydrophobic, helical, membrane-spanning domains plus a cytosolic site for binding to specific G proteins. G proteins are heterotrimeric and consist of α, β, and γ subunits (7,8). Each α subunit has intrinsic guanosine triphosphatase (GTPase) activity at the guanine nucleotide-binding site, plus specific binding sites for the receptor and for effector proteins such as phospholipase C (PLC), adenylate cyclase, or other hydrolases. When a ligand binds to its specific G-protein–coupled receptor, guanosine diphosphate (GDP) is rapidly exchanged for GTP. This causes the G protein to dissociate from the receptor and the α subunit to dissociate from the β-γ complex. The α and β-γ complex each may then activate effector proteins in different biochemical pathways (7,9). When GTP is hydrolyzed by GTPase, the heterotrimeric G-protein complex reassociates and can be reactivated again. A wide range of heterotrimeric G proteins are expressed in mammalian cells (1,7), only some of which initiate InsP3 formation and Ca_i^{2+} signaling (see below).

Growth factor receptors represent another class of plasma membrane receptors. These receptors exhibit ligand-activated protein kinase activity and have only one membrane-spanning domain. Activation of these receptors stimulates several signal transduction pathways, including regulatory proteins of phosphatidylinositol metabolism, the arachidonic acid cascade, and mitogen-activated protein (MAP) kinase (1,10).

Yet another class of plasma membrane receptors comprises those with endogenous guanylate cyclase activity. Once activated, these receptors lead to increases in $3',5'$-cyclic guanosine monophosphate (cGMP) levels (11,12). Some of these receptors behave as ligand-gated ion channels. Members of this family include the atrial natriuretic peptide receptor, the nicotinic acetylcholine receptor, and the serotonin receptor subtype 5-HT3.

Several G-protein–coupled receptors in the liver have been particularly well studied. These include the V_{1a} vasopressin receptor, the α_{1B}-adrenergic receptor, several subtypes of the P2Y class of purinergic receptors, and the angiotensin receptors. Tyrosine kinase receptors for several types of growth factors are expressed in liver as well. Upon activation, each of these receptors initiates signaling events that lead to an increase in Ca_i^{2+} (1). The binding of Ca^{2+} mobilizing hormones and growth factors to their specific plasma membrane receptors activates PLC, which is membrane-associated. α, β, and γ subtypes of PLC are recognized (13). Many isoforms of these subtypes have been identified; $PLC\beta_1$ and $PLC\beta_2$ are the isoforms activated by G proteins, while PLCγ is activated by receptor tyrosine kinases (1,13). Activation of PLC hydrolyzes the membrane phospholipid phosphatidylinositol-4-5-bisphosphate (PIP_2). The hydrolysis of PIP_2 by PLC results in the formation of diacylglycerol (DAG) and InsP3. DAG remains at the plasma membrane to activate protein kinase C (PKC), while InsP3 diffuses into the cytosol to release Ca^{2+} from intracellular stores via its interaction with the InsP3 receptor (InsP3R). The InsP3R generally resides in the membrane of the endoplasmic reticulum (14) and the nuclear envelope (15,16), although InsP3Rs have been localized to the plasma membrane in certain tissues (17).

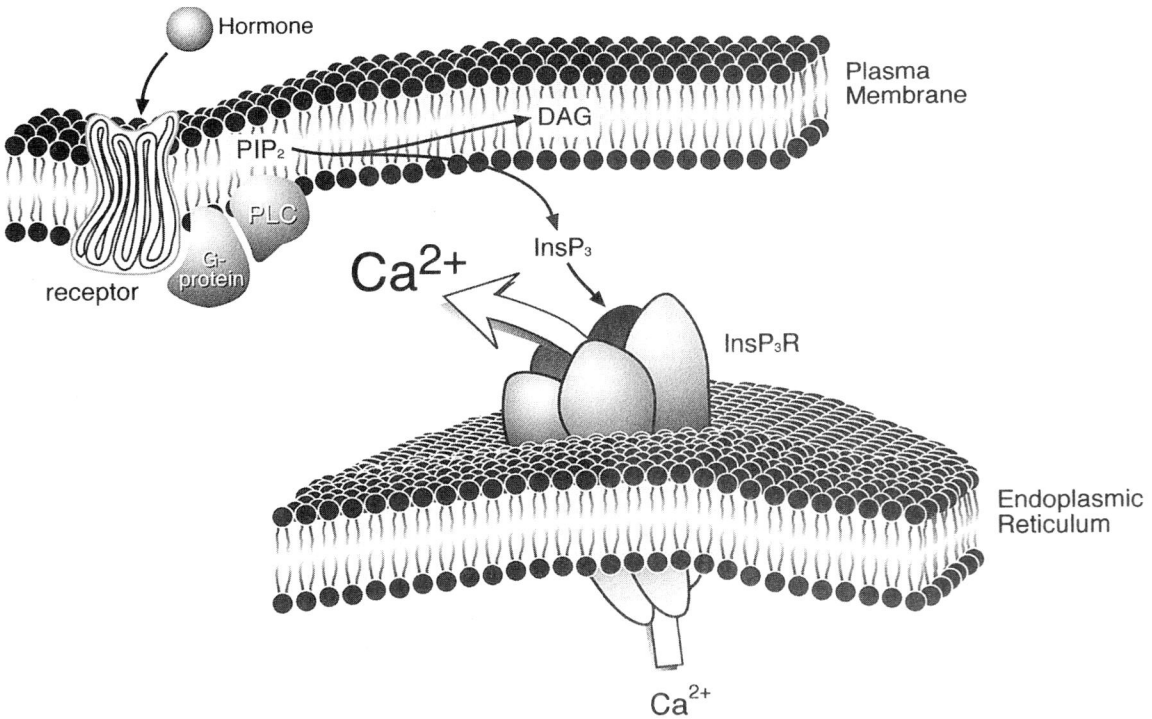

FIGURE 38.1. Mechanism of hormone-induced Ca^{2+} signaling in hepatocytes. Upon binding to its specific G-protein–coupled plasma membrane receptor, a hormone induces phospholipase C (*PLC*) to hydrolyze phosphatidyinositol bisphosphate (PIP_2) to form diacylglycerol (*DAG*) and inositol 1,4,5-trisphosphate (*InsP3*). InsP3 then binds to its tetrameric receptor (*InsP3R*) in the endoplasmic reticulum, which acts as a Ca^{2+} channel to allow Ca^{2+} to enter the cytosol.

The sequence of events linking hormone receptors to Ca_i^{2+} signaling is summarized in Fig. 38.1.

Like the plasma membrane, the nuclear envelope is a site for both synthesis and hydrolysis of the phosphorylated forms of phosphatidylinositol (18). PLCβ₁ in particular is localized both to the nucleus and the plasma membrane (19). Modulation of PLCβ₁ expression in cell lines suggests that this enzyme plays a functional role in the nucleus. Nuclear PLCβ₁ has been implicated in mitogen-activated cell growth and differentiation (19). Current evidence thus suggests that the nucleus possesses separate machinery for inositide metabolism and InsP3-dependent Ca^{2+} signaling (see Nuclear Ca^{2+} Signaling, below).

Inositol 1,4,5-Trisphosphate Receptor

The InsP3 receptor is an InsP3-gated Ca^{2+} channel located on the endoplasmic reticulum (20). In hepatocytes, increases in cytosolic Ca^{2+} (Ca_i^{2+}) are initiated by binding of InsP3 to the InsP3R (3). Three isoforms of the InsP3R have been identified and are denoted types I, II, III. Full-length sequences for these distinct InsP3R genes have been determined (21–23). Two additional isoforms, type IV and V, are proposed to exist based on partial sequence information (24). InsP3R isoforms share considerable sequence homology, but each subtype is expressed and regulated in a distinct fashion. There also are isoform-specific differences in tissue expression and subcellular distribution, suggesting that the various isoforms serve distinct roles in Ca_i^{2+} signaling.

InsP3Rs are homotetramers consisting of 313-, 307-, or 304-kd subunits, corresponding to the type I, II, or III isoform, respectively (25). There is limited evidence that heterotetramers can form as well (26,27). The InsP3R has six membrane-spanning domains, and is oriented so that the C-terminus of the protein is in the cytoplasm. Deletion analysis studies have identified three regions within the InsP3R: an N-terminal InsP3-binding domain, a Ca^{2+} channel-forming C-terminal domain, and a regulatory domain flanked by the InsP3-binding domain and the channel region (25,28). The C-terminal region also contains an ankyrin-binding domain, which is likely required for anchoring the InsP3R to the cytoskeleton (29).

The InsP3 binding domain includes multiple sequences scattered throughout the N-terminal region of the protein (28), suggesting that tertiary structure plays a role in forming the InsP3 binding site. Upon InsP3 binding, the receptor undergoes a large conformational change (28). This results in opening of the Ca^{2+} channel, so Ca^{2+} in the endoplasmic reticulum is released into the cytosol. Although each of the three InsP3R isoforms acts as an InsP3-gated Ca^{2+} channel (20,30,31), the isoforms are not uniformly sensitive to InsP3. The relative order of affinity is type II > type I > type III (32). The dissociation constant (K_d) for the type II InsP3R is 27 nM, which is twice as great as the affinity of the type I isoform, and ten times the affinity of the type III isoform (32). InsP3 is absolutely required for Ca^{2+} release via the InsP3R, but the concentration of Ca^{2+} in the cytosol modulates the open probability of the Ca^{2+} channel (20,30,31). This dependence of the InsP3R on the cytosolic Ca^{2+} concentration is important for organizing the spatial and temporal pattern of Ca_i^{2+} signals. For example, the open probability of the type I InsP3R exhibits a bell-shaped dependence on Ca_i^{2+} (20). Thus, Ca_i^{2+} concentrations less than 1 to 2 μM exhibit a positive feedback effect on the InsP3R, while higher concentrations become progressively inhibitory. This relationship is responsible for regenerative Ca_i^{2+} release and Ca_i^{2+} oscillations (33), which can occur even in the presence of constant amounts of InsP3 (34). In contrast to the type I InsP3R, the open probability of the type III InsP3R exhibits a sigmoidal dependency on Ca_i^{2+}, which lacks an inhibitory phase (30,35). Thus, Ca_i^{2+} signaling via the type III InsP3R tends to be all-or-none, and activation of this isoform results in rapid and complete emptying of Ca^{2+} stores (30). The type III InsP3R is found in the apical region of epithelia, where Ca_i^{2+} signals originate (36–39), and thus it may serve as the isoform that triggers Ca^{2+} release (30). The role of the type II InsP3R in Ca_i^{2+} signaling is less clear. Single channel recordings of this isoform suggest it displays a sigmoidal dependence on Ca_i^{2+} (31), similar to what is observed with the type III InsP3R. However, cells expressing only the type II isoform exhibit sustained Ca_i^{2+} oscillations, similar to what is observed in cells expressing only the type I InsP3R (40). Inhibition of the type I InsP3R by high Ca_i^{2+} concentrations results from interactions with calmodulin (41), so it is possible that calmodulin or other cofactors similarly interact with the type II InsP3R but were omitted from single channel studies. Further work will be needed to clarify the relationship between the single channel properties of the type II InsP3R and its behavior in intact cells. Calmodulin also may affect the binding of InsP3 to its receptor (42,43). This has been examined using peptides consisting of the N-terminal 581 amino acids of InsP3R isoforms, which contain the full InsP3-binding domain. In this system, calmodulin decreases the binding affinity of InsP3 to the type I and III InsP3R, but only minimally affects binding to the type II InsP3R. These effects were observed in both the presence and absence of Ca^{2+} (43). Together, these observations suggest that distinct InsP3R isoforms may be involved in different intracellular functions.

Cells can express different InsP3R isoforms, and many cell types express more than one isoform. For example, cerebellar Purkinje neurons express almost exclusively type I InsP3R, whereas the type II and III isoforms predominate in AR4-2j and RINm5F cells, respectively (44). B-lymphocytes and pancreatic acinar cells express all three isoforms, while hepatocytes express only type I and type II InsP3R (44). The type III InsP3R is not detected in hepatocytes, but is expressed in bile duct epithelia (45). Moreover, isoforms may be expressed in distinct subcellular locations. Pancreatic acinar cells express all three isoforms in the apical region (38,39), while the nonpigmented ciliary epithelium of the eye expresses the type I InsP3 basolaterally and the type III isoform apically, without expressing the type II isoform to a measurable extent (37). Although it has been reported that the InsP3R is most concentrated in the apical region of hepatocytes (46)(Fig. 38.2), the subcellular distribution of InsP3R isoforms in hepatocytes and in bile duct epithelia are topics of active investigation.

The InsP3R has approximately 2,000 amino acids and includes sites for phosphorylation by kinases such as 3',5'-cyclic adenosine monophosphate (cAMP)-dependent protein kinase (PKA), cGMP-dependent kinase (PKG), protein kinase C (PKC), and Ca^{2+}-calmodulin–dependent protein kinase II (CamKII). InsP3R activity is further modulated by adenosine triphosphate (ATP) (35), accessory proteins such as phosphoinositol bisphosphate (PIP$_2$) (47) and FK 506 binding protein (FKBP) (48), and Ca^{2+} (20,30). The effects of InsP3R phosphorylation by PKA are tissue-specific. PKA augments InsP3-inducing Ca^{2+} mobilization by increasing the sensitivity of the receptor to cytosolic Ca^{2+} in liver (49), but PKA is inhibitory in other tissues (25). PKG and PKC both phosphorylate the InsP3R and alter its function as well (25,50), but whether there are liver-specific effects of these kinases is not established. In cerebellar microsomes, which predominantly express the type I InsP3R (44), phosphorylation by CaMKII increases

the sensitivity to Ca^{2+} efflux. ATP increases the open probability of the types I and III InsP3R up to a concentration of 2 mM, while ATP is inhibitory at concentrations above 4 mM (35). Degradation of the InsP3R can occur through the proteosome pathway (51), and provides yet another level of regulation of this Ca^{2+} release channel.

Ryanodine Receptor

The other major class of intracellular Ca^{2+} release channels is the ryanodine receptor (RyR). Like the InsP3R, the RyR has three family members, and these channels contribute to Ca_i^{2+} signaling by releasing Ca^{2+} from the lumen of sarcoplasmic or endoplasmic reticulum into the cytosol (1). RyR is a homotetramer consisting of four identical subunits, each of which contains approximately 5,000 amino acids (52). The C-terminal regions of the RyR tetramer cooperate to form a Ca^{2+} channel, while the N-terminal regions project into the cytosol to form the so-called foot domain. RyR and InsPR share some sequence homology, especially in the C-terminal Ca^{2+} channel-forming region (53).

RyR isoforms have functional similarities as well as differences. All three isoforms autocatalytically release Ca^{2+} via a process known as Ca^{2+}-induced Ca^{2+} release (CICR). The type II and III RyR also are sensitive to cyclic adenosine diphosphate (ADP)-ribose (cADPR), while the type I RyR is not (54,55). The Ca^{2+}-mobilizing properties of cADPR were first demonstrated in sea urchin eggs. It is now appreciated that cADPR mobilizes Ca^{2+} via the RyR in a wide range of mammalian cell types as well, including smooth (56) and cardiac (55) muscle, neuroendocrine cells (57), lymphocytes (58), and pancreatic acini (59). In addition, the enzyme that catalyzes the formation of cADPR from the oxidized form of nicotinamide adenine dinucleotide (NAD$^+$) (ADP-ribosyl cyclase or CD38) is expressed in many tissues, including liver (60). However, a direct role for cADPR-mediated Ca_i^{2+} signaling in hepatocytes has not been established.

RyR is of primary importance for Ca_i^{2+} signaling in muscle, including vascular smooth muscle. Many other cell types express RyR as well, but there is conflicting evidence regarding the presence and role of RyR in hepatocytes. Molecular studies suggest that none of the three RyR isoforms is expressed in liver (61). However, pharmacologic inhibition of the RyR reduces the speed of hormone-induced Ca_i^{2+} waves (46). In addition, ryanodine-binding sites have been identified in hepatic microsomes (62), and ryanodine releases Ca^{2+} from hepatic microsomal vesicles as well (63). Finally, cADPR induces the release of Ca^{2+} from the nuclear envelope of isolated rat liver nuclei (16). Therefore, a novel RyR isoform or an RyR-like protein may contribute to Ca_i^{2+} signaling in hepatocytes.

Nicotinic acid adenine dinucleotide phosphate (NAADP) is another second messenger that mediates release of Ca^{2+} from intracellular stores. Like cADPR, this messenger molecule was discovered in sea urchin eggs (64) and has now been

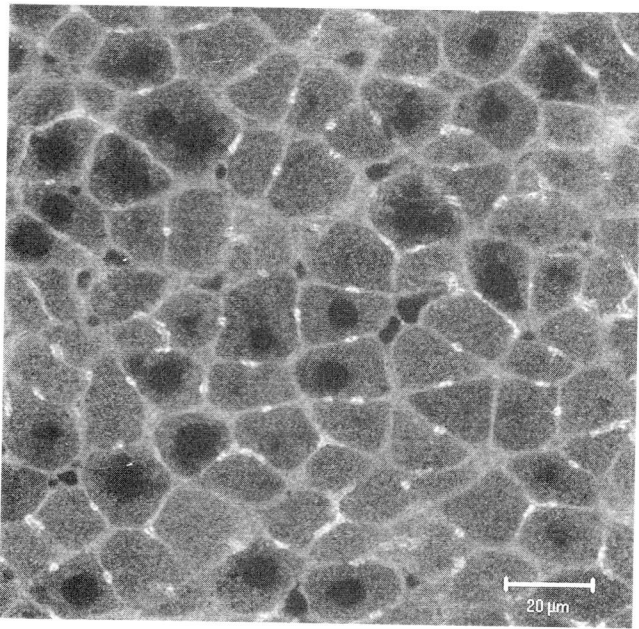

FIGURE 38.2. Distribution of the InsP3 receptor (InsP3R) in the liver. A confocal immunofluorescence image of rat liver shows the distribution of the InsP3R (*green*). The specimen also is labeled with rhodamine phalloidin (*red*) to identify canaliculi. The InsP3R is most concentrated in the pericanalicular regions, with lesser staining elsewhere in the cytosol. See Color Plate 13.

found to induce Ca_i^{2+} signaling in mammalian cells as well (65). However, the subcellular location of NAADP-sensitive Ca^{2+} stores and their relation to Ca^{2+} stores gated by InsP3R and RyR remain to be investigated. The role of NAADP in hepatocyte Ca_i^{2+} signaling is unknown as well.

Mitochondria

Mitochondria are best known for the metabolic and respiratory role they play in cells. However, it is now clear that mitochondria strongly influence Ca_i^{2+} signaling as well, by actively taking Ca^{2+} up from, and releasing Ca^{2+} back into, the cytosol (66,67). Mitochondria have their own Ca^{2+} transport machinery, involving Ca^{2+} influx through a uniporter, and Ca^{2+} efflux via both a Na^+ exchanger (68) and an H^+ exchanger (69). The uniporter is driven by the potential gradient across the mitochondrial membrane, while the Ca^{2+} efflux mechanisms are active transport systems (70). Ca^{2+} efflux from mitochondria also can occur through the permeability transition pore (PTP). Formation of this pore results in a sudden, marked increase in the permeability of the mitochondrial inner membrane to ions and small molecules. Irreversible formation of the PTP can dissipate the potential gradient across the mitochondrial membrane, leading to mitochondrial swelling and irreversible cell injury (70), including necrosis (71). However, the PTP also can form in a reversible fashion. This occurs in normal mitochondrial function and plays a role in Ca_i^{2+} signaling (70,72,73). Formation of the PTP is enhanced by factors including increases in mitochondrial free Ca^{2+}, membrane depolarization, and alkaline matrix pH (70,74). Activation of the PTP leads to rapid release of large amounts of mitochondrial Ca^{2+} into the cytosol (72,75). Formation of the PTP is inhibited by antioxidants, reducing agents, PLA₂ inhibitors, and the cyclic immunosuppressive peptide cyclosporin A (70,76). Endogenous inhibitors of the permeability transition include ADP, Mg^{2+}, and increased mitochondrial membrane potential (70). Current evidence suggests that reversible formation of the PTP typically is involved in Ca_i^{2+} signaling through the following sequence of events (72): (a) elevations in Ca_i^{2+} are taken up by mitochondria through their uniporter, as a result of the mitochondrial membrane potential gradient; (b) H^+ efflux occurs to compensate for this influx of cations, resulting in increased mitochondrial pH; (c) this increased pH activates formation of the PTP, which alters the membrane potential gradient; (d) Ca^{2+} thus is released from the mitochondria, triggering mitochondrial Ca^{2+}-induced Ca^{2+} release (mCICR). Thus, mCICR depends on the transient depolarization of mitochondria that results from the H^+ conductive pathway provided by opening of the PTP. Ca^{2+} waves can propagate across the cytosol via mCICR in regions where mitochondria are densely distributed (72,77). Mitochondria are densely distributed in hepatocytes (Fig. 38.3), and participate in hepatocyte Ca_i^{2+} signaling (77,78).

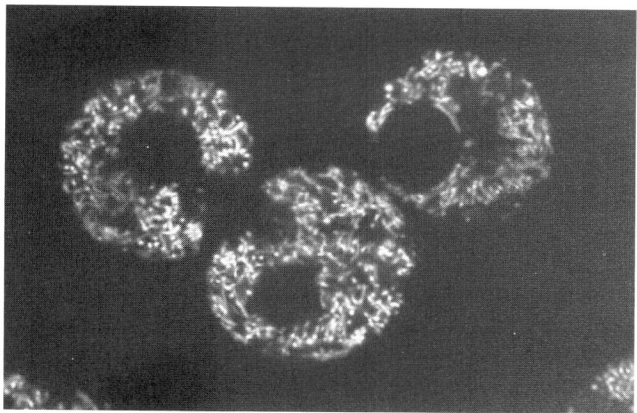

FIGURE 38.3. Distribution of mitochondria in hepatocytes. A confocal image of isolated rat hepatocytes loaded with the mitochondrial dye rhodamine 123 demonstrates that mitochondria are densely distributed throughout each cell. Mitochondria influence cytosolic Ca^{2+} signaling in hepatocytes by taking up Ca^{2+} from nearby InsP3 receptors, then releasing it back into the cytosol.

Mitochondria are able to sequester significant amounts of Ca^{2+} from the cytosol. Free mitochondrial Ca^{2+} was first monitored in cells by targeting the Ca^{2+}-sensitive photoprotein aequorin to mitochondria (79,80). It was observed that mitochondrial Ca^{2+} can closely parallel the cytosolic Ca^{2+} increase induced by receptor activation. It also was observed that the increase in mitochondrial Ca^{2+} following release of Ca^{2+} from intracellular stores is faster and larger than the increase that follows influx of extracellular Ca^{2+} (80). Based on this, it was hypothesized that mitochondria are close to intracellular Ca^{2+} release sites, and thus are exposed to local concentrations of Ca^{2+} much higher than those measured elsewhere in the cytosol. This hypothesis is consistent with electron microscopy data that show a close proximity between mitochondria and the endoplasmic reticulum (81). Subsequent work has provided further functional evidence for microdomains where mitochondria and InsP3Rs are in close apposition, so that mitochondria take up a significant fraction of the Ca^{2+} released by the InsP3R (77,78).

There also is evidence of microheterogeneity among mitochondria. It has been estimated that approximately 30% of the total cellular mitochondrial pool is located in microdomains of high Ca_i^{2+} (82). In addition, subcellular regions that contain fewer mitochondria show greater sensitivity to InsP3 (77). Since the uptake of Ca^{2+} by mitochondria decreases the positive feedback that Ca^{2+} may exert on the InsP3R, mitochondria can locally modulate InsP3R sensitivity and thus define the threshold for InsP3 to trigger Ca_i^{2+} signals in different subcellular regions (77).

The uptake of Ca^{2+} by mitochondria affects multiple factors in cell metabolism, including the mitochondrial proton motive force, electron transport, and the activity of dehydrogenases associated with the tricarboxylic acid (TCA) cycle, adenine nucleotide translocase, the F_1-ATPase, and pyruvate dehydrogenase (PDH) phosphorylase (83,84). Studies in isolated hepatocytes have revealed that slow or small Ca_i^{2+} elevations are not transmitted effectively into mitochondria, and therefore are unable to activate mitochondrial metabolism (84). In contrast, Ca_i^{2+} oscillations trigger mitochondrial Ca^{2+} oscillations and sustained reduced nicotinamide adenine dinucleotide (phosphate) [NAD(P)H] formation (85). Thus, the frequency rather than the amplitude of Ca_i^{2+} oscillations regulates mitochondrial metabolism (84,85). A recent study using the ATP-sensitive phosphoprotein luciferase to monitor the mitochondrial ATP concentration has shown that increases in mitochondrial Ca^{2+} furthermore trigger a long-term memory of the Ca^{2+} signal (86). This allows ATP production to persist beyond the time period that mitochondrial Ca^{2+} is elevated (86). Thus, Ca^{2+} signaling in the cytosol and mitochondria are interdependent and together regulate cell metabolism in a complex fashion (73,75,83).

ORGANIZATION OF Ca^{2+} SIGNALS

Detection of Ca^{2+} Signals in Hepatocytes

Our understanding of the way in which Ca_i^{2+} signals are organized has evolved dramatically over the past 20 years, in large part as a result of two parallel technical advances. First, development of Ca^{2+}-sensitive fluorescent dyes has permitted Ca_i^{2+} to be monitored continuously in live cells. Second, improvements in fluorescence imaging techniques have permitted Ca_i^{2+} to be detected not only in populations of cells but in single cells and in distinct subcellular regions of individual cells as well (3). As observations move from cell populations to single cells to subcellular regions, the complexity of Ca_i^{2+} signaling patterns increases, and the time scale of signaling events decreases (Fig. 38.4). It is now appreciated that Ca_i^{2+} signaling is regulated at the subcellular level, and that this level of regulation is necessary for Ca_i^{2+} in turn to act as a second messenger that regulates multiple cell functions simultaneously.

The first Ca^{2+}-sensitive fluorescent dye to receive widespread use was Quin-2, which was developed 20 years ago (87). An important innovation introduced at that time was the coupling of the dye to an acetoxymethyl ester, which rendered the dye cell-permeant and thus permitted it to be loaded easily into live cells (87,88). Other Ca^{2+} dyes were developed subsequently that provided additional advantages. For example, fura-2 and indo-1 could be used for ratiometric measurements of Ca_i^{2+}, which permitted improved quantification of Ca^{2+} concentrations in cytosol (89). Other Ca^{2+} dyes have been developed that allow preferential measurement of Ca^{2+} in organelles such as the mitochondria or endoplasmic reticulum (84,90).

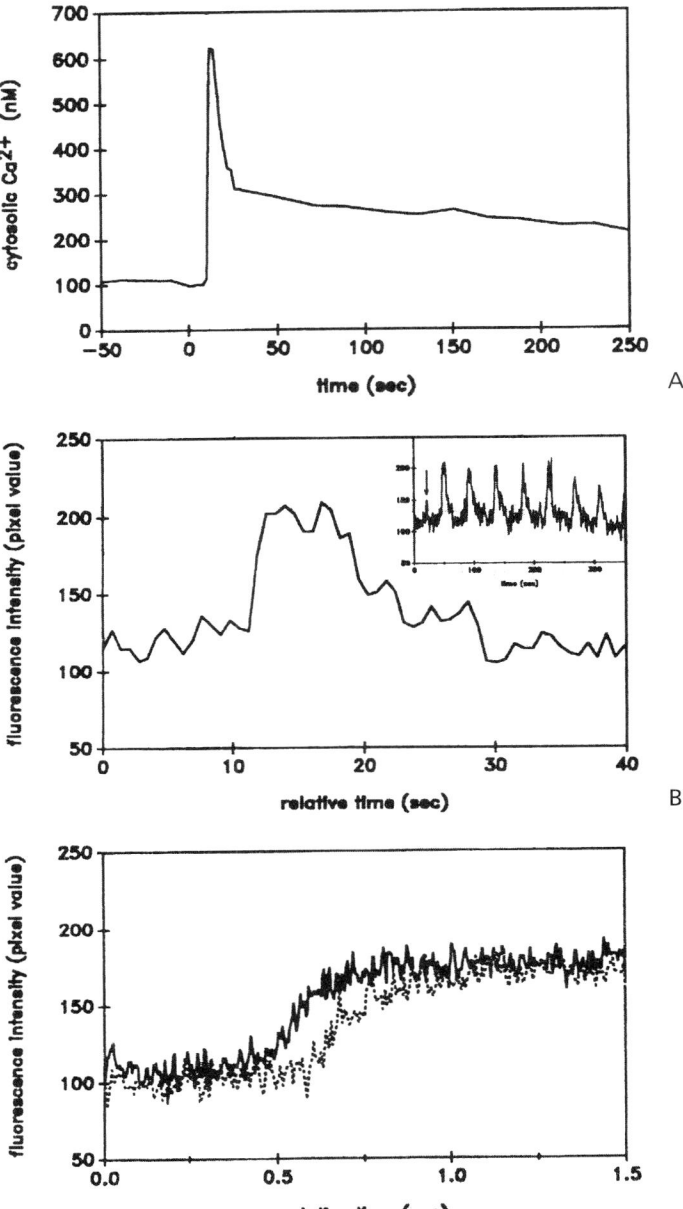

FIGURE 38.4. Different views of cytosolic Ca^{2+} signaling in hepatocytes. In each case, isolated rat hepatocytes were stimulated with the α_{1B}-adrenergic agonist phenylephrine. **A:** In a population of hepatocytes, a single transient peak is observed, followed by a sustained elevation. **B:** In a single hepatocyte, a series of repetitive peaks (oscillations) are observed. **C:** In different regions of the same hepatocyte, the increase in Ca^{2+} occurs at different times. This represents a Ca^{2+} wave. Notice that these Ca^{2+} signaling events occur over progressively shorter time intervals as the level of focus moves from populations to single cells to subcellular regions. (From Nathanson MH. Cellular and subcellular calcium signaling in gastrointestinal epithelium. *Gastroenterology* 1994;106:1349–1364, with permission.)

Fluorescence detection systems also have evolved considerably over the past 20 years. Initial studies used spectrofluorimetry to examine Ca_i^{2+} in cell populations (88). Improvements in low light level cameras, computers, and image processing then permitted fluorescence studies to be performed at the single cell level (91,92). Further improvements in these technologies, along with the introduction of confocal microscopy, permitted subcellular Ca_i^{2+} signals and Ca_i^{2+} gradients to be appreciated (93–95). The relative advantages of each of these imaging modalities have been reviewed (3).

Although Ca^{2+} signaling usually is studied with Ca^{2+}-sensitive fluorescent dyes, other approaches have been applied. These include $^{45}Ca^{2+}$ efflux studies, electrophysiologic (patch clamp) studies that use Ca^{2+}-dependent Cl^- currents as a surrogate marker for Ca_i^{2+}, and bioluminescence studies using the photoprotein aequorin. In fact, the first description of Ca_i^{2+} oscillations in hepatocytes was based on luminescence measurements of microinjected aequorin (96). More recently, recombinant aequorin has been expressed in a targeted fashion to selectively detect Ca^{2+} signals in cellular compartments such as the mitochondria (79), endoplasmic reticulum (97), nucleus (98), or beneath the plasma membrane (99). These alternative methods of monitoring Ca_i^{2+} have been reviewed as well (3).

Ca²⁺ Signaling Patterns in Hepatocytes

Peptide hormones such as vasopressin or angiotensin generally induce biphasic increases in Ca_i^{2+} in populations of isolated hepatocytes (Fig. 38.4). These increases typically consist of two components. The first component is the rapid peak and then fall in Ca_i^{2+}, which takes place over a period of seconds. This is due to release of Ca^{2+} from InsP3-sensitive stores and occurs even in Ca^{2+}-free medium (92,100). The second component is the sustained plateau in Ca_i^{2+}, which follows the rapid peak. This occurs only in the presence of extracellular Ca^{2+} and is due to influx of that Ca^{2+} to replenish depleted intracellular stores (101). This biphasic Ca_i^{2+} signaling pattern is highly reproducible among cell preparations. In contrast, Ca^{2+} signaling patterns vary markedly among single hepatocytes. Different stimuli evoke distinct responses (102), and additional variation can be seen among hepatocytes that are stimulated under identical conditions (92,103). The range of signaling patterns seen among single hepatocytes includes single transient or sustained Ca_i^{2+} increases and repetitive Ca_i^{2+} spikes (i.e., oscillations). For example, lower concentrations of vasopressin induce Ca_i^{2+} oscillations, while higher concentrations induce sustained increases in Ca_i^{2+} (92). In contrast, stimulation of hepatocytes with phenylephrine typically evokes Ca_i^{2+} oscillations, but the oscillation frequency is dose-dependent (92). The duration of individual Ca_i^{2+} spikes also depends on the agonist. For example, Ca_i^{2+} spikes induced by phenylephrine are short (approximately 7 sec-

onds) compared to the duration of spikes induced by vasopressin (approximately 10 seconds) or angiotensin (approximately 15 seconds)(96,102). The frequency of vasopressin-induced Ca_i^{2+} oscillations tends to be greater than that of phenylephrine-induced oscillations as well. Differences in the frequency of Ca_i^{2+} oscillations have been shown to regulate gene transcription in some cell systems (6,104,105), although this has not yet been demonstrated in hepatocytes.

The mechanism responsible for Ca_i^{2+} oscillations is not completely understood. It was proposed initially that Ca_i^{2+} oscillations result from oscillations in the concentration of InsP3. However, nonhydrolyzable InsP3 analogues can generate Ca_i^{2+} oscillations (34), and thapsigargin, which releases Ca^{2+} from the endoplasmic reticulum through an InsP3-independent mechanism, also triggers Ca_i^{2+} oscillations (106). Thus, it currently is thought that Ca_i^{2+} oscillations do not depend upon InsP3 oscillations. Instead, oscillations are thought to result from the bell-shaped dependence of the open probability of the InsP3R on Ca_i^{2+} (see above). Experimental studies that suggest this are further supported by mathematical models that predict that bimodal dependence of the InsP3R would result in Ca_i^{2+} oscillations (33). Extracellular Ca^{2+} contributes to Ca_i^{2+} oscillations in hepatocytes, since Ca_i^{2+} oscillations gradually dissipate in Ca^{2+}-free medium (100). Extracellular Ca^{2+} thus serves to maintain internal Ca^{2+} stores, which are the primary source of Ca^{2+} for oscillations in hepatocytes (100).

Subcellular Ca²⁺ Signals and Ca²⁺ Waves

Ca_i^{2+} signals in single cells vary not only over time but over space as well. For example, increases in Ca_i^{2+} in epithelia may occur as polarized waves (93,107), or they may be restricted to specific subcellular regions (108,109). Increases in Ca_i^{2+} typically begin near the apical membrane, where the InsP3R is most concentrated (36,110). The first evidence of Ca_i^{2+} waves was obtained in the medaka egg during fertilization (111). Subsequently, Ca_i^{2+} waves also were observed in nonpolarized preparations of hepatocytes, and it was noted that the site of origin remained constant irrespective of the agonist (94). Both vasopressin and phenylephrine induced Ca_i^{2+} waves that began at a single locus, and these waves furthermore spread in a nondiminishing fashion across the cell. Since these hormones increase Ca_i^{2+} through InsP3 mobilization, it has been proposed that the InsP3R would be concentrated in the region where Ca_i^{2+} waves begin. Immunofluorescence studies in rat liver and in isolated rat hepatocyte couplets now have demonstrated that the InsP3R is concentrated in the pericanalicular region (46)(Fig. 38.2), and examination of Ca_i^{2+} signaling in polarized preparations of isolated hepatocytes has suggested that this is the region where Ca_i^{2+} waves originate (46). Thus, the subcellular distribution of InsP3Rs in hepatocytes may serve to organize the spatial pattern of Ca_i^{2+} signals.

Several studies have examined the mechanism by which Ca_i^{2+} waves spread from their initiation site near the canalicular membrane to the rest of the cell. Apical-to-basal propagation of Ca_i^{2+} waves has been observed in other polarized epithelia, including lacrimal and pancreatic acinar cells (93,107,112). As in hepatocytes, the InsP3R is concentrated in the apical region of these cells as well. Unlike hepatocytes, though, these epithelia express RyR (59,113,114). Several lines of evidence indicate that the RyR in these cells is distributed through most of the cell, but is excluded from the extreme apex where the InsP3R is located (113). Furthermore, inhibition of the RyR serves to inhibit the spread of Ca_i^{2+} waves into the basolateral region (107). Thus, the RyR may facilitate the spread of Ca_i^{2+} waves away from their initiation point near the apical membrane. Since the presence of RyR in hepatocytes remains controversial, a role for RyR in the propagation of Ca^{2+} waves in liver awaits further investigation. The speed of Ca_i^{2+} waves in hepatocytes is not altered in Ca^{2+}-free medium (46), nor does the amplitude of Ca_i^{2+} waves decrease (46). These observations suggest that the spread of Ca_i^{2+} waves across the hepatocyte depends only on release of Ca^{2+} from intracellular stores. Although the InsP3R is concentrated apically in hepatocytes, lower level expression of the receptor throughout the cell or even expression of a novel low-affinity

InsP3R isoform could account for the spread of Ca_i^{2+} waves into the basolateral region. Alternatively, InsP3 could merely serve to initiate the Ca^{2+} release process at the canalicular region, followed by activation of neighboring Ca^{2+} stores through an as yet unidentified mechanism.

Spread of Ca²⁺ Signals from Cell to Cell

Ca_i^{2+} signals occur asynchronously among isolated hepatocytes. For example, the lag time between stimulation with vasopressin and initiation of Ca_i^{2+} signaling varies among isolated hepatocytes by up to several seconds, while the frequency of Ca^{2+} oscillations can vary by up to 50% among isolated hepatocytes stimulated with phenylephrine (103). However, hepatocytes that communicate via gap junctions are able to coordinate their Ca_i^{2+} signals. For example, stimulation of an isolated hepatocyte couplet with vasopressin induces a single Ca_i^{2+} wave that crosses both of the cells, while stimulation with phenylephrine induces Ca_i^{2+} oscillations that are synchronized in the two cells (103). In the isolated perfused rat liver, Ca_i^{2+} signaling displays an even higher level of organization, since vasopressin induces Ca_i^{2+} waves that cross the entire lobule (115–117)(Fig. 38.5). Ca_i^{2+} waves cross individual hepatocytes at the same speed, regardless of

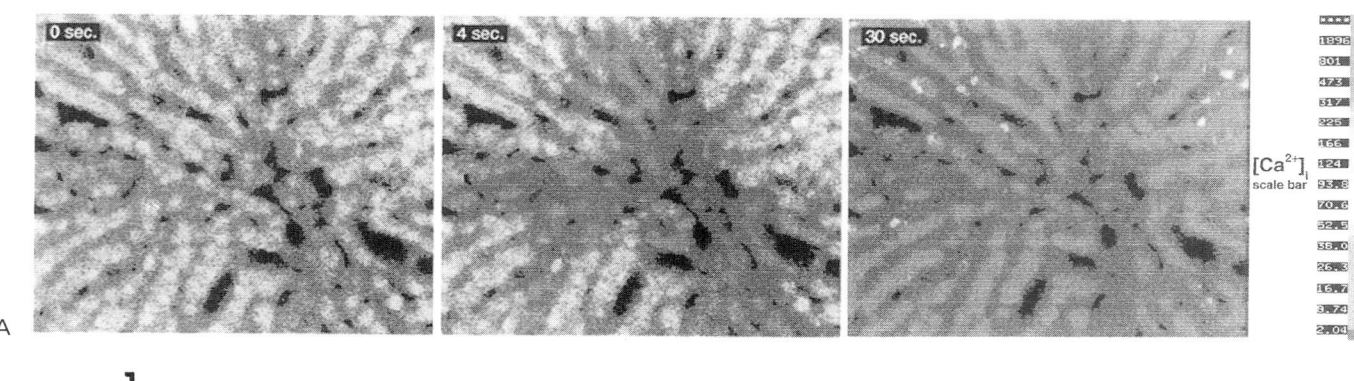

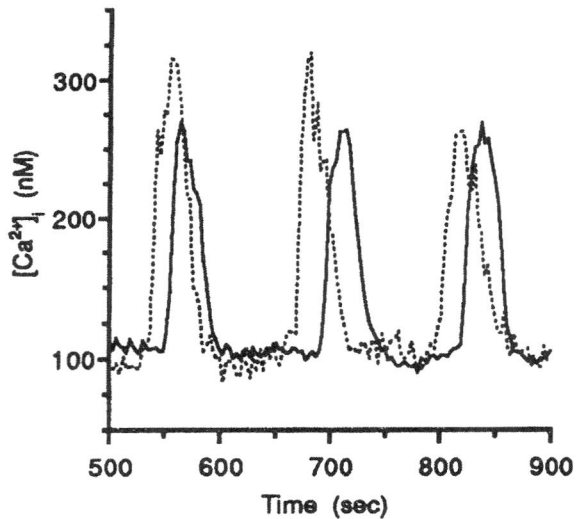

FIGURE 38.5. Organization of Ca²⁺ signals in the intact liver. **A:** Serial confocal images of a vasopressin-induced Ca²⁺ wave in the isolated perfused rat liver demonstrates that the increase in Ca²⁺ begins in the pericentral region, then spreads as a wave toward the periportal regions. Images were obtained at baseline and after 4 and 30 seconds of stimulation with vasopressin (20 nM). (From Motoyama K, Karl IE, Flye MW, et al. Effect of Ca2+ agonists in the perfused liver: determination via laser scanning confocal microscopy. *Am J Physiol Regul Integr Comp Physiol* 1999; 276:R575–R585, with permission.) See Color Plate 14. **B:** Ca²⁺ signals in individual hepatocytes within an isolated perfused rat liver stimulated with vasopressin (100 pM). Tracing shows Ca²⁺ oscillations detected in two hepatocytes separated by a distance of 40 μm. The phase difference between the two cells is due to the time needed for a Ca²⁺ wave to spread from one cell to the other. (From Robb-Gaspers LD, Thomas AP. Coordination of Ca²⁺ signaling by intercellular propagation of Ca²⁺ waves in the intact liver. *J Biol Chem* 1995;270:8102–8107, with permission.)

whether the hepatocytes are isolated or within the liver (115). Vasopressin-induced Ca_i^{2+} waves cross the hepatic lobule in a pericentral-to-periportal direction (115,117), presumably since the V_{1a} vasopressin receptor is most heavily expressed among pericentral hepatocytes (115). In contrast, ATP induces Ca_i^{2+} signals in a random fashion across the hepatic lobule (117), consistent with evidence that there is no P2Y receptor gradient across the lobule (118). Thus, sophisticated patterns of Ca_i^{2+} signaling are induced in the intact liver, and these patterns appear to be agonist-specific. This may permit different Ca^{2+} agonists to have distinct effects in liver even though Ca_i^{2+} signals induced by these agonists may appear similar in isolated hepatocytes.

The basis for organization of Ca_i^{2+} signals in liver has been studied in multicellular systems of hepatocytes. Ca_i^{2+} waves can spread from hepatocyte to hepatocyte (103,119), and this type of communication depends critically on gap junctions. Studies in isolated rat hepatocyte couplets demonstrate that hepatocytes communicate via gap junctions, and that both Ca^{2+} and InsP3 can cross these gap junctions (119). In addition, hormone-induced Ca_i^{2+} signaling is highly coordinated in such couplets, and this coordination depends on gap junction conductance as well (103). Hepatocytes express two gap junction isoforms, connexin32 and connexin26 (120). Expression of both of these isoforms is dramatically reduced after bile duct ligation, and coordination of Ca_i^{2+} signals is impaired under this condition as well (120). Furthermore, cell-to-cell spread of InsP3 and Ca_i^{2+} waves is markedly impaired in hepatocytes isolated from connexin32 knockout mice (121). Thus, gap junctions play an essential role in organizing Ca_i^{2+} signals among adjacent hepatocytes.

Organization of cell-to-cell Ca_i^{2+} waves depends on other factors in addition to gap junctions. For example, increases in InsP3 are required in each cell across which a Ca^{2+} wave spreads (122). Moreover, neither InsP3 nor Ca^{2+} alone is sufficient to support the spread of a Ca_i^{2+} wave across an hepatocyte (123). The presence of agonist binding to its specific receptor at the surface of the cell also is required to support the spread of Ca_i^{2+} waves. This condition was demonstrated in experiments in which one or both cells of a hepatocyte couplet were microperfused with norepinephrine. Stimulation of individual cells evoked Ca_i^{2+} oscillations only in the cell being perfused, and perfusion of the entire couplet was necessary to evoke Ca_i^{2+} oscillations in both cells (123). Thus, the presence of hormone at each cell ensures that the cell generates sufficient levels of intracellular messengers to reach a level of excitability necessary for supporting the propagation of a Ca_i^{2+} wave. This concept of cytosol as an excitable medium was initially demonstrated in *Xenopus* oocytes (124), but likely accounts for Ca_i^{2+} signaling patterns observed in hepatocytes as well (116).

Other studies have focused on the mechanism by which intercellular Ca_i^{2+} waves become oriented within the hepatic acinus. Vasopressin-induced waves begin in the region of the central venule, where the V_{1a} vasopressin receptor is most heavily expressed, then spread to the portal region, where the receptor is less heavily expressed (115,117). In contrast, ATP-induced Ca_i^{2+} waves begin in a seemingly random pattern across the hepatic acinus (117). Studies in isolated hepatocytes similarly show that pericentral hepatocytes are more sensitive to vasopressin but not to ATP (118). Moreover, studies in isolated hepatocyte couplets and triplets stimulated with vasopressin or norepinephrine show that one cell generally has increased sensitivity to a particular hormone and acts as a pacemaker to drive Ca_i^{2+} oscillations in neighboring cells. This increased sensitivity appears to be due to increased expression of hormone receptor rather than differences in downstream signaling components such as G proteins or InsP3R (125,126). Cells with increased expression of hormone receptor produce higher concentrations of InsP3, so they respond sooner than other cells stimulated with the same concentration of hormone. As a result, cells with the greatest level of hormone receptor expression act as pacemakers for that hormone. Furthermore, different cells can act as the pacemaker for different hormones (126). Thus, the pattern of Ca_i^{2+} waves and oscillations in the intact liver depends upon multiple factors, which include (a) the establishment of pacemaker cells by virtue of increased expression of hormone receptors, (b) simultaneous stimulation of both pacemaker and nonpacemaker cells, and (c) communication of second messengers among these cells via gap junctions (127).

The liver also possesses paracrine mechanisms for generating and regulating Ca_i^{2+} signals. Hepatocytes are able to secrete ATP (128), and both hepatocytes and bile duct cells express P2Y ATP receptors (129–131). Since P2Y receptors are G-protein–coupled receptors that link to InsP3-mediated Ca_i^{2+} signaling, secretion of ATP by hepatocytes stimulates Ca_i^{2+} signaling in neighboring hepatocytes and bile duct cells (128). This paracrine signaling mechanism thus permits increases in Ca_i^{2+} to spread among neighboring cells independent of communication via gap junctions. Ca_i^{2+} signaling in liver also can be modified rather than initiated by paracrine pathways. For example, bradykinin does not mobilize Ca_i^{2+} in isolated hepatocytes, yet in the intact liver it modifies the propagation of Ca_i^{2+} waves induced by vasopressin (132). Work in cocultures of sinusoidal endothelial cells and hepatocytes and studies in the perfused liver suggest this occurs through a nitric oxide (NO)-dependent mechanism. Specifically, bradykinin induces NO release from endothelial cells, which diffuses to hepatocytes where it stimulates generation of cGMP. In hepatocytes, cGMP activates cGMP dependent kinase, which in turn may phosphorylate and thus modulate the InsP3R (132). This last step is controversial, since some investigators have reported that NO donors and cGMP analogues potentiate InsP3-induced Ca^{2+} mobilization in hepatocytes (133), while others have observed no such effect (134). In any case, these studies demonstrate that there are various paracrine pathways for regulation of Ca_i^{2+} signaling in liver.

Nuclear Ca²⁺ Signaling

The nucleus is separated from the cytosol by the nuclear envelope, which is a specialized region of the endoplasmic reticulum (135). Like the endoplasmic reticulum, the nuclear envelope is able to store and release Ca^{2+}. The nuclear envelope accumulates Ca^{2+} via a Ca^{2+}-ATPase pump (136,137), and releases Ca^{2+} via channels that are sensitive to InsP3 (16,138) or cADPR (16,139). These Ca^{2+} storage pumps and release channels have distinct distributions within the nuclear envelope. The Ca^{2+}-ATPase pump is located only in the outer leaflets of the envelope (15), while the InsP3R is located only in the inner membrane (15). Cyclic ADP ribose-sensitive channels appear to be present on both sides of the nuclear envelope (18).

Several lines of evidence suggest that InsP3 releases Ca^{2+} directly from the nuclear envelope into the nucleus. InsP3 releases $^{45}Ca^{2+}$ into isolated hepatocyte nuclei (140), and InsP3 increases free nuclear Ca^{2+} (16) even if the nucleus is surrounded by a Ca^{2+} chelator (141). Similarly, direct injection of InsP3 into the nucleus of *Xenopus laevis* oocytes results in increased nuclear Ca^{2+}, even if cytosolic InsP3Rs are blocked (142). Photorelease of caged InsP3 in the nuclei of starfish oocytes (141) increases nuclear Ca^{2+} as well. The nuclear envelope possesses the machinery necessary to produce InsP3, including PIP2 and phospholipase C (19), and this machinery may be activated selectively through tyrosine kinase pathways (143). In one study, IGF-1 and integrins caused PIP2 breakdown in the nucleus but not at the plasma membrane (143), while activation of G-protein–linked receptors caused breakdown of PIP2 in the cytosol, but not in the nucleus (144). It also has been hypothesized that relocation of MAP kinase to the nucleus activates nuclear phospholipase C to generate InsP3 in the nucleus (18).

Like InsP3, cADPR can elevate Ca^{2+} in isolated hepatocyte nuclei (16,139). Photorelease of caged cADPR furthermore induces nuclear Ca^{2+} oscillations in starfish oocyte nuclei (141). These findings suggest that the machinery needed for production of cADPR exists in the nucleus. More recently, it has been demonstrated directly that ADP-ribosyl cyclase (CD38) is located on the inner membrane of the nuclear envelope, where it colocalizes with the RyR (139). Thus, the nucleus has the independent capacity to generate both InsP3- and cADPR-mediated Ca^{2+} signals.

Nuclear Ca^{2+} signaling also may occur by transmission of cytosolic Ca^{2+} signals into the nucleus. The nuclear envelope contains pores that are permeable to molecules up to 60 kd in size (145). In the absence of a gating mechanism, a pore of this size would allow rapid equilibration of Ca^{2+} between the nucleus and cytosol. Under certain circumstances, free diffusion of Ca^{2+} through the nuclear pore indeed occurs (98,146). However, a nuclear-cytosolic Ca^{2+} gradient has been demonstrated in a number of cell types (141,147), suggesting that the permeability of nuclear pores can be regulated. Moreover, electrophysiologic studies (135) suggest that Ca^{2+} permeability through the nuclear pores is severely restricted. Atomic force microscopy studies similarly suggest that nuclear pore permeability is regulated, and that depletion of Ca^{2+} within the nuclear envelope closes the pores (148). Other work using fluorescent dyes (149) or aequorin (150) also demonstrates that depletion of Ca^{2+} attenuates the permeability of the pores to intermediate-sized molecules that lack the nuclear localization sequence. Since EF-hand Ca^{2+}-binding motifs are present in the nuclear pore, it is possible that these function as Ca^{2+} gating sensors for the pore (18).

Although nuclear Ca^{2+} signals can originate inside the nucleus, and the permeability of nuclear pores to Ca^{2+} is regulated, there is considerable evidence that nuclear Ca^{2+} can passively follow Ca_i^{2+} (142,151). For example, stimulation of basophilic leukemia cells with antigen or photoreleased InsP3 results in a Ca^{2+} wave that appears to spread from the cytosol into the nucleus (146). Similar observations have been made in hepatocytes stimulated with vasopressin (152). Moreover, a mathematical analysis of Ca^{2+} waves in hepatocytes stimulated with vasopressin suggests that nuclear Ca^{2+} signals can be described simply by diffusion of Ca^{2+} inward from the nuclear envelope (153).

Nuclear Ca^{2+} also can contribute to Ca^{2+} signals in the cytosol. For example, localized increases of Ca^{2+} in the cytosol (Ca^{2+} puffs) can spread across the cell by diffusing across the nucleus. Ca^{2+} puffs are highly transient and localized Ca_i^{2+} signals that result from the coordinated opening of small clusters of InsP3Rs (154). Puffs can be triggered by a subthreshold concentration of agonist, and the resulting Ca_i^{2+} signal rapidly dissipates by diffusion in the cytosol and sequestration of Ca^{2+} into intracellular stores. However, since the range of diffusion of Ca^{2+} in the nucleus can be much greater than in cytosol (153), Ca^{2+} puffs generated near the nuclear envelope can spread into and across the nucleus in order to spread to other, more distant regions of the cytosol (151). Thus, the nucleus may function as a tunnel that helps distribute Ca^{2+} to the cytosol.

Ca²⁺ Signaling in Bile Duct Cells

Ca_i^{2+} signaling has been examined to a limited extent in bile duct epithelia. ATP and uridine triphosphate (UTP) both increase Ca_i^{2+} in the Mz-ChA-1 cholangiocarcinoma cell line, a model for bile duct epithelium (131). ATP and UTP also increase Ca_i^{2+} in primary cultures of rat bile duct epithelia, and acetylcholine (ACh) increases Ca_i^{2+} in these cells as well (129). As in hepatocytes and other epithelia, the range of patterns of agonist-induced Ca_i^{2+} signals includes sustained and transient Ca_i^{2+} increases and Ca_i^{2+} oscillations. Ca_i^{2+} spikes induced by ACh are longer in duration and lower in frequency than those induced by ATP (129).

Ca_i^{2+} signaling is mediated by InsP3 in bile duct cells, since increases in Ca_i^{2+} are blocked by InsP3R antagonists. Limited evidence suggests that the type I and III but not the type II InsP3R is expressed in this cell type (45). Ca_i^{2+} regulates certain types of Cl^- channels in bile duct cells (155,156), and potentiates the effects of adenylyl cyclase and cAMP via a calcineurin-dependent pathway (157). Indirect evidence suggests Ca_i^{2+} may affect growth and apoptosis as well (158). Other effects of this second messenger in bile duct cells are topics of investigation.

FUNCTIONAL EFFECTS OF Ca²⁺ SIGNALS

Ca^{2+} regulates a wide range of functions in liver and in other tissues. The following subsections provide illustrative examples of the different ways in which Ca^{2+} regulates liver function. This is not an exhaustive list of Ca^{2+}-mediated functions.

Glucose Metabolism

Storage and release of glucose was among the first functions of the liver shown to be regulated by Ca_i^{2+}. Synthesis of glycogen is regulated by glycogen synthase, while phosphorylase is the rate-limiting enzyme for glycogenolysis. Both enzymes are regulated by phosphorylation and dephosphorylation (159), and an increase in Ca_i^{2+} is one of the most important signals for regulating these events (160). For example, hormones such as vasopressin and angiotensin increase InsP3 in hepatocytes, which mobilizes Ca^{2+}, leading to phosphorylation and activation of glycogen phosphorylase, and then glycogenolysis. Similarly, in both rat and human hepatocytes, nucleotides activate glycogen phosphorylase and thus stimulate glycogenolysis by binding to P2Y nucleotide receptors (161). Glucagon and β-adrenergic agonists also stimulate glycogen phosphorylase activity in liver, but through an alternative, cAMP-dependent pathway. Ca^{2+}-mobilizing bile acids such as ursodeoxycholic acid (UDCA), taurolithocholic acid (TLCA), and lithocholic acid (LCA) activate phosphorylase to the same extent as hormones such as vasopressin (162). These bile acids activate phosphorylase through a Ca^{2+}-dependent but InsP3-independent mechanism (162), consistent with the observation that they increase Ca_i^{2+} in an InsP3-independent fashion (163,164).

Gluconeogenic enzymes are preferentially located in the periportal region (165), although other factors also may be involved in regional differences in glycogenolytic capacity. ATP mobilizes glucose mainly from the periportal zone, while norepinephrine and vasopressin preferentially release glucose from pericentral hepatocytes. This may in part reflect the fact that pericentral hepatocytes are more sensitive than periportal hepatocytes to vasopressin and norepinephrine (118). When hepatocytes are not uniformly sensitive to a particular hormone, then intercellular communication via gap junctions enhances glucose release. For example, glucose release is impaired in perfused livers from connexin32-deficient mice upon stimulation with either norepinephrine or glucagon (166). Similarly, vasopressin- or glucagon-induced glucose release is impaired in perfused rat livers treated with the gap junction blocker 18α-glycyrrhetinic acid (αGA)(167). However, glucose release is not altered in αGA-treated livers stimulated with dibutyryl cAMP or 2,5-di(*tert*-butyl)-1,4-benzohydroquinone (*t*BuBHQ), both of which stimulate glucose release in a receptor-independent fashion (167). Hormone-induced glucose release also is impaired if gap junctions are blocked in isolated rat hepatocytes, or if hepatocytes are dispersed (168). Therefore, hepatocytes may contribute differently to glucose metabolism across the hepatic lobule, although there is some integration of metabolic activity via gap junctions.

Bile Flow and Paracellular Permeability

Ca_i^{2+} regulates fluid and electrolyte secretion in many types of epithelia (3). For example, in pancreatic acinar cells apical-to-basal Ca_i^{2+} waves direct vectorial transport of Cl^- and Na^+ (93,169). Although polarized Ca_i^{2+} waves also occur in hepatocytes (46), the effects of these waves on bile secretion is not yet established. Nonetheless, it is established that Ca_i^{2+} has multiple effects on bile flow. The net effect of Ca_i^{2+} on bile acid–independent bile flow is inhibitory (170). Studies in the isolated perfused rat liver have shown that a range of Ca^{2+} agonists, including vasopressin, the Ca^{2+} ionophore A23187, and the Ca^{2+}-ATPase inhibitor *t*BuBHQ, decrease bile flow. This inhibitory effect occurs independently of protein kinase C activation or vasoconstriction (170). Ca_i^{2+} may inhibit bile flow in part by increasing tight junction permeability, which would allow reflux of biliary constituents into the sinusoidal space, thereby dissipating the osmotic gradient that drives bile flow (171). Evidence that Ca_i^{2+} increases paracellular permeability comes from studies in both isolated perfused rat livers and isolated rat hepatocyte couplets. In the isolated perfused rat liver, Ca^{2+} agonists such as vasopressin, angiotensin, and phenylephrine increase paracellular permeability (172). Subsequent studies in hepatocyte couplets confirmed that vasopressin increases paracellular permeability, but suggested that this effect actually is mediated by protein kinase C (171). Nitric oxide (NO) also increases paracellular permeability in isolated rat hepatocyte couplets, but this effect is mediated by a direct effect of NO on protein kinase C and occurs without any increase in Ca_i^{2+} (134). Thus, Ca_i^{2+} signals may increase paracellular permeability in hepatocytes, but they appear to do so only by activating protein kinase C.

Canalicular Contraction

Hepatocytes secrete bile across their apical membrane into a canalicular network that drains into the bile ducts. Time lapse microscopy has demonstrated that bile canalicular segments within this network repeatedly expand and contract (173,174). Canalicular contraction is a Ca^{2+} dependent process. Microinjection of Ca^{2+} into isolated rat hepatocyte couplets or stimulation of couplets with Ca^{2+} agonists such as vasopressin induces canalicular contraction (171,175). In permeabilized hepatocytes, Ca^{2+} plus ATP also induces canalicular contraction (176). Canalicular contraction involves actin and calmodulin activation as well (176). In hepatocytes, actin filaments are located beneath the cell membrane, and are most concentrated in the pericanalicular region (Fig. 38.2). Increases in Ca_i^{2+} lead to phosphorylation of myosin light chain kinase (177), which in turn induces the pericanalicular actin network to contract. These pericanalicular filaments induce periodic contractions in individual pairs of hepatocytes (173), and these contractions are organized to form peristaltic waves within the hepatic lobule (174). Canalicular peristalsis is necessary to maintain bile flow, and agents such as phalloidin are thought to induce cholestasis in part by preventing contractions of pericanalicular actin (178). Canalicular peristalsis occurs at a frequency of approximately 1.5 to 3.0 contractions/minute and in a pericentral to periportal direction (174), which matches the frequency and direction of Ca_i^{2+} waves in the liver (46,115,116). Based on these observations it has been suggested that canalicular peristalsis *in vivo* may be directed by propagating Ca_i^{2+} waves (4,115).

Exocytosis

Ca_i^{2+} regulates exocytosis directly in certain cell types. For example, presynaptic increases in Ca_i^{2+} are associated with release of neurotransmitters in squid axons (179). Also, localized apical increases in Ca_i^{2+} induce exocytic release of zymogen granules in pancreatic acinar cells (169). Interestingly, not every apical increase in Ca_i^{2+} induces exocytosis in the acinar cell. Only Ca_i^{2+} signals that reach a concentration of 5 to 10 μM are sufficient to trigger exocytosis (169). Current evidence suggests Ca_i^{2+} plays a less direct role in regulating exocytosis in liver. For example, vasopressin stimulates biliary exocytosis in the isolated perfused rat liver (IPRL)(180). However, this effect appears to be mediated by PKC and can be reproduced by PKC agonists that do not increase Ca^{2+} (171,180). Moreover, Ca^{2+} ionophores increase Ca_i^{2+} yet decrease exocytosis in IPRL. Thus PKC activation rather than Ca_i^{2+} may serve to stimulate exocytosis in liver, although hormone-induced Ca^{2+} influx can activate PKC in hepatocytes (171).

Tauroursodeoxycholic acid (TUDCA) also stimulates exocytosis in IPRL (181). As with hormones such as vasopressin, TUDCA-induced exocytosis is thought to occur by inducing Ca^{2+} influx, which then leads to activation of the α isoform of PKC (181,182). TUDCA does not stimulate exocytosis after common bile duct ligation, even though the choleretic effect of TUDCA is maintained under these cir-

cumstances. However, Ca^{2+} influx is selectively impaired after bile duct ligation (181). This provides additional evidence that Ca^{2+} influx plays a role in exocytosis in liver, and furthermore suggests that impairment of Ca^{2+} influx mechanisms may contribute to cholestasis.

Ca^{2+} Signaling Induced by Bile Acids

Certain bile acids can induce Ca_i^{2+} signaling. Hydrophobic bile acids that increase Ca_i^{2+} are LCA and TLCA. Relatively low concentrations of these bile acids cause a rapid, prolonged increase in Ca_i^{2+} in hepatocytes (163,164). Bile acids such as taurodeoxycholic acid and taurochenodeoxycholic acid also can increase Ca_i^{2+}, but much higher concentrations are required. In contrast, cholic acid and taurocholic acid do not affect Ca_i^{2+}, even when these bile acids are present in millimolar amounts (164,183). LCA- and TLCA-induced Ca_i^{2+} signaling occurs independently of extracellular Ca^{2+}. In addition, these bile acids mobilize Ca^{2+} from the same pool as InsP3, but without InsP3 formation (163). Therefore, it is thought that these bile acids increase Ca_i^{2+} by permeabilizing the endoplasmic reticulum, which may in part account for their toxicity. Although LCA and TLCA do not increase Ca_i^{2+} in most cell types, this is likely because most types of cells lack a mechanism to take up bile acids. For example, TLCA does not increase Ca_i^{2+} in either platelets or neuroblastoma cells, but it potently increases Ca_i^{2+} in both of these cell types once they are permeabilized (184). Both LCA and TLCA are cholestatic, but it is unclear whether this is due to their effect on Ca_i^{2+} (170,185). The therapeutic bile acids UDCA and TUDCA also increase Ca_i^{2+} in hepatocytes, and promote rather than inhibit bile flow, suggesting that increases in Ca_i^{2+} do not necessarily induce cholestasis. TUDCA induces a more prolonged increase in Ca_i^{2+} than does TLCA, and the sustained phase of the TUDCA-induced Ca_i^{2+} signal depends on the influx of extracellular Ca^{2+} (186). TUDCA and TLCA both activate PKC in hepatocytes as well, but each of these bile acids preferentially activates distinct PKC isoforms (182,187). It remains to be established whether this differential activation of specific PKC isoforms may in part explain the different effects of these two bile acids on hepatocyte function.

Regulation of Cell Volume

Many cells have the ability to regulate their volume. Since hepatocytes and biliary epithelia frequently are exposed to osmotic stress, the ability to regulate cell volume is particularly important in liver. Indirect evidence suggests that Ca_i^{2+} may be involved in volume regulation in two ways. First, regulatory volume changes in liver are mediated by extracellular ATP (188). Specifically, cell swelling induces release of ATP, which then activates hepatocyte P2Y receptors. This leads to activation of Cl^- channels, which are responsible for regulatory volume decreases (188). Stimulation of P2Y receptors likely activates these Cl⁻ channels via increases in Ca_i^{2+} (131,155), although this has not yet been demonstrated directly. This autocrine pathway for cell volume regulation has been demonstrated in primary hepatocytes (189) as well as in liver cell lines (188). In addition, both swelling-induced and constitutive ATP release occurs in the Mz-ChA-1 bile duct cell line (190). ATP release in this cell line similarly is responsible for P2Y receptor-mediated activation of Cl⁻ channels and volume regulation (155,156,190). In addition, though, inhibition of P2Y receptors under isotonic conditions leads to cell swelling in these cells (190). Stimulation of bile duct cells with ATP or other Ca^{2+} agonists under isotonic conditions does not induce a change in cell volume, though (129). Thus, Ca_i^{2+} may be important for autocrine regulation as well as maintenance of cell volume in hepatocytes and bile duct epithelia.

Hypo-osmotic cell swelling also activates a number of MAP kinase (MAPK) signaling pathways in the liver (191). Cell swelling has been associated with activation of Erk-1 and Erk-2, p38^{MAPK}, and the c-*Jun*–N-terminal kinases (JNK). Ca_i^{2+} plays an intermediate step in this MAPK activation in certain cell types. For example, Erk activation in astrocytes requires Ca^{2+} influx (192). It is less clear whether Ca_i^{2+} similarly is involved in hepatocytes (191).

CONCLUSION

The importance of Ca^{2+} as a second messenger in liver and in other tissues is well known. Most of the cellular components that are involved in generating Ca_i^{2+} signals have been identified and were reviewed here. It is now becoming apparent, however, that Ca_i^{2+} signaling also depends on interactions between these components. Thus, Ca_i^{2+} signaling in one region of the cytosol is dependent on Ca_i^{2+} signaling in other subcellular regions, as well as on interactions between the cytosol and organelles, and among neighboring cells. Future advances in this field likely will result from an increased understanding of how these various aspects of Ca_i^{2+} signaling are integrated to regulate signaling in the intact liver. This in turn may increase our understanding of the complex way in which liver function is regulated by Ca^{2+} in health and disease.

REFERENCES

1. Berridge MJ. Inositol trisphosphate and calcium signalling. *Nature* 1993;361:315–325.
2. Clapham DE. Calcium signaling. *Cell* 1995;80:259–268.
3. Nathanson MH. Cellular and subcellular calcium signaling in gastrointestinal epithelium. *Gastroenterology* 1994;106:1349–1364.
4. Nathanson MH, Schlosser SF. Calcium signaling mechanisms in liver in health and disease. In: Boyer JL, Ockner RK, eds. Progress in liver diseases. Philadelphia: WB Saunders, 1996:1–27.
5. Nathanson MH, O'Neill AF, Burgstahler AD. Primitive organization of cytosolic Ca^{2+} signals in hepatocytes from the little skate *Raja erinacea*. *J Exp Biol* 1999;202:3049–3056.
6. Berridge MJ. The AM and FM of calcium signalling. *Nature* 1997;386:759–760.
7. Simon MI, Strathmann MP, Gautam N. Diversity of G proteins in signal transduction. *Science* 1991;252:802–808.
8. Wu D, Katz A, Lee C-H, et al. Activation of phospholipase C by α₁-adrenergic receptors is mediated by the α subunits of Gq family. *J Biol Chem* 1992;267:25798–25802.
9. Katz A, Wu D, Simon MI. Subunits beta gamma of heterotrimeric G protein activate beta 2 isoform of phospholipase C. *Nature* 1992;360:686–689.
10. Lev S, Moreno H, Martinez R, et al. Protein tyrosine kinase PYK2 involved in Ca^{2+}-induced regulation of ion channel and MAP kinase functions. *Nature* 1995;376:737–745.
11. Hobbs AJ, Ignarro LJ. Nitric oxide-cyclic GMP signal transduction system. *Methods Enzymol* 1996;269:134–148.
12. Wedel BJ, Garbers DL. New insights on the functions of the guanylyl cyclase receptors. *FEBS Lett* 1997;410:29–33.
13. Rhee SG, Choi KD. Regulation of inositol phospholipid-specific phospholipase C isozymes. *J Biol Chem* 1992;267:12393–12396.
14. Streb H, Irvine RF, Berridge MJ, et al. Release of Ca^{2+} from a nonmitochondrial intracellular store in pancreatic acinar cells by inositol-1,4,5-trisphosphate. *Nature* 1983;306:67–68.
15. Humbert JP, Matter N, Artault JC, et al. Inositol 1,4,5-trisphosphate receptor is located to the inner nuclear membrane vindicating regulation of nuclear calcium signaling by inositol 1,4,5-trisphosphate—discrete distribution of inositol phosphate receptors to inner and outer nuclear membranes. *J Biol Chem* 1996;271:478–485.
16. Gerasimenko OV, Gerasimenko JV, Tepikin AV, et al. ATP-dependent accumulation and inositol trisphosphate- or cyclic ADP-ribose-mediated release of Ca^{2+} from the nuclear envelope. *Cell* 1995;80:439–444.
17. Khan AA, Soloski MJ, Sharp AH, et al. Lymphocyte apoptosis: Mediation by increased type 3 inositol 1,4,5-trisphosphate receptor. *Science* 1996;273:503–507.
18. Santella L, Carafoli E. Calcium signaling in the cell nucleus. *FASEB J* 1997;11:1091–1109.
19. Divecha N, Rhee S-G, Letcher AJ, et al. Phosphoinositide signalling enzymes in rat liver nuclei: phosphoinositidase C isoform β1 is specifically, but not predominantly, located in the nucleus. *Biochem J* 1993;289:617–620.
20. Bezprozvanny I, Watras J, Ehrlich BE. Bell-shaped calcium-response curves of Ins(1,4,5)P₃- and calcium-gated channels from endoplasmic reticulum of cerebellum. *Nature* 1991;351:751–754.
21. Furuichi T, Yoshikawa S, Miyawaki A, et al. Primary structure and functional expression of the inositol 1,4,5-trisphosphate-binding protein P400. *Nature* 1989;342:32–38.
22. Maranto AR. Primary structure, ligand binding, and localization of the human type 3 inositol 1,4,5-trisphosphate receptor expressed in intestinal epithelium. *J Biol Chem* 1994;269:1222–1230.
23. Sudhof TC, Newton CL, Archer BT, et al. Structure of a novel InsP₃ receptor. *EMBO J* 1991;10:3199–3206.
24. Ross CA, Danoff SK, Schell MJ, et al. Three additional inositol 1,4,5-trisphosphate receptors: molecular cloning and differential localization in brain and peripheral tissues. *Proc Natl Acad Sci USA* 1992;89:4265–4269.
25. Mikoshiba K. The InsP3 receptor and intracellular Ca^{2+} signaling. *Curr Opin Neurobiol* 1997;7:339–345.
26. Joseph SK, Lin C, Pierson S, et al. Heteroligomers of type-I and

type-III inositol trisphosphate receptors in WB rat liver epithelial cells. *J Biol Chem* 1995;270:23310–23316.

27. Monkawa T, Miyawaki A, Sugiyama T, et al. Heterotetrameric complex formation of inositol 1,4,5-trisphosphate receptor subunits. *J Biol Chem* 1995;270:14700–14704.

28. Mignery GA, Sudhof TC. The ligand binding site and transduction mechanism in the inositol-1,4,5-triphosphate receptor. *EMBO J* 1990;9:3893–3898.

29. Bourguignon LYW, Jin H. Identification of the ankyrin-binding domain of the mouse T-lymphoma cell inositol 1,4,5-trisphosphate (IP$_3$) receptor and its role in the regulation of IP$_3$-mediated internal Ca^{2+} release. *J Biol Chem* 1995;270:7257–7260.

30. Hagar RE, Burgstahler AD, Nathanson MH, et al. Type III InsP3 receptor channel stays open in the presence of increased calcium. *Nature* 1998;396:81–84.

31. Ramos-Franco J, Fill M, Mignery GA. Isoform-specific function of single inositol 1,4,5-trisphosphate receptor channels. *Biophys J* 1998;75:834–839.

32. Newton CL, Mignery GA, Südhof TC. Co-expression in vertebrate tissues and cell lines of multiple inositol 1,4,5-trisphosphate (InsP$_3$) receptors with distinct affinities for InsP$_3$. *J Biol Chem* 1994;269:28613–28619.

33. De Young GW, Keizer J. A single-pool inositol 1,4,5-trisphosphate-receptor-based model for agonist-stimulated oscillations in Ca^{2+} concentration. *Proc Natl Acad Sci USA* 1992;89:9895–9899.

34. Wakui M, Potter BVL, Petersen OH. Pulsatile intracellular calcium release does not depend on fluctuations in inositol trisphosphate concentration. *Nature* 1989;339:317–320.

35. Hagar RE, Ehrlich BE. Regulation of the type III InsP3 receptor by InsP3 and ATP. *Biophys J* 2000;79:271–278.

36. Nathanson MH, Fallon MB, Padfield PJ, et al. Localization of the type 3 inositol 1,4,5-trisphosphate receptor in the Ca^{2+} wave trigger zone of pancreatic acinar cells. *J Biol Chem* 1994;269:4693–4696.

37. Hirata K, Nathanson MH, Burgstahler AD, et al. Relationship between inositol 1,4,5-trisphosphate receptor isoforms and subcellular Ca^{2+} signaling patterns in nonpigmented ciliary epithelia. *Invest Ophthalmol Vis Sci* 1999;40:2046–2053.

38. Lee MG, Xu X, Zeng WZ, et al. Polarized expression of Ca^{2+} channels in pancreatic and salivary gland cells—Correlation with initiation and propagation of $[Ca^{2+}]_i$ waves. *J Biol Chem* 1997;272:15765–15770.

39. Yule DI, Ernst SA, Ohnishi H, et al. Evidence that zymogen granules are not a physiologically relevant calcium pool—defining the distribution of inositol 1,4,5-trisphosphate receptors in pancreatic acinar cells. *J Biol Chem* 1997;272:9093–9098.

40. Miyakawa T, Maeda A, Yamazawa T, et al. Encoding of Ca^{2+} signals by differential expression of IP3 receptor subtypes. *EMBO J* 1999;18:1303–1308.

41. Michikawa T, Hirota J, Kawano S, et al. Calmodulin mediates calcium-dependent inactivation of the cerebellar type 1 inositol 1,4,5-trisphosphate receptor. *Neuron* 1999;23:799–808.

42. Cardy TJ, Taylor CW. A novel role for calmodulin: Ca2+-independent inhibition of type-1 inositol trisphosphate receptors. *Biochem J* 1998;334:447–455.

43. Vanlingen S, Sipma H, De Smet L, et al. Ca^{2+} and calmodulin differentially modulate myo-inositol 1,4,5-trisphosphate (IP3)-binding to the recombinant ligand-binding domains of the various IP3 receptor isoforms. *Biochem J* 2000;346:275–280.

44. Wojcikiewicz RJH. Type I, II, and III inositol 1,4,5-trisphosphate receptors are unequally susceptible to down-regulation and are expressed in markedly different proportions in different cell types. *J Biol Chem* 1995;270:11678–11683.

45. Dufour J-F, Luthi M, Forestier M, et al. Expression of inositol 1,4,5-trisphosphate receptor isoforms in rat cirrhosis. *Hepatology* 1999;30:1018–1026.

46. Nathanson MH, Burgstahler AD, Fallon MB. Multi-step mechanism of polarized Ca^{2+} wave patterns in hepatocytes. *Am J Physiol Gastrointest Liver Physiol* 1994;267:G338–G349.

47. Lupu VD, Kaznacheyeva E, Krishna UM, et al. Functional coupling of phosphatidylinositol 4,5-bisphosphate to inositol 1,4,5-trisphosphate receptor. *J Biol Chem* 1998;273:14067–14070.

48. Cameron AM, Steiner JP, Sabatini DM, et al. Immunophilin FK506 binding protein associated with inositol 1,4,5-trisphosphate receptor modulates calcium flux. *Proc Natl Acad Sci USA* 1995;92:1784–1788.

49. Joseph SK, Ryan SV. Phosphorylation of the inositol trisphosphate receptor in isolated rat hepatocytes. *J Biol Chem* 1993;268:23059–23065.

50. Schlossmann J, Ammendola A, Ashman K, et al. Regulation of intracellular calcium by a signalling complex of IRAG, IP3 receptor and cGMP kinase I beta. *Nature* 2000;404:197–201.

51. Wojcikiewicz RJH, Ernst SA, Yule DI. Secretagogues cause ubiquitination and down-regulation of inositol 1,4,5-trisphosphate receptors in rat pancreatic acinar cells. *Gastroenterology* 1999;116:1194–1201.

52. McPherson PS, Campbell KP. The ryanodine receptor/Ca^{2+} release channel. *J Biol Chem* 1993;268:13765–13768.

53. Mignery GA, Sudhof TC, Takei K, et al. Putative receptor for inositol 1,4,5-trisphosphate similar to ryanodine receptor. *Nature* 1989;342:192–195.

54. Sonnleitner A, Conti A, Bertocchini F, et al. Functional properties of the ryanodine receptor type 3 (RyR3) Ca^{2+} release channel. *EMBO J* 1998;17:2790–2798.

55. Mészáros LG, Bak J, Chu A. Cyclic ADP-ribose as an endogenous regulator of the non-skeletal type ryanodine receptor Ca^{2+} channel. *Nature* 1993;364:76–79.

56. Kuemmerle JF, Makhlouf GM. Agonist-stimulated cyclic ADP ribose—Endogenous modulator of Ca^{2+}-induced Ca^{2+} release in intestinal longitudinal muscle. *J Biol Chem* 1995;270:25488–25494.

57. Clementi E, Riccio M, Sciorati C, et al. The type 2 ryanodine receptor of neurosecretory PC12 cells is activated by cyclic ADP-ribose—role of the nitric oxide cGMP pathway. *J Biol Chem* 1996;271:17739–17745.

58. Guse AH, Da Silva CP, Berg I, et al. Regulation of calcium signalling in T lymphocytes by the second messenger cyclic ADP-ribose. *Nature* 1999;398:70–73.

59. Cancela JM, Petersen OH. The cyclic ADP ribose antagonist 8-NH$_2$-cADP-ribose blocks cholecystokinin-evoked cytosolic Ca^{2+} spiking in pancreatic acinar cells. *Pflugers Arch* 1998;435:746–748.

60. Rusinko N, Lee HC. Widespread occurrence in animal tissues of an enzyme catalyzing the conversion of NAD^+ into a cyclic metabolite with intracellular Ca^{2+}-mobilizing activity. *J Biol Chem* 1989;264:11725–11731.

61. Giannini G, Conti A, Mammarella S, et al. The ryanodine receptor/calcium channel genes are widely and differentially expressed in murine brain and peripheral tissues. *J Cell Biol* 1995;128:893–904.

62. Shoshan-Barmatz V. High affinity ryanodine binding sites in rat liver endoplasmic reticulum. *FEBS Lett* 1990;263:317–320.

63. Lilly LB, Gollan JL. Ryanodine-induced calcium release from hepatic microsomes and permeabilized hepatocytes. *Am J Physiol Gastrointest Liver Physiol* 1995;268:G1017–G1024.

64. Lee HC, Aarhus R. A derivative of NADP mobilizes calcium stores insensitive to inositol trisphosphate and cyclic ADP-ribose. *J Biol Chem* 1995;270:2152–2157.

65. Cancela JM, Churchill GC, Galione A. Coordination of ago-

nist-induced Ca2+ signalling patterns by NAADP in pancreatic acinar cells. *Nature* 1999;398:74–76.

66. Pozzan T, Rizzuto R. High tide of calcium in mitochondria. *Nature Cell Biol* 2000;2:E25–E27.

67. Rutter GA, Rizzuto R. Regulation of mitochondrial metabolism by ER Ca²⁺ release: an intimate connection. *Trends Biochem Sci* 2000;25:215–221.

68. Crompton M, Capano M, Carafoli E. 1976. The sodium induced efflux of calcium from heart mitochondria. A possible mechanism for the regulation of mitochondrial calcium. *Eur J Biochem* 1976;69:453–462.

69. Gunter TE, Chace JH, Puskin JS, et al. Mechanism of sodium independent calcium efflux from rat liver mitochondria. *Biochemistry* 1983;22:6341–6351.

70. Gunter TE, Gunter KK, Sheu SS, et al. Mitochondrial calcium transport: physiological and pathological relevance. *Am J Physiol Cell Physiol* 1994;267:C313–C339.

71. Nazareth W, Nasser Y, Crompton M. Inhibition of anoxia-induced injury in heart myocytes by cyclosporin A. *J Mol Cell Cardiol* 1991;23:1351–1354.

72. Ichas F, Jouaville LS, Mazat JP. Mitochondria are excitable organelles capable of generating and conveying electrical and calcium signals. *Cell* 1997;89:1145–1153.

73. Ichas F, Jouaville LS, Sidash SS, et al. Mitochondrial calcium spiking: A transduction mechanism based on calcium-induced permeability transition involved in cell calcium signalling. *FEBS Lett* 1994;348:211–215.

74. Petronilli V, Cola C, Massari S, et al. Physiological effectors modify voltage sensing by the cyclosporin A-sensitive permeability transition pore of mitochondria. *J Biol Chem* 1993;268: 21939–21945.

75. Jouaville LS, Ichas F, Holmuhamedov EL, et al. Synchronization of calcium waves by mitochondrial substrates in *Xenopus laevis* oocytes. *Nature* 1995;377:438–441.

76. Nicolli A, Basso E, Petronilli V, et al. Interactions of cyclophilin with the mitochondrial inner membrane and regulation of the permeability transition pore, a cyclosporin A-sensitive channel. *J Biol Chem* 1996;271:2185–2192.

77. Hajnóczky G, Hager R, Thomas AP. Mitochondria suppress local feedback activation of inositol 1,4,5-trisphosphate receptors by Ca²⁺. *J Biol Chem* 1999;274:14157–14162.

78. Csordas G, Thomas AP, Hajnóczky G. Quasi-synaptic calcium signal transmission between endoplasmic reticulum and mitochondria. *EMBO J* 1999;18:96–108.

79. Rizzuto R, Simpson AWM, Brini M, et al. Rapid changes of mitochondrial Ca²⁺ revealed by specifically targeted recombinant aequorin. *Nature* 1992;358:325–327.

80. Rizzuto R, Brini M, Murgia M, et al. Microdomains with high Ca²⁺ close to IP₃-sensitive channels that are sensed by neighboring mitochondria. *Science* 1993;262:744–747.

81. Satoh T, Ross CA, Villa A, et al. The inositol 1,4,5,-trisphosphate receptor in cerebellar Purkinje cells: quantitative immunogold labeling reveals concentration in an ER subcompartment. *J Cell Biol* 1990;111:615–624.

82. Rizzuto R, Bastianutto C, Brini M, et al. Mitochondrial Ca²⁺ homeostasis in intact cells. *J Cell Biol* 1994;126:1183–1194.

83. Robb-Gaspers LD, Burnett P, Rutter GA, et al. Integrating cytosolic calcium signals into mitochondrial metabolic responses. *EMBO J* 1998;17:4987–5000.

84. Hajnóczky G, Robb-Gaspers LD, Seitz MB, et al. Decoding of cytosolic calcium oscillations in the mitochondria. *Cell* 1995; 82:415–424.

85. Pralong W-F, Spät A, Wollheim CB. Dynamic pacing of cell metabolism by intracellular Ca²⁺ transients. *J Biol Chem* 1994; 269:27310–27314.

86. Jouaville LS, Pinton P, Bastianutto C, et al. Regulation of mitochondrial ATP synthesis by calcium: Evidence for a long-term metabolic priming. *Proc Natl Acad Sci USA* 1999;96: 13807–13812.

87. Tsien RY. A non-disruptive technique for loading calcium buffers and indicators into cells. *Nature* 1981;290:527–528.

88. Tsien RY, Pozzan T, Rink TJ. Calcium homeostasis in intact lymphocytes: cytoplasmic free calcium monitored with a new, intracellularly trapped fluorescent indicator. *J Cell Biol* 1982;94:325–334.

89. Grynkiewicz G, Poenie M, Tsien RY. A new generation of Ca⁺ indicators with greatly improved fluorescence properties. *J Biol Chem* 1985;260:3440–3450.

90. Hofer AM, Machen TE. Technique for *in situ* measurement of calcium in intracellular inositol 1,4,5-trisphosphate-sensitive stores using the fluorescent indicator mag-fura-2. *Proc Natl Acad Sci USA* 1993;90:2598–2602.

91. Harootunian AT, Kao JPY, Paranjape S, et al. Generation of calcium oscillations in fibroblasts by positive feedback between calcium and IP₃. *Science* 1991;251:75–78.

92. Rooney TA, Sass EJ, Thomas AP. Characterization of cytosolic calcium oscillations induced by phenylephrine and vasopressin in single Fura-2 loaded hepatocytes. *J Biol Chem* 1989;264: 17131–17141.

93. Kasai H, Augustine GJ. Cytosolic Ca²⁺ gradients triggering unidirectional fluid secretion from exocrine pancreas. *Nature* 1990;348:735–738.

94. Rooney TA, Sass EJ, Thomas AP. Agonist-induced cytosolic calcium oscillations originate from a specific locus in single hepatocytes. *J Biol Chem* 1990;265:10792–10796.

95. Nathanson MH, Burgstahler AD. Subcellular distribution of cytosolic Ca²⁺ in isolated rat hepatocyte couplets: evaluation using confocal microscopy. *Cell Calcium* 1992;13:89–98.

96. Woods NM, Cuthbertson KR, Cobbold PH. Repetitive transient rises in cytoplasmic free calcium in hormone-stimulated hepatocytes. *Nature* 1986;319:600–602.

97. Montero M, Brini M, Marsault R, et al. Monitoring dynamic changes in free Ca²⁺ concentration in the endoplasmic reticulum of intact cells. *EMBO J* 1995;14:5467–5475.

98. Brini M, Murgia M, Pasti L, et al. Nuclear Ca²⁺ concentration measured with specifically targeted recombinant aequorin. *EMBO J* 1993;12:4813–4819.

99. Marsault R, Murgia M, Pozzan T, et al. Domains of high Ca²⁺ beneath the plasma membrane of living A7r5 cells. *EMBO J* 1997;16:1575–1581.

100. Kawanishi T, Blank LM, Harootunian AT, et al. Ca²⁺ oscillations induced by hormonal stimulation of individual fura-2-loaded hepatocytes. *J Biol Chem* 1989;264:12859–12866.

101. Hansen CA, Yang L, Williamson JR. Mechanisms of receptor-mediated Ca²⁺ signaling in rat hepatocytes. *J Biol Chem* 1991;266:18573–18579.

102. Woods NM, Cuthbertson KSR, Cobbold PH. Agonist-induced oscillations in cytoplasmic free calcium concentration in single rat hepatocytes. *Cell Calcium* 1987;8:79–100.

103. Nathanson MH, Burgstahler AD. Coordination of hormone-induced calcium signals in isolated rat hepatocyte couplets: demonstration with confocal microscopy. *Mol Biol Cell* 1992; 3:113–121.

104. Dolmetsch RE, Xu K, Lewis RS. Calcium oscillations increase the efficiency and specificity of gene expression. *Nature* 1998; 392:933–936.

105. Li W, Llopis J, Whitney M, et al. Cell-permeant caged InsP3 ester shows that Ca²⁺ spike frequency can optimize gene expression. *Nature* 1998;392:936–941.

106. Foskett JK, Roifman CM, Wong D. Activation of calcium oscillations by thapsigargin in parotid acinar cells. *J Biol Chem* 1991; 266:2778–2782.

107. Nathanson MH, Padfield PJ, O'Sullivan AJ, et al. Mechanism of Ca^{2+} wave propagation in pancreatic acinar cells. *J Biol Chem* 1992;267:18118–18121.

108. Thorn P, Lawrie AM, Smith PM, et al. Local and global cytosolic Ca^{2+} oscillations in exocrine cells evoked by agonists and inositol trisphosphate. *Cell* 1993;74:661–668.

109. Kasai H, Li YX, Miyashita Y. Subcellular distribution of Ca^{2+} release channels underlying Ca^{2+} waves and oscillations in exocrine pancreas. *Cell* 1993;74:669–677.

110. Yamamoto-Hino M, Miyawaki A, Segawa A, et al. Apical vesicles bearing inositol 1,4,5-trisphosphate receptors in the Ca^{2+} initiation site of ductal epithelium of submandibular gland. *J Cell Biol* 1998;141:135–142.

111. Gilkey JC, Jaffe LF, Ridgway EB, et al. A free calcium wave traverses the activated egg of the medaka, *Oryzias latipes*. *J Cell Biol* 1978;76:448–466.

112. Toescu EC, Lawrie AM, Petersen OH, et al. Spatial and temporal distribution of agonist-evoked cytoplasmic Ca^{2+} signals in exocrine acinar cells analysed by digital image microscopy. *EMBO J* 1992;11:1623–1629.

113. Leite MF, Dranoff JA, Gao L, et al. Expression and subcellular localization of the ryanodine receptor in rat pancreatic acinar cells. *Biochem J* 1999;337:305–309.

114. DiJulio DH, Watson EL, Pessah IN, et al. Ryanodine receptor type III (Ry_3R) identification in mouse parotid acini—properties and modulation of [^{3}H]ryanodine-binding sites. *J Biol Chem* 1997;272:15687–15696.

115. Nathanson MH, Burgstahler AD, Mennone A, et al. Ca^{2+} waves are organized among hepatocytes in the intact organ. *Am J Physiol Gastrointest Liver Physiol* 1995;269:G167–G171.

116. Robb-Gaspers LD, Thomas AP. Coordination of Ca^{2+} signaling by intercellular propagation of Ca^{2+} waves in the intact liver. *J Biol Chem* 1995;270:8102–8107.

117. Motoyama K, Karl IE, Flye MW, et al. Effect of Ca2+ agonists in the perfused liver: determination via laser scanning confocal microscopy. *Am J Physiol Regul Integr Comp Physiol* 1999;276: R575–R585.

118. Tordjmann T, Berthon B, Combettes L, et al. The location of hepatocytes in the rat liver acinus determines their sensitivity to calcium-mobilizing hormones. *Gastroenterology* 1996;111: 1343–1352.

119. Saez JC, Connor JA, Spray DC, et al. Hepatocyte gap junctions are permeable to the second messenger, inositol 1,4,5-triphosphate, and to calcium ions. *Proc Natl Acad Sci USA* 1989;86:2708–2712.

120. Fallon MB, Nathanson MH, Mennone A, et al. Altered expression and function of hepatocyte gap junctions after common bile duct ligation in the rat. *Am J Physiol Cell Physiol* 1995;268:C1186–C1194.

121. Niessen H, Willecke K. Strongly decreased gap junctional permeability to inositol 1,4,5-trisphosphate in connexin32 deficient hepatocytes. *FEBS Lett* 2000;466:112–114.

122. Boitano S, Dirksen ER, Sanderson MJ. Intercellular propagation of calcium waves mediated by inositol trisphosphate. *Science* 1992;258:292–295.

123. Tordjmann T, Berthon B, Claret M, et al. Coordinated intercellular calcium waves induced by noradrenaline in rat hepatocytes: dual control by gap junction permeability and agonist. *EMBO J* 1997;17:5398–5407.

124. Lechleiter J, Girard S, Peralta E, et al. Spiral calcium wave propagation and annihilation in *Xenopus laevis* oocytes. *Science* 1991;252:123–126.

125. Tordjmann T, Berthon B, Jacquemin E, et al. Receptor-oriented intercellular calcium waves evoked by vasopressin in rat hepatocytes. *EMBO J* 1998;17:4695–4703.

126. Combettes L, Tran D, Tordjmann T, et al. Ca^{2+}-mobilizing hormones induce sequentially ordered Ca^{2+} signals in multicellular systems of rat hepatocytes. *Biochem J* 1994;304:585–594.

127. Burgstahler AD, Nathanson MH. Coordination of calcium waves among hepatocytes: teamwork gets the job done. *Hepatology* 1998;27:634–635.

128. Schlosser SF, Burgstahler AD, Nathanson MH. Isolated rat hepatocytes can signal to other hepatocytes and bile duct cells by release of nucleotides. *Proc Natl Acad Sci USA* 1996;93: 9948–9953.

129. Nathanson MH, Burgstahler AD, Mennone A, et al. Characterization of cytosolic Ca^{2+} signaling in rat bile duct epithelia. *Am J Physiol Gastrointest Liver Physiol* 1996;271:G86–G96.

130. Kitamura T, Brauneis U, Gatmaitan Z, et al. Extracellular ATP, intracellular calcium and canalicular contraction in rat hepatocyte doublets. *Hepatology* 1991;14:640–647.

131. McGill J, Basavappa S, Mangel AW, et al. Adenosine triphosphate activates ion permeabilities in biliary epithelial cells. *Gastroenterology* 1994;107:236–243.

132. Patel S, Robb-Gaspers LD, Stellato KA, et al. Coordination of calcium signalling by endothelial-derived nitric oxide in the intact liver. *Nature Cell Biol* 1999;1:467–471.

133. Rooney TA, Joseph SK, Queen C, et al. Cyclic GMP induces oscillatory calcium signals in rat hepatocytes. *J Biol Chem* 1996; 271:19817–19825.

134. Burgstahler AD, Nathanson MH. NO modulates the apicolateral cytoskeleton of isolated hepatocytes by a PKC-dependent, cGMP-independent mechanism. *Am J Physiol Gastrointest Liver Physiol* 1995;269:G789–G799.

135. Dale E, DeFelice LJ, Kyozuka K, et al. Voltage clamp of the nuclear envelope. *Philos Trans R Soc Lond [Biol]* 1995;255: 119–124.

136. Nicotera P, McConkey DJ, Jones DP, et al. ATP stimulates Ca^{2+} uptake and increases the free Ca^{2+} concentration in isolated rat liver nuclei. *Proc Natl Acad Sci USA* 1989;86:453–457.

137. Lanini L, Bachs O, Carafoli E. The calcium pump of the liver nuclear membrane is identical to that of endoplasmic reticulum. *J Biol Chem* 1992;267:11548–11552.

138. Nicotera P, Orrenius S, Nisson T, et al. An inositol 1,4,5-trisphosphate-sensitive Ca^{2+} pool in liver nuclei. *Proc Natl Acad Sci USA* 1990;87:6858–6862.

139. Adebanjo OA, Anandatheerthavarada HK, Koval AP, et al. A new function for CD38/ADP-ribosyl cyclase in nuclear Ca^{2+} homeostasis. *Nature Cell Biol* 1999;1:409–414.

140. Malviya AN, Rogue P, Vincendon G. Stereospecific inositol 1,4,5-[^{32}P]trisphosphate binding to isolated rat liver nuclei: evidence for inositol trisphosphate receptor-mediated calcium release from the nucleus. *Proc Natl Acad Sci USA* 1990;87:9270–9274.

141. Santella L, Kyozuka K. Calcium release into the nucleus by 1,4,5-trisphosphate and cyclic ADP-ribose gated channels induces the resumption of meiosis in starfish oocytes. *Cell Calcium* 1997;22:1–10.

142. Hennager DJ, Welsh MJ, DeLisle S. Changes in either cytosolic or nucleoplasmic inositol 1,4,5-trisphosphate levels can control nuclear Ca^{2+} concentration. *J Biol Chem* 1995;270:4959–4962.

143. Clark EA, Brugge JS. Integrins and signal transduction pathways: the road taken. *Science* 1995;268:233–239.

144. Plevin R, Palmer S, Gardner SD, et al. Regulation of bombesin-stimulated inositol 1,4,5-trisphosphate generation in Swiss 3T3 fibroblasts by a guanine-nucleotide-binding protein. *Biochem J* 1990;268:605–610.

145. Gerace L, Burke B. Functional organization of the nuclear envelope. *Annu Rev Cell Biol* 1988;4:335–374.

146. Allbritton NL, Oancea E, Kuhn MA, et al. Source of nuclear calcium signals. *Proc Natl Acad Sci USA* 1994;91: 12458–12462.

147. Waybill MM, Yelamarty RV, Zhang Y, et al. Nuclear calcium

gradients in cultured rat hepatocytes. *Am J Physiol Endocrinol Metab* 1990;261:E49–E57.

148. Perez-Terzic C, Jaconi M, Clapham DE. Nuclear calcium and the regulation of the nuclear pore complex. *BioEssays* 1997;19: 787–792.

149. Stehno-Bittel L, Perez-Terzic C, Clapham DE. Diffusion across the nuclear envelope inhibited by depletion of the nuclear Ca^{2+} store. *Science* 1995;270:1835–1838.

150. Badminton MN, Campbell AK, Rembold CM. Differential regulation of nuclear and cytosolic Ca^{2+} in HeLa cells. *J Biol Chem* 1996;271:31210–31214.

151. Lipp P, Thomas D, Berridge MJ, et al. Nuclear calcium signalling by individual cytoplasmic calcium puffs. *EMBO J* 1997;16:7166–7173.

152. Lin C, Hajnóczky G, Thomas AP. Propagation of cytosolic calcium waves into the nuclei of hepatocytes. *Cell Calcium* 1994; 16:247–258.

153. Fox JL, Burgstahler AD, Nathanson MH. Mechanism of long-range Ca^{2+} signalling in the nucleus of isolated rat hepatocytes. *Biochem J* 1997;326:491–495.

154. Yao Y, Choi J, Parker I. Quantal puffs of intracellular Ca^{2+} evoked by inositol trisphosphate in *Xenopus* oocytes. *J Physiol (Lond)* 1995;482:533–553.

155. Schlenker T, Fitz JG. Ca^{2+}-activated Cl^- channels in a human biliary cell line: regulation by Ca^{2+}/calmodulin-dependent protein kinase. *Am J Physiol Gastrointest Liver Physiol* 1996;271: G304–G310.

156. Schlenker T, Romac J, Sharara AI, et al. Regulation of biliary secretion through apical purinergic receptors in cultured rat cholangiocytes. *Am J Physiol Gastrointest Liver Physiol* 1997; 273:G1108–G1117.

157. Alvaro D, Alpini G, Jezequel AM, et al. Role and mechanisms of action of acetylcholine in the regulation of rat cholangiocyte secretory function. *J Clin Invest* 1997;100:1349–1362.

158. Alpini G, Glaser SS, Ueno Y, et al. Heterogeneity of the proliferative capacity of rat cholangiocytes after bile duct ligation. *Am J Physiol Gastrointest Liver Physiol* 1998;274:G767–G775.

159. Krebs EG. Role of the cyclic AMP-dependent protein kinase in signal transduction. *JAMA* 1989;262:1815–1818.

160. Blackmore PF, Strickland WG, Bocckino SB, et al. Mechanism of hepatic glycogen synthase in activation induced by Ca^{2+}-mobilizing hormones. *Biochem J* 1986;237:235–242.

161. Keppens S, DeWulf H. Characterization of the liver P_2-purinoceptor involved in the activation of glycogen phosphorylase. *Biochem J* 1986;240:367–371.

162. Bouscarel B, Fromm H, Nussbaum R. Ursodeoxycholate mobilizes intracellular Ca^{2+} and activates phosphorylase *a* isolated hepatocytes. *Am J Physiol Gastrointest Liver Physiol* 1993;264: G243–G251.

163. Combettes L, Berthon B, Doucet E, et al. Characteristics of bile acid-mediated Ca^{2+} release from permeabilized liver cells and liver microsomes. *J Biol Chem* 1989;264:157–167.

164. Combettes L, Dumont M, Berthon B, et al. Release of calcium from the endoplasmic reticulum by bile acids in rat liver cells. *J Biol Chem* 1988;263:2299–2303.

165. Jungermann K, Katz N. Functional specialization of different hepatocyte populations. *Physiol Rev* 1989;69:708–764.

166. Stumpel F, Ott T, Willecke K, et al. Connexin 32 gap junctions enhance stimulation of glucose output by glucagon and noradrenaline in mouse liver. *Hepatology* 1998;28:1616–1620.

167. Nathanson MH, Rios-Velez L, Burgstahler AD, et al. Communication via gap junctions modulates bile secretion in the isolated perfused rat liver. *Gastroenterology* 1999;116: 1176–1183.

168. Eugenin EA, Gonzalez H, Saez CG, et al. Gap junctional communication coordinates vasopressin-induced glycogenolysis in rat hepatocytes. *Am J Physiol Gastrointest Liver Physiol* 1998;37:G1109–G1116.

169. Ito K, Miyashita Y, Kasai H. Micromolar and submicromolar Ca^{2+} spikes regulating distinct cellular functions in pancreatic acinar cells. *EMBO J* 1997;16:242–251.

170. Nathanson MH, Gautam A, Bruck R, et al. Effects of Ca^{2+} agonists on cytosolic Ca^{2+} in isolated hepatocytes and on bile secretion in the isolated perfused rat liver. *Hepatology* 1992;15: 107–116.

171. Nathanson MH, Gautam A, Ng OC, et al. Hormonal regulation of paracellular permeability in isolated rat hepatocyte couplets. *Am J Physiol Gastrointest Liver Physiol* 1992;262: G1079–G1086.

172. Lowe PJ, Miyai K, Steinbach JH, et al. Hormonal regulation of hepatocyte tight junctional permeability. *Am J Physiol Gastrointest Liver Physiol* 1988;255:G454–G461.

173. Oshio C, Phillips MJ. Contractility of bile canaliculi: Implications for liver function. *Science* 1981;212:1041–1042.

174. Watanabe N, Tsukada N, Smith CR, et al. Motility of bile canaliculi in the living animal: implications for bile flow. *J Cell Biol* 1991;113:1069–1080.

175. Watanabe S, Smith CR, Phillips MJ. Coordination of the contractile activity of bile canaliculi: evidence from calcium microinjection of triplet hepatocytes. *Lab Invest* 1985;53: 275–279.

176. Watanabe N, Tsukada N, Smith CR, et al. Permeabilized hepatocyte couplets: adenosine triphosphate-dependent bile canalicular contractions and a circumferential pericanalicular microfilament belt demonstrated. *Lab Invest* 1991;65:203–213.

177. Yamaguchi Y, Dalle Molle E, Hardison WGM. Vasopressin and A23187 stimulate phosphorylation of myosin light chain-1 in isolated rat hepatocytes. *Am J Physiol Gastrointest Liver Physiol* 1991;261:G312–G319.

178. Phillips MJ, Poucell S, Oda M. Mechanisms of cholestasis. *Lab Invest* 1986;54:593–608.

179. Llinas R, Sugimori M, Silver RB. Microdomains of high calcium concentration in a presynaptic terminal. *Science* 1992; 256:677–679.

180. Bruck R, Nathanson MH, Roelofsen H, et al. Effects of protein kinase C and cytosolic Ca^{2+} on exocytosis in the isolated perfused rat liver. *Hepatology* 1994;20:1032–1040.

181. Beuers U, Nathanson MH, Isales CM, et al. Tauroursodeoxycholic acid stimulates hepatocellular exocytosis by mobilization of extracellular $Ca^+ {}^+$, a mechanism defective in cholestasis. *J Clin Invest* 1993;92:2984–2993.

182. Beuers U, Throckmorton DC, Anderson MS, et al. Taurorsodeoxycholic acid activates protein kinase C in isolated rat hepatocytes. *Gastroenterology* 1996;110:1553–1563.

183. Anwer MS, Engelking LR, Nolan K, et al. Hepatotoxic bile acids increase cytosolic Ca^{2+} activity of isolated rat hepatocytes. *Hepatology* 1988;8:887–891.

184. Coquil JF, Berthon B, Chomiki N, et al. Effects of taurolithocholate, a Ca^{2+}-mobilizing agent, on cell Ca^{2+} in rat hepatocytes, human platelets and neuroblastoma NG108-15 cell line. *Biochem J* 1991;273:153–160.

185. Farrell GC, Duddy SK, Kass GEN, et al. Release of Ca^{2+} from the endoplasmic reticulum is not the mechanism for bile acid-induced cholestasis and hepatotoxicity in the intact rat liver. *J Clin Invest* 1990;85:1255–1259.

186. Beuers U, Nathanson MH, Boyer JL. Effects of tauroursodeoxycholic acid on cytosolic Ca^{2+} signals in isolated rat hepatocytes. *Gastroenterology* 1993;104:604–612.

187. Beuers U, Probst I, Soroka CJ, et al. Modulation of protein kinase C by taurolithocholic acid in isolated rat hepatocytes. *Hepatology* 1999;29:477–482.

188. Wang Y, Roman R, Lidofsky SD, et al. Autocrine signaling

through ATP release represents a novel mechanism for cell volume regulation. *Proc Natl Acad Sci USA* 1996;93:12020–12025.

189. Feranchak AP, Fitz JG, Roman RM. Volume-sensitive purinergic signaling in human hepatocytes. *J Hepatol* 2000;33:174–182.

190. Roman RM, Feranchak AP, Salter KD, et al. Endogenous ATP release regulates Cl⁻ secretion in cultured human and rat biliary epithelial cells. *Am J Physiol Gastrointest Liver Physiol* 1999;276:G1391–G1400.

191. Haussinger D, Schliess F. Osmotic induction of signaling cascades: role in regulation of cell function. *Biochem Biophys Res Commun* 1999;255:551–555.

192. Schliess F, Kurz AK, Vom Dahl S, et al. Mitogen-activated protein kinases mediate the stimulation of bile acid secretion by tauroursodeoxycholate in rat liver. *Gastroenterology* 1997;113:1306–1314.

39

NITRIC OXIDE IN THE LIVER

MARK G. CLEMENS

Nitric oxide (NO) is a pluripotent gaseous free radical that has been identified as an important signaling molecule in virtually every tissue in the body. In the liver, like many other organs, NO has many actions and can be derived from multiple cellular sources. As a result, the exact role of NO in regulating cell or organ function is complex, and experimental evidence often appears to be contradictory. Moreover, the wealth of information concerning the role of NO in the liver is growing at a rapid rate. Prior to 1994, when the previous edition of this book was published, Medline listed 4,731 publications on NO, of which 205 matched for *nitric oxide* and *liver*. In 2000, Medline listed 33,556 publications on NO, with 1,584 of them matching for *nitric oxide* and *liver*. In spite of the proliferation of published studies, the exact role of NO in biologic regulation remains controversial. Because of the liver's complex complement of cell types, all of which are likely to be important sources of NO, the role of NO in the liver can be particularly confusing. Nitric oxide is clearly involved in normal regulation of liver function; moreover, a selective review of the literature can result in compelling evidence that NO is a primary mediator of liver cell injury. An equally compelling case can be made for the hypothesis that NO generation constitutes a potent protective mechanism in the face of potentially injurious stimuli. These apparently discrepant findings appear to be largely the result of diverse effects of NO depending on the microenvironment in which it is generated as well as the variable activity of the nitric oxide synthases. These enzymes can produce either nitric oxide or superoxide under different conditions of availability of substrate and cofactors. Since this chapter specifically summarizes the role of NO in the liver, an exhaustive treatment of the basic chemistry and biochemistry of NO and the nitric oxide synthases is not presented. Nevertheless, some basic properties of both NO and the enzymes that generate it are pertinent to the understanding of its role in regulating hepatic function and will be summarized to provide a context for the discussion of the role of NO in regulating liver function.

CHEMISTRY AND BIOCHEMISTRY OF NITRIC OXIDE AND NITRIC OXIDE SYNTHASES

NO is a gaseous radical, the majority of which is produced by a family of enzymes, the nitric oxide synthases (NOSs). All three isoforms of NOS are found in the liver (1–5). Of these, the inducible (inflammatory) NOS (iNOS, NOS-2) and the endothelial constitutive (eNOS, NOS-3) are the most important. The neuronal constitutive (nNOS, NOS-1) form appears to be restricted to nerve endings found in the larger blood vessels, and the functional implications of this isoform remain to be elucidated (2). Thus, this chapter focuses on the role of NO produced by eNOS and iNOS, with the recognition that future work may identify an important function for nNOS in the liver.

Chemistry of Nitric Oxide

Somewhat paradoxically, the very simple chemical structure of NO constituted a major barrier to the elucidation of its

M. G. Clemens: Department of Biology, University of North Carolina at Charlotte, Charlotte, North Carolina 28223.

very important function as an important endogenous biologic regulator. It was unprecedented that such a simple, carbonless gas produced by an enzymatic reaction could exert such important signaling functions. This is especially true in the context that the vast majority of signaling functions are mediated by noncovalent binding based on specific molecular shape properties. NO, on the other hand, interacts with target molecules via covalent redox reactions (6). In spite of its chemical simplicity, its specific reactivity with biologic molecules confers upon NO the potential to regulate cellular function at multiple levels. Moreover, the simplicity of NO is overcome by the complex regulation of the enzymes responsible for its synthesis.

Probably the most important of the reactions of NO from the point of view of biologic regulation is the reaction with iron in heme proteins to form nitrosyl complexes (7–9). This reaction can be an important modulator of the function of the heme proteins. On the one hand, such an interaction with a heme protein can cause activation. A common example is in the activation of guanyl cyclase by NO. NO binding results in activation of the enzyme and 3',5'-cyclic guanosine monophosphate (cGMP) production. On the other hand, NO binding to mitochondrial aconitase results in inactivation of enzyme activity. Alternatively, NO binding to hemoglobin results in either scavenging (inactivation) of NO, thus limiting the biologic half-life of NO, or transport of NO to remote tissues where it can be released and exert biologic actions (9). The significance of these binding properties for hepatic regulation is described below. Finally, NO may serve to reduce heme iron in the Fe^{4+} state to Fe^{3+}. In doing so, NO can limit the oxidizing potential of pro-oxidant iron (6). Thus, the reactions of NO with iron proteins alone are complex, with the functional result depending on the protein.

Second to its ability to react with metal complexes in proteins, the reaction of NO with other radicals, especially superoxide (O_2^-), is likely to be the most important (10,11) (see Chapters 18 and 19 and website chapter 💻 W-13). The significance of this reaction is also complicated. On the one hand, reaction with O_2^- has been proposed to be a major mechanism of the antiinflammatory action of NO in

that it scavenges superoxide. On the other hand, the product of this reaction, peroxynitrite ($ONOO^-$) is potentially more toxic than either of its precursors. Finally, NO can react directly with thiol groups or, following generation of $ONOO^-$, with tyrosine hydroxyl groups on cellular enzymes (8). In either case, these interactions typically result in inhibition of enzyme activity.

Enzymatic Production on Nitric Oxide

The vast majority of NO produced in biologic systems is the result of the enzymatic conversion of L-arginine to L-citrulline by NOSs. Although the different isozymes are encoded by different genes located on different chromosomes, there is considerable sequence homology in the NOS proteins (12). Most notably, several regions essential for catalytic activity are highly conserved. These include binding sites for reduced nicotinamide adenine dinucleotide phosphate (NADPH), flavin adenine dinucleotide (FAD), flavin mononucleotide (FMN), and calmodulin, as well as dependence on tetrahydrobiopterin (BH_4) as a cofactor. As such, all three forms consume oxygen and receive electrons from NADPH, which are then transferred to L-arginine to form NO plus L-citrulline:

$$\text{L-Arginine} + 2O_2 + 1.5 \text{ NADPH/H}^+ \rightarrow$$
$$\text{L-citrulline} + \cdot NO + 1.5 \text{ NADP.}$$

This reaction involves the formation of several intermediates resulting from sequential electron transfer steps. It is significant that the transfer of the electron from NADPH to O_2 is fairly independent of BH_4 or substrate (L-arginine) availability, while the completion of the transfer of electrons to L-arginine is highly dependent on the presence of adequate BH_4 and L-arginine (13–16) (Fig. 39.1). This property of the NOS enzymes has potentially very important implications for modulation of liver function since the reduction of O_2 by NADPH generates O_2^- (superoxide). Thus in the absence of sufficient L-arginine or BH_4, activated NOS will produce O_2^- rather than NO. In reality, it is unlikely that, under *in vivo* conditions, NOS will completely switch over from an NO to an O_2^- generating system. Instead, cogeneration of

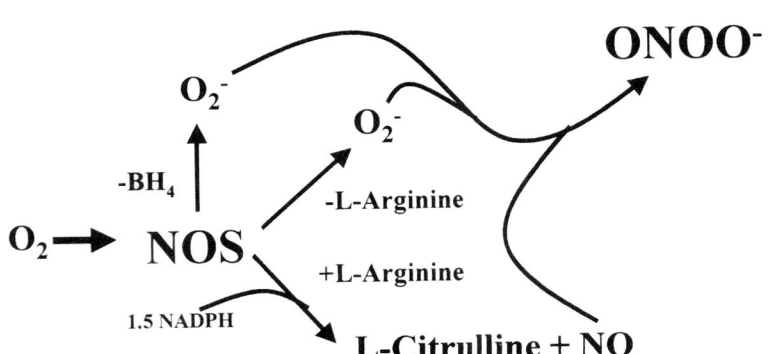

FIGURE 39.1. Generation of superoxide and peroxynitrite by nitric oxide (*NO*) synthases (*NOS*) in conditions of substrate or cofactor limitation. (Based on refs. 12, 14, and 15.)

NO and O_2^- is the likely result. As described above, the combination of NO and O_2^- results in the formation of peroxynitrite, which can be extremely toxic.

REGULATION OF NITRIC OXIDE SYNTHASE ACTIVITY

Transcriptional Regulation

Although iNOS and eNOS are commonly differentiated as inducible and constitutive forms, respectively, both forms are subject to regulation at the level of gene expression. Regulation by gene expression is most important for iNOS, as it constitutes the principal mechanism for regulation. Originally identified as being induced in macrophages, iNOS is now known to be induced in a wide range of cells. In the liver these include not only the Kupffer cells, but also hepatocytes, vascular endothelial cells, smooth muscle cells, and hepatic stellate cells. In general, iNOS is induced by inflammatory mediators (17). While iNOS can be induced by individual mediators, the level of induction is synergistically affected by combinations of extracellular stimuli such as the so-called cytomix [tumor necrosis factor-α (TNF-α) + interleukin-1β (IL-1β) + interferon-γ (IFN-γ) + endotoxin]. This synergism reflects the complexity of the promoter region of the human iNOS gene. Interestingly, in spite of the homology of NOS proteins between species, the iNOS promoter shows substantial variation between the human and murine genes (17). The human iNOS gene has a 5′ flanking region of approximately 16 kilobases (kb) and is dependent primarily on the binding of nuclear factor κB (NFκB), activating protein (AP-1), and signal transducer and activator of transcription 1α (STAT-1α) to their respective consensus sequences. In contrast, the murine 5′ flanking region is approximately 1 kb yet it contains additional sequences for IFN-stimulated response elements (ISREs) and hypoxia response elements (HREs). These differences may account for some of the differential results reported in studies in mice versus those using human cells. Nevertheless, in both species, activation of gene transcription by signaling pathways associated with inflammation is the primary mechanism for positive regulation of iNOS activity.

It is noteworthy that inflammatory mediators such as endotoxin and cytokines constitute far more potent inducers of the iNOS gene than does oxidative stress such as is associated with ischemia or reperfusion. iNOS transcription is also inhibited by transforming growth factor-β (TGF-β), which further contributes to decreased gene expression by destabilizing iNOS messenger RNA (mRNA).

Although eNOS is commonly considered to be a constitutive enzyme that is regulated posttranslationally by Ca^{2+} and calmodulin, enzyme levels are also regulated. Levels of eNOS are upregulated by stimuli such as shear stress (18). Levels are also upregulated in response to certain cholesterol-lowering drugs such as simvastatin (19). Conversely, eNOS levels have been reported to be decreased during inflammatory states such as endotoxemia (20,21).

Posttranslational Regulation

Unlike iNOS, which is primarily regulated by altering the amount of enzyme present, eNOS is exquisitely sensitive to posttranslational regulation (22). This degree of regulation is the result of the nature of the interaction between the NOS enzyme and calmodulin. While iNOS binds calmodulin and thus is active even at Ca^{2+} concentrations below that in resting cells, eNOS requires that calmodulin be bound to Ca^{2+} before binding. As a result, eNOS activity is primarily regulated by fluctuations in intracellular Ca^{2+}. This Ca^{2+} dependence allows eNOS to be regulated with a very short time constant and to be responsive to the presence of endothelium-dependent vasodilators [e.g., acetylcholine or adenosine triphosphate (ATP)] as well as physical factors such as shear stress.

Recent studies have also demonstrated that binding of calmodulin to eNOS can also be regulated by interactions with membrane-associated proteins such as caveolin-1 (22,23). eNOS is found in the particulate fraction of tissue homogenates, indicating that it normally exists as a membrane bound protein. Immunoprecipitation studies indicate that eNOS is associated with the specific membrane subdomain of the caveolae, where it is bound to caveolin-1. Binding to caveolin-1 maintains the eNOS in an inactive state until it is displaced by Ca^{2+} calmodulin, at which point it moves to the cytoplasm in an active state and generates NO. The significance of this interaction is that overexpression of caveolin-1 has been reported in conditions such as cirrhosis (24). Moreover, increased expression of caveolin-1 decreases the interaction of eNOS with calmodulin. This level of regulation may contribute significantly to the microvascular deficits observed in cirrhosis (see Blood Flow Regulation, below).

The association of eNOS with caveolae is related to its posttranslational regulation by fatty acylation (25). This involves the addition of two molecules of myristic acid during translation. This step is thought to be irreversible and is necessary for targeting to the caveolar membrane domain. An additional site can also be palmitoylated in a reversible manner. Both types of acylation serve to help anchor the NOS enzyme in the membrane, where it is held in an inactive state bound to caveolin. Palmitoylation is sensitive to signaling molecules and may serve as an additional mechanism to regulate the release of the eNOS from the membrane during agonist stimulation (22).

NITRIC OXIDE IN NORMAL REGULATION

Blood Flow Regulation

The significance of NO as an endogenous biologic signaling molecule was originally recognized in the context of its role as a vasodilator serving as the endothelium-dependent relaxing factor (26). In this capacity, NO is well recognized as an important regulator of local blood flow in many vascular beds. The role of NO in regulation of the hepatic circulation, however, has been less clear. Although a role for NO in the control of basal resistance in the hepatic artery has been easily identified (27–29), a functional role for eNOS in the portal circulation has been more controversial (30–32). On the other hand, iNOS is virtually absent in the normal liver, but highly upregulated in response to a variety of inflammatory or oxidative stresses. This led to the common postulate that iNOS, but not eNOS, contributed to maintaining sinusoidal perfusion following stress conditions (32). While very logical, the experimental results suggest that the situation is more complicated. Treatment of rats with nonspecific NOS or primarily eNOS inhibitors results in a rapid exacerbation of injury following stresses such as endotoxin injection (33,34). This exacerbation of injury is associated with local failure of microvascular perfusion (32) and the development of patchy necrosis (33). At the same time, in spite of marked upregulation of iNOS under these conditions, specific iNOS antagonists have little effect on liver perfusion and typically result in amelioration of injury if any effect is observed (35,36). Improvement in organ function appears to be more a function of support of the systemic circulation than of a direct effect on liver function (37). These results suggest that NO is necessary to maintain the sinusoidal perfusion, but that the relatively small amount generated by eNOS is adequate. The specific compartmentalization in the endothelial cells may also be significant in maintaining perfusion in that NO generated by endothelial cells or hepatic stellate cells, even at low levels, is capable of diffusing to the sites of action for vasoregulation (38).

Altered activity of eNOS may also be important in the development of increased intrahepatic resistance during the development of injury that leads to cirrhosis. Sinusoidal endothelial cells isolated from livers of rats subjected to CCl_4 or bile duct ligation exhibit a specific decrease in the enzymatic activity of eNOS without a decrease in total eNOS protein expression (4). A probable mechanism for this apparent posttranslational event that serves to functionally downregulate eNOS activity has recently been reported (24). As described above, eNOS is normally localized in caveolar subdomains of the plasma membrane of endothelial cells where it is found bound to the membrane protein caveolin-1 (22). A similar localization of eNOS associated with caveolae has been reported in cardiac myocytes in which eNOS binds to caveolin-3. There are two characteristics of this interaction that are of major importance: (a) binding of caveolin and Ca^{2+}-calmodulin by eNOS are mutually exclusive, and (b) binding of eNOS to caveolin maintains the eNOS in an inactive state. The mechanism of this inhibition appears to be the inhibition of the eNOS reductase domain by caveolin-binding (38a).

This mechanism may be highly significant in that caveolin binding inhibits not only the generation of NO but also the acceptance of electrons from NADPH. This would serve to prevent the caveolin-bound eNOS from synthesizing O_2^-. It is also significant that the caveolin-binding domain of eNOS does not appear to be present in iNOS, although it may be present in nNOS (22). Moreover, iNOS activity does not require Ca^{2+} binding to calmodulin. Therefore, caveolin-1 upregulation is not likely to affect NO production from iNOS.

This mechanism of regulation of eNOS activity appears to be of functional significance in the liver in light of the recent report by Shah et al. (24) demonstrating that caveolin-1 expression is upregulated in livers of rats with experimental cirrhosis. What is more, even though the total amount of calmodulin found in cell lysates was not changed with cirrhosis, the amount of calmodulin that could be coprecipitated with eNOS was dramatically diminished. In contrast, the amount of caveolin-1 that coprecipitated with eNOS was substantially increased. These results would suggest that overexpression of caveolin-1 in vascular endothelial cells of cirrhotic livers serves to functionally impair eNOS activity. This interpretation is further supported by the observation that NO production was decreased in these livers and vascular resistance was increased. Interestingly, preliminary results from our lab indicate that caveolin-1 is also upregulated in endotoxemia, a condition that also leads to increased portal resistance. This observation provides at least preliminary evidence that altered regulation of caveolin may be a common mechanism for the development of vascular deficits in the liver during inflammatory states.

There is reason to believe that NO may be involved in limiting the progression of liver diseases that involve vascular alterations such as in cirrhosis. Recent work from Rockey's group (39) showed that the portal hypertension that accompanies cirrhosis can be substantially ameliorated by transient transduction of the liver with nNOS. Hepatic stellate cells relax in response to NO both *in vitro* (40) and *in situ* (31) (see Chapter 39). In Rockey's group's (39) experiments, the adenovirus vector preferentially transduced the hepatic stellate cells. As a result, local production of NO would limit the vasoconstrictive effects of stellate cell activation, thus limiting perfusion deficits. Indeed, Rockey's group found that the transduced livers had a significantly lower portal pressure. Interestingly, the major effect on resistance was on the pressure at zero flow, which is an indicator of sinusoidal sites of action. This finding is consistent with action of NO on the hepatic stellate cells to limit the resistance to flow. In addition, the antiinflammatory actions of NO may serve to limit the activation of the stellate cells. These areas warrant further investigation.

The exact mechanisms by which eNOS regulates sinusoidal perfusion is not clear. Sinusoidal endothelial cells respond to shear stress with increased NO release (5,41), but the portal circulation does not dilate in response to the classic endothelium-dependent vasodilator ATP (42). However, endothelin acting through endothelin (ET)$_{B1}$ receptors is coupled to NO production, while putative ET$_{B2}$ receptors cause constriction (43). Many studies have shown that endothelin and its receptors are altered in response to injurious or inflammatory stimuli in the liver. ET$_B$ receptors are upregulated in cirrhosis (44) and following inflammatory or oxidative stress (45). This change in receptor expression may contribute to the changes in vascular response in these stress conditions (46). Recent work from our lab has shown that ET$_B$ receptors are upregulated during endotoxemia. Concurrently, the portal pressure and sinusoid constrictor responses to ET$_B$ agonists as well as liver injury are markedly potentiated by pretreatment with L-NAME (47). Indeed, in the absence of L-NAME, the ET$_B$ agonist IRL 1620 did not cause sinusoidal constriction while in the presence of L-NAME; contraction of the stellate cells resulting in constriction of the sinusoid was clearly demonstrated (47). These results suggest a compensatory upregulation of eNOS stimulation via increased coupling to ET$_B$ receptors. Such a response would contribute to the protection of sinusoidal perfusion during upregulation of endothelins. One caveat that must be considered in interpreting results reporting the effects of NOS inhibitors on liver perfusion is that initiation of inflammation in the liver typically results in systemic effects that give rise to induction of iNOS in peripheral vascular tissue. This is certainly the case in endotoxemia or sepsis, in which the circulatory collapse that results in septic shock has been ascribed to the gross overexpression of iNOS in resistance vessels (48). As such, treatment *in vivo* with NOS inhibitors is likely to produce significant changes in hepatic perfusion just by virtue of the fact that systemic hemodynamics are disrupted.

Although NO was originally identified as a modulator of blood flow via its vasodilatory properties, it also has an important impact on injury-related blood flow regulation by virtue of its effect on neutrophil adhesion to vascular endothelium as well as platelet aggregation. Considerable evidence now indicates that neutrophil accumulation following inflammatory or oxidative stress in the liver contributes to hepatocyte injury (49,50). In such cases, administration of NOS antagonists significantly increases the accumulation of neutrophils and exacerbates liver injury to a similar extent (34,51). Interestingly, NOS inhibition in this study also inhibited the generation of peroxynitrite but still exacerbated injury (52). These results suggest that NO exerts an antiinflammatory effect by attenuating adhesion of neutrophils. The mechanism of this inhibitory effect on neutrophil adhesion is likely the result of inhibition of expression of vascular adhesion molecules p-selectin and intercellular adhesion molecule-1 (ICAM-1) (53). Of these, ICAM-1 is probably the more important since it is required for emigration of the neutrophils from the vascular space, and blocking ICAM-1 attenuates injury without decreasing sinusoidal neutrophil sequestration (54). NO may also

serve to antagonize sinusoidal constriction, thus attenuating physical trapping of neutrophils in the sinusoids (55). Additionally, NO released from endothelial cells inhibits platelet aggregation, thus further contributing to the maintenance of microvascular perfusion (33). In summary, NO, especially that derived from the eNOS localized in sinusoidal endothelial cells, is required to maintain perfusion of the hepatic microcirculation. This effect is mediated by a combination of (a) vasodilatory effects that counter the increased vasoconstrictor tone resulting from upregulation of endothelin, (b) inhibition of neutrophil adhesion or emigration, and (c) inhibition of platelet aggregation.

Carbon Monoxide in Hepatic Regulation

The role of NO in regulating microvascular perfusion in the liver is further complicated by the reports that carbon monoxide (CO) generated by heme oxygenase also contributes to the regulation of hepatic perfusion (56,57). Similar to the NOSs, heme oxygenases exist in constitutive and inducible forms. Heme oxygenase-1 (HO-1) is a stress-inducible isoform of HO also known as heat shock protein 32. It is induced by oxidative stress and heat shock as well as other potentially injurious stimuli, including NO (29,58). Heme oxygenase-2 is a constitutive enzyme that serves as an important step in the catabolism of heme from heme-containing proteins such as hemoglobin and the cytochromes. Both enzymes catalyze the conversion of heme to biliverdin and CO. Biliverdin is subsequently converted to bilirubin. Under normal conditions, HO-2 is the dominant isoform in the liver expressed primarily in hepatocytes. HO-1 is expressed at only low levels, primarily in Kupffer cells. CO, like NO, binds to heme proteins and can thus activate guanyl cyclase in a manner similar to NO. Although the binding affinity of CO for heme is much less than that of NO, the estimated concentrations in the microenvironment of the vasculature is much higher than that of NO. In certain injuries such as that which accompanies hemorrhagic shock and resuscitation, inhibition of HO-1, but not NOS, impairs sinusoidal perfusion and exacerbates injury (29). HO-1 induction has also been reported to be protective in sepsis (59). This suggests that NO and CO may act as redundant mechanisms to help protect sinusoidal perfusion following injury. The relative importance of each is most likely related to the specific injury, especially with respect to the relative degrees of upregulation of HO-1 vs. NOS.

While the generation of CO by HO-1 appears to be an important regulator of vascular tone, it is also necessary to consider that generation of CO by heme oxygenase also cogenerates antioxidant capacity in the form of the biliverdin–bilirubin system (Fig. 39.2). Although this has been considered to be a theoretical contributor to vascular protection, recent work has suggested that this property may account for the entire protective capacity as assessed by

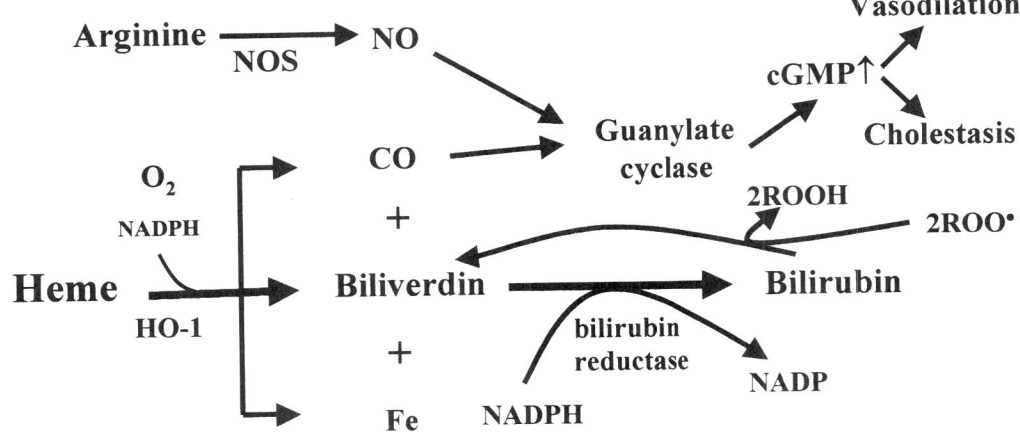

FIGURE 39.2. Mechanisms of production of carbon monoxide (*CO*) and biliverdin by heme oxygenase. In addition to the interaction between CO and nitric oxide (*NO*) in activating guanyl cylcase, the reaction produces bilirubin catalyzed by biliverdin reductase. Bilirubin is reconverted to biliverdin in scavenging reactive oxygen. The system is regenerated by biliverdin reductase in the presence of reduced nicotinamide adenine dinucleotide phosphate (*NADPH*).

inhibition of p-selectin expression (60). This will be an important area of investigation for the near future.

In addition to its effects on the vasculature, CO has been proposed to be an important modulator of other cell functions (61). While many of these effects are likely mediated by the antioxidant properties of bilirubin, recent studies have shown that CO modulates biliary function at least partly via a cGMP-dependent mechanism. Inhibition of heme oxygenase with Zn protoporphyrin IX exerts a choleretic effect that is reversed by exogenous CO and partly reversed by 8-bromo-cGMP. This effect correlates with a decrease in the spontaneous rate of bile canaliculus contraction in response to CO. Additionally, exogenous CO opens paracellular pathways between blood and bile. The functional implications of these responses are not yet well elucidated.

REGULATION OF METABOLISM

In 1985, West et al. (62) reported that conditioned medium from Kupffer cells inhibited protein synthesis in hepatocytes. This effect was subsequently found to be dependent on induction of iNOS in the hepatocytes (63). Ultimately, this discovery led to the cloning of the human iNOS from hepatocytes (64,65). Since that time, NO has been implicated in a myriad of mechanisms regulating liver metabolism. These include inhibition of protein synthesis (66,67), gluconeogenesis (68,69), and mitochondrial respiration as well as metabolic inhibition resulting from depletion of pyridine nucleotides as a result of activation of the polyadenylate ribose synthase (PARS) pathway (70). Typically, these effects require relatively high levels of NO and

may also require sufficient oxidant production (e.g., superoxide) to produce significant amounts of peroxynitrite.

It is well known that hepatic gluconeogenic response is downregulated during inflammatory states such as sepsis or endotoxemia. Moreover, the time course of changes in gluconeogenesis is similar to the appearance of iNOS induction. Exogenous NO also inhibits gluconeogenesis. The contribution of NO to the suppression of gluconeogenesis is only partial since NO specifically inhibits the activity of glyceraldehyde-3-phosphate dehydrogenase via sulfhydryl interaction (68,69) while the decrease in gluconeogenesis in sepsis is largely dependent on the transcriptional downregulation of phosphoenol pyruvate carboxykinase (71,72). This suggests that NO-mediated inhibition of gluconeogenesis may be present, but is not the primary mechanism for decreased gluconeogenesis.

The effects of NO on mitochondrial respiration are likely to be of greater significance. NO interacts with the heme groups of the cytochromes of the electron transport chain, resulting in decreased respiratory activity (73–76). The net effect of these actions is a decrease in the metabolic rate of the hepatocytes. Although it is clear that NO interaction with these enzymes causes decreased oxidative capacity of the mitochondria, it is not clear that this decreased capacity significantly contributes to development of liver injury. NO can also affect mitochondrial permeability.

Since many of the metabolic effects of NO appear to be regulated directly by peroxynitrite rather than NO itself, it is important to consider conditions in which peroxynitrite formation might be enhanced. While temporal association of NOS activity with the presence of oxidative stress (e.g., via xanthine oxidase activation) has been considered as a primary source of peroxynitrite, it is now recognized that all three isoforms of NOS are capable of generating superoxide instead of NO when substrate (arginine) or cofactor (tetrahydro-biopterin) are inadequately available (13). The result is cogeneration of NO and O_2^- by the same enzyme. This mechanism is likely to be particularly significant in inflammatory states in which highly upregulated levels of iNOS consume substantial quantities of both arginine and BH_4. The exact functional implications remain to be elucidated.

NITRIC OXIDE IN APOPTOSIS

Perhaps the most significant direct cellular effect of NO with respect to hepatic injury is via its effect on apoptosis. Many reports have indicated that high levels of NO induce apoptosis in many cell types. This effect appears to be mediated primarily by the effect of peroxynitrite on increases in mitochondrial permeability either directly (77,78,78a) or through DNA damage with subsequent activation of the PARS pathway (79,80). This mitochondrial permeability transition results in the release of cytochrome *c* from the mitochondria, which constitutes a signal for apoptosis (72,78,81,82). More recently it has been recognized that NO can exert biphasic effects on apoptosis (83). In addition to being proapoptotic, studies indicate that even relatively low levels of NO can effectively inhibit apoptosis (84–86). At very low levels of NO, apoptosis is inhibited by inhibiting caspase-3–like activity. This effect appears to be mediated by S-nitrosylation of the enzyme (85,87). Moreover, even prolonged exposure to relatively high levels of NO can protect from TNF-α–induced apoptosis by inducing heat shock protein 70 (HSP 70) (86). It has been shown that apoptosis is a significant mechanism leading to hepatic cell death during inflammatory states. Since the same stimuli also induce iNOS in hepatocytes, this may constitute a self-limiting mechanism to control the rate of apoptosis. The notion that this is part of a regulated system is supported by the observation that p53, which leads to apoptosis in cells with DNA damage, also downregulates expression of iNOS (88,89). Thus cells responding to inflammatory stimuli for apoptosis but not those undergoing apoptosis in response to DNA damage can be salvaged by the effect of NO. Such a mechanism may provide protection against excessive cell death during inflammatory responses without preventing the elimination of cells with damaged DNA (88,89). It may also contribute to the role of iNOS induction in liver regeneration (89,90). Failure of this mechanism may be responsible for the proposed tumorigenic actions of NO (91–93). As is the case in the capacity for NO to regulate metabolic response in the liver, the effect of NO generation on apoptosis is likely to be modulated by the degree of coupling of the enzyme to NO production rather than generation of O_2^-. Thus, in the absence of adequate substrate or cofactor, activation of NOS would be predicted to lead to enhanced mitochondrial and DNA damage mediated by peroxynitrite

generation. The exact impact of uncoupling of NOS activity from NO synthesis *in vivo* remains to be elucidated.

CONCLUSION

NO plays important and diverse roles in the liver with the potential for both protection of the liver cells from injury as well as exacerbation of injury. The most important factors in determining whether NO will be protective or injurious are the localization of NO production, the amount of NO being produced, and the relative amounts of superoxide anion being produced in the same location as the NO. The small amounts of NO produced by eNOS in endothelial cells appear to be necessary and perhaps sufficient to maintain perfusion and to provide the necessary antiinflammatory and antithrombotic effects. Moreover, it is not likely that endothelial cell–derived NO exerts any injurious effect in the liver. Indeed, functional downregulation of eNOS by overexpression of and binding to caveolin-1 has been implicated as a probable mechanism for vascular impairment in experimental cirrhosis. Although upregulation of iNOS was originally considered to be part of the host defense by increasing the killing capacity of macrophages, iNOS function in the liver has focused largely on induction in hepatocytes. When the conditions are right for peroxynitrite generation, NO, via formation of peroxynitrite, can damage cellular components including DNA by its strong oxidizing effect. The probability for significant peroxynitrite synthesis is increased by inadequate arginine or BH_4 availability. This situation results in an electron being transferred to O_2 to form superoxide without completion of the transfer of the oxygen to arginine. In addition, NO can directly inhibit enzyme activities by interaction with sulfhydryl groups and metal-centered groups such as heme. Although these interactions result in inhibition of specific metabolic pathways, it is not clear that metabolic inhibition necessarily leads to cell injury but rather may constitute a normal regulatory mechanism. Indeed in the case of inhibition of caspase activity, enzyme inhibition results in protection from apoptotic cell death. Thus, although NO in very high concentrations induces cell injury under some conditions, the preponderance of evidence would suggest that under most conditions endogenous NO exerts protective effects in the liver.

REFERENCES

1. Knowles RG, Merrett M, Salter M, et al. Differential induction of brain, lung and liver nitric oxide synthase by endotoxin in the rat. *Biochem J* 1990;270:833–836.
2. Esteban FJ, Pedrosa JA, Jimenez A, et al. Distribution of neuronal nitric oxide synthase in the rat liver. *Neurosci Lett* 1997; 226:99–102.
3. Clemens MG. Does altered regulation of ecNOS in sinusoidal endothelial cells determine increased intrahepatic resistance

leading to portal hypertension? *Hepatology* 1998;27: 1745–1747.

4. Rockey DC, Chung JJ. Reduced nitric oxide production by endothelial cells in cirrhotic rat liver: endothelial dysfunction in portal hypertension. *Gastroenterology* 1998;114:344–351.

5. Shah V, Haddad FG, Garcia-Cardena G, et al. Liver sinusoidal endothelial cells are responsible for nitric oxide modulation of resistance in the hepatic sinusoids. *J Clin Invest* 1997;100: 2923–2930.

6. Nathan C, Xie QW. Nitric oxide synthases: roles, tolls, and controls. *Cell* 1994;78:915–918.

7. Grisham MB, Jourd'Heuil D, Wink DA. Nitric oxide. I. Physiological chemistry of nitric oxide and its metabolites: implications in inflammation. *Am J Physiol* 1999;276:G315–G321.

8. Miller MJ, Sandoval M. Nitric Oxide. III. A molecular prelude to intestinal inflammation. *Am J Physiol* 1999;276: G795–G799.

9. Stamler JS, Singel DJ, Loscalzo J. Biochemistry of nitric oxide and its redox-activated forms [see comments]. *Science* 1992; 258:1898–1902.

10. Beckman JS, Koppenol WH. Nitric oxide, superoxide, and peroxynitrite: the good, the bad, and ugly. *Am J Physiol* 1996;271: C1424–C1437.

11. Crow JP, Beckman JS. The importance of superoxide in nitric oxide-dependent toxicity: evidence for peroxynitrite-mediated injury. *Adv Exp Med Biol* 1996;387:147–161.

12. Knowles RG, Moncada S. Nitric oxide synthases in mammals. *Biochem J* 1994;298:249–258.

13. Vasquez-Vivar J, Kalyanaraman B, Martasek P, et al. Superoxide generation by endothelial nitric oxide synthase: the influence of cofactors. *Proc Natl Acad Sci USA* 1998;95:9220–9225.

14. Vasquez-Vivar J, Hogg N, Martasek P, et al. Tetrahydrobiopterin-dependent inhibition of superoxide generation from neuronal nitric oxide synthase. *J Biol Chem* 1999;274:26736–26742.

15. Schmidt HH, Hofmann H, Schindler U, et al. NO from NO synthase. *Proc Natl Acad Sci USA* 1996;93:14492–14497.

16. Xia Y, Tsai AL, Berka V, et al. Superoxide generation from endothelial nitric-oxide synthase. A Ca2+/calmodulin-dependent and tetrahydrobiopterin regulatory process. *J Biol Chem* 1998;273:25804–25808.

17. Taylor BS, Geller DA. Molecular regulation of the human inducible nitric oxide synthase (iNOS) gene [In Process Citation]. *Shock* 2000;13:413–424.[MEDLINE record in process 13:413–424.]

18. Topper JN, Cai J, Falb D, et al. Identification of vascular endothelial genes differentially responsive to fluid mechanical stimuli: cyclooxygenase-2, manganese superoxide dismutase, and endothelial cell nitric oxide synthase are selectively up-regulated by steady laminar shear stress. *Proc Natl Acad Sci USA* 1996;93:10417–10422.

19. Pruefer D, Scalia R, Lefer AM. Simvastatin inhibits leukocyte-endothelial cell interactions and protects against inflammatory processes in normocholesterolemic rats. *Arterioscler Thromb Vasc Biol* 1999;19:2894–2900.

20. Chen K, Inoue M, Wasa M, et al. Expression of endothelial constitutive nitric oxide synthase mRNA in gastrointestinal mucosa and its downregulation by endotoxin. *Life Sci* 1997;61: 1323–1329.

21. Liu SF, Adcock IM, Old RW, et al. Differential regulation of the constitutive and inducible nitric oxide synthase mRNA by lipopolysaccharide treatment in vivo in the rat. *Crit Care Med* 1996;24:1219–1225.

22. Michel T, Feron O. Nitric oxide synthases: which, where, how, and why? *J Clin Invest* 1997;100:2146–2152.

23. Michel JB, Feron O, Sase K, et al. Caveolin versus calmodulin.

24. Shah V, Toruner M, Haddad F, et al. Impaired endothelial nitric oxide synthase activity associated with enhanced caveolin binding in experimental cirrhosis in the rat. *Gastroenterology* 1999; 117:1222–1228.

25. Feron O, Michel JB, Sase K, et al. Dynamic regulation of endothelial nitric oxide synthase: complementary roles of dual acylation and caveolin interactions. *Biochemistry* 1998;37: 193–200.

26. Coccheri S, Nazzari M. Defibrotide as a possible anti-ischemic drug. *Semin Thromb Hemost* 1996;22(suppl 1):9–14.

27. Ayuse T, Brienza N, Revelly JP, et al. Role of nitric oxide in porcine liver circulation under normal and endotoxemic conditions. *J Appl Physiol* 1995;78:1319–1329.

28. Mathie RT, Ralevic V, Alexander B, et al. Nitric oxide is the mediator of ATP-induced dilatation of the rabbit hepatic arterial vascular bed. *Br J Pharmacol* 1991;103:1602–1606.

29. Pannen BH, Bauer M. Differential regulation of hepatic arterial and portal venous vascular resistance by nitric oxide and carbon monoxide in rats. *Life Sci* 1998;62:2025–2033.

30. Mittal MK, Gupta TK, Lee FY, et al. Nitric oxide modulates hepatic vascular tone in normal rat liver. *Am J Physiol* 1994; 267:G416–G422.

31. Zhang JX, Pegoli WJ, Clemens MG. Endothelin-1 induces direct constriction of hepatic sinusoids. *Am J Physiol* 1994;266: G624–G632.

32. Shibayama Y, Nakata K. Role of septal fibrosis in development of hepatic circulatory disturbance in the presence of liver cell enlargement. *Liver* 1992;12:84–89.

33. Harbrecht BG, Billiar TR, Stadler J, et al. Inhibition of nitric oxide synthesis during endotoxemia promotes intrahepatic thrombosis and an oxygen radical-mediated hepatic injury. *J Leukoc Biol* 1992;52:390–394.

34. Harbrecht BG, Wu B, Watkins SC, et al. Inhibition of nitric oxide synthase during hemorrhagic shock increases hepatic injury. *Shock* 1995;4:332–337.

35. Saetre T, Gundersen Y, Thiemermann C, et al. Aminoethylisothiourea, a selective inhibitor of inducible nitric oxide synthase activity, improves liver circulation and oxygen metabolism in a porcine model of endotoxemia. *Shock* 1998;9:109–115.

36. Thiemermann C, Ruetten H, Wu CC, et al. The multiple organ dysfunction syndrome caused by endotoxin in the rat: attenuation of liver dysfunction by inhibitors of nitric oxide synthase. *Br J Pharmacol* 1995;116:2845–2851.

37. Wray GM, Millar CG, Hinds CJ, et al. Selective inhibition of the activity of inducible nitric oxide synthase prevents the circulatory failure, but not the organ injury/dysfunction, caused by endotoxin. *Shock* 1998;9:329–335.

38. Ou J, Carlos TM, Watkins SC, et al. Differential effects of nonselective nitric oxide synthase (NOS) and selective inducible NOS inhibition on hepatic necrosis, apoptosis, ICAM-1 expression, and neutrophil accumulation during endotoxemia. *Nitric Oxide* 1997;1:404–416.

38a. Ghosh S, Gachhui C, Crooks C, et al. Interaction between caveolin-1 and reductase domain of endothelial nitric-oxide synthase. Consequences for catalysis. *J Biol Chem* 1998;273:22267–22271.

39. Yu Q, Shao R, Qian HS, et al. Gene transfer of the neuronal NO synthase isoform to cirrhotic rat liver ameliorates portal hypertension. *J Clin Invest* 2000;105:741–748.

40. Rockey DC, Chung JJ. Inducible nitric oxide synthase in rat hepatic lipocytes and the effect of nitric oxide on lipocyte contractility. *J Clin Invest* 1995;95:1199–1206.

41. Macedo MP, Lautt WW. Shear-induced modulation of vasoconstriction in the hepatic artery and portal vein by nitric oxide. *Am J Physiol* 1998;274:G253–G260.

42. Lee JW, Filkins JP. Exogenous ATP and hepatic hemodynamics in the perfused rat liver. *Circ Shock* 1988;24:99–110.

43. Higuchi H, Satoh T. Endothelin-1 induces vasoconstriction and nitric oxide release via endothelin ET(B) receptors in isolated perfused rat liver. *Eur J Pharmacol* 1997;328:175–182.

44. Gandhi CR, Sproat LA, Subbotin VM. Increased hepatic endothelin-1 levels and endothelin receptor density in cirrhotic rats. *Life Sci* 1996;58:55–62.

45. Sonin NV, Garcia-Pagan JC, Nakanishi K, et al. Patterns of vasoregulatory gene expression in the liver response to ischemia/reperfusion and endotoxemia. *Shock* 1999;11:175–179.

46. Clemens MG, Bauer M, Pannen BH, et al. Remodeling of hepatic microvascular responsiveness after ischemia/reperfusion. *Shock* 1997;8:80–85.

47. Bauer M, Bauer I, Sonin NV, et al. Functional significance of endothelin B receptors in mediating sinusoidal and extrasinusoidal effects of endothelins in the intact rat liver [see comments]. *Hepatology* 2000;31:937–947.

48. Vallance P, Moncada S. Role of endogenous nitric oxide in septic shock. *New Horiz* 1993;1:77–86.

49. Saarela J, Rehn M, Oikarinen A, et al. The short and long forms of type XVIII collagen show clear tissue specificities in their expression and location in basement membrane zones in humans. *Am J Pathol* 1998;153:611–626.

50. Liu P, McGuire GM, Fisher MA, et al. Activation of Kupffer cells and neutrophils for reactive oxygen formation is responsible for endotoxin-enhanced liver injury after hepatic ischemia. *Shock* 1995;3:56–62.

51. Fukatsu K, Saito H, Han I, et al. Nitric oxide donor decreases neutrophil adhesion in both lung and peritoneum during peritonitis. *J Surg Res* 1998;74:119–124.

52. Liu P, Yin K, Nagele R, et al. Inhibition of nitric oxide synthase attenuates peroxynitrite generation, but augments neutrophil accumulation in hepatic ischemia-reperfusion in rats. *J Pharmacol Exp Ther* 1998;284:1139–1146.

53. Liu P, Xu B, Hock CE, et al. NO modulates P-selectin and ICAM-1 mRNA expression and hemodynamic alterations in hepatic I/R. *Am J Physiol* 1998;275:H2191–H2198.

54. Farhood A, McGuire GM, Manning AM, et al. Intercellular adhesion molecule 1 (ICAM-1) expression and its role in neutrophil-induced ischemia-reperfusion injury in rat liver. *J Leukoc Biol* 1995;57:368–374.

55. Jaeschke H, Smith CW, Clemens MG, et al. Mechanisms of inflammatory liver injury: adhesion molecules and cytotoxicity of neutrophils. *Toxicol Appl Pharmacol* 1996;139:213–226.

56. Suematsu M, Kashiwagi S, Sano T, et al. Carbon monoxide as an endogenous modulator of hepatic vascular perfusion. *Biochem Biophys Res Commun* 1994;205:1333–1337.

57. Suematsu M, Goda N, Sano T, et al. Carbon monoxide: an endogenous modulator of sinusoidal tone in the perfused rat liver. *J Clin Invest* 1995;96:2431–2437.

58. Bauer M, Pannen BHJ, Bauer I, et al. Evidence for a functional link between stress response and vascular control in hepatic portal circulation. *Am J Physiol* 1996;271:G929–G935.

59. Downard PJ, Wilson MA, Spain DA, et al. Heme oxygenase-dependent carbon monoxide production is a hepatic adaptive response to sepsis. *J Surg Res* 1997;71:7–12.

60. Vachharajani TJ, Work J, Issekutz AC, et al. Heme oxygenase modulates selectin expression in different regional vascular beds. *Am J Physiol Heart Circ Physiol* 2000;278:H1613–H1617.

61. Suematsu M, Ishimura Y. The heme oxygenase-carbon monoxide system: a regulator of hepatobiliary function. *Hepatology* 2000;31:3–6.

62. West MA, Keller GA, Hyland BJ, et al. Hepatocyte function in sepsis: Kupffer cells mediate a biphasic protein synthesis response in hepatocytes after exposure to endotoxin or killed *Escherichia coli*. *Surgery* 1985;98:388–395.

63. Billiar TR, Curran RD, Ferrari FK, et al. Kupffer cell: hepatocyte cocultures release nitric oxide in response to bacterial endotoxin. *J Surg Res* 1990;48:349–353.

64. Chartrain NA, Geller DA, Koty PP, et al. Molecular cloning, structure, and chromosomal localization of the human inducible nitric oxide synthase gene. *J Biol Chem* 1994;269:6765–6772.

65. Ferrante A, Jenkin CR, Reade PC. Changes in the activity of the reticulo-endothelial system of rats during an infection with *T. lewisi*. *Aust J Exp Biol Med Sci* 1978;56:47–59.

66. Curran RD, Ferrari FK, Kispert PH, et al. Nitric oxide and nitric oxide-generating compounds inhibit hepatocyte protein synthesis. *FASEB J* 1991;5:2085–2092.

67. Thelen M, Schulz D, Schild H, et al. [Changes in liver haemodynamics after mesenterico-caval dacron prosthesis anastomosis ("H-shunt") in portal hypertension (author's transl)]. Anderungen der Leberhamodynamik nach mesenterikokavaler Dacron-Prothesen-Anastomose (sog. "H-Shunt") bei portaler Hypertension. *ROFO* 1978;128:423–431.

68. Ou J, Molina L, Kim YM, et al. Excessive NO production does not account for the inhibition of hepatic gluconeogenesis in endotoxemia. *Am J Physiol* 1996;271:G621–G628.

69. Mahnke PF, Keitel R, Otto U. [Morphological studies on swine livers after extracorporeal perfusion]. Morphologische Untersuchungen an Schweinelebern nach extrakorporaler Perfusion. *Z Exp Chir* 1978;11:95–102.

70. Szabo C. Potential role of the peroxynitrate-poly(ADP-ribose) synthetase pathway in a rat model of severe hemorrhagic shock. *Shock* 1998;9:341–344.

71. Wang K, Deutschman CS, Clemens MG, et al. Reciprocal expression of phosphoenolpyruvate carboxykinase and acute phase genes during acute inflammation. *Shock* 1995;3:204–209.

72. Fraser R, Bosanquet AG, Day WA. Filtration of chylomicrons by the liver may influence cholesterol metabolism and atherosclerosis. *Atherosclerosis* 1978;29:113–123.

73. Fisch C, Robin MA, Letteron P, et al. Cell-generated nitric oxide inactivates rat hepatocyte mitochondria in vitro but reacts with hemoglobin in vivo. *Gastroenterology* 1996;110:210–220.

74. Giulivi C. Functional implications of nitric oxide produced by mitochondria in mitochondrial metabolism. *Biochem J* 1998;332:673–679.

75. Kantrow SP, Taylor DE, Carraway MS, et al. Oxidative metabolism in rat hepatocytes and mitochondria during sepsis. *Arch Biochem Biophys* 1997;345:278–288.

76. Kurose I, Kato S, Ishii H, et al. Nitric oxide mediates lipopolysaccharide-induced alteration of mitochondrial function in cultured hepatocytes and isolated perfused liver. *Hepatology* 1993;18:380–388.

77. Balakirev MY, Khramtsov VV, Zimmer G. Modulation of the mitochondrial permeability transition by nitric oxide. *Eur J Biochem* 1997;246:710–718.

78. Hortelano S, Dallaporta B, Zamzami N, et al. Nitric oxide induces apoptosis via triggering mitochondrial permeability transition. *FEBS Lett* 1997;410:373–377.

78a. Balakirev MY, Khramtsov VV, Zimmer G. Modulation of the mitochondrial permeability transition by nitric oxide. *Eur J Biochem* 1997;246:710–718.

79. Szabo C, Ohshima H. DNA damage induced by peroxynitrite: subsequent biological effects. *Nitric Oxide* 1997;1:373–385.

80. Szabo C. DNA strand breakage and activation of poly-ADP ribosyltransferase: a cytotoxic pathway triggered by peroxynitrite. *Free Radic Biol Med* 1996;21:855–869.

81. Costantini P, Petronilli V, Colonna R, et al. On the effects of paraquat on isolated mitochondria. Evidence that paraquat

causes opening of the cyclosporin A-sensitive permeability transition pore synergistically with nitric oxide. *Toxicology* 1995;99: 77–88.

82. Packer MA, Murphy MP. Peroxynitrite causes calcium efflux from mitochondria which is prevented by cyclosporin A. *FEBS Lett* 1994;345:237–240.

83. Kim YM, Bombeck CA, Billiar TR. Nitric oxide as a bifunctional regulator of apoptosis. *Circ Res* 1999;84:253–256.

84. Kim YM, Talanian RV, Billiar TR. Nitric oxide inhibits apoptosis by preventing increases in caspase-3–like activity via two distinct mechanisms. *J Biol Chem* 1997;272:31138–31148.

85. Duca C, Duca S, Uray Z, et al. Improvement of perfusion flow in the isolated rat liver under the influence of streptase. Autohistoradiographic aspects of 125I-labelled fibrinogen deposition. *Arzneimittelforschung* 1978;28:407–409.

86. Kim YM, de Vera ME, Watkins SC, et al. Nitric oxide protects cultured rat hepatocytes from tumor necrosis factor-alpha-induced apoptosis by inducing heat shock protein 70 expression. *J Biol Chem* 1997;272:1402–1411.

87. Li J, Billiar TR, Talanian RV, et al. Nitric oxide reversibly inhibits seven members of the caspase family via S-nitrosylation. *Biochem Biophys Res Commun* 1997;240:419–424.

88. Ambs S, Ogunfusika MO, Merriam WG, et al. Up-regulation of inducible nitric oxide synthase expression in cancer-prone p53 knockout mice. *Proc Natl Acad Sci USA* 1998;95: 8823–8828.

89. Storch W. [About the differentiation of antibodies against the connective tissue (author's transl)].Zur Differenzierung von Antikorpern gegen Bindegewebe. *Acta Histochem* 1978;62:57–67.

90. Rai RM, Lee FY, Rosen A, et al. Impaired liver regeneration in inducible nitric oxide synthase-deficient mice. *Proc Natl Acad Sci USA* 1998;95:13829–13834.

91. Bartsch H, Ohshima H, Pignatelli B, et al. Endogenously formed N-nitroso compounds and nitrosating agents in human cancer etiology. *Pharmacogenetics* 1992;2:272–277.

92. Kew MC, Minick OT, Bahu RM, et al. Ultrastructural changes in the liver in heatstroke. *Am J Pathol* 1978;90:609–618.

93. Ohshima H, Bartsch H. Chronic infections and inflammatory processes as cancer risk factors: possible role of nitric oxide in carcinogenesis. *Mutat Res* 1994;305:253–264.

The Liver: Biology and Pathobiology, Fourth Edition, edited by I. M. Arias, J. L. Boyer, F. V. Chisari, N. Fausto, D. Schachter, and D. A. Shafritz.
Lippincott Williams & Wilkins, Philadelphia © 2001.

INTERLEUKIN-6 SIGNALING DURING THE ACUTE-PHASE RESPONSE OF THE LIVER

JOHANNES G. BODE
PETER C. HEINRICH

Recent reviews on the subject of cytokines and the acute phase response have been published (1–6) (see Chapter 41). This chapter focuses on the acute-phase response of the liver with emphasis on interleukin-6 (IL-6) signal transduction regulating acute-phase protein (APP) expression.

J. G. Bode: Department of Internal Medicine, Division of Gastroenterology Hepatology and Infectiology, Laboratory of Experimental Hepatology, Heinrich-Heine University, Düsseldorf, 40225 Düsseldorf, Germany.

P. C. Heinrich: Department of Biochemistry, University Hospital of the Rheinisch Westfälische Technische Hochschule Aachen, D-52074 Aachen, Germany.

ACUTE-PHASE RESPONSE OF THE ORGANISM

Neoplasm, tissue injury, infection, or inflammation are accompanied by a number of changes within the organism, representing an immediate set of inflammatory reactions counteracting these challenges, aiming at the isolation and neutralization of pathogens and the prevention of further pathogen entry. The resulting minimization of tissue damage and promotion of repair processes permits the homeostatic mechanisms of the organism to rapidly restore normal physiologic function. The inflammatory cascade is initiated through activated blood monocytes and tissue macrophages at the sites of injury by the release of a set of primary inflammatory mediators, such as histamine, leukotrienes, prostaglandins, and the proinflammatory cytokines IL-1β

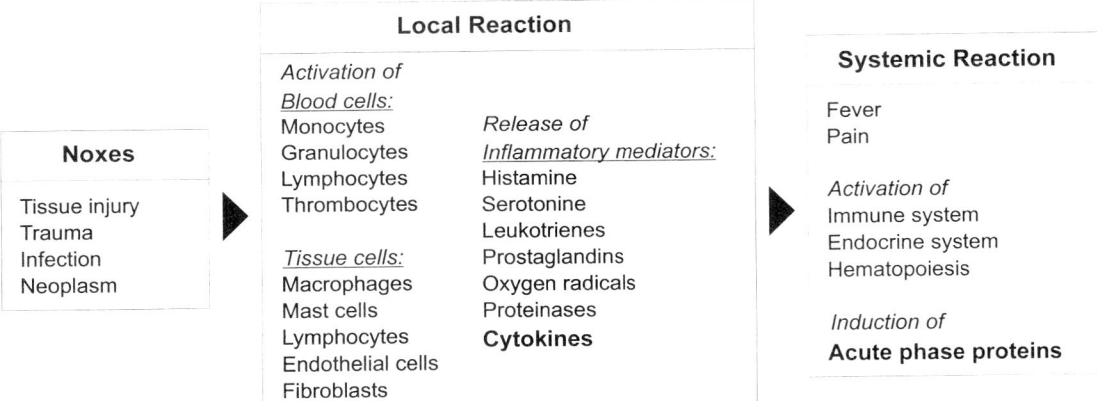

FIGURE 40.1. The acute inflammation process.

and tumor necrosis factor-α (TNF-α) (Fig. 40.1) (reviewed in refs. 1–6). These again induce the synthesis of a range of secondary cytokines and chemokines such as IL-6 and IL-8 from macrophages, monocytes, endothelial cells, and fibroblasts. The chemotactic activities of some of these molecules in turn lead to the attraction of neutrophils and other immune effector cells, e.g., lymphocytes, to the site of inflammation, where the immigrated cells release further inflammatory cytokines. This process rapidly enhances the local inflammatory response to counteract the inflammatory stimulus and to tidy up the cellular debris generated by any associated tissue damage.

This local response may escalate into a systemic reaction of the organism characterized by the induction of neuroendocrine changes such as, for example, pain, fever, somnolence, and increased release of such systemically acting mediators as arginine, vasopressin, insulin-like growth factor, corticotropin-releasing hormone, corticotropin, and others. Furthermore, hematopoietic alterations such as leukocytosis and thrombocytosis, metabolic disturbances such as cachexia, and modifications of the lipid metabolism and decreased gluconeogenesis belong to the characteristic, systemic phenomena observed during the acute-phase reaction.

Apart from these systemic alterations, changes of plasma levels of several different proteins, known as the acute-phase proteins have been recognized as a characteristic feature of the acute-phase response (Table 40.1). Increases or decreases in concentrations of these proteins are mainly attributed to modifications of their synthesis by hepatocytes. The extent of these changes varies largely and depends on the species investigated. Thus, α_2-macroglobulin and α_1-acid glycoprotein are major APPs in rats with increases of about 100-fold during inflammation, whereas the plasma concentrations of these proteins do not change in humans (7,8). The main acute-phase reactants in humans are C-reactive protein and serum amyloid A; their *in vivo* concentrations rise as much as 1,000-fold during an inflammatory response (9,10).

TABLE 40.1. MAJOR HUMAN AND RAT ACUTE-PHASE PLASMA PROTEINS

Human
  C-reactive protein
  Serum amyloid A
  LPS-binding protein
  Fibrinogen
  Haptoglobin
  α_1-Antichymotrypsin
Rat
  α_2-Macroglobulin
  LPS-binding protein
  α_1-Acid glycoprotein
  Cysteine proteinase inhibitor
  Serine proteinase inhibitor 2.3
  Tissue inhibitor of metalloproteinases-1

LPS, lipopolysaccharide.

ACUTE-PHASE RESPONSE OF THE LIVER AND INVOLVEMENT OF THE NEUROENDOCRINE AXIS

The liver plays a pivotal role in the acute-phase response of the organism. Its importance for the systemic reaction toward pathogens is emphasized by the fact that it contains the largest pool of macrophages (Kupffer cells) of the body at a strategically important anatomic and physiologic position (11,12).

As already mentioned, hepatocytes are the major sites of APP synthesis. The list of cytokines capable of inducing APP production in the liver is extensive and still increasing. It includes the members of the IL-6–type cytokine family: IL-6, leukemia inhibitory factor (LIF), IL-11, oncostatin M (OSM), ciliary neurotrophic factor (CNTF), cardiotrophin-1 (CT-1), and other mediators of growth regulation, differentiation, or inflammation such as glucocorticoids, epidermal growth factor (EGF), hepatocyte growth factor (HGF), IL-1, and TNF-α. Among these cytokines, IL-6 has been identified as the major stimulator of APP synthesis in parenchymal cells of the liver. These *in vitro* observations have been confirmed by the phenotype of IL-6 knockout mice, where IL-6 has been shown to be crucial for the acute-phase response during sterile experimental inflammation (13).

As schematically shown in Fig. 40.2, the inflammatory cascade leading to induction of APP synthesis is primed by inflammatory stimuli such as viruses, bacteria/lipopolysaccharide (LPS), or tissue injury acting on blood monocytes and resident tissue macrophages such as Kupffer cells. In turn, these cells release the proinflammatory mediators IL-1 and TNF-α into the circulation, and subsequently induce IL-6 through an autocrine loop. The IL-6 serum levels are further increased by IL-6 produced by IL-1– and TNF-α–stimulated endothelial cells, fibroblasts, and other stromal cells. Moreover, IL-6 is also produced by cells from the anterior pituitary gland (14). As depicted in Fig. 40.2, IL-6 and IL-1 stimulate the secretion of adrenocorticotropic hormone (ACTH) from the anterior pituitary gland via the

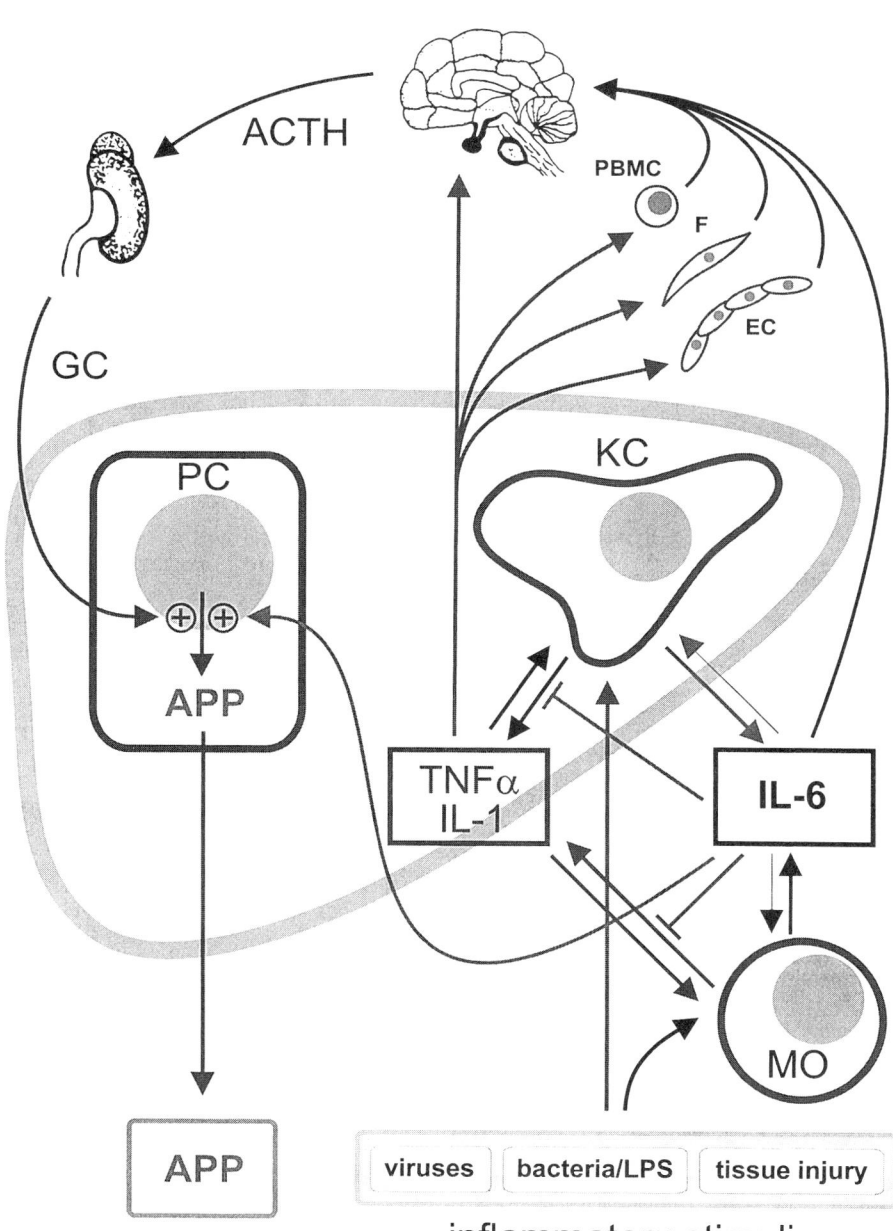

FIGURE 40.2. Involvement of the neuroendocrine axis in the acute-phase response of the liver. *ACTH*, adrenocorticotropic hormone; *APP*, acute-phase protein; *EC*, endothelial cells; *F*, fibroblasts; *GC*, glucocorticoids; *IL*, interleukin; *KC*, Kupffer cells; *MO*, monocytes; *PBMC*, peripheral blood mononuclear cells; parenchymal cells; *TNF*, tumor necrosis factor.

induction of corticotropin-releasing hormone (CRH), released from the hypothalamus. Furthermore, despite the induction of ACTH via CRH, IL-6 can directly induce the release of ACTH, prolactin, growth hormone, and luteinizing hormone from the anterior pituitary gland (4,15). ACTH subsequently leads to the release of glucocorticoids from the adrenal glands. Glucocorticoids are important regulators modulating the inflammatory response, since they have been shown to upregulate the production of cytokine receptors in hepatocytes, as for example IL-6 or interferon-γ (IFN-γ) receptors sensitizing these cells to the respective cytokines (4,16,17). Moreover, in certain species, glucocorticoids directly upregulate the production of a number of APPs by hepatocytes (18,19). On the other hand, glucocorticoids display an important inhibitory activity against inflammatory cytokine production by monocytes, macrophages, and other immune effector cells (not shown in Fig. 40.2). In summary, these facts reflect a complex regulatory feedback mechanism between the neuroendocrine and immune system involved in the control of inflammatory responses of the organism.

RELEVANCE OF THE ACUTE-PHASE RESPONSE IN RELATION TO METABOLIC FUNCTIONS

It is interesting that not only the well-known secreted APPs change during the hepatic acute-phase response, but also key enzymes of liver-specific metabolic functions. Thus, it has been shown in rat hepatocyte primary cultures that the glucagon-mediated expression of the gluconeogenic key enzyme phosphoenolpyruvate-carboxykinase is inhibited by IL-6, IL-1β, and TNF-α (20,21). Surprisingly, the expression of the key enzyme of the glycolytic pathway, glucokinase—induced by insulin—is also impaired by IL-6, IL-1β, and TNF-α (20,21). Based on these observations, the authors conclude that the liver—disturbed in its homeostasis—gives priority to the synthesis of APPs instead of important metabolic enzymes in order to cope with the limited amounts of amino acids for protein biosynthesis.

INTERLEUKIN-6–INDUCED ACUTE-PHASE PROTEIN SYNTHESIS IN HEPATOCYTES THROUGH THE JAK/STAT PATHWAY

Interleukin-6–Type Cytokines and Their Receptors

IL-6 belongs to a family of cytokines characterized by a four-alpha-helix bundle topology. Besides IL-6, the cytokines IL-11, LIF, CNTF, CT-1, OSM, and the recently discovered B-cell stimulatory factor-3/novel neurotrophin-1 are members of this family. With the exception of CNTF and CT-1, IL-6–type cytokines are classic secretory proteins

synthesized with N-terminal signal peptides (reviewed in ref. 3).

The tertiary structure of IL-6 has been solved by nuclear magnetic resonance (NMR) spectroscopy (22) and x-ray crystallography (23). As shown in Fig. 40.3, helix A (red) is connected by a long loop with helix B (green) in such a way that helix B lies parallel to helix A. Helix B is separated from helix C (yellow) by a very short loop allowing only an antiparallel packaging. Helix C is again joined by a long loop with helix D (blue), resulting in parallel packaging of the C-terminal helices. As a consequence the overall fold shows an up-up-down-down topology of the four long alpha-helices. Some biochemical properties of human IL-6 are listed in Table 40.2.

IL-6 exerts its action via a specific surface receptor complex on hepatocytes consisting of an α-receptor subunit, gp80, and a signal transducing subunit, gp130. Both receptor chains are type I membrane proteins characterized by an extracellular N-terminus and one transmembrane domain. Gp80 and gp130 both belong to the cytokine receptor class I family defined by the presence of at least one cytokine-binding module consisting of two fibronectin type III–like domains of which the N-terminal domain contains a set of four conserved cysteine residues and the C-terminal domain, a WSXWS motif (24).

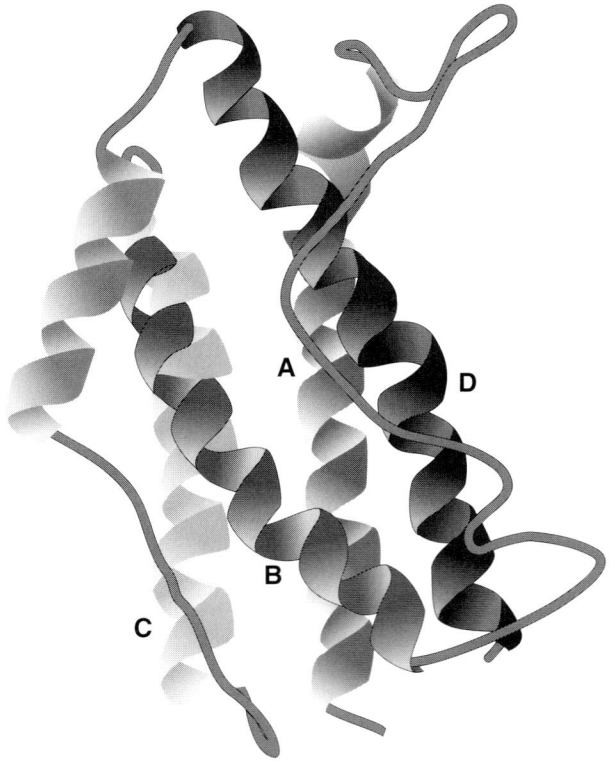

FIGURE 40.3. The three-dimensional structure of interleukin-6 (IL-6) (*ribbon representation*). The four long α-helices (*A, B, C,* and *D*) and the connecting loops (*gray*), as far as they have been defined, are shown. The Brookhaven Databank accession number is 1IL6.

TABLE 40.2. BIOCHEMICAL PROPERTIES OF HUMAN INTERLEUKIN-6 (IL-6) AND ITS RECEPTOR SUBUNITS

Property	IL-6	IL-6R	gp130
Number of amino acids			
Precursor	212	468	918
Mature protein	184	449	896
Extracellular domain		339	597
Transmembrane domain		28	22
Intracellular domain		82	277
Molecular mass (kd)			
Predicted	20.8	49.9	101
Observed	21–28	80	130–150
Glycosylation			
Potential *N*-glycosylation sites	2	5	10
N-glycosylation demonstrated	Yes 1–2	Yes	Yes
Number of cysteine residues	4		
Number of S-S bridges	2		
mRNA size (kb)	1.3	5	7
Number of exons	5	n.d.	17
Chromosomal localization	7p21-p14	n.d.	5,17
Soluble forms		Yes[a,b]	Yes[a]

[a]Generated by alternative splicing.
[b]Generated by shedding.
mRNA, messenger RNA.

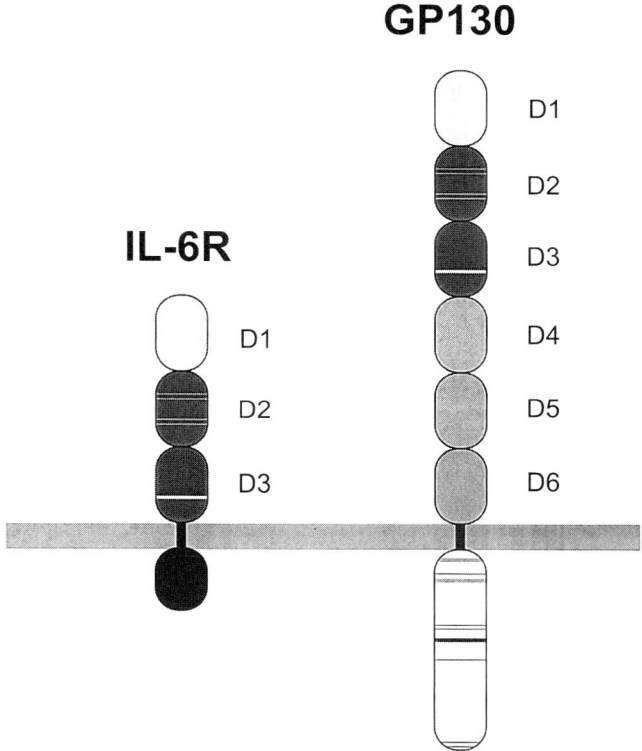

FIGURE 40.4. Domain composition of IL-6 receptor subunits. Predicted immunoglobulin (Ig)-like domains are shown in *light gray*, fibronectin type III–like domains in *medium gray*, and cytokine-binding modules (CBMs) in *dark gray*. The *horizontal bars* in the CBMs define the conserved cysteine residues (*thin white lines*) or the WSXWS motif (*broad white bars*). The lengths of the cytoplasmic parts correspond to the respective numbers of amino acids. Tyrosine residues in the cytoplasmic domain of gp130 are represented as *dark lines*, box 1 and box 2 as *gray bars*, and the di-leucine motif as a *dark gray bar*.

Figure 40.4 shows the domain structures of the two IL-6 receptor chains and Table 40.2 their biochemical properties. Both IL-6 receptor subunits contain an Ig-like domain located at the N-terminus. Gp130 has three additional membrane-proximal fibronectin type III–like domains.

The binding of IL-6 to its α-receptor gp80 has been studied in great detail. Whereas the Ig-like domain of gp80 is dispensable for biologic activity, the residues crucial for ligand binding are located in the cytokine-binding module. Mutagenesis studies have shown that residues in the loops near the hinge region between the domains of the cytokine-binding module are involved in ligand recognition (25,26). The IL-6/gp80 complex forms a ternary complex with two signal transducing receptor subunits gp130. Based on the growth hormone–growth hormone receptor complex structure (27), a model for the IL-6/gp80/gp130 ternary complex has been proposed and used for mutagenesis studies. In this model (Fig. 40.5) domains D2 and D3 of gp130 (Fig. 40.4) are in contact with IL-6. Point mutations of tyrosine 190 and phenylalanine 191 in D2 and valine 252 in D3 led to the loss of binding of gp130 to IL-6/IL-6R complexes as well as to impaired signal transduction (28,29). Most interestingly, also the N-terminal domain D1 of gp130 turned out to be crucial for ligand binding and signaling (29,30).

The role of the membrane-proximal domains D4, D5, and D6 of gp130 in receptor activation has been investigated by construction of deletion mutants lacking D4, D5, and D6. Deletion of D5 did not alter the affinity of the receptor to its ligand, but this mutant did not transduce any signal in response to IL-6. Thus, it has been concluded that

high-affinity ligand binding is not sufficient for receptor activation, but an adjustment of a well-defined gp130 dimer conformation is required for gp130 activation and signal transduction (31).

Due to the lack of a three-dimensional (3D) structure of a comparable cytokine-receptor complex, no molecular model that shows the binding of the second gp130 molecule to the IL-6/IL-6R complex is presently available.

Interleukin-6 Signaling

The major steps in IL-6 signal transduction have been worked out independently in two laboratories (32,33). The first event in IL-6 signaling is the binding of the ligand to its α-receptor, followed by the homodimerization of the signal transducer gp130 by formation of a ternary complex. The IL-6–induced dimerization of gp130 initiates a phosphorylation cascade (Fig. 40.6). The first step in this cascade is the autophosphorylation of tyrosine kinases of the Janus (Jak) family. The Janus kinases Jak1, Jak2, and

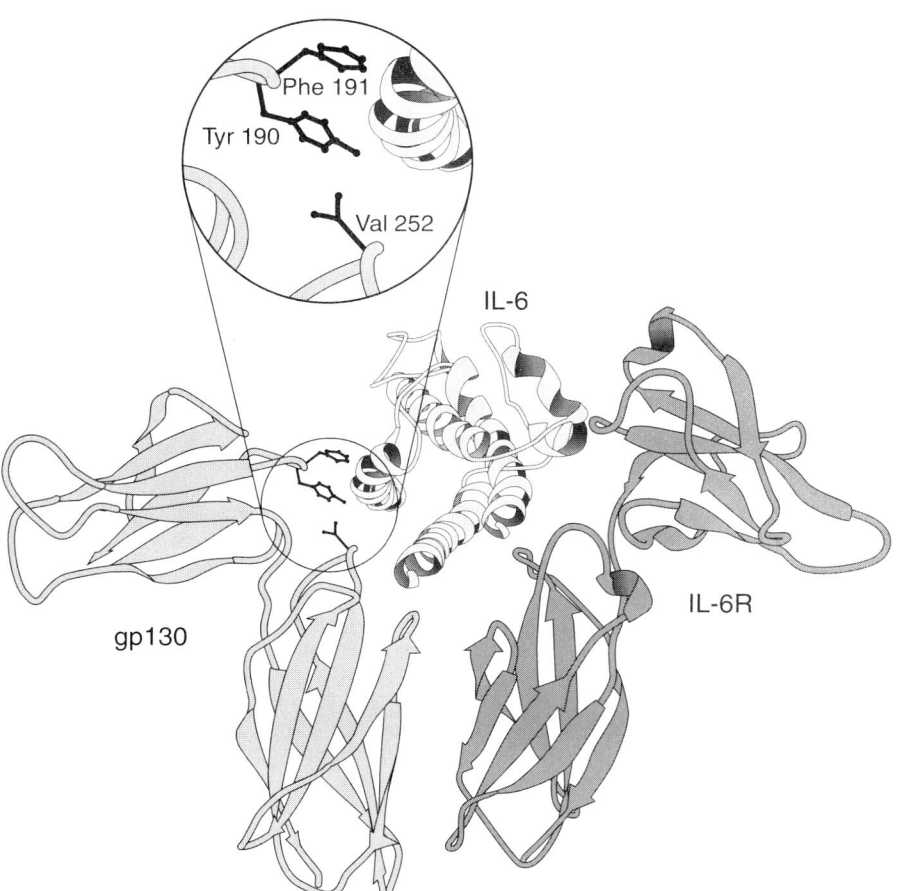

FIGURE 40.5. Model of the Interleukin (*IL*)-6–IL-6R-gp130 ternary complex. Amino acid side chains analyzed by mutagenesis are depicted in the insert and labeled in *orange*: tyrosine 190, phenylalanine 191, and valine 252.

Tyk2—all constitutively bound to the membrane-proximal part of the cytoplasmic tail of gp130—become tyrosine-phosphorylated and thus enzymatically active. Subsequently, tyrosine residues in the cytoplasmic part of gp130 are phosphorylated. These phosphotyrosines function as docking sites for transcription factors of the STAT (signal transducers and activators of transcription) family recruiting unphosphorylated predimerized STAT factors (34,35) via their Src homology 2 (SH2) domains. In turn, the STAT factors are also phosphorylated at tyrosine residues near their C-termini and released from the receptor complex. Phosphorylated homo- or heterodimeric STATs are translocated to the nucleus where they bind to IL-6–responsive elements in the 5′-flanking regions of target genes, e.g., acute-phase protein genes.

The importance of these signaling components not only for IL-6 but also for the signal transduction of other cytokines is emphasized by the fact that gene knockouts of STAT3 (36), gp130 (37), and Jak1 (38) showed lethal phenotypes, whereas the phenotypes of mice deficient for only one IL-6–type cytokine displayed relatively mild defects.

In the following subsections the different steps and the key players involved in IL-6 signaling are discussed in more detail.

Janus Kinases

Janus kinases (Jaks) are intracellular tyrosine kinases with molecular masses of 120 to 140 kd. Four members are known in mammalian cells: Jak1, Jak2, and Tyk2 are widely expressed, and Jak3 is mainly found in cells of hematopoietic origin. The structural organization of Jaks is shown in Fig. 40.7. A typical kinase domain, also called JH1 (Jak homology-1) domain, is located at the C-terminus. It is preceded by a kinase-like domain (JH2). The N-terminal half of the Jaks contains five additional regions with high sequence similarity between the different Jaks (JH3 to JH7) (reviewed in refs. 39–41).

Within the kinase domain, Jaks show considerable similarity to other kinases with respect to an activation loop implicated in regulation of kinase activity (reviewed in ref. 42). Ligand-induced receptor dimerization is thought to bring the associated Jaks into close proximity, leading to their activation via inter- or intramolecular phosphorylation at sites necessary for catalytic activity (40,41). The significance of the kinase-like domain is not clear. This domain has been described to have an influence on the kinase activity, although no clear picture emerges from the

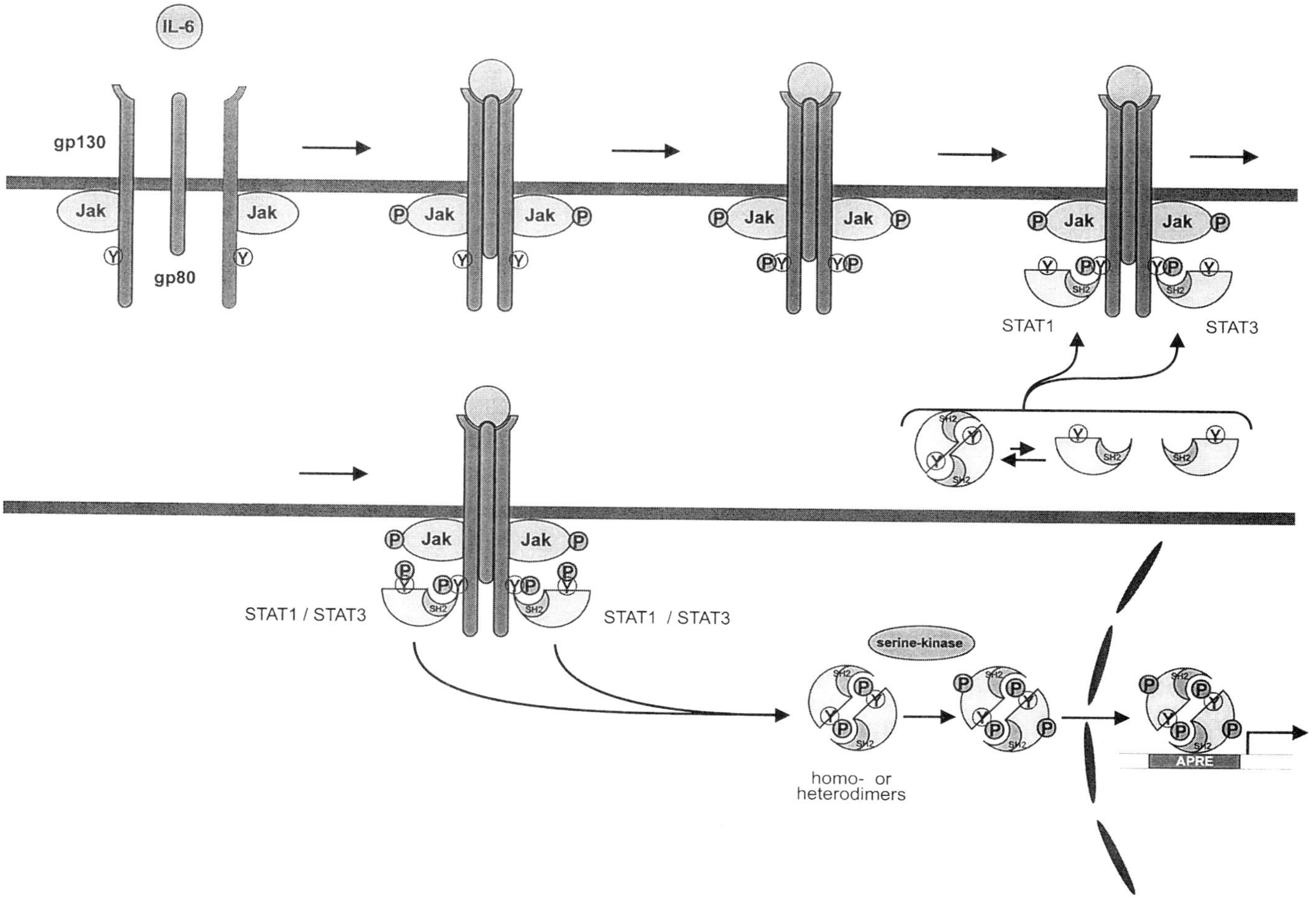

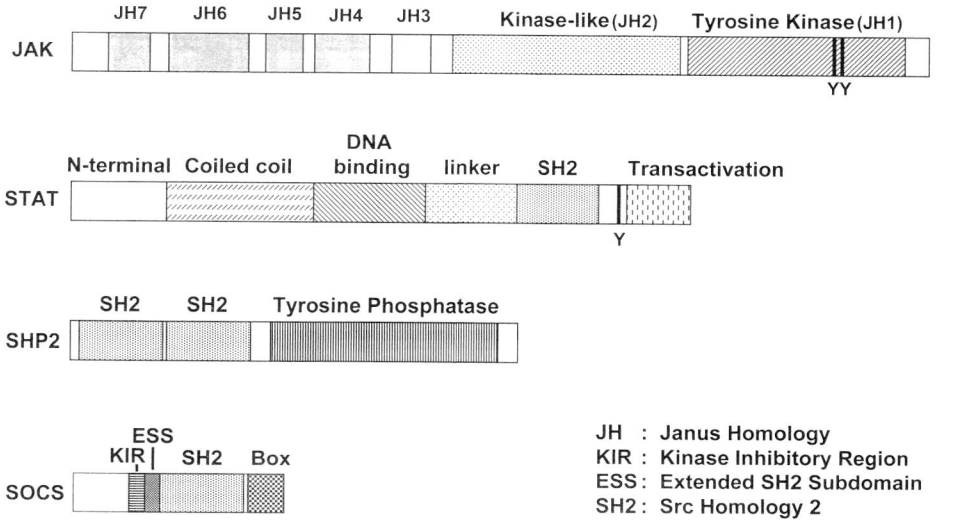

FIGURE 40.6. Interleukin-6 (*IL-6*) signal transduction through the gp130/Jak/STAT pathway. *APRE*, acute phase response element; *encircled Y*, tyrosine; *black P* in *gray circle*, phosphate; *Jak*, Janus kinases; *STAT*, signal transducer and activator of transcription; *SH2*, Src homology domain 2.

FIGURE 40.7. Structural organization of Janus kinases (*JAK*), *STAT* (signal transducer and activator of transcription) factors, SH2-domain–containing tyrosine phosphatase (*SHP2*), and suppressors of cytokine signaling (*SOCS*) proteins.

literature as to whether this is a positive or a negative one. The N-terminal half of the Jak regions JH7 to JH3 (Fig. 40.7) is involved in receptor association (40,41).

It should be noted that Jaks, apart from being receptor-associated enzymes, may fulfill further functions. For Tyk2 a structural role has been demonstrated: it is necessary for surface expression of the IFNARI receptor as well as for high-affinity binding of IFN-α (43,44).

IL-6 leads to the activation of Jak1, Jak2, and Tyk2 (32,33,45). This holds true also for the other IL-6–type cytokines IL-11, LIF, OSM, CT-1, and CNTF. Which kinases and to what extent a certain kinase is activated varies between cells (33,46) and possibly reflects different expression levels of Jaks. Among the Jaks, Jak1 plays a crucial role for signal transduction of IL-6–type cytokines as demonstrated by studies with Jak1-deficient fibrosarcoma cells and with cells derived from Jak1 knockout animals (38,47).

STAT Family of Transcription Factors

Seven mammalian STAT genes have been cloned so far and localized in three chromosomal clusters, suggesting that this family of proteins has evolved by gene duplication. The mammalian STAT factors are designated as STAT1, 2, 3, 4, 5a, 5b, and 6 (reviewed in ref. 40). Except for STAT2, alternatively spliced forms have been described. In the case of STAT4 and STAT6, the corresponding isoforms could not be identified.

With the exception of STAT4, STAT factors are ubiquitously expressed. STAT 4 expression is more restricted to myeloid cells and testis (48). The regulation of synthesis of STATs does not seem to play a major role in cytokine signaling. STAT activity is predominantly regulated by post-translational modifications, i.e., tyrosine and serine phosphorylation. STATs are mainly activated after stimulation of cytokine receptors. However, there are a growing number of reports demonstrating STAT activation also via receptor tyrosine kinases: EGR receptor (EGF-R), fibroblast growth factor receptor (FGF-R), c-*met*, platelet-derived growth factor receptor (PDGF-R), colony-stimulating factor-1 receptor (CSF-1-R), c-*kit*, and insulin-R (49–58), and G-protein–coupled receptors (angiotensin-R) (59). Ligands signaling through the same class of receptor complexes activate usually the same set of STAT factors (49); e.g., all IL-6–type cytokines activate STAT3 and STAT1.

STATs are proteins with a conserved structural organization (Fig. 40.7). They consist of 750 to 850 amino acids (e.g., STAT1, 750 aa; STAT3, 770 aa). Various domains within the STAT molecules have been defined: a tetramerization domain at the N-terminus, a DNA-binding domain in the middle, an SH2-domain, and a transactivation domain at the C-terminal end. In all STATs a tyrosine residue near the C-terminus is phosphorylated upon activation (tyrosine 701 for STAT1 and tyrosine 705 for STAT3) (reviewed in refs. 3 and 40).

The function of the highly conserved SH2-domain is well established. This domain is responsible for the binding of the STATs to tyrosine-phosphorylated receptor motifs (60–62) and also for homo- and heterodimerization. A preassociation of unphosphorylated STAT factors has been described (34,35). The mechanism responsible for this interaction, however, needs to be elucidated.

The activity of the C-terminal transactivation domain of STATs is at least partially regulated by a serine phosphorylation (S727 in STAT1 and STAT3) (63–66). Recent experiments of Jain et al. (67) have shown that STAT3 serine phosphorylation after IL-6 stimulation is due to the action of protein kinase Cδ (PKCδ).

The tyrosine phosphorylated STAT dimers translocate from the cytoplasm to the nucleus (Fig. 40.6); upon IL-6 treatment of liver cells, nuclear translocation of STAT3 occurs within minutes. The translocation is transient. The mechanism by which STAT factors enter the nucleus is unknown. A nuclear localization sequence (NLS) responsible for the transport of proteins to the cell nucleus has not been identified in any of the STAT molecules cloned so far. Therefore, nuclear translocation of STATs might be achieved either via an untypical NLS or via an NLS-containing shuttle protein that associates with activated STATs. In this respect it should be noted that activated STAT5 (68) as well as STAT3 (69) form complexes with the glucocorticoid receptor known to contain two NLS (70).

After nuclear translocation, STATs bind to specific enhancer sequences and stimulate—and in certain cases possibly also repress—transcription of respective target genes. During the past few years new target genes for IL-6 have been identified and functional STAT binding sites have been found in the promoter regions of these genes. STAT3 involvement in the transcriptional regulation of many of the well-known APPs such as C-reactive protein, α_1-antichymotrypsin, α_2-macroglobulin, lipopolysaccharide-binding protein, and tissue inhibitor of metalloproteinases-1 has been shown in hepatocytes *in vitro* and *in vivo* (71–75).

Besides APPs, a variety of STAT-activated genes has been described: *Jun* B, c-*Fos*, interferon regulatory factor-1, CCAAT enhancer binding protein-β (C/EBPβ), intestinal collagenase, vasoactive intestinal peptide, proopiomelanocortin, heat shock protein (hsp)90, and IL-6 signal transducer gp130 (reviewed in ref. 3). The promoter analysis of STAT-regulated genes revealed that STATs often associate with other transcription factors, resulting in a cooperative action. It has been shown, for example, that STAT3—the major transcription factor activated in liver cells upon IL-6 treatment—interacts with C/EBPβ/nuclear factor (NF)-IL-6 (74,76), NFκB (77), activating protein (AP)-1 (74,75,78,79), and glucocorticoid receptor (69).

Moreover, tandem arrangement of STAT binding sites has been reported for rat α_2-macroglobulin and human α_1-antichymotrypsin promoters, suggesting that STAT dimers might form multimers on clustered binding sites. Such a multimerization has been demonstrated for STAT1. For this process the N-terminus has been shown to be crucial (80,81). These two modes of cooperative action support the notion that gene regulation of IL-6–responsive genes is an integrative process in which several transcription factors together modulate the rate of transcription of a target gene.

Although much detailed information on STAT enhancer interaction became available during the last years, it is still not known how STAT factors and their cooperating transcription factors communicate to the basal transcription machinery. In the case of STAT1, an interaction with cyclic AMP response-element–binding protein (CBP) and p300 has been described (82,83). Also STAT3 has been found to interact with CBP, resulting in an enhanced transcription of the human α_1-antichymotrypsin gene (Schniertshauer, thesis Aachen 1998).

NEGATIVE REGULATION OF INTERLEUKIN-6 SIGNALING

In most systems STAT activation is transient, suggesting the existence of efficient mechanisms for STAT inactivation. Various mechanisms of STAT inactivation have been proposed:

- gp130-, Jak-kinase-, and STAT-dephosphorylation by tyrosine phosphatases;
- induction of feedback inhibitors inactivating Janus kinases;
- complex formation of activated STAT-dimers with specific protein inhibitors.

Tyrosine Phosphatases

Among various tyrosine phosphatases known, SH2-domain–containing tyrosine phosphatase (SHP-2) seems to play a pivotal role in IL-6 signaling. After IL-6–type cytokine stimulation, not only Jaks and STATs but also the tyrosine phosphatase SHP-2 is recruited to gp130 and subsequently phosphorylated. Whereas the role of the activated STATs in signaling is well established, that of SHP-2 is less clear.

SHP-2 is a ubiquitously expressed tyrosine phosphatase of 585 amino acids and a molecular mass of about 65 kd. SHP-2, like its homologue SHP-1, contains two SH2 domains at its N-terminus (Fig. 40.7). Both SH2-domains are required for the recruitment of SHP-2 to the phosphotyrosine motif of the activated gp130.

SHP-2 binds to phosphotyrosine 759 of gp130 (60,84). SHP-2 also interacts with Grb2 and very likely links the

gp130/Jak/STAT pathway to the Ras/Raf/MAP kinase pathway (85). Exchange of Y759 by phenylalanine in gp130 abrogates SHP-2 tyrosine phosphorylation (60,86) and in turn leads to elevated and prolonged STAT1- and STAT3-activation, resulting in an enhanced APP gene induction (87–89).

SHP-2 can be phosphorylated by many tyrosine kinases such as Src (90), bcr-abl (91), and Jaks. A Jak/SHP-2 interaction and the phosphorylation of SHP-2 by Jaks have been demonstrated (92). Although several reports on the role of SHP-2 in IL-6 signaling have been published, further clarification is needed.

Feedback Inhibitors: Suppressors of Cytokine Signaling

A new family of feedback inhibitors of cytokine signaling has been discovered in three different laboratories. These proteins are referred to as suppressors of cytokine signaling (SOCS) (93), Jak-binding proteins (JAB) (94), and STAT-induced STAT inhibitors (SSIs) (95). The proteins of this family are relatively small molecules, about 200 amino acids in length, containing a central SH2-domain, a kinase inhibitory region (KIR), and a carboxy-terminal domain called the SOCS box (Fig. 40.7). The SOCS box plays an important role in the regulation of degradation of these proteins (96). The SH2-domain was shown to directly interact with the kinase domain of Jak1, Jak2, and Tyk2, thereby preventing receptor phosphorylation and activation of the STAT-factors (97–99). SOCS proteins are rapidly induced by a variety of cytokines, particularly through the Jak/STAT pathway. Due to their potent action on Jak kinase activity, SOCS proteins represent powerful feedback inhibitors of the Jak/STAT pathway (Fig. 40.8). Recently, it has been found that inhibition of tyrosine phosphorylation of the phosphatase SHP-2 correlates with an enhanced induction of SOCS3 messenger RNA (mRNA). On the other hand, overexpression of SOCS3 protein decreased the level of tyrosine phosphorylated SHP-2 after IL-6 stimulation. Interestingly, SOCS3, but not SOCS1, requires and binds to the SHP-2 recruitment site of the cytoplasmic region (Y759) of gp130 to exert its negative function on IL-6 signaling (100).

Protein Inhibitors of Activated STATs

In various human tissues protein inhibitors of activated STATs (designated as PIASs) have been discovered (101,102). It is speculated that there may exist a specific PIAS for each phosphorylated STAT factor. For example, STAT3, but not STAT1, activity is regulated by PIAS3 (Fig. 40.8). However, it is still not understood how PIAS proteins are regulated.

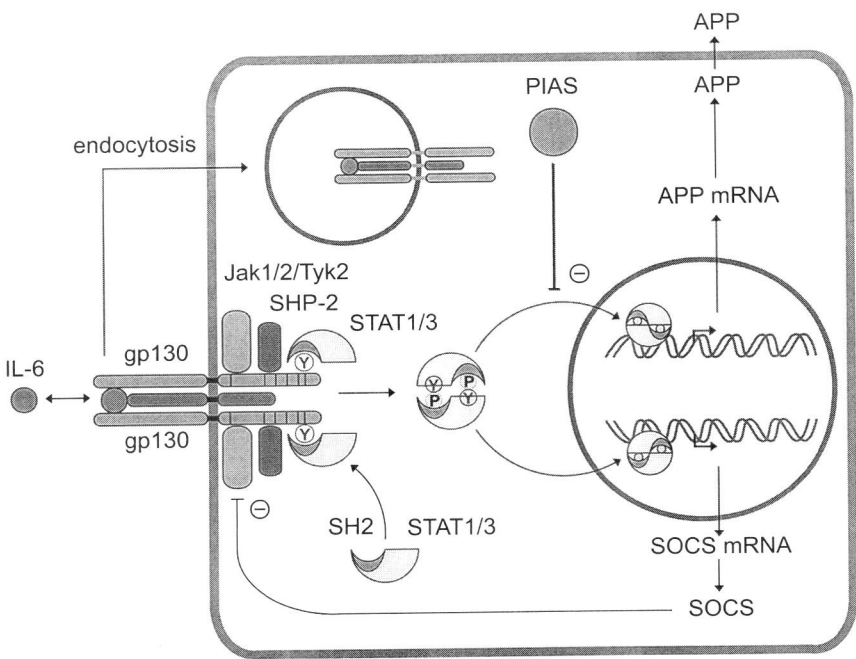

FIGURE 40.8. Negative regulation of the interleukin-6 (*IL-6*)–type cytokine signal transduction pathway. *APP*, acute-phase protein; *PIAS*, protein inhibitors of activated STATs; *SH2*, Src homology 2; *SOCS*, suppressors of cytokine signaling.

Modulation of the Jak/STAT Pathway Through the Availability of the Signaling Components

Modulation of the Jak/STAT pathway occurs in the following ways:

- escape from overstimulation by ligand/receptor internalization;
- regulation of the availability of the signaling molecules by different half-lives.

Endocytosis of the Interleukin-6/ Interleukin-6 Receptor Complex

Most cells escape from being overstimulated by surface receptor internalization. After binding to its receptor, IL-6 is efficiently internalized and the α-receptors/gp80 are downregulated (Fig. 40.8), resulting in a complete depletion of IL-6 surface binding sites within 30 to 60 minutes (103,104). To replenish IL-6 binding sites, *de novo* protein synthesis is required, suggesting that ligand and gp80 have been degraded after internalization, most likely in the lysosomal compartment. It has been previously demonstrated that the IL-6 signal transducer gp130 contains a di-leucine internalization motif within its cytoplasmic tail necessary for the endocytosis of the IL-6 receptor complex (105). Since gp80 *per se* is internalized very inefficiently, the observed downregulation of the IL-6 α-receptor can be explained by the formation of a ternary receptor complex consisting of IL-6/gp80 and gp130 in which gp130 not only mediates signal transduction, but also promotes efficient endocytosis of the IL-

6/IL-6 receptor complex (Fig. 40.8). Recently, the activation of the Jak/STAT pathway via the IL-6 receptor complex or agonistic antibodies against gp130 have been shown not to be required for efficient endocytosis to occur (106), suggesting that signaling and endocytosis are independent processes. Interestingly, the signal transducer gp130 undergoes constitutive endocytosis independent of the presence of IL-6. Internalization of gp130 occurs most likely via clathrin-coated pits, since a constitutive interaction between gp130 and the plasma membrane adaptor protein complex AP-2 has been observed (107).

Half-Lives of Signaling Components

Whereas considerable information has been accumulated concerning the time course of activation for the individual signaling molecules, data on the availability of the proteins involved in IL-6–type cytokine signal transduction are scarce. Nevertheless, the availability of these molecules, determined by the balance of protein synthesis and degradation, also influences IL-6 signal transduction. The turnover rates for the various proteins differ substantially (108). Three groups of signaling proteins can be discriminated; whereas the feedback inhibitors SOCS1, SOCS2, and SOCS3 are very short-lived (1 to 1.5 hours), STAT1, STAT3, and SHP2 have an extremely low turnover (8.5 to 20 hours). The Janus kinases Jak1, Jak2, Tyk2, and gp130 show intermediate half-lives (2 to 3 hours). Based on these observations it is concluded that signaling components activated by posttranslational modifications are long-lived, whereas the activities of short-lived proteins is mainly regulated at the transcriptional level.

MODULATION OF INTERLEUKIN-6 SIGNALING THROUGH THE JAK/STAT PATHWAY BY CROSS-TALKS WITH OTHER SIGNALING CASCADES

Preactivation of Erk-Type Mitogen-Activated Protein Kinases Inhibits Interleukin-6–Induced STAT Activation

A number of mediators has been reported to downregulate Jak/STAT activation, e.g., transforming growth factor-β (TGF-β), granulocyte/macrophage colony-stimulating factor (GM-CSF), and angiotensin II (109–111). The protein kinase C activator phorbol 12-myristate 13-acetate (PMA) was recently shown to inhibit IL-6–induced STAT3 activation via Erk/MAP kinases (112,113). These studies have been extended by the use of the Erk activators basic FGF (bFGF) and constitutively active raf (113a). Moreover, phosphotyrosine-759 of gp130—the docking site for SHP2 (see Tyrosine Phosphatases, above) and SOCS3—is crucial for the inhibitory effect of PMA-induced mitogen-activated protein (MAP) kinases on IL-6 signaling. Both PMA and bFGF rapidly stimulate SOCS3 mRNA expression. These findings are schematically summarized in Fig. 40.9. As mentioned above (Fig. 40.8) SOCS3 in turn inhibits IL-6

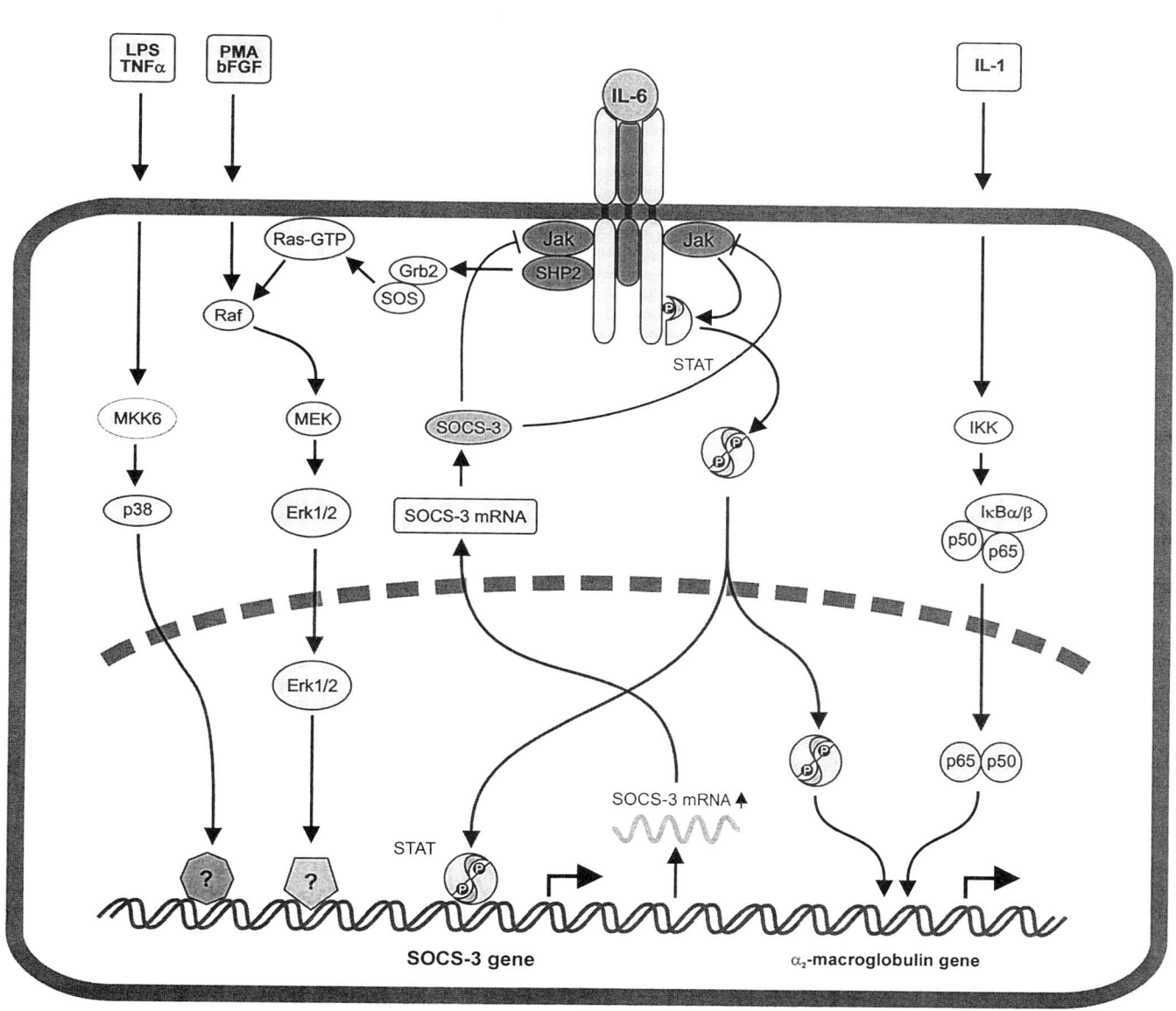

FIGURE 40.9. Modulation of interleukin-6 (*IL-6*) signaling through the Jak/STAT pathway by cross-talks with other signaling cascades. *bFGF*, basic fibroblast growth factor; *Jak*, Janus kinases; *LPS*, lipopolysaccharide; *PMA*, phorbol 12-myristate 13-acetate; *STAT*, signal transducer and activator of transcription; *SOCS*, suppressors of cytokine signaling; *TNF*, tumor necrosis factor.

signaling via inactivation of Jak kinases and thereby APP induction. Accordingly, the IL-6–induced SOCS3 expression is impaired.

In conclusion, it is intriguing that preactivation of the MAP kinase cascade by PMA or bFGF impairs the IL-6–dependent stimulation of the gp130/Jak/STAT pathway via induction of the negative feedback inhibitor SOCS3 (Fig. 40.9). This cross-talk between the Jak/STAT- and the MAP-kinase pathways is even more complicated, since Erk-type MAP-kinases are activated through gp130-associated SHP-2.

Interleukin-6 Signaling Is Down-Modulated by Pretreatment with Proinflammatory Mediators

Pretreatment of rat Kupffer cells as well as human macrophages with the proinflammatory mediators TNF-α

or LPS largely decreases or even completely abolishes STAT3 activation after IL-6 stimulation (114). This inhibition closely correlates with the induction of SOCS3 mRNA by LPS or TNF-α. Since neither LPS nor TNF-α influences IL-6–induced STAT3-activation in HepG2 cells or rat hepatocytes, this effect might be macrophage-specific. Both LPS and TNF-α are well-known activators of the p38 MAP kinase (115,116). Interestingly, inhibition of the p38 activity not only neutralizes particularly the TNF-α action on IL-6–induced STAT3-activation, but also suppresses TNF-α–mediated induction of SOCS3 mRNA. Therefore, it can be concluded that inhibition of STAT3-activation and induction of SOCS3 mRNA are functionally linked (Fig. 40.9).

Another remarkable mechanism for the modulation of IL-6 signaling has recently been observed. IL-1—but not TNF-α—has been shown to inhibit dose-dependently IL-

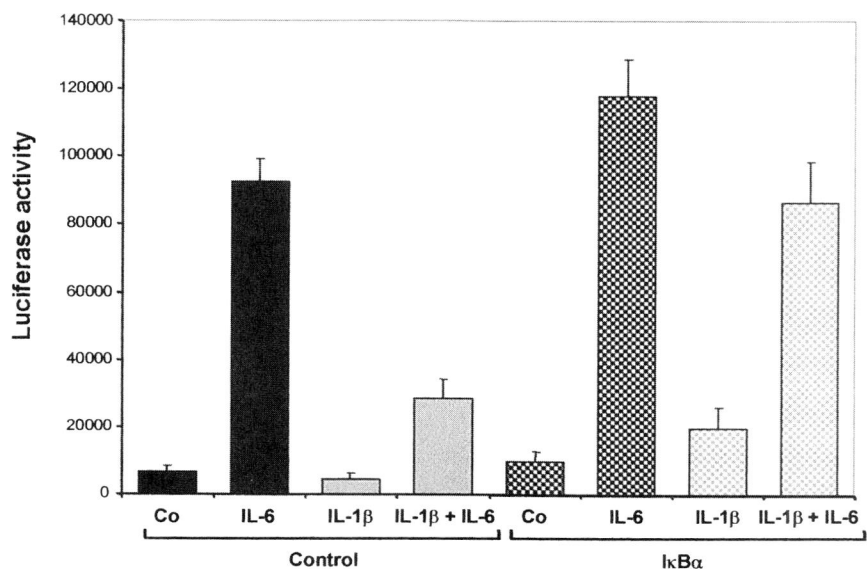

FIGURE 40.10. Inhibition of interleukin-6 (*IL-6*)–induced luciferase activity by IL-1β in HepG2 cells. **A:** HepG2 cells were transiently cotransfected with complementary DNAs (cDNAs) coding for the α₂-macroglobulin promoter luciferase and IκBα and subsequently stimulated with IL-6, IL-1β, or IL-6 and IL-1β. After cell lysis, luciferase activity was determined and normalized to cotransfected β-galactosidase activity. **B:** Promoter region of the rat α₂-macroglobulin gene. The two STAT3 binding sites (distal and proximal APREs) are underlined, the two putative overlapping NFκB binding sites are represented as hatched bars.

6–induced APP synthesis in and secretion by primary cultures of hepatocytes (117). As shown in Fig. 40.10, overexpression of IκBα and consequently prevention of NFκB activation blocks the inhibitory effect of IL-1β on IL-6–induced α$_2$-macroglobulin promoter activation (Bode et al., unpublished data). This observation might be explained by a competition of NFκB and STAT3 for overlapping binding elements in the α$_2$-M promoter (118) (Figs. 40.9, and 40.10 lower panel).

INTEGRATIVE VIEW ON THE CROSS-TALK BETWEEN THE SIGNALING PATHWAYS OF INTERLEUKIN-6 AND PROINFLAMMATORY MEDIATORS

As mentioned above, LPS as well as TNF-α inhibit IL-6–stimulated STAT3 activation in macrophages. This inhibition correlates with the induction of SOCS-3. Furthermore, IL-1 interferes with the α$_2$-macroglobulin promoter activation through STAT3 induced by IL-6 (Fig. 40.9).

With respect to these observations, it is important to note that IL-6—besides its proinflammatory properties—also exerts antiinflammatory actions. For example, IL-6 does not upregulate other inflammatory mediators, it does not induce cyclooxygenase activity leading to the production of prostaglandins, and it does not induce metalloproteinases responsible for tissue degradation (119). In contrast to IL-1 and TNF-α, which are poorly tolerated by mammals since they cause shock, IL-6 has no such effect (120).

An important antiinflammatory property of IL-6 is its potency to inhibit the synthesis of TNF-α and IL-1, both *in vitro* and *in vivo* (121). It is also of interest to note that IL-6 acts on human monocytes leading to the release of IL-1 receptor antagonist (122). Moreover, it was shown that IL-6 suppresses macrophage colony-stimulating factor–induced proliferation and differentiation of both tissue and bone marrow macrophages (123). Considering these antiinflammatory properties of IL-6, it is attractive to speculate that the STAT3-dependent IL-6 signaling cascade needs to be down-regulated by the proinflammatory mediators LPS, IL-1, or TNF-α in vivo in order to enforce the inflammatory response. Subsequently, the proinflammatory phase is terminated through the IL-6–dependent inhibition of IL-1 and TNF-α production. This inhibition of proinflammatory cytokine synthesis is reinforced by the induction of glucocorticoids resulting in a most likely STAT3-dependent dominating antiinflammatory response (Fig. 40.2).

ACKNOWLEDGMENTS

We thank Gerhard Müller-Newen, Iris Behrmann, and Fred Schaper for their critical reading of this manuscript, Peter Freyer for his help with the artwork, and Silvia Cottin for secretarial assistance. The experimental work performed in the Department of Biochemistry in Aachen and mentioned in this chapter has been supported by grants from the Deutsche Forschungsgemeinschaft (Bonn), and the Fonds der Chemischen Industrie (Frankfurt).

REFERENCES

1. Gabay C, Kushner I. Acute-phase proteins and other systemic responses to inflammation. *N Engl J Med* 1999;340:448–454.
2. Ramadori G, Christ B. Cytokines and the hepatic acute-phase response. *Semin Liver Dis* 1999;19:141–155.
3. Heinrich PC, Behrmann I, Müller-Newen G, et al. Interleukin-6–type cytokine signalling through the gp130/Jak/STAT pathway. *Biochem J* 1998;334:297–314.
4. Mackiewicz A. Acute phase proteins and transformed cells. *Int Rev Cytol* 1997;170:225–300.
5. Moshage H. Cytokines and the hepatic acute phase response. *J Pathol* 1997;181:257–266.
6. Baumann H, Gauldie J. The acute phase response. *Immunol Today* 1994;15:74–80.
7. van Gool J, Boers W, Sala M, et al. Glucocorticoids and catecholamines as mediators of acute phase proteins, especially rat alpha-macrofoetoprotein. *Biochem J* 1984;220:125–132.
8. Marinkovic S, Jahreis GP, Wong GG, et al. IL-6 modulates the synthesis of a specific set of phase plasma proteins in vivo. *J Immunol* 1989;142:808–812.
9. Kushner I. The phenomenon of the acute phase response. *Ann NY Acad Sci* 1982;389:39–48.
10. Kushner I, Mackiewicz A. Acute phase proteins as disease markers. *Dis Markers* 1987;5:1–11.
11. Wisse E. Kupffer cell reactions under various conditions as observed in the electron microscope. *J Ultrastruct Res* 1974;46:499–520.
12. Decker K. Biologically active products of stimulated liver macrophages (Kupffer cells). *Eur J Biochem* 1990;192:245–261.
13. Kopf M, Baumann H, Freer G, et al. Impaired immune and acute-phase responses in interleukin-6–deficient mice. *Nature* 1994;368:339–342.
14. Spangelo BL, Jarvis WD, Judd AM, et al. Induction of interleukin-6 release by interleukin-1 in rat anterior pituitary cells in vitro: evidence for an eicosanoid-dependent mechanism. *Endocrinology* 1991;129:2886–2894.
15. Navarra P, Tsagarakis S, Faria MS, et al. Interleukins-1 and -6 stimulate the release of corticotropin-releasing hormone-41 from rat hypothalamus in vitro via the eicosanoid cyclooxygenase pathway. *Endocrinology* 1991;128:37–44.
16. Rose-John S, Schooltink H, Lenz D, et al. Studies on the structure and regulation of the human hepatic interleukin-6–receptor. *Eur J Biochem* 1990;190:79–83.
17. Schooltink H, Schmitz-van de Leur H, Heinrich PC, et al. Upregulation of the interleukin-6–signal transducing protein (gp 130) by interleukin-6 and dexamethasone in HepG2 cells. *FEBS Lett* 1992;297:263–265.
18. Baumann H, Firestone GL, Burgess TL, et al. Dexamethasone regulation of alpha 1-acid glycoprotein and other acute phase reactants in rat liver and hepatoma cells. *J Biol Chem* 1983;258:563–570.
19. Baumann H, Richards C, Gauldie J. Interaction among hepatocyte-stimulating factors, interleukin 1, and glucocorticoids for regulation of acute phase plasma proteins in human hepatoma (HepG2) cells. *J Immunol* 1987;139:4122–4128.
20. Christ B, Nath A, Heinrich PC, et al. Inhibition by recombi-

nant human interleukin-6 of the glucagon-dependent induction of phosphoenolpyruvate carboxykinase and of the insulin-dependent induction of glucokinase gene expression in cultured rat hepatocytes: regulation of gene transcription and messenger RNA degradation. *Hepatology* 1994;20:1577–1583.

21. Christ B, Nath A. Impairment by interleukin 1 beta and tumour necrosis factor alpha of the glucagon-induced increase in phosphoenolpyruvate carboxykinase gene expression and gluconeogenesis in cultured rat hepatocytes. *Biochem J* 1996;320:161–166.

22. Xu GY, Yu HA, Hong J, et al. Solution structure of recombinant human interleukin-6. *J Mol Biol* 1997;268:468–481.

23. Somers W, Stahl M, Seehra JS. 1.9 Å crystal structure of interleukin 6: implications for a novel mode of receptor dimerization and signaling. *EMBO J* 1997;16:989–997.

24. Bazan JF. Structural design and molecular evolution of a cytokine receptor superfamily. *Proc Natl Acad Sci USA* 1990;87:6934–6938.

25. Yawata H, Yasukawa K, Natsuka S, et al. Structure-function analysis of human IL-6 receptor: dissociation of amino acid residues required for IL-6–binding and for IL-6 signal transduction through gp130. *EMBO J* 1993;12:1705–1712.

26. Kalai M, Montero-Julian FA, Grötzinger J, et al. Participation of two Ser-Ser-Phe-Tyr repeats in interleukin-6 (IL-6)-binding sites of the human IL-6 receptor. *Eur J Biochem* 1996;238:714–723.

27. de Vos AM, Ultsch M, Kossiakoff AA. Human growth hormone and extracellular domain of its receptor: crystal structure of the complex. *Science* 1992;255:306–312.

28. Horsten U, Müller-Newen G, Gerhartz C, et al. Molecular modeling-guided mutagenesis of the extracellular part of gp130 leads to the identification of contact sites in the interleukin-6 (IL-6).IL-6 receptor.gp130 complex. *J Biol Chem* 1997;272:23748–23757.

29. Kurth I, Horsten U, Pflanz S, et al. Activation of the signal transducer glycoprotein 130 by both IL-6 and IL-11 requires two distinct binding epitopes. *J Immunol* 1999;162:1480–1487.

30. Hammacher A, Richardson RT, Layton JE, et al. The immunoglobulin-like module of gp130 is required for signaling by interleukin-6, but not by leukemia inhibitory factor. *J Biol Chem* 1998;273:22701–22707.

31. Kurth I, Horsten U, Pflanz S, et al. Importance of the membrane-proximal extracellular domains for activation of the signal transducer glycoprotein 130. *J Immunol* 2000;164:273–282.

32. Lütticken C, Wegenka UM, Yuan J, et al. Association of transcription factor APRF and protein kinase Jak1 with the interleukin-6 signal transducer gp130. *Science* 1994;263:89–92.

33. Stahl N, Boulton TG, Farruggella T, et al. Association and activation of Jak-Tyk kinases by CNTF-LIF-OSM-IL-6 beta receptor components. *Science* 1994;263:92–95.

34. Stancato LF, David M, Carter-Su C, et al. Preassociation of STAT1 with STAT2 and STAT3 in separate signalling complexes prior to cytokine stimulation. *J Biol Chem* 1996;271:4134–4137.

35. Haan S, Kortylewski M, Behrmann I, et al. Cytoplasmic STAT proteins associate prior to activation. *Biochem J* 2000;345:417–421.

36. Takeda K, Noguchi K, Shi W, et al. Targeted disruption of the mouse Stat3 gene leads to early embryonic lethality. *Proc Natl Acad Sci USA* 1997;94:3801–3804.

37. Yoshida K, Taga T, Saito M, et al. Targeted disruption of gp130, a common signal transducer for the interleukin 6 family of cytokines, leads to myocardial and hematological disorders. *Proc Natl Acad Sci USA* 1996;93:407–411.

38. Rodig SJ, Meraz MA, White JM, et al. Disruption of the Jak1

gene demonstrates obligatory and nonredundant roles of the Jaks in cytokine-induced biologic responses. *Cell* 1998;93:373–383.

39. Leonard WJ, O'Shea JJ. JAKS and STATS: Biological implications. *Annu Rev Immunol* 1998;16:293–322.

40. Pellegrini S, Dusanter-Fourt I. The structure, regulation and function of the Janus kinases (JAKs) and the signal transducers and activators of transcription (STATs). *Eur J Biochem* 1997;248:615–633.

41. Duhé RJ, Farrar WL. Structural and mechanistic aspects of Janus kinases: how the two-faced god wields a double-edged sword. *J Interferon Cytokine Res* 1998;18:1–15.

42. Johnson LN, Noble MEM, Owen DJ. Active and inactive protein kinases: structural basis for regulation. *Cell* 1996;85:149–158.

43. Velazquez L, Mogensen KE, Barbieri G. Distinct domains of the protein tyrosine kinase tyk2 required for binding of interferon-alpha/beta and for signal transduction. *J Biol Chem* 1995;270:3327–3334.

44. Gauzzi MC, Barbieri G, Richter MF, et al. The amino-terminal region of Tyk2 sustains the level of interferon alpha receptor 1, a component of the interferon alpha/beta receptor. *Proc Natl Acad Sci USA* 1997;94:11839–11844.

45. Narazaki M, Witthuhn BA, Yoshida K, et al. Activation of JAK2 kinase mediated by the interleukin 6 signal transducer gp130. *Proc Natl Acad Sci USA* 1994;91:2285–2289.

46. Matsuda T, Yamanaka Y, Hirano T. Interleukin-6–induced tyrosine phosphorylation of multiple proteins in murine hematopoietic lineage cells. *Biochem Biophys Res Commun* 1994;200:821–828.

47. Guschin D, Rogers N, Briscoe J, et al. A major role for the protein tyrosine kinase JAK1 in the JAK/STAT signal transduction pathway in response to interleukin-6. *EMBO J* 1995;14:1421–1429.

48. Zhong Z, Wen Z, Darnell JE Jr. Stat3 and Stat4: members of the family of signal transducers and activators of transcription. *Proc Natl Acad Sci USA* 1994;91:4806–4810.

49. Briscoe J, Guschin D, Muller M. Signal transduction. Just another signalling pathway. *Curr Biol* 1994;4:1033–1035.

50. Park OK, Schaefer TS, Nathans D. In vitro activation of Stat3 by epidermal growth factor receptor kinase. *Proc Natl Acad Sci USA* 1996;93:13704–13708.

51. Novak U, Mui A, Miyajima A, et al. Formation of STAT5–containing DNA binding complexes in response to colony-stimulating factor-1 and platelet-derived growth factor. *J Biol Chem* 1996;271:18350–18354.

52. Yamamoto H, Crow M, Cheng L, et al. PDGF receptor-to-nucleus signaling of p91 (STAT1 alpha) transcription factor in rat smooth muscle cells. *Exp Cell Res* 1996;222:125–130.

53. Novak U, Nice E, Hamilton JA, et al. Requirement for Y706 of the murine (or Y708 of the human) CSF-1 receptor for STAT1 activation in response to CSF-1. *Oncogene* 1996;13:2607–2613.

54. Deberry C, Mou S, Linnekin D. Stat1 associates with c-kit and is activated in response to stem cell factor. *Biochem J* 1997;327:73–80.

55. Ceresa BP, Pessin JE. Insulin stimulates the serine phosphorylation of the signal transducer and activator of transcription (STAT3) isoform. *J Biol Chem* 1996;271:12121–12124.

56. Chen XH, Patel BK, Wang LM, et al. Jak1 expression is required for mediating interleukin-4–induced tyrosine phosphorylation of insulin receptor substrate and Stat6 signaling molecules. *J Biol Chem* 1997;272:6556–6560.

57. Chuang LM, Wang PH, Chang HM, et al. Novel pathway of insulin signaling involving Stat1alpha in Hep3B cells. *Biochem Biophys Res Commun* 1997;235:317–320.

58. Schaper F, Siewert E, Gomez-Lechon MJ, et al. Hepatocyte

growth factor/scatter factor (HGF/SF) signals via the STAT3/APRF transcription factor in human hepatoma cells and hepatocytes. *FEBS Lett* 1997;405:99–103.

59. Bhat GJ, Thekkumkara TJ, Thomas WG, et al. Activation of the STAT pathway by angiotensin II in T3CHO/AT1A cells. Cross-talk between angiotensin II and interleukin-6 nuclear signaling. *J Biol Chem* 1994;269:31443–31449.

60. Stahl N, Farruggella TJ, Boulton TG, et al. Choice of STATs and other substrates specified by modular tyrosine-based motifs in cytokine receptors. *Science* 1995;267:1349–1353.

61. Greenlund AC, Farrar MA, Viviano BL, et al. Ligand-induced IFN gamma receptor tyrosine phosphorylation couples the receptor to its signal transduction system (p91). *EMBO J* 1994; 13:1591–1600.

62. Heim MH, Kerr IM, Stark GR, et al. Contribution of STAT SH2 groups to specific interferon signaling by the Jak-STAT pathway. *Science* 1995;267:1347–1349.

63. Lütticken C, Coffer P, Yuan J, et al. Interleukin-6–induced serine phosphorylation of transcription factor APRF: evidence for a role in interleukin-6 target gene induction. *FEBS Lett* 1995; 360:137–143.

64. Zhang X, Blenis J, Li HC, et al. Requirement of serine phosphorylation for formation of STAT-promoter complexes. *Science* 1995;267:1990–1994.

65. Wen Z, Zhong Z, Darnell JE Jr. Maximal activation of transcription by Stat1 and Stat3 requires both tyrosine and serine phosphorylation. *Cell* 1995;82:241–250.

66. Wen Z, Darnell JE Jr. Mapping of Stat3 serine phosphorylation to a single residue (727) and evidence that serine phosphorylation has no influence on DNA binding of Stat1 and Stat3. *Nucleic Acids Res* 1997;25:2062–2067.

67. Jain N, Zhang T, Kee WH, et al. Protein kinase C delta associates with and phosphorylates Stat3 in an interleukin-6–dependent manner. *J Biol Chem* 1999;274:24392–24400.

68. Stöcklin E, Wissler M, Gouilleux F, et al. Functional interactions between Stat5 and the glucocorticoid receptor. *Nature* 1996;383:726–728.

69. Zhang Z, Jones S, Hagood JS, et al. STAT3 acts as a co-activator of glucocorticoid receptor signaling. *J Biol Chem* 1997; 272:30607–30610.

70. Picard D, Yamamoto KR. Two signals mediate hormone-dependent nuclear localization of the glucocorticoid receptor. *EMBO J* 1987;6:3333–3340.

71. Zhang D, Sun M, Samols D, et al. STAT3 participates in transcriptional activation of the C-reactive protein gene by interleukin-6. *J Biol Chem* 1996;271:9503–9509.

72. Kordula T, Rydel RE, Brigham EF, et al. Oncostatin M and the interleukin-6 and soluble interleukin-6 receptor complex regulate alpha-1-antichymotrypsin expression in human cortical astrocytes. *J Biol Chem* 1998;273:4112–4118.

73. Wegenka UM, Buschmann J, Lütticken C, et al. Acute-phase response factor, a nuclear factor binding to acute-phase response elements, is rapidly activated by interleukin-6 at the posttranslational level. *Mol Cell Biol* 1993;13:276–288.

74. Schumann RR, Kirschning CJ, Unbehaun A, et al. The lipopolysaccharide-binding protein is a secretory class 1 acute-phase protein whose gene is transcriptionally activated by APRF/STAT/3 and other cytokine-inducible nuclear proteins. *Mol Cell Biol* 1996;16:3490–3503.

75. Bugno M, Graeve L, Gatsios P, et al. Identification of the interleukin-6/oncostatin M response element in the rat tissue inhibitor of metalloproteinases-1 (TIMP-1) promoter. *Nucleic Acids Res* 1995;23:5041–5047.

76. Stephanou A, Isenberg DA, Akira S, et al. The nuclear factor interleukin-6 (NF-IL6) and signal transducer and activator of transcription-3 (STAT-3) signalling pathways co-operate to mediate the activation of the hsp90beta gene by interleukin-6 but have opposite effects on its inducibility by heat shock. *Biochem J* 1998;330:189–195.

77. Brown RT, Ades IZ, Nordan RP. An acute phase response factor/NF-kappa B site downstream of the junB gene that mediates responsiveness to interleukin-6 in a murine plasmacytoma. *J Biol Chem* 1995;270:31129–31135.

78. Korzus E, Nagase H, Rydell R, et al. The mitogen-activated protein kinase and JAK-STAT signaling pathways are required for an oncostatin M-responsive element-mediated activation of matrix metalloproteinase 1 gene expression. *J Biol Chem* 1997; 272:1188–1196.

79. Symes A, Gearan T, Eby J, et al. Integration of Jak-Stat and AP-1 signaling pathways at the vasoactive intestinal peptide cytokine response element regulates ciliary neurotrophic factor-dependent transcription. *J Biol Chem* 1997;272:9648–9654.

80. Xu X, Sun YL, Hoey T. Cooperative DNA binding and sequence-selective recognition conferred by the STAT amino-terminal domain. *Science* 1996;273:794–797.

81. Vinkemeier U, Cohen SL, Moarefi I, et al. DNA binding of in vitro activated Stat1 alpha, Stat1 beta and truncated Stat1: interaction between NH2-terminal domains stabilizes binding of two dimers to tandem DNA sites. *EMBO J* 1996;15: 5616–5626.

82. Zhang JJ, Vinkemeier U, Gu W, et al. Two contact regions between Stat1 and CBP/p300 in interferon gamma signaling. *Proc Natl Acad Sci USA* 1996;93:15092–15096.

83. Horvai AE, Xu L, Korzus E, et al. Nuclear integration of JAK/STAT and Ras/AP-1 signaling by CBP and p300. *Proc Natl Acad Sci USA* 1997;94:1074–1079.

84. Fuhrer DK, Feng GS, Yang YC. Syp associates with gp130 and Janus kinase 2 in response to interleukin-11 in 3T3-L1 mouse preadipocytes. *J Biol Chem* 1995;270:24826–24830.

85. Fukada T, Hibi M, Yamanaka Y, et al. Two signals are necessary for cell proliferation induced by a cytokine receptor gp130: involvement of STAT3 in anti-apoptosis. *Immunity* 1996;5: 449–460.

86. Schaper F, Gendo C, Eck M, et al. Activation of SHP2 via the IL-6 signal transducing receptor protein gp130 requires JAK1 and limits acute-phase protein expression. *Biochemical J* 1998; 335:557–565.

87. Schmitz J, Dahmen H, Grimm C, et al. The cytoplasmic tyrosine motifs in full-length gp130 have different roles in IL-6 signal transduction. *J Immunol* 2000;164:848–854.

88. Symes A, Stahl N, The protein tyrosine phosphatase SHP-2 negatively regulates ciliary neurotrophic factor induction of gene expression. *Curr Biol* 1997;9:697–700.

89. Kim H, Hawley TS, Hawley RG, et al. Protein tyrosine phosphatase 2 (SHP-2) moderates signaling by gp130 but is not required for the induction of acute-phase plasma protein genes in hepatic cells. *Mol Cell Biol* 1998;18:1525–1533.

90. Feng GS, Hui CC, Pawson T. SH2-containing phosphotyrosine phosphatase as a target of protein-tyrosine kinases. *Science* 1993;259:1607–1611.

91. Tauchi T, Feng GS, Shen R, et al. SH2-containing phosphotyrosine phosphatase Syp is a target of p210bcr-abl tyrosine kinase. *J Biol Chem* 1994;269:15381–15387.

92. Yin T, Shen R, Feng GS, et al. Molecular characterization of specific interactions between SHP-2 phosphatase and JAK tyrosine kinases. *J Biol Chem* 1997;272:1032–1037.

93. Starr R, Willson TA, Viney EM, et al. A family of cytokine-inducible inhibitors of signalling. *Nature* 1997;387:917–921.

94. Endo TA, Masuhara M, Yokouchi M, et al. A new protein containing an SH2 domain that inhibits JAK kinases. *Nature* 1997;387:921–924.

95. Naka T, Narazaki M, Hirata M, et al. Structure and function of

a new STAT-induced STAT inhibitor. *Nature* 1997;387: 924–929.

96. Narazaki M, Fujimoto M, Matsumoto T, et al. Three distinct domains of SSI-1/SOCS-1/JAB protein are required for its suppression of interleukin 6 signaling. *Proc Natl Acad Sci USA* 1998;95:13130–13134.

97. Yasukawa H, Misawa H, Sakamoto H, et al. The JAK-binding protein JAB inhibits Janus tyrosine kinase activity through binding in the activation loop. *EMBO J* 1999;18:1309–1320.

98. Nicholson SE, Willson TA, Farley A, et al. Mutational analyses of the SOCS proteins suggest a dual domain requirement but distinct mechanisms for inhibition of LIF and IL-6 signal transduction. *EMBO J* 1999;18:375–385.

99. Sasaki S, Yasukawa A, Suzuki A, et al. Cytokine-inducible SH2 protein-3 (CIS3/SOCS3) inhibits Janus tyrosine kinase by binding through the N-terminal kinase inhibitory region as well as SH2 domain. *Genes Cells* 1999;4:339–351.

100. Schmitz J, Weissenbach M, Heinrich PC, et al. ·SOCS 3 exerts its inhibitory function on interleukin-6 signal transduction through the SHP2 recruitment site of gp130. *J Biol Chem* 2000;275:12848–12856.

101. Chung CD, Liao J, Liu B, et al. Specific inhibition of Stat3 signal transduction by PIAS3. *Science* 1997;278:1803–1805.

102. Liu B, Liao J, Rao X, et al. Inhibition of Stat1-mediated gene activation by PIAS1. *Proc Natl Acad Sci USA* 1998;95: 10626–10631.

103. Zohlnhofer D, Graeve L, Rose-John S, et al. The hepatic interleukin-6 receptor. Down-regulation of the interleukin-6 binding subunit (gp80) by its ligand. *FEBS Lett* 1992;306:219–222.

104. Nesbitt JE, Fuller GM. Dynamics of interleukin-6 internalization and degradation in rat hepatocytes. *J Biol Chem* 1992;267: 5739–5742.

105. Dittrich E, Renfrew-Haft C, Muys L, et al. A di-leucine motif and an upstream serine in the interleukin-6 (IL-6) signal transducer gp130 mediate ligand-induced endocytosis and down-regulation of the IL-6 receptor. *J Biol Chem* 1996;271:5487–5494.

106. Thiel S, Behrmann I, Dittrich E, et al. Internalization of the interleukin 6 signal transducer gp130 does not require activation of the Jak/STAT pathway. *Biochem J* 1998;330:47–54.

107. Thiel S, Dahmen H, Martens A, et al. Constitutive internalization and association with adaptor protein-2 of the interleukin-6 signal transducer gp130. *FEBS Lett* 1998;441: 231–234.

108. Siewert E, Müller-Esterl W, Starr R, et al. Different protein turnover of interleukin-6–type cytokine signalling components. *Eur J Biochem* 1999;265:251–257.

109. Bright JJ, Sriram S. TGFβ inhibits IL-12–induced activation of Jak-STAT pathway in T lymphocytes. *J Immunol* 1998;161: 1772–1777.

110. Sengupta TK, Schmitt EM, Ivashkiv LB. Inhibition of cytokines and Jak-STAT activation by distinct signaling pathways. *Proc Natl Acad Sci USA* 1996;93:9499–9504.

111. Bhat GJ, Abraham ST, Baker KM. Angiotensin II interferes with interleukin-6–induced STAT3 signaling by a pathway involving mitogen-activated protein kinase kinase 1. *J Biol Chem* 1996;271:22447–22452.

112. Jain N, Zhang T, Fong SL, et al. Repression of Stat3 activity by activation of mitogen-activated protein kinase (MAPK). *Oncogene* 1998;17:3157–3167.

113. Sengupta TK, Talbot ES, Scherle PA, et al. Rapid inhibition of interleukin-6 signaling and STAT3 activation mediated by mitogen-activated protein kinases. *Proc Natl Acad Sci USA* 1998;95:11107–11112.

113a. Terstegen L, Gatsios P, Bode JG, et al. The inhibition of interleukin-6-dependent STAT activation by mitogen-activated protein kinases depends on tyrosine 759 in the cytoplasmic tail of glycoprotein 130. *J Biol Chem* 2000;275:18810–18817.

114. Bode JG, Nimmesgern A, Schmitz J, et al. LPS and TNFα induce SOCS3 mRNA and inhibit IL-6–induced activation of STAT3 in macrophages. *FEBS Lett* 1999;463:365–370.

115. Han J, Lee JD, Bibbs L, et al. A MAP kinase targeted by endotoxin and hyperosmolarity in mammalian cells. *Science* 1994; 265:808–811.

116. Lee JC, Laydon JT, McDonnell PC, et al. A protein kinase involved in the regulation of inflammatory cytokine biosynthesis. *Nature* 1994;372:739–746.

117. Andus T, Geiger T, Hirano T, et al. Action of recombinant human interleukin-6, interleukin-1β and tumor necrosis factor α on the mRNA induction of acute-phase proteins. *Eur J Immunol* 1988;18:739–746.

118. Zhang Z, Fuller GM. The competitive binding of STAT3 and NF-kappaB on an overlapping DNA binding site. *Biochem Biophys Res Commun* 1997;237:90–94.

119. Barton BE. The biological effects of interleukin-6. *Med Res Rev* 1996;16:87–109.

120. Neta R, Vogel SN, Sipe JD, et al. Comparison of in vivo effects of human recombinant IL 1 and human recombinant IL 6 in mice. *Lymphokine Res* 1988;7:403–412.

121. Ulich TR, Guo KZ, Remick D, et al. Endotoxin-induced cytokine gene expression in vivo. III. IL-6 mRNA and serum protein expression and the in vivo hematologic effects of IL-6. *J Immunol* 1991;146:2316–2323.

122. Tilg H, Trehu E, Atkins MB, et al. Interleukin-6 (IL-6) as an anti-inflammatory cytokine: induction of circulating IL-1 receptor antagonist and soluble tumor necrosis factor receptor p55. *Blood* 1994;83:113–118.

123. Riedy MC, Stewart CC. Inhibitory role of interleukin-6 in macrophage proliferation. *J Leukocyte Biol* 1992;52:125–127.

INNATE IMMUNE SENSING AND THE TOLL-LIKE RECEPTORS

BRUCE BEUTLER

Placed in the path of portal blood draining the gut and other enteric structures, the liver is often the first organ to encounter microbes or their molecular constituents, and has developed an immune function that coexists with its metabolic function. Immunity is subserved largely by Kupffer cells lining the hepatic sinusoids. As such, it is innate immunity rather than acquired immunity that dominates in the detection of foreign molecules. Among inducers of innate immune responses, lipopolysaccharide (LPS, or endotoxin; a product of gram-negative organisms), lipopeptides, peptidoglycan, unmethylated DNA, zymosan, and many other agents have been described. LPS is perhaps the most powerful of these. The mechanism by which it is detected long eluded understanding but has come into sharp focus with the identification of Toll-like receptor 4 as the plasma membrane protein that binds LPS and mediates all LPS responses. This receptor, and others like it, are presumed to be the principal exponents of innate immune sensing.

B. Beutler: Department of Immunology, Scripps Research Institute, La Jolla, California 92037.

THE GENERAL STRATEGIES OF INNATE AND ACQUIRED IMMUNITY

Vertebrates alone possess an acquired immune system, that is, one that requires exposure to an antigen to develop its full potency. The acquired immune response takes days or weeks to become fully effective, and grows stronger with repeated exposure to the inciting antigen. It is mediated by lymphocytes, which arose only recently in metazoan evolution. Lymphocytes are collectively endowed with the extraordinary ability to generate millions of different receptor molecules through rearrangements of their own genomic DNA. As such, one lymphocyte or another is likely to react with any foreign macromolecule the host encounters. In the course of development, autoreactive clones are eliminated, and it is at this point that a distinction between self and nonself is made.

Remarkable as acquired immunity may be, it is insufficient to protect the host. So much is obvious from the fact that neutropenic individuals are severely immunocompromised, despite the continued presence of functional lymphocytes. Furthermore, the acquired immune system cannot operate without supporting cells, notably macrophages and dendritic cells, which present antigens to lymphocytes in a recognizable molecular format. These cells also stimulate lymphocytes to divide by activating specific mitogenic receptors through the elaboration of soluble and membrane-bound ligands (cytokines). Without the assistance of myeloid cells, acquired immunity would be an impossibility.

In a sense, this is not surprising. The "newer" acquired immune system (also variously referred to as the "adaptive" or "specific" immune system) was built atop the older system of innate immunity (also called "natural" immunity). First recognized as an important protective mechanism by Metchnikoff more than 100 years ago, phagocytes are more than they appear. While the ameboid cells that patrol the body are not sentient beings, they behave with what seems a kind of intelligence. They are discriminating in their behavior, attacking only microbial invaders and tolerating cells and tissues of the host. Hence, long before the acquired immune system evolved, the innate immune system was fully capable of distinguishing self from nonself. Furthermore, though lacking the immense repertoire of receptors for which the lymphoid compartment is famous, innate immune cells nonetheless cope with an immense variety of pathogens.

How do they accomplish this? The inescapable conclusion is that innate immune cells must utilize receptors of a very special type. These receptors must never react with healthy host tissues, but must somehow react with virtually all pathogens. The receptors must not be of numerous types: enough is known of the genome to realize that a huge array of receptor genes (comparable, for example, to the repertoire of rearranged immunoglobulins) is not present in the germline. Therefore, only a limited number of microbial determinants must be targeted by the innate immune system. These determinants might be presumed to be indispensable for the pathogens, since mutation and selection among pathogens would otherwise bring about their loss.

THE RESPONSE TO LIPOPOLYSACCHARIDE AS A PARADIGM OF INNATE IMMUNE SENSING

The receptors of innate immunity trigger what we have come to call the inflammatory response. They lead to the release of cytokine mediators that activate other innate immune cells at a distance, preparing the host for the spread of infection in the event that immediate containment is unsuccessful. This is much in evidence in the response to LPS.

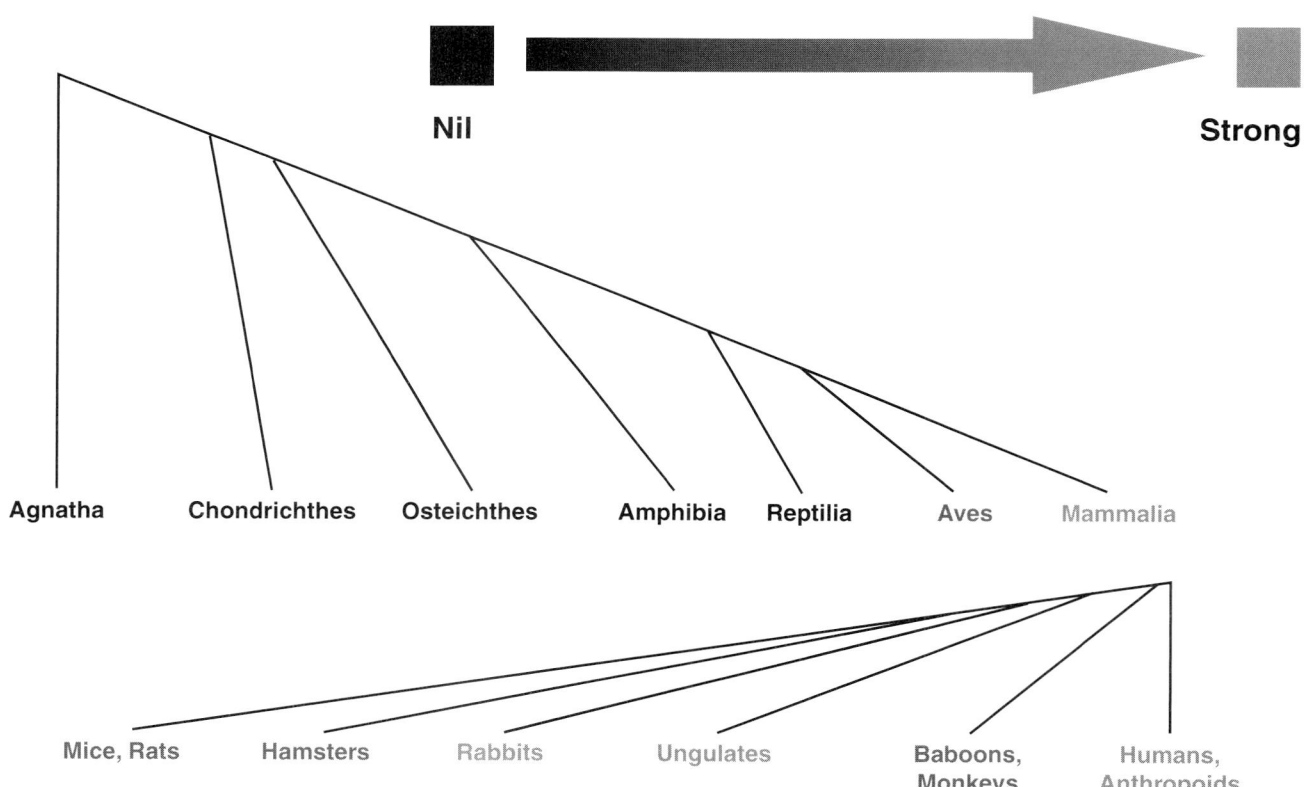

FIGURE 41.1. The phylogeny of lipopolysaccharide (LPS) responses. *Light gray* color indicates an intense response; *black* indicates no response; *shading* in between indicates responses of intermediate intensity. Only mammals show pronounced sensitivity to LPS, and among mammals, great variability is observed.

LPS fulfills the criterion of indispensability. It is present on nearly all gram-negative bacteria, and is an important structural component of the outer membrane. It has indeed become a target of the innate immune system, and macrophages react violently to it, releasing tumor necrosis factor (TNF), interleukin-1 (IL-1), and many other cytokines when they encounter it. These cytokines, if over-produced, can cause shock and death. However, at lower levels, they are known to mediate protective effects, against gram-negative organisms and also against unrelated infectious agents of gram-positive, fungal, or protozoal taxa. The fact that cross-protection occurs may indicate that the innate immune system deals with many pathogens in a similar manner. Among the end effects of cytokine release are the induction of fever, the synthesis and release of acute-phase reactants, and vasodilation with a fall in blood pressure. Interestingly, the response to LPS is phylogenetically erratic (Fig. 41.1). While some invertebrates respond to LPS in some fashion (witness the gelation response of *Limulus* amebocyte lysates), most are quite indifferent to it, as are most vertebrates. Indeed, birds are minimally susceptible to LPS toxicity, and among mammals, a great deal of variability exists, so that even rather closely related families of *Mammalia* (e.g., the lower primates vs. the anthropoid apes) show very different patterns of response. This fact in itself could be taken to suggest that a few, critical determinants of the LPS response might exist in mammals.

There has been considerable mystery as to how LPS triggers macrophage responses. In 1990, a partial answer came to light with the finding that the LPS is immobilized on the macrophage surface by CD14 (1), a glycosylinositolphosphate-linked protein with a leucine-rich structure. It was found to be transferred to CD14 by the action of LPS binding protein (LBP) (2–5), a plasma protein produced by the liver and now known to offer protection against certain gram-negative bacteria (6). However, these findings did not reveal the mechanism by which a transmembrane signal was generated. CD14 has no cytoplasmic component, and cannot evoke such a signal.

Many attempts were made to identify a second "signaling" receptor for LPS. Direct efforts at purifying such a receptor through the use of affinity methods, or by cross-linking CD14 to other proteins on the cell surface, were fruitless. Many candidates were proposed, but none survived rigorous experimental analysis.

THE SEARCH FOR THE *Lps* GENE

The signaling component of the LPS receptor was identified through genetic studies undertaken with mice that were unresponsive to LPS. In 1965, C3H/HeJ mice were found to be resistant to the lethal effect of LPS (7). Resistance was ultimately ascribed to a spontaneous mutation, occurring at a single locus on chromosome 4 (8,9). This locus was termed *Lps*, and the particular allele present in C3H/HeJ mice was termed *Lps^d*, to denote a defective or deficient response to LPS. The mutation conferred total or near-total insensitivity to LPS, and in future analyses of signal transduction using cytokine production as an end point, it became very clear that the LPS dose-response curve was displaced by three to four orders of magnitude in cells derived from C3H/HeJ mice. Interestingly, C3H/HeJ mice were found to be hypersusceptible to authentic gram-negative infections (10,11). Therefore, it became clear that timely detection of a gram-negative infection via the LPS signaling pathway was essential for an effective host response.

In 1978, a second mutation at the *Lps* locus was reported in an unrelated *Mus musculus* strain. C57BL/10ScCr mice were noted to be similarly unresponsive to LPS, and when crossed to C3H/HeJ mice, produced unresponsive progeny (12). However, the defect in these animals was recessive, while the C3H/HeJ defect was codominant. This implied that the mutations at *Lps* involved the same gene, but were structurally dissimilar.

Among the speculations concerning the *Lps* locus, and the critical gene it contained, were that a component of the interferon-α/β complex (also on chromosome 4) might be the gene; that a signaling protein such as protein kinase C might be encoded by it; and that it might code for a microtubule-associated protein (since taxol, a weak LPS mimetic, is known to associate with microtubules). Complementary DNA (cDNA) cloning approaches failed to identify the *Lps* gene product, though it was claimed on the basis of weak evidence that the guanosine triphosphate (GTP)-binding protein Ran/TC4 was encoded by the gene in question (13). In fact, Ran/TC4 is encoded by a gene that resides on mouse chromosome 17, and is thus entirely unrelated to the *Lps* locus.

In the end, the *Lps* mutations were identified through positional cloning efforts by Poltorak et al. (14), who refined the location of the mutation in C3H/HeJ mice on 2,093 meioses, sequenced the major part of a large (2.6 megabases) critical region, and found that only a single gene was present in the entire interval. This gene coded for the orphan receptor, Toll-like receptor 4 (Tlr4). C3H/HeJ mice were found to have a point mutation of *Tlr4*, whereas the gene was deleted entirely in C57BL/10ScCr mice (15,16).

EVOLUTIONARY ORIGINS OF TLR4

As noted earlier, the innate immune system is phylogenetically older than the acquired immune system. Moreover, it is the only immune system in invertebrate organisms. Basic studies of invertebrate immunity therefore provide a template for the understanding of immunity in higher organisms. In 1996, it was reported that the *Drosophila* Toll protein, previously known to have a developmental function in the embryo (17,18), was required for an effective response to fungal infection in the adult fly (19). The existence of such a function was guessed from the fact that fungal growth is ordinarily controlled by drosomycin, an antifungal protein under the control of a promoter driven by members of the Rel family of transcription factors. Two such factors, Dif and Dorsal, are activated as a result of Toll ligation (20), which occurs in embryo when the prohormone Spätzle is cleaved to its mature form by the proteolytic enzyme Snake.

Mutational studies demonstrated that viable Toll-defective flies (bearing loss-of-function mutations of Toll) were susceptible to infection by the fungus *Aspergillus fumigatus*. Similarly, impairment of signaling intermediates (Pelle, Tube, or Dif) would prevent an effective response to fungal infection. The entire axis of the innate immune response to fungus was thus solved in a very short period of time. At least one other member of the Toll family in *Drosophila* has subsequently been shown to mediate resistant to bacterial infection (21). It is noteworthy that these responses occur in the *Drosophila* fat body, the functional equivalent of the vertebrate liver.

MAMMALIAN TLRS AND THEIR SPECIFICITY

It was not obvious that this same system actually applied in vertebrates, which have diverged from *Drosophila* for approximately 500 million years. It was known that homologues of *Drosophila* Toll were present in mammals, as representatives of the family had been found among expressed sequence tag (EST) databases, and on this basis five Tlr cDNAs were cloned before the function of any Tlr was assigned (22–24). Moreover, ligation of at least one of the Tlrs (Tlr4) could cause NFκB translocation in transfected cell lines (23). But the true ligands of each Tlr could not be identified through transfection studies, and all remained orphan receptors. Indeed, a concerted search for an LPS transducer among known members of the Toll-like receptor family in vertebrates ended with embarrassment, in that it was incorrectly claimed that Tlr2 was responsible for such a function, whereas Tlr4 was not (25,26). This work caused considerable confusion in the field during its earliest days.

The fact that Tlr4 (and not Tlr2) was responsible for LPS signal transduction was underscored by the knockout of *Tlr2* in mice. Animals lacking *Tlr2* were entirely normal in their response to LPS. Notably, however, they did not respond to muramyldipeptide (the smallest unit of peptidoglycan) (27) or to certain bacterial lipopeptides (28). It was also pointed out that *Tlr4* defects create resistance to lipoteichoic acid (*Tlr2* defects do not) (27). Hence, while the function of most Tlrs remains undeciphered, the two Tlrs for which at least some functions have been assigned present a picture in which oligospecific reactivity to microbial products is the rule.

At present writing, nine mammalian Tlr cDNAs have been cloned (28a). Two subgroups of Tlrs are apparent from analyses of sequence alignments. All have a leucine-rich ectodomain and display varying numbers of leucine-rich repeat motifs. All have well-conserved Toll-like domains on the cytoplasmic side. All but Tlr2 and Tlr4 remain orphan receptors, although a common theme of innate immune response is strongly suspected.

OTHER RECEPTORS WITH TOLL-LIKE DOMAINS

In 1991, with the cloning of one subunit of the IL-1 receptor cDNA, it was recognized that strong homology existed between the *Drosophila* Toll and IL-1R cytoplasmic domains (for which reason the Toll-like domain is sometimes referred to as a Toll-IL-1R–like domain, or TIR) (29). The other chain of the IL-1R (IL-1RAcP) and both chains of the IL-18R were also found to have Toll-like domains, though both chains of both receptors have immunoglobulin-repeat ectodomains. More recently, an orphan receptor termed SIGIRR has also been identified through EST database searches, which has a well-conserved Toll-like domain and a single immunoglobulin (Ig)-repeat ectodomain (30).

The proinflammatory nature of IL-1 and IL-18 receptors is well understood. So, too, are some details of the signaling pathways that serve both of these receptors (see below). The presence of Toll-like cytoplasmic domains may be seen as an evolutionary attempt to enhance the signal elicited by an infectious organism, wherein IL-1 is elicited by the primary stimulus, and may serve to generate a greatly amplified response. Hence, a single LPS molecule might potentially cause the activation of many cells, at anatomic sites far beyond the locus of the infection.

LIPOPOLYSACCHARIDE IS A DIRECT LIGAND FOR TLR4

In *Drosophila*, the protein Spätzle is generated in response to infection, through the action of unknown protease(s) activated by pathogen molecules yet to be identified. Spätzle is the proximal ligand for Toll receptor activation, and Toll does not have direct contact with the pathogen or any of its components.

In mammals, the situation is different, in that Tlr4 (and by implication, other Tlrs) interacts directly with a component of the pathogen (in this case, LPS). The fact of direct contact was inferred from genetic complementation studies (31) in which advantage was taken of species-dependent selectivity in response to different LPS partial structures. While lipid A, the toxic center of LPS, is capable of activating both human and mouse macrophages, stimulating them to produce TNF, tetra-acyl lipid A (which lacks secondary acyl chains) is only capable of stimulating mouse macrophages; when applied to human cells, it antagonizes activation by lipid A or intact LPS (Fig. 41.2).

By transducing an immortalized macrophage cell line derived from C3H/HeJ macrophages to express the normal mouse or human Tlr4 proteins, it was demonstrated that the species origin of Tlr4 is the sole determinant of selectivity in the response to tetra-acyl lipid A. Cells expressing human Tlr4 would not respond to tetra-acyl lipid A, though their response to intact lipid A was normal. Insofar as the Tlr4 protein "reads" the structure of lipid A and determines whether secondary acyl chains are present, it may be concluded that close physical contact between Tlr4 and the agonist must exist. Furthermore, it is clear that structural differences between different Tlr4 molecules influence reactivity with a given molecular species of LPS.

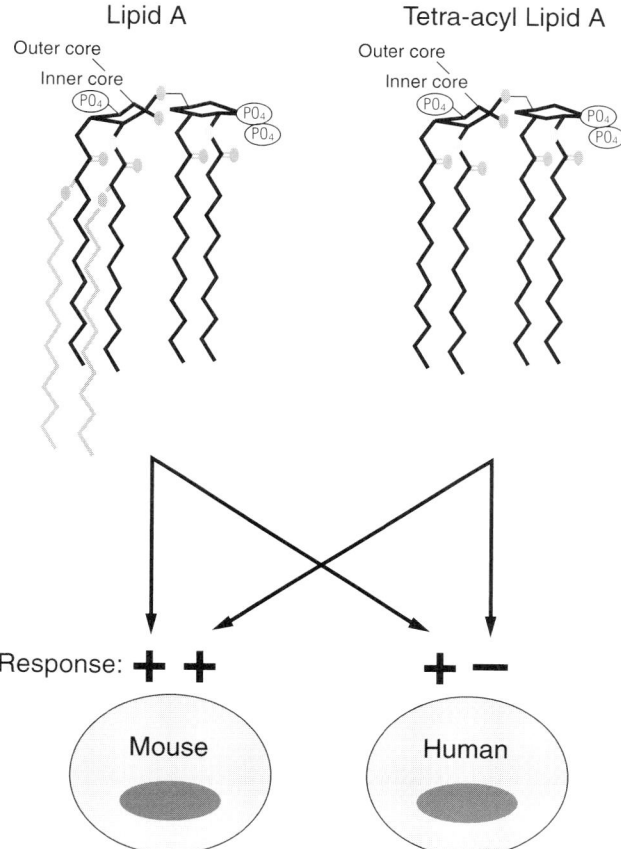

FIGURE 41.2. Interspecies differences in responses to lipopolysaccharide (LPS) partial structures. While both human and mouse macrophages show vigorous responses to lipid A, the toxic center of LPS, human macrophages fail to respond to tetra-acyl lipid A (lacking secondary acyl chains). By contrast, mouse macrophages respond strongly to tetra-acyl lipid A. This species difference was ascribed solely to the species origin of Tlr4. Hence, it is Tlr4 that interprets the structure of an LPS molecule, and differences in Tlr4 primary structure (as, for example, the difference between human and mouse Tlr4) can determine whether response to a particular LPS molecule will occur.

Similar conclusions were sustained by studies of LPS response in hamster cells transduced to express the human Tlr4 protein (32). Such differences, manifested at the level of polymorphisms occurring within a species, might influence susceptibility to specific gram-negative organisms.

It has also been shown that overexpression of Tlr4 on the macrophage surface leads to exaggerated sensitivity to LPS (approximately 30-fold lower concentrations of LPS are required to induce half-maximal secretion of TNF). It is therefore supposed that Tlr4 is a limiting factor in the transduction complex, though it is quite certain that accessory proteins are required as well. Consistent with the codominant suppressive phenotype associated with the $Tlr4^{\text{Lps-d}}$ allele, overexpression of this mutant form of the protein will strongly suppress LPS signaling, essentially abolishing it in most clones examined (33).

POLYMORPHISM AT THE TLR4 LOCUS

The genes encoding human and mouse Tlr4 are placed at a considerable distance from any known neighbors, and lie in the midst of a region rich in retroviral repeats (Fig. 41.3). The human locus is in the cytogenetic interval 9q33-9q34, while the mouse locus is placed in the distal third of chromosome 4. Both human and murine forms of the gene have been sequenced to completion, and the exons of several other mammalian species have also been sequenced for the purpose of phylogenetic comparison.

Among mice, considerable variability is observed at the *Tlr4* locus. In addition to the mutations that create LPS resistance in C3H/HeJ and C57BL/10ScCr strains, a considerable amount of coding polymorphism has been observed, with 11 amino acid substitution sites observed among 35 strains, most in the ectodomain of the protein. At present, no clear phenotypic effect has been ascribed to any murine polymorphism, though potentially, such an analysis might be carried out using the same transfection system used to infer physical contact between LPS and Tlr4 (31).

Among human populations, Tlr4 also shows impressive structural variation. In Caucasians, a variant allele (TLR4-B; Gb:AF177766) in which two amino acid substitutions modify the mid-ectodomain is present at a frequency of approximately 14% in the population at large. TLR4-B is extremely rare among African Americans, and presumably arose in the European population. However, an African allele has been identified in which substitution at one of the two sites altered in the European population has occurred. This would suggest that the European allele arose upon an African background, through mutation or crossover. Moreover, among African Americans and Africans, mutation at Tlr4 is more abundant than it is among Caucasians. The difference between these populations might reflect the effects of selective pressures exerted by microbial pathogens that differed between the two geographic locations

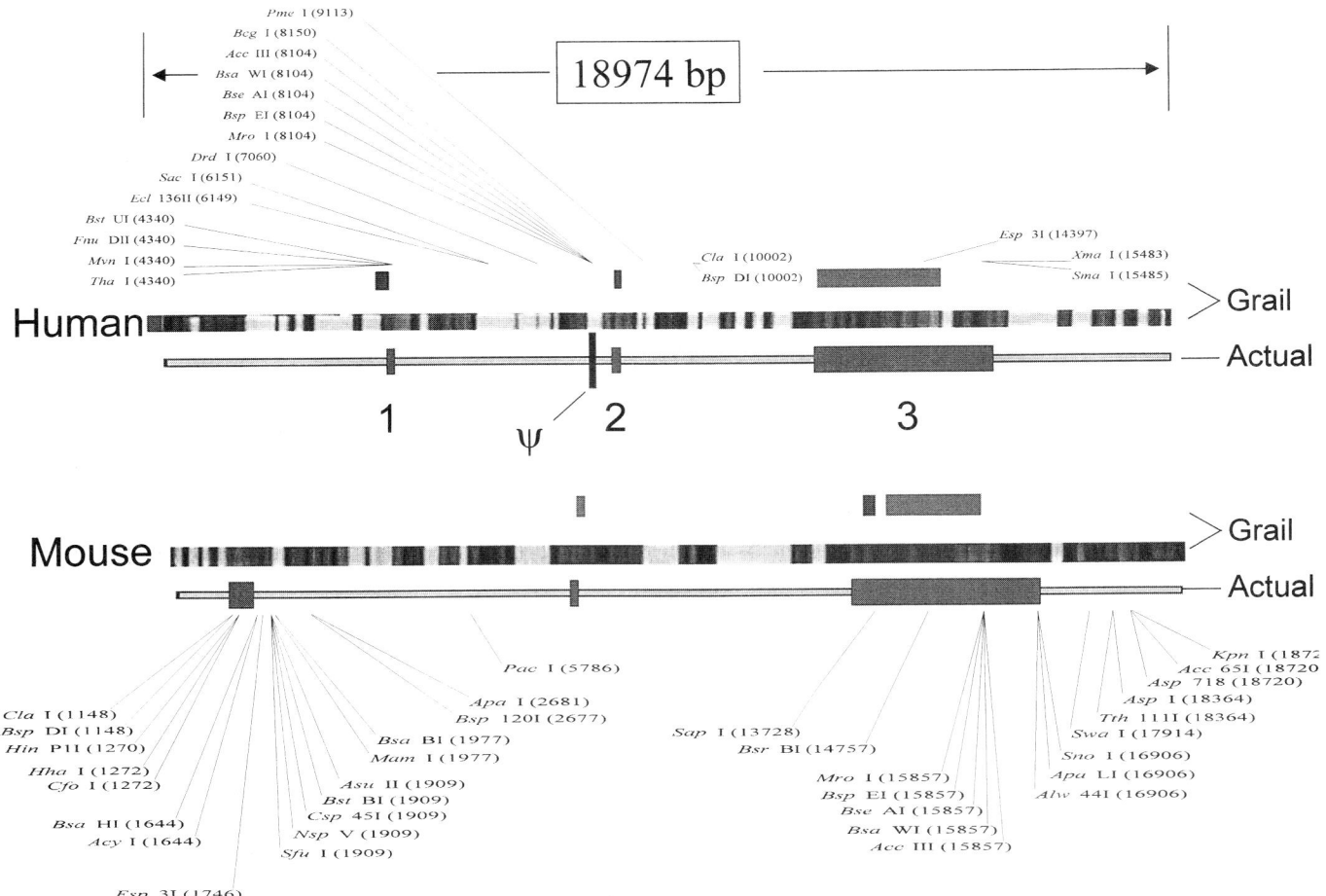

FIGURE 41.3. The genomic structure of *Tlr4* and TLR4, the human and mouse Toll-like receptor 4 genes, illustrated using the gene prediction program GRAIL. *Gray-scale image* portrays the G/C content of genomic DNA in a region spanning both genes (*darker areas* are G/C rich; *lighter areas* are A/T rich). The *light gray* regions of genomic sequence denote areas that are composed of repetitive DNA (chiefly of retroviral origin). The location of exons encoding the processed messenger RNA (mRNA) is shown as *bars* adjacent to each sequence. The actual locations of the exons are well predicted by GRAIL (*top gray bars*), which efficiently recognizes genes in anonymous DNA sequences.

(Smirnova et al., in preparation). However, in humans as in mice, phenotypic significance has yet to be assigned to the TLR4 polymorphisms that have been identified.

THE STRUCTURE OF THE LIPOPOLYSACCHARIDE SIGNALING COMPLEX

Shimazu and co-workers (34) recently reported that the small, secreted protein MD-2 may be coprecipitated from the macrophage surface together with Tlr4. Moreover, coexpression of MD-2 and Tlr4 imparts LPS responsiveness to 293 cells, which are otherwise insensitive to LPS. Although transfection-based analyses have proved misleading in the past, it is possible that MD-2 is indeed essential for LPS sig-

naling, and knockout of the MD-2 gene is eagerly awaited for this reason.

Assuming that Tlr4 requires MD-2 for effective responses to LPS, and assuming that CD14 is also essential, a tripartite protein complex may be envisioned, wherein LPS would necessarily bind to Tlr4 to elicit a signal. It cannot, at this point, be said that other proteins are not also involved. Moreover, cofactors for signaling on the cytoplasmic side have not yet been fully deciphered.

Kawai et al. (35) showed that MyD88, a cytoplasmic protein with a Toll-like domain, is required for LPS toxicity, insofar as knockout mutations greatly diminish the lethal effect of LPS. MyD88 is also required for signaling from other receptors that have a Toll-like domain (notably the IL-1 and IL-18 receptors) (36). It is presumed that this protein is recruited to Tlr4, wherein it undergoes heterotypic interaction with the receptor Toll-like domain to initiate a signal. Signaling may also involve phosphorylation of the receptor, though at present writing this has not been shown to occur.

Acting in conjunction with MyD88, the IL-1 receptor associated kinase (IRAK) is involved in transducing the LPS signal to the level of NFκB (37,38). TRAF-6 is also required for this purpose, and a "bridge" between TRAF-6 and MEKK-1 is reportedly formed by ECSIT, a protein with binding affinity for TRAF-6 (39).

It must be acknowledged, however, that understanding of the LPS signal transduction cascade remains quite sketchy, as complex and as highly ramified as the pathway seems to be. For example, the events that lead to mitogen-activated protein (MAP) kinase activation, p38 activation, and phosphatidylinositol-3 (PI3) kinase activation—all of which certainly occur as a result of LPS activation (40–43)—are quite mysterious. Do other proteins engage Tlr4 directly to achieve these ends?

Mutational evidence suggests that this may be the case. In humans, a single instance of co-resistance to LPS and IL-1 has been reported in a young girl who suffered from a severe immunodeficiency (44). It would appear that this patient suffered from a global defect in Tlr signal transduction. Yet MyD88 expression and structure were normal, implying that other cofactors for signal transduction remain to be discovered.

THE ROLE OF OTHER MEMBERS OF THE TLR FAMILY

Knockout work appears to be leading the way in analysis of Tlr receptor function. Targeted mutation of the Tlr4 gene in mice confirmed the phenotype known to exist in C3H/HeJ animals and C57BL/10ScCr animals (45). Moreover, it ruled out a role for Tlr2 in LPS signal transduction (27). Importantly, however, it established that Tlr2 does play a role in peptidoglycan signaling (27) and in bacterial lipopeptide signaling (28), so that it may now be inferred that oligospecificity of Tlr receptor function is the rule. It is widely guessed that other bacterial determinants (for example, CpG dinucleotides, presented in the correct sequence context) may be sensed through other Tlrs. Such well-known inducing molecules as lipoarabinomannan (a constituent of mycobacteria) are being investigated to determine Tlr specificity. However, it is well to be mindful of the potential failure of transfection as a tool in such studies, and the gold standard for assessment of signal transducing potential must henceforth be mutational deletion of the Tlr involved.

Remarkably, CD14 shows broad specificity in its ability to engage microbial products ranging from LPS to peptidoglycan to lipopeptides. It is not yet known whether the role played by CD14 is a universal one, or whether other pro-

teins served to concentrate the signal carried by other inducers. But it is likely that the Tlrs are the principal (and perhaps the only) receptor pathway by which microbes are sensed.

CONCLUSION: THE ADMIXTURE OF INNATE AND ACQUIRED IMMUNE FUNCTIONS IN IMMUNITY AND IMMUNOPATHOLOGY

The acquired immune system came into existence in the context of the innate immune system that predated it. As lymphocytes share a common ontogenic origin with macrophages, it is not surprising that they should be endowed with Tlrs just as the latter cells are. Hence, in mice, the mitogenic effect of LPS is a direct one, and is mediated by Tlr4. Beyond the fact that innate immune and acquired immune responses are not fully separable, it might be guessed that each system might influence the other.

In the case of the innate immune system exerting an effect on the acquired immune system, there is ample evidence of such an influence. Acquired immunity could not exist without the innate immune system. Not only do the innate immune cells themselves (macrophages and dendritic cells) support an acquired immune response through the vital function of antigen presentation, but they elaborate cytokines that are indispensable for an acquired immune response to occur.

It is also clear that cooperativity occurs in the opposite direction. The output of an acquired immune response is, at one level, the production of antibody, and antibody opsonizes microbial targets so as to cause their elimination by innate immune cells. Lymphokines (most strikingly interferon-γ) can also influence the behavior of macrophages.

In proposing the occurrence of "horror autotoxicus," Ehrlich envisioned a problem in which antitoxins (antibodies) might attack tissues of the host, leading to an autoimmune catastrophe. We know very well that this can occur. We know also that in its purest form, sepsis represents another type of autoimmune catastrophe, one in which the host is damaged by an overly exuberant innate immune response. We are left to wonder whether interplay between these two forms of immunity might exist, and specifically, whether innate immune activation via the Tlrs could contribute to various autoimmune diseases (Fig. 41.4).

It has recently been shown that antibodies against Tlr4 may have strong agonist properties if cross-linked by a secondary antibody (46). In certain autoimmune diseases, antibodies against Tlrs might actually exist. If so, it is possible that they might induce cytokine synthesis to the detriment of the host. It is also possible that certain polymorphisms of Tlrs might predispose to autoimmune disease, or that defects of signaling within the Tlr pathway could augment such disease. Awareness of the Tlrs as the principal

When the Immune Systems Overreact

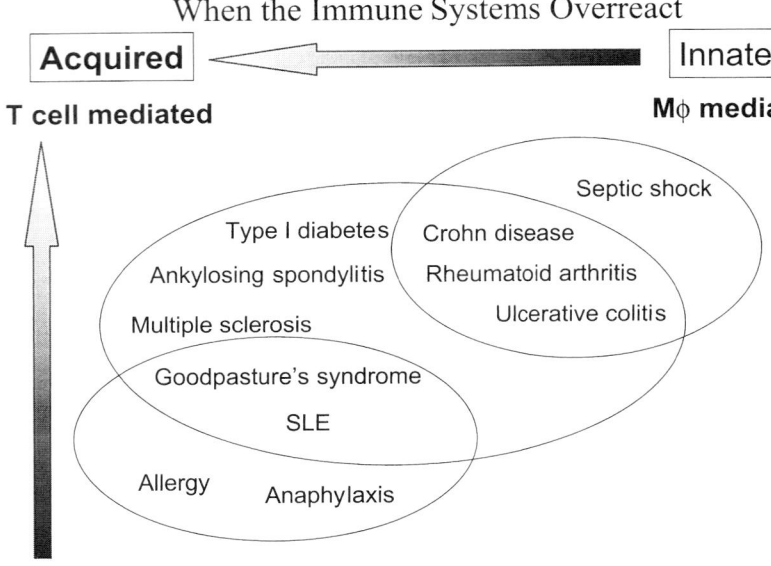

FIGURE 41.4. The spectrum of autoimmune diseases. Both innate and acquired immune dysfunction can cause disease in humans. While some autoimmune diseases involve principally cells of the acquired immune system, and at that, may be initiated by errors in B-cell or T-cell function, the innate immune system is frequently involved in pathogenesis as well, if only because of the close interplay that has evolved among cellular components of the immune system. Endotoxic shock may be taken as an example of autoimmunity in which the innate immune system alone plays a prominent role. *SLE*, systemic lupus erythematosus.

exponent of innate immune sensing may place us in a position to understand such diseases.

REFERENCES

1. Wright SD, Ramos RA, Tobias PS, et al. CD14, a receptor for complexes of lipopolysaccharide (LPS) and LPS binding protein. *Science* 1990;249:1431–1433.
2. Hailman E, Lichenstein HS, Wurfel MM, et al. Lipopolysaccharide (LPS)-binding protein accelerates the binding of LPS to CD14. *J Exp Med* 1994;179:269–277.
3. Tobias PS, Mathison JC, Ulevitch RJ. A family of lipopolysaccharide binding proteins involved in responses to gram-negative sepsis. *J Biol Chem* 1988;263:13479–13481.
4. Tobias PS, Soldau K, Ulevitch RJ. Isolation of a lipopolysaccharide-binding acute phase reactant from rabbit serum. *J Exp Med* 1986;164:777–793.
5. Tobias PS, Soldau K, Ulevitch RJ. Identification of a lipid A binding site in the acute phase reactant lipopolysaccharide binding protein. *J Biol Chem* 1989;264:10867–10871.
6. Jack RS, Fan X, Bernheiden M, et al. Lipopolysaccharide-binding protein is required to combat a murine gram-negative bacterial infection. *Nature* 1997;389:742–745.
7. Heppner G, Weiss DW. High susceptibility of strain A mice to endotoxin and endotoxin-red blood cell mixtures. *J Bacteriol* 1965;696–703.
8. Watson J, Kelly K, Largen M, et al. The genetic mapping of a defective LPS response gene in C3H/HeJ mice. *J Immunol* 1978; 120:422–424.
9. Watson J, Riblet R, Taylor BA. The response of recombinant inbred strains of mice to bacterial lipopolysaccharides. *J Immunol* 1977;118:2088–2093.
10. O'Brien AD, Rosenstreich DL, Scher I, et al. Genetic control of susceptibility to *Salmonella typhimurium* in mice: role of the LPS gene. *J Immunol* 1980;124:20–24.
11. Rosenstreich DL, Weinblatt AC, O'Brien AD. Genetic control of resistance to infection in mice. *CRC Crit Rev Immunol* 1982;3:263–330.
12. Coutinho A, Meo T. Genetic basis for unresponsiveness to lipopolysaccharide in C57BL/10Cr mice. *Immunogenetics* 1978; 7:17–24.
13. Kang AD, Wong PM, Chen H, et al. Restoration of lipopolysaccharide-mediated B-cell response after expression of a cDNA encoding a GTP-binding protein. *Infect Immun* 1996;64: 4612–4617.
14. Poltorak A, Smirnova I, He XL, et al. Genetic and physical mapping of the Lps locus—identification of the toll-4 receptor as a candidate gene in the critical region. *Blood Cells Mol Dis* 1998; 24:340–355.
15. Poltorak A, He X, Smirnova I, et al. Defective LPS signaling in C3H/HeJ and C57BL/10ScCr mice: mutations in *Tlr4* gene. *Science* 1998;282:2085–2088.
16. Poltorak A, Smirnova I, Clisch R, et al. Limits of a deletion spanning *Tlr4* in C57BL/10ScCr mice. *J Endotoxin Res* 2000;6:51–56.
17. Anderson KV, Bokla L, Nusslein-Volhard C. Establishment of dorsal-ventral polarity in the Drosophila embryo: the induction of polarity by the Toll gene product. *Cell* 1985;42:791–798.
18. Hashimoto C, Hudson KL, Anderson KV. The Toll gene of Drosophila, required for dorsal-ventral embryonic polarity, appears to encode a transmembrane protein. *Cell* 1988;52:269–279.
19. Lemaitre B, Nicolas E, Michaut L. et al. The dorsoventral regulatory gene cassette spatzle/Toll/cactus controls the potent antifungal response in Drosophila adults. *Cell* 1996;86:973–983.
20. Manfruelli P, Reichhart JM, Steward R, et al. A mosaic analysis in Drosophila fat body cells of the control of antimicrobial peptide genes by the Rel proteins dorsal and DIF. *EMBO J* 1999; 18:3380–3391.
21. Williams MJ, Rodriguez A, Kimbrell DA, et al. The 18-wheeler mutation reveals complex antibacterial gene regulation in Drosophila host defense. *EMBO J* 1997;16:6120–6130.
22. Chaudhary PM, Ferguson C, Nguyen V, et al. Cloning and characterization of two Toll/interleukin-1 receptor-like genes TIL3 and TIL4: evidence for a multi-gene receptor family in humans. *Blood* 1998;91:4020–4027.

23. Medzhitov R, Preston-Hurlburt P, Janeway CA Jr. A human homologue of the Drosophila Toll protein signals activation of adaptive immunity. *Nature* 1997;388:394–397.
24. Rock FL, Hardiman G, Timans JC, et al. A family of human receptors structurally related to Drosophila Toll. *Proc Natl Acad Sci USA* 1998;95:588–593.
25. Kirschning CJ, Wesche H, Merrill Ayres T, et al. Human toll-like receptor 2 confers responsiveness to bacterial lipopolysaccharide. *J Exp Med* 1998;188:2091–2097.
26. Yang R-B, Mark MR, Gray A, et al. Toll-like receptor-2 mediates lipopolysaccharide-induced cellular signalling. *Nature* 1998;395:284–288.
27. Takeuchi O, Hoshino K, Kawai T, et al. Differential roles of TLR2 and TLR4 in recognition of gram-negative and gram-positive bacterial cell wall components. *Immunity* 1999;11;443–451.
28. Takeuchi O, Kaufmann A, Grote K, et al. Cutting edge: preferentially the R-stereoisomer of the mycoplasmal lipopeptide macrophage-activating lipopeptide-2 activates immune cells through a Toll-like receptor 2– and MyD88-dependent signaling pathway. *J Immunol* 2000;164:554–557.
28a. Du X, Poltorak A, Wei Y, Beutler B. Three novel mammalian toll-like receptors: gene structure, expression, and evolution. *Ear Cytok Netw* 2000;11:362–371.
29. Gay NJ, Keith FJ. Drosophila Toll and IL-1 receptor [letter]. *Nature* 1991;351:355–356.
30. Thomassen E, Renshaw BR. Identification and characterization of SIGIRR, a molecule representing a novel subtype of the IL-1R superfamily. *Cytokine* 1999;11:389–399.
31. Poltorak A, Ricciardi-Castagnoli P, Citterio A, et al. Physical contact between LPS and Tlr4 revealed by genetic complementation. *Proc Natl Acad Sci USA* 2000;97:2163–2167.
32. Lien E, Means TK, Heine H. et al. Toll-like receptor 4 imparts ligand-specific recognition of bacterial lipopolysaccharide. *J Clin Invest* 2000;105:497–504.
33. Du X, Poltorak A, Silva M. et al. Analysis of Tlr4-mediated LPS signal transduction in macrophages by mutational modification of the receptor. *Blood Cells Mol Dis* 1999;25:328–338.
34. Shimazu R, Akashi S, Ogata H, et al. MD-2, a molecule that confers lipopolysaccharide responsiveness on Toll-like receptor 4. *J Exp Med* 1999;189:1777–1782.
35. Kawai T, Adachi O, Ogawa T, et al. Unresponsiveness of MyD88-deficient mice to endotoxin. *Immunity* 1999;11:115–122.
36. Adachi O, Kawai T, Takeda K, et al. Targeted disruption of the MyD88 gene results in loss of IL-1– and IL-18–mediated function. *Immunity* 1998;9:143–150.
37. Medzhitov R, Preston-Hurlburt P, Kopp E. et al. MyD88 is an adaptor protein in the hToll/IL-1 receptor family signaling pathways. *Mol Cell* 1998;2:253–258.
38. Muzio M, Ni J, Feng P, et al. IRAK (Pelle) family member IRAK-2 and MyD88 as proximal mediators of IL-1 signaling. *Science* 1997;278:1612–1615.
39. Kopp E, Medzhitov R, Carothers J, et al. ECSIT is an evolutionarily conserved intermediate in the Toll/IL-1 signal transduction pathway. *Genes Dev* 1999;13:2059–2071.
40. Hambleton J, Weinstein SL, Lem L, et al. Activation of c-Jun N-terminal kinase in bacterial lipopolysaccharide-stimulated macrophages. *Proc Natl Acad Sci USA* 1996;93:2774–2778.
41. Han J, Bohuslav J, Jiang Y, et al. CD14 dependent mechanisms of cell activation. *Prog Clin Biol Res* 1998;397:157–168.
42. Han J, Lee JD, Bibbs L, et al. A MAP kinase targeted by endotoxin and hyperosmolarity in mammalian cells. *Science* 1994;265:808–811.
43. Rosoff PM, Cantley LC. Lipopolysaccharide and phorbol esters induce differentiation but have opposite effects on phosphatidylinositol turnover and Ca2+ mobilization in 70Z/3 pre-B lymphocytes. *J Biol Chem* 1985;260:9209–9215.
44. Kuhns DB, Long Priel DA, Gallin JI. Endotoxin and IL-1 hyporesponsiveness in a patient with recurrent bacterial infections. *J Immunol* 1997;158:3959–3964.
45. Hoshino K, Takeuchi O, Kawai T, et al. Cutting edge: Toll-like receptor 4 (TLR4)-deficient mice are hyporesponsive to lipopolysaccharide: evidence for TLR4 as the Lps gene product. *J Immunol* 1999;162:3749–3752.
46. Natterman J, Du X, Wei Y, et al. Endotoxin-mimetic effect of antibodies against toll-like receptor 4. *J Endotoxin Res* 2000;6:257–264.

42

LIVER REGENERATION

NELSON FAUSTO

MAIN BIOLOGIC FEATURES

The liver has the unique capacity to regulate its growth and mass, a property that is particularly remarkable because the liver is normally a quiescent organ. Hepatocytes in animals and humans have very low proliferative activity, negligible rates of apoptosis, and a long life span. In the rat liver, less than 1 in 10,000 hepatocytes replicate at any one time. However, as it is well known, hepatocytes do not lose the capacity to proliferate and replicate readily in response to loss of tissue caused by partial hepatectomy (PH) or a reduction in the number of cells, most commonly caused by toxic agents or viruses (1–4). After PH or necrogenic injury, hepatocytes replicate in a quasi-synchronous manner to compensate for the decreased functional mass (either tissue or cell loss). The standard partial hepatectomy involves the

removal of two-thirds of the liver, leading to restoration of tissue mass by 10 to 14 days (5). Smaller resections cause growth responses that are proportional to the amount of tissue removed. In adult rat liver, but not in liver of newborns, there is a threshold for tissue deficiency (approximately 30% deficit) below which growth is slow and hepatocyte replication is asynchronous (6). At the other extreme, hepatectomies involving the resection of 80% or more of liver tissue do not elicit efficient regeneration and are associated with high mortality.

In both rats and mice, liver growth ceases when the regenerated liver mass reaches approximately 10% (plus or minus) of the original hepatic mass before PH. In rodents, the operation consists of the removal of the median and left lateral lobes, also referred to as anterior lobes, leaving intact the right lateral and caudate lobes (posterior lobes). Importantly, tissue growth takes place by expansion of the posterior lobes through hepatocyte proliferation but does not involve the regrowth of the anterior lobes. Since the first

N. Fausto: Department of Pathology, University of Washington School of Medicine, Seattle, Washington 98195-7705.

decade of the 20th century, the hepatic growth after PH has been universally referred to as "liver regeneration," but it is more accurately described as a process of compensatory hyperplasia. Thus, the cessation of growth after PH is not determined by restoration of anatomic form, as would be the case in limb regeneration in amphibians, but depends on the restoration of full functional capacity in the regenerated organ.

As discussed in Chapters 2 and 61 and website chapter 🖳 W-31, the liver contains progenitor cells that can proliferate and differentiate under certain experimental conditions. However, these cells are not responsible for liver regeneration after PH or chemical injury induced by carbon tetrachloride (CCl_4). In both of these situations, hepatocyte replication accounts for liver growth and restoration of mass. In a young adult rat or mouse, approximately 95% of hepatocytes replicate during the first 3 days after PH (7). This proportion drops to approximately 80% in senescent rats (8). The newborn liver contains only diploid hepatocytes but polyploidization and binuclearity develop rapidly (8,9). At 3 months of age the rat liver contains at most 10% to 20% diploid hepatocytes. At this age the majority of the hepatocytes are either mono- or binucleated tetraploid, but a small component of binucleated octoploid cells is present (4× nuclei). All of these cell types are capable of replicating after PH. Surprisingly, diploid tetraploid and octoploid hepatocytes have equal capacity to repopulate damaged livers, indicating that hepatocytes retain replicative capacity regardless of the level of ploidy (10). In the regenerated liver of both rats and mice, the proportion of binucleate cells decreases from the normal level of 25% to 30% to approximately 10% with a corresponding increase in the level of polyploidy, both for tetraploid and octoploid cells (11). An important conclusion derived from these data is that all classes of hepatocytes participate in liver regeneration and do so by either mitotic division of mononucleated cells or by cytokinesis of binucleated cells after DNA replication in both nuclei.

Two other aspects of the biology of replication in the regenerating liver warrant special consideration: the synchrony of the process and the spatial distribution of replicating hepatocytes. Considering that the liver of rodents contains approximately 10^7 hepatocytes, it is remarkable that cell replication is synchronized during liver regeneration after PH or toxic injury. In the murine liver, hepatocyte DNA replication after PH is slower than in rats and does not start for about 30 hours after PH, reaching a maximum at 40 to 44 hours (12,13). In contrast, in the regenerating rat liver, replication starts at 12 to 14 hours after the operation and reaches a peak at 24 hours (7). At the peak of DNA replication in rats, approximately 40% of hepatocytes may be involved. This value is similar for mice, although there are wide variations depending on the strain and experimental conditions. Despite the delayed start of hepatocyte replication in mice, the activation of immediate early genes after PH has a similar timing in rats and mice.

The spatial distribution of proliferating hepatocytes in the regenerating liver has a predictable pattern that varies according to the time after the operation. Initially cell proliferation is highest in cells located in zone 1 of the lobule, particularly in those situated near to but not adjacent to the portal tracts (14,15). Cells immediately adjacent to the portal triads have lower levels of replication compared to cells located further down in zone 1. Hepatocytes with the lowest levels of replication are located in zone 3 of the lobule, surrounding central veins but, as regeneration progresses (16,17) there is a more random distribution of proliferating cells throughout the lobule. It has been suggested that the pattern of spatial distribution of hepatocyte proliferation after PH reflects a streaming process in which only zone 1 cells replicate but then migrate or "stream" through the lobule as liver regeneration progresses. This view is not supported by observations that indicate that hepatocytes have the capacity to proliferate regardless of location and ploidy and do so after PH (14,18). Moreover, if the spatial pattern of hepatocyte replication after PH were due to the streaming of a localized proliferative component, it has to be assumed that a hepatocyte located near the portal space migrates to a position adjacent to the central vein in 24 hours or less, an assumption that is not compatible with experimental observations. The most likely explanation for the zonal distribution of cell proliferation in the regenerating liver is that cells of zone 1 have a shorter G_1 interval than cells in zones 2 and 3 (19). Analysis of the expression of immediate early genes after PH indicates that activation of these genes at the start of liver regeneration occurs more or less simultaneously in cells throughout the lobule. This suggests that the stimuli that initiate regeneration reach hepatocytes randomly and prepare the cells for replication (see Integration of Cytokine and Growth Factor Pathways: Priming and Progression Stages of Liver Regeneration, below). The variable length of the G_1 phase of the cell cycle associated with the cell's position in the lobule may be a consequence of differential activation of cyclins and cyclin-dependent kinases.

Newly replicated hepatocytes form clusters, first in periportal areas and subsequently in the centrolobular region (20). Endothelial cells invade these clusters to restore one-cell-thick cords that have two surfaces lined by sinusoids. Early as well as late changes in the expression of extracellular matrix components after PH have been reported. Increases in urokinase-type plasminogen activator and plasmin as well as fibrinogen degradation occur rapidly and persist for several hours after PH (21,22). Transcripts of the tissue inhibitor of metalloproteinase TIMP-1 increase greatly at the time of the peak of DNA replication and are localized mostly in portal and perisinusoidal mesenchymal cells (23). Upregulation of procollagen α_1 and α_2 transcripts occurs after the cessation of DNA replication and is associated with increased serum aminoterminal procollagen type III peptide (PIIINP). The changes in the expression of extracellular matrix components suggest that remodeling of the extracellular matrix precedes and accompanies cell proliferation and that matrix synthesis coincides with the restoration of quiescence. The reported increase TIMP-1 messenger RNA (mRNA) in the absence of major changes in metalloproteinase activity suggests that TIMP-1 may have other functions besides metalloproteinase inhibition (23).

Changes in hepatocyte cell volume occur very rapidly after PH. Volume increases of hepatocytes are associated with the activation of system A amino acid transport, and increased intracellular alanine and water influx counterbalanced by chloride efflux (24–26). Blockage of system A transport activity inhibited DNA replication after PH without altering protein synthesis (26). Changes in hepatocyte membrane potential occur almost immediately after PH and have been described as hyperpolarization or depolarization. Prevention of depolarization did not alter the expression of immediate early genes after PH (27).

During liver regeneration after PH or CCl_4 administration, hepatocytes replicate once or twice to replenish hepatocytes lost, respectively, by surgical removal of tissue or cell death. Repopulation and serial transplantation studies have demonstrated that hepatocytes have a remarkable proliferative capacity (see Chapter 61) and can undergo as many as 80 population doublings (28–31). Given this replicative potential, it may no longer be surprising that hepatocytes do proliferate after PH. Perhaps more puzzling is that despite their replicative potential, hepatocytes are normally quiescent cells. This implies that hepatocyte replication is actively suppressed in the normal liver and that repressor mechanisms are lifted after PH. Moreover, the strictly regulated and self-limited nature of hepatocyte replication after PH indicates that there is a strong selective pressure favoring replicative repression. Unfortunately, despite the progress in understanding the initiation of liver regeneration, due to a great extent to the availability of knockout and transgenic animals, little is known about the mechanisms that signal the cessation of growth in the regenerating liver.

LIVER REGENERATION IN HUMANS

The principles that regulate liver growth deduced from experimental observations in rodents also guide the regeneration of human liver. These principles are clearly illustrated by the outcomes of "small for size" and "large for size" orthotopic liver transplantation in humans (32). Transplantation of a liver of small relative mass for a particular host results in liver growth that stops when the hepatic mass has reached an optimal liver/body mass ratio for the recipient. In contrast, a liver of large relative mass for a particular recipient will not grow in the new host and may even decrease in mass by apoptosis. Thus for healthy livers, free of accumulations of fat, glycogen, or other types of abnor-

malities, the optimal liver/body mass ratio constitutes the end point of processes that correct a deficit or an excess of hepatic mass.

Two important procedures used clinically in liver transplantation rely on the capacity of the liver to regulate its growth: split liver transplantation and living donor transplantation (33). In split transplantation, after removal from the donor, the liver is divided into two large fragments, each containing the complete set of arteries, veins, and bile ducts needed to establish necessary vascular and biliary connections in the new host. In this manner, two "mini-livers" obtained from a single organ can be transplanted into two recipients. Transplantation of liver lobes from living donors is being used with increased frequency both for pediatric and adult patients. In this procedure 30% to 60% of the liver is resected from the donor and used for transplantation (Fig. 42.1). The rate of regeneration in both donor and recipient after right-lobe adult-to-adult transplantation is remarkably fast as estimated by volumetric magnetic resonance imaging (MRI) (34,35). Liver volume doubles at 7 days after PH (donor) and in 7 to 14 days after transplantation (recipient). By 60 days after the procedures, liver volumes have almost reached their original values. An equally rapid increase in hepatic mass of both donor and recipient livers has been obtained after left lobe transplantation from living donors (36,37).

The minimal ratio of right lobe graft mass to the recipient body weight that permits optimal growth of the transplant is estimated to be 0.8% to 1%. These results are remarkable in that they show that a human hepatic segment, which is 200- to 400-fold larger than a mouse liver, grows only slightly slower than the murine liver after PH. This conclusion needs to be drawn with caution because clinical measurements of liver growth in living donor transplantation have been based on volumetric determinations by MRI-enhanced computer tomography (CT) (34). It has not yet been shown that there is a strong correlation between MRI-estimated volume increases and indices of cell proliferation. One concern is that the rapid increase in volume observed in the liver of the donor and recipient might reflect the presence of edema. However, liver function is also very rapidly restored during the period of time in which there is maximal volume increase and the enlarged liver shows no abnormalities on MRI images. Thus, despite the need for further data, it can be concluded that hepatic enlargement in liver donors and recipients after the surgical procedures represents the growth of fully functional liver tissue.

GENE EXPRESSION DURING LIVER REGENERATION

A very large number of genes are activated after PH at the transcriptional or posttranscriptional level (38,39).

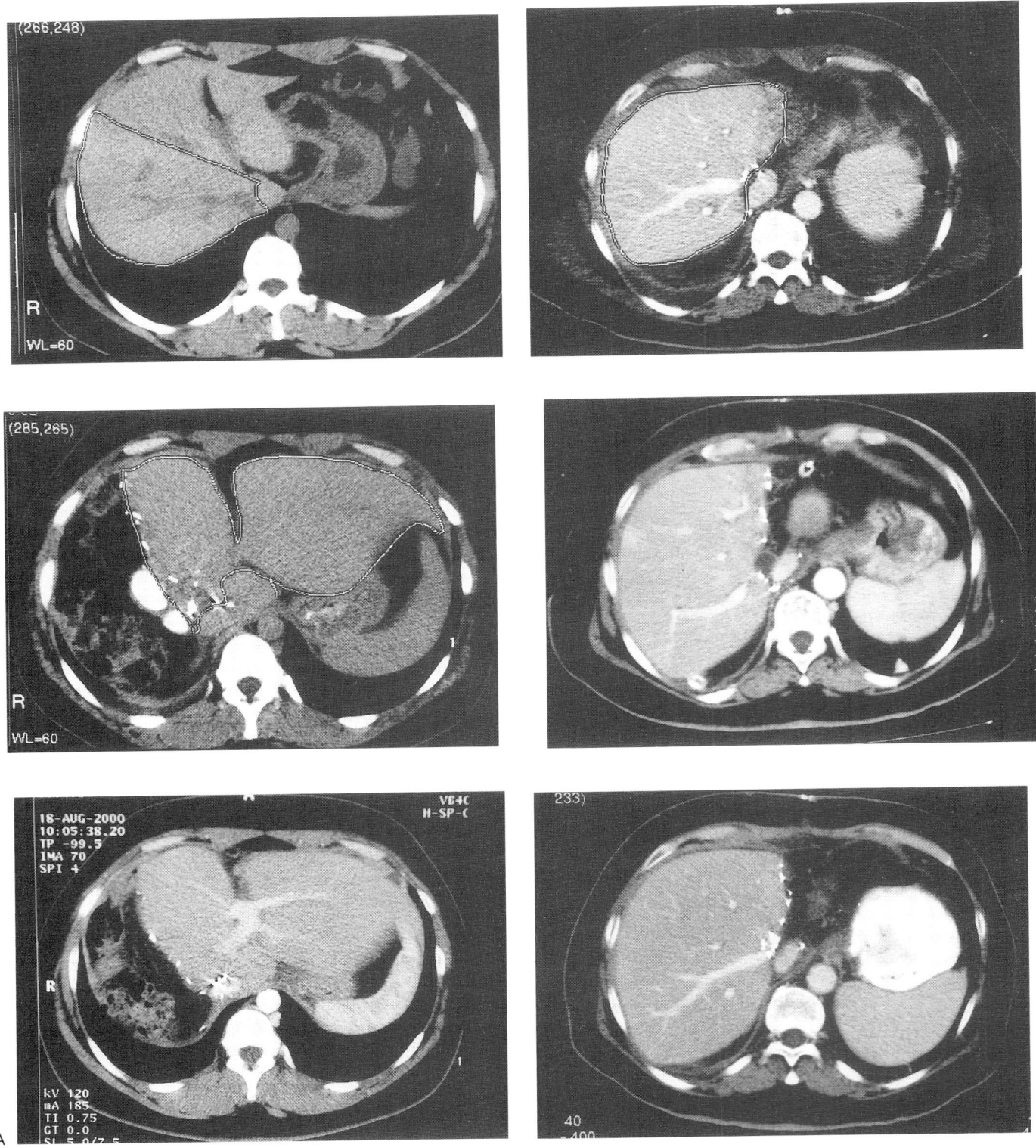

FIGURE 42.1. Liver regeneration in living donor transplantation. **A:** Donor liver. **Top image** shows the donor liver with the right lobe (to be used as the graft) outlined; **middle** and **lower images**, left lobe regeneration 1 week (left lobe outlined) and 3 weeks after partial hepatectomy, respectively. **B:** Recipient liver. **Top, middle,** and **lower** images are, respectively, graft regeneration at 1 (graft outlined), 2, and 3 weeks after transplantation. (Courtesy of Dr. R. Troisi, Ghent University Hospital; see ref. 35.)

Involved in this process are cell cycle genes, metabolic genes, genes coding for extracellular matrix proteins, growth factors, cytokines, and transcription factors, to name some of the key players. Gene expression during liver regeneration can be divided into phases that include the expression of (a) immediate early genes, (b) delayed early genes, and (c) cell cycle genes (2,3). Expression of these genes is controlled by transcription factors, cytokines, and growth factors, which themselves are modulated by signal transduction pathways that receive and transduce stimuli necessary for cell replication and tissue regeneration (40,41).

The Immediate Early Phase of Gene Activation

Immediate early genes are activated very rapidly after PH (1 to 3 hours) in mice and rats, and their activation does not require protein synthesis. Other than that, these genes do not share common sequences or physiologic functions. The first described components of this response were the proto-oncogenes c-*fos*, c-*jun*, and c-*myc* (42–44). Subsequent analysis of gene expression at the start of liver regeneration by subtractive hybridization revealed that more than 70 genes may participate in the immediate early response (45,46). This number will likely increase as powerful complementary DNA (cDNA) microarray technologies capable of detecting 5,000 to 20,000 RNAs are applied to the study of liver regeneration. In addition to c-*fos*, c-*jun*, junB, c-*myc*, and c-*ets*, immediate early genes include, among others, IκBα, insulin-like growth factor (IGF)-binding protein-1, phosphatases (PRL-1, a nuclear protein tyrosine phosphatase), as well as metabolic genes such as phosphoenolpyruvate carboxykinase (PEPCK) and glucose-6-phophatase (47,48). A very important goal in studies of liver regeneration is determining which among these many genes are essential for hepatocyte proliferation. It is likely that a large proportion of immediate early genes are metabolic genes unrelated to or not directly connected with DNA replication.

The regulation of c-*myc* expression has been particularly well studied in both liver regeneration and hepatic development (44,49). Although c-*myc* regulation after PH has a transcriptional component, the major mechanisms of c-*myc* regulation in regeneration and development are posttranscriptional, as demonstrated in studies using transgenic mice (50). Analysis of knockout mice lacking c-*myc*, c-*fos*, or c-*jun* showed that deficiency of these genes have different effects on liver regeneration and development (51). Both c-*myc* and c-*jun* knockouts are embryonic lethals, animals dying between 9 and 13 days [embryonic day 9 (E9) to E13] of development (52,53). Although lack of c-*myc* expression produced cardiac and neural tube defects in mouse embryos, c-*jun* deficiency caused a major defect in hepatogenesis. Moreover, homozygous c-*jun* deficient

embryonic stem cells failed to colonize the liver in chimeric mice, demonstrating that c-*jun* has an essential function in liver development (53). In contrast with these findings, c-*fos* deficiency caused only partial lethality (54). Surviving animals deficient in c-*fos* develop normally and have no defects in liver regeneration after PH.

Transcription Factor Activation and the Immediate Early Gene Response

The transcription factors that are rapidly activated after PH include NFκB, STAT3 (signal transducer and activator of transcription), activator protein-1 (AP-1), and CCAAT enhancer binding protein-β (C/EBPβ) (3,38). The importance of these factors lies in their capacity to bind to multiple genes that contain specific recognition sequences and consequently activate the transcription of the target genes. As a consequence, a single stimulus acting on a transcription factor can lead to transcriptional activation of multiple genes. Of particular importance for immediate early genes is the activation of the transcription factors NFκB and STAT3. Moreover c-*fos* and c-*jun*, which are transcribed in the immediate early gene response, code for protein subunit components of AP-1. STAT3 activation and its relationships with the interleukin-6 (IL-6) family of cytokines is described in detail in Chapters 40 and 41. In addition to the four transcription factors listed above, two others, cAMP-responsive promoter element modulator (CREM) and X-box–binding protein (XBP)-1, have recently been identified as being important components of the regenerative response (55,56). CREM and other 3′,5′-cyclic adenosine monophosphate (cAMP) responsive transcription factors are discussed in Chapters 37 and 40.

NFκB and STAT3 Activation

NFκB and STAT3 are activated during the first few hours after PH. NFκB binding is increased within 30 minutes after PH in rats and mice and returns to normal by 3 hours. STAT3 increase follows NFκB by about 1 hour (57–59). NFκB is a heterodimeric protein composed of two subunits p65 (rel A) and p50 (NFκB1). In the liver as in other tissues, NFκB is bound to an inhibitor (IκB) through its rel A component. There are three isoforms of this inhibitor, IκBα being the most active form in the liver. Activation of NFκB (Fig. 42.2) and its translocation to the nucleus requires the inactivation of IκB through phosphorylation and ubiquitination followed by proteasome degradation (60–62). Tumor necrosis factor (TNF) is one of the major activators of NFκB in the liver (57). Binding of TNF to its receptor type 1 (TNFR1) initiates a cascade of events consisting of the binding of the adapter proteins TRADD (TNF receptor associated death domain) and TRAF2 (TNF receptor associated factor 2), which in turn activate NIK (NFκB-inducing kinase). NIK forms a complex that con-

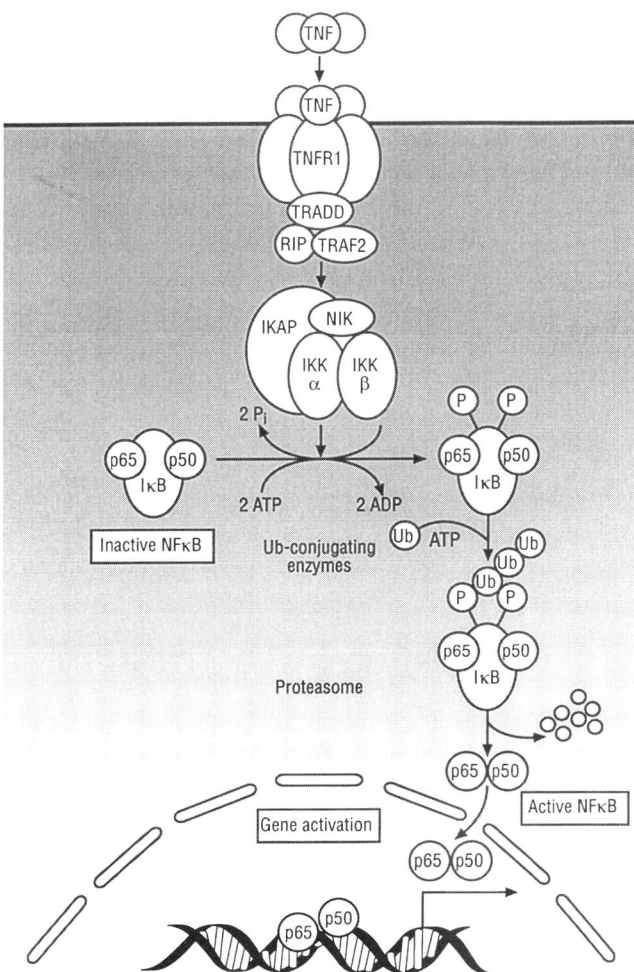

FIGURE 42.2. Steps involved in the activation of NFκB by tumor necrosis factor (*TNF*). The diagram shows the binding of TNF to trimeric TNF receptor type 1 (*TNFR1*) and subsequent binding of the acceptor protein TRADD (*TNF receptor–associated death domain protein*) to the "death domain" of TNFR1. A complex is formed with the acceptor proteins RIP and TRAF2 leading to the activation of NFκB-inducing kinase (*NIK*) and the IκB kinases (*IKKα* and *IKKβ*). Inactive NFκB with its subunits p65 and p50 and the inhibitor IκB is shown on the **left**. Phosphorylation and ubiquitination (*Ub*) of IκB leads to its degradation in the proteasome, releasing active NFκB, shown on the **lower right**. Active NFκB enters the nucleus, binds to recognition sequences, and initiates gene activation. (Redrawn from Baeuerle PA. Reactive oxygen species as costimulatory signals of cytokine-induced NF-κB activation pathways. In: Sen C-K, Sies H, Bauerle P, eds. *Antioxidant and redox regulation of genes.* San Diego: Academic Press, 2000:181–201, with permission.)

tains the IκB kinases IKKα and IKKβ. These kinases phosphorylate serine residues in the N-terminal region of IκB, initiating the process of IκB degradation (63–65). The activity of kinases involved in the IκB degradation are enhanced by ROS (reactive oxygen species) that can be generated by TNF and many other agents and cellular processes.

NFκB translocation to the nucleus and DNA binding leads to the expression of more than a dozen genes likely to be involved in the immediate early gene response. NFκB activation is required for both liver development and liver regeneration. Rel A–deficient mice develop normally up to E14, but all mice die between E14 and E16 with massive hepatocyte apoptosis (66). Interestingly, these animals can be rescued by crossing them with TNFR1 knockouts (67,68). Double transgenics lacking both Rel A and TNFR1 survive through the embryonic period and are born with normal livers. However, these animals perish within the first month of life with massive acute hepatitis. Work with these NFκB/TNFR1 double knockouts established that (a) NFκB is required for liver development and its main activator in the liver is TNF, (b) NFκB deficiency in the developing liver is lethal and causes apoptosis, (c) livers develop normally in the absence of both NFκB and signaling through TNFR1, and (d) animals lacking both NFκB and TNF die with overwhelming liver infection during the neonatal period (67). In hepatocytes and oval cells in culture, blockage of NFκB by a dominant IκBα gene caused apoptosis in cells exposed to TNF (69–72). Inhibition of NFκB binding during liver regeneration by an adenovirus vector expressing a dominant IκBα repressor caused massive apoptosis and inhibited cell replication (73). Despite the strong evidence showing that inhibition of NFκB binding causes apoptosis, this is not an obligatory finding. In liver cells exposed to (*N*-tosyl-*L*-phenylalanine chloromethyl ketone (TPCK), inhibition of NFκB binding by the drug caused cell cycle arrest in G_0 for at least 4 days without evidence of apoptosis (71).

The essential role of NFκB in liver regeneration has been highlighted by studies with mice that lack either type 1 or type 2 TNF receptors (13,74,75). Lack of TNFR2 caused no change in NFκB binding, IL-6 synthesis, STAT3 activation, and hepatocyte DNA replication after PH. In contrast, animals that lack TNFR1 showed deficient NFkB binding, low IL-6 production, decreased STAT3 binding, and low levels of hepatocyte DNA replication. In these animals a single injection of IL-6 restored the STAT3 activation and corrected the DNA replication defect. Studies with liver cells in culture using a NFκB repressor showed that specific blockage of NFκB causes inhibition of STAT3 (71).

IL-6 is a NFκB target gene that is a strong inducer of STAT3 activation (see Chapter 40). IL-6 knockout mice have a severe deficit of liver regeneration and show high mortality after PH (76). An injection of IL-6 immediately before PH corrected the deficit in liver regeneration and restored STAT3 activation. Taken together, these results suggest that signaling through TNFR1 leading to the activation of NFκB and subsequent IL-6 production and STAT3 activation is a mechanism by which liver regeneration after PH is initiated (3). Although IL-6 and STAT3 appear to play an essential role in DNA replication after PH, it remains to be shown that specific inhibition of STAT3 activation after PH prevents DNA replication.

Activator Protein-1 Activation at the Initiation of Liver Regeneration

The AP-1 transcription factor is composed of c-*fos*/c-*jun* heterodimers and c-*jun* hemodimers (77). In the regenerating liver AP-1 may also contain *jun*B and liver regeneration factor-1 (LRF-1), which, like c-*fos* and c-*jun*, are induced as immediate early genes. However, c-*fos* and c-*jun* are rapidly induced (30 to 60 minutes after PH), while *jun*B and LRF-1 are induced later (78). It has been proposed that the components of the AP-1 complex change during the first 12 hours after PH and that these changes result in differential gene activation during the early stages of liver regeneration. Delayed early genes are regulated by the later AP-1 complexes, which can bind to cAMP response elements (CREs). In this manner, genes induced in the immediate early response assemble to form the AP-1 complex, which then regulates the expression of a set of delayed early genes (79). To be noted also is that while the expression of c-*fos*, c-*jun*, and *jun*B is rapid and transient after PH, persisting for no more than 4 to 5 hours, the AP-1 complexes formed by homo- or heterodimers of the proteins coded by these genes persist for a much longer period of time.

AP-1 production in the regenerating liver is at least in part dependent on TNF activity. Jun N-terminal kinase (JNK) is activated rapidly after PH, remains high for 8 to 10 hours and can be blocked by anti-TNF antibodies (80,81). Similarly, AP-1 binding activity is delayed after PH in TNFR1 and TNFR2 knockout mice (13,75). Nevertheless, hepatocytes isolated from mice lacking TNFR1 and placed in primary culture show strong AP-1 binding, suggesting that there are other pathways unrelated to TNF that may control AP-1 production and binding. However, if both TNF receptors participate in TNF signaling leading to AP-1 activation, and the activation is solely dependent on TNF, AP-1 activity would be entirely blocked only in TNF knockouts or in double knockout mice that lack both TNFR1 and TNFR2.

Regulation of CCAAT Enhancer Binding Protein in the Regenerating Liver

C/EBP are CCAATT enhanced binding transcription factors that contain a leucine zipper and DNA-binding domains. Three C/EBP isoforms, α, β, and γ, are constitutively expressed in the liver. Although electrophoretic mobility shift assays (EMSAs) show little change in the extent of overall C/EBP DNA binding after PH, there are important changes in the proportions of C/EBPα and C/EBPβ contained in the C/EBP complex (82–85). These changes have important consequences for the regulation of hepatocyte replication because C/EBPα has a negative effect on proliferation (86–88) whereas C/EBPβ may be required for proliferation (89). C/EBPα mRNA and protein decreases by 50% or more at 1 to 3 hours after PH (82,83). The decrease in C/EBPα mRNA appears to be reg-

ulated at the level of transcription and is blocked by treatment with cycloheximide. In contrast, C/EBPβ mRNA increases during the first 4 hours after partial hepatectomy in parallel with the increase of C/EBPβ protein. As a result, there is an approximately eightfold increase in the ratio of C/EBPβ to C/EBPα in the C/EBP complexes that bind to DNA at 16 hours after PH (41).

The three C/EBP isoforms are known to be mediators of the hepatic acute-phase response to inflammation (90). However, both C/EBPα and β participate in cell cycle regulation. C/EBPα has been reported to block hepatocyte replication through at least two mechanisms: blockage of proteolytic degradation of p21 protein, a cell cycle inhibitor, and reduction of E2F complexes containing the retinoblastoma protein p107 (86,91). Interestingly, the effect of C/EBPα on p21 involves an increase in protein stability without alteration in mRNA levels. Although C/EBPα is decreased after PH in young rats, the reduction of the level of C/EBPα after PH is much delayed in the regenerating liver of old rats in which DNA synthesis is slow. In knockout animals lacking C/EBPα, E2F complexes and S-phase specific proteins continue to be expressed for much longer periods in neonatal mice relative to control animals.

Data suggesting that C/EBPβ is required for liver regeneration derives mostly from experiments with C/EBPβ knockout mice (89). These animals are markedly hypoglycemic after PH and had decreased DNA replication, which was apparently unrelated to the activity of gluconeogenic enzymes. Although the precise mechanism of action of C/EBPβ in hepatocyte replication has not been established, lack of C/EBPβ is associated with decreased expression of several immediate early genes such as MKP-1 [mitogen-activated protein (MAP) kinase protein phosphatase] and the Egr-1 transcription factor as well as the cell cycle proteins cyclin B and E. Although TNF signaling may participate in the regulation of C/EBP expression after PH, alterations observed in C/EBPβ knockout mice appear to be independent of IL-6 activity.

cAMP-Responsive Promotor Element Modulator and X-Box–Binding Protein 1 Transcription Factors

The transcription factor CREM (CRE modulator) belongs to a family of basic leucine zipper (bZIP) proteins that bind to cAMP-responsive promoter elements (CREs) located in cAMP inducible genes. CREM activity requires phosphorylation at SER-117 through the effect of protein A (PKA) and other kinases (see Chapter 37). CREM knockout mice have reduced and delayed DNA replication after PH, a defect that is associated with alterations in various cyclins (55). X-box–binding protein 1 (XBP-1) is another member of the family of transcription factors that act as cAMP activators and inhibitors. Deletion of XBP-1 caused liver apoptosis and hypoplasia during embryonic development and lethality at E14 to E16 (56). XBP-1 induction after PH starts within 30 minutes after the operation and lasts for at least 16 hours. It is presumed that CREM and XBP-1 participate in the regulation of liver regeneration through their effect on cAMP responsive genes.

Delayed Early Genes

This group of genes is transcribed after the immediate early gene response but before expression of cell cycle genes reaches their maximum. Most of these genes were detected in RNA subtraction experiments and remain uncharacterized. Delayed early genes include *HRS/SRp40*, a member of the family of Arg-Ser–rich proteins (SR proteins) that function as splicing factors and modulate RNA alternative splicing (48).

An interesting delayed early gene expressed in regenerating mouse liver is *bcl-x*, the main antiapoptotic gene in the liver. Expression of *bcl-x* mRNA exhibits a peak 4 to 6 hours after PH in mice, while the protein, detected by immunohistochemistry and Western blot analysis, shows maximal expression at 12 hours (92). The increase in *bcl-x* transcripts in the regenerating liver results at least in part from posttranscriptional changes in mRNA stability (39,92a). Consistent with the patterns of expression of delayed early genes, *bcl-x* expression after PH can be blocked by cycloheximide. Expression of *bcl-x* mRNA shows a second peak at 48 hours, while the mRNAs for the proapoptotic genes *BAK*, *BAD*, and *BAX* decline early after PH and show increases at later times after the operation (92). These studies demonstrate that *bcl-x* expression has a cell-cycle–dependent regulation in the regenerating liver, but it is not known whether the increased expression correlates with enhanced antiapoptotic activity.

EXPRESSION OF CELL CYCLE GENES

This group of genes, which includes the cyclins and cyclin dependent kinases (cdks), are expressed during cell cycle progression from G_1 to S and finally to mitosis (M) (see Chapter 64). During the G_1 phase of cell cycle progression, cdks phosphorylate the retinoblastoma proteins (pRb and p107) and release members of the E2F family, which are helix–loop–helix leucine zipper transcription factors (Fig. 42.3). Phosphorylation of pRb causes its dissociation from E2F, eliminating the repression of gene transcription caused by the binding of pRb to gene promoter sites. To date, five main types and several subtypes of cyclins and six members of the E2F family have been described. In liver regeneration, most studies have focused on the roles of cyclin D1 and E2F1 in hepatocyte cell cycle progression. E2F1 interacts exclusively with pRb, and its overexpression promotes cell proliferation *in vivo* and *in vitro* (93). The timing of

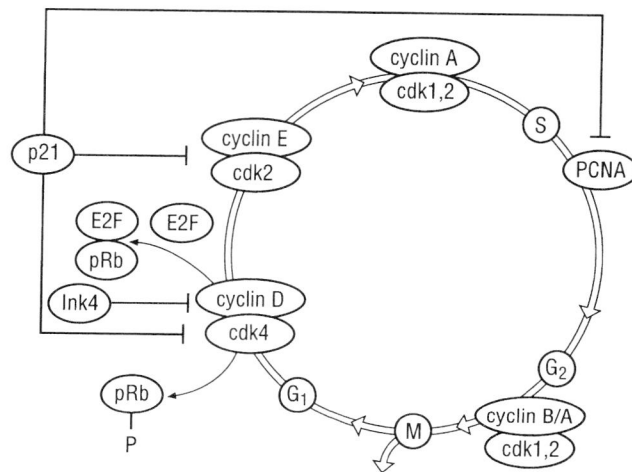

FIGURE 42.3. Cyclins and the cell cycle. The diagram indicates the phases of the cell cycle (G_1, S, G_2, and M), the expression of Cyclins D, E, A, and B, and the expression of inhibitors of the cell cycle (*pRb*, *INK4*, and *p21*). Phosphorylation of the pRb/E2F complex in G_1 by cyclin-dependent kinase 4 (*cdk4*) causes the dissociation of E2F from the complex and the activation of cyclin E/cdk2. Expression of cyclin D and E precede the start of DNA replication. Cyclins A and B expression occur later in the cell cycle (S, G_2). p21 also inhibits DNA replicatin by binding to proliferating cell nuclear antigen (PCNA). (Redrawn from Schönthal AH, Mueller S, Cadena E. Redox regulation of p21, role of reactive oxygen and nitrogen species in cell cycle progression. In: Sen C-K, Sies H, Baeuerle P, eds. Antioxidant and redox regulation of genes. San Diego: Academic Press, 2000:311–336, with permission.)

E2F1 expression in regenerating mouse liver varies among different strains. In C3H mice E2F1 and its target gene dihydrofolate reductase (*Dhfr*) are induced at the G_1/S boundary, while in C57BL/6S the induction of these genes follows the peak of DNA replication (94). Surprisingly, deficiency of E2F1 in knockout mice had no effect on DNA replication during liver regeneration and did not alter hepatocarcinogenesis induced by diethylnitrosamine (93). E2F1 might not be required for liver regeneration, but it is also possible that its loss is compensated for by another member of the E2F family, most likely E2F4, which is abundant in normal and regenerating liver. This issue can be resolved by the analysis of liver regeneration and cell cycle progression in E2F1/E2F4 double knockout mice.

Cyclins are differentially expressed during liver regeneration. In regenerating mouse liver, increased expression of cyclin D1 mRNA and protein precede the start of DNA replication, but their expression remains elevated for several days after the peak of DNA synthesis. Cyclin E expression broadly coincides with the period of DNA replication, while cyclins A and B are expressed very transiently after the first peak of hepatocyte replication (95). Transcription rate analysis using nuclear runoff assays suggest that the changes in cyclin D1 and E mRNA as well as in other cyclin mRNAs during liver regeneration are regulated at the posttranscriptional level, through the modulation of mRNA stability. Cyclin D1 forms a complex with cdk4, which causes phosphorylation of pRb and E2F activation. Both cdk2 and cdk4 increase after partial hepatectomy. Additionally cyclin D1 may sequester the cell cycle inhibitor p27 promoting cdk2 activation (96). Hepatocytes in primary culture and most likely also during liver regeneration *in vivo* can reach the G_1 phase even in the absence of growth factor stimulation. However, growth factors as well as cyclin D1 and E are required for the progression through a restriction point in mid/late G_1 (97). Cyclin D1 expression increases after cells go through the G_1 restriction point and is a marker for a stage in late G_1, in which progression to replication becomes autonomous and no longer depends on growth factor activity (98). Increased cyclin D1 expression in mid/late G_1 is associated with the activation of extracellular regulated kinases (ERKs). DNA replication in the regenerating rat liver is inhibited by drugs (PD98059 inhibitor) that block ERK activity, and in hepatocyte cultures, the inhibitor blocks MEK-1, the kinase upstream from ERK1, cyclin D1 accumulation, as well as DNA replication. Conversely, transient transfection of ERK1 in cultured hepatocytes increases cyclin D1 mRNA expression (99).

An essential role for cyclin E in hepatocyte proliferation after PH has recently been demonstrated in mice with a conditional deletion of the 40S ribosomal protein S6 (100). Deficiency of S6 did not impair the liver response to fasting and refeeding, but greatly inhibited DNA replication and increase in tissue mass after PH. Cyclin E expression after PH was not detectable in S6 knockouts, and DNA synthesis was impaired despite formation of active cyclin D/cdk4 complexes. These results suggest that ribosome biogenesis is somehow linked with a checkpoint step in G_1 that requires cyclin E.

INTEGRATION OF CYTOKINE AND GROWTH FACTOR PATHWAYS: PRIMING AND PROGRESSION STAGES OF LIVER REGENERATION

Although the precise contribution of cytokines and growth factors to the multiple pathways activated during liver regeneration remains to be elucidated, the available data support the notion that liver regeneration is a multistep process involving multiple mediators (Fig. 42.4) (see website chapter

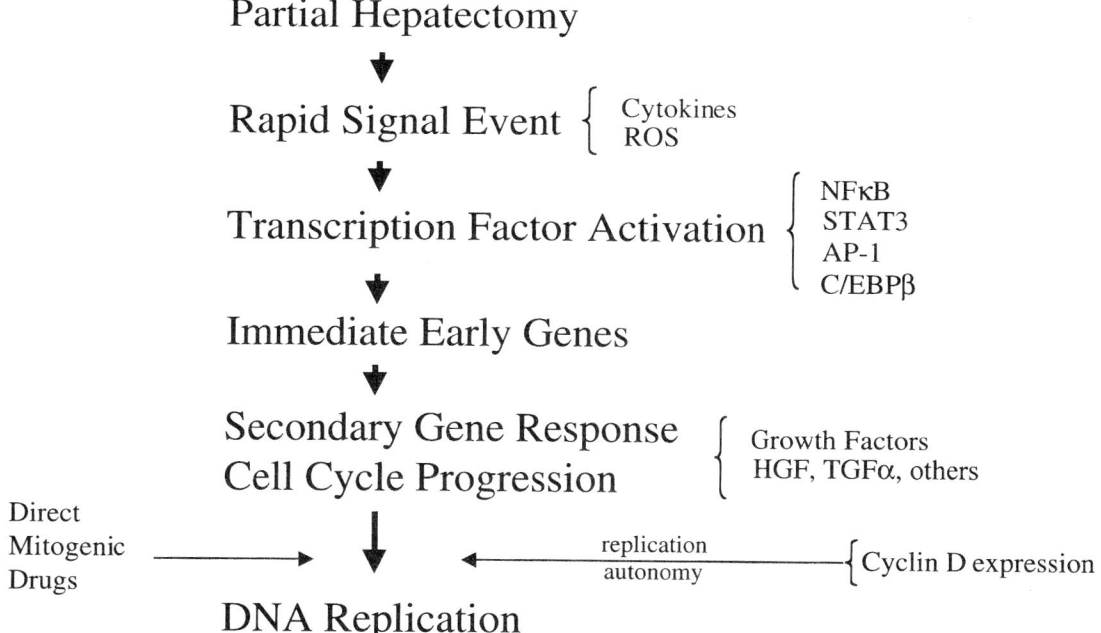

FIGURE 42.4. Sequence of events during liver regeneration. The early events after partial hepatectomy are regulated mostly by cytokines [tumor necrosis factor (TNF) and interleukin-6 (IL-6)] and can be modulated by reactive oxygen species (*ROS*). The priming phase of liver regeneration involves the activation of transcription factors [hepatocyte growth factor (*HGF*) and transforming growth factor-α (*TGF-α*)] and a large number of immediate early genes. Cell cycle progression and the secondary gene response are under the control of growth factors. Cyclin D1 maximal expression corresponds to a phase in which replication can progress even in the absence of growth factors. Direct mitogens may act at this stage and bypass the earlier activation phases. *AP-1*, activator protein-1; *C/EBPβ*, CCAAT enhancer binding protein-β; *STAT*, signal transducer and activator of transcription.

W-31). We have divided liver regeneration into two major phases—priming and cell cycle progression (3,40). Priming is a reversible process in which quiescent hepatocytes (G_0) move into the cell cycle (G_1) through the effect of the cytokines TNF and IL-6 (and perhaps other cytokines). During the priming stage there is activation of the transcription factors NFκB and STAT3 as well as AP-1 and C/EBP, and the triggering of the immediate early gene response after PH. Priming events sensitize cells to growth factors, but the events, although necessary, are not sufficient for hepatocyte replication. Progression through the cell cycle leading to DNA replication ($G_1 - S$) requires hepatocyte growth factor (HGF) and transforming growth factor-α (TGF-α), which are the major agents, as well as cyclins D1 and E, which can move the cell beyond a restriction point in G_1. Maximal cyclin D1 expression corresponds to a point in the cell cycle at which cells gain replication autonomy and can progress into DNA replication independently of growth factors. Cyclins A and B expression coincides with DNA replication and mitosis (S, G_s/M phases of the cycle).

GROWTH FACTORS

Hepatocytes from adult humans and rodents show little replicative activity in serum-free cultures but can be induced to replicate by several growth factors. The most important of these factors are HGF, TGF-α, and epidermal growth factor (EGF). Both HGF and TGF-α levels increase after PH (4,40), but it has not been firmly established that EGF production increases in the liver after the operation, although this has been reported in the literature (101). In addition to these factors, acidic FGF, heparin-binding EGF (HB-EGF), and keratinocyte growth factor (KGF) also stimulate DNA replication in cultured hepatocytes (102–104). Other agents such as growth-hormone thyroid and parathyroid hormones may be "permissive" for liver regeneration, while norepinephrine and insulin are important adjuvant factors.

The basic information about growth factors that participate in liver regeneration can be found in Chapter 56 of the third edition of this book (105), now available in website chapter W-31. HGF effects in liver growth and development are discussed in Chapter 43, and a detailed discussion of the role of HGF, TGF-α, and EGF in liver regeneration can be found in ref. 40. In this section we present a brief summary of new information about growth factor activity in liver growth and development, focusing on TGF-α.

Transforming Growth Factor-α Expression During Liver Growth and Regeneration

TGF-α expression correlates well with hepatocyte proliferation during the neonatal period, in the regenerating liver after PH or chemical injury, and in hepatocarcinogenesis (40). TGF-α peptide as well as the mRNA are high in livers of newborn animals and increase up to 1 to 2 weeks after birth.

After that time TGF-α levels decrease drastically, and by 3 weeks after birth, reach very low values that persist throughout the life of the animal. The changes in TGF-α expression detected in the newborn period parallel the level of replicative activity of hepatocytes and the establishment of hepatocyte quiescence. TGF-α production increases during liver regeneration after PH, or chemical injury induced by CCl_4 or galactosamine (106). In each experimental condition the increase in TGF-α coincides with DNA replication. Several reports have suggested that hepatocyte DNA replication correlates better with TGF-α than HGF expression. This is the case for hepatocyte replication induced by galactosamine, phenobarbital, and dimethyl nitrosamine as well as after transplantation of human livers (107,108). Analysis of liver regeneration in dexamethasone-treated and hypophysectomized rats revealed that these procedures delay DNA replication and that TGF-α mRNA expression paralleled the shift in the timing of proliferation. In contrast, expression of HGF, TGF-β1, as well as proto-oncogenes were not delayed, suggesting that TGF-α has an important role in regulating hepatocyte proliferation after PH (109).

Constitutive expression of TGF-α in the liver of transgenic mice as well as in cultured hepatocytes makes the normally quiescent hepatocyte become a continuously replicating cell. *In vivo*, constitutive TGF-α proliferation leads to tumor development in almost 90% of animals at 12 to 15 months of life (110–113). TGF-α is synthesized as a 160 amino acid precursor that is an integral membrane protein. A 50 amino acid sequence in the ectodomain flanked by proteolytic cleavage sites constitutes the soluble, diffusable TGF-α (113a). However, the plasma membrane-anchored form is active and can bind to an EGF receptor in an adjacent cell. Both anchored and diffuse TGF-α bind to the EGF receptor and initiate a well-described signal transduction pathway that involves tyrosine phosphorylation of the receptor and activation of the MAP kinases ERK1 and 2. The binding affinity of TGF-α to the EGF receptor is approximately 20-fold lower than that of EGF, but TGF-α causes a more sustained stimulation of ERK1 and 2 and higher levels of DNA replication in hepatocytes (114,115). In this regard, EGF has been thought to act as a partial agonist in TGF-α–mediated hepatocyte DNA replication.

TGF production is highly sensitive to regulation by TGF-α and EGF, which function as enhancers of an autocrine loop for TGF production. The promoter region of the TGF-α gene contains an EGF/TGF-α response element that regulates both the basal gene activity as well as responses to EGF and TGF-α (116). Another autocrine loop that enhances TGF-α production is through the defective cleavage of membrane-bound TGF-α, which can increase EGF receptor activation (117). The autocrine self-inducing pathway is active in the regenerating liver, but it is not known to what extent activation of the TGF-α gene is dependent on EGF/TGF-α transcription effects or differential cleavage of membrane bound TGF-α. Studies in cultured colon carcinoma cells indicate that TGF-α expression provides growth advantage, facilitates reentry into the cell cycle, and contributes to autonomy of replication (118).

Although there is good information about the mechanisms of action of TGF-α in the regenerating liver, little is known about TGF-α inducing signals after PH or chemical injury. TNF can greatly increase TGF-α–induced hepatocyte DNA replication in rat liver (see below), suggesting that priming events during liver regeneration enhance the responsiveness of hepatocytes to TGF-α (119). The mechanism by which TNF enhances TGF-α mitogenicity is not known. TNF can stimulate TGF-α mRNA production in cultured mouse hepatocytes by both transcriptional and posttranscriptional mechanisms and caused a sixfold increase in TGF-α mRNA after injection into mice. Moreover, TNF antibodies significantly decreased expression of TGF-α mRNA and peptide during liver regeneration induced by CCl$_4$ chemical injury (120). These experiments imply that the priming effect of TNF on TGF-α mitogenicity is the result of a direct stimulation of TGF-α production. However, in our own experiments, the priming effect occurred independently of changes in TGF-α levels and are more likely due to the activation of MAP kinase downstream pathways.

Growth Factor Redundancy in the Regenerating Liver

HGF and TGF-α activate similar signal transduction pathways in cultured hepatocytes, but these factors have an additive effect in stimulating hepatocyte replication both *in vivo* and in culture (106). It has been suggested that there is crosstalk between c-*met* and TGF-α (121) and that HGF acts by stimulating TGF-α production (108). On the other hand, it is conceivable that HGF and TGF-α may act preferentially in different sets of hepatocytes. This would be the case if the c-*met* and EGF receptors had a differential distribution among hepatocytes in the hepatic lobule (122), an issue that could in principle be resolved by the analysis of liver regeneration in mice lacking either HGF or TGF-α. However, these experiments are complex because HGF, c-*met*, and EFF receptor knockout mice are embryonic lethals. To study the role of HGF in the regenerating liver it is necessary to produce conditional knockouts for either HGF or c-*met*, that is, using a system that would prevent activation of either of these genes after PH. In contrast, TGF-α knockouts develop normally and have no obvious abnormalities in liver regeneration (123), probably because the deficit is compensated by EGF activity. To overcome this problem, a system that would permit the conditional ablation of the EGF receptor during liver regeneration needs to be devised.

CYTOKINES

Tumor necrosis factor-α (TNF-α), referred to here as TNF, is a cytokine with multiple effects including tumor cell cyto-

toxicity and gene-inducing effects, which are important in immune as well as proliferative responses. TNF (as well as IL-1 and IL-8) acts as an early cytokine to initiate the acute-phase response in the liver, both directly and through IL-6 activation (124). Although until recently TNF was not generally considered to be a liver mitogen, several reports suggested that TNF may have a proliferative effect on parenchymal and nonparenchymal cells and may participate in liver regeneration. Earlier observations showed that endotoxin [lipopolysaccharide (LPS)], an agent that releases TNF, stimulates liver regeneration through the secretion of a mitogenic agent (125). Subsequently it was determined that regeneration after PH in LPS-resistant mice, germ-free mice, and athymic nude mice is slow and that cyclin D1 mRNA increases after PH are greatly delayed in athymic nude mice (126,127). Other data demonstrated that TNF injected into rats at relatively high doses induced DNA replication in both parenchymal and nonparenchymal cells (128). In these experiments, nonparenchymal cell labeling by bromodeoxyuridine (BrdU) reached a peak 24 hours after TNF injection, while maximal hepatocyte labeling occurred 12 hours later, suggesting that activation of nonparenchymal cells may be necessary for TNF-induced hepatocyte DNA replication.

More direct evidence for the involvement of TNF in liver regeneration was obtained in work using anti-TNF antibodies (129). Injection of the antibodies into rats decreased DNA replication after PH and inhibited activation of signal transduction pathways involving JNK and C/EBP (81,130). It was also demonstrated that blood TNF concentration increases within 1 hour after PH in rats and mice and is followed by an equally large increase in blood IL-6 (131). The role of TNF and IL-6 in liver regeneration was firmly established in studies of knockout mice that lacked either TNF receptors or cytokine IL-6 (13,76). TNF signal transduction is initiated by the binding of the cytokine to two separate receptors that do not heterodimerize. These receptors, which bind trimeric TNF, are referred to as type 1 and type 2 receptors (TNFR1 and TNFR2, respectively) or as p55 (TNFR1) and p75 (TNFR2) receptors. DNA synthesis after PH was severely impaired in TNFR1 knockouts but not in mice lacking TNFR2. In TNFR1-deficient mice the expected increases in NFκB and STAT3 were greatly diminished, AP-1 binding was decreased, and C/EBP binding was not altered after PH. In addition, plasma IL-6 and liver IL-6 mRNA were low in TNFR1 knockouts. A single injection of IL-6 shortly before PH restored DNA replication, STAT3, and AP-1 binding after PH. In contrast to these results, liver regeneration after PH in TNFR2 knockouts was not altered, although AP-1 and C/EBP binding as well as c-*jun* and c-*myc* mRNA expression after PH were delayed by about 4 hours (13,74).

Mice lacking IL-6 have a high mortality after PH, and the survivors have deficient hepatocyte DNA replication and delayed mass restoration (76). In these animals, STAT3 activation was very low after PH, but a single injection of IL-6 restored STAT3 binding, prevented mortality, and corrected the defect in DNA replication. The data obtained in these various experimental systems established that one of the pathways by which liver regeneration after PH is initiated involves signaling through TNFR-1 and the downstream sequence TNFR1 → NFκB → IL-6 → STAT3. Activation of STAT3 may cause an increase in cyclin D1 and consequent cell cycle progression, but definitive experiments need to be conducted to demonstrate that specific blockage of STAT3 inhibits cyclin D1 activation after PH. IL-6 can induce hepatocyte DNA replication depending on the experimental condition. In primary cultures of mouse hepatocytes maintained in 10% serum, IL-6 stimulates DNA replication but is inactive in serum-free cultures (Campbell and Fausto, unpublished data). Coexpression of IL-6 with soluble IL-6 receptor can cause regenerative hyperplasia and adenomas, as well as severe liver injury in transgenic mice (132,133). On the other hand, IL-6 can also inhibit growth factor and TNF-induced DNA replication in cultured hepatocytes (134,135). Thus, IL-6 can be either stimulatory or inhibitory for hepatocyte replication depending on dosage, presence of its soluble receptor, and culture conditions. Hepatocytes *in vivo* are apparently not capable of producing IL-6, but biliary cells secrete IL-6 and show a large increase of DNA replication after IL-6 exposure with maximal levels achieved 24 hours after exposure (136).

It is unlikely that the initiation of liver regeneration after PH through a cytokine pathway is a linear sequence of events as outlined above. It is known that inducible nitric oxide synthase (iNOS) production increases shortly after PH, and that hepatic injury rather than regeneration occurs after PH in iNOS knockout mice (137). In these animals induction of TNF, NFκB, IL-6, and STAT3 after PH is not altered, suggesting that nitric oxide may protect against cytokine-mediated injury in the regenerating liver. Another system that suppresses cytokine activity may become active during liver regeneration (137a). SOCS3, a component of a family of proteins that suppress cytokine activity (SOCS, suppressors of cytokine synthesis) is activated after PH. SOCS3 is a STAT3 target gene, but through a feedback mechanism it inhibits IL-6 signaling by binding to the gp130 receptor (138). In the regenerating liver, SOCS3 probably prevents excess production of cytokines and protects against cytokine-mediated liver injury. In addition to TNF and IL-6, CXC chemokines have also been shown to have proliferative effects in hepatocytes, although a role for these chemokines in liver regeneration has not yet been established (139).

PRIMING IS REQUIRED FOR HEPATOCYTE REPLICATION AFTER PARTIAL HEPATECTOMY

The notion that hepatocyte replication in the regenerating liver is a multistep process was originally proposed by Bucher and her colleagues (140,141), who showed that growth hormone injections and surgical stress, which are not mitogenic by themselves, can shorten the replicative period of hepatocytes after PH. Experiments in rats and mice involving the induction of hepatocyte proliferation by nutritional shifts also suggested that priming was necessary for hepatocytes to acquire replicative competence (142, 143).

Although HGF, TGF-α, and EGF induce a significant level of DNA replication in hepatocytes in primary cultures, infusion of these growth factors for 24 hours directly into the portal circulation of rats *in vivo* induces DNA replication in less than 10% of hepatocytes (144). Prolonged infusion or repeated injection of very large doses of HGF can increase hepatocyte DNA replication, but the doses used in these experiments are well above the physiologic range (145,146). However, a strong hepatocyte response to physiologic doses of growth factors is obtained when HGF, TGF-α, or EGF is infused into the portal circulation of rats with a 30% hepatectomy (144). This type of operation by itself has only a small effect on DNA replication and does not show the sharp peak of replication observed 24 hours after a 70% hepatectomy (1). However, infusion of growth factors into 30% hepatectomized rats enhances and synchronizes the replicative response and increases hepatocyte DNA replication to the level observed after 70% hepatectomy. Priming of hepatocytes to respond to growth factors *in vivo* was also shown to occur in livers perfused with small doses of collagenase (147).

The demonstration of the role of TNF in liver regeneration after PH led to studies to determine whether TNF could serve as a priming agent to initiate liver regeneration and could make hepatocytes capable of fully responding to HFG and/or TGF-α (119). A single injection of TNF given to nonhepatectomized rats before infusion of either growth factor caused NFκB and STAT3 activation and increased by approximately fourfold the proliferative response of hepatoctyes to HGF or TGF-α. TNF injection followed by the combined infusion of HGF and TGF-α into nonhepatectomized rats increased hepatocyte DNA replication from 15% (HGF plus TGF-α infusion only) to 40%, a level of replication comparable to that obtained after 70% hepatectomy. These experiments established that TNF can function as a priming agent for DNA replication *in vivo* and suggest that it plays this role at the initiation of liver regeneration.

TUMOR NECROSIS FACTOR INCREASE AT THE START OF LIVER REGENERATION: ROLE OF LIPOPOLYSACCHARIDE AND INTERACTIONS BETWEEN HEPATOCYTES AND NONPARENCHYMAL CELLS

Kupffer cells, stellate cells, and endothelial cells produce TNF, HGF, TGF-β, activin, and other factors involved in liver regeneration that act through a paracrine mechanism. The exception to this rule is TGF-α, which is produced by hepatocytes and acts through autocrine mechanisms. The mechanisms by which hepatic and plasma TNF rise rapidly after PH are unknown (13,74,129,131). It has been suggested that gut-derived endotoxin (LPS) could be the agent that induces TNF production from Kupffer cells at the start of liver regeneration. Note, however, that LPS is normally released from gram-negative intestinal flora. Thus, if LPS plays a role in modulating TNF levels at the start of liver regeneration, mechanisms must exist to sensitize Kupffer cells to LPS. LPS forms a complex with LPS-binding protein (LBP) that interacts with membrane-bound CD14 receptors. Activation of CD14 transduces intracellular signals through a Toll-like (Tlr4) receptor (148). LPS also interacts with a soluble form of CD14 (sCD14), which can be produced by hepatocytes. Mechanisms that enhance Kupffer cell sensitivity to LPS at the start of liver regeneration might include increased expression of the CD14 and Tlr4 receptors, release of sCD14 by hepatocytes, and increased production of LBP. Alternatively, because of the reduced size of the liver after PH, LPS activity per Kupffer cell may increase above a threshold that induces TNF production.

C3H/HeJ and C57BL/10ScCr mice, which are much less sensitive to LPS compared to C3H/HeN mice, have, respectively, a missense and a null mutation of Tlr4 (148). Compared to C3H/HeN mice, C3H/HeJ mice have decreased TNF release and delayed hepatocyte proliferation after PH (125,126). This observation is consistent with a role of LPS in the initiation of liver regeneration. The involvement of LPS in the initiation of liver regeneration requires steps occurring in both nonparenchymal cells and hepatocytes under the following potential sequence Fig. 42.5:

Kupffer cell events: LPS → (ROS) → TNF → ROS → NFκB → IL-6 release

Hepatocyte: IL-6 released from Kupffer cells → STAT3 → Cyclin D1 → DNA

However, experiments with cultured hepatocytes and oval cell, suggest that this is a simplistic schema because these cells can respond to TNF directly in the absence of Kupffer cells (71). For instance, in AML12 murine hepatocytes, TNF has a proliferative effect and activates multiple signal transduction pathways including NFκB, STAT3, ERK1 and 2, JNK, and p38. Although cytokine release

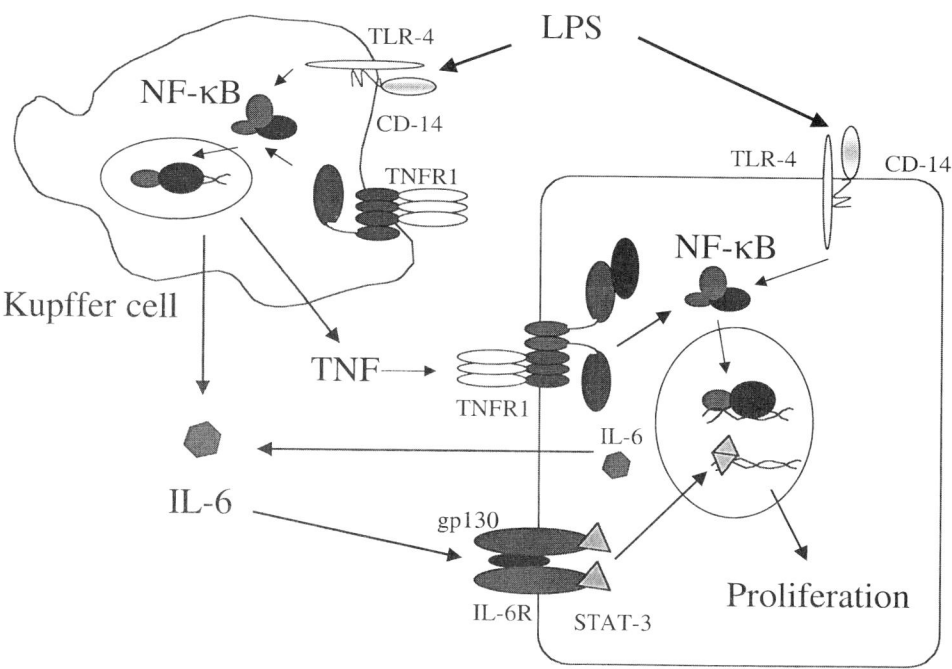

FIGURE 42.5. Involvement of lipopolysaccharide (*LPS*) and cytokines during liver regeneration. The diagram shows activation of NFκB and production of interleukin-6 (*IL-6*) in Kupffer cells under the stimulus of LPS and tumor necrosis factor (*TNF*). TNF and LPS can also stimulate hepatocytes directly causing NFκB activation. IL-6 produced in Kupffer cells stimulates DNA replication through the activation of STAT3. The receptors for LPS (*TLR-4* and *CD-14*), TNF (*TNFR1*), and IL-6 (*gp130* and *IL-6R*) are shown in the diagram. *STAT*, signal transducer and activator of transcription.

from Kupffer cells may be required to initiate liver regeneration, it is not known whether the role of Kupffer cells in stimulating hepatocyte replication depends on the release of TNF, IL-6, both cytokines, and/or additional cytokines (149).

SIGNALING THROUGH TUMOR NECROSIS FACTOR RECEPTOR TYPE 1: PROLIFERATION OR APOPTOSIS

Signaling through TNFR1 plays an important role in liver regeneration but signaling through this receptor may also cause hepatocyte apoptosis (Fig. 42.6). Cell death rather than proliferation as a consequence of TNF exposure can occur by blockage of NFκB activation or by impaired antioxidant defenses generally related to glutathione deficiency. Inhibition of NFκB activation by NFκB antibodies or expression of a dominant IκB repressor modifies the TNF effect on hepatocytes from proliferation to apoptosis. Two experimental situations in mouse liver *in vivo* also demonstrate the requirement for NFκB activation to protect hepatocytes against TNF injury. As already mentioned,

Rel A knockout mice die at E14 to E16 with massive hepatocyte apoptosis. Double knockout animals deficient in both TNFR1 signaling and NFκB activation are rescued from embryonic lethality (67,68), demonstrating that TNF is responsible for the liver apoptosis in Rel A knockouts. Another situation in which inhibition of NFκB activation led to hepatocyte apoptosis *in vivo* was obtained in partially hepatectomized rats that were injected with an adenovirus vector expressing a IκB "superrepressor" gene (73). Surprisingly, DNA replication after PH was not altered in these animals, but there was cell cycle blockage at the G$_2$ phase of the cell cycle, decreased mitogenesis, and hepatocyte apoptosis occurring 24 to 48 hours after the operation.

Although the inhibition of NFκB binding changes the TNF effect from proliferation into apoptosis, an intact NFκB-binding response to TNF is by itself not sufficient to prevent TNF-induced hepatocyte apoptosis. This condition occurs both *in vivo* and in cultured hepatocytes by pretreating the animals or cells with a small dose of actinomycin D before TNF exposure. Under these conditions the inhibitor blocks the transcription of genes related to antioxidant defenses and interferes with glutathione production (150). This model has been extrapolated to explain potential inter-

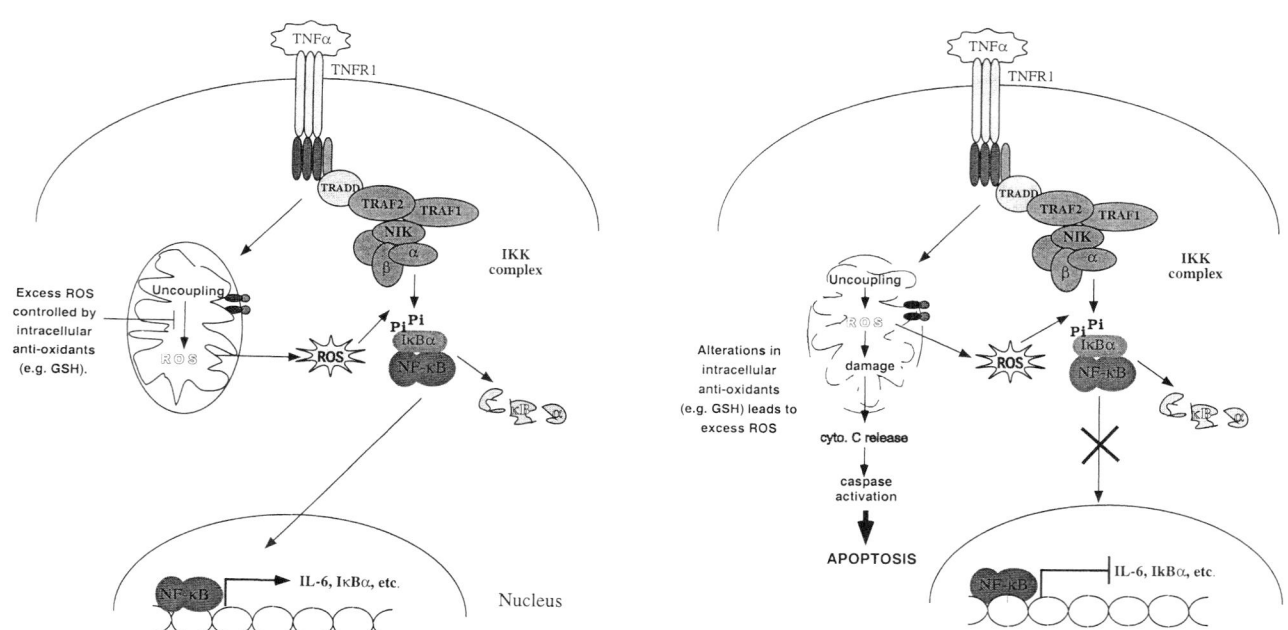

FIGURE 42.6. Apoptosis and DNA replication through tumor necrosis factor receptor type 1 (*TNFR1*) signaling. **Left:** Apoptosis produced by TNF signaling through TNFR1. Apoptosis is caused by excess production of reactive oxygen species (*ROS*), causing mitochondrial damage, cytochrome C release, and caspase activation. Blockage of NFκB activity may also lead to apoptosis. **Right:** Gene activation produced by TNF signaling through TNFR1. In this case, excess ROS formation is prevented by reduced glutathione (*GSH*) and other intracellular antioxidants. ROS formed in mitochondria may stimulate NFκB activation through an effect on IκB phosphorylation. *IKK*, IκB kinase; *IL-6*, interleukin-6. *TRADD*, TNF receptor–associated death domain protein. (See fig. 42.2 for detailed pathways of signaling through TNFRI.)

relationships between the TNF-dependent proliferative and apoptotic pathways at the start of liver regeneration. Both in its proliferative and apoptotic effects TNF generates excess ROS (151,152). Oxidant production by mitochondria increases during the first hour after PH, and the effect is partially blocked by anti-TNF antibodies (152). Excess ROS at the start of liver regeneration is rapidly neutralized by antioxidant defenses (153), and ROS may be directed toward the activation of NFκB by enhancing IκBα degradation. In the absence of protective mechanisms, ROS accumulates, and causes mitochondrial injury, caspase activation, and subsequent apoptosis (150).

MECHANISMS OF LIVER REGENERATION AFTER CHEMICAL INJURY

Liver regeneration after toxic injury differs from regeneration after PH in that hepatocyte replication takes place in response to extensive cell death induced by the toxic agent. In contrast, liver regeneration after PH unfolds in a liver of reduced mass but with intact cellular and tissue structure. It could be expected that the mechanisms of hepatocyte replication after PH and toxic injury would be very dissimilar (154). However, studies of liver regeneration after toxic injury using CCl4 as the toxic agent reveal that the mechanisms of hepatic replication after this type of injury do not appear to differ in major ways from those described after PH. An immediate early gene response occurs during the first few hours after CCl4 administration, and both HGF and TGF-α are involved in regeneration after injury (106,155). The major difference between CCl4- and PH-induced regeneration is in the timing of DNA replication. In both rats and mice given CCl4, maximum levels of DNA replication occur approximately 1 day later than after PH. Given that the timing of the immediate early gene response is similar in the two types of regenerative processes, cell cycle progression through the G1 phase of the cell cycle is slower in injury-induced hepatocyte replication. The mechanisms for the prolonged G1 phase after hepatocyte injury have not been determined.

Several studies have examined whether TNF plays a stimulatory role in liver regeneration induced by toxic agents. Hepatic toxins such as ethanol and CCl4 induce an increase of TNF in both liver and blood (75,156–158). Anti-TNF antibodies greatly inhibited liver regeneration after PH in rats receiving ethanol for 5 weeks (156), and deficient liver regeneration after CCl4 injury occurred in mice lacking TNFR1 (75). In TNFR1 knockouts there was little increase in NFκB and STAT3 binding after CCl4, IL-6 levels were lower than in wild-type mice, and DNA replication was greatly delayed. The extent of injury caused by CCl4 in TNFR1 and control mice was similar as assessed by histologic examination and transaminase activity. Thus, signaling through TNFR1 is important for efficient regeneration after CCl4, as is the case for PH-induced hepatic regeneration. An apparently conflicting result was obtained in experiments in which rats exposed to CCl4 received recombinant soluble TNF receptor to block TNF signaling (157). Animals receiving the soluble receptor had reduced liver injury and mortality, suggesting that under these conditions TNF may have had a cytotoxic effect. Other studies using anti-TNF antibodies showed that TNF modulates liver repair after CCl4 through an effect on immediate early genes and AP-1 binding (159). Taken together, the available evidence is consistent with the notion that TNF may not participate in the development of injury after CCl4 administration, but that signaling through TNFR1 is required for recovery from injury and efficient hepatocyte replication. Similar to the observations on liver regeneration after PH, IL-6–deficient mice have defective regeneration after CCl4 treatment. In these animals NFκB and STAT3 binding after PH was diminished and DNA replication and mitosis were decreased. In addition, more severe hepatocellular injury and apoptosis occurred in IL-6 knockout mice (160), indicating that IL-6 has an important role in protection against injury and in liver repair.

MECHANISMS OF HEPATOCYTE PROLIFERATION IN COMPENSATORY RESPONSES AND DIRECT MITOGENESIS

This chapter has focused on the mechanisms of hepatocyte proliferation in compensatory processes, that is, proliferation elicited by a tissue deficit or in response to cell death. However, a large number of agents, referred to as direct mitogens, can cause hepatocyte proliferation in the absence of either tissue or cell deficit (161). Among these are lead nitrate, ethylene dibromide, 9-cis-retinoic acid, triiodothyronine, various peroxisomal proliferators, as well as TNF at high doses. These agents have little in common besides their shared ability to induce hepatocyte replication in rat liver. More recently, another agent (the mitogen 1,4-bis[z-(3,5-dichlorophyridyloxy)] benzene) was identified as being capable of inducing replication in mouse liver (162). The mechanisms by which direct hepatocyte mitogens act differ among different agents. For instance, lead nitrate and ethylene dibromide require TNF for its proliferative effects and cause an immediate early gene response (128). However, increased HGF or TGF-α activity was not detected in animals injected with these agents, suggesting that in this situation TNF acts as a complete mitogen for hepatocytes. It has been reported that TNF may participate in hepatocyte replication induced by peroxisome proliferators (163); but other work did not provide evidence for TNF involvement (164). In 9-cis-retinoic acid- or triiodothyronine-injected rats, transcription factor activation, TNF increas, the immediate early gene response, and growth factor activity were not detectable (161). It is possible, but unlikely, that the mitogenesis produced by these agents is not sufficiently synchronized to permit the detection of such changes. The more plausible explanation for the effect of these two agents as well as TCPOBOP is that they act as cell cycle promoters at the level of cyclin D1 stimulation (162) through nuclear hormone receptors, and thus bypass the priming phase of liver regeneration (Fig. 42.4). This would explain why hepatocyte replication induced by these drugs does not depend on cytokines and growth factors.

ACKNOWLEDGMENTS

The author thanks members of his lab for their work and dedication, and Patricia Fern for her assistance in preparing the manuscript. The research described was supported in part by National Cancer Institute grant CA23226.

REFERENCES

1. Bucher NLR. Regeneration of mammalian liver. *Int Rev Cytol* 1963;15:245–300.
2. Fausto N. Hepatic regeneration. In: Bircher J, Benhamou J-P, McIntyre N, et al., eds. *Oxford textbook of clinical hepatology*, 2nd ed, vol 1. Oxford: Oxford Medical, 1999:189–202.
3. Fausto N. Liver regeneration. *J Hepatol* 2000;32:19–31.
4. Michalopoulos GK, DeFrances MC. Liver regeneration. *Science* 1997;276:60–66.
5. Higgins GM, Anderson RM. Experimental pathology of the liver. I. Restoration of the liver of the white rat following partial surgical removal. *Arch Pathol* 1931;12:186–202.
6. Bucher NLR, Swaffield MN. The rate of incorporation of labeled thymidine into the deoxyribonucleic acid of regenerating rat liver in relation to the amount of liver excised. *Cancer Res* 1964;24:1611–1625.
7. Grisham JW. A morphologic study of deoxyribonucleic acid synthesis and cell proliferation in regenerating rat liver; autoradiography with thymidine-H³. *Cancer Res* 1962;22:842–849.
8. Tsanev R. Cell cycle and liver function. In: Reinert J, Holtzer H, eds. *Cell cycle and cell differentiation*. New York: Springer-Verlag, 1975:197–248.
9. Nadal C, Zajdela F. Polyploidie somatique dans le foie de rat. I. Le role des cellules binucleees dans la genese des cellules polyploides. *Exp Cell Res* 1966;42:99–116.
10. Weglarz TC, Deglan JL, Sandgren EP. Hepatocyte transplantation into diseased mouse liver: kinetics of parenchymal repopulation and identification of the proliferative capacity of tetraplois and octaploid hepatocytes. *Am J Pathol* 2000;157:1963–1974.
11. Gerhard H. A quantitative model of cellular regeneration in rat liver after partial hepatectomy. In: Lesch R, Reutter W, eds. Liver regeneration after experimental injury. New York: Stratton Intercontinental Medical, 1973:340–346.
12. Wright N, Alison M. The liver. In: Wright N, Alison M, eds. *The biology of epithelial cell populations*, vol 2. Oxford: Clarendon Press, 1984:880–980.
13. Yamada Y, Kirillova I, Peschon JJ, et al. Initiation of liver growth by tumor necrosis factor: deficient liver regeneration in mice lacking type I tumor necrosis factor receptor. *Proc Natl Acad Sci USA* 1997;94:1441–1446.
14. Rabes H. Kinetics of hepatocellular proliferation after partial resection of the liver. *Prog Liver Dis* 1976;5:83–99.

15. Rabes H. Kinetics of hepatocellular proliferation as a function of the microvascular structure and functional state of the liver. *Ciba* 1978;55:31–60.
16. Zajicek G, Ariel I, Arber N. The streaming liver III. Littoral cells accompany the streaming hepatocyte. *Liver* 1988;8: 213–218.
17. Sigal SH, Brill S, Fiorino AS, et al. The liver as a stem cell and lineage system. *Am J Physiol* 1992;263:G139–G148.
18. Gebhardt R. Different proliferative activity in vitro of periportal and perivenous hepatocytes. *Scand J Gastroenterol* 1988;23: 8–18.
19. Gebhardt R. Metabolic zonation of the liver: regulation and implications for liver function. *Pharmacol Ther* 1992;53: 275–354.
20. Martinez-Hernandez A, Amenta PS. The extracellular matrix in hepatic regeneration. *FASEB J* 1995;9:1401–1410.
21. Mars WM, Liu ML, Kitson RP, et al. Immediate early detection of urokinase receptor after partial hepatectomy and its implications for initiation of liver regeneration. *Hepatology* 1995;21: 1695–1701.
22. Kim TH, Mars WM, Stolz DB, et al. Extracellular matrix remodeling at the early stages of liver regeneration in the rat [see comments]. *Hepatology* 1997;26:896–904.
23. Rudolph KL, Trautwein C, Kubicka S, et al. Differential regulation of extracellular matrix synthesis during liver regeneration after partial hepatectomy in rats. *Hepatology* 1999;30:1159–1166.
24. Wang K, Wondergem R. Redistribution of hepatocyte chloride during L-alanine uptake. *J Membr Biol* 1993;135:237–244.
25. Schliess F, HS, Kubitz R, et al. Osmosignalling in the liver. In: Haeussinger HPD, ed. *Signalling in the liver*, 1st ed. Dordrecht: Kluwer Academic, 1998:129–151.
26. Freeman TL, Ngo HQ, Mailliard ME. Inhibition of system A amino acid transport and hepatocyte proliferation following partial hepatectomy in the rat. *Hepatology* 1999;30:437–444.
27. Minuk GY, Kren BT, Xu R, et al. The effect of changes in hepatocyte membrane potential on immediate-early proto-oncogene expression following partial hepatectomy in rats. *Hepatology* 1997;25:1123–1127.
28. Sandgren EP, Palmiter RD, Heckel JL, et al. Complete hepatic regeneration after somatic deletion of an albumin-plasminogen activator transgene. *Cell* 1991;66:245–256.
29. Rhim JA, Sandgren EP, Degen JL, et al. Replacement of diseased mouse liver by hepatic cell transplantation. *Science* 1994; 263:1149–1152.
30. Rhim JA, Sandgren EP, Palmiter RD, et al. Complete reconstitution of mouse liver with xenogeneic hepatocytes. *Proc Natl Acad Sci USA* 1995;92:4942–4946.
31. Overturf K, al-Dhalimy M, Ou CN, et al. Serial transplantation reveals the stem-cell-like regenerative potential of adult mouse hepatocytes. *Am J Pathol* 1997;151:1273–1280.
32. Francavilla A, Zeng Q, Polimeno L, et al. Small-for-size liver transplanted into larger recipient: a model of hepatic regeneration. *Hepatology* 1994;19:210–216.
33. Kremer BC, Henne-Bruns D, Koonstra G, et al. *Atlas of liver, pancreas, and kidney transplantation*. New York: Thieme, 1994.
34. Marcos A, Fisher RA, Ham JM, et al. Liver regeneration and function in donor and recipient after right lobe adult to adult living donor liver transplantation. *Transplantation* 2000;69: 1375–1379.
35. Troisi R, Cuomo O, De Hemptinne B. Adult-to-adult living-related liver transplantation using the right lobe. *Dig Liver Dis* 2000;32:238–242.
36. Nakagami M, Morimoto T, Itoh K, et al. Patterns of restoration of remnant liver volume after graft harvesting in donors for living related liver transplantation. *Transplant Proc* 1998;30: 195–199.

37. Kawasaki S, Makuuchi M, Matsunami H, et al. Living related liver transplantation in adults. *Ann Surg* 1998;227:269–274.

38. Taub R. Transcriptional control of liver regeneration. *FASEB J* 1996;10:413–427.

39. Kren BT, Steer CJ. Posttranscriptional regulation of gene expression in liver regeneration: role of mRNA stability. *FASEB J* 1996;10:559–573.

40. Fausto N, Laird AD, Webber EM. Liver regeneration. 2. Role of growth factors and cytokines in hepatic regeneration. *FASEB J* 1995;9:1527–1536.

41. Diehl AM, Rai RM. Regulation of signal transduction during liver regeneration. *FASEB J* 1996;10:215–227.

42. Thompson NL, Mead JE, Braun L, et al. Sequential protooncogene expression during rat liver regeneration. *Cancer Res* 1986;46:3111–3117.

43. Alcorn J, Feitelberg S, Brenner D. Transient induction of c-*jun* during hepatic regeneration. *Hepatology* 1990;11:909–915.

44. Morello D, FitzGerald MJ, Babinet C, et al. c-*myc*, c-*fos*, and c-*jun* regulation in the regenerating livers of normal and H-2K/c-*myc* transgenic mice. *Mol Cell Biol* 1990;10:3185–3193.

45. Haber BA, Mohn KL, Diamond RH, et al. Induction patterns of 70 genes during nine days after hepatectomy define the temporal course of liver regeneration. *J Clin Invest* 1993;91:1319–1326.

46. Mohn K, Laz TM, Hsu J-C, et al. The immediate-early growth response in regenerating liver and insulin-stimulated H-35 cells; comparison with serum-stimulated 3T3 cells and identification of 41 novel immediate-early genes. *Mol Cell Biol* 1991;11:381–390.

47. Peng Y, Du K, Ramirez S, et al. Mitogenic up-regulation of the PRL-1 protein-tyrosine phosphatase gene by Egr-1. Egr-1 activation is an early event in liver regeneration. *J Biol Chem* 1999;274:4513–4520.

48. Du K, Leu JI, Peng Y, et al. Transcriptional up-regulation of the delayed early gene HRS/SRp40 during liver regeneration. Interactions among YY1, GA-binding proteins, and mitogenic signals. *J Biol Chem* 1998;273:35208–35215.

49. Lavenu A, Pistoi S, Pournin S, et al. Both coding exons of the c-*myc* gene contribute to its posttranscriptional regulation in the quiescent liver and regenerating liver and after protein synthesis inhibition. *Mol Cell Biol* 1995;15:4410–4419.

50. Pistoi S, Morello D. Liver regeneration 7. Prometheus' myth revisited: transgenic mice as a powerful tool to study liver regeneration. *FASEB J* 1996;10:819–828.

51. Fausto N. Lessons from genetically engineered animal models. V. Knocking out genes to study liver regeneration: present and future. *Am J Physiol* 1999;277:G917–921.

52. Davis AC, Wims M, Spotts GD, et al. A null c-*myc* mutation causes lethality before 10.5 days of gestation in homozygotes and reduced fertility in heterozygous female mice. *Genes Dev* 1993;7:671–682.

53. Hilberg F, Aguzzi A, Howells N, et al. c-*jun* is essential for normal mouse development and hepatogenesis. *Nature* 1993;365:179–181.

54. Johnson RS, Spiegelman BM, Papaioannou V. Pleiotropic effects of a null mutation in the c-*fos* proto-oncogene. *Cell* 1992;71:577–586.

55. Servillo G, Della Fazia MA, Sassone-Corsi P. Transcription factor CREM coordinates the timing of hepatocyte proliferation in the regenerating liver. *Genes Dev* 1998;12:3639–3643.

56. Reimold AM, Etkin A, Clauss I, et al. An essential role in liver development for transcription factor XBP-1. *Genes Dev* 2000;14:152–157.

57. FitzGerald MJ, Webber EM, Donovan JR, et al. Rapid DNA binding by nuclear factor kappa B in hepatocytes at the start of liver regeneration. *Cell Growth Differ* 1995;6:417–427.

58. Cressman DE, Diamond RH, Taub R. Rapid activation of the Stat3 transcription complex in liver regeneration. *Hepatology* 1995;21:1443–1449.

59. Cressman DE, Greenbaum LE, Haber BA, et al. Rapid activation of post-hepatectomy factor/nuclear factor kappa B in hepatocytes, a primary response in the regenerating liver. *J Biol Chem* 1994;269:30429–30435.

60. Ashkenazi A, Dixit VM. Death receptors: signaling and modulation. *Science* 1998;281:1305–1308.

61. Ghosh S, May MJ, Kopp EB. NF-kB and Rel proteins: evolutionarily conserved mediators of immune responses. *Annu Rev Immunol* 1998;16:225–260.

62. Baeuerle PA, Baltimore D. NF-kappa B: ten years after. *Cell* 1996;87:13–20.

63. Maniatis T. Catalysis by a multiprotein IkappaB kinase complex [comment]. *Science* 1997;278:818–819.

64. Li N, Karin M. Signaling pathways leading to nuclear factor-kappa B activation [In Process Citation]. *Methods Enzymol* 2000;319:273–279.

65. Karin M. How NF-kappaB is activated: the role of the IkappaB kinase (IKK) complex. *Oncogene* 1999;18:6867–6874.

66. Beg AA, Sha WC, Bronson RT, et al. Embryonic lethality and liver degeneration in mice lacking the RelA component of NF-κB. *Nature* 1995;376:167–170.

67. Rosenfeld ME, Prichard L, Shiojiri N, et al. Prevention of hepatic apoptosis and embryonic lethality in RelA/TNFR-1 double knockout mice. *Am J Pathol* 2000;156:997–1007.

68. Doi TS, Marino MW, Takahashi T, et al. Absence of tumor necrosis factor rescues RelA-deficient mice from embryonic lethality. *Proc Natl Acad Sci USA* 1999;96:2994–2999.

69. Bellas RE, FitzGerald MJ, Fausto N, et al. Inhibition of NF-kappa B activity induces apoptosis in murine hepatocytes. *Am J Pathol* 1997;151:891–896.

70. Arsura M, FitzGerald MJ, Fausto N, et al. Nuclear factor-kappaB/Rel blocks transforming growth factor beta1-induced apoptosis of murine hepatocyte cell lines. *Cell Growth Differ* 1997;8:1049–1059.

71. Kirillova I, Chaisson M, Fausto N. Tumor necrosis factor induces DNA replication in hepatic cells through nuclear factor kappaB activation. *Cell Growth Differ* 1999;10:819–828.

72. Xu Y, Bialik S, Jones BE, et al. NF-kappaB inactivation converts a hepatocyte cell line TNF-alpha response from proliferation to apoptosis. *Am J Physiol* 1998;275:C1058–1066.

73. Iimuro Y, Nishiura T, Hellerbrand C, et al. NFkappaB prevents apoptosis and liver dysfunction during liver regeneration. *J Clin Invest* 1998;101:802–811.

74. Yamada Y, Webber EM, Kirillova I, et al. Analysis of liver regeneration in mice lacking type 1 or type 2 tumor necrosis factor receptor: requirement for type 1 but not type 2 receptor. *Hepatology* 1998;28:959–970.

75. Yamada Y, Fausto N. Deficient liver regeneration after carbon tetrachloride injury in mice lacking type 1 but not type 2 tumor necrosis factor receptor. *Am J Pathol* 1998;152:1577–1589.

76. Cressman DE, Greenbaum LE, DeAngelis RA, et al. Liver failure and defective hepatocyte regeneration in interleukin-6–deficient mice. *Science* 1996;274:1379–1383.

77. Karin M, Liu Z, Zandi E. AP-1 function and regulation. *Curr Opin Cell Biol* 1997;9:240–246.

78. Hsu J-C, Bravo R, Taub R. Interactions among LRF-a, JunB, c-*jun*, and c-*fos* define a regulatory program in the G₁ phase of liver regeneration. *Mol Cell Biol* 1992;12:4654–4665.

79. Westwick JK, Brenner DA. Proto-oncogenes/transcription factors. In: *Liver growth and repair*, London: Chapman & Hall, 1998:297–310.

80. Westwick J, Weitzel C, Leffert H, et al. Activation of jun kinase

is an early event in hepatic regeneration. *J Clin Invest* 1995;95: 803–810.

81. Westwick JK, Weitzel C, Minden A, et al. Tumor necrosis factor alpha stimulates AP-1 activity through prolonged activation of the c-*jun* kinase. *J Biol Chem* 1994;269:26396–26401.

82. Mischoulon D, Rana B, Bucher NLR, et al. Growth-dependent inhibition of CCAAT enhancer-binding protein (C-EBPα) gene expression during hepatocyte proliferation in the regenerating liver and in culture. *Mol Cell Biol* 1992;12:2553–2560.

83. Flodby P, Antonson P, Barlow C, et al. Differential patterns of expression of three C/EBP isoforms, HNF-1, and HNF-4 after partial hepatectomy in rats. *Exp Cell Res* 1993;208:248–256.

84. Greenbaum LE, Cressman DE, Haber BA, et al. Coexistence of C/EBP alpha, beta, growth-induced proteins and DNA synthesis in hepatocytes during liver regeneration. Implications for maintenance of the differentiated state during liver growth. *J Clin Invest* 1995;96:1351–1365.

85. Diehl AM, Yang SQ. Regenerative changes in C/EBPα C/EBPβ expression modulate binding to the C/EBP site in the c-*fos* promoter. *Hepatology* 1994;19:447–456.

86. Timchenko NA, Harris TE, Wilde M, et al. CCAAT/enhancer binding protein alpha regulates p21 protein and hepatocyte proliferation in newborn mice. *Mol Cell Biol.* 1997;17: 7353–61.

87. Soriano HE, Kang DC, Finegold MJ, et al. Lack of C/EBP alpha gene expression results in increased DNA synthesis and an increased frequency of immortalization of freshly isolated mice [correction of rat] hepatocytes [published erratum appears in *Hepatology* 1998;27:1457]. *Hepatology* 1998;27:392–401.

88. Timchenko NA, Wilde M, Kosai KI, et al. Regenerating livers of old rats contain high levels of C/EBPalpha that correlate with altered expression of cell cycle associated proteins. *Nucleic Acids Res* 1998;26:3293–3299.

89. Greenbaum LE, Li W, Cressman DE, et al. CCAAT enhancer-binding protein beta is required for normal hepatocyte proliferation in mice after partial hepatectomy. *J Clin Invest* 1998;102: 996–1007.

90. Burgess-Beusse BL, Darlington GJ. C/EBPalpha is critical for the neonatal acute-phase response to inflammation. *Mol Cell Biol* 1998;18:7269–7277.

91. Timchenko NA, Wilde M, Darlington GJ. C/EBPalpha regulates formation of S-phase-specific E2F-p107 complexes in livers of newborn mice. *Mol Cell Biol* 1999;19:2936–2945.

92. Tzung SP, Fausto N, Hockenbery DM. Expression of Bcl-2 family during liver regeneration and identification of Bcl-x as a delayed early response gene. *Am J Pathol* 1997;150:1985–1995.

92a. Fan G, Kren BT, Steer CJ. Regulation of apoptosis-associated genes in the regenerating liver. *Semin Liver Dig* 1998;18: 123–140.

93. Lukas ER, Bartley SM, Graveel CR, et al. No effect of loss of E2F1 on liver regeneration or hepatocarcinogenesis in C57BL/6J or C3H/HeJ mice. *Mol Carcinogen* 1999;25: 295–303.

94. Bennett LM, Farnham PJ, Drinkwater NR. Strain-dependent differences in DNA synthesis and gene expression in the regenerating livers of CB57BL/6J and C3H/HeJ mice. *Mol Carcinogen* 1995;14:46–52.

95. Albrecht JH, Hoffman JS, Kren BT, et al. Cyclin and cyclin-dependent kinase 1 mRNA expression in models of regenerating liver and human liver diseases. *Am J Physiol* 1993;265: G857–864.

96. Albrecht JH, Rieland BM, Nelsen CJ, et al. Regulation of G(1) cyclin-dependent kinases in the liver: role of nuclear localization and p27 sequestration. *Am J Physiol* 1999;277:G1207–1216.

97. Loyer P, Cariou S, Glaise D, et al. Growth factor dependence of progression through G1 and S phases of adult rat hepatocytes in

vitro. Evidence of a mitogen restriction point in mid-late G1. *J Biol Chem* 1996;271:11484–11492.

98. Albrecht JH, Hansen LK. Cyclin D1 promotes mitogen-independent cell cycle progression in hepatocytes. *Cell Growth Differ* 1999;10:397–404.

99. Talarmin H, Rescan C, Cariou S, et al. The mitogen-activated protein kinase kinase/extracellular signal-regulated kinase cascade activation is a key signalling pathway involved in the regulation of G(1) phase progression in proliferating hepatocytes. *Mol Cell Biol* 1999;19:6003–6011.

100. Volarevic S, Stewart MJ, Ledermann B, et al. Proliferation, but not growth, blocked by conditional deletion of 40S ribosomal protein S6. *Science* 2000;288:2045–2047.

101. Mullhaupt B, Feren A, Fodor E, et al. Liver expression of epidermal growth factor RNA. Rapid increases in immediate-early phase of liver regeneration. *J Biol Chem* 1994;269: 19667–19670.

102. Tanahashi T, Imamura T, Suzuki M. Re-evaluation of FGF-1 as a potent mitogen for hepatocytes. *In Vitro Cell Dev* 1994; 30A:139–141.

103. Housley RM, Morris CF, Boyle W, et al. Keratinocyte growth factor induces proliferation of hepatocytes and epithelial cells throughout the rat gastrointestinal tract. *J Clin Invest* 1994;94: 1764–1777.

104. Ito N, Kawata S, Tamura S, et al. Heparin-binding EGF-like growth factor is a potent mitogen for rat hepatocytes. *Biochem Biophys Res Commun* 1994;198:25–31.

105. Fausto N, Webber EM. Liver regeneration. In: Arias I, Boyer J, Fausto N, et al., eds. *The liver biology and pathobiology*, 3rd ed. New York: Raven Press, 1994:1059–1084.

106. Webber EM, FitzGerald MJ, Brown PI, et al. TGFα expression during liver regeneration after partial hepatectomy and toxic injury, and potential interactions between TGFα and HGF. *Hepatology* 1993;18:1422–1431.

107. Tomiya T, Ogata I, Fujiwara K. Transforming growth factor alpha levels in liver and blood correlate better than hepatocyte growth factor with hepatocyte proliferation during liver regeneration. *Am J Pathol* 1998;153:955–961.

108. Tomiya T, Ogata I, Yamaoka M, et al. The mitogenic activity of hepatocyte growth factor on rat hepatocytes is dependent upon endogenous transforming growth factor alpha. *Am J Pathol* 2000;157:1693–1701.

109. Nagy P, Bisgaard HC, Schnur J, et al. Studies on hepatic gene expression in different liver regenerative models [In Process Citation]. *Biochem Biophys Res Commun* 2000;272:591–595.

110. Lee GH, Merlino G, Fausto N. Development of liver tumors in transforming growth factor alpha transgenic mice. *Cancer Res* 1992;52:5162–5170.

111. Takagi H, Sharp R, Hammermeister C, et al. Molecular and genetic analysis of liver oncogenesis in transforming growth factor transgenic mice. *Cancer Res* 1992;52:5171–5177.

112. Webber EM, Wu JC, Wang L, et al. Overexpression of transforming growth factor-alpha causes liver enlargement and increased hepatocyte proliferation in transgenic mice. *Am J Pathol* 1994;145:398–408.

113. Jhappan C, Stahle C, Harkins RN, et al. TGF-alpha overexpression in transgenic mice induces liver neoplasia and abnormal development of the mammary gland and pancreas. *Cell* 1990;61:1137–1146.

113a. Shum L, Miettinen PJ, Derynk R. Transforming growth factor-α: In: Aggarwal BB, Gutterman JV, eds. *Human cytokines*. Cambridge: Blackwell Science, 1966:384–421.

114. Thoresen GH, Guren TK, Sandnes D, et al. Response to transforming growth factor alpha (TGFalpha) and epidermal growth factor (EGF) in hepatocytes: lower EGF receptor affinity of TGFalpha is associated with more sustained activation of

p42/p44 mitogen-activated protein kinase and greater efficacy in stimulation of DNA synthesis. *J Cell Physiol* 1998;175:10–18.

115. Guren TK, Thoresen GH, Dajani OF, et al. Epidermal growth factor behaves as a partial agonist in hepatocytes: effects on DNA synthesis in primary culture and competition with transforming growth factor alpha. *Growth Factors* 1996;13:171–179.

116. Awwad R, Humphrey LE, Periyasamy B, et al. The EGF/TGFalpha response element within the TGFalpha promoter consists of a multi-complex regulatory element. *Oncogene* 1999;18:5923–5935.

117. Yang H, Jiang D, Li W, et al. Defective cleavage of membrane bound TGFalpha leads to enhanced activation of the EGF receptor in malignant cells. *Oncogene* 2000;19:1901–1914.

118. Jiang D, Yang H, Willson JK, et al. Autocrine transforming growth factor alpha provides a growth advantage to malignant cells by facilitating re-entry into the cell cycle from suboptimal growth states. *J Biol Chem* 1998;273:31471–31479.

119. Webber EM, Bruix J, Pierce RH, et al. Tumor necrosis factor primes hepatocytes for DNA replication in the rat. *Hepatology* 1998;28:1226–1234.

120. Gallucci RM, Simeonova PP, Toriumi W, et al. TNF-alpha regulates transforming growth factor-alpha expression in regenerating murine liver and isolated hepatocytes. *J Immunol* 2000; 164:872–878.

121. Jo M, Kim TH, Seol DW, et al. Apoptosis induced in normal human hepatocytes by tumor necrosis factor-related apoptosis-inducing ligand. *Nat Med* 2000;6:564–567.

122. Gebhardt R, Jonitza D. Different proliferative responses of periportal and perivenous hepatocytes to EGF. *Biochem Biophys Res Commun* 1991;181:1201–1207.

123. Russell WE, Carver RS. *The EGF/TGFalpha family of growth factors and their receptors.* London: Chapman & Hall, 1998: 185–218.

124. Heinrich P, Behrmann I, Graeve L, et al. The acute-phase response of the liver: molecular mechanism of IL-6 signalling from the plasma membrane to the nucleus. In: Haussinger D, Heinrich P, eds. *Signalling in the liver.* Dordrecht: Kluwer Academic, 1998:55–71.

125. Cornell R. Restriction of gut-derived endotoxin impairs DNA synthesis for liver regeneration. *Am J Physiol* 1985;18: R563–R569.

126. Cornell RP, Liljequist BL, Bartizal KF. Depressed liver regeneration after partial hepatectomy of germ free, athymic and lipopolysaccharide-resistant mice. *Hepatology* 1990;11:916–922.

127. Albrecht JH, Hoffman JS, Kren BT, et al. Cyclin and cyclin-dependent kinase 1 mRNA expression in models of regenerating liver and human liver diseases. *Am J Physiol* 1993;265: G857–864.

128. Shinozuka H, Ohmura T, Katyal SL, et al. Possible roles of nonparenchymal cells in hepatocyte proliferation induced by lead nitrate and by tumor necrosis factor alpha. *Hepatology* 1996;23: 1572–1577.

129. Akerman P, Cote P, Yang SQ, et al. Antibodies to tumor necrosis factor-alpha inhibit liver regeneration after partial hepatectomy. *Am J Physiol* 1992;263:G579–585.

130. Diehl AM, Yin M, Fleckenstein J, et al. Tumor necrosis factor-a induces c-*jun* during the regenerative response to liver injury. *Am J Physiol* 1994;267:G552–G561.

131. Trautwein C, Rakemann T, Niehof M, et al. Acute-phase response factor, increased binding, and target gene transcription during liver regeneration. *Gastroenterology* 1996;110:1854–1862.

132. Maione D, Di Carlo E, Li W, et al. Coexpression of IL-6 and soluble IL-6R causes nodular regenerative hyperplasia and adenomas of the liver. *EMBO J* 1998;17:5588–5597.

133. Schirmacher P, Peters M, Ciliberto G, et al. Hepatocellular hyperplasia, plasmacytoma formation, and extramedullary

hematopoiesis in interleukin (IL)-6/soluble IL-6 receptor double-transgenic mice. *Am J Pathol* 1998;153:639–648.

134. Nakamura T, Arakaki R, Ichihara A. Interleukin-1 beta is a potent growth inhibitor of adult rat hepatocytes in primary culture. *Exp Cell Res* 1998;179:488–497.

135. Satoh M, Yamazaki M. Tumor necrosis factor stimulates DNA synthesis of mouse hepatocytes in primary culture and is suppressed by transforming growth factor beta and interleukin 6. *J Cell Physiol* 1992;150:134–139.

136. Matsumoto K, Fujii H, Michalopoulos G, et al. Human biliary epithelial cells secrete and respond to cytokines and hepatocyte growth factors in vitro: interleukin-6, hepatocyte growth factor and epidermal growth factor promote DNA synthesis in vitro. *Hepatology* 1994;20:376–382.

137. Rai RM, Lee FYJ, Rosen A, et al. Impaired liver regeneration in inducible nitric oxide synthase-deficient mice. *Proc Natl Acad Sci USA* 1998;95:13829–13834.

137a. Campbell, et al. Expression of suppressors of cytokine signaling during liver regeneration. *J Clin Invest*, in press.

138. Heinrich PC, Behrmann I, Muller-Newen G, et al. Interleukin-6–type cytokine signalling through the gp130/Jak/STAT pathway. *Biochem J* 1998;334:297–314.

139. Colletti LM, Green M, Burdick MD, et al. Proliferative effects of CXC chemokines in rat hepatocytes in vitro and in vivo. *Shock* 1998;10:248–257.

140. Moolten FL, Oakman NJ, Bucher NLR. Accelerated response of hepatic DNA synthesis to partial hepatectomy in rats pretreated with growth hormone or surgical stress. *Cancer Res* 1970;30:2353–2357.

141. Bucher NLR, Farmer SR. Liver regeneration following partial hepatectomy: genes and metabolism. In: Strain AJ, Diehl AM, eds. *Liver growth and repair.* London: Chapman & Hall, 1998: 3–27.

142. Leduc EH. Mitotic activity in the liver of the mouse during inanition followed by refeeding with different levels of protein. *Am J Anat* 1949;84:397–430.

143. Mead JE, Braun L, Martin DA, et al. Induction of replicative competence ("priming") in normal liver. *Cancer Res* 1990;50: 7023–7030.

144. Webber EM, Godowski PJ, Fausto N. In vivo response of hepatocytes to growth factors requires an initial priming stimulus. *Hepatology* 1994;19:489–497.

145. Ishiki Y, Ohnishi H, Muto Y, et al. Direct evidence that hepatocyte growth factor is a hepatotrophic factor for liver regeneration and has a potent antihepatitis effect in vivo. *Hepatology* 1992;16:1227–1235.

146. Patijn GA, Lieber A, Schowalter DB, et al. Hepatocyte growth factor induces hepatocyte proliferation in vivo and allows for efficient retroviral-mediated gene transfer in mice. *Hepatology* 1998;28:707–716.

147. Liu M-L, Mars WM, Zarnegar R, et al. Collagenase pretreatment and the mitogenic effects of hepatocyte growth factor and transforming growth factor-α in adult rat liver. *Hepatology* 1994;19:1521–1527.

148. Poltorak A, He X, Smirnova I, et al. Defective LPS signaling in C3H/HeJ and C57BL/10ScCr mice: mutations in Tlr4 gene. *Science* 1998;282:2085–2088.

149. Meijer C, Wiezer MJ, Diehl AM, et al. Kupffer cell depletion by CI2MDP-liposomes alters hepatic cytokine expression and delays liver regeneration after partial hepatectomy. *Liver* 2000;20:66–77.

150. Pierce RH, Campbell JS, Stephenson AB, et al. Disruption of redox homeostasis in tumor necrosis factor-induced apoptosis in a murine hepatocyte cell line [In Process Citation]. *Am J Pathol* 2000;157:221–236.

151. Goossens V, Grooten J, De Vos K, et al. Direct evidence for

tumor necrosis factor-induced mitochondrial reactive oxygen intermediates and their involvement in cytotoxicity. *Proc Natl Acad Sci USA* 1995;92:8115–8119.

152. Lee FY, Li Y, Zhu H, et al. Tumor necrosis factor increases mitochondrial oxidant production and induces expression of uncoupling protein-2 in the regenerating mouse liver. *Hepatology* 1999;29:677–687.

153. Huang ZZ, Li H, Cai J, et al. Changes in glutathione homeostasis during liver regeneration in the rat. *Hepatology* 1998; 27:147–153.

154. Czaja MJ. Liver regeneration following hepatic injury. In: Strain AJ, Diehl AM, eds. *Liver growth and repair*. London: Chapman & Hall, 1998:28–49.

155. Schmiedeberg P, Biempica L, Czaja MJ. Timing of protooncogene expression varies in toxin-induced liver regeneration. *J Cell Physiol* 1993;154:294–300.

156. Akerman PA, Cote PM, Yang SQ, et al. Long-term ethanol consumption alters the hepatic response to the regenerative effects of tumor necrosis factor-alpha. *Hepatology* 1993;17:1066–1073.

157. Czaja MJ, Xu J, Alt E. Prevention of carbon tetrachloride-induced rat liver injury by soluble tumor necrosis factor receptor. *Gastroenterology* 1995;108:1849–1854.

158. Diehl AM. Cytokine regulation of liver injury and repair [In Process Citation]. *Immunol Rev* 2000;174:160–171.

159. Bruccoleri A, Gallucci R, Germolec DR, et al. Induction of early-immediate genes by tumor necrosis factor alpha contribute to liver repair following chemical-induced hepatotoxicity. *Hepatology* 1979;25:133–141.

160. Kovalovich K, DeAngelis RA, Li W, et al. Increased toxin-induced liver injury and fibrosis in interleukin-6–deficient mice. *Hepatology* 2000;31:149–159.

161. Columbano A, Shinozuka H. Liver regeneration versus direct hyperplasia. *FASEB J* 1996;10:1118–1128.

162. Ledda-Columbano GM, Pibiri M, Loi R, et al. Early increase in cyclin-D1 expression and accelerated entry of mouse hepatocytes into S phase after administration of the mitogen 1, 4-Bis[2- (3,5-Dichloropyridyloxy)] benzene. *Am J Pathol* 2000;156:91–97.

163. Bojes HK, Germolec DR, Simeonova P, et al. Antibodies to tumor necrosis factor alpha prevent increases in cell replication in liver due to the potent peroxisome proliferator, WY-14,643. *Carcinogenesis* 1997;18:669–674.

164. Ledda-Columbano GM, Curto M, Piga R, et al. In vivo hepatocyte proliferation is inducible through a TNF and IL-6–independent pathway. *Oncogene* 1998;17:1039–1044.

The Liver: Biology and Pathobiology, Fourth Edition, edited by I. M. Arias, J. L. Boyer, F. V. Chisari, N. Fausto, D. Schachter, and D. A. Shafritz.
Lippincott Williams & Wilkins, Philadelphia © 2001.

43

HEPATOCYTE GROWTH FACTOR: ITS ROLE IN HEPATIC GROWTH AND PATHOBIOLOGY

REZA ZARNEGAR
MARIE C. DEFRANCES
GEORGE K. MICHALOPOULOS

A decade after its discovery in the context of liver regeneration, hepatocyte growth factor (HGF) is now recognized as a multifunctional cytokine involved in growth regulation and differentiation of multiple tissues. The accumulated literature shows that, in addition to liver, HGF has effects on brain growth and development, lung, kidney, intestine, breast, smooth and skeletal muscle, myocardium, and reproductive and genitourinary tissues. The effects of HGF on cellular populations of the above tissues are mitogenic and motogenic. This chapter focuses on general aspects of HGF and its receptor, and on the role of HGF in liver growth and differentiation. The available evidence indicates that HGF has regulatory control of liver embryonic growth and development, adult liver regeneration and differentiation of hepatocytes, bile duct epithelium, and sinusoidal endothelial cells. Adult liver regeneration occurs as a result of injury to the liver resulting in acute or chronic loss of hepatic parenchyma (1). Injury to the liver can be caused by surgery (such as partial hepatectomy), by chemical toxicity [such as carbon tetrachloride (CCl_4) administration], by viral infection (e.g., hepatitis B or C virus), accumulation of toxic metabolites from genetic diseases, autoimmune mechanisms, etc. Any injury resulting in loss of hepatic parenchyma triggers hepatic regeneration. HGF has been shown to have potential impact on regeneration induced by any of the above mechanisms (2) (see Chapter 42 and website chapter 🖥 W-31).

Studies on the mechanisms of liver regeneration in the early 1960s demonstrated the presence of humoral factor(s) in the circulating blood as the trigger of the regenerative

R. Zarnegar, M. C. DeFrances, and G. K. Michalopoulos: Department of Pathology, Division of Cellular and Molecular Pathology, University of Pittsburgh, School of Medicine, Pittsburgh, Pennsylvania 15261.

response in hepatocytes (3). Subsequent investigations utilizing primary cultures of rat hepatocytes in chemically defined media supported this observation by showing that sera from hepatectomized animals contained a substance that stimulated hepatocyte replication *in vitro* (4,5). With the revolutionary advances in the techniques for protein purification and microsequencing as well as complementary DNA (cDNA) cloning, a serum protein was purified that was directly mitogenic in primary cultures of hepatocytes (6–9) and its gene was molecularly cloned in the late 1980s. This substance was named originally hepatopoietin A (5) and subsequently hepatocyte growth factor (HGF) (10,11). During the years that led to the discovery of the circulating factor in serum as HGF, other nonhumoral substances were found to induce DNA replication in hepatocytes *in vitro* and *in vivo*. These can be classified as "direct mitogens" and include epidermal growth factor (EGF), transforming growth factor-α (TGF-α), and acidic fibroblast growth factor (aFGF) (12–15). In addition, since the discovery of HGF, many other factors have been found to be critical in liver regeneration and to increase in plasma after partial hepatectomy. These substances include tumor necrosis factor-α (TNF-α) (17–19), interleukin-6 (IL-6) (16), and norepinephrine (20). Since these substances are not direct mitogens for hepatocytes, they could not have been detected by the assay that led to the discovery of HGF, as that assay was geared toward isolation of direct mitogens. The simultaneous elevation in the plasma, following partial hepatectomy, of many substances (TNF-α, IL-6, norepinephrine) having regulatory effects on liver regeneration and hepatocyte growth suggests that the plasma circulating regenerative stimulus described above is more complex than originally thought and probably includes other substances besides the mitogen HGF. These substances, even though not directly mitogenic in culture, may have stimulatory effects *in vivo* that would not have been detected by the cell culture bioassay.

GENERAL ASPECTS OF HEPATOCYTE GROWTH FACTOR STRUCTURE AND FUNCTION

Biochemical and Structural Properties of Hepatocyte Growth Factor Protein

HGF purified from rabbit serum, rat platelets, or human plasma is a heparin-binding heterodimeric glycoprotein consisting of a heavy chain (α) and a light chain (β) with molecular masses of 58,000 to 69,000 and 30,000 to 34,000, respectively (6–8) as determined by sodium dodecylsulfate-polyacrylamide gel electrophoresis (SDS-PAGE). HGF isolated from the conditioned medium of a human embryonic lung fibroblast cell line or from human placenta exists predominantly as an unprocessed single-chain pro-HGF polypeptide with a molecular mass of 87,000 to

92,000 (21,22). Analysis of the cDNA nucleotide sequence of HGF revealed that the two polypeptide chains of HGF are encoded in a single open reading frame to yield the pre-pro-HGF molecule coding for 728 amino acids (10,11). The signal peptide of 31 amino acids at the amino terminus of pre-pro-HGF is removed in the endoplasmic reticulum to yield the pro-HGF precursor (11).

Comparison of the amino acid sequence of HGF to those of other known proteins showed homology to factors involved in the blood coagulation cascade or in fibrinolysis. Several of these factors contain varying numbers of polypeptide structures known as kringles, which are composed of a stretch of approximately 90 amino acids forming a double-looped structure held together by three disulfide bonds. For example, factor XII and urokinase-type plasminogen activator (u-PA) each contain one kringle domain; prothrombin and tissue-type plasminogen activator (t-PA) each contain two kringle domains, while plasminogen contains five (11,23). Although each kringle generally has a unique amino acid sequence, a short seven amino acid sequence (Asp-Tyr-Cys-Arg-Asp-Pro-Asp) is common in most kringle domains at a specific location. By comparing the amino acid sequences of HGF and these other kringle-containing proteins, the highest degree of homology (39%) was found to exist between HGF and plasminogen (11). The α chain of HGF contains four kringle domains with substantial amino acid sequence similarity to the kringles 1, 4, and 5 of plasminogen. The β chain of HGF is also unusual in that it possesses homology to the serine protease domains present in several of the enzymes mentioned above. HGF does not, however, have any known enzymatic (proteolytic) activity likely due to substitution of two out of three amino acids required in the catalytic triad (serine by tyrosine, and histidine by glutamine).

Pathways of Activation of Hepatocyte Growth Factor

HGF is synthesized as a precursor (pro-HGF) molecule, and this is the predominant form by which HGF is present in the matrix of most tissues (21,22). Conversion of the single chain pro-HGF to the heterodimeric form is an essential step for HGF function. *In vitro* mutagenesis studies in which an amino acid at the cleavage site between the α and β chains was altered by introducing a single nucleotide substitution in the coding region of the HGF cDNA at this region clearly have demonstrated that pro-HGF binds to the HGF receptor but does not elicit a mitogenic stimulus (24). This argues for a mechanism of HGF activation whereby HGF is cleaved by proteolysis to the mature heterodimeric form (see below). As predicted from the deduced amino acid sequence of pro-HGF as well as by direct N-terminal amino acid sequencing of the β chain of HGF, the cleavage site is at Arg494-Val495, which, when cleaved, generates the α and β chains of mature active heterodimeric HGF.

The first described pathway involved in HGF activation involves u-PA. This enzyme is known for its capacity to convert inactive plasminogen into its active form, plasmin. The cleavage site employed for conversion of plasminogen to plasmin has the same sequence (Arg-Val-Val) as that employed for activation of HGF. Incubation of pro-HGF with purified u-PA resulted in HGF activation (25,26). In addition, activation of pro-HGF by tissue homogenates from regenerating liver was substantially inhibited by addition of anti–u-PA antibodies (27). The precise stoichiometry of the reaction is not clear. Studies by Comoglio's group (28) suggest that u-PA and HGF may be forming a one-to-one complex with each other of relatively longer life than commonly seen in enzymatic reactions. On the other hand, this may reflect the artificiality of *in vitro* reactions utilizing u-PA. Results of the interaction of purified u-PA with its substrates in pure reaction are difficult to extrapolate to the true *in vivo* situation, in which u-PA carries out its enzymatic function bound to its cellular receptor. Typically, u-PA itself exists in two forms—single-chain u-PA (scu-PA) and two-chain u-PA (tcu-PA)—each of which possesses activity. Either of them has their activity dramatically enhanced by binding to a specific glycoprotein known as the u-PA receptor (u-PA-R). The latter is a glycosylphosphatidyl inositol (GPI) linked glycoprotein with no apparent function other than that of binding u-PA and enhancing its activity, though some studies have suggested that u-PA-R has signaling capabilities by virtue of its lateral association with other membrane bound signaling molecules, such as integrins and caveolin (29–32). u-PA-R is concentrated in specific locations on plasma membrane or in submembrane vesicles known as caveolae. Recent studies have also demonstrated association or close proximity of the HGF receptor with either u-PA or u-PA-R on the plasma membrane of hepatocytes during liver regeneration (33). Hepatocytes in culture do produce u-PA and activate pro-HGF (34). Significantly, antibodies against the u-PA-R diminish this effect. HGF itself has been shown to increase urokinase gene expression in cultures of epithelial cells (35,36).

Another pathway involved in activation of HGF is that involving a protein with substantial homology to coagulation factor XII (37). This protein was named HGF activator (HGFA) but subsequent studies demonstrated that factor XII itself can also activate HGF to a certain extent (37). Relatively specific inhibitors of HGFA were also recently described, themselves subject to proteolytic activation, suggesting that a complex regulatory pathway employing HGFA may be involved (38). HGFA is produced by hepatocytes and other cell types and appears to function as a soluble protein in tissue fluids (39). Expression of HGFA mRNA in hepatocytes increases following liver or kidney injury (39). Other studies have shown a coordinated regulation of HGF, HGFA and c-*met* in fetal intestinal mucosa (40).

Structure–Function Analysis of the Hepatocyte Growth Factor Molecule

Detailed site-directed mutagenesis studies have been carried out by several laboratories to determine the role of each kringle domain in the HGF molecule. At the N-terminus of pro-HGF, deletion of the amino acids forming a hairpin loop (before kringle one) abrogates binding of HGF to its receptor, and thus abolishes its biologic activity. A novel fold seen at the amino-terminal domain and prior to kringle one also confers binding of HGF to heparin (41). Removal of kringles one or two also has a similar effect, indicating that they too are required for interaction of HGF with its cell surface receptor. Deletion of kringle three or four, although substantially reducing HGF bioactivity, did not totally diminish it. As expected, when the entire α chain of HGF was deleted, complete loss of bioactivity occurred due to the inability of HGF to associate with its receptor. On the other hand, eliminating the entire β chain of HGF did not affect the association of HGF with its receptor, but it did completely block mitogenic stimulation of hepatocytes (24,42,43). This has led some to speculate that the β chain of HGF is responsible for activating the HGF receptor. However, at the present time, a controversy regarding the role of the β chain of HGF in receptor activation exists. For example, some studies suggest that deletion of the β chain of HGF, although abolishing its mitogenic activity, has no effect on HGF-induced motogenicity (44). The proteins known as HGF/NK1 and HGF/NK2 are derived from splicing variation of the full-length HGF messenger RNA (mRNA) and retain the amino-terminal hairpin loop as well as the first kringle (NK1) or the first two kringles (NK2). Several reports have described agonistic effects of these molecules on the HGF receptor (45–49). Transgenic mice overexpressing the HGF splicing variants NK1 and NK2 (see below) have some properties of the phenotype seen with complete HGF transgenics (45). Cooperative effects between the α chain and the β chain added as separated proteins on stimulation of the HGF receptor have also been described (50). The preponderance of evidence suggests that even though some residual functions of HGF may be expressed in the absence of the β chain, the complete biologic effects of HGF are only seen with molecular forms in which the β chain is preserved.

Hepatocyte Growth Factor Gene Organization

Southern blot analysis has revealed the presence of a single copy gene for human HGF, which is located on the long arm of chromosome 7 at q21.1 (51,52). [This region of chromosome 7 (7q21-31) harbors the gene for the HGF receptor as well (53).] The structural organization of the human HGF gene has been determined by several overlapping clones isolated from lambda phage genomic libraries and is estimated to span approximately 70 kilobases (kb) of genomic DNA comprising 18 exons interrupted by 17 introns. The first exon contains the 5′-untranslated region of the mRNA and codes for the signal peptide (54,55). The α chain, which consists of four kringle domains, is encoded by the next ten exons. Each kringle domain of the α chain is encoded by two exons, in similarity to the genes encoding other kringle-containing proteins. The spacer region between the α and β chains is found in the 12th exon, while the remaining six exons code for the serine protease-like domain of the β chain. The transcription initiation site for the HGF gene was determined to be at 76 base pairs (bp) upstream of the translation start codon.

Hepatocyte Growth Factor Gene and Its Transcriptional Control

HGF gene encompasses approximately 70 kb of genomic DNA and contains 18 exons interrupted by 17 introns, and is under tight transcriptional regulation (56). Understanding the molecular mechanisms governing the transcriptional control of this gene is an important area of investigation for several reasons. First, under normal conditions the HGF gene is permanently silenced in most epithelial cells such as hepatocytes and bile duct epithelial cells in the liver, while it is transcribed in the stromal compartment of the liver such as in Ito cells (or stellate cells) and endothelial cells. HGF expression in the mesenchymal cells is inducible by extracellular cues such as hormones and cytokines, and regulation is mainly at the transcriptional level. Second, HGF is aberrantly expressed in some epithelial tumors and in other pathologic conditions such as cirrhosis of the liver (56). Therefore, functional studies on the HGF gene promoter have been carried out to identify the *cis*-acting DNA elements and their cognate transcription factors using *in vitro* and *in vivo* analyses of the transgenic mouse models. The *in vivo* studies have revealed that the proximal promoter (~100 bp, which has a TATA-like box at −30 bp) and its upstream 5′-flanking sequences (at least 600 bp) are absolutely essential for the basal and inducible expression of the HGF gene (57). Moreover, the *in vivo* studies also show that the HGF promoter and its upstream region contain the necessary elements to dictate the cell-type–specific pattern of HGF gene expression (57). Fine mapping of the promoter region using *in vitro* and *in vivo* DNase I footprinting, gel shift, and functional assays has identified several important regulatory elements. A *cis*-acting element at position −16 to +11 bp in the mouse HGF promoter bp was identified as a novel regulatory site through which members of the CCAAT enhancer binding protein (C/EBP) family of transcription factors, especially C/EBPβ (also known as

NF-IL-6), bind and confer responsiveness to serum, TNF-α, IL-1, IL-6, and EGF (58). Cotransfection studies using expression vectors encoding any of the three isoforms of the C/EBP transcription factor (α, β, and δ) resulted in a marked induction of HGF promoter activity (58). This C/EBP site (TTGCAA) is located in the core promoter and overlaps a unique palindrome site (ACCGGT) to which a repressor factor (yet to be identified) binds and represses the HGF gene promoter (59). Another *cis*-acting element in the upstream region of the HGF promoter at position −872 to −860 bp was characterized as an estrogen responsive element (ERE) (an RGGTCA, IR3) to which the nuclear orphan receptor chicken ovalbumin upstream promoter transcription factor (COUP-TF) binds avidly. Estrogen receptor (ER) can compete with COUP-TF and relieves the repressive function of COUP-TFs on the HGF promoter through binding to the same imperfect ERE element (60). Further characterization of the HGF promoter identified an enhancer element as an Sp1 site (−328 to −297 bp), which has a CTCCC motif to which Sp1 and Sp3 bind and activate the HGF promoter (61). Additional studies on the HGF promoter have uncovered a composite multifunctional regulatory element at position −260 to −230 bp from the transcription start site to which members of the nuclear factor 1 (NF1) and upstream stimulatory factor (USF) bind to the HGF promoter and regulate its transcription. Gel mobility shift and electrophoretic mobility shift assays as well as mutational analyses revealed that the binding sites of

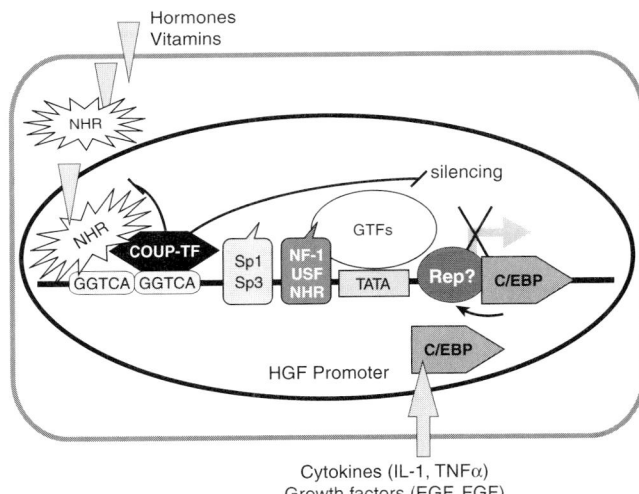

FIGURE 43.1. Schematic representation of the hepatocyte growth factor (*HGF*) gene promoter region. The diagram depicts the various cis elements and their cognate transcription factors that have been functionally implicated in the regulation of HGF gene transcription. *C/EBP*, CCAAT enhancer-binding protein; *COUP-TF*, chicken ovalbumin upstream transcription factor; *EGF*, epidermal growth factor; *FGF*, fibroblast growth factor; *GTF*, general transcription factors; *IL-1*, interleukin 1; *NHR*, nuclear hormone receptor; *NF-1*, nuclear factor-1; *Rep?*, an unknown repressor; *TNFα*, tumor necrosis factor α; *USF*, upstream stimulatory factor.

the two different transcription factor families overlap one another and that NF1 suppresses HGF gene promoter activity, while USF has an activating function. Interestingly, during activation of the HGF gene in liver regeneration after partial hepatectomy, it was noted that the binding activity of USF to the HGF promoter element increases, while that of the NF1 decreases. Other studies have shown that the wild-type but not the mutant p53 binds to and activates the HGF promoter (62). Interestingly, the HGFR gene promoter is also upregulated by the wild-type but not the mutant form of p53 (63), which may indicate a common pathway for concerted regulation of the receptor and its ligand expression (see Transitional Regulation of the Hepatocyte Growth Factor Receptor (*c-met*) Gene, below). Studies on the HGF promoter point to a complex pattern of gene regulation involving multiple positive and negative elements through which extracellular and intracellular cues can exert their modulatory functions. A diagram of the HGF promoter and its functional elements and their cognate regulatory factors are shown in Fig. 43.1.

Hepatocyte Growth Factor Gene Expression and Generation of Splicing Variants

The HGF mRNA and protein have been detected in a variety of adult and embryonic tissues (64–66). Among these are blood, brain, liver, lung, kidney, placenta, and spleen. In general, HGF mRNA is expressed in nonepithelial cells such as fibroblasts in connective tissues, Ito cells and Kupffer cells of the liver, macrophages and endothelial cells in the lung, mesangial cells in the kidney, and leukocytes and megakaryocytes (67–70). The major transcript for human and rat HGF mRNA extracted from placenta, liver, or MRC-5 cells has been reported as 6 kb in size (10,11), which encodes 134 nucleotides of the 5′-untranslated region, 2,184 nucleotides of the HGF coding region, and 3.6 kb of the 3′-untranslated region (10). In addition to the 6-kb transcript, a truncated variant of the HGF transcript (1.5 kb) was detected in placenta that codes for the N-terminal portion of HGF, including either the first kringle or the first two kringles with a putative molecular weight of about 30,000 (71). The proteins encoded by these altered transcripts have been called NK1 and NK2, correspondingly. It was determined that these shorter HGF transcripts are generated by an alternative splicing event. Analysis of conditioned medium from MRC-5 cells as well as cloning and sequencing the truncated cDNA prepared from these cells has revealed that the truncated HGF protein forms exist naturally (72,73). NK2 is unable to stimulate DNA synthesis in target cells normally activated by full-length HGF. However, it competed efficiently with full-length HGF for binding to the HGF receptor (72). The significance of the presence of these abbreviated HGF forms is not clear. Transgenic mice for NK1 exhibit the full biologic

spectrum of the complete HGF transgenics (45). Weaker biologic effects are seen with NK2 transgenics. These effects include enhancement of metastasis in induced melanoma tumors (45). On the other hand, combined bitransgenic mice for both HGF and NK2 have diminished effects compared to the HGF transgenics, suggesting a true *in vivo* role of competition between HGF and the NK2 variant (45). Weaker effects of NK2 as compared to NK1 have also been described in cell cultures (47). Heparin induces dimerization of either NK1 or NK2 and dramatically enhances their biologic effects (49).

Another naturally occurring variant of HGF also exists in relatively high abundance. This variant was isolated from cDNA libraries prepared from MRC-5 cells (21), human leukocyte (74), and human placenta, and results from alternative splicing. This deleted form of HGF differs from full-length HGF by lacking five amino acids (Phe-Lys-Pro-Ser-Ser) in the first kringle domain (21). It is biologically more potent than the undeleted form (43).

Factors that modulate HGF gene expression have been studied *in vitro* utilizing either embryonic lung fibroblast cells or human foreskin fibroblasts, which normally produce relatively substantial amounts of HGF mRNA and protein. Agents that so far are known to upregulate HGF mRNA expression in this system include the cytokine IL-1, and the phorbol ester TPA (tetradecanoylphorbol acetate), a skin tumor promoter (75,76). Factors that negatively modulate HGF gene expression in the cultured fibroblasts include TGF-β1 and the glucocorticoid analogue dexamethasone (77,78). *In vivo*, HGF mRNA expression has been induced experimentally in damaged tissues as well as in distal organs by a variety of injuries such as partial hepatectomy, CCl_4 treatment, nephrectomy, ischemia, or pneumonectomy (79–81). What triggers HGF mRNA expression after such treatments is not clear, but it appears that IL-1 may play an important role in this process. Norepinephrine, a substance that exerts regulatory effects on both HGF and EGF receptors, also increases HGF in embryonic human lung fibroblasts (82,83). This effect of norepinephrine, however, appears to be mediated though the β-adrenergic receptor. It is also not clear whether the increase in HGF mRNA expression in various damaged tissues is controlled at the transcriptional level or regulated posttranscriptionally. For regulation of HGF gene expression, see Hepatocyte Growth Factor Gene and its Transcriptional Control, above.

THE HEPATOCYTE GROWTH FACTOR RECEPTOR

General Aspects of c-*met* Structure and Function

The receptor for HGF has been identified as c-*met*, a proto-oncogene product that is a transmembrane protein with tyrosine kinase activity in its cytoplasmic portion. Ironically, an oncogene was cloned and sequenced before HGF itself had been cloned and was initially discovered based on its ability to transform normal fibroblast cell lines if introduced to these cells. This transforming oncogene was isolated from the genomic DNA prepared from a human osteosarcoma cell line (HOS) that had been treated with the carcinogen (*N*-methyl-*N'*-nitro-*N*-nitrosoguanidine, MMNG). Genomic DNA isolated from this treated cell line caused normal, non-tumorigenic NIH-3T3 fibroblasts to become transformed and produce tumors. The activated oncogene responsible for this transformation was named the *Met* oncogene (84,85). It was shown that the activation of the oncogene involved a chromosomal rearrangement that linked a sequence known as the translocated promoter region (tpr) on chromosome 1 to the C-terminal portion of the *Met* gene located on chromosome 7 (53). This translocation resulted in a truncated receptor (65 kd, also called p65tpr-Met) having a constitutively active tyrosine kinase. The cellular counterpart of the activated *Met* oncogene was later isolated, and its cDNA was cloned and sequenced from human and mouse cDNA libraries (86,87). The deduced amino acid sequence of this cDNA revealed structures characteristic of polypeptide growth factor receptors consisting of an extracellular ligand-binding domain rich in cysteine, a transmembrane domain, and an intracellular C-terminal domain with a protein tyrosine kinase (88). The normal counterpart of the activated *Met* oncogene is called the *c-met* proto-oncogene and is now known to be expressed in most epithelial cells, some mesenchymal cells, central nervous system neurons, and muscle cells (89).

An exhausting search for the ligand of this putative growth factor receptor was conducted using every purified and well-characterized polypeptide growth factor available; however, all failed to stimulate the tyrosine kinase activity of c-*met*. In the late 1980s and early 1990s when information on the biochemical characterization of the HGF protein and its broad spectrum of target cells became available, it prompted investigators to test whether HGF is the ligand for c-*met*, and in fact HGF activated the tyrosine kinase of c-*met* (90,91).

The mature c-*met* receptor is a heterodimer held together by disulfide bonds and consists of a large polypeptide chain with a molecular mass of 145,000 d containing the transmembrane domain and the intracellular tyrosine kinase domain (called the β chain), and an α chain that is approximately 45,000 d (92). Both polypeptide chains of c-*met* are derived from a single chain precursor posttranslationally modified by proteolytic cleavage at a potential cleavage site (Lys303-Arg-Lys-Lys-Arg-Ser308). Similar cleavage sites are also present in the insulin and insulin-like growth factor I receptors. Site-directed mutational analysis of the cleavage site in c-*met* utilizing a hybrid soluble form of c-*met* in which the extracellular domain of the receptor was fused to the constant region of immunoglobulin G

(IgG) heavy chain has shown that substitution of Arg and Lys with Ala totally abolishes the conversion of the c-*met* precursor to a heterodimer (93). Single amino acid substitutions with Ala at positions 304, 306, or 307 also had similar effects. The uncleavable c-*met* binds to mature heterodimeric HGF and to single chain pro-HGF (93). In these studies, however, the effects of modification of the proteolytic cleavage site on the tyrosine kinase activity of c-*met* receptor could not be examined, and it remains to be clarified whether proteolytic processing to the heterodimeric form is required for c-*met* activation and signal transduction. Studies on a human colon carcinoma cell line have shown that the c-*met* precursor was not cleaved to a heterodimer despite its conserved cleavage site (94). This single chain c-*met* retained its tyrosine kinase activity and was constitutively autophosphorylated *in vivo*. Interestingly, the precursor for the insulin receptor was also not processed in the same cell line, suggesting that a common defect may exist in the secretory pathway of this cell line. It is not clear whether a lack of c-*met* processing contributed to the transformation of these cells or whether altered processing merely resulted from other unrelated cellular defects in the cells. C-terminally truncated versions of c-*met* (both membrane bound and soluble forms) that lack the tyrosine kinase domain have also been detected in the culture supernatants from several carcinoma cell lines, but it is unclear whether these forms of c-*met* actually have a physiologic role. It has been postulated that they may interfere with receptor signal transduction by directly competing with the full-length receptor for binding to HGF (95).

Transcriptional Regulation of the Hepatocyte Growth Factor Receptor (c-*met*) Gene

In contrast to the HGF gene, the HGFR gene is transcribed in both epithelial and mesenchymal cells; however, similar to the HGF gene, the expression of the HGFR gene is inducible and tightly regulated through transcription mechanisms. The HGFR spans approximately 120 kb in size and consists of 21 exons interrupted by 20 introns (96). The HGFR promoter region lacks a TATA box but is guanosine-cytosine (GC) rich and contains several functional SP sites to which SP1 and SP3 proteins bind (97,98). Similar to the HGF gene, the HGFR gene is strongly induced by various extracellular stimuli such as TPA, IL-1, IL-6, TNF-α, EGF, and HGF (99,100).

In the murine HGFR promoter region, potential regulatory elements such as AP-1, Myb, Myc, IL-6-RE, WT1/EGR1 C/EBP, p53, NFκB, HNF3, ERE, AhRARNT, MyoD, ETS, GATA, and several others exist (97). The functionality of some of these sites and their cognate transcription factors have been confirmed. p53, for example, was shown to induce the HGFR promoter in response to ultraviolet (UV) light irradiation and DNA damage (63). AP-1 was found to mediate the stimulatory effects of HGF on the HGFR promoter in hepatic cells (98). Ets (101) and Pax3 (102) have also been shown to functionally upregulate the HGFR gene promoter. The functional role of other sites/factors awaits future analysis.

It appears that the promoters of the HGF and HGFR genes are modulated by a complex and combinatorial effect of various genetic and perhaps epigenetic (i.e., DNA methylation) phenomena. Although these two promoters are different, they share some common pathways for regulation at the extracellular levels (i.e., both genes are inducible by cytokines such as IL-1 and TNF-α) and both promoters have common functional *cis*-acting elements (such as p53, C/EBP, Sp1, and AP-1).

Hepatocyte Growth Factor Receptor and Neoplasia

The gene encoding the c-*met* proto-oncogene has been estimated to be at least 100 kb in size. Northern blot analysis of RNA prepared from normal human, mouse, and rat tissues has shown that c-*met* mRNA and protein are expressed at relatively low levels in a variety of tissues such as breast, liver, lung, kidney, large and small intestine, placenta, skin, stomach, and thyroid as well as in most human carcinoma cell lines (103). These studies have shown that many cell lines and tissues contain a single 9-kb transcript (104); although some tumor cell lines such as a human gastric carcinoma cell line, in which the gene for c-*met* is amplified and overexpressed, contain c-*met* mRNA species with sizes of 9, 8, 7, 5, and 3.4 kb (104). Transfection studies of NIH-3T3 fibroblasts (which normally do not express c-*met* but do express HGF) with a cDNA encoding normal c-*met* resulted in an autocrine loop that led to the transformation of these cells and tumor formation when injected to nude mice (105). Investigation of tissues from human colorectal adenoma and carcinoma primary tumors recently revealed that the c-*met* proto-oncogene is significantly overexpressed in 70% of these tumors as compared to the adjacent normal mucosa (106). A major transcript of 8 kb and a minor transcript of 5 kb were detected in most of these tumors. Amplification of the c-*met* proto-oncogene has also been reported for gastric carcinoma cell lines and for gastric carcinoma tissues, indicating that c-*met* gene amplification may contribute to neoplasia (107). Overexpression of both c-*Neu* and c-*met* has been observed in cholangiocarcinogenesis. Increased expression of both mRNA and protein was seen for these genes in the metaplastic intestinal epithelium, which appears as a precancerous lesion in relation to this process (108). As mentioned, the activated oncogene *tpr-Met* results from gene rearrangement. The size of the transcript encoding the rearranged Met product in MMNG-treated HOS cells is reported as 5 kb. Utilizing a very sensitive reverse-transcriptase polymerase chain reaction (RT-PCR) assay, the expression of the rearranged mRNA

for *tpr-Met* was detected at very low levels in several human carcinoma cell lines derived from pancreas, colon, bladder, and stomach, as well as in the biopsy samples of human gastric mucosa showing cancer or precursor lesions (109). Recently, mutations in the kinase domain of c-*met* were described in familial forms of renal neoplasia (papillary tumors). The mutation pattern in members of the same family strongly suggested that the mutations were associated with the pathogenesis of the neoplasms (110).

Several studies suggest that c-*met* is contributing to the phenotype or to the genesis of hepatocellular carcinomas. Mutations in the kinase domain of c-*met* occur in childhood hepatoblastomas, whereas such mutations were not present in hepatocellular carcinomas of adults. The mutations may be the cause for the appearance of these tumors early in childhood in hepatitis B virus (HBV) carriers (111). Other studies have shown overexpression of c-*met* in variable percentages of hepatocellular cancer (112–116). These findings are not unique to liver cancers and suggest that overexpression of c-*met*, though perhaps contributory to the phenotype, is not a stable feature of the pathogenesis of hepatocellular cancer in adults.

It should be noted that the role of HGF and its receptor in pathogenesis of liver tumors often appears contradictory. There is no evidence from the existing studies in the literature that HGF per se is expressed in hepatocellular carcinomas. On the other hand, hepatocellular carcinomas were seen in transgenic mice in which HGF was overexpressed in hepatocytes. One study demonstrated severe cytologic abnormalities preceding development of hepatocellular carcinomas in mice in which mouse HGF was expressed under the influence of the metallothionein promoter (117). In another study, overexpression of human HGF under the influence of the albumin promoter also enhanced the appearance of hepatocellular carcinomas in mice treated with diethylnitrosamine. The increase in liver neoplasia was more dramatic in the female mice (118). In contrast to these observations, mice bitransgenic for both c-*myc* and HGF under the influence of the albumin promoter showed a decrease in neoplasia when compared to the c-*myc* transgenic mice (119). The effect was associated with enhanced apoptosis in mice in which hepatocytes were expressing HGF. Studies with hepatocellular carcinoma cell lines showed that HGF often fails to stimulate DNA synthesis, and in many instances it may actually cause a decrease in cell proliferation (120,121), and other studies related this effect to prolonged and sustained induction of p21 (122). Injection of HGF in rats bearing preexisting tumors induced by diethylnitrosamine resulted in suppression of DNA synthesis in more than 80% of the early neoplasms, whereas an increase in DNA synthesis was noted in about 5% of the tumors (123). The latter studies suggest that the effect of exogenous HGF and its receptor on existing liver neoplasms may often result in suppression of proliferation of the neoplastic cells. Clearly the effects of stimulation of

HGF receptor are not uniform in liver tumors and may be more suppressive than stimulatory when HGF is administered as an exogenous agent. These pathways are obviously different from when HGF is expressed as an internal factor, as with transgenic mice in which HGF is expressed in hepatocytes. It should be noted that HGF transgenic mice have a much smaller tumor burden and overall much less cytologic effects compared to similar transgenic mice with TGF-α (124). The mixed stimulatory and inhibitory effects of HGF depending on its mode of administration are also compatible with the original isolation of HGF as tumor cytotoxic factor based on its cytotoxic effects on sarcomas and other neoplastic cells (125,126).

Hepatocyte Growth Factor Receptor Activation and Its Substrates

Binding of the active heterodimeric form of HGF to the Met protein causes dimerization of the receptors and activation of the tyrosine kinase catalytic site. Sites of the HGF molecule responsible for the binding to the receptor are discussed above. The cytoplasmic tail of the receptor is composed of a multifunctional docking site made of the tandemly arranged degenerate sequence Y1349VHVXXXY1356VNV. Two adjacent tyrosine residues (Y1234 and Y1235) are also essential for the activation of the catalytic site of the receptor (127). Unique to the Met receptor (and its homologues c-Ron and c-Sea) is that there is only one docking site for the interaction with downstreaxem substrates (128). As is typical for tyrosine kinase receptors, activation of the catalytic site is associated with docking of many proteins with SH2 and SH3 homology domains. Such signal transducers include phosphatidylinositol-3 (PI3) kinase, phospholipase Cγ, pp60c-src, and the GRB-2-Sos complex (129). Activation of the HGF receptor also induces activation of STAT3 (signal transducer and activator of transcription), though not as rapidly as IL-6 or EGF (130,131). Following activation and downstream signaling events, the Met receptor protein is subject to polyubiquitination and degradation in proteasomes (132). Studies have shown that a major direct target of the Met receptor is the adaptor molecule Gab-1, a docking protein with functional similarity to the IRS1 substrate of the insulin receptor (133,134). Gab-1 is also a target of phosphorylation by the EGF receptor (135). The precise interaction of Gab-1 with the Met receptor has not been fully characterized, and it appears that Grb2 is involved (134). It should be noted that while there are many distinct differences in the effects of HGF and those of other receptor tyrosine kinase ligands, such as EGF and FGF1, there is no obvious unique signaling pathway associated with the HGF receptor that is not seen with the other receptor tyrosine kinases. Any differences described are incremental and quantitative rather than qualitative. This reflects our lack of full understanding of the signaling pathways of receptor tyrosine kinases in general. A good example of this issue are the different effects induced in cells bearing the EGF receptor by the EGF-R ligands EGF and TGF-α. Use of site-directed mutagenesis and transgenic models has provided some understanding of the contributions of the different signaling pathways to the end results of HGF action. As mentioned above, the two tyrosines (Y1349 and Y1356) in the cytoplasmic tail are essential for the function of the receptor. Mutation of the two tyrosines results in loss of biologic function, as shown by loss of the transforming activity in susceptible cell lines (134). In whole animals, mutation of both tyrosine residues of the catalytic site in the mouse genome resulted in embryonic death, with placenta, liver, and limb muscle defects, mimicking the phenotype of met null mutant mice (see below). In contrast, disrupting the consensus site for Grb2 binding allowed development to proceed to term without affecting placenta and liver. There was, however, a striking reduction in limb muscle and a generalized deficit of secondary fibers (136). These data show that the different components of the Met signaling pathway are differentially crucial for different end points of the action of HGF, with late myogenesis being more critical to the association of Grb2 binding than other phenomena. Activation of c-*met* receptor may also be affected by lateral effects mediated by other adjacent tyrosine kinases, at least in neoplastic cells. Overexpression of TGF-α leads to tyrosine phosphorylation of the HGF receptor in several cell lines (137). The effect is blocked by antibodies to TGF-α or the EGF receptor. The mechanisms for the phenomenon are not clear, and it has not been shown to occur in normal epithelial cells; thus, it may be related to changes associated with the neoplastic phenotype (138).

GENERAL BIOLOGIC ASPECTS OF HEPATOCYTE GROWTH FACTOR

Hepatocyte Growth Factor Uptake and Clearance *In Vivo*

Following injection into the penile vein, HGF disappears from the blood in a biphasic fashion consisting of a rapid phase (half-life of 4 minutes) followed by a slow phase where high levels of HGF remain in the peripheral blood (terminal half-life of 85 minutes). The major organ for HGF uptake in the rat is liver and, to a lesser extent, the kidney (139,140). In contrast to the large amount of ^{125}I-HGF in the peripheral blood after systemic injection, administration of radiolabeled HGF into the portal vein resulted in the appearance of much less radioactivity in the peripheral blood (more than 70% of the injected HGF did not leave the liver), implicating liver as a major site of HGF uptake. This is further supported by the drastic reduction in plasma clearance of HGF when it was injected into rats after treatment with carbon tetrachloride (141). A small portion of HGF (less than 5%) was detected in the bile soon after HGF administration, indicating that HGF either remained in the liver or more likely reentered the blood compartment (139). When HGF sequestration is expressed per gram of tissue, spleen and adrenal glands were also efficient in taking up HGF (139,140). Clearance of HGF complexed to heparin is much slower that that of the native protein alone (142,143). Whether the uptake of HGF is mediated through c-*met* or through other binding sites such as mannose or galactose receptors, asialoglycoprotein receptors, or other cell-associated heparin-like molecules is unclear. Studies by Liu et al. have shown that hepatic uptake of HGF was reduced in the presence of excess unlabeled ligand, indicating a saturation of binding/removal phenomenon (184). Receptor-mediated HGF internalization in perfused rat liver was shown to be only partially inhibited by agents known to interfere with receptor-mediated peptide uptake, suggesting that internalization of HGF may occur by both receptor- and nonreceptor- (low-affinity sites) mediated mechanisms (140). *In vitro* studies using isolated rat hepatocytes as well as *in vivo* experiments with rats have revealed the presence of two binding sites for HGF: one sensitive to the presence of excess heparin and one resistant, probably representing the HGF receptor (144). In addition, other studies have shown that a relatively large amount of HGF in the rat liver is sequestered in the extracellular matrix in the subendothelial space, which could be eluted by *in situ* perfusion using 1 M NaCl (145). The cell types that are responsible for HGF uptake in the liver or other organs, however, remain to be determined. Since the liver is the major site for HGF uptake, it is possible that a disturbance in HGF clearance from the circulation by liver or kidney may account for high levels of HGF noted in various liver diseases such as fulminant hepatic failure and chronic renal failure (see below). In addition to heparinoids and glycosaminoglycans, recent studies have shown a remarkable affinity of HGF for binding to thrombospondin and different types of collagen forms, including collagen IV (146).

Biologic Effects on Cellular Targets

There are currently more than 13,000 publications in the Medline stored literature related to effects of HGF on different cellular types. Targets of the biologic effects of HGF include all normal epithelial cells, many neoplastic cell lines, skeletal, and smooth muscle, and several neuronal cell types. The effects of HGF on epithelial cells include stimulation of duct formation *in vivo* and *in vitro* and support of branching morphogenesis. In general, in addition to its mitogenic effects, HGF is also a strong motogen. HGF was independently purified and characterized from the culture medium of MRC-5 human embryonic lung fibroblasts, based on its ability to induce motility and migration of a variety of normal epithelial and carcinoma cells and was named scatter factor (SF) by Stoker et al. in the 1980s (147–150). After the amino acid sequence of SF became available from its cDNA nucleotide sequence, it was noted that these two activities (mitogenesis of HGF and motoge-

nesis of SF) are caused by the same molecular entity. In general, HGF is produced by mesenchymal and stromal cells, and it stimulates the growth and/or motility of a variety of epithelial cells in a paracrine and possibly an endocrine fashion. HGF was found to have strong trophic effects for motor neurons of the spinal cord (151). HGF is also expressed in many neurons of the central nervous system, including frontal lobe and temporal lobe (152). A distinct pattern of HGF expression was seen in the hippocampus, in which one is populated by neurons expressing HGF, whereas an adjacent portion contains neurons expressing the HGF receptor (153). The functions of HGF in the adult central nervous system are not clear at this point.

In liver, HGF is produced by the stellate cells (Ito cells) (154,155), and it has effects on cells expressing the Met receptor, such as hepatocytes, bile duct cells, and sinusoidal endothelial cells (see Chapters 30 and 65). HGF stimulates motogenesis and mitogenesis in primary cultures of rat, mouse, and human hepatocytes (156–158) and bile duct epithelium (157). Other studies have demonstrated angiogenic effects of HGF, but to date there are no studies available on the direct effects of HGF on sinusoidal endothelial cells. HGF stimulates both motogenesis and mitogenesis in cultures of hepatocytes in collagen gels (159), resulting in formation of hepatocellular plates. The mitogenic effects of HGF are suppressible by both complex matrix (type I collagen gels, Matrigel) and TGF-β1 (159). The same agents, however, do not affect the motogenic effects of HGF (158). HGF and EGF have synergistic effects promoting growth of hepatocytes in long-term cultures allowing for clonogenic growth of hepatocytes (160). Of interest, addition of HGF alone in such cultures in the presence of collagen gels stimulated arrangement of the hepatocytes in acinar and ductular configurations (160). In three dimensional cultures, HGF (as well as EGF) was essential for the formation of histiotypic organization of the hepatocytes and these effects were antagonized by TGF-β1 (161). HGF has stimulatory effects on liver growth and regeneration (see Hepatocyte Growth Factor Role in Liver Regeneration, below). Complex metabolic effects of HGF on hepatocytes include stimulation of fatty acid and triglyceride synthesis and lipoprotein secretion (162).

Role of Hepatocyte Growth Factor in Embryogenesis

Complementary patterns of expression of HGF and its receptor are seen in embryogenesis (163) (see Chapter 2). In general, HGF is expressed by mesenchymal cell types, whereas expression of the receptor is seen in developing epithelial cell populations. Transient HGF and c-*met* expression is seen in areas of muscle formation and in developing motor neurons. In kidney, mesenchymal cells expressing HGF develop expression of the Met receptor at the time when the kidney mesenchyme undergoes epithelial conversion (164). Deletion mutants of HGF or its receptor Met resulted in similar phenotypes. Both conditions were associated with embryonic lethality (165–167). In both conditions there were defects in development of liver, placenta, and skeletal muscle. Livers were overall atrophic with a decreased number of hepatocytes. The reasons for the hepatic effects are not clear, but they attest to the overall trophic and growth-stimulating effects of HGF in liver. Of interest, HGF and c-*met* expression are maximally enhanced in liver during embryogenesis at a time when hepatocytes are arranged in acinar and hemiacinar configurations (160). Previous studies have shown that this stage is essential for hepatic development and that it precedes formation of the hepatic plates. In view of the above-mentioned effects of HGF inducing acinar configurations in hepatocyte cultures in collagen gels (160) and similar effects on tubulogenesis in other cell types, it is tempting to speculate that the presence of HGF is crucial for the completion of these complex stages of histologic morphogenesis.

HEPATOCYTE GROWTH FACTOR–RELATED MOLECULES

In addition to plasminogen, which shares significant sequence and structural homology with HGF, a cDNA clone encoding another product with similar structure and overall sequence homology to that of HGF has also been described. The putative product of this cDNA clone was named HGF-like protein (HGFL). It contains four kringle domains in the α chain and a serine protease-like domain in the β chain, and has 40% overall amino acid sequence homology to HGF. Its mRNA was detected in high levels in the liver, and to a lesser degree in lung, adrenal, and placenta (168,169). In contrast to HGF, which is synthesized primarily by mesenchymal cells, HGFL is produced predominantly by hepatocytes, and it is secreted into the plasma as the inactive single chain precursor. Also, in contrast to HGF, whose cleavage appears to be mediated by two predominant pathways, cleavage of HGFL to its active heterodimeric form is mediated by a variety of proteases (168). The gene for the HGF-like molecule was localized to human chromosome 3, and it consists of the same numbers of introns and exons as HGF, although the overall size of HGF-like gene is approximately one-tenth of that of HGF. Comparison of a partial amino acid sequence of a plasma protein known as macrophage stimulating factor (MSP) with that of the HGFL molecule suggests that the HGFL gene product is identical to a protein known as MSP (170) that has been reported to stimulate the responsiveness of mouse peritoneal resident macrophages to chemoattractants and to activate their phagocytic activity. Activities associated with HGFL and its receptor c-*Ron* (see below) include stimulating proliferation of mammary duct epithelial cells and keratinocytes, maturation of megakaryocytes, motility

of keratinocytes, and bone resorption and contraction of osteoclasts. Even though the effects of HGF and HGFL overlap in some epithelial systems, HGFL has no essential role in embryogenesis. Disruption of the HGFL gene was compatible with embryogenesis (171). Adult mice homozygous for the HGFL deletion developed microvesicular steatosis in hepatocytes. The receptor of HGFL was identified as the product of the human proto-oncogene c-*Ron* (172). The protein encoded for the HGFL receptor is very similar to the Met protein, including similar tyrosine kinase activation domains and docking sites composed of two tyrosines (see above). Homozygous deletion of the mouse stk receptor (the murine homologue of the human c-*ron*) is associated with early embryonic lethality. Embryos fail to implant and do not progress beyond the blastocyst stage (173). The discrepancy between the severe effects on embryogenesis following deletion of the HGFL receptor and the complete absence of effects following deletion of the ligand HGFL raises the possibility that other ligands for c-*Ron* might also exist. Such ligands, however, have not been identified as yet. The remarkable similarities of the structures of HGF and HGFL and those of their receptors suggest that the two receptor/ligand systems evolved in parallel from another ancestral receptor/ligand gene set, not identified so far. Homologues of both c-*met*, c-*Ron*, and of the avian homologue c-*Sea* were recently identified in the teleost puffer fish (*Fugu rubripes*), suggesting that the HGF and HGFL ligand/receptor systems emerged early on in vertebrate evolution (174).

ROLE OF HEPATOCYTE GROWTH FACTOR IN THE LIVER REGENERATION AND CHRONIC LIVER INJURY

More information is available on the expression of HGF in animals with experimentally induced liver injuries and liver diseases than for any other diseased tissue or organ. Most of the liver-related studies have focused on the role of HGF in liver regeneration, its effects in chronic liver injury, and changes related to HGF and its receptor in fulminant hepatitis.

Hepatocyte Growth Factor Role in Liver Regeneration

In experimental animals treated with hepatotoxins that induce hepatocyte necrosis (such as treatment with CCl_4), or other kinds of liver injuries such as ischemia, physical crushing, or two-thirds partial hepatectomy (PHx), the levels of HGF protein and HGF activity in the plasma increase very rapidly during the early phase of liver regeneration, implying that HGF may be involved in the overall process, leading the hepatocytes to enter the cell cycle (175,176). The amount of the HGF transcript also rises not only in the livers of injured animals but also in the lung, spleen, and kidney, suggesting endocrine as well as paracrine functions for HGF in liver regeneration (79–81,177). The role of inflammatory cytokines and norepinephrine as signaling agents for this phenomenon was discussed above. As mentioned, HGF was originally isolated from plasma of partially hepatectomized rats and was considered to be the agent primarily responsible for the transmission of the mitogenic signals to hepatocytes during liver regeneration. Subsequent studies using anti-HGF antibodies demonstrated a rise of HGF in the plasma within 1 to 2 hours after partial hepatectomy (79). More prolonged changes in plasma HGF after partial hepatectomy were also noted after human liver resection (178), persisting up to 2 weeks after partial hepatectomy. The origin of the HGF rising in the plasma is not clear. Direct measurements of HGF clearance during liver regeneration did not demonstrate significant differences in HGF clearance between normal and regenerating liver (139).

In view of the direct mitogenic effects of HGF on hepatocytes in culture and the early rise of HGF in the plasma, it was logical to postulate a direct link between this event and stimulation of hepatocyte DNA synthesis. Direct infusion of moderate doses of HGF systemically or into the portal circulation in normal rats or mice has direct mitogenic effects on hepatocytes. DNA synthesis is induced in zone 1 (periportal) hepatocytes (179). This effect is enhanced by preinfusion of TNF-α (17). When HGF is infused in larger amounts, it causes a dramatic increase in liver weight associated with enhanced mitogenesis in hepatocytes. This was observed both in normal as well as IL-6–deficient mice (180). Withdrawal of the infused HGF is followed by marked hepatocyte apoptosis and a decrease in overall hepatic DNA back to normal levels (181). Infusion of smaller amounts of HGF following prior treatment of the animals with small amounts of collagenase (179) also leads to enhancement of the effect of HGF. The peculiar effect of collagenase raises the possibility that infusion of HGF *in vivo* is likely to be less effective in a normal matrix environment but would be more effective in an environment of matrix remodeling. This would imply that matrix remodeling may be part of the early stages of the regenerative process, causing enhanced sensitivity of hepatocytes to mitogenic stimuli such HGF. This hypothesis is also supported by findings in hepatocyte cultures. Stimulation of DNA synthesis by either EGF or HGF is suppressed when hepatocytes are maintained in collagen type I gels and extracts from the EHS mouse sarcoma cell line (Matrigel) (159,182). Additional studies had shown that, during isolation of hepatocytes by collagenase perfusion of the liver, hepatocytes enter into the cell cycle, as evidenced by increased expression of cell cycle marker proteins (182,183). This suggests that the effect of matrix degradation and release of matrix bound products (which include HGF) may be sufficient to induce hepatocytes to enter into

the cell cycle. As mentioned above, HGF is present in large amounts in the matrix of normal liver (145). Infusion of radiolabeled HGF demonstrates accumulation of HGF in periportal sites (184). Processes associated with matrix degradation have the potential of releasing HGF and making it available to hepatocytes either directly in their local environment, or via release in the plasma and reuptake by the hepatocytes. Pathways leading to matrix remodeling involve urokinase or membrane-type matrix metalloproteinases (MT-MMPs) initiated protease cascades (185,186). Urokinase is also involved in activation of HGF (see Pathways of Activation of Hepatocyte Growth factor, above). Urokinase activity is rapidly upregulated following partial hepatectomy, primarily due to translocation of the urokinase receptor from cytoplasm to the plasma membrane (27). Direct evidence that urokinase is actually involved in activation of HGF during liver regeneration was provided by the demonstration that single-chain HGF processing to the active two-chain form by regenerating liver homogenates is inhibited by addition of antiurokinase antibodies (27). Further studies have shown that increased urokinase activity immediately after PHx leads to activation of all the expected subsequent steps in matrix remodeling, such as activation of plasminogen to plasmin and activation of MMP-9 (187,188), increased expression of MMP-9 on hepatocytes, as well as degradation of biomatrix proteins. Of relevance to these findings, mice with homozygous deletions of the plasminogen gene have defective regenerative responses following chemical injury (189). In addition to the activation of the urokinase-initiated matrix remodeling cascade, there is also activation of the pathway initiated by MT-MMP. The latter pathway proceeds to activation of MMP-2 and also involves tissue inhibitor of metalloproteinase-2 (TIMP-2). Activation of this pathway occurs later than the activation of the urokinase pathway (187). While the above studies demonstrate that there is active matrix remodeling occurring during liver regeneration, they do not directly prove that HGF rising in the plasma is derived from hepatic matrix. Given the high concentrations of HGF in hepatic matrix, however, and the active remodeling of matrix in periportal sites, this is an attractive possibility that warrants further investigation. Other substances associated with biomatrix are also elevated in the plasma with the same kinetics as HGF. These include hyaluronic acid and TGF-β1 (190). Elimination of the mito-inhibitory TGF-β1 protein from the ambient environment of the hepatocytes via matrix remodeling may be the reason why only hepatocytes, of the many potential epithelial cell targets, respond to the elevated levels of plasma HGF during the early stages of liver regeneration. It also should be noted that HGF itself may be a secondary later contributor to the activation of the matrix remodeling cascades via effects on hepatocyte gene expression. It has been shown that HGF induces MMP gene expression in cultures of epithelial cells (191). A schematic picture of the interaction between urokinase, matrix remodeling, and HGF release and local activation in the early stages of liver regeneration is shown in Fig. 43.2.

Other converging observations also support the importance of HGF released from preexisting stores during the early stages of liver generation. Tyrosine phosphorylation of the HGF receptor occurs at 30 and 60 minutes after partial hepatectomy, coinciding with the rise of HGF in the plasma (33). Mice deficient in urokinase, the initiator of both matrix remodeling and HGF activation, show retarded and decreased regenerative activity following partial hepatectomy (192). The importance of the plasma HGF as well as HGF present in the ambient environment of hepatocytes in the early stages of liver generation was directly demonstrated by infusion of anti-HGF antibodies prior to partial hepatectomy. It was noted that hepatocyte proliferation was suppressed for more than 72 hours, whereas proliferation of nonparenchymal cells was not affected (193).

The signal transduction pathways associated with activation of HGF receptor have been extensively studied in many different cell types (see Chapter 35). In the context of liver regeneration and hepatocyte mitogenesis, key events associated with proliferation of hepatocytes include activa-

tion of transcription factors NFκB, AP-1, and STAT3. Defective activation of these transcription factors is seen in knockout mice for IL-6 and TNF-α receptor I (16,18). Mice deficient for HGF or its receptor do not survive embryogenesis. Thus, the contribution of HGF to the signaling events associated with hepatocyte proliferation at the early stages of liver regeneration cannot be directly assessed, other than by use of blocking antibodies. Studies with hepatocyte cultures, however, have demonstrated that HGF alone (as well as EGF alone) can stimulate a complete mitogenic pathway in resting quiescent rat or human hepatocytes, including activation of AP-1, STAT3, and NFκB (130,131). Since HGF is a complete mitogen for hepatocytes both *in vivo* (179) and *in vitro* (159), and since the HGF receptor is activated within 30 to 60 minutes after partial hepatectomy (33), it is highly likely that HGF contributes to the activation of these specific signaling events or other signaling events associated with mitogenesis in hepatocytes. It is also highly likely that key signaling events related to hepatocyte mitogenesis may be subject to the control of multiple cytokines, creating overlapping and redundant pathways via which entry of hepatocytes into the cell cycle is guaranteed, even in the absence of some of the

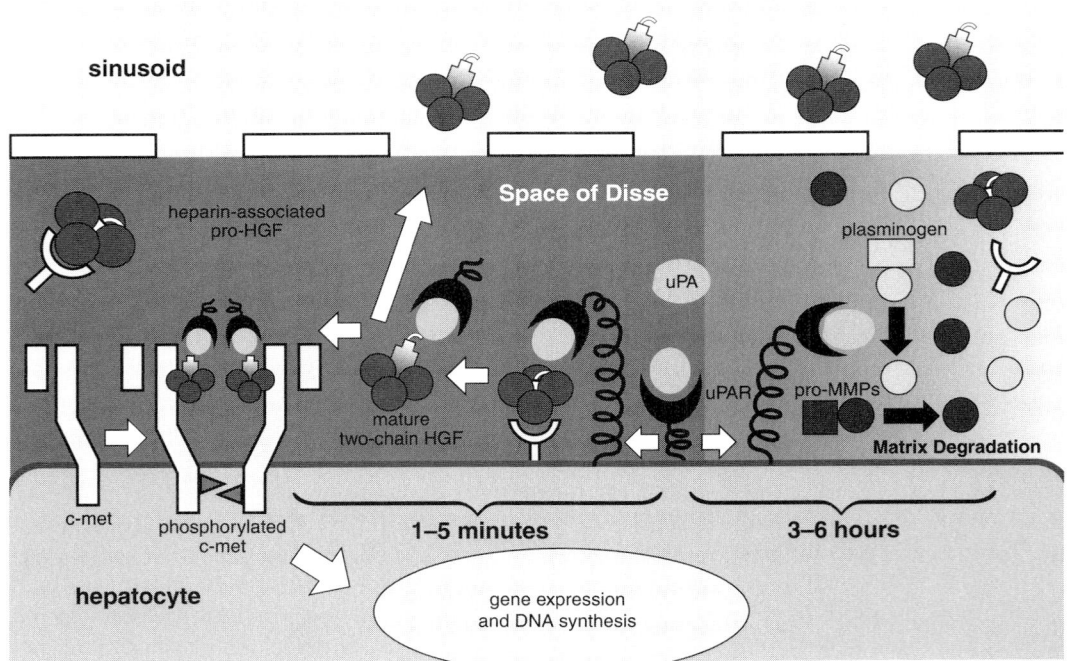

FIGURE 43.2. Schematic cartoon of hepatocyte growth factor (*HGF*)-related immediate early events occurring in the hepatocyte microenvironment following partial hepatectomy. The scheme shows proteolytic activation of inactive pro-HGF and matrix degradation via the urokinase-type plasminogen activator (*u-PA*) u-PA receptor (*u-PAR*) system, plasmin, and metalloproteinases (*MMPs*) after partial hepatectomy. Activation of HGF appears to be an early event, since phosphorylation of the HGF receptor occurs by 30 minutes. The events related to HGF thought to occur in the first 5 minutes are depicted on the **left** of the schematic cartoon. Matrix degradation and proteolysis events occurring later are shown on the **right**.

key extracellular signals. Mice deficient in IL-6 or TNF-α receptor I eventually restore most if not all of the hepatic mass. The same observations relate to rats subjected to blockade of the α1-adrenergic (norepinephrine) receptor (20) or following infusion of TGF-β1 (194) or administration of *N*-acetylaminofluorene (AAF) (195). The only blockade that appears to completely block the regenerative response is the permanent inactivation of NFκB (196). The inability to permanently block liver regeneration by eliminating specific nonmitogenic cytokines clearly associated with the regenerative response suggests that there is considerable redundancy in the pathways generated by the mitogens (HGF and EGF) and nonmitogenic cytokines. It also suggests that the multiplicity of signaling pathways activated in hepatocytes is crucial not only for the initiation of the mitogenic signals but also for the timing and the precision of the regenerative response. As mentioned above, with the exception of the elimination of the intracellular NFκB signaling, all defects associated with extracellular signals (homozygous deletions in IL-6, TNF-α receptor I, or u-PA, blockade of the norepinephrine α1-adrenergic receptor, infusion of TGF-β1, etc.) only delay and do not abolish liver regeneration. This suggests that these extracellular signals are crucial for the timing and precision of liver regeneration but operate in a redundant fashion with receptor tyrosine kinase ligands (HGF, EGF, TGF-α) and are not absolutely essential for the completion of the response. This may be difficult to sort out, as mentioned above, unless conditional deletion mutant strains of mice for either HGF or its receptor become available in the future.

Hepatocyte Growth Factor and Chronic Liver Injury

Several reports have shown that administration of HGF during and/or after exposure of the liver to a variety of chronic injury models has ameliorative effects on hepatic histology and retards or prevents fibrosis (197). The effects on injury caused by chemicals may be due to effects of HGF on metabolic activation of the toxic chemical, resulting in less liver injury, when HGF is administered during the time of the administration of the chemical. Convincing results have also been presented, however, showing effects of HGF after the chemical had already induced a certain degree of liver injury and fibrosis (197). Other reports have shown similar effects of HGF in chronic models of injury of kidney (198) and lungs (199). HGF also prevented massive hepatic failure induced by lipopolysaccharide (LPS) and galactosamine, suggesting that the protective effects of HGF against liver injury are more general and not limited to directly toxic chemical agents (200). In other studies, HGF abrogated the severe apoptosis and liver failure induced by the agonist anti-fas antibody both in culture and in whole animals, while inducing the antiapoptotic protein bcl-xL (201). The mechanisms leading to these

effects are not entirely clear, but they raise the possibility that HGF may be used as part of a therapeutic regimen to prevent chronic injury to the liver induced by a variety of agents, such as alcoholism and chronic hepatitis. In a recent report (202) HGF was used in a gene therapy protocol in which vectors expressing HGF were given by intramuscular injection to mice with liver fibrosis induced by chemical injury. The expression of the HGF in the vector led to increased levels of HGF in the plasma and was associated with substantial improvement of the histologic picture of the fibrotic livers, raising the issue of using HGF as part of a gene therapy protocol for treatment of liver fibrosis and prevention of cirrhosis. The 5 amino acid deletion variant of HGF has been specifically investigated in this regard, and it appears to be more effective as an antifibrogenic agent than the complete HGF molecule (203,204).

Hepatocyte Growth Factor and Fulminant Hepatitis

When HGF was first discovered, it was thought that it could be used as a therapeutic agent in situations such as fulminant hepatitis, in which massive death of hepatocytes is not accompanied by compensatory regenerative activity. It was soon shown, however, that levels of HGF in plasma are very high during fulminant hepatitis. In fact, this condition is associated with the highest levels of HGF than any other disease state (205–207). Elevated levels of plasma HGF are also seen in chronic liver disease and liver failure (207). These findings are in apparent contradiction to the protective effects of HGF against acute and chronic liver injury, discussed above, and suggest that HGF, while apparently useful in chronic injury models, may not be of use for therapy in the catastrophic environment of fulminant hepatic failure. The reasons for the paradox are not clear. While levels of HGF in the plasma appear very high, probably due to massive release of HGF from the hepatic biomatrix, the status of HGF activation (two chain active versus single chain inactive) has not been investigated. Recent preliminary studies suggest that the apparent inability of HGF to stimulate hepatocyte replication and prevent death of hepatocytes may be due to severe downregulation of the HGF receptor induced by simultaneous elevation of IL-6 and TGF-β1 in the plasma (208).

CONCLUSION

In the last ten years since their discovery, HGF and its receptor have emerged as major regulators of cell growth, motility, and morphogenesis. Despite the multiple targets of HGF, the embryonic lethality associated with placenta, muscle, and liver dysmorphogenesis in HGF and c-*met* knockout mice clearly suggests that liver is a major overall target of the HGF/c-*met* system. The multiplicity of effects on several tissues and the new evidence for the emergence of the HGF receptor in early vertebrates suggest that HGF may have evolved as a signaling molecule in response to the need for complex cell movement and morphogenesis associated with vertebrate embryonic growth. In that sense, since liver regeneration may be viewed as an example of the most complex new tissue formation in an adult animal, the crucial need of HGF for liver regeneration is not surprising. More refined animal genetic models may be able to further elucidate the complex effects of the HGF/c-*met* system, not only on liver growth and regeneration but on overall liver function, maintenance, and physiology.

ACKNOWLEDGMENTS

Work performed in the authors' laboratories have been supported in parts by grants from the American Cancer Society (ACS) (CN-55) and National Institute of Environmental Health Sciences (R01 ES06109–01) awarded to R.Z., and in parts by grants from the National Institutes of Health (R01 CA35373 and R01 CA30241) awarded to G.K.M.

REFERENCES

1. Grisham JW. A morphological study of deoxyribonucleic acid synthesis and cell proliferation in regenerating liver, autoradiography with 3H-thymidine. *Cancer Res* 1962;22:842–849.
2. Michalopoulos GK, DeFrances M. Liver regeneration. *Science* 1997;276:60–71.
3. Moolten FL, Bucher NLR. Regeneration of rat liver: transfer of humoral agents by cross circulation. *Science* 1967;158:272–274.
4. Michalopoulos GK, Cianciulli HD, Novotny AR, et al. Liver regeneration studies with rat hepatocytes in primary culture. *Cancer Res* 1982;42:4673–4678.
5. Michalopoulos GK, Houck KA, Dolan M, et al. Control of hepatocyte proliferation by two serum factors. *Cancer Res* 1984;44:4414–4441.
6. Nakamura T, Nawa K, Ichihara A, et al. Subunit structure of hepatocyte growth factor from rat platelets. *FEBS Lett* 1987;224:311–318.
7. Gohda E, Tsubouchi H, Nakayama H, et al. Partial purification and characterization of hepatocyte growth factor from plasma of patients with fulminant hepatic failure. *J Clin Invest* 1988;81:414–419.
8. Zarnegar R, Michalopoulos GK. Purification and biological characterization of human Hepatopoietin A:A polypeptide growth factor for hepatocytes. *Cancer Res* 1989;49:3314–3320.
9. Zarnegar R, Muga S, Enghild J, et al. NH2-terminal amino acid sequence of rabbit hepatopoietin A: a heparin-binding polypeptide growth factor for hepatocytes. *Biochem Biophys Res Commun* 1989;163:1370–1376.
10. Miyazawa K, Tsubouchi H, Naka D, et al. Molecular cloning and sequence analysis of cDNA for human hepatocyte growth factor. *Biochem Biophys Res Commun* 1989;163:967–973.
11. Nakamura T, Nishizawa T, Hagiya M, et al. Molecular cloning and expression of hepatocyte growth factor. *Nature* 1989;342:440–443.
12. McGowan JA, Strain AJ, Bucher NLR. DNA synthesis in primary cultures of adult rat hepatocytes in a defined medium: effects of epidermal growth factor, insulin, glucagon, and cyclic-AMP. *J Cell Physiol* 1981;180:353–363.
13. McGowan JA, Bucher NLR. Pyruvate promotion of DNA synthesis in serum-free primary cultures of adult rat hepatocytes. *In Vitro Cell Dev Biol* 1983;19:159–166.
14. Mead JE, Fausto N. Transforming growth factor TGFa may be a physiological regulator of liver regeneration by means of an autocrine mechanism. *Proc Natl Acad Sci USA* 1989;86:1558–1562.
15. Kan M, Huan J, Mansson P, et al. Heparin-binding growth factor type 1 (acidic fibroblast growth factor): a potential biphasic autocrine and paracrine regulator of hepatocyte regeneration. *Proc Natl Acad Sci USA* 1989;86:7432–7436.
16. Cressman DE, Greenbaum LE, DeAngelis RA, et al. Liver failure and defective hepatocyte regeneration in interleukin-6–deficient mice. *Science* 1996;274:1379–1383.
17. Webber EM, Bruix J, Pierce RH, et al. Tumor necrosis factor primes hepatocytes for DNA replication in the rat. *Hepatology* 1998;28:1226–1234.
18. Yamada Y, Webber EM, Kirillova I, et al. Analysis of liver regeneration in mice lacking type 1 or type 2 tumor necrosis factor receptor: requirement for type 1 but not type 2 receptor. *Hepatology* 1998;28:959–970.
19. Yamada Y, Kirillova I, Peschon JJ, et al. Initiation of liver growth by tumor necrosis factor: deficient liver regeneration in mice lacking type I tumor necrosis factor receptor. *Proc Natl Acad Sci USA* 1997;18:94:1441–1446.
20. Cruise JL, Knechtle SJ, Bollinge RR, et al. α 1-adrenergic effects and liver regeneration. *Hepatology* 1987;7:1189–1194.
21. Rubin JS, Chan ML, Bottaro D, et al. A broad-spectrum human lung fibroblast-derived mitogen is a variant of hepatocyte growth factor. *Proc Natl Acad Sci USA* 1991;88:415–419.
22. Hernandez J, Zarnegar R, Strom S, et al. Characterization of the effects of human placental HGF on rat hepatocytes. *J Cell Physiol* 1992;150:116–121.
23. Deleted.
24. Lokker NA, Mark MR, Luis EA, et al. Structure-function analysis of hepatocyte growth factor: identification of variants that lack mitogenic activity yet retain high affinity receptor binding. *EMBO J* 1992;11:2503–2510.
25. Mars WM, Zarnegar R, Michalopoulos GK. Activation of hepatocyte growth factor by the plasminogen activators u-PA and t-PA. *Am J Pathol* 1993;143:949–958.
26. Naldini L, Tamagnone L, Vigna E, et al. Extracellular proteolytic cleavage by urokinase is required for activation of hepatocyte growth factor/scatter factor. *EMBO J* 1992;11:4825–4833.
27. Mars WM, Liu ML, Kitson RP, et al. Immediate early detection of urokinase receptor after partial hepatectomy and its implications for initiation of liver regeneration. *Hepatology* 1995;21:1695–1701.
28. Naldini L, Vigna E, Bardelli A, et al. Biological activation of pro-HGF (hepatocyte growth factor) by urokinase is controlled by a stoichiometric reaction. *J Biol Chem* 1995;270:603–611.
29. Reuning U, Magdolen V, Wilhelm O, et al. Multifunctional potential of the plasminogen activation system in tumor invasion and metastasis (review). *Int J Oncol* 1998;13:893–906.
30. Koshelnick Y, Ehart M, Stockinger H, et al. Mechanisms of signaling through urokinase receptor and the cellular response. *Thromb Haemost* 1999;82:305–311.
31. Chapman HA, Wei Y, Simon DI, et al. Role of urokinase receptor and caveolin in regulation of integrin signaling. *Thromb Haemost* 1999;82:291–297.
32. Preissner KT, Kanse SM, Chavakis T, et al. The dual role of the urokinase receptor system in pericellular proteolysis and cell

adhesion: implications for cardiovascular function. *Basic Res Cardiol* 1999;94:315–321.

33. Stolz DB, Mars WM, Petersen BE, et al. Growth factor signal transduction immediately after two-thirds partial hepatectomy in the rat. *Cancer Res* 1999;59:3954–3960.

34. Mars WM, Kim TH, Beer-Stolz D, et al. The presence of urokinase in serum free primary rat hepatocyte cultures and its role in activating hepatocyte growth factor. *Cancer Res* 1996;56:2837–2843.

35. Ried S, Jager C, Jeffers M, et al. Activation mechanisms of the urokinase-type plasminogen activator promoter by hepatocyte growth factor/scatter factor. *J Biol Chem* 1999;274:16377–86.

36. Webb CP, Hose CD, Koochekpour S, et al. The geldanamycins are potent inhibitors of the hepatocyte growth factor/scatter factor-met-urokinase plasminogen activator-plasmin proteolytic network. *Cancer Res* 2000;60:342–349.

37. Shimomura T, Miyazawa K, Komiyama Y, et al. Activation of hepatocyte growth factor by two homologous proteases, blood-coagulation factor XIIa and hepatocyte growth factor activator. *Eur J Biochem* 1995;229:257–261.

38. Shimomura T, Denda K, Kawaguch T, et al. Multiple sites of proteolytic cleavage to release soluble forms of hepatocyte growth factor activator inhibitor type 1 from a transmembrane form. *J Biochem (Tokyo)* 1999;126:821–828.

39. Okajima A, Miyazawa K, Naitoh Y, et al. Induction of hepatocyte growth factor activator messenger RNA in the liver following tissue injury and acute inflammation. *Hepatology* 1997;25:97–102.

40. Matsubara Y, Ichinose M, Yahagi N, et al. Hepatocyte growth factor activator: a possible regulator of morphogenesis during fetal development of the rat gastrointestinal tract. *Biochem Biophys Res Commun* 1998;253:477–484.

41. Chirgadze DY, Hepple J, Byrd RA, et al. Insights into the structure of hepatocyte growth factor/scatter factor (HGF/SF) and implications for receptor activation. *FEBS Lett* 1998;23:126–129.

42. Okigaki M, Komada M, Uehara Y, et al. Functional characterization of HGF mutants obtained by deletion of structural domains. *Biochemistry* 1992;31:9555–9561.

43. Matsumoto K, Takehara T, Inoue H, et al. Deletion of kringle domains or the N-terminal hairpin structure in HGF results in marked decreases in related biological activities. *Biochem Biophys Res Commun* 1991;181:691–699.

44. Hartmann G, Naldini L, Weidner KM, et al. A functional domain in the heavy chain of SF/HGF binds the c-*met* receptor and induces cell dissociation but not mitogenesis. *Proc Natl Acad Sci USA* 1992;89:11574–11578.

45. Otsuka T, Jakubczak J, Vieira W, et al. Disassociation of met-mediated biological responses in vivo: the natural hepatocyte growth factor/scatter factor splice variant NK2 antagonizes growth but facilitates metastasis. *Mol Cell Biol* 2000;20:2055–2065.

46. Day RM, Cioce V, Breckenridge D, et al. Differential signaling by alternative HGF isoforms through c-*met*: activation of both MAP kinase and PI 3-kinase pathways is insufficient for mitogenesis. *Oncogene* 1999;18:3399–3406.

47. Montesano R, Soriano JV, Malinda KM, et al. Differential effects of hepatocyte growth factor isoforms on epithelial and endothelial tubulogenesis. *Cell Growth Differ* 1998;9:355–365.

48. Cioce V, Csaky KG, Chan AML, et al. Hepatocyte growth factor (HGF)/NK1 is a naturally occurring HGF/scatter factor variant with partial agonist/antagonist activity. *J Biol Chem* 1996;271:13110–13115.

49. Schwall RH, Chang LY, Godowski PJ, et al. Heparin induces dimerization and confers proliferative activity onto the hepatocyte growth factor antagonists NK1 and NK2. *J Cell Biol* 1996;133:709–718.

50. Matsumoto K, Kataoka H, Date K, et al. Cooperative interaction between α- and β-chains of hepatocyte growth factor on c-*met* receptor confers ligand-induced receptor tyrosine phosphorylation and multiple biological responses. *J Biol Chem* 1998;273:22913–22920.

51. Zarnegar R, Petersen B, DeFrances MC, et al. Localization of hepatocyte growth factor (HGF) gene on human chromosome 7. *Genomics* 1992;12:147–150.

52. Fukuyama R, Ichijoh Y, Minoshima S, et al. Regional localization of the HGF gene to human chromosome 7 band q21.1. *Genomics* 1992;11:410–415.

53. Dean M, Park M, LeBeau MM, et al. The human met oncogene is related to tyrosine kinase oncogenes. *Nature* 1985;318:385–388.

54. Seki T, Hagiya M, Shimonishi M, et al. Organization of the HGF encoding gene. *Gene* 1991;102:213–219.

55. Miyazawa K, Kitamura A, Kitamura N. Structural organization and the transcriptional initiation site of the human HGF gene. *Biochemistry* 1991;30:9170–9176.

56. Zarnegar R. Regulation of HGF and HGFR gene expression. *EXS* 1995;74:33–49.

57. Bell AW, Jiang JG, Chen Q, et al. The upstream regulatory regions of the hepatocyte growth factor gene promoter are essential for its expression in transgenic mice. *J Biol Chem* 1998;273:6900–6908.

58. Jiang JG, Zarnegar R. A novel transcriptional regulatory region within the core promoter of the hepatocyte growth factor gene is responsible for its inducibility by cytokines via the C/EBP family of transcription factors. *Mol Cell Biol* 1997;17:5758–5770.

59. Liu Y, Beedle AB, Lin L, et al. Identification of a cell-type-specific transcriptional repressor in the promoter region of the mouse hepatocyte growth factor gene. *Mol Cell Biol* 1994;14:7046–7058.

60. Jiang JG, Bell A, Liu Y, et al. Transcriptional regulation of the hepatocyte growth factor gene by the nuclear receptors chicken ovalbumin upstream promoter transcription factor and estrogen receptor. *J Biol Chem* 1997;272:3928–3934.

61. Jiang JG, Chen Q, Bell A, et al. Transcriptional regulation of the hepatocyte growth factor (HGF) gene by the Sp family of transcription factors. *Oncogene* 1997;14:3039–3049.

62. Metcalfe AM, Dixon RM, Radda GK. Wild-type but not mutant p53 activates the hepatocyte growth factor/scatter factor promoter. *Nucleic Acids Res* 1997;25:983–986.

63. Seol DW, Chen Q, Smith ML, et al. Regulation of the c-*met* proto-oncogene promoter by p53. *J Biol Chem* 1999;274:3565–3572.

64. Tashiro K, Hagiya M, Hishizawa T, et al. Deduced primary structure of rat hepatocyte growth factor and expression of the mRNA in rat tissues. *Proc Natl Acad Sci USA* 1990;87:3200–3204.

65. Okajima A, Miyazawa K, Kitamura N. Primary structure of rat Hepatocyte growth factor and induction of its mRNA during liver regeneration following hepatic injury. *Eur J Biochem* 1990;193:375–381.

66. Zarnegar R, Muga S, Rahija R, et al. Tissue distribution of hepatopoietin A: a heparin binding polypeptide growth factor for hepatocytes. *Proc Natl Acad Sci USA* 1990;87:1252–1256.

67. DeFrances MC, Wolf H, Michalopoulos GK, et al. The presence of hepatocyte growth factor in the developing rat. *Development* 1992;116:387–395.

68. Kinoshita T, Tashiro K, Nakamura T. Marked increase of HGF mRNA in non-parenchymal liver cells of rats treated with hepatotoxins. *Biochem Biophys Res Commun* 1989;165:1229–1234.

69. Noji S, Tashiro K, Koyama E, et al. Expression of Hepatocyte growth factor gene in endothelial and Kupffer's cells of damaged

rat livers as revealed by in situ hybridization. *Biochem Biophys Res Commun* 1990;173:42–47.

70. Schirmacher P, Geerts A, Pietrangelo A, et al. Hepatocyte growth factor/hepatopoietin A is expressed in fat-storing cells from rat liver but not myofibroblast-like cells derived from fat-storing cells. *Hepatology* 1992;15:5–11.

71. Miyazawa K, Kitamura A, Naka D, et al. An alternatively processed mRNA generated from human hepatocyte growth factor gene. *Eur J Biochem* 1991;197:15–22.

72. Chan AM-L, Rubin JS, Bottaro DP, et al. Identification of a competitive HGF antagonist encoded by an alternative transcript. *Science* 1991;254:1382–1385.

73. Cioce V, Csaky KG, Chan AML, et al. Hepatocyte growth factor (HGF)/NK1 is a naturally occurring HGF/scatter factor variant with partial agonist/antagonist activity. *J Biol Chem* 1996;271:13110–13115.

74. Seki T, Ihara I, Sugimura A, et al. Isolation and expression of cDNA for different forms of hepatocyte growth factor from human leukocyte. *Biochem Biophys Res Commun* 1990;172:321–327.

75. Gohda E, Kataoka H, Tsubouchi H, et al. Phorbol ester-induced secretion of human hepatocyte growth factor by human skin fibroblasts and its inhibition by dexamethasone. *FEBS Lett* 1992;301:107–110.

76. Matsumoto K, Okazaki H, Nakamura T. Up-regulation of HGF gene expression by IL-1 in human skin fibroblasts. *Biochem Biophys Res Commun* 1992;188:235–243.

77. Matsumoto K, Tajima H, Okazaki H, et al. Negative regulation of HGF gene expression in human lung fibroblasts and leukemic cells by transforming growth factor b and glucocorticoids. *J Biol Chem* 1992;267:24917–24920.

78. Ota S, Tanaka Y, Bamba H, et al. Nonsteroidal anti-inflammatory drugs may prevent colon cancer through suppression of hepatocyte growth factor expression. *Eur J Pharmacol* 1999;367:131–138.

79. Zarnegar R, DeFrances MC, Kost D, et al. Expression of Hepatocyte Growth Factor (HGF) in regenerating rat liver after partial hepatectomy. *Biochem Biophys Res Commun* 1991;177:559–565.

80. Kono S, Nagaike M, Masumoto K, et al. Marked induction of HGF mRNA in intact kidney and spleen in response to injury of distant organs. *Biochem Biophys Res Commun* 1992;186:991–998.

81. Hamanoue M, Kawaida K, Takao S, et al. Rapid and marked induction of HGF during liver regeneration after ischemic or crush injury. *Hepatology* 1992;16:1485–1492.

82. Cruise JL, Houck KA, Michalopoulos GK. Induction of DNA synthesis in cultured rat hepatocytes through stimulation of α 1 adrenoreceptor by norepinephrine. *Science* 1985;227:749–751.

83. Broten J, Michalopoulos G, Petersen B, et al. Adrenergic stimulation of hepatocyte growth factor expression. *Biochem Biophys Res Commun* 1999;262:76–79.

84. Cooper CS, Park M, Blair D, et al. Molecular cloning of a new transforming gene from a chemically transformed human cell line. *Nature* 1984;311:29–33.

85. Park M, Dean M, Cooper CS, et al. Mechanism of met oncogene activation. *Cell* 1986;45:895–904.

86. Park M, Dean M, Kaul K, et al. Sequence of Met protooncogene cDNA has features characteristic of the tyrosine kinase family of growth factor receptors. *Proc Natl Acad Sci USA* 1987;84:6379–6383.

87. Chan AM, King HWS, Deakin EA, et al. Characterization of the mouse met protooncogene. *Oncogene* 1988;2:593–599

88. Tempest PR, Stratton MR, Cooper CS. Structure of the met protein kinase activity among human tumor cell lines. *Br J Cancer* 1988;58:3–7.

89. Vigna E, Naldini L, Tamagnone L, et al. Hepatocyte growth factor and its receptor, the tyrosine kinase encoded by the c-*met* proto-oncogene. *Cell Mol Biol (Noisy-le-grand)* 1994;40:597–604.

90. Bottaro DP, Rubin JS, Faletto DL, et al. Identification of the hepatocyte growth factor receptor as the c-*met* proto-oncogene product. *Science* 1991;251:802–804.

91. Naldini L, Vigna E, Narsimhan R, et al. Hepatocyte growth factor stimulates the tyrosine kinase activity of the receptor encoded by the proto-oncogene, c-*met*. *Oncogene* 1991;6:501–504.

92. Giordano S, DiRenzo MF, Narsimhan RP, et al. Biosynthesis of the protein encoded by the proto-oncogene. *Oncogene* 1989;4:1383–1388.

93. Mark MR, Lokker NA, Zioncheck TF, et al. Expression and characterization of hepatocyte growth factor receptor-IgG fusion protein. *J Biol Chem* 1992;267:26166–26171.

94. Mondino A, Giordano S, Comoglio P. Defective posttranslational processing activates the tyrosine kinase encoded by the Met proto-oncogene (hepatocyte growth factor receptor). *Mol Cell Biol* 1991;11:6084–6092.

95. Prat M, Crepaldi T, Gandino L, et al. C-terminal truncated forms of Met, the hepatocyte growth factor receptor. *Mol Cell Biol* 1991;11:5954–5962.

96. Liu Y. The human hepatocyte growth factor receptor gene: complete structural organization and promoter characterization. *Gene* 1998;215:159–169.

97. Seol DW, Zarnegar R. Structural and functional characterization of the mouse c-*met* proto-oncogene (hepatocyte growth factor receptor) promoter. *Biochim Biophys Acta* 1998;1395:252–258.

98. Seol DW, Chen Q, Zarnegar R. Transcriptional activation of the hepatocyte growth factor receptor (c-met) gene by its ligand (hepatocyte growth factor) is mediated through AP-1. *Oncogene* 2000;19:1132–1137.

99. Moghul A, Lin L, Beedle A, et al. Modulation of c-*met* proto-oncogene (HGF receptor) mRNA abundance by cytokines and hormones: evidence for rapid decay of the 8 kb c-*met* transcript. *Oncogene* 1994;9:2045–2052.

100. Chen Q, Seol DW, Carr B, et al. Co-expression and regulation of Met and Ron proto-oncogenes in human hepatocellular carcinoma tissues and cell lines. *Hepatology* 1997;26:59–66.

101. Gambarotta G, Boccaccio C, Giordano S, et al. Ets up-regulates MET transcription. *Oncogene* 1996;13:1911–1917.

102. Epstein JA, Shapiro DN, Cheng J, et al. Pax3 modulates expression of the c-*met* receptor during limb muscle development. *Proc Natl Acad Sci USA* 1996;93:4213–4218.

103. Prat M, Narsimhan RP, Crepaldi T, et al. The receptor encoded by the human c-*met* oncogene is expressed in hepatocytes, epithelial cells and solid tumors. *Int J Cancer* 1991;49:323–328.

104. Giordano L, Ponzetto C, DiRenzo MF, et al. Tyrosine kinase receptor indistinguishable from in-Met protein. *Nature* 1989;339:155–156.

105. Rong S, Bodescot M, Blair D, et al. Tumorigenicity of the met proto-oncogene, and the gene for HGF. *Mol Cell Biol* 1992;12:5152–5158.

106. Liu C, Park M, Tsao MS. Overexpression of proto-oncogene but EGF receptor or c-erbB-2 in primary human colorectal carcinomas. *Oncogene* 1992;7:181–185.

107. Kuniyasu H, Yasui W, Kitadai Y, et al. Frequent amplification of the gene in scirrhous type stomach cancer. *Biochem Biophys Res Commun* 1992;189:227–232.

108. Radaeva S, Ferreira-Gonzalez A, Sirica AE. Overexpression of C-NEU and C-*MET* during rat liver cholangiocarcinogenesis: a link between biliary intestinal metaplasia and mucin-producing cholangiocarcinoma. *Hepatology* 1999;29:1453–1462.

109. Soman NR, Corriea P, Ruiz BA, et al. The TPR-Met oncogenic

rearrangement is present and expressed in human gastric carcinoma and precursor lesions. *Proc Natl Acad Sci USA* 1991; 88:4892–4896.

110. Schmidt L, Duh FM, Chen F, et al. Germline and somatic mutations in the tyrosine kinase domain of the MET proto-oncogene in papillary renal carcinomas. *Nat Genet* 1997;16: 68–73.

111. Park WS, Dong SM, Kim SY, et al. Somatic mutations in the kinase domain of the Met/hepatocyte growth factor receptor gene in childhood hepatocellular carcinomas. *Cancer Res* 1999; 59:307–310.

112. Ueki T, Fujimoto J, Suzuki T, et al. Expression of hepatocyte growth factor and its receptor c-*met* proto-oncogene in hepatocellular carcinoma. *Hepatology* 1997;25:862–866.

113. Ljubimova JY, Petrovic LM, Wilson SE, et al. Expression of HGF, its receptor c-*met*, c-myc, and albumin in cirrhotic and neoplastic human liver tissue. *J Histochem Cytochem* 1997;45: 79–87.

114. D'Errico A, Fiorentino M, Ponzetto A, et al. Liver hepatocyte growth factor does not always correlate with hepatocellular proliferation in human liver lesions: its specific receptor c-*met* does. *Hepatology* 1996;24:60–64.

115. Selden C, Farnaud S, Ding SF, et al. Expression of hepatocyte growth factor mRNA, and c-*met* mRNA (hepatocyte growth factor receptor) in human liver tumors. *J Hepatol* 1994;21: 227–234.

116. Boix L, Rosa JL, Ventura F, et al. c-*met* mRNA overexpression in human hepatocellular carcinoma. *Hepatology* 1994;19: 88–91.

117. Sakata H, Takayama H, Sharp R, et al. Hepatocyte growth factor/scatter factor overexpression induces growth, abnormal development, and tumor formation in transgenic mouse livers. *Cell Growth Differ* 1996;7:1513–1523.

118. Bell A, Chen Q, DeFrances MC, et al. The five amino acid-deleted isoform of hepatocyte growth factor promotes carcinogenesis in transgenic mice. *Oncogene* 1999;18:887–895.

119. Santoni-Rugiu E, Preisegger KH, Kiss A, et al. Inhibition of neoplastic development in the liver by hepatocyte growth factor in a transgenic mouse model. *Proc Natl Acad Sci USA* 1996;93: 9577–9582.

120. Ogasawara H, Hiramoto J, Takahashi M, et al. Hepatocyte growth factor stimulates DNA synthesis in rat preneoplastic hepatocytes but not in liver carcinoma cells. *Gastroenterology* 1998;114:775–781.

121. Shiota G, Kawasaki H, Nakamura T, et al. Inhibitory effect of hepatocyte growth factor on metastasis of hepatocellular carcinoma in transgenic mice. *Res Commun Mol Pathol Pharmacol* 1996;91:33–39.

122. Shima N, Stolz DB, Miyazaki M, et al. Possible involvement of p21/waf1 in the growth inhibition of HepG2 cells induced by hepatocyte growth factor. *J Cell Physiol* 1998;177:130–136.

123. Liu ML, Mars WM, Michalopoulos GK. Hepatocyte growth factor inhibits cell proliferation in vivo of rat hepatocellular carcinomas induced by diethylnitrosamine. *Carcinogenesis* 1995; 16:841–843.

124. Jhappan C, Stahle C, Harkins RN, et al. TGFα overexpression in transgenic mice induces liver neoplasia and abnormal development of the mammary gland and pancreas. *Cell* 1990;61: 1137–1146.

125. Higashio K, Shima N, Goto M, et al. Identity of a tumor cytotoxic factor from human fibroblasts and hepatocyte growth factor. *Biochem Biophys Res Commun* 1990;170:397–404.

126. Amicone L, Spagnoli FM, Spath G, et al. Transgenic expression in the liver of truncated Met blocks apoptosis and permits immortalization of hepatocytes. *EMBO J* 1997;16:495–503.

127. Longati P, Bardelli A, Ponzetto C, et al. Tyrosines 1234–1235 are critical for activation of the tyrosine kinase encoded by the MET proto-oncogene (HGF receptor). *Oncogene* 1994;9: 49–57.

128. Ponzetto C, Bardelli A, Zhen Z, et al. A multifunctional docking site mediates signaling and transformation by the hepatocyte growth factor/scatter factor receptor family. *Cell* 1994;77: 261–271.

129. Comoglio PM, Boccaccio C. The HGF receptor family: unconventional signal transducers for invasive cell growth. *Genes Cells* 1996;1:347–354.

130. Runge DM, Runge D, Foth H, et al. STAT 1α/1β, STAT 3 and STAT 5: expression and association with c-*met* and EGF-receptor in long-term cultures of human hepatocytes. *Biochem Biophys Res Commun* 1999;265:376–381.

131. Schaper F, Siewert E, Gomez-Lechon MJ, et al. Hepatocyte growth factor/scatter factor (HGF/SF) signals via the STAT3/APRF transcription factor in human hepatoma cells and hepatocytes. *FEBS Lett* 1997;405:99–103.

132. Jeffers M, Taylor GA, Weidner KM, et al. Degradation of the Met tyrosine kinase receptor by the ubiquitin-proteasome pathway. *Mol Cell Biol* 1997;17:799–808.

133. Birchmeier W, Brinkmann V, Niemann C, et al. Role of HGF/SF and c-*met* in morphogenesis and metastasis of epithelial cells. *Ciba Found Symp* 1997;212:230–240.

134. Bardelli A, Longati P, Gramaglia D, et al. Gab1 coupling to the HGF/Met receptor multifunctional docking site requires binding of Grb2 and correlates with the transforming potential. *Oncogene* 1997;15:3103–3111.

135. Lehr S, Kotzka J, Herkner A, et al. Identification of tyrosine phosphorylation sites in human Gab-1 protein by EGF receptor kinase in vitro. *Biochemistry* 1999;38:151–159.

136. Maina F, Casagranda F, Audero E, et al. Uncoupling of Grb2 from the Met receptor in vivo reveals complex roles in muscle development. *Cell* 1996;87:531–542.

137. Presnell SC, Stolz DB, Mars WM, et al. Modifications of the hepatocyte growth factor/c-*met* pathway by constitutive expression of transforming growth factor-α in rat liver epithelial cells. *Mol Carcinogen* 1997;18:244–255.

138. Jo M, Stolz DB, Esplen JE, et al. Cross-talk between epidermal growth factor receptor and c-*met* signal pathways in transformed cells. *J Biol Chem* 2000;275:8806–8811.

139. Appasamy R, Tanabe M, Murase N, et al. Pharmacokinetics of HGF blood clearance, organ uptake and biliary excretion in normal and partially hepatectomized rat. *J Lab Invest* 1993; 68:270–276.

140. Liu KX, Kato Y, Narukawa M, et al. Importance of the liver in plasma clearance of hepatocyte growth factor in rats. *Am J Physiol* 1992;263:G642–G649.

141. Liu KX, Kato Y, Yamazaki M, et al. Decrease in the hepatic clearance of hepatocyte growth factor in carbon tetrachloride-intoxicated rats. *Hepatology* 1993;17:651–660.

142. Kato Y, Liu KX, Nakamura T, et al. Heparin-hepatocyte growth factor complex with low plasma clearance and retained hepatocyte proliferating activity. *Hepatology* 1994;20:417–424.

143. Schwall RH, Chang LY, Godowski PJ, et al. Heparin induces dimerization and confers proliferative activity onto the hepatocyte growth factor antagonists NK1 and NK2. *J Cell Biol* 1996;133:709–718.

144. Zarnegar R, DeFrances MC, Oliver L, et al. Identification and partial characterization of receptor binding sites for HGF on rat hepatocytes. *Biochem Biophys Res Commun* 1990;173: 1179–1185.

145. Masumoto A, Yamamoto N. Sequestration of a hepatocyte growth factor in extracellular matrix in normal adult rat liver. *Biochem Biophys Res Commun* 1991;174:90–95.

146. Lamszus K, Joseph A, Jin L, et al. Scatter factor binds to throm-

bospondin and other extracellular matrix components. *Am J Pathol* 1996;149:805–819.

147. Stoker M, Gherardi E, Perryman M, et al. Scatter factor is a fibroblast-derived modulator of epithelial cell mobility. *Nature* 1987;327:239–242.

148. Gherardi E, Gray J, Stoker M, et al. Purification of scatter factor, a fibroblast-derived basic protein that modulates epithelial interactions and movement. *Proc Natl Acad Sci USA* 1989;86:5844–5848.

149. Gherardi E, Stoker M. Hepatocytes and scatter factor. *Nature* 1990;346:228.

150. Weidner KM, Behrens J, Vandekerckhove J, et al. Scatter factor: molecular characteristics and effect on the invasiveness of epithelial cells. *J Cell Biol* 1990;111:2097–2108.

151. Ebens A, Brose K, Leonardo ED, et al. Hepatocyte growth factor/scatter factor is an axonal chemoattractant and a neurotrophic factor for spinal motor neurons. *Neuron* 1996;17:1157–1172.

152. Jung W, Castren E, Odenthal M, et al. Expression and functional interaction of hepatocyte growth factor-scatter factor and its receptor c-*met* in mammalian brain. *J Cell Biol* 1994;126:485–494.

153. Achim CL, Katyal S, Wiley CA, et al. Expression of HGF and cMet in the developing and adult brain. *Brain Res Dev* 1997;102:299–303.

154. Schirmacher P, Geerts A, Jung W, et al. The role of Ito cells in the biosynthesis of HGF-SF in the liver. *EXS* 1993;65:285–299.

155. Schirmacher P, Geerts A, Pietrangelo A, et al. Hepatocyte growth factor/hepatopoietin A is expressed in fat-storing cells from rat liver but not myofibroblast-like cells derived from fat-storing cells. *Hepatology* 1992;15:5–11.

156. Strain AJ, Ismail T, Tsubouchi H, et al. Native and recombinant human hepatocyte growth factors are highly potent promoters of DNA synthesis in both human and rat hepatocytes. *J Clin Invest* 1991;87:1853–1857.

157. Joplin R, Hishida T, Tsubouchi H, et al. Human intrahepatic biliary epithelial cells proliferate in vitro in response to human hepatocyte growth factor. *J Clin Invest* 1992;90:1284–1289.

158. Petersen B, Yee CJ, Bowen W, et al. Distinct morphological and mito-inhibitory effects induced by TGF-β 1, HGF and EGF on mouse, rat and human hepatocytes. *Cell Biol Toxicol* 1994;10:219–230.

159. Michalopoulos GK, Bowen W, Nussler AK, et al. Comparative analysis of mitogenic and morphogenic effects of HGF and EGF on rat and human hepatocytes maintained in collagen gels. *J Cell Physiol* 1993;156:443–452.

160. Block GD, Locker J, et al. Population expansion, clonal growth and specific differentiation patterns in primary cultures of hepatocytes induced by HGF/SF, EGF and TGFa in a chemically defined (HGM) medium. *J Cell Biol* 1996;132:1133–1149.

161. Michalopoulos GK, Bowen WC, Zajac VF, et al. Morphogenetic events in mixed cultures of rat hepatocytes and nonparenchymal cells maintained in biological matrices in the presence of hepatocyte growth factor and epidermal growth factor. *Hepatology* 1999;29:90–100.

162. Kaibori M, Kwon AH, Oda M, et al. Hepatocyte growth factor stimulates synthesis of lipids and secretion of lipoproteins in rat hepatocytes. *Hepatology* 1998;27:1354–1361.

163. Sonnenberg E, Meyer D, Weidner KM, et al. Scatter factor/hepatocyte growth factor and its receptor, the c-*met* tyrosine kinase, can mediate a signal exchange between mesenchyme and epithelia during mouse development. *J Cell Biol* 1993;123:223–235.

164. Tsarfaty I, Rong S, Resau JH, et al. The Met proto-oncogene mesenchymal to epithelial cell conversion. *Science* 1994;263:98–101.

165. Schmidt C, Bladt F, Goedecke S, et al. Scatter factor/hepatocyte growth factor is essential for liver development. *Nature* 1995;373:699–702.

166. Uehara Y, Minowa O, Mori C, et al. Placental defect and embryonic lethality in mice lacking hepatocyte growth factor/scatter factor. *Nature* 1995;373:702–705.

167. Bladt F, Riethmacher D, Isenmann S, et al. Essential role for the c-*met* receptor in the migration of myogenic precursor cells into the limb bud. *Nature* 1995;376:768–771.

168. Degen SJ, Stuart LA, Han S, et al. Characterization of the mouse cDNA and gene coding for a hepatocyte growth factor-like protein: expression during development. *Biochemistry* 1991;30:9781–9791.

169. Han S, Stuart LA, Degen SJ. Characterization of the DNF15S2 locus on human chromosome 3: identification of a gene coding for four kringle domains with homology to hepatocyte growth factor. *Biochemistry* 1991;30:9768–9780.

170. Skeel A, Yoshimura T, Showalter SD, et al. Macrophage stimulating protein: purification, partial amino acid sequence, and cellular activity. *J Exp Med* 1991;173:1227–1234.

171. Bezerra JA, Carrick TL, Degen JL, et al. Biological effects of targeted inactivation of hepatocyte growth factor-like protein in mice. *J Clin Invest* 1998;101:1175–1183.

172. Waltz SE, Toms CL, McDowell SA, et al. Characterization of the mouse Ron/Stk receptor tyrosine kinase gene. *Oncogene* 1998;16:27–42.

173. Muraoka RS, Sun WY, Colbert MC, et al. The Ron/STK receptor tyrosine kinase is essential for peri-implantation development in the mouse. *J Clin Invest* 1999;103:1277–1285.

174. Cottage A, Clark M, Hawker K, et al. Three receptor genes for plasminogen related growth factors in the genome of the puffer fish Fugu rubripes. *FEBS Lett* 1999;443:370–374.

175. Lindroos P, Zarnegar R, Michalopoulos GK. Hepatocyte growth factor (hepatopoietin A) rapidly increases in plasma before DNA synthesis and liver regeneration stimulated by partial hepatectomy and carbon tetrachloride administration. *Hepatology* 1991;13:743–750.

176. Kinoshita T, Hirao S, Matsumoto K, et al. Possible endocrine control by hepatocyte growth factor of liver regeneration after partial hepatectomy. *Biochem Biophys Res Commun* 1991;177:330–335.

177. Yanagita K, Nagaike M, Ishibashi H, et al. Lung may have an endocrine function producing hepatocyte growth factor in response to injury of distal organs. *Biochem Biophys Res Commun* 1992;182:802–809.

178. Tomiya T, Tani M, Yamada S, et al. Serum hepatocyte growth factor levels in hepatectomized and nonhepatectomized surgical patients. *Gastroenterology* 1992;103:1621–1624.

179. Liu ML, Mars WM, Zarnegar R, et al. Collagenase pretreatment and the mitogenic effects of hepatocyte growth factor and transforming growth factor-α in adult rat liver. *Hepatology* 1994;19:1521–1527.

180. Patijn GA, Lieber A, Schowalter DB, et al. Hepatocyte growth factor induces hepatocyte proliferation in vivo and allows for efficient retroviral-mediated gene transfer in mice. *Hepatology* 1998;28:707–716.

181. Nagoshi S, Yasuda H, Suda J, et al. Hepatocyte apoptosis and hepatic expression of transforming growth factor-β1 mRNA during involution of hyperplastic rat liver induced by hepatocyte growth factor. *J Gastroenterol Hepatol* 1998;13:786–793.

182. Rana B, Mischoulon D, Xie Y, et al. Cell-extracellular matrix interactions can regulate the switch between growth and differentiation in rat hepatocytes: reciprocal expression of C/EBP α and immediate-early growth response transcription factors. *Mol Cell Biol* 1994;14:5858–5869.

183. Kost DP, Michalopoulos GK. Effect of epidermal growth factor on the expression of protooncogenes c-myc and c-Ha-ras in

short-term primary hepatocyte culture. *J Cell Physiol* 1990;144:122–127.

184. Liu ML, Mars WM, Zarnegar R, et al. Uptake and distribution of hepatocyte growth factor in normal and regenerating adult rat liver. *Am J Pathol* 1994;144:129–140.

185. Dano K, Romer J, Nielsen BS, et al. Cancer invasion and tissue remodeling—cooperation of protease systems and cell types. *APMIS* 1999;107:120–127.

186. Seiki M. Membrane-type matrix metalloproteinases. *APMIS* 1999;107:137–143.

187. Kim TH, Mars WM, Stolz DB, et al. Extracellular matrix remodeling at the early stages of liver regeneration in the rat. *Hepatology* 1997;26:896–904.

188. Kim TH, Mars WM, Stolz DB, et al. Expression and activation of pro-MMP-2 and pro-MMP-9 during rat liver regeneration. *Hepatology* 2000;31:75–82.

189. Bezerra JA, Bugge TH, Melin-Aldana H, et al. Plasminogen deficiency leads to impaired remodeling after a toxic injury to the liver. *Proc Natl Acad Sci USA* 1999;96:15143–15148.

190. Michalopoulos GK. Hepatocyte growth factor (HGF) and its receptor (Met) in liver regeneration, neoplasia and disease. In: Jirtle RL, ed. *Liver regeneration and carcinogenesis.* New York: Academic Press, 1995:27–49.

191. Dunsmore SE, Rubin JS, Kovacs SO, et al. Mechanisms of hepatocyte growth factor stimulation of keratinocyte metalloproteinase production. *J Biol Chem* 1996;271:24576–24582.

192. Roselli HT, Su M, Washington K, et al. Liver regeneration is transiently impaired in urokinase-deficient mice. *Am J Physiol* 1998;275:G1472–1479.

193. Burr AW, Toole K, Chapman C, et al. Anti-hepatocyte growth factor antibody inhibits hepatocyte proliferation during liver regeneration. *J Pathol* 1998;185:298–302.

194. Russell WE, Coffey RJ Jr, Ouellette AJ, et al. Type β transforming growth factor reversibly inhibits the early proliferative response to partial hepatectomy in the rat. *Proc Natl Acad Sci USA* 1988;85:5126–5130.

195. Solt DB, Medline A, Farber E. Rapid emergence of carcinogen-induced hyperplastic lesions in a new model for the sequential analysis of liver carcinogenesis. *Am J Pathol* 1977;88:595–618.

196. Iimuro Y, Nishiura T, Hellerbrand C, et al. NFkappaB prevents apoptosis and liver dysfunction during liver regeneration. *J Clin Invest* 1998;101:802–811.

197. Matsuda Y, Matsumoto K, Yamada A, et al. Preventive and therapeutic effects in rats of hepatocyte growth factor infusion on liver fibrosis/cirrhosis. *Hepatology* 1997;26:81–89.

198. Mizuno S, Kurosawa T, Matsumoto K, et al. Hepatocyte growth factor prevents renal fibrosis and dysfunction in a mouse model of chronic renal disease. *J Clin Invest* 1998;101:1827–1834.

199. Yaekashiwa M, Nakayama S, Ohnuma K, et al. Simultaneous or delayed administration of hepatocyte growth factor equally represses the fibrotic changes in murine lung injury induced by bleomycin. A morphologic study. *Am J Respir Crit Care Med* 1997;156:1937–1944.

200. Kosai K, Matsumoto K, Funakoshi H, et al. Hepatocyte growth factor prevents endotoxin-induced lethal hepatic failure in mice. *Hepatology* 1999;30:151–159.

201. Kosai K, Matsumotom K, Nagata S, et al. Abrogation of Fas-induced fulminant hepatic failure in mice by hepatocyte growth factor. *Biochem Biophys Res Commun* 1998;244:683–690.

202. Ueki T, Kaneda Y, Tsutsui H, et al. Hepatocyte growth factor gene therapy of liver cirrhosis in rats. *Nat Med* 1999;5:226–230.

203. Masunaga H, Fujise N, Shiota A, et al. Preventive effects of the deleted form of hepatocyte growth factor against various liver injuries. *Eur J Pharmacol* 1998;342:267–279.

204. Yasuda H, Imai E, Shiota A, et al. Antifibrogenic effect of a deletion variant of hepatocyte growth factor on liver fibrosis in rats. *Hepatology* 1996;24:636–642.

205. Tsubouchi H, Horono S, Gohda E, et al. Clinical significance of human hepatocyte growth factor in blood from patients with fulminant hepatic failure. *Hepatology* 1989;9:875–881.

206. Tsubouchi H, Hirono S, Gohda E, et al. Human hepatocyte growth factor in blood of patients with fulminant hepatic failure. I. Clinical aspects. *Dig Dis Sci* 1991;36:780–784.

207. Tsubouchi H, Niitani Y, Hirono S, et al. Levels of the human hepatocyte growth factor in serum of patients with various liver diseases determined by an enzyme-linked immunosorbent assay. *Hepatology* 1991;13:1–5.

208. Mizuguchi T, Hui T, Kamohara Y, et al. IL-6 and TGF-β 1 downregulate *c-met* expression through suppression of Sp-1 DNA binding activity. Abstract 928, *Hepatology* 1999;30:392A.

The Liver: Biology and Pathobiology, Fourth Edition, edited by I. M. Arias, J. L. Boyer, F. V. Chisari, N. Fausto, D. Schachter, and D. A. Shafritz. Lippincott Williams & Wilkins, Philadelphia © 2001.

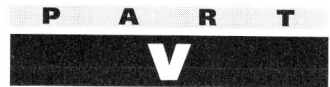

RELATION TO OTHER ORGANS

HEPATIC ENCEPHALOPATHY

ROGER F. BUTTERWORTH

Hepatic encephalopathy (HE) occurs as one of two major forms:

1. Portal–systemic encephalopathy (PSE), the most commonly encountered form of HE, accompanies the development of portal–systemic collaterals that arise from portal hypertension, most often due to cirrhosis. Neurologically, PSE develops slowly, starting with abnormalities of sleep patterns, shortened attention span, and muscular incoordination progressing through lethargy to stupor and ultimately to coma. Repeated episodes of PSE precipitated by gastrointestinal bleeding, constipation, or sedative drugs are common. In addition, PSE is commonly encountered following surgical decompression of the portal hypertensive state, and more recently following transjugular intrahepatic portosystemic shunts (TIPS).

2. HE associated with acute liver failure is a clinical syndrome resulting from severe inflammatory and/or necrotic liver disease, of rapid onset. The neurologic disorder progresses from altered mental status to coma generally within hours or days. Death frequently results from brain herniation caused by increased intracranial pressure as a consequence of massive brain edema. HE accompanying acute liver failure differs fundamentally from PSE whether assessed neurologically, neuropathologically, or neurochemically.

This chapter focuses on recent developments in our understanding of pathophysiologic mechanisms and the impact of these developments on current therapies for HE. New findings derived from studies in postmortem brain samples from patients with acute or chronic liver disease, from animal models of HE, as well as from noninvasive approaches such as positron emission tomography (PET), magnetic resonance imaging (MRI), and spectroscopy (MRS) are included.

Recent studies in both human and experimental HE reveal that, when liver fails, alterations in expression of many genes occur in the brain. Several of these genes have been identified and include monoamine oxidase (MAO-A isoform), the peripheral-type benzodiazepine receptor, neuronal nitric oxide synthase, the astrocytic glutamate transporter (GLT-1), and aquaporin-4 (1,2). These genes code for proteins with key roles in the maintenance of cerebral excitability, cerebral blood flow, and water homeostasis. Changes in their expression could contribute to the pathogenesis of HE in acute or chronic liver failure.

R. F. Butterworth: Neuroscience Research Unit, Hôpital Saint-Luc, University of Montreal, Montreal, Quebec H2X 3J4 Canada.

PORTAL–SYSTEMIC ENCEPHALOPATHY

Neuropathology

Portal–Systemic encephalopathy (PSE) is characterized neuropathologically by alterations of astrocytic morphology. These morphologic changes are known as Alzheimer type II astrocytosis, a typical example of which is shown in Fig. 44.1.

The Alzheimer type II astrocyte has a large, swollen nucleus with a prominent nucleolus and margination of the chromatin pattern. Alzheimer type II cells are seen in both gray and white matter structures in PSE.

Brain Energy Metabolism

Brain energy metabolism as assessed either by cerebral oxygen consumption [cerebral metabolic rate $(CMR)_{O_2}$] or cerebral glucose utilization $(CMR_{glucose})$ is reduced in patients with PSE. Such reductions parallel the onset of overt clinical symptoms of HE and decrease further with deteriorating neurologic status. Decreased brain glucose utilization in early PSE is most likely the consequence of decreased energy demand rather than the cause of PSE [i.e., reduced neuronal activity in brain in PSE results in decreased energy requirements and, consequently, reduced fuel (glucose) consumption]. Evidence in support of this conclusion is derived from studies in both human and experimental PSE. Portacaval anastomosis in the rat results in modest neurologic impairment (reduced activity, altered

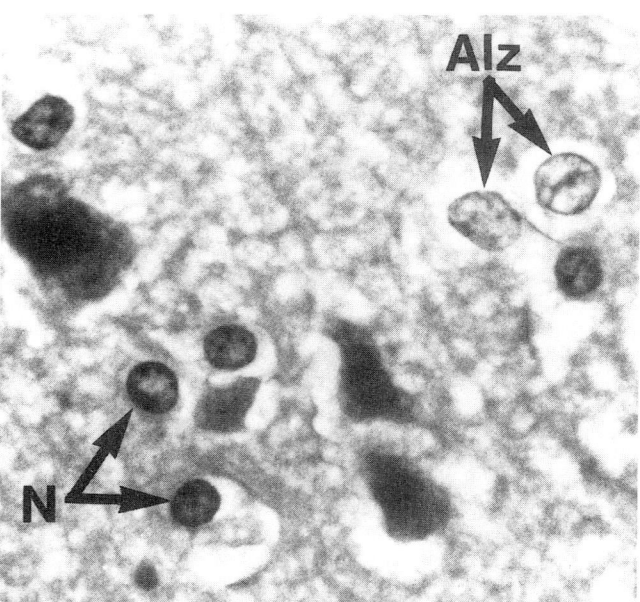

FIGURE 44.1. Alzheimer type II astrocytosis in prefrontal cortex of a 51-year-old cirrhotic patient who died in hepatic coma. *Arrows* indicate characteristic Alzheimer type II astrocyte with large pale nucleus and margination of chromatin pattern (*Alz*) compared to normal astrocytes (*N*) with normal chromatin pattern.

TABLE 44.1. POSSIBLE MECHANISMS INVOLVED IN NEUROTRANSMISSION FAILURE IN PORTAL–SYSTEMIC ENCEPHALOPATHY

Direct effects of the ammonium ion (NH_4^+) on:
  Inhibitory neurotransmission
  Excitatory neurotransmission
Indirect effects of hyperammonemia:
  astrocytic modifications leading to glutamatergic synaptic
    regulation defect
  accumulation of neuroactive and neurotoxic metabolites of
    tryptophan in brain
  activation of peripheral-type benzodiazepine receptors
    resulting in increased neurosteroid synthesis
Presence of substances that bind to the GABA–benzodiazepine
  receptor complex

GABA, γ-aminobutyric acid.

sleep patterns, abnormal reflexes) and in decreased brain glucose utilization (3). However, direct measurements in the brains of portacaval-shunted rats reveal no changes of high-energy phosphates whether assessed biochemically (4) or using nuclear magnetic resonance (NMR) methods (5). NMR studies in cirrhotic patients with mild PSE likewise do not reveal significant reductions of brain levels of adenosine triphosphate (ATP) (6). On the other hand, deep coma resulting from the administration of ammonium salts to portacaval-shunted rats ultimately results in reductions of brain ATP concentrations and accumulation of brain lactate (4,7). These findings suggest that altered brain energy metabolism may play a role in the pathogenesis of PSE at late (deep coma) stages.

An increasing body of evidence suggests that neurologic dysfunction in early PSE results from neurotransmission failure. Possible neurotransmission defects in PSE are listed in Table 44.1 and include direct neurotoxic effects mediated by the ammonium ion (NH_4^+) on inhibitory and excitatory neurotransmission, the accumulation of neuroactive and neurotoxic metabolites of tryptophan, as well as altered glutamatergic synaptic regulation and activation of peripheral-type benzodiazepine receptors. In addition, there is evidence to suggest that PSE may be the consequence, at least in part, of the action of substances that bind to the γ-aminobutyric acid (GABA)-benzodiazepine receptor complex in brain.

Ammonia

Evidence of an association between PSE and ammonia dates back over a century to the pioneering studies of Eck, who described the effects of portacaval anastomosis in dogs. Feeding of meat to shunted dogs resulted in severe neurologic impairment progressing to coma. Subsequent studies in the 1950s that attempted to treat ascites in cirrhotic patients using ammonium ion-exchange resins led to reduction of ascitic volume, but also to the precipitation of neurologic symptoms that were indistinguishable from PSE (8). Arterial blood ammonia concentrations are frequently (but not always) increased in patients with PSE, and brain ammonia may reach millimolar concentrations at coma stages of encephalopathy in experimental PSE (4). A more recent report described findings using PET to investigate brain ammonia metabolism using $^{13}NH_3$ in cirrhotic patients (9). A significant increase in the cerebral metabolic rate for ammonia (CMR_A) was observed in patients with mild PSE. This increase of CMR_A was accompanied by an increase in brain ammonia utilization and by an increase in the apparent permeability–surface area product (PS) in PSE patients (Fig. 44.2). This increased ease with which ammonia appears to move into brain in these patients could account for:

1. the hypersensitivity of cirrhotic patients to ammoniagenic conditions such as protein loading, gastrointestinal bleeding, and constipation;
2. the occurrence of neurologic impairment in some patients with near-normal arterial ammonia levels.

There is evidence of a pathogenetic link between sustained hyperammonemia and the presence of Alzheimer type II astrocytes. For example, Alzheimer type II astrocytosis has been described in (a) human hyperammonemic syndromes associated with congenital urea cycle enzyme defects, (b) experimental animals with urease-induced hyperammonemia, and (c) primary cultures of astrocytes exposed to pathophysiologically relevant (millimolar) concentrations of ammonia. For a more complete description of these and other aspects of astrocytic pathology in PSE, the reader is referred to a review article on the subject (10).

Concentrations of ammonia in the low millimolar range cause deleterious effects on central nervous system (CNS) function by both direct and indirect mechanisms. Direct effects of NH_4^+ on both inhibitory and excitatory neurotransmission have been reported (11,12). Millimolar concentrations of ammonia impair postsynaptic inhibition in brain by inactivation of the extrusion of Cl^- from neurons (11). This inactivation of Cl^- extrusion abolishes the concentration gradient for Cl^- across the neuronal membrane. Consequently, the opening of Cl^- channels by the inhibitory neurotransmitter no longer takes place and the inhibitory postsynaptic potential (IPSP) is abolished. It has been estimated that brain ammonia concentrations as low as 0.5 mM may exert this adverse effect on inhibitory neu-

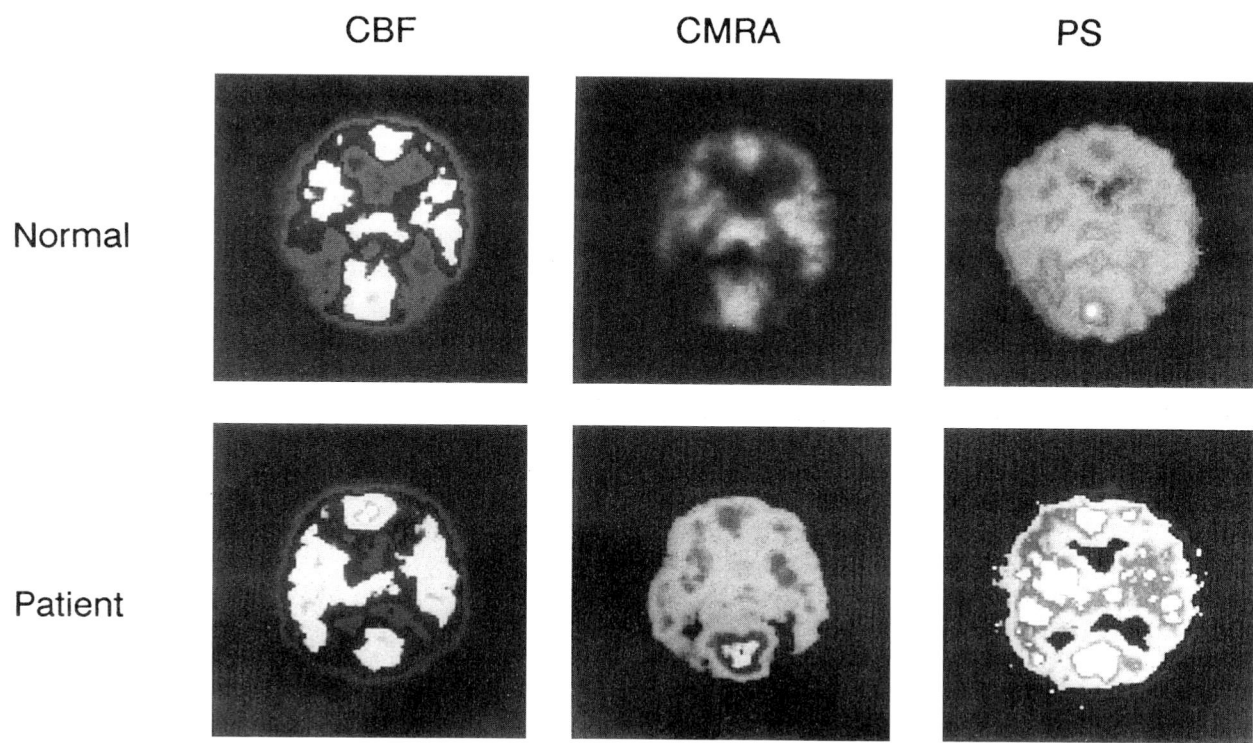

FIGURE 44.2. Positron emission tomography (PET) images of cerebral blood flow (*CBF*), cerebral metabolic rate for ammonia (*CMR$_A$*), and permeability–surface area product (*PS*) from a normal subject with an arterial ammonia concentration of 26 μM compared to a patient with liver disease, mild encephalopathy, and an arterial ammonia concentration of 66 μM. (From Lockwood AH, Yap EWH, Wong W-H. Cerebral ammonia metabolism in patients with severe liver disease and minimal hepatic encephalopathy. *J Cereb Blood Flow Metab* 1991;11:337–341, with permission.)

rotransmission (11). Brain ammonia concentrations within this range are encountered in early PSE in experimental animals (4).

Ammonia also has deleterious effects on excitatory neurotransmission. Effects on both presynaptic and postsynaptic neuronal membranes have been demonstrated (12). NH_4^+ ions, in pathologically relevant concentrations, interfere with excitatory neurotransmission by preventing the action of glutamate at the postsynaptic receptor (12). In addition, NH_4^+ depolarizes neurons to a variable degree without consistently changing membrane resistance, probably by reducing K^+ concentrations (12).

In addition to direct effects of ammonia on neurotransmission in the CNS, there is evidence to suggest that indirect mechanisms resulting from the effects of ammonia on blood–brain barrier amino acid transport systems and on astrocytic function are also implicated in the pathogenesis of PSE. These mechanisms and their possible roles in mediation of the neurologic symptoms of PSE are discussed in subsequent sections of this chapter.

As already mentioned, ammonia-precipitated PSE in rats, at coma stages of encephalopathy, may be ultimately associated with impaired brain energy metabolism (4). Possible mechanisms responsible for this include inhibitory effects of ammonia on the tricarboxylic acid cycle enzyme α-ketoglutarate dehydrogenase (13) and on the malate-aspartate shuttle (4). In addition, ammonia appears to stimulate glycolysis at the level of phosphofructokinase (14). These metabolic effects of ammonia would be expected to result in increased lactate/pyruvate ratios in brain. Such changes are indeed observed in experimental PSE in rats (4) and cerebrospinal fluid (CSF) lactate concentrations correlate well with the deterioration and subsequent recovery of neurologic status in portacaval-shunted rats in which severe PSE was precipitated by ammonia administration (7), as well as in cirrhotic patients with mild to moderate PSE (15).

Ammonia Removal by Brain—Glutamine Formation

Brain is devoid of a urea cycle. It relies instead on glutamine formation for effective removal of ammonia. The enzyme responsible, glutamine synthetase, has a nonneuronal, almost exclusively astrocytic, localization, and it is thus the astrocyte and not the neuron that is responsible for ammonia removal by brain.

CSF glutamine concentrations are increased and correlate well with the severity of neurologic impairment in PSE patients (16). Glutamine concentrations are elevated two- to fivefold in CSF and brain tissue from experimental animals with PSE (17,18), and increased brain glutamine has also been described in NMR studies in both human and experimental PSE (5,6,19). Glutamine concentrations in autopsied brain tissue from cirrhotic patients who died in hepatic coma are increased two- to fivefold (20), suggesting

that the brains of these patients had been exposed to increased concentrations of ammonia.

Glutamate

A report in 1990 by Schmidt et al. (21) described a dose-dependent inhibition of D-aspartate uptake into rat hippocampal slices by blood extracts from patients with varying degrees of severity of PSE. D-aspartate is routinely used as a nonmetabolizable analogue for the study of high-affinity glutamate uptake into brain. In the study by Schmidt et al., the relative potency of inhibition of D-aspartate uptake correlated with blood ammonia concentrations in patients with PSE. Earlier studies had demonstrated inhibition of high-affinity glutamate uptake into rat synaptosomal preparations following exposure to 5 mM ammonia (22), and treatment of cultured rat astrocytes with 2 mM ammonia for 4 days resulted in a 35% decrease in capacity for glutamate uptake by these cells (23).

Subsequent studies revealed that electrically stimulated Ca^{2+}-dependent release of glutamate (i.e., release of glutamate from the neurotransmitter pool in presynaptic nerve terminals) from superfused hippocampal slices from rats following portacaval anastomosis is significantly increased (24). *In vivo* studies using either the "cortical cup" approach or cerebral microdialysis likewise demonstrated increased extracellular glutamate in brain in experimental PSE (25,26). The findings of reduced capacity for glutamate uptake into neurons and astrocytes following exposure to pathophysiologic concentrations of ammonia (described above) together with the consistent observations of increased extracellular glutamate following portacaval anastomosis suggest that extracellular (synaptic) concentrations of glutamate are increased in PSE due to a failure of mechanisms responsible for its uptake.

Decreased densities of postsynaptic glutamate-binding sites have been reported in the brains of rats following portacaval anastomosis (27) and in the brains of dogs with PSE resulting from congenital portal–systemic shunts (28). Although in both cases, *reductions* of glutamate-binding sites were observed, the subclass of binding site involved was not identical in the two reports. Glutamate-binding sites in preparations from mammalian brain have been subdivided according to their pharmacologic characteristics into the *N*-methyl-D-aspartate (NMDA) and non-NMDA subclasses. These subclasses have distinct neurobiologic properties and neuroanatomic distribution in the CNS. Whereas portacaval shunting in the rat led to a generalized loss of the NMDA subclass of glutamate-binding sites (27), studies in the congenital dog model of PSE (28) revealed losses of the non-NMDA subclass. These discrepancies could result from species differences or could relate to the more advanced stage of PSE in the dog studies compared to the portacaval-shunted rat. The finding of decreased densities of glutamate-binding sites in PSE is consistent with downregulation of these sites as a result of their exposure to increased extracellular concentrations of endogenous ligand (glutamate).

Tryptophan and Its Neuroactive and Neurotoxic Metabolites

Administration of large doses of tryptophan to dogs with Eck fistulas results in a neuropsychiatric syndrome resembling PSE (29), and CSF tryptophan concentrations are increased in patients in hepatic coma (30). Portacaval anastomosis results in increased blood–brain barrier transport of tryptophan into brain (31), and there is convincing evidence to suggest that this enhanced brain uptake of tryptophan is directly linked to increased brain ammonia metabolism, and more specifically to increased brain glutamine synthesis (32). Since tryptophan is the obligate precursor of the monoamine neurotransmitter serotonin (5-HT) and since tryptophan hydroxylation (the rate-limiting step in brain 5-HT synthesis) is not saturated at normal blood and brain tryptophan concentrations, increased availability of tryptophan has the potential to result in increased 5-HT synthesis in brain. Evidence consistent with 5-HT synthesis and turnover in brain in human and experimental PSE has been accumulating in recent years. For example, increased concentrations of the 5-HT metabolite 5-hydroxyindoleacetic acid (5-HIAA) have consistently been reported in CSF of cirrhotic patients in hepatic coma (30), in autopsied brain tissue from patients with PSE (33), and in the brains of rats following portacaval anastomosis (34). The magnitude of the 5-HIAA/5-HT concentration ratio (a parameter considered to reflect 5-HT turnover in brain) is elevated in brain tissue from cirrhotic patients who died in hepatic coma (33) and in the brains of portacaval-shunted rats administered ammonium salts to precipitate severe encephalopathy (34). Furthermore, direct assessment of 5-HT turnover in brain using an *in vivo* decarboxylase inhibition assay revealed significantly increased 5-HT turnover in the brains of portacaval-shunted animals (35). Serotonin plays a key role in the regulation of sleep mechanisms, and alterations of 5-HT neurotransmission have been implicated in psychiatric disorders in humans. Thus, the early changes in 5-HT turnover in brain in experimental PSE could relate to the signs and symptoms characteristic of early PSE in humans such as altered sleep patterns and personality changes.

In fact, there is direct evidence for altered 5-HT metabolism and function in *human* PSE. Increased activities of monoamine oxidase MAO_A and of MAO_A messenger RNA (mRNA) have been described in autopsied brain tissue from cirrhotic patients who died in hepatic coma (36) (in human brain, MAO_A is responsible for 5-HT degradation). Furthermore, concentrations of the 5-HT metabolite, 5-HIAA, were found to be increased in the same material (33). In a parallel series of studies in autopsied brain tissue

from patients with PSE, densities of postsynaptic serotonin (5-HT_2) receptors, measured using ^{3}H-ketanserin, were found to be significantly increased (37). These findings, when taken in conjunction with the MAO_A increase and increased 5-HIAA in these brains, suggest that a synaptic *deficit* of 5-HT may occur in human PSE. Further evidence consistent with the notion that diminished 5-HT neurotransmission is implicated in the pathogenesis of human PSE is provided by the results of a study published in 1989 in which cirrhotic patients were treated with the 5-HT_2 receptor antagonist ketanserin in an effort to reduce portal hypertension. Although beneficial effects on portal pressure were observed, 25% of patients developed severe (grade II-III) PSE (38). Encephalopathy was reversed when ketanserin treatment was stopped and blood concentrations of ketanserin in those patients who developed PSE were not significantly different from those who did not. These findings suggest increased brain sensitivity of some patients with chronic liver disease to 5-HT blockade and are consistent with the proposal that a central serotonergic deficit may be a significant contributory cause of early PSE in humans.

In addition to alterations of the 5-HT system, other neuroactive or neurotoxic metabolites of tryptophan are also increased in brain in chronic liver disease. One such example is quinolinic acid (QUIN) synthesized from tryptophan via the kynurenine pathway. QUIN appears to be particularly sensitive to increased availability of tryptophan (39). QUIN has been identified in both rodent and human brain extracts, and cerebral cortical QUIN concentrations are elevated in rats following portacaval anastomosis (40). Furthermore, QUIN concentrations are increased up to sevenfold in CSF and autopsied frontal cortex of cirrhotic patients with PSE (41).

Another neuroactive tryptophan metabolite is the trace amine tryptamine. Tryptamine content of CSF is increased in cirrhotic patients with PSE (42), and a significant loss of ^{3}H-tryptamine–binding sites (consistent with downregulation of these sites) has been described in autopsied brain tissue from PSE patients (43).

Endogenous Benzodiazepines

Throughout the 1980s a great deal of attention was focused on the notion that HE was the result of alterations of the GABA neurotransmitter system in brain. Abnormalities of the brain GABA system were reported in experimental animal models of acute liver failure (44). However, in animal models of PSE, no alterations of the GABA system were observed whether reflected by studies of GABA content, its related enzymes, or its binding sites (45,46). Furthermore, autopsied brain samples from cirrhotic patients who died in hepatic coma contained normal activities of GABA-related enzymes (47) and unchanged densities and affinities of GABA-binding sites (48).

During this period, two preliminary reports appeared describing amelioration of the neurologic status in patients with HE following administration of the benzodiazepine antagonist Ro 15-1788 (flumazenil) (49,50). The link to the GABA theory of HE is immediately evident; benzodiazepine-binding sites in the central nervous system form part of the GABA–benzodiazepine–chloride ionophore complex. Stimulation of the benzodiazepine-binding site "facilitates" the action of GABA on the functionally linked GABA-A site of the complex. In this way, chloride channel opening is increased and hyperpolarization and inhibition occur. The process is generally referred to as positive allosteric modulation of the GABA-A receptor by the benzodiazepine. It was suggested by one group of investigators (49) that the ameliorative action of flumazenil in HE was due either to inhibition of increased densities of benzodiazepine-binding sites or by inhibition of the action of an "endogenous" ligand at these sites. Subsequent investigations revealed no alterations of densities or affinities of these sites in either experimental (51) or human (48) PSE, leaving open the possibility that the beneficial effects of flumazenil in PSE were the result of the blocking of the action of endogenous benzodiazepine receptor ligands.

Following these reports, intensive investigations were undertaken to measure concentrations of substances that bind to brain benzodiazepine receptors in brain in HE. Initial reports demonstrated that CSF from patients with advanced HE contained significant amounts of substances with benzodiazepine binding capacity (52). Furthermore, this activity appeared to reside in two known 1,4-benzodiazepines, namely diazepam and its NN-desmethyl metabolite, both of which are positive allosteric modulators (i.e., facilitators) of GABA neurotransmission. An independent study of benzodiazepine receptor ligands confirmed the presence of these two benzodiazepines in both serum and CSF of humans with PSE (53). On the other hand, no increases of these benzodiazepines were observed in the brains of portacaval-shunted rats.

Unfortunately, the interest generated by these reports has been tempered by other reports casting doubt on the relative importance of endogenous benzodiazepines in the pathogenesis of PSE. The concentrations of benzodiazepines reported in blood, CSF, and brain extracts in HE are low. Rarely have blood concentrations of benzodiazepines in PSE been reported to attain even those in the therapeutic (anxiolytic) range. Brain levels of diazepam in experimental HE in the rat are in the 20- to 30-nM range, some 100- to 200-fold lower than brain concentrations of diazepam described in diazepam-induced sedation in the same animal species (54). Clinical trials with benzodiazepine receptor antagonists (described in a later section) have yielded mixed results.

In a further development in the GABA–benzodiazepine theory, it has been reported that endogenous peptides with high affinity for GABA-related benzodiazepine receptors are increased in experimental and human PSE. In one study, diazepam-binding inhibitor (DBI), a negative allosteric modulator of GABAergic neurotransmission (i.e., it has the potential to reduce GABAergic neurotransmission resulting in increased arousal), was found to be elevated threefold in the CSF of patients with chronic liver disease and PSE (55). Clinical stages correlated well with CSF DBI concentrations, and patients with liver disease but no neurologic symptoms had CSF DBI levels within the normal range. However, it is not evident how elevated CSF or brain DBI could be implicated in the pathogenesis of PSE in view of its arousal properties.

Peripheral-Type Benzodiazepine Receptors

Mammalian brain contains two distinct types of benzodiazepine receptors: the type referred to in the previous section of this chapter, forming part of the GABA-benzodiazepine receptor complex, situated on the postsynaptic neuronal membrane, and a second type, the "peripheral-type" benzodiazepine receptor (PTBR), so-called due to its initial discovery in peripheral tissues such as kidney. The PTBR does not form part of the GABA receptor complex; rather, it is localized on the outer mitochondrial membrane, particularly of astrocytes and appears to be implicated in cellular metabolism and cell proliferation. There is strong evidence to suggest that PTBRs and their endogenous ligands may play an important role in the cellular response in several tissues to chronic liver disease and portal–systemic shunting. Increased densities of PTBRs have been reported in autopsied brain tissue from cirrhotic patients who died in hepatic coma (56), and increased PTBR-binding sites and PTBR mRNA have been described in the brains of rats following portacaval anastomosis (57,58).

Endogenous ligands for the PTBR include the neuropeptide octadecaneuropeptide (ODN) and, using an immunocytochemical technique and an antibody of high specific activity to synthetic ODN, it was demonstrated that portacaval anastomosis results in increased ODN-immunolabeling in astrocytes of several brain regions (59). Exposure to PTBR ligands results in proliferation and swelling of mitochondria in cultured glioma cells (60), and, since mitochondrial proliferation and swelling are observed in astrocytes of the brains of rats following portacaval anastomosis, it is possible that PTBRs play a role in the pathogenesis of this astrocytic response to portal–systemic shunting.

Increased densities of PTBRs in brain in clinical and experimental PSE could result from the effects of ammonia. In line with this possibility, increased densities of PTBRs have been reported in the brains of mice with chronic hyperammonemia resulting from a congenital urea-cycle enzyme defect (61).

It has been suggested that activation of PTBRs in brain in chronic liver failure could result in increased synthesis of neurosteroids (57,58), some of which have potent neuroinhibitory properties (10).

Manganese

A highly consistent finding on MRI of cirrhotic patients is bilateral symmetrical hyperintensities in globus pallidus on T1-weighted imaging (6). A representative example of these hyperintensities is shown in Fig. 44.3.

A convincing body of evidence suggests that these images are the result of pallidal manganese deposition. Manganese is normally eliminated via the hepatobiliary route, and blood manganese concentrations are increased in cirrhotic patients who manifest pallidal signal hyperintensities on MRI (62). Furthermore, similar pallidal signals have been reported in a patient with Alagille syndrome, a disorder characterized by cholestasis, intrahepatic bile duct paucity, and increased blood manganese (63). Pallidal signal hyperintensities have also been reported in patients during total parenteral nutrition where it was proposed that the cause was again manganese deposition in the brain (64).

Direct studies using neutron activation analysis reveal up to sevenfold increases in manganese content of dissected pallidum obtained at autopsy from cirrhotic patients who died in hepatic coma (65). More recent studies in experimental animals with either surgical portacaval shunts or biliary cirrhosis also revealed selective accumulation of manganese in pallidum and other basal ganglia structures (66) (Table 44.2).

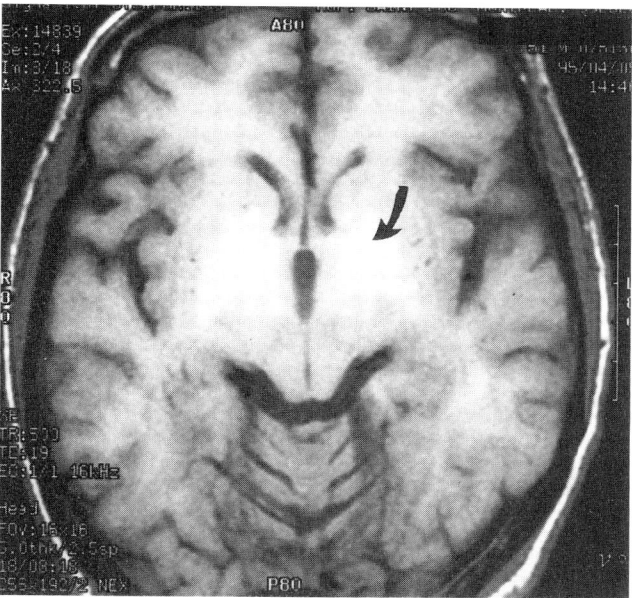

FIGURE 44.3. Magnetic resonance image (MRI) of a cirrhotic patient showing bilateral T1-weighted signal hyperintensities in globus pallidus (*arrow*). Such signal hyperintensities are observed in over 80% of cases. (From Spahr L, Butterworth RF, Fontaine S, et al. Increased blood manganese in cirrhotic patients: relationship to pallidal magnetic resonance signal hyperintensity and neurological symptoms. *Hepatology* 1996;24:1116–1120, with permission.)

TABLE 44.2. BRAIN MANGANESE CONCENTRATIONS IN DISSECTED PALLIDAL TISSUE FROM CIRRHOTIC PATIENTS WHO DIED IN HEPATIC COMA AND FROM RATS WITH EXPERIMENTAL ACUTE OR CHRONIC LIVER FAILURE

Subjects	Pallidal Manganese Concentrations (μg/g)
Patients	
Controls (n)	1.41 ± 0.91 (8)
Cirrhotics (n)	4.04 ± 1.54[b] (8)
Rats	
Controls (sham-operated) (n)	0.54 ± 0.02 (6)
Portacaval-shunted (n)	1.05 ± 0.07[b] (6)
Bile-duct ligated (cirrhosis) (n)	0.85 ± 0.06[a] (6)
Hepatic devascularization (acute liver failure) (n)	0.72 ± 0.07 (6)

Values represent mean ± S.E. of determinations in dissected pallidal tissue; n, number of samples; values significantly different from the appropriate control group indicated by [a]$p < 0.05$, [b]$p < 0.01$ by analysis of variance.

Nitric Oxide

Following portacaval shunting in the rat, activities of the constitutive (neuronal) form of nitric oxide synthase (nNOS) are significantly increased in brain (67). These increased activities are accompanied by increased nNOS protein and mRNA (68). Although the precise mechanism has not been definitely established, there is evidence to suggest that ammonia may be implicated, since exposure of nerve terminal (synaptosomal) preparations to ammonia results in increased uptake of L-arginine, the obligate precursor for NOS (69). These increases in nNOS expression and activity and the consequent increases in nitric oxide production could be implicated in the alterations of cerebral perfusion characteristic of chronic liver failure.

ACUTE LIVER FAILURE

Neuropathology

In contrast to the Alzheimer type II astrocytosis characteristic of PSE, the neuropathologic hallmark of acute liver failure is cytotoxic brain edema, with astrocytic swelling being consistently reported (Fig. 44.4) (70).

Brain Energy Metabolism

Studies using ^{1}H-NMR have failed to detect measurable changes in brain levels of high-energy phosphates in acute liver failure (71).

Ammonia

Patients with acute liver failure who develop intracranial hypertension and cerebral herniation manifest arterial

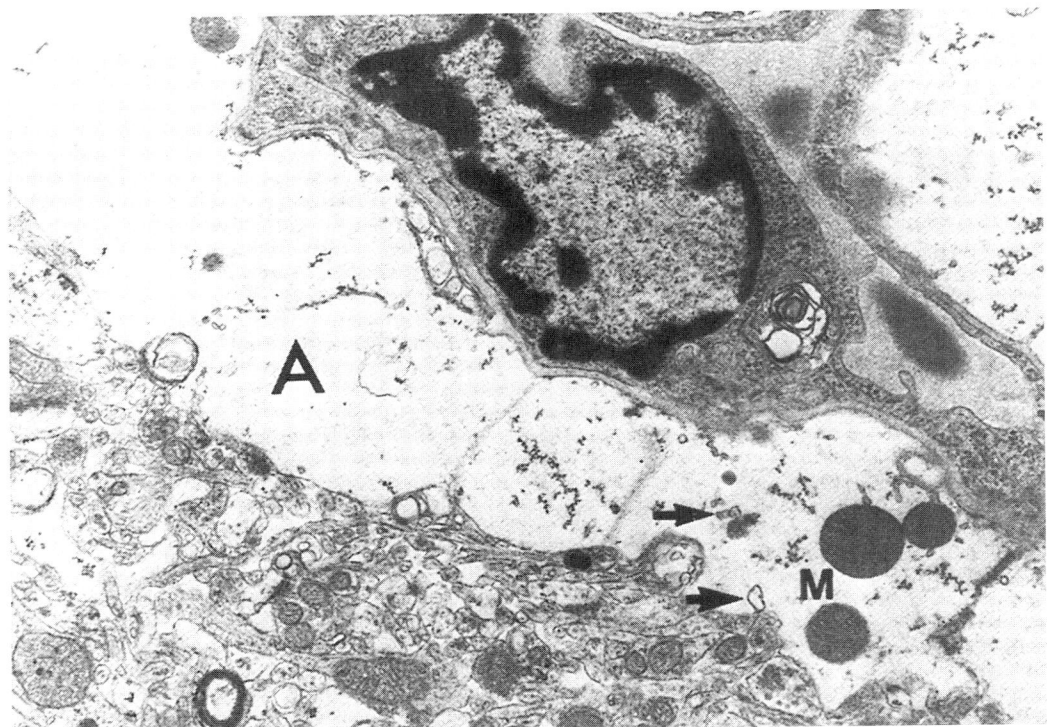

FIGURE 44.4. Cytotoxic brain edema in a patient with acute liver failure due to acetaminophen overdose. Perivascular astrocyte (*A*) is markedly swollen. The endoplasmic reticulum is dilated (*arrow*) and mitochondria (*M*) are swollen. Original magnification ×6000. (From Kato M, Hughes RD, Keays RT, et al. Electron microscopic study of brain capillaries in cerebral edema from fulminant hepatic failure. *Hepatology* 1992;15:1060–1066, with permission.)

ammonia levels significantly higher than patients who did not develop this complication (72) (Fig. 44.5). Brain concentrations of ammonia may reach millimolar levels in acute liver failure, and it is therefore likely that direct multiple effects of ammonia on brain inhibitory and excitatory neurotransmission (described earlier in this chapter) contribute significantly to the spectrum of neurologic symptoms of acute liver failure, which may include seizures as well as cognitive and motor deficits.

Increased brain ammonia concentrations may also be causally related to the phenomenon of cerebral edema in acute liver failure. Brain ammonia concentrations are in the 1- to 5-mM range at coma and edematous stages of encephalopathy in experimental animal models of acute liver failure (73), and treatment of isolated cerebral cortical slices with ammonia in concentrations equivalent to those reported in brain in experimental acute liver failure results in significant swelling and in concomitant reductions of inulin space (74). It is interesting to note that swelling of cerebral cortical astrocytes is observed following ammonia infusions to primates (75), and exposure of primary cultures of astrocytes to millimolar concentrations of ammonia also results in significant cell swelling (76).

Recent evidence suggests that this ammonia-induced swelling may be mediated via a metabolite of ammonia rather than ammonia *per se*. As outlined in an earlier section of this chapter, ammonia removal in brain depends on glutamine synthesis, and a significant correlation has been demonstrated between the rise in brain glutamine and brain water concentrations in normal rats receiving ammonia infusions, leading to the suggestion that the ammonia-induced increase in brain water content was mediated by the osmotic effects of increased glutamine (77). In favor of this possibility, treatment of hyperammonemic animals with methionine sulfoximine, an inhibitor of glutamine synthesis in brain, prevented the increases of both glutamine and water content of the brains of these animals. Ammonia infusion in rats 24 hours after portacaval anastomosis results in brain edema of a sufficient magnitude to raise intracranial pressure (78), and, once again, inhibition of glutamine synthesis in the brains of these animals inhibits water accumulation and prevents intracranial hypertension. Studies in postmortem brain tissue from patients who died in acute liver failure reveal significantly increased glutamine concentrations (79), and brain glutamine concentrations are increased sixfold in experimental

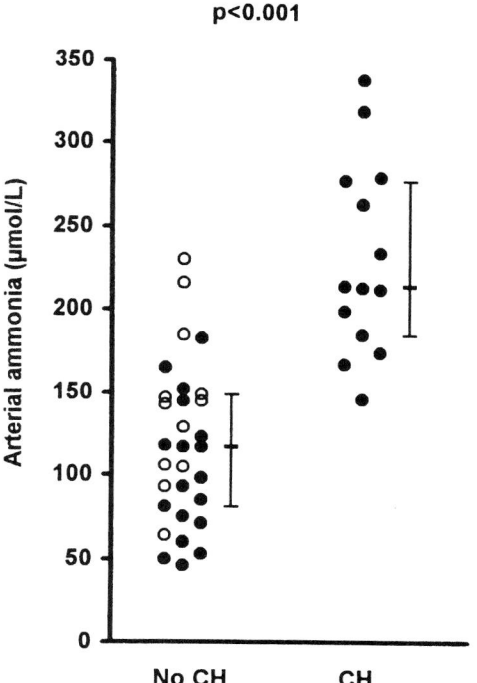

p<0.001

FIGURE 44.5. Arterial ammonia concentrations in 30 patients with acute liver failure who did not develop cerebral herniation (*No CH*) compared to 14 patients who died from cerebral herniation (*CH*). *Error bars* represent median values. *Open circles* represent patients who underwent liver transplantation. (From Clemmensen JO, Larsen FS, Kondrup J, et al. Cerebral herniation in patients with acute liver failure is correlated with arterial ammonia concentration. *Hepatology* 1999;29:648–653, with permission.)

ischemic liver failure (73) in parallel with increasing brain water content in these animals. Taken together, these findings represent a consistent body of evidence supporting a major role of ammonia via its metabolite glutamine in the pathogenesis of brain edema in acute liver failure.

Glutamate

Brain concentrations of glutamate are significantly reduced in experimental ischemic liver failure (73,80) and in thioacetamide-induced liver failure (80) in the rat in parallel with the deterioration of neurologic status in these animals. CSF glutamate concentrations in these animals are concomitantly increased (80), and using the technique of *in vivo* brain dialysis, increased extracellular brain concentrations of glutamate have been consistently reported in experimental acute liver failure (81,82).

Evidence of glutamatergic synaptic dysfunction in brain in acute liver failure has been accumulating in recent years (83). Such evidence includes reductions in expression of the high-affinity astrocytic glutamate transporter GLT-1 in the brains of rats with acute liver failure (84). This loss of glutamate transported expression offers a plausible explanation

for the findings of increased extracellular glutamate concentrations in the brains of these animals (82). Decreased uptake of glutamate into nerve terminal preparation from rats with thioacetamide-induced liver failure has also been described (85).

Reductions in the AMPA/kainate (non-NMDA) subclass of glutamate receptors were reported in brain in experimental acute liver failure (86), and it was suggested that this reduction in receptors and the consequent relative increase in the other subclass (NMDA) of glutamate receptors could be implicated in the pathogenesis of HE in acute liver failure. Consistent with this possibility, administration of the NMDA receptor antagonist memantine was shown to improve neurologic status in rats with acute liver failure due to hepatic devascularization (87).

The γ-Aminobutyric Acid System and Endogenous Benzodiazepines

Permeability of the blood–brain barrier to GABA is not increased in experimental acute liver failure (88), and GABA content of autopsied brain tissue from patients with acute liver failure is within normal limits (89). Furthermore, CSF GABA concentrations are unchanged at all stages of neurologic impairment in experimental acute liver failure (80).

However, galactosamine-induced acute liver failure in rabbits is associated with increased densities of GABA-related benzodiazepine-binding sites in brain (90). Furthermore, administration of the benzodiazepine receptor antagonist flumazenil resulted in amelioration of neurologic status in these animals (91). On the other hand, HE resulting from ischemic liver failure in the rat was not reversed by administration of a benzodiazepine receptor antagonist (92). Similar negative findings were reported using benzodiazepine receptor antagonists in a rabbit model of ischemic liver failure (93).

Monoamines

Alterations of both noradrenergic and serotonergic systems have been described in acute liver failure. For example, studies in several animal models including hepatectomy (94), liver devascularization (95), and thioacetamide-induced toxic liver injury (96) in the rat have consistently reported decreased brain noradrenaline. Hepatectomy results in increased noradrenaline release into ventriculocisternal perfusates (97), and *in vivo* cerebral microdialysis studies reveal increased extracellular brain concentrations of noradrenaline in rats with acute (ischemic) liver failure (98). A subsequent report suggested that this latter phenomenon was the result of a loss of noradrenaline transporter sites in the brains of these animals (99). Consistent with increased extracellular (synaptic) concentrations of noradrenaline were the findings of a selective loss of noradrenaline α and β receptor sites in the brains of rats with acute liver failure (98). As a consequence of these findings, it was suggested that a deficit in central noradrenergic function could be responsible for the cognitive and neuropsychiatric symptoms associated with acute liver failure.

Alterations of serotonin receptors have also been described in the brains of rats with thioacetamide-induced liver failure (100). Furthermore, in both thioacetamide-induced hepatic damage as well as in experimental hepatic devascularization, increased extracellular brain concentrations of serotonin and of its acid metabolite 5-HIAA have been reported (96,101). A subsequent study revealed significant losses of serotonin transporter sites in the brains of rats with acute liver failure (102). Increased brain concentrations of 5-HIAA were also reported in autopsied brain tissue from patients with acute liver failure who died in hepatic coma (103), suggesting that alterations of serotonergic function are also implicated in the pathogenesis of HE in acute liver failure in humans.

Summary

Major pathophysiologic findings in PSE and in acute liver failure are summarized in Table 44.3. There can be little doubt, given the overwhelming body of evidence from both clinical and experimental studies, that ammonia plays a major role. Ammonia is increased in brain in both acute and chronic liver failure to attain millimolar concentrations at coma stages of encephalopathy. Levels of the ammonia-detoxification product glutamine are increased in brain and correlate with the degree of neurologic impairment in chronic liver disease. The ultimate neuropathologic feature characteristic of PSE, Alzheimer type II astrocytosis, as well as the associated increased densities of astrocytic "peripheral-type" benzodiazepine-bindings sites, are also encountered in chronic hyperammonemic syndromes of nonhepatic origin. Millimolar concentrations of ammonia have direct toxic effects on both CNS inhibition and excitation. Prolonged exposure of brain to increased ammonia results in disruption of neuron-astrocyte metabolic interactions, and, in particular, may result in a defect in glutamatergic synaptic regulation. Ammonia-induced accumulation of brain glutamine leads to increased brain uptake of tryptophan, which in turn results in increased synthesis of neuroactive (tryptamine) and neurotoxic (quinolinic acid) metabolites of serotonin, and increased activities of monoamine oxidase and of serotonin receptor densities are consistent with a synaptic deficit of serotonin in human PSE. Precipitous increases of brain ammonia appear to be implicated, via glutamine synthesis and accumulation in brain, in the pathogenesis of brain edema in acute liver failure.

There is little convincing evidence that primary alterations of brain energy metabolism are the cause of hepatic encephalopathy in either acute or chronic liver failure at least until late (preterminal) stages.

TABLE 44.3. PATHOPHYSIOLOGY OF PORTAL–SYSTEMIC ENCEPHALOPATHY AND ACUTE LIVER FAILURE: A SUMMARY

	PSE	Acute Liver Failure
Neuropathology	Alzheimer type II astrocytosis	Brain edema
PET findings	Increased brain ammonia uptake	
MRI findings	Pallidal hyperintensity	
Brain energy metabolism	Unchanged until terminal stages	
Brain ammonia	Increased (0.2 to 1.0 mM)	Increased (1 to 5 mM)
Brain amino acids		
Glutamine	Increased	Increased
Glutamate	Increased (extracellular)	Increased (extracellular)
GABA	Unchanged	Unchanged
Astrocytic function		
GFAP immunostaining	Decreased	
Peripheral-type BZ receptors	Increased	
Neurotransmitter function		
Glutamate system	Decreased NMDA and non–NMDA-binding sites	Decreased non–NMDA-binding sites
	Increased quinolinic acid	Loss of GLT-1 transporter expression
Serotonin (5-HT) system	Increased 5-HIAA	Increased 5-HIAA
	Increased MAO$_A$	Loss of serotonin uptake sites
	Increased 5HT$_2$ receptors	
Noradrenaline system	Unchanged	Loss of noradrenaline uptake sites
GABA system	Unchanged	Altered in galactosamine models
Endogenous benzodiazepine-receptor ligands	1,4-Benzodiazepines increased	1,4-Benzodiazepines increased
	DBI, increased	

BZ, benzodiazepine; GABA, γ-aminobutyric acid; GFAP, glial fibrillary acidic protein; 5-HIAA, hydroxyindoleacetic acid; MAO, monoamine oxidase; MRI, magnetic resonance imaging; NMDA, *N*-methyl-D-aspartate; PET, positron emission tomography.

It is unlikely, however, that ammonia's direct and indirect effects on brain function are the sole cause of neurologic dysfunction in liver failure. Other neurotoxic substances such as manganese as well as mercaptans, short-chain fatty acids and neuroactive substances that bind to the GABA-related benzodiazepine receptor (substances that are normally removed by liver), could gain entry to brain in liver failure and act synergistically with ammonia-related mechanisms.

THERAPEUTIC IMPLICATIONS

The maintenance of normal levels of consciousness and neurologic function depends on a delicate balance between excitatory and inhibitory mechanisms in the CNS. This chapter has illustrate some aspects of the diversity and complexity of neurochemical mechanisms that may contribute to an imbalance between excitation and inhibition and, in this way, be implicated in the pathogenesis of HE in acute and chronic liver failure. Effects of ammonia and other substances generated in liver failure on both excitatory and inhibitory systems in brain have been demonstrated. The severity and duration of hyperammonemia coupled with other precipitating factors, such as the use of sedatives, add a further dimension to the complexity, making a single therapeutic approach to HE difficult, if not impossible. Strategies aimed at the prevention and treatment of HE are of two major types, namely ammonia-lowering strategies and the use of neuroactive drugs (104).

Ammonia-Lowering Strategies

Colonic cleansing reduces the luminal ammonia content and lowers blood ammonia in cirrhotic patients (105). Nonabsorbable disaccharides such as lactulose and lactitol are still routinely used to decrease ammonia production in the gut (106). In the case of lactulose, the ammonia-lowering effect appears to involve increased fecal nitrogen excretion by facilitation of the incorporation of ammonia into bacteria as well as a cathartic effect (104). Antibiotics such as neomycin are also used to lower blood ammonia by inhibition of ammonia production by intestinal bacteria. However, neomycin therapy is associated with significant toxic side effects.

Restriction of dietary protein remains an important means of prevention of PSE in cirrhotic patients. However, long-term nitrogen restriction is potentially harmful, and a positive nitrogen balance is essential to promote liver regeneration and to increase the capacity for ammonia removal by muscle (107). Protein intake in the 1- to 2-g/kg/day range is generally recommended to maintain an adequate nitrogen balance (108).

An alternative means of lowering blood ammonia in acute or chronic liver failure is the stimulation of ammonia fixation. Ammonia is normally removed by urea formation (periportal hepatocytes) as well as by glutamine formation (perivenous hepatocytes, muscle, and brain). Strategies aimed at stimulating residual urea or glutamine synthesis have emerged in recent years, and one of the most successful, L-ornithine L-aspartate, has been shown in controlled clinical trials to be effective in lowering blood ammonia and concomitantly improving neuropsychiatric status in cirrhotic patients (109). Studies in experimental animals reveal that, in chronic liver failure, this beneficial effect is due to the stimulation of urea and glutamine formation in the liver and in the stimulation of glutamine formation by skeletal muscle (110). In experimental acute liver failure, the ammonia-lowering effect of L-ornithine L-aspartate appears to be due predominantly to the stimulation of muscle glutamine synthetase (111). Successful lowering of blood ammonia concentrations in cirrhotic patients has also been accomplished using sodium benzoate (112).

Use of Neuroactive Drugs

As the precise neurobiologic mechanisms and alterations in neurotransmitter systems responsible for the pathogenesis of HE become more clearly defined, it is anticipated that novel pharmacologic approaches will emerge.

A number of controlled clinical trials have been performed to evaluate the efficacy of the central (GABA-related) benzodiazepine receptor antagonist flumazenil in patients with PSE (113,114). In a subset of HE patients, improvements following flumazenil have been spectacular (113). However, enthusiasm for this approach has been tempered by the possible confounding effects of prior exposure of patients to pharmaceutical benzodiazepines (used as sedatives or as part of an endoscopic workup) and by the poor correlation between the clinical response and blood levels of benzodiazepines in these patients (113,115). Adding to these difficulties is the lack of an oral formulation for flumazenil.

Both levodopa (L-DOPA) and the dopamine receptor agonist bromocriptine have been used in clinical trials in patients with PSE. While results were not encouraging in terms of overall cognitive improvement (116,117), it is possible that they had a beneficial effect on motor performance.

In experimental animal models of acute and chronic liver failure, various other experimental approaches have been tried, and in some cases beneficial effects were observed. For example, antagonists of certain serotonin receptor subtypes appear to be beneficial in thioacetamide-induced liver failure (118), and, more recently, administration of the glutamate (NMDA) receptor antagonist memantine was reported to ameliorate the CNS effects of experimental acute liver failure (87).

Mild Hypothermia

Hypothermia extends the survival time and prevents the development of brain edema in rats with acute liver failure caused by hepatic devascularization (119) and mild hypothermia (33° to 35°C) reduces ammonia-induced brain swelling and increased intracranial pressure in porta-caval-shunted rats administered ammonium salts (120). These findings have led to the successful use of mild hypothermia for the treatment of uncontrolled intracranial hypertension in patients with acute liver failure (121,122). Possible mechanisms underlying the beneficial effect of hypothermia in acute liver failure include reduced blood–brain transfer of ammonia (121,123) and normalization of extracellular brain amino acid patterns (123). Moderate hypothermia may thus serve as an effective bridge to liver transplantation in patients with acute liver failure.

REFERENCES

1. Butterworth RF. Alterations of neurotransmitter-related gene expression in human and experimental portal-systemic encephalopathy. *Metab Brain Dis* 1998;13:337–349.
2. Margulies JE, Thompson RC, Demetriou AA. Aquaporin-4 water channel is up-regulated in the brain in fulminant hepatic failure. *Hepatology* 1999;30:395A (#938).
3. Hawkins RA, Mans AM. Brain energy metabolism in hepatic encephalopathy. In: Butterworth RF, Pomier Layrargues G, eds. *Hepatic encephalopathy: pathophysiology and treatment*. Clifton, NJ: 1989:159–176.
4. Hindfelt B, Plum F, Duffy TE. Effects of acute ammonia intoxication on cerebral metabolism in rats with portacaval shunts. *J Clin Invest* 1977;59:386–396.
5. Fitzpatrick SM, Behar KL, Shulman RG. In vivo NMR spectroscopy studies of cerebral metabolism in rats after portacaval shunting. In: Butterworth RF, Pomier Layrargues G, eds. *Hepatic encephalopathy: pathophysiology and treatment*. Clifton, NJ: 1989:177–187.
6. Morgan MY. Noninvasive neuroinvestigation in liver disease. *Semin Liver Dis* 1996;16:293–314.
7. Therrien G, Giguère JF, Butterworth RF. Increased cerebrospinal fluid lactate reflects deterioration of neurological status in experimental portal-systemic encephalopathy. *Metab Brain Dis* 1991;6:225–231.
8. Gabuzda G Jr, Philips GB, Davidson CS. Reversible toxic manifestations in patients with cirrhosis of the liver given cation-exchange resins. *N Engl J Med* 1952;246:124–130.
9. Lockwood AH, Yap EWH, Wong W-H. Cerebral ammonia metabolism in patients with severe liver disease and minimal hepatic encephalopathy. *J Cereb Blood Flow Metab* 1991;11:337–341.
10. Norenberg MD. Astrocytic-ammonia interactions in hepatic encephalopathy. *Semin Liver Dis* 1996;16:245–253.
11. Raabe W. Synaptic transmission in ammonia intoxication. *Neurochem Pathol* 1987;6:145–166.
12. Szerb JC, Butterworth RF. Effect of ammonium ions on synaptic transmission in the mammalian central nervous system. *Prog Neurobiol* 1992;39:135–153.
13. Lai JCK, Cooper AJL. Brain α-ketoglutarate dehydrogenase: kinetic properties, regional distribution and effects of inhibitors. *J Neurochem* 1986;47:1376–1386.
14. Lowry OH, Passonneau JV. Kinetic evidence for multiple binding sites on phosphofructokinase. *J Biol Chem* 1966;241:2268–2279.
15. Yao H, Sadoshima S, Fujii K, et al. Cerebrospinal fluid lactate in patients with hepatic encephalopathy. *Eur Neurol* 1987;27:182–187.
16. Butterworth RF, Giguère JF, Michaud J, et al. Ammonia: key factor in the pathogenesis of hepatic encephalopathy. *Neurochem Pathol* 1987;6:1–12.
17. Giguère JF, Butterworth RF. Amino acid changes in regions of the CNS in relation to function in experimental portal-systemic encephalopathy. *Neurochem Res* 1984;9:1309–1319.
18. Therrien G, Butterworth RF. Cerebrospinal fluid amino acids in relation to neurological status in experimental portal-systemic encephalopathy. *Metab Brain Dis* 1992;6:65–74.
19. Laubenberger J, Haussinger D, Boyer S, et al. Proton magnetic resonance spectroscopy of brain in symptomatic and asymptomatic patients with liver cirrhosis. *Gastroenterology* 1997;112:1610–1616.
20. Lavoie J, Giguère JF, Pomier Layrargues G, et al. Amino acid changes in autopsied brain tissue from cirrhotic patients with hepatic encephalopathy. *J Neurochem* 1987;49:692–697.
21. Schmidt W, Wolf G, Grungreiff K, et al. Hepatic encephalopathy influences high affinity uptake of transmitter glutamate and aspartate into the hippocampal formation. *Metab Brain Dis* 1990;5:19–32.
22. Mena EE, Cotman CW. Pathologic concentrations of ammonium ions block L-glutamate uptake. *Exp Neurol* 1985;59:259–263.
23. Bender AS, Norenberg MD. Effect of ammonia on L-glutamate uptake in cultured astrocytes. *Neurochem Res* 1996;21:567–573.
24. Butterworth RF, Le O, Lavoie J, et al. Effect of portacaval anastomosis on electrically-stimulated release of glutamate from rat hippocampal slices. *J Neurochem* 1991;56:1481–1484.
25. Moroni F, Lombardi G, Moneti G, et al. The release and neosynthesis of glutamic acid are increased in experimental models of hepatic encephalopathy. *J Neurochem* 1983;40:850.
26. Tossman U, Delin A, Eriksson LS, et al. Brain cortical amino acids measured by intracerebral dialysis in portacaval shunted rats. *Neurochem Res* 1987;12:265.
27. Peterson C, Giguère JF, Cotman CW, et al. Selective loss of N-methyl-D-aspartate-sensitive L-^{3}H-glutamate binding sites in rat brain following portacaval anastomosis. *J Neurochem* 1990;55:386.
28. Maddison JE, Watson WEJ, Dodd PR, et al. Alterations in cortical ^{3}H-kainate and α^{3}H-amino-3-hydroxy-5-methyl-4-isoxazolepropionic acid binding in a spontaneous canine model of chronic hepatic encephalopathy. *J Neurochem* 1991;56:1881–1888.
29. Ogihara K, Mozai T, Hirai SN. Tryptophan as a cause of hepatic coma. *N Engl J Med* 1966;275:1255.
30. Young SN, Lal S, Feldmuller F, et al. Relationships between tryptophan in serum and CSF and 5-hydroxyindoleacetic acid in CSF of man: effects of cirrhosis of the liver and probenecid administration. *J Neurol Neurosurg Psychiatry* 1975;38:322–330.
31. Huet PM, Pomier Layrargues G, Duguay L, et al. Blood-brain barrier transport of tryptophan and phenylalanine: effect of portacaval shunt in dogs. *Am J Physiol* 1981;4:163–169.
32. James JH, Ziparo V, Jeppsson B, et al. Hyperammonemia, plasma amino acid imbalance and blood-brain amino acid transport: a unified theory of portal-systemic encephalopathy. *Lancet* 1979;2:772–775.
33. Bergeron M, Reader TA, Pomier Layrargues G, et al. Monoamines and metabolites in autopsied brain tissue from cir-

Hepatic Encephalopathy 645

rhotic patients with hepatic encephalopathy. *Neurochem Res* 1989;14:853–859.

34. Bergeron M, Swain MS, Reader TA, et al. Effect of ammonia on brain serotonin metabolism in relation to function in the portacaval shunted rat. *J Neurochem* 1990;55:222–229.

35. Bengtsson F, Bugge M, Johansen KH, et al. Brain tryptophan hydroxylation in the portacaval shunted rat: a hypothesis for the regulation of serotonin turnover *in vivo. J Neurochem* 1991;56: 1069–1074.

36. Mousseau DD, Baker GB, Butterworth RF. Increased density of catalytic sites and expression of brain monoamine oxidase A in humans with hepatic encephalopathy. *J Neurochem* 1997;68: 1200–1208.

37. Raghavendra Rao VL, Butterworth RF. Alterations of [³H]8-OH-DPAT and [³H]-ketanserin binding sites in autopsied brain tissue from cirrhotic patients with Hepatic Encephalopathy. *Neurosci Lett* 1994;182:69–72.

38. Vorobioff J, Garcia-Tsao G, Groszmann R, et al. Long-term hemodynamic effects of ketanserin, a 5-hydroxytryptamine blocker, in portal hypertensive patients. *Hepatology* 1989;9: 88–91.

39. During MJ, Heyes MP, Freese A, et al. Quinolinic acid concentrations in striatal extracellular fluid reach potentially neurotoxic levels following systemic L-tryptophan loading. *Brain Res* 1989;476:384–387.

40. Moroni F, Lombardi G, Carla V, et al. Content of quinolinic acid and other tryptophan metabolites increases in brain regions of rats used as experimental models of hepatic encephalopathy. *J Neurochem* 1986;46:869–874.

41. Moroni F, Lombardi G, Carla V, et al. Increase in the content of quinolinic acid in cerebrospinal fluid and frontal cortex of patients with hepatic failure. *J Neurochem* 1986;47:1667–1671.

42. Young SN, Lal S. CNS tryptamine metabolism in hepatic coma. *J Neural Transm* 1980;47:153–161.

43. Mousseau DD, Pomier Layrargues G, Butterworth RF. Region-selective decreases in densities of [³H]-tryptamine binding sites in autopsied brain tissue from cirrhotic patients with Hepatic Encephalopathy. *J Neurochem* 1994;61:621–625.

44. Schafer DF, Jones EA. Hepatic encephalopathy and the γ-aminobutyric acid system. *Lancet* 1982;1:18–20.

45. Butterworth RF, Giguère JF. Cerebral amino acids in portal-systemic encephalopathy: lack of evidence for altered γ-aminobutyric acid (GABA) function. *Metab Brain Dis* 1986;1:221–228.

46. Roy S, Pomier Layrargues G, Butterworth RF, et al. Hepatic encephalopathy in cirrhotic and portacaval shunted dogs: lack of changes in brain GABA uptake, brain GABA levels, brain glutamic acid decarboxylase and brain postsynaptic GABA receptors. *Hepatology* 1988;8:845–849.

47. Lavoie J, Giguère JF, Pomier Layrargues G, et al. Activities of neuronal and astrocytic marker enzymes in autopsied brain tissue from patients with hepatic encephalopathy. *Metab Brain Dis* 1987;2:283–290.

48. Butterworth RF, Lavoie J, Giguère JF, et al. Affinities and densities of high affinity ³H-muscimol (GABA-A) binding sites and central benzodiazepine receptors are unchanged in autopsied brain tissue from cirrhotic patients with hepatic encephalopathy. *Hepatology* 1988;8:1084–1088.

49. Scollo-Lavizzari G, Steinmann E. Reversal of hepatic coma by benzodiazepine antagonist Ro15-1788. *Lancet* 1985;1: 1324–1325.

50. Grimm G, Ferenci P, Katzenschlager R, et al. Improvement of hepatic encephalopathy treated with flumazenil. *Lancet* 1988;1:1392–1394.

51. Mans AM, Kukulka KM, McAvoy KJ, et al. Regional distribution and kinetics of three sites on the GABA_A receptor: lack of

effect of portacaval shunting. *J Cereb Blood Flow Metab* 1992; 12:334–346.

52. Mullen KD, Szauter KM, Kaminsky-Russ K. "Endogenous" benzodiazepine activity in body fluids of patients with hepatic encephalopathy. *Lancet* 1990;336:81–83.

53. Olasmaa M, Rothstein JD, Guidotti A, et al. Endogenous benzodiazepine receptor ligands in human and animal hepatic encephalopathy. *J Neurochem* 1990;55:2015–2023.

54. Caccia S, Carli M, Garattini S, et al. Pharmacological activities of clobazam and diazepam in the rat: relation to drug brain levels. *Arch Int Pharmacodyn* 1980;243:275–283.

55. Rothstein JD, McKhann G, Guarneri P, et al. Hepatic encephalopathy and cerebrospinal fluid content of diazepam binding inhibitor (DBI). *Ann Neurol* 1989;26:57–62.

56. Lavoie J, Pomier Layrargues G, Butterworth RF. Increased densities of peripheral-type benzodiazepine receptors in brain autopsy samples from cirrhotic patients with hepatic encephalopathy. *Hepatology* 1990;11:874–878.

57. Giguère JF, Hamel E, Butterworth RF. Increased densities of binding sites for the "peripheral-type" benzodiazepine receptor ligand ³H-PK11195 in rat brain following portacaval anastomosis. *Brain Res* 1992;585:295–298.

58. Desjardins P, Bandeira P, Raghavendra Rao VL, et al. Increased expression of the peripheral-type benzodiazepine receptor-isoquinoline carboxamide binding protein in mRNA brain following portacaval anastomosis. *Brain Res* 1997;758:255–258.

59. Butterworth RF, Tonon MC, Désy L, et al. Increased brain content of the endogenous benzodiazepine receptor ligand octadecaneuropeptide (ODN) following portacaval anastomosis in the rat. *Peptides* 1991;12:119–125.

60. Shiraishi T, Black KL, Ikesaki K. Peripheral benzodiazepine receptor ligands induce morphological changes in mitochondria of cultured glioma cells. *Soc Neurosci Abstr* 1990;16:214–216.

61. Raghavendra Rao VL, Qureshi IA, Butterworth RF. Increased densities of binding sites for the "peripheral-type" benzodiazepine receptor ligand [³H]-PK 11195 in congenital ornithine transcarbamylase deficient sparse-fur mouse. *Pediatr Res* 1993; 34:777–780.

62. Spahr L, Butterworth RF, Fontaine S, et al. Increased blood manganese in cirrhotic patients: relationship to pallidal magnetic resonance signal hyperintensity and neurological symptoms. *Hepatology* 1996;24:1116–1120.

63. Devenyi AG, Barron TF, Mamourian AC. Dystonia, hyperintense basal ganglia, and high whole blood manganese levels in Alagille's syndrome. *Gastroenterology* 1994;106:1068–1071.

64. Mirowitz SA, Westrich TJ, Hirsch JD. Hyperintense basal ganglia on T₁-weighted MR images in patients receiving parenteral nutrition. *Radiology* 1991;191:117–120.

65. Pomier Layrargues G, Spahr L, Butterworth RF. Increased manganese concentrations in pallidum of cirrhotic patients: cause of magnetic resonance hyperintensity? *Lancet* 1995;345:735.

66. Rose C, Butterworth RF, Zayed J, et al. Manganese deposition in basal ganglia structures results from both portal-systemic shunting and liver dysfunction. *Gastroenterology* 1999;117:640–644.

67. Raghavendra Rao VL, Audet RM, Butterworth RF. Increased nitric oxide synthase activities and L-[³H]arginine uptake in brain following portacaval anastomosis. *J Neurochem* 1995;65: 677–681.

68. Raghavendra Rao VL, Audet RM, Butterworth RF. Increased neuronal nitric oxide synthase expression in brain following portacaval anastomosis. *Brain Res* 1997;765:169–172.

69. Raghavendra Rao VL, Audet RM, Butterworth RF. Portacaval shunting and hyperammonemia stimulate the uptake of L-³H-arginine but not of L-³H-nitroarginine into rat brain synaptosomes. *J Neurochem* 1997;68:337–343.

70. Kato M, Hughes RD, Keays RT, et al. Electron microscopic study of brain capillaries in cerebral edema from fulminant hepatic failure. *Hepatology* 1992;15:1060–1066.

71. Bates TE, Williams SR, Kauppinen RA, et al. Observation of cerebral metabolites in an animal model of acute liver failure *in vivo*: ^{1}H and ^{31}P nuclear magnetic resonance study. *J Neurochem* 1978;53:102–110.

72. Clemmensen JO, Larsen FS, Kondrup J, et al. Cerebral herniation in patients with acute liver failure is correlated with arterial ammonia concentration. *Hepatology* 1999;29:648–653.

73. Swain M, Butterworth RF, Blei AT. Ammonia and related amino acids in the pathogenesis of brain edema in acute ischemic liver failure in rats. *Hepatology* 1992;15:449–453.

74. Ganz R, Swain M, Traber P, et al. Ammonia-induced swelling of rat cerebral cortical slices: implications for the pathogenesis of brain edema in acute hepatic failure. *Metab Brain Dis* 1989;4: 213–223.

75. Voorhoies TM, Ehrlich ME, Duffy TE, et al. Acute hyperammonemia in the young primate: physiologic and neuropathologic correlates. *Pediatr Res* 1983;17:970–975.

76. Norenberg MD, Baker L, Norenberg LOB, et al. Ammonia-induced astrocyte swelling in primary culture. *Neurochem Res* 1991;16:833–836.

77. Takahashi H, Koehler RC, Brusilow SW, et al. Inhibition of brain glutamine accumulation prevents cerebral edema in hyperammonemia rats. *Am J Physiol* 1991;281:H826–H829.

78. Blei, AT, Olafsson S, Therrien G, et al. Ammonia-induced brain edema and intracranial hypertension in rats after portacaval anastomosis. *Hepatology* 1994;19:1437–1444.

79. Record CO, Buxton B, Chase R, et al. Plasma and brain amino acids in fulminant hepatic failure and their relationship to hepatic encephalopathy. *Eur J Clin Invest* 1976;6:387–394.

80. Swain MS, Bergeron M, Audet R, et al. Monitoring of neurotransmitter amino acids by means of an indwelling cisterna magna catheter. A comparison of two rodent models of fulminant hepatic failure. *Hepatology* 1992;16:1028–1035.

81. Bossman DK, Deutz NEP, Maas MAW, et al. Amino acid release from cerebral cortex in experimental acute liver failure, studied by in vivo cerebral cortex microdialysis. *J Neurochem* 1992;59:591–599.

82. Michalak A, Rose C, Butterworth J, et al. Neuroactive amino acids and glutamate (NMDA) receptors in frontal cortex of rats with experimental acute liver failure. *Hepatology* 1996;24: 908–913.

83. Butterworth RF. Hepatic encephalopathy and brain edema in acute hepatic failure: Does glutamate play a role? *Hepatology* 1997;25:1032–1034.

84. Knecht K, Michalak A, Rose C, et al. Decreased glutamate transporter (GLT-1) expression in frontal cortex of rats with acute liver failure. *Neurosci Lett* 1997;229:201–203.

85. Oppong KNW, Bartlett K, Record CO, et al. Synaptosomal glutamate transport in thioacetamide-induced hepatic encephalopathy in the rat. *Hepatology* 1995;22:553–558.

86. Michalak A, Butterworth RF. Selective loss of binding sites for the glutamate receptor ligands [^{3}H]kainate and (S)-[^{3}H]5-fluorowillardiine in the brains of rats with acute liver failure. *Hepatology* 1997;24:631–635.

87. Vogels BAPM, Mass MAW, Daalhuisen J, et al. Memantine, a non-competitive NMDA-receptor antagonist improves hyperammonemia-induced encephalopathy and acute hepatic encephalopathy in rats. *Hepatology* 1997;25:820–827.

88. Knudsen GM, Poulson HE, Paulson OB. Blood-brain barrier permeability in galactosamine-induced hepatic encephalopathy: no evidence for increased GABA transport. *J Hepatol* 1988; 6:187–192.

89. Swain M, Butterworth RF, Blei AT. Ammonia and related amino acids in the pathogenesis of brain edema in acute ischemic liver failure in rats. *Hepatology* 1992;15:449–453.

90. Schafer DF, Fowler JM, Munson PJ, et al. Gamma-aminobutyric acid and benzodiazepine receptors in an animal model of fulminant hepatic failure. *J Lab Clin Med* 1983;102:870–880.

91. Bassett ML, Mullen KD, Skolnick P, et al. Amelioration of hepatic encephalopathy by pharmacologic antagonism of the GABA$_A$-benzodiazepine receptor complex in a rabbit model of fulminant hepatic failure. *Gastroenterology* 1987;93:1069–1077.

92. Zieve L, Ferenci P, Rzepczynski D, et al. A benzodiazepine antagonist does not alter the course of hepatic encephalopathy or neural γ-aminobutyric acid (GABA) binding. *Metab Brain Dis* 1987;2:201–205.

93. van der Rijt CCD, de Knegt RJ, Schalm SW, et al. Flumazenil does not improve hepatic encephalopathy associated with acute ischemic liver failure in the rabbit. *Metab Brain Dis* 1990;5:131–141.

94. Hadesman R, Wiesner RH, Go VLW, et al. Concentrations of 3,4-dihydroxyphenylalanine and catecholamines and metabolites in brain in an hepatic model of hepatic encephalopathy. *J Neurochem* 1995;65:1166–1175.

95. Murakami N, Saito K, Kato T, et al. Changes in brain monoamine metabolism in rats with acute ischemic hepatic failure under artificial cardiopulmonary management. *Gastroenterol Jpn* 1992;27:191–198.

96. Yurdaydin C, Hörtnagl H, Steindl P, et al. Increased serotoninergic and noradrenergic activity in hepatic encephalopathy in rats with thioacetamide-induced acute liver failure. *Hepatology* 1990;12:695–700.

97. McKinzie SL, Hammond DL, Grabau C, et al. Releases of norepinephrine and dopamine in vestriculocisternal perfusions in hepatectomized and laparotomized rats. *J Neurochem* 1996;66: 569–578.

98. Michalak M, Rose C, Buu PNT, et al. Evidence for altered central noradrenergic function in experimental acute liver failure in the rat. *Hepatology* 1998;27:362–368.

99. Michalak A, Rose C, Butterworth RF. Loss of noradrenaline transporter sites in frontal cortex of rats with acute (ischemic) liver failure. *Neurochem Int* 2000;38:25–30.

100. Kaneko K, Kurumaji A, Watanabe A, et al. Changes in high K$^+$-evoked serotonin release and serotonin 2A/2C receptor binding in the frontal cortex of rats with thioacetamide-induced hepatic encephalopathy. *J Neural Transm* 1998;105:13–30.

101. Bergqvist PB, Vogels BA, Bosman DK, et al. Neocortical dialysate monoamines of rats after acute, subacute, and chronic liver shunt. *J Neurochem* 1995;64:1238–1244.

102. Michalak A, Chataurct N, Butterworth RF. Evidence for a serotonin transporter deficit in experimental acute liver failure. *Neurochem Int* 2001;38:163–168.

103. Al-Mardini H, Harrison EJ, Ince PG, et al. Brain indoles in human hepatic encephalopathy. *Hepatology* 1993;17:1033–1040.

104. Ferenci P, Herneth A, Steindl P. Newer approaches to therapy of hepatic encephalopathy. *Semin Liver Dis* 1996;16:329–338.

105. Wolpert E, Phillips SF, Summerskill WH. Ammonia production in the human colon: effects of cleansing, neomycin and acetohydroxamic acid. *N Engl J Med* 1970;283:159–164.

106. Morgan MY, Hawley KE. Lactitol vs lactulose in the treatment of acute hepatic encephalopathy in cirrhotic patients: a double-blind randomized trial. *Hepatology* 1987;7:1278–1284.

107. Lockwood AM, McDonald JM, Rieman RE. The dynamics of ammonia metabolism in men: effects of liver disease and hyperammonemia. *J Clin Invest* 1979;63:449–460.

108. Swart GR, van den Berg JWO, van Vuure JK, et al. Minimum protein requirements in liver cirrhosis determined by nitrogen

balance measurements at three levels of protein intake. *Clin Nutr* 1989;8:329–336.

109. Kircheis G, Nilius R, Held C, et al. Therapeutic efficacy of L-ornithine-L-aspartate infusions in patients with cirrhosis and hepatic encephalopathy: results of a placebo-controlled, double-blind study. *Hepatology* 1997;25:1351–1360.

110. Rose C, Michalak A, Pannunzio P, et al. Orthinine-L-aspartate in experimental portal-systemic encephalopathy: therapeutic efficacy and mechanism of action. *Metab Brain Dis* 1998;13: 147–157.

111. Rose C, Michalak A, Rama Rao KV, et al. L-Ornithine-L-Aspartate lowers plasma and cerebrospinal fluid ammonia and prevents brain edema in rats with acute liver failure. *Hepatology* 1999;30:636–640.

112. Sushma S, Dasarathy S, Tandon RK, et al. Sodium benzoate in the treatment of acute hepatic encephalopathy: a double-blind randomized trial. *Hepatology* 1992;16:138–144.

113. Pomier Layrargues G, Giguère JF, Lavoie J, et al. Clinical efficacy of benzodiazepine antagonist RO 15-1788 (flumazenil) in cirrhotic patients with hepatic coma: results of a randomized double-blind placebo-controlled cross-over trial. *Hepatology* 1994;19:32–37.

114. Gyr K, Meier R, Haussler J, et al. Evaluation of the efficacy and safety of flumazenil in the treatment of portal systemic encephalopathy: a double blind, randomised, placebo controlled multicentre study. *Gut* 1996;39:319–324.

115. Butterworth RF, Wells J, Pomier Layrargues G. Detection of benzodiazepines in hepatic encephalopathy: reply. *Hepatology* 1995;2:605.

116. Morgan MY, Jakobovits AW, James IM, et al. Successful use of bromocriptine in the treatment of chronic hepatic encephalopathy. *Gastroenterology* 1980;78:663–670.

117. Uribe M, Farca A, Marquez MA, et al. Treatment of chronic portal systemic encephalopathy with bromocriptine: a double-blind controlled trial. *Gastroenterology* 1979;76:1347–1351.

118. Herneth AM, Steindl P, Ferenci P. Central acting (5-HT) ligands which ameliorate hepatic encephalopathy (HE) require partial 5-HT$_{1A}$ agonistic properties. *Hepatology* 1994;20:108A.

119. Traber P, DalCanto M, Granger D, et al. Effect of body temperature on brain edema and encephalopathy in the rat after hepatic devascularization. *Gastroenterology* 1989;96:888–891.

120. Cordoba J, Crespin J, Gottstein J, et al. Mild hypothermia modifies ammonia-induced brain edema in rats after portacaval anastomosis. *Gastroenterology* 1999;116:686–693.

121. Jalan R, Olde Damink SWM, Deutz NEP, et al. Moderate hypothermia for uncontrolled intracranial hypertension in acute liver failure. *Lancet* 1999;35:1164–1168.

122. Roberts RDR, Mamas D. Induced hypothermia in the management of cerebral oedema secondary to fulminant liver failure. *Clin Transplant* 1999;13:546–548.

123. Rose C, Michalak A, Pannunzio M, et al. Mild hypothermia delays the onset of coma and prevents brain edema and extracellular brain glutamate accumulation in rats with acute liver failure. *Hepatology* 2000;31:872–877.

The Liver: Biology and Pathobiology, Fourth Edition, edited by I. M. Arias, J. L. Boyer, F. V. Chisari, N. Fausto, D. Schachter, and D. A. Shafritz.
Lippincott Williams & Wilkins, Philadelphia © 2001.

45

ALTERATIONS OF THE KIDNEY IN LIVER DISEASE

PAOLO GENTILINI
GIACOMO LAFFI
MASSIMO PINZANI
GIORGIO LA VILLA

Certain physiologic and pathologic situations suggest that the liver and kidney present some similarities in their function, especially in eliminating toxic molecules and maintaining salt and water and metabolic equilibrium. Although physiologic research provides evidence of this complementary function, the relationship between liver and kidney is studied most commonly in the course of liver disease.

During acute liver disease, the kidney may manifest toxic or hemodynamic damages similar to those observed during cirrhosis. Generally, renal impairment is related to the severity of liver damage, and its worsening or improvement reflects the course of hepatic injury. Renal impairment is most accurately studied during chronic liver disease, which provides more opportunity for treatment than does acute liver injury.

Although morphologic renal alterations have been studied for several years, most research is currently directed to renal functional impairment (RFI) and hepatorenal syndrome (HRS), which, in many respects, depend on hemodynamic derangement, which in turn is usually accompanied by positive sodium balance and ascites. The same hemodynamic modifications can compromise local hemo-

dynamic and oxygen support for other organs, such as the heart and lungs, although the principal target is the kidney.

This chapter addresses the following subjects: (a) the physiologic relationship between liver and kidney, considering more specifically the presence and activity of intrahepatic receptors, which contribute to the regulation of renal salt and water excretion; (b) organic renal impairment, principally due to precipitation of immunoglobulins and cryoglobulins in glomeruli, and development of cirrhotic glomerulonephritis, such as membranous glomerulonephritis (MGN) or membranoproliferative glomerulonephritis (MPGN); (c) metabolic renal damage, as represented by renal tubular acidosis (RTA); (d) RFI, due to renal impairment and hemodynamic alterations with hyperdynamic circulation resulting in ascites and edema; and (e) pathogenesis of the HRS.

PHYSIOLOGIC RELATIONSHIP BETWEEN LIVER AND KIDNEY

Experimental and clinical evidence indicates that the liver plays an important role in body fluid handling both in physiologic and pathologic conditions (see website chapter 🖳 W-34). The liver participates through receptors that detect changes in osmolality and ion concentration. Three types of receptors have been identified in the liver that

P. Gentilini, M. Pinzani, and G. La Villa: Department of Internal Medicine, University of Florence, Florence, 50134 Italy.
G. Laffi: Department of Internal Medicine, University of Florence; U.O. Medical Pathology I, Azienda Hospital Careg, Florence, 50139, Italy.

directly or indirectly influence renal function: hepatic osmoreceptors, sodium receptors, and low-pressure baroreceptors (1–3).

Hepatic Osmoreceptors

In animals, the administration of hypotonic solutions in the portal vein elicits water diuresis, whereas infusion of hypertonic solutions results in water retention, even if plasma osmolality is unaffected. These renal responses are abolished by section of the hepatic vagus nerve. The concept of hepatic osmoreceptors was further supported by electrophysiologic studies and data obtained in unanesthetized, chronically instrumented animals, which revealed that stimulation of hepatic osmoreceptors by intraportal infusion of sodium chloride solutions of different osmolality induces changes in plasma arginine vasopressin (AVP) levels that mediated the antidiuretic response (4).

Hepatic osmoreceptors may provide a mechanism whereby challenges to extracellular fluid osmolality are rapidly buffered. Indeed, experimental animals submitted to hepatic vagotomy have an impaired ability to adjust water excretion rapidly in response to an oral water load or deprivation, but do not alter overall regulation of renal water handling (5). These considerations are contrary to the possibility that hepatic osmoreceptors play a role in the pathogenesis of AVP hypersecretion and water retention in pathologic conditions.

Hepatic Sodium Receptors

Perlmutt et al. (6) administered isotonic saline into the portal vein and vena cava of conscious rats, which enhanced diuretic and natriuretic response in the absence of changes in glomerular filtration rate (GFR). Section of the hepatic branch of the right vagus did not affect natriuretic response, indicating that a humoral factor of hepatic origin may be the mediator. Impulses from afferent hepatic nerves are sensitive to NaCl (7,8).

Stimulation of the hepatic NaCl receptor by intraportal infusion of hypertonic saline in conscious rabbits decreases efferent renal sympathetic nerve activity (ERSNA), which was abolished by hepatic denervation. Suppression of ERSNA by intraportal infusion of hypertonic saline is dose-dependent, involving AVP action via the area postrema, since both pretreatment with a vasopressin V1 antagonist and lesion of the area postrema blunted the effects (9). An increase in hepatic afferent nerve activity by hypertonic NaCl was suppressed in a dose-dependent manner by ouabain, furosemide, or bumetamide, indicating that the hepatic sodium receptors sense Na^+ concentration through the bumetamide-sensitive Na^+,K^+ $2Cl^-$ cotransporter.

Some studies also evaluated ERSNA and sodium excretion in response to an oral sodium load in chronically instrumented conscious dogs. NaCl-free food intake had no effect on renal nerve activity or sodium excretion, whereas high-NaCl food intake decreased ERSNA and increased sodium excretion. Postprandial natriuresis was abolished by hepatic or renal denervation. A hepatorenal reflex was proposed, which is activated by NaCl delivered to the liver via the portal vein, reducing ERSNA and renal sodium reabsorption without influencing renal hemodynamics or GFR. This reflex plays a significant role in regulating sodium balance in physiologic conditions (6–9).

Hepatic Baroreceptors

Nijima (10) demonstrated that hepatic afferent nerve activity is stimulated by receptors located in the portal venous rather than the arterial side of the hepatic circulation, and that these receptors are baroreceptors and not volume receptors. The reflex increase in ERSNA, which was induced by thoracic vena cava constriction, was abolished by hepatic denervation, and was active in rats with cirrhosis (11). The effects of increased ERSNA on renal hemodynamics and function include reduced renal blood flow (RBF), enhanced sodium reabsorption, and renin release. In experimental animals, increments in portal pressure were associated with renal vasoconstriction and sodium retention, whereas reduced portal pressure induced diuretic response. These effects were abolished by renal denervation.

Infusion of glutamine or serine (but not of glutamate) into the superior mesenteric vein of anesthetized rats decreased RBF, GFR, and urinary flow rate. Spinal transection, renal denervation, or section of the vagal hepatic nerves eradicated the effects of mesenteric glutamine administration. Infusion of glutamine into the jugular vein had no deleterious effect on renal hemodynamics. These data provide evidence that hepatorenal depressor reflex can impair renal hemodynamics and function. Lang et al. (12) proposed that glutamine causes hepatocyte swelling and that the consequent increment in sinusoidal pressure is the afferent stimulus of this hepatorenal reflex. The renal effects of mesenteric glutamine were mimicked by mesenteric infusion of serotonin and abolished by methysergide, suggesting involvement of hepatic serotonergic nerves. It was also speculated that this hepatorenal reflex might explain the renal vasoconstriction that characterizes HRS. In cirrhotic rats with hepatic denervation, cumulative sodium retention was significantly attenuated. Cirrhotic rats with intact hepatic innervation decreased creatinine clearance by 70%.

More recently, the role of hepatic baroreceptors in determining renal dysfunction in cirrhosis was investigated using transjugular intrahepatic portal systemic shunt (TIPS). Improvement in systemic hemodynamics induced by TIPS was without effect on RBF. In contrast, transient occlusion of TIPS was associated with sudden decrement in RBF, which was attributed to activation of the hepatorenal reflex.

ORGANIC RENAL IMPAIRMENT

Independently of the severity of liver damage, many liver diseases are associated with microhematuria and proteinuria. The principal conditions capable of inducing simultaneous alterations in both the liver and kidney are presented in Table 45.1. In the the past, numerous studies were performed in cirrhotic patients postmortem, and revealed varying degrees of renal damage in up to 100% of cases. However, these reports suffer from autolysis due to profound hemodynamic derangement and other factors (13). Subsequent studies described findings from living patients submitted to renal biopsy. These alterations mainly consisted in mesangial matrix hypertrophy, capillary wall thickening, and immunoglobulin deposits in the mesangial area and capillary walls (14,15).

Immunofluorescent observations revealed deposition of immunoglobulin (Ig)A, IgG, IgM, and C3 (16,17). In cirrhotic patients showing glomerulonephritis, 80% had glomerular deposition of IgA (16).

An important hypothesis concerning the pathogenesis of renal damage is based on deposition of immunocomplexes

TABLE 45.1. PATHOLOGIC CONDITIONS CHARACTERIZED BY LIVER AND KIDNEY INVOLVEMENT

Simultaneous hepatic and renal involvement
  Congenital
    Polycystic disease
    Caroli's syndrome
    Sickle cell anemia
    Hemochromatosis
  Acquired
    Systemic diseases
      Collagen diseases
      Hemodynamic alterations (heart failure, shock)
      Infections (sepsis, miliary tuberculosis,
        Waterhouse–Friederichsen syndrome, hepatitis B virus
        infection, hepatitis C virus infection, human
        immunodeficiency virus infection, infectious mono-
        nucleosis, yellow fever, malaria, leptospirosis,
        schistosomiasis)
      Disease of unknown etiology (sarcoidosis, amyloidosis,
        Reye's syndrome)
    Pregnancy
      Toxemia
      Acute fatty liver
    Toxic agents
      Drugs (tetracyclines, acetaminophen, sulfonamides,
        streptomycin, halothane)
      Vegetable toxins (toadstool toxins)
      Industrial toxins (carbon tetrachloride, copper sulfate,
        chromium, methoxyflurane, iproniazid)
Primary liver disease with secondary renal involvement
  Chronic liver disease with immunocomplex-mediated
    glomerulonephritis
  Chronic liver disease with renal tubular acidosis
  Cholestasis with renal tubular involvement
  Acute liver failure with renal functional impairment
  Hepatorenal syndrome

within the kidney (16,18). During hepatitis B virus (HBV)-related chronic liver disease, immunocomplexes containing HBV antigen were often accompanied by hepatitis B antigen (HBeAg) in the glomerular capillary wall (17). When immunocomplexes are deposited within the kidney, serum levels of C3 and C4 are reduced. Renal deposits contain all types of immunoglobulins with prevalence of IgG in the subepithelial space (17).

Viral particles capable of inducing severe renal damage have been found more frequently in patients with hepatitis C virus (HCV)-related chronic active hepatitis (CAH) than in patients with cirrhosis (19). Typical alterations of the kidney during HCV-related liver disease include MPGN, especially in patients who show high serum levels of rheumatoid factor or typical mixed cryoglobulinemia (MC) (20,21). Thus MPGN is related to deposition of immunocomplexes and IgM, C3, and C1q complement in the capillary wall. The deposition of immunocomplexes is generally followed by activation of the complement system with cellular proliferation and intraglomerular infiltration of cells with phagocytic activity. Proteases and oxidizing agents are released with consequent cellular damage. However, it is uncertain whether HCV antigens independently induce glomerular damage in the absence of MC or whether B-lymphocyte activation and consequent production of IgM result in renal damage (22) and increased permeability (23).

Morphologic alterations of the kidney occurring during HCV-related cirrhosis appear strictly related to viral infection since MPGN was partially reversed in patients who underwent liver transplant, but worsened over time with the same severity as glomerulonephritis observed prior to transplantation (24). Primary biliary cirrhosis (PBC) may also be associated with MPGN characterized by mesangial cell proliferation and deposition of IgG, C3, and C1q on glomerular basement membranes (25).

METABOLIC RENAL DAMAGE

Acute renal failure with anuria and signs of tubular impairment is observed in patients with ascending cholangitis or extrahepatic cholestasis. The most important histologic alterations are tubular necrosis and deposition of pigmented casts in tubular cells and obstructed tubuli (26).

RTA represents a deficit in renal acidification capacity in the presence of normal GFR. The site of deficit can be distal tubuli, collecting ducts, or proximal tubuli. Typical biochemical signs of RTA occur during acute and chronic liver disease, particularly in cholestasis. Abnormal function of H–adenosine triphosphatase (ATPase) and H-K-ATPases, which are involved in terminal nephron acidification, may determine different forms of RTA. Three principal types of RTA have been described (27). RTA type I is based on a distal tubular gradient defect, and is defective in excretion of titratable acidity, maintenance of ammoniogenic capacity, and serum acidosis. All types of RTA may be incomplete or complete. The complete form of RTA type I is rare in liver disease and is frequently accompanied by nephrocalcinosis, whereas the incomplete form is most common and occurs in autoimmune liver disease, CAH, or cryptogenic cirrhosis. The clinical relevance of the incomplete form is slight.

In patients with autoimmune liver disease, hepatic damage is often associated with the hypokalemia, acidosis, and osteomalacia. In our experience, patients with extrahepatic cholestasis and chronic postviral liver diseases, as well as those affected by PBC, often present typical signs of RTA type I (28). Since PBC represents one of the most frequent diseases characterized by a copper excretion defect that may be complicated by RTA, and, in light of a similar association described in patients with Wilson's disease, copper may be responsible for inducing tubular lesions (28,29). Administration of penicillamine reduces renal abnormalities by decreasing copper availability within the kidney (30). During RTA, hypouricemia may also occur due to renal tubular damage.

Incomplete type I RTA also occurs with alcoholic liver disease (38%), especially in patients with a higher degree of liver dysfunction (31).

Type II RTA is caused by proximal tubular dysfunction characterized by bicarbonate wasting and has been observed in CAH.

Several mechanisms have been proposed to explain the occurrence of RTA in chronic liver disease. In the past, a critical role was ascribed to bile acids, conjugated bilirubin, and endotoxinemia due to gram-negative sepsis. Other authors suggested that increased renal sodium retention and low sodium diet may be responsible for decreased availability of sodium at the distal tubules, a phenomenon that may delay or block the normal acidifying capacity of the kidney. However, abnormal sodium retention and consequent renal impairment with hemodynamic modifications do not correlate with RTA (32). Alcohol abuse may itself lead to RTA (33). Finally, although immunologic mechanisms could not be excluded, especially in light of renal excretion of Tamm–Horsfall protein in patients with RTA (34), a mechanism leading to metabolic acidosis remains unclear and may be based on multifactorial mechanisms that modify proton ATPase activity.

RENAL FUNCTIONAL IMPAIRMENT

RFI may occur during acute or chronic liver disease, although accurate descriptions are rare during acute liver damage. Acute liver failure is generally characterized by jaundice and encephalopathy. Different kinds of renal damage have been reported in patients with severe liver damage due to paracetamol overdose (35), although similar renal alterations occur in patients without liver damage. RFI influences survival of patients awaiting liver transplanta-

tion. In other cases of acute liver failure, RFI may be present in 40% of cases (36). The principal mechanism leading to renal impairment may be a decrease in RBF due to systemic hypotension and renal vasoconstriction. The vasoactive substances responsible for hemodynamic derangement are the same as those implicated in RFI occurring in liver cirrhosis (37). In cases with a prolonged course, ATN can supervene (38).

During the long course of chronic liver disease, the kidneys generally maintain physiologic function as evidenced by return to normal sodium and water excretion observed in some patients with decompensated cirrhosis. The only dysfunction may be a delay in eliminating a water load. During the early stages of CAH, decreased renal clearances occur even in the absence of portal hypertension or ascites (38). We found a decrease of over 50% in renal clearances in 15% to 20% of patients affected by CAH and in the early stage of cirrhosis. Subsequently, renal hypoperfusion becomes greater (39,40). The majority of patients eventually have signs of fluid accumulation, ascites being the major complication during cirrhosis that can be followed by decreased sensitivity to diuretics (refractory ascites), spontaneous bacterial peritonitis (SBP), or HRS (41).

Hemodynamic Alterations and Ascites

During the course of liver disease, several hemodynamic, hormonal, and functional modifications occur according to the different stages of the disease. The pathogenesis of ascites is not completely understood. Several hypotheses have been formulated to explain positive sodium balance and fluid accumulation. Hemodynamic alterations and ascites generally occur after the onset of portal hypertension. These phenomena may be the principal cause of other complications, such as bleeding and encephalopathy. Portal hypertension is mainly due to an increase in intrahepatic resistance as a consequence of nodular regeneration and activation of hepatic stellate cells (42–44) (see Chapter 31).

Kowalski and Abelman (45) described almost 50 years ago a hyperdynamic circulatory syndrome in patients with advanced liver disease. This syndrome, characterized by vasodilation, decreased peripheral vascular resistance (PVR), and increased cardiac output, also occurs in animals with extensive portal–systemic shunting, liver failure, or both (see Chapter 47). Fluid retention and ascites formation are intimately related to deranged systemic hemodynamics and affect abnormal distribution of blood flow (see Chapter 47 and website chapter 🖳 W-32). Schrier et al. (46) emphasized the importance of both splanchnic and peripheral vasodilation in determining renal sodium and water reabsorption. This specific hypothesis, the peripheral arterial vasodilation theory, suggests that patients with advanced cirrhosis have a persistent tendency toward a decrease in PVR and blood pressure, together with an increase in cardiac output, heart rate, and total blood volume, and a decrease in effective arterial blood volume (EABV). These phenomena are also observed during sepsis, arteriovenous shunts, and pregnancy (46). The decrease in EABV, sensed by high-pressure baroreceptors, leads to rapid stimulation of the major vasoactive systems, the sympathetic nervous system (SNS), and the renin-angiotensin-aldosterone system (RAAS). Such activation is followed by nonosmotic hypersecretion of AVP and other natriuretic hormones (47–49). According to Schrier et al. (46), in the early stages of cirrhosis moderate arterial vasodilation is balanced by transient sodium and water retention, leading to the so-called hyperdynamic circulation. This provisional plasma expansion could contribute to suppressing antinatriuretic systems. Over time, however, progressive and fatal vasodilation increases and an ongoing decrease in EABV continues to stimulate the vasoactive systems. Consequently, fluid accumulates, and plasma renin activity (PRA) and serum and urinary catecholamines continue to increase.

However, according to other experimental and clinical evidence, positive sodium balance occurs prior to hemodynamic derangement. Unikowsky et al. (50) observed that sodium retention in cirrhotic dogs was counteracted by lowering portal pressure without other hemodynamic modifications. Increase in presinusoidal pressure in animals was without effect in determining positive sodium balance. Lewis et al. (51) found that cardiac output increased in cirrhotic patients before any reduction in PVR, and appeared to be related to enhanced cardiac preload caused by total blood volume expansion. The hyperdynamic circulatory syndrome appears only in the supine position, which is associated with translocation of blood volume toward the central area (52). In this setting, EABV is expanded with a consequent suppression of PRA and a subsequent increase in sodium excretion. Central blood volume (CBV), as measured by radionuclide angiography, increases (53).

These basic observations suggest that total blood volume, including EABV, may be expanded according to the overflow theory. Other researchers demonstrated lower natriuretic response to a saline load and higher plasma levels of atrial natriuretic peptide (ANP) due to spontaneous right atrial distention. Patients who received 20 mM of sodium diet/day achieved sodium balance within 2 rather than in 5 days (controls), and sodium balance was achieved following a diet of 100 mmol/day of sodium, but with an increase in ANP levels (54). Furthermore, a sodium-restricted diet may prevent ascitic formation, and administration of spironolactone is effective in maintaining optimal sodium excretion together with lowering portal pressure (see Chapter 47). Finally, circulating vasoactive substances do not always correlate with the level of fluid accumulation (55).

Considering all these data, the underfilling theory, first proposed by Witte et al. in 1971, can still be considered valid, especially with Schrier's more recent completion, which underlines the importance of hyperdynamic circulation leading to sodium and water retention. However, this pathogenetic mechanism, which is present during decompensation, may be preceded by a period during which, theoretically, abnormal stimuli in the hepatorenal reflex, through activation of hepatic sodium receptors, may provoke primary sodium retention. Because of altered Starling forces in splanchnic and hepatic compartments, fluid accumulates within the liver leading to overproduction of lymph, resulting in its accumulation in the peritoneal cavity (56). Due to portosystemic shunts, a lower amount of ingested sodium could reach the liver and activate these receptors. In addition, derangement of the liver structure may also impair the function of intrahepatic osmoreceptors and/or afferent hepatic nerves. Rats with cirrhosis exhibited reduced activity of hepatic afferent nerves (57) and blunted natriuresis in response to high NaCl intake.

During the course of cirrhosis, the pathogenesis of ascites may be divided into two major stages. First, in the preascitic stage, renal abnormal retention of sodium and water with positive sodium balance becomes effective without evidence of hemodynamic derangement. Second, in the ascitic stage, which is characterized by decompensation and peripheral edema, signs of hyperdynamic circulation are evident and, although total plasma volume continues to be increased, EABV is decreased. In this setting, the progressive decrease in PVR and mean arterial pressure (MAP) may continue to stimulate the kidney to retain sodium and water. Reduction in cardiovascular reactivity to vasopressor agents also occurs in the first stage possibly because of increased production of nitric oxide (NO) and other vasodilating substances that modify peripheral α1-adrenoreceptor activity (58) (see below). The two principal mechanisms are variably mixed, with one or the other being prevalent in different stages of cirrhosis.

Local Hemodynamics

Observations in decompensated cirrhotic patients reveal that blood flow is not increased in all organs. Increased splanchnic blood flow occurs in cirrhotic patients and experimental animals with portal obstruction (59), and contributes to maintenance and aggravation of the portal hypertension syndrome. Cutaneous and muscular circulation may be increased in patients with cirrhosis. Palmar erythema and spider nevi are early clinical signs of cutaneous hyperperfusion. Plethysmography studies confirm increased forearm blood flow in advanced cirrhosis. Recent investigations using the duplex Doppler ultrasound reveal that brachial and femoral arterial blood flow in absolute terms or as a fraction of cardiac output are reduced in patients with RFI when compared to patients with ascites or healthy controls, indicating that vascular resistance is increased in some extrarenal vascular beds. In cirrhotic patients, renal perfusion correlates directly with brachial or femoral artery blood flow, indicating that changes in blood flow in these vascular beds parallel renal circulation. Epstein et al. (60) observed that renal hemodynamic disturbances are reversible. Similar hemodynamic modifications in the kidney were reported by using the washout technique with ^{133}Xe. Arteriovenous shunts, probably located between the inner cortex and medulla, appear in patients with postviral chronic liver disease (61). Renal arterial resistance increases in the preascitic stage of cirrhosis and is greater in the ascitic phase, particularly during diuretic treatment. Even cerebral autoregulation is impaired in cirrhosis (62), and cerebral vascular resistance, as indicated by the resistive index in the middle cerebral artery, is increased in patients with RFI.

During chronic liver disease, subclinical cardiac impairment may worsen hemodynamics and renal function. Cirrhotic cardiomyopathy has been described in alcoholic cirrhotic patients possibly due to a toxic effect of alcohol. However, nonalcoholic cardiomyopathy was postulated on the basis of an impaired myocardial function in patients with postviral cirrhosis (63). These abnormalities may only become evident in response to maneuvers associated with increased cardiac activity such as volume expansion, agonist stimulation, tilting, or exercise (52).

In a group of cirrhotic patients, dextran infusion produced a constant and progressive increase in right and left atrial pressures without a proportional increase in cardiac index; analysis of the left ventricular function curve indicated an impairment of left ventricular function (64). Bernardi et al. (65) evaluated systolic time intervals in cirrhotic patients at rest and after exercise, and observed reduced left ventricular contractile function parallel to the severity of cirrhosis. Grose et al. (63) confirmed an insufficient increment in cardiac output in cirrhotic patients during maximal exercise.

Downregulation of β_2-receptors may be responsible for depressed myocardial contractility. After tilting, cirrhotic patients showed heart rates similar to those in healthy subjects, despite remarkably higher values of plasma norepinephrine (NE), suggesting an impaired response of the heart to sympathetic stimulation.

In a hyperdynamic circulation, the heart is overloaded by a persistent increase in cardiac output associated with the expansion of the circulating blood volume and eventual impairment in cardiac contractility (66). Cirrhotic cardiomyopathy is a silent consequence of the hyperdynamic circulation, but may contribute to further circulatory derangement and renal dysfunction in advanced liver disease. Vagal dysfunction in patients with ascitic cirrhosis is positively correlated with heart rate and cardiac index, and inversely related to peripheral vascular resistances (66). Deranged hemodynamics may also compromise pulmonary circulation because of arterial vasodilation and/or the opening of arteriovenous shunts. This derangement, called the hepatopulmonary syndrome, is a consequence of systemic vasodilation. It usually does not compromise survival in patients, but may be an indication for liver transplantation.

Role of Vasoactive, Natriuretic, and Antinatriuretic Factors in Determining Renal Dysfunction

Many of the following factors maintain the systemic circulation and to renal function in cirrhosis:

1. SNS, with increased production of NE;
2. RAAS, with increased production of renin, angiotensin II (AG II), and aldosterone;
3. vasoactive diuretic or antidiuretic hormones AVP, ANP, brain natriuretic peptide (BNP), C-type natriuretic peptide (CNP), calcitonin gene-related peptide (CGRP), and others;
4. renal autocrine and paracrine factors (prostaglandins (PGs), prostacyclins (PGIs), kallikrein–kinin system, platelet activating factor (PAF), endothelins (ETs), vasoactive intestinal peptide (VIP), nitric oxide (NO), serotonin, histamine, and others).

Most of these substances determine vasoconstriction or dilation, which favors either diuresis or antidiuresis, respectively. Their production is usually increased during HRS (67). The continuous activation of the SNS is demonstrated by increased levels of NE in plasma and urine, leading to arterial vasoconstriction and decreased RBF and GFR. Renin is overproduced with the consequent greater availability of AG II, which inhibits renin release through negative feedback and induces PG synthesis. Moreover, AG II maintains efferent glomerular tone, which is counteracted by bradykinin (68). The maintenance of efferent glomerular tone contributes to sustain GFR, even in the presence of abnormal sodium and water reabsorption. Administration of a single low dose of captopril, an angiotensin-converting enzyme (ACE) inhibitor, which is insufficient to modify mean arterial pressure (MAP), reduces GFR and filtration fraction (FF) and decreases sodium and water excretion (69). Administration of saralazin, an AG II antagonist, or ACE inhibitors, which reduce MAP, are dangerous to renal function in patients with ascitic cirrhosis. Overstimulation of the major vasoactive systems is unable to maintain normal vascular resistance, and is insufficient to blunt an increase in total blood volume in the presence of decreased CBV (70). Head-out water immersion provoked a rapid increase in sodium and urinary excretion after CBV expansion in patients with decompensated cirrhosis. Moreover, the response to diuretics in decompensated cirrhosis improves during plasma expansion (71). Different responses occur in patients, possibly because the response depends on the degree of decompensation, which ultimately leads to vessel underfilling (72). Hyperdynamic circulation is observed only in the supine position (73). Since the SNS and RAAS are activated throughout the course of decompensated cirrhosis, sodium and water retention are required to increase total blood volume, although this phenomenon results in ascites and peripheral edema.

During decompensated cirrhosis, there is a constant increase in AVP release, which is the principal cause of hyponatremia. The hypersecretion of AVP is not due to osmotic stimuli since it is not sensitive to changes in blood tonicity. However, rapid plasma volume expansion, such as after LeVeen shunt insertion, is generally followed by partial block of AVP production. AVP overproduction may also occur after rapid volume depletion because of diarrhea, vomiting, sodium restricted diet, or overaggressive diuretic treatment (74), which can cause renal ischemia and prerenal azotemia. AVP is an important vasoconstrictor that stimulates V1 receptors, inhibits sympathetic efferent stimuli, and potentiates baroreflexes. Furthermore, it influences PVR and may act as a renal vasodilating factor influencing V2 receptors, possibly through NO release (75). During cirrhosis in animal models, administration of V2 antagonists or niravoline, a k-opioid agonist that inhibits AVP production, increases water excretion during ascites (76).

A continuous tendency toward positive sodium balance and increased water reabsorption may also be due to decreased production of natriuretic factors. The most important and well-known factor is ANP; its release is physiologically related to expansion of CBV and increased intracardiac pressure. During cirrhosis, the production of ANP increases in cirrhotic patients with or without renal dysfunction. These findings support the overflow theory, although patients with decreased EABV also have CBV. During cirrhosis, ANP continues to have a natriuretic function, especially when CBV is further expanded. In decompensated cirrhotic patients, head-out water immersion persists in an increase in CBV, followed by increased urinary sodium and $3',5'$-cyclic guanosine monophosphate (cGMP) excretion. A similar effect occurs following the insertion of TIPS (77). The nearly constant increase in ANP is followed by overexcretion of sodium and water, but these phenomena are not related, and increased renal secretion of cGMP is not always followed by increased renal sodium and water excretion in patients with decompensated cirrhosis (78). The effective response of the kidney to ANP overproduction may also be overproduction of antinatriuretic factors, such as AVP, dopamine, NE, or AG II, which increase proximal reabsorption by tubular cells.

Other physiologic diuretic factors include BNP, which is increased in patients with cirrhosis with or without RFI, as well as during head-out water immersion and peritoneovenous shunt insertion (79). However, intravenous administration of low doses of BNP to patients with positive sodium balance and ascites generally does not provoke natriureses (80).

CNP, a third natriuretic peptide first isolated from porcine brain, induces arterial vessel dilation through a PG-NO path-

way (81). CNP and ANP together are capable of a concentration-dependent increase in cGMP availability in human cortical collecting ducts, suggesting the presence of specific natriuretic peptide receptors in these renal cells. Infusion of pharmacologic doses of BNP and CNP induces a natriuretic response in normal but not in cirrhotic rats (82). ANP, BNP, and CNP are the principal elements of the physiologic natriuretic system, which regulates sodium and water balance and counteracts vasoconstricting systems, which are activated in patients with portal hypertension (83).

Other natriuretic factors are adrenomedullin (AM), CGRP, and urodilatin (URO). AM, an endothelial-derived relaxing peptide found in glomerular structures and distal tubular cells, increases renin release, thereby influencing sodium and water excretion (84). This factor, acting through PG release, also induces vasodilation followed by hypotension (85). Its plasma concentration in patients with decompensated cirrhosis is related to the severity of liver disease and plasma levels of renin, aldosterone, and NE, and may influence the hyperdynamic circulation in patients with decompensated cirrhosis (86).

CGRP, like AM, increases urinary flow rate and sodium and potassium excretion (87). URO, recently discovered in human urine, is produced by renal collecting tubuli. Direct infusion of URO in cirrhotic patients increases GFR, decreases RBF, and increases the distal fractional reabsorption of sodium. Moreover, URO excretion, together with GFR, sodium, and cGMP excretion, increase following head-out water immersion in normal subjects. However, in patients with compensated or decompensated cirrhosis, URO was normal, suggesting that its production does not play a critical role in provoking ascites and renal dysfunction in cirrhotic patients (88).

Renal autocrine systems include arachidonic acid metabolites, the kallikrein–kinin system, ETs, and PAF. Some of these factors partially act outside the kidney. Most vasoactive molecules derive from arachidonic acid metabolism through intermediate endoperoxides. Endoperoxide synthase (PES) produces PGs (PGE_1, PGE_2), PGIs (PGI_1, PGI_2), thromboxane (TxA_2), and leukotrienes (LTs), which are present in arteriolar endothelium and released by neutrophils and platelets in response to other vasoactive molecules, such as AG II, catecholamines, PAF, and kinins (89). They play an important role in regulating hemodynamics, GFR, sodium, and water handling in normal subjects and in patients with cirrhosis. All arachidonic acid metabolites are increased in the urine of decompensated cirrhotics including PGs, PGIs, and TxB_2, the stable nonenzymatic metabolite of TxA_2 (89) (Figure 45.1). Activation of the autocrine systems with production of PGs and PGIs may play a protective role, in which vasodilating activity counteracts the vasoconstricting action of TxA_2, $PGF_{1\alpha}$, PAF, etc.

During the long course of chronic liver disease, balance between vasodilation and vasoconstriction in the kidney ensures a sufficient supply of oxygen even in the presence of

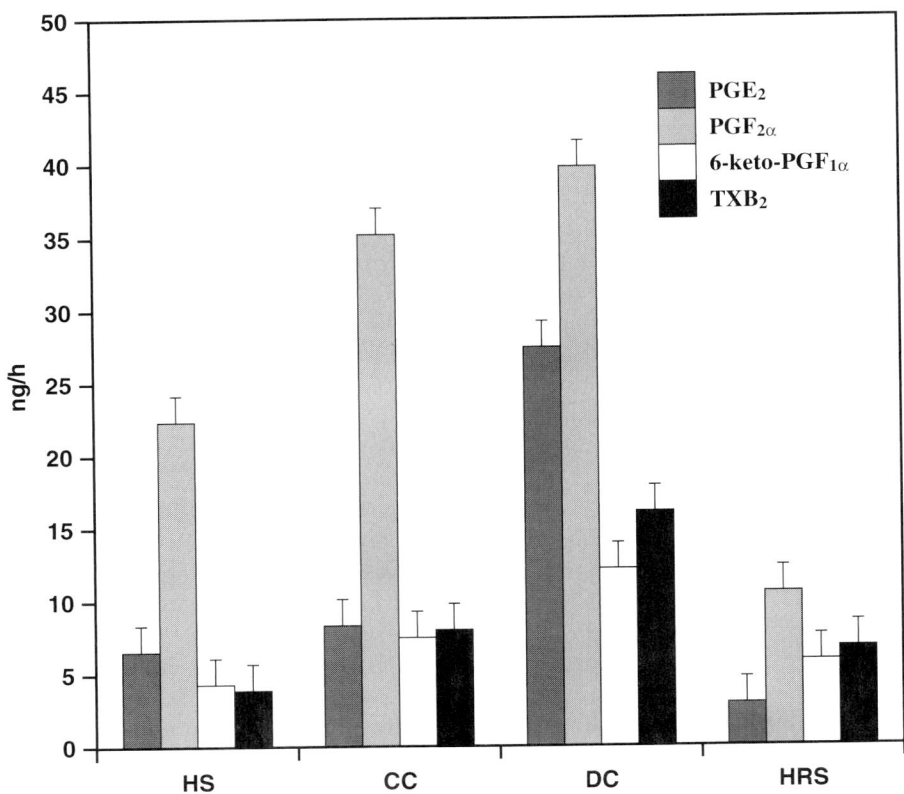

FIGURE 45.1. Urinary excretion of arachidonic acid metabolites in healthy subjects (*HS*) and patients with compensated cirrhosis (*CC*), decompensated or ascitic cirrhosis (*DC*), and hepatorenal syndrome (*HRS*).

a sustained tendency to vasoconstriction in the outer renal cortex. Administration of nonsteroidal antiinflammatory drugs (NSAIDs) inhibits cyclooxygenase activity, PG release, renal function, and sodium and water excretion in patients with decompensated cirrhosis (90). Administration of drugs capable of blunting or inhibiting TxA_2 improves renal function through relative overproduction of PGs. In advanced liver disease, the administration of drugs capable of blocking Tx synthase activity, such as OKY 046, or Tx receptors, such as ONO 3807, leads to a significant improvement in GFR and sodium excretion (91).

In advanced cirrhosis, especially during HRS, urinary excretion of LTE_4, an expression of LT renal production, increases (89). PAF production is provoked by endotoxins and may play a supplemental role in influencing GFR and RBF and decreasing sodium and water excretion. Activity of the kallikrein–kinin system is strictly related to the PG system, and maintains intrarenal vasodilation. In patients with cirrhosis, urinary excretion of kinins is increased in correlation with RBF and GFR levels.

ET_1 and other ETs also play a role in hemodynamic equilibrium within the kidney and are vasoconstrictive. Administration of antibodies against ET_1 receptors

improved renal postischemic vasoconstriction (92,93). Administration of the calcium-channel blocker nifedipine to animals subsequently treated with ET_1 blocked vasoconstriction from the latter molecule. ET_1 influences the release of ANP, partially blunting the water-retaining activity of AVP. ET_1 is elevated in serum and renal veins of patients with decompensated cirrhosis. Although ET_1 appears to be related to endotoxemia, its plasma levels are unmodified in varying positions, following physical exercise and after administration of albumin or ornipressin, or insertion of TIPS (94,95).

Finally, another vasoactive substance, NO, a local vasodilator, which counterbalances humoral and paracrine vasoconstricting substances (see Chapter 39). NO induces hyporesponsiveness to vasoconstrictor molecules such as NE, metoxamine, vasopressin, and ET_1. NO may be responsible for peripheral hyporesponsiveness to methoxamine, an α_1-adrenergic agonist, although other unknown factors probably play a role in splanchnic and systemic vasodilation (96,97). Deficiency in NO production increases intravascular resistance and impairs the response to a NO agonist (98). This phenomenon is related to the degree of hepatic failure.

Increased production of NO with overproduction of nitrites and nitrates occurs in animals and patients with cirrhosis in relation to endotoxin production (99). Administration of NO antagonists in cirrhotic rats corrects splanchnic and peripheral vasodilation. Decreased sensitivity of α_1-adrenoreceptors of peripheral vessel to catecholamines and AG II occurs in cirrhotic patients. NO appears to play a major role in sustaining the hyperdynamic circulation during cirrhosis, with and without ascites, and favors the opening of peripheral shunts (see Chapter 39).

Most of these investigations were conducted by venous occlusion plethysmography, although measurement of forearm blood flow with this technique is less sensitive than direct invasive techniques. In patients with alcoholic cirrhosis, forearm blood flow is increased and vascular resistance is decreased when compared to results in healthy subjects. Brachial infusion of N^G-monomethyl-L-arginine (L-NMMA), a nonselective NOS inhibitor, decreases forearm blood flow; the vasoconstrictor response is greater in decompensated than in compensated patients.

Release of NO and other vasoactive molecules in patients with cirrhosis results from circulating endotoxins. During cirrhosis, endotoxemia is a consequence of the loss of Kupffer cells and hepatocyte function as well as overgrowth of intestinal bacteria (100). Endotoxemia is indirectly responsible for splanchnic and peripheral vasodilation with hyperdynamic circulation (101). Endotoxemia may be the most important reason for overproduction of NO. In addition to endothelial cells, circulating neutrophils and monocytes can produce large amounts of NO. Administration of antibiotics in portal hypertensive rats did not improve the hyperdynamic circulation (102). Nevertheless, endotoxemia remains an important, though not exclusive, pathogenetic factor for splanchnic vasodilation (103).

Tumor necrosis factor-α (TNF-α) (see Chapter 41) may also induce hemodynamic derangement in portal hypertensive rats. Inhibition of TNF-α improves the hyperdynamic circulation and reduces NO production in decompensated cirrhotic rats (104).

DEFINITION OF REFRACTORY ASCITES, RENAL FUNCTIONAL IMPAIRMENT, AND HEPATORENAL SYNDROME

Refractory ascites is an accumulation of ascites, in spite of a sodium-restricted diet (40 mmol/d) and high doses of diuretics (400 mg/d of spironolactone plus 160 mg/d of furosemide). According to Arroyo et al. (105), there are two subtypes of refractory ascites:

■ diuretic-resistant ascites—significantly reduced or absent response to the treatment cited above; and
■ diuretic-intractable ascites—ascites that cannot be controlled due to complications induced by diuretics.

The progression from treatable to nontreatable ascites (refractory ascites) may be due to severity of liver disease, progressive increment in portal hypertension, progressive peripheral vasodilation with hyperdynamic circulation and decrease in EABV, imbalance of extrarenal and intrarenal vasoactive substances, including the prevailing activation of the RAAS, and/or progressive increase in sodium reabsorption in the proximal tubule.

The diuretic response depends on the Child-Pugh class in liver cirrhosis. Patients with alcoholic liver disease often have a spontaneous decrease in portal pressure and an improvement in diuretic responsiveness. Progression of decompensated cirrhosis is characterized by worsening in hemodynamics, increasing signs of hyperdynamic circulation, and reduced MAP. These phenomena are related to decreased EABV. Immersion of ascitic patients in warm water (head-out water immersion) provokes a greater increase in ANP serum levels and natriuresis when compared to results in control subjects. Patients who have overexpanded CBV and increased diuresis are considered hyperresponsive, whereas patients with greater hyperdynamic circulation have greater reduction in renal clearances and more elevated levels of PRA and aldosterone, and do not respond to immersion. The RAAS and SNS are more activated, whereas autocrine intrarenal systems appear less so and, to some extent, are exhausted in advanced liver disease, resulting in progressive prevalence of vasoconstricting factors over vasodilating ones. In this setting, sodium reabsorption in the proximal tubule becomes prominent, reducing the availability of sodium at Henle's loop and the distal tubuli, thus blunting the effect of antialdosterone diuretics. The continuous use of high doses of diuretics may independently decrease renal clearance and diuretic response.

RFI during cirrhosis is divided into two stages. The first stage is reversible, and may last for months in patients with cirrhosis who are decompensated. This stage corresponds to the second type of HRS and may be followed by a more severe renal impairment typical of HRS during which creatinemia and blood urea nitrogen (BUN) rapidly increase, and urine is practically sodium free. These types may occur sequentially (106).

The classic concept of RFI and HRS is based on the functional derangement of renal hemodynamics and the consequences of renal clearance. Such interpretation is principally based on the fact that when the kidney from a decompensated cirrhosis patient with renal dysfunction is transplanted to another patient, the kidney may show rapid recovery and reversal of vasoconstriction (107). However, in patients with HRS submitted to the liver transplantation, the recovery of renal function is often delayed and incomplete and prognosis is poorer (108).

The explanation for progression from RFI to open HRS is based on studies in humans in whom the activation of renal autocrine systems was followed by progressive exhaustion. During this final stage, vasodilating substances, such as PGs or PGI$_2$, progressively decrease, whereas vasocon-stricting substances, especially TxA$_2$ and LTs, are overpro-duced. The progressive prevalence of vasoconstricting fac-tors within the ischemic kidney may explain the final stage of irreversible vasoconstriction and progressive decrease in GFR, and sodium and water excretion. Thus, HRS is the last episode of a continuing functional derangement within the kidney without excluding the possibility of final renal tubular damage in the form of ATN.

Continuous administration of diuretics, often accompa-nied by antibiotics or other nephrotic agents, may also lead to pathologic alterations within the kidney. Mild alterations occur in the first stage. During HRS, frequent alterations occur at the tubular level. Renal biopsy in patients with cir-rhosis and HRS often reveals tubular degeneration and interstitial leukocyte infiltration, similar to that observed in patients with ATN (109). Since tubular damage may occur without modifications in urinary excretion, it is often diffi-cult to transfer from a functional to a pathologic complica-tion.

REFERENCES

1. Friedman MI. Hepatic nerve function. In: Arias IM, Jakoby WB, Popper H, et al., eds. *The liver: biology and pathobiology*, 2nd ed. New York: Raven Press, 1988:949–959.
2. Kostreva DR. Venous low-pressure baroreceptor reflexes arsing from the liver, spleen, mesenteric bed, and hindlimb veins. In: Epstein M, ed. *The kidney in liver disease*, 3rd ed. Baltimore: Williams and Wilkins, 1988:456–468.
3. Lang F, Ottl I, Haussinger D, et al. Renal hemodynamic response to intravenous and oral amino acids in animals. *Semin Nephrol* 1995;15:415–418.
4. Baertschi AJ, Vallet PG. Osmosensitivity of the portal vein area and vasopressin release in rats. *J Physiol (Lond)* 1981;315:217–230.
5. Adachi A, Niijima A, Jacobs HL. An hepatic osmoreceptor mechanism in the rat: electrophysiological and behavioural studies. *Am J Physiol* 1976;231:1043–1049.
6. Perlmutt JH, Azz O, Haberich FJ. A comparison of sodium excretion in response to infusion of isotonic saline into the vena porta and vena cava of conscious rats. *Pflugers Arch* 1975;357:1–14.
7. Andrews WHH, Orbach J. Sodium receptors activating some nerves of perfused rabbit livers. *Am J Physiol* 1974;227:1273–1275.
8. Tyryshkina EM, Ivanova LN, Finkinstein YaD, et al. Participa-tion of the liver receptors in the regulation of ion composition, osmolality and extracellular fluid volume. *Pflugers Arch* 1981;390:270–277.
9. Nishida Y, Sugimoto I, Morita H, et al. Suppression of renal sympathetic nerve activity during portal vein infusion of hyper-tonic saline. *Am J Physiol* 1998;274:R97–R103.
10. Nijima A. Afferent discharges from venous pressoreceptors in liver. *Am J Physiol* 1977;232:C76–C81.
11. Di Bona GF, Sawin LL. Hepatorenal baroreflex in cirrhotic rats. *Am J Physiol* 1995;269:G29–G33.
12. Lang F, Tschernko E, Schulze E, et al. Hepatorenal reflex regu-lating kidney function. *Hepatology* 1991;14:590–594.
13. Eknoyan G. Glomerular abnormalities in liver disease. In: Epstein M, ed. *The kidney in liver disease*, 4th ed. Philadelphia: Hanley & Belfus, 1996:123–150.
14. Axelsen RA, Crawford DH, Endre ZH, et al. Renal glomerular lesions in unselected patients with cirrhosis undergoing ortho-topic liver transplantation. *Pathology* 1995;27:237–246.
15. Altraif IH, Abdulla AS, Sebayel MI, et al. Hepatitis C associated glomerulonephritis. *Am J Nephrol* 1995;15:407–410.
16. Woodroffe AJ, Gormly AA, McKenzie PE, et al. Immunologic studies in IgA nephropathy. *Kidney Int* 1980;18:366–378.
17. Johnson RJ, Couser WG. Hepatitis B infection and renal dis-ease: clinical, immunopathogenic and therapeutic considera-tions. *Kidney Int* 1990;37:663–676.
18. Crawford DH, Endre ZH, Axelsen RA, et al. Universal occur-rence of glomerular abnormalities in patients receiving liver transplants. *Am J Kidney Dis* 1992;4:339–344.
19. Johnson RJ, Wilson R, Yamabe H, et al. Renal manifestations of hepatitis C virus infection. *Kidney Int* 1994;46:1255–1263.
20. D'Amico G, Colasanti G, Ferrario F, et al. Renal involvement in essential mixed cryoglobulinemia. *Kidney Int* 1989;35:1004–1014.
21. Couser WG, Johnson RJ. Postinfectious glomerulonephritis. In: Neilson EG, Couser WG, eds. *Immunological renal disease*. Philadelphia: Lippincott-Raven, 1997:915–943.
22. Johnson RJ, Gretch DR, Yamabe H, et al. Membranoprolifera-tive glomerulonephritis associated with hepatitis C virus infec-tion. *N Engl J Med* 1993;328:465–470.
23. Pasquariello A, Ferri C, Moriconi L, et al. Cryoglobulinemic membranoproliferative glomerulonephritis associated with hepatitis C virus. *Am J Nephrol* 1993;13:300–304.
24. Brunkhorst R, Klein V, Koch K. Recurrence of membranopro-liferative glomerulonephritis after renal transplantation in a patient with chronic hepatitis C. *Nephron* 1996;72:465–467.
25. Vlassopoulos D, Divari E, Savva S, et al. Membranous glomeru-lonephritis associated with primary biliary cirrhosis. *Nephrol Dial Transplant* 1998;13(2):459–461.
26. Allison ME, Moss MG, Fraser MM, et al. Renal function in chronic obstructive jaundice: a micropuncture study in rats. *Clin Sci Mol Med* 1978;54:649–659.
27. Oster JR, Perez GO. Derangements of acid-base homeostasis in liver disease. In: Epstein M, ed. *The kidney in liver disease*, 4th ed. Philadelphia: Hanley & Belfus, 1996:109–122.
28. Gentilini P, La Villa G, Romanelli RG, et al. Renal impairment in chronic liver disease with and without cholestasis. In: Gentilini P, Arias IM, McIntyre N, Rodes J, eds. *Cholestasis*. Amsterdam: Elsevier Science, 1994:213–226.
29. Golding PL, Smith M, Williams R. Multisystem involvement in chronic liver disease. Studies on the incidence and pathogenesis. *Am J Med* 1973;55:772–782.
30. Leu ML, Strickland GT. Renal tubular acidosis in Wilson's dis-ease: characteristics, mechanisms and implications. *Taiwan I Hsueh Hui Tsa Chih* 1977;76:829–842.
31. Parè P, Reynolds TB. Impaired renal acidification in alcoholic liver disease. *Arch Intern Med* 1984;144:941–944.
32. Caregaro L, Lauro S, Ricci G, et al. Distal renal tubular acido-sis in hepatic cirrhosis: clinical and pathogenetic study. *Clin Nephrol* 1981;15:143–147.
33. De Marchi S, Cecchin E, Basile A, et al. Renal tubular dys-function in chronic alcohol abuse—effects of abstinence. *N Engl J Med* 1993;329:1927–1934.
34. Tsantoulas DC, McFarlane IG, Portmann B, et al. Cell-medi-ated immunity to human Tamm–Horsfall glycoproteins in autoimmune liver disease with renal tubular acidosis. *Br Med J* 1974;1:527–530.
35. Makin AJ, Wendon J, Williams R. A 7-year experience of severe acetaminophen-induced hepatotoxicity (1987–1993). *Gastroen-terology* 1995;109:1907–1916.

36. Ellis AJ, Saleh M, Smith H, et al. Late-onset hepatic failure: clinical features, serology and outcome following transplantation. *J Hepatol* 1995;23:363–372.

37. Ellis AJ, O'Grady JG. Clinical disorders of renal function in acute liver failure. In: Arroyo V, Ginès P, Rodés P, et al., eds. *Ascites and renal dysfunction in liver disease.* Oxford: Blackwell Scientific, 1999:63–78.

38. Gentilini P, Laffi G, Buzzelli G, et al. Renal functional impairment and sodium retention in liver cirrhosis. *Digestion* 1980;20:73–78.

39. Platt JF, Marn CS, Baliga PK, et al. Renal dysfunction in hepatic disease: early identification with renal duplex Doppler ultrasonography in patients who undergo liver transplantation. *Radiology* 1992;183:801–806.

40. Maroto A, Ginès A, Salò J, et al. Diagnosis of functional kidney failure of cirrhosis with Doppler sonography: prognostic value of resistive index. *Hepatology* 1994;20:839–844.

41. Gentilini P, Laffi G, La Villa G, et al. Long course and prognostic factors of virus-induced cirrhosis of the liver. *Am J Gastroenterol* 1997;92:66–72.

42. Pinzani M, Failli P, Ruocco C, et al. Fat-storing cells as liver-specific pericytes. Spatial dynamics of agonist-stimulated intracellular calcium transients. *J Clin Invest* 1992;90:642–646.

43. Rockey DC. The cellular pathogenesis of portal hypertension: stellate cell contractility, endothelin, and nitric oxide. *Hepatology* 1997;25:2–5.

44. Pinzani M, Gentilini P. Biology of the hepatic stellate cells and their possible relevance in the pathogenesis of portal hypertension in cirrhosis. *Semin Liver Dis* 1999;19:397–410.

45. Kowalski JF, Abelman WH. The cardiac output at rest in Laennec's cirrhosis. *J Clin Invest* 1953;32:1025–1033.

46. Schrier RW, Arroyo V, Bernardi M, et al. Peripheral arteriolar vasodilation hypothesis: a proposal for the initiation of renal sodium and water retention in cirrhosis. *Hepatology* 1988;8:1151–1157.

47. Laffi G, Pinzani M, Meacci E, et al. Renal hemodynamic and natriuretic effects of human atrial natriuretic factor infusion in cirrhosis with ascites. *Gastroenterology* 1989;96:167–177.

48. La Villa G, Asbert M, Jimenez W, et al. Natriuretic hormone activity in the urine of cirrhotic patients. *Hepatology* 1990;12:467–475.

49. Ginès P, Jimenez W, Arroyo V, et al. Atrial natriuretic factor in cirrhosis with ascites. Plasma levels, cardiac release and splanchnic extraction. *Hepatology* 1988;8:636–642.

50. Unikowsky B, Wexler MJ, Levy M. Dogs with experimental cirrhosis of the liver but without intrahepatic hypertension do not retain sodium or form ascites. *J Clin Invest* 1983;72:1594–1604.

51. Lewis FW, Adair O, Rector WG Jr. Arterial vasodilation is not the cause of increased cardiac output in cirrhosis. *Gastroenterology* 1992;102:1024–1029.

52. Laffi G, Barletta G, La Villa G, et al. Altered cardiovascular responsiveness to active tilting in nonalcoholic cirrhosis. *Gastroenterology* 1997;113:891–898.

53. Wong F, Liu P, Tobe S, et al. Central blood volume in cirrhosis: measurement by radionuclide angiography. *Hepatology* 1994;19:312–321.

54. Wong F, Liu P, Allidina Y, et al. Pattern and consequences of sodium handling in preascitic cirrhosis. *Gastroenterology* 1995;108:1820–1827.

55. Epstein M, Levinson R, Sancho J. Characterisation of the renin-aldosterone system in decompensated cirrhosis. *Circ Res* 1997;41:818–829.

56. Levy M. Pathophysiology of ascites formation. In: Epstein M, ed. *The kidney in liver disease,* 4th ed. Philadelphia: Hanley & Belfus, 1996:179–220.

57. Tanaka K, Matsuda T, Morita H, et al. Depressed sensitivity of

58. the hepatoportal NaCl receptors in rats in carbon tetrachloride-induced cirrhosis. *Am J Physiol* 1995;R1390–R1395.

58. Pinzani M, Marra F, Fusco BM, et al. Evidence for α1-adrenoceptor hyperresponsiveness in hypotensive cirrhotic patients with ascites. *Am J Gastroenterol* 1991;86:711–714.

59. Vorobioff J, Bredfeldt JE, Groszmann R. Hyperdynamic circulation in portal hypertensive rat model: a primary factor for maintenance of chronic portal hypertension. *Am J Physiol* 1983;244:G652–G657.

60. Epstein M, Berk DP, Hollenberg NK, et al. Renal failure in the patient with cirrhosis. The role of active vasoconstriction. *Am J Med* 1970;49:175–185.

61. Gentilini P, Laffi G, Stefani P, et al. Early functional modifications of the kidney in chronic active hepatitis. In: Gentilini P, Popper H, Teodori U, eds. *Chronic hepatitis.* Basil: Karger, 1976:69–76.

62. Lagi A, La Villa G, Barletta G, et al. Cerebral autoregulation in cirrhotic patients with ascites. A transcranial doppler study. *J Hepatol* 1997;27:114–120.

63. Grose RD, Nolan J, Dillon JF, et al. Exercise-induced left ventricular dysfunction in alcoholic and non-alcoholic cirrhosis. *J Hepatol* 1995;26:326–332.

64. Gentilini P, Laffi G, Fantini F, et al. Systemic haemodynamics and renal function in cirrhotic patients during plasma volume expansion. *Digestion* 1983;27:138–145.

65. Bernardi M, Rubboli A, Trevisan F, et al. Systemic haemodynamics and renal function in cirrhotic patients during plasma volume expansion. *Digestion* 1983;27:138–145.

66. Trevisani F, Sica G, Mainquà P, et al. Autonomic dysfunction and hyperdynamic circulation in cirrhosis with ascites. *Hepatology* 1999;30:1387–1392.

67. Gentilini P, Laffi G. Pathophysiology and treatment of ascites and the hepatorenal syndrome. *Baillieres Clin Gastroenterol* 1992;3:581–607.

68. Goodfriend TL, Elliott ME, Catt KJ. Angiotensin receptors and their antagonists. *N Engl J Med* 1996;334:1649–1654.

69. Gentilini P, Romanelli RG, La Villa G, et al. Effects of low-dose captopril on renal hemodynamics and function in patients with cirrhosis of the liver. *Gastroenterology* 1993;104:588–594.

70. Wong F, Liu P, Aliidina Y, et al. The effect of posture on central blood volume in patients with preascitic cirrhosis on a sodium-restricted diet. *Hepatology* 1996;23:1141–1147.

71. Gentilini P, Casini-Raggi V, Di Fiore G, et al. Albumin improves the response to diuretics in patients with cirrhosis and ascites: result of a randomized, controlled trial. *J Hepatol* 1999;30:646–652.

72. Epstein M. Renal effects to head-out water immersion in humans: a 15-year update. *Physiol Rev* 1992;72:563–621.

73. Bernardi M, Fornale L, Di Marco C, et al. Hyperdynamic circulation of advanced cirrhosis: a re-appraisal based on posture induced changes in nonalcoholic cirrhosis. *J Hepatol* 1995;22:309–318.

74. Vaamonde C. Renal water handling in liver disease. In: Epstein M, ed. *The kidney in liver disease,* 4th ed. Philadelphia: Hanley & Belfus, 1996:33–74.

75. Aki Y, Tamaki T, Kiyomoto H, et al. Nitric oxide may participate in V2 vasopressin-receptor-mediated renal vasodilation. *J Cardiovasc Pharmacol* 1994;23:331–336.

76. Bosch-Marce M, Jimenez W, Angeli P, et al. Aquaretic effect of the k-opioid agonist RU 51599 in cirrhotic rats with ascites and water retention. *Gastroenterology* 1995;109:217–233.

77. Lebrec D, Giuily N, Hadengue A, et al. Transjugular intrahepatic portosystemic shunts: comparison with paracentesis in patients with cirrhosis and refractory ascites: a randomized trial. French Group of Clinicians and a Group of Biologists. *J Hepatol* 1996;25:135–144.

78. Abraham WT, Lauwaars ME, Kim JK, et al. Reversal of atrial natriuretic peptide resistance by increasing distal tubular sodium delivery in patients with decompensated cirrhosis. *Hepatology* 1995;22:737–743.
79. Moller S, Bendtsen F, Henriksen JH. Effects of volume expansion on systemic hemodynamics and central and arterial blood volume in cirrhosis. *Gastroenterology* 1995;109:1917–1925.
80. La Villa G, Riccardi D, Lazzeri C, et al. Blunted natriuretic response to low-dose natriuretic peptide infusion in nonazotemic cirrhotic patients with ascites and avid sodium retention. *Hepatology* 1995;22:1745–1750.
81. Amin J, Carretero OA, Ito S. Mechanisms of action of atrial natriuretic factor and C-type natriuretic peptide. *Hypertension* 1996;27:684–687.
82. Komeicki H, Moreau R, Cailmail S, et al. Blunted natriuresis and abnormal systemic hemodynamic responses to C-type and brain natriuretic peptides in rats with cirrhosis. *J Hepatol* 1995;22:319–325.
83. Wong F, Blendis LM. Natriuretic peptides: are these new links in the hepatorenal connections? *Gut* 1997;40:151–152.
84. Guevara M, Ginès P, Jimenez W, et al. Increased adrenomedullin levels in cirrhosis: relationship with hemodynamic abnormalities and vasoconstrictor systems. *Gastroenterology* 1998;114:336–343.
85. Fernandez-Rodriguez CM, Prada IR, Prieto J, et al. Circulating adrenomedullin in cirrhosis: relationship to hyperdynamic circulation. *J Hepatol* 1998;29:250–256.
86. Kojima H, Tsujimoto T, Uemura M, et al. Significance of increased plasma adrenomedullin concentration in patients with cirrhosis. *J Hepatol* 1998;28:840–846.
87. Elhawary AM, Pang CC. Renal vascular and tubular actions of calcitonin gene-related peptide: effect of NG-nitro-L-arginine methyl ester. *J Pharmacol Exp Ther* 1995;273:56–63.
88. Salo J, Jimenez W, Kuhn M, et al. Urinary excretion of urodilatin in patients with cirrhosis. *Hepatology* 1996;24:1428–1432.
89. Laffi G, La Villa G, Pinzani M, et al. Lipid-derived autocoids and renal function in liver cirrhosis. In: Epstein M, ed. *The kidney in liver disease.* Philadelphia: Hanley & Belfus, 1996:307–337.
90. Gentilini P. Cirrhosis, renal function and NSAIDs. *J Hepatol* 1993;19:200–203.
91. Gentilini P, Laffi G, Meacci E, et al. Effects of OKY 046, a thromboxane-synthase inhibitor, on renal function in nonazotemic cirrhotic patients with ascites. *Gastroenterology* 1988;94:1470–1477.
92. Chan L, Chittinandana A, Shapiro JL, et al. Effect of an endothelin-receptor antagonist on ischemic acute renal failure. *Am J Physiol* 1994;266:F135–F138.
93. Vane JR, Anggard EE, Botting RM. Regulatory function of the vascular endothelium. *N Engl J Med* 1990;323:27–36.
94. Guevara M, Ginès P, Fernandez-Esparrach G, et al. Reversibility of hepatorenal syndrome by prolonged administration of ornipressin and plasma volume expansion. *Hepatology* 1998;27:35–41.
95. Guevara M, Ginès P, Bandi JC, et al. Transjugular intrahepatic portosystemic shunt in hepatorenal syndrome: effects on renal function and vasoactive systems. *Hepatology* 1998;28:416–422.
96. Laffi G, Foschi M, Masini E, et al. Increased production of nitric oxide by neutrophils and monocytes from cirrhotic patients with ascites and hyperdynamic circulation. *Hepatology* 1999;522:1666–1673.
97. Bandi JC, Fernàndez M, Bernadich C, et al Hyperkinetic circulation and decreased sensitivity to vasoconstrictors following portacaval shunt in the rat. Effects of chronic nitric oxide inhibition. *J Hepatol* 1999;31:719–724.
98. Gupta TKTM, Chung MK. Endothelial dysfunction in the intrahepatic microcirculation of cirrhotic rats. *Hepatology* 1998;28:926–931.
99. Guarner C, Soriano G, Tomas A, et al. Increased serum nitrite and nitrate levels in patients with cirrhosis: relationship to endotoxemia. *Hepatology* 1993;18:1139–1143.
100. Guarner C, Runyon BA, Young S, et al. Intestinal bacterial overgrowth and bacterial translocation in cirrhotic rats with ascites. *J Hepatol* 1997;26:1372–1378.
101. Martin PY, Ginès P, Schrier RW. Nitric oxide as a mediator of hemodynamic abnormalities and sodium and water retention in cirrhosis. *N Engl J Med* 1998;339:533–541.
102. Chu CJ, Lee FY, Wang SS, et al. Evidence against a role for endotoxin in the hyperdynamic circulation of rats with prehepatic portal hypertension. *J Gastroenterol Hepatol* 1999;11:152–158.
103. Van de Castelle M, Hösli M, Sägesser H, et al. Intraportal administration of glyceryl trinitrate or nitroprusside exerts more systemic intrahepatic effects in anaesthetised cirrhotic rats. *J Hepatol* 1999;31:300–305.
104. Lopez-Talavera JC, Levitzki A, Martinez M, et al. Tyrosine kinase inhibition ameliorates the hyperdynamic state and decreases nitric oxide production in cirrhotic rats with portal hypertension and ascites. *J Clin Invest* 1997;100:664–670.
105. Arroyo V, Ginès P, Gerbes AL, et al. Definition and diagnostic criteria of refractory ascites and hepatorenal syndrome in cirrhosis. International Ascites Club. *Hepatology* 1996;23:164–176.
106. Gentilini P, Laffi G, La Villa G, et al. Ascites and hepatorenal syndrome during cirrhosis: two entities or the continuation of the same complication? *J Hepatol* 1999;31:1088–1097.
107. Iwatsuki S, Corman J, Popovtzer M, et al. Recovery from hepatorenal syndrome after orthotopic liver transplantation. *N Engl J Med* 1973;289:1155–1159.
108. Gonwa TA, Morris CA, Goldstein RM, et al. Long-term survival and renal function following liver transplantation in patients with and without hepatorenal syndrome—experience in 300 patients. *Transplantation* 1991;51:428–430.
109. Gentilini P. Hepatorenal syndrome: differential diagnosis and therapy. In: Schmid R, Gerok W, Bianchi L, et al., eds. *Extrahepatic manifestation in liver diseases.* Falk Symposium 69. Dordrecht: Kluwer Academic, 1993:193–212.

The Liver: Biology and Pathobiology, Fourth Edition, edited by I. M. Arias, J. L. Boyer, F. V. Chisari, N. Fausto, D. Schachter, and D. A. Shafritz. Lippincott Williams & Wilkins, Philadelphia © 2001.

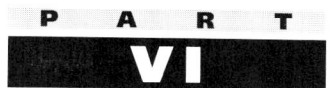

PATHOBIOLOGIC ANALYSIS

MOLECULAR PATHOPHYSIOLOGY OF MEMBRANE TRANSPORT FUNCTION IN CHOLESTASIS

JAMES L. BOYER

Advances in understanding the pathophysiology of cholestasis have progressed rapidly since expression and positional cloning have identified many of the major genes that encode for the transport proteins that produce bile. The major membrane transport systems that result in the formation of bile are illustrated in Figure 46.1, and their functions are briefly summarized in Table 46.1. The molecular basis of bile formation is reviewed in Chapters 24, 25, and 27 and website chapters 🖳 W-22 through W-24, and is the subject of several reviews (1–3).

In general, cholestasis results from defects in the regulation and expression of the membrane transporters that generate bile secretion and from cellular events that impair signal transduction pathways, cytoskeletal structures, tight and gap junctional proteins and the targeting of intracellular vesicles. This chapter focuses primarily on defects in membrane transporters in hepatocytes and cholangiocytes that contribute to the pathogenesis of cholestatic liver disease and is based on experimental work with animal models of cholestasis and on discoveries of the genetic basis of several hereditary and acquired human cholestatic disorders (Table 46.2) (see Chapter 26).

EXPERIMENTAL MODELS AND HEREDITARY CHOLESTATIC DISORDERS

Much information has been obtained through the use of several experimental models in rats that resemble acquired cholestatic disorders in humans. Several animal models where the genes have either been knocked out or spontaneously mutated, as well as the discovery of the genetic basis of several rare hereditary disorders of cholestasis, have provided the most direct evidence for the critical role that specific transport proteins play in the production of bile and the pathogenesis of cholestasis. Animal models that are most frequently used to study acquired cholestatic disorders are listed in Table 46.3. Models that result in acquired disturbances of transport systems in hepatocytes and cholan-

J. L. Boyer: Department of Internal Medicine and Liver Center, Yale University School of Medicine, New Haven, Connecticut 06520-8019; and Department of Medicine, Yale New Haven Hospital, New Haven, Connecticut 06510.

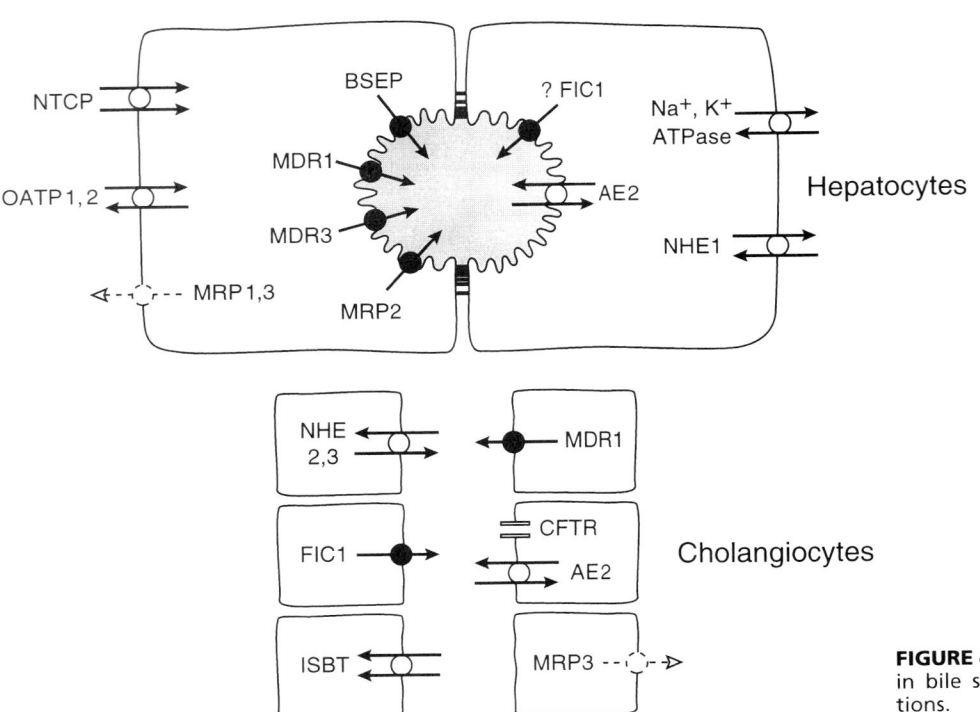

FIGURE 46.1. Location of major transporters in bile secretion. See Table 46.1 for definitions.

TABLE 46.1. NOMENCLATURE, LOCATION, AND FUNCTION OF THE MAJOR HEPATOCYTE AND CHOLANGIOCYTE MEMBRANE TRANSPORTERS INVOLVED IN BILE SECRETION

Name	Abbreviation	Location	Function
Chloride-bicarbonate anion exchanger isoform 2	AE2	Canalicular membrane	Acid loader-excretes bicarbonate into bile and stimulates bile flow independent of bile salts
Sodium-taurocholate cotransporter	NTCP	Basolateral membrane of hepatocytes	Primary carrier for conjugated bile-salt uptake from portal blood
Organic-anion–transporting polypeptides	OATP (1,2)	Basolateral membrane of hepatocytes	Broad substrate carriers for sodium-independent uptake of bile salts, organic anions, and other amphipathic organic solutes from portal blood
Multidrug-resistance-1 P-glycoprotein[a]	MDR1	Canalicular and cholangiocyte apical membrane	ATP-dependent excretion of various organic cations, xenobiotics, and cytotoxins into bile; barrier function in cholangiocytes
Multidrug-resistance-3 P-glycoprotein (phospholipid export pump)[a]	MDR3	Canalicular membrane	ATP-dependent translocation of phosphatidylcholine from inner to outer leaflet of membrane bilayer
Multidrug-resistance-associated protein (canalicular multispecific organic-anion transporter)[a]	MRP2 (cMOAT)	Canalicular membrane	Mediates ATP-dependent multispecific organic-anion transport (e.g., bilirubin diglucuronide) into bile; contributes to bile-salt–independent bile flow by GSH transport
Canalicular bile-salt-export pump[a] (sister of P-glycoprotein)	BSEP (SPGP)	Canalicular membrane	ATP-dependent bile-salt transport into bile; stimulates bile salt dependent bile flow
Cystic fibrosis transmembrane regulator[a]	CFTR	Apical (luminal) membrane of cholangiocyte	Chloride channel; facilitates chloride entry into bile
Chloride-bicarbonate anion exchanger isoform 2	AE2	Apical (luminal) membrane of cholangiocyte	Facilitates bicarbonate secretion into bile and contributes to bile flow independent of bile salts
Familial intrahepatic cholestasis-1	FIC1	Apical membrane of cholangiocyte and intestine, also expressed in canalicular membrane	A P-type ATPase that may function as an aminophospholipid transferase
Ileal sodium dependent bile salt transporter	ISBT	Apical membrane of cholangiocyte and intestine	Primary carrier for sodium dependent bile salt uptake from intestine by ileum and cholangiocytes
Multidrug-resistance–associated protein-3[a]	MRP3	Basolateral membrane of hepatocytes and cholangiocytes	Expression induced in cholestasis. Transports all bile salts and may facilitate their cholehepatic shunting

[a]These transporters are members of the ATP-binding cassette family.

TABLE 46.2. HEREDITARY AND ACQUIRED MOLECULAR CHANGES OF HEPATOCELLULAR TRANSPORT SYSTEMS IN HUMANS

Disease	Molecular Change
Hereditary:	
Progressive familial intrahepatic cholestasis (PFIC)	
PFIC-1 (low γ-GT)	Mutation of *FIC1* gene (chromosome 18q21–22); low γ-GT
PFIC-2 (low γ-GT)	Mutation of *BSEP* gene (chromosome 2q24); low γ-GT
PFIC-3 (high γ-GT)	Canalicular BSEP protein absent.
	Mutation of *MDR3* gene (chromosome 7q21); high γ-GT.
	Canalicular MDR3 protein absent
Benign recurrent intrahepatic cholestasis (BRIC)	Mutation of *FIC1* gene (chromosome 18q21–22)
Dubin–Johnson syndrome	Mutation of *MRP2* gene (10q23–24).
	Canalicular MRP2 protein absent.
Acquired:	
Primary biliary cirrhosis	AE2 mRNA and protein reduced; hepatocytes and cholangiocytes are affected. MDR3 mRNA levels unchanged.
Extrahepatic biliary atresia	NTCP mRNA reduced. Inverse correlation with serum bilirubin levels; increase after successful Kasai procedure. BSEP protein maintained at canalicular membrane.
Primary sclerosing cholangitis	OATP mRNA increased, possibly diminishing hepatic retention of organic anions.
Extrahepatic biliary obstruction	MDR1 and MDR3 mRNA increased. Direct correlation with serum bilirubin levels.

giocytes include common bile duct ligation (CBDL) and administration of α-napthlyisothiocyanate (ANIT) in rats as a model of obstructive cholestasis associated with proliferation of cholangiocytes; estrogen (ethinyl estradiol) (EE) treatment as an example of cholestasis of pregnancy and pill-induced cholestasis; and administration of lipopolysaccharide (LPS) as a model of cholestasis of sepsis. References to these models can be found elsewhere (3,4). Several genetically altered rat and mouse models have also been of interest, including the TR-/Gronigen/EHBR rat as a model of Mrp2 deficiency and knockout mouse models where several other transporters have been deleted. Genetically altered animal models will be used increasingly in the future.

HEREDITARY DEFECTS IN BILE TRANSPORT PROTEINS

Hepatocytes

Progressive Familial Intrahepatic Cholestasis

Advances in positional cloning have led to the discovery of the genes that are mutated in several familial disorders of cholestasis. These progressive familial intrahepatic cholestatic disorders (PFICs) are also reviewed in greater detail elsewhere (Chapters 24 and 26). Although rare diseases, their phenotypes provide proof of principle for the important role that specific transport proteins play in the production of bile and the development of cholestatic liver injury. Table 46.2 summarizes these disorders, including the specific genes involved and their chromosome location. PFIC-1, also known as Byler's disease, results from mutations in *FIC1*, a gene that encodes for a P-type ATPase that functions as an aminophospholipid transferase in other cell types (5). The gene is highly expressed in the intestine and also the cholangiocyte. However, it remains to be determined how mutations in this gene can account for cholestasis in both PFIC-1 and benign recurrent cholestasis in the adult. PFIC-2 results from mutations in the canalicular membrane bile salt export pump (*BSEP*), formerly known as the sister of P-glycoprotein, and provides compelling evidence for the importance of this member of the ATP binding cassette gene family in determining bile salt-dependent bile flow (6–8). More then ten mutations have been described in families with this familial disorder (7). PFIC-3

TABLE 46.3. EXPERIMENTAL MODELS OF CHOLESTATIC LIVER DISEASE

Model	Clinical Correlates
Common bile duct ligation in the rat (CBDL)	Extrahepatic bile duct obstruction; biliary atresia; vanishing bile duct
α-napthyl isothiocyanate administration in the rat (ANIT)	Extrahepatic bile duct obstruction with bile duct proliferation
Ethinyl estradiol administration in the rat (EE)	Cholestasis of pregnancy; contraceptive pill-induced cholestasis
Lipopolysaccharide administration in the rat (LPS)	Cholestasis of sepsis
Mdr2 knockout mouse	MDR3 mutations (PFIC-3)
Bile salt export pump knockout mouse	BSEP mutations (PFIC-2)
Ferrochelatase knockout mouse	Erythropoietic protoporphyria
TR-/Gronigen/Eisai hyperbilirubinemic rat (EHBR)	MRP2 deficiency/Dubin–Johnson syndrome

results from mutations in *MDR3*, which encodes for a phospholipid flippase (9,10). The knockout mouse of the MDR homologue, Mdr2, is unable to excrete phospholipid into bile (11). In the absence of biliary phospholipids, bile salts do not form mixed micelles in bile and thus their detergent properties are unbuffered (12–15). Over time, damage to the lipid membranes in the cholangiocytes results in the development of biliary fibrosis and cirrhosis. Heterozygotes in Mdr2(−/−) mice have a partial deficiency in phospholipid excretion and are phenotypically normal. Mothers of MDR3 homozygous-deficient children with PFIC-3 also have normal phenotypes but can develop cholestasis of pregnancy when exposed to increasing levels of estrogens as the pregnancy develops (16).

Cholangiocytes

Cystic Fibrosis

Mutations in *CFTR* can result in cholestatic liver injury. CFTR is normally expressed on the luminal membrane of cholangiocytes, where it functions as a chloride channel to secrete chloride (17). Defects in CFTR may result in an impaired secretory response to hormones such as secretin, VIP and bombesin which normally stimulate bicarbonate excretion via a chloride/bicarbonate anion exchanger (AE2) that is dependent on a chloride channel to recycle chloride across the luminal membrane of the cholangiocyte (18).

Alagille's Syndrome

Mutations in the gene *JAGGED*1, which encodes for an unknown ligand of the notch receptor, result in a cholestatic disorder known as Alagille's syndrome, manifested by a number of developmental defects including hypoplasia of the interlobular bile ducts (19,20). The notch receptor is important in the differentiation of tissues during development.

ACQUIRED DEFECTS IN BILE TRANSPORT PROTEINS — GENERAL OVERVIEW

The molecular characterization of transport systems that determine the formation of bile has made it possible to assess their responses to cholestatic liver injury at the genetic level. Although the picture is still incomplete, a common pattern of expression has begun to emerge. Results obtained from cholestatic animal models as well as human cholestatic liver disorders suggest that the expression of specific membrane transporters adapts to a variety of forms of cholestatic liver injury in a manner that tends to diminish the hepatic uptake of bile salts from portal blood, while at the same time maintaining or in some instances upregulating mechanisms that may help to facilitate the exit of bile salts and other toxic substances from hepatocytes (3). Thus, transport proteins on the

basolateral sinusoidal membrane which normally function to selectively remove bile salts and other cholephiles from portal blood are usually downregulated during cholestatic liver injury, in some instances by transcriptional and in others by posttranscriptional mechanisms. In contrast, some canalicular transport proteins, particularly the Mdr homologues, are either not severely impaired or may actually be upregulated; these include Mdr1, Bsep/BSEP and Mdr2 (21–23). These later findings suggest that the cholestatic hepatocyte attempts to maintain canalicular export function. Furthermore, Mrp1 and MRP3/Mrp3, homologues of Mrp2 that are expressed at the sinusoidal membrane at low levels in normal liver, are substantially upregulated in Mrp2-deficient and bile duct-ligated rats and may facilitate the removal of hydrophobic bile salts and other products from the cholestatic hepatocyte (24–26).

Less is known concerning molecular responses in cholangiocytes during cholestasis. However, bile duct proliferation is characteristic of many cholestatic disorders, particularly those that result in both intrahepatic and extrahepatic bile duct obstruction. The ileal sodium-dependent bile salt transporter (Isbt) is also located on the luminal membrane of cholangiocytes, and there is evidence that this cholangiocyte transporter can function to remove bile salts from bile (27,28). Since the cholestatic hepatocyte continues to excrete bile salts, albeit at a reduced rate, Isbt could function to remove bile salts from an obstructed cholestatic biliary tree. MRP3 is also located on the blood side of the cholangiocyte and is upregulated in the cholestatic liver (25,29). MRP3/Mrp3 is capable of transporting bile salts and might function to return bile salts to the systemic circulation during cholestasis (26,29,30). Mrp3 has a particularly high affinity for sulfated bile salts, and sulfated bile salt conjugates are formed in the cholestatic liver (26). Recent studies suggest that renal bile salt transporters may also undergo adaptive regulation in animal models of cholestasis, resulting in diminished reabsorption of bile acids from the glomerular filtrate, thereby facilitating an extrahepatic pathway for the disposal of bile salts (31). Thus, a pattern of adaptive regulatory responses in organic anion transporter expression is emerging in several different tissues including the liver, biliary epithelial cells and kidney that can be interpreted as an attempt to mitigate tissue damage from the retention of bile salts.

These responses in gene expression are reviewed in more detail below.

TRANSPORTERS ON THE BASOLATERAL MEMBRANE OF THE HEPATOCYTE

Ion Transporters: (Na⁺/K⁺-ATPase and Na⁺/H⁺ Exchange)

Several major ion transport proteins are located on the basolateral membrane and regulate important homeostatic housekeeping functions in the hepatocyte, including maintenance of cell volume and intracellular pH. These transporters include Na^+K^+-ATPase, and the Na^+/H^+ exchanger–isoform 1 (NHE-1). Although many cholestatic agents have been shown to inhibit the sodium pump *in vitro*, the molecular expression of the sodium pump is not only unimpaired but is actually upregulated in several animal models of cholestasis (32–35). This adaptive response could result from an attempt to counteract increased sodium entry and cell swelling that may result from the detergent properties of retained bile salts.

Na^+/H^+ exchange is also upregulated at both transcriptional and posttranscriptional levels following common bile duct ligation in the rat, resulting in an increase in intracellular pH. This response may also contribute to sodium entry and cell swelling in the cholestatic liver (36).

Organic Anion Transporters (NTCP/Ntcp, Oatps/OATPs, Mrps/MRPS)

NTCP/ntcp

Ntcp and its human homologue NTCP are the major determinant of the selective hepatic uptake of conjugated bile salts from the portal circulation and are substantially downregulated in cholestasis (21,32–35,37,38). Transcription of Ntcp is impaired in the bile duct-obstructed rat, and the protein disappears rapidly from the sinusoidal membrane throughout the hepatic lobule (32). NTCP mRNA has also been evaluated in patients with biliary atresia and is diminished. However, NTCP mRNA increases toward normal values if biliary drainage is restored by a successful portoenterostomy (Kasai procedure) (39). Levels of hepatic NTCP mRNA correlate inversely with the level of the total serum bilirubin in these patients, a finding also observed for Ntcp mRNA in the bile duct-obstructed rat model (32). In the rat model, retention of biliary constituents, but not the depletion of bile, regulates mRNA levels of Ntcp (37).

Significant progress has been made in understanding the transcriptional regulation of Ntcp. The promoter region of *Ntcp* in the rat contains several regulatory response elements including binding regions for the transactivators, HNF1 and retinoid receptors (RXR) (40,41). Several additional upstream regions are involved in cytokine responses. Cholestasis produced by administration of endotoxin (LPS) results in loss of HNF1 and footprint B, a previously uncharacterized binding protein, now identified as an RXRa:RARa heterodimer (41), which decreases Ntcp expression that parallels the reductions in bile flow (38). LPS also results in a release of cytokines (TNF-α and IL-1β) that may contribute to the diminished Ntcp expression (35). The hepatic retention of bile salts would also be expected to influence the expression of transporters like Ntcp if they interact with other nuclear receptors such as the farsenoid X receptor (FXR), which is a bile salt response

element (41–44). Although impairment of Ntcp and NTCP can explain the reduced Na^+-dependent uptake of conjugated bile salts, sodium-independent mechanisms for hepatic bile salt uptake persist due to the continued expression of several other sinusoidal membrane organic anion transporters (45).

Oatp1,2, Lst1/OATP1,2

Organic anion transporting polypeptides represent a growing family of transporters with broad substrate specificity that are capable of translocating a wide range of organic anions, including unconjugated and conjugated bile salts, bulky organic cations and even certain uncharged organic substrates (46–54). These proteins (Oatps) appear to function as anion exchangers, exchanging the extracellular anion with either intracellular bicarbonate or glutathione (55,56). Several of these liver Oatp homologues are expressed in other tissues as well, including the brain and renal epithelium (52,57–60). However, human OATP2 and its rat homologue, Lst1 (also known as Oatp4) (51), are specifically expressed only in hepatic parenchymal cells (49,53,54). Several cholestatic animal models have been used to evaluate the expression of Oatp1, Oatp2 and the liver-specific Lst1 (51). CBDL, EE and LPS all result in downregulation of Oatp1, although mRNA levels remain unchanged after EE treatment, suggesting that the mechanism of EE cholestasis is mainly posttranscriptional (22,34,61,62). Oatp2, which is expressed predominantly in the brain and in lower amounts in the liver, is not reduced by CBDL in the rat (61). However, the liver-specific Lst1 (Oatp-4) is markedly diminished after CBDL and in a rat model of sepsis (51). Nevertheless, functional studies indicate that sodium-independent bile salt uptake is relatively unaffected in these animal models (45). Studies in patients with sclerosing cholangitis suggest that OATP1 mRNA expression is actually increased, raising the possibility that OATP1 can function to extrude organic anions from the cholestatic human hepatocyte (63). Thus, at present it is not possible to generalize about the functional role of changes in the molecular expression of Oatp/OATPs in cholestasis.

Mrp1,3/MRP1/MRP3

Mrp1 and 3 are homologues of the canalicular membrane multidrug-resistant associated protein Mrp2 and are only expressed at very low levels at the basolateral membrane in normal liver (64,65). However, Mrp1, Mrp-like proteins (66) and Mrp3 are upregulated during cholestasis produced by LPS and bile duct ligation in the rat (22,29,67). Human MRP3 has also been located on the basolateral membrane of cholangiocytes in addition to the hepatocyte (25,29), and its expression is increased in both the Dubin–Johnson syndrome, where canalicular MRP2 is genetically absent (24) and in a patient with primary biliary cirrhosis (PBC) (24). Mrp3 is also upregulated in the Eisai hyperbilirubinemic rat (67). These observations suggest that Mrp3 and MRP3 might function to facilitate the efflux of substrates normally extruded into bile by Mrp2/MRP2. Divalent organic anions such as sulfated and glucuronide bile salt conjugates are high-affinity substrates for this MRP homologue (64). Functional expression of Mrp3 in LLC–PK1 cells indicate that Mrp3 has the highest affinity for sulfated bile salts compared to other conjugated bile salts (26). Since sulfated bile salt conjugates are synthesized in the liver when it becomes cholestatic, it seems likely that basolateral Mrps/MRPs in hepatocytes and cholangiocytes may be upregulated to function as efflux pumps during cholestasis. Several other MRPs have been described in human liver (MRP4-6), but their function remains to be determined (65,68,69).

TRANSPORTERS ON THE CANALICULAR MEMBRANE OF THE HEPATOCYTE (Mdr1A,B/MDR1, Mdr2/MDR3, Mrp2/MRP2, Bsep/BSEP)

While the downregulation of basolateral transporters that function as hepatic uptake mechanisms in the hepatocyte can be viewed as adaptive responses that retard the accumulation of potential toxic substrates, hepatic levels of bile acids and other choliphiles continue to accumulate in the cholestatic liver. Furthermore, the canalicular excretion of these substrates by the bile export pumps is rate-limiting in the overall process of clearance from blood to bile. Thus it is likely that the regulation of the expression of these important export pumps is a major determinant of the molecular response to cholestatic liver injury and determines the cholestatic phenotype.

Canalicular Organic Solute Transporters

Mdr1a,b/MDR1

The multidrug-resistant gene *MDR* encodes for the drug efflux pump P-glycoprotein 170 (Pgp-170). In contrast to most of the transport systems for the hepatic uptake of organic substrates, cholestasis results in a significant upregulation of Pgp-170 in both animal models and humans. CBDL (23,70,71), LPS (22,70), and ANIT (23) all increase the expression of Mdr1a/b mRNA, and the level of expression correlates with the severity of the cholestasis as reflected by the levels of plasma bilirubin and alkaline phosphatase (23). The expression of Mdr1a/b is also increased in models of liver regeneration (72). Similar findings are reported for MDR1 mRNA levels in biopsies from patients with bile duct obstruction (73). Although it is known that several exogenous stimuli such as heat shock, UV light, chemotherapeutic agents and carcinogens increase the transcription of the Mdr1 gene promoter (72), the factor(s) that

regulate the transcription of this gene in cholestatic liver remain to be identified. Upregulation of Mdr1 in cholestasis is associated with an increase in the excretion of Mdr1 substrates (23,74).

To date, no genetic defect in MDR P-glycoprotein 170 has been described. In addition, the Mdr1a(−/−) knockout mouse has normal rates of bile flow and only modest impairment in organic cation excretion (75). Double knockout mice, Mdr1a,b(−/−), also demonstrate normal bile flow, but organic cation transport is significantly impaired (76). However, substrates for Mdr1a,b such as cyclosporin A can inhibit ATP-dependent bile salt transport in rat (77) and human canalicular membrane vesicles (78). Cyclosporin competitively inhibits bile salt transport when Bsep is expressed in Sf9 insect cells. (79). Thus, genetic polymorphisms in the hepatic expression of human Pgp-170 might predispose to cholestatic injury by limiting the excretion of conventional MDR substrates such as cyclosporin and thereby facilitate inhibition of BSEP.

Mdr2/MDR3

The importance of this phospholipid export pump in the pathogenesis of cholestasis is dramatically demonstrated by mutations in the *MDR3/Mdr2 gene* which result in progressive familiar intrahepatic cholestasis (PFIC) type 3 in children (9,10) and biliary cirrhosis in the mouse knockout model, Mdr2(−/−) (11). In the absence of the canalicular Mdr2/MDR3 gene product, a phospholipid flippase, phosphatidyl choline, cannot be excreted into bile, and bile salts, which continue to be excreted normally, cannot form mixed micelles. The consequence of this genetic defect in both animals and humans is progressive injury to the bile duct epithelium (12–15). The function of Mdr2/MRP3 was established in the Mdr2 knockout mouse, which has a complete deficiency of phospholipid in the bile and which develops portal inflammation and bile ductular proliferation, characteristic of nonsuppurative cholangitis. With time, fibrosis occurs and these animals develop a biliary-type cirrhosis and, in some cases, hepatocellular carcinoma (15). Proof that MDR3 encodes for the phospholipid transferase came from studies where the human *MDR3* was expressed as a transgene in the Mdr2(−/−) animals and restored the ability of the mice to excrete phospholipid and regain the normal phenotype (80). Mdr2 deficiency in the mouse model can also be corrected by transplantation of MDR3 transgenic hepatocytes (81). Other studies in bile duct-obstructed Mdr2(−/−) mice revealed that lipoprotein X (LPX) was absent in serum. LPX is a lipoprotein normally found in the serum of patients with cholestatic liver disease. These findings demonstrated that (a) phospholipids must first be excreted into bile for this abnormal serum lipoprotein to be formed, and (b) LPX must develop from the regurgitation of bile into plasma during bile duct obstruction (82).

Children with PFIC-type 3 also have defective phospholipid excretion in bile, bile duct proliferation by histologic exam and an elevated level of γ-glutamyl transferase, thus distinguishing these patients from those with PFIC-1 or -2, where bile duct proliferation is absent and γ-glutamyl transferase is normal (83).

Heterozygotes for *Mdr2* or *MDR3* demonstrate partial deficiencies in phospholipid excretion but under normal conditions do not have a cholestatic phenotype (10,13,84). However, mothers of PFIC-3 patients are obligate heterozygotes, *MDR3* (+/−), and are at risk to develop cholestasis during the third trimester of pregnancy, when high levels of estrogens are present (16). These findings suggest that polymorphisms in the expression of MDR3 might predispose patients to cholestatic liver injury if they are exposed to other potential cholestatic agents including drugs and environmental toxins. Patients with PBC have normal MDR3 mRNA levels (85); however, further studies are needed to determine the role that MDR3 heterozygosity plays in idiosyncratic human cholestatic disorders. Mdr2 is upregulated after bile duct obstruction (71), ANIT (23), partial hepatectomy (72), griseofulvin, or 1,4 diethoxy-carobonyl-1,4-dihydrocollodine administration in the rat (86).

Mrp2/MRP2

Mrp2/MRP2 encode for the conjugate drug export pump, also known as the canalicular multidrug organic anion transporter, cMOAT (64). Mutations in the *Mrp2* gene result in a stop codon and premature termination of protein translocation in mutant TR−/GY (87) and EHBR rats (88). Mutations in the *MRP2* gene in humans result in the Dubin–Johnson syndrome (89–91). These mutations are a genetically determined cause of conjugated hyperbilirubinemia. Although not a cholestatic disorder by definition, since bile salt excretion is normal, this mutation results in impaired excretion of a variety of amphipathic organic anions, including leukotrienes, conjugated bilirubin, divalent bile acids, and coproporphyrin isomer series 1, as well as a variety of other compounds including BSP, indocyanine green, and oral cholecystographic agents (64). Antibiotics such as ampicillin and cephtriaxone and heavy metals are also excreted by Mrp2. Although it is not known if bile secretion is impaired in Dubin–Johnson syndrome, bile salt-independent bile flow is reduced in the rat model as a result of impaired glutathione excretion (92). Current evidence suggests that glutathione is a low-affinity substrate for Mrp2 and that Mrp2 is the major pathway for excretion of glutathione as well as oxidized GSSG and glutathione conjugates (93). Since the excretion of glutathione is a major determinant of bile salt-independent bile flow (94), deficiencies in the Mrp2/MRP2 transporter which result in diminished glutathione excretion may contribute to or predispose to other forms of cholestatic injury. Therefore, it is

noteworthy that the expression of Mrp2 at both the mRNA and protein levels is markedly downregulated in several experimental animal models of cholestasis including CBDL, EE, and LPS (22,70,95). This impairment is particularly noted following administration of LPS, providing an experimental explanation for the increases in conjugated bilirubin in serum that are characteristic of sepsis-induced jaundice (21,22,70). Retrieval of Mrp2 from the canalicular membrane to a subcellular localization may precede changes in mRNA expression after LPS (96,97) as well as phalloidin (98) and represents early posttranscriptional events that may contribute to cholestasis. Like Ntcp, the promoter region of *Mrp2* contains response elements to the nuclear receptor heterodimer RXRa:RARa, which is regulated by cytokines (41). As previously mentioned, the downregulation of Mrp2 in cholestasis also explains the impairment in the biliary excretion of a variety of substrates including glutathione, bilirubin diglucuronide, cysteinyl leukotrienes, antibiotics and bile acid sulfates and glucuronides. Since glutathione is an antioxidant, its hepatic retention in cholestasis may be protective.

Little information exists concerning the expression of MRP2 in human cholestatic liver diseases. However, preliminary reports suggest that MRP2 RNA is downregulated in PBC (99), but is not significantly reduced in patients with cholestatic alcoholic hepatitis (100).

Bsep/BSEP

These genes encode for the sister of P-glycoprotein, the canalicular membrane bile salt export pump. Mutations in *BSEP* result in PFIC type 2, also known as Byler's syndrome (6–8). More than ten different mutations have been described in families with this pediatric cholestatic disorder which resembles the Byler's disease (PFIC-1) phenotype, with absence of bile duct proliferation and normal γ-glutamyl transferase levels in serum, findings perhaps explained by a primary defect in excretion of bile salts from hepatocytes into bile. Functional expression of rat liver Bsep in an Sf9 insect cell expression system demonstrates ATP-dependent bile salt transport with a Km for taurocholate that is identical to one determined from transport studies in isolated rat canalicular membrane vesicles (101). Preliminary unpublished studies in a knockout mouse model also demonstrate impaired bile salt transport into bile (V. Ling and I. Yousef, personal communication, 2000). Together these findings provide compelling evidence that Bsep/BSEP is the major if not sole canalicular transport protein for determining bile salt excretion and bile salt-dependent bile formation.

Therefore, it is surprising to find that the expression of Bsep in several rat models of cholestasis is only moderately impaired (21,22). Although a variety of cholestatic agents profoundly inhibit ATP-dependent bile salt transport *in vitro* in isolated rat liver canalicular membrane vesicles, including LPS (33,102), EE (103), and cyclosporin A (77), downregulation *in vivo* is less pronounced. While three days of CBDL results in inhibition of Bsep mRNA and protein expression by about 30% and 50%, respectively, after 7 to 14 days, mRNA and protein expression recover to about 60% and 80% of control values, respectively, and immuno-fluorescence studies indicate that the transporter remains at the canalicular membrane (21). Furthermore, bile salt excretion continues in the face of complete obstruction, albeit at a reduced rate (21). LPS and EE administration *in vivo* to rats also resulted in only partial inhibition of Bsep expression (21,22). Preliminary clinical studies in patients with biliary atresia also find that the BSEP protein is maintained in its normal amount and location in this cholestatic disorder (104). Together these experimental observations suggest that, as is the case for Pgp-170, the expression of this sister of P-glycoprotein is relatively well preserved during cholestatic liver injury compared to canalicular transport proteins such as Mrp2 or basolateral membrane bile salt transporters. Bsep mRNA and protein are also well maintained and even upregulated following partial hepatectomy in the rat (105). Nevertheless, taurocholate transport is competitively *cis*-inhibited by various cholestatic drugs including cyclosporin A, rifamycin, rifamycin SV and glibenclamide in Sf9 cells expressing rat Bsep (79). Altogether, these findings suggest that the cholestatic effects of these compounds may be determined in part by the extent to which the canalicular export pumps continue to function as export pumps. Interestingly, the cholestatic metabolite estradiol-17β-glucuronide inhibited ATP-dependent taurocholate transport only when Mrp2 was coexpressed in Sf9 cells, suggesting that this compound results in trans-inhibition of Bsep-mediated bile salt transport only after excretion into the bile canaliculi by Mrp2 (79). Thus, some drugs may produce cholestasis by inhibiting the bile salt export pump only after excretion into bile.

Canalicular Ion Transporters (AE2)

AE2

This transporter encodes for the canalicular Cl^-/HCO_3^- exchanger that regulates the excretion of bicarbonate, a partial determinant of canalicular bile salt-independent bile formation (18,106). AE2 is also expressed on the luminal membrane of the cholangiocyte (see below) and is a determinant of bicarbonate excretion from this epithelium (107). Thus, impairment of AE2 would be expected to reduce bile flow. Whether this predisposes to cholestasis is not known. However, reduced levels of liver AE2 mRNA expression and immunoreactivity at the canaliculus and bile ducts have been described in patients with PBC but not in other cholestatic and noncholestatic liver diseases, suggesting that they might be primary rather then secondary changes (108–110). Treatment of patients with ursodeoxycholic acid normalized the expression of AE2 mRNA and

partially restored immunoreactivity to the protein (108,109). Reduced expression of AE2 mRNA was also observed in salivary glands of patients with PBC and the sicca syndrome, suggesting that there may be a generalized deficiency in this transporter in this disease (111). Only one study of AE2 activity has been performed in a cholestatic animal model after EE treatment; the activity was found to be normal (112).

Transporters on the Cholangiocyte Luminal Membrane Involved in Bile Secretory Function (AE2; CFTR; NHE-2,3; Isbt; FIC1; JAG1; and Mdr1a)

Cholangiocytes modify the primary secretion from hepatocytes by functioning as both a secretory and absorptive epithelium. Net secretion from this epithelium varies but may account for as little as 5% to 10% in rodents to as much as 40% in human liver following a meal (106).

Ion Transporters (AE2, CFTR, and NHE2,3)

As discussed above, this secretion is composed mainly of HCO_3^- anions that are exchanged for Cl^- by AE2, a Cl^-/HCO_3^- exchanger on the luminal membrane and facilitated by the luminal entry of chloride via CFTR, a Cl^- channel also known as the cystic fibrosis transmembrane regulator (106). Opening of the Cl^- channel is regulated by cAMP in response to secretin, but bombesin and VIP also stimulate AE2, although the second message is not known (113,115). Mutations in the *CFTR* gene can result in inspissated bile and progressive cholestatic liver disease, emphasizing the importance of this Cl^- channel in cholangiocyte secretion (116). Whether polymorphisms in CFTR predispose to cholestatic liver injury from other agents is not clear. Fluid reabsorption also occurs across the cholangiocyte luminal membrane, mediated in part by NHE-2 and or -3 isoforms (117). A more detailed discussion of the role of these ion transporters in bile secretion can be found elsewhere (106,118).

To date, there are few studies on the effects of cholestatic agents and cholestatic liver disorders on these processes. As mentioned previously, impaired AE2 mRNA and immunoreactivity have been described in patients with PBC who classically manifest bile ductopenia (108,109). However, obstructive cholestasis in the rat, which is associated with bile duct epithelial proliferation rather than ductopenia, actually results in increased expression of secretin receptors and an enhancement of cholangiocyte cAMP levels and secretory capacity that parallels the degree of cholangiocyte proliferation (118,119). This proliferation during obstructive jaundice may be due in part to the presence of retained bile salts (120). Secretin receptors are upregulated on the basolateral membrane after bile duct ligation (119), a phenomenon that is markedly downregulated if cholangiocyte proliferation is diminished in the bile duct ligated rat by vagotomy (121) or by prior bile salt depletion (122). Bile duct proliferation in the bile duct-obstructed rat is also inhibited by somatostatin and gastrin, a process mediated by SSTR$_2$ receptors for somatostatin on large cholangiocytes (123). Although gastrin does not inhibit bile flow in normal or bile duct-ligated rats, it depresses secretin receptor gene expression and thus inhibits secretin-induced bicarbonate secretion (124). Endothelin-1 is another peptide that blocks the effects of secretin-induced secretion in the bile duct-ligated rat by interacting with ET$_A$ receptors (125).

Isbt

This gene product for the ileal sodium-dependent bile salt transporter is also expressed on the cholangiocyte luminal membrane and on the luminal membrane of the proximal tubule of the kidney (27,28,126). Its function is to reabsorb bile salts. Whether cholangiocyte Isbt has a function in the normal liver is not known, but its expression is upregulated following bile duct proliferation in the bile duct-obstructed rat (31). In these circumstances it is possible that Isbt functions to remove bile salts from the obstructed biliary lumen when they continue to be excreted into canalicular bile by Bsep. A bile salt anion exchange mechanism has been functionally described on the basolateral membrane of rat cholangiocytes and could function together with Mrp3 to return the reabsorbed bile salts to the systemic circulation where they may be excreted in part by the kidney (29,127). Preliminary studies indicate that Isbt is downregulated on the luminal membrane of the proximal tubule of the rat kidney, a change that would diminish the capacity of the kidney to reabsorb bile salts from the glomerular filtrate (31). In contrast, Mrp2, which is also expressed on the apical membrane of the proximal tubule (128), is upregulated, an adaptation that should facilitate the excretion of bile salt sulfates (31). It remains to be determined whether changes in the regulation of these transporters account in part for the increase in renal bile salt excretion that occurs during cholestasis.

Mutations in the *Isbt* gene in humans result in primary bile salt malabsorption, but the effects of these mutations on cholangiocyte or renal handling of bile salts are not known (129).

Fic1

This gene encodes for a P-type ATPase which is thought to function as an aminophospholipid transferase that maintains phosphatidylserine and phosphatidyl ethanolamine within the inner bilayer of the plasma membrane (5). Although its function in the liver is not yet known, mutations in this gene result in two cholestatic disorders, PFIC1 (Byler's disease) in childhood and benign recurrent intra-

hepatic cholestasis (BRIC) in adults (83). Both disorders result in intrahepatic cholestasis, yet the gene product appears to be expressed primarily in the intestine and to some extent in the bile duct epithelium. Preliminary studies also suggest that there is aminophospholipid transferase activity in isolated rat canalicular membranes (130). PFIC1 is a progressive, ultimately fatal, pediatric cholestatic disorder characterized by intermittent episodes of diarrhea, normal γ-glutamyl transferase levels in the serum, a lack of bile duct proliferation and the absence of bile salts in the bile (131). Electron microscopy reveals gross distortion of the canalicular membrane and the accumulation of hepatic organelles within the canalicular lumen ("Byler's bile"). Thus, it is likely that this gene defect results in impaired excretion of bile salts across the bile canaliculus. While there is considerable phenotypic heterogeneity in PFIC1 and BRIC, it is puzzling that mutations in the same regions of the gene result in both a nonprogressive benign recurrent cholestatic disorder in adults and progressive disease in children. Some members of BRIC families have the gene defect but do not express the cholestatic phenotype, suggesting that other genetic or environmental factors may be required to express the disease (132).

JAGGED1

This gene encodes for an unknown ligand for the notch1 receptor that is important for cell differentiation (19,20). Mutations in *JAGGED1* result in Alagille's syndrome, an autosomal dominant disorder associated with more than 50 different mutations that result in neonatal cholestasis, bile duct paucity and a number of extrahepatic developmental defects (133,134). The latter include congenital heart disease, butterfly vertebra, a distinctive facial appearance with frontal bossing and pointed chin, and retinal posterior embryotoxon. During human fetal liver development, JAGGED1 is first expressed on ductal plate cells that give rise to the biliary epithelium (20). Signs of cholestatic liver disease usually present before one year of age in the majority of patients. However, the clinical course is quite variable. As many as 20% may die from advanced cirrhosis; most survive into adulthood without disease progression, when the cholestasis often resolves. Liver biopsies characteristically demonstrate a paucity of interlobular bile ducts. It is not known why cholestasis in most patients spontaneously improves.

Mdr1a

This gene product is also expressed in cholangiocytes as well as hepatocytes (135). This P-glycoprotein functions to excrete organic cations in hepatocytes, but in cholangiocytes like the intestine, Mdr gene products may serve as a barrier to prevent the accumulation of toxic lipophilic substrates that are excreted into bile by hepatocytes and which might diffuse into these cells during their passage down the biliary tree. Mutations or altered patterns of expression of this cholangiocyte transporter would reduce the capacity of the cholangiocyte to protect itself from toxic compounds and theoretically could contribute to the development of bile duct injury.

SUMMARY

This chapter has focused on the roles that membrane transporters in hepatocytes and cholangiocytes play in inherited as well as acquired forms of cholestasis. There are a number of other structural and functional defects that also contribute to the development of bile secretory failure. While a discussion of these cellular processes is beyond the scope of this review, they will be mentioned briefly for further reference.

Cytoskeletal Changes

Profound changes in the cytoskeleton of the hepatocytes occur as secondary consequences of cholestatic injury, including disruption of microtubules, increases in intermediate filaments and an accumulation of actin microfilaments that become particularly prominent in and around the pericanalicular cytoplasm and beneath the junctional contacts (136). Changes in these structural proteins are generally considered a secondary response to cholestasis. However, a severe form of familial cholestasis has been described in Canadian Indians (North American Indian childhood cirrhosis) where there is a striking accumulation of actin filaments in hepatocytes, reminiscent of phalloidin toxicity in animal models (137). Dysfunction of the cell cytoskeleton results in altered canalicular contractility and a reduction in "microperistalsis" that may contribute to stasis in cholestatic disorders (see Chapter 24 and website chapters 🖥 W-1 and W-2).

Tight Junctions

These structures form the only major permeability barrier between blood and bile and form the seals between adjacent hepatocytes that define the lumen of the bile canaliculus (138) (see Chapter 24). Thus, their structural integrity is critical to the maintenance of osmotic gradients within the canalicular space that provide the driving force for the forward movement of bile. Physical as well as functional disruptions to this permeability barrier have been described in a variety of experimental models of cholestasis and cholestatic disorders in humans and thus contribute in a major way to dissipation of the osmotic gradients that are necessary for bile production (139–143). Considerable advances have been made in understanding the molecular basis of tight junctions, and proteins such as occludens and claudens are known to be important in forming this junctional barrier (See Chapter 3).

Many forms of cholestasis result in loss or rearrangement of these proteins and functional increases in junctional permeability in the tight junction, but it remains to be determined whether mutations in genes that code for these proteins are a primary cause of cholestatic liver disease (142,144). Because these gene products form important barrier functions for many different epithelia, such mutations may be lethal to the embryo. Knockout animal models should help elucidate their role in the pathogenesis of cholestasis.

Gap Junctions

Gap junction channels form sites of intercellular communication between hepatocytes and are formed from proteins called connexins (145) (see Chapter 3). Although connexins are coded for by a multigene family, only connexins 26 and 32 are expressed in the liver. Connexins function to permit small molecules (less than 1 kd) to move between cells. Regulation of the opening and closing of these channels is important for the intercellular coordination of a variety of signal transduction mechanisms. In liver cells, the intercellular movement of small ions like calcium may help to coordinate canalicular contractions within the lobule and thus facilitate the forward flow of bile (146,147). However, it is not yet clear how important connexins are for normal bile production or whether abnormalities in their expression might predispose to cholestasis. Here again, studies in knockout animal models will be of interest. Cholestasis imposed by CBDL in the rat results in downregulation of connexins 26 and 32 as detected by Western blot analysis and immunofluorescence studies, possibly reducing the migration of calcium waves or IP_3 between hepatocytes (148). Loss of the connexin proteins might also be a protective mechanism in cholestasis by isolating hepatocytes from their neighbors, thereby preventing exposure to toxic levels of calcium and other molecules that would normally diffuse through these channels.

Transcytosis and Exocytosis

Basolateral and canalicular transport proteins target their respective plasma membrane domains after synthesis in the endoplasmic reticulum and Golgi apparatus (see Chapter 9 and website chapter 🖥 W-6). This process involves movement in lipid vesicles along microtubules powered by the molecular motors dynein and kinesin (149,150). Normally, the movement of these vesicles on microtubules and their fusion with early and late endosomal compartments in the liver is a highly regulated process involving active phosphorylation and dephosphorylation reactions dependent on a series of protein and lipid kinases and phosphatases (151–154). Cholestatic liver injury disrupts vesicular transcytosis and exocytosis, leading to the accumulation of vesicles within the pericanalicular region of hepatocytes (155–159). High concentrations of bile salts inhibit the functions of dynein and kinesin and possibly other critical enzymes (160). The expression and subcellular localization of heterotrimeric G proteins is affected (161), resulting in altered cyclic AMP-mediated signal transduction, which normally facilitates targeting of vesicles to the canalicular domain (162). Failure of vesicles to target the bile canaliculus results in a decreased number of functional transport proteins at the canalicular membrane, further contributing to the cholestatic process.

REFERENCES

1. Müller M, Jansen PLM. Molecular aspects of hepatobiliary transport. *Am J Physiol* 1997;35:G1285–G1303.
2. Trauner M, Meier PJ, Boyer JL. Molecular pathogenesis of cholestasis. *N Engl J Med* 1998;339:1217–1227.
3. Trauner M, Meier PJ, Boyer JL. Molecular regulation of hepatocellular transport systems in cholestasis. *J Hepatol* 1999; 31:165–178.
4. Duffy MC, Boyer JL. Pathophysiology of intrahepatic cholestasis and biliary obstruction. In: Ostrow JD, ed. *Bile pigments and jaundice*. 1st ed. New York: Marcel Dekker Inc, 1986:333–372.
5. Bull LN, van Eijk MJT, Pawlikowska L, et al. A gene encoding a P-type ATPase mutated in two forms of hereditary cholestasis. *Nat Genet* 1998;18:219–224.
6. Strautnieks SS, Kagalwalla AF, Tanner MS, et al. Identification of a locus for progressive familial intrahepatic cholestasis PFIC2 on chromosome 2q24. *Am J Hum Genet* 1997;61:630–633.
7. Strautnieks SS, Bull L, Knisely AS, et al. A gene encoding a liver-specific ABC transporter is mutated in progressive familial intrahepatic cholestasis. *Nat Genet* 1998;20:233–238.
8. Jansen PL, Strautnieks SS, Jacquemin E, et al. Hepatocanalicular bile salt export pump deficiency in patients with progressive familial intrahepatic cholestasis. *Gastroenterology* 1999;117:1370–1379.
9. deVree JML, Jacquemin E, Sturm E, et al. Mutations in the MDR3 gene cause progressive familial intrahepatic cholestasis. *Proc Natl Acad Sci U S A* 1998;95:282–287(abst).
10. Deleuze JF, Jacquemin E, Dubuisson C, et al. Defect on multidrug-resistance 3 gene expression in a subtype of progressive familial intrahepatic cholestasis. *Hepatology* 1996;23:904–908.
11. Smit JJM, Schinkel AH, Elferink RPJO, et al. Homozygous disruption of the murine mdr2 P-glycoprotein gene leads to a complete absence of phospholipid from bile and to liver disease. *Cell* 1993;75:451–462.
12. Mauad TH, van Nieuwkerk CMJ, Dingemans KP, et al. Mice with homozygous disruption of the *mdr*2 p-glycoprotein gene. A novel animal model for studies of nonsuppurative inflammatory cholangitis and hepatocarcinogenesis. *Am J Pathol* 1994; 145:1237–1245.
13. Oude Elferink RPJ, Ottenhoff R, van Wijland M, et al. Regulation of biliary lipid secretion by mdr2 P-glycoprotein in the mouse. *J Clin Invest* 1995;95:31–38.
14. Oude Elferink RPJ, Groen AK. The role of mdr2 P-glycoprotein in biliary lipid secretion. Cross-talk between cancer research and biliary physiology. *J Hepatol* 1995;23:617–625.
15. Oude Elferink RPJ, Tytgat GNJ, et al. The role of mdr2 P-glycoprotein in hepatobiliary lipid transport. *FASEB J* 1997;11:19–28.
16. Jacquemin E, Cresteil D, Manouvrier S, et al. Heterozygous non-sense mutation of the MDR3 gene in familial intrahepatic cholestasis of pregnancy. *Lancet* 1999;353:210–211.
17. Cohn JA, Strong TV, Picciotto MR, et al. Localization of the cystic fibrosis transmembrane conductance regulator in human bile duct epithelial cells. *Gastroenterology* 1993;105:1857–1864.
18. Boyer JL. Bile duct epithelium: frontiers in transport physiology. *Am J Physiol* 1996;270:G1–G5.
19. Spinner NB. Alagille syndrome and the notch signaling pathway: new insights into human development. *Gastroenterology* 1999;116:1257–1260.
20. Louis AA, Van EP, Haber BA, et al. Hepatic jagged1 expression studies. *Hepatology* 1999;30:1269–1275.
21. Lee JM, Trauner M, Soroka CJ, et al. Expression of the bile salt export pump is maintained after chronic cholestasis in the rat. *Gastroenterology* 2000;118:163–172.
22. Vos TA, Guido J, Hooiveld EJ, et al. Up-regulation of the multidrug resistance genes, Mrp1 and Mdr1b, and down-regulation of the organic anion transporter, Mrp2, and the bile salt transporter, Spgp, in endotoxemic rat liver. *Hepatology* 1998;28:1637–1644.
23. Schrenk D, Gant TW, Preisegger K-H, et al. Induction of multidrug resistance gene expression during cholestasis in rats and nonhuman primates. *Hepatology* 1993;17:854–860.
24. Konig J, Rost D, Cui Y, et al. Characterization of the human multidrug resistance protein isoform MRP3 localized to the basolateral hepatocyte membrane. *Hepatology* 1999;29:1156–1163.
25. Kool M, van der Linden M, deHaas M, et al. MRP3, an organic anion transporter able to transport anticancer drugs. *Proc Natl Acad Sci U S A* 1999;96:6914–6919.
26. Hirohashi T, Suzuki H, Takikawa H, et al. ATP-dependent transport of bile salts by rat multidrug resistance-associated protein 3 (Mrp3). *J Biol Chem* 2000;275:2905–2910.
27. Alpini G, Glaser SS, Rodgers R, et al. Functional expression of the apical Na⁺-dependent bile acid transporter in large but not small rat cholangiocytes. *Gastroenterology* 1997;113:1734–1740.
28. Lazaridis KN, Pham L, Tietz P, et al. Rat cholangiocytes absorb bile acids at their apical domain via the ileal sodium-dependent bile acid transporter. *J Clin Invest* 1997;100:2714–2721.
29. Ogawa K, Suzuki H, Hirohashi T, et al. Characterization of inducible nature of MRP3 in rat liver. *Am J Physiol Gastrointest Liver Physiol* 2000;278:G438–G446.
30. Hirohashi T, Suzuki H, Sugiyama Y. Characterization of the transport properties of cloned rat multidrug resistance-associated protein 3 (MRP3). *J Biol Chem* 1999;274:15181–15185.
31. Lee JM, Azzaroli F, Gigliozzi A, et al. Adaptive regulation of the ileal sodium-dependent bile salt transporter (ISBT), and the multispecific organic anion transporter (MRP2), in kidney and cholangiocytes in chronic cholestasis—alternative pathways for bile salt excretion. *Hepatology* 1999;30:417A(abst).
32. Gartung C, Ananthanarayanan M, Rahman MA, et al. Down-regulation of expression and function of the rat liver Na⁺/bile acid cotransporter in extrahepatic cholestasis. *Gastroenterology* 1996;110:199–209.
33. Moseley RH, Wang W, Takeda H, et al. Effect of endotoxin on bile acid transport in rat liver: a potential model for sepsis-associated cholestasis. *Am J Physiol* 1996;271:G137–G146.
34. Simon FR, Fortune J, Iwahashi M, et al. Ethinyl estradiol cholestasis involves alterations in expression of liver sinusoidal transporters. *Am J Physiol* 1996;34:G1043–G1052.
35. Green RM, Beier D, Gollan JL. Regulation of hepatocyte bile salt transporters by endotoxin and inflammatory cytokines in rodents. *Gastroenterology* 1996;111:193–198.
36. Elsing C, Reichen J, Marti U, et al. Hepatocellular Na⁺/K⁺ exchange is activated at transcriptional and posttranscriptional levels in rat biliary cirrhosis. *Gastroenterology* 1994;107:468–478.
37. Gartung C, Schuele S, Schlosser SF, et al. Expression of the rat liver Na⁺/taurocholate cotransporter is regulated in vivo by

retention of biliary constituents but not their depletion. *Hepatology* 1997;25:284–290.

38. Trauner M, Arrese M, Lee H, et al. Endotoxin downregulates rat hepatic ntcp gene expression via decreased activity of critical transcription factors. *J Clin Invest* 1998;101:2092–2100.

39. Shneider BL, Fox VL, Schwarz KB, et al. Hepatic basolateral sodium-dependent bile acid transporter expression in two unusual cases of hypercholanemia and in extrahepatic biliary atresia. *Hepatology* 1997;25:1176–1183.

40. Karpen SJ, Sun A, Kudish B, et al. Multiple factors regulate the rat liver basolateral sodium-dependent bile acid cotransporter gene promoter. *J Biol Chem* 1996;271:15211–15221.

41. Denson LA, Auld KL, Schiek DS, et al. Interleukin-1β suppresses retinoid transactivation of two hepatic transporter genes involved in bile formation. *J Biol Chem* 2000;275:8835–8843.

42. Makishima M, Okamoto AY, Repa JJ, et al. Identification of a nuclear receptor for bile acids. *Science* 1999;284:1362–1365.

43. Parks DJ, Blanchard SG, Bledsoe RK, et al. Bile acids: natural ligands for an orphan nuclear receptor. *Science* 1999;284:1365–1368.

44. Wang H, Chen J, Hollister K, et al. Endogenous bile acids are ligands for the nuclear receptor FXR/BAR. *Mol Cell* 1999;3:543–553.

45. Gartung C, Trauner M, Schlosser SF, et al. Sodium-independent uptake of bile acids is unaffected by down-regulation of an organic anion transporter (oatp) in rat liver during cholestasis produced by common bile duct ligation (CBDL). *Hepatology* 1996;24:369A(abst).

46. Kullak-Ublick G-A, Hagenbuch B, Stieger B, et al. Functional characterization of the basolateral rat liver organic anion transporting polypeptide. *Hepatology* 1994;20:411–416.

47. Kullak-Ublick GA, Hagenbuch B, Stieger B, et al. Molecular and functional characterization of an organic anion transporting polypeptide cloned from human liver. *Gastroenterology* 1995;109:1274–1282.

48. Eckhardt U, Schroeder A, Stieger B, et al. Polyspecific substrate uptake by the hepatic organic anion transporter Oatp1 in stably-tranfected CHO cells. *Am J Physiol* 1999;276:G1037–G1042.

49. Abe T, Kakyo M, Tokui T, et al. Identification of a novel gene family encoding human liver-specific organic anion transporter LST-1. *J Biol Chem* 1999;274:17159–17163.

50. Reichel C, Gao B, Van Montfoort J, et al. Localization and function of the organic anion-transporting polypeptide oatp2 in rat liver. *Gastroenterology* 1999;117:688–695.

51. Kakyo M, Unno M, Tokui T, et al. Molecular characterization and functional regulation of a novel rat liver-specific organic anion transporter rlst-1. *Gastroenterology* 1999;117:770–775.

52. Kullak-Ublick G-A, Fisch T, Oswald M, et al. Dehydroepiandrosterone sulfate (DHEAS): identification of a carrier protein in human liver and brain. *FEBS Lett* 1998;424:173–176.

53. Hsiang B, Zhu Y, Wang Z, et al. A novel human hepatic organic anion transporting polypeptide (OATP2). Identification of a liver-specific human organic anion transporting polypeptide and identification of rat and human hydroxymethylglutaryl-CoA reductase inhibitor transporters. *J Biol Chem* 1999;274:37161–37168.

54. Konig J, Cui Y, Nies AT, et al. A novel human organic anion transporting polypeptide localized to the basolateral hepatocyte membrane. *Am J Physiol* 2000;278:G156–G164.

55. Li L, Lee TK, Meier PJ, et al. Identification of glutathione as a driving force and leukotriene C4 as a substrate for oatp1, the hepatic sinusoidal organic solute transporter. *J Biol Chem* 1998;273:16184–16191.

56. Satlin LM, Amin V, Wolkoff AW. Organic anion transporting polypeptide mediates organic anion/HCO₃⁻ exchange. *J Biol Chem* 1997;272:26340–26345.

57. Noe B, Hagenbuch B, Stieger B, et al. Isolation of a multispecific organic anion and cardiac glycoside transporter from rat brain. *Proc Natl Acad Sci U S A* 1997;94:10346–10350.

58. Abe T, Kakyo M, Sakagami H, et al. Molecular characterization and tissue distribution of a new organic anion transporter subtype (oatp3) that transports thyroid hormones and taurocholate and comparison with oatp2. *J Biol Chem* 1998;273:22395–22401.

59. Kanai N, Lu R, Satriano JA, et al. Identification and characterization of a prostaglandin transporter. *Science* 1995;268:866–869.

60. Saito H, Masuda S, Inui K. Cloning and functional characterization of a novel rat organic anion transporter mediating basolateral uptake of methotrexate in the kidney. *J Biol Chem* 1996;271:20719–20724.

61. Gartung C, Matern S. Molecular regulation of organic anion transport in cholestasis. In: Manns M, Boyer JL, Jansen PLM, et al., eds. *Falk Symposium 102: cholestatic liver diseases.* Dordrecht, The Netherlands, Kluwer Academic Publishers, 1998:21–28.

62. Green RM, Gollan JL, Hagenbuch B, et al. Regulation of hepatocyte bile salt transporters during hepatic regeneration. *Am J Physiol* 1997;36:G621–G627.

63. Kullak-Ublick G-A, Beuers U, Fahney C, et al. Identification and functional characterization of the promoter region of the human organic anion transporting polypeptide gene. *Hepatology* 1997;26:991–997.

64. Konig J, Nies AT, Cui Y, et al. Conjugate export pumps of the multidrug resistance protein (MRP) family: localization, substrate specificity, and MRP2-mediated drug resistance. *Biochim Biophys Acta* 1999;1461:377–394.

65. Borst P, Evers R, Kool M, et al. The multidrug resistance protein family. *Biochim Biophys Acta* 1999;1461:347–357.

66. Hirohashi T, Suzuki H, Ito K, et al. Hepatic expression of multidrug resistance-associated protein-like proteins maintained in Eisai hyperbilirubinemic rats. *Mol Pharmacol* 1998;53:1068–1075.

67. Hirohashi T, Suzuki H, Ito K, et al. Hepatic expression of multidrug resistance-associated protein-like proteins maintained in Eisai hyperbilirubinemic rats. *Mol Pharmacol* 1998;53:1068–1075.

68. Kool M, De Haas GL, Scheffer GL, et al. Analysis of expression of cMOAT (MRP2), MRP3, MRP4, and MRP5, homologs of the multidrug resistance-associated protein gene (MRP1), in human cancer cell lines. *Cancer Res* 1997;57:3537–3547.

69. Kool M, van der Linden M, De Haas M, et al. Expression of human MRP6, a homologue of the multidrug resistance protein gene MRP1, in tissues and cancer cells. *Cancer Res* 1999;59:175–182.

70. Trauner M, Arrese M, Soroka C, et al. The rat canalicular conjugate export pump (mrp 2) is down-regulated in intrahepatic and obstructive cholestasis. *Gastroenterology* 1997;113:255–264.

71. Kagawa T, Watanabe N, Sato M, et al. Differential expression of multidrug resistance (mdr) and canalicular multispecific organic anion transporter (cMOAT) genes following extrahepatic biliary obstruction in rats. *Biochem Mol Biol Int* 1998;44:443–452.

72. Nakatsukasa H, Silverman JA, Gant TW, et al. Expression of multidrug resistance genes in rat liver during regeneration and after carbon tetrachloride intoxication. *Hepatology* 1993;18:1202–1207.

73. Nozawa S, Miyazaki M, Tou HI, et al. Human MDR1 and MDR3 gene expression in the liver with obstructive jaundice. *Gastroenterology* 1997;112:A1349(abst).

74. Takikawa H, Takamori Y, Sano N, et al. Changes in biliary excretory mechanisms in rats with ethinyl estradiol-induced cholestasis. *J Gastroenterol Hepatol* 1998;13:186–191.

75. Smit JW, Schinkel AH, Muller M, et al. Contribution of the murine mdr1a P-glycoprotein to hepatobiliary and intestinal elimination of cationic drugs as measured in mice with an mdr1a gene disruption. *Hepatology* 1998;27:1056–1063.

76. Schinkel AH, Mayer U, Wagenaar E, et al. Normal viability and altered pharmacokinetics in mice lacking mdr1-type (drug-transporting) P-glycoproteins. *Proc Natl Acad Sci U S A* 1997; 94:4028–4033.

77. Boehme M, Mueller M, Leier I, et al. Cholestasis caused by inhibition of the adenosine triphosphate-dependent bile salt transport in rat liver. *Gastroenterology* 1994;107:255–265.

78. Kadmon M, Klünemann C, Böhme M, et al. Inhibition by cyclosporin A of adenosine triphosphate-dependent transport from the hepatocyte into bile. *Gastroenterology* 1993;104: 1507–1514.

79. Stieger B, Fattinger K, Madon J, et al. Drug- and estrogen-induced cholestasis through inhibition of the hepatocellular bile salt export pump (Bsep) of rat liver. *Gastroenterology* 2000;118: 422–430.

80. Smith AJ, de Vree JML, Ottenhoff R, et al. Hepatocyte-specific expression of the human MDR3 P-glycoprotein gene restores the biliary phosphatidylcholine excretion absent in Mdr2 (−/−). *Hepatology* 1998;28:530–536.

81. de Vree JML, Ottenhoff R, Smith AJ, et al. Rapid correction of Mdr2 deficiency by transplantation of MDR3 transgenic hepatocytes. *Hepatology* 1998;28:387A(abst).

82. Oude Elferink RPJ, Ottenhoff R, Van Marle J, et al. Class III P-glycoproteins mediate the formation of lipoprotein X in the mouse. *J Clin Invest* 1998;102:1749–1757.

83. Bull LN, Carlton VEH, Stricker NL, et al. Genetic and morphological findings in progressive familial intrahepatic cholestasis (Byler disease [PFIC-1] and Byler syndrome): evidence for heterogeneity. *Hepatology* 1997;26:155–164.

84. de Vree JML, Jacquemin E, Sturm E, et al. Mutations in the MDR3 gene cause progressive familial intrahepatic cholestasis. *Proc Natl Acad Sci U S A* 1998;95:282–287.

85. Dumoulin FL, Reichel C, Sauerbruch T, et al. Semiquantitation of intrahepatic MDR3 mRNA levels by reverse transcription/competitive polymerase chain reaction. *J Hepatol* 1997;26: 852–856.

86. Preisegger K-H, Stumptner C, Riegelnegg D, et al. Experimental mallory body formation is accompanied by modulation of the expression of multidrug-resistance genes and their products. *Hepatology* 1996;24:248–252.

87. Buechler M, Koenig J, Brom M, et al. cDNA cloning of the hepatocyte canalicular isoform of the multidrug resistance protein, cMrp, reveals a novel conjugate export pump deficient in hyperbilirubinemic mutant rats. *J Biol Chem* 1996;271: 15091–15098.

88. Ito K, Suzuki H, Hirohashi T, et al. Molecular cloning of canalicular multispecific organic anion transporter defective in EHBR. *Am J Physiol* 1997;272:G16–G22.

89. Kartenbeck J, Leuschner U, Mayer R, et al. Absence of the canalicular isoform of the MRP gene-encoded conjugate export pump from the hepatocytes in Dubin-Johnson syndrome. *Hepatology* 1996;23:1061–1066.

90. Paulusma CC, Kool M, Bosma PJ, et al. A mutation in the human canalicular multispecific organic anion transporter gene causes the Dubin-Johnson syndrome. *Hepatology* 1997;25: 1539–1542.

91. Wada M, Toh S, Taniguchi K, et al. Mutations in the canalicular multispecific organic anion transporter (cMOAT) gene, a novel ABC transporter, in patients with hyperbilirubinemia II/Dubin-Johnson syndrome. *Hum Mol Genet* 1998;7: 203–207.

92. Oude Elferink RPJ, Ottenhoff R, Liefting W, et al. Hepatobil-iary transport of glutathione and glutathione conjugate in rats with hereditary hyperbilirubinemia. *J Clin Invest* 1989;84: 478–483.

93. Paulusma C, van Geer M, Evers R, et al. Canalicular multispecific organic anion transporter/multidrug resistance protein 2 mediates low-affinity transport of reduced glutathione. *Biochem J* 1999;338:393–401.

94. Ballatori N, Truong AT. Relation between biliary glutathione excretion and bile acid-independent bile flow. *Am J Physiol* 1989;256:G22–G30.

95. Koopen NR, Wolters H, Havinga R, et al. Impaired activity of the bile canalicular organic anion transporter (Mrp2/cmoat) is not the main cause of ethinylestradiol-induced cholestasis in the rat. *Hepatology* 1998;27:537–545.

96. Kubitz R, Wettstein M, Warskulat U, et al. Regulation of the multidrug resistance protein 2 in the rat liver by lipopolysaccharide and dexamethasone. *Gastroenterology* 1999;116:401–410.

97. Paulusma C, Kothe MJC, Bakker CTM, et al. Zonal down-regulation and redistribution of the multidrug resistance protein 2 during bile duct ligation in rat liver. *Hepatology* 2000;31: 684–693.

98. Rost D, Kartenbeck J, Keppler D. Changes in the localization of the rat canalicular conjugate export pump Mrp2 in phalloidin-induced cholestasis. *Hepatology* 1999;29:814–821.

99. Oswald M, Kullak-Ublick G-A, Beuers U, et al. Expression of the hepatocyte canalicular multidrug resistance associated protein 2 (MRP2) in primary biliary cirrhosis. *Hepatology* 1998;28: 544A(abst).

100. Zollner G, Fickert P, Zens R, et al. Hepatobiliary transporter expression in percutaneous liver biopsies of patients with cholestatic liver diseases. *Hepatology* 2001;33:633–646.

101. Gerloff T, Stieger B, Hagenbuch B, et al. The sister of P-glycoprotein represents the canalicular bile salt export pump of mammalian liver. *J Biol Chem* 1998;273:10046–10050.

102. Bolder U, Huong-Thu T, Schteingart CD, et al. Hepatocyte transport of bile acids and organic anions in endotoxemic rats: impaired uptake and secretion. *Gastroenterology* 1997;112: 214–225.

103. Bossard R, Stieger B, O'Neill B, et al. Ethinylestradiol treatment induces multiple canalicular membrane transport alterations in rat liver. *J Clin Invest* 1993;91:2714–2720.

104. Kogan D, Ananthanarayanan M, Emre S, et al. The bile salt excretory pump (BSEP/SPGP) is not down-regulated in human cholestasis associated with extrahepatic biliary atresia (EHBA). *Hepatology* 1999;30:468A(abst).

105. Gerloff T, Geier A, Stieger B, et al. Differential expression of basolateral and canalicular organic anion transporters during regeneration of rat liver. *Gastroenterology* 1999;117:1408–1415.

106. Boyer JL, Nathanson MH. Bile formation. In: Schiff ER, Sorrell MF, Maddrey WC, eds. *Schiff's diseases of the liver*. 8th ed. Philadelphia, Lippincott–Raven Publishers, 1999:119–146.

107. Martinez-Anso E, Castillo JE, Diez J, et al. Immunohistochemical detection of chloride/bicarbonate anion exchangers in human liver. *Hepatology* 1994;19:1400–1406.

108. Prieto J, Qian C, Garcia N, et al. Abnormal expression of anion exchanger genes in primary biliary cirrhosis. *Gastroenterology* 1993;105:572–578.

109. Medina JF, Martinez-Anso E, Vazquez JJ, et al. Decreased anion exchanger 2 immunoreactivity in the liver of patients with primary biliary cirrhosis. *Hepatology* 1997;25:12–17.

110. Prieto J, Garcia N, Marti-Climent JM, et al. Assessment of biliary bicarbonate secretion in humans by positron emission tomography. *Gastroenterology* 1999;117:167–172.

111. Vazquez JJ, Vazquez M, Idoate MA, et al. Anion exchanger immunoreactivity in human salivary glands in health and Sjögren's syndrome. *Am J Pathol* 1995;146:1422–1432.

112. Alvaro D, Gigliozzi A, Piat C, et al. Inhibition of biliary bicarbonate secretion in ethinyl estradiol-induced cholestasis is not associated with impaired activity of the Cl^-/HCO_3^- exchanger in the rat. *J Hepatol* 1997;26:146–157.

113. McGill JM, Basavappa S, Gettys TW, et al. Secretin activates Cl^- channels in bile duct epithelial cells through a cAMP-dependent mechanism. *Am J Physiol* 1994;29:G731–G736.

114. Alvaro D, Cho WK, Mennone A, et al. Effect of secretin on intracellular pH regulation in isolated rat bile duct epithelial cells. *J Clin Invest* 1993;92:1314–1325.

115. Cho WK, Boyer JL. Vasoactive intestinal polypeptide is a potent regulator of bile secretion from rat cholangiocytes. *Gastroenterology* 1999;117:420–428.

116. Colombo C, Crosignani A, Battezzati PM. Liver involvement in cystic fibrosis. *J Hepatol* 1999;31:946–954.

117. Mennone A, Biemersderfer D, Negoianu D, et al. Role of sodium/hydrogen exchanger isoform NME3 in fluid secretion and absorption in mouse and rat hepatocytes. *Am J Physiol* 2001;280:6247–6254.

118. Baiocchi L, LeSage G, Glaser S, et al. Regulation of cholangiocyte bile secretion. *J Hepatol* 1999;31:179–191.

119. Alpini G, Ulrich CD II, Phillips JO, et al. Upregulation of secretin receptor gene expression in rat cholangiocytes after bile ligation. *Am J Physiol* 1994;266:G922–G928.

120. Alpini G, Glaser SS, Ueno Y, et al. Bile acid feeding induces cholangiocyte proliferation and secretion: evidence for bile acid-regulated ductal secretion. *Gastroenterology* 1999;116:179–186.

121. LeSage G, Alvaro D, Benedetti A, et al. Cholinergic system modulates growth, apoptosis, and secretion of cholangiocytes from bile duct-ligated rats. *Gastroenterology* 1999;117:191–199.

122. Alpini G, Glaser S, Phinizy JL, et al. Bile acid depletion decreases cholangiocyte proliferative capacity and secretin-stimulated ductal bile secretion in bile duct-ligated (BDL) rats. *Gastroenterology* 1997;112:1210A(abst).

123. Alpini G, Glaser SS, Ueno Y, et al. Heterogeneity of the proliferative capacity of rat cholangiocytes after bile duct ligation. *Am J Physiol* 1998;274:G767–G775.

124. Glaser SS, Rodgers RED, Phinizy JL, et al. Gastrin inhibits secretin-induced ductal secretion by interaction with specific receptors on rat cholangiocytes. *Am J Physiol* 1997;36:G1061–G1070.

125. Caligiuri A, Glaser S, Rodgers R, et al. Endothelin-1 inhibits secretin-stimulated ductal secretion by interacting with ET_A receptors on large cholangiocytes. *Am J Physiol* 1998;275:G835–G846.

126. Craddock AL, Love MW, Daniel RW, et al. Expression and transport properties of the human ileal and renal sodium-dependent bile acid transporter. *Am J Physiol* 1998;37:157–169.

127. Benedetti A, DiSario A, Marucci L, et al. Carrier-mediated transport of conjugated bile acids across the basolateral membrane of biliary epithelial cells. *Am J Physiol* 1997;35:G1416–G1424.

128. Schaub TP, Kartenbeck J, Konig J, et al. Expression of the MRP2 gene-encoded conjugate export pump in human kidney proximal tubules and in renal cell carcinoma. *J Am Soc Nephrol* 1999;10:1159–1169.

129. Love MW, Dawson PA. New insights into bile acid transport. *Curr Opin Lipidol* 1998;9:225–229.

130. Ujhazy P, Ortiz DF, Misra S, et al. ATP-dependent aminophospholipid translocase activity in rat canalicular membrane vesicles and its relationship to FIC1. *Hepatology* 1999;30:462A (abst).

131. Clayton RJ, Iber FL, Ruebner BH, et al. Byler disease: fatal familial intrahepatic cholestasis in an Amish kindred. *Am J Dis Child* 1969;117:112–124.

132. Tygstrup N, Steig BA, Juijn JA, et al. Recurrent familial intra-hepatic cholestasis in the Faeroe Islands. phenotypic heterogeneity but genetic homogeneity. *Hepatology* 1999;29:506–508.

133. Oda T, Elkahloun AG, Pike BL, et al. Mutations in the human *Jagged1* gene are responsible for Alagille syndrome. *Nat Genet* 1997;16:235–242.

134. Li L, Kranta ID, Deng Y, et al. Alagille syndrome is caused by mutations in human *Jagged1*, which encodes a ligand for *Notch1*. *Nat Genet* 1997;16:243–251.

135. Gigliozzi A, Fraioli F, Sundaram P, et al. Molecular identification and functional characterization of mdr1a in rat cholangiocytes. *Gastroenterology* 2000;19:1113–1122.

136. Phillips MJ, Poucell S, Oda M. Mechanisms of cholestasis. *Lab Invest* 1986;54:593–608.

137. Weber AM, Tuchweber B, Yousef I, et al. Severe familial cholestasis in North American Indian children—a microfilament dysfunction. *Gastroenterology* 1981;81:653–662.

138. Boyer JL. Tight junctions in normal and cholestatic liver: Does the paracellular pathway have functional significance? *Hepatology* 1983;3:614–617.

139. Anderson JM. Leaky junctions and cholestasis: a tight correlation. *Gastroenterology* 1996;110:1662–1665.

140. Rahner C, Stieger B, Landmann L. Structure-function correlation of tight junctional impairment after intrahepatic and extrahepatic cholestasis in rat liver. *Gastroenterology* 1996;110:1564–1578.

141. Fallon MB, Brecher AR, Balda MS, et al. Altered hepatic localization and expression of occludin after common bile duct ligation. *Am J Physiol* 1995;269:C1057–C1062.

142. Fallon MB, Mennone A, Anderson JM. Altered expression and localization of the tight junction protein ZO-1 after common bile duct ligation. *Am J Physiol* 1993;264:C1439–C1447.

143. Lora L, Mazzon E, Martines D, et al. Hepatocyte tight-junctional permeability is increased in rat experimental colitis. *Gastroenterology* 1997;113:1347–1354.

144. Anderson JM, Glade JL, Stevenson BR, et al. Hepatic immunohistochemical localization of the tight junction protein ZO-1 in rat models of cholestasis. *Am J Pathol* 1989;134:1055–1062.

145. Spray DC, Bai S, Burk RD, et al. Regulation and function of liver gap junctions and their genes. In: Boyer JL, Ockner RK, eds. *Progress in liver diseases*. 12th ed. Philadelphia: WB Saunders, 1994:1–18.

146. Beuers U, Nathanson MH, Isales CM, et al. Tauroursodeoxycholic acid stimulates hepatocellular exocytosis and mobilizes extracellular Ca^{++} mechanisms defective in cholestasis. *J Clin Invest* 1993;92:2984–2993.

147. Nathanson MH, Rios-Velez L, Burgstahler A, et al. Communication via gap junctions modulates bile secretion in the isolated perfused rat liver. *Gastroenterology* 1999;116:1176–1183.

148. Fallon MB, Nathanson MH, Mennone A, et al. Altered expression and function of hepatocyte gap junctions after common bile duct ligation in the rat. *Am J Physiol* 1995;268:C1186–C1194.

149. Hamm-Alvarez SF, Sheetz MP. Microtubule-dependent vesicle transport: Modulation of channel and transporter activity in liver and kidney. *Physiol Rev* 1998;78:1109–1129.

150. Zegers MMP, Hoekstra D. Mechanisms and functional features of polarized membrane traffic in epithelial and hepatic cells. *Biochem J* 1998;336:257–269.

151. Misra S, Ujhazy P, Varticovski L, et al. Phosphoinositide 3-kinase lipid products regulate ATP-dependent transport by sister of P-glycoprotein and multidrug resistance-associated protein 2 in bile canalicular membrane vesicles. *Proc Natl Acad Sci U S A* 1999;96:5814–5819.

152. Misra S, Ujhazy P, Gatmaitan Z, et al. The role of phosphoinositide 3-kinase in taurocholate-induced trafficking of ATP-dependent canalicular transporters in rat liver. *J Biol Chem* 1998;273:26638–26644.

153. Ihrke G, Martin GV, Shanks MR, et al. Apical plasma membrane proteins and endolyn-78 travel through a subapical compartment in polarized WIF-B hepatocytes. *J Cell Biol* 1998;141: 115–133.

154. Tuma PL, Finnegan CM, Yi JH, et al. Evidence for apical endocytosis in polarized hepatic cells: Phosphoinositide 3-kinase inhibitors lead to the lysosomal accumulation of resident apical plasma membrane proteins. *J Cell Biol* 1999;145:1089–1102.

155. Larkin JM. Vesicle-mediated transcytosis — insights from the cholestatic rat liver. *Gastroenterology* 1993;105:594–610.

156. Larkin JM, Palade GE. Transcytotic vesicular carriers for polymeric IgA receptors accumulate in rat hepatocytes after bile duct ligation. *J Cell Sci* 1991;98:205–216.

157. Stieger B, Landmann L. Effects of cholestasis on membrane flow and surface polarity in hepatocytes. *J Hepatol* 1996;24: 128–134.

158. Stieger B, Meier PJ, Landmann L. Effect of obstructive cholestasis on membrane traffic and domain-specific expression of plasma membrane proteins in rat liver parenchymal cells. *Hepatology* 1994;20:201–212.

159. Jones AL, Schmucker DL, Mooney JS, et al. Morphometric analysis of rat hepatocytes after total biliary obstruction. *Gastroenterology* 1976;71:1050–1060.

160. Marks DL, LaRusso NF, McNiven MA. Isolation of the microtubule-vesicle motor kinesin from rat liver: selective inhibition by cholestatic bile acids. *Gastroenterology* 1995;108:824–833.

161. Rodriguez-Henche N, Guijarro LG, Couvineau A, et al. G proteins in rat liver proliferation during cholestasis. *Hepatology* 1994;20:1041–1047.

162. Boyer JL, Soroka CJ. Vesicle targeting to the apical domain regulates bile excretory function in isolated rat hepatocyte couplets. *Gastroenterology* 1995;109:1600–1611.

THE BIOLOGY OF PORTAL HYPERTENSION

ROBERTO J. GROSZMANN
MAURICIO R. LOUREIRO-SILVA
MING-HUNG TSAI

A grasp of the biological mechanisms involved in the pathogenesis of portal hypertension is essential to an understanding of the devastating complications of chronic liver disease and to the development of rational therapies. Ascites, gastroesophageal varices, gastropathy and portosystemic encephalopathy all result from this important syndrome. This chapter is an overview of the basic pathophysiological mechanisms of the intrahepatic, splanchnic and systemic circulatory derangements which lead to portal hypertension and cause the portosystemic collateral system to develop. The comprehension of basic hemodynamic principles (1) is essential for a better understanding of these pathophysiological mechanisms.

THE ROLE OF INCREASED RESISTANCE IN PORTAL HYPERTENSION

Anatomical Components

Portal hypertension is associated with increased resistance to the flow of portal blood; however, there is little resistance

R. J. Groszmann: Department of Internal Medicine (Digestive Diseases), Yale University School of Medicine, New Haven, Connecticut 06520; Department of Medicine, Digestive Disease Section, Veterans Affairs Connecticut Healthcare System, West Haven, Connecticut 06516.
M. R. Loureiro-Silva and M.-H. Tsai: Department of Medicine (Digestive Diseases), Yale University School of Medicine, New Haven, Connecticut 06520; Section of Digestive Diseases, VA Medical Center, West Haven, Connecticut 06516.

in the normal liver and portal pressure remains low (4 to 8 mmHg) over a wide range of portal flows. It is extremely important to recognize that flow into the portal system is actively regulated by changes in vascular resistance at the level of the splanchnic arterioles and not by the liver itself (2,3). Portal hypertensive syndromes have been classified according to the major site of resistance to portal blood flow, which may be prehepatic, posthepatic, or intrahepatic (presinusoidal, sinusoidal or postsinusoidal) (4,5).

Different anatomical lesions have been implicated in the development of increased intrahepatic resistance in chronic liver diseases. Fibrosis, hepatocyte enlargement, sinusoidal collapse, defenestration of endothelial sinusoidal cells, development of basement membrane in the space of Disse and regenerative nodule formation, individually or in a group, impair the mechanisms that compensate for changes in portal flow in order to maintain a normal portal pressure.

Liver fibrosis represents the hepatic tissue repair reaction that results from a disturbed balance between production and degradation of connective tissue in response to a chronic injury (6). Although activated hepatic stellate cells are believed to represent the principal fibroblastic cell type involved in liver fibrogenesis, fibroblast cells (a different liver cell population) present within the portal field or around central veins play an important role in scar formation (7).

Although the amount of extracellular matrix in the liver is similar in different forms of injury, its distribution within the liver lobule depends on the nature of the pathogen (8).

However, as the liver disease develops, the distribution pattern of fibrosis may change. For example, portal hypertension in hepatic schistosomiasis is often said to result from a granulomatous reaction to parasite eggs in the portal venules that results in periportal fibrosis (9). However, in late schistosomiasis, an elevated wedge hepatic venous pressure gradient may be observed, reflecting increased sinusoidal resistance due to deposition of collagen in the space of Disse (perisinusoidal fibrosis) and consequent sinusoidal narrowing (10). Correlation and lack of correlation between portal hypertension and different types of liver fibrosis have been reported (11–16).

In advanced cirrhosis, collagen in the space of Disse (perisinusoidal fibrosis) may resemble a basement membrane and serve as a barrier between the sinusoid and the liver cell, hindering transfer of oxygen and nutrients. The transition from the permeable perisinusoidal space to an impermeable collagenous membrane associated with endothelial defenestration has been described as capillarization by Schaffner and Popper (17). With capillarization, the thickened space of Disse causes narrowing of the sinusoids and results in increased vascular resistance (18,19). Endothelial fenestration is an important determinant of transinusoidal exchange and may also play a role in modulating intrahepatic resistance. Endotoxemia, commonly observed in cirrhotic patients, can by itself produce a reversible and significant decrease in the porosity of the sinusoidal endothelium (20). Bhunchet and Fujieda (21) have described capillarization as an intermediate process towards venulization of the sinusoids, which represents a defense mechanism to maintain the blood flow in the cirrhotic liver.

The hepatocyte enlargement is the only anatomical factor that can be effectively ameliorated resulting in portal pressure decrease. With abstinence from alcohol, portal hypertension may resolve (22), along with hepatomegaly, liver cell enlargement and steatosis. Shibayama et al. have studied the sinusoidal microcirculatory effects of liver cell enlargement in rats with cirrhosis induced by a diet deficient in choline (23). In this model, sinusoidal stenoses are caused by liver cell enlargement due to fat droplets, and are correlated with increased sinusoidal vascular resistance, portal hypertension and the presence of ascites. With a normal diet, hepatocyte size normalizes with disappearance of sinusoidal stenoses and a marked decrease in vascular resistance. Similar conclusions were reported using a carbon tetrachloride-induced cirrhotic model in which the major sites of increased resistance are in the intrahepatic portal vein, possibly resulting from distortion of its peripheral branches, and in the sinusoids. The increase in sinusoidal resistance was correlated with the encroachment of enlarged hepatocytes on the sinusoidal space (24). In another study, septal fibrosis in the rat was shown to have a significant impact on portal pressure only in the presence of deformation of the sinusoids induced by hepatocyte enlargement due to steatosis (25).

It has been postulated that at a critical point (50% over the normal hepatocyte size), the liver can no longer compensate for the hepatocyte enlargement due to the restriction of the hepatic cytoskeleton, resulting in portal pressure increase (26). In fact, no correlation between portal hypertension and a 45% enlargement of hepatocytes was observed (27).

Portal hypertension is frequently observed in acute liver failure and in acute hepatitis, and is probably caused by sinusoidal obstruction as well. Dropout of hepatocytes results in sinusoidal collapse, which can be assessed by reticulin staining with Sirius red. There is a direct correlation between the degree of reticulin collapse and portal pressure in acute liver failure (28). In addition, the severity of acute hepatitis, the hepatic venous pressure gradient and the fractional area of sinusoidal collapse also demonstrate close correlation (29).

A variety of other nonalcoholic liver diseases cause portal hypertension due to increased sinusoidal vascular resistance. In hepatic amyloidosis, portal pressure is correlated with compression of the sinusoids by massive amyloid deposits in the space of Disse (30). All of the above findings support the hypothesis that portal hypertension results from decreased intrahepatic vascular space of many causes; the location of the main obstruction varies with the etiology of the disease process.

Functional Components

The morphological changes occurring in chronic liver diseases are undoubtedly the most important factor involved in the increase in intrahepatic resistance. However, functional factors play an important role in the maintenance of increased vascular resistance. Bhatal et al. (31) were the first to show that nitroprusside and papaverine reduce perfusion resistance up to 15% in *in vitro* perfused cirrhotic rat liver, representing up to 28% of the magnitude by which hepatic vascular resistance of the liver exceeded normal values. Interestingly, the magnitude of the effect in the diseased liver seems to be similar for different vasodilators and is almost negligible in the normal liver. This demonstrates the presence of an enhanced intrinsic vascular tone in the intrahepatic microvascular bed of the cirrhotic liver, which is lacking in the normal controls.

It is a common dogma of vascular tone regulation that resistance to blood flow through a tissue is determined by the caliber of resistance vessels containing abundant vascular smooth muscle. Capillaries, on the other hand, being devoid of vascular smooth muscle, are thought to function solely as exchange vessels with no involvement in blood flow regulation. Numerous recent reports suggest that this paradigm may not be valid in the liver (32).

Normally, there is a step pressure gradient between the portal venules and central vein, demonstrating that the highest vascular resistance occurs in the sinusoidal microvasculature (33). In addition, liver sinusoids have been demonstrated to contract and relax in response to different vasoactive agents (34,35). Although sinusoidal endothelial cells posses contractile proteins (36), changes in sinusoidal lumen were found to be predominant at sites colocalizing with hepatic stellate cells (HSCs) (34).

HSCs are located in the space of Disse in close contact with hepatocytes and sinusoidal endothelial cells. Cytoplasmatic processes that rise from a multiform cell body project vertically toward the nearby sinusoids through the intercellular space or emit laterally, encircling the sinusoidal wall (37). This peculiar structure is reminiscent of tissue pericytes that control microcirculation by constricting capillaries (38,39). The contractile properties of HSCs have been demonstrated in normal livers (34,39,40) and with great enhancement after liver injury (41), leading to activation of this cell type. Activated HSCs express the cytoskeletal alpha smooth muscle actin gene, characteristic of vascular smooth muscle, whose amount seems to correlate with their capacity to contract (41,42). The contractility of HSCs can be modulated by vasoactive substances, such as nitric oxide (NO), endothelin, carbon monoxide (CO), prostaglandin F_{2a}, thrombin, angiotensin II, thromboxane A2, substance P, arginine vasopressin, etc. (39,41,43–46). Hence, the status of HSC activation and the ratio of vasoconstrictive/vasodilative agents present in the hepatic microcirculation could affect hepatic vascular resistance in liver cirrhosis.

Role of Endothelins in Normal and Cirrhotic Liver

Endothelins (ETs) constitute a family of 21-amino-acid peptides with potent vasoactive properties occurring in at least four isoforms, named ET-1, -2, -3 and β. Different cell types, including sinusoidal endothelial cells and HSCs, synthesize ETs (47). As major inducers of HSC contractility, ETs have emerged as possible candidates involved in the increased hepatic vascular resistance in liver cirrhosis (39,45,48). ET-1 is the most extensively studied of these peptides since it is, in equimolar terms, the most potent vasoconstrictor known so far (49). Two types of G-protein coupled receptors, ET_a and ET_b, mediate the vascular response to ETs, which thus depends on the ratio of different receptor subtypes on the local vasculature (50). On vascular smooth muscles both receptors are present and produce a sustained vasoconstriction. Thereby, ET-1 preferentially activates ET_a receptors due to the high receptor affinity (51). Endothelial cells, however, express only ET_b receptors, which bind ET-1 with lower affinity than ET_a receptors, mediating vasodilation by the release of NO and prostacyclins (51). ET receptors are expressed in the liver mainly on HSC and sinusoidal endothelial cells (SECs), but also to a lesser extend on Kupffer cells and hepatocytes (48,52).

In normal liver, ET-1 causes an increase in portal pressure in vivo as well as in isolated perfused liver, suggesting a contributory role of ET-1 for modulating hepatic vascular resistance (34,53–55). The site of action is controversial; several reports suggest a mainly sinusoidal effect being mediated predominantly by the contraction of HSC (39,42,44). On the other hand, Kaneda et al. have located the point of maximal contraction in response to ET-1 at the distal segment of preterminal portal venules and thus at a pre-sinusoidal level (56). However, neither acute nor chronic blockade of endothelin receptors has shown significant effects on portal pressure in normal rats (57–59). This argues against a major role of endogenous ET-1 in physiologic regulation of hepatic vascular tone.

In liver cirrhosis, arterial and venous plasma concentrations of ET-1 (and ET-3) are elevated, and a hepatosplanchnic release of ETs, which seems to correlate with sinusoidal pressure, has been reported (60–63). Moreover, gene expression of ET-1 is largely enhanced in cirrhotic liver whereby activated HSCs and SECs appear as major sites of ET-1 synthesis (62,64,65). Additionally, binding studies have shown an increased ET receptor density in cirrhotic rat liver (66). Correspondingly, increased ET receptor gene expression is found in liver tissue of cirrhotic patients, and seems to correlate with the degree of portal hypertension (65). Since ET-1 receptor density is higher on HSCs than on other hepatic cell types (67) and upregulation of ET receptors on HSCs occurs in liver cirrhosis (59), the enhanced ET receptor expression and density in the cirrhotic liver appears at least in part to be attributed to HSCs. With progression of liver injury, the degree of activation and ET-induced contractility of isolated HSCs increases proportionally (41). This might be reflected in the finding of a significant correlation between the extent of HSC activation and the level of portal vascular resistance in alcoholic patients (15). However, in the rat, ET-1-induced sinusoidal constriction is enhanced in the ethanol-induced fatty liver (68) but not in the cirrhotic liver, where ET-1 effects on hepatic hemodynamics have been reported to be blunted (41,62). The latter phenomenon could be explained by the higher basal contractile tone in advanced liver cirrhosis, allowing less room for a further increase in vascular resistance by ET-1 administration. The role of ET in modulating portal pressure in conditions of chronic liver disease and increased hepatic vascular resistance has been addressed in several studies by using ET receptor antagonists (41,57–59,62,69). Short-term administration of the nonselective ET_a and ET_b receptor blockers bosentan and TAK-044 decreased portal pressure in experimental cirrhosis to different degrees between 11% and 40% (57–59). This suggests a specific role for ET in the maintenance of increased intrahepatic vascular tone in liver cirrhosis. Chronic blockade of ET receptors so far, however, failed to prevent the development of portal hypertension and hyperdynamic circulation in cirrhotic rats (69), rendering the exact role of ETs in the pathogenesis of portal hypertension in liver cirrhosis open to further investigation.

Interestingly, NO donors or endogenous NO oppose or even completely abolish the vasoconstrictive effect of ET-1 on *in vitro* perfused liver or activated HSCs in culture (34,44,70,71). Additionally, it has been demonstrated that NO has a blocking effect on ET generation (72). Therefore, NO production in the microcirculatory unit of the liver is of crucial importance for counterbalancing at least the enhanced contractility of HSCs to different stimuli.

Endothelial Dysfunction and Nitric Oxide Deficiency (see Chapters 39 and 65 and Website Chapter ⌨ W-32)

Sinusoidal endothelial cells (SECs), although anatomically and biologically distinct from endothelial cells in other vasculature (e.g., lack of basement membrane and fenestration) are analogous to those cells in respect to the production and release of vasodilators such as NO (besides prostacyclins, carbon monoxide, hyperpolarizing factor, etc.) and vasoconstrictors such as ETs (73,74). Thereby, SECs modulate locally intrahepatic vascular tone, and a delicate balance exists between endothelial vasodilators and vasoconstrictors. Isolated SECs have been demonstrated to express endothelial nitric oxide-synthase (eNOS, a constitutive isoform associated with regulatory physiological mechanisms) protein and to increase the release of NO in response to flow and subsequently shear stress, the unique stimulus for the synthesis of NO by eNOS (75). Also in the intact *in vitro* perfused liver, incremental increases in flow, leading to an increase in perfusion pressure, contemporaneously activate eNOS, thereby increasing NO production, serving to limit the increase in perfusion pressure (76). Livers from cirrhotic rats with ascites showed no vasorelaxation or paradoxically vasoconstriction in response to acetylcholine (Fig. 47.1) (77). This paradoxic vasoconstriction is similarly observed in other vascular beds in conditions of hypertension and/or after the development of atherosclerosis and has also been attributed to the loss of counterbalancing vasodilatory effects of endothelium-derived NO (78,79). The reduction in NO release in the cirrhotic liver microcirculation also leads to greater increases in perfusion pressure in response to incremental increases in flow and subsequently shear stress (76). It has to be emphasized at this point that presumably in the cirrhotic liver due to rareness of the sinusoidal population, narrowing of the existing sinusoids by mechanical compression, regenerative nodules and fibrosis, extremely high blood velocities and wall shear forces affect the SECs. Considering that shear stress is the most potent physiologic regulator of eNOS (80–82), it is tempting to speculate that eNOS-derived NO production in the cirrhotic vasculature does not increase appropriately in response to the increased shear stress. Consequently, the impairment in the flow regulation promotes a further increase in portal vascular resistance.

NO influences vascular homeostasis not only by modulation of vasomotion. NO inhibits platelet aggregation,

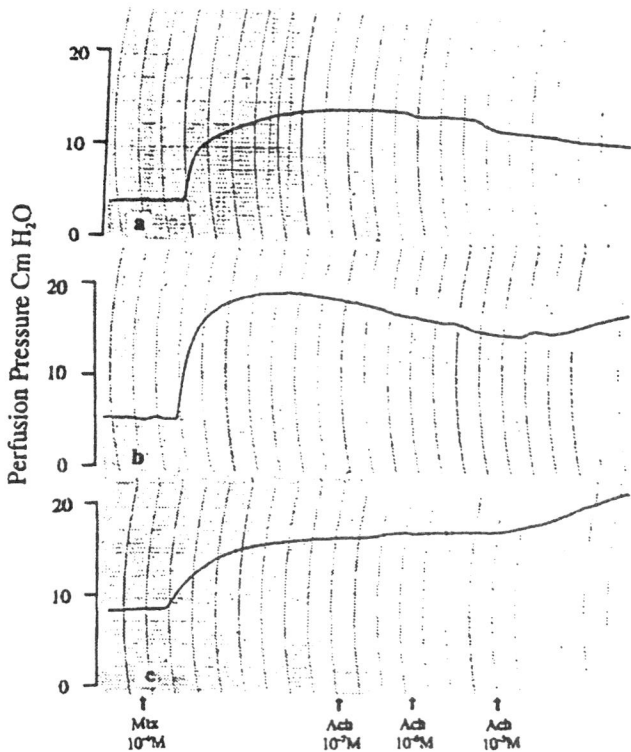

FIGURE 47.1. Representative tracings of response to cumulative doses of acetylcholine (*Ach*) after preconstriction of intrahepatic microcirculation with methoxamine (*Mtx*) in normal liver (*a*), cirrhotic liver from nonascitic rat (*b*), and cirrhotic liver from ascitic rat (*c*). The vasorelaxing response to Ach (nitric oxide-medicated) is significantly diminished in cirrhotic livers. (From Gupta TK, Toruner M, Chung MK et al. Endothelial dysfunction and decreased production of nitric oxide in the intrahepatic microcirculation of cirrhotic rats. *Hepatology* 1998;28:926–931, with permission.)

adhesion, and activation and keeps platelets in a resting stage, counteracting the direct platelet-activating effect of high shear stress levels likely to be present in the microcirculation of the cirrhotic liver (83,84). Consequently, decreased bioavailability of NO by injury to the endothelium is accompanied by increased thrombogenesis (85). In fact, thrombosis of medium and large portal veins and hepatic veins is a frequent occurrence in liver cirrhosis, which may contribute to the progression of portal hypertension (86). Cugno et al. (87) have shown in cirrhotic patients a decreased plasma concentration of both low and high molecular weight kininogen that could contribute also to the imbalance in coagulation and fibrinolysis.

Additionally, NO can alter extracellular matrix generation and decreases collagen synthesis in vascular smooth muscle cells (88). Therefore, it is reasonable to speculate that NO deficiency in cirrhotic liver may be involved in enhanced synthesis and deposition of collagen. Although this hypothesis still has to be proven, chronic treatment with L-arginine has been reported to protect the liver partially from the elevation of collagen content (89). Moreover, NO maintains the anti-adhesive nature of the endothelium by suppression of specific adhesion molecules, leading to inhibition of leukocyte and monocyte adhesion (83,90), which are known key events in the development of atherosclerosis and thus endothelial dysfunction (83,91). Finally, NO scavenges free oxygen radicals and directly interferes with enzyme systems producing oxygen radicals (92,93), thereby protecting the endothelium from oxidative stress. Indeed, NO inhibition has been demonstrated to increase lipid peroxidation induced by carbon tetrachloride (89). Taken together, these anti-atherogenic and antithrombotic properties of NO imply that the endothelial dysfunction associated with liver cirrhosis is one of the main factors that participate in the process of increasing hepatic vascular resistance.

This endothelial dysfunction in cirrhotic livers seems to manifest despite normal eNOS gene and protein expression (76,94) and has been suggested to be due to abnormalities in the posttranslational modification of eNOS in injured SECs. Caveolin-1, coat protein of intracellular transport vesicles and putative signaling molecule, decreases catalytic eNOS activity (95). This inhibitory effect is reversed by the stimulatory calcium-binding protein calmodulin (96). Shah et al. recently showed that (a) the catalytic activity of eNOS is reduced in cirrhotic liver despite normal eNOS protein levels, and (b) this reduction is associated with both an enhanced interaction of eNOS with caveolin-1 and a diminished interaction with calmodulin (76). Intriguingly, the expression of the inhibitory binding protein caveolin-1 is markedly increased in endothelial cells of cirrhotic livers.

In addition to a reduction in the production of NO, a decrease in the ability of the effector mechanism to respond fully to NO in cirrhotic rat livers was recently reported (97) in a comparative study of vasorelaxation induced by nitroglycerin and S-adenosyl-N-nitrosopenicillamine.

A deficit of other vasodilators, different from NO, could also be partly responsible for the increased hepatic vascular resistance in chronic liver diseases. By using N$^\omega$-nitro-L-arginine (NNA) for blockade of NO formation in the *in vitro* perfused cirrhotic liver, it has been shown that about 50% of the impairment in agonist-induced vasorelaxation are mediated by NO. The questions of what other vasodilators are involved and to what extent mechanical components participate in increased vascular resistance in cirrhosis remain to be answered. The vasodilator prostaglandin does not appear to be important for the regulation of hepatic vascular resistance (77,98). Most likely, the enhanced intrahepatic vascular tone in liver cirrhosis is multifactorial. However, a major contribution seems to be mediated by the deficit of NO. Therefore, pharmacological reduction of increased hepatic vascular resistance, for example by restoring NO, may open a new avenue of therapy. In fact, this is the most causative and primary pharmacological approach for the treatment of portal hypertension of intrahepatic ori-

gin at a given timepoint of existing liver fibrosis/cirrhosis. Presumably, restoring NO bioavailability in the liver microcirculation may in fact not only reverse the direct intrahepatic effects of NO deficiency but also prevent indirect complications that are associated with portal hypertension. Besides NO-donor molecules (97), transduction of liver with recombinant adenovirus carrying the neuronal NOS gene induces a reduction in intrahepatic vascular resistance and portal pressure in different models of cirrhosis and portal hypertension (99).

Carbon Monoxide as a Modulator of Hepatic Vascular Tone (see Chapter 39)

Carbon monoxide (CO), besides biliverdin and free iron, is a product of degradation of iron-protoporphyrin IX by the enzyme heme-oxygenase (HO). Like NO, CO is able to activate soluble guanylcyclase, inducing several regulation processes, including vasorelaxation (100). HO exists in three isoforms: the inducible HO-1, the constitutive HO-2 (100), and the recently discovered HO-3 (101). HO-1, which is identical to heat shock protein 32, is induced by different stimuli such as cytokines, heavy metals and oxidants. The HO substrate iron-protoporphyrin can also upregulate the inducible isoform (100).

The liver is one of the major organs in which the heme molecules are degraded by HO. Using immunohistochemical techniques, Goda et al. (102) have studied the distribution of HO-1 and HO-2 in rat livers. The inducible isoform HO-1 was observed only in Kupffer cells, while the constitutive isoform HO-2 was present in parenchymal cells but not in Kupffer cells. HO-2 in parenchymal cells appears to play a major role in the regulation of microvascular tone in physiological condition (102). However, the induction of HO-1 also increases CO generation, resulting in a vascular resistance decrease in perfused rat livers (103). In both conditions, the decrease in hepatic vascular resistance occurs through CO release in the perisinusoidal space, resulting in sinusoidal relaxation. Although both isoforms were undetectable in HSCs (102), the participation of these cells in the CO-mediated sinusoidal relaxation has been suggested (43).

Fernandes and Bonkovsky (104) have studied the expression of the HO isoforms in partial portal vein-ligated (PVL) and sham-operated (SO) rats. They assessed the expression of HO mRNA and protein by reverse-transcription polymerase chain reaction (RT-PCR) and Western blot analysis, and observed that (a) the HO-1 expression in hepatocytes and splanchnic organs was significantly higher in PVL (portal hypertensive) animals than in SO controls, and (b) HO-2 is expressed in all liver cell types and splanchnic organs of both PVL and SO animals.

Whether HO-1-mediated CO plays a role in the modulation of hepatic vascular resistance in cirrhotic animals (103) and whether the diseased vascular system does not relax in response to CO modulation remains to be clarified.

In summary, there are multiple intrahepatic lesions that may lead to increased resistance to blood flow. Some of them are at this point irreversible, such as fibrosis and capillarization of the space of Disse. Other lesions, particularly hepatocyte enlargement with sinusoidal encroachment, may be slowly reversible. Finally, functional factors that may modulate intrahepatic resistance are quite dynamic, including endothelial factors, sympathetic tone, possible activity of sinusoidal fenestrae and stellate cell activation. Ongoing study of reversible components carries with it the hope that therapeutic agents will eventually be developed which reduce portal pressure and improve liver perfusion in portal hypertension by lowering intrahepatic resistance.

PORTOSYSTEMIC COLLATERAL RESISTANCE

Portosystemic collaterals develop as a result of portal hypertension. Although they decompress the portal circulation, they also lead to important complications. The most lethal of these complications are gastroesophageal varices with variceal hemorrhage and portosystemic encephalopathy. In advanced disease, splanchnic blood flow is diverted almost entirely through the collateral system, bypassing the liver and depriving it of portal flow. Gastroesophageal collaterals are both a conduit through which toxins escape hepatic metabolism, and also a cause of significant morbidity and mortality due to their propensity to bleed.

Although the collateral circulation begins as a consequence of portal hypertension, it evolves into an important mediator of the circulatory derangements of portal hypertension in its own right. The vascular resistance of the collateral bed, although lower than that of the obstructed portal system, is nevertheless higher than normal portal resistance (105–110). Hence, portosystemic collaterals do not permit complete portal decompression, and portal hypertension persists even in the extreme situation in which all portal flow escapes through collaterals. The factors which modulate the development of the collateral system and regulate flow through it should be multiple. However, since portosystemic collaterals receive much of the splanchnic blood flow in portal hypertension, it follows that factors affecting this system will have a great impact on the vascular response of the entire portal circulation.

In the PVL rat, the collateral system is fully established within six to eight days following portal vein stenosis (111). Reduction in portal pressure by propranolol and clonidine has been shown to ameliorate the development of portosystemic shunting, indicating portal pressure as a major component in collateral formation (112,113). However, it has been shown that there is a strong positive correlation between portal pressure and mesenteric-systemic shunting one day after portal vein ligation (114). Nevertheless, this correlation disappears at three and seven days after ligation, suggesting that (a) portal hypertension is an important driving force for the initial development of portosystemic shunting, and (b) factors other than portal hypertension may be also involved in the later period. Furthermore, reduction of portosystemic shunting has also been reported by preventing an increase in splanchnic blood flow without any decrease in portal pressure (115). This demonstrates that a reduction in portal pressure is not an absolutely necessary requirement to ameliorate the collateral circulation. Therefore, propranolol and clonidine may prevent collateral formation at least in part by decreasing flow, and not only because of their effects on portal pressure. It has been shown that in portal hypertensive rats, the collateral vessels probably arise from the passive dilatation of the preexisting venous system (116). However, there is evidence indicating the possibility that NNA prevents the formation of new collateral vessels (115). In fact, NO may be directly involved in the development of collaterals. NO may act as an autocrine regulator of the microvascular events necessary for angiogenesis (117). Sumanovski et al. showed increased angiogenesis in chronic portal hypertension and inhibition of NO formation significantly preventing angiogenesis (118). Portal hyperemia leads to increased portocollateral blood flow and shear stress. These factors serve as a driving force to increase NO release from the collateral endothelium. Moreover, cyclic strain has been reported to upregulate endothelial NOS expression and subsequently NO production and endothelial proliferation, a process occurring within 24 hours of cyclic distention (119). This phenomenon might explain the positive correlation between portal pressure and mesenteric-systemic shunting on the first day after portal vein ligation, when increased shear stress in collateral circulation is not evident. Additionally, NO is an important regulator of vascular wall remodeling with luminal expansion (120). Taken together, it is attractive to hypothesize that portal vein ligation enhances immediately cyclic strain on splanchnic venous vasculature and preexisting collateral vessels, leading to endothelial NO release and resultant vasodilation and proliferation. Increased shear stress subsequently contributes to the ongoing development and maintenance of this collateral circulation. In addition, bacterial translocation, known to be a stimulus to upregulate NO production, takes place in most PVL rats in the early days after ligation (121). Its role in the development of collateral circulation and hyperdynamic circulation in this animal model needs to be clarified.

It is noteworthy to point out that portocaval anastomosis and portosystemic shunting are associated with similar systemic circulatory disturbance as observed in portal hypertension (122). Moreover, the graded diversion of portal blood flow to the systemic circulation has been shown to cause a systemic vasodilatory response in portal hypertensive and particularly in normal rats, indicating that portosystemic shunting per se may contribute to arterial vasodilatation in portal hypertension (123).

The development of an isolated perfused portosystemic collateral circulation in a rat model has permitted direct investigation of this important circulatory bed (124). A role for the endothelium-derived relaxing factor NO is demonstrated in studies using this model. Following acetylcholine-induced vasodilatation (a phenomenon known to be mediated by NO secretion), the infusion of NNA is shown to prevent this vasodilatation. Likewise, removal of endothelium also prevents acetylcholine-induced vasodilatation. The vasodilators isoproterenol (a β_2-adrenoreceptor agonist) and sodium nitroprusside, a NO donor, which have endothelium-independent mechanisms of action, are not blocked by NNA or by removal of endothelium. These findings support a role for endothelium-derived NO in modulating vascular resistance in the portal collateral system. Additionally, prostaglandin has recently been suggested to modulate responses to vasoconstrictor in the collateral circulation (125).

Isoproterenol induces vasodilatation of the isolated perfused portosystemic collateral bed, suggesting the presence of β-adrenoreceptors. This is supported by the fact that propranolol, a nonspecific β-adrenoreceptor blocker, prevents isoproterenol-induced vasodilatation (124). It is not yet known which β-adrenoreceptor subtype (β_1 or β_2) mediates vasodilatation, although the presence of both subtypes in the superior mesenteric vein and of only β_2-adrenoreceptors in the rat portal vein is already reported (126).

Studies using the vasoconstrictor norepinephrine suggest the presence of α-adrenoreceptors in the portal collateral system, although it is not yet known which subtype of α-adrenoreceptors predominates. An important vasoconstrictor role for 5-hydroxytryptamine (5-HT) is also demonstrated in this vascular bed; selective blockade of 5-HT-mediated vasoconstriction by ICI 169,369 provides evidence that the receptors involved may be of the 5-HT_2 type (124). In addition, Chan et al. recently reported that vasopressin produces a direct vasoconstrictive effect on the portosystemic collateral vessels through the vasopressin V_1 receptor (125).

THE HYPERDYNAMIC CIRCULATION IN PORTAL HYPERTENSION

As the understanding of resistance has become more detailed in recent years, other factors in the pathogenesis of portal hypertension have also been examined. By now the so-called hyperdynamic circulation in portal hypertension has become well accepted, and has relegated to a position of largely historical interest the once prevalent "backward flow theory" (see Chapter 45 and website chapter 🖵 W-34).

In the normal state, the flow of portal blood through the liver accounts for nearly all the blood entering the splanchnic system (portal venous inflow). In portal hypertension, perfusion of the liver by portal blood is decreased and may be negligible. Despite hepatic hypoperfusion with portal blood, the portal venous inflow is actually greatly increased.

In portal hypertension, portal venous inflow is therefore comprised of (diminished) portohepatic blood flow plus the large amount of blood that bypasses the liver through portosystemic collaterals (110).

Identification of the hyperdynamic circulatory state, including increased portal venous inflow, led to the recognition of the importance of the increased inflow into the portal system as a major factor in the development and maintenance of portal hypertension (127–129).

The clinical manifestations of the hyperdynamic circulation are rapid pulse, warm, well-perfused extremities and low blood pressure. Hemodynamic studies reveal high cardiac index, low systemic vascular resistance and expanded blood volume (129,130). Its characteristics have been studied in humans (128,130–132) as well as laboratory animals (109,133,134). The presence of a hyperdynamic circulation has been shown to be independent of the site of increased resistance to blood flow in humans, and is well-documented in various types of portal hypertension (129–132,135,136). A widely studied animal model is the rat with portal vein stenosis, which develops a syndrome with many similarities to the circulatory derangements seen in humans. These include elevated portal pressure, portosystemic shunting, and a hyperdynamic splanchnic and systemic circulation (127,133,137).

The hyperdynamic circulation is characterized by an elevated cardiac index with generalized vasodilatation due to decreased arteriolar resistance in many regional vascular territories. Increased flow is observed in peripheral beds such as skeletal muscle (131,138) and visceral organs such as the kidneys (110,127). Flow to the splanchnic organs (intestines, spleen, pancreas, stomach) is increased by approximately 50% in comparison with normal controls (110,127,134,139).

The hyperdynamic circulation is now recognized to play a role in elevating the portal pressure and in maintaining portal hypertension, despite the presence of a portosystemic collateral system. However, normalization of increased portal venous inflow reduces portal pressure by no more than 15% to 20% (106,107,109). Therefore, the pathogenesis of portal hypertension is now viewed as interplay between elevated resistance and hyperdynamic flow (107,109,128, 140).

Although the hyperdynamic circulation plays a secondary role in the pathogenesis of portal hypertension, it has been the focus of intensive research. One important reason is that the presence of collateral circulation and vasodilatation which is part of the hyperdynamic splanchnic and systemic circulation contributes directly to the clinical consequences of portal hypertension, including portosystemic encephalopathy, ascites, and hemorrhage from gastroesophageal varices. Moreover, the mechanisms of action of most of the pharmacologic agents clinically available for the treatment of portal hypertension involve modulation of the hyperdynamic circulation.

PATHOGENESIS OF THE HYPERDYNAMIC CIRCULATION

Increased Circulating Levels of Vasodilators in Chronic Liver Disease (Fig. 47.2)

Much attention has been focused on the search for humoral mediators of the hyperdynamic syndrome. Investigators have postulated that endogenous vasodilators which are present in portal blood and cleared by the normal liver may be bypassing the liver through portosystemic collaterals and/or escaping extraction and inactivation due to hepatocellular dysfunction. Experimental data have lent support to the hypothesis that a transferrable humoral factor is present in the blood of portal hypertensive donor animals (138,141). However, in a parabiotic rat model with extensive cross-circulation between portal vein stenosed and control animals, the latter do not develop a hyperdynamic circulation (142). Rather than refuting the existence of a transferable factor, these data may indicate that extraction and inactivation of the vasodilator(s) by the normal liver and/or dilution prevent vasodilatation in this model.

Glucagon has served as the prototype among endogenous vasodilators found in increased concentrations in portal hypertension. Increased circulating glucagon has been demonstrated in portal hypertensive animals and humans (143–146).

By infusing glucagon into normal rats to achieve levels seen in portal hypertensive controls, Benoit and coworkers demonstrate that this peptide significantly decreases splanchnic vascular resistance (141). Moreover, an antiserum directed against glucagon ameliorates the hyperdynamic splanchnic circulation in portal hypertensive animals (147). These investigators estimate that glucagon could account for up to 40% of the splanchnic hyperemia observed in portal hypertension. However, Sikuler and Groszmann report no correlation between blood glucagon levels and portal venous inflow, and therefore question a major role for glucagon in mediating the hyperdynamic circulation (148).

Some experimental data suggest that the vasoconstrictive action of somatostatin is in part due to inhibition of glucagon release and support a role for glucagon in maintaining splanchnic hyperemia in portal hypertension (149,150). However, recent data seem to suggest a minor role in the vasodilatation observed in cirrhotic patients (151) and suggest a different mechanism for the vasoconstrictive activity of somatostatin (152).

Postprandial splanchnic circulatory response in cirrhosis could shed light on some of the hemodynamic derangements that characterize the portal hypertensive state. In fact, postprandial hyperemia could be a risk factor for variceal bleeding in cirrhotic patients. Octreotide, a long-acting synthetic analogue of somatostatin, has been reported to blunt postprandial hyperemia in cirrhotic patients (153,154). These findings suggest that vasointestinal peptides are important factors leading to postprandial hyperemia and a target for treatment in this setting. Inter-

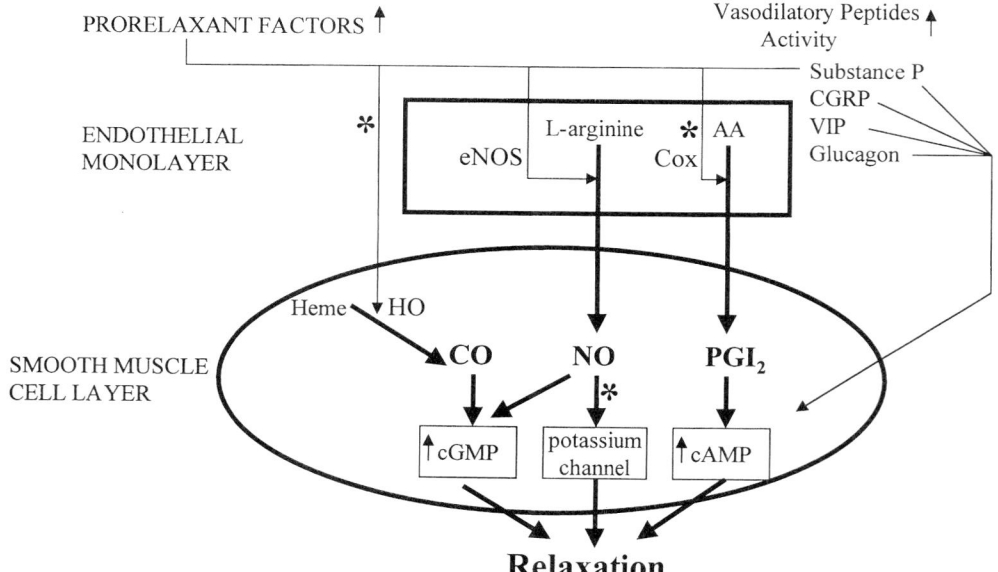

FIGURE 47.2. Various possible pathways that may induce vasodilatation in chronic liver diseases. *Asterisks* represent possible mechanisms that need to be confirmed in portal hypertensive states. *CGRP*, calcitonin gene-related peptide; *eNOS*, endothelial nitric oxide synthase; *NO*, nitric oxide; *CO*, carbon monoxide; *Cox*, cyclooxygenase; *HO*, heme oxygenase; *PGI₂*, prostacyclin; *AA*, arachidonic acid.

estingly, the potent vasodilator NO may also contribute to postprandial hyperemia (155,156).

Although somatostatin infusion decreases hyperdynamic portal venous inflow and portal hypertension, it does not reduce them to normal, indicating that additional factors must be at work. Moreover, somatostatin also inhibits the release of several other splanchnic peptide vasodilators such as vasoactive intestinal peptide and substance P. Hence, the effect of somatostatin on the hyperdynamic circulation may be mediated by other peptides in addition to glucagon. However, roles for these substances are purely conjectural at this time (149). Furthermore, a study recently released from our laboratory suggests that octreotide potentiates local vasoconstriction in superior mesenteric arteries by a mechanism involving the activation of protein kinase C that is consistent with our recent observation in cirrhotic patients (151,152).

It may be noteworthy that the splanchnic circulation in cirrhosis appears to have greater glucagon sensitivity than the systemic circulation. In cirrhosis, doses which cause only minimal systemic effects cause significant increases in portal pressure and azygos blood flow (an index of collateral blood flow) resulting from splanchnic vasodilatation and increased portal venous inflow (144). However, evidence is mounting against an important role for glucagon in the hyperdynamic circulation of cirrhosis.

A role for prostacyclin in mediating the hyperdynamic splanchnic circulation in portal vein-stenosed rabbits has also been proposed (157). In these animals, increased mesenteric blood flow, decreased vascular resistance and increased splenic pulp pressure (an approximation of portal pressure) are associated with significant (27%) increases in the systemic arterial concentration of prostacyclin. On the other hand, patients with liver cirrhosis have been reported to have increased levels of 6-keto-PGF, a stable metabolite of prostacyclin (158). Cyclooxygenase blockade with indomethacin results in a decrease in prostacyclin levels and significant amelioration of the hyperdynamic circulation in experimental animals and cirrhotic patients (157,159,160). This in turn is reversed, with relapse of splanchnic hyperemia and exacerbation of portal hypertension, when prostacyclin is infused into indomethacin-treated animals. The splanchnic hemodynamic effects of prostacyclin are also demonstrated in normal rabbits, in which dose-related increases are observed in blood flow in the superior mesenteric artery and portal vein. Prostacyclin may also be a systemic vasodilator in chronic portal hypertension, attaining high circulating levels by bypassing the liver (its main site of degradation) via portosystemic collaterals (159). Cyclooxygenase blockade results in improved vascular response to vasoconstrictors (161,162). Cyclooxygenase can be either constitutive or inducible. Either type has been reported to be stimulated by the same physicochemical factors that regulate its NO counterpart (163–166). Investigators have shown increased constitutive cyclooxygenase I expression in

the superior mesenteric artery of portal vein-stenosed rats two days after surgery (167). In addition, inhibition of prostaglandin has been shown to improve splanchnic hemodynamics independent of NO in portal hypertensive rabbits (168). Finally, experiments exploring the interaction between these two vasodilators showed a possible compensatory mechanism between the two vasoactive substances that promote splanchnic hyperemia (169). A conflicting report argues against the role of prostaglandin (170).

CO has been reported to interact with other vasodilators such as NO and glucagon in various pathophysiological conditions (171–175). Increased inducible HO-1 isoform expression in the splanchnic organ and liver in portal vein-stenosed rat has been observed (104). Its pathophysiological significance in the vasodilation observed in cirrhosis and the relevance to other vasodilators need to be clarified.

A number of other endogenous vasodilators have been tested in the search for humoral mediators of the hyperdynamic circulation. For example, bile acids circulate in increased levels in portal hypertensive states and possess vasodilatory properties. In one study using portal vein-stenosed rats, reduction to normal of circulating bile acid levels was not accompanied by amelioration of the hyperdynamic circulation (176). Hence, the role of bile acids in mediating the hyperdynamic circulation is not well defined. The role of the capsaicin-calcitonin gene-related peptide (CGRP) vasodilation pathway is still controversial (177–179). A number of other candidate vasodilators have been studied without demonstration of a significant role for any of them.

Vasoconstriction activated by most vasoconstrictors involves several steps. They consist of interaction of the agonist with the receptor, and then a signal transduction pathway involving guanine nucleotide regulatory proteins (G protein), membrane phosphoinositide hydrolysis, protein kinase C and mobilization of intracellular and extracellular calcium (180). Interaction between endogenous vasodilators and this signal transduction system has also been reported (181,182). Abnormalities of this signal transduction mechanism have been shown in cirrhotics and portal hypertensive animals (182,183). Studies investigating signal transduction anomaly in denuded mesenteric vasculature and aorta have yielded different localizations of alteration in this signal cascade (184,185). However, these studies may provide another explanation for the persistently (although improved) blunt response to vasopressor after de-endothelization or incubation with NNA that has been attributed to structural change or presence of other vasodilators (186–188).

Attention has been focused on the role of local vasodilators produced by the endothelium of resistance vessels, which play a major role in the intrinsic modulation of vascular tone (189,190). The discovery of endothelium-derived relaxing factors and the identification of NO as the most important of these factors (191,192) have provided an important opportunity for further exploration of the hyperdynamic circulation.

Acute administration of the nonspecific NO synthase inhibitor NNA in portal hypertensive rats has been shown to normalize the splanchnic and systemic hemodynamics with reduction in portal venous inflow, cardiac output, improved mean arterial pressure and an increase in both splanchnic and systemic vascular resistance (193,194). Chronic inactivation of overproduced NO by increasing blood hemoglobin that scavenges NO was demonstrated to improve splanchnic vasodilatation in portal hypertension (195). Likewise, chronic inhibition of NO production by L-arginine analogues corrects peripheral vasodilation and prevents the development of systemic hyperdynamic ciculation in portal vein-ligated rats (196,197). This vasodilatation is characterized by hyporeactivity to various vasoconstrictors including norepinephrine, angiotensin, methoxamine, vasopressin and endothelin (198–202). The impaired responsiveness to vasoconstrictors is independent of the type of receptor and is not due to altered number or affinity to receptors (198, 203). Furthermore, non-receptor-mediated vasoconstriction is also impaired (204,205). This vasoresponsiveness defect is found not only in mesenteric vasculature but also in aortic vessels (206–209) and has been localized to the endothelium, since removal of endothelium corrects in large part the hyporeactivity (186). NO has been shown to be responsible for the endothelium-derived hyporeactivity by the demonstration of inhibition of NO biosynthesis restoring vascular reactivity to normal levels (199,200,204, 205,210). Thereby, endothelial NO overproduction plays an important role in both splanchnic and systemic vasodilation. Since the use of high doses of NO inhibitors in these investigations could have potentially led to maximal blockade of normal NO synthesis rather than exact inhibition of overproduced NO, Niederberger et al. used low doses of L-NAME titrated to achieve levels of vascular NO production in cirrhotic rats comparable to those in normal rats. Normalization of vascular NO synthesis, estimated by aortic concentration of cGMP, resulted in normalization of arterial pressure, cardiac index, and systemic vascular resistance in experimental cirrhosis (211). In patients with alcoholic cirrhosis, forearm blood flow is increased and vascular resistance is decreased compared to healthy controls. Brachial infusion of L-NMMA dose-dependently decreases forearm blood flow, with the vasoconstrictor response being greater in decompensated patients than in compensated patients (212). In response to methacholine, which stimulates eNOS-derived NO release, the increase in forearm blood flow has been shown to be enhanced in cirrhotic patients compared to normal subjects, whereas the effect of sodium nitroprusside, an endothelium-independent vasodilator, was found unaltered (213). It is widely known that NO exerts its vasodilation effect through cGMP, an intracellular second messenger that has been used as an index of NO production (214). Investigators have reported

increased cGMP in tissue homogenates of superior mesenteric arteries and aorta of portal hypertensive rats (211,215), and *in vitro* in a reporter cell line coincubated with mesenteric arteries of cirrhotic rats stimulated with bradykinin (216). However, it is notable that cGMP is not the exclusive mediator activated by NO. It is known that NO can directly activate potassium channels (217). Atucha et al. showed that a combined administration of a guanylate cyclase inhibitor and a nonspecific potassium channel blocker potentiates the pressure response to vasoconstrictors in superior mesenteric arteries as compared to treatment with either inhibitor (218). Finally, direct demonstration of enhanced production of NO in splanchnic vasculature was shown in *in vitro* perfused mesenteric arteries, with monitoring of endothelial NO release by chemiluminescence (187,219) (Fig. 47.3). The predominant splanchnic origin of increased NO production in cirrhotic patients is reflected by higher plasma concentrations of NO in portal venous plasma than in peripheral venous plasma (220).

Vallance and Moncada proposed the hypothesis that endotoxemia of liver cirrhosis upregulates induced NO synthase (iNOS) in vessel walls, leading to sustained NO release and hyperdynamic circulation (221). However, a strong line of evidence over the past years suggests the eNOS isoform as the main enzymatic source of NO overproduction. A unique function of eNOS is the production of NO in response to blood flow and shear stress (222). Flow-mediated vasodilatation is proportional to shear stress induced by flow and is independent of intraluminal pressure. This is the normal constitutive mechanism that mediates vascular dilatation secondary to increased blood flow. Chronic elevation in blood flow by exercise or arteriovenous fistula leads to an increased production of endothelial NO (223). Mesenteric arteries of portal hypertensive rats which are exposed to chronic high blood flow are found to upregulate eNOS protein (224–226). Additionally, the enzyme activity is enhanced, as evidenced by a calcium-dependent increase in L-arginine conversion to L-citruline in the particulate fraction but not in the cytosolic fraction from superior mesenteric arteries of portal hypertensive rats and rabbits (215,227). Finally, endothelial production and release of NO in response to flow and shear stress is enhanced in superior mesenteric arteries of portal hypertensive rats (219). This increased synthesis of NO is easily explainable as a normal chronic adaptive mechanism of the endothelium in response to chronically increased splanchnic blood flow and subsequently enhanced shear stress (222). However, it has recently been demonstrated that in the mesenteric vasculature, eNOS upregulation and thus increased eNOS-derived NO release precede the development of the hyperdynamic splanchnic circulation in portal hypertensive rats (228). Therefore, shear stress alone is not responsible for eNOS upregulation; other factors are involved.

Comparable to the splanchnic circulation, a growing number of studies support eNOS as the major enzymatic source for the vascular NO overproduction responsible for

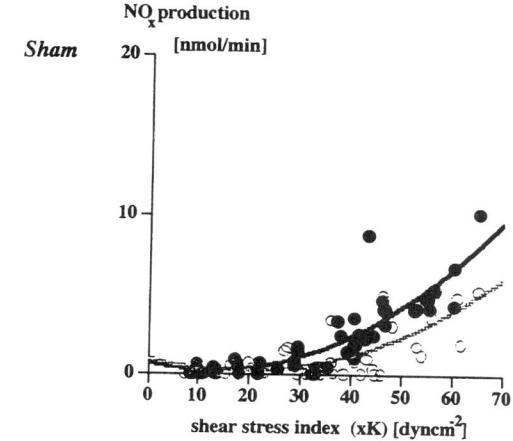

Sham

A

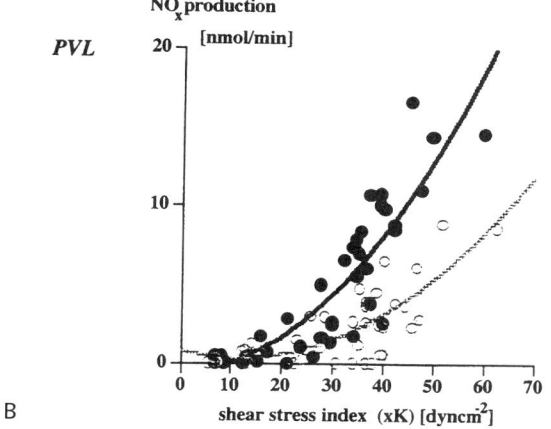

PVL

B

FIGURE 47.3. Regression coefficients between the amount of NOx (nitric oxide metabolite) production and shear stress index. Experiments in **(A)** sham and **(B)** portal vein-ligated (PVL) rats. Note the significantly higher slope of NOx production versus shear stress index in PVL rats compared with sham rats during the first perfusion cycle [$P < 0.0001$, analysis of variance (ANOVA) with repeated measurements]. Incubation with L-NMMA decreased the slopes in both treatment groups, the decrease being significantly greater in the PVL rats. *filled circles*, 1st perfusion cycle (Krebs alone); *open circles*, 2nd perfusion cycle (after L-NMMA). (From Hori N, Wiest R, Groszmann RJ. Enhanced release of nitric oxide in response to changes in flow and shear stress in the superior mesenteric arteries of portal hypertensive rats. *Hepatol* 1998;28:1467–1473, with permission.)

systemic arterial vasodilation. The hyporesponsiveness to vasoconstrictors in aortic rings of portal hypertensive rats is endothelium-dependent and reversed by nonspecific inhibition of NO formation (207–209). This demonstrates that endothelium-derived NO is the major vasodilator responsible for this manifestation of systemic arterial vasodilation. This endothelial NO production has been shown to be calcium-dependent and inhibitable by selective calmodulin inhibitors (207). Additionally, aminoguanidine, a preferential inhibitor of iNOS, was found to have no effect on aortic hyporeactivity in experimental cirrhosis, not supporting

iNOS induction as the source of NO in this vasculature (208,209). Moreover, vasodilator response to substances exerting their effect by eNOS-derived NO release is enhanced in aortic rings of portal hypertensive rats (207,229). These findings are consistent with eNOS upregulation and eNOS-derived NO overproduction in the systemic circulation being responsible for arterial vasodilation and reduction in vascular resistance. However, enhanced iNOS activity was reported in aortic tissue in the very early phase after portal vein ligation (210). Its appearance seems transient, and its pathophysiological significance in this animal model needs to be defined.

On the other hand, endotoxemia is a common finding in liver cirrhosis, particularly with progressive severity of disease and predominantly in the portal circulation (230–232). Endotoxin and lipopolysaccharides are potent stimuli for NO synthesis directly and via proinflammatory cytokines (233). However, investigators have failed to convincingly link endotoxemia and iNOS production. So far, no clear iNOS protein expression has been detected in the splanchnic vasculature of different animal models of portal hypertension (224,226,227). However, transcriptional expression of iNOS has been reported (224,234), leaving the possibility of low-level vascular iNOS in operation. Nevertheless, the high sensitivity of RT-PCR for the detection of iNOS mRNA in these studies has to be taken into consideration in the interpretation of these results, particularly in respect to the hemodynamic significance of the low level of iNOS-mediated NO. Additionally, the development of hyperdynamic circulation and associated vascular hyporesponsiveness in portal hypertension could not be prevented by inhibition of iNOS by dexamethasone or aminoguanidine (235,236). These findings do not support a major role of iNOS-mediated NO synthesis in the splanchnic vasodilatation and hyperdynamic circulation in portal hypertension.

However, several studies found a correlation between serum levels of endotoxin and NO in liver cirrhosis (237,238), suggesting a causative role of endotoxemia for the observed NO overproduction. Recently, Wiest et al. disclosed enhanced eNOS expression in mesenteric tissue in the presence of bacterial translocation in ascitic cirrhotic rats, supporting such a link (187). Moreover, tumor necrosis factor alpha (TNF-α), a known stimulus of NO release (233), is noted in increased levels in portal hypertension (238,239). Antagonism of TNF-α with antibodies or thalidomide blunts the development of the hyperdynamic circulation in prehepatic portal hypertensive or cirrhotic rats (239,240). Furthermore, another study showed that tyrosine kinase inhibition, and thus blocking the signaling events induced by TNF-α, ameliorates the hyperdynamic state and decreases NO production in cirrhotic rats with ascites (241). However, the TNF-α level is not consistently correlated with hemodynamic impairment (187,239). This discrepancy may be due to the method of analysis or simply a reflection of different roles in different animal models. It is noteworthy to point out that several studies failed to find significant endotoxemia in PVL rats (231,242), thus making the connection between endotoxemia and TNF-α only conjectural in this model at this point. Bacterial translocation to mesenteric lymph node is a common finding in cirrhotic animals (243). Recent evidence has suggested a link between bacterial translocation and elevated TNF-α and enhanced eNOS-derived NO production and thus further hemodynamic impairment (187). It is likely that this confined harboring of bacteria triggers the immunity system, producing cytokines including TNF-α that in turn contribute to the hemodynamic impairment. Analysis of endotoxin in the infected lymph node might help solve this issue. It is conceivable that bacterial translocation can aggravate vasodilatation by upregulating the TNF-α-stimulated cofactor tetrahydrobiopterin, which in turn upregulates eNOS-derived NO biosynthesis (187). However, the exact mechanism remains to be clarified. Finally, some authors proposed that the increased TNF-α and NO levels in the portal hypertension state tend to create oxidative stress, which might in turn contribute to hyperdynamic circulation. Those authors showed that hyperdynamic circulation could be prevented in different animal models by the administration of an antioxidant such as lipoic acid and N-acetylcysteine (244,245). However, further investigations of the mechanism and the effects of antioxidants in well-established portal hypertensive models should be performed to confirm this finding.

Plasma Volume

The hyperdynamic circulation is mediated in large part by vasodilatation, but this alone is not sufficient to cause the circulation to become hyperdynamic. Many vasodilators lower vascular resistance in normal humans or animals, but also cause underfilling of the circulation due to increased vascular capacitance. In this situation, the cardiac index either decreases or remains unchanged, rather than becoming hyperkinetic (246–248).

For many years, plasma volume expansion has been recognized in a wide variety of portal hypertensive liver diseases (130,249). In conditions of constant peripheral vascular resistance, an increase in circulatory blood volume results in increased venous return and cardiac output (250). However, an acute expansion of blood volume leads to stress relaxation of the vasculature and cardiac output after the initial increase returns to normal. This demonstrates that blood volume expansion alone is not sufficient to maintain a hyperkinetic circulatory state. It is the combination of arterial vasodilation and blood volume expansion that makes optimal conditions for maintaining the hyperdynamic circulatory state in portal hypertension. Sodium retention is the earliest and the most frequent abnormality of renal function associated with portal hypertension (251–253) and is the pathophysiological hall-

mark for plasma volume expansion. Studies using the portal vein-stenosed rat have explored the role of plasma volume expansion in the hyperdynamic circulation (254). Major hemodynamic differences are observed between portal vein-stenosed rats fed a sodium-restricted diet, in which plasma volume fails to expand, compared with controls fed a normal diet. The dramatic increases in systemic and splanchnic blood flow as well as portal pressure seen in the normal diet group are significantly attenuated in the sodium-restricted group. Moreover, the fully developed hyperdynamic circulation is found to be nearly reversible by sodium restriction, with decreases towards normal in portal venous inflow and portal pressure, as well as increases in systemic and splanchnic vascular resistance. In contrast, sodium restriction in the normal rat has little hemodynamic effect (254).

Subsequent studies have demonstrated that in the portal vein-stenosed rat, vasodilatation, expansion of the plasma volume by sodium retention, and development of the hyperdynamic circulation follow each other in a stepwise sequence (251,255). Resistance in the systemic circulation drops significantly within one day of partial portal vein ligation, followed on day 2 by parallel increases in plasma volume and a progressive increase in systemic and regional blood flows. The fully expanded plasma volume is observed on day 4 and coincides with a maximally hyperkinetic cardiac index and regional blood flows. In PVL rats, it has been shown that central blood volume is the responsible signal triggering sodium retention (256). Peripheral vasodilation occurs within one day after portal vein ligation (251), leading to a decrease in central blood volume, probably due to an impairment in venous return to the heart. This relative underfilling of arterial circulation is the physiological stimulus for baroreceptor, for activating the sympathetic nervous system, renin–angiotensin system, and for release of antidiuretic hormone. Mediators from these systems then result in sodium and water retention by the kidneys. Sodium retention is mainly due to increased tubular reabsorption of sodium mediated by receptors for angiotensin, aldosterone and α-adrenergic stimuli (257,258). The impairment in water excretion is more complex and involves an increased secretion of antidiuretic hormone, reduced delivery of filtrate to the ascending limb of the loop of Henle, and reduced renal synthesis of prostaglandins (253). In prehepatic portal hypertension, the avidity for sodium retention ceases with the normalization of the central volume (256). In liver cirrhosis, however, more complex mechanisms probably take place. Myocardial reserve function is also impaired, complicating the response to blood volume load (259). Moreover, the development of ascites leads to an additional fluid shift, perpetuating the relative circulatory underfilling and acting as a constant stimulus for sodium retention.

Short-term inhibition of NO synthesis results in a significant increase in urine volume and sodium excretion in rats with cirrhosis and ascites, but not in normal rats (260,261). This effect is not likely to be due to a direct renal effect of the

NOS inhibitor since its intrarenal infusion increases renal blood flow but does not affect natriuresis (262). The mechanism of natriuresis induced by NO inhibition is multifactorial. Inhibition of NO synthesis in nonpressor doses improves renal excretion of sodium and water mainly via a decrease in tubular reabsorption (261). Additionally, in the presence of an arterial hypertensive response, the natriuretic effect occurs predominantly by a pressure-induced increase in filtered sodium load (260). Subsequently, the prolonged inhibition of NO synthesis not only restores systemic hemodynamics by correcting peripheral vasodilation but also ameliorates sodium retention and plasma volume expansion in PVL rats (196). Thereby, the observed negative correlation between arterial pressure and plasma volume and sodium space further supports the causal relationship between peripheral vasodilation and sodium retention and plasma volume expansion in experimental portal hypertension. Indeed, studies that examined the role of vasodilatation and plasma volume expansion in the hyperdynamic circulation provide support for the peripheral arterial vasodilatation hypothesis (252,263). This theory offers a unifying explanation of the salient clinical features of the portal hypertensive syndrome, namely the hyperdynamic circulatory state, renal sodium retention and, in the presence of intrahepatic sinusoidal hypertension, also the accumulation of ascites. Finally, normalization of hemodynamics by normalizing vascular NO production improves sodium and water handling in ascitic cirrhotic rats (211). These changes take place in the setting of a decrease in plasma concentrations of renin, aldosterone, and vasopressin to normal levels with no change in the glomerular filtration rate. These findings are consistent with a reversal of arterial underfilling secondary to systemic vasodilation, leading to a downregulation of baroreceptors and volume receptors and thus a decrease in sympathetic firing and release of vasopressin, as well as increased renal perfusion pressure with subsequent deactivation of the renin–angiotensin–aldosterone system.

For further discussion of this important topic, the reader is referred to the discussion of the pathogenesis of ascites in Chapter 45 and website chapter 🖥 W-34.

ACKNOWLEDGMENTS

M.R.L-A. was supported by FAPESP 98114790-1. M-H.T. was supported by Chang Gung Medical Research Fund, Chang Gung Memorial Hospital, Taiwan. This research was supported by the U.S. Veterans Administration Merit Review. The authors gratefully acknowledge Maryann Vergato for excellent secretarial assistance.

REFERENCES

1. Genecin P, Groszmann RJ. The biology of portal hypertension. In: Arias IM, Popper H, Jakoby WB, et al., eds. *The liver: biology and pathobiology.* 3rd ed. New York: Raven Press, 1994; 1327–1341.
2. Genecin P, Groszmann RJ. Hepatic blood flow, measurement and physiological regulation. In: McIntyre N, Benhamou J-P, Bircher J, et al., eds. *Oxford textbook of clinical hepatology.* Oxford: Oxford University Press, 1991;31–37.
3. Greenway CV, Stark RD. Hepatic vascular bed. *Physiol Rev* 1971;51:23–65.
4. Groszmann RJ, Atterbury CE. The pathophysiology of portal hypertension. A basis for classification. *Semin Liver Dis* 1982;2:177–186.
5. Groszmann RJ, de Franchis R. Portal hypertension. In: Schiff E, Sorrel M, Maddrey C, eds. *Schiff's diseases of the liver.* Philadelphia: Lippincott-Raven Publishers, 1999:387–442.
6. Knittel T, Ramadori G. Current concepts of liver fibrosis. Forum trends. *Exp Clin Med* 1994;4:236–257.
7. Knittel T, Kobold D, Saile B, et al. Rat liver myofibroblasts and stellate cells: different cell populations of the fibroblast lineage with fibrogenic potential. *Gastroenterology* 1999;117:1205–1221.
8. Friedman S. Hepatic fibrosis—Mechanisms and treatment strategies. *N Engl J Med* 1993;328:1828–1835.
9. Beker S, Valencia-Parparcen J. Portal hypertension syndrome. A comparative analysis of bilharzial fibrosis and hepatic cirrhosis. *Am J Dig Dis* 1968;13:1047–1054.
10. Ramos OL, Saad F, Leser WP. Portal hemodynamics and liver cell function in hepatic schistosomiasis. *Gastroenterology* 1964; 47:241–247.
11. Goodman ZD, Ishak KG. Occlusive venous lesions in alcoholic liver disease. A study of 200 cases. *Gastroenterology* 1982;83: 786–796.
12. Lieber CS, Zimmon DS, Kessler RE, et al. Portal hypertension in experimental alcoholic liver injury. *Clin Res* 1976;24:478(a).
13. Shibayama Y, Nakata K. The role of pericentral fibrosis in experimental portal hypertension in rats. *Liver* 1991;11:94–99.
14. Miyakawa H, Iida S, Leo MA, et al. Pathogenesis of precirrhotic portal hypertension in alcohol-fed baboons. *Gastroenterology* 1985;88:143–150.
15. Orrego H, Blendis LM, Crossley IR, et al. Correlation of intrahepatic pressure with collagen in the Disse space and hepatomegaly in humans and in the rat. *Gastroenterology* 1981; 80:546–556.
16. Shibayama Y, Nakata K. Significance of septal fibrosis for disturbance of hepatic circulation. *Liver* 1992;12:22–25.
17. Schaffner F, Popper H. Capillarization of the hepatic sinusoids in man. *Gastroenterology* 1963;44:239–251.
18. Orrego H, Medline A, Blendis LM, et al. Collagenization of the Disse space in alcoholic liver disease. *Gut* 1979;20:673–679.
19. Popper H, Paronetto F, Schaffner F, et al. Studies on hepatic fibrosis. *Lab Invest* 1961;10:265–278.
20. Dobbs BR, Rogers WT, Xing H-Y, et al. Endotoxin-induced defenestration of the hepatic endothelium: a factor in the pathogenesis of cirrhosis? *Liver* 1994;14:230–233.
21. Bhunchet E, Fujieda K. Capillarization and venularization of hepatic sinusoids in porcine serum-induced rat liver fibrosis: a mechanism to maintain liver blood flow. *Hepatology* 1993;18: 1450–1458.
22. Reynolds TB, Geller HM, Kuzma OT. Spontaneous decrease in portal pressure with clinical improvement in cirrhosis. *N Engl J Med* 1960;263:734–739.
23. Shibayama Y, Nakata K. The role of sinusoidal stenoses in portal hypertension of liver cirrhosis. *J Hepatol* 1989;8:60–66.
24. Shibayama Y. On the pathogenesis of portal hypertension in cirrhosis of the liver. *Liver* 1988;8:95–99.
25. Shibayama Y, Nakata K. Role of septal fibrosis in development of hepatic circulatory disturbance in the presence of liver cell enlargement. *Liver* 1992;12:84–89.

26. Colman JC, Britton RS, Orrego H. Relation between osmotically-induced hepatocyte enlargement and portal hypertension. *Am J Physiol* 1983;245:G382–G387.

27. Mastaï R, Huet PM, Brault A, et al. The rat liver microcirculation in alcohol-induced hepatomegaly. *Hepatology* 1989;10:941–945.

28. Navasa M, Garcia-Pagan JC, Bosch J, et al. Portal hypertension in acute liver failure. *Gut* 1992;33:965–968.

29. Valla D, Flejou JF, Lebrec D, et al. Portal hypertension and ascites in acute hepatitis: clinical, hemodynamic and histological correlations. *J Hepatol* 1989;10:482–487.

30. Bion E, Brenard R, Pariente EA, et al. Sinusoidal portal hypertension in hepatic amyloidosis. *Gut* 1991;32:227–230.

31. Bhathal PS, Grossman HJ. Reduction of the increased portal vascular resistance of the isolated perfused cirrhotic rat liver by vasodilators. *J Hepatol* 1985;1:325–337.

32. Clemens MG. Does altered regulation of ec-NOS in sinusoidal endothelial cells determine increased inthahepatic resistance leading to portal hypertension? *Hepatology* 1998;27:1745–1747.

33. Nakata K, Leong GF, Brauer RW. Direct measurement of blood pressures in minute vessels of the liver. *Am J Physiol* 1960;199:1181–1188.

34. Zhang JX, Pegoli W Jr, Clemens MG. Endothelin-1 induces direct constriction of hepatic sinusoids. *Am J Physiol* 1994;266:G624–G632.

35. McCuskey RS. A dynamic and static study of hepatic arterioles and hepatic sphincters. *Am J Anat* 1966;119:455–477.

36. McCuskey RS, Reilly FD. Hepatic microvasculature: dynamic structure and its regulation. *Semin Liver Dis* 1993;13:1–12.

37. Wake K. Perisinusoidal fat-storing cells of the liver. In: Surrenti C, Casini A, Milani S, et al., eds. *Fat-storing cells in liver fibrosis.* Dordrecht: Kluwer Academic Publishers, 1994:1–10.

38. Sims DE. The pericyte—a review. *Tissue Cell* 1986;18:153–174.

39. Pinzani M, Failli P, Ruocco C, et al. Fat-storing cells as liver-specific pericytes—spatial dynamics of agonist-stimulated intracellular calcium transients. *J Clin Invest* 1992;90:642–646.

40. Bauer M, Zhang JX, Bauer I, et al. ET-1-induced alterations of hepatic microcirculation: sinusoidal and extrasinusoidal sites of action. *Am J Physiol* 1994;267:G143–G149.

41. Rockey DC, Weisiger RA. Endothelin-induced contractility of stellate cells from normal and cirrhotic rat liver: implications for regulation of portal pressure and resistance. *Hepatology* 1996;24:233–240.

42. Housset CN, Rockey DC, Friedman SL, et al. Hepatic lipocytes: a major target for endothelin-1. *J Hepatol* 1995;22:55–60.

43. Suematsu M, Goda N, Sano T, et al. Carbon monoxide: an endogenous modulator of sinusoidal tone in the perfused rat liver. *J Clin Invest* 1995;96:2431–2437.

44. Kawada N, Tran-Thi TA, Klein H, et al. The contraction of hepatic stellate (Ito) cells stimulated with vasoactive substances. Possible involvement of endothelin 1 and nitric oxide in the regulation of the sinusoidal tonus. *Eur J Biochem* 1993;213:815–823.

45. Sakamoto M, Ueno T, Kin M, et al. Ito cell contraction in response to endothelin-1 and substance P. *Hepatology* 1993;18:978–983.

46. Bataller R, Nicolas JM, Gines P, et al. Arginine vasopressin induces contraction and stimulates growth of cultured human hepatic stellate cells. *Gastroenterology* 1997;113:615–624.

47. Simonson MS, Dunn MJ. Endothelins: a family of regulatory peptides. *Hypertension* 1991;17:856–863.

48. Housset C, Rockey DC, Bissell DM. Endothelin receptors in rat liver: lipocytes as a contractile target for endothelin 1. *Proc Natl Acad Sci U S A* 1993;90:9266–9270.

49. Yanagisawa M, Kurihara H, Kimura S, et al. A novel potent vasoconstrictor peptide produced by vascular endothelial cells. *Nature* 1988;332:411–415.

50. Sokolovsky M. Endothelin receptor subtypes and their role in transmembrane signaling mechanisms. *Pharmacol Ther* 1995;68:435–471.

51. Webb DJ, Monge JC, Rabelink TJ, et al. Endothelin: new discoveries and rapid progress in the clinic. *Trends Pharmacol Sci* 1998;19:5–8.

52. Stephenson K, Gupta A, Mustafa SB, et al. Endothelin-stimulated nitric oxide production in the isolated Kupffer cell. *J Surg Res* 1997;73:149–154.

53. Oshita M, Takei Y, Kawano S, et al. Roles of endothelin-1 and nitric oxide in the mechanism for ethanol-induced vasoconstriction in rat liver. *J Clin Invest* 1993;91:1337–1342.

54. Okumura S, Takei Y, Kawano S, et al. Vasoactive effect of endothelin-1 on rat liver *in vivo*. *Hepatology* 1994;19:155–161.

55. Gandhi CR, Stephenson K, Olson MS. Endothelin, a potent peptide agonist in the liver. *J Biol Chem* 1990;265:17432–17435.

56. Kaneda K, Ekataksin W, Sogawa M, et al. Endothelin-1-induced vasoconstriction causes a significant increase in portal pressure of rat liver: localized constrictive effect on the distal segment of preterminal portal venules as revealed by light and electron microscopy and serial reconstruction. *Hepatology* 1998;27:735–747.

57. Reichen J, Gerbes AL, Steiner MJ, et al. The effect of endothelin and its antagonist Bosentan on hemodynamics and microvascular exchange in cirrhotic rat liver. *J Hepatol* 1998;28:1020–1030.

58. Sogni P, Moreau R, Gomola A, et al. Beneficial hemodynamic effects of bosentan, a mixed ET(A) and ET(B) receptor antagonist, in portal hypertensive rats. *Hepatology* 1998;28:655–659.

59. Gandhi CR, Nemoto EM, Watkins SC, et al. An endothelin receptor antagonist TAK 044 ameliorates carbon-tetrachloride-induced acute liver injury and portal hypertension in rats. *Liver* 1998;18:39–48.

60. Moller S, Gülberg V, Henriksen JH, et al. Endothelin-1 and endothelin-3 in cirrhosis: relations to systemic and splanchnic haemodynamics. *J Hepatol* 1995;23:135–144.

61. Gülberg V, Gerbes AL, Vollmar AM, et al. Endothelin-3-like immunoreactivity in plasma of patients with cirrhosis of the liver. *Life Sci* 1992;51:1165–1169.

62. Leivas A, Jimenez W, Lamas S, et al. Endothelin 1 does not play a major role in the homeostasis of arterial pressure in cirrhotic rats with ascites. *Gastroenterology* 1995;108:1842–1848.

63. Gerbes AL, Moller S, Gülberg V, et al. Endothelin-1 and -3 plasma concentrations in patients with cirrhosis: role of splanchnic and renal passage and liver function. *Hepatology* 1995;21:735–739.

64. Pinzani M, Milani S, De Franco R, et al. Endothelin 1 is overexpressed in human cirrhotic liver and exerts multiple effects on activated hepatic stellate cells. *Gastroenterology* 1996;110:534–548.

65. Leivas A, Jimenez W, Bruix J, et al. Gene expression of endothelin-1 and ETa and ETb receptors in human cirrhosis: Relationship with hepatic hemodynamics. *J Vasc Res* 1998;35:186–193.

66. Gandhi CR, Sproat LA, Subbotin VM. Increased hepatic endothelin-1 levels and endothelin receptor density in cirrhotic rats. *Life Sci* 1996;58:55–62.

67. Furuya S, Naruse S, Nakayama T. Binding of ^{125}I-endothelin to fat-storing cells in rat liver revealed by electron microscopic radioautography. *Anat Embryol* 1992;185:97–100.

68. Bauer M, Paquette NC, Zhang JX, et al. Chronic ethanol consumption increases hepatic sinusoidal contractile response to endothelin-1 in the rat. *Hepatology* 1995;22:1565–1576.

69. Poo JL, Jimenez S, Munoz RM, et al. Chronic blockade of endothelin receptors in cirrhotic rats: hepatic and hemodynamic effects. *Gastroenterology* 1999;116:161–167.

70. Rockey DC, Chung JJ. Inducible nitric oxide synthase in rat hepatic lipocytes and the effect of nitric oxide on lipocyte contractility. *J Clin Invest* 1995;95:1199–1206.

71. Tran-Thi TA, Kawada N, Decker K. Regulation of endothelin-1 action on the perfused rat liver. *FEBS Lett* 1993;318:353–357.

72. Boulanger C, Luscher TF. Release of endothelin from the porcine aorta. Inhibition by endothelium-derived nitric oxide. *J Clin Invest* 1990;85:587–590.

73. Rubanyi GM. Endothelium-derived relaxing and contracting factors. *J Cell Biochem* 1991;46:27–36.

74. Vane JR, Anggard EE, Botting RM. Regulatory functions of the vascular endothelium. *N Engl J Med* 1990;323:27–36.

75. Shah V, Haddad FG, Garcia-Cardena G, et al. Liver sinusoidal endothelial cells are responsible for nitric oxide modulation of resistance in the hepatic sinusoids. *J Clin Invest* 1997;100:2923–2930.

76. Shah V, Toruner M, Haddad F, et al. Impaired endothelial nitric oxide synthase activity associated with enhanced caveolin binding in experimental liver cirrhosis. *Gastroenterology* 1999;117:1222–1228.

77. Gupta TK Toruner M, Chung MK, et al. Endothelial dysfunction and decreased production of nitric oxide in the intrahepatic microcirculation of cirrhotic rats. *Hepatology* 1998;28:926–931.

78. Ludmer PL, Selwyn AP, Shook TL, et al. Paradoxical vasoconstriction induced by acetylcholine in atherosclerotic coronary arteries. *N Engl J Med* 1986;315:1046–1051.

79. Conraads VM, Bosman JM, Clayes MJ, et al. Paradoxic pulmonary vasoconstriction in response to acetylcholine in patients with pulmonary hypertension. *Chest* 1994;106:385–390.

80. Buga GM, Gold ME, Fukuto JM, et al. Shear stress-induced release of nitric oxide from endothelial cells grown on beads. *Hypertension* 1991;17:187–193.

81. Kuchan MJ, Frangos JA. Role of calcium and calmodulin in flow-induced nitric oxide production in endothelial cells. *Am J Physiol* 1994;266:C628–C636.

82. Ranjan V, Xiao Z, Diamond SL. Constitutive NOS expression in cultured endothelial cells is elevated by fluid shear stress. *Am J Physiol* 1995;269:H550–H555.

83. Busse R, Fleming I. Endothelial dysfunction in atherosclerosis. *J Vasc Res* 1996;3:181–194.

84. Radomski MW, Palmer RMJ, Moncada S. An L-arginine/nitric oxide pathway present in human platelets regulates aggregation. *Proc Natl Acad Sci U S A* 1990;87:5193–5197.

85. Diodati JG, Dakak N, Gilligan DM, et al. Effect of. atherosclerosis on endothelium-dependent inhibition of platelet activation in humans. *Circulation* 1998;98:17–24.

86. Wanless IR, Wong F, Blendis LM, et al. Hepatic and portal vein thrombosis in cirrhosis: possible role in development of parenchymal extinction and portal hypertension. *Hepatology* 1995;21:1238–1247.

87. Cugno M, Scott CF, Salerno F, et al. Parallel reduction of plasma levels of high and low molecular weight kininogen in patients with cirrhosis. *Thromb Haemost* 1999;82:1428–1432.

88. Myers PR, Tanner MA. Vascular endothelial cell regulation of extracellular matrix collagen: role of nitric oxide. *Arterioscler Thromb Vasc Biol* 1998;18:717–722.

89. Muriel P. Nitric oxide protection of rat liver form lipid peroxidation, collagen accumulation, and liver damage induced by carbon tetrachloride. *Biochem Pharmacol* 1998;56:773–779.

90. Kubes P, Suzuki M, Granger DN. Nitric oxide: an endogenous modulator of leukocyte adhesion. *Proc Natl Acad Sci U S A* 1991;88:4651–4655.

91. Böger RH, Bode-Böger SM, Frölich JC. The L-arginine-nitric oxide pathway: role in atherosclerosis and therapeutic implications. *Atherosclerosis* 1996;127:1–11.

92. Keaney JF, Vita JA. Atherosclerosis oxidative stress, and antioxidant protection in endothelium-derived relaxing factor action. *Prog Cardiovasc Dis* 1995;38:129–154.

93. Clancy RM, Leszczynska-Piziak J, Abramson SB. Nitric oxide, an endothelial cell relaxation factor, inhibits neutrophil superoxide anion production via a direct action on the NADPH oxidase. *J Clin Invest* 1992;90:1116–1121.

94. Rockey DC, Chung JJ. Reduced nitric oxide production by endothelial cells in cirrhotic rat liver: endothelial dysfunction in portal hypertension. *Gastroenterology* 1998;114:344–351.

95. Michel JB, Feron O, Sase K, et al. Caveolin versus calmodulin. Counterbalancing allosteric modulators of endothelial nitric oxide synthase. *J Biol Chem* 1997;272:25907–25912.

96. Michel JB, Feron O, Sacks D, et al. Reciprocal regulation of endothelial nitric-oxide synthase by Ca2+-calmodulin and caveolin. *J Biol Chem* 1997;272:15583–15586.

97. Dudenhoerf A, Toruner M, Cadelina G, et al. Bioactivation of nitroglycerin and vasomotor response to nitric oxide is impaired in cirrhotic rat livers. *Hepatology* 1999;30:230A(abst).

98. Mittal MK, Gupta TK, Lee FY, et al. Nitric oxide modulates hepatic vascular tone in normal rat liver. *Am J Physiol* 1994;267:G416–G422.

99. Yu Q, Shao R, Qian HS, et al. Gene transfer of the neuronal NO synthase isoform to cirrhotic rat liver ameliorates portal hypertension. *J Clin Invest* 2000;105:741–748.

100. Maines MD. Heme oxygenase: function, multiplicity, regulatory mechanisms, and clinical applications. *FASEB J* 1988;2:2557–2568.

101. McCoubrey K, Huang TJ, Maines MD. Isolation and characterization of a cDNA from the rat brain that encodes hemoprotein heme oxygenase-3. *Eur J Biochem* 1997;247:725–735.

102. Goda N, Suzuki K, Naito M, et al. Distribution of heme oxygenase isoforms in rat liver. *J Clin Invest* 1998;101:604–612.

103. Wakabayashi Y, Takamiya R, Mizuki A, et al. Carbon monoxide overproduced by heme oxygenase-1 causes a reduction of vascular resistance in perfused rat liver. *Am J Physiol* 1999;277:G1088–G1096.

104. Fernandez M, Bonkovsky HL. Increased heme oxygenase-1 gene expression in liver cells and splanchnic organs from portal hypertensive rats. *Hepatology* 1999;29:1672–1679.

105. Blei AT, Gottstein J. Isosorbide dinitrate in experimental portal hypertension. A study of factors that modulate the hemodynamic response. *J Hepatol* 1986;6:107–111.

106. Kroeger RJ, Groszmann RJ. Increased portal venous resistance hinders portal pressure reduction during the administration of b-adrenergic blocking agents in a portal hypertensive model. *J Hepatol* 1985;5:97–101.

107. Benoit JN, Womack WA, Hernandez L, et al. "Forward" and "backward" flow mechanisms of portal hypertension. Relative contributions in the rat model of portal vein stenosis. *Gastroenterology* 1985;89:1092–1096.

108. Groszmann RJ. Pathophysiology of cirrhotic portal hypertension. In: Boyer JL, Bianchi L, eds. *Liver cirrhosis. Falk Foundation, 44*. Lancaster:MTP Press Ltd., 1987:279–291.

109. Sikuler E, Groszmann RJ. Interaction of flow and resistance in maintenance of portal hypertension in a rat model. *Am J Physiol* 1986;250:G205–G212.

110. Vorobioff J, Bredfeldt JE, Groszmann RJ. Increased blood flow through the portal system in cirrhotic rats. *Gastroenterology* 1984;87:1120–1126.

111. Sikuler E, Kravetz D, Groszmann RJ. Evolution of portal hypertension and mechanisms involved in its maintenance in a rat model. *Am J Physiol* 1985;248:G618–G625.

112. Sarin SK, Groszmann RJ, Mosca PG, et al. Propranolol ameliorates the development of portal-systemic shunting in a chronic murine schistosomiasis model of portal hypertension. *J Clin Invest* 1991;87:1032–1036.

113. Lin HC, Sarbrane O, Lebrec D. Prevention of portal hypertension and portosystemic shunts by early chronic administration of clonidine in conscious portal vein stenosed rats. *J Hepatol* 1991;14:325–330.

114. Geraghty JG, Angerson WJ, Carter DC. Portal venous pressure and portosystemic shunting in experimental portal hypertension. *Am J Physiol* 1989;257:G52–G56.

115. Lee FY, Colombato LA, Albillos A, et al. Administration of N-omega-nitro-L-arginine ameliorates portal-systemic shunting in portal hypertensive rats. *Gastroenterology* 1993;105:1464–1470.

116. Halvorsen JF, Myking AO. The portosystemic collateral pattern in the rat. *Eur Surg Res* 1974;6:183–195.

117. Ziche M, Morbidelli L, Masini E, et al. Nitric oxide mediates angiogenesis in vivo and endothelial cell growth and migration in vitro promoted by substance P. *J Clin Invest* 1994;94:2036–2044.

118. Sumanovski LT, Battegay E, et al. Increased angiogenesis in portal hypertensive rats: role of nitric oxide. *J Hepatol* 1999;29:1044–1049.

119. Awolesi MA, Sessa WC, Sumpio BE. Cyclic strain upregulates nitric oxide synthase in cultured bovine aortic endothelial cells. *J Clin Invest* 1995;96:1449–1454.

120. Rudic RD, Shesely EG, Maeda N, et al. Direct evidence for the importance of endothelium-derived nitric oxide in vascular remodeling. *J Clin Invest* 1998;101:731–736.

121. Garcia-Tsao G, Albillos A, Barden GE, et al. Bacterial translocation in acute and chronic portal hypertension. *J Hepatol* 1993;17:1081–1085.

122. Kravetz D, Arderiu M, Bosch J, et al. Hyperglucagonemia and hyperkinetic circulation after portocaval shunt in the rat. *Am J Physiol* 1987;252:G257–G261.

123. Bernadich C, Bandi JC, Piera C, et al. Circulatory effects of graded diversion of portal blood flow to the systemic circulation in rats: role of nitric oxide. *J Hepatol* 1997;26:262–267.

124. Mosca P, Lee F-Y, Kaumann AJ, et al. Pharmacology of portal-systemic collaterals in portal hypertensive rats: role of endothelium. *Am J Physiol* 1992;263:G544–G550.

125. Chan CC, Lee FY, Wang SS, et al. Effects of vasopressin on portal-systemic collaterals in portal hypertensive rats: role of nitric oxide and prostaglandin. *J Hepatol* 1999;30:630–635.

126. Kaumann AJ, Groszmann RJ. Catecholamines relax portal and mesenteric veins from normal and portal hypertensive rats. *Am J Physiol* 1989;257:G977–G981.

127. Vorobioff J, Bredfeldt JE, Groszmann RJ. Hyperdynamic circulation in portal-hypertensive rat model: a primary factor for maintenance of chronic portal hypertension. *Am J Physiol* 1983;244:G52–G57.

128. Cohn JN, Khatri IM, Groszmann RJ, et al. Hepatic blood flow in alcoholic liver disease measured by an indicator dilution technique. *Am J Med* 1972;53:704–714.

129. Kowalski HJ, Abelmann WH. The cardiac output at rest in Laennec's cirrhosis. *J Clin Invest* 1953;32:1025–1033.

130. Murray JF, Dawson AM, Sherlock S. Circulatory changes in chronic liver disease. *Am J Med* 1958;24:358–367.

131. Kontos HH, Shapiro W, Mauck HP, et al. General and regional circulatory alterations in cirrhosis of the liver. *Am J Med* 1964;37:526–535.

132. Sabba C, Ferraioli G, Genecin P, et al. Evaluation of postprandial hyperemia in superior mesenteric artery and portal vein in healthy and cirrhotic humans in an operator-blind echo-Doppler study. *J Hepatol* 1991;13:714–718.

133. Benoit JN, Womack WA, Korthuis RJ, et al. Chronic portal hypertension: effects on gastrointestinal blood flow distribution. *Am J Physiol* 1986;250:G535–G538.

134. Lee SS, Girod C, Broullon A, et al. Hemodynamic characterization of chronic bile duct-ligated rats: effect of pentobarbital sodium. *Am J Physiol* 1986;251:G176–G180.

135. Braillon A, Moreau R, Hadengue A, et al. Hyperkinetic circulatory syndrome in patients with presinusoidal portal hypertension. Effect of propranolol. *J Hepatol* 1989:312–318.

136. Harada A, Nonami T, Kasai Y, et al. Systemic hemodynamics in noncirrhotic portal hypertension—a clinical study of 19 patients. *Jpn J Surg* 1988;18:620–625.

137. Blanchet L, Lebrec D. Changes in splanchnic blood flow in portal hypertensive rats. *Eur J Clin Invest* 1982;12:327–330.

138. Korthuis RJ, Benoit JN, Kvietys PR, et al. Humoral factors may mediate increased rat hindquarter blood flow in portal hypertension. *Am J Physiol* 1985;249:H827–H833.

139. Bosch J, Storer EH, Enriquez R, et al. Chronic bile duct ligation in the dog. Hemodynamic characterization of a portal hypertensive model. *J Hepatol* 1983;3:1002–1007.

140. Witte CL, Witte MH, Bair G, et al. Experimental study of hyperdynamic vs. stagnant mesenteric blood flow in portal hypertension. *Ann Surg* 1974;179:304–310.

141. Benoit JN, Barrowman JA, Harper SL, et al. Role of humoral factors in the intestinal hyperemia associated with chronic portal hypertension. *Am J Physiol* 1984;247:G486–G493.

142. Sikuler E, Groszmann RJ. Hemodynamic studies in a parabiotic model of portal hypertension. *Experientia* 1985;41:1323–1325.

143. Sherwin R, Joshi P, Hendler R, et al. Hyperglucagonemia in Laennec's cirrhosis: the role of portal-systemic shunting. *N Engl J Med* 1974;290:239–242.

144. Silva G, Navasa M, Bosch J, et al. Hemodynamic effects of glucagon in portal hypertension. *J Hepatol* 1990;11:668–673.

145. Sherwin RS, Fisher M, Bessoff J, et al. Hyperglucagonemia in cirrhosis: altered secretion and sensitivity to glucagon. *Gastroenterology* 1978;74:1224–1228.

146. Gomis R, Fernandez-Alvarez J, Pizcueta MP, et al. Impaired function of pancreatic islets from rats with portal hypertension resulting from cirrhosis and portal vein ligation. *J Hepatol* 1994;19:1257.

147. Benoit JN, Zimmermann B, Premen AJ, et al. Role of glucagon in splanchnic hyperemia of chronic portal hypertension. *Am J Physiol* 1986;251:G674–G677.

148. Sikuler E, Groszmann RJ. Hemodynamic studies in long- and short-term portal hypertensive rats: the relation of systemic glucagon levels. *J Hepatol* 1986;41:4–18.

149. Kravetz D, Bosch J, Arderiu MT, et al. Effects of somatostatin on splanchnic hemodynamics and plasma glucagon in portal hypertensive rats. *Am J Physiol* 1988;254:G322–G328.

150. Pizcueta MP, Garcia-Pagan JC, Fernandez M, et al. Glucagon hinders the effects of somatostatin on portal hypertension. A study in rats with partial portal vein ligation. *Gastroenterology* 1991;101:1710–1715.

151. Chatila R, Ferayorni L, Gupta T, et al. Local arterial vasoconstriction by octreotide in patients with cirrhosis. *J Hepatol* 2000;31:572–576.

152. Wiest R, Tsai M-H, Groszmann RJ. Octreotide potentiates local vasoconstriction in superior mesenteric arteries: mechanism and pharmacodynamics in portal hypertensive and control rats. *Gastroenterology* 2000;118:A963.

153. Buonamico P, Carlo S, Garcia-Tsao G, et al. Octreotide blunts postprandial splanchnic hyperemia in cirrhotic patients: A double blind randomized echo-doppler study. *J Hepatol* 1995;21: 134–139.

154. McCormick PA, Biagini MR, Dick R, et al. Octreotide inhibits the meal-induced increases in the portal venous pressure of cirrhotic patients with portal hypertension: a double-blind, placebo-controlled study. *J Hepatol* 1992;16:1180–1186.

155. Alemany CA, Oh W, Stronestreet BS. Effects of nitric oxide synthesis inhibition on mesenteric perfusion in young pigs. *Am J Physiol* 1997;272:G612–G616.

156. Matheson PJ, Spain DA, Harris PD, et al. Glucose and glutamine gavage increase portal vein nitric oxide metabolite via adenosine A2b activation. *J Surg Res* 1999;84:57–63.

157. Sitzmann JV, Bulkley GB, Mitchell MC, et al. Role of prostacyclin in the splanchnic hyperemia contributing to portal hypertension. *Ann Surg* 1989;209:322–327.

158. Guarner C, Soriano G, Such J, et al. Systemic prostacyclin in cirrhotic patients. Relationship with portal hypertension and changes after intestinal decontamination. *Gastroenterology* 1992;102:303–309.

159. Sitzmann JV, Li SS, Adkinson NF. Evidence for role of prostacyclin as a systemic hormone in portal hypertension. *Surgery* 1991;109:149–153.

160. Bruix J, Bosch J, Kravetz D, et al. Effects of prostaglandin inhibition on systemic and hepatic hemodynamics in patients with cirrhosis of the liver. *Gastroenterology* 1985;88:430–435.

161. Sitzmann JV, Li SS, Lin PW. Prostacyclin mediates splanchnic vascular response to norepinephrine in portal hypertension. *J Surg Res* 1989;47:208–211.

162. Wu Y, Li SS, Campbell KA, et al. Modulation of splanchnic vascular sensitivity to angiotensin II. *Surgery* 1991;110:162–168.

163. Masferrer JL, Seibert K, Zweifel B, et al. Endogenous glucocorticoids regulate an inducible cyclooxygenase enzyme. *Proc Natl Acad Sci U S A* 1992;89:3917–3921.

164. Hecker M, Mulsch A, Bassenge E, et al. Vasoconstriction and increased flow: two principal mechanisms of shear stress-dependent endothelial autocoid release. *Am J Physiol* 1993;265: H828–H833.

165. De Nucci G, Gryglewski RJ, Warner TD, et al. Receptor-mediated release of endothelium-derived relaxing factor and prostacyclin from bovine aortic endothelial cells is coupled. *Proc Natl Acad Sci U S A* 1988;85:2334–2338.

166. Knowles RG, Salter M, Brooks SL, et al. Antiinflammatory glucocorticoids inhibit the induction by endotoxin of nitric oxide synthase in the lung, liver, and aorta of the rat. *Biochem Biophys Res Commun* 1990;172:1042–1048.

167. Hou MC, Cahill PA, Zhang S, et al. Enhanced cyclooxygenase I expression within superior mesenteric artery of portal hypertensive rats: role in the hyperdynamic circulation. *J Hepatol* 1998;27:20–27.

168. Wu Y, Cartland Burns R, Sitzmann JV. Effects of nitric oxide and cyclooxygenase inhibition on splanchnic hemodynamics in portal hypertension. *J Hepatol* 1993;18:1416–1421.

169. Fernandez M, Garcia Pagan JC, Casadevall M, et al. Acute and chronic cyclooxygenase blockade in portal hypertensive rats: influence on nitric oxide biosynthesis. *Gastroenterology* 1996; 110:1529–1535.

170. Blanchard A, Hernando N, Fernandez-Nunez D, et al. Lack of effect of indomethacin on systemic and splanchnic hemodynamics in portal hypertensive rats. *Clin Sci* 1985;68:605–607.

171. Wagner CT, Durante W, Christodoulides N, et al. Hemodynamic forces induce the expression of heme oxygenase in cultured vascular smooth muscle cells. *J Clin Invest* 1997;100: 589–596.

172. Yet SF, Pellacani A, Patterson C, et al. Induction of heme oxygenase I expression in vascular smooth muscle cells. A link to endotoxic shock. *J Biol Chem* 1997;272:4295–4301.

173. Terry CM, Clikeman JA, Hoidal JR, et al. Effect of tumor necrosis factor-α and interleukin-1 α on heme oxygenase-1 expression in human endothelial cells. *Am J Physiol* 1998; 274:H883–H891.

174. Durante W, Kroll MH, Christodoulides N, et al. Nitric oxide induces heme oxygenase-1 gene expression and carbon monoxide production in vascular smooth muscle cells. *Circ Res* 1997; 80:557–564.

175. Bakken AF, Thaler MM, Schmid R. Metabolic regulation of heme catabolism and bilirubin production: hormonal control of hepatic heme oxygenase activity. *J Clin Invest* 1972;51: 530–536.

176. Genecin P, Polio J, Colombato LA, et al. Bile acids do not mediate the hyperdynamic circulation in portal hypertensive rats. *Am J Physiol* 1990;259:G21–G25.

177. Fernandez M, Casadevall M, Schuligoi R, et al. Neonatal capsaicin treatment does not prevent splanchnic vasodilatation in portal hypertensive rats. *Hepatol* 1994;20:1609–1614.

178. Lee SS, Sharkey KA. Capsaicin treatment blocks development of hyperkinetic circulation in portal hypertensive rats. *Am J Physiol* 1993;264:G868–G873.

179. Hori N, Okanoue T, Sawa Y, et al. Role of calcitonin generelated peptide in the vascular system on the development of hyperdynamic circulation in conscious cirrhotic rats. *J Hepatol* 1997;26:1111–1119.

180. Lee MW, Severson DL. Signal transduction in vascular smooth muscle: diacylglycerol second messenger and PKA action. *Am J Physiol* 1994;267:C659–C678.

181. Jeremy JY, Mikhailidis DP, Karatapanis S, et al. Altered prostaglandin synthesis by aorta from hepatic portal vein-constricted rats: evidence for effects on protein kinase C and calcium. *J Hepatol* 1994;21:1017–1022.

182. Laffi G, Marra F, Failli P, et al. Defective signal transduction in platelet from cirrhotics is associated with increased cyclic nucleotide. *Gastroenterology* 1993:105:148–156.

183. Cahill PA, Wu Y, Sitzmann JV. Altered adenylyl cyclase activities and G-protein abnormalities in portal hypertensive rabbits. *J Clin Invest* 1994;93:2691–2700.

184. Trombino C, Tazi KA, Gadano A, et al. Protein kinase C alteration in aortic vascular smooth muscle cells from rats with cirrhosis. *J Hepatol* 1998;28:670–676.

185. Atucha NM, Ortiz MC, Martinez C, et al. Role of protein kinase C in mesenteric pressor response of rats with portal hypertension. *Br J Pharmacol* 1996;118;227–282.

186. Atucha NM, Shah V, Garcia-Cardena G, et al. Role of endothelium in the abnormal response of mesenteric vessels in rats with portal hypertension and liver cirrhosis. *Gastroenterology* 1996; 111:1627–1632.

187. Wiest R, Das S, Cadelina G, et al. Bacterial translocation in cirrhotic rats stimulates eNOS-derived NO production and impairs mesenteric vascular contractility. *J Clin Invest* 1999; 104:1223–1233.

188. Tsoporis J, Fields N, Lee RM, et al. Arterial vasodilation and cardiovascular structural changes in normotensive rats. *Am J Physiol* 1991;260:H1944–H1952.

189. Furchgott RF. Role of endothelium in responses of vascular smooth muscle. *Circ Res* 1983;53:557–573.

190. Vanhoutte PM, Rubanyi GM, Miller VM, et al. Modulation of vascular smooth muscle contraction by the endothelium. *Annu Rev Physiol* 1986;48:307–320.

191. Palmer RMJ, Ferrige AG, Moncada S. Nitric oxide release accounts for the biological activity of endothelium-derived relaxing factor. *Nature* 1987;327:524–526.

192. Kelm M, Feelisch M, Spahr R, et al. Quantitative and kinetic

characterization of nitric oxide and EDRF released from endothelial cells. *Biochem Biophys Res Commun* 1988;154: 236–244.

193. Pizcueta P, Pique JM, Fernandez M, et al. Modulation of the hyperdynamic circulation of cirrhotic rats by nitric oxide inhibition. *Gastroenterology* 1992;103:1909–1915.

194. Pizcueta P, Pique JM, Bosch J, et al. Effects of inhibiting nitric oxide biosynthesis on the systemic and splanchnic circulation of rats with portal hypertension. *Br J Phamacol* 1992;105: 184–190.

195. Casadevall M, Pique JM, Cirera I, et al. Increased blood hemoglobin attenuates splanchnic vasodilatation in portal hypertensive rats by nitric oxide inactivation. *Gastroenterology* 1996;110:1156–1165.

196. Lee FY, Colombato LA, Albillos A, et al. N-omega-nitro-L-arginine administration corrects peripheral vasodilation and systemic capillary hypotension and ameliorates plasma volume expansion and sodium retention in portal hypertensive rats. *J Hepatol* 1993;17:84–90.

197. Garcia-Pagan JC, Fernandez M, Bernadich C, et al. Effects of continued NO inhibition on portal hypertensive syndrome after portal vein stenosis in rat. *Am J Physiol* 1994;267: G984–G990.

198. Murray BM, Paller MS. Decreased pressor reactivity to angiotensin II in cirrhotic rats. Evidence for a post-receptor defect in angiotensin action. *Circ Res* 1985;57:424–431.

199. Sieber CC, Groszmann RJ. in vitro hyporeactivity to methoxamine in portal hypertensive rats: reversal by nitric oxide blockade. *Am J Physiol* 1992;262:G996–G1001.

200. Sieber CC, Groszmann RJ. Nitric oxide mediates hyporeactivity to vasopressors in mesenteric vessels of portal hypertensive rats. *Gastroenterology* 1992;103:235–239.

201. Kiel JW, Pitts V, Benoit JN, et al. Reduced vascular sensitivity to norepinephrine in portal hypertensive rats. *Am J Physiol* 1985;248:G192–G195.

202. Hartleb M, Moreau R, Cailmail S, et al. Vascular hyporesponsiveness to endothelin I in rats with cirrhosis. *Gastroenterology* 1994;107:1085–1093.

203. Liao JF, Yu PC, Lin HC, et al. Study on the vascular reactivity and α1 adrenoceptors of portal hypertensive rats. *Br J Pharmacol* 1994;111:439–444.

204. Sieber CC, Lopez-Talavera JC, Groszmann RJ. Role of nitric oxide in the in vitro splanchnic vascular hyporeactivity in ascitic cirrhotic rats. *Gastroenterology* 1993;104:1750–1754.

205. Sieber CC, Sumanovski LT, Moll-Kaufmann C, et al. Hyposensitivity to nerve stimulation in portal hypertensive rats: role of nitric oxide. *Eur J Clin Invest* 1997;27:902–907.

206. Castro A, Jimenez W, Claria J, et al. Impaired responsiveness to angiotensin II in experimental cirrhosis: Role of nitric oxide. *J Hepatol* 1993;18:367–372.

207. Gadano AC, Sogni P, Yang S, et al. Endothelial calcium-calmodulin-dependent nitric oxide synthase in the in vitro vascular hyporeactivity of portal hypertensive rats. *J Hepatol* 1997; 26:678–686.

208. Ortiz MC, Fortepiani LA, Martinez C, et al. Vascular hyporesponsiveness in aortic rings from cirrhotic rats: role of nitric oxide and endothelium. *Clin Sci* 1996;91:733–738.

209. Weigert AL, Martin PY, Niederberger M, et al. Endothelium-dependent vascular hyporesponsiveness without detection of nitric oxide synthase induction in aorta of cirrhotic rats. *J Hepatol* 1995;22:1856–1862.

210. Gadano AC, Sogni P, Heller J, et al. Vascular nitric oxide production during the development of two experimental models of portal hypertension. *J Hepatol* 1999;30:896–903.

211. Niederberger M, Martin PY, Gines P, et al. Normalization of nitric oxide production corrects arterial vasodilation and hyperdynamic circulation in cirrhotic rats. *Gastroenterology* 1995; 109:1624–1630.

212. Campillo B, Chabrier PE, Pelle G, et al. Inhibition of nitric oxide synthesis in forearm arterial bed of patients with advanced cirrhosis. *J Hepatol* 1995;22:1423–1429.

213. Albillos A, Rossi I, Cacho G, et al. Enhanced endothelium-dependent vasodilation in patients with cirrhosis. *Am J Physiol* 1995;268:G459–G464.

214. Murad F. Cyclic guanosine monophosphate as a mediator of vasodilation. *J Clin Invest* 1986;78:1–5.

215. Cahill PA, Redmond EM, Hodges R, et al. Increased endothelial nitric oxide synthase activity in the hyperemic vessels of portal hypertensive rats. *J Hepatol* 1996;25:370–378.

216. Ros J, Jimenez W, Lamas S, et al. Nitric oxide production in arterial vessels of cirrhotic rats. *J Hepatol* 1995;21:554–560.

217. Bolotina VM, Najibi S, Palacino JJ, et al. Nitric oxide directly activates calcium-dependent potassium channels in vascular smooth muscle. *Nature* 1994;368:850–853.

218. Atucha NM, Ortiz MC, Fortepiani LA, et al. Role of cyclic guanosine monophosphate and potassium channels as mediators of the mesenteric vascular hyporesponsiveness in portal hypertensive rats. *J Hepatol* 1998;27:900–905.

219. Hori N, Wiest R, Groszmann RJ. Enhanced release of nitric oxide in response to changes in flow and shear stress in the superior mesenteric arteries of portal hypertensive rats. *J Hepatol* 1998;28:1467–1473.

220. Battista S, Bar F, Mengozzo G, et al. Hyperdynamic circulation in patients with cirrhosis: direct measurement of nitric oxide levels in hepatic and portal veins. *J Hepatol* 1997;26:75–80.

221. Vallance P, Moncada S. Hyperdynamic circulation in cirrhosis: a role for nitric oxide? *Lancet* 1991;337:776–778.

222. Forstermann U, Boissel JP, Kleinert H. Expressional control of the constitutive isoforms of nitric oxide synthase (NOS I and NOS III). *FASEB J* 1998;12:773–790.

223. Sessa WC, Prichard K, Seyedi N, et al. Chronic exercise in dogs increase coronary vascular nitric oxide production and endothelial cell nitric oxide synthase gene expression. *Circ Res* 1994; 74:349–353.

224. Martin PY, Xu DL, Niederberger M, et al. Upregulation of endothelial constitutive NOS: a major role in the increased NO production in cirrhotic rats. *Am J Physiol* 1996;270:F494–F499.

225. Martin PY, Ohara M, Gines P, et al. Nitric oxide synthase (NOS) inhibition for one week improves renal sodium and water excretion in cirrhotic rats with ascites. *J Clin Invest* 1998;101:235–242.

226. Niederberger M, Gines P, Martin PY, et al. Comparison of vascular nitric oxide production and systemic hemodynamics in cirrhotic versus prehepatic portal hypertension in rats. *J Hepatol* 1996:24:947–951.

227. Cahill PA, Foster C, Redmon EM, et al. Enhanced nitric oxide synthase activity in portal hypertensive rabbits. *J Hepatol* 1995;22:598–606.

228. Wiest R, Shah V, Sessa WC, et al. Nitric oxide overproduction by eNOS precedes hyperdynamic splanchnic circulation in portal hypertensive rats. *Am J Physiol* 1999;276:G1043–G1051.

229. Claria J, Jimenez W, Ros J, et al. Increased nitric oxide-dependent vasorelaxation in aortic rings of cirrhotic rats with ascites. *J Hepatol* 1994;20:1615–1621.

230. Lin RS, Lee FY, Lee SD, et al. Endotoxemia in patients with chronic liver diseases: relationship to severity of liver diseases, presence of esophageal varices, and hyperdynamic circulation. *J Hepatol* 1995;22:165–172.

231. Lee FY, Wang SS, Yang MC, et al. Role of endotoxemia in hyperdynamic circulation in rats with extrahepatic or intrahepatic portal hypertension. *J Gastroenterol Hepatol* 1996;11: 152–158.

232. Lumsden AB, Henderson JM, Kutner MH. Endotoxin level measured by a chromogenic assay in portal, hepatic and peripheral venous blood in patients with cirrhosis. *J Hepatol* 1988;8:232–236.

233. Kilbourn RG, Belloni P. Endothelial cell production of nitric oxide in response to interferon γ in combination with tumor necrosis factor, interleukin 1, or endotoxin. *J Natl Cancer Inst* 1990;82:772–776.

234. Morales-Ruiz M, Jimenez W, Perez-Sala D, et al. Increased nitric oxide synthase expression in arterial vessels of cirrhotic rats with ascites. *J Hepatol* 1996;24:1481–1486.

235. Fernandez M, Garcia-Pagan JC, Casadevall M, et al. Evidence against a role for inducible nitric oxide synthase in the hyperdynamic circulation of portal hypertensive rats. *Gastroenterology* 1995;108:1487–1495.

236. Heinemann A, Stauber RE. The role of inducible nitric oxide synthase in vascular hyporeactivity of endotoxin-treated and portal hypertensive rats. *Eur J Pharmacol* 1995;278:87–90.

237. Guarner C, Soriano G, Tomas A, et al. Increased serum nitrite and nitrate levels in patients with cirrhosis: relationship to endotoxemia. *J Hepatol* 1993;18:1139–1143.

238. Chu CJ, Lee FY, Wang SS, et al. Hyperdynamic circulation of cirrhotic rats with ascites: role of endotoxin, tumor necrosis factor-α and nitric oxide. *Clin Sci* 1997;93:219–225.

239. Lopez-Talavera JC, Merrill W, Groszmann RJ. Tumor necrosis factor α: a major contributor to the hyperdynamic circulation in prehepatic portal hypertension rats. *Gastroenterology* 1995;108:761–767.

240. Lopez-Talavera JC, Cadelina G, Olchowski J, et al. Thalidomide inhibits tumor necrosis factor α, decreases nitric oxide synthesis, and ameliorates the hyperdynamic circulatory syndrome in portal hypertensive rats. *J Hepatol* 1996;23:1616–1621.

241. Lopez-Talavera JC, Levitzki A, Martinez M, et al. Tyrosine kinase inhibition ameliorates the hyperdynamic state and decreases nitric oxide production in cirrhotic rats with portal hypertension and ascites. *J Clin Invest* 1997;100:664–670.

242. Mehta R, Gottstein J, Zeller PW, et al. Endotoxin and the hyperdynamic circulation of portal vein-ligated rats. *J Hepatol* 1990;12:1152–1156.

243. Garcia-Tsao G, Lee FY, Barden GE, et al. Bacterial translocation to mesenteric lymph nodes is increased in cirrhotic rats with ascites. *Gastroenterology* 1995;108:1835–1841.

244. Fernando B, Marley R, Holt S, et al. N-Acetylcysteine prevents development of hyperdynamic circulation in portal hypertensive rat. *J Hepatol* 1998;28:689–694.

245. Marley R, Holt S, Fernando B, et al. Lipoic acid prevents development of the hyperdynamic circulation in anesthetized rats with biliary cirrhosis. *J Hepatol* 1999;29:1358–1363.

246. Graham RM, Pettinger WA. Drug therapy-prazosin. *N Engl J Med* 1979;300:232–236.

247. Pagani M, Vatner SF, Braunwald E. Hemodynamic effects of intravenous nitroprusside in the conscious dog. *Circulation* 1978;57:144–157.

248. Styles M, Coleman AJ, Leary WP. Some hemodynamic effects of sodium nitroprusside. *Anesthesiol* 1973;38:173–176.

249. Maddrey WC, Boyer JL, Sen NN. Plasma volume expansion in portal hypertension. *Johns Hopkins Med J* 1969;125:171–182.

250. Guyton AC, Lindsey AW, Kaufmann B. Effect of mean circulatory filling pressure and other peripheral circulatory factors on cardiac output. *Am J Physiol* 1955;180:463–468.

251. Colombato LA, Albillos A, Groszmann RJ. Temporal relationship of peripheral vasodilatation, plasma volume expansion and the hyperdynamic circulatory state in portal-hypertensive rats. *J Hepatol* 1992;15:323–328.

252. Schrier RW, Arroyo V, Bernardi M, et al. Peripheral arterial vasodilatation hypothesis: a proposal for the initiation of renal sodium and water retention in cirrhosis. *Hepatology* 1988;8:1151–1157.

253. Gines P, Martin PY, Niederberger M. Prognostic significance of renal dysfunction in cirrhosis. *Kidney Int Suppl* 1997;61:S77–S82.

254. Genecin P, Polio J, Groszmann RJ. Na restriction blunts expansion of plasma volume and ameliorates hyperdynamic circulation in portal hypertension. *Am J Physiol* 1990;259:G498–G503.

255. Albillos A, Colombato LA, Groszmann RJ. Vasodilatation and sodium retention in prehepatic portal hypertension. *Gastroenterology* 1992;102:931–935.

256. Colombato LA, Albillos A, Groszmann RJ. The role of central blood volume in the development of sodium retention in portal hypertensive rats. *Gastroenterology* 1996;110:193–198.

257. Bosch J, Arroyo V, Rodes J. Hepatic and systemic hemodynamics and the renin–angiotension–aldosterone system in cirrhosis. In: Epstein M, ed. *The kidney and liver disease.* Elsevier Biomedical, 1983:423–439.

258. Schrier RW, De Wardener HE. Tubular reabsorption of sodium ion: influence of factors other than aldosterone and glomerular filtration rate. *N Engl J Med* 1971;285:1231–1243.

259. Ingles AC, Hernandez I, Garcia-Estan J, et al. Limited cardiac preload reserve in conscious cirrhotic rats. *Am J Physiol* 1991;260:H1912–H1917.

260. Claria J, Jimenez W, Ros J, et al. Pathogenesis of arterial hypotension in cirrhotic rats with ascites: role of endogenous nitric oxide. *J Hepatol* 1992;15:343–349.

261. Atucha NM, Garcia-Estan J, Ramirez A, et al. Renal effects of nitric oxide synthesis inhibition in cirrhotic rats. *Am J Physiol* 1994;267:R1454–R1460.

262. Lahera V, Salom MG, Fiksen-Olsen MJ, et al. Effects of NG-monomethyl-L-arginine and L-arginine on acetylcholine renal response. *Hypertension* 1990;15:659–663.

263. Arroyo V, Gines P. Arteriolar vasodilation and the pathogenesis of the hyperdynamic circulation and renal sodium and water retention in cirrhosis (editorial). *Gastroenterology* 1992;102:1077–1079.

48

α1-ANTITRYPSIN DEFICIENCY

DAVID H. PERLMUTTER

The classical form of α1-antitrypsin (α1-AT) deficiency, homozygous for the mutant α1-ATZ allele, is a relatively common disease. It affects approximately 1 in 1,600 to 1 in 2,000 live births in most populations of Northern European ancestry (1,2). Although only a subgroup of deficient individuals develop liver disease, it represents the most common metabolic cause of liver disease in children (3) and can be associated with chronic liver disease and hepatocellular carcinoma in adults (4). This deficiency also causes premature development of pulmonary emphysema in adults.

The α1-AT molecule is a single-chain secretory glycoprotein that inhibits destructive neutrophil proteases including elastase, cathepsin G and proteinase 3. It is often referred to as a hepatic acute phase reactant in that plasma α1-AT is predominantly derived from the liver and plasma levels increase 3- to 5-fold during the host response to tissue injury/inflammation. It is the archetype of a family of structurally related circulating serine protease inhibitors termed SERPINS. In the deficient state, there is an approximately 85% to 90% reduction in serum concentrations of α1-AT. A single amino acid substitution results in a mutant protein that is unable to traverse the secretory pathway. This α1-ATZ protein is retained in the endoplasmic reticulum (ER) rather than secreted into the blood and body fluids.

The classical deficient state is also unique as a genetic disease in that it causes injury to one target organ, lung, by a loss-of-function mechanism and injury to another target organ, liver, by what appears to be a gain-of-function mechanism. Most of the data in the literature indicate that emphysema results from a decreased number of α1-AT molecules within the lower respiratory tract, allowing unregulated elastolytic attack on the connective tissue matrix of the lung (5,6). Oxidative inactivation of residual α1-AT as a result of cigarette smoking accelerates lung injury (7). Moreover, the elastase–antielastase theory for the pathogenesis of emphysema is based on the concept that oxidative inactivation of α1-AT as a result of cigarette smoking plays a key role in the emphysema of α1-AT-sufficient individuals, the vast majority of cases of emphysema (5,8). It has been more difficult to explain the pathogenesis of liver injury in this deficiency. Results of transgenic animal experiments have provided further evidence that the liver disease does not result from a deficiency in antielastase activity (9,10). Most of the data in the literature corroborate the concept that liver injury in α1-AT deficiency results from the hepatotoxic effects of retention of the mutant α1-ATZ molecule in the ER of liver cells.

Although it is a single gene defect, there is extraordinary variation in the phenotypic expression of disease in the classical form of α1-AT deficiency. For instance, nationwide prospective screening studies done by Sveger in Sweden

D. H. Perlmutter: Departments of Pediatrics, Cell Biology, and Physiology, Washington University School of Medicine; Division of Gastroenterology and Nutrition, St. Louis Children's Hospital, St. Louis, Missouri 63110.

have shown that only 10% to 15% of the PIZZ[1] population develop clinically significant liver disease over the first 20 years of life (1,11). These data indicate that other genetic traits and/or environmental factors predispose a subgroup of PIZZ individuals to liver injury. There is also variation in incidence and severity of lung injury among α1-AT-deficient individuals. Environmental factors, such as cigarette smoking, obviously play an important role in the phenotypic expression of lung disease (12,13). However, there are well documented examples of siblings and other relatives of deficient individuals with severe emphysema who have the same genotype, a history of heavy cigarette smoking and only mild, subclinical pulmonary function abnormalities even at advanced ages (14). This suggests that there are other genetic traits that play a role in determining the phenotypic expression of lung disease as well as liver disease in this genetic disorder.

The diagnosis of α1-AT deficiency is based on the altered migration of the abnormal α1-ATZ molecule in serum specimens subjected to isoelectric focussing gel analysis. Treatment of α1-AT deficiency-associated liver disease is mostly supportive. Liver replacement therapy has been used successfully for severe liver injury. Although the clinical efficacy has not been demonstrated, many patients with emphysema due to α1-AT deficiency are currently being treated by intravenous and intratracheal aerosol administration of purified plasma α1-AT. An increasing number of patients with severe emphysema have undergone lung transplantation.

Recent studies of other genetic diseases have shown that α1-AT deficiency is a prototype of diseases in which mutant proteins accumulate in an inappropriate subcellular compartment. Studies of the basic cell biology of protein folding and trafficking have also shown ancient pathways within cells that constitute protective mechanisms for responding to the presence of mutant proteins in specific organelles. These "quality control" pathways are mediated by molecular chaperones, folding catalysts and translocation processes by which mutant proteins may be delivered to degradative systems within the cell. In some cases, it appears that cells attempt to protect themselves from mutant proteins by facilitating aggregation and then sequestering protein aggregates within specific locations to limit potential damage. There are also now well described protective signal transduction pathways such as the unfolded protein response in which the cell can produce more chaperones, folding catalysts and components of membrane structure to prevent damage from mutant or unassembled proteins. An understanding of these "quality control" mechanisms and cellular response pathways has already resulted in several new genetic and pharmacologic strategies for the prophylaxis of both liver and lung disease in α1-AT deficiency, currently under development for clinical application. However, further studies of these pathways will be needed to more clearly understand the variation in disease among affected patients and to develop the most effective strategies for prophylaxis and treatment.

CLINICAL MANIFESTATIONS OF LIVER DISEASE

Liver involvement is often first noticed at 1 to 2 months of age, because of persistent jaundice. Conjugated bilirubin levels in the blood and serum transaminase levels are mildly to moderately elevated (15,16). A few infants are recognized initially because of a cholestatic clinical syndrome characterized by pruritus and hypercholesterolemia. The clinical picture in these infants resembles extrahepatic biliary atresia, but histologic examination shows paucity of intrahepatic bile ducts (17).

Liver disease may be first discovered in late childhood or early adolescence when the affected individual is seen with abdominal distention from hepatosplenomegaly and/or ascites or has upper intestinal bleeding caused by esophageal variceal hemorrhage. In some of these cases, there is a history of unexplained prolonged obstructive jaundice during the neonatal period. In others, there is no evidence of any previous liver injury, even when the neonatal history is carefully reviewed.

The incidence and natural history of liver disease in α1-AT deficiency has been determined by Sveger, who carried out a nationwide screening study of newborn infants in Sweden (1). From 200,000 infants, 127 PIZZ newborns were identified and have been followed prospectively until 18 years of age at the time of the last report (11). The results show that more than 85% of these children have persistently normal serum transaminases with no evidence of liver dysfunction. One issue not addressed by the Sveger study is whether 18-year-olds with α1-AT deficiency have persistent subclinical histologic abnormalities, despite a lack of clinical or biochemical evidence of liver injury, and whether liver disease will eventually become clinically evident during adulthood.

α1-AT deficiency should be considered in the differential diagnosis of any adult who presents with chronic hepatitis, cirrhosis, portal hypertension, or hepatocellular carcinoma of unknown origin. An autopsy study in Sweden shows a higher risk of cirrhosis and primary liver cancer in adults with α1-AT deficiency than was previously suspected (4). In many of these cases, cirrhosis or hepatocellular carcinoma was found incidentally without any evidence of clinical liver disease during an entire lifetime. In many cases, however, there was no evidence of significant liver injury in α1-AT-deficient individuals at autopsy. Cases in which cirrhosis and/or hepatocellular carcinoma are found incidentally at autopsy also represent examples of the hepatic effects of α1-AT deficiency that are in striking contrast to other cases in which liver disease is severe enough to require liver transplantation by 6 to 24 months of age for

---

[1]Nomenclature for the Protease Inhibitor genotype, homozygous for the Z allele.

survival. Thus, the overwhelming clinical experience with this disease indicates that there is wide variation in liver disease phenotype among PIZZ α1-AT-deficient individuals, with many "protected" from liver disease, or having very slowly progressing liver disease.

It is still not clear whether liver injury results from the heterozygous α1-AT MZ state by itself. Studies of liver biopsy collections (18) and liver transplant databases (19) have identified heterozygous patients with severe liver disease and no other explanation. However, these studies are biased in ascertainment and one is never assured about the exclusion of environmental causes of liver disease. A cross-sectional study of patients with α1-AT deficiency in a referral-based Austrian university hospital who were reexamined with the most sophisticated and sensitive assays available suggests that liver disease in heterozygotes can be accounted for, to a great extent, by infections with hepatitis B or C virus or autoimmune disease (20).

Liver disease has been described for several other allelic variants of α1-AT. Children with compound heterozygosity type PISZ are affected by liver injury in a manner similar to PIZZ children (1). There are several reports of liver disease in α1-AT deficiency type PIM$_{malton}$(21,22). These are particularly interesting associations because the abnormal PIM$_{malton}$ α1-AT molecule has been shown to undergo polymerization and retention within the ER (23), and the α1-ATS molecule has been shown to form heteropolymers with the α1-ATZ molecule (24). Liver disease has been detected in single patients with several other α1-AT allelic variants (3), but it is not clear whether other causes of liver injury for which we now have more sophisticated diagnostic assays, such as infection with hepatitis C and autoimmune hepatitis, have been completely excluded in these cases.

Diagnosis is established by a serum α1-AT phenotype determination in isoelectric focusing or by agarose electrophoresis at acid pH. Liver histology is characterized by periodic acid–Schiff-positive, diastase-resistant globules in the ER of hepatocytes. These globules are most prominent in periportal hepatocytes, but may also be seen in Kupffer cells and cells of biliary ductular lineage (25). There may be evidence of variable degrees of hepatocellular necrosis, inflammatory cell infiltration, periportal fibrosis, and/or cirrhosis. There is often evidence of bile duct epithelial cell destruction, and occasionally there is a paucity of intrahepatic bile ducts. Our recent study has shown that there may also be an intense autophagic reaction detected by electron microscopic examination of liver biopsies with a full array of nascent and degradative-type autophagic vacuoles (26).

STRUCTURE, FUNCTION, AND PHYSIOLOGY

α1-AT is encoded by a single approximately 12.2-kb gene on human chromosome 14q31-32.3 (27,28). The α1-AT gene is organized in 7 exons and 6 introns. The first three exons and a short 5′ segment of the fourth exon code for 5′ untranslated regions of the α1-AT mRNA. The first two exons and a short 5′ segment of the third exon are included in the primary transcript in macrophages but not in hepatocytes, accounting for a slightly longer mRNA. There are, in fact, two mRNA species in macrophages, depending on alternative posttranscriptional splicing pathways involving one of the two most 5′ exons (29,30). Most of the fourth exon and the remaining three exons encode the protein sequence of α1-AT.

The α1-AT protein is a single-chain, approximately 55-kd polypeptide with 394 amino acids and 3 asparagine-linked complex carbohydrate side chains. There are two major isoforms in serum, depending on the presence of a biantennary or triantennary configuration for the carbohydrate side chains. X-ray crystallography studies have shown that α1-AT has a globular shape and a highly ordered internal domain composed of two central β sheets surrounded by a small β sheet and nine α helices (31,32). The dominant structure is the 5-stranded β-pleated sheet termed the A sheet (Fig. 48.1).

α1-AT is the archetype of a family of structurally related proteins called *SERPINS*, including antithrombin III, α-antichymotrypsin, C1 inhibitor, α2-antiplasmin, protein C inhibitor, heparin cofactor II, plasminogen activator inhibitors, protease nexin I, ovalbumin, angiotensinogen, corticosteroid-binding globulin, and thyroid-binding globulin (3,32). These proteins share about 25% overall homology, with higher degrees of regional homology in functional domains. Most SERPINS function as suicide inhibitors by forming complexes with a specific target protease. Other SERPINS are not inhibitory. For instance, corticosteroid and thyroid hormone-binding globulins, which are thought to represent carriers for corticosteroid and thyroid hormones, respectively, form complexes but do not inactivate their hormone ligands.

A comparison of α1-AT with other members of the SERPIN supergene family has generated several important concepts about the structure and function of α1-AT. For instance, the reactive site, P1 residue, of α1-AT is localized to a mobile loop which rises above the gap in the center of the A sheet (33,34). The P1 residue itself is the most important determinant of functional specificity for each SERPIN molecule. This concept was dramatically confirmed by the discovery of α1-AT Pittsburgh, a variant in which the P1 residue of α1-AT, Met 358, is replaced by Arg 358. In this variant, α1-AT functions as a thrombin inhibitor, and severe bleeding diathesis results (35).

α1-AT is an inhibitor of serine proteases in general, but under physiologic conditions its targets are probably only neutrophil elastase, cathepsin G and proteinase 3, proteases released by activated neutrophils. The kinetics of association of α1-AT and these enzymes are more favorable, by several orders of magnitude, than those for α1-AT and any other serine protease (36).

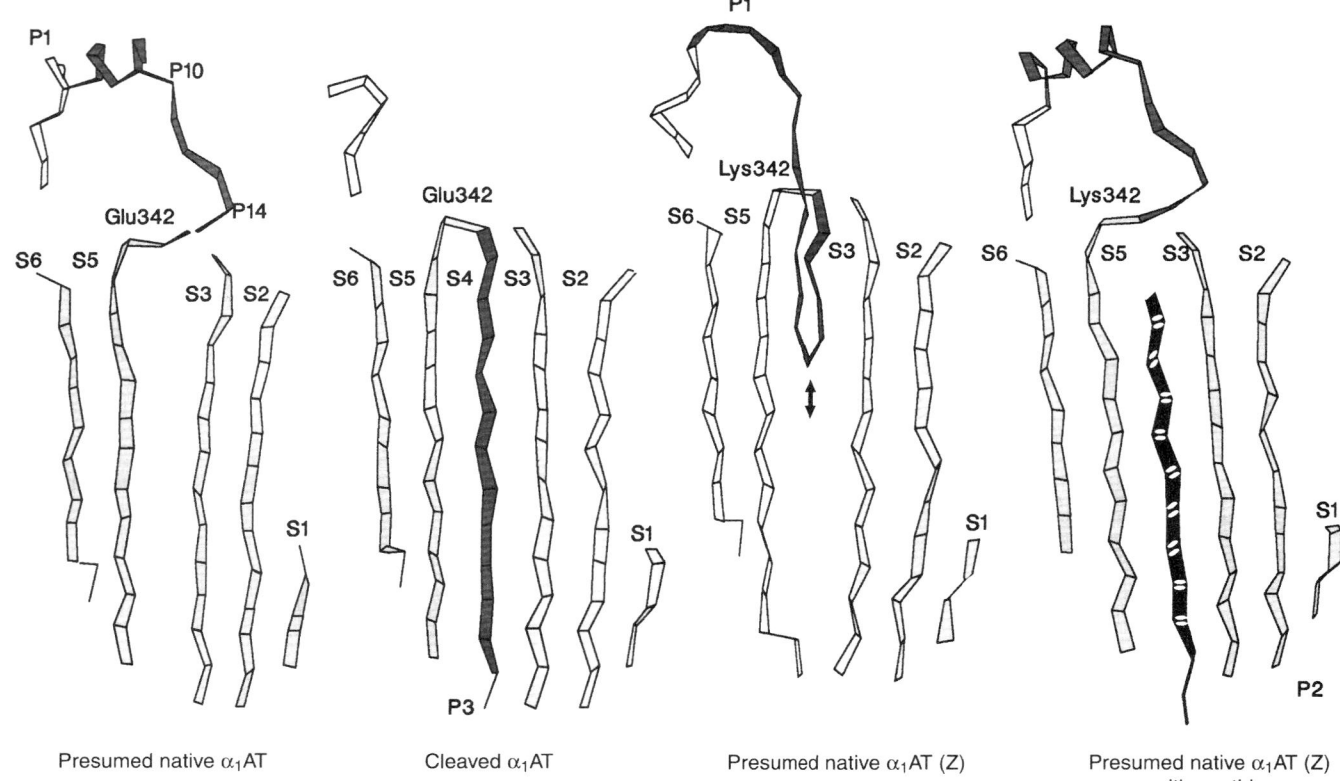

Presumed native α₁AT   Cleaved α₁AT   Presumed native α₁AT (Z)   Presumed native α₁AT (Z)
with peptide

A–D

FIGURE 48.1. Ribbon diagrams of the A-sheet and reactive-site loop of α1-AT in several different states. The positions of the residue P₁ in the reactive site loop and of glutamate 342 are indicated. **A:** Presumed native α1-AT. This state is presumed because it has not been crystallized. However, it is generated by computer models based on the crystal structures of cleaved α1-AT and native ovalbumin. The reactive-site loop is shown in *dark gray* with residues P₁₀, P₁₄ numbered from the reactive-site methionine P₁. The carboxyl-terminal fragment is shown as an *open ribbon*. α-helices of the A-sheet are shown in *light gray* and referred to as S₁, S₂, S₃, S₅ and S₆. The position of glutamate 342 is indicated. There is a gap in the A-sheet between S₃ and S₅. **B:** Cleaved α1-AT. The reactive-site loop in *dark gray* is cleaved and inserts into the A-sheet. It is referred to as S₄ in between α helices S₁–S₃ and S₅–S₆ of the A sheet shown in *light gray*. The positions of the P₃ residue of the reactive site loop and of glutamate 342 are indicated. **C:** Presumed native α1-AT (Z). The reactive-site loop simultaneously collapses into the gap in the A-sheet but because of the substitution of lysine at residue 342, it cannot fully insert. **D:** Presumed native α1-AT (Z) with peptide. A synthetic peptide that mimics the insertion of a reactive site loop from an adjacent α1-AT is shown in black. The insertion of peptide would prevent insertion from an adjacent α1-AT molecule and therein prevent polymerization. (From Carrell RW, Evans DL, Stein DE. Mobile reactive centre of serpins and the control of thrombosis. *Nature* 1991;353:576–578.)

α1-AT acts competitively by allowing target enzymes to bind directly to its reactive loop, a substrate-like region within the carboxyl-terminal region of the inhibitor molecule. This reaction between enzyme and inhibitor is essentially second-order, and the resulting complex contains one molecule of each of the reactants. A peptide bond in the inhibitor is hydrolyzed during formation of the enzyme–inhibitor complex. However, hydrolysis of this reactive-site peptide bond does not proceed to completion. An equilibrium, near unity, is established between complexes in which the reactive-site peptide bond of α1-AT is intact (native inhibitor) and those in which this peptide bond is cleaved (modified inhibitor). The complex of α1-AT and ser-

ine protease is a covalently stabilized structure, resistant to dissociation by denaturing compounds including sodium dodecyl sulfate and urea. The interaction between α1-AT and serine protease is suicidal in that the modified inhibitor is no longer able to bind and/or inactivate enzyme. Studies have now shown that the irreversible trapping of target enzyme is mediated by a profound conformational change in α1-AT, such that the cleaved reactive loop, binding enzyme, inserts into the gap in A sheet (37). Carrell and Lomas have likened the inhibitory mechanism to a "mousetrap, with the active inhibitor circulating in the metastable stressed-form and then springing into the stable, relaxed form to lock the complex with its target protease" (37).

The functional activity of α1-AT *in vivo* may be regulated by several factors. For one, it may be rendered inactive as an elastase inhibitor by active oxygen products, intermediates of activated neutrophils and macrophages that can oxidize the reactive-site methionine of α1-AT (7). This effect is thought to constitute the basis for increased susceptibility to emphysema in smokers, whether deficient in α1-AT or not. The α1-AT molecule may also be inactivated *in vivo* by the proteolytic action of thiol proteases as well as metalloproteases, such as collagenase and pseudomonas elastase (38).

Several studies have indicated that α1-AT protects experimental animals from the lethal effects of tumor necrosis factor (TNF) (39,40). Most of the evidence from these studies indicates that this protective effect is due to inhibition of the synthesis and release of platelet-activating factor from neutrophils (40,41), presumably through the inhibition of neutrophil-derived proteases.

α1-AT also appears to have functional activities that do not involve the inhibition of neutrophil proteases. The carboxyl-terminal fragment of α1-AT, which can be generated during the formation of a complex with serine protease or during proteolytic inactivation by thiol- or metalloproteases, is a potent neutrophil chemoattractant (42,43).

The predominant site of synthesis of plasma α1-AT is the liver (44).Tissue-specific expression of α1-AT in human hepatoma cells is directed by structural elements within a 750-nucleotide region upstream of the hepatocyte transcriptional start site in exon Ic. Within this region, there are structural elements that are recognized by nuclear transcription factors including HNF-1α and HNF-1β, C-EBP, HNF-4, and HNF-3 (45). HNF-1α and HNF-4 appear to be particularly important for expression of the human α1-AT gene (46,47).

Plasma concentrations of α1-AT increase 3- to 5-fold during the host response to inflammation and/or tissue injury (3). The source of this additional α1-AT has always been considered the liver; thus, α1-AT is known as a positive hepatic acute phase reactant. Synthesis of α1-AT in human hepatoma cells (HepG2, Hep3B) is upregulated by interleukin 6 (IL-6) but not by interleukin 1 (IL-1) or TNF (48). Plasma concentrations also increase during oral contraceptive therapy and pregnancy (49).

α1-AT is also synthesized and secreted in primary cultures of human blood monocytes as well as bronchoalveolar and breast milk macrophages (50). Expression of α1-AT in monocytes and macrophages is profoundly influenced by products generated during inflammation (48,51). Synthesis of α1-AT in liver cells and mononuclear phagocytes is also regulated by a feed-forward mechanism. In this regulatory loop, elastase-α1-AT complexes mediate an increase in the synthesis of α1-AT through the interaction of a pentapeptide domain in the carboxylterminal tail of α1-AT with a novel cell surface receptor (52). This class of receptor molecules is now referred to as serpin-enzyme complex (SEC) receptors because they recognize the highly conserved domains of several other serpin–enzyme complexes (53,54).

α1-AT mRNA has been isolated from multiple tissues in transgenic mice (55,56), but only in some cases have studies distinguished whether such α1-AT mRNA is in ubiquitous tissue macrophages or other cell types. For instance, α1-AT is synthesized in enterocytes and intestinal paneth cells, as determined by studies in intestinal epithelial cell lines, ribonuclease protection assays of human intestinal RNA, and *in situ* hybridization analysis in cryostat sections of human intestinal mucosa (30,57). Expression of α1-AT in enterocytes increases markedly as they differentiate from crypt to villus, in response to IL-6, and during inflammation *in vivo*. α1-AT is also synthesized by pulmonary epithelial cells (58,59). Synthesis of α1-AT in pulmonary epithelial cells is less responsive to IL-6 than to a related cytokine, oncostatin M (59).

The half-life of α1-antitrypsin in plasma is approximately 5 days (60). It is estimated that the daily production rate of α1-AT is 34 mg per kilogram of body weight, with 33% of the intravascular pool of α1-AT degraded daily. Several physiologic factors may affect the rate of α1-AT catabolism. First, desialylated α1-AT is cleared from the circulation in minutes (3), probably via hepatic asialoglycoprotein receptor-mediated endocytosis. Second, α1-AT in complex with elastase or proteolytically modified is cleared more rapidly than native α1-AT (61). Because its ligand specificity is similar to that required for *in vivo* clearance of serpin-enzyme complexes, the SEC receptor may also be involved in the clearance and catabolism of α1-AT-elastase and other serpin-enzyme complexes (54,62). The low-density protein receptor-related protein (LRP) can also mediate clearance and catabolism of α1-AT-elastase complexes (63,64). α1-AT diffuses into most tissues and is found in most body fluids (5).

VARIANTS OF α1-ANTITRYPSIN

Variants of α1-AT in humans are classified according to the protease inhibitor (PI) phenotype system as defined by agarose electrophoresis or isoelectric focusing of plasma in polyacrylamide at acid pH (65). The PI classification assigns a letter to variants, according to migration of the major isoform, using alphabetic order from anode to cathode, or from low to high isoelectric point. For example, the most common normal variant migrates to an intermediate isoelectric point, designated M. Individuals with the most common severe deficiency have a α1-AT allelic variant that migrates to a high isoelectric point, designated Z.

In recent years it has become possible to identify greater polymorphic variation of α1-AT by direct DNA sequence analysis. Using these techniques in addition to isoelectric focusing, more than 100 allelic variants have been reported (66).

Normal Allelic Variants

The most common *normal variant* of α1-AT is termed M$_1$ and is found in 65% to 70% of Caucasians in the United States (67). The M$_2$ allele, characterized by an additional base change from the M$_3$ sequence, occurs in 15% to 20% of the Caucasian population (66). Each of the normal allelic variants are associated with serum concentrations of, and functional activity for, α1-AT within the normal range.

Null Allelic Variants

α1-AT variants in which α1-AT is not detectable in serum are called *null allelic variants* and, when inherited with another null variant or deficiency variant, are associated with premature development of emphysema (8). Several types of defects, including insertions and deletions, appear to be responsible for these variants (3,8,68). A single-base substitution has been discovered in the Null$_{Ludwigshafen}$ allele (69). A recent study suggests that this mutant α1-AT molecule is synthesized and secreted in transfected heterologous cells, but there is a slight decrease in its rate of secretion and it completely lacks functional activity (70). It is not yet known whether instability or accelerated catabolism *in vivo* are the explanation for the inability to detect this mutant α1-AT molecule in serum specimens.

Dysfunctional Variants

Dysfunctional variants of α1-AT include α1-AT Pittsburgh (35). There also is a decrease in serum concentration and functional activity for α1-AT M$_{Mineral Springs}$ (71).

Deficiency Variants

Several variants of α1-AT associated with a reduction in serum concentrations of α1-AT have been described and are called *deficiency variants*. Some of these variants are not associated with clinical disease, such as the S variant (27, 72). Other deficiency variants are associated with emphysema such as M$_{Heerlen}$ (73), M$_{Procida}$ (74), M$_{Malton}$ (21), M$_{Duarte}$ (3), M$_{Mineral Springs}$ (71), P$_{Lowell}$ (75), and W$_{Bethesda}$ (76). In two persons with M$_{Malton}$ and one with M$_{Duarte}$, hepatocyte α1-AT inclusions and liver disease have been reported (3,21,22). In one person with the deficiency variant S$_{Iiyama}$, emphysema and hepatocyte inclusions were reported but this person did not have liver disease (77).

MECHANISM OF DEFICIENCY

A point mutation results in the substitution of lysine for glutamate 342 (37) and a mutant α1-ATZ molecule which is retained in the ER rather than secreted (78). Defective secretion is observed in liver cells, macrophages and transfected cell lines (3). Site-directed mutagenesis studies have shown that the single amino acid substitution (E342K) is sufficient to produce the defect in secretion (79–81). The mutant α1-ATZ molecule is partially functionally active, having about 50% to 80% of the elastase inhibitory capacity of wild-type α1-ATM (82–84). There is a modest increase in the rate of *in vivo* clearance/catabolism of radiolabeled α1-ATZ compared with wild-type α1-ATM when infused into normal individuals, but this difference does not account for the decrease in blood levels of α1-AT in deficient individuals (60).

A series of studies by Carrell and colleagues have provided a mechanistic explanation for misfolding of α1-ATZ in the ER (37). Apparently, substitution of Glu 342 by Lys in the α1-ATZ variant reduces the stability of the molecule in its monomeric form and increases the likelihood that it will form polymers by means of a so-called "loop-sheet" insertion mechanism (85). In this mechanism, the reactive center loop of one α1-AT molecule inserts into a gap in the β-pleated A sheet of another α1-AT molecule. Carrell and co-workers were the first to notice that the site of the amino acid substitution in the α1-ATZ variant was at the base of the reactive center loop, adjacent to the gap in the A sheet (Fig. 48.1). These investigators predicted that a change in the charge at this residue, as occurs with the substitution of Lys for Glu, would prevent the insertion of the reactive-site loop into the gap in the A sheet during interaction with enzyme; therefore, the mutant α1-ATZ would be susceptible to the insertion of the reactive center loop of adjacent molecules into the gap in its A sheet. This would, in turn, cause the mutant α1-ATZ to be more susceptible to polymerization than the wild-type α1-AT. In fact, their experiments showed that α1-ATZ undergoes this form of polymerization to a certain extent spontaneously and to a greater extent during relatively minor perturbations, such as a rise in temperature. Presumably, an increase in body temperature during systemic inflammation would exacerbate this tendency *in vivo*. Polymers could also be detected by electron microscopy in the ER of hepatocytes in a liver biopsy specimen from a PIZZ individual (85). Similar polymers have been found in the plasma of patients with the PIS$_{Iiyama}$ α1-AT variant and the PIM$_{Malton}$ α1-AT variant (23,86). The mutation in α1-AT PIS$_{Iiyama}$ (Ser 53 to Phe) (77), and in α1-ATPIM$_{Malton}$ (Phe 52 deletion) (21) affect residues that provide a ridge for the sliding movement that opens the A sheet. Thus, these mutations would be expected to interfere with the insertion of the reactive center loop into the gap in the A sheet, and therefore leave the gap in the A sheet available for spontaneous loop-sheet polymerization. It is indeed interesting that the hepatocytic α1-AT globules have been observed in a few patients with these two variants. Recent observations suggest that the α1-ATS variant also undergoes loop-sheet polymerization (24) and that this may account for its retention in the ER, albeit a milder degree of retention than that for α1-ATZ (72). Moreover, α1-ATS can apparently form heteropolymers with α1-ATZ (24), providing a potential explanation for liver disease in patients with the SZ phenotype. The precise mechanism for loop-sheet insertion for each of these mutant proteins is currently under further investigation (86,87).

A complementary study by Yu et al. comparing the folding kinetics of mutant α1-ATZ to wild-type α1-ATM in transverse urea gradient gels (88) has provided further understanding of the mechanism for misfolding in the ER. This study shows that α1-ATZ folds at an extremely slow rate, unlike the wild-type α1-ATM which folds in minutes. The delay in folding leads to an accumulation of an intermediate which has a high tendency to polymerize, presumably by the loop-sheet insertion mechanism.

By themselves, however, these data do not prove that the polymerization of α1-ATZ results in retention in the ER. In fact, many polypeptides must assemble into oligomeric or polymeric complexes to traverse the ER and reach their destination within the cell, at the surface of the plasma membrane, or into the extracellular fluid (89). However, evidence that polymerization results in the retention of α1-ATZ in the ER has been provided by studies in which the fate of α1-ATZ is examined after the introduction of additional mutations into the molecule. For instance, Kim et al. (90) introduced a mutation into the α1-AT molecule at amino acid 51, F51L. This mutation is remote from the Z mutation, E342K, but apparently impedes loop-sheet polymerization and prevents insertion of synthetic peptide into the gap in the A sheet, implying that the mutation leads to closing of this gap. The double-mutated F51L α1-ATZ molecule was less prone to polymerization and folded more efficiently *in vitro* than α1-ATZ. Moreover, the introduction of the F51L mutation partially corrected the intracellular retention properties of α1-ATZ in microinjected *Xenopus* oocytes (91) and in yeast (92).

Further evidence has recently come from studies of two families with autosomal dominantly inherited dementia (93). This dementia was associated with a histological picture of unique neuronal inclusion bodies and characterized biochemically by polymers of a neuron-specific member of the SERPIN family, neuroserpin. Moreover, the mutation in neuroserpin in one family is homologous to the mutation in the α1-AT S$_{liyama}$ allele that is associated with polymerization and inclusions in the ER of liver cells. Taken together, these studies provide relatively strong evidence that the polymerization of α1-ATZ results in its retention with the ER.

However, it is still unclear what proportion of the newly synthesized mutant α1-ATZ molecules is converted to the polymeric state in the ER. It is also not known whether polymeric molecules are degraded in the ER less rapidly than their monomeric counterpart or whether polymeric molecules, when retained in the ER, are more hepatotoxic than their monomeric counterparts. Indeed, recent studies on the effect of temperature on the fate of α1-ATZ have

indicated the high degree of complexity involved in these issues. Although Lomas et al. showed that a rise in temperature to 42°C increases the polymerization of purified α1-ATZ *in vitro* (85), Burrows et al. found that a rise in temperature to 42°C resulted in increased secretion of α1-ATZ as well as decreased intracellular degradation of α1-ATZ in a model cell culture system (94). In contrast, lowering the temperature to 27°C resulted in diminished intracellular degradation of α1-ATZ without any change in the small amount of α1-ATZ secreted (94).

PATHOGENESIS OF LIVER DISEASE

There are several theories for the pathogenesis of liver injury in α1-AT deficiency. According to the *immune theory*, liver damage results from an abnormal immune response to liver antigens (95). This theory is based on an increase in the HLA DR3-DW25 haplotype observed in α1-AT-deficient individuals with liver disease (96). However, there is no difference in the expression of class II major histocompatibility complex (MHC) antigen in the livers of these individuals compared with normal controls (97). Moreover, an increase in the prevalence of a particular HLA DR haplotype in the affected population does not by itself imply altered immune function. In fact, because of the linkage disequilibrium displayed by genes within the MHC, it is possible that increased susceptibility is caused by the products of unrelated but linked genes. For instance, the MHC contains genes for several heat shock/stress proteins (98) which play an important role in the folding/translocation of polypeptides and could therefore theoretically affect the fate and hepatotoxicity of α1-ATZ in the ER (see Fate of Mutant α1-ATZ in the Endoplasmic Reticulum, below).

The *accumulation theory*, in which liver damage is thought to be caused by an accumulation of mutant α1-AT molecules in the ER of liver cells, is the most widely accepted. Experimental results in transgenic mice are most consistent with this theory and completely exclude the possibility that liver damage is caused by "proteolytic attack" as a consequence of diminished serum α1-AT concentrations. Transgenic mice carrying the mutant human α1-ATZ allele develop periodic acid–Schiff-positive, diastase-resistant intrahepatic globules and liver injury (9,10). Because there are normal levels of antielastases in these animals, as directed by endogenous genes, the liver injury cannot be attributed to "proteolytic attack."

Some have argued that the histologic characteristics of the liver in the transgenic mouse model are not identical to those in humans. Detailed histologic characterization of the liver in one transgenic mouse model by Geller and colleagues has shown that there are focal areas of liver cell necrosis, microabscesses with an accumulation of neutrophils and regenerative activity in the form of multicellular liver plates, and focal nodule formation during the neonatal period (99). Nodular clusters of altered hepatocytes that lack α1-AT-immunoreactivity are also seen during the neonatal period. With aging, there is a decrease in the number of hepatocytes containing α1-ATZ globules; there is also an increase in the number of nodular aggregates of α1-AT-negative hepatocytes and development of periosinusoidal fibrosis. Within 6 weeks, there are dysplastic changes in these aggregates. Adenomas occur within 1 year, and invasive hepatocellular carcinoma is seen between 1 and 2 years of age (99). The relationship between the α1-ATZ globules and inflammation or dysplasia is, however, not yet apparent from these animal studies. The histopathology of the α1-ATZ transgenic mice is remarkably similar to that of hepatitis B virus surface antigen in transgenic mice, and is particularly interesting because hepatitis B virus is retained in the ER, or in the ER-Golgi intermediate compartment of hepatocytes, often called "ground-glass hepatocytes" (100). It is still unclear why the liver injury in this transgenic mouse model is somewhat milder and less fibrogenic than that seen in children with α1-AT-deficiency-associated liver disease. It is possible that there are strain-specific factors that condition the response to injury in the mouse. There are certainly host-specific factors that determine the amount of liver injury in α1-AT deficiency (see below), and we find that the amount of inflammation and fibrosis varies widely among our patients with liver disease from α1-AT deficiency.

Data from individuals who have null alleles of α1-AT have also been used as evidence against the "proteolytic attack" theory. These individuals do not develop liver injury —at least not enough liver injury to result in clinical detection. However, only a few individuals with null alleles have been reported, each has a different allele, and based on data in PIZZ individuals in which about 10% to 15% of the population develops clinically significant liver injury, it might be necessary to evaluate seven to eight individuals with each null allele before detecting one with liver injury.

The recognition that several other naturally occurring variant alleles of α1-AT associated with deficiency can undergo polymerization has provided some support for the *accumulation theory*. The most important of these is the compound heterozygous α1-ATSZ phenotype. Recent work by Lomas and colleagues has shown that α1-ATS and α1-ATZ may form heteropolymers (24). We know from the nationwide study of α1-AT deficiency in Sweden that the incidence of liver disease among individuals with the PISZ phenotype is similar to that of individuals with the PIZZ phenotype (1,11). We also now know that the PIMMalton allele undergoes polymerization, and liver injury has been reported in several patients with this allele (21,22). However, there is a report of an individual with PIS_Iiyama allele having hepatocyte α1-AT globules but no liver injury (77). Moreover, a recent report by Ray and Brown has indicated that PIM_Heerlen and PIM_Procidia undergo aggregation

and that the PIM_Mineral Springs and PINull_Ludwigshafen may undergo aggregation, but there are no reports of liver disease in individuals carrying these alleles (70). However, there are only a few patients with the M_Malton, S_Iiyama, M_Heerlen, M_Procida, M_Mineral springs and Null_Ludwigshafen that have been identified. It is also not clear how many of these patients have been thoroughly examined for liver disease. Again, on the basis of what we know about the PIZZ and PISZ phenotype, at least seven to eight individuals with each of these alleles would need to be examined to detect one with liver injury.

It has been difficult to reconcile the accumulation theory with the observations of Sveger, which show that only a subset of PIZZ α1-AT-deficient individuals develop significant liver damage. We have made the prediction that a subset of the PIZZ population is more susceptible to liver injury by virtue of one or more additional inherited traits or environmental factors that exaggerate the intracellular accumulation of the mutant α1-AT Z protein or exaggerate the cellular pathophysiological consequence of mutant α1-AT accumulation. To address this prediction experimentally, we transduced skin fibroblasts from PIZZ individuals, with or without liver disease, with amphotropic recombinant retroviral particles designed for constitutive expression of the mutant α1-ATZ gene (101). The PIZZ individuals were carefully selected to ensure appropriate representation. Susceptible hosts were defined as having severe liver disease by clinical criteria. Protected hosts were discovered incidentally and never had clinical or biochemical evidence of liver disease. Human skin fibroblasts do not express the endogenous α1-AT gene but, presumably, express other genes involved in the postsynthetic processing of secretory proteins. The results show that expression of the human α1-AT gene was conferred on each fibroblast cell line. Compared with the same cell line transduced with the wild-type α1-ATM gene, there was selective intracellular retention of the mutant α1-ATZ protein in each case. However, there was a marked delay in degradation of the mutant α1-ATZ protein after it accumulated in the fibroblasts from PIZZ individuals with liver disease (susceptible hosts) as compared with those without liver disease (protected hosts) (Fig. 48.2). Thus, these data provide evidence that other factors that affect the fate of the mutant α1-ATZ molecule, such as a lag in ER degradation, at least in part determine susceptibility to liver disease.

Data from our most recent studies of different susceptible hosts have suggested that there are several mechanisms by which ER degradation may be delayed, each affecting a separate step in the pathway (see Fate of Mutant α1-ATZ in the Endoplasmic Reticulum, below). Carrell and Lomas have suggested that differences in the incidence or severity of febrile illnesses which could affect the relative degree of polymerization of α1-ATZ provide an explanation for differences in the development of liver disease (85). There are, however, no data to substantiate this hypothesis. We have

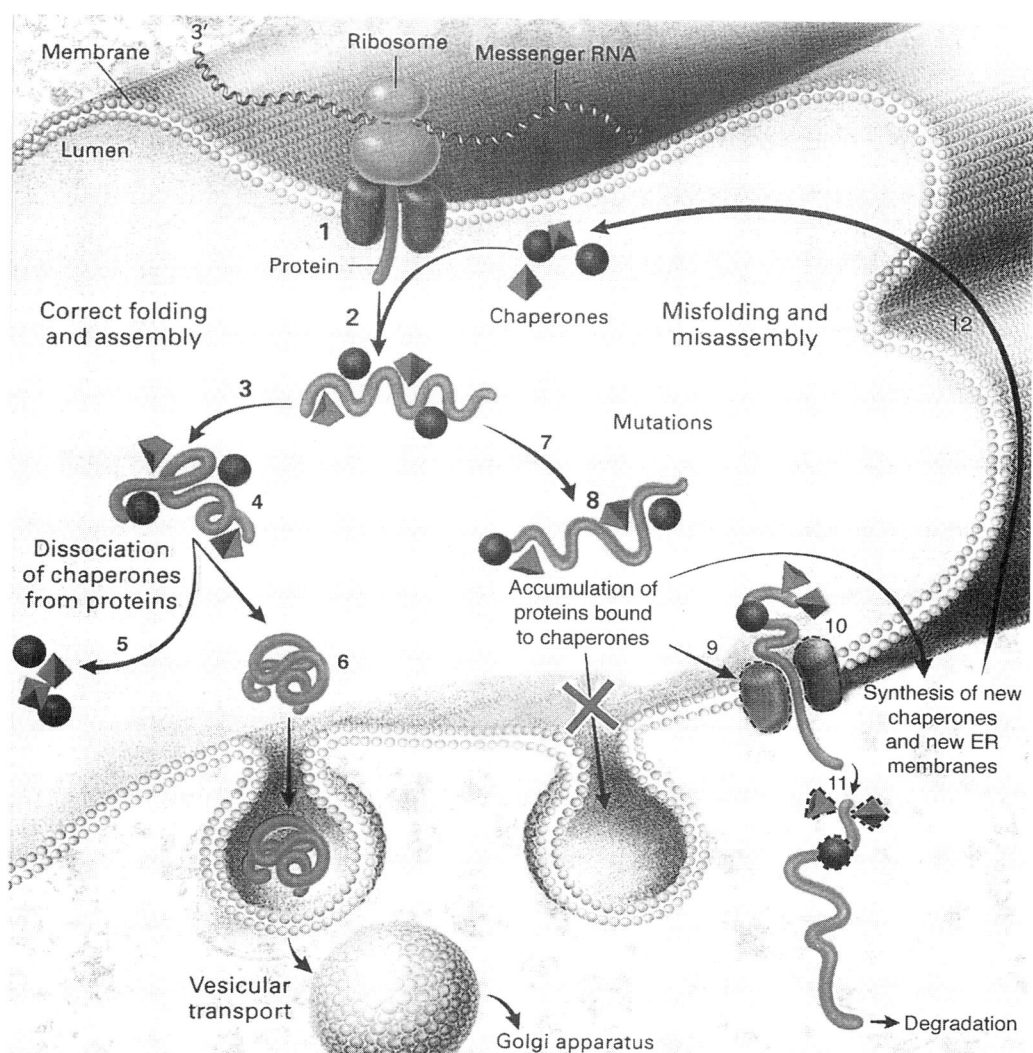

FIGURE 48.2. Fate of secretory proteins in the endoplasmic reticulum (*ER*). Secretory proteins are cotranslationally translocated into the lumen of the ER through the import channel (*1*). These polypeptides transiently interact with several different chaperones (*2*) to facilitate folding (*3*). Once folding is completed (*4*), there is dissociation of chaperones (*5*) and vesicular transport out of the ER (*6*). In the case of mutant proteins (*7*) which remain mutant even after interaction with chaperones (*8*), there is an accumulation of mutant proteins bound to their chaperones. The quality control apparatus of the ER mediates transport of these mutant proteins, free or bound to chaperones, to the ER membrane (*9*) or through a channel, perhaps even through the import channel (*10*), into the cytoplasm (*11*) for degradation. The accumulation of mutant proteins also induces the synthesis of new chaperones (*12*) and new ER membrane to accommodate the increased load of mutant proteins and thereby protect the cells. (From Kuznetsov G, Nigam SK. Folding of secretory and membrane proteins. *N Engl J Med* 1998;339:1688–1695, with permission.)

not seen any differences in the incidence or severity of febrile illnesses between our susceptible and protected hosts. Furthermore, recent studies have suggested that in addition to its effect on polymerization of α1-ATZ, enhanced temperature may have independent effects on the fate of mutant α1-ATZ which are potentially protective (94).

FATE OF THE MUTANT α1-ATZ IN THE ENDOPLASMIC RETICULUM

It now appears that the key processes for determining the folding of secretory proteins during biogenesis and the fate of mutant secretory proteins occur in the ER. In fact, these processes have been referred to as the "quality control mechanism" of the cell. After translocation into the lumen of the ER, nascent secretory polypeptide chains undergo a series of post-translational modifications, including glycosylation formation of disulfide bonds, oligomerization and folding. These modifications and transport through the ER to the Golgi is facilitated by transient and sequential interactions with ER proteins, termed molecular chaperones.

Several families of ER chaperones have been identified. One has been referred to as the polypeptide chain-binding protein family and includes several heat-shock/stress proteins, GRP78/BiP and GRP94, protein disulfide isomerase, and ERp72 (102). Several calcium-binding phosphoproteins of the ER, most notably calnexin and calreticulin, have also been implicated as having molecular chaperone activity within the ER. Calnexin is an approximately 88-kd transmembrane ER resident phosphoprotein (103) now known to facilitate the folding and assembly of many membrane and secretory glycoproteins (104). In addition to its chaperone activity (105), calnexin uses a lectin-like mechanism to bind the innermost glucose residue of the asparagine-linked oligosaccharide side chains present on most glycoproteins (106). The innermost glucose residue becomes accessible almost immediately after the secretory glycoprotein has undergone the initial stages of oligosaccharide side chain trimming in the lumen of the ER, including the removal of the two outermost glucose residues by the action of glucosidases I and II (Fig. 48.3). Once bound to calnexin, monoglucosylated glycoproteins are retained in the ER until properly folded. Once folding

is complete, the glycoprotein can dissociate from calnexin for vesicular transport out of the ER. Two studies have indicated that a unique reglucosylating enzyme, uridine diphosphate-glucose:glycoprotein glucosyltransferase (UDGGT), can transfer glucose onto unfolded or denatured, deglucosylated proteins in the ER (107,108). In fact, the binding of glycoproteins to calnexin during folding in the ER is now thought to depend on a cycle of glucosidase II activity, producing the deglucosylated form of a protein and reglucosylation by ER luminal UDGGT, leading to regeneration of the monoglucosylated form. The glucosyltransferase acts preferentially on unfolded or denatured proteins. Thus, the repeated cycles of binding to and dissociation from calnexin are designed to maximize the possibility that a given unfolded or denatured protein will undergo proper folding for transport out of the ER.

As a part of its quality control functions, the ER also possesses machinery whereby it can degrade any mutant or unassembled polypeptides that is unable to fold properly even after interaction with the ER chaperones (Fig. 48.4). This machinery has come to be called the "ER degradation pathway" (109). Although the ER degradation pathway was originally thought to involve a distinct proteolytic system, it now appears to be mediated in large part from the cytoplasmic aspect of the ER by the ubiquitin system (110) and the proteasome (111). The role of the proteasome was originally shown for the mutant membrane protein CFTRΔF508 (112,113) as well as for α1-ATZ (114,115). Although it is relatively easy to conceptualize how a trans-

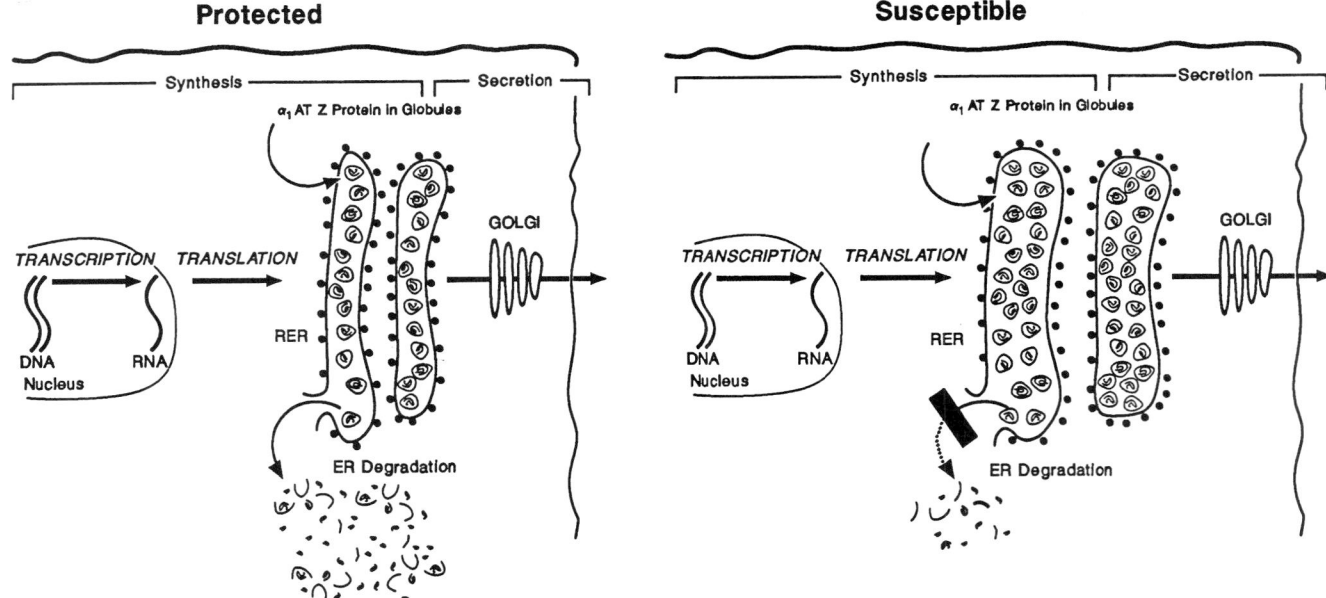

FIGURE 48.3. Differences in endoplasmic reticulum (*ER*) degradation of α1-ATZ in protected and susceptible hosts. The block in ER degradation in susceptible hosts is represented by a *small dark bar*. RER, rough ER. (From Teckman JH and Perlmutter DH. Conceptual advances in pathogenesis and treatment of childhood metabolic liver disease. *Gastroenterology* 1995;108:1263, with permission.)

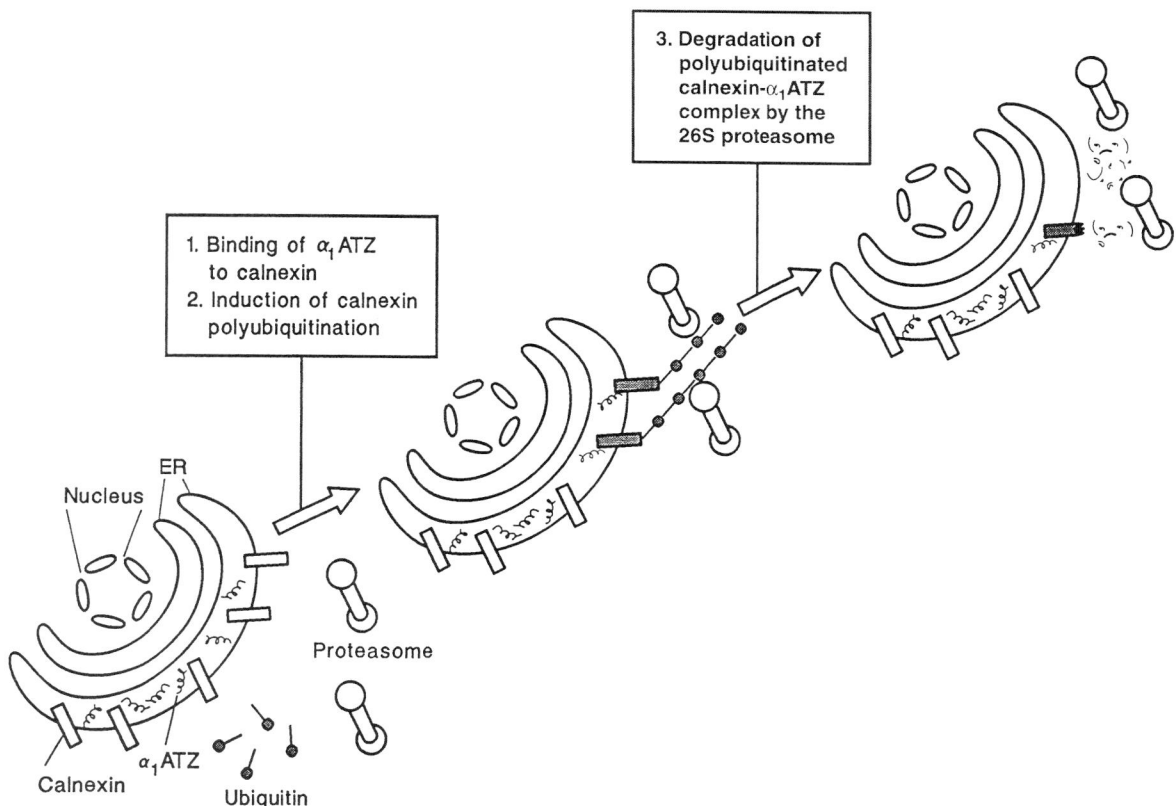

FIGURE 48.4. Endoplasmic reticulum (*ER*) degradation of α1-ATZ. In one pathway for ER degradation, α1-ATZ in the lumen of the ER binds to the transmembrane chaperone calnexin. Calnexin molecules bound by α1-ATZ are then polyubiquitinated, presumably on their cytoplasmic tail. The polyubiquitinated calnexin-α1-ATZ complexes are degraded by the proteasome. There are many calnexin molecules still present to provide chaperone activity for endogenous wild-type proteins. This figure does not show the ubiquitin-independent proteasomal and nonproteasomal mechanisms for ER degradation of α1-ATZ.

membrane protein such as CFTRΔF508 might be accessible on the cytoplasmic aspect of the ER membrane for ubiquitination and degradation by the proteasome, it is more difficult to conceptualize how this might occur for a luminal polypeptide such as α1-ATZ. To address this issue, we used a cell-free microsomal translocation system and found that α1-ATZ must interact with the transmembrane molecular chaperone calnexin in order to be degraded. The results showed that degradation of the α1-ATZ-calnexin complex by the proteasome involves both ubiquitin-dependent and -independent mechanisms (115,116). The ubiquitin-dependent mechanism requires recruitment of the ubiquitin conjugating enzyme E2-F1 from the cytoplasm onto the ER membrane and polyubiquitination of the cytoplasmic tail of calnexin (117). Degradation of the mutant secretory protein carboxypeptidase Y in yeast also requires recruitment of Ubc7p (the yeast homologue of E2-F1) from the cytoplasm by the ER membrane protein Cue1p to generate a *ubiquitin conjugation platform* at the surface of the ER (117). Taken together, these studies show that there are

at least two pathways and several steps in each pathway involved in ER degradation of α1-ATZ: binding to calnexin; induction of calnexin ubiquitination by a *ubiquitin conjugation platform* at the surface of the ER that includes E2-F1; and degradation of α1-ATZ-calnexin and α1-ATZ-polyubiquitinated calnexin complexes by the 26S proteasome (Fig. 48.5). Studies of α1-ATZ expressed in yeast (114) and of the truncated mutant α1-AT$_{Hong Kong}$ in transfected mouse hepatoma cells (118) have also shown that calnexin and the proteasome are involved in the ER degradation of these molecules.

We do not yet know exactly how the entire α1-ATZ-calnexin complex, including the luminal domain of calnexin associated with α1-ATZ, is degraded. The proteasome may initiate a process that is completed by other enzymes within the ER membrane or within the ER lumen. Several other mechanisms by which the ubiquitin system and the proteasome gain access to membrane-bound and lumenal substrates of the ER degradation pathway have been discussed in the literature. The retrograde translocation mechanism in

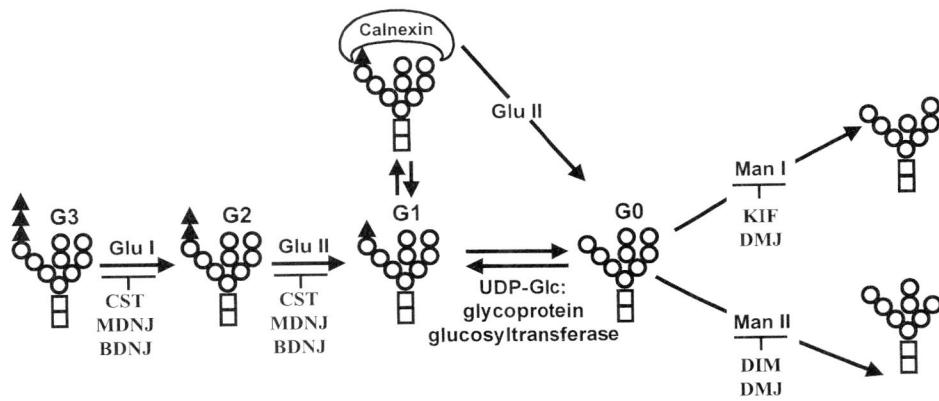

FIGURE 48.5. Oligosaccharide side chain trimming in the endoplasmic reticulum (ER). There are two N-acetyl glucosamine (*open squares*), nine mannose (*open circles*) and three glucose residues (*filled triangles*) on each asparagine-linked oligosaccharide side chain. Trimming involves removal of the outermost glucose by glucosidase I and the second glucose by glucosidase II. Calnexin binds glycoproteins by recognizing the innermost glucose. However, this glucose residue can still be removed by glucosidase II when the glycoprotein is bound to calnexin. The glycoprotein then dissociates from calnexin. If the polypeptide is mutant or unassembled, it can be recognized by the reglycosylating enzyme, *UPD-Glc*:glycoprotein glucosyltransferase, to add back a glucose molecule in a manner that leads to re-association with calnexin. Glucosidase I and II activities can be inhibited by castanospermine (*CST*), N-methyl deoxynojirimicin (*MDNJ*), and N-butyl deoxnojirimicin (*BDNJ*). There are also α mannosidases in the ER. Mannosidase I can remove a single mannose residue from the inner branch. It is inhibited by kifunensine (*KIF*) and deoxymannojirimicin (*DMJ*). Mannosidase II can remove a single mannose from the outer branch. It is inhibited by 1,4 dideoxy-1,4-imino-O-mannitol hydrochloride (*DIM* and *DMJ*).

which substrates are transported from the ER lumen or membrane through the Sec61p translocon has received the most attention (119–126). Recently, Mayer et al. have shown that a chimeric ER membrane protein may be dislocated and degraded directly at the ER membrane by a membrane-bound assembly of the ubiquitin-dependent proteasomal system (127). This "membrane extraction" mechanism, or "dislocation" mechanism, may be particularly relevant to degradation of α1-ATZ because ER degradation of this substrate appears to involve polyubiquitination on the cytoplasmic tail of the transmembrane ER chaperone calnexin only when it has bound α1-ATZ at the luminal surface of the ER membrane. It is also possible that the proteasome gains access to α1-ATZ and/or the α1-ATZ-polyubiquitinated calnexin during the formation of autophagic vacuoles. Our recent studies have shown that retention of α1-ATZ in the ER is associated with the induction of an autophagic response (26). The autophagic response is thought to be a general mechanism by which intracellular organelles, or parts of organelles, are degraded. It is a highly evolutionarily conserved process that occurs in many cell types, especially during stress states, such as nutrient deprivation, and during the cellular remodeling that accompanies morphogenesis, differentiation and senescence. Several studies have suggested that autophagic vacuoles are derived in part from subdomains of ER (128). Autophagosomes initially form as invaginations from ribosome-free areas of the ER membrane. Together with con-

stituents of the ER, autophagosomes engulf cytosolic constituents including components of the ubiquitin system and the proteasome (129,130). Thus, it is possible that degradation of α1-ATZ is mediated by proteasomal machinery engulfed during formation of the autophagosome. Indeed, in our recent studies an intense autophagic response was demonstrated in cell culture model systems with ER retention of mutant α1-ATZ and in liver biopsy specimens from patients with α1-AT deficiency (26). Moreover, α1-AT and calnexin were colocalized within autophagosomes as well as within the ER. Finally, degradation of α1-ATZ in the cell culture model system is partially abrogated by inhibitors of autophagy including wortmannin, 3-methyladenine and LY294002. However, it is also possible that α1-ATZ molecules taken up into autophagosomes are degraded by a nonproteasomal mechanism when the autophagosomes merge/fuse with the lysosomal pathway, and that the autophagic and proteasomal pathways constitute completely independent mechanisms for degradation of α1-ATZ.

A study by Van Leyen et al. has suggested the possibility that a certain, very specialized type of autophagic response, termed programmed organelle degradation, allows access of cytoplasmic proteases to both luminal and integral membrane proteins (131). Whole organelles are degraded during differentiation of specific cell types. In the central fiber cells of the eye lens, organelles are degraded so that the cell can become transparent to incoming light. In reticulocytes, organelles are degraded to accommodate the sole need for globin synthesis by a mechanism that leaves the plasma membrane intact. These processes appear to involve the highly regulated recruitment of 15-lipoxygenase from the cytoplasm to the ER membrane where it presumably oxygenates membrane phospholipids, in turn releasing proteins from the ER lumen and membrane. A mechanism like this could possibly account for the ER degradation pathway of some substrates.

Together, these studies indicate that degradation of α1-ATZ is a complex process that may involve more than one pathway and at least several sequential steps in each pathway. Theoretically, each of these pathways or its individual steps may be affected in an α1-AT-deficient patient who is "susceptible" to liver disease — that is, there may be heterogeneity among susceptible hosts in the mechanism by which ER degradation is delayed. Indeed, there is already some evidence for distinct mechanisms of delayed ER degradation among susceptible hosts. In one susceptible host, the retained α1-ATZ interacts poorly with calnexin (101). In the liver cells of this host, there is likely to be only a very little polyubiquitinated calnexin-α1-ATZ complex that can be recognized for proteolysis by the proteasome. In several other susceptible hosts, the retained α1-ATZ interacts well with calnexin but is degraded slowly (Teckman J, Qu D, and Perlmutter DH, *unpublished observations*). These hosts may have a defect in calnexin that prevents its ubiquitination or a defect in the ubiquitin system or the proteasome. Hosts with the latter defect would also be more likely to respond to a pharmacological agent such as interferon-γ (132) that enhances the activity of the ubiquitin-dependent proteasomal system. Recent studies involving yeast which have identified at least 30 putative recessive mutants and seven complementation groups of strains defective in ER degradation of α1-ATZ (133), are likely to lead to the recognition of other mechanisms for excessive ER retention of α1-ATZ.

MECHANISM OF LIVER CELL INJURY

There is still relatively limited information about the mechanism by which ER retention of α1-ATZ leads to liver cell injury. In the transgenic mice that express human α1-ATZ, there is mild inflammation and necrosis, formation of adenomas and ultimately hepatocellular carcinoma (99), but this animal model has not yet provided any clues for understanding the mechanism of hepatotoxicity. There is also relatively little information about the short-term and long-term effects of ER retention of α1-ATZ in cell culture systems. In one report a number of years ago (134), the accumulation of α1-ATZ in *Xenopus* oocytes was associated with the release of lysosomal enzymes, but there has not been any follow-up study of this potential mechanism. Several more recent studies using model systems have provided

interesting and perhaps relevant information. Raposo and colleagues used a novel approach to establish cell lines with marked retention of MHC class I molecules in the ER (135). This led to a marked alteration in the structure of the ER into an expanded network of tubular and fenestrated membranes. Marker studies suggest that this altered network is derived from the ER and ER-Golgi intermediate compartment. Electron-dense compartments resembling lysosomes appear to bud off from this altered network. Because ubiquitin and ubiquitin-activating enzymes were associated with the cytosolic aspect of the electron-dense bodies, the bodies were thought to represent compartments in which ER degradation takes place. The electron-dense bodies also resemble the autophagic vacuoles that we observed in liver biopsies from α1-AT-deficient patients and in genetically engineered cell culture model systems (26).

Work in several labs has shown that a novel structure called the aggresome is formed in cells when the expression of mutant membrane proteins, such as CFTRΔF508, other mutant membrane proteins and mutant viral proteins exceeds the capacity of the proteasome to degrade them (136,137). The aggresome is a pericentriolar membrane-free cytoplasmic inclusion containing mutant, ubiquitinated protein ensheathed in a case of vimentin and perhaps other intermediate filaments. Formation of these structures requires an intact microtubular system that presumably plays a role in moving the aggregate to the pericentriolar location. Indeed, formation of aggresomes is now thought to be a mechanism by which the cell can sequester aggregated proteins to prevent them from having toxic effects on critical structures within the cell. Because autophagosomes have been seen in the vicinity of the aggresomes (136), it is possible that the cell uses the autophagic machinery to ultimately degrade aggresomes. Our recent studies indicate that retention of α1-ATZ induces an expansion of, and alteration in the structure of, the ER and the formation of autophagic vesicles but does not cause aggresome formation (26). Thus, there is specificity in the response of the cell to different types of protein aggregates, but autophagy may represent, at least in part, a final common pathway.

The unfolded protein response (UPR) is also induced by the accumulation of unfolded proteins in the ER (Fig. 48.4). It results in the induction, or upregulation, of a repertoire of genes encoding chaperones such as BiP, GRP94, and enzymes that facilitate disulfide bond formation including protein disulfide isomerase, ERp72 and ERO1 (138,139). Enzymes in the phospholipid biosynthetic pathway are also induced, permitting the synthesis of new ER membrane to accommodate the increased load (138). These target genes have a common upstream activating sequence in their promoters, the unfolded protein response element (UPRE), which directs that transcription as a part of the response pathway. Studies in the laboratory of Peter Walter using yeast have shown that the UPR involves the oligomerization and transautophosphorylation of a novel ER transmembrane serine/threonine kinase, Ire1p. Once activated, Ire1p has endonuclease activity and, together with tRNA ligase, mediates a unique posttranscriptional splicing pathway to generate Hac1p[i], a transcription factor capable of binding to the UPRE (139). In mammalian cells, there appears to be a homologue of yeast Ire1p (140). Moreover, another protein, ATF6, appears to be involved in the mammalian UPR (141). ATF6 is a type II transmembrane glycoprotein that resides in the ER and is expressed constitutively. When mutant or unassembled proteins accumulate in the ER, the cytoplasmic tail of ATF6 is cleaved and translocates into the nucleus, where it functions as a transcription factor capable of binding to the UPRE.

The presence of mutant proteins in the ER also leads to reduced translation of endogenous proteins. Harding et al. have characterized a novel gene called PERK which encodes a type 1 transmembrane ER resident protein and appears to initiate a signal transduction pathway for inhibition of protein translation (142). PERK has a luminal domain that resembles that of Ire1p and a cytoplasmic tail with a protein kinase domain that resembles the eukaryotic initiation factor-2α (E1F2α) kinases. Accumulation of mutant proteins in the ER is associated with increased protein kinase activity of PERK, phosphorylation of a key serine residue on E1F2α, and inhibition of translation.

Two other signal transduction pathways activated by mutant proteins in the ER have recently been characterized and may be relevant to α1-AT deficiency. The ER overload pathway is a signaling pathway that appears to be distinct from the UPR, and involves activation of NFκB and release of active oxygen intermediates (143). So far, this pathway has only been described in experimental conditions associated with ER overload of mutant or unassembled membrane proteins. Recent studies in the Morimoto lab have shown that the heat shock factor HSF2 may be activated by the accumulation of ubiquitinated proteins (144). The downstream effect of HSF2 activation by ubiquitinated protein is induction of the classical heat shock response including cytoplasmic and nuclear chaperones HSP90, HSP70, HSC70, HSP27, an ER chaperone GRP78/BiP, and mitochondrial chaperone HSP60.

It is not yet known whether one or all of these signaling pathways are induced by ER retention of α1-ATZ or whether there is any alteration in their activation in the subgroup of α1-AT-deficient patients who are susceptible to liver disease. Because these are considered response pathways that are designed to protect the cell, it is presumed that they must be overwhelmed by the concentration or intrinsic toxic potential of a particular mutant protein before cell injury occurs. However, the consequences of prolonged activation of these response pathways are entirely unknown and could potentially include cytotoxic and/or oncogenic effects.

OTHER DISORDERS WITH ENDOPLASMIC RETICULUM RETENTION OF MUTANT OR UNASSEMBLED PROTEINS

There are many other examples of disorders in which mutant or unassembled proteins are retained in the ER (Table 48.1). For example, in most cases of cystic fibrosis, a partially active but mutant CFTR molecule (CFTRΔF508) is retained and degraded in the ER rather than transported to the apical plasma member from which it ordinarily functions as a chloride transporter (145). Recent studies have indicated that about 37% of Wilson disease (WD) alleles have the H1069Q mutation that is associated with retention and degradation of the WD ATPase in the ER (146). Some patients with Fabry's disease are characterized by a mutant galactosidase that does not reach its final destination in the lysosome but rather forms aggregates in the ER (147).

A study of the combined deficiency of coagulation factors V and VIII has provided some extraordinary information about folding in the secretory pathway (148). It is an autosomal recessive disorder that has been described in 58 families and linked to a gene on chromosome 18q. Nichols et al. used positional cloning techniques to identify mutations in ERGIC-53, a transmembrane protein localized to the ER-Golgi intermediate compartment that has mannose-specific lectin properties. The results therefore imply that ERGIC-53 mediates cargo-selective ER-to-Golgi transport for the two coagulation proteins. Because there is complete loss of ERGIC-53 but residual levels of factors V and VIII in the blood, it is likely that ERGIC-53 facilitates the transport of this subset of proteins but is not absolutely required for their secretion. A recent study with cell lines expressing genetically engineered dominant-negative forms of ERGIC-53 have in fact shown that the ERGIC-53 cycling pathway facilitates secretion of the two coagulation proteins (149). Thus, the interaction between factors V and VIII and ERGIC-53 constitutes one of the first examples of selective packaging of secretory proteins as cargo for export from the ER.

There are also several examples of infectious diseases in which mutant or unassembled proteins accumulate in the ER of liver cells. Hepatitis B virus infection is one of the most well-characterized of these. Ground-glass hepatocytes which are seen in individuals infected with hepatitis B virus are thought to arise from the accumulation of the large form of the hepatitis B virus surface antigen and empty virions in the ER (100). Recent studies have suggested that this process is associated with alterations in the morphology of the ER with the formation of large cisternae and budding tubules (150), in some ways similar to what we have seen in liver biopsy specimens from α1-AT-deficient patients and in cell culture model systems of α1-AT deficiency (26). It is not yet clear whether this process is cytopathic, whether it involves an apop-

TABLE 48.1. EXAMPLES OF INBORN ERRORS OF METABOLISM IN WHICH ABNORMAL PROTEINS ARE RETAINED IN ENDOPLASMIC RETICULUM

Proteins	Type of Protein	Related Disease
α1-Antitrypsin	Secreted	Emphysema, liver disease
α1-Antichymotrypsin	Secreted	α1-antichymotrypsin deficiency
Complement component C2	Secreted	Type II complement C2 deficiency
Complement component factor H	Secreted	Factor H deficiency
Fibrinogen	Secreted	Familial hypofibrinogenemia
α2-plasmin inhibitor	Secreted	α2-plasmin inhibitor deficiency
Protein C deficiency	Secreted	Hereditary protein C
LDL Receptor	Membrane	Familial hypercholesterolemia
CFTR	Membrane	Cystic fibrosis
β-Hexosaminidase	Lysosomal	Tay–Sachs disease
Microsomal triglyceride transfer protein	Secreted	Abetalipoproteinemia, Hypolipoproteinemia
Palmitoyl protein thioesterase	Secreted	Infantile neuronal ceroid lipofuscinosis
Sucrase-isomaltase	Membrane	Congenital sucrase-isomaltase deficiency
Thyroglobulin	Secreted	Congenital hypothyroid
Type I procollagen	Secreted	Osteogenesis imperfecta type II
Vasopressin precursor	Secreted	Central diabetes insipidus
Proteolipid protein	Membrane	Pelizaeus–Merzbacher disease
Vasopressin receptor	Secreted	Congenital nephrogenic diabetes insipidus
Water channel (aquaporin)	Secreted	Congenital nephrogenic diabetes insipidus
Unknown	Secreted/Membrane	Carbohydrate-deficient glycoprotein syndrome
ERGIC-53	Membrane	Combined deficiency of coagulation factors V and VIII
Von Willebrand	Secreted	Von Willebrand's disease
Factor VII	Secreted	Hereditory factor VII deficiency
Glycoprotein GPIIb/IIIa	Membrane	Glanzmann's thrombasthenia
Rhodopsin	Membrane	Autosomal dominant retinitis pigmentosa
Fibrillin	Secreted	Marfan's syndrome
Wilson disease ATPase	Membrane	Wilson disease
α-Galactosidase A	Lysosomal	Fabry disease
Myeloperoxidase	Granular	Hereditary myeloperoxidase deficiency
HFE	Membrane	Hemochromatosis

totic mechanism, or, conversely, whether it induces resistance to apoptosis and a tendency toward malignant transformation. Transgenic mice which overexpress hepatitis B virus surface antigen have ground-glass hepatocytes (100) and have a hepatic histopathology that is remarkably similar to that in mice transgenic for α1-ATZ (99). Two of the envelope glycoproteins of hepatitis C virus also accumulate in the ER of infected cells (151), and it has been speculated that the retention of hepatitis C virus envelope proteins in the ER results in apoptosis.

In some of the metabolic diseases associated with an "ER storage" state, a mutant protein is retained in the ER of liver cells, and yet there is no evidence that these disorders are associated with liver injury — for example, complement C2 and factor H deficiency. When compared to what we know about α1-AT deficiency, this observation has important implications. It may indicate that α1-ATZ has intrinsic hepatotoxic properties. Alternatively, the hepatotoxic effect may be dependent on the relative concentration of mutant protein that is retained in the ER. Because α1-AT is one of the most abundant products of the liver cell, α1-ATZ is likely to reach particularly high levels in the ER.

TREATMENT

The most important principle in the treatment of α1-AT deficiency is avoidance of cigarette smoking. Cigarette smoking markedly accelerates the destructive lung disease that is associated with α1-AT deficiency, reduces the quality of life, and significantly shortens the longevity of these individuals (12,13).

There is no specific therapy for α1-AT deficiency-associated liver disease. Therefore, clinical care largely involves supportive management of symptoms due to liver dysfunction and for the prevention of complications. Progressive liver dysfunction in α1-AT-deficient patients has been treated by orthotopic liver transplantation, with survival rates approaching 90% at 1 year and 80% at 5 years (152).

Several studies have shown that a class of compounds called chemical chaperones can reverse the cellular mislocalization or misfolding of mutant plasma membrane, lysosomal, nuclear and cytoplasmic proteins including CFTRΔF508, prion proteins, mutant aquaporin molecules associated with nephrogenic diabetes insipidus, and mutant galactosidase A associated with Fabry disease (153–155). These compounds include glycerol, trimethylamine oxide, deuterated water and 4-phenylbutyric acid (PBA). We recently found that glycerol and PBA mediate a marked increase in the secretion of α1-ATZ in a model cell culture system (94). Moreover, oral administration of PBA was well tolerated by PiZ mice (transgenic for the human α1-ATZ gene) and consistently mediated an increase in blood levels of human α1-AT, reaching 20% to 50% of the levels present in PiM mice and normal humans. PBA did not affect the synthesis or intracellular degradation of α1-ATZ. The α1-ATZ secreted in the presence of PBA was functionally active, in that it could form an inhibitory complex with neutrophil elastase. Because PBA has been used safely for years in children with urea cycle disorders as an ammonia scavenger and because clinical studies have suggested that only partial correction of the deficiency state is needed for the prevention of both liver and lung injury in α1-AT deficiency (3,8,156), PBA constitutes an excellent candidate for chemoprophylaxis of target organ injury in α1-AT deficiency.

It also now appears that several iminosugar compounds (Fig. 48.3) may be potentially useful for chemoprophylaxis of liver and lung disease in α1-AT deficiency. These compounds are designed to interfere with oligosaccharide side chain trimming of glycoproteins and are now being examined as potential therapeutic agents for viral hepatitis and other types of infections (157,158). We have examined several of these compounds initially to determine the effect of inhibiting glucose or mannose trimming from the carbohydrate side chain of mutant α1-ATZ on its fate in the ER, but found to our surprise that one glucosidase inhibitor, castanospermine (CST) and 2 α mannosidase I inhibitors, kifunensine (KIF) and deoxymannojirimicin (DMJ), actually mediate increased secretion of α1-ATZ (159). The α1-ATZ that is secreted in the presence of these drugs is partially functionally active. KIF and DMJ are less attractive candidates for chemoprophylactic trials because they delay degradation of α1-ATZ in addition to increasing its secretion and therefore have the potential to exacerbate susceptibility to liver disease. However, CST has no effect on the degradation of α1-ATZ and, therefore, may be targeted for development as a chemoprophylactic agent. The mechanism of action of CST on α1-ATZ secretion is unknown. An interesting hypothesis for the mechanism of action of KIF and DMJ has mutant α1-ATZ interacting with ERGIC-53 for transport from ER to Golgi when mannose trimming is inhibited.

Novoradovskaya et al. have suggested that inhibition of ER degradation of α1-ATZ by proteasome inhibitor lactacystin and by protein synthesis inhibitor cycloheximide is associated with increased secretion of α1-ATZ (160). We have been unable to confirm this result (94). Moreover, there are now several lines of evidence indicating that there is not a simple relationship between ER degradation of α1-ATZ and its secretion such that perturbations that delay degradation are automatically accompanied by increased

secretion. Some physiologic and pharmacologic perturbations are associated with delayed degradation without any change in secretion. Other perturbations increase secretion without any change in degradation. Increased temperature is associated with both delayed degradation and increased secretion (94).

Some patients with α1-AT deficiency and emphysema are currently receiving replacement therapy with purified and recombinant plasma α1-AT either by intravenous or intratracheal aerosol administration (8). This therapy is associated with improvement in serum concentrations of α1-AT and in α1-AT and neutrophil elastase inhibitory capacity in bronchoalveolar lavage fluid without significant side effects. Although initial studies have suggested that there is a slower decline in forced expiratory volume in patients on replacement therapy, this only occurred in a subgroup of patients and the study was not randomized (161). Protein replacement therapy is designed only for individuals with established and progressive emphysema. It is not being considered for individuals with liver disease, because there is no information to support the notion that deficient serum levels of α1-AT are mechanistically related to liver injury.

A number of patients with severe emphysema from α1-AT deficiency have undergone lung transplantation in the past ten years. The latest data from the St. Louis International Lung Transplant Registry shows actuarial survival for patients in this category who underwent transplantation between 1987 and 1994 at approximately 50% for 5 years. Lung function and exercise tolerance are significantly improved (162).

Replacement of α1-AT by somatic gene therapy has also been discussed in the literature (163). This strategy is potentially less expensive than replacement therapy with purified protein. Again, this therapeutic strategy would only be useful in ameliorating emphysema. It would be helpful to know that replacement therapy with purified α1-AT, as it is currently applied, is effective in ameliorating emphysema in this deficiency before embarking on clinical trials involving gene therapy. Several novel types of gene therapy, such as repair of mRNA by trans-splicing ribozymes (164) and chimeric RNA/DNA oligonucleotides (165), are theoretically attractive alternative strategies for liver disease in α1-AT deficiency because they would prevent the synthesis of mutant α1-ATZ protein and ER retention. In fact, a chimeric RNA/DNA oligonucleotide based on the sequence of coagulation factor IX in complex with lactose so that it could be taken up by asialoglycoprotein receptor-mediated endocytosis was delivered to hepatocytes with high efficiency after intravenous administration (165).

Other studies have shown that transplanted hepatocytes can repopulate the diseased liver in several mouse models (166,167), including a mouse model of a childhood metabolic liver disease termed hereditary tyrosinemia. Replication of the transplanted hepatocytes occurs only when there is injury and/or regeneration in the liver. The results provide evidence that it may be possible to use hepatocyte transplantation techniques to treat hereditary tyrosinemia and, perhaps, other metabolic liver diseases in which the defect is cell-autonomous. For instance, α1-AT deficiency involves a cell-autonomous defect and would be an excellent candidate for this strategy.

Alternative strategies for at least partial correction of α1-AT deficiency may result from a more detailed understanding of the fate of the α1-ATZ molecule in the ER. For instance, delivery of synthetic peptides to the ER to insert into the gap in the A-sheet or into a particular hydrophobic pocket of the α1-AT molecule (34) and prevent polymerization of α1-AT might result in release of the mutant α1-ATZ molecules into the extracellular fluid and prevent accumulation in the ER. Although it is not yet entirely clear, there is some evidence from studies on the assembly of MHC class I molecules that synthetic peptides may be delivered to the ER from the extracellular medium of cultured cells (168). There is also evidence that certain molecules may be transported retrograde to the ER by receptor-mediated endocytosis (169). Second, elucidation of the biochemical mechanism by which abnormally folded α1-AT undergoes intracellular degradation might allow pharmacological manipulation of this degradative system, such as enhancing proteasomal activity with interferon γ in the subpopulation of the PIZZ individuals predisposed to liver injury.

ACKNOWLEDGMENTS

The author is indebted to Mary Pichler for preparing this manuscript and to the support from the U.S. National Institutes of Health (HL37784, DK52526, DK56783).

REFERENCES

1. Sveger T. Liver disease in α$_1$-antitrypsin deficiency detected by screening of 200,000 infants. *N Engl J Med* 1976;294: 1316–1321.
2. Silverman EK, Miletich HP, Pierce JA, et al. α1-antitrypsin deficiency: prevalence estimation from direct population screening. *Am Rev Respir Dis* 1989;140:961–966.
3. Teckman JH, Qu D, Perlmutter DH. Molecular pathogenesis of liver disease in α1-antitrypsin deficiency. *Hepatology* 1996; 24:1504–1516.
4. Eriksson S, Carlson J, Velez R. Risk of cirrhosis and primary liver cancer in α-1-antitrypsin deficiency. *N Engl J Med* 1986; 314:736–739.
5. Gadek JE, Fells GA, Zimmerman RL, et al. Antielastases of the human alveolar structure: implications for the protease-antiprotease theory of emphysema. *J Clin Invest* 1981;68:889–898.
6. Perlmutter DH, Pierce JA. The α-1-antitrypsin gene and emphysema. *Am J Physiol* 1989; L147–L162.
7. Janoff A. Elastases and emphysema: current assessment of the protease-antiprotease hypothesis. *Am Rev Respir Dis* 1985;132: 417–433.
8. Crystal RG. Alpha-1-antitrypsin deficiency, emphysema and liver disease: genetic basis and strategies for therapy. *J Clin Invest* 1990;95:1343–1352.
9. Carlson JA, Rogers BB, Sifers RN, et al. Accumulation of PiZ antitrypsin causes liver damage in transgenic mice. *J Clin Invest* 1989;83:1183–1190.
10. Dycaico MJ, Grant SG, Felts K, et al. Neonatal hepatitis induced by α-1-antitrypsin: a transgenic mouse model. *Science* 1988;242:1409–1412.
11. Sveger T. The natural history of liver disease in α-1-antitrypsin deficient children. *Acta Paediatr Scand* 1995;77:847–851.
12. Larsson C. Natural history and life expectancy in severe α-1-antryspin deficiency, PiZ. *Acta Med Scand* 1978;204: 345–351.
13. Janus ED, Phillips NT, Carrell RW. Smoking, lung function and α-1-antitrypsin deficiency. *Lancet* I 1985; I:152–154.
14. Silverman EK, Province MA, Rao DC, et al. A family study of the variability of pulmonary function in α1-antitrypsin deficiency: quantitative phenotypes. *Am Rev Resp Dis* 1990;142: 1015–1021.
15. Sharp HL, Bridges RA, Krivit W, et al. Cirrhosis associated with α-1-antitrypsin deficiency: a previously unrecognized inherited disorder. *J Lab Clin Med* 1969;73:934–939.
16. Ibarguen E, Gross CR, Savik SK, et al. Liver disease in α-1-antitrypsin deficiency: prognostic indicators. *J Pediatr* 1990; 117:864–870.
17. Hadchouel M, Gautier M. Histopathologic study of the liver in the early cholestatic phase of α-1-antitrypsin deficiency. *J Pediatr* 1976;89:211–215.
18. Hodges JR, Millward Sadler GH, Barbatis C, et al. Heterozygous MZ α1-antitrypsin deficiency in adults with chronic active hepatitis and cryptogenic cirrhosis. *N Engl J Med* 1981; 304:357–360.
19. Graziadei IW, Joseph JJ, Wiesner RH, et al. Increased risk of chronic liver failure in adults with heterozygous α$_1$-antitrypsin deficiency. *Hepatology* 1998;28:1058–1063.
20. Propst T, Propst A, Dietze O, et al. High prevalence of viral infections in adults with homozygous and heterozygous α1-antitrypsin deficiency and chronic liver disease. *Ann Intern Med* 1992;117:641–645.
21. Curiel DT, Holmes MD, Okayama H, et al. Molecular basis of the liver and lung disease associated with α1-antitrypsin deficiency allele M$_{malton}$. *J Biol Chem* 1989;264:13938–13945.
22. Reid CL, Wiener GJ, Cox DW, et al. Diffuse hepatocellular dysplasia and carcinoma-associated with the M$_{malton}$ variant of α1-antitrypsin. *Gastroenterology* 1987;93:181–187.
23. Lomas DA, Elliott PR, Sidhar SK, et al. α1-antitrypsin M$_{malton}$ (Phe^{52deleted}) forms loop-sheet polymers *in vivo*: evidence for the C-sheet mechanism of polymerization. *J Biol Chem* 1995;270: 16864–16874.
24. Mahadeva R, Change W-SW, Dafforn TR, et al. Heteropolymerization of S, I, and Z α1-antitrypsin and liver cirrhosis. *J Clin Invest* 1999;103:999–1006.
25. Yunis EJ, Agostini RM, Glew RH. Fine structural observations of the liver in α1-antitrypsin deficiency. *Am J Clin Pathol* 1976;82:265–286.
26. Teckman JH, Perlmutter DH. Retention of the mutant secretory protein α-1-antitrypsin Z in the endoplasmic reticulum induces autophagy. *Mol Biol Cell* (in review).
27. Long GL, Chandra T, Woo SL, et al. Complete nucleotide sequence of the cDNA for human α$_1$-antitrypsin and the gene for the S variant. *Biochemistry* 1984;23:4828–4837.
28. Lai EC, Kao FT, Law ML, et al. Assignment of the α$_1$-antitrypsin gene and sequence-regulated gene to human chromosome 14 by molecular hybridization. *Am J Hum Genet* 1983;35: 385–392.

29. Perlino E, Cortese R, Ciliberto G. The human α_1-antitrypsin gene is transcribed from two different promoters in macrophages and hepatocytes. *EMBO J* 1987;6:2767–2771.

30. Hafeez W, Ciliberto G, Perlmutter DH. Constitutive and modulated expression of the human α_1-antitrypsin gene: Different transcriptional initiation sites used in three different cell types. *J Clin Invest* 1992;89:1214–1222.

31. Loebermann H, Tokuoka R, Deisenhofer J, et al. Human α-1-proteinase inhibitor: crystal structure analysis of two crystal modifications, molecular model and preliminary analysis of the implications for function. *J Mol Biol* 1984;177:531–556.

32. Huber R, Carrell RW. Implications of the three-dimensional structure of α-1-antitrypsin for structure and function of serpins. *Biochemistry* 1990;28:8951–8966.

33. Elliott PR, Lomas DA, Carrell RW, et al. Inhibitory conformation of the reactive loop of α_1-antitrypsin. *Nat Struct Biol* 1996;3:676–681.

34. Elliott PR, Abrahams J-P, Lomas DA. Wild-type α_1-antitrypsin is in the cannonical inhibitory conformation. *J Mol Biol* 1998;275:419–425.

35. Owen MC, Brennan SO, Lewis JH, et al. Mutation of antitrypsin to antithrombin: α-1-antitrypsin Pittsburgh (358 Met-Arg), a fatal bleeding disorder. *N Engl J Med* 1983;309:694–698.

36. Travis J, Salveson GS. Human plasma proteinase inhibitors. *Annu Rev Biochem* 1983;52:655–709.

37. Carrell RW, Lomas DA. Conformational disease. *Lancet* 1997;350:134–138.

38. Mast AE, Enghild JJ, Nagase H, et al. Kinetics and physiologic relevance of the inactivation of α_1-proteinase inhibitor, α_1-antichymotrypsin, and antithrombin III by matrix metalloproteinases-1 (tissue collagenase), -1 (72-kDa gelatinase/type IV collagenase), and -3 (stromelysin). *J Biol Chem* 1991;266:15810–15816.

39. Libert C, Van Molle W, Brouckaert P, et al. α_1-antitrypsin inhibits the lethal response to TNF in mice. *J Immunol* 1996;157:5126–5129.

40. Van Molle W, Libert C, Fiers W, et al. α_1-acid glycoprotein and α_1-antitrypsin inhibit TNF-induced, but not anti-Fas-induced apoptosis of hepatocytes in mice. *J Immunol* 1997;59:3555–3564.

41. Camussi G, Tetta C, Bussolino F, et al. Synthesis and release of platelet-activating factor is inhibited by plasma α_1-proteinase inhibitor or α_1-antichymotrypsin and is stimulated by proteinases. *J Exp Med* 1988;168:1293–1306.

42. Banda MJ, Rice AG, Griffin GL, et al. The inhibitory complex of human α-1-proteinase inhibitor and human leukocyte elastase is a neutrophil chemoattractant. *J Exp Med* 1988;167:1608–1615.

43. Joslin G, Griffin GL, August AM, et al. The serpin-enzyme complex (SEC) receptor mediate the neutrophil chemotactic effect of α_1-antitrypsin-elastse complexes and amyloid-β peptide. *J Clin Invest* 1992;90:1150–1154.

44. Hood JM, Koep LJ, Peters RL, et al. Liver transplantation for advanced liver disease with α_1-antitrypsin deficiency. *N Engl J Med* 1980;302:272–276.

45. DeSimone V, Cortese R. Transcription factors and liver-specific genes. *Biochim Biophys Acta* 1992;1132:119–126.

46. Tripodi M, Abbott C, Vivian N, et al. Disruption of the LF-A1 and LF-B1, binding sites in the human α-1-antitrypsin gene, has a differential effect during development in transgenic mice. *EMBO J* 1991;10:3177–3182.

47. Hu C, Perlmutter DH. Regulation of α_1-antitrypsin gene expression in human intestinal epithelial cell line Caco2 by HNF1α and HNF4. *Am J Physiol* 1999;276:G1181–G1194.

48. Perlmutter DH, May LT, Sehgal PB. Interferon ($_2$/interleukin-6 modulates synthesis of α1-antitrypsin in human mononuclear phagocytes and in human hepatoma cells. *J Clin Invest* 1989;264:9485–9490.

49. Laurell C-B, Rannevik G. A comparison of plasma protein changes induced by danazol, pregnancy and estrogens. *J Clin Endocrinol Metab* 1979;49:719–725.

50. Perlmutter DH, Cole FS, Kilbridge P, et al. Expression of the α_1-proteinase inhibitor gene in human monocytes and macrophages. *Proc Natl Acad Sci U S A* 1985;82:795–799.

51. Barbey-Morel C, Pierce JA, Campbell EJ, et al. Lipopolysaccharide modulates the expression of α_1-proteinase inhibitor and other serine proteinase inhibitors in human monocytes and macrophages. *J Exp Med* 1987;166:1041–1054.

52. Perlmutter DH, Glover GI, Rivetna M, et al. Identification of a serpin-enzyme complex (SEC) receptor on human hepatoma cells and human monocytes. *Proc Natl Acad Sci U S A* 1990;87:3753–3757.

53. Joslin G, Fallon RJ, Bullock J, et al. The SEC receptor recognizes a pentapeptide neo-domain of α1-antitrypsin-protease complexes. *J Biol Chem* 1991;266:11281–11288.

54. Joslin G, Wittwer A, Adams S, et al. Cross-competition for binding of α1-antitrypsin (α-1-AT)-elastase complexes to the serpin-enzyme complex receptor by other serpin-enzyme complexes and by proteolytically-modified α-1-AT. *J Biol Chem* 1993;268:1886–1893.

55. Kelsey GD, Povey S, Bygrave AE, et al. Species- and tissue-specific expression of human γ-1-antitrypsin in transgenic mice. *Genes Dev* 1987;1:161–171.

56. Carlson JA, Rogers BB, Sifers RN, et al. Multiple tissues express α-1-antitrypsin in transgenic mice and man. *J Clin Invest* 1988;82:26–36.

57. Molmenti EP, Perlmutter DH, Rubin DC. Cell-specific expression of α_1-antitrypsin in human intestinal epithelium. *J Clin Invest* 1993;92:2022–2034.

58. Venembre P, Boutten A, Seta N, et al. Secretion of α1-antitrypsin by alveolar epithelial cells. *FEBS Lett* 1994;346:171–174.

59. Cichy J, Potempa J, Travis J. Biosynthesis of α1-proteinase inhibitor by human lung-derived epithelial cells. *J Biol Chem* 1997;272:8250–8255.

60. Laurell C-B, Nosslin B, Jeppsson J-O. Catabolic rate of α_1-antitrypsin of PI type M and Z in man. *Clin Sci Mol Med* 1977;52:457–461.

61. Mast AE, Enghild JJ, Pizzo SV, et al. Analysis of the plasma elimination kinetics and conformational stabilities of native, proteinase-complexed, and reactive site-cleaved serpins: comparison of α 1-proteinase inhibitor, α1-antichymotrypsin, antithrombin III, α 2-antiplasmin, angiotensinogen, and ovalbumin. *Biochemistry* 1991;30:1723–1730.

62. Perlmutter DH, Joslin G, Nelson P, et al. Endocytosis and degradation of α-1-antitrypsin-proteinase complexes is mediated by the SEC receptor. *J Biol Chem* 1990;265:16713–16716.

63. Poller W, Willnow TE, Hilpert J, et al. Differential recognition of α1-antitrypsin-elastase and α_1-antichymotrypsin-cathespin G complexes by the low density lipoprotein receptor-related protein. *J Biol Chem* 1995;270:2841–2845.

64. Kounnas MZ, Church FC, Argraves WS, et al. Cellular internalization and degradation of antithrombin-III-thrombin, heparin cofactor II-thrombin, and α1-antitrypsin-trypsin complexes is mediated by the low density lipoprotein receptor-related protein. *J Biol Chem* 1996;271:6523–6529.

65. Pierce JA, Eradio BG. Improved identification of antitrypsin phenotypes through isoelectric focusing with dithioerythritol. *J Lab Clin Med* 1979;94:826–831.

66. Barker A, Brantly M, Campbell E, et al. α1-antitrypsin deficiency: Memorandum from a WHO meeting. *Bull World Health Organ* 1997;75:397–415.

67. Nukiwa T, Brantly M, Ogushi F, et al. Characterization of the M1 (ala 213) type of α_1-antitrypsin, a newly recognized common "normal" α_1-antitrypsin haplotype. *Biochemistry* 1987;26: 5259–5267.

68. Brantly M, Brashears-Macatee S, Kidd VJ, et al. α1-antitrypsin gene mutation hot spot associated with the formation of a retained and degraded null variant. *Am J Respir Cell Mol Biol* 1997;16:224–231.

69. Frazier GC, Siewertsen MA, Hofker MH, et al. A null deficiency allele of α-1-antitrypsin, QO ludwigshafen, with altered tertiary structure. *J Clin Invest* 1990;86:1878–1884.

70. Ray S, Brown JL. Comparison of the properties of rare variants of α_1-Proteinase inhibitor expressed in COS-1 cells and assessment of their potential as risk factors in human disease. *Biochim Biophys Acta (in press)*.

71. Curiel DT, Vogelmeier C, Hubbard RC, et al. Molecular basis of α-1-antitrypsin deficiency and emphysema associated with α-1-antitrypsin M mineral springs allele. *Mol Cell Biol* 1990;10: 47–56.

72. Teckman JH, Perlmutter DH. The endoplasmic reticulum degradation pathway for mutant secretory proteins α1-antitrypsin Z and S is distinct from that for an unassembled membrane protein. *J Biol Chem* 1996;271:13215–13220.

73. Kramps JA, Brouwers JW, Maesen F, et al. PiM$_{heerlen}$ a PiM allele resulting in very low α-1-antitrypsin serum levels. *Hum Genet* 1981;59:104–107.

74. Takahashi H, Nukiwa T, Satoh K, et al. Characterization of the gene and protein of the α-1-antitrypsin "deficiency" allele M procida. *J Biol Chem* 1988;263:15528–15534.

75. Holmes MD, Brantly ML, Crystal RG. Molecular analysis of the heterogeneity among the P-family of α-1-antitrypsin alleles. *Am Rev Respir Dis* 1990;142:1185–1192.

76. Holmes MD, Brantly ML, Fells GA, et al. Alpha-1-antitrypsin W$_{Bethesda}$: molecular basis of an unusual α-1-antitrypsin deficiency variant. *Biochem Biophys Res Commun* 1990;170: 1013–1022.

77. Seyama K, Nukiwa T, Takabe K, et al. S$_{iiyama}$ serine 53 (TCC) to phenylalanine 53 (TTC): a new α-1-antitrypsin deficient variant with mutation on a predicted conserved residue of the serpin backbone. *J Biol Chem* 1991;266:12627–12632.

78. Perlmutter DH, Kay RM, Cole FS, et al. The cellular defect in α1-proteinase inhibitor deficiency is expressed in human monocytes and xenopus oocytes injected with human liver mRNA. *Proc Natl Acad Sci U S A* 1985;82:6918–6921.

79. McCracken AA, Kruse KB, Brown JL. Molecular basis for defective secretion of variants having altered potential for salt bridge formation between amino acids 240 and 242. *Mol Cell Biol* 1989;9:1408–1414.

80. Sifers RN, Hardick CP, Woo SLC. Disruption of the 240-342 salt bridge is not responsible for the defect of the PIZ α1-antitrypsin variant. *J Biol Chem* 1989;264:2997–3001.

81. Wu Y, Foreman RC. The effect of amino acid substitutions at position 342 on the secretion of human α1-antitrypsin from xenopus oocytes. *FEBS Lett* 1990;268:21–23.

82. Bathurst IC, Travis J, George PM, et al. Structural and functional characterization of the abnormal Z α_1-antitrypsin isolated from human liver. *FEBS Lett* 1984;177:179–183.

83. Ogushi F, Fells GA, Hubbard RC, et al. Z-type α_1-antitrypsin is less competent than M1-type α_1-antitrypsin as an inhibitor of neutrophil elastase. *J Clin Invest* 1987;89:1366–1374.

84. Lomas DA, Evans DL, Stone SR, et al. Effect of the Z mutation on the physical and inhibitory properties of α1-antitrypsin. *Biochemistry* 1993;32:500–508.

85. Lomas DA, Evans DL, Finch JJ, et al. The mechanism of Z α1-antitrypsin accumulation in the liver. *Nature* 1992;357: 605–607.

86. Lomas DA, Finch JT, Seyama K, et al. α1-antitrypsin S$_{iiyama}$ (SER53®Phe): further evidence for intracellular loop-sheet polymerization. *J Biol Chem* 1993;268:15333–15335.

87. Dafforn TR, Mahadeva R, Elliott PR, et al. A kinetic mechanism for the polymerization of α-antitrypsin. *J Biol Chem* 1999;274:9548–9555.

88. Yu M-H, Lee KN, Kim J. The Z type variation of human α1-antitrypsin causes a protein folding defect. *Nat Struct Biol* 1995; 2:363–367.

89. Hurtley SM, Helenius A. Protein oligomerization in the endoplasmic reticulum. *Annu Rev Cell Biol* 1989;5:277–307.

90. Kim J, Lee KN, Yi G-S, et al. A thermostable mutation located at the hydrophobic core of α1-antitrypsin suppresses the folding defect of the Z-type variant. *J Biol Chem* 1995;270: 8597–8601.

91. Sidhar SK, Lomas DA, Carrell RW, et al. Mutations which impede loop-sheet polymerization enhance the secretion of human α1-antitrypsin deficiency variants. *J Biol Chem* 1995;270:8393–8396.

92. Kang HA, Lee KN, Yu M-H. Folding and stability of the Z and S$_{iiyama}$ genetic variants of human α1-antitrypsin. *J Biol Chem* 1997;272:510–516.

93. Davis RL, Shrimpton AE, Holohan PD, et al. Familial dementia caused by polymerization of mutant neuroserpin. *Nature* 1999;401:376–379.

94. Burrows JAJ, Willis LK, Perlmutter DH. Chemical chaperones mediate increased secretion of mutant α1-antitrypsin (α1-AT) Z. A potential pharmacological strategy for prevention of liver injury and emphysema in α1-AT deficiency. *Proc Natl Acad Sci USA* 2000;97:1796–1801.

95. Povey S. Genetics of α1-antitrypsin deficiency in relation to neonatal liver disease. *Mol Biol Med* 1990;7:161–162.

96. Doherty DG, Donaldson PT, Whitehouse DB, et al. HLA phenotype and gene polymorphism in juvenile liver disease associated with α1-antitrypsin deficiency. *Hepatology* 1990;12:218–223.

97. Lobo-Yeo A, Senaldi G, Portmann B, et al. Class I and class II major histocompatibility complex antigen expression on hepatocytes: a study in children with liver disease. *Hepatology* 1990; 12:223–232.

98. The MHC Sequencing Consortium. Complete sequence and gene map of a human major histocompatibility complex. *Nature* 1999;401:921–923.

99. Geller SA, Nichols WS, Kim S, et al. Hepatocarcinogenesis is the sequel to hepatitis in Z #2 α1-antitrypsin transgenic mice: histopathological and DNA ploidy studies. *Hepatology* 1994; 9:389–397.

100. Chisari FV. Hepatitis B virus transgenic mice: insights into the virus and the disease. *Hepatology* 1995;22:1317–1325.

101. Wu Y, Whitman I, Molmenti E, et al. A lag in intracellular degradation of mutant α1-antitrypsin correlates with the liver disease phenotype in homozygous PiZZ α1-antitrypsin deficiency. *Proc Natl Acad Sci U S A* 1994;91:9014–9018.

102. Kuznetsov G, Nigam SK. Folding of secretory and membrane proteins. *New Engl J Med* 1998;339:1688–1695.

103. Helenius A, Trombetta ES, Hebert DN, et al. Calnexin, calreticulin and the folding of glycoproteins. *Trends Cell Biol* 1997;7: 193–200.

104. Ou W-J, Cameron PH, Thomas DY, et al. Association of folding intermediates of glycoproteins with calnexin during protein maturation. *Nature* 1993;364:771–776.

105. Ihara Y, Cohen-Doyle MF, Saito Y, et al. Calnexin discriminates between protein conformational states and functions as a molecular chaperone *in vitro*. *Mol Cell* 1999;4:331–341.

106. Zapun A, Petrescu SM, Rudd PM, et al. Conformation-independent binding of monoglycosylated ribonuclease B to calnexin. *Cell* 1997;88:29–38.

107. Sousa MC, Ferrero-Garcia MA, Parodi AJ. Recognition of the oligosaccharide and protein moieties of glycoproteins by the UDP-glucose: glycoprotein glucosyltransferase. *Biochemistry* 1992;31:97–105.

108. Hebert DN, Foellmer B, Helenius A. Glucose trimming and reglycosylation determine glycoprotein association with calnexin in the endoplasmic reticulum. *Cell* 1995;81:425–453.

109. Bonifacino JS, Suzuki CK, Lippincott-Schwartz J, et al. Pre-golgi degradation of newly-synthesized T-cell antigen receptor chains: intrinsic sensitivity and the role of subunit assembly. *J Cell Biol* 1989;109:73–83.

110. Hershko A, Ciechanover A. The ubiquitin system. *Annu Rev Biochem* 1998;67:425–479.

111. Elgaard L, Molinari M, Helenius A. Setting the standards: quality control in the secretory pathway. *Science* 1999;286:1882–1888.

112. Ward CL, Omura S, Kopito RR. Degradation of CFTR by the ubiquitin-proteasome pathway. *Cell* 1995;83:121–127.

113. Jensen TJ, Loo MA, Pind S, et al. Multiple proteolytic systems, including the proteasome, contribute to CFTR processing. *Cell* 1995;83:129–135.

114. Werner ED, Brodsky JL, McCracken AA. Proteasome-dependent endoplasmic reticulum-associated protein degradation: an unconventional route to a familiar fate. *Proc Natl Acad Sci U S A* 1996;93:13797–13801.

115. Qu D, Teckman JH, Omura S, et al. Degradation of mutant secretory protein, α1-antitrypsin Z, in the endoplasmic reticulum requires proteasome activity. *J Biol Chem* 1996;271:22791–22795.

116. Teckman JH, Marcus N, Perlmutter DH. The role of ubiquitin in proteasomal degradation of mutant α1-antitrypsin Z in the endoplasmic reticulum. *Am J Physiol* 2000;278:G39–G48.

117. Biederer T, Volkwein C, Sommer T. Role of Cue1p in ubiquitination and degradation at the ER surface. *Science* 1997;278:1806–1809.

118. Liu Y, Choudhury P, Cabral C, et al. Intracellular disposal of incompletely folded human α1-antitrypsin involves release from calnexin and post-translational trimming of asparagine-linked oligosaccharides. *J Biol Chem* 1997;272:7946–7951.

119. Wiertz EJ, Tortorella D, Bogyo M, et al. SEC61-mediated transfer of a membrane protein from the endoplasmic reticulum to the proteasome for destruction. *Nature* 1996;384:432–438.

120. Hughes EA, Hammond C, Cresswell P. Mutant major histocompatibility complex class I heavy chains are translocated into the cytoplasm and degraded by the proteasome. *Proc Natl Acad Sci U S A* 1997;94:1896–1901.

121. Yang M, Omura S, Bonifacino JC, et al. Novel aspects of degradation of T cell receptor subunits from the endoplasmic reticulum (ER) in T cells—importance of oligosaccharide processing, ubiquitination, and proteasome-dependent removal from ER membranes. *J Exp Med* 1998;187:835–846.

122. Liao W, Yeung S-CJ, Chan L. Proteasome-mediated degradation of apolipoprotein B targets both nascent peptides cotranslationally before translocation and full-length apolipoprotein B after translocation into the endoplasmic reticulum. *J Biol Chem* 1998;273:27225–27230.

123. De Virgilio M, Weninger H, Ivessa NE. Ubiquitination is required for the retrotranslocation of a shortlived luminal endoplasmic reticulum glycoprotein to the cytosol for degradation by the proteasome. *J Biol Chem* 1998;273:9734–9743.

124. Loayza D, Tam A, Schmidt WK, et al. Ste6p mutants defective in exit from the endoplasmic reticulum (ER) reveal aspects of an ER quality control pathway in saccharomyces cerevisiae. *Mol Cell Biol* 1998;18:2767–2784.

125. Plemper RK, Bohmler S, Bordallo J, et al. Mutant analysis links the translocon and BIP to retrograde protein transport for ER degradation. *Nature* 1997;388:891–895.

126. Pilon M, Schekman R, Romisch K. Sec61p mediates export of a mutant secretory protein from the endoplasmic reticulum to the cytosol for degradation. *EMBO J* 1997;16:4540–4548.

127. Mayer T, Braun T, Jentsch S. Role of the proteasome in membrane extraction of a shortlived ER-transmembrane protein. *EMBO J* 1998;17:3251–3257.

128. Dunn WA. Studies on the mechanism of autophagy: formation of autophagic vacuole. *J Cell Biol* 1991;110:1923–1933.

129. Kopitz J, Kisen GO, Gordon PB, et al. Nonselective autophagy of cytosolic enzymes by isolated rat hepatocytes. *J Cell Biol* 1990;111:941–953.

130. Lenk SE, Dunn Jr WA, Trausch JS, et al. Ubiquitin-activating enzyme, E1, is associated with maturation of autophagic vacuoles. *J Cell Biol* 1992;118:301–308.

131. Van Leyen K, Duvoisin R, Engelhardt H, et al. A function for lipoxygenase in programmed organelle degradation. *Nature* 1998;395:392–395.

132. Gaczynska M, Rock KL, Goldber AL. Gamma-interferon and expression of MHC genes regulate peptide hydrolysis by proteasomes. *Nature* 1993;365:264–267.

133. McCracken AA, Karpichev IV, Ernaga JE, et al. Yeast mutants deficient in ER-associated degradation of the Z variant of α-1-protease inhibitor. *Genetics* 1996;144:1355–1362.

134. Bathurst IC, Errington DM, Foreman RC, et al. Human Z α-1-antitrypsin accumulates intracellularly and stimulates lysosomal activity when synthesized in the xenopus oocyte. *FEBS Lett* 1985;183:304–308.

135. Raposo G, van Santen HM, Leijendekker R, et al. Mutant major histocompatibility complex class I molecules accumulate in an expanded ER-Golgi intermediate compartment. *J Cell Biol* 1995;131:1403–1419.

136. Johnston JA, Ward CL, Kopito RR. Aggresomes: a cellular response to mutant proteins. *J Cell Biol* 1998;143:1883–1898.

137. Anton LC, Schubert U, Bacik I, et al. Intracellular localization of proteasomal degradation of a viral antigen. *J Cell Biol* 1999;146:113–124.

138. Sidrauski C, Chapman R, Walter P. The unfolded protein response: An intracellular signaling pathway with many surprising features. *Trends Cell Biol* 1998;8:245–249.

139. Frand AR, Kaiser CA. The ERO1 gene of yeast is required for oxidation of protein dithiols in the endoplasmic reticulum. *Mol Cell* 1998;1:161–170.

140. Tirasophon W, Welihinda AA, Kaufman RJ. A stress response pathway from the endoplasmic reticulum to the nucleus requires a novel bifunctional protein kinase/endoribonuclease (Ire1p) in mammalian cells. *Genes Dev* 1998;12:1812–1824.

141. Haze K, Yoshida H, Yanagi H, et al. Mammalian transcription factor ATF6 is synthesized as a transmembrane protein and activated by proteolysis in response to endoplasmic reticulum stress. *Mol Biol Cell* 1999;10:3787–3799.

142. Harding HP, Zhang Y, Ron D. Protein translation and folding are coupled by an endoplasmic-reticulum-resident kinase. *Nature* 1999;397:271–274.

143. Pahl HL, Baeuerle PA. Endoplasmic-reticulum-induced signal transduction and gene expression. *Trends Cell Biol* 1997;7:50–55.

144. Mathew A, Mathur SK, Morimoto RI. Heat shock response and protein degradation: regulation of HSF2 by the ubiquitin-proteasome pathway. *Mol Cell Biol* 1998;18:5091–5098.

145. Welsh MJ, Smith AE. Molecular mechanisms of CFTR chloride channel dysfunction in cystic fibrosis. *Cell* 1993;73:1251–1254.

146. Payne AS, Kelly EJ, Gitlin JD. Functional expression of the

Wilson disease protein reveals mislocalization and impaired copper-dependent trafficking of the common H1069Q mutation. *Proc Natl Acad Sci U S A* 1998;95:10854–10859.

147. Fan J-Q, Ishii S, Asano N, et al. Accelerated transport and maturation of lysosomal α-galactosidase A in Fabry lymphoblasts by an enzyme inhibitor. *Nat Med* 1999;5:112–115.

148. Nichols WC, Seligsohn U, Zivelin A, et al. Mutations in the ER-Golgi intermediate compartment protein ERGIC-53 cause combined deficiency of coagulation factors V and VIII. *Cell* 1998;93:61–70.

149. Moussalli M, Pipe SW, Hauri H-P, et al. Mannose-dependent endoplasmic reticulum (ER)-golgi intermediate compartment-53-mediated ER to golgi trafficking of coagulation factors V and VIII. *J Biol Chem* 1999;274:32539–32542.

150. Roingeard P, Sureau C. Ultrastructural analysis of hepatitis B virus in HepG2-transfected cells with special emphasis on subviral filament morphogenesis. *Hepatology* 1998;28:1128–1133.

151. Dubuisson J, Rice CM. Hepatitis C virus glycoprotein folding: Disulfide bond formation and association with calnexin. *J Virol* 1996;70:778–786.

152. United Network for Organ Sharing Data Request Service, 1999, *in preparation.*

153. Sato S, Ward CL, Krouse ME, et al. Glycerol reverses the misfolding phenotype of the most common cystic fibrosis mutation. *J Biol Chem* 1996;271:635–638.

154. Tamarappoo B, Verkman AS. Defective aquaporin-2 trafficking in nephrogenic diabetes insipidus and correction by chemical chaperones. *J Clin Invest* 1998;101:2257–2267.

155. Brown CR, Hong-Brown LQ, Welch WJ. Correcting temperature-sensitive protein folding defects. *J Clin Invest* 1997;99:1432–1444.

156. Campbell EJ, Campbell MA, Boukedes SS, et al. Quantum proteolysis by neutrophils: implications for pulmonary emphysema in α1-antitrypsin deficiency. *J Clin Invest* 1999;104:337–344.

157. Jacob GS. Glycosylation inhibitors in biology and medicine. *Curr Opin Struct Biol* 1995;5:605–611.

158. Zitzmann N, Mehta AS, Carrouee S, et al. Imino sugars inhibit the formation and secretion of bovine viral diarrhea virus, a pestvirus model of hepatitis C virus: Implications for the development of broad spectrum antihepatitis virus agents. *Proc Natl Acad Sci U S A* 1999;96:11878–11882.

159. Marcus NY, Perlmutter DH. Glucosidase and mannosidase inhibitors mediate increased secretion of mutant α1 antitrypsin Z. *J Biol Chem* 2000;275:1987–1992.

160. Novoradovskaya N, Lee J, Yu ZX, et al. Inhibition of intracellular degradation increases secretion of a mutant form of α-1-antitrypsin associated with profound deficiency. *J Clin Invest* 1998;101:2693–2701.

161. The Alpha-1-Antitrypsin Deficiency Registry Study Group. Survival and FEV$_1$ decline in individuals with severe deficiency of α$_1$-antitrypsin. *Am J Respir Crit Care Med* 1998;158:49–59.

162. Trulock EP. Lung transplantation for α$_1$-antitrypsin deficiency emphysema. *Chest* 1996;110:284S–294S.

163. Anderson WF. Human gene therapy. *Nature* 1998;392:25–30.

164. Lan N, Howrey RP, Lee SW, et al. Ribozyme-mediated repair of sickle β-globin mRNAs in erythrocyte precursors. *Science* 1998; 280:1593–1596.

165. Kren BT, Bandyopadhyay P, Steer CJ. *In vivo* site-directed mutagenesis of the factor IX gene by chimeric RNA/DNA oligonucleotides. *Nat Med* 1998;4:285–290.

166. Rhim JA, Sandgen EP, Degen JL, et al. Replacement of disease mouse liver by hepatic cell transplantation. *Science* 1994;263: 1149–1152.

167. Overturf K, Al-Dhalimy M, Tanguay R, et al. Hepatocytes corrected by gene therapy are selected *in vivo* in a murine model of hereditary tyrosinaemia type I. *Nat Genet* 1996;12:266–273.

168. Day PM, Yewdell JW, Porgador A, et al. Direct delivery of exogenous MHC class I molecule-binding oligopeptides to the endoplasmic reticulum of viable cells. *Proc Natl Acad Sci U S A* 1997;94:8064–8069.

169. Lord JM, Roberts LM. Toxin entry: retrograde transport through the secretory pathway. *J Cell Biol* 1998;140:733–736.

The Liver: Biology and Pathobiology, Fourth Edition, edited by I. M. Arias, J. L. Boyer, F. V. Chisari, N. Fausto, D. Schachter, and D. A. Shafritz. Lippincott Williams & Wilkins, Philadelphia © 2001.

PATHOPHYSIOLOGY OF LIVER FIBROSIS

MARCOS ROJKIND
PATRICIA GREENWEL

Liver fibrosis is a dynamic process resulting in excess deposition of extracellular matrix components (see website chapter 🖥 W-27). It is a multifunctional process that involves several cell types, cytokines, chemokines and growth factors and results from a dysregulation of the homeostatic mechanisms that maintain the liver ecosystem. Although all cell types within the liver play individual roles in the host's response to injury, and as such produce multiple factors that activate the fibrogenic cascade, mainly one cell type, the hepatic stellate cell (HSC), is responsible for excess deposition of connective tissue components, including type I collagen (1–5) (see Chapter 31). The extracellular matrix itself plays an important role in liver fibrosis, and its role as a source of stimuli that regulate gene expression has been established (see Chapter 37 and website chapter 🖥 W-27). Moreover, the extracellular matrix serves as a storage site for cytokines and growth factors, and thus tissue injury could induce their release. This event may be responsible for providing the initial signal for tissue repair, prior to the activation of cells within the liver and/or the arrival of inflammatory cells (1,2).

Liver fibrosis is an important component of cirrhosis. Excess collagen deposition results from the imbalance between its synthesis and degradation. Thus, in this chapter we discuss key elements of both processes. We analyze some important local and systemic factors that upregulate collagen gene expression in HSCs. In addition, because impor-

tant aspects pertaining to the activation of HSCs and Kupffer cells (KCs), and the upregulation of collagen gene expression in HSCs involves the production and/or accumulation of reactive oxygen intermediates, we summarize important molecular mechanisms whereby connections between oxidative stress and cell injury, inflammation and fibrosis are established (Fig. 49.1).

THE FIBROGENIC CASCADE

To facilitate studies pertaining to liver fibrosis, the fibrogenic cascade can be artificially divided into the following six steps: (a) activation of HSCs and KCs, (b) migration and proliferation of HSCs, (c) synthesis and deposition of extracellular matrix components, (d) remodeling of scar tissue, (e) wound contraction, and (f) apoptosis of HSCs. However, the cascade is complex and multiple cell types within the liver participate in the overall process. Moreover, while these events occur in a time-dependent manner, it is yet to be determined whether they represent a continuum or are independent but interconnected phenomena triggered by one or multiple factors. Because the biology of HSCs and KCs, key participants of the fibrogenic cascade, is discussed in great detail in Chapter 31 and website chapter 🖥 W-26 respectively, here we review fibrogenesis as a whole and integrate the cascade of key events leading to cirrhosis. However, when necessary, we briefly discuss the role of HSCs and KCs in fibrogenesis and refer the readers to the chapters in which these topics are covered; in these instances few or no references are provided.

Multiple chemical and biological agents induce liver fibrosis. Although each agent has a unique mechanism to

M. Rojkind: Departments of Medicine and Pathology, Albert Einstein College of Medicine, Bronx, New York 10461.

P. Greenwel: Departments of Biochemistry and Molecular Biology, Mount Sinai School of Medicine, New York, New York 10029.

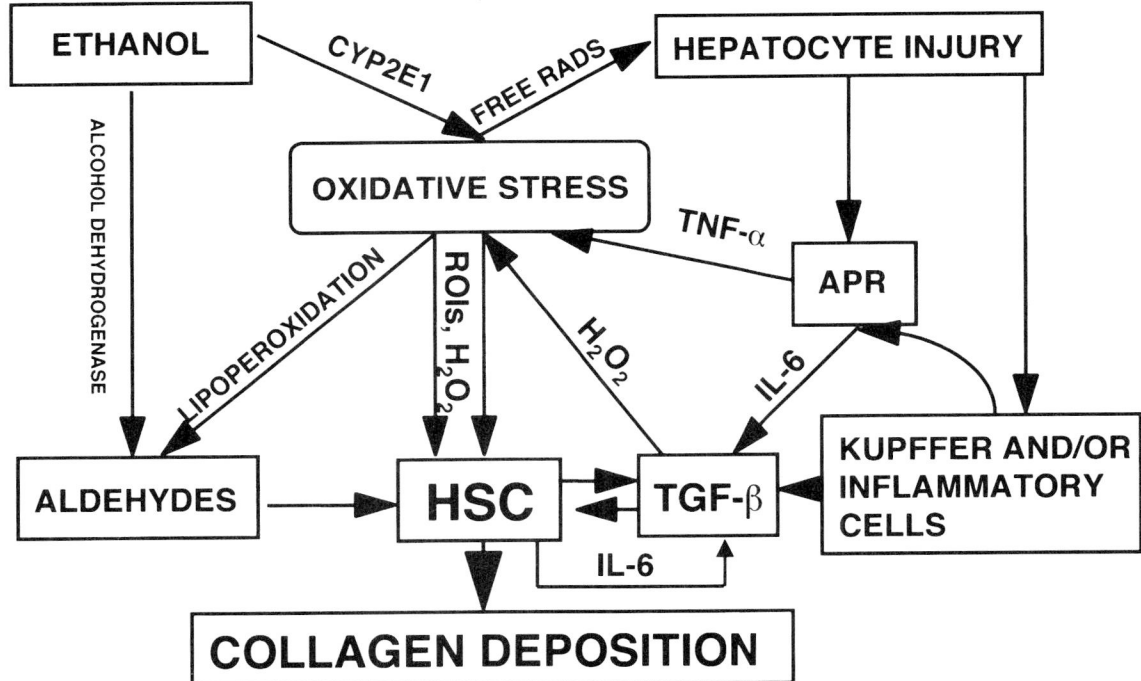

FIGURE 49.1. Schematic representation of key pathogenic mechanisms involved in ethanol-mediated upregulation of the type I collagen genes in hepatic stellate cells (*HSCs*). The figure illustrates that oxidative stress in general, and H_2O_2 in particular, are key elements of the fibrogenic cascade. This reactive oxygen species is a second messenger of the aldehyde- and transforming growth factor (*TGF*)-β1-mediated upregulation of the α1(I) collagen gene. Moreover, H_2O_2 is also involved in the activation of HSCs and enhances their production of TGF-β1. The figure also shows that Kupffer and inflammatory cells contribute to the fibrogenic cascade by producing TGF-β1 and acute-phase cytokines. *APR*, acute-phase response; *IL-6*, interleukin-6; *ROIs*, reactive oxygen intermediates; *TNF-α*, tumor necrosis factor α.

induce cell injury and/or trigger the fibrogenic cascade, all initial responses converge into a common pathway that eventually upregulates the expression of extracellular matrix components in HSCs. Thus, rather than describing the multiple mechanisms of cytotoxicity, we concentrate here on the fibrogenic mechanisms and emphasize molecular events leading to enhanced production of scar tissue, particularly with regard to type I collagen.

Based on current knowledge of the biology of HSCs, we postulate that the signals that trigger the fibrogenic response by inducing the activation of HSCs are "suicidal," and thus are programmed to destroy activated HSCs upon completion of the command. According to this hypothesis, an initial signal "turns on" the program in HSCs, and then multiple secondary signals, such as those provided by KCs and inflammatory cells, sustain the survival of HSCs and allow them to complete their "mission," that is, to produce collagen at the injured site, remodel and contract the scar prior to their death. Thus, when the stimulus that induced the fibrogenic response ceases, the program of HSCs is rerouted to apoptosis (6,7). This hypothesis has important implications regarding whether liver fibrosis is a reversible process and whether therapeutic interventions to remove

scar tissue will be successful without inducing a regenerative response and/or reactivating inflammation (see the section entitled Antifibrogenic Therapy below).

According to this hypothesis, fibrosis is conditionally reversible, based on the fact that HSCs produce multiple matrix metalloproteinases (MMPs) which degrade interstitial and basement membrane collagens (8–10). Thus, when the fibrogenic stimulus is singular, or multiple stimuli have not induced a state in which the excess deposition of extracellular matrix components is accompanied by a distortion of liver architecture, the process may be completely reversible (11,12). At this stage of liver fibrosis, discontinuation of the fibrogenic stimulus results in HSC death, and MMPs that have been secreted by them and remain bound to collagen may suffice to remove fibrous tissue (13). Moreover, the small amounts of MMPs produced for normal tissue remodeling enter the scar tissue and participate in its removal (14). However, when the fibrogenic process is already associated with formation of connective tissue septa, distortion of liver architecture and formation of vascular shunts, fibrosis becomes irreversible, unless one finds the means to prevent apoptosis of HSCs, and at the same time, stimulate production and activation of MMPs, downregulate the expression of tissue inhibitors of metalloproteinases (TIMPs) and inhibit the production of collagen.

Activation of Kupffer Cells and Hepatic Stellate Cells

Activation of Kupffer Cells

Liver fibrosis results from alterations in the homeostatic mechanisms that maintain the liver ecosystem (1,2). Thus, although HSCs are the main producers of extracellular matrix components in normal and diseased livers, other cells provide signals necessary to maintain homeostasis and to start and/or sustain the cascade of events required for proper healing. KCs from normal liver are known to produce factors that prevent proliferation and/or collagen synthesis by HSCs *in vitro* (1,2,4,5). *In vivo*, they prevent endotoxin from reaching high blood levels and play a key role in the pathogenesis of liver cirrhosis (15–21). KCs obtained from injured livers produce cytokines and growth factors that induce the proliferation of HSCs and hepatocytes, and/or are chemotactic for inflammatory cells and HSCs. Moreover, they are more phagocytic than are normal KCs and their capacity to remove endotoxin is impaired (see website chapter 🖥 W-26). Accordingly, in patients with liver injury, blood endotoxin levels are increased, as well as levels of several induced cytokines, such as tumor necrosis factor-α (TNF-α), interleukin-6 (IL-6), interleukin-1 (IL-1) and oncostatin M (OSM) (22). Since these cytokines increase during the acute-phase response (APR) and exert important regulatory effects on collagen gene expression by HSCs, the role of the APR in liver fibrogenesis will be discussed in the section below entitled Role of Systemic Factors (see also Chapters 40 and 41). Overall, the above data support the view that KCs play a role in activating HSCs and/or in enhancing their capacity to produce extracellular matrix components. Indeed, the inactivation of KCs with gadolinium chloride results in a significant reduction of the hypermetabolic state induced by ethanol, and decreases the rate of oxygen consumption in alcohol-fed rats (17). Likewise, administration of gadolinium chloride decreased pig serum-induced rat liver fibrosis, in part by enhancing the production of MMP-13 by KCs (19).

KCs also play a role in alcohol-induced hepatocyte damage and alcohol elimination. Inactivation of KCs decreases the extent of liver damage (steatosis, inflammation, and necrosis) and lowers the high elimination rates of ethanol observed in alcohol-fed rats (23). Because KCs appear to be involved in inducing cytochrome P-450 enzymes in hepatocytes, including CYP2E1, cross-talk between these two cell types may result in the induction of CYP2E1 in hepatocytes (24,25). This enzyme metabolizes ethanol with formation of acetaldehyde and free radicals (see the section below entitled Fibrogenic Actions of Ethanol and Acetaldehyde). In addition, because CYP2E1 is induced in hepatocytes, alcohol metabolism is enhanced and its elimination

is increased (25). It has also been postulated that ethanol induces CYP2E1 in KCs (24). Accordingly, we cannot exclude the possibility that KCs participate in ethanol metabolism, increased formation of lipoperoxides and reactive oxygen intermediates which produce hepatocyte injury and/or activate HSCs. Further studies are needed to establish the extent of involvement of KCs in ethanol metabolism and the molecular mechanisms whereby ethanol-related products induce damage and/or activation of HSCs.

In addition to producing acute-phase cytokines, activated KCs produce the fibrogenic cytokine transforming growth factor (TGF)-β1 (4,5) (see Chapter 31), which results in the formation of autocrine and paracrine loops which sustain high cytokine levels in injured liver. The autocrine loop may continue to upregulate levels of this cytokine in KCs, whereas the paracrine loop targets HSCs and induces the expression of TGF-β1 (4,5). Moreover, TGF-β1 induces accumulation of H_2O_2 in various cells types (26–29), and this reactive oxygen species is involved in the activation of HSCs (28) and upregulating the expression of α1(I) collagen mRNA (29–31).

In several chronic liver diseases, there is no overt inflammatory response of the host liver (32). Thus, autocrine and paracrine cytokine loops generated by the injurious agents, and release of cytokines and growth factors that are bound to extracellular matrix components, are sufficient to trigger and sustain an activation of KCs and HSCs (1,2). Cytokines and chemokines, such as IL-8, colony stimulating factor-1, monocyte chemoattractant protein-1 and leukotrienes play a key role in recruiting neutrophils and monocytes into the injured site (33–37). These inflammatory cells, together with activated KCs, produce cytokines and growth factors which are needed to sustain the fibrogenic response.

Activation of Hepatic Stellate Cells

In normal livers, HSCs are found within the space of Disse and beneath the endothelial cells (5,38) (see Chapter 30 and website chapter 🖥 W-32). They emit multiple star-like projections and establish direct contact, via gap junctions with other HSCs (39) and hepatocytes (46) and perhaps also with endothelial cells. HSCs play a role in vitamin A metabolism, which together with triglycerides are stored as fat droplets (3–5). HSCs cultured *in vitro* or following liver injury undergo a phenotypic transformation that is referred to as activation. This process is characterized by depletion in vitamin A stores and a decrease in retinol-binding proteins (3–5). There are also important morphological and functional changes in activated HSCs characterized by increased expression of myogenic and neurogenic proteins (3,41–45) and transformation into highly contractile myofibroblasts (44) (see Chapter 31). It is important, however, to emphasize that HSCs are heterogeneous and that not all cells simultaneously express all markers. Quiescent cells express mainly desmin and sarcomeric myosin, whereas activated cells upregulate the expression of most other markers (3,5,41–45).

HSC activation is complex, involving transcriptional and posttranscriptional events. Unfortunately, the molecular mechanisms involved remain to be elucidated. Although it has been accepted that the expression of alpha-smooth muscle actin (αSMA) reflects the activation status of HSCs, we still need to establish whether changes in vitamin A stores, increased expression of myogenic and neurogenic proteins and upregulation of the expression of type I collagen and other extracellular matrix components represent a continuous and integrated flow of events, or whether these are independent phenomena that occur during activation. Moreover, we need to establish whether activation which occurs *in vivo* in injured livers is the same process as that occurring *in vitro* (see Chapter 31).

Initial studies to determine changes in the transcriptional apparatus of HSCs during activation revealed that the expression and DNA binding activity of c-Myb is increased in activated HSCs (46,47). This transcription factor plays an important role in cell differentiation and proliferation (48). In HSCs, c-Myb binds to a proximal box (Box E) of the αSMA promoter and enhances transcription of the gene (47). While overexpression of c-Myb upregulates αSMA, a dominant negative form of c-Myb or an antisense DNA prevents HSC activation (47). It has been proposed that cysteine 43 of c-Myb is a sensor that detects redox changes in HSCs (47). Thus, changes in the c-Myb redox state may alter its DNA affinity, and induce significant changes in HSC gene expression. Expression and/or activity of several other transcription factors, including NFκB, KLF6 and Sp1, are also increased during HSCs activation (46,49,50) (see Chapter 31).

Sp1 is a ubiquitously expressed sequence-specific DNA binding protein which enhances RNA polymerase II-mediated gene transcription (51). During *in vitro* HSC activation, the transcriptional activity of Sp1 increases via a yet uncharacterized posttranscriptional mechanism (50). This transcription factor plays a key role in basal expression, and in the TGF-β1-induced upregulation of type I collagen genes in HSCs (50,52).

NFκB is a transcription factor whose nuclear translocation and DNA-binding capacity are sensitive to changes in redox and/or oxidative stress status (53). However, the target genes whose transcriptional activity is altered in HSCs remain to be identified. NFκB is induced by multiple cytokines, some of which contain functional NFκB binding sites in their promoter regions (54). Thus, enhanced production and/or activity of NFκB may induce cytokine transcription, some of which are fibrogenic (39,55,56).

KLF6 (also known as COPEB or Zf9) is a poorly characterized member of the Krüppel-like family of transcription factors which is upregulated *in vivo* in HSCs at early timepoints after CCl$_4$-induced liver injury. KLF6 is a ubiq-

uitous transcription factor that binds to GC-rich regions in DNA. This transcription factor may play a role in upregulating *col1a1* and TGF-β1 gene expression in HSCs. Unfortunately, the exact role of KLF6 in HSC activation remains unclear. KLF6 activates latent TGF-β1 in aortic endothelial cells by upregulating the expression and activity of urokinase plasminogen activator.

With regard to posttranscriptional mechanisms involved in HSC activation, upregulation of α1(I) collagen mRNA is exerted primarily through an increase in mRNA stability (1.5 hours half-life in quiescent vs. 24 hours in activated HSCs) (57). Unknown factors which bind to a C-rich sequence in the α1(I) collagen mRNA 3' untranslated region, including αCP, play a key role in increasing mRNA stability in activated HSCs (58).

Migration and Proliferation of Hepatic Stellate Cells

Activated HSCs migrate to injured sites and are organized in a pattern reminiscent of the collagen fibers which eventually form fibrous septa (59). HSC migration and proliferation respond to multiple growth factors, primarily platelet-derived growth factor-BB (PDGF-BB) (5,60,61). PDGF-mediated proliferation is activated by a specific signal transduction pathway (5,60).

Synthesis and Deposition of Extracellular Matrix Components

Although HSCs are the main producers of extracellular matrix components in the liver, other cell types contribute significantly to the synthesis of one or more of these macromolecules. Altogether, these proteins, irrespectively of their cellular origin, form the complex network of loose connective tissue, basement membranes and scar tissue of the liver. Basic aspects of extracellular matrix synthesis and deposition have been reviewed (62,63). Because type I collagen is the main collagen in scar tissue, we summarize below the knowledge of mechanisms involved in its upregulation during liver fibrogenesis.

Role of Local Factors

Fibrogenic Actions of Ethanol and Acetaldehyde
Ethanol is fibrogenic *per se* and induces collagen gene expression independently of nutritional status (64). However, some nutrients, in particular high-fat diets, enhance fibrogenesis (65). Accordingly, supplementation of an alcohol-containing diet with high amounts of fat accelerates and/or enhances alcohol-induced liver fibrosis, whereas supplementation with a soybean-derived polyunsaturated lecithin ameliorates the disease (66).

Direct fibrogenic actions of ethanol require its metabolism by alcohol dehydrogenase and/or CYP2E1 (25,64).

Thus, irrespective of whether levels of CYP2E1 are normal or increased, ethanol metabolites induce collagen gene expression (Fig. 49.1). Acetaldehyde is the main metabolite of ethanol produced by alcohol dehydrogenase (64,67). *In vitro*, at a 175 μmolar concentration, it induces the production of type I collagen by cultured HSCs (64,67). This effect is mediated by a *de novo* protein synthesis-dependent mechanism and involves the transcriptional activation of both type I collagen genes (67). Recent studies with cultured mouse HSCs revealed that acetaldehyde-induced transcriptional activation of the α1(I) collagen gene (*col1a1*) involves the accumulation of H_2O_2 and can be prevented by the addition of catalase (30). The molecular events whereby H_2O_2 accumulates in acetaldehyde-treated HSCs and/or how this reactive oxygen species enhances

col1a1 transcription remain to be established. However, both acetaldehyde and H_2O_2 enhance nuclear translocation and DNA binding activity of p35C/EBPβ to the -370 to -345 region of the *col1a1* promoter and transactivates gene expression (29,30). (Fig. 49.2).

When ethanol is metabolized via CYP2E1, in addition to acetaldehyde, there is formation of free radicals which induces an oxidative stress response, activates lipoperoxidation and generates 4-hydroxy-2-nonenal (HNE) and malonyl dialdehyde (64) (see Chapter 50 and website chapter 🖳 W-41). These aldehydes, similar to acetaldehyde, induce the transcriptional activation of the type I collagen genes (68) (Fig. 49.3). Although the molecular mechanisms whereby HNE activates collagen gene expression remain to be fully elucidated, this aldehyde exerts its action at least in

α1(I) COLLAGEN GENE

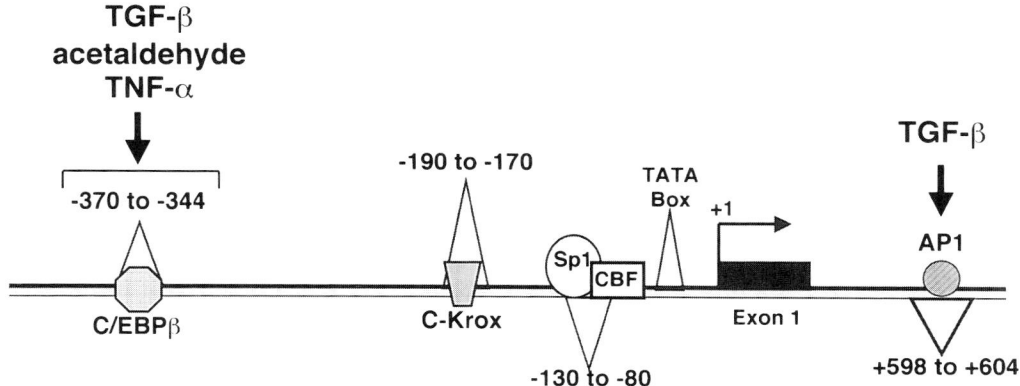

α2(I) COLLAGEN GENE

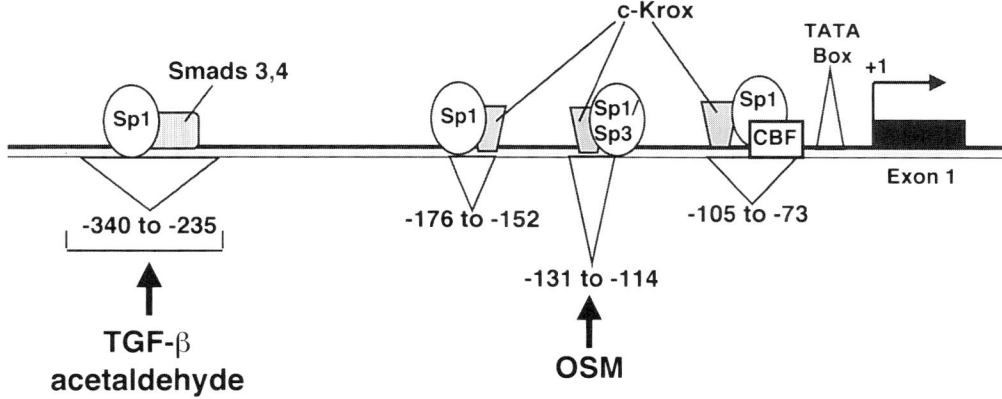

FIGURE 49.2. Schematic representation of *cis-* and *trans-*regulatory elements of the 5′ proximal region of the α1(I) and α2(I) collagen promoters. The multiple regulatory sites that have been mapped to these promoters are shown, as are some of the transcription factors that bind to them. *C/EBP*, CCAAT/enhancer binding protein, *OSM*; oncostatin M; *TGF-β*, transforming growth factor-β.

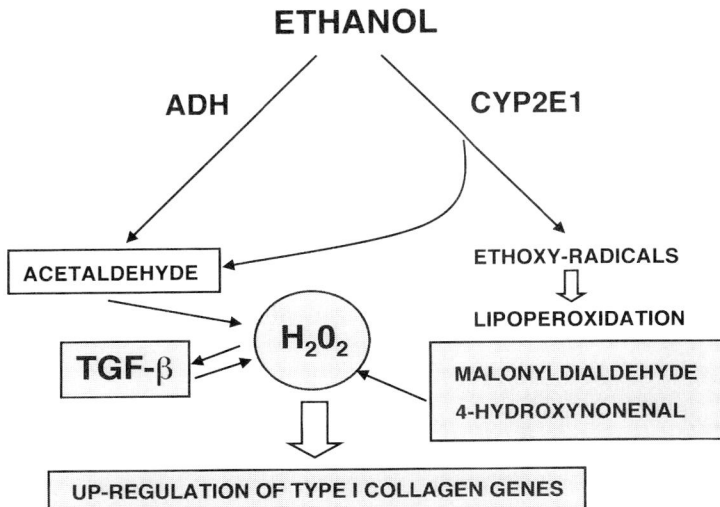

FIGURE 49.3. This figure illustrates that irrespective of whether ethanol is metabolized by alcohol dehydrogenase (*ADH*) or by CYP2E1, the aldehydes generated directly (i.e., acetaldehyde) or after free radical formation and lipoperoxidation [i.e., malonyldialdehyde and 4-hydroxy-2-nonenal (HNE)] upregulate the expression of the collagen genes via increased formation of H_2O_2. The figure also shows that transforming growth factor β (*TGF-β*) 1 further enhances liver fibrogenesis by contributing to H_2O_2 formation.

part via an oxidative stress response. HNE induces an accumulation of H_2O_2 in HSCs and increases the binding of the transcription factor AP1 by a mechanism that involves the activation of c-Jun N-terminal kinase and p38MAPK (69).

Fibrogenic Actions of Transforming Growth Factor-β1

The TGF-β superfamily comprises a large number of structurally related cytokines that include, among others, the TGF-βs, activins and decapentaplegic/Vg-related factors (70). These cytokines possess numerous biological activities and play important roles during development, differentiation and tissue remodeling (70).

TGF-β1, the prototype member of the family, is a strong modulator of cell proliferation and increases extracellular matrix deposition by two major mechanisms. It increases the production of extracellular matrix proteins and protease inhibitors, and downregulates the expression of various metalloproteinases (71) (Fig. 49.4). In the liver, several cell types are capable of synthesizing TGF-β1 (72). Hepatocytes

contain significant amounts of latent TGF-β1 protein, but do not express TGF-β mRNA (73,74). Thus, in these cells TGF-β1 is not generated *de novo*, but from uptake into hepatocytes (73,74). In normal liver, TGF-β1 and TGF-β2 mRNAs are predominantly expressed by KCs, while TGF-β3 is detected only in HSCs. During fibrogenesis, the expression of TGF-β2 and TGF-β3 is downregulated, whereas that of TGF-β1 significantly increases in HSCs and endothelial cells (72).

TGF-β is overexpressed during liver regeneration and fibrosis (see Chapter 42 and website chapter 🖥 W-31). However, there are significant differences regarding its spatiotemporal expression. In CCl₄-induced acute liver damage, TGF-β mRNA rises significantly after 24 hours post-injury, peaks at 48 hours (after the major wave of hepatocyte cell division and mitosis occur) and returns to normal values by 72 hours (see Chapter 42 and website chapter 🖥 W-31). Since this cytokine is a potent inhibitor of hepatocyte proliferation, it may regulate hepatocyte growth during regeneration. How-

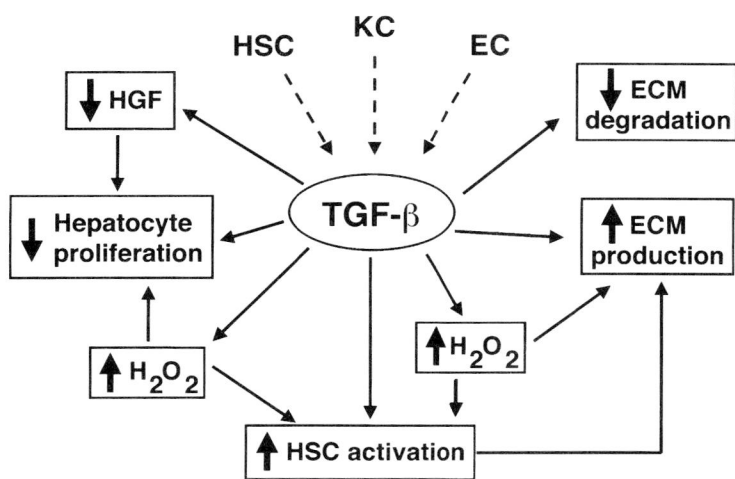

FIGURE 49.4. The pluripotential actions of transforming growth factor (*TGF*)-β1 and probable mechanisms whereby this cytokine contributes to liver fibrosis and cirrhosis. TGF-β1 is produced by hepatic stellate cells (*HSCs*), Kuppfer cells (*KCs*) and endothelial cells (*ECs*). Because TGF-β1 induces the formation of H_2O_2 and this reactive oxygen species activates HSCs and further enhances their expression of TGF-β1, there is formation of autocrine and paracrine loops that assure the continuous production of this fibrogenic cytokine. TGF-β1 induces liver fibrosis by dual mechanisms. It induces the expression of type I collagen and enhances collagen deposition and accumulation in the tissue by preventing its degradation. It also inhibits the production of hepatocyte growth factor, a growth factor required for hepatocyte proliferation with recently demonstrated antifibrogenic properties.

ever, during fibrogenesis, the production of TGF-β is sustained for prolonged periods of time. Steady-state levels of TGF-β mRNA are increased in livers from animals with schistosomiasis, in those treated with CCl_4, as well as in those fed alcohol (5) (see Chapters 50 and 51). Likewise, KCs obtained from ethanol-fed rats secrete higher levels of TGF-β than do those obtained from control animals (75). Consistent with these results, a direct correlation between steady-state levels of α1(I) collagen and TGF-β mRNAs has been demonstrated in patients with chronic hepatitis and cirrhosis. Furthermore, treatment with interferon-α decreases the expression of α1(I) collagen mRNA and downregulates the expression of TGF-β mRNA (76). Moreover, overexpression of TGF-β1 in mice using a recombinant replication-deficient adenovirus encoding this cytokine leads to a significant increase in the number of activated HSCs and in steady-state levels of α1(I) collagen mRNA in the liver (77). Conversely, in TGF-β1-deficient mice, HSC activation occurring after the induction of an acute liver injury with CCl_4 is significantly delayed compared with that observed in CCl_4-injured normal wild-type mice (77).

TGF-β is a potent inhibitor of hepatocyte proliferation, arresting cells at the G1 phase of the cell cycle. This TGF-β-mediated effect is due, at least in part, to its ability to inhibit the phosphorylation of the protein product of the retinoblastoma susceptibility gene. In some cell types, TGF-β-dependent inhibition of cell proliferation is mediated via H_2O_2, resulting from an inhibition in enzymes responsible for elimination of reactive oxygen intermediates (26). TGF-β is an inhibitor of the expression of hepatocyte growth factor (HGF), an important stimulator of hepatocyte proliferation during regeneration, and induces apoptosis *in vitro* and *in vivo* (78,79). Treatment of animals with a recombinant form of HGF may revert liver cirrhosis (80). Accordingly, if confirmed, this could provide an additional mechanism whereby TGF-β enhances fibrogenesis.

TGF-β1 can activate HSCs by a direct mechanism involving a paracrine loop. Treatment of HSCs with this cytokine enhances the expression of αSMA and results in a loss of retinylpalmitate (4,5).

The mechanisms whereby TGF-β1 induces all of these activities are only partially understood. The first step involves dimerization of two types of transmembrane receptors, named types I and II, with serine/threonine phosphorylation of the type I receptor. This phosphorylation allows the type I receptor to propagate the signal to downstream

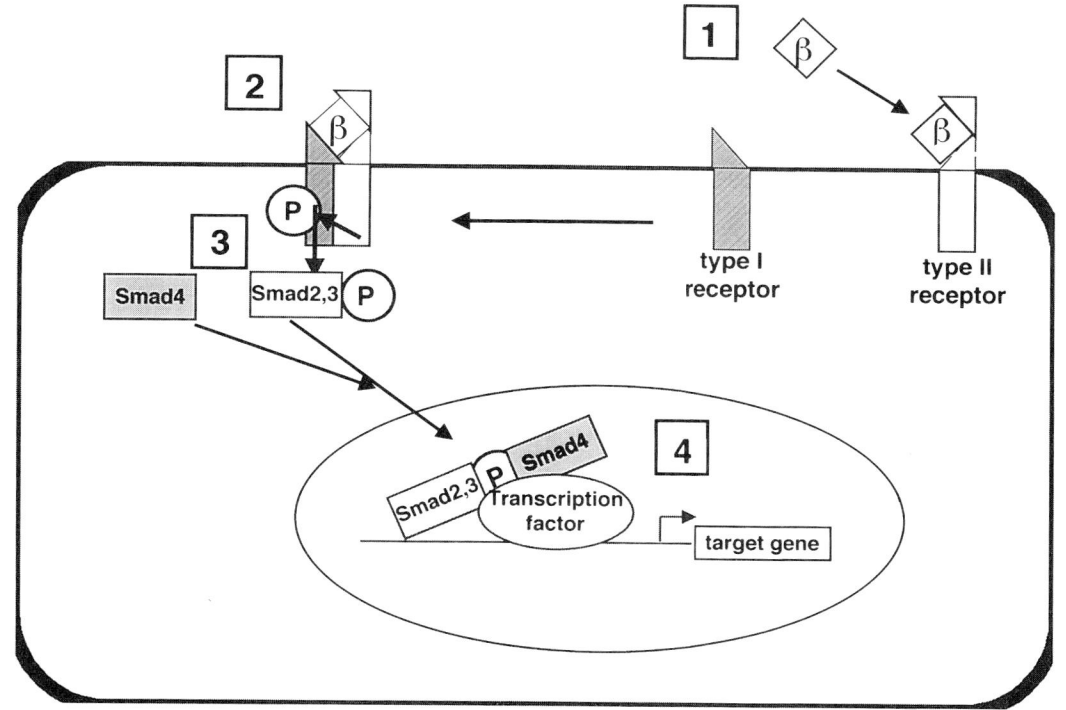

FIGURE 49.5. Schematic representation of some molecular mechanisms whereby transforming growth factor (TGF)-β1 induces the transcription of target genes. Upon interaction of TGF-β1 with the type II receptor (*Step 1*), TGF-β1 induces dimerization of the type II receptor with, and concomitant phosphorylation of the type I receptor (*Step 2*). Downstream propagation of the signal transduction occurs when the TGF-β1 receptor complex facilitates the phosphorylation of Smad 2 and Smad 3, which form heterocomplexes with Smad 4 (*Step 3*) and are translocated into the nucleus (*Step 4*). These Smad complexes form multimeric complexes with other transcription factors and induce the transcription of target genes. (Modified from Massague J, Wotton D. Transcriptional control by the TGF-β/Smad signaling system. *EMBO J* 2000;19:1745–1754, with permission.)

substrates (81) (Fig. 49.5). The TGF-β-elicited pathway is complex and involves activation and/or inactivation of many kinases and other proteins. Members of the Smad family of proteins, specifically Smads 2, 3 and 4, are essential components of the TGF-β1 signaling pathway. After phosphorylation, Smad 2 and Smad 3 form heterooligomers with Smad 4 that translocate to the nucleus. Smad complexes regulate transcription by binding directly to defined DNA sequences or without binding to DNA (81)(Fig. 49.5).

TGF-β stimulates collagen production mainly at the transcriptional level by a mechanism that does not require *de novo* protein synthesis (82). In HSCs, TGF-β1-responsive elements have been localized in the promoter region of the human α2(I) collagen gene (nucleotides −333 to −255), and within the first intron of the human α1(I) collagen gene (nucleotides +598 to +604) (52,83). In the former, TGF-β1 induces transcription by enhancing the binding of complexes containing Sp1/Sp3 and/or Smad3/4; in the latter, AP-1, is the responsible transactivator (Fig. 49.2). In transgenic mice, only 440 bp of the immediate 5′ flanking sequence of the COL1A1 gene or 313 bp of the proximal promoter region of the COL1A2 gene are required for high-level transgene expression in HSCs from CCl4-treated animals *in vivo* (84,85). Recently, *in vitro* studies using rat HSCs transfected with reporter vectors driven by different segments of the mouse *col1a1* promoter localized a functional TGF-β1-responsive element in the area spanning nucleotides −370 to −344 (29). This area is also essential for acetaldehyde-responsiveness (30). TGF-β1, as well as acetaldehyde, enhance the nuclear concentration and binding of members of the C/EBPβ family of transcription factors to this DNA element by an H_2O_2-dependent mechanism (29,30) (Fig. 49.2). Thus, this region of the *col1a1* promoter may be a site of convergence of many stimuli which regulate collagen gene expression.

Other Fibrogenic Cytokines
Other novel cytokines, including fibrosin (86–90) and connective tissue growth factor (CTGF) (91–100), may play a role in liver fibrogenesis.

Fibrosin (also known as fibroblast-stimulating factor 1), a 60 kd cytokine produced by CD4+ lymphocytes (87), was first isolated and purified from culture medium conditioned by egg granulomas obtained from livers of mice infected with *Schistosoma mansoni* (86,87) (see Chapter 51). It is similar to other fibroblast growth factors regarding its capacity to bind heparin. Its nucleotide and amino acid sequences are unique, and thus, fibrosin represents a new class of fibroblast growth factors. Fibrosin production can be stimulated in cultured fibroblasts by physiologic concentrations of ethanol (90). In rats with liver injury induced by intragastric infusion of ethanol, the expression of fibrosin is upregulated (90).

Fibrosin stimulates proliferation of fibroblasts and HSCs (88). Although this growth factor increases collagen produc-

tion in fibroblasts, it has no effect on the levels of expression of α1(I) collagen mRNA, suggesting that fibrosin may act at a posttranscriptional level (88). Fibrosin upregulates the expression of fibronectin mRNA by cultured HSCs (88).

CTGF is a 38 kd cysteine-rich secreted growth factor originally isolated from human umbilical vein endothelial cell cultures by affinity chromatography using antibodies to PDGF peptides (91). CTGF protein has high homology to CEF 10 mRNA expressed in chick fibroblasts (91). In mice, the expression of CTGF increases by day 14.5 of development in many tissues including liver. Expression was particularly elevated in secretory and absorptive epithelial cells and hepatocytes (92).

CTGF stimulates fibroblast proliferation and extracellular matrix synthesis, and its expression is elevated in diseases characterized by excess deposition of connective tissue, including scleroderma and pulmonary and kidney fibrosis (93–95). This factor is also expressed in fibrotic human liver and in animal models of liver cirrhosis (96). In the former, concentrations of CTGF correlate with the extent of fibrosis. HSCs are the main producers of this factor in the liver (97).

The production of CTGF is inhibited by TNF-α (98). Its expression is enhanced in fibroblasts treated with TGF-β, but not by other growth factors (99). CTGF appears to be an important autocrine growth factor produced by TGF-β (100).

Role of Systemic Factors

Depending on the extent of injury, the response of the host can be local and/or systemic. When events are localized to the liver, they are confined to activation of KCs and HSCs, or result in recruitment of inflammatory cells, which, together with KCs, produce cytokines and growth factors required for healing (1,2).

When the extent of injury is greater than the capacity of local events to control it, there is a systemic response which is common to all inflammatory processes irrespective of the injurious agent. This systemic reaction corresponds to the APR.

The Acute-Phase Response
The APR is a systemic response of the organism to nonspecific inflammatory stimuli (see Chapter 40). It is characterized by increased production of cytokines which include TNF-α, IL-6, IL-1 and OSM and alterations in the expression of a group of hepatocyte-specific proteins named acute-phase proteins (101). While some of these proteins are upregulated (e.g., fibrinogen), others are downregulated (e.g., albumin). However, the nature of the proteins whose expression is altered during the APR varies with the animal species.

Patients with alcoholic hepatitis have many manifestations of the APR and have elevated blood levels of TNF-α, IL-6 and IL-1 (22), which play a key role in hepatocyte proliferation after partial hepatectomy and participate in connective tissue production and remodeling (39,55,102) (see Chapter 42 and website chapter ⌨ W-31). Although it has been postulated that the APR is beneficial for the host, data indicate that the APR and IL-6, in particular, enhance fibrogenesis (55,56). Although the APR is not fibrogenic *per se*, when repeated APR episodes are superimposed on rats receiving CCl₄ to produce cirrhosis, the deposition of liver collagen and the expression of α1(I) collagen and TIMP-1 mRNAs are upregulated above levels observed in animals receiving only CCl₄ (56). Thus, in alcoholic patients who already have liver injury and in whom fibrosis is present, the superimposition of repeated episodes of alcoholic hepatitis and a concomitant APR may be detrimental and enhance the fibrogenic cascade.

Interleukin-6

IL-6 is a pleiotropic cytokine that plays important roles during many biological processes including the APR, cell differentiation, development, liver regeneration, immune response and hematopoiesis (103) (see Chapter 40). This cytokine can be induced by a wide variety of agents in many cell types, including HSCs, KCs and sinusoidal endothelial cells (39,104) (see Chapter 31). Depending on the cell type, its molecular weight can range from 23 to 45 kd due to differences in posttranslational modifications (103).

During tissue injury, IL-6 is a major systemic alarm signal which leads to major changes in the biochemical, physiological and immunological status of the host. Although these changes are aimed at limiting tissue injury, IL-6 overexpression can lead to disease, including liver fibrosis (103,105). In liver, IL-6 is a profibrogenic cytokine which enhances extracellular matrix deposition through the upregulation of α1(I) collagen and fibronectin gene transcription (39); stimulation of expression of other fibrogenic cytokines, such as fibrosin and TGF-β (39,55,56,90); and by enhancing the production of MMP inhibitors including α2macroglobulin and TIMP-1 (106,107).

The mechanisms whereby IL-6 exerts its activities are only partially understood (108) (see Chapter 40). In HSCs, IL-6 upregulates α1(I) collagen gene transcription via a protein synthesis-dependent mechanism (55). However, the *cis-* and *trans-* regulatory elements of the gene involved in this IL-6-elicited effect are presently unknown. In hepatocytes, an IL-6/OSM-responsive element has been located in the 5′ flanking region of the rat TIMP-1 gene, between nucleotides −64 and −36 and binds the transcription factors AP-1 and STAT3 (109). Although the binding of AP-1 is constitutive, IL-6 enhances TIMP-1 transcription, at least in part through the activation and binding of STAT3 to this element (109).

Oncostatin M

OSM is a multifunctional cytokine of the IL-6 family that is produced by many cell types including T-lymphocytes and monocytes (110). Similar to other APR cytokines, OSM is increased during the APR, and its expression in the liver is increased in cirrhotic patients (111). Thus, OSM is another APR cytokine that could play an important role in liver fibrogenesis. In liver, OSM is produced by hematopoietic cells (CD45+), although the receptor protein for OSM, gp130, is expressed mainly in hepatocytes (112). In conjunction with glucocorticoids, OSM induces differentiation of hepatocytes and suppresses hematopoiesis (112). In mice, the expression of OSM occurs around embryonic day 18.5, and therefore its production results in cessation of hematopoiesis in the liver. Because OSM shares the same receptor as IL-6, namely gp 130, the differentiation of hepatocytes is altered in gp130-deficient mice (112).

Similar to IL-6, OSM induces the expression of type I collagen in cultured fibroblasts and human HSCs (111). However, in contrast to IL-6, OSM modulates type I collagen gene expression in human HSCs at the posttranscriptional level (111). These results are in contrast with findings obtained with cultured human fibroblasts in which OSM induces transcription of the COL1A2 gene (113). In these cells, an OSM-responsive element was identified to a TCCTCC motif located between nucleotides −128 and −123 of the COL1A2 promoter. This motif binds transcriptional complexes containing Sp1 and Sp3 and is important for basal as well as OSM-stimulated COL1A2 expression (113) (Fig. 49.2).

OSM receptors are expressed in several cell types, and therefore this cytokine can induce multiple biological activities that include extracellular matrix biosynthesis as well as cell survival and differentiation. Although the OSM receptor lacks an intrinsic tyrosine kinase domain present in many growth factor receptors, its signal transduction is elicited through the JAK/STAT tyrosine kinase pathway (110).

TGF-β is a major mediator of fibrogenesis. However, other cytokines and growth factors contribute to the maintenance of homeostasis and are involved in excess collagen production during liver fibrogenesis. Thus, relative changes in the ratios of these factors, rather than individual changes in a particular cytokine or growth factor, are responsible for alterations in disease.

Tissue Remodeling

The liver contains a relatively small amount of connective tissue components, of which collagens are the most abundant and have been more widely investigated (see website chapter ⌨ W-32). Liver collagens are mainly localized to vascular spaces such as portal tracts and perivenular areas, and in general, only small amounts of these proteins are present within the parenchyma. This is due in part to the structure of the sinusoids which are lined by fenestrated endothelial cells. Thus, there is no continuous basement membrane, and only small amounts of connective tissue components are sparsely scattered in the space of Disse (see website chapters 🖳 W-32 and W-33). However, in cirrhotic livers, there is a 5- to 10-fold increase in liver collagen (2). Although most collagen is deposited within septa that surround nodules of hepatocytes, there is also increased deposition within the space of Disse (2), and in some instances, there is formation of a continuous basement membrane. These alterations in the liver ecosystem may be responsible for many functional disturbances.

The liver differs from other tissues in its general response to injury. If the injury is single and of great intensity as to remove a significant mass of functional parenchyma, there is regeneration with full restoration of structure and function. However, when the injury is repetitive and of small intensity, and is insufficient to trigger a strong regenerative response, there is scar formation. In both types of responses there is increased collagen synthesis and deposition; however, they differ in the type of collagen produced, sites of deposition and intensity of the remodeling process (114). While in the regenerative response the collagens produced are those required to make new sinusoids and restore the ecosystem, in fibrotic liver, the main collagens are those present in scar tissue, mainly type I collagen. In the regenerative response, there is active remodeling; in the cirrhotic liver, extracellular

matrix remodeling is the limiting step. Thus, a better understanding of the molecular events involved in collagen synthesis, deposition and remodeling may result in novel and efficient means to treat liver cirrhosis.

Although increased collagen synthesis is a key element of liver fibrosis, the disease process is more complex and other factors need to be taken into consideration if one is to develop an integral approach to therapy. At least initially, cirrhosis is a silent disease. At late stages of the disease, when the patient is seen by a physician, collagen synthesis may be normal or even absent. However, the scar tissue that accumulated during the disease remains in the liver and is responsible for many complications. Hence, although we need therapy directed at protecting hepatocytes from the injurious agent, inhibiting the inflammatory response and blocking the release and/or activity of fibrogenic cytokines and growth factors that activate HSCs, and intervening at various steps of collagen synthesis to abort the process, we also need to be concerned with inducing production and/or activation of MMPs involved in collagen degradation and/or in eliminating the inhibitors that prevent their activity. Therefore, we will review knowledge of the roles of MMPs and their inhibitors in liver fibrogenesis (Table 49.1).

TABLE 49.1. MATRIX METALLOPROTEINASES IN THE LIVER

Matrix Metalloproteinase	Cellular Source	ECM Substrates	Changes Occurring During Fibrosis/Cirrhosis
MMP-1 (collagenase-1)	Stellate cells	Native type I, III and V collagens	Very low expression in normal liver. No major change during fibrogenesis.
MMP-13 (collagenase-3)	Stellate cells Kupffer cells (?)	Same as MMP-1	Very low expression in normal liver. Transient upregulation after acute liver injury. No major changes during fibrogenesis.
MMP-2 (72 kd gelatinase, gelatinase A, type IV collagenase)	Stellate cells	Denatured collagens, laminin, fibronectin, nidogen	Low expression in normal liver. Upregulated during fibrogenesis, reaching maximum levels at intermediate stages of fibrosis.
MMP-9 (92 kd gelatinase, gelatinase B)	Kupffer cells	Type IV collagen, laminin, nidogen	Low levels in normal liver. Upregulated during early phases of fibrosis.
MMP-3 (stromelysin-1, transin)	Stellate cells Hepatocytes (?)	Basement membrane components, i.e., type IV collagen, laminin, nidogen, fibronectin	Very low expression in normal liver. Increased during early phases of acute liver injury.
MMP-10 (stromelysin-2)	Stellate cells	Same as MMP-3	Not determined.
MMP-14 (MT1-MMP)	All liver types, but predominantly stellate cells	Denatured collagens, laminin, fibronectin, nidogen, collagens I and III. Activates MMP-2 and MMP-13.	Upregulated during chronic hepatitis.
MMP-15 (MT2-MMP)	Hepatocytes, biliary epithelial cells	Same as MMP-14	Not determined.

MMP, matrix metalloproteinase; ECM, extracellular matrix.

Pioneer studies performed in the 1970s demonstrated increased activity of interstitial collagenase in early stages of hepatic fibrosis in rats, in baboons fed alcohol chronically and in patients with alcoholic fibrosis (12). As the severity of the disease progressed, interstitial collagenase activity decreased (12). Moreover, immunocytochemical studies revealed that the MMPs are colocalized with collagen fibers in normal liver and scar tissue of the cirrhotic liver (12,14). During the past few years, knowledge achieved in the general area of study of MMPs has been put to use to investigate how the extracellular matrix is remodeled in normal and fibrotic liver. Extracellular matrix degradation in the liver is a complex process involving various hepatic cell types, several MMPs, and TIMPs 1 and 2.

Matrix Metalloproteinase (MMP)-1 and MMP-13

MMP-1 and MMP-13 (also known as collagenases 1 and 3, respectively) are the major secreted neutral proteinases capable of initiating the degradation of native types I, III and V collagens (115). The individual contribution of these MMPs to extracellular matrix degradation in normal liver and during hepatic fibrogenesis is unclear, because mice and rats possess only a homologue of MMP-13. Primates express both genes (115).

HSCs of human origin express MMP-1 mRNA *in vitro*. However, while basal levels of expression are hardly detectable, they are upregulated by TNF-α (9). Likewise, *in vivo*, the expression of this mRNA in normal liver is very low. Despite the increase in collagenolytic activity observed during early stages of liver fibrogenesis, the levels of MMP-1 mRNA are not significantly altered in liver obtained from patients with fibrosis (10).

With regard to MMP-13, in rats, during CCl$_4$- and galactosamine-induced acute liver injury, MMP-13 mRNA is transiently upregulated between 6 hours and 1 day after injury, returning to normal values by day 2 (116). Likewise, levels of TIMP-1 mRNA increase but with different kinetics, reaching their maximum only after the peak of MMP-13 mRNA expression has occurred (116). In contrast, during CCl$_4$-induced chronic liver injury or after bile duct ligation, the expression of MMP-13 mRNA remains similar to control values throughout both models of liver injury (10). Likewise, in an experimental model of spontaneous recovery from liver fibrosis, levels of MMP-13 mRNA remain comparable to those observed at peak fibrosis, unlike TIMPs 1 and 2, which increase during fibrogenesis and decrease during spontaneous resolution of rat liver fibrosis (117). The major source of MMP-13 mRNA is HSCs, although KCs may also contribute to its expression (8,10,19). During HSC *in vitro* activation, MMP-13 mRNA is expressed at early stages in culture (less than 4 days), but becomes undetectable in more activated cells (8).

Based on these findings, the expression of MMP-13 appears to be an early event that precedes increased type I collagen production. This is consistent with data obtained

in other experimental systems (14). Altogether, these findings suggest that this MMP plays a key role in removing matrix debris while HSCs are getting prepared to migrate and/or lay down collagen fibrils. Accordingly, MMP-13 participates in early remodeling and not in late stages of the disease when required for the removal of scar tissue.

Matrix Metalloproteinase (MMP)-2

MMP-2, also known as 72-kd gelatinase, gelatinase A, or type IV collagenase, is capable of degrading denatured interstitial collagens (gelatin), fibronectin, laminin and nidogen (115). In the liver, MMP-2 transcripts are detected predominantly in HSCs and myofibroblasts (118). In rats, during CCl$_4$-induced liver fibrosis, MMP-2 mRNA increases several-fold, reaching its maximum during intermediate stages of fibrosis (119). Likewise, this mRNA significantly increases in livers of patients with chronic hepatitis, but is only slightly elevated in those with cirrhosis. Concomitant to these changes in mRNA expression, levels of latent and active MMP-2 increase (119). *In vitro*, activated HSCs synthesize this MMP mainly as the latent, inactive form (pro-MMP-2) (8). However, when these cells are cocultured with hepatocytes, enhanced production of active MMP-2 is observed. This effect is reproduced by the addition of plasma membrane-enriched fractions from hepatocytes with conditioned medium from pure HSC cultures (120). Thus, these data suggest that cell–cell interactions play an important role in MMP-2 activation in HSCs. On the other hand, cell–matrix interactions can also modulate the activation of MMP-2 in these cells. HSCs cultured on plastic, fibronectin, laminin, collagen VI or Matrigel predominantly express inactive pro-MMP-2 (121,122). In contrast, HSCs cultured on type I collagen markedly secrete the active enzyme. This effect is exerted in part through interactions with α2β1 integrin, a collagen receptor, and is mediated via activation of MT1-MMP, a membrane-type MMP (121,122). MMP-2 may be an autocrine factor for the proliferation of HSCs (123); however, the underlying mechanisms are presently unknown.

Matrix Metalloproteinase (MMP)-3 and MMP-10

MMP-3 (stromelysin-1 or transin) and MMP-10 (stromelysin-2) are capable of degrading basement membrane components, including type IV collagen, nidogen and fibronectin (115). In the liver, they are expressed mainly by HSCs (8,9). With regard to MMP-3, this enzyme is synthesized and secreted during early phases of HSCs activation *in vitro*, but not in quiescent cells or fully activated HSCs (8). In cultured HSCs, MMP-3 mRNA can be up-regulated by fibronectin, IL-1α or TNF-α, through a MAPK- and AP-1-dependent signal transduction pathway (124). *In vivo*, increased expression of MMP-3 mRNA is observed in nonparenchymal cells during early phases of rat liver regeneration following CCl$_4$-induced injury (125). Hepatocytes also appear to express this transcript, particularly in areas subsequently eliminated by necrosis (126).

Matrix Metalloproteinase (MMP)-9

MMP-9, also known as gelatinase B or 92-kd gelatinase, is capable of degrading gelatin, type IV collagen, laminin and nidogen, thus facilitating cellular migration across basement membranes (115). *In vivo*, in an experimental model of biliary fibrosis, MMP-9 proteolytic activity gradually increases, reaching a plateau 10 days after ligation (126). The major source of this enzyme in the liver is KCs (9). Indeed, *in vitro* studies have demonstrated that pro-MMP-9 is synthesized and released by human and rat KCs stimulated with phorbol esters (8). OK-432, a macrophage-activating agent, induces a marked increase in MMP-9 activity in rats with dimethylnitrosamine-induced liver cirrhosis. Concomitantly, a significant decrease in the degree of fibrosis is observed (127).

Membrane-Type Matrix Metalloproteinases (MT-MMPs)

Membrane-type MMPs (MT-MMPs) play a dual role in extracellular matrix remodeling through activation of MMP-2 and MMP-13, and via direct cleavage of some connective tissue proteins such as gelatin, collagen types I and III, fibronectin, laminin, vitronectin and aggrecan (115). In the liver, two members of this class of MMPs have been studied, namely MT1-MMP and MT2-MMP. With regard to MT-1-MMP (also known as MMP-14), it has been demonstrated that in chronic hepatitis, and to a lesser degree in liver cirrhosis, the expression of hepatic MT-1-MMP mRNA increases, mainly in HSCs (118). On the other hand, hepatocytes as well as endothelial and Kupffer cells may also contribute, but to a lesser extent, to the production of this enzyme *in vivo* (9).

The regulation of MT1-MMP expression has been investigated in cultured HSCs. During plastic-induced activation, these cells significantly upregulate MT1-MMP mRNA over 5 to 14 days (123). Likewise, increased MT1-MMP protein is observed in HSCs cultured on type I collagen (121). Concomitant to these changes, pro-MMP-2 becomes activated, thus suggesting that MT1-MMP plays a key role in MMP-2 activation (120). With regard to MT2-MMP (also known as MMP-15), very little is known except that hepatocytes and biliary epithelial cells appear to be the major producers of this MMP in the liver (128).

Tissue Inhibitors of Metalloproteinases (TIMPs)

TIMP-1 mRNA expression increases at early points after liver injury in several experimental models including CCl_4, galactosamine, and bile duct ligation, and remains elevated as the liver becomes fibrotic (10,116). Elevation in TIMP-1 mRNA precedes that of $\alpha1(I)$ collagen mRNA. Likewise,

TIMP-1 expression is increased several-fold in samples obtained from livers of patients with biliary atresia, primary biliary cirrhosis, primary sclerosing cholangitis, and cirrhosis (116). Moreover, levels of TIMP-1 closely correlate with the degree of periportal necrosis, portal inflammation, and liver fibrosis (10). Similar to TIMP-1, the expression of TIMP-2 and TIMP-3 is also increased during liver fibrogenesis. However, in some studies, their kinetics of induction are different from that of TIMP-1, with the latter appearing at earlier timepoints after liver injury (126). The major source of TIMP-1 in the liver is HSCs (9,10); however, hepatocytes also contribute to its expression (107). Regarding TIMP-2, both HSCs and KCs express it, while hepatocytes are the major producers of TIMP-3 (9). During spontaneous recovery from liver fibrosis, there is a rapid decrease in the expression of TIMP-1 and TIMP-2 mRNAs, whereas the expression of MMP-13 mRNA remains at levels comparable to peak fibrosis. Collagenase activity in liver homogenates increases, with a concomitant decrease in total liver collagen (117). These data further support the importance of TIMPs in regulating collagen degradation during liver fibrogenesis.

Several cytokines, including TGF-β, OSM and TNF-α, upregulate TIMP-1 expression by cultured HSCs (9,111, 129). TIMP-1 and TIMP-2 expression is upregulated during *in vitro* HSC activation (10,129). With regard to TIMP-1, the increase is mediated at the transcriptional level, and involves two areas of the promoter region of the human TIMP-1 gene. One is located between nucleotides −93 and −87 and binds an AP-1-containing complex. The other localizes to the area spanning nucleotides −63 to −53 and binds a 30 kd transcriptional factor (130).

Wound Contraction

HSCs are firmly adhered to liver endothelial cells and play a key role in regulating portal blood flow, and consequently in regulating portal pressure. However, because they express multiple muscle and nonmuscle myosins and actins, when transformed into myofibroblasts, they have the capacity to contract the scar tissue and fibrous septa in which they are embedded (see Chapter 31).

Apoptosis

Apoptosis may play an important role in determining the fate of HSCs. In the *in vitro* model of HSC activation, progression of this event is accompanied by an increased number of cells undergoing spontaneous apoptosis. Concomitantly, there is an increase in the expression of Fas (APOI/CD95) and its ligand. *In vivo*, apoptotic HSCs are observed in the recovery phase after acute liver damage induced by CCl_4 (131). Likewise, in a model of spontaneous recovery from liver fibrosis, apoptosis contributes to the elimination of this cell population (117). Thus, these data suggest that apoptosis may be involved in eliminating excess HSCs as acute injury is repaired, or during resolution of fibrosis. The mechanisms whereby HSCs can overcome apoptotic induction during liver fibrogenesis remain obscure. TGF-β, and to a lesser extent TNF-α, may play a role in this process (7).

ROLE OF OXIDATIVE STRESS IN LIVER FIBROGENESIS

In living organisms in which oxygen consumption is vital to support cellular functions, the formation of reactive oxygen intermediates (ROIs) such as superoxide anion and hydrogen peroxide is a naturally occurring process (see Chapters 18 and 19 and website chapter 🖳 W-13). However, because of the potential toxicity of such ROIs, cells posses several enzymatic mechanisms to eliminate them and transform them into less harmful substances. Under normal physiological conditions, ROIs are formed and actively eliminated. However, when the production of ROIs exceeds the capacity of the cells to eliminate them, their accumulation induces a state of oxidative stress (132,133) which is responsible for multiple metabolic alterations resulting in excess collagen deposition and/or cell death.

Ethanol metabolism induces changes in the cellular redox state and alters the ratios of NAD/NADH and NADP/NADPH (66) (see Chapter 50 and website chapter 🖳 W-41). These alterations in turn trigger multiple metabolic disturbances that include, among others, the production and accumulation of lactic acid, a metabolite known to induce collagen synthesis (64). A few years ago a direct relationship between oxidative stress and collagen gene expression by HSCs was demonstrated (46,134). More recently, a direct connection between the formation of H_2O_2 and NADPH was established. Patients lacking NADPH oxidase or those with a deficiency in glucose-6-phosphate dehydrogenase have an impaired capacity to generate nitric oxide, superoxide ion and H_2O_2 (135). While the former enzyme is directly involved in the formation of H_2O_2 in various cell types, the latter has as a key function in NADPH formation (27). The molecular mechanisms whereby ROIs are fibrogenic are currently under investigation. In addition to the direct stimulation of collagen signal transduction pathways by ROIs (29–31), there are several transcription factors, including AP-1, NFκB, Sp1 and c-Myb whose transcriptional activities are modulated by changes in the redox state of the cell (53,136,137).

In addition to changing the cellular redox state, ethanol metabolism via CYP2E1 generates free radicals and gives rise to several lipoperoxides (138), of which HNE and malonyldialdehyde have been shown to activate the conversion of HSCs to myofibroblasts and to induce the expression of type I collagen genes (68) (Fig. 49.3). Although the signal transduction pathways whereby oxidative stress activates HSCs remain to be elucidated, c-Myb appears to play a key role in this activation (47). Indeed, the use of antioxidants, such as tocopherols, prevent HSC activation, inhibit collagen synthesis and ameliorate liver fibrosis induced by CCl_4 (139,140). Recently, the direct fibrogenic action of H_2O_2 was demonstrated. This ROI functions as a second messenger in TGF-β- and acetaldehyde-mediated *col1a1* gene upregulation (29-31). Moreover, H_2O_2 is involved in activation of KCs and HSCs and in their production of TGF-β1 and other fibrogenic cytokines (28). These paracrine and autocrine loops further perpetuate the initial fibrogenic cascade (4,5,17).

ANTIFIBROGENIC THERAPY

Although the field of antifibrogenic therapy has expanded rapidly, the concept is not new (Table 49.2). Pioneering work demonstrated that interference with the process of collagen synthesis using the proline analogue L-azetidine-2-carboxylic acid prevented collagen deposition, ameliorated liver fibrosis and restored hepatic function in rats treated with CCl_4 to produce cirrhosis (11). Shortly thereafter, it was demonstrated that the antiinflammatory drug colchicine prevented liver fibrosis in rats, ameliorated liver cirrhosis in humans, and, in some instances, reverted fibrosis (11,141). Although its mechanism of action remains to be fully elucidated, colchicine may act by modulating the inflammatory and immunological responses of the host and/or by affecting plasma membrane composition and fluidity (11).

With the advent of molecular biology to study the regulation of gene expression and the development of procedures for the isolation and culture of HSCs, progress has been made in understanding the inflammatory response of the host, mechanisms of activation of KCs and HSCs, and molecular events leading to excess collagen production. Thus, the field of antifibrogenic therapy has been brought into a new dimension of therapeutic possibilities that include, among others, gene therapy (11,66,80,142–149). Table 49.2 summarizes strategies utilized to prevent, ameliorate and/or revert liver fibrosis. However, most of these strategies are based on preventing active collagen deposition and have been quite successful in animal studies in which therapy is administered simultaneously and/or during the course of induction of liver fibrosis. Unfortunately, human liver fibrosis is a silent disease, and therefore many patients have undetected advanced disease with septa and distortion of liver architecture. Hence, we need to develop new strategies aimed at removing old fibrous septa and stimulating regeneration. This is the challenge for the 21st century.

TABLE 49.2. HEPATIC FIBROSIS: THERAPEUTIC STRATEGIES

Drug/Therapy	Observed Effect	Proposed Mechanism
Colchicine	Prevents CCl$_4$-induced liver fibrosis. Ameliorates and/or reverts liver cirrhosis in humans.	Inhibits cytokine production and/or secretion. Immunomodulator. Modifies plasma membrane composition and fluidity.
Hepatocyte growth factor	Ameliorates dimethylnitrosamine-induced liver fibrosis.	Enhances hepatocyte regeneration. Decreases TGF-β expression and HSC activation.
HOE 077	Prevents liver fibrogenesis in several animals.	Inhibits collagen synthesis and HSC activation.
Interferons (α,β,γ)	Prevent liver fibrosis in several experimental models. Decrease liver fibrosis in humans.	Antiviral agents. Inhibit collagen synthesis and HSC activation.
Liver growth factor	Ameliorates CCl$_4$-induced liver cirrhosis.	Enhances hepatocyte proliferation.
Pentoxifylline	Protects against CCl$_4$ or bile-duct ligation-induced fibrosis.	Inhibits phosphodiesterases, HSC activation and PDGF-induced proliferation.
Polyunsaturated lecithin	Protects against alcohol-induced fibrosis in baboons.	Decreases oxidative stress. Inhibits HSC activation. Stimulates collagenase activity.
Rapamycin	Prevents CCl$_4$-induced fiber fibrosis.	Immunosuppressive agent.
Sho-saiko (TJ9) (Baicalin, baicalein?)	Protects against dimethylnitrosamine-induced fibrosis.	Blocks HSC activation.
Soluble TGF-β type II receptor/ Dominant negative type II TGF-β receptor	Protects against hepatic fibrosis induced by bile duct ligation and dimethylnitrosamine.	Blocks TGF-β signaling. Decreases HSC activation.
Telomerase gene delivery	"Rescues" CCl$_4$-induced liver fibrogenesis in telomerase-deficient mice.	Stimulates hepatocyte proliferation.

HSC, hepatic stellate cells; PDGF, platelet-derived growth factor.

ACKNOWLEDGMENTS

Part of this work was supported by Grants RO1 AA09231, RO1 AA10541 (M.R.), and RO1 AA12196 (P.G.) from the National Institute of Alcohol Abuse and Alcoholism and Grants from the Alcohol Medical Beverage Research Foundation to MR and PG.

REFERENCES

1. Rojkind M, Greenwel P. The liver as a bioecological system. In: Arias IM, Jakoby WB, Popper H, eds. *The liver: biology and pathobiology.* New York: Raven Press, 1988:707–716.
2. Greenwel P, Geerts A, Ogata I, et al. Liver fibrosis. In: Arias IM, Boyer JL, Fausto N, eds. *The liver: biology and pathobiology.* Raven Press, New York. 1994:1367–1381.
3. Hautekeete ML, Geerts A. The hepatic stellate (Ito) cell: its role in human liver disease. *Virchows Arch* 1997;430:195–207.
4. Gressner AM. Transdifferentiation of hepatic stellate cells (Ito cells) to myofibroblasts: a key event in hepatic fibrogenesis. *Kidney Int Suppl* 1996;54:S39–S45.
5. Friedman SL. Cytokines and fibrogenesis. *Semin Liver Dis* 1999;19:129–140.
6. De Bleser PJ, Niki T, Xu G, et al. Localization and cellular sources of activins in normal and fibrotic rat liver. *Hepatology* 1997;26:905–912.
7. Saile B, Matthes N, Knittel T, et al. Transforming growth factor-β and tumor necrosis factor-α inhibit both apoptosis and proliferation of activated rat hepatic stellate cells. *Hepatology* 1999;30:196–202.
8. Arthur MJ. Fibrosis and altered matrix degradation. *Digestion* 1998;59:376–380.
9. Knittel T, Mehde M, Kobold D, et al. Expression patterns of matrix metalloproteinases and their inhibitors in parenchymal

10. and nonparenchymal cells of rat liver: regulation by TNF-α and TGF-β1. *J Hepatol* 1999;30:48–60.
10. Arthur MJ, Iredale JP, Mann DA. Tissue inhibitors of metalloproteinases: role in liver fibrosis and alcoholic liver disease. *Alcohol Clin Exp Res* 1999;23:940–943.
11. Rojkind M. Fibrogenesis in cirrhosis. Potential for therapeutic intervention. *Pharmacol Ther* 1992;53:81–104.
12. Okazaki I, Watanabe T, Hozawa S, et al. Molecular mechanism of the reversibility of hepatic fibrosis: with special reference to the role of matrix metalloproteinases. *J Gastroenterol Hepatol* 2000;15:D26–D32.
13. Montfort I, Perez-Tamayo R, Alvizouri AM, et al. Collagenase of hepatic and sinusoidal liver cells in the reversibility of experimental cirrhosis of the liver. *Virchows Arch B Cell Pathol* 1990;59:281–289.
14. Rojkind M. Role of metalloproteinases in liver fibrosis. *Alcohol Clin Exp Res* 1999;23:934–939.
15. Thurman RG. II. Alcoholic liver injury involves activation of Kupffer cells by endotoxin. *Am J Physiol* 1998;275:G605–G611.
16. Enomoto N, Ikejima K, Bradford BU, et al. Role of Kupffer cells and gut-derived endotoxins in alcoholic liver injury. *J Gastroenterol Hepatol* 2000;15:D20–D25.
17. Rivera CA, Bradford BU, Seabra V, et al. Role of endotoxin in the hypermetabolic state after acute ethanol exposure. *Am J Physiol* 1998;275:G1252–G1258.
18. Knolle PA, Gerken G. Local control of the immune response in the liver. *Immunol Rev* 2000;174:21–34.
19. Hironaka K, Sakaida I, Matsumura Y, et al. Enhanced interstitial collagenase (matrix metalloproteinase-13) production of Kupffer cell by gadolinium chloride prevents pig serum-induced rat liver fibrosis. *Biochem Biophys Res Commun* 2000;267:290–295.
20. Parlesak A, Schafer C, Schutz T, et al. Increased intestinal permeability to macromolecules and endotoxemia in patients with chronic alcohol abuse in different stages of alcohol-induced liver disease. *J Hepatol* 2000;32:742–747.

21. Tamai H, Kato S, Horie Y, et al. Effect of acute ethanol administration on the intestinal absorption of endotoxin in rats. *Alcohol Clin Exp Res* 2000;24:390–394.

22. McClain CJ, Barve S, Deaciuc I, et al. Cytokines in alcoholic liver disease. *Semin Liver Dis* 1999;19:205–219.

23. Adachi Y, Bradford BU, Gao W, et al. Inactivation of Kupffer cells prevents early alcohol-induced liver injury. *Hepatology* 1994;20:453–460.

24. Koivisto T, Mishin VM, Mak KM, et al. Induction of cytochrome P-4502E1 by ethanol in rat Kupffer cells. *Alcohol Clin Exp Res* 1996;20:207–212.

25. Lieber CS. Microsomal ethanol-oxidizing system (MEOS): the first 30 years (1968–1998)—a review. *Alcohol Clin Exp Res* 1999;23:991–1007.

26. Kayanoki Y, Fujii J, Suzuki K, et al. Suppression of antioxidative enzyme expression by transforming growth factor-β1 in rat hepatocytes. *J Biol Chem* 1994;269:15488–15492.

27. Thannickal VJ, Aldweib KD, Fanburg BL. Tyrosine phosphorylation regulates H_2O_2 production in lung fibroblasts stimulated by transforming growth factor-β1. *J Biol Chem* 1998;273:23611–23615.

28. De Bleser PJ, Xu G, Rombouts K, et al. Glutathione levels discriminate between oxidative stress and transforming growth factor-β signaling in activated rat hepatic stellate cells. *J Biol Chem* 1999;274:33881–33887.

29. Garcia-Trevijano ER, Iraburu MJ, Fontana L, et al. Transforming growth factor-β1 induces the expression of α1(I) procollagen mRNA by a hydrogen peroxide-C/EBPβ-dependent mechanism in rat hepatic stellate cells. *Hepatology* 1999;29:960–970.

30. Greenwel P, Domínguez-Rosales JA, Mavi G, et al. Hydrogen peroxide: A link between acetaldehyde-elicited α1(I) collagen gene upregulation and oxidative stress in mouse hepatic stellate cells. *Hepatology* 2000;31:109–116.

31. Dominguez-Rosales JA, Mavi G, Levenson SM, et al. H_2O_2 is an important mediator of physiological and pathological healing responses. *Arch Med Res* 2000;31:15–20.

32. Popper H, Lieber CS. Histogenesis of alcoholic fibrosis and cirrhosis in the baboon. *Am J Pathol* 1980;98:695–716.

33. Dong W, Simeonova PP, Gallucci R, et al. Cytokine expression in hepatocytes: role of oxidant stress. *J Interferon Cytokine Res* 1998;18:629–638.

34. Sato E, Simpson KL, Grisham MB, et al. Reactive nitrogen and oxygen species attenuate interleukin-8-induced neutrophil chemotactic activity *in vitro*. *J Biol Chem* 2000;275:10826–10830.

35. Chapoval AI, Kamdar SJ, Kremlev SG, et al. CSF-1 (M-CSF) differentially sensitizes mononuclear phagocyte subpopulations to endotoxin *in vivo*: a potential pathway that regulates the severity of gram-negative infections. *J Leukoc Biol* 1998;63:245–252.

36. Xu Y, Rojkind M, Czaja MJ. Regulation of monocyte chemoattractant protein 1 by cytokines and oxygen free radicals in rat hepatic fat-storing cells. *Gastroenterology* 1996;110:1870–1877.

37. Shirley MA, Reidhead CT, Murphy RC. Chemotactic LTB4 metabolites produced by hepatocytes in the presence of ethanol. *Biochem Biophys Res Commun* 1992;185:604–610.

38. Wake K. Cell–cell organization and functions of 'sinusoids' in liver microcirculation system. *J Electron Microsc (Tokyo)* 1999;48:89–98.

39. Greenwel P, Rubin J, Schwartz M, et al. Liver fat-storing cell clones obtained from a CCl4-cirrhotic rat are heterogeneous with regard to proliferation, expression of extracellular matrix components, interleukin-6, and connexin 43. *Lab Invest* 1993;69:210–216.

40. Rojkind M, Novikoff PM, Greenwel P, et al. Characterization and functional studies on rat liver fat-storing cell line and freshly isolated hepatocyte coculture system. *Am J Pathol* 1995;146:1508–1520.

41. Ogata I, Saez CG, Greenwel P, et al. Rat liver fat-storing cell lines express sarcomeric myosin heavy chain mRNA and protein. *Cell Motil Cytoskeleton* 1993;26:125–132.

42. Niki T, De Bleser PJ, Xu G, et al. Comparison glial fibrillary acidic protein and desmin staining in normal and CCl4-induced fibrotic rat livers. *Hepatology* 1996;23:1538–1545.

43. Mayer DC, Leinwand LA. Sarcomeric gene expression and contractility in myofibroblasts. *J Cell Biol* 1997;139:1477–1484.

44. Gabbiani G. Some historical and philosophical reflections on the myofibroblast concept. *Curr Top Pathol* 1999;93:1–5.

45. Niki T, Pekny M, Hellemans K, et al. Class VI intermediate filament protein nestin is induced during activation of rat hepatic stellate cells. *Hepatology* 1999;29:520–527.

46. Lee KS, Buck M, Houglum K, et al. Activation of hepatic stellate cells by TGF-α and collagen type I is mediated by oxidative stress through c-myb expression. *J Clin Invest* 1995;96:2461–2468.

47. Buck M, Kim DJ, Houglum K, et al. c-Myb modulates transcription of the α-smooth muscle actin gene in activated hepatic stellate cells. *Am J Physiol Gastrointest Liver Physiol* 2000;278:G321–G328.

48. Oh IH, Reddy EP. The myb gene family in cell growth, differentiation and apoptosis. *Oncogene* 1999;18:3017–3033.

49. Hellerbrand C, Jobin C, Licato LL, et al. Cytokines induce NF-κB in activated but not in quiescent rat hepatic stellate cells. *Am J Physiol* 1998;275:G269–278.

50. Rippe RA, Almounajed G, Brenner DA. SP1 binding activity increases in activated Ito cells. *Hepatology* 1995;22:241–251.

51. Suske G. The Sp-family of transcription factors. *Gene* 1999;238:291–300.

52. Inagaki Y, Truter S, Greenwel P, et al. Regulation of the α2(I) collagen gene transcription in fat-storing cells derived from a cirrhotic liver. *Hepatology* 1995;22:573–579.

53. Sen CK, Packer L. Antioxidant and redox regulation of gene transcription. *FASEB J* 1996;10:709–720.

54. Akira S, Kishimoto T. NF-IL6 and NF-κB in cytokine gene regulation. *Adv Immunol* 1997;65:1–46.

55. Greenwel P, Iraburu MJ, Reyes-Romero M, et al. The induction of an acute phase response in rats stimulates the expression of α1(I) procollagen mRNA in their livers. Possible role of interleukin-6. *Lab Invest* 1995;72:83–91.

56. Greenwel P, Rojkind M. Accelerated development of liver fibrosis in CCl4-treated rats by the weekly induction of acute phase response episodes: upregulation of α1(I) procollagen and tissue inhibitor of metalloproteinase-1 mRNAs. *Biochim Biophys Acta* 1997;1361:177–184.

57. Stefanovic B, Hellerbrand C, Holcik M, et al. Posttranscriptional regulation of collagen α1(I) mRNA in hepatic stellate cells. *Mol Cell Biol* 1997;17:5201–5209.

58. Stefanovic B, Hellerbrand C, Brenner DA. Regulatory role of the conserved stem-loop structure at the 5′ end of collagen α1(I) mRNA. *Mol Cell Biol* 1999;19:4334–4342.

59. Geerts A, Lazou JM, De Bleser P, et al. Tissue distribution, quantitation and proliferation kinetics of fat-storing cells in carbon tetrachloride-injured rat liver. *Hepatology* 1991;13:1193–1202.

60. Pinzani M, Marra F, Carloni V. Signal transduction in hepatic stellate cells. *Liver* 1998;18:2–13.

61. Ikeda K, Wakahara T, Wang YQ, et al. *In vitro* migratory potential of rat quiescent hepatic stellate cells and its augmentation by cell activation. *Hepatology* 1999;29:1760–1767.

62. Nimni ME. Collagen: structure, function, and metabolism in normal and fibrotic tissues. *Semin Arthritis Rheum* 1983;13:1–86.

63. Prockop DJ, Kivirikko KI. Collagens: molecular biology, diseases, and potentials for therapy. *Annu Rev Biochem* 1995;64:403–434.

64. Lieber CS. Ethanol metabolism, cirrhosis and alcoholism. *Clin Chim Acta* 1997;257:59–84.

65. French SW, Takahashi H, Wong K, et al. Ito cell activation induced by chronic ethanol feeding in the presence of different dietary fats. *Alcohol Alcohol Suppl* 1991;1:357–361.

66. Lieber CS. Prevention and treatment of liver fibrosis based on pathogenesis. *Alcohol Clin Exp Res* 1999;23:944–949.

67. Greenwel P. Acetaldehyde-mediated collagen regulation in hepatic stellate cells. *Alcohol Clin Exp Res* 1999;23:930–933.

68. Bedossa P, Houglum K, Trautwein C, et al. Stimulation of collagen α1(I) gene expression is associated with lipid peroxidation in hepatocellular injury: a link to tissue fibrosis? *Hepatology* 1994;19:1262–1271.

69. Uchida K, Shiraishi M, Naito Y, et al. Activation of stress signaling pathways by the end product of lipid peroxidation. 4-Hydroxy-2-nonenal is a potential inducer of intracellular peroxide production. *J Biol Chem* 1999;274:2234–2242.

70. Massague J. The transforming growth factor-β family. *Annu Rev Cell Biol* 1990;6:597–641.

71. Border WA, Noble NA. Transforming growth factor-β in tissue fibrosis. *N Engl J Med* 1994;331:1286–1292.

72. De Bleser PJ, Niki T, Rogiers V, et al. Transforming growth factor-β gene expression in normal and fibrotic rat liver. *J Hepatol* 1997;26:886–893.

73. Roth S, Michel K, Gressner AM. (Latent) transforming growth factor-β in liver parenchymal cells, its injury-dependent release, and paracrine effects on rat hepatic stellate cells. *Hepatology* 1998;27:1003–1012.

74. Roth-Eichhorn S, Kuhl K, Gressner AM. Subcellular localization of (latent) transforming growth factor-β and the latent TGF-β binding protein in rat hepatocytes and hepatic stellate cells. *Hepatology* 1998;28:1588–1596.

75. Kamimura S, Tsukamoto H. Cytokine gene expression by Kupffer cells in experimental alcoholic liver disease. *Hepatology* 1995;22:1304–1309.

76. Castilla A, Prieto J, Fausto N. Transforming growth factor-β1 and -α in chronic liver disease. Effects of interferon-α therapy. *N Engl J Med* 1991;324:933–940.

77. Hellerbrand C, Stefanovic B, Giordano F, et al. The role of TGF-β1 in initiating hepatic stellate cell activation *in vivo*. *J Hepatol* 1999;30:77–87.

78. Ramadori G, Neubauer K, Odenthal M, et al. The gene of hepatocyte growth factor is expressed in fat-storing cells of rat liver and is downregulated during cell growth and by transforming growth factor-β. *Biochem Biophys Res Commun* 1992; 183:739–742.

79. Oberhammer FA, Pavelka M, Sharma S, et al. Induction of apoptosis in cultured hepatocytes and in regressing liver by transforming growth factor-β 1. *Proc Natl Acad Sci U S A* 1992; 89:5408–5412.

80. Ueki T, Kaneda Y, Tsutsui H, et al. Hepatocyte growth factor gene therapy of liver cirrhosis in rats. *Nat Med* 1999;5:226–230.

81. Massague J, Wotton D. Transcriptional control by the TGF-β/Smad signaling system. *EMBO J* 2000;19:1745–1754.

82. Greenwel P, Inagaki Y, Hu W, et al. Sp1 is required for the early response of α2(I) collagen to transforming growth factor-β1. *J Biol Chem* 1997;272:19738–19745.

83. Armendariz-Borunda J, Simkevich CP, Roy N, et al. Activation of Ito cells involves regulation of AP-1 binding proteins and induction of type I collagen gene expression. *Biochem J* 1994; 304:817–824.

84. Houglum K, Buck M, Alcorn J, et al. Two different *cis*-acting regulatory regions direct cell-specific transcription of the collagen α1(I) gene in hepatic stellate cells and in skin and tendon fibroblasts. *J Clin Invest* 1995;96:2269–2276.

85. Inagaki Y, Truter S, Bou-Gharios G, et al. Activation of pro-α-

2(I) collagen promoter during hepatic fibrogenesis in transgenic mice. *Biochem Biophys Res Commun* 1998;250:606–611.

86. Prakash S, Wyler DJ. Fibroblast stimulation in schistosomiasis. XI. Purification to apparent homogeneity of fibroblast-stimulating factor-1, an acidic heparin-binding growth factor produced by schistosomal egg granulomas. *J Immunol* 1991;146: 1679–1684.

87. Prakash S, Wyler DJ. Fibroblast stimulation in schistosomiasis. XII. Identification of CD4+ lymphocytes within schistosomal egg granulomas as a source of an apparently novel fibroblast growth factor (FsF-1). *J Immunol* 1992 148:3583–3587.

88. Greenwel P, Wyler DJ, Rojkind M, et al. Fibroblast-stimulating factor-1, a novel lymphokine produced in schistosomal egg granulomas, stimulates liver fat-storing cells *in vitro*. *Infect Immun* 1993;61:3985–3987.

89. Prakash S, Robbins PW, Wyler DJ. Cloning and analysis of murine cDNA that encodes a fibrogenic lymphokine, fibrosin. *Proc Natl Acad Sci U S A* 1995;92:2154–2158.

90. Prakash S, Nanji AA, Robbins PW. Fibrosin: a novel lymphokine in alcohol-induced fibrosis. *Exp Mol Pathol* 1999;67: 40–49.

91. Bradham DM, Igarashi A, Potter RL, et al. Connective tissue growth factor: a cysteine-rich mitogen secreted by human vascular endothelial cells is related to the SRC-induced immediate early gene product CEF-10. *J Cell Biol* 1991;114:1285–1294.

92. Surveyor GA, Brigstock DR. Immunohistochemical localization of connective tissue growth factor (CTGF) in the mouse embryo between days 7.5 and 14.5 of gestation. *Growth Factors* 1999;17:115–124.

93. Frazier K, Williams S, Kothapalli D, et al. Stimulation of fibroblast cell growth, matrix production, and granulation tissue formation by connective tissue growth factor. *J Invest Dermatol* 1996;107:404–411.

94. Mori T, Kawara S, Shinozaki M, et al. Role and interaction of connective tissue growth factor with transforming growth factor-β in persistent fibrosis: a mouse fibrosis model. *J Cell Physiol* 1999;81:153–159.

95. Sato S, Nagaoka T, Hasegawa M, et al. Serum levels of connective tissue growth factor are elevated in patients with systemic sclerosis: association with extent of skin sclerosis and severity of pulmonary fibrosis. *J Rheumatol* 2000;27:149–154.

96. Paradis V, Dargere D, Vidaud M, et al. Expression of connective tissue growth factor in experimental rat and human liver fibrosis. *Hepatology* 1999;30:968–976.

97. Williams EJ, Gaca MD, Brigstock DR, et al. Increased expression of connective tissue growth factor in fibrotic human liver and in activated hepatic stellate cells. *J Hepatol* 2000;32: 754–761.

98. Abraham DJ, Shiwen X, Black CM, et al. Tumor necrosis factor α suppresses the induction of connective tissue growth factor by transforming growth factor-β in normal and scleroderma fibroblasts. *J Biol Chem* 2000;275:15220–15225.

99. Kothapalli D, Hayashi N, Grotendorst GR. Inhibition of TGF-β-stimulated CTGF gene expression and anchorage-independent growth by cAMP identifies a CTGF-dependent restriction point in the cell cycle. *FASEB J* 1998;12:1151–1161.

100. Duncan MR, Frazier KS, Abramson S, et al. Connective tissue growth factor mediates transforming growth factor-β-induced collagen synthesis: down-regulation by cAMP. *FASEB J* 1999; 13:1774–1786.

101. Gabay C, Kushner I. Acute-phase proteins and other systemic responses to inflammation. *N Engl J Med* 1999;340:448–454.

102. Solis-Herruzo JA, Brenner DA, Chojkier M. Tumor necrosis factor-α inhibits collagen gene transcription and collagen synthesis in cultured human fibroblasts. *J Biol Chem* 1988;263: 5841–5845.

103. Heinrich PC, Castell JV, Andus T. Interleukin-6 and the acute phase response. *Biochem J* 1990;265:621–636.

104. Greenwel P, Schwartz M, Rosas M, et al. Characterization of fat-storing cell lines derived from normal and CCl4-cirrhotic livers: differences in the production of interleukin-6. *Lab Invest* 1991;65:644–653.

105. Choi I, Kang HS, Yang Y, et al. IL-6 induces hepatic inflammation and collagen synthesis *in vivo*. *Clin Exp Immunol* 1994; 95:530–535.

106. Horn F, Wegenka UM, Lutticken C, et al. Regulation of α-2-macroglobulin gene expression by interleukin-6. *Ann N Y Acad Sci* 1994;737:308–323.

107. Roeb EL, Graeve R, Hoffmann K, et al. Regulation of tissue inhibitor of metalloproteinases-1 gene expression by cytokines and dexamethasone in rat hepatocyte primary cultures. *Hepatology* 1993;18:1437–1442.

108. Hirano T. Interleukin 6 and its receptor: ten years later. *Int Rev Immunol* 1998;16:249–284.

109. Bugno M, Graeve L, Gatsios P, et al. Identification of the interleukin-6/oncostatin M response element in the rat tissue inhibitor of metalloproteinases-1 (TIMP-1) promoter. *Nucleic Acids Res* 1995;23:5041–5047.

110. Gomez-Lechon MJ. Oncostatin M: signal transduction and biological activity. *Life Sci* 1999;65:2019–2030.

111. Levy MT, Trojanowska M, Reuben A. Oncostatin M: a cytokine upregulated in human cirrhosis, increases collagen production by human hepatic stellate cells. *J Hepatol* 2000;32:218–226.

112. Kamiya A, Kinoshita T, Ito Y, et al. Fetal liver development requires a paracrine action of oncostatin M through the gp130 signal transducer. *EMBO J* 1999;18:2127–2136.

113. Ihn H, LeRoy EC, Trojanowska M. Oncostatin M stimulates transcription of the human α2(I) collagen gene via the Sp1/Sp3-binding site. *J Biol Chem* 1997;272:24666–24672.

114. Rojkind M, Mourelle M. The liver as a bioecological system: Modifications during regeneration and repair. In: Nimni M, ed. *Collagen: chemistry, biology and technology.* Vol. I. Boca Raton: CRC Press, 1988:137–160.

115. Westermarck J, Kahari VM. Regulation of matrix metalloproteinase expression in tumor invasion. *FASEB J* 1999;13:781–792.

116. Yata Y, Takahara T, Furui K, et al. Expression of matrix metalloproteinase-13 and tissue inhibitor of metalloproteinase-1 in acute liver injury. *J Hepatol* 1999;30:419–424.

117. Iredale JP, Benyon RC, Pickering J, et al. Mechanisms of spontaneous resolution of rat liver fibrosis. Hepatic stellate cell apoptosis and reduced hepatic expression of metalloproteinase inhibitors. *J Clin Invest* 1998;102:538–549.

118. Takahara T, Furui K, Yata Y, et al. Dual expression of matrix metalloproteinase-2 and membrane-type 1-matrix metalloproteinase in fibrotic human livers. *Hepatology* 1997;26: 1521–1529.

119. Takahara T, Furui K, Funaki J, et al. Increased expression of matrix metalloproteinase-II in experimental liver fibrosis in rats. *Hepatology* 1995;21:787–795.

120. Theret N, Musso O, L'Helgoualc'h A, et al. Activation of matrix metalloproteinase-2 from hepatic stellate cells requires interactions with hepatocytes. *Am J Pathol* 1997;150:51–58.

121. Preaux AM, Mallat A, Nhieu JT, et al. Matrix metalloproteinase-2 activation in human hepatic fibrosis regulation by cell-matrix interactions. *Hepatology* 1999;30:944–950.

122. Theret N, Lehti K, Musso O, et al. MMP2 activation by collagen I and concanavalin A in cultured human hepatic stellate cells. *Hepatology* 1999;30:462–468.

123. Benyon RC, Hovell CJ, Da Gaca M, et al. Progelatinase A is produced and activated by rat hepatic stellate cells and promotes their proliferation. *Hepatology* 1999;30:977–986.

124. Poulos JE, Weber JD, Bellezzo JM, et al. Fibronectin and cytokines increase JNK, ERK, AP-1 activity, and transin gene expression in rat hepatic stellate cells. *Am J Physiol* 1997;273: G804–G811.

125. Herbst H, Heinrichs O, Schuppan D, et al. Temporal and spatial patterns of transin/stromelysin RNA expression following toxic injury in rat liver. *Virchows Arch B Cell Pathol Incl Mol Pathol* 1991;60:295–300.

126. Kossakowska AE, Edwards DR, Lee SS, et al. Altered balance between matrix metalloproteinases and their inhibitors in experimental biliary fibrosis. *Am J Pathol* 1998;153:1895–1902.

127. Ueno T, Sujaku K, Tamaki S, et al. OK-432 treatment increases matrix metalloproteinase-9 production and improves dimethyl-nitrosamine-induced liver cirrhosis in rats. *Int J Mol Med* 1999; 3:497–503.

128. Theret N, Musso O, L'Helgoualc'h A, et al. Differential expression and origin of membrane-type 1 and 2 matrix metalloproteinases (MT-MMPs) in association with MMP2 activation in injured human livers. *Am J Pathol* 1998;153:945–954.

129. Herbst H, Wege T, Milani S, et al. Tissue inhibitor of metalloproteinase-1 and -2 RNA expression in rat and human liver fibrosis. *Am J Pathol* 1997;150:1647–1659.

130. Trim JE, Samra SK, Arthur MJ, et al. Upstream tissue inhibitor of metalloproteinases-1 (TIMP-1) element-1, a novel and essential regulatory DNA motif in the human TIMP-1 gene promoter, directly interacts with a 30-kd nuclear protein. *J Biol Chem* 2000;275:6657–6663.

131. Saile B, Knittel T, Matthes N, et al. CD95/CD95L-mediated apoptosis of the hepatic stellate cell. A mechanism terminating uncontrolled hepatic stellate cell proliferation during hepatic tissue repair. *Am J Pathol* 1997;151:1265–1272.

132. Kaplowitz N, Tsukamoto H. Oxidative stress and liver disease. *Prog Liver Dis* 1996;14:131–159.

133. Storz G, Imlay JA. Oxidative stress. *Curr Opin Microbiol* 1999; 2:188–194.

134. Houglum K, Brenner DA, Chojkier M. D-α-tocopherol inhibits collagen α1(I) gene expression in cultured human fibroblasts. Modulation of constitutive collagen gene expression by lipid peroxidation. *J Clin Invest* 1991;87:2230–2235.

135. Tsai KJ, Hung IJ, Chow CK, et al. Impaired production of nitric oxide, superoxide, and hydrogen peroxide in glucose-phosphate–dehydrogenase-deficient granulocytes. *FEBS Lett* 1998;436:411–414.

136. Dalton TP, Shertzer HG, Puga A. Regulation of gene expression by reactive oxygen. *Annu Rev Pharmacol Toxicol* 1999;39: 67–101.

137. Bowie A, O'Neill LA. Oxidative stress and nuclear factor-κB activation: a reassessment of the evidence in the light of recent discoveries. *Biochem Pharmacol* 2000;59:13–23.

138. Dupont I, Bodenez P, Berthou F, et al. Cytochrome P-450 2E1 activity and oxidative stress in alcoholic patients. *Alcohol Alcohol* 2000;35:98–103.

139. Liu SL, Degli Esposti S, Yao T, et al. Vitamin E therapy of acute CCl4-induced hepatic injury in mice is associated with inhibition of nuclear factor-κB binding. *Hepatology* 1995;22:1474–1481.

140. Chojkier M, Houglum K, Lee KS, Buck M. Long- and short-term D-α-tocopherol supplementation inhibits liver collagen α1(I) gene expression. *Am J Physiol* 1998;275:G1480–G1485.

141. Kershenobich D, Vargas F, Garcia-Tsao G, et al. Colchicine in the treatment of cirrhosis of the liver. *N Engl J Med* 1988;318: 1709–1713.

142. Schuppan D, Strobel D, Hahn EG. Hepatic fibrosis—therapeutic strategies. *Digestion* 1998;59:385–390.

143. Shimizu I, Ma YR, Mizobuchi Y, Liu F, et al. Effects of Sho-saiko-to, a Japanese herbal medicine, on hepatic fibrosis in rats. *Hepatology* 1999;29:149–160.

144. Diaz-Gil JJ, Munoz J, Albillos A, et al. Improvement in liver

fibrosis, functionality and hemodynamics in CCl₄-cirrhotic rats after injection of the liver growth factor. *J Hepatol* 1999;30: 1065–1072.

145. Zhu J, Wu J, Frizell E, et al. Rapamycin inhibits hepatic stellate cell proliferation *in vitro* and limits fibrogenesis in an *in vivo* model of liver fibrosis. *Gastroenterology* 1999;117:1198–1204.

146. Qi Z, Atsuchi N, Ooshima A, et al. Blockade of type β transforming growth factor signaling prevents liver fibrosis and dysfunction in the rat. *Proc Natl Acad Sci U S A* 1999;96:2345–2349.

147. George J, Roulot D, Koteliansky VE, et al. *In vivo* inhibition of rat stellate cell activation by soluble transforming growth factor-β type II receptor: a potential new therapy for hepatic fibrosis. *Proc Natl Acad Sci U S A* 1999;96:12719–12724.

148. Ueno H, Sakamoto T, Nakamura T, et al. A soluble transforming growth factor-β receptor expressed in muscle prevents liver fibrogenesis and dysfunction in rats. *Hum Gene Ther* 2000;11: 33–42.

149. Rudolph KL, Chang S, Millard M, et al. Inhibition of experimental liver cirrhosis in mice by telomerase gene delivery. *Science* 2000;287:1253–1258.

The Liver: Biology and Pathobiology, Fourth Edition, edited by I. M. Arias, J. L. Boyer, F. V. Chisari, N. Fausto, D. Schachter, and D. A. Shafritz.
Lippincott Williams & Wilkins, Philadelphia © 2001.

50

ALCOHOLIC AND NONALCOHOLIC STEATOHEPATITIS

ANNA MAE DIEHL

HISTOPATHOLOGY

Steatohepatitis (SH) is a liver disease characterized by hepatic steatosis, inflammation, and increased hepatocyte death (1). SH is believed to be an intermediate stage in the spectrum of fatty liver disease (FLD), which ranges from simple steatosis (fatty liver) on one extreme, to cirrhosis on the opposite end of the spectrum. Steatosis is rapidly reversible, and, even when chronic, it is typically associated with few clinical problems. In contrast, SH seldom reverts to normal hepatic histology, even when the precipitating condition is removed (2). Rather, patients with SH often develop increased hepatic fibrosis and, with time, cirrhosis occurs in a substantial fraction of these individuals (3–6). Liver-related morbidity and mortality occur in patients with SH (6,7). These outcomes are significantly increased in those with associated hepatic fibrosis or cirrhosis (6). Thus, the transition from simple steatosis to SH appears to represent a rate-limiting step in the progression to cirrhosis and clinical liver disease in patients with FLD.

Associated Conditions

FLD is one of the most common causes of elevated serum liver enzymes in Western Europe, Japan, and the U.S. (8–11). In these parts of the world, ultrasound surveys of

the general population indicate that almost one quarter of the adult population has hepatic steatosis (12). Habitual alcohol consumption and obesity are the two most common conditions that are associated with FLD (10,13). Demographic surveys (11) and autopsy studies (14) indicate that the prevalence of cirrhosis is greatest in obese alcohol consumers, prompting speculation that chronic alcohol ingestion and obesity have additive, and perhaps synergistic, effects on FLD pathogenesis (15).

Tables 50.1 to 50.3 demonstrate that many conditions have been associated with FLD (also reviewed in ref. 16). As with alcohol and obesity, most of these conditions generally lead to simple hepatic steatosis (fatty liver) and only infrequently result in SH or cirrhosis. Interestingly, emerging evidence suggests that some conditions that lead to fatty liver (e.g., alcohol use, obesity) also increase the probability of developing cirrhosis from virus-mediated chronic liver injury (17,18). Similarly, hepatocytes in alcohol- or obesity-related fatty livers are also extremely vulnerable to necrosis after transient, acute ischemia and reperfusion (19,20). This is exemplified by the high incidence of primary graft non-function (i.e., massive, acute hepatic necrosis) in liver transplant recipients who receive a fatty liver graft that was functioning well in the donor before the organ was procured (21,22).

Clinical Features

In patients with FLD, as in most patients with other chronic liver diseases, symptoms and signs of liver damage correlate imperfectly with histologic stage. For example,

A. M. Diehl: Department of Medicine, The Johns Hopkins University School of Medicine, The Johns Hopkins University; Department of Medicine, Johns Hopkins Hospital, Baltimore, Maryland 21205.

TABLE 50.1. DRUGS/TOXINS ASSOCIATED WITH STEATOSIS

Metals	Antibiotics	Cytotoxic/Cytostatic Drugs	Other Drugs
Antimony	Azaserine	L-Asparaginase	Amiodarone
Barium Salts	Bleomycin	Azacytidine	Coumadin
Borates	Puromycin	Azauridine	Dichloroethylene
Carbon disulfide	Tetracycline	Methotrexate	Ethionine
Chromates			Ethyl bromide
Phosphorus			Estrogens
Rare earths of low atomic numbers			Flectol H
Thallium compounds			Glucocorticoids
Uranium compounds			Hydrazine
			Hypoglycin
			Orate
			Perhexilene maleate
			Safrole

TABLE 50.2. INBORN ERRORS OF METABOLISM ASSOCIATED WITH STEATOSIS

Abetalipoproteinemia
Familial hepatosteatosis
Galactosemia
Glycogen storage disease
Hereditary fructose intolerance
Homocystinuria
Systemic carnitine deficiency
Tyrosinemia
Resfum's disease
Schwachman's syndrome
Weber–Christian syndrome
Wilson's disease

TABLE 50.3. ACQUIRED METABOLIC DISORDERS ASSOCIATED WITH STEATOSIS

Antiviral therapy for HIV infection
Diabetes mellitus
Inflammatory bowel disease
Jejuno-ileal bypass
Kwashiorkor and marasmus
Obesity
Serum lipid abnormalities
Starvation and cachexia
Severe anemia
Total parenteral nutrition

HIV, human immunodeficiency virus.

most individuals with simple hepatic steatosis are entirely asymptomatic, with only mild hepatomegaly, good hepatic function, and normal–slightly increased serum aminotransferase values (12,23,24). However, a paucity of clinical symptoms and signs of liver disease at a single point in time does not assure a good long-term prognosis, because many patients with SH or cirrhosis have equally benign clinical features for years before overt hepatic decompensation develops (6,25). Conversely, although liver failure is much

more common in patients with SH and, especially, cirrhosis (5,6, 26), it may (albeit rarely) complicate acute hepatic steatosis (27).

Because clinical manifestations of liver damage do not reliably predict the extent of hepatic fibrosis (which provides the best indication of irreversible underlying liver damage), liver biopsy is required to distinguish patients with early disease (i.e., steatosis) from other individuals with more advanced liver damage (i.e., SH or cirrhosis) before clinical complications of hepatic dysfunction become problematic. However, advocacy for this invasive diagnostic approach has been timid and, consequently, knowledge about the natural history of FLD is limited. Nevertheless, recent retrospective analyses of clinical-pathologic data from large cohorts of patients with FLD provide convincing evidence that a sizable proportion (15% to 30%) of individuals with steatosis develop cirrhosis (6,7). Furthermore, these studies also demonstrate that patients with advanced stages of FLD have a substantial rate of liver-related mortality (11% within a decade of diagnosis). Recent recognition that the prognosis of FLD resembles that of chronic alcoholic, autoimmune, or viral liver disease has spawned interest in defining the mechanisms that mediate the initiation and progression of FLD.

PATHOGENESIS — GENERAL CONCEPTS

A "multiple-hit" model for FLD pathogenesis is consistent with patient data which suggest that steatosis is common, generally well tolerated and an important, but incomplete, stimulus for the inflammatory and fibrotic responses that cause irreversible liver damage. According to this model (Fig. 50.1), many insults cause hepatocytes to accumulate lipid. If appropriate protective (adaptive) responses to these insults do not occur, hepatocyte dysfunction and liver failure ensue relatively immediately. Massive hepatic infiltration with inflammatory cells is not required for this type of acute liver failure

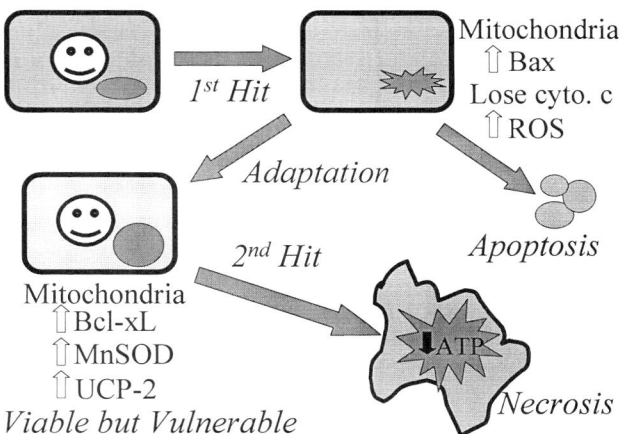

FIGURE 50.1 Two-hit model for fatty liver disease (FLD) pathogenesis. Many insults (i.e., 1st hits) threaten hepatocyte survival by increasing mitochondrial production of reactive oxygen species (*ROS*) and enhancing the formation of pores, such as those that contain the channel protein Bax, which permit the escape of mitochondrial factors (e.g., cytochrome c) that promote programmed cell death (i.e., apoptosis). Unless hepatocytes induce mechanisms to limit these potentially lethal signals, they go on to die by apoptosis. However, hepatocytes that adapt to apoptotic stress by upregulating defensive mechanisms that reduce mitochondrial permeability (e.g., induction of the antiapoptotic channel protein *Bcl-xL*), detoxify superoxide anion [e.g., manganese superoxide dismutase (*MnSOD*)], and inhibit the formation of ROS during mitochondrial respiration [e.g., uncoupling protein-2 (*UCP-2*)] can survive. Although these and other adaptations permit the fatty hepatocytes to remain viable, some of the adaptive responses (such as the induction of mitochondrial uncoupling proteins) might inadvertently enhance their vulnerability to adenosine triphosphate (*ATP*) depletion. Thus, adapted hepatocytes might be more vulnerable to 2nd "hits" that cause cellular necrosis.

because it reflects massive hepatocyte apoptosis. On the other hand, if adaptation occurs, hepatic function is preserved and the fatty hepatocytes remain viable. Apparently, protective adaptations normally occur when the liver is challenged by pro-steatotic insults, because fatty liver usually has a benign clinical course. However, because some of the adaptive responses enhance vulnerability to other types of stress, hepatocyte death can also be triggered by subsequent exposure to one of these other insults (i.e., a "second hit") (Fig. 50.2).

At this point, it is not clear whether these secondary stresses primarily promote the accumulation of inflammatory cells within the hepatic parenchyma, and these cells, in turn, kill hepatocytes (Fig. 50.2A), or whether the insults kill the unusually vulnerable hepatocytes directly and then, inflammatory cell infiltration occurs secondarily to clear the cellular debris (Fig. 50.2B). Either scenario might promote a self-perpetuating cycle of inflammation and hepatocyte death (i.e., SH). Moreover, the resultant increase in inflammatory mediators is likely to activate fibrogenesis by hepatic stellate cells. Scarring (cirrhosis) will develop in the liver unless the inflammation–death cycle can be reversed, permitting matrix degradation to exceed matrix formation (a "third hit" might prevent this).

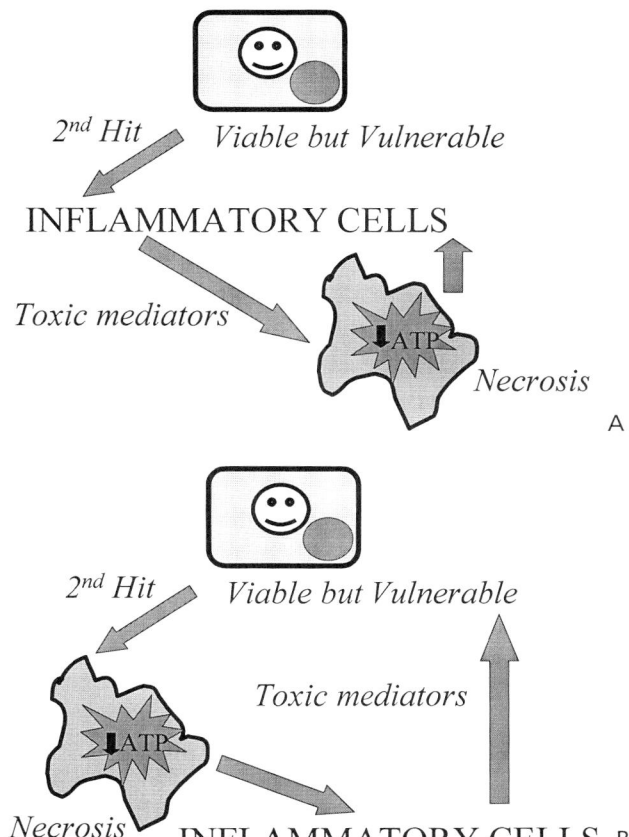

FIGURE 50.2. Potential mechanisms for the progression of steatosis to steatohepatitis (SH) **A:** Insults that cause inflammatory cells to accumulate within the liver might increase hepatocyte exposure to noxious inflammatory cell products. Fatty hepatocytes are more vulnerable to the lethal actions of these inflammatory mediators and undergo necrosis, which in turn provokes a subsequent inflammatory response that kills even more hepatocytes. **B:** Hepatocytic death increases, either because cells fail to adapt to the "1st hit," or because adapted hepatocytes in the liver experiences "2nd hits" that cause viable but vulnerable, adapted hepatocytes to undergo necrosis. In either case, the increased hepatocyte death triggers an inflammatory response that recruits immune cells to the liver, resulting in an increased local release of toxic inflammatory mediators that kills even more hepatocytes, inciting an additional inflammatory response. Chronic inflammation, in turn, stimulates fibrogenesis and can eventually result in cirrhosis.

Thus, the "multiple-hit" model for FLD pathogenesis predicts that primary, pro-steatotic insults rarely kill hepatocytes or cause acute liver failure, but commonly compromise hepatocyte viability. Whether or not liver failure and portal hypertension ever develop (and the time course of their evolution) depends upon exposure to secondary insults, as well as the duration and intensity of these secondary stresses. The latter, in turn, are likely to be influenced by host, as well as environmental, factors. Given that the transition from steatosis to SH is generally required for FLD to produce clinically significant, adverse outcomes, it is important to identify the mechanisms that permit hepatocytes to survive chronically in an environment that promotes hepatic steatosis and to understand how these adaptive responses might enhance hepatocyte lethality.

PATHOGENESIS — ANIMAL MODELS OF FATTY LIVER DISEASE

Animal models should be helpful in delineating the mechanisms that mediate the initiation and progression of FLD. At the present time, FLD pathogenesis has been studied most extensively in two small animal models (mice and rats that are genetically obese or that have been fed ethanol chronically). Thus, the work in these model systems will be emphasized here. However, this approach is not intended to minimize the important contributions that have resulted from the evaluation of other experimental models, some of which are listed in Table 50.4. Ultimately, it will be necessary to compare the abnormalities in all of these different models to determine whether common mechanisms are fundamentally involved in FLD pathogenesis.

Genetically Obese Mice and Rats

Our group has studied genetically obese mice and rats that have naturally occurring mutations that lead to deficiency of the appetite-suppressing hormone, leptin (the product of the ob gene) (28), or defects in its receptor, ob-R (29,30). Because normal satiety signals are inhibited in these rodents, they overeat and become obese. Both leptin-defi-

TABLE 50.4. ANIMAL MODELS OF FATTY LIVER DISEASE

Toxin-induced
  Alloxan
  Carbon tetrachloride
  Ethanol
  Ethionine
  Lipopolysaccharide + aspirin
  Tetracycline
Nutritionally induced
  Choline and/or methionine-deficient diets
  Energy dense diets (sucrose, fats)
Associated with Genetic Obesity
  Leptin deficient ob/ob mice
  Leptin-resistant fa/fa rats, db/db mice
Occurring in Transgenic Mice
  with lipodystrophy secondary to:
    Adipose-specific over-expression of SREBP-1c
    Adipose-specific disruption of C/EBP α
    Adipose-specific disruption of PPAR γ
  with disruption of PPARα and certain PPARα-regulated genes:
    PPARα-null
    fatty acyl CoA oxidase (AOX)-null
    PPARα-null/AOX null double knockout

cient ob/ob mice and fa/fa rats (which have defective leptin receptors) spontaneously develop fatty livers (31). Interestingly, both strains also exhibit several other characteristics that are commonly associated with FLD in humans, including hyperinsulinemia and hyperglycemia (i.e., insulin resistance) and hyperlipidemia (reviewed in ref. 204). Thus, these animals provide a convenient model to test the "multiple-hit" theory of FLD progression.

Vulnerability to Endotoxin-Mediated Damage

Because gut-derived bacterial products have been implicated in the pathogenesis of FLD associated with chronic alcohol ingestion (32,33) and also with liver damage following jejuno-ileal bypass surgery for obesity (34,35), we asked whether rats or mice with obesity-related fatty livers would exhibit enhanced vulnerability to endotoxin-mediated liver damage. In order to address this question, adult, obese fa/fa rats and ob/ob mice and their lean litter mates were treated with small doses of lipopolysaccharide (LPS). Both obese strains developed significantly more liver injury, as evidenced by greater increases in serum liver enzymes and extensive areas of hepatic inflammation and liver cell death histologically (31). These findings have been reproduced subsequently by at least two other groups (20,36). Thus, the fatty livers of these obese rodents are sensitized to endotoxin-mediated injury. The next task is to identify the mechanisms that are responsible for this sensitization.

Hepatocyte Sensitization to Tumor Necrosis Factor Lethality

Similar to obese humans (37), even in the absence of exposure to exogenous LPS, ob/ob mice are known to have increased expression of the LPS-inducible cytokine, TNFα, in white adipose tissues and blood (38,39). Because TNFα is known to be a proximal mediator of LPS-induced liver damage (40), we suspected that the increased severity of LPS-related liver damage in obese rodents might reflect a super-induction of TNFα in response to treatment with exogenous LPS. To our surprise, this did not occur. In fact, serum TNFα concentrations were actually lower in obese animals than in lean controls following LPS injection (31,41). These observations demonstrated that obesity-related increases in LPS-liver damage do not require an extraordinary induction of TNFα. Rather, hepatocytes in fatty livers appear to be unusually likely to die when exposed to "ordinary" concentrations of TNFα.

Immunologic Mechanisms for Sensitization to Lipopolysaccharide Toxicity

Non-Obese Animal Models
Interestingly, chronic ethanol consumption, another common cause of steatosis, is also known to enhance hepatic sen-

sitivity to TNF-mediated damage (42,43). Drugs that inhibit RNA and protein synthesis have a similar effect (44,45), as does infection with the bacterium *Propionibacterium acnes* (46). The immunologic mechanisms that mediate *P. acnes*-related sensitization to LPS hepatotoxicity have been well characterized by Matsui and colleagues (46). The bacterium infects hepatic macrophages, activating them and increasing the local production of interluekin (IL)-12 and IL-18. These cytokines interact and affect a selective reduction in liver CD4NK1.1 T cells, a specific subpopulation of liver lymphocytes that are the predominant hepatic source of IL-4. When IL-4 production is decreased, TH-1 (pro-inflammatory) cytokine responses to LPS predominate because antiinflammatory (TH-2) cytokines are reduced. A relative excess of TH-1 cytokines, such as interferon (IFN)-γ, ensues and kills hepatocytes, although the precise molecular and cellular mechanisms involved are not well understood.

Obese Animal Models

Given similarities in the sensitivity to LPS-induced liver damage between *P. acnes*-primed mice and ob/ob mice with fatty livers, we wondered whether the two models might also share similar immunologic deficits. To address this question, we isolated liver mononuclear cells from obese, ob/ob mice and age- and gender-matched lean control mice. Similar to *P. acnes*-infected mice, obese, ob/ob mice had a selective reduction in liver CD4NK1.1 T cells (47). Efforts are being directed towards delineating the mechanism(s) responsible for the obesity-related reduction in this subpopulation of liver lymphocytes.

Macrophage Abnormalities

In the *P. acnes* model, lymphocyte depletion occurs secondary to macrophage activation and increased production of IL-12 and IL-18. *In vivo* and *in vitro* studies of macrophages from fa/fa rats and ob/ob mice and their lean litter mates demonstrate that the obese animals also have abnormal macrophages. For example, peritoneal macrophages from ob/ob mice have an impaired ability to phagocytose *Candida albicans in vitro*, a defect that can be improved when the cells are pretreated with leptin (41). Similarly, the hepatic uptake of intraperitoneally injected fluorescent-labeled microspheres (31) or radiolabeled bacteria (41) is inhibited in obese, leptin-resistant fa/fa rats. Northern blot analysis of liver RNA from these animals reveals profoundly reduced expression of the Kupffer cell-specific gene, KCR (31). LPS injection produces a similar inhibition of KCR expression in lean controls (31), suggesting that constitutive phenotype of Kupffer cells in the obese animals may reflect chronically increased exposure to LPS.

Consistent with this possibility, cultured peritoneal macrophages from leptin-deficient ob/ob mice exhibit abnormal cytokine induction after acute LPS challenge, producing significantly less TNFα mRNA, but much more IL-6 mRNA than cells from their lean litter mates (48). Compared to macrophages from lean mice, macrophages from ob/ob mice also release significantly more H_2O_2, both before and after LPS treatment (48). The basal and LPS-induced activities of cyclooxygenase (COX)-2, the cytokine-inducible enzyme that regulates macrophage prostanoid release, are also significantly greater in ob/ob macrophages than in lean mouse macrophages (48). Finally, RNAase protection assays demonstrate significantly greater induction of IL-12 and IL-18 mRNAs in the livers of ob/ob mice compared to lean controls following LPS challenge (47).

Because IL-12 expression is regulated predominantly at the transcriptional level (49), it is likely that ob/ob mice produce more IL-12 protein than lean mice. However, because IL-18 expression has considerable posttranscriptional regulation (50), direct measurement of IL-18 protein is necessary to determine whether increases in IL-18 mRNA lead to increases in the biological activity of this cytokine. ELISA assays demonstrate that serum concentrations of IL-18 protein are significantly greater in ob/ob mice than in lean controls both before and after LPS injection (47). Thus, similar to *P. acnes*-primed mice, obese mice with fatty livers have abnormal macrophages, increased production of IL-12 and IL-18, and selective depletion of CD4NK1.1 T cells.

Changes in the Cytokine Microenvironment

Because CD4NK1.1 T cells are the major source of hepatic IL-4 (51), ELISPOT assays were performed with mononuclear cells harvested from lean and obese livers to determine whether IL-4 production had been effected. Consistent with the decreased numbers of CD4NK1.1 T cells in ob/ob mice, liver mononuclear cells from these animals produce less IL-4 than do mononuclear cells from the livers of lean control mice (47). This decrease in IL-4-producing liver lymphocytes is predicted to favor a predominance of TH-1 cytokines in response to LPS challenge (46,51,52). This outcome was observed; that is, compared to LPS-treated lean mice, in LPS-treated ob/ob mice the hepatic expression of the TH-1 cytokine, IFN-γ, is enhanced, while hepatic expression of the TH-2 cytokine, IL-10, is inhibited (47). These changes in hepatic cytokine production are likely to contribute to the reduced serum levels of IL-10 in LPS-treated ob/ob mice that have been reported by Faggioni and coworkers (20). Studies are in progress to clarify whether, and how, these changes in the cytokine microenvironment potentiate TNF-mediated hepatocyte death.

Tumor Necrosis Factor α and Hepatocyte Viability—General Concepts

As mentioned earlier, healthy adult hepatocytes normally do not die when they are exposed to TNFα (53). Indeed, both *in vivo* and *in vitro*, TNF generally promotes hepatocyte proliferation (54–58). Comparison of the proliferative responses in mice that lack type-1 or type-2 TNF receptors demonstrates that the hepatotrophic actions of TNFα are mediated predominately via the type-1 receptor (59). This is intriguing because the same receptor contains a Fas-like death domain and is known to initiate TNF-mediated apoptosis in hepatocytes (60). Indeed, there is no doubt that TNF is a critical mediator of hepatocyte death in many types of experimentally induced liver injury (reviewed in refs. 45 and 40). Of particular relevance to FLD is work by Thurman's group, who used TNF receptor type 1 (TNFR-1)-deficient mice to prove that TNFα is required for ethanol-induced liver damage (61). Taken together, these observations suggest that TNFα mediates FLD and causes hepatocyte death instead of hepatocyte proliferation because the transduction of intracellular signals downstream from TNFR-1 has been altered.

A detailed discussion of TNFα signal transduction can be found in several recent reviews (see refs. 62–65) and will not be repeated in this chapter. Briefly, mitochondria are now known to be critical targets for TNFα (66,67). In cells that are sensitive to TNF killing, the mitochondrial release of reactive oxygen species (ROS) and cytochrome c increase within minutes of TNFα exposure. This is quickly followed by the activation of effector caspases, including caspase 3, and completion of cellular apoptosis within an hour (68–71). TNFα also evokes cellular responses that inhibit apoptosis (72–74). The activation of the redox-sensitive transcription factor, NFκβ, plays a central role in the TNF-survival response, because various experimental strategies that abrogate NFκβ induction potentiate TNF lethality (75,76). Presumably, NFκβ activation prevents apoptosis by increasing the transcription of survival genes, such as bcl-2, bcl-xL (74), bfl-1 (77), inducible nitric oxide synthase (iNOS) (78), and manganese superoxide dismutase (MnSOD)(79), that can abort apoptosis. However, while NFκβ induction is necessary for cells to survive TNF-initiated apoptosis, it is not always sufficient to assure this outcome, because increases in NFκβ-DNA binding activity precede apoptosis in some types of cells (60,69,73,80,81).

Tumor Necrosis Factor α and Hepatocyte Viability in Obesity-Related Fatty Livers

Our studies of FLD in ob/ob mice suggest that hepatocytes in these animals are experiencing apoptotic stress constitutively, but manage to survive because various survival factors have been upregulated. The evidence for increased apoptotic stress in ob/ob fatty livers includes increased mitochondrial production of superoxide anion and hydrogen peroxide (82), increased expression of the proapoptotic mitochondrial protein, bax (83), and decreased mitochondrial content of cytochrome c (82). Balancing these potentially noxious responses are increased expression of the antiapoptotic mitochondrial proteins, bcl-2 and bcl-xL (83), and upregulated antioxidant defenses, including increased mitochondrial MnSOD activity and enhanced mitochondrial accumulation of reduced glutathione (GSH) (82). Although hepatocytes in fatty livers are viable, these cells are

clearly more vulnerable to the lethal effects of various secondary insults, including endotoxin challenge and transient ischemia (19,20). This suggests that the adaptive response might be only partially successful or that certain adaptations might even be harmful in other contexts.

With reference to the first possibility, preliminary work in our laboratory suggests that NFκβ activation is inhibited and iNOS induction is attenuated in ob/ob livers following LPS exposure. Given evidence that maximal induction of iNOS expression requires NFκβ (84) and that iNOS activation generates nitric oxide, which protects hepatocytes from TNF-mediated killing (85), inhibition of iNOS in ob/ob fatty livers provides a mechanism that might help to explain their enhanced sensitivity to LPS toxicity. The possibility that certain adaptations in fatty livers might potentiate the lethality of secondary insults also merits consideration. Serum and liver concentrations of fatty acids are increased in ob/ob mice (86–88), and unsaturated fatty acids induce the expression of the mitochondrial uncoupling protein (UCP)-2 in cultured hepatocytes (89). Mitochondria in ob/ob fatty livers express unusually high levels of UCP-2 (19). This inner mitochondrial transmembrane protein reduces the electrochemical gradient that results from electron transport chain activity, partially depolarizing the inner mitochondrial membrane and limiting the efficiency of mitochondrial adenosine triphosphate (ATP) synthesis (90,91). Thus, mitochondria with increased UCP-2 activity are predicted to be more vulnerable to collapse of the inner membrane potential with consequent interruption of mitochondrial ATP synthesis and cell death by necrosis (91). Consistent with this possibility, preliminary studies in our laboratory indicate that freshly isolated hepatocytes from ob/ob mice have less ATP than freshly isolated hepatocytes from normal control mice, and unlike control hepatocytes, exhibit a dose-related increase in LDH release (a measure of cellular necrosis) when incubated with TNFα.

Endogenous Ethanol Production and Obesity

As mentioned earlier, the histopathology of obesity-associated (nonalcoholic) FLD is identical to the FLD that is associated with chronic alcohol ingestion (2). Recent studies in mice that are genetically deficient for the type-1 TNF receptor prove that TNF is required for ethanol to produce FLD because, unlike control mice, TNFR-1 knockout mice do not develop steatosis or SH when fed ethanol (61). Intestinally derived bacterial products are the presumed stimulus for TNFα production in ethanol-fed rodents, because oral antibiotics and other treatments that reduce the intestinal bacterial flora inhibit ethanol-related increases in TNFα production by hepatic macrophages and provide protection from ethanol-induced liver damage (32,33). TNFα mRNA levels are increased constitutively in the livers of adult ob/ob mice. Recent work in our laboratory suggests that intestinal bacterial products might also provide the stimulus for increased TNFα expression in obese mice.

Analysis of the exhaled breath from ob/ob mice and their lean litter mates revealed a significant increase in the breath ethanol content of the obese group, although the animals had never been fed ethanol. Further studies demonstrated that in ob/ob mice, breath ethanol content increases with age and exhibits striking diurnal variation, being greatest after the dark period, which is when the mice feed. Treatment of ob/ob mice with neomycin, a poorly absorbed oral antibiotic, significantly reduces their breath ethanol content, suggesting that their intestinal flora are the most likely source of ethanol (92).

Decades ago, other workers showed that the intestinal flora of humans and rats can produce ethanol during the fermentation of dietary carbohydrates (93,94). Moreover, gut bacteria can also metabolize ethanol to its toxic metabolite, acetaldehyde (94). Given this information, the highest concentrations of ethanol and acetaldehyde in ob/ob mice are expected to exist within the lumen of the gastrointestinal tract. This may injure the intestinal epithelial barrier, enhancing its permeability to other bacterial products, such as LPS endotoxin. Preliminary experiments by our group suggest that neomycin treatment at least partially restores the hepatic population of CD4(+)NK1.1 T cells in ob/ob mice to normal levels. This observation is intriguing because this lymphocyte population modulates the balance between TH-1 (proinflammatory) and TH-2 (antiinflammatory) cytokine responses in the liver (51).

Thus, if confirmed, our findings suggest a unifying pathogenic mechanism for obesity- and alcohol-associated FLD; that is, high concentrations of ingested or endogenously produced ethanol within the gastrointestinal tract may increase intestinal permeability and permit the escape of bacterial endotoxins that activate the innate immune system and induce excessive, local production of TNFα and other proinflammatory cytokines. Increases in these cytokines, in turn, are likely to have many consequences, including the inhibition of insulin-initiated signals (39,95,96). The resultant insulin-resistant state might alter intermediary metabolism and promote hepatic lipid accumulation (97). Because insulin is also a viability factor for hepatocytes (98), the impaired propagation of insulin signals may also potentiate apoptosis in fatty hepatocytes.

Insulin-Resistance and Obesity-Related Fatty Liver Disease (see Chapter 36)

The potential importance of insulin-resistance in the FLD pathogenesis is supported by a growing body of clinical evidence (11,99). In addition, SH is strongly associated with increased TNFα and insulin resistance in transgenic mice that develop FLD and lipodystrophy due to adipocyte-specific overexpression of truncated form of sterol-regulatory element binding protein (SREBP)-1c, a transcription factor that regulates many facets of hepatic lipid metabolism (100). Interestingly, these lipodystrophic mice produce very little leptin, an adipose-specific gene product (28). Moreover,

treatment with recombinant leptin improves both insulin resistance and FLD in these mice (101). Taken together, these results suggest that leptin and TNFα differentially modulate insulin-dependent signaling. This, in turn, might help to explain why absolute or relative deficiency of leptin (as occurs in ob/ob mice and fa/fa rats) is associated with extremely severe consequences of insulin resistance.

Recent experiments with the oral hypoglycemic drug metformin confirm the importance of insulin resistance in the pathogenesis of FLD in ob/ob mice. Metformin is known to improve hepatic sensitivity to insulin (102–104). To determine whether improved hepatic insulin sensitivity affects the evolution of obesity-related FLD, we compared liver histology and serum aminotransferases in three groups of ob/ob mice (104a). One group was treated with metformin; one untreated control group was pair-fed the same amount of diet as the metformin group (to control for the known anorexogenic effects of metformin); the other untreated control group was permitted *ad libitum* consumption of the same chow that was given to the metformin and pair-fed groups (to control for the effects of caloric restriction). Metformin treatment significantly improved liver enzyme abnormalities and virtually abolished hepatic steatosis in ob/ob mice, whereas merely reducing caloric ingestion had little impact on these endpoints. The mechanism(s) underlying metformin's benefits are being investigated. To date, we have evidence for metformin-related decreases in the hepatic expression of TNFα mRNA and an associated downregulation of UCP-2, a TNFα-regulated gene (105). As expected, decreases in hepatocyte UCP-2 content were associated with increases in hepatocyte ATP content. Improved hepatic energy homeostasis, in turn, likely contributes to the metformin-induced normalization of the hepatocyte phenotype. Although preliminary, these results in ob/ob mice (which are incapable of expressing the leptin protein) suggest that leptin is not required to overcome hepatic insulin resistance. Rather, inhibition of TNFα-regulated events appears to be important for FLD to regress. Given these insights, it will be important to evaluate the respective roles of insulin (and insulin resistance), TNFα, and leptin (and leptin resistance) in the pathogenesis of FLD due to alcohol, other toxins, and inherited metabolic disorders.

Small Animal Models of Chronic Ethanol Ingestion

Similar to adult humans and baboons, rats and mice that are fed ethanol-containing diets develop hepatic steatosis within days to weeks. Although chronic voluntary ingestion of ethanol typically results in slight increases in serum aminotransferase values, hepatic infiltration with inflammatory cells is not conspicuous and cirrhosis does not develop in normal adult rats despite 1 to 2 years of ethanol exposure (106). In contrast, significant SH and hepatic fibrosis have been noted in baboons that ingested nutritionally replete liquid diets containing ethanol for periods of months to years (106). Thus, more advanced stages of liver damage tend to follow chronic ethanol ingestion in baboons than in rats. However, hepatic inflammation and fibrosis can be increased somewhat in adult rats (and mice) by administering ethanol continuously via an indwelling gastric cannula (107). Differences in the degree of SH and fibrosis between the two rat models of ethanol administration are felt to reflect, at least in part, the higher blood ethanol levels that are achieved when ethanol is given by the gastric cannulation method. Several theories have been forwarded to explain why higher levels of ethanol exposure might be more likely to cause SH (and consequent fibrosis).

Increased Production of Toxic Ethanol Metabolites

In the liver, ethanol is oxidized by three major enzyme systems: cytosolic alcohol dehydrogenase/mitochondrial aldehyde dehydrogenase, microsomal cytochrome P-450 isoenzymes (e.g., Cyp 2E1), and peroxisomal catalase. Without chronic stimulation to induce microsomal ethanol oxidizing enzymes, most ethanol is metabolized to acetaldehyde by cytosolic alcohol dehydrogenase (ADH). Acetaldehyde is a reactive byproduct of this reaction, and there is evidence that acetaldehyde adducts of cellular macromolecules form when acetaldehyde generation is increased. Aldehyde dehydrogenase (ALDH), a mitochondria-associated enzyme, oxidizes acetaldehyde to acetate. The latter serves as a carbon source for several intermediate metabolic pathways and is ultimately converted to CO_2 and H_2O (108). Genetic polymorphisms of ADH and/or ALDH can create imbalances in the relative activities of these enzymes and lead to acetaldehyde accumulation during ethanol oxidation. The latter has been associated with a tendency to develop alcohol-induced SH and cirrhosis in certain human populations (109).

In addition, sustained increases in blood ethanol concentrations are important because they promote the induction of microsomal ethanol oxidizing enzymes, such as cytochrome P-450-2E1 (Cyp 2E1), which generate not only acetaldehyde, but also other reactive metabolites, including the 1-hydroxyethyl radical, superoxide radical and H_2O_2 (110). Similar to acetaldehyde, the latter intermediates are believed to kill hepatocytes by damaging vital cellular macromolecules (109,111). In patients and baboons, the zonal distribution of Cyp 2E1 expression matches the zonal distribution of alcohol-induced liver injury (108). Cyp 2E1 expression and activity are also induced in rat liver during continuous intragastric administration of ethanol and correlate with lipid peroxidation and liver damage in that model (112). Moreover, unlike normal cultured hepatocytes which have little endogenous Cyp 2E1 activity and are relatively insensitive to ethanol-induced lethality, hepatocyte cell lines that have been engineered to overexpress

Cyp 2E1 die when exposed to ethanol (113). In addition, Cyp 2E1 is a heme-containing enzyme, and increases in the hepatic iron content (which enhance the microsomal production of ROS (114)) potentiate alcohol-related liver damage (115). All of these observations support the importance of this enzyme system in alcoholic liver disease pathogenesis. There are also data suggesting that Cyp 2E1 induction might contribute to the pathogenesis of nonalcoholic steatohepatitis (NASH). For example, one group of investigators reported increased hepatocyte expression of Cyp 2E1 in acinar zones 2 and 3 in rats with diet-induced hepatic steatosis. In that model, increases in Cyp 2E1 expression correlated positively with liver malondialdehyde content and negatively with superoxide dismutase, reduced GSH and vitamin E content, suggesting that diet-induced steatosis increases Cyp 2E1, which, in turn, leads to oxidative stress in the liver (116). Immunohistochemistry has also demonstrated increases in hepatic Cyp 2E1 expression in some patients with NASH (117). Thus, an upregulation of Cyp 2E1 by ethanol or dietary factors might provide a common mechanism for SH due to alcohol and obesity.

Other data negate the importance of Cyp2E1 induction for FLD pathogenesis. For example, although Cyp2E1 is induced in rats treated chronically with intragastric alcohol, gadolinium chloride prevents alcohol-dependent liver toxicity in this model (118). Conversely, Wistar rats develop fatty livers after ingesting high-carbohydrate diets, although the diets repress Cyp 2E1 expression and activity (119). High-carbohydrate diets also inhibit ethanol-induction of Cyp 2E1, but not ethanol-induced FLD, in Sprague-Dawley rats (120). Cyp 2E1 induction does not occur in two obesity-related models of FLD: adult male ob/ob mice (121,122) and Zucker fa/fa rats (122). Moreover, IL-1 depresses Cyp 2E1 in normal mice, suggesting that this enzyme is not likely to contribute to liver damage once an inflammatory cytokine response is in progress (123). Thus, although Cyp 2E1 activation might potentiate the evolution of alcoholic FLD, it appears that induction of this enzyme is neither an absolute prerequisite for, nor a predictable consequence of, hepatic steatosis or SH in general. This suggests that other factors might have a more important role in the genesis of alcohol-related FLD than Cyp 2E1 induction *per se.*

Potentially pertinent in this regard is growing evidence that the ingestion of polyunsaturated fatty acids (PUFAs) potentiate alcohol-related liver damage in several experimental model systems (107,120). Peroxisomes are known to play an important role in PUFA metabolism, and ethanol is also a substrate for peroxisomal catalase, which can generate potentially toxic fatty acid ethyl esters (111). Diets enriched with unsaturated fatty acids, such as linoleic or oleic acid (124,125), or situations (e.g., type II diabetes) that increase circulating levels of free fatty acids (126) also increase the DNA binding activity of the peroxisome proliferator alpha receptor (PPARα) in the livers of rats and mice. Increases in PPARα in turn induce hepatic expression of the PPARα-regulated microsomal enzymes Cyp 4A1 and Cyp 4A2 (124). Thus, it is conceivable that increases in these other P-450 isoenzymes might "substitute" for Cyp 2E1 induction and produce equally noxious outcomes as those that have been attributed to Cyp 2E1 activation. Indeed, increased Cyp 4A-mediated omega-oxidation of long chain fatty acids to toxic dicarboxylic acids is one of the mechanisms that has been proposed to explain the association of SH with increased PPARα activity in fatty acyl CoA oxidase (AOX)-null mice (127).

Studies of these animals and other mice with genetic disruption of PPARα, which regulates the transcription of hepatocyte genes involved in fatty acid uptake, esterification, and oxidation (128) demonstrate that PPARα activity fundamentally influences the evolution of FLD: PPARα-knockout mice exhibit enhanced sensitivity to fasting-induced hepatic steatosis (129), while AOX knockout mice develop steatosis and SH spontaneously (130). The mechanisms by which PPARα modulates murine sensitivity to FLD are complex. Because double knockout mice with disruptions of both the PPARα and AOX genes have less severe hepatic steatosis than AOX-null mice, it has been suggested that FLD results from the accumulation of endogenous activators of PPARα that are ordinarily metabolized by AOX (127). The livers of AOX −/− mice also exhibit spontaneous peroxisomal proliferation and eventually develop hepatocellular carcinomas (130). This observation suggests that mechanisms that are initiated when peroxisome proliferators induce hepatocarcinogenesis, such as the inhibition of TGFβ-1-induced hepatocyte apoptosis (131), might also occur during FLD. Evidence that neutralization of TNFα with anti-TNFα antibodies prevents the antiapoptotic effects of peroxisome proliferators in mice suggests that PPARα activation might enhance some TNFα-dependent survival signal (132). However, if true, the latter possibility is also somewhat paradoxical, because PPARα is known to inhibit the DNA binding activity of NFκβ (133), an important TNFα-regulated survival factor for hepatocytes (134). Moreover, there is considerable evidence that fatty livers are unusually vulnerable to damage from various insults that increase hepatic TNFα expression (19,20,31,36). Some of these conflicting observations might be attributable to time- and/or species-dependent variability in PPARα–TNFα interactions. For example, there is one report that the expression of PPARα and several PPARα-regulated genes was decreased in rat livers 16 hours after the systemic administration of recombinant TNFα (135). Moreover, because human livers have considerably less PPARα-DNA binding activity than rodent livers (136), it is not clear whether, or how, the effects of PPARα on lipid homeostasis and cellular survival are important for the pathogenesis of FLD in humans. One report indicates that chronic ethanol ingestion decreases liver levels of PPARα mRNA in rats and correlates this response with decreased hepatic concentrations of

PUFA (137). However, it is not clear whether chronic ethanol ingestion also inhibits PPARα activity or the expression of PPARα-regulated genes, such as AOX. Thus, it is not known to what extent, if any, that alcohol-induced FLD is mediated by PPARα.

Increases in Intestinal Permeability and Endotoxin Exposure

As mentioned earlier, a number of investigators have speculated that products derived from intestinal bacteria (particularly LPS endotoxins) are involved in the pathogenesis of ethanol-associated SH (reviewed in ref. 138), because SH is inhibited by administering lactobacillus (32) or poorly absorbed oral antibiotics (33) to rats receiving ethanol-containing diets. Higher intraintestinal concentrations of ethanol and acetaldehyde are expected when ethanol is delivered by continuous intragastric infusion than after intermittent, voluntary ingestion of ethanol-containing liquid diets. The former might damage the intestinal mucosal barrier and permit the egress of gut-derived bacterial products (139), including LPS which, in turn, can induce cytokine gene expression in hepatic macrophages (40). Consistent with this possibility, TNFα expression is increased in macrophages isolated from the livers of rats that develop SH during intragastric administration of ethanol with a high-fat diet (140). As discussed in the previous sections, the importance of TNFα in the pathogenesis of ethanol-induced fatty liver is demonstrated by recent evidence that FLD does not develop in ethanol-fed rats that have been treated with neutralizing anti-TNF antibodies (141) or in genetically engineered mice with targeted disruption of the type 1 TNF receptor gene (61).

Insulin-Resistance and Alcoholic Fatty Liver Disease

The association between increases in hepatic TNFα, hepatic insulin resistance and FLD in ob/ob mice suggests the possibility that TNFα-related inhibition of insulin-dependent signal transduction might also play a role in the genesis of alcohol-induced FLD. Wands and colleagues have shown that insulin-dependent tyrosyl-phosphorylation of IRS-1 is inhibited in rats that have been fed ethanol-containing diets (142,143). This effect appears to play a major role in the antiproliferative actions of ethanol because chronic ethanol consumption is able to repress "spontaneous" increases in hepatocyte proliferation that occur in transgenic mice that overexpress IRS-1 in the liver (144). Interestingly, TNFα is also known to inhibit insulin-initiated IRS-1 phosphorylation (39). Thus, some of the *in vivo* effects of ethanol on insulin signaling may be mediated indirectly, via ethanol-induced cytokines. The beneficial effects of TNFα neutralization on experimentally induced alcoholic liver disease support this possibility. However, recent evidence that ethanol also suppresses insulin-induced proliferation of NIH3T3 cell lines that overexpress IRS-1 suggest that the drug itself may mediate at least some of these inhibitory effects on insulin signaling (145). However, there is no information available concerning the utility of other insulin-sensitizing strategies on the evolution of alcohol-related FLD.

Leptin and Alcoholic Fatty Liver Disease (see Chapter 17)

Interestingly, a few groups have reported that leptin levels are increased in rats that have ingested alcohol chronically (146), as well as in some patients with alcoholic cirrhosis (147,148). The benefits of leptin administration in lipodystrophic mice with insulin resistance and FLD (101) suggest that such alcohol-related increases in leptin might reflect the body's efforts to counterbalance the antiinsulin actions of TNFα. However, it is not clear whether alcohol also alters leptin receptor expression or function. If chronic alcohol exposure causes leptin resistance, then increases in leptin levels might be relatively inconsequential.

Indeed, indirect evidence suggests that alcohol-related increases in leptin expression are probably not accompanied by increases in leptin activity because despite increased leptin expression, rats that have ingested ethanol chronically are unusually vulnerable to LPS-induced liver injury (42). Thus, in this regard, ethanol-fed rats resemble both mice that are spontaneously leptin-deficient (20,31,36) and normal mice that are rendered leptin-resistant by treatment with leptin receptor antagonists. The possibility that leptin resistance might be one of the mechanisms that contributes to ethanol-related sensitivity to LPS is further supported by recent evidence that exogenous leptin protects leptin-deficient mice from LPS lethality (36).

THERAPY

Current treatment for FLD predominantly involves efforts to remove or reduce the two most obvious risk factors (i.e., alcohol abuse and obesity) that are commonly associated with this histopathology. Abstinence from alcohol is a cen-

tral component of treatment for all stages of alcohol-induced FLD. Indeed, sobriety improves the survival of both noncirrhotic and cirrhotic patients with alcoholic FLD (149,150). However, abstinence does not assure a good outcome for all patients with FLD caused by alcohol abuse. Complete recovery from hepatic steatosis occurs within 1 to 2 weeks of discontinuing alcohol ingestion. Liver damage resolves much more gradually (over months) in a minority of patients with alcohol-induced SH. However, in most patients who stop drinking after developing SH, hepatitis persists. At least one quarter of these individuals become cirrhotic within 5 years (150).

Similarly, weight loss is an imperfect "cure" for obesity-related FLD. Weight reduction is known to decrease serum aminotransferase values in some obese patients (151–153). However, rapid or extreme weight loss appears to promote the transition from steatosis to cirrhosis in others (34,154). Moreover, nutritional supplements have been shown to improve the rapid progression of FLD that occurs when jejuno-ileal bypass surgery is done to provoke weight loss in obese individuals (155,156). Thus, although there is little doubt that obesity is a risk factor for FLD, weight reduction is not always an effective treatment, and may even exacerbate this problem.

As discussed in previous sections, work with experimental animal models of FLD is beginning to suggest new therapeutic targets. In those systems, various strategies that decrease the absorption of intestinal endotoxin (32,33) or which prevent increases in the activity of TNFα (61,141), an endotoxin-inducible cytokine, inhibit alcohol-induced FLD (Table 50.5). However, apart from the proven utility of corticosteroids in highly selected subsets of patients with severe, acute alcohol-induced SH (reviewed in ref. 157), there is little information about the efficacy of any other antiinflammatory/anticytokine treatment in the prevention or treatment of alcoholic- or obesity-related FLD in humans. Nevertheless, it is important to acknowledge that oral antibiotics were reported to improve cholestasis in surgical patients receiving total parenteral nutrition (158), a known cause of FLD (159).

Increases in the hepatic production of ROS occur in experimental models of liver damage due to alcohol inges-

TABLE 50.5. POTENTIAL TREATMENTS FOR FATTY LIVER DISEASE

Rationale	Therapy
Prevent gut-derived endotoxemia	Antibiotics, lactobacillus
Inhibit TNFα activity	Anti-TNF antibodies, TNF receptor antagonists
Generalized inhibition of inflammation	Corticosteroids
Decrease ROS	GSH prodrugs (S-adenosyl-methionine, betaine, choline), vitamin E, silymarin, propylthiouracil
Reduce liver lipid content	Ursodeoxycholic acid, gemfibrozil
Improve insulin sensitivity	Leptin, troglitazone, metformin

GSH, glutathione; ROS, reactive oxygen species; TNFα, tumor necrosis factor α.

tion, endotoxin treatment, and obesity (see earlier sections). Treatment with various antioxidants (Table 50.5) decreases experimental, alcohol-induced liver damage (160–165) and improves the FLD that develops in rats fed choline- and methionine-deficient diets (160,166), but benefits have been inconsistent in the small groups of alcoholic patients with FLD who have been treated with similar agents (167–174). Fatty livers provide increased substrates for lipid peroxidation by ROS. Thus, treatments to reduce hepatic lipid content might be beneficial in patients with FLD. Benefits were reported in two patients with NASH who were treated with ursodeoxycholic acid (175), which is expected to increase the biliary excretion of lipids by improving bile flow. A small trial of the triglyceride-lowering agent gemfibrozil also showed some benefits in patients with nonalcoholic FLD (176).

As discussed earlier, insulin resistance is a prominent feature of many experimental models of FLD, and correlations between the severity of insulin resistance and FLD have been documented in humans (99). Moreover, treatments that improve hepatic insulin resistance reverse FLD in experimental animals (101) (Table 50.5). These results have encouraged clinicians to consider insulin-sensitizing drugs as potential treatments for NASH (177). On the other hand, enthusiasm is tempered by more widespread evidence that at least one of these agents (i.e., troglitazone) causes idiosyncratic acute liver failure (178).

CONCLUSION

FLD encompasses a spectrum of hepatic histopathology. Steatosis is the most common, earliest, and most benign stage of FLD. Although hepatocytes in fatty livers are viable, these cells have become more vulnerable to lethality from various secondary stresses. The cellular and molecular mechanisms underlying the vulnerability of fatty hepatocytes are not well understood, but appear to involve immunologic responses that modify the cytokine microenvironment within the liver. Changes in the cytokine milieu interfere with the actions of both exogenous factors, including insulin, and endogenous factors, such as the transcription factors PPARα and NFκβ, that are necessary for hepatocyte survival. This provokes adaptations in cellular organelles, such as peroxisomes and mitochondria, that regulate hepatic redox and energy homeostasis. Hepatocyte ATP depletion and necrosis are potentiated, and SH (hepatocyte death and an accompanying inflammatory response) develops following trivial challenges that are innocuous to nonsteatotic livers. The acute, clinical outcome of SH is dictated by the extent of hepatocyte loss and the severity of the associated inflammatory response. This more advanced stage of FLD is rarely fatal. In fact, SH is generally accompanied by only modest clinical and laboratory abnormalities. However, even when clinical evidence of liver damage

is quite subtle, smoldering SH promotes a fibrogenic response that gradually leads to cirrhosis in many individuals. Consequently, FLD is a common cause of cirrhosis. A better understanding of the mechanisms that are responsible for the initiation and progression of FLD is necessary to develop effective treatments for this type of liver disease.

REFERENCES

1. Ludwig J, Viggiano RT, McGill DB. Nonalcoholic steatohepatitis. Mayo Clinic experiences with a hitherto unnamed disease. *Mayo Clin Proc* 1980;55:342–348.
2. Sheth SG, Gordon FD, Chopar S. Nonalcoholic steatohepatitis. *Ann Intern Med* 1997;126:137–145.
3. Powell EE, Cooksley GE, Hanson R, et al. The natural history of nonalcoholic steatohepatitis: a follow-up study of 42 patients for up to 21 years. *Hepatology* 1990;11:74–80.
4. Bacon B, Faravash MJ, Janney CG, et al. Nonalcoholic steatohepatitis: an expanded clinical entity. *Gastroenterology* 1994;107:1103–1106.
5. Caldwell SH, Oelsner DH, Iezzoni JC, et al. Cryptogenic cirrhosis: clinical characterization and risk factors for underlying disease. *Hepatology* 1999;29:664–669.
6. Matteoni C, Younossi ZM, McCullough A. Nonalcoholic fatty liver disease: A spectrum of clinical pathological severity. *Gastroenterology* 1999;116:1413–1419.
7. Angulo P, Deach JC, Batts KP, et al. Independent predictors of liver fibrosis in patients with nonalcoholic steatohepatitis. *Hepatology* 1999;30(406A).
8. Nomura H, Kashiwagi S, Hayashi J, et al. Prevalence of fatty liver in a general population of Okinawa, Japan. *Jpn J Med* 1988;27:142–149.
9. Bizzaro N, Tremolada F, Casarin C, et al. Serum alanine aminotransferase levels among volunteer blood donors: effect of sex, alcohol intake and obesity. *Ital J Gastroenterol* 1992;24:237–241.
10. Bellentani S, Tiribelli C, Saccoccio G, et al. Prevalence of chronic liver disease in the general population of northern Italy: the Dyonisos study. *Hepatology* 1994;20:1442–1449.
11. Marchesini G, Brizi M, Morselli-Labate AM, et al. Association of nonalcoholic fatty liver disease with insulin resistance. *Am J Med* 1999;107:450–455.
12. el-Hassan AY, Ibrahim EM, al-Mulhim FA, et al. Fatty infiltration of the liver: analysis of prevalence, radiological and clinical features and influence on patient management. *Br J Radiol* 1992;65:774–778.
13. Hodgson M, Van Thiel DH, Goodman-Klein B. Obesity and hepatotoxin risk factors for fatty liver disease. *Br J Ind Med* 1991;48:690–695.
14. Wanless IR, Lentz JS. Fatty liver hepatitis (steatohepatitis) and obesity: an autopsy study with analysis of risk factors. *Hepatology* 1990;12:1106–1110.
15. Giraud NS, Borotto E, Aubert A, et al. Excess weight risk factor for alcoholic liver disease. *Hepatology* 1997;25:108–111.
16. Okolo PI, Diehl AM. Nonalcoholic steatohepatitis and focal fatty liver. In: Feldman M, Scharschmidt BF, Sleisenger MH, eds. *Sleisenger and Fordtran's gastrointestinal and liver disease,* 6th ed. Philadelphia: WB Saunders, 1998:1215–1220.
17. Czaja AJ, Carpenter HA, Santrach PJ, et al. Host- and disease-specific factors affecting steatosis in chronic hepatitis C. *J Hepatol* 1998;29:198–206.
18. Poupon RY, Serfaty LD, Amorim M, et al. Combination of steatosis and alcohol intake is the main determinant of fibrosis progression in patients with hepatitis C. *Hepatology* 1999;30:406A.

19. Chavin K, Yang SQ, Lin HZ, et al. Obesity induces expression of uncoupling protein-2 in hepatocytes and promotes liver ATP depletion. *J Biol Chem* 1999;274:5692–5700.

20. Faggioni R, Fantuzzi G, Gabay C, et al. Leptin deficiency enhances sensitivity to endotoxin-induced lethality. *Am J Physiol* 1999;276:R136–R142.

21. D'Alessandro AM, Kalayoglu M, Sollinger HW, et al. The predictive value of donor liver biopsy on the development of primary nonfunction after orthotopic liver transplantation. *Transplant Proc* 1991;23:1536–1537.

22. Gao W, Connor HD, Lemasters JJ, et al. Primary nonfunction of fatty livers produced by alcohol is associated with a new, antioxidant-insensitive free radical species. *Transplantation* 1995;59:674–679.

23. Leevy CM. Fatty liver: a study of 270 patients with biopsy proven fatty liver and a review of the literature. *Medicine (Baltimore)* 1962;4:249–258.

24. Teli M, James OF, Burt AD, et al. A natural history of nonalcoholic fatty liver: a follow-up study. *Hepatology* 1995;22:1714–1717.

25. Adler M, Schaffner F. Fatty liver hepatitis and cirrhosis in obese patients. *Am J Med* 1979;67:811–816.

26. Watanabe A, Kobayashi M, Yoshitomi S, et al. Liver fibrosis in obese patients with fatty liver. *J Med* 1989;20:357–362.

27. Randall B. Fatty liver and sudden death. a review. *Hum Pathol* 1980;11:167–173.

28. Campfield LA, Smith FJ, Burn P. The OB protein (leptin) pathway—a link between adipose tissue mass and central neural networks. *Horm Metab Res* 1996;28:619–632.

29. Lee GH, Proenca R, Montez JM, et al. Abnormal splicing of the leptin receptor in diabetic mice. *Nature* 1996;379:632–635.

30. Phillips MS, Liu Q, Hammond HA, et al. Leptin receptor missense mutation in the fatty Zucker rat. *Nat Genet* 1996;13:18–19.

31. Yang SQ, Lin HZ, Lane MD, et al. Obesity increases sensitivity to endotoxin liver injury: implications for pathogenesis of steatohepatitis. *Proc Natl Acad Sci U S A* 1997;94:2557–2562.

32. Nanji AA, Khettry U, Sadrzadeh SM. Lactobacillus feeding reduces endotoxemia and severity of experimental alcoholic liver disease. *Proc Soc Exp Biol Med* 1994;205:243–247.

33. Adachi Y, Moore LE, Bradford BU, et al. Antibiotics prevent liver injury in rats following longterm exposure to ethanol. *Gastroenterology* 1995;108:218–224.

34. Vyberg M, Ravn V, Andersen B. Patterns of progression of liver injury following jejunoileal bypass for morbid obesity. *Liver* 1987;7:271–276.

35. Requarth JA, Burchard KW, Colacchio TA, et al. Longterm morbidity following jejunoileal bypass. The continuing potential need for surgical reversal. *Arch Surg* 1995;130:318–325.

36. Takahashi N, Waelput W, Guisez Y. Leptin is an endogenous protective protein against the toxicity exerted by tumor necrosis factor. *J Exp Med* 1999;189:207–212.

37. Kern PA, Saghizadeh M, Ong JM, et al. The expression of tumor necrosis factor in human adipose tissue. Regulation by obesity, weight loss, and relationship to lipoprotein lipase. *J Clin Invest* 1995;95:2111–2119.

38. Yamakawa T, Tanaka S-I, Yamakawa T, et al. Augmented production of tumor necrosis factor α in obese mice. *Clin Immunol Immunopathol* 1995;75:51–56.

39. Hotamisligil GS, Peraldi SP, Budavari A, et al. IRS-1-mediated inhibition of insulin receptor tyrosine kinase activity in TNF-α- and obesity-induced insulin resistance. *Science* 1996;271:665–668.

40. Tracey KJ, Cerami A. Tumor necrosis factor, other cytokines and disease. *Annu Rev Cell Biol* 1993;9:317–343.

41. Loffreda S, Yang SQ, Lin HZ, et al. Leptin regulates proinflammatory immune responses. *FASEB J* 1998;12:57–65.

42. Honchel R, Ray RB, Marsano L, et al. Tumor necrosis factor in alcohol-enhanced endotoxin liver injury. *Alcohol Clin Exp Res* 1992;16:665–669.

43. Hansen J, Cherwitz DL, Allen JI. The role of tumor necrosis factor α in acute endotoxin-induced hepatotoxicity in ethanol-fed rats. *Hepatology* 1994;20:461–474.

44. Hishinuma I, Nagakawa J, Hirota K, et al. Tumor necrosis factor-α in galactosamine-induced hepatitis. *Hepatology* 1990;12:1187–1191.

45. Vassalli P. The pathophysiology of tumor necrosis factor. *Annu Rev Immunol* 1992;10:411–452.

46. Matsui K, Yoshimoto T, Tsutsui H, et al. Propionibacterium acnes treatment diminishes CD4+NK1.1+ T cells but induces type 1 T cells in the liver by induction of IL-12 and IL-18 production from Kupffer cells. *J Immunol* 1997;159:97–106.

47. Guebre-Xabier M, Yang SQ, Lin HZ, et al. Altered hepatic lymphocyte subpopulations in obesity-related fatty livers. *Hepatology* 1999;30:376A.

48. Lee F-Y, Li Y, Yang EK, et al. Phenotypic abnormalities in macrophages from leptin-deficient, obese mice. *Am J Physiol Cell Physiol* 1999;276:C386–C394.

49. Trinchieri G. Interleukin-12: A proinflammatory cytokine with immunoregulatory functions that bridge innate resistance and antigen-specific adaptive immunity. *Annu Rev Immunol* 1995;13:251–276.

50. Dinarello CA. IL-18: A TH1-inducing, proinflammatory cytokine and new member of the IL-1 family. *J Allergy Clin Immunol* 1999;103:11–24.

51. Emoto M, Emoto Y, Kaufmann SH. IL-4 producing CD4+TCR α β int liver lymphocytes: influence of thymus, β 2-microglobulin and NK1.1 expression. *Int Immunol* 1995;7:1729–1739.

52. Kawamura T, Takeda K, Mendiratta SK, et al. Critical role of NK1+T cells in IL-12-induced immune responses *in vivo. J Immunol* 1998;160:16–19.

53. Leist M, Cantner F, Bohlinger I, et al. Murine hepatocyte apoptosis induced *in vitro* and *in vivo* by TNF-α requires transcriptional arrest. *J Immunol* 1994;153:1778–1788.

54. Feingold KR, Soued M, Grunfeld C. Tumor necrosis factor stimulates DNA synthesis in the liver of intact rats. *Biochem Biophys Res Commun* 1988;153:576–582.

55. Beyer HS, Stanley M, Theologides, A. Tumor necrosis factor-α increases hepatic DNA and RNA and hepatocyte mitosis. *Biochem Int* 1990;22:405–410.

56. Akerman P, Cote P, Yang SQ, et al. Antibodies to tumor necrosis factor α inhibit liver regeneration after partial hepatectomy. *Am J Physiol* 1992;263:G579–G585.

57. Diehl AM, Yin M, Fleckenstein J, et al. Tumor necrosis factor α induces c-jun during the regenerative response to liver injury. *Am J Physiol* 1994;267:G552–G561.

58. Yamada Y, Kirillova I, Peschon JJ, et al. Initiation of liver growth by tumor necrosis factor: deficient liver regeneration in mice lacking type I tumor necrosis factor receptor. *Proc Natl Acad Sci* 1997;94:1441–1446.

59. Yamada Y, Weber EM, Kirillova I, et al. Analysis of liver regeneration in mice lacking type 1 or type 2 tumor necrosis factor receptor: requirement for type 1 but not type 2 receptor. *Hepatology* 1998;28:959–970.

60. Leist M, Gantner F, Jilg S, et al. Activation of the 55 kd TNF receptor is necessary and sufficient for TNF-induced liver failure, hepatocyte apoptosis, and nitrite release. *J Immunol* 1995;154:1307–1316.

61. Yin M, Wheeler MD, Kono H, et al. Essential role of tumor

necrosis factor α in alcohol-induced liver injury in mice. *Gastroenterology* 1999;117:942–952.

62. Smith CA, Farrah T, Goodwin RG. The TNF receptor superfamily of cellular and viral proteins: activation, costimulation, and death. *Cell* 1994;76:959–962.

63. Heller RA, Kronke M. Tumor necrosis factor receptor-mediated signaling pathways. *J Cell Biol* 1994;126:5–9.

64. Baker SJ, Reddy EP. Transducers of life and death: TNF receptor superfamily and associated proteins. *Oncogene* 1996;12:1–9.

65. Magnusson C, Vaux DL. Signaling by CD95 and TNF receptors: not only life and death. *Immunol Cell Biol* 1999;77:41–46.

66. Goossens V, Grooten J, De Vos K, et al. Direct evidence for tumor necrosis factor-induced mitochondrial reactive oxygen intermediates and their involvement in cytotoxicity. *Proc Natl Acad Sci U S A* 1995;92:8115–8119.

67. Kroemer G, Dallaporta B, Resche-rignon M. The mitochondrial death/life regulator in apoptosis and necrosis. *Ann Rev Physiol* 1998;60:619–642.

68. Schulze-Osthoff K, Bakker AC, Vanhaesebroeck B, et al. Cytotoxic activity of tumor necrosis factor is mediated by early damage of mitochondrial functions. Evidence for the involvement of mitochondrial radical generation. *J Biol Chem* 1992;267:5317–5323.

69. Schulze-Osthoff K, Beyaert R, Vandevoorde V, et al. Depletion of the mitochondrial electron transport abrogates the cytotoxic and gene-inductive effects of TNF. *EMBO J* 1993;12:3095–3104.

70. Pastorino JG, Simbula G, Yamamoto K, et al. The cytotoxicity of tumor necrosis factor depends on induction of the mitochondrial permeability transition. *J Biol Chem* 1996;271:29792–29798.

71. Higuchi M, Aggarwal BB, Yeh ET. Activation of CPP32-like protease in tumor necrosis factor-induced apoptosis is dependent on mitochondrial function. *J Clin Invest* 1997;99:1751–1758.

72. Beg AA, Finco TS, Nantermet PV, et al. Tumor necrosis factor and interleukin-1 lead to phosphorylation and loss of I κ B α: a mechanisms for NF κ B activation. *Mol Cell Biol* 1993;13:3301–3310.

73. Kelliher MA, Grimm S, Ishida Y, et al. The death domain kinase RIP mediates the TNF-induced NF-κB signal. *Immunity* 1998;8:297–303.

74. Tamatani M, Che YH, Matsuzaki H, et al. Tumor necrosis factor induces Bcl-2 and Bcl-x expression through NFκB activation in primary hippocampal neurons. *J Biol Chem* 1999;274:8531–8538.

75. Van Antwerp DJ, Martin SJ, Kafri T, et al. Suppression of TNF-α-induced apoptosis by NF-κ B. *Science* 1996;274:784–787.

76. Wang CY, Mayo MW, Baldwin ASJ. TNF- and cancer therapy-induced apoptosis: potentiation by inhibition of NF-κ B. *Science* 1996;274:784–787.

77. Zong WX, Edelstein LC, Chen C, et al. The prosurvival Bcl-2 homolog Bfl-1/A1 is a direct transcriptional target of NF-κB that blocks TNFα-induced apoptosis. *Genes Dev* 1999;13:382–387.

78. Bohlinger I, Leist M, Barsig J, et al. Interleukin-1 and nitric oxide protect against tumor necrosis factor α-induced liver injury through distinct pathways. *Hepatology* 1995;22:1829–1837.

79. Manna SK, Zhang HJ, Yan T, et al. Overexpression of manganese superoxide dismutase suppresses tumor necrosis factor-induced apoptosis and activation of nuclear transcription factor-κ B and activated protein-1. *J Biol Chem* 1998;273:13245–13254.

80. Schutze S, Potthoff K, Machleidt T, et al. TNF activates NF-kB by phosphatidylcholine-specific phospholipase C-induced "acidic" sphygomyelin breakdown. *Cell* 1992;71:765–776.

81. Yeh WC, Shahinian A, Speiser D, et al. Early lethality, functional NF-κ B activation, and increased sensitivity to TNF-induced cell death in TRAF-2-deficient mice. *Immunity* 1997;7:715–725.

82. Yang SQ, Li Y, Lin HZ, et al. Mitochondrial adaptations to chronic oxidative stress in obesity-related fatty livers. *Arch Biochem Biophys* 2000;378:259–268.

83. Rashid A, Wu T-C, Huang CC, et al. Mitochondrial proteins that regulate apoptosis and necrosis are induced in mouse fatty liver. *Hepatology* 1999;29:1131–1138.

84. Kim YM, Lee BS, Yi KY, et al. Upstream Nf-κB site is required for the maximal expression of mouse inducible nitric oxide synthase gene in interferon-γ plus lipopolysaccharide-induced RAW 264.7 macrophages. *Biochem Biophys Res Commun* 1997;236:655–660.

85. Kim YM, Talanian RV, Billiar TR. Nitric oxide inhibits apoptosis by preventing increases in caspase-3-like activity via two distinct mechanisms. *J Biol Chem* 1997;272:31138–31148.

86. Surwit RS, Wang S, Petro AE, et al. Diet-induced changes in uncoupling proteins in obesity-prone and obesity-resistant strains of mice. *Proc Natl Acad Sci U S A* 1998;95:4061–4065.

87. Boss O, Bobbioni-Harsch E, Assimacopoulos-Jeannet F, et al. Uncoupling protein-3 expression in skeletal muscle and free fatty acids in obesity. *Lancet* 1998;351:1933.

88. Wiegle DS, Selfridge LI, Schwartz MW, et al. Elevated free fatty acids induce uncoupling protein 3 expression in muscle: a potential explanation for the effect of fasting. *Diabetes* 1998;47:298–302.

89. Cortez-Pinto H, Lin HZ, Yang SQ, et al. Lipids upregulate uncoupling protein-2 expression in hepatocytes. *Gastroenterology* 1999 (in press).

90. Ricquier D, Casteilla L, Bouillaud F. Molecular studies of the uncoupling protein. *FASEB J* 1991;5:2237–2242.

91. Boss O, Muzzin P, Giacobino JP. The uncoupling proteins, a review. *Eur J Endocrinol* 1998;139:1–9.

92. Cope K, Risby T, Diehl AM. Increased gastrointestinal ethanol production in obese mice: implications for fatty liver disease pathogenesis. *Gastroenterology* 2000;119:1340–1347.

93. Mezey E, Imbembo AL, Potter JJ, et al. Endogenous ethanol production and hepatic disease following jejunoileal bypass for morbid obesity. *Am J Clin Nutr* 1975;28:1277–1283.

94. Baraona E, Julkunen R, Tannenbaum L, et al. Role of intestinal bacterial overgrowth in ethanol production and metabolism in rats. *Gastroenterology* 1986;90:103–110.

95. Uysal KT, Wiesbrock SM, Marino MW, et al. Protection from obesity-induced insulin-resistance in mice lacking TNF α function. *Nature* 1997;389:610–614.

96. Valverde AM, Teruel T, Navarro P, et al. Tumor necrosis factor-α causes insulin receptor substrate-2-mediated insulin resistance and inhibits insulin-induced adipogenesis in fetal brown adipocytes. *Endocrinology* 1998;139:1229–1238.

97. Moller DE, Flier JS. Insulin resistance. Mechanisms, syndromes, and implications. *N Engl J Med* 1991;325:938–948.

98. Diamond RH, Du HK, Lee V, et al. Novel delayed-early and highly insulin-induced growth response genes. *J Biol Chem* 1993;268:15185–15192.

99. Marceau P, Biron S, Hould FS, et al. Liver pathology and the metabolic syndrome X in severe obesity. *J Clin Endocrinol Metab* 1999;84:1513–1517.

100. Shimomura I, Hammer RE, Richardson JA, et al. Insulin resistance and diabetes mellitus in transgenic mice expressing nuclear SREP-1c in adipose tissue: model for congenital generalized lipodystrophy. *Genes Dev* 1998;12:3182–3194.

101. Shimomura I, Hammer RE, Ikemoto S, et al. Leptin reverses insulin resistance and diabetes mellitus in mice with congenital lipodystrophy. *Nature* 1999;401:73–76.

102. Dagogo-Jack S, Santiago JV. Pathophysiology of type 2 diabetes and modes of action of therapeutic interventions. *Arch Intern Med* 1997;157:1802–1807.

103. Wiernsperger NF, Bailey CJ. The antihyperglycaemic effect of metformin: therapeutic and cellular mechanisms. *Drugs* 1999; 58:31–39.

104. Shulman GI. Cellular mechanisms of insulin resistance in humans. *Am J Cardiol* 1999;84:3J–10J.

104a. Lin HZ, Yang SQ, Chuckaree C, et al. Metformin treatment reverses fatty liver disease in obese, leptin-deficient mice. *Nature Medicine* 2000;6:998–1003.

105. Cortez-Pinto H, Yang SQ, Lin HZ, et al. Bacterial lipopolysaccharide induces uncoupling protein-2 in hepatocytes via a tumor necrosis α-dependent mechanism. *Biochem Biophys Res Commun* 1998;251:313–319.

106. Lieber CS, DeCarli LM. The feeding of alcohol in liquid diets: two decades of applications and 1982 update. *Alcohol Clin Exp Res* 1982;6:523–531.

107. Tsukamoto H, Towner SJ, Ciofalo LM, et al. Ethanol-induced liver fibrosis in rats fed high-fat diets. *Hepatology* 1986;6: 814–822.

108. Lieber C. Hepatic, metabolic and toxic effect of ethanol. 1991 update. *Alcohol Clin Exp Res* 1991;15:573–592.

109. Crabb DW. Ethanol oxidizing enzymes: roles in alcohol metabolism and alcoholic liver disease. *Prog Liver Dis* 1995;13: 151–172.

110. Gergel D, Misik V, Riesz P, Cederbaum AI. Inhibition of rat and human cytochrome P4502E1 catalytic activity and reactive oxygen radical formation by nitric oxide. *Arch Biochem Biophys* 1997;337:239–250.

111. Lieber CS. Biochemical factors in alcoholic liver disease. *Semin Liver Dis* 1993;13:136–147.

112. Nanji AA, Zhao S, Sadrzadeh SMH, et al. Markedly enhanced cytochrome P450 2E1 induction and lipid peroxidation is associated with severe liver injury in fish oil-ethanol-fed rats. *Alcohol Clin Exp Res* 1994;18:1280–1285.

113. Wu D, Cederbaum AI. Ethanol-induced apoptosis to stable HepG2 cell lines expressing human cytochrome P-4502E1. *Alcohol Clin Exp Res* 1999;23:67–76.

114. Puntarulo S, Cederbau AI. Role of cytochrome P-450 in the stimulation of microsomal production of reactive oxygen species by ferritin. *Biochim Biophys Acta* 1996;1289:238–246.

115. Tsukamoto H, Horne W, Kamimura S, et al. Experimental liver cirrhosis induced by alcohol and iron. *J Clin Invest* 1995;96: 620–630.

116. Dai N, Zeng M, Li J. Correlation between hepatocyte cytochrome P450IIE1 expression and oxidation, antioxidation in rat nonalcoholic steatosis model. *Chung Hua Kan Tsang Ping Tsa Chih* 1999;7:104–106.

117. Weltman MD, Farrell GC, Hall P, et al. Hepatic cytochrome P450 2E1 is increased in patients with nonalcoholic steatohepatitis. *Hepatology* 1998;27:128–133.

118. Koop DR, Klopfenstein B, Iimuro Y, et al. Gadolinium chloride blocks alcohol-dependent liver toxicity in rats treated chronically with intragastric alcohol despite the induction of Cyp2E1. *Mol Pharmacol* 1997;51:944–950.

119. Leclercq I, Horsmans Y, Desager JP, et al. Reduction in hepatic cytochrome P-450 is correlated to the degree of liver fat content in animal models of steatosis in the absence of inflammation. *J Hepatol* 1998;28:410–416.

120. Tsukada H, Wang PY, Kaneko T, Wang Y, Nakano M, Sato A. Dietary carohydrate intake plays an important role in preventing alcoholic fatty liver in the rat. *J Hepatol* 1998;29:715–724.

121. Roe AL, Howard G, Blouin R, et al. Characterization of cytochrome P450 and glutathione S-transferase activity and expression in male and female ob/ob mice. *Int J Obese Relat Metab Disord* 1999;23:48–53.

122. Enriquez A, Leclercq I, Farrell GC, et al. Altered expression of hepatic Cyp2E1 and Cyp4A in obese, diabetic ob/ob mice, and

fa/fa Zucker rats. *Biochem Biophys Res Commun* 1999;255: 300–306.

123. Shedlofsky SL, Swim AT, Robinson JM, et al. Interelukin-1 (IL-1) depresses cytochrome P450 levels and activities in mice. *Life Sci* 1987;40:2331–2336.

124. Jump DB, Thelen A, Mater M. Dietary polyunsaturated fatty acids and hepatic gene expression. *Lipids* 1999;34:S209–S212.

125. Moya-Camarena SY, Van den Heuvel JP, Belury MA. Conjugated linoleic acid activates peroxisome proliferator-activated receptor α and β subtypes but does not induce hepatic peroxisome proliferation in Sprague–Dawley rats. *Biochim Biophys Acta* 1999;1436:331–342.

126. Asayama K, Sandhir R, Sheikh FG, et al. Increased peroxisomal fatty acid β-oxidation and enhanced expression of peroxisome proliferator-activated receptor-α in diabetic rat liver. *Mol Cell Biochem* 1999;194:227–234.

127. Hashimoto T, Fujita T, Usuda N, et al. Peroxisomal and mitochondrial fatty acid β-oxidation in mice nullizygous for both peroxsome proliferator-activated receptor α and peroxisomal fatty acyl-CoA oxidase. Genotype correlation with fatty liver phenotype. *J Biol Chem* 1999;273:19228–19236.

128. Motojima K, Passilly P, Peters JM, et al. Expression of putative fatty acid transporter genes are regulated by peroxisome proliferator-activated receptor α and γ activators in a tissue- and inducer-specific manner. *J Biol Chem* 1998;273:16710–16714.

129. Leone TC, Weinheimer CJ, Kelly DP. A critical role for the peroxisome proliferator-activated receptor α (PPARα) in the cellular fasting response: the PPARα-null mouse as a model of fatty acid oxidation disorders. *Proc Natl Acad Sci U S A* 1999;96: 7473–7478.

130. Fan CY, Pan J, Chu R, et al. Hepatocellular and hepatic peroxisomal alterations in mice with a disrupted peroxisomal fatty acyl-coenzyme A oxidase gene. *J Biol Chem* 1996;271:24698–24710.

131. Roberts RA, James NH, Woddyatt NJ, et al. Evidence for the suppression of apoptosis by the peroxisome proliferator-activated receptor α (PPAR α). *Carcinogenesis* 1998;19:43–48.

132. Rolfe M, James NH, Roberts RA. Tumour necrosis factor α (TNF α) suppresses apoptosis and induces DNA synthesis in rodent hepatocytes: a mediator of the hepatocarcinogenicity of peroxisome proliferators? *Carcinogenesis* 1997;18:2277–2280.

133. Delerive P, De bosscher K, Besnard S, et al. Peroxisome proliferator-activated receptor α negatively regulates the vascular inflammatory gene response by negative cross-talk with transcription factors NF-κ B and AP-1. *J Biol Chem* 1999;274:32048–32054.

134. Iimuro Y, Nishiura T, Hellerbrand C, et al. NF κ B prevents apoptosis and liver dysfunction during liver regeneration. *J Clin Invest* 1998;101:802–811.

135. Beier K, Volkl A, Fahimi HD. TNF-α downregulates the peroxisome peroliferator-activated receptor-α and the mRNAs encoding peroxomal proteins in rat liver. *FEBS Lett* 1997;412:385–387.

136. Palmer CN, Hsu MH, Griffin KJ, et al. Peroxisome proliferator-activated receptor-α expression in human liver. *Mol Pharmacol* 1998;53:14–22.

137. Wan YJ, Morimoto M, Thurman RG, et al. Expression of the peroxisome proliferator-activated receptor gene is decreased in experimental alcoholic liver disease. *Life Sci* 1995;56:307–317.

138. McClain CJ, Hill DB, Schmidt J, et al. Cytokines and alcoholic liver disease. *Semin Liver Dis* 1993;13:170–182.

139. Bjarnason I, Waard K, Peters TJ. The leaky Gut of alcoholism: possible route of entry for toxic compounds. *Lancet* 1984;1: 179–182.

140. Kamimura S, Tsukamoto H. Cytokine gene expression by Kupffer cells in experimental alcoholic liver disease. *Hepatology* 1995;22:1304–1309.

141. Iimuro Y, Gallucci RM, Luster MI, et al. Antibodies to tumor necrosis factor α attenuates hepatic necrosis and inflammation

caused by chronic exposure to ethanol in the rat. *Hepatology* 1997;26:1530–1537.

142. Sasaki Y, Hayashi N, Ito T, et al. Influence of ethanol on insulin receptor substrate-1-mediated signal transduction during rat liver regeneration. *Alcohol Alcohol* 1994;29:99–106.

143. Sasaki Y, Wands JR. Ethanol impairs insulin receptor substrate-1 mediated signal transduction during rat liver regeneration. *Biochem Biophys Res Commun* 1994;199:403–409.

144. Mohr L, Tanaka S, Wands JR. Ethanol inhibits hepatocyte proliferation in insulin receptor substrate 1 transgenic mice. *Gastroenterology* 1998;115:1158–1165.

145. de la Monte SM, Ganju N, Tanaka S, et al. Differential effects of ethanol on insulin-signaling through the insulin receptor substrate-1. *Alcohol Clin Exp Res* 1999;23:770–777.

146. Lin HZ, Yang SQ, Zeldin G, et al. Chronic ethanol consumption induces the production of tumor necrosis factor-α and related cytokines in liver and adipose tissue. *Alcohol Clin Exp Res* 1998;22:231S–247S.

147. Henriksen JH, Holst JJ, Moller S, et al. Increased circulating leptin in alcoholic cirrhosis: relation to release and disposal. *Hepatology* 1999;29:1818–1824.

148. McCullough AJ, Bugianesi E, Marchesini G, Kalhan SC. Gender-dependent alterations in serum leptin in alcoholic cirrhosis. *Gastroenterology* 1998;115:947–953.

149. Galambos J. Natural history of alcoholic hepatitis III: histologic changes. *Gastroenterology* 1972;56:515–522.

150. Pares A, Caballeria J, Brugera M. Histologic course of alcoholic hepatitis: influence of abstinence, sex, and extent of hepatic damage. *J Hepatol* 1986;2:33–38.

151. Eriksson S, Eriksson KF, Bondesson L. Nonalcoholic steatohepatitis in obesity: a reversible condition. *Acta Med Scand* 1986;220:83–88.

152. Palmer M, Schaffner F. Effect of weight reduction on hepatic abnormalities in overweight patients. *Gastroenterology* 1990;99:1408–1411.

153. Ueno T, Sugawara H, Sujaku K, et al. Therapeutic effects of restricted diet and exercise in obese patients with fatty liver. *J Hepatol* 1997;27:103–107.

154. Capron JP, Delamarre M, Dupas JL, et al. Fasting in obesity: another cause of liver injury with alcoholic hyaline? *Dig Dis Sci* 1982;54:374–377.

155. Moxley RT, Posefsky T, Lockwood DH. Protein nutrition and liver disease after jejunoileal bypass for morbid obesity. *N Engl J Med* 1974;290:921–925.

156. Heimburger SL, Seiger E, Logerfo P, et al. Reversal of severe fatty hepatic infiltration after jejunoileal bypass for morbid obesity by calorie-free amino acid infusion. *Am J Surg* 1975;129:70–78.

157. Imperiale TF, McCullough AJ. Do corticosteroids reduce mortality from alcoholic hepatitis? A meta-analysis of the randomized trials. *Ann Intern Med* 1990;113:299–300.

158. Capron JP, Herve MA, Ginestron JL, et al. Metronidazole in prevention of cholestasis associated with total parenteral nutrition. *Lancet* 1983;1:446–449.

159. Fouin-Fortenet H, LeQuernec L, Erlinger S, et al. Hepatic alterations during total parenteral nutrition in patients with inflammatory bowel disease: A possible consequence of lithocholate toxicity. *Gastroenterology* 1982;82:932–938.

160. Feo F, Pascale R, Garcea R, et al. Effect of the variations of S-adenosyl-L-methionine liver content on fat accumulation and ethanol metabolism in ethanol-intoxicated rats. *Toxicol Appl Pharmacol* 1986;83:331–341.

161. Lieber SC, Casini A, DeCarli LM, et al. S-adenosyl-L-methionine attenuates alcohol-induced liver injury in the baboon. *Hepatology* 1990;11:165–172.

162. Garcia-Ruiz C, Morales A, Coleli A, et al. Feeding S-Adenosyl-L-Methionine attenuates both ethanol-induced depletion of mitochondrial glutathione and mitochondrial dysfunction in perioportal and perivenous rat hepatocytes. *Hepatology* 1995;21:207–214.

163. Nanji AA, Yang EK, Fogt F, et al. Medium chain triglycerides and vitamin E reduce the severity of established experimental alcoholic liver disease. *J Pharmacol Exp Ther* 1996;277:1694–1700.

164. Barak AJ, Beckenhauer HC, Badakhsh S, et al. The effect of betaine in reversing alcoholic steatosis. *Alcohol Clin Exp Res* 1997;21:1100–1102.

165. Sadrzadeh SM, Nanji AA. The 21-aminosteroid 16-desmethyl tirilazad mesylate prevents necroinflammatory changes in experimental alcoholic liver disease. *J Pharmacol Exp Ther* 1998;284:406–412.

166. Weltman MD, Farrell GC, Liddle C. Increased hepatocyte CYP2E1 expression in a rat nutritional model of hepatic steatosis with inflammation. *Gastroenterology* 1996;111:1645–1653.

167. Orrego H, Kalant H, Israel Y, et al. Effect of shortterm therapy with propylthiouracil in patients with alcoholic liver disease. *Gastroenterology* 1979;75:105–112.

168. Orrego H, Blade JE, Blendis LM, et al. Longterm treatment of alcoholic liver disease with propylthiouracil. *N Engl J Med* 1987;317:1421–1425.

169. Ferenci P, Dragosics B, Dittrich H, et al. Randomized controlled trial of silymarin treatment in patients with cirrhosis of the liver. *J Hepatol* 1989;9:105–113.

170. Vendemiale G, Altomare E, Trizio T, et al. Effects of oral S-adenosyl-L-methionine on hepatic glutathione in patients with liver disease. *Scand J Gastroenterol* 1989;24:407–415.

171. de la Maza MP, Petermann M, Bunout D, et al. Effects of longterm vitamin E supplementation in alcoholic cirrhotics. *J Am Coll Nutr* 1995;14:192–196.

172. Feher J, Lengyel G, Blazovics A. Oxidative stress in the liver and biliary tract diseases. *Scand J Gastroenterol* 1998;228:38–46.

173. Velussi M, Cernigoi AM, De monte A, et al. Longterm treatment with an antioxidant drug (silymarin) is effective on hyperinsulinemia, exogenous insulin need and malondialdehyde levels in cirrhotic diabetic patients. *J Hepatol* 1997;26:871–879.

174. Pares A, Planas R, Torres M, et al. Effects of silymarin in alcoholic patients with cirrhosis of the liver: results of a controlled, double-blind, randomized and multicenter trial. *J Hepatol* 1998;28:615–621.

175. Abdelmalek M, Ludwig J, Lindor K. Two cases from the spectrum of nonalcoholic steatohepatitis. *Clin Gastroenterology* 1995;20:127–130.

176. Basaranoglu M, Acbay O, Sonsuz A. A controlled trial of gemfibrozil in the treatment of patients with nonalcoholic steatohepatitis. *J Hepatol* 1999;31:384.

177. Krentz AJ. Nonalcoholic steatohepatitis. *Lancet* 1999;354:1300.

178. Kohlroser J, Mathai J, Reichheld J, et al. Hepatotoxicity due to troglitazone: report of two cases and review of adverse events reported to the United States Food and Drug Administration. *Am J Gastroenterol* 2000;95:272–276.

SCHISTOSOMIASIS: A MODEL OF IMMUNOLOGICALLY MEDIATED LIVER DISEASE

MIGUEL J. STADECKER
HECTOR J. HERNANDEZ

Schistosomes, the causative agents of schistosomiasis, are blood-dwelling trematode helminths which possess a complex life cycle that makes use of humans, among many vertebrates, as permanent hosts, and aquatic snails as intermediate hosts. Schistosomiasis is a major tropical infectious parasitic disease that rightly earned its place in books on liver pathobiology because some schistosome species precipitate a fierce, potentially lethal immunopathological reaction in the hepatic microvasculature.

There is an exquisite species specificity in schistosomiasis, in that individual schistosome species can only successfully complete their life cycles and produce pathology in the appropriate permanent or intermediate hosts. There is also rigorous anatomic specificity in that the final habitat of the adult parasites and site of pathology are predetermined in each case. Thus, *Schistosoma mansoni* and *Schistosoma japonicum* are the two major pathogenic hepatotropic species in humans.

THE PATHOBIOLOGY OF SCHISTOSOMIASIS

Infection with schistosomes occurs in contaminated fresh waters where free-swimming cercariae, emanating from parasitized snails, actively penetrate the human skin. Over the next several weeks, and without causing symptoms, the developing parasites (schistosomula) migrate to the lung, gain access to the systemic circulation and, responding to as yet completely unknown signals, reach and recognize their final habitat in the portal–mesenteric venous circulation. Here female and male schistosomes acquire sexual maturity, leading to copious oviposition for prolonged periods of time. The resulting parasite eggs can exit the vascular stream and, taking advantage of the host's granulomatous inflammatory reaction, perforate the debilitated neighboring intestinal wall with the purpose of returning to the bodies of fresh water and perpetuating the life cycle; alternatively, eggs are swept downstream into the liver, where they lodge in the small portal vein radicals and die within a few days. In the liver, the eggs precipitate an even stronger inflammatory granulomatous response. Granulomas are more or less circumscribed spheroidal perioval aggregates of inflammatory cells, composed chiefly of macrophages, lymphocytes and eosinophils, all embedded in an increasingly collagenized extracellular matrix. The progressive accumulation of broad bands of scar tissue, sometimes adopting the form of "clay-pipe stem" fibrosis, gradually restricts the blood flow through the liver, leading to portal hypertension and the development of splenomegaly, portal-systemic shunting and significant collateral circulation. Eventually there is ascites, cachexia, gastrointestinal bleeding, and death. It becomes obvious that whereas the worms themselves elicit little if any tissue reaction, it is the eggs that are responsible for the severe pathology and characteristic clinical picture in schistosomiasis.

M. J. Stadecker: Department of Pathology, Tufts University School of Medicine, Department of Pathology, New England Medical Center, Boston, Massachusetts 02111.

H. J. Hernandez: Department of Pathology, Tufts University School of Medicine, Boston, Massachusetts 02111.

Interestingly, not all patients with schistosomiasis undergo the ominous course described above; in fact, only a minority does. Most patients instead suffer from a milder disease, characterized by intermittent abdominal pain and diarrhea, which is compatible with a relatively productive life. Clinically there is a spectrum of disease; however, there are two relatively well-recognized polar forms. The severe form of disease has been termed hepatosplenic schistosomiasis, and the milder form is known as intestinal schistosomiasis. The reason for the wide range of disease severity is not known precisely, but apparently depends mostly on host genetic factors (1,2) rather than on the load of infecting schistosomes (worm

burden) or their strains, or on environmental factors. The key issue is that individuals with mild intestinal schistosomiasis seem to be able to effectively curtail the magnitude of the immunopathological damage triggered by the parasite eggs.

THE BASIS OF THE EGG-INDUCED IMMUNOPATHOLOGY

Important for the understanding of schistosomal disease is the notion that the inflicted tissue damage is caused by an immunopathological reaction against highly immunogenic

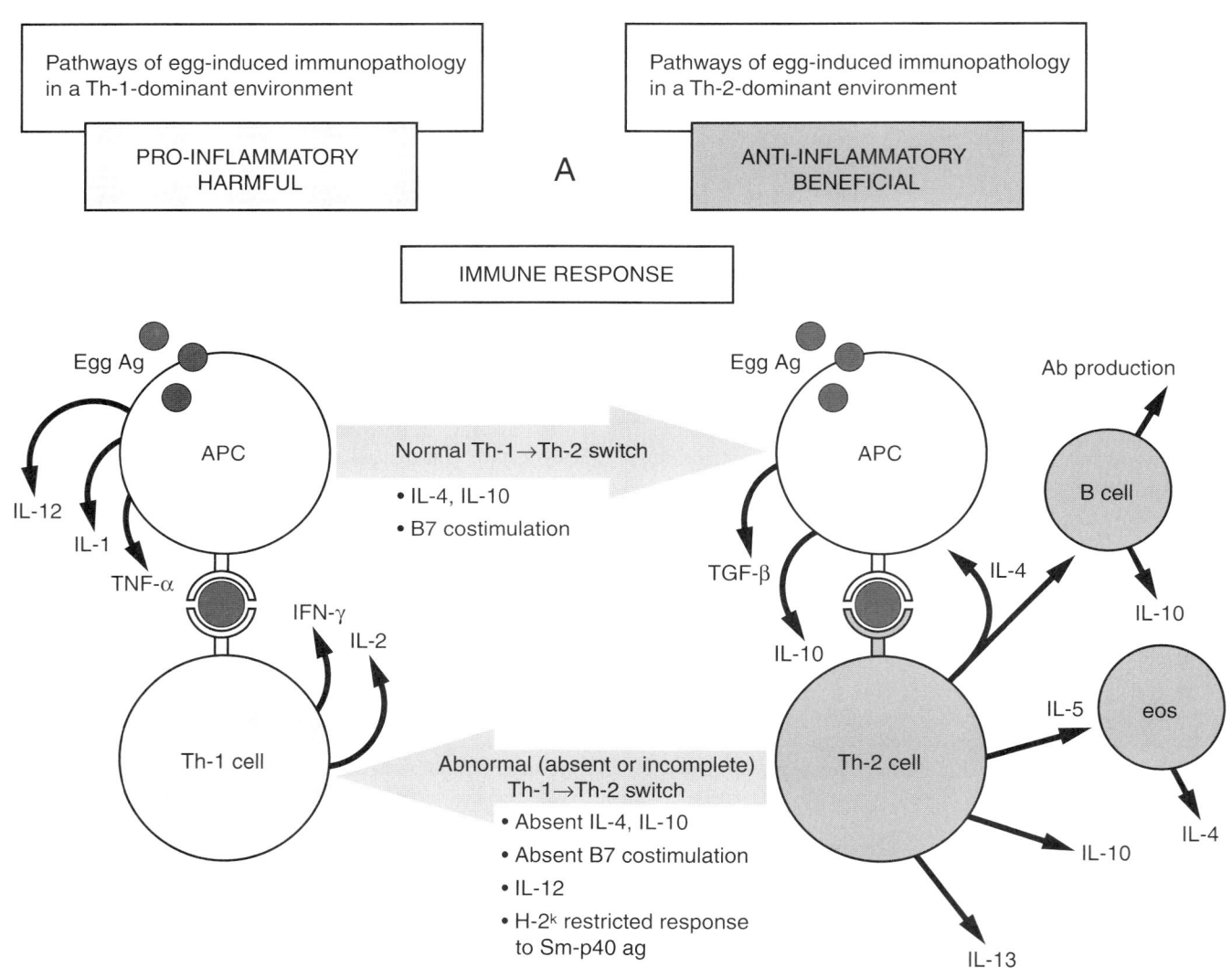

A

FIGURE 51.1. Pathways of schistosome egg-induced immunopathology in Th-1 or Th-2-dominant environments. **A:** Cells and signature cytokines characteristic of the initial immune response, which is of the Th-1-type (**left**). Normally, the Th-1 response switches to a Th-2 response, similarly marked by characteristic cells and cytokines (**right**). In certain circumstances, the Th-1 → Th-2 switch fails, or materializes incompletely. Factors facilitating or opposing the switch are indicated. **B:** The pathology in mice and humans, with examples, that results in each case. *APC*, antigen-presenting cell; *eos*, eosinophil; *egg ag*, egg antigen; *ab*, antibody.

egg products. By comparison, the immune response against the helminths themselves, remarkably, is as ineffective as it is nonpathogenic, allowing each worm virtually unperturbed parasitism for many years. As is the case in humans, the mouse is also susceptible to infection with *S. mansoni* or *S. japonicum* and similarly develops hepato-intestinal egg granulomas and several of the other subsequent manifestations of pathology. This established an invaluable model to document and study the immune basis of the pathological events. In particular, the experimental murine infection with *S. mansoni* has facilitated the examination, with great detail, of some of the cellular, subcellular and humoral components of the host's immune and inflammatory responses against the parasite eggs, as well as some of the egg molecules that are the target of the host's immunopathogenic response.

Since the 1970s it has been known that athymic mice fail to develop egg granulomas (3), which pointed at T lymphocytes as mediators of granuloma formation. Subsequently, as subpopulations of T cells were discovered, it became apparent that granulomas are mediated by MHC

class II-restricted CD4+ T helper (Th) cells sensitized to typically "exogenous" egg antigens (4,5); CD8+ T cells, as well as γδ-T cells are ineffective (5,6). Granuloma formation cannot singly be attributed to either the Th-1-type [interferon-γ (IFN-γ) and interleukin (IL-2)-producing], or the Th-2-type (IL-4, IL-5, IL-10 and IL-13-producing) CD4+ Th cells, as both subpopulations can respond to stimulation with schistosomal egg antigens (SEA). In fact, there is presently abundant evidence suggesting that egg granulomas can be formed in environments dominated by either Th-1- or Th-2-type cytokines (7–9) (Fig. 51.1A,B and Fig. 51.2).

As do humans, mouse strains exhibit considerable variation in immune response and immunopathology to infection with schistosomes (see later). Nevertheless, as a rule, following egg laying, there is an early temporary prevailing Th-1-type cytokine response which lasts less than two weeks and is normally superseded by a Th-2-polarized response (10) (Fig. 51.1A). Egg laying by itself promotes the Th-1 → Th-2 cytokine switch (8); however, other forces involved in the immune response also play a

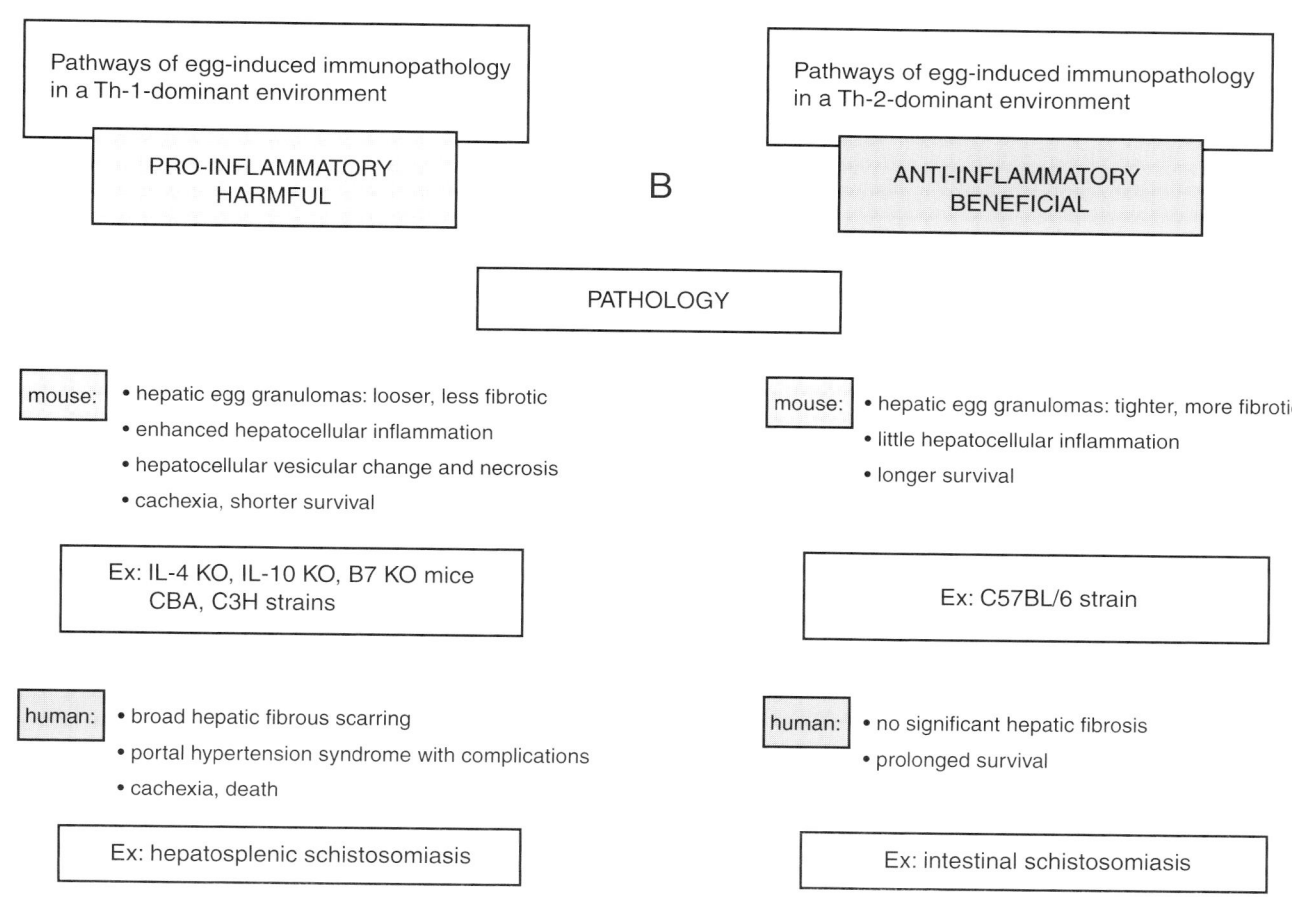

FIGURE 51.1. B. See legend on page 756.

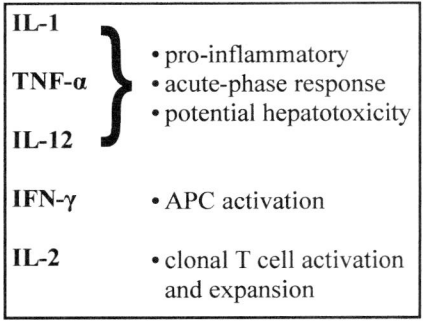

Th-1-type pro-inflammatory
cytokines

IL-1	}	• pro-inflammatory • acute-phase response • potential hepatotoxicity
TNF-α		
IL-12		
IFN-γ	• APC activation
IL-2	• clonal T cell activation and expansion

Th-2-type anti-inflammatory
cytokines

IL-10	• anti-inflammatory • down-regulates immune response
TGF-ß	• anti-inflammatory • profibrotic
IL-4	• anti-inflammatory • protects hepatic parenchyma
IL-5	• eosinophil recruitment
IL-13	• profibrotic

FIGURE 51.2. Main role of cytokines involved in the Th-1-type and Th-2-type immunopathology of schistosomiasis. *IL*, interleukin; *TNF-α*, tumor necrosis factor α; *IFN-γ*, interferon-γ; *TGF-β*, transforming growth factor-β.

decisive role. For example, in schistosome-infected mice lacking B7 costimulatory molecules, CD4+ Th cell responses against SEA are of the Th-1 type and fail to switch to a Th-2 response (11); a similar phenomenon has been observed in mice deficient in B cells (12). Interestingly, in circumstances where the development of a normal Th-2 response is impaired, as occurs in mice deficient in B7 costimulatory molecules or IL-4 (11,13), hepatic granulomas can be surrounded by variable to severe hepatocellular microvesicular change and necrosis, often resulting in death. The reason for the hepatic damage is not precisely known but has been attributed to toxic egg products or proinflammatory Th-1-type cytokines, such as tumor necrosis factor α (TNF-α), (13) (Fig. 51.1A, *left* and Fig. 51.2) reaching the hepatic parenchyma through poorly circumscribed, leaky granulomas (Fig. 51.1B, *left*). In contrast, mice developing normal Th-2 responses display tighter, more fibrotic and eosinophil-rich granulomas along with little, if any, hepatocellular injury (Fig. 51.1B, *right*). Several Th-2-type antiinflammatory cytokines have been implicated in this contained host-protective granulomatous response. IL-13, a cytokine related to IL-4, has recently been identified as a fibrogenic factor (14,15), whereas the presence of IL-4 itself primarily serves to prevent the hepatotoxicity (15); IL-5 acts as a chemoattractant for eosinophils (16), which themselves are a significant source of IL-4 (17). The role of IL-10 is discussed later (Fig. 51.1A, *right* and Fig. 51.2).

Another function that depends on Th-2 cells is to provide help for B cells in the production of antibodies against egg antigens, although a clear-cut impact of specific antibodies on the disease has yet to be demonstrated in *S. mansoni* infection. However, such antibodies have been postu-

lated to bear immunogenic idiotopes capable of engendering downregulatory antiidiotypic networks (18). This idea was originally derived from the observation that children suffer from less severe disease if born of mothers who are also infected, and that this could be due to transplacental passage of antischistosome antibodies.

The above findings suggest that granuloma formation in a Th-2 environment has an overall beneficial effect and is host-protective, whereas granulomatous inflammation in a milieu dominated by Th-1-type cytokines may be harmful and potentially life-threatening. The paradigm that has emerged from the murine model indeed correlates well with recent findings in human schistosomiasis patients, in whom a Th-2-like profile has been detected in patients with mild intestinal schistosomiasis (see later), whereas a Th-1-like profile is associated with the severe hepatosplenic disease (19). However, the association in the murine model of fibrosis with Th-2-type cytokines, such as IL-13 and possibly transforming growth factor β (TGF-β), raises the question about the pathogenesis of the hepatic fibrosis observed in the Th-1-related human hepatosplenic schistosomiasis. This severe form of fibrosis could well be stimulated by other fibrogenic mediators; on the other hand, it could be totally unrelated to preexisting granulomas and due to other events, such as episodes of hepatocellular necrosis, as is the case in other liver diseases. In any case, enhanced fibrosis within a granuloma appears to serve the useful function of sealing its contents, whereas fibrosis spanning extended areas has obvious deleterious effects on the intrahepatic hemodynamics. The implications from these findings are that complex immunopathological reactions, such as granulomatous inflammation and fibrosis, can be orchestrated through different pathways, which can, in turn, lead to dissimilar biological and clinical outcomes.

THE HETEROGENEITY AND SPECIFICITY OF THE PATHOGENIC ANTI-EGG CD4+ T CELL RESPONSE

The severity of the egg-induced hepatic pathology varies significantly amongst inbred mouse strains (20,21). Polar examples are the CBA or C3H mice, which produce large granulomas, and the C57BL/6 mice, in which the granulomas are significantly smaller. Although the effector pathways of the genetically determined cause for their enhanced pathology have not been fully elucidated, it is known that schistosome-infected CBA and C3H mice display increased T cell proliferation with a lingering Th-1-type cytokine profile in response to SEA (22,23).

Another striking difference between these mice is their immune response to schistosomal egg antigen Sm-p40, a 40 kd glycoprotein of 354 amino acids and clearly the most abundant soluble egg component (24,25). The CBA and C3H high pathology mouse strains (both of the H-2^k haplotype) mount strong T cell responses against Sm-p40, whereas H-2^b low pathology C57BL/6 mice do not. Moreover, in C3H mice, all clonal T cell hybridoma responses derived from egg antigen-sensitized T cell populations were specific for Sm-p40, whereas in C57BL/6 mice none of them were (22). The H-2^k-restricted T cell response to Sm-p40 has been extensively investigated. Sm-p40 was found to have three T cell epitopes (23), of which the one residing in peptides 234 to 246 (PKSDNQIKAVPAS) is immunodominant (23,26); alanine-monosubstituted synthetic analog peptides allowed further identification of D237 as the primary MHC class II (I-A^k) anchor residue and of N238, Q239 and K241 as the main T cell receptor (TCR) contact residues (27).

Of considerable interest is the intriguing observation that the Sm-p40 antigen predominantly stimulates Th-1-type (IFN-γ and IL-2) cytokine production by CD4+ Th cells, which may, at least in part, account for a persistent Th-1 component in the anti-SEA response of infected CBA and C3H mice (23,28). One reason for this bias may have to do with Sm-p40's poor glycosylation, although this needs to be further researched. Another important point regarding the Sm-p40 antigen is that it elicits a strong T cell response in high-pathology mouse strains. This raises the possibility of a direct role in the enhanced immunopathology, an issue that is currently under investigation.

The degree of CD4+ Th cell-mediated immunopathology in schistosomiasis is likely related to the extent of activation of specific T cell clones reacting to the corresponding egg antigens. This spurs the search for, and identification of, other important egg immunogens, a task that has been made feasible with the help of SEA-specific T cell hybridomas derived from sensitized individuals. Using this approach, our laboratory recently described *Schistosoma mansoni* phosphoenolpyruvate carboxykinase (Sm-PEPCK), a 62 kd egg component that induces a relatively prominent T cell response in the C57BL/6 mouse (29). Sm-PEPCK has been cloned, and a T cell epitope has been mapped (30).

THE REGULATION OF EGG IMMUNOPATHOLOGY: IMMUNOMODULATION

It has been long appreciated that eggs embolizing in the liver during the acute phase of schistosomiasis elicit a substantially greater granulomatous reaction than those arriving at later times in the disease (31). This lesional downregulation, known as "immunomodulation," has greatly intrigued researchers, who over the years have advanced several theories to explain it. The suppressive action of CD8+ T cells (32–34) and of the aforementioned antiidiotypic networks (18) are some of the postulated mechanisms. While it now appears that there is no single regulatory mechanism underlying immunomodulation, it is believed that the severe clinical forms of schistosomiasis (see above) are somehow linked to a deficient immunomodulatory process.

Our laboratory has for many years advocated a key role for IL-10 in the immunomodulation phenomenon (35). IL-10 is a powerful Th-2-type antiinflammatory cytokine of multicellular origin (36) (Fig. 51.1A, *right*). Its likely role in immunomodulation is suggested by the observation that macrophages isolated from granulomas do not stimulate CD4+ Th cells, but rather induce unresponsiveness, which can be abrogated following neutralization of macrophage-derived IL-10 (37,38). IL-10 has been shown to inhibit the production of proinflammatory monokines (39), including IL-12 (40), and downregulate B7 costimulatory molecule expression (38,41) thereby inhibiting T cell activation. Moreover, when administered *in vivo* to schistosome-infected mice, a long-lasting IL-10 fusion protein can downmodulate granuloma formation (42). In support of IL-10's pivotal downmodulatory function, we recently found that in schistosome-infected IL-10 knockout mice there is markedly enhanced acute hepatic perioval granulomatous inflammation, and that after 15 weeks of infection, there is virtually no immunomodulation (C. Sadler, L. Rutitzky, R. A. Wilson and M. J. Stadecker, unpublished observation).

Several studies in humans strongly support the biological effects of IL-10 observed in the experimental murine system. For example, high levels of IL-10 have been detected in patients with the benign forms of schistosomiasis (43,44) and related filariasis (45). Moreover, in human schistosomiasis and filariasis, IL-10 can similarly induce a state of T-cell unresponsiveness/anergy (46,47). Importantly, in an *in vitro* model, granuloma formation is significantly enhanced following neutralization of IL-10, which is produced by lymphoid cells from patients with mild intestinal schistosomiasis, but not with severe acute or hepatosplenic schistosomiasis (48). All in all, these studies convincingly demonstrate that effective immunomodulation of granuloma formation is intimately related to, and dependent on, a firmly established Th-2 cytokine environment, in which IL-10 plays a critical role (Fig. 51.1A, *right*).

PERSPECTIVES FOR IMMUNO-INTERVENTION IN SCHISTOSOMIASIS

Despite the availability of drugs for treatment and significant progress in sanitation and education, schistosomiasis is still a formidable public health problem in many areas of the third world and shows no signs of retreat. Effective immunotherapy is, therefore, an ideal theoretical approach towards a long-lasting decline in the devastating impact of schistosomiasis, both at the individual and population levels.

There are two obvious opportunities for possible immuno-intervention in schistosomiasis. The first one is the classical approach of immunization (vaccination) with the pathogen's antigens for the purpose of bolstering the host's specific defenses at the time of infection. With this idea in mind, several worm antigens have been identified and have provided limited protection in the experimental infection. The interested reader can examine different views on this topic (49,50), as it is not further developed in the present article.

The other approach to immuno-intervention is the downregulation of excessive, harmful CD4+ T-cell-mediated immunopathology. This concept is based on the assumption that induction of specific T-cell unresponsiveness to sufficient egg antigens will result in an overall decrease of the magnitude of the inflammatory response. There are currently several strategies to induce T-cell unresponsiveness to peptides and proteins *in vivo*. They are based on the administration of the protein, or of relevant immunodominant (wild-type) peptides, or of analog peptides with demonstrated antagonist properties; alternatively or additionally they can make use of agents that prevent or inhibit T-cell activation, such as IL-10 or blockers of co-stimulation. Some of these regimens have been employed successfully in the amelioration of T-cell-mediated autoimmune disease. Regardless, whether such strategies will succeed in experimental schistosomiasis, or can be implemented in human schistosomiasis, remains to be investigated; in any case, their realization will in part depend on the identification of the critical egg immunogens and their T-cell epitopes.

CONCLUSION

The principal disease manifestations of schistosomiasis are the result of an immune-mediated pathogenic clash between schistosome egg antigens and specifically sensitized CD4+ T cells, which, in the cases of *S. mansoni* and *S. japonicum* infection, takes place in the liver and intestine. This article

attempts to synthesize and summarize the current views on the cellular basis and regulation of the immunopathology in schistosomiasis. Undoubtedly, as is the case in any complex biological system, pressing questions remain to be answered and conflicting issues need to be addressed.

It is clear that for the success of their millennial coevolution, this immunopathological reaction against the eggs must have played useful roles for host and parasite alike. For the host, the immunopathology is in most cases limited and probably beneficial, as it walls off potentially injurious egg products and proinflammatory mediators, but in a minority of cases it can be harmful and potentially lethal. For the parasite, however, the immunopathology is essential: it facilitates intestinal transmural egg migration and thus is crucial for the perpetuation of the species. Clear proof of this is the reduction of fecal egg counts in individuals with decreased CD4+ Th cell counts (51). Given the seemingly inevitable endurance of this host–parasite relationship, future basic research is needed to shed further light on the intricacies of their interaction, at the same time attempting to devise long-term strategies for amelioration of disease in those most gravely afflicted or at risk.

ACKNOWLEDGMENTS

We gratefully acknowledge Hiroko Asahi, Silas Chikunguwo and Pedro Flores Villanueva, who critically contributed to the work in our laboratory, as well as National Institutes of Health and World Health Organization for providing the grant support.

REFERENCES

1. Marquet S, Abel L, Hillaire D, et al. Genetic localization of a locus controlling the intensity of infection by *Schistosoma mansoni* on chromosome 5q31-q33. *Nat Genet* 1996;2:181–184.
2. Secor WE, del Corral H, dos Reis MG, et al. Association of hepatosplenic schistosomiasis with HLA-DQB1*0201. *J Infect Dis* 1996;174:1131–1135.
3. Phillips SM, DiConza JJ, Gold JA, et al. Schistosomiasis in the congenitally athymic (nude) mouse. I. Thymic dependency of eosinophilia, granuloma formation, and host morbidity. *J Immunol* 1977;118:594–599.
4. Mathew RC, Boros DL. Anti-L3T4 antibody treatment suppresses hepatic granuloma formation and abrogates antigen-induced interleukin-2 production in *Schistosoma mansoni* infection. *Infect Immun* 1986;54:820–826.
5. Hernandez HJ, Wang Y, Tzellas N, et al. Expression of class II, but not class I, major histocompatibility complex molecules is required for granuloma formation in infection with *Schistosoma mansoni. Eur J Immunol* 1997;27:1170–1176.
6. Iacomini J, Ricklan D, Stadecker M. T cells expressing the γδ T cell receptor are not required for egg granuloma formation in schistosomiasis. *Eur J Immunol* 1997;25:884–888.
7. Chikunguwo S, Kanazawa T, Dayal Y, et al. The cell-mediated response to schistosomal antigens at the clonal level. *In vivo* functions of cloned murine egg antigen-specific CD4+ T helper type 1 lymphocytes. *J Immunol* 1991;147:3921–3925.

8. Pearce E, Caspar P, Grzych J, et al. Downregulation of Th1 cytokine production accompanies induction of Th2 responses by a parasitic helminth, *Schistosoma mansoni. J Exp Med* 1991;173:159–166.

9. Stadecker MJ. The development of granulomas in schistosomiasis: genetic backgrounds, regulatory pathways, and specific egg antigen responses that influence the magnitude of disease. *Microbes Infect* 1999;1:505–510.

10. Stadecker MJ, Hernandez HJ. The immune response and immunopathology in infection with *Schistosoma mansoni*: a key role of major egg antigen Sm-p40. *Parasite Immunol* 1998;20:217–221.

11. Hernandez HJ, Sharpe AH, Stadecker MJ. Experimental murine schistosomiasis in the absence of B7 costimulatory molecules: reversal of elicited T cell cytokine profile and partial inhibition of egg granuloma formation. *J Immunol* 1999;162:2884–2889.

12. Hernandez HJ, Wang Y, Stadecker MJ. In infection with *Schistosoma mansoni*, B cells are required for T helper type 2 cell responses but not for granuloma formation. *J Immunol* 1997;158:4832–4837.

13. Brunet LR, Finkelman FD, Cheever AW, et al. IL-4 protects against TNF-α-mediated cachexia and death during acute schistosomiasis. *J Immunol* 1997;159:777–785.

14. Chiaramonte MG, Donaldson DD, Cheever AW, et al. An IL-13 inhibitor blocks the development of hepatic fibrosis during a T-helper type 2-dominated inflammatory response. *J Clin Invest* 1999;104:777–785.

15. Fallon PG, Richardson EJ, McKenzie GJ, et al. Schistosome infection of transgenic mice defines distinct and contrasting pathogenic roles for IL-4 and IL-13: IL-13 is a profibrotic agent. *J Immunol* 2000;164:2585–2591.

16. Sher A, Coffman RL, Hieny S, et al. Interleukin 5 is required for the blood and tissue eosinophilia but not granuloma formation induced by infection with *Schistosoma mansoni. Proc Natl Acad Sci U S A* 1990;87:61–65.

17. Rumbley CA, Sugaya H, Zekavat SA, et al. Activated eosinophils are the major source of Th2-associated cytokines in the schistosome granuloma. *J Immunol* 1999;162:1003–1009.

18. Colley DG, Montesano MA, Freeman GL, et al. Infection-stimulated or perinatally initiated idiotypic interactions can direct differential morbidity and mortality in schistosomiasis. *Microbes Infect* 1999;1:517–524.

19. Mwatha JK, Kimani G, Kamau T, et al. High levels of TNF, soluble TNF receptors, soluble ICAM-1, and IFN-γ, but low levels of IL-5 are associated with hepatosplenic disease in human schistosomiasis mansoni. *J Immunol* 1998;160:1992–1999.

20. Cheever A, Duvall R, Hallack T Jr, et al. Variation of hepatic fibrosis and granuloma size among mouse strains infected with *Schistosoma mansoni. Am J Trop Med Hyg* 1987;37:85–97.

21. Fanning M, Peters P, Davis R, et al. Immunopathology of murine infection with *Schistosoma mansoni*: Relationship of genetic background to hepatosplenic disease and modulation. *J Infect Dis* 1981;144:148–153.

22. Hernandez HJ, Trzyna WC, Cordingley JS, et al. Differential antigen recognition by T cell populations from strains of mice developing polar forms of granulomatous inflammation in response to eggs of *Schistosoma mansoni. Eur J Immunol* 1997;27:666–670.

23. Hernandez HJ, Edson CM, Harn DA, et al. *Schistosoma mansoni*: genetic restriction and cytokine profile of the CD4+ T helper cell response to dominant epitope peptide of major egg antigen Sm-p40. *Exp Parasitol* 1998;90:122–130.

24. Nene V, Dunne D, Johnson K, et al. Sequence and expression of a major egg antigen from *Schistosoma mansoni*. Homologies to heat shock proteins and α-crystallins. *Mol Biochem Parasitol* 1986;21:179–188.

25. Chikunguwo S, Quinn S, Harn D, et al. The cell-mediated

26. Chen Y, Boros DL. Identification of the immunodominant T cell epitope of p38, a major egg antigen, and characterization of the epitope-specific Th responsiveness during murine *schistosomiasis mansoni. J Immunol* 1998;160:5420–5427.

27. Hernandez HJ, Stadecker MJ. Elucidation and role of critical residues of immunodominant peptide associated with T cell-mediated parasitic disease. *J Immunol* 1999;163:3877–3882.

28. Cai Y, Langley J, Smith D, et al. A cloned major *Schistosoma mansoni* egg antigen with homologies to small heat shock proteins elicits Th1 responsiveness. *Infect Immun* 1996;64:1750–1755.

29. Asahi H, Hernandez HJ, Stadecker MJ. A novel 62-kilodalton egg antigen from *Schistosoma mansoni* induces a potent CD4(+) T helper cell response in the C57BL/6 mouse. *Infect Immun* 1999;67:1729–1735.

30. Asahi H, Osman A, Cook RM, et al. *Schistosoma mansoni* phosphoenolpyruvate carboxykinase (Sm-PEPCK), a novel egg antigen: immunological properties of the recombinant protein and identification of T cell epitope. *Infect Immun* 2000 *(in press)*.

31. Andrade Z, Warren K. Mild prolonged schistosomiasis in mice: alteration in host response with time and the development of portal fibrosis. *Trans R Soc Trop Med Hyg* 1964;58:53–57.

32. Boros DL. Immunoregulation of granuloma formation in murine *schistosomiasis mansoni. Ann N Y Acad Sci* 1986;465:313–323.

33. Chensue SW, Warmington KS, Hershey SD, et al. Evolving T cell responses in murine schistosomiasis. Th2 cells mediate secondary granulomatous hypersensitivity and are regulated by CD8+ T cells *in vivo. J Immunol* 1993;151:1391–1400.

34. Pedras-Vasconcelos JA, Pearce EJ. Type 1 CD8+4 T cell responses during infection with the helminth *Schistosoma mansoni. J Immunol* 1996;157:3046–3053.

35. Stadecker MJ, Flores Villanueva P. Accessory cell signals regulate Th-cell responses: from basic immunology to a model of helminthic disease. *Immunol Today* 1994;15:571–574.

36. Moore KW, O'Garra A, de Waal R, et al. Interleukin-10. *Annu Rev Immunol* 1993;11:165–190.

37. Flores Villanueva PO, Harris TS, Ricklan DE, et al. Macrophages from schistosomal egg granulomas induce unresponsiveness in specific cloned Th-1 lymphocytes *in vitro* and down-regulate schistosomal granulomatous disease *in vivo. J Immunol* 1994;152:1847–1855.

38. Flores Villanueva PO, Reiser H, Stadecker MJ. Regulation of T helper cell responses in experimental murine schistosomiasis by IL-10. Effect on expression of B7 and B7-2 costimulatory molecules by macrophages. *J Immunol* 1994;153:5190–5199.

39. de Waal Malefyt R, Abrams J, Bennett B, et al. Interleukin 10 (IL-10) inhibits cytokine synthesis by human monocytes: an autoregulatory role of IL-10 produced by monocytes. *J Exp Med* 1991;174:1209–1220.

40. Aste-Amezaga M, Ma X, Sartori A, et al. Molecular mechanisms of the induction of IL-12 and its inhibition by IL-10. *J Immunol* 1998;160:5936–5944.

41. Ding L, Linsley PS, Huang LY, et al. IL-10 inhibits macrophage costimulatory activity by selectively inhibiting the up-regulation of B7 expression. *J Immunol* 1993;151:1224–1234.

42. Flores-Villanueva PO, Zheng XX, Strom TB, et al. Recombinant IL-10 and IL-10/Fc treatment down-regulate egg antigen-specific delayed hypersensitivity reactions and egg granuloma formation in schistosomiasis. *J Immunol* 1996;156:3315–3320.

43. Araujo MI, de Jesus AR, Bacellar O, et al. Evidence of a T helper type 2 activation in human schistosomiasis. *Eur J Immunol* 1996;26:1399–1403.

44. Malaquias LC, Falcao PL, Silveira AM, et al. Cytokine regula-

tion of human immune response to *Schistosoma mansoni*: analysis of the role of IL-4, IL-5 and IL-10 on peripheral blood mononuclear cell responses. *Scand J Immunol* 1997;46: 393–398.

45. Mahanty S, Nutman TB. Immunoregulation in human lymphatic filariasis: the role of interleukin 10. *Parasite Immunol* 1995;17:385–392.

46. King CL, Medhat A, Malhotra I, et al. Cytokine control of parasite-specific anergy in human urinary schistosomiasis. IL-10 modulates lymphocyte reactivity. *J Immunol* 1996;156: 4715–4721.

47. Mahanty S, Mollis SN, Ravichandran M, et al. High levels of spontaneous and parasite antigen-driven interleukin-10 production are associated with antigen-specific hyporesponsive-

ness in human lymphatic filariasis. *J Infect Dis* 1996;173: 769–773.

48. Falcao PL, Malaquias LC, Martins-Filho OA, et al. Human *Schistosomiasis mansoni*: IL-10 modulates the *in vitro* granuloma formation. *Parasite Immunol* 1998;20:447–454.

49. Bergquist NR. Schistosomiasis vaccine development: progress and prospects. *Mem Inst Oswaldo Cruz* 1998;93:95–101.

50. Gryseels B. 2000. Schistosomiasis vaccines: a devil's advocate view. *Parasitol Today* 16:46–48.

51. Karanja DM, Colley DG, Nahlen BL, et al. Studies on schistosomiasis in western Kenya: I. Evidence for immune-facilitated excretion of schistosome eggs from patients with *Schistosoma mansoni* and human immunodeficiency virus coinfections. *Am J Trop Med Hyg* 1997;56:515–521.

The Liver: Biology and Pathobiology, Fourth Edition, edited by I. M. Arias, J. L. Boyer, F. V. Chisari, N. Fausto, D. Schachter, and D. A. Shafritz. Lippincott Williams & Wilkins, Philadelphia © 2001.

IMMUNE MECHANISMS OF VIRAL CLEARANCE AND DISEASE PATHOGENESIS DURING VIRAL HEPATITIS

CARLO FERRARI
FRANCIS V. CHISARI

Hepatocellular injury can occur in the context of a wide variety of diseases of variable etiology, including viral infections in which the immune response is believed to play a central role in viral clearance and disease pathogenesis. Much has been learned during the last few years about these immune mechanisms thanks to the development of animal models of infection and liver disease and the discovery of new molecular tools to finely dissect the capacity of the immune response to induce both tissue injury and viral clearance. In particular, molecular cloning of the immunoglobulin and T-cell receptor genes, resolution of the three-dimensional structure of the human class I histo-compatibility leukocyte antigen (HLA), sequence analysis of the antigen fragments bound to HLA molecules *in vivo*, fine molecular dissection of the intracellular pathways of antigen processing and presentation to T cells, the development of new methods to identify and quantitate antigen-specific T cells, and the functional and molecular characterization of a wide set of cytokines as the molecular mediators of many T-cell functions now provide a fundamental framework for studies designed to elucidate the complex network of specific immune responses involved in disease progression and viral clearance in infected individuals. In this chapter we discuss the immune mechanisms thought to be operative in hepatitis B and C virus infections in light of recent important discoveries that have clarified hitherto obscure aspects of the immune response involved in termination of infection in those patients who successfully deal with these viruses, and responsible for viral persistence and chronic liver disease in those who do not.

C. Ferrari: Department of Infectious Diseases, University Hospital of Parma, 43100 Parma, Italy.

F. V. Chisari: Department of Molecular and Experimental Medicine, The Scripps Research Institute, La Jolla, California 92037.

IMMUNE RECOGNITION OF INFECTED CELLS

Viruses are obligatory intracellular pathogens that depend on the host cell synthetic machinery for their replication and growth. Indeed, at the earliest stage of the encounter between virus and host, viruses frequently use normal cell surface molecules to bind to the target cell (1). An important aspect of the defense against virus infections is the neutralization of the circulating virus and the interference with its entry into the host cell. These functions are carried out primarily by antibodies specifically directed against viral antigens that can enhance the phagocytic clearance of viral particles by opsonization or can inhibit infection by blocking attachment and penetration of the virus into the cell. The second fundamental step of antiviral protective immunity is the elimination of intracellular virus by the cellular immune response. Traditionally, this has been thought to require the immune destruction of infected cells by cytotoxic T lymphocytes (CTL). Recently, it has become clear that the cellular immune response can also purge certain viruses from infected cells without killing the infected cells, by secreting antiviral cytokines that inhibit viral gene expression and replication, thereby curing infections without destroying the infected organ or killing the host.

It is clear, from studies in other viral systems, that CD8+ CTLs are the principal effectors of virus-induced immunopathology; however, CD4+ T cells, cells of the innate immune response, such as macrophages, polymorphonuclear cells, leukocytes, natural killer (NK) cells, and natural killer T (NKT) cells, as well as lymphokines, chemokines and complement can also contribute to virus-induced tissue injury. In addition, it is clear that all of these cells, as well as antibody-producing B lymphocytes, can be involved in viral clearance by triggering the destructive and noncytopathic antiviral events described above. Thus, viral clearance and disease pathogenesis can be viewed as two sides of the same coin, with injury being the price paid for resolution of the infection. In this vein, if most cells of a large vital organ, such as the liver, are infected by a noncytopathic virus, such as HBV or HCV, and if the only way to eliminate the virus is by killing all of the infected cells, there can be two outcomes: viral persistence with varying degrees of chronic disease, if the immune response isn't robust enough to find and destroy all of the infected cells; or destruction of the organ and the death of the host if it is. On the other hand, if the cellular immune system can also eliminate a virus noncytopathically after antigen recognition by secreting antiviral cytokines that can diffuse and reach many more infected cells, another outcome is possible: viral clearance without massive tissue injury. These concepts will be discussed in more detail later in this chapter.

Major Histocompatibility Complex Class I-Restricted CD8+ T Cells

While B cells recognize sequential or conformational epitopes on native antigen molecules, CD4+ and CD8+ T cells recognize processed antigenic peptides associated with major histocompatibility complex (MHC) molecules (human lymphocyte antigens, HLA, in humans). Peptides recognized by HLA class I-restricted CD8+ CTL are usually produced in the intracellular cytosolic compartment by degradation of viral proteins synthesized endogenously within infected cells (2–5). Newly synthesized proteins are degraded by cytoplasmic proteases (proteasomes) into peptides which are delivered to transmembrane peptide transporters that transfer them across the membrane of the endoplasmic reticulum (ER) from the cytoplasm to the ER lumen (6). Here they bind to HLA class I molecules, causing a conformational change that stabilizes the assembly of the class I heavy chain with β-2-microglobulin (7–9). The solution of the crystal structure of different HLA class I molecules (10–13) has revealed a peptide-binding groove located between the α-1 and α-2 domains of the heavy chain, consisting of two adjacent helical regions on top of an eight-stranded β sheet (14,15). This cleft can accommodate peptides of 8 to 10 amino acids in a fully extended conformation or slightly longer species in a helical form (15). Indeed, naturally processed peptides eluted from purified HLA class I molecules are usually 8 to 10 amino acids long (13,16–26) and they have been shown to bind to HLA class I molecules with high affinity (27–28). This conservation of length may be assured either by specific selection operated by the transmembrane transporter molecules or by preferential generation of octamers, nonamers, and decamers by the proteasome. Exceptions to this length constraint are the longer peptides eluted from HLA class I molecules that derive from protein signal sequences and that can probably enter the ER by the classical signal-dependent mechanism required for protein translocation into the lumen of the ER (29–30). Although the general rule is that endogenously synthesized antigens enter the intracellular pathway of antigen processing for association with HLA class I molecules, some exogenous antigens, such as hepatitis B surface antigen (HBsAg), that enter antigen-presenting cells by endocytosis can reach the cytosol for endogenous processing even if they are not synthesized within the cell where processing takes place (2).

Major Histocompatibility Complex Class II-Eestricted CD4+ T Cells

In contrast to CD8+ CTL, HLA class II-restricted CD4+ T cells generally recognize peptide fragments derived from extracellular antigens which are proteolytically processed in acidified endosomes after endocytosis by specialized antigen-presenting cells, especially dendritic cells, macrophages, and B cells (31). Following synthesis in the ER, transport of class II molecules to the proper peptide binding compartment (endosomes) and prevention of endogenous antigen binding in the ER (where cytosolic peptides are delivered for HLA class I binding) are functions of the invariant chain (32). While the HLA class I groove appears to accommodate 8 to 10 mers, being closed at both ends (13,14), the HLA class II cleft seems to be open, thereby allowing accommodation of larger peptides of variable length and with heterogeneous sites of terminal truncation (33–36).

The specificity of the interaction between the exogenous peptide/HLA class II molecule complex and the CD4 cell is provided by the T-cell receptor, and its avidity is strengthened by the direct binding of the CD4 molecule with the β-2 domain of the HLA class II molecule (37,38). The CD4+ T-cell response to exogenous antigens is principally regulatory in its function by secreting lymphokines that modulate the activity of antigen-specific B cells and CD8+ T cells, and can also inhibit viral replication, similar to the function of the same cytokines secreted by CD8+ T cells. However, cytotoxic activity expressed by CD4+, HLA class II-restricted T cells has been reported (39–44), and recognition of endogenous peptides derived from intracellular processing of newly synthesized antigen within HLA class II-positive virus-infected cells has also been observed, although infrequently (45–51).

Peptide discrimination between HLA class I and class II binding mostly depends upon the intracellular compartmentalization of the antigen. Endogenous synthesis of antigen takes place within infected cells that must be identified and destroyed or purged of viruses by the immune system. As a general rule, cytosolic processing of endogenous antigen generates peptides for association with HLA class I in the ER, and the molecular complex HLA class I/endogenous peptide eventually expressed at the surface of the infected cell provides the appropriate signal for CTL recognition of intracellular virus. Preferential interaction of CD8+ CTL with HLA class I molecules is due to the direct binding of CD8 with the α-3 domain of the class I molecule needed to stabilize the interaction between effector and target cell (52,53). In accordance with this role of the HLA class I molecules in endogenous antigen presentation, empty class I heterodimers assembled in the absence of endogenous peptide are highly unstable and quickly dissociate (54–57), thereby limiting the availability of free HLA class I in the compartment of exogenous antigen processing and thus the possibility of binding to exogenous peptides, which would make innocent uninfected cells susceptible to lysis by CD8+ CTL.

Natural Killer Cells and Natural Killer T Cells

Early in the course of infection, before activation and expansion of virus-specific HLA class I- and class II-restricted T cells, cytokines released by infected cells or cells of the innate immune system can elicit responses mediated by NK cells and by NKT cells. NK cells are believed to play an important

role in host defense against viruses by killing virus-infected cells without HLA restriction or apparent specificity for viral antigens, and by secreting antiviral cytokines (58). Classical NK cells do not rearrange immunoglobulin or T-cell receptor genes, are CD3-negative, and develop normally in athymic nude mice and apparently also in immunodeficient SCID mice. They can mediate perforin-dependent lysis and secrete a wide array of cytokines and chemokines, including IFNγ and TNFα. Moreover, NK cells are the principal effectors of antibody-dependent cell-mediated cytotoxicity (ADCC), which is mediated by the recognition of antibody-coated target cells by the NK Fc receptor, CD16 (58).

Cytotoxic activity and release of cytokines by NK cells appear to be regulated by a balance between positive and negative signals delivered by families of receptors recently identified and responsible for initiation or suppression of cell activation (59). Inhibitory NK receptors include the human KIR molecules that are members of the Ig-superfamily and contain either two or three Ig domains in the extracellular region, and the human CD94/NKG2A and the mouse Ly49 that are members of the C-type lectin-superfamily and possess carbohydrate recognition domains in the extracellular region (59). All these molecules have been implicated in NK recognition of polymorphic MHC class I ligands, and all contain ITIM sequences in their cytoplasmic domain, indicating a common mechanism of NK cell inhibition. Inhibition appears to be transient, and there is no evidence that engagement of inhibitory receptors leads to deletion or long-lived anergy of the cell. A puzzling discovery is that the NK receptors that activate cytotoxicity are isoforms of the inhibitory receptors; they possess similar external binding domains but have shorter cytoplasmic tails lacking critical elements for negative signaling, such as the ITIM sequences (58,59). This raises the issue, still unsolved, of how NK cells can distinguish between stimulatory and inhibitory signals deriving from the external environment.

Available data favor the idea that expression of HLA class I inhibits NK cell activation. Recognition of an appropriate HLA class I molecule by NK receptors would lead to the delivery of a negative signal causing inhibition of NK killing. Therefore, attempts by a virus to evade immune recognition by CTLs by suppressing HLA class I expression would increase the visibility of the target cells by NK cells, an obvious survival strategy with great benefits for the host.

Many features of NK cells are shared by a population of T cells called NKT cells that have an extremely limited T-cell receptor (TCR) repertoire with predominant TCR α/β expression (58). They depend on nonclassical, MHC class I-like CD1 molecules for their development, and they recognize mainly glycolipids presented by CD1. Their proliferation is supported by IL2, and stimulation of their CD3 complex can lead to production of IFNγ and IL4. Interestingly, these cells have been described at high frequency in unchallenged livers, suggesting a possible role for these cells in the pathogenesis of hepatic infections (58).

THE IMMUNE RESPONSE TO HEPATITIS B VIRUS

The antibody response to HBV envelope antigens is a T-cell-dependent process (60) that plays a critical role in viral clearance by complexing with free viral particles, preventing the infection of susceptible cells. The role of antibodies to the capsid and nonstructural proteins in HBV immunobiology is less clear, although passively administered anti-HBe antibodies have been reported to protect chimpanzees against HBV infection (61). The T-cell response to HBV is vigorous, polyclonal and multispecific in patients with acute hepatitis who ultimately clear the virus, and it is weak or barely detectable in patients with chronic hepatitis, except during acute exacerbations of chronic disease (62) or after spontaneous or interferon-α-induced viral clearance (63). Many T-cell epitopes have been defined in the various HBV proteins with the HLA class II-restricted, CD4-positive helper T-cell response being focused principally on the nucleocapsid antigens of HBV, while all of the viral proteins are targeted by the class I-restricted, CD8-positive CTL response in acutely infected patients (64).

Despite the vigor of the T-cell response to HBV during acute viral hepatitis, however, very low levels of virus remain present in the circulation for several decades following complete clinical and serological resolution of disease (65). Recent studies indicate that long-term persistence of trace amounts of viral DNA is associated with equally long-term persistence of HBV-specific CTLs that display activation markers, suggesting that the transcriptionally active virus is able to produce viral antigens that actively maintain the CTL response indefinitely, perhaps for life (66). This implies that acute and chronic HBV infection may represent ends of a quantitative spectrum rather than qualitatively different conditions. The ability of HBV to persist at a low level after recovery from acute infection and to simultaneously maintain and evade the immune response might yield insight into the immunological and virological basis for high-level viral persistence in patients with chronic hepatitis. The subject of viral persistence will be considered in greater detail later in this review.

A large body of evidence suggests that the vigor of the CTL response to HBV is the principal determinant of viral clearance in acutely infected patients (64). It is widely believed that the CTL response clears viral infections by killing infected cells. This is certainly true for many viruses, especially those that do not infect large numbers of cells. CTL-killing is an inefficient process, however, requiring direct physical contact between the CTL and the infected cells. Thus, it may not be possible for CTLs to kill all infected cells if the CTLs are greatly outnumbered such as during HBV and HCV infec-

tion, which can involve virtually all of the hepatocytes in the liver (see Hepatitis B Viral Clearance and Disease Pathogenesis, below). Thus, although the liver disease in viral hepatitis is certainly due to the cytopathic activity of the CTL response, viral clearance may require more efficient CTL functions than the one-on-one process of killing. This new concept will be discussed in more detail below.

HEPATITIS B VIRAL CLEARANCE AND DISEASE PATHOGENESIS

Destruction of Infected Cells

Since viruses are intracellular parasites, antiviral CTL are believed to play a major role in the eradication of infection by virtue of their capacity to identify virus-infected cells through recognition of viral peptides derived from intracellular processing of endogenously synthesized antigens. It is generally assumed that CTL activation leads to the destruction of infected cells and that this is an essential step for eradication of intracellular virus. Therefore, in infections with noncytopathic viruses, such as HBV and HCV, immunopathology is thought to be due to a destructive mechanism that terminates the infection when it is efficient, or causes a persistent necroinflammatory disease when it is not. According to these concepts, acute self-limited hepatitis B virus infection is the result of a coordinated efficient cellular and humoral antiviral response consisting of (a) CTL-mediated elimination of infected cells, (b) antibody-mediated neutralization of free circulating viral particles, and (c) inhibition of liver cell reinfection. Chronic hepatitis B is thought to reflect diminished CTL activity that is able to destroy some but not all of the infected cells, whereas a lack of CTL activity is assumed to be responsible for chronic HBV infection without liver disease, that is, the "healthy carrier state."

While the notion that the destructive activity of the cytotoxic T cells is primarily responsible for the elimination of intracellular virus is attractive, it is difficult to reconcile with the fact that all liver cells would have to be destroyed because 100% of the hepatocytes are infected during the early stages of HBV infection. This would imply that massive hepatic necrosis should represent a frequent outcome of an acute HBV infection, unless liver cell destruction by CTL is a slowly progressive event, involving only a limited proportion of liver cells at a time. It would also imply that the immune system has the capacity to destroy more than a kilogram of tissue (10^{11} hepatocytes) in the space of a few weeks, an unlikely possibility given the fact that there are only 10^{12} lymphocytes in the entire body. Recent studies carried out in animal models of HBV infection (such as transgenic mice and infected chimpanzees) and in HBV-infected patients using the most advanced technological tools permit reinterpretation of the nature of the cell-mediated immune events occurring during acute and chronic HBV infection and lead to a new paradigm in viral immunology, that is, the concept that HBV-specific CTLs can purge this virus from infected cells without killing them.

Nondestructive Purging of Virus from Infected Cells

Important new insights into the pathogenetic and noncytopathic antiviral capacity of the CTL response to HBV have been forthcoming from studies in HBV transgenic mice that develop an acute necroinflammatory liver disease following adoptive transfer of HBsAg-specific CTL lines and clones (67,68). As illustrated in Figure 52.1, the earliest

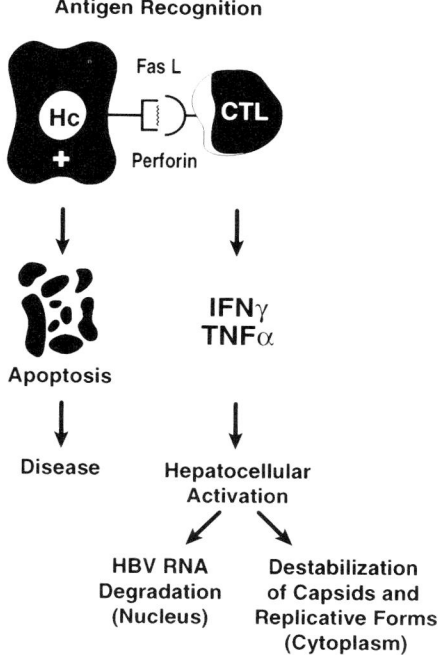

FIGURE 52.1. Noncytolytic clearance of hepatitis B virus (*HBV*) from the hepatocyte by T-cell-derived cytokines. Upon antigen recognition, CD8+ cytotoxic T lymphocytes (*CTLs*) deliver an apoptotic signal to their target cells, killing them. They also secrete interferon-γ (*IFNγ*) and tumor necrosis factor-α (*TNFα*), cytokines that abolish HBV gene expression and viral replication *in vivo*, curing them. The curative effect of the CTL response is more efficient than its destructive effect. The outcome of an infection may depend on the relative balance of these two effects with a predominantly curative response leading to viral clearance, and a predominantly destructive response leading to viral persistence and chronic liver disease. Importantly, if the curative process only partially inhibits viral gene expression and replication, it could paradoxically lead to viral persistence by reducing the immunological visibility of the virus without removing it. Note that antiviral cytokines produced by non-T cells during acute infection or by HBV-nonspecific T cells in the event of a superinfection could also inhibit HBV replication by a bystander mechanism. This is common during hepatitis delta virus superinfection of patients chronically infected by HBV, and it has been described during hepatitis A virus and hepatitis C virus superinfection as well.

event in this disease is recognition of hepatocellular antigen by the CTLs, which trigger the hepatocytes to undergo apoptosis (67). Subsequently, the release of chemokines by the activated CTLs causes an influx of antigen-nonspecific inflammatory cells into the vicinity of each CTL, leading to an amplification of their destructive potential and the killing of neighboring hepatocytes as bystanders. Nonetheless, the overall magnitude of CTL-mediated hepatocellular injury is quite modest in this transgenic mouse model (69–71), yet HBV gene expression and replication are abolished in all of the hepatocytes, most of which are not killed by the CTLs or the recruited inflammatory cells (71). During this remarkable antiviral process, the viral nucleocapsids disappear from the cytoplasm of the hepatocytes and the viral RNAs are destroyed soon after they are synthesized in the nucleus, yet the hepatocytes remain perfectly healthy (72). As a result, all of the viral gene products and virions disappear from the liver and the serum (69). This antiviral process is completely blocked by the administration of antibodies to interferon γ (IFNγ) and tumor necrosis factor α (TNFα) before the CTLs are injected, and it is not induced by HBsAg-specific CTL derived from IFNγ-knockout mice, indicating that IFNγ is responsible for this antiviral effect. Furthermore, HBsAg-specific Fas ligand-deficient and perforin-deficient CTL clones that do not cause hepatitis in these animals do inhibit viral replication, proving genetically that the cytopathic and antiviral functions of CTLs are completely independent of each other. The identity of the cytokine-induced cellular genes that mediate this process and the target elements in the virus that are susceptible to control by this process are under investigation.

These results suggest that a strong intrahepatic immune response to HBV can suppress viral gene expression and replication and perhaps even "cure" infected hepatocytes of the virus *without killing them.* Importantly, this illustrates that infected cells can become active participants in the antiviral response by responding to cytokine-induced signals and activating specific intracellular signal transduction pathways that interrupt the viral life cycle. Additionally, the data suggest that a weak immune response could contribute to viral persistence and chronic liver disease by reducing the expression of viral antigens sufficiently for the infected cells to escape immune recognition, but not enough for the virus to be eliminated, or by failing to eliminate the viral transcriptional template in the infected cells.

One might predict from the foregoing that superinfection of the HBV-infected liver by other pathogens might facilitate the clearance of HBV if they induce the local production of antiviral cytokines to which HBV is susceptible. Precisely these events have been shown to occur in the HBV transgenic mice during lymphocytic choriomeningitis virus infection of the liver (70) as well as adenovirus- and cytomegalovirus-induced hepatitis (F.V. Chisari, unpublished observations, 2000). Intriguingly, isolated case reports have been published suggesting that superinfection by HAV or HCV is sometimes associated with clearance of HBV in chronically infected patients (73,74).

If these observations are applicable to HBV infection, it would suggest that viral clearance in hepatitis B might be primarily caused by a cytokine-mediated noncytopathic mechanism rather than by the destruction of infected liver cells. The evidence that transgenic mice are not infected by HBV and do not produce the episomal covalently closed circular HBV DNA (cccDNA) transcriptional template (74), however, limits the applicability of these results to natural HBV infection in humans.

Acute Hepatitis B Virus Infection in Chimpanzees and Humans

These questions were resolved by studying the early events occurring in HBV-infected chimpanzees, since these animals develop acute hepatitis and mount immune responses to HBV proteins similar to those observed in humans (75). In this animal model, all HBV DNA forms, including the cccDNA, peak in the liver approximately 8 weeks after infection and decline rapidly thereafter. In contrast, serum alanine aminotransferase (ALT) activity doesn't start to increase and histological evidence of hepatitis doesn't appear until 10

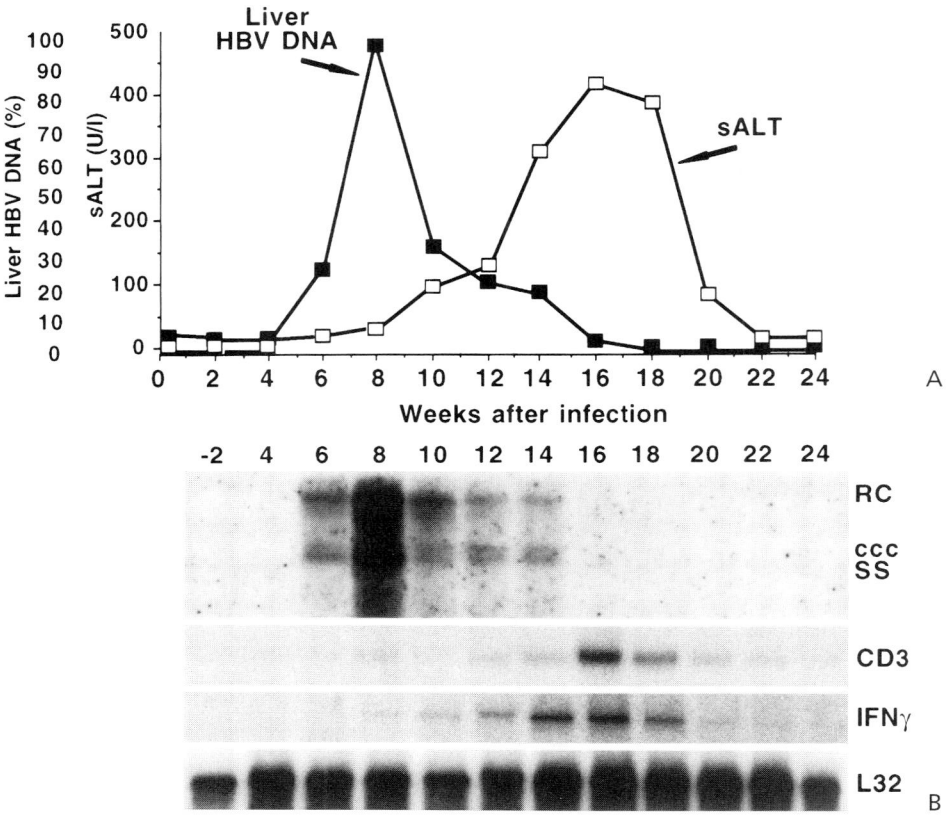

FIGURE 52.2. Noncytolytic clearance of hepatitis B virus (*HBV*) in an acutely infected chimpanzee. In this experiment, serum and needle liver biopsies were obtained on a weekly basis after inoculation of a chimpanzee with HBV-positive plasma from an HBV transgenic mouse. The chimpanzee became transiently infected as indicated by the appearance and eventual clearance of HBV DNA from the liver. The chimpanzee also developed an episode of acute hepatitis as seen by the transient elevation of serum alanine aminotransferase (*sALT*) activity. Note that the kinetics of viral clearance [determined by competitive polymerase chain reaction (PCR), **A** and by Southern blot, **B**] preceded the kinetics of disease activity by several weeks, indicating that the two events are independent during acute HBV infection in this model, similar to the observations in the HBV transgenic mice. Note also that the covalently closed circular (*ccc*) DNA species as well as the viral replicative intermediates disappeared from the liver with similar kinetics, suggesting that the cccDNA is susceptible to noncytolytic clearance mechanisms as well as the replicative intermediates. Finally, note that the decrease in viral DNA coincides with the appearance of interferon-γ (*IFNγ*) messenger RNA in the liver while the liver disease correlates primarily with the appearance of CD3 mRNA, a T-cell marker. This suggests that antiviral inflammatory cytokines produced by non-T cells may play an important role in the early viral clearance process, while the disease is more closely related to the influx of T cells into the liver. *RC*, relaxed circular; *SS*, single-standard.

to 12 weeks after infection, and they reach a peak between weeks 16 and 21. Therefore, there is no evidence of liver cell injury at the time when HBV replication is decreasing most rapidly (Fig. 52.2). Importantly, the disappearance of viral DNA was associated with the appearance of interferon γ in the liver and not with classical T-cell markers which appeared later, coincident with elevated serum ALT activity, that is, liver disease. Thus, the decline of HBV DNA from serum and liver preceded the influx of T cells and the associated acute viral hepatitis. This suggests that most viral DNA (at least 90% in the chimpanzee model) is eliminated by T-cell-independent, noncytolytic processes that do not require the destruction of liver cells (75).

The nature of the non-T cell(s) responsible for the early noncytolytic clearance of HBV is currently unknown, but the likely candidates are NK cells and NKT cells because of their abundance in the liver (76–78) and because they are rich sources of cytokines like IFNγ and TNFα that are known to have antiviral activity against HBV. The NK cell is a particularly attractive candidate because of its ability to recognize infected cells that express low levels of HLA class I molecules. If this proves to be correct, the early NK cell response to HBV could have a dual effect during the infection by secreting antiviral cytokines. First, it would inhibit HBV replication, thereby reducing the viral load and the number of infected cells. Second, it would upregulate HLA class I expression on the hepatocyte, thereby making it more visible to conventional class I-restricted T cells that then recognize, kill and secrete their own antiviral cytokines, thereby curing the remaining infected cells. This scenario is compatible with the sequence of events observed in the infected chimpanzees.

These concepts are supported by immunological analysis of the early incubation phase of HBV infection in recent unpublished studies in acutely infected humans that provide new insight into the HBV-specific CD4 and CD8 T-cell responses before clinical onset. As in the chimpanzee studies, HBV replication is controlled before the onset of clinical symptoms when serum ALT levels are still normal (79). This provides further evidence that HBV infection can be controlled without a biochemically detectable destruction of infected liver cells.

Interestingly, HBV-specific CD4 and CD8 T cells are detectable in the peripheral blood of acutely infected chimpanzees as early as 2 weeks after infection, long before they appear in the liver and the induction of liver disease (R. Thimme and F.V. Chisari, unpublished observation, 2000). Furthermore, the same T-cell responses are detectable in the circulation during the early incubation phase (8 to 10 weeks after infection) in humans (79). Furthermore, the peak frequency of circulating HBV-specific CTLs in humans (80) and intrahepatic CTLs in chimpanzees coincides with clinical onset and ALT elevation.

Taken together, the most recent results derived from animal and human studies allow a more accurate picture to be drawn of the virologic and immunologic events occurring after HBV infection and the mechanisms responsible for viral control and liver damage (Fig. 52.3). The most striking observation emerging from these studies is that control of viral replication and elimination of most HBV DNA molecules occur before the onset of liver damage and clinical symptoms. This event is therefore independent of the immune destruction of infected hepatocytes and is probably due to the suppression of viral gene expression and replication by soluble factors, including IFNγ and TNFα, released by liver-infiltrating T and non-T cells.

Using new, highly sensitive techniques to quantitate the number of virus-specific T cells, it has recently been shown that the maximal frequency of HBV-specific CD8 cells in the circulation generally coincides with the peak of liver damage, confirming the chimpanzee experiment (75) and suggesting an important role for these cells in the pathogenesis of liver disease (80).

Chronic Hepatitis B Virus Infection in Humans

The concept that an effective HBV-specific CD8+ T-cell response can inhibit virus replication without evidence of liver damage can also be applied to chronic healthy carriers of HBV. Patients with chronic HBV infection without signs of liver damage have generally been considered to lack an active CTL response against HBV. Recent studies carried out by tetramer staining and functional analysis of circulating and intrahepatic CTLs show that functionally active HBV-specific CD8+ T cells are present in the circulation and the liver of these patients, despite the absence of liver damage (81). HBV-specific CTLs present in the circulation in these patients express the phenotype of antigen-primed resting T cells, expand efficiently, display cytolytic activity and secrete antiviral cytokines *in vitro* upon stimulation with viral antigen. Moreover, a high fraction of liver-infiltrating CD8+ T cells are HBV-specific in these patients. Although these results do not rule out the possibility that some degree of liver cell lysis (not detectable as serum ALT elevation) caused by HBV-specific CTLs may occur in healthy carriers, the sparsely scattered pattern of CD8+ cells within the liver parenchyma suggests that control of virus replication in these patients may occur primarily through the secretion of cytokines by HBV-specific CTLs. In this scenario, liver cell destruction by direct cell-to-cell contact would be limited to few hepatocytes at most, and viral control would be almost exclusively exerted by soluble cytokines which can diffuse through the parenchyma, keeping viral replication under control.

In striking contrast to chronic healthy carriers who are able to control virus replication, a reservoir of functionally active HBV-specific CTLs is not detectable in patients with chronic active hepatitis, who are unable to control the virus and display a high degree of liver damage and high levels of HBV replication (81). In these patients, HBV-specific

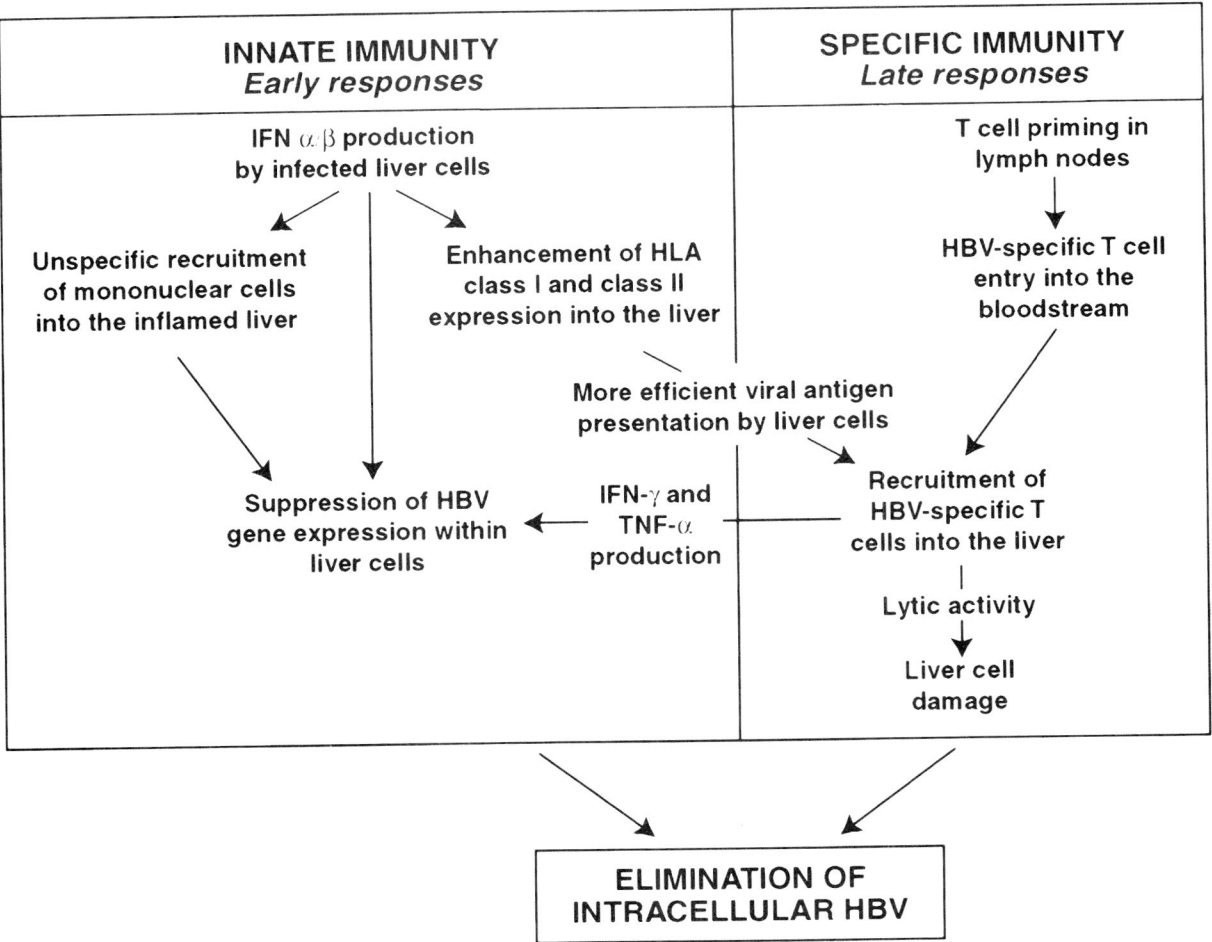

FIGURE 52.3. Role of innate and virus-specific immunity in the pathogenesis of liver cell damage and viral clearance in hepatitis B virus (*HBV*) infection. Recent studies in human and chimpanzee infection (see text) suggest a pathogenic model in which the innate immunity plays a crucial role in suppression of viral gene expression within infected liver cells. Based on this model, α and β interferons (*IFN*) produced by infected liver cells would be primarily responsible for early intrahepatic recruitment of virus-nonspecific immune mononuclear cells. In concert with the effect of cytokines produced by these cells, type I interferons would cause initial suppression of HBV genes within infected hepatocytes. Moreover, they would enhance the expression of histocompatibility leukocyte antigen (*HLA*) class I molecules and would induce *de novo* synthesis of HLA class II molecules on the surface of liver cells. Only after this event, HBV-specific T cells, previously primed in the local lymph nodes, would recognize efficiently infected liver cells displaying efficient effector function (lytic activity and production of anti-viral cytokines). This would enhance the inhibition of intracellular HBV genes and would induce liver cell destruction, thereby complementing the effect of the innate immunity and allowing final elimination of intracellular virus. Liver cell damage would result from the combined effect of HBV-specific T cells and virus nonspecific mononuclear cells, which represent the major component of the intrahepatic infiltrates. *TNF-α*, tumor necrosis factor α.

CTLs are detectable only within the liver, where their frequency is low because they are diluted among a large number of virus-nonspecific T cells that may play an important role in the pathogenesis of liver cell damage (81).

The behavior of the CTL response in patients with chronic HBV infection supports the notion that control of HBV replication may be exerted by HBV-specific CTLs without causing cell destruction. Indeed, the presence of functionally active CTLs in the liver and circulation of

healthy carriers is associated with inhibition of virus replication and lack of liver damage. Moreover, control of virus replication seems to require the capacity to rapidly mount strong CD8-mediated effector mechanisms, as shown by comparing the features of HBV-specific CTLs in healthy HBV carriers and patients who successfully recover from acute hepatitis B with those of patients with a chronic active infection, persistent liver damage, and active virus replication. Therefore, restoration of the CTL capacity to expand vigorously and to exert efficient effector function after antigen stimulation represents one of the main objectives of antiviral therapies in patients with chronic hepatitis B, to make their CTLs functionally similar to those of individuals who are able to control virus replication (healthy carriers and individuals recovered from acute HBV infection). Recent studies show that this objective can be achieved by lamivudine therapy that is able to restore virus-specific helper (82) and CTL functions (82a) and to render HBV-specific CTLs susceptible to exogenous stimulation. Despite this, however, most patients relapse when lamivudine therapy is stopped, suggesting that CTL responses must be further boosted to achieve viral clearance in this setting. These results are also consistent with the hypothesis that the CTL response alone is not sufficient to eradicate the infection. This may imply that in patients with chronic hepatitis, something else besides the capacity of T cells to expand and express effector function upon antigen re-encounter is missing and needs to be restored.

HEPATITIS C VIRAL CLEARANCE AND DISEASE PATHOGENESIS

Mechanisms for Control of Hepatitis C Virus Infection

Although hepatitis B and C viruses can cause a similar spectrum of acute and chronic liver diseases, with possible evolution to cirrhosis and hepatocellular carcinoma, the different natural histories of HBV and HCV infections, with different rates of chronic progression and a different association with extrahepatic manifestations and autoimmune disorders, suggest that the immune system deals with the two viruses through distinct mechanisms, and that HBV and HCV may use different strategies to evade immune control and to persist in the infected host. Indeed, approximately 5% to 10% of adults infected by HBV develop a chronic infection, whereas more than 70% of patients become persistently infected with HCV. This high rate of chronic evolution makes human acute hepatitis C an ideal model to characterize the mechanisms that are critical for viral control and liver cell injury, because of the possibility to compare, from the early clinical stages of disease, patients who resolve infection with those who do not (83,84). An important contribution to our understanding of the mechanisms responsible for termination of infection also comes from prospective studies of the HCV-specific immune response in chimpanzees infected with HCV, the only animal species known to support HCV replication and to develop an acute disease similar to natural hepatitis C in humans (85).

Chimpanzees that succeed in spontaneously terminating HCV infection mount an early, strong, and multispecific CTL response against multiple HCV epitopes (85). In contrast, animals that develop a chronic infection show weaker CTL responses, especially at the very early stages of disease

(85). The vigorous CTL response associated with control of infection contrasts with the poor antibody responses detected in the same animals (85). These findings suggest that antiviral CTLs rather than the antibody response are crucial for protection against HCV. Concerns about the role of the antibody response in control of HCV infection were initially raised by the observation that chimpanzees who had successfully recovered from acute hepatitis C could be reinfected with the same inoculum used for the original infection (86,87). Moreover, it is well known that anti-E2 antibodies are constantly detectable in chronic hepatitis C and that resolution of HCV infection can occur in the absence of antibodies, as shown by the outcome of HCV infection in agammaglobulinemic children who can terminate infection in a proportion of cases similar to the general population (88–90).

Despite this apparent lack of correlation between antibody responses and control of infection, several lines of evidence suggest that neutralizing antibodies are produced during natural HCV infection: (a) sera derived from patients with chronic HCV infection can inhibit HCV infection of susceptible lymphoid lines *in vitro* (91); (b) chimpanzees can be successfully protected by hyperimmune sera derived from immunization of rabbits with a synthetic peptide of the hypervariable region 1 from infection with the homologous viral strain (92); (c) these hyperimmune sera can also prevent HCV infection in cell culture (93); and (d) sera from patients with acute and chronic HCV infection contain antibodies that can inhibit the binding of envelope antigens to hepatocyte lines *in vitro* (94). The main target of the neutralizing activity is the HVR1 region of the E2 protein, and its variability may reflect, at least in part, the selective pressure imposed by the antibody response (95–97). This is also suggested by the lack of variability of the HVR1 region when the antibody response is absent (agammaglobulinemic patients) (98) and by the evidence that anti-HVR1 antibodies can precipitate HCV (91), inhibit viral attachment (99), and reduce or inhibit viral infectivity *in vitro* (100) and *in vivo* (92,101).

Concurrently with the CTL response, early multispecific, CD4-mediated responses are also mounted by infected individuals who recover from HCV infection, indicating that these responses are associated with, and may contribute to, resolution of infection (83,84). This is indicated by sequential studies of the HLA class II-restricted response to HCV antigens carried out from the early stages of disease in patients with acute hepatitis C and different outcome of infection. Not only the strength but also the quality of the CD4-mediated responses differ in relation to the final outcome, the responses being significantly stronger and more Th1-oriented in those patients who resolve infection compared to those who develop chronic disease (102).

Similar to what was described previously for hepatitis B, both HLA class I- and class II-restricted T-cell responses remain detectable in the peripheral blood following resolution of hepatitis C, even in the absence of apparent reexposure to the virus (103,104). The features of these long-lasting T-cell responses suggest that they may actually represent effector rather than memory responses and that they may be crucial to control the traces of virus that persist. This suggests that clinical resolution of HCV infection does not necessarily imply eradication of HCV, and it suggests that long-lasting T-cell memory following hepatitis C can be maintained by the chronic production of minute amounts of antigen.

The Immune Response in Chronic Hepatitis C

A puzzling observation is that HCV-specific HLA class II-restricted T-cell responses appear to be stronger in patients with chronic HCV infection than in the acute stage of infection in patients who subsequently develop a chronic disease (105–108). This may suggest that the T-cell response progressively increases as a function of the duration of infection, but longitudinal studies have not been performed yet. CD4+ T cells from chronically infected patients are characteristically polyclonal and multispecific. A clear hierarchy of T-cell responsiveness to HCV proteins has been defined in these patients. Specifically, core and NS4 are recognized by most patients, whereas the putative envelope proteins (E1 and E2/NS1) and NS5 are immunogenic for a small proportion of patients. However, these findings must be interpreted cautiously, because envelope proteins are highly variable and the lack of T-cell response *in vitro* may be related to the lack of appropriate reagents to study the response to these proteins, that is, the lack of complete sequence homology between recombinant proteins used *in vitro* and proteins of the infecting virus that prime the immune response *in vivo*.

Also, the HLA class I-restricted T-cell response against HCV is readily detectable in the peripheral blood of a good proportion of patients with chronic HCV infection following stimulation of T cells with HCV-derived peptides (107–110). The frequency of circulating HCV-specific CTL assessed by tetramer staining has been reported to range between 0.01% and 1.2% of the total pool of peripheral CD8+ cells, and their phenotype is consistent with the features of resting memory T cells (111). These findings represent an important difference in the pathobiology of chronic HCV and HBV infections, because CTL responses are generally undetectable in the peripheral blood of patients with chronic hepatitis B.

In patients with chronic HCV infection, HCV-specific helper and cytotoxic T cells able to recognize structural and nonstructural HCV proteins in the context of several different HLA molecules have also been detected within the liver (112–116). Different HCV proteins can be simultaneously recognized by intrahepatic T cells of individual patients. The high immunogenicity of core and NS4 at the HLA class II-restricted T-cell level has been confirmed by the isolation of core- and NS4-specific T cells from liver infiltrates. Remark-

ably, HCV-specific CD4+ T cells sequestered within the inflamed liver can be functionally and clonotypically different from HCV-specific T cells present in the peripheral blood, suggesting a specific compartmentalization of some T cells at the site of infection (117). HCV-specific T-cell sequestration within the infected liver is also suggested by the observation that the frequency of HCV-specific CTL within the liver is significantly higher than in the peripheral blood (111), but the evidence that only 1% to 2% of the total infiltrating CD8 cells is HCV-specific indicates that nonvirus-specific mononuclear cells represent the major component of the intrahepatic cellular infiltrate. Most virus-specific and nonspecific T cells are activated and able to predominantly produce Th1 cytokines. Among these infiltrates, there is an enrichment of lymphocytes typical of innate immunity, such as NK cells, natural T (NT) cells, and NKT cells that may play an important role in maintaining chronic liver damage (118,119).

Sequence of Immune Events After Hepatitis C Virus Infection

Current evidence suggests that control of infection is strictly dependent upon the vigor, the breadth, and the quality of the early cell-mediated immune responses (Fig. 52.4). The capacity of infected individuals to mount a wide spectrum of CTL responses with different specificities during the early stages of infection is probably the most critical factor to successfully control the heterogeneous infecting viral quasispecies. Effective control cannot occur without a concurrent multispecific CD4 response that enhances and maintains the CTLs and produces, in concert with CTLs, Th1 cytokines that could have an antiviral effect at the site of infection, although the susceptibility of HCV to control by inflammatory cytokines has not been established. In the presence of these multispecific and Th1-oriented cellular responses, the likelihood of viral escape from immune surveillance and persistence is negligible. Based on the results in the chimpanzee model of infection, antibody responses seem to be less critical for initial virus control, although they certainly contribute to spontaneous resolution of infection.

The primary mechanisms responsible for the differential strength and quality of the early cellular responses associated with resolution or chronic evolution of infection remain undefined, although host and viral factors have been implicated. Recent studies provide evidence that the HLA class II alleles DRB1*1101 and DQB1*0301 are associated with spontaneous viral clearance (120). Moreover, dose of the virus, route of infection, genotype, and heterogeneity of the infecting inoculum have been suggested to influence the outcome of infection.

Escape from antibody and CTL responses or interference with other host immune functions as a result of viral mutations may play an important role in view of the extremely high variability of this virus. Although studies in patients

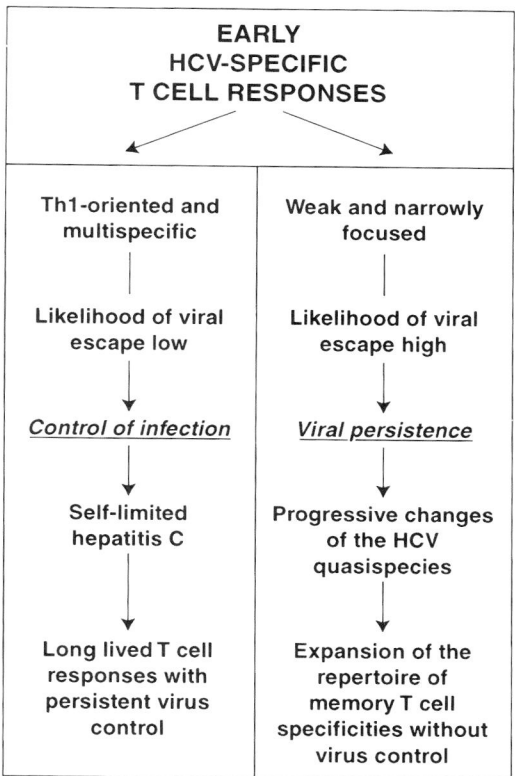

FIGURE 52.4. Role of the hepatitis C virus (*HCV*)-specific T-cell response in the control of HCV infection. Analysis of the immune response in human and chimpanzee HCV infection suggests that the vigor, breadth, and quality of the early cell-mediated immune response influence the outcome of infection. CD4- and CD8-mediated HCV-specific T-cell responses oriented towards the preferential production of the Th1 cytokines and characterized by a wide spectrum of viral peptide specificities are associated with successful control of infection. In contrast, weak and more narrowly focused HCV-specific T-cell responses are associated with HCV persistence. In this condition, the likelihood of viral escape from T-cell surveillance would he higher. Once persistence has been established, progressive changes of the viral quasi-species may lead to expansion of the repertoire of memory T-cell specificities. Although able to express effector function *in vitro*, a proportion of these cell populations may be functionally ineffective *in vivo* because of the loss of their target sequence as a result of the continuous changes of the HCV.

with chronic HBV and HIV infections establish the principle that escape through mutational inactivation of protective epitopes may occur when the CTL response is narrowly focused on a single or a few immundominant epitopes (121–123), as previously suggested by studies in chimpanzees (124), no definitive data are available at present to confirm that these mechanisms are really operative in human HCV infection (125). Since weaker HCV-specific CD4 and CD8 responses at the early stages of chimpanzee and human infections are associated with chronic evolution, escape from protective T-cell responses may occur in principle more easily in these patients by virtue of the narrowly focused nature of their responses directed against a limited number of epitopes. Further studies must define, however, whether the require-

ments for virus selection and escape are actually met during HCV infection and whether escape mechanisms may represent a primary cause of viral persistence.

Given the heterogeneous nature of the viral population that infects individual patients, it is likely that different evasion strategies have been evolved by HCV and can act simultaneously to interfere with the host's defensive mechanisms at different levels. The potential ability of HCV to circumvent the antiviral effect of IFN by the interaction of E2 with protein kinase PKR (126) and its potential to interfere with TNF-induced apoptosis through the binding of the core protein to members of the TNF receptor family represent described mechanisms that may be involved in the pathogenesis of both liver cell damage and viral persistence (127–129). Moreover, it has been suggested that production of neutralizing antibodies able to efficiently inhibit HCV binding to host cells could be limited by the high affinity of E2 for CD81 (130).

Why the virus can survive in chronic patients even in the presence of multiple populations of HCV-specific CTLs with different specificities, able to efficiently expand and to express their effector function *in vitro* following antigen re-encounter remains unknown. It is possible that results of *in vitro* studies overestimate the actual antiviral efficiency of HCV-specific CTLs in chronic patients. Indeed, the evolution of the viral quasispecies during the course of a viral infection may cause the sequential priming of a wide array of CTL populations able to recognize new emerging epitopes. This phenomenon can lead to the progressive expansion of the repertoire of memory T-cell specificities circulating in individual patients. However, a proportion of the memory cells will persist and expand upon *in vitro* stimulation despite the loss of the corresponding epitope. Although able to express effector function *in vitro*, these cell populations may be functionally ineffective *in vivo* because of the loss of their target sequence.

Finally, the recent observation that HCV can bind to CD81 (131) has important pathogenetic implications. Indeed, costimulatory signals may be delivered to B cells (and perhaps other cell types) upon appropriate engagement of CD81, since this molecule is a component of a molecular complex with CD21 and CD19 that participates in B-cell activation (132). Engagement of this complex by HCV may lower the B-cell activation threshold (133), thereby facilitating autoantibody production, similar to what has been reported for EBV that binds CD21 (134). This may explain why extrahepatic manifestations caused by autoimmune reactions with the presence of circulating autoantibodies are frequently associated with HCV infection.

Moreover, the possibility that a costimulatory signal is delivered by the E2-CD81 interaction, together with other undefined mechanisms, may also contribute to the activation and expansion of non–virus-specific cell populations in the infected organ. This may in turn contribute to the dilution of liver infiltrating HCV-specific lymphocytes, causing interference with the expression of their antiviral effector function.

MECHANISMS OF HEPATITIS B VIRUS AND HEPATITIS C VIRUS PERSISTENCE

For a noncytopathic virus to persist it must either overwhelm or not induce an effective antiviral immune response, or it must be able to evade it. All of these scenarios could be operative in patients chronically infected by HBV and HCV. Indeed, neonatal tolerance is probably responsible for both the lack of an antiviral immune response and for viral persistence following mother–infant transmission, which is the most common antecedent of persistent HBV infection worldwide (64). The immunological basis for viral persistence during adult onset infection is not well understood. Perhaps the simplest explanation is quantitative, based on the kinetics of infection relative to the induction of a CTL response during the early days of an infection. For example, viral persistence would be predicted if the size of the inoculum or the replication rate of an incoming virus exceeds the kinetics of the immune response such that the effector-to-target cell ratio favors the virus even when the CTL response is fully in place. However, since the CTL response is much less vigorous in chronically infected patients than it is during acute infection (135,136–138), other factors must be involved as well. Reasonable candidates are the induction of peripheral tolerance or exhaustion of the T-cell response by the high viral load that characterizes most persistently infected patients. Additionally, virus-specific CTLs that might otherwise become activated by antigen recognition in the immunostimulatory context of secondary lymphoid organs might be inactivated if antigen is presented in the absence of costimulatory signals in the liver.

Other candidate mechanisms that could contribute to viral persistence include infection of immunologically privileged sites, viral inhibition of antigen presentation, selective immune suppression, downregulation of viral gene expression, and viral mutations that abrogate, anergize or antagonize antigen recognition by virus specific T cells (reviewed in ref. 64). There is some evidence that privileged sites may play a role since HBV and HCV do infect extrahepatic tissues. Also, we have shown that circulating HBV-specific CTLs can cause hepatitis, but not nephritis, in HBV transgenic mice that express the virus in the liver and the kidney, due to the limited access of the CTLs to antigen-positive cells present on the other side of microvascular barriers that exist in the kidney but are not present in the liver sinusoid (67). Additionally, it has been suggested that infected cells that express Fas ligand can protect themselves against CTL-mediated injury by actively destroying the CTLs via the same Fas ligand–Fas receptor pathway that CTLs use to kill their target cells, but in reverse (139). Importantly, it appears that hepatocytes can be induced to express Fas ligand during an inflammatory response (140). If so, individuals whose hepatocytes express Fas ligand most efficiently would be most likely to delete their HBV- or HCV-specific CTLs and, therefore, become chronically

infected. An interesting correlate of this scenario is the theoretical possibility that HBV or HCV might be able to induce Fas ligand expression by the hepatocytes, thereby deleting the virus-specific CTL population when it enters the liver. In either case, Fas ligand induction would have to occur without inducing hepatocyte fratricide by virtue of Fas ligand–Fas interactions between adjacent cells (140). Alternatively, HBV or HCV could theoretically downregulate Fas expression, rendering the infected hepatocyte relatively resistant to destruction by the CTL. All of these theories are testable, but they are strictly speculative at present.

Certain viruses (e.g. poxviruses, adenoviruses, herpesviruses, etc.) have evolved the ability to inhibit antigen presentation, or to suppress or neutralize antiviral cytokines extracellularly as survival strategies (reviewed in refs.141 and 142). Thus far, however, there is no evidence that these processes are operative during HBV or HCV infection. As discussed earlier, however, inflammatory cytokines, especially IFNγ, suppress HBV gene expression and replication, which could contribute to viral persistence if the effect is incomplete or if the virus infects an individual whose immune response to HBV does not produce this cytokine. Indeed, the cytopathic potential of the CTLs in these individuals would trigger hepatitis, whereas the failure of their CTLs to produce the appropriate cytokines might contribute to viral persistence. Analysis of cytokine expression in the liver of patients with chronic HBV infection should clarify this interesting hypothesis. Whether these events occur during HCV infection remains to be determined.

The role of viral escape mutations as a cause of viral persistence has attracted considerable interest in recent years. Many conditions must be fulfilled, however, for a mutant virus to be selected by CTL-mediated immune pressure (reviewed in ref. 64). Perhaps the most important condition is the occurrence of a strong CTL response that is focused on a single viral epitope. This scenario would favor the outgrowth of variant viruses because they would not be otherwise visible to the immune system. This type of CTL response is unusual, however, during HBV infection where the CTL response is typically vigorous and multispecific during acute hepatitis and weak or undetectable during chronic hepatitis (136,137,142,63). Accordingly, mutational inactivation of CTL epitopes is uncommon during chronic HBV infection (143).

Nonetheless, strong, narrowly focused CTL responses do occur occasionally in these patients, and in this setting viral escape mutations can occur (121, 122). Vigorous oligoclonal expansions of T cells have been described in other persistent viral infections, especially HIV (145) and EBV (146). Even in these infections, however, viral mutations that affect recognition of an epitope by some CTL clones do not automatically affect all CTL clones specific for the same epitope, since different T-cell clones can bind different residues in the same epitope (147,148). While CTL escape can confer a strong survival advantage, it is important to emphasize that selection of escape variants in all of these infections occurs in the setting of a preexisting persistent infection; that is, viral persistence probably leads to the selection of escape variants, not the reverse.

The situation may be somewhat different in early chronic HIV infection, where the CTL response is characteristically very strong yet unable to clear the virus (145). The incredibly high rate of HIV production and the exceptionally high mutation rate of this virus may cause so many different viruses to be generated each day that they exceed the capacity of the immune system to respond effectively simply on a numerical basis (148). In this regard, the ostensibly vigorous immune response HIV appears to be unable to compete with the capacity of the virus to generate mutants. Mutational inactivation of CTL epitopes might thus play an earlier and more important role in the establishment of viral persistence for HIV than for HBV (149). It is important to emphasize, however, that the overwhelming rates of viral replication and spread relative to the ability of the immune system to produce enough CTLs to reach and destroy all of the infected cells, plus the immunosuppressive effects of the virus itself, are more important than viral mutation for the development of persistent infection.

The situation may be different again during chronic HCV infection, where an extensive quasispecies of viral variants can coexist with a multispecific CTL response (150–152) that is intermediate in strength between the response of patients chronically infected by HBV and HIV. Unlike HBV and HIV, where the viral load is high, the viral titer is very low during chronic HCV infection (153), so viral persistence cannot easily be blamed on an overwhelming infection in this instance. Therefore, escape mutants may play a greater role in the primary establishment of HCV persistence than is likely for HBV. Importantly, CTL escape has been observed in a chronically HCV-infected chimpanzee (154); however, the extent to which the mutation contributed to or was a consequence of persistent HCV infection in this case remains to be determined.

In view of the multispecificity of the CTL response to most persistent viruses, current data favor the notion that negative selection of CTL escape mutants is most likely to occur after a persistent infection is already established. In this setting, viral mutations could solidify the chronicity of the infection and perhaps even make it irreversible. Whether such mutations can also serve as the primary cause of viral persistence in the context of a multispecific T-cell response remains to be proven.

IMMUNE PATHOGENESIS OF HEPATOCELLULAR CARCINOMA

The mechanisms responsible for malignant transformation in chronic HBV and HCV infection are not well defined,

and both viral and host factors have been implicated in the process. On the one hand, all cases of hepatocellular carcinoma (HCC) occur after many years of chronic hepatitis which could, theoretically, provide the mitogenic and mutagenic environment to precipitate random genetic and chromosomal damage and lead to the development of HCC. On the other hand, in chronic HBV infection, most tumors contain clonally integrated HBV DNA and microdeletions in the flanking cellular DNA which could, theoretically, deregulate cellular growth control mechanisms (155). Furthermore, the HBV X gene product has been shown to transactivate cellular genes associated with cellular growth control (156–158) and inhibit p53 gene function *in vitro* (159), suggesting that deregulated X gene expression from integrated fragments of subviral DNA could play a role in hepatocarcinogenesis (160). Similarly, C-terminally truncated viral envelope proteins expressed from integrated subviral DNA may have transactivating activity (161,162) and could potentially contribute to carcinogenesis in chronic HBV infection. Like retroviruses, however, HBV integration does not occur in resting hepatocytes; so if HBV integration plays a role in hepatocarcinogenesis, antecedent events must occur that trigger hepatocellular turnover. These mechanisms can't be operative in chronic HCV infection, because this virus doesn't replicate in the nucleus or integrate into the cellular genome. Certain HCV gene products may have procarcinogenic activity, however, and these aspects of HCV biology are discussed by Brechot et al. in Chapter 54.

In an effort to clarify the carcinogenic potential of chronic hepatitis, we previously showed that transgenic mice that produce hepatotoxic quantities of the HBV large envelope polypeptide (163–166) display hepatocellular injury, regenerative hyperplasia, chronic inflammation, Kupffer cell hyperplasia, oxygen radical production, glutathione depletion, oxidative DNA damage, transcriptional deregulation, and aneuploidy that inexorably progresses to HCC (165–170). While those studies demonstrated that HBV can cause hepatocellular carcinoma in the absence of insertional mutagenesis, X gene expression or genotoxic chemicals, they did not prove that chronic immune-mediated hepatitis was a procarcinogenic stimulus in itself. The current study was undertaken, therefore, to determine whether hepatocellular carcinoma can be triggered by a chronic, virus-specific immune response in HBV transgenic mice.

To test this hypothesis, we developed a model of chronic immune-mediated liver disease using transgenic mice that express nontoxic concentrations of the large, middle, and small envelope proteins in the hepatocyte. Similar to human chronic HBsAg carriers, these mice are immunologically tolerant to HBsAg and they develop no evidence of liver disease except ground glass hepatocytes during their lifetime. They were thymectomized, lethally irradiated and reconstituted with bone marrow and spleen cells either from syngeneic nontransgenic donors that were previously immunized with a recombinant vaccinia virus that expresses HBsAg and displayed HBsAg-specific CTLs and anti-HBs antibodies, or from immunologically tolerant transgenic donors. All results were compared with unmanipulated age- and sex-matched transgenic mice. All of the mice that were reconstituted with immunologically primed nontransgenic immune systems developed acute hepatitis and cleared HBsAg from their serum. Subsequently, all of these mice developed chronic hepatitis and HCC (171).

The pathogenetic importance of immune-mediated hepatocellular injury in hepatocarcinogenesis in this study is strengthened by the fact that hepatocellular carcinoma occurs in the context of necrosis, inflammation, and regeneration (cirrhosis) in several human liver diseases other than hepatitis B, including chronic hepatitis C (reviewed in ref. 172), alcoholism (173), hemochromatosis (174), glycogen storage disease (175), α-1-antitrypsin deficiency (176,177), and primary biliary cirrhosis (178). Irrespective of etiology or pathogenesis, therefore, it would appear that chronic liver cell injury is a premalignant condition that initiates a cascade of events characterized by increased rates of cellular DNA synthesis and production of endogenous mutagens coupled with compromised cellular detoxification and repair functions. If these processes are sustained for a sufficiently long period of time, they would be expected to cause the multiple genetic and chromosomal changes necessary to trigger the development of hepatocellular carcinoma (Fig. 52.5). This notion is supported by the close correlation between chronic inflammation and carcinogenesis in animal models of wounding and inflammation that lead to skin cancer (179–181), and in humans where continuous

oral irritation leads to oral cancer (181), chronic inflammatory bowel disease predisposes to bowel cancer (183–186), chronic cystitis precedes bladder cancer (187–191), and reflux esophagitis leads to esophageal cancer (192,193).

While these associations strongly suggest that chronic necroinflammation may be procarcinogenic in regenerative tissues, they do not constitute proof of this concept. The current results, however, provide definitive evidence that HBV-specific chronic immune-mediated liver cell injury is sufficient to initiate and sustain the process of hepatocarcinogenesis in this model. Furthermore, they demonstrate that the immune response is procarcinogenic despite the absence of cofactors such as viral integration, X gene expression or genotoxic agents that have been proposed to contribute to the development of HCC in humans. Since the immunological, virological, and histological features of this model closely resemble human chronic hepatitis, the results suggest that an ineffective immune response is the principal oncogenic factor during chronic HBV infection in humans. It is ironic that the same T-cell response that can eradicate HBV from the liver when it is strong can be procarcinogenic by triggering a chronic necroinflammatory liver disease when it is unable to completely terminate the infection. If this is correct, therapeutic enhancement of the T-cell response to HBV in chronically infected patients should prevent HCC.

CONCLUSION

The diversity of clinical syndromes and disease manifestations associated with HBV and HCV infections strongly

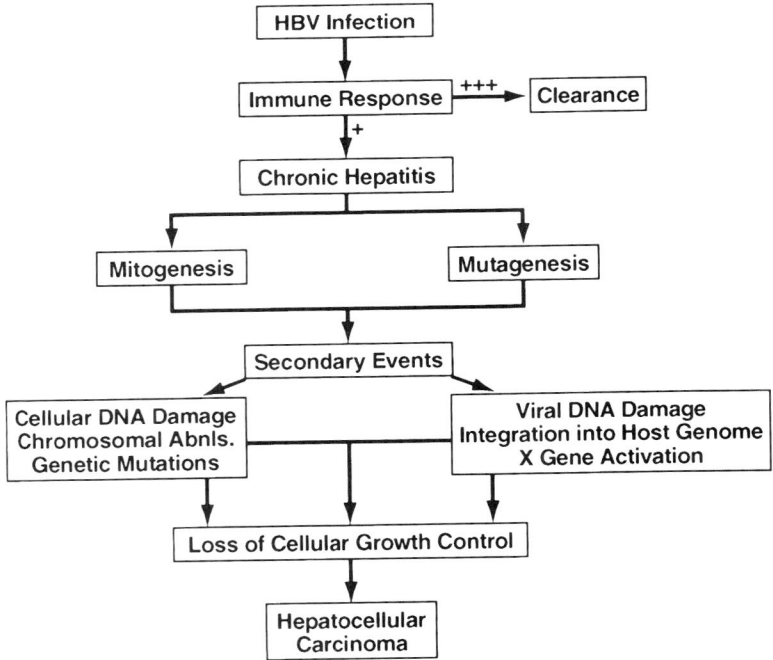

FIGURE 52.5. The chronic injury → hepatocellular carcinoma (HCC) hypothesis. According to this hypothesis, a vigorous (+++) immune response to hepatitis B virus (HBV) leads to viral clearance while an absent (–) immune response leads to the "healthy" carrier state, and an intermediate (+) immune response produces chronic hepatitis. This indolent necroinflammatory liver disease is characterized by chronic liver cell necrosis which stimulates a sustained regenerative response. The inflammatory component includes activated macrophages that are a rich source of free radicals. The collaboration of these mitogenic and mutagenic stimuli has the potential to cause cellular and viral DNA damage, chromosomal abnormalities, genetic mutations, etc., that deregulate cellular growth control in a multistep process that eventually leads to hepatocellular carcinoma.

suggests that the clinical outcome of these infections is determined by the quality and vigor of the antiviral immune response produced by the infected host. NK cells probably recognize infected cells first, secreting inflammatory cytokines that can greatly reduce the burden of virus (at least for HBV) and upregulate class I and class II expression, thereby facilitating antigen processing and presentation to CD4+ and CD8+ T cells that are induced in peripheral lymphoid organs. CD4+ helper T cells serve a critically important regulatory function by secreting a variety of cytokines that can facilitate B cell maturation, expression, and antibody secretion, and foster the development of a strong CTL response. CD8+ CTLs can kill infected cells by direct contact, triggering them to undergo apoptosis, and by recruiting antigen-nonspecific inflammatory cells that amplify their cytopathic potential. They also secrete cytokines when they recognize antigen in the infected tissue, some of which have the potential to inhibit the expression and replication of HBV in the hepatocytes. Antibodies to antigens expressed at the surface of virus particles can provide protection from initial infection and can prevent viral spread from cell to cell once infection is established. Antibody-mediated immune complex formation can contribute to extrahepatic syndromes in these patients and may even play a role in liver disease if they can bind to the surface of antigen-positive hepatocytes and recruit Fc-receptor-positive killer cells, thereby mediating antibody-dependent cellular cytotoxicity. All limbs of the immune response must cooperate productively to terminate a viral infection. Individual differences in the efficiency of viral antigen processing by hepatocytes and professional antigen-presenting cells, or at the level of antigen recognition and responsiveness by B and T lymphocytes, will affect the strength of the antiviral immune response and the extent to which it contributes to viral clearance and liver disease.

At the effector level, it would appear that the CTL response can activate two different pathways to eliminate a virus, either by killing the infected cells or by eliminating the virus from within the cell without killing it. These alternate scenarios can be activated simultaneously as a consequence of antigen recognition. According to this view, viral clearance depends on the development of a vigorous intrahepatic immune response, with the severity of the associated liver disease being determined by the number of infected hepatocytes and the balance between the cytopathic and antiviral regulatory effects of the intrahepatic inflammatory cells. If the T-cell response is strong and the number of infected cells is low, viral clearance should occur, rapidly and efficiently, with little evidence of liver disease, simply by killing the infected cells. Even a strong T-cell response may not be able to clear a massive viral infection, however, unless the curative limb of the response is called into play. In the absence of this component, the cytopathic function of the immune response may not be able to eliminate all of the infected cells, leading to persistent infection

and chronic liver disease. On the other hand, if the T-cell response is quantitatively suboptimal, the virus could persist even if the appropriate antiviral cytokines are produced and the virus is susceptible to their control, since, at insufficient levels, they will suppress viral gene expression without eliminating it, thereby making the virus less visible to the immune system.

It is important to emphasize that these principles need not extend to all viral infections (e.g., HCV), or even to the same virus when it infects different cells, since multiple factors must cooperate for intracellular viral inactivation by the immune response to occur. First, the appropriate cytokines must be secreted in sufficient amounts in the environment of the infected cells. Second, the infected cells must be able to respond to the cytokines by activating antiviral signaling pathways appropriate for the resident virus. Finally, the viral transcriptional template must be eradicated as well as its products. Based on these concepts, strategies designed to boost the specific immune response (e.g., CTL immunotherapy) to a virus or to alter the balance between the cytopathic and the regulatory components of the response (e.g., targeted cytokine immunotherapy) could terminate persistent viral infections of the liver and ameliorate the severity and consequences of the associated chronic liver disease. These concepts have been established primarily by studies carried out in HBV-related systems. Whether these principles apply to the rest of the hepatitis viruses, especially HCV, remains to be determined.

ACKNOWLEDGMENTS

Sections of this chapter have been previously published in *Hepatology* 1995;22:1316–325, *Springer Semin Immunopathol* 1995;17:261–281, *Am J Pathol* 2000;156:1117–1132, *Molecular Genetic Medicine* 1992;67–104, *Curr Top in Microbiol* 1991;168, and *Annu Rev Immunol* 1995;13:29–60, and have been modified and reproduced with permission from the publishers. This work was supported by National Insitutes of Health grants AI-20001, CA-40489, CA-54560, and CA-76403 to F.V.C.; RR00833 to the Scripps General Clinical Research Center; BioMed grant BMH4-98-2239, grants from the Instituto Superiore di Sanità, Italy (Viral Hepatitis Project), Schering-Plough S.p.A, and Fondazione Corsi, Italy to C.F.

REFERENCES

1. Knipe DM. Virus-host cell interaction. In: Fields BN, Knipe DV, et al. eds. *Fundamental Virology.* New York: Raven Press, 1991;267–290.
2. Rock KL, Goldberg AL. Degradation of cell proteins and generation of MHC class I-presented peptides. *Annu Rev Immunol* 1999;17:739–779.
3. Moore MW, Carbone FR, Bevan MJ. Introduction of soluble

protein into the class I pathway of antigen processing and presentation. *Cell* 1988;54:777–785.

4. Morrison LA, Lukacher AE, Braciale VL, et al. Differences in antigen presentation to MHC class I- and class II-restricted influenza virus specific cytolytic T lymphocyte clones. *J Exp Med* 1986;163:903–921.

5. Townsend AR, Rothbard MJ, Gotch FM, et al. The epitopes of influenza nucleoprotein recognized by cytotoxic T lymphocytes can be defined with short synthetic peptides. *Cell* 1986;44:959–968.

6. Monaco JJ. A molecular model of MHC class I-restricted antigen processing. *Immunol Today* 1992;13:173–179.

7. Silver ML, Parker KC, Wiley DC. Reconstitution by MHC-restricted peptides of HLA-A2 heavy chain with β-microglobulin, *in vitro*. *Nature* 1991;350:619–622.

8. Townsend A, Ohlén C, Bastin J, et al. Association of class I major histocompatibility heavy and light chains induced by viral peptides. *Nature* 1989;340:443–448.

9. Townsend A, Elliott T, Cerundolo V, et al. Assembly of MHC class I molecules analyzed *in vitro*. *Cell* 1990;62:285–295.

10. Bjorkman PJ, Saper MA, Samroui B, et al. Structure of the human class I histocompatibility antigen, HLA-A2. *Nature* 1987;329:506–512.

11. Bjorkman PJ, Saper MA, Samroui B, et al. The foreign antigen binding site and T cell recognition regions of class I histocompatibility antigens. *Nature* 1987;329:512–518.

12. Garrett TPJ, Saper MA, Bjorkman PJ, et al. Specificity pockets for the side chains of peptide antigens in HLA-Aw68. *Nature* 1989;342:692–696.

13. Madden DR, Gorga JC, Strominger JL, et al. The structure of HLA-B27 reveals nonamer self-peptides bound in an extended conformation. *Nature* 1991;353:321–325.

14. Bjorkman PJ. Structure, function, and diversity of class I major histocompatibility complex molecules. *Ann Rev Biochem* 1990;59:253–258.

15. Saper MA, Bjorkman PJ, Wiley DC. Refined structure of the human histocompatibility antigen HLA-A2 at 2.6 A resolution. *J Mol Biol* 1991;219:277–319.

16. Rotzschke O, Falk K, Deres K, et al. Isolation and analysis of naturally processed viral peptides as recognized by cytotoxic T cells. *Nature* 1990;348:252–254.

17. Van Bleek GM, Nathenson SG. Isolation of an endogenously processed immunodominant viral peptide from the class I H-2Kb molecule. *Nature* 1990;348:213–216.

18. Jardetzky TS, Lane VS, Robinson RA, et al. Identification of self peptides bound to purified HLA-B27. *Nature* 1991;353:326–328.

19. Falk K, Rotzschke O, Stevanovic S, et al. Allele-specific motifs revealed by sequencing of self-peptides eluted from MHC molecules. *Nature* 1991;351:290–296.

20. Jardetzky TS, Lane WS, Robinson RA, et al. Identification of self peptides bound to purified HLA-B27. *Nature* 1991;353:326–329.

21. Hunt DF, Henderson RA, Shabanowitz J, et al. Characterization of peptides bound to the class I MHC molecule HLA-A2.1 by mass spectrometry. *Science* 1992;255:1261–1263.

22. Fremont DH, Matsumara M, Stura EA, et al. Crystal structures of two viral peptides in complex with murine MHC class I H-2Kb. *Science* 1992;257:919–927.

23. Matsumara M, Fremont DH, Peterson PA, et al. Emerging principles for the recognition of peptide antigens by MHC class I moledules. *Science* 1992;257:927–934.

24. Zhang W, Young ACM, Imarai M, et al. Crystal structure of the major histocompatibility complex class I H-2Kb molecule containing a single viral peptide: implications for peptide binding and T cell receptor recognition. *Proc Natl Acad Sci U S A* 1992;89:8403–8408.

25. Silver ML, Guo H-C, Strominger JL, et al. Atomic structure of a human MHC molecule presenting an influenza virus peptide. *Nature* 1992;360:367–369.

26. Guo H-C, Jardetzky TS, Garrett TPJ, et al. Different length peptides bind to HLA-Aw68 similarly at their ends but bulge out in the middle. *Nature* 1992;360:364–366.

27. Cerundolo V, Elliott T, Elvin J, et al. The binding affinity and dissociation rates of peptides for class I major histocompatibility complex molecules. *Eur J Immunol* 1991;21:2069–2075.

28. Christinck ER, Luscher MA, Barber BH, et al. Peptide binding to class I MHC on living cells and quantitation of complexes required for CTL lysis. *Nature* 1991;352:67–70.

29. Wei M, Cresswell P. HLA-A2 molecules in an antigen-processing mutant cell contain signal sequence-derived peptides. *Nature* 1992;356:443–447.

30. Henderson RA, Michel H, Sakaguchi K, et al. HLA-A2.1-associated peptides from a mutant cell line: a second pathway of antigen presentation. *Science* 1992;255:1264–1266.

31. Germain RN. MHC-dependent antigen processing and peptide presentation: providing ligands for T lymphocyte activation. *Cell* 1994.76:287–299.

32. Teyton L, O'Sullivan D, Dickson PW, et al. Invariant chain distinguishes between the exogenous and endogenous antigen presentation pathway. *Nature* 1990;348:39–44.

33. Rudensky AY, Preston-Hurlburt P, Hong S-C, et al. Sequence analysis of peptides bound to MHC class II molecules. *Nature* 1991;353:622–627.

34. Hunt DF, Michel H, Dickinson TA, et al. Peptides presented to the immune system by the murine class II major histocompatibility complex molecule I-Ad. *Science* 1992;256:1817–1820.

35. Rudensky AY, Preston-Hurlburt P, Al-Ramadi BK, et al. Truncation variants of peptides isolated from MHC class II molecules suggest sequence motifs. *Nature* 1992;359:429–431.

36. Chicz RM, Urban RG, Lane WS, et al. Predominant naturally processed peptides bound to HLA-DR1 are derived from MHC-related molecules and are heterogeneous in size. *Nature* 1992;358:764–768.

37. Konig R, Huang L-Y, Germain RN. MHC class II interaction with CD4 mediated by a region analogous to the MHC class I binding site for CD8. *Nature* 1992;356:796–798.

38. Cammarota G, Scheirle A, Takacs B, et al. Identification of a CD4 binding site of the β2 domain of HLA-DR molecules. *Nature* 1992;356:799–801.

39. Braciale TJ, Morrison LA, Sweetser MT, et al. Antigen presentation pathway to class I and II MHC-restricted T lymphocytes. *Immunol Rev* 1987;98:95–114.

40. Browning M, Reiss CS, Huang A. The soluble viral glycoprotein of vesicular stomatitis virus efficiently sensitized target cells for lysis by CD4+ T lymphocytes. *J Virol* 1990;64:3810–3816.

41. Kaplan DR, Griffith R, Braciale VL, et al. Influenza virus-specific human cytotoxic T cell clones: heterogeneity in antigen specificity and restriction by class II MHC products. *Cell Immunol* 1984;88:193–206.

42. Jacobson S, Sekaly RP, Jacobson CL, et al. HLA class II-restricted presentation of cytoplasmic measles virus antigens to cytotoxic T cells. *J Virol* 1989;63:1756–1762.

43. Yasukawa M, Zarling JM. Human cytotoxic T cell clones directed against herpes simplex virus infected cells. *J Immunol* 1984;133:422–427.

44. Muller D, Koller BH, Whitton JL, et al. LCMV-specific, class II-restricted cytotoxic T cells in β2-microglobulin-deficient mice. *Science* 1992;255:1576–1578.

45. Jaraquemada D, Marti M, Long EO. An endogenous processing pathway in vaccinia virus infected cells for presentation of cytoplasmic antigens to class II-restricted T cells. *J Exp Med* 1990;172:947–953.

46. Jin Y, Shih W-K, Berkower I. Human T cell response to the surface antigen of hepatitis B virus (HBsAg). *J Exp Med* 1988;168: 293–306.

47. Nuchtern JG, Biddison WE, Klausner RD. Class II MHC molecules can use endogenous pathway of antigen presentation. *Nature* 1990;343:74–76.

48. Thomas DB, Hodgson J, Riska PF, et al. The role of the endoplasmic reticulum in antigen processing. *J Immunol* 1990;144: 2789–2794.

49. Weiss S, Bogen B. MHC class II-restricted antigen presentation of intracellular antigen. *Cell* 1991;64:767–776.

50. Penna A, Fowler P, Bertoletti A, et al. Hepatitis B virus (HBV)-specific cytotoxic T cell (CTL) response in humans: characterization of HLA class II-restricted CTLs that recognize endogenously synthesized HBV envelope antigens. *J Virol* 1992;66: 1193–1198.

51. Mainati MS, Marti M, LaVaute T, et al. Processing pathways for presentation of cytosolic antigen to MHC class II-restricted T cells. *Nature* 1992;357:702–704.

52. Potter TA, Rajan TV, Dick RF, et al. Substitution at residue 227 of H-2 class I molecules abrogates recognition by CD8-dependent, but not CD8-independent, cytotoxic T lymphocytes. *Nature* 1989;337:73–75.

53. Salter RD, Benjamin RJ, Wesley PK, et al. A binding site for T-cell co-receptor CD8 on the α-3 domain of HLA-A2. *Nature* 1990;345:41–46.

54. Kvist S, Hamann U. A nucleoprotein peptide of influenza A virus stimulates assembly of HLA-B27 class I heavy chains b2-microglobulin translated *in vitro*. *Nature* 1990;348:446–448.

55. Ljunggren HG, Stam NJ, Ohlén C, et al. Empty MHC class I molecules come out in the cold. *Nature* 1990;346:476–480.

56. Hosken NA, Bevan MJ Defective presentation of endogenous antigen by a cell line expressing class I molecules. *Science* 1990;248:367–370.

57. Ortiz-Navarette V, Hammerling GJ. Surface appearance and instability of empty H-2 class I molecules under physiological conditions. *Proc Natl Acad Sci U S A* 1991;88:3594–3597.

58. Biron CA, Nguyen KB, Pien GC, et al. Natural killer cells in antiviral defense. *Annu Rev Immunol* 1999;17:189–220.

59. Lanier, LL. NK Cell receptors. *Annu Rev Immunol* 1998;16: 359–393.

60. Milich DR, McLachlan A. The nucleocapsid of hepatitis B virus is both a T-cell-independent and a T-cell-dependent antigen. *Science* 1986;234:1398–1401.

61. Stephan W, Prince AM, Brotman B. Modulation of hepatitis B infection by intravenous application of an immunoglobulin preparation that contains antibodies to hepatitis B e and core antigens but not to hepatitis B surface antigen. *J Virol* 1984;51: 420–424.

62. Tsai SL, Chen PJ, Lai MY, et al. Acute exacerbations of chronic type B hepatitis are accompanied by increased T cell responses to hepatitis B core and e antigens. Implications for hepatitis e antigen seroconversion. *J Clin Invest* 1992;89:87–96.

63. Rehermann B, Lau D, Hoofnagle JH, et al. Cytotoxic T lymphocyte responsiveness after resolution of chronic hepatitis B virus infection. *J Clin Invest* 1996;97:1655–1665.

64. Chisari FV, Ferrari C. Hepatitis B virus immunopathogenesis. *Annu Rev Immunol* 1995;13:29–60.

65. Michalak TI, Pasquinelli C, Guilhot S, et al. Hepatitis B virus persistence after recovery from acute viral hepatitis. *J Clin Invest* 1994;93:230–239.

66. Rehermann B, Ferrari C, Pasquinelli C, et al. The hepatitis B virus persists for decades after recovery from acute viral hepatitis despite active maintenance of a cytotoxic T lymphocyte response. *Nature Med* 1996;2:1104–1108.

67. Ando K, Guidotti LG, Wirth S, et al. Class I restricted cytotoxic

68. Moriyama T, Guilhot S, Klopchin R, et al. Immunobiology and pathogenesis of hepatocellular injury in hepatitis B virus transgenic mice. *Science* 1990;248:361–364.

69. Guidotti LG, Ishikawa T, Hobbs MV, et al. Intracellular inactivation of the hepatitis B virus by cytotoxic T lymphocytes. *Immunity* 1996;1:25–36.

70. Guidotti LG, Borrow P, Hobbs MV, et al. Viral cross talk: intracellular inactivation of the hepatitis B virus during an unrelated viral infection of the liver. *Proc Natl Acad Sci U S A*; May 14;93: 4589–4594.

71. Guidotti LG, Borrow P, Brown A, et al. Noncytopathic clearance of lymphocytic choriomeningitis virus from the hepatocyte. *J Exp Med* 1999;189:1555–1564.

72. Heise T, Guidotti LG, Cavanaugh VJ, et al. Hepatitis B virus RNA-binding proteins associated with cytokine-induced clearance of viral RNA from the liver of transgenic mice. *J Virol* 1999;73(1):474–481.

73. McClary H, Koch R, Chisari FV, et al. Relative sensitivity of hepatitis B virus and other hepatotropic viruses to the antiviral effects of cytokines. *J Virol* 2000;74:2255–2264.

74. Guidotti LG, Matzke B, Schaller H, et al. High-level hepatitis B virus replication in transgenic mouse. *J Virol* 1995;69:6158–6168.

75. Guidotti LG, Rochford R, Chung J, et al. Viral clearance without destruction of infected cells during acute HBV infection. *Science* 1999;284:825–829.

76. MacDonald HR. NK1.1+ T cell receptor-a/b + cells: new clues to their origin, specificity and function. *J Exp Med* 1995;182: 633–638.

77. Ohteki T, MacDonald HR. Major histocompatibility complex class I-related molecules control and development of CD4+ and CD4− subsets of natural killer 1.1+ T cell receptor a/b+ cells in the liver of mice. *J Exp Med* 1994;180:699–704.

78. Doherty DG, Norris S, Madrigal-Estebas L, et al. The human liver contains multiple populations of NK cells, T cells and CD3+CD56+ natural T cells with distinct cytotoxic activities and Th 1, Th 2 and Th 0 cytokine secretion patterns. *J Immunol* 1999;163:2314–2321.

79. Webster GJM, Reignat S, Maini MK, et al. Incubation phase of acute hepatitis B in man: dynamic of cellular immune mechanisms. *Hepatology* 2000;32:1117–1124.

80. Maini M, Boni C, Ogg G, et al. Direct *ex vivo* analysis of hepatitis B virus-specific CD8+ T cells associated with the control of infection. *Gastroenterology* 1999;117:1–13.

81. Maini M, Boni C, Lee CK. The role of virus-specific CD8+ cells in liver damage and viral control during persistent hepatitis B virus (HBV) infection. *J Exp Med* 2000;191:1269–1280.

82. Boni C, Bertoletti A, Penna A, et al. Lamivudine treatment can restore T cell responsiveness in chronic hepatitis B. *J Clin Invest* 1998;102:968–975.

82a. Boni C, Penna A, Ogg GS, et al. Lamivudine treatment can overcome cytotoxic T-cell hyporesponsiveness in chronic hepatitis: new perspectives for immune therapy. *Hepatology* 2001;33: 963–971.

83. Missale G, Bertoni R, Lamonaca V, et al. Different clinical behaviors of acute hepatitis C virus infection are associated with different vigor of the antiviral cell-mediated immune response. *J Clin Invest* 1996;98(3):706–714.

84. Diepolder HM, Zachoval R, Hoffmann RM, et al. Possible mechanism involving T-lymphocyte response to nonstructural protein 3 in viral clearance in acute hepatitis C virus infection. *Lancet* 1995;346(8981):1006–1007.

85. Cooper S, Erikson AL, Adams EJ, et al. Analysis of a successful immune response against hepatitis C virus. *Immunity* 1999; 10:439–449.

T lymphocytes are directly cytopathic for their target cells *in vivo*. *J Immunol* 1994;152:3245–3253.

86. Farci P, Alter HJ, Govindarajan S. Lack of protective immunity against reinfection with hepatitis C virus. *Science* 1992;258: 135–140.

87. Prince AM, Brotman B, Huima T, et al. Immunity in hepatitis C infection. *J Infect Dis* 1992;165:438–443.

88. Bijoro K, Froland SS, Yun Z, et al. Hepatitis C infection in patients with primary hypogammaglobulinemia after treatment with contaminated immune globulin. *N Engl J Med* 1994;331: 1607–1611.

89. Adams G, Kuntz S, Rabalais G, et al. Natural recovery from acute hepatitis C virus infection by agammaglobulinemic twin children. *Pediatr Infect Dis J* 1997;16:533–534.

90. Christie JM, Healey CJ, Watson J, et al. Clinical outcome of hypogammaglbulinaemic patients following outbreak of acute hepatitis C: 2 year follow up. *J Exp Immunol* 1997;110:4–8.

91. Shimizu YK, Hijikata M, Iwamoto A, et al. Neutralizing antibodies against hepatitis C virus and the emergence of neutralization escape mutant viruses. *J Virol* 1994;68:1494–1500.

92. Farci P, Shimoda A, Wong D. Prevention of hepatitis C virus infection in chimpanzees by hyperimmune serum against the hypervariable region 1 of the envelope 2 protein. *Proc Natl Acad Sci U S A* 1996;93:15394–15399.

93. Shimizu YK, Igarashi H, Kiyohara T, et al. A hyperimmune serum against a synthetic peptide corresponding to the hypervariable region 1 of hepatitis C virus can prevent viral infection in cell cultures. *Virology* 1996;223:409–412.

94. Rosa D, Campagnoli S, Moretto C. A quantitative test to estimate neutralizing antibodies to the hepatitis C virus: cytofluorimetric assessment of envelope glycoprotein 2 binding to target cells. *Proc Natl Acad Sci U S A* 1996;93:1759–1763.

95. Mondelli MU. Is there a role for immune responses in the pathogenesis of hepatitis C? *J Hepatol* 1996;25:232–238.

96. Weiner AJ, Geysen HM, Christopherson C, et al. Evidence for immune selection of hepatitis C (HCV) putative envelope glycoprotein variants: potential role in chronic HCV infection. *Proc Natl Acad Sci U S A* 1992;89:3468–3472.

97. Kato N, Sekiya H, Ootsuyama Y. Humoral immune response to hypervariable region 1 of the putative envelope glycoprotein (gp 70) of hepatitis C virus. *J Virol* 1993;67:3923–3930.

98. Kumar U, Monjardino J, Thomas HC. Hypervariable region of hepatitis C virus envelope glycoprotein (E2/NS1) in an agammaglobulinemic patient. *Gastroenterology* 1994;106:1072–1075.

99. Zibert A, Schreier E, Roggendorf M. Antibodies in human sera specific to hypervariable region 1 of hepatitis C virus can block viral attachment. *Virology* 1995;208:653–661.

100. Shimizu YK, Purcell RH, Yoshikura H. Correlation between the infectivity of hepatitis C virus *in vivo* and its infectivity *in vitro*. *Proc Natl Acad Sci U S A* 1993;90:6037–6041.

101. Kojima M, Osuga T, Tsuda F, et al. Influence of antibodies to the hypervariable region of E2/NS1 glycoprotein on the selective replication of hepatitis C virus in chimpanzees. *Virology* 1994;204:665–672.

102. Tsai SL, Liaw YF, Chen MH, et al. Detection of type 2-like T-helper cells in hepatitis C virus infection: implications for hepatitis C virus chronicity. *Hepatology* 1997;25:449–458.

103. Ferrari C, Valli A, Galati L, et al. T-cell response to structural and nonstructural hepatitis C virus antigens in persistent and selflimited hepatitis C virus infections. *Hepatology* 1994;19:286–295.

104. Takaki A, Wiese M, Maertens G, et al. A strong cellular, not humoral immune response distinguishes recovered from chronic patients 18 years after a single source outbreak of hepatitis C. *Hepatology* 1998;28 (4) Abs n.630 .

105. Botarelli P, Brunetto MR, Minutello MA, et al. T-lymphocyte response to hepatitis C virus in different clinical courses of infection. *Gastroenterology* 1993;104:580–587.

106. Hoffmann RM, Diepolder HM, Zachoval R, et al. Mapping of immunodominant CD4+ T lymphocytes epitope of hepatitis C virus antigens and their relevance during the course of chronic infection. *Hepatology* 1995;21:632–636.

107. Battegay M, Fikes J, Di Biscieglie AM, et al. Patients with chronic hepatitis C have circulating cytotoxic T cells which recognize hepatitis C virus encoded peptides binding to HLA-A2.1 molecule. *J Virol* 1995;69:2462–2470.

108. Cherny A, Mc Hutchison JG, Pasquinelli C, et al. Cytotoxic T lymphocyte response to hepatitis C virus derived peptides containing the HLA-A2.1 binding motif. *J Clin Invest* 1995;95: 521–530.

109. Shirai M, Arichi T, Nishioka M, et al. CTL Responses of HLA-A2.1-transgenic mice specific for Hepatitis C viral peptides predict epitopes for CTL of humans carrying HLA-A2.1. *J Immunol* 1995;154:2733–2742.

110. Kita H, Morijama T, Kaneko T, et al. HLA B44-restricted cytotoxic T lymphocytes recognizing an epitope on Hepatitis C virus nucleocapsid protein. *Hepatology* 1993;18:1039–1043.

111. He XS, Rehermann B, Lopez-Labrador FX, et al. Quantitative analysis of hepatitis C virus-specific CD8+ T cells in peripheral blood and liver using peptide-MHC tetramers. *Proc Natl Acad Sci U S A* 1999;96:5692–5697.

112. Koziel MJ, Dudley D, Wong J, et al. Intrahepatic cytotoxic T lymphocytes specific for hepatitis C virus in persons with chronic hepatitis. *J Immunol* 1992;149:3339–3344.

113. Koziel MJ, Dudley D, Afdhal N, et al. HLA class I restricted cytotoxic T lymphocytes specific for hepatitis C virus: identification of multiple epitopes and characterization of patterns of cytokines release. *J Clin Invest* 1995;96:2311–2315.

114. Wong DKH, Dudley DD, Afdhal NH, et al. Liver derived CTL in Hepatitis C virus infection: breadth and specificity of responses in a cohort of persons with chronic infection. *J Immunol* 1998;160:1479–1488.

115. Nelson DR, Marousis CG, Davis GL, et al. The role of hepatitis C virus specific cytotoxic T lymphocytes in chronic hepatitis C. *J Immunol* 1997;158:1473–1481.

116. Nelson DR, Marousis CG, Ohno T, et al. Intrahepatic Hepatitis C virus-specific cytotoxic T lymphocyte activity and response to interferon α therapy in chronic Hepatitis C. *Hepatology* 1998; 28:225–230.

117. Minutello MA, Pileri P, Unutmaz D, et al. Compartmentalization of T-lymphocytes to the site of the disease: intrahepatic CD4+ T cells specific for the protein NS4 of hepatitis C virus in patients with chronic hepatitis C. *J Exp Med* 1993;178:17–26.

118. Nuti S, Rosa D, Valiante NM, et al. Dynamics of intrahepatic lymphocytes in chronic hepatitis C: enrichment for Va24+ T cells and rapid elimination of effector cells by apoptosis. *Eur J Immunol* 1998;28:3448–3455.

119. Valiante NM, D' Andrea A, Crotta S, et al. Life, activation and death of intrahepatic lymphocytes in chronic hepatitis C. *Immunol Rev* 2000;174;77–89.

120. Thursz M, Yallop R, Goldin R, et al. Influence of MHC class II genotype on outcome of infection with hepatitis C virus. *Lancet* 1999;354:2119–2124.

121. Bertoletti A, Costanzo A, Chisari FV, et al. Cytotoxic T lymphocyte response to a wild type hepatitis B virus epitope in patients chronically infected by variant viruses carrying substitutions within the epitope. *J Exp Med* 1994;180:933–943.

122. Bertoletti A, Sette A, Chisari FV, et al. Natural variants of cytotoxic epitopes are T cell receptor antagonists for anti-viral cytotoxic T cells. *Nature* 1994;369:407–410.

123. Meier UC, Klenerman P, Griffin P, et al. Cytotoxic T lymphocytes lysis inhibited by viable HIV mutants. *Science* 1995;270: 1360–1362.

124. Weiner A, Erickson AL, Kansopon J, et al. Persistent hepatitis C virus infection in a chimpanzee is associated with emergence

of a cytotoxic T lymphocyte escape variant. *Proc Natl Acad Sci U S A* 1995;92:2755–2759.

125. Tsai SL, Chen YM, Chen MH, et al. Hepatitis C virus variants circumventing cytotoxic T lymphocyte activity as a mechanism of chronicity. *Gastroenterology* 1998;115:954–966.

126. Taylor DR, Shi ST, Romano PR, et al. Inhibition of the interferon-inducible protein kinase PKR by HCV E2 protein. *Science* 1999;285:107–110.

127. Chen CM, You LR, Hwang LH, et al. Direct interaction of hepatitis C virus core protein with the cellular lymphotoxin-β receptor modulates the signal pathway of lymphotoxin-β receptor. *J Virol* 1997;71:9417–9426.

128. Zhu N, Khoshnan A, Schneider R, et al. Hepatitis C virus core protein binds to the cytoplasmic domain of tumor necrosis factor (TNF) receptor 1 and enhances TNF-induced apoptosis. *J Virol* 1998;72:3691–3697.

129. Ray RB, Meyer K, Steele R, et al. Inhibition of tumor necrosis factor (TNFα)-mediate apoptosis by hepatitis C virus core protein. *J Biol Chem* 1998;273:2256–2259.

130. You LR, Chen CM, Wu Lee YH. Hepatitis C virus core protein enhances NF-kB signal pathway triggering by lymphotoxin-β receptor ligand and tumor necrosis factor α. *J Virol* 1999; 1672–1681.

131. Pileri P, Uematsu Y, Campagnoli S, et al. Binding of hepatitis C virus to CD81. *Science* 1998;282:938–941.

132. Bradbury LE, Kansas GS, Levy S, et al. The CD19/CD21 signal transducing complex of human B lymphocytes includes the target of antiproliferative antibody-1 and Leu-13 molecules. *J Immunol* 1992;149:2841–2850.

133. Fearon DT, Carter RH. The CD19/CR2/TAPA-1 complex of B lymphocytes: linking natural to acquired immunity. *Annu Rev Immunol* 1995;13:127–149.

134. Cooper NR, Moore MD, Nemerow GR. Immunobiology of CR2, the B lymphocyte receptor for Epstein–Barr virus and the C3d complement fragment. *Annu Rev Immunol* 1988;6:85–113.

135. Penna A, Chisari FV, Bertoletti A, et al. Cytotoxic T lymphocytes recognize an HLA A2-restricted epitope within the hepatitis B virus nucleocapsid antigen. *J Exp Med* 1991;174:1565–1570.

136. Missale G, Redeker A, Person J, et al. HLA-A31 and HLA-Aw68 restricted cytotoxic T cell responses to a single hepatitis B virus nucleocapsid epitope during acute viral hepatitis. *J Exp Med* 1993;177:751–762.

137. Nayersina R, Fowler P, Guilhot S, et al. HLA-A2-restricted cytotoxic T lymphocyte responses to multiple hepatitis B surface antigen epitopes during hepatitis B virus infection. *J Immunol* 1993;150:4659–4671.

138. Rehermann B, Fowler P, Sidney J, et al. The cytotoxic T lymphocyte response to multiple hepatitis B polymerase epitopes during and after acute viral infection. *J Exp Med* 1995;181: 1047–1058.

139. Griffith TS, Brunner T, Fletcher SM, et al. Fas ligand-induced apoptosis as a mechanism of immune privilege. *Science* 1995; 270:1189–1192.

140. Galle PR, Hofmann WJ, Walczak H, et al. Involvement of the CD95 (APO-1/Fas) receptor and ligand in liver damage. *J Exp Med* 1995;182:1223–1230.

141. Gooding LR. Virus proteins that counteract host immune defenses. *Cell* 1992;71:5–7.

142. Alcami A, Smith GL. Cytokine receptors encoded by poxviruses: a lesson in cytokine biology. *Immunol Today* 1995;16:474–478.

143. Rehermann B, Pasquinelli C, Mosier SM, et al. Hepatitis B virus (HBV) sequence variation in cytotoxic T lymphocyte epitopes is not common in patients with chronic HBV infection. *J Clin Invest* 1995;96:1527–1534.

144. Deleted.

145. Kalams SA, Johnson RP, Trocha AK, et al. Longitudinal analysis of

T cell receptor (TCR) gene usage by human immunodeficiency virus 1 envelope-specific cytotoxic T lymphocyte clones reveals a limited TCR repertoire. *J Exp Med* 1994;179:1261–1271.

146. Argaet VPC, Schmidt CW, Burrows SR, et al. Dominant selection of an invariant T cell antigen receptor in response to persistent infection by Epstein-Barr virus. *J Exp Med* 1994;180: 2335–2340.

147. Kuchroo VK, Greer JM, Kaul D, et al. A single TCR antagonist peptide inhibits experimental allergic encephalomyelitis by a diverse T cell repertoire. *J Immunol* 1994;153:3326–3336.

148. Ho DD, Newmann AU, Perelson AS, Chen W, et al. Rapid turnover of plasma virions and CD4 lymphocytes in HIV-1 infection. *Nature* 1995;373:123–126.

149. Borrow P, Lewicki H, Wei X, et al. Antiviral pressure exerted by HIV-1-specific cytotoxic T lymphocytes (CTLs) during primary infection demonstrated by rapid selection of CTL escape virus. *Nat Med* 1997;3:205–211.

150. Koziel MJ, Dudley D, Afdhal N, et al. Hepatitis C virus (HCV)-specific cytoxic T lymphocytes recognize epitopes in the core and envelope proteins of HCV. *J Virol* 1993;67:7522–7532.

151. Pantaleo G, Demarest JF, Soudeyns H, et al. Major expansion of CD8+ cells with a predominant V-β usage during the primary immune response to HIV. *Nature* 1994;370:463–467.

152. Simmonds P. Variability of hepatitis C virus. *Hepatology* 1995; 21:570–583.

153. Choo Q-L, Weiner AJ, Overby LR, et al. Hepatitis C virus: the major causative agent of viral non-A, non-B hepatitis. *Br Med Bull* 1990;46:423–441.

154. Weiner A, Erickson AL, Kansopon J, et al. Persistent hepatitis C virus infection in a chimpanzee is associated with emergence of a cytotoxic T lymphocyte escape variant. *Proc Natl Acad Sci U S A* 1995;92:2755–2759.

155. Matsubara K, Tokina T. Integration of hepatitis B virus DNA and its implications for hepatocarcinogenesis. *Mol Biol Med* 1990;7:243–260.

156. Maguire HF, Hoeffler JP, Siddiqui A. HBV X protein alters the DNA binding specificity of CREB and ATF-2 by protein–protein interactions. *Science* 1991;252:842–844.

157. Kekule AS, Lauer U, Weiss L, et al. Hepatitis B virus transactivator HBx uses a tumour promoter signaling pathway. *Nature* 1993;361:742–745.

158. Natoli G, Avantaggiati ML, Chirillo P, et al. Induction of the DNA-binding activity of c-jun/c-fos heterodimers by the hepatitis B virus transactivator pX. *Mol Cell Biol* 1994;14: 989–998.

159. Wang XW, Forrester K, Yeh H, et al. Hepatitis B virus X protein inhibits p53 sequence-specific DNA binding, transcriptional activity, and association with transcription factor ERCC3. *Proc Natl Acad Sci U S A* 1994;91:2230–2234.

160. Koike K, Moriya K, Iino S, et al. High level expression of hepatitis B virus HBx gene and hepatocarcinogenesis in transgenic mice. *Hepatology* 1994;19:810–819.

161. Hildt E, Saher G, Bruss V, et al. The hepatitis B virus large surface protein (LHBs) is a transcriptional activator. *Virology* 1996; 225:235–239.

162. Meyer M, Caselmann WH, Schluter V, et al. Hepatitis B virus transactivator MHBst: activation of NF-κB, selective inhibition by antioxidants and integral membrane localization. *EMBO J* 1992;11:2991–3001.

163. Chisari FV, Pinkert CA, Milich DR, et al. A transgenic mouse model of the chronic hepatitis B surface antigen carrier state. *Science* 1985;230:1157–1160.

164. Chisari FV, Filippi P, McLachlan A, et al. Expression of hepatitis B virus large envelope polypeptide inhibits hepatitis B surface antigen secretion in transgenic mice. *J Virol* 1986;60:880–887.

165. Chisari FV, Filippi P, Buras J, et al. Structural and pathological

effects of synthesis of hepatitis B virus large envelope polypeptide in transgenic mice. *Proc Natl Acad Sci U S A* 1987;84: 6909–6913.

166. Chisari FV, Klopchin K, Moriyama T, et al. Molecular pathogenesis of hepatocellular carcinoma in hepatitis B virus transgenic mice. *Cell* 1989;59:1145–1156.

167. Dunsford HA, Sell S, Chisari FV. Hepatocarcinogenesis due to chronic liver cell injury in hepatitis B virus transgenic mice. *Cancer Res* 1990;50:3400–3407.

168. Pasquinelli C, Bhavani K, Chisari FV. Multiple oncogenes and tumor suppressor genes are structurally and functionally intact during hepatocarcinogenesis in hepatitis B virus transgenic mice. *Cancer Res* 1992;52:2823–2829.

169. Hagen TM, Wehr C, Huang S-N, et al. Extensive oxidative DNA damage in hepatocytes of transgenic mice with chronic active hepatitis destined to develop hepatocellular carcinoma. *Proc Natl Acad Sci U S A* 1994;91:12808–12812.

170. Huang S-N, Chisari FV. Strong, sustained hepatocellular proliferation precedes hepatocarcinogenesis in hepatitis B surface antigen transgenic mice. *Hepatology* 1995;21:620–626.

171. Nakamoto Y, Guidotti LG, Kuhlen CV, et al. Immune pathogenesis of hepatocellular carcinoma. *J Exp Med* 1998;188: 341–350.

172. Alter HJ. Transfusion-associated non-A, non-B hepatitis: the first decade. In: Zuckerman AJ, ed. *Viral hepatitis and liver disease.* New York: Alan R. Liss, 1988:534–542.

173. Lieber CS, Garro A, Leo MA, et al. Alcohol and cancer. *Hepatology* 1986;6:1005–1019.

174. Niederau C, Fischer R, Sonnenberg A, et al. Survival and causes of death in cirrhotic and in noncirrhotic patients with primary hemochromatosis. *N Engl J Med* 1985;313:1256–1262.

175. Limmer J, Fleig WE, Leupold D, et al. Hepatocellular carcinoma in type 1 glycogen storage disease. *Hepatology* 1988;8: 531–537.

176. Carlson J, Eriksson S. Chronic "cryptogenic" liver disease and malignant hepatoma in intermediate α-1-antitrypsin deficiency identified by a pi 2-specific monoclonal antibody. *Scand J Gastroenterol* 1985;20:835–841.

177. Eriksson S, Carlson J, Velez RN. Risk of cirrhosis and primary liver cancer in α-1-antitrypsin deficiency. *N Engl J Med* 1986; 314:736–740.

178. Melia WM, Wilkinson ML, Portmann BC, et al. Hepatocellular carcinoma in the noncirrhotic liver: a comparison with that complicating cirrhosis. *Q J Med* 1984;53:391–400.

179. Dolberg DS, Hollingsworth R, Hertle M, et al. Wounding and

its role in RSV-mediated tumor formation. *Science* 1985;230: 676–678.

180. Sieweke MH, Stoker AW, Bissell MJ. Evaluation of the cocarcinogenic effect of wounding in Rous sarcoma virus tumorigenesis. *Cancer Res* 1989;49:6419–6424.

181. Lacey M, Alpert S, Hanahan D. Bovine papillomavirus genome elicits skin tumours in transgenic mice. *Nature* 1986;322: 609–612.

182. Konstantinidis A, Smulow JB, Sonnenschein C. Tumorigenesis at a predetermined oral site after one intraperitoneal injection of N-nitroso-N-methylurea. *Science* 1982;216:1235–1237.

183. Korelitz BI. Carcinoma of the intestinal tract in Crohn's disease: results of a survey conducted by the National Foundation for Ileitis and Colitis. *Am J Gastroenterol* 1983;78:44–46.

184. Collins RH Jr, Feldman M, Fordtran JS. Colon cancer, dysplasia, and surveillance in patients with ulcerative colitis: a critical review. *N Engl J Med* 1987;316:1654–1658.

185. D'Argenio G, Cosenza V, Delle Cave M, et al. Butyrate enemas in experimental colitis and protection against large bowel cancer in a rat model. *Gastroenterology* 1996;110:1727–1734.

186. Johnson LD, Ausman LM, Sehgal PK, et al. A prospective study of the epidemiology of colitis and colon cancer in cotton-top tamarins (*Saguinus oedipus*). *Gastroenterology* 1996;110:102–115.

187. Locke JR, Hill DE, Walzer Y. Incidence of squamous cell carcinoma in patients with longterm catheter drainage. *J Urol* 1985;133:1034–1035.

188. Kantor AF, Hartge P, Hoover RN, et al. Epidemiological characteristics of squamous cell carcinoma and adenocarcinoma of the bladder. *Cancer Res* 1988;48:3853–3855.

189. Yamamoto M, Wu HH, Momose H, et al. Marked enhancement of rat urinary bladder carcinogenesis by heat-killed *Escherichia coli*. *Cancer Res* 1992;52:5329–5333.

190. Kawai K, Yamamoto M, Kameyama S, et al. Enhancement of rat urinary bladder tumorigenesis by lipopolysaccharide-induced inflammation. *Cancer Res* 1993;53:5172–5175.

191. Kawai K, Kawamata H, Kemeyama S, et al. Persistence of carcinogen-altered cell population in rat urothelium which can be promoted to tumors by chronic inflammatory stimulus. *Cancer Res* 1994;54:2630–2632.

192. Dahms BB, Rothstein FC. Barrett's esophagus in children: a consequence of chronic gastroesophageal reflux. *Gastroenterology* 1984;86:318–323.

193. Cameron AJ, Ott BJ, Payne WS. The incidence of adenocarcinoma in columnar-lined (Barrett's) esophagus. *N Engl J Med* 1985;313:857–859.

53

EPIDEMIOLOGY, NATURAL HISTORY, AND PREVENTION OF VIRAL HEPATITIS

MIRIAM J. ALTER
BETH P. BELL

Viral hepatitis refers to a primary infection of the liver caused by at least five unrelated viruses, and acute and chronic liver disease due to viral hepatitis accounts for substantial morbidity and mortality worldwide. Two of these viruses, hepatitis A virus (HAV) and hepatitis E virus (HEV), are primarily transmitted by the fecal-oral route and cause acute self-limited disease. The other three viruses, hepatitis B virus (HBV), hepatitis C virus (HCV), and hepatitis D virus (HDV), are transmitted by percutaneous or permucosal exposures to blood or body fluids that contain blood. All three can result in a chronic infection that places the individual at risk for chronic liver disease or primary hepatocellular carcinoma. The serologic exclusion of the known hepatitis viruses continues to leave cases of hepatitis that clinically appear to be viral in origin. The majority of these cases of "non-ABCDE" hepatitis appear to be parenterally transmitted. Several new viruses have been recently identified and proposed as the putative agents of non-ABCDE hepatitis, but to date, studies of these viruses have failed to show an association with either acute or chronic liver disease.

M. J. Alter: Epidemiology Section, Hepatitis Branch, Centers for Disease Control and Prevention, Atlanta, Georgia 30333.
B. P. Bell: Hepatitis Branch, Centers for Disease Control and Prevention, Atlanta, Georgia 30333.

HEPATITIS A VIRUS

In 1973, HAV was identified by immune electron microscopy (IEM) in stool samples of patients with hepatitis A (1). This discovery led to the development of serologic tests that differentiated acute and resolved infections, characterization of the virus, definition of pathogenetic events during infection, and further definition of the epidemiology of HAV infection. In contrast to the other hepatitis viruses, HAV has been propagated in cell culture, which has facilitated the development of effective vaccines (2–4).

Natural History and Diagnosis

HAV can produce either asymptomatic or symptomatic infection in humans after an average incubation period of 28 days (range: 15 to 50 days). The likelihood of having symptoms with HAV infection is related to the person's age. In children less than 6 years of age, most (70%) infections are asymptomatic; among older children and adults, infection is usually symptomatic, with jaundice occurring in more than 70% of patients. Signs and symptoms usually last less than 2 months, although 10% to 15% of symptomatic persons have prolonged or relapsing disease lasting up to 6 months.

In infected persons, HAV replicates in the liver, is excreted in bile, and is shed in the stool. Peak infectivity of infected persons occurs during the 2-week period before onset of jaundice or elevation of liver enzymes, when the concentration of virus in stool is highest (up to 10^8 infectious particles/mL) (5). The concentration of virus in stool declines after jaundice appears. Children and infants can shed HAV for longer periods than do adults, up to several months after the onset of clinical illness (6); however, for practical purposes, both children and adults with hepatitis A can be assumed to be noninfectious 1 week after jaundice appears. Chronic shedding of HAV in feces does not occur, although shedding may occur in persons who have relapsing illness. Viremia occurs soon after infection and persists through the period of liver enzyme elevation (7).

Although the case-fatality rate for acute liver failure among reported hepatitis A cases of all ages is approximately 0.3%, the rate is higher (1.8%) among adults greater than 50 years of age. Persons with chronic liver disease who acquire hepatitis A are at increased risk of acute liver failure.

Serologic testing to detect immunoglobulin M (IgM) antibody to the capsid proteins of HAV (IgM anti-HAV) is required to confirm a diagnosis of acute HAV infection. Immunoglobulin G (IgG) anti-HAV, which appears early in the course of infection, remains detectable for the person's lifetime and confers lifelong protection against the disease.

HAV RNA can be detected in the blood and stool of most persons during the acute phase of infection by using nucleic acid amplification methods, and nucleic acid sequencing has been used to determine the relatedness of HAV isolates (5,8,9). Such sequencing has been particularly useful in linking sporadic cases of hepatitis A identified in different geographic areas to a common source outbreak (8). The detection of HAV antigen or HAV RNA in the stool of infected persons by enzyme immunoassays (EIA) and polymerase chain reaction (PCR) cannot delineate whether a person is infectious because these assays may detect defective as well as infectious viral particles. Nucleic acid amplification by immunocapture PCR (IC-PCR) requires the presence of intact virus.

Epidemiology

Modes of Transmission and Persons at Risk

Because of the high concentration of virus in the stool of infected persons, HAV infection is acquired primarily by the fecal-oral route. This occurs most commonly by person-to-person transmission in households and extended family settings and between sexual contacts. Person-to-person transmission results in high rates of infection in young children in developing countries and is the predominant mode of transmission in the United States, where most disease occurs in the context of communitywide outbreaks. In experimentally infected nonhuman primates, HAV has been detected in saliva during the incubation period; however, transmission by saliva has not been demonstrated.

HAV can remain infectious in the environment, and fecal contamination of food or water can occur, particularly in areas where sanitation is poor and HAV is endemic. In the United States, foodborne or waterborne hepatitis A outbreaks are recognized relatively infrequently. Recognized foodborne outbreaks usually are associated with contamination of food during preparation by a food handler with HAV infection (10,11), but have also been associated with food contaminated before retail distribution, such as shellfish harvested from polluted water and lettuce or fruits contaminated at the growing or processing stage (8,11). Waterborne hepatitis A outbreaks are rare, but have been reported in association with sewage contamination or inadequate treatment of water (11).

In the U.S. and other parts of the developed world, outbreaks in child care centers have been recognized for several decades (12). During the past two decades, outbreaks among users of injection and noninjection drugs have been reported with increasing frequency in the U.S. and Europe (4,11). Transmission among injection drug users likely occurs through percutaneous and fecal-oral routes (e.g., sharing needles or other paraphernalia, and having household or other close personal contact with infected persons).

HAV, like other predominantly enteric infections, may be transmitted during sexual activity. Virus transmission between sexual partners is facilitated by sexual practices involving oral-anal contact, and hepatitis A outbreaks among men who have sex with men (MSM) have been reported frequently.

On rare occasions, HAV infection has been transmitted by transfusion of blood or blood products collected from donors during the viremic phase of their infection (11). In addition, outbreaks have been reported in Europe and the U.S. among patients who received factor VIII and factor IX concentrates prepared using solvent–detergent treatment to inactivate lipid-containing viruses (4,11). Hepatitis A has also been reported in adult cancer patients treated with lymphocytes incubated in serum from a donor with HAV infection.

The risk of transmission from pregnant women who develop hepatitis A in the third trimester of pregnancy to newborns appears to be low. IgG anti-HAV is passively transferred across the placenta.

Geographic Patterns of Transmission

Worldwide, the endemicity of HAV infection differs markedly among and within countries (Fig. 53.1) (11). Four patterns of HAV infection can be differentiated, each characterized by the age groups in which the majority of transmission occurs, distinct age-specific profiles of anti-HAV prevalence and hepatitis A incidence, and prevailing environmental (hygienic and sanitary) and socioeconomic conditions (Table 53.1) (11).

In areas with a high endemic pattern of infection, represented by the least developed countries (i.e., parts of Africa, Asia, Central and South America), poor socioeconomic conditions allow HAV to spread readily. Most persons are

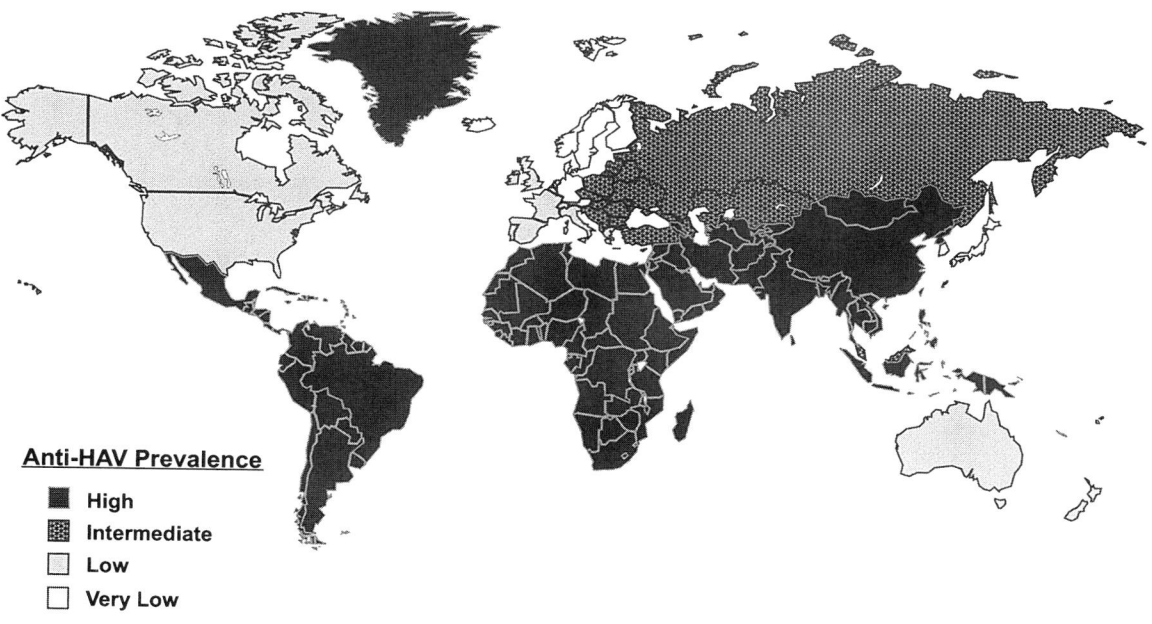

Anti-HAV Prevalence

- ■ **High**
- ▓ **Intermediate**
- � **Low**
- □ **Very Low**

FIGURE 53.1. Worldwide distribution and endemicity of hepatitis A virus infection (*HAV*). (From Bell BP, Shapiro CN, Margolis HS. Hepatitis A virus. In: Feigan RD, Cherry JD, eds. *Textbook of Pediatric Infectious Diseases*. 4th ed. Philadelphia: WB Saunders, 1997:1865–1881, with permission.)

infected as young children and essentially the entire population becomes infected before reaching adolescence.

An intermediate endemicity of HAV infection is found in Eastern Europe and parts of the former Soviet Union, Western Europe, the Americas (including parts of the U.S.), and Asia. With improved sanitary conditions in these areas, HAV is not transmitted as readily, and the predominant age of infection is older than in high endemic areas. Paradoxically, as the socioeconomic level of a country increases and the endemicity of HAV infection decreases, the overall incidence and average age of reported cases of disease often

increase because HAV transmission can occur in age groups in which symptomatic infection is more common. Large common source outbreaks can also occur because of the relatively high rate of virus transmission and large numbers of susceptible persons, especially among those of higher socioeconomic level. Nevertheless, person-to-person transmission in communitywide epidemics continues to account for much of the disease in these countries. These outbreaks often show a cyclic pattern; they subside when the susceptible population is depleted, but recur when a new cohort of susceptible children reach an age at which clinical disease

TABLE 53.1. EPIDEMIOLOGIC CHARACTERISTICS OF ENDEMIC PATTERNS OF HEPATITIS A VIRUS INFECTION

Endemicity of Infection	Prevalence of Hepatitis A Virus Infection (%)							Geographic areas[a]
	Age Group (years)							
	0–5	6–10	11–15	16–20	21–30	31–40	>40	
High	40	50–100	80–100	80–100	>85	>85	>85	Africa, Middle East, most of Asia, South America, Central America
Intermediate	20	20–30	30–40	40–50	50–65	75–80	>80	Eastern Europe and former Soviet Union, most Caribbean islands
Low	0–5	2–5	5–10	5–15	15–20	20–40	>40	Western Europe, Australia, New Zealand, Japan, Canada, United States
Very Low	0	0	0–1	1–3	5–10	10–15	15–35	Scandinavian countries

[a]See Figure 53.1.
From Bell BP, Shapiro CN, Margolis HS. Hepatitis A Virus. In: Feigan RD, Cherry JD, eds. *Textbook of pediatric infectious diseases,* 4th ed., Philadelphia: WB Saunders, 1997, 1865–1881, with permission.

occurs more commonly. This pattern can be seen in parts of the U.S., such as in American Indian communities that experience large outbreaks approximately every 7 years, during which most reported cases occur among children aged 5 to 15 years.

In most areas of North America and Western Europe, sanitary and hygienic conditions are such that the endemicity of HAV infection is low. Relatively fewer children are infected, and disease often occurs in the context of communitywide and child care center outbreaks, and occasionally as common-source outbreaks. In some countries (i.e., Scandinavia) the endemicity of HAV infection is very low, and disease occurs almost exclusively among defined risk groups such as travelers returning from areas with a high or intermediate endemicity of infection or injection drug users.

In the U.S., large nationwide epidemics have occurred approximately every 10 years, with the most recent peaking in 1989 (4). However, even between these epidemics, disease rates are relatively high and many communities experience periodic epidemics. In 1997, 31,032 cases were reported to the Centers for Disease Control and Prevention (CDC), which, after correcting for underreporting, represent an estimated 90,000 cases.

In the U.S., hepatitis A incidence varies by age, race/ethnicity, and geographic region. The highest rates occur among children 5 to 14 years of age, and almost 30% of cases occur among children less than 15 years of age (13). Since many children have unrecognized asymptomatic infection, they likely represent a major reservoir for HAV transmission. Among racial/ethnic groups, rates among American Indians and Alaska Natives are highest, and more than ten times that in other racial/ethnic groups. Rates among Hispanics are approximately three times higher than among non-Hispanics. Disease rates are substantially higher in the Western and Southwestern U.S. compared with other regions.

As determined by the Third National Health and Nutrition Examination Survey (NHANES III) conducted from 1988 to 1994, 31.3% of the general population in the U.S. has serologic evidence of prior HAV infection (4) (CDC, unpublished data). Anti-HAV prevalence is directly related to age, ranging from 9.4% among children less than 12 years of age to 74.6% among persons over 70 years of age. Anti-HAV prevalence is highest among Mexican-Americans (70.2%), compared with non-Hispanic blacks (39.1%) and whites (23.3%). Factors related most strongly with anti-HAV positivity are age, race/ethnicity and birthplace outside of the U.S.

Data from disease surveillance systems indicate that the most commonly reported source for infection is household or sexual contact with a person who has hepatitis A (15% to 30% of reported cases) (Fig. 53.2) (13). An additional 10% to 15% of reported cases occur among children and employees of child care centers and members of their households. International travel (5% to 7%) and suspected food- or waterborne outbreaks (2% to 5%) each account for a small proportion of cases, and vary little by year. In

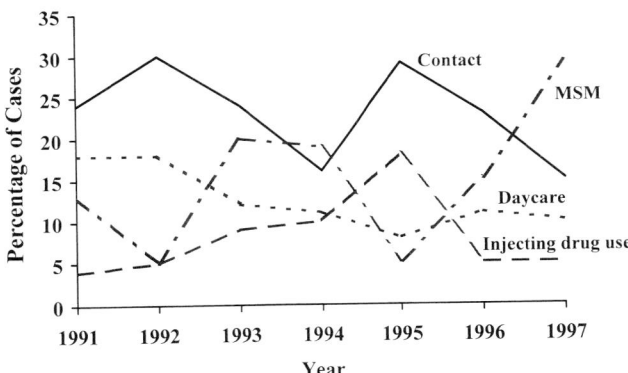

FIGURE 53.2. Trends in risk factors for reported cases of hepatitis A, Sentinel Counties, U.S., 1991–1997. *Contact*, personal contact with hepatitis A case; *MSM*, men who have sex with men. (From Bell BP, Shapiro CN, Alter MJ, et al. The diverse patterns of hepatitis A epidemiology in the U.S.—implications for vaccination strategies. *J Infect Dis* 1998;178:1579–1584, with permission.)

contrast, the proportions of cases associated with MSM activity or injection drug use vary widely (5% to 30% of cases) as a result of periodic outbreaks occurring in these subgroups in some communities (Fig. 53.2).

Nearly 50% of patients with hepatitis A do not have a recognized source for infection. Many of these patients may have acquired their infection from household contact with persons, especially children, with asymptomatic or unrecognized infection. In one study of adults without an identified source of infection, 52% of their households included a child less than 6 years old, and the presence of a young child was associated with HAV transmission within the household (14). In studies where serologic testing of the household contacts of adults without an identified source of infection was performed, 25% to 40% of their contacts less than 6 years old had serologic evidence of acute HAV infection (IgM anti-HAV) (14) (CDC, unpublished data).

Prevention

Hepatitis A can be prevented by: (a) general measures of good personal hygiene, particularly hand washing, provision of safe drinking water, and proper disposal of sanitary waste; (b) preexposure immunization with hepatitis A vaccine; and (c) pre- or postexposure immunization with immune globulin (IG).

Active Immunization

Inactivated hepatitis A vaccines have been evaluated for efficacy in controlled clinical trials and licensed in the U.S. and other countries (2,3). In extensive studies in children and adults, these vaccines have been found to be highly immunogenic; 95% to 100% of children over 2 years old and adults respond with levels of antibody considered to be protective after one dose of vaccine. A second dose is necessary to boost antibody levels for long-term protection (15,16). Studies in children less than 2 years of age are limited, but suggest that passively transferred maternal antibody interferes with the immune response.

Inactivated hepatitis A vaccine is 94% to 100% efficacious in preventing clinically apparent disease (2,3). Protective levels of anti-HAV have been shown to persist in adult vaccine recipients for at least 6 years after vaccination. Estimates based on kinetic models of antibody decline suggest that the duration of protection could be 20 years or longer (17).

In the U.S., vaccination against hepatitis A is recommended for persons at increased risk of hepatitis A (Table 53.2) (4). Vaccination of persons with chronic liver disease, including those who are awaiting or have received liver transplants, is also recommended because of the increased risk of fulminant hepatitis A.

Vaccination of persons at increased risk for hepatitis A will have little effect on national disease rates, because most cases do not occur among persons in these groups. To achieve a sustained reduction in national incidence of hepatitis A, widespread routine vaccination is needed. In the U.S., routine vaccination of children beginning at or after 2 years of age is recommended in communities with persistently elevated rates of hepatitis A (approximately twice the national average) and should be considered in communities with rates greater than (but less than twice) the national average (4). Vaccination of successive cohorts of young children should significantly lower the incidence of hepatitis A over time and eventually provide the opportunity to eliminate HAV transmission. To achieve this goal, children throughout the U.S. will need to be vaccinated against hepatitis A. This effort would be facilitated by the availability of a vaccine for use in

infants or children in the second year of life and combination vaccines that include hepatitis A vaccine.

Several lines of evidence indicate that hepatitis A vaccines may have some efficacy in providing postexposure protection. Limited studies in chimpanzees suggest that active postexposure immunization initiated soon after exposure may provide some protection, including the elimination of virus shedding. In one randomized trial of preexposure hepatitis A vaccine efficacy, no cases of hepatitis A occurred in vaccine recipients beginning 17 days after vaccination, indicating that vaccine may have some effectiveness when administered after exposure (2). In one small randomized trial of postexposure hepatitis A vaccine efficacy, the vaccine was 79% efficacious in preventing IgM anti-HAV positivity compared to no intervention (18); however, the efficacy of vaccine in providing postexposure protection compared to IG has not been evaluated.

Passive Immunization

When administered before exposure or within 2 weeks after exposure, IG is more than 85% effective in preventing hepatitis A by passive transfer of anti-HAV. Whether IG completely prevents infection or leads to asymptomatic infection and the development of persistent anti-HAV (passive-active immunity) is probably related to the amount of time that has elapsed between exposure and IG administration (19). Persons who have been recently exposed to HAV and who have not previously received hepatitis A vaccine should be administered IG as soon as possible, but not more than two weeks after exposure (Table 53.2) (4). IG also may be given to persons who are traveling internation-

TABLE 53.2. RECOMMENDATIONS FOR USE OF HEPATITIS A VACCINE AND IMMUNE GLOBULIN, UNITED STATES

Group/Setting	Children[a]	Adolescents	Adults
Preexposure protection with hepatitis A vaccine			
Routine Vaccination			
International travelers[b]	+[c]	+	+
Residents of communities with elevated rates	+	+/–	
Men who have sex with men	na[d]	+	+
Illicit drug users	na[d]	+	+
Persons with chronic liver disease	+	+	+
Persons receiving clotting factors	+	+	+
Persons who work with hepatitis A virus in research laboratory settings	na[d]	na[d]	+
Postexposure protection with immune globulin[e]			
Close personal contact with persons with hepatitis A[f]	+	+	+
Child care centers	+/–	+/–	+/–
Common source exposure[f]	+	+	+

Source: adapted from reference 4.
[a]Hepatitis A vaccine is not licensed for children <2 years old.
[b]Immune globulin may be given in addition to or instead of hepatitis A vaccine.
[c]Children <2 years old should receive immune globulin.
[d]Not applicable.
[e]Hepatitis A vaccine can be given simultaneously if indicated.
[f]If immune globulin can be given within 2 weeks of exposure.

ally to countries with high or intermediate endemicity of HAV infection instead of, or in addition to, hepatitis A vaccine. IG should be given to children less than 2 years of age who are traveling to such countries, since hepatitis A vaccine is not licensed for children in this age group.

When indicated, hepatitis A vaccine can be given at the same time as IG, at a separate injection site. Although the concurrent administration of IG results in reduced immunogenicity of hepatitis A vaccine, this effect is not likely to be clinically significant because the final antibody concentrations achieved are at least 100 times above the level considered protective (20).

HEPATITIS B VIRUS

In 1965, Blumberg and colleagues described an isoprecipitin in the serum of Australian Aborigines (21), termed Australia antigen, that was later shown to be related to HBV infection. Within a decade following the discovery of Australia antigen, which was ultimately shown to be the surface antigen of HBV, the virus was fully characterized, various antigen and antibody systems were described, and immunoassays for their detection were developed. The availability of serological tests for hepatitis B surface antigen (HBsAg) expanded the understanding of the epidemiology and consequences of HBV infection. Worldwide, an estimated 300 million persons are chronically infected with HBV.

The realization that HBsAg could serve as an immunogen for the production of anti-HBs, and that this antibody was protective against HBV infection, led to the development of hepatitis B vaccines, which were produced and licensed in a number of countries beginning in the 1980s. By 1990, there was a worldwide effort to eliminate the transmission of HBV and HBV-related chronic liver disease and primary hepatocellular carcinoma (PHC) through routine vaccination of all infants.

Natural History and Diagnosis

HBV infection can cause a broad spectrum of disease ranging from asymptomatic acute infection to fulminant liver failure and death, and individuals with persistent infection can remain asymptomatic or progress to chronic liver disease, liver failure or develop PHC. The incubation period for acute HBV infection ranges from 45 to 160 days (mean, 120 days), and the onset of acute disease is usually insidious. Extrahepatic manifestations of disease (e.g., skin rashes, arthralgias, and arthritis) can also occur (22).

A direct relationship exists between age at infection and the likelihood of symptomatic HBV infection. Infections in infants and children less than 5 years of age rarely produce signs or symptoms consistent with viral hepatitis, while 10% of older children and 30% of adults may be become jaundiced, and a higher proportion may have additional signs or symptoms consistent with viral hepatitis. Fulminant hepatitis occurs in up to 1% of adults with acute hepatitis B and rarely in infected infants; however, fulminant hepatitis in infants may be more frequently associated with infections due to hepatitis B e antigen (HBeAg)-negative variants (23).

The risk of chronic HBV infection has been shown to be inversely related to age and averages 90% for infants infected at birth, 30% for children infected before age 5 years, and 2% to 6% among adults. The majority of persons chronically infected with HBV remain healthy and do not suffer the consequences of HBV-related chronic liver disease or PHC, especially if they became infected as adults. However, moderate to severe chronic hepatitis, cirrhosis, or PHC may occur in about one-third of chronically infected persons (24), with premature mortality rates of 25% in those infected as infants or young children (25).

Several well defined antigen–antibody systems are associated with HBV infection, including HBsAg and antibody to HBsAg (anti-HBs); hepatitis B core antigen (HBcAg) and antibody to HBcAg (anti-HBc); and HBeAg and antibody to HBeAg (anti-HBe) (26). Serologic assays are commercially available for all of these except HBcAg, because no free HBcAg circulates in blood. In newly infected individuals, HBsAg is identified in serum 30 to 60 days after exposure to HBV and persists for variable periods. The presence of HBsAg is indicative of ongoing HBV infection and potential infectiousness. Anti-HBc develops in all HBV infections and indicates previous or ongoing infection with HBV. It appears at the onset of symptoms or liver test abnormalities in acute HBV infection, rapidly rises to high levels, and persists for life. Acute or recently acquired infection can be distinguished by the presence of the IgM class of anti-HBc, which is detected at the onset of acute hepatitis B and persists for about 6 months.

In persons who recover from HBV infection, HBsAg is eliminated from the blood, usually in 2 to 3 months, and anti-HBs develops during convalescence. The presence of anti-HBs is generally interpreted as indicating recovery and immunity from HBV infection. After recovery from natural infection, most persons will be positive for both anti-HBs and anti-HBc, whereas only anti-HBs develops in persons who are successfully vaccinated against hepatitis B. In persons who do not recover from HBV infection and become chronically infected with HBV, HBsAg (and anti-HBc) remain detectable.

A third antigen, HBeAg, can be detected in serum of persons with acute or chronic HBV infection. The presence of HBeAg correlates with viral replication and high levels of virus (i.e., high infectivity). Antibody to HBeAg (anti-HBe) correlates with the loss of replicating virus and with lower levels of virus. However, all HBsAg-positive persons should be considered potentially infectious, regardless of their HBeAg or anti-HBe status.

HBV DNA in serum can be detected by nucleic acid hybridization or PCR amplification following extraction or immunocapture of HBV. These diagnostic methods are primarily used in research; however, monitoring of HBV DNA has proven useful in the evaluation and management of patients on antiviral therapy for chronic HBV infection. HBV DNA can be detected in tissue by *in situ* hybridization or following PCR amplification; methods primarily relegated to research situations. In addition, nucleic acid sequence analysis has been used to identify genetic variants of HBV. Such analysis has proven useful in determining the relatedness of HBV isolates in unusual situations of disease transmission or outcome (27,28).

Epidemiology

Modes of Transmission and Persons at Risk

HBV is transmitted by percutaneous and mucous membrane exposures to infectious blood and body fluids that contain blood. Although HBsAg has been detected in a wide variety of body fluids, only serum, semen, and saliva have been demonstrated to be infectious. The presence of HBeAg in serum correlates with higher titers of HBV (up to 10^9 particles/mL) and greater infectivity. Percutaneous exposures that have resulted in HBV transmission include transfusion of blood or blood products from infectious donors, contaminated equipment used for therapeutic injections, other healthcare-related and cosmetic (e.g., tattooing) procedures, illegal injection drug use, and needle

sticks or other injuries from sharp instruments sustained by healthcare personnel (29–35). Because HBV is stable on environmental surfaces (36), indirect inoculation of HBV can also occur via inanimate objects, and contaminated environmental surfaces have been a major source for HBV transmission among chronic hemodialysis patients.

Mucous membrane exposures to infectious blood or serum-derived body fluids through sexual and perinatal exposures are extremely efficient modes for HBV transmission (37,38). No infections have been demonstrated in susceptible persons orally exposed to HBsAg-positive saliva, although transmission by saliva has been demonstrated to animals by subcutaneous inoculation.

Person-to-person spread of HBV can occur in settings involving nonsexual interpersonal contact over a long period of time, such as among household contacts of a chronically infected person (37). The precise mechanisms of transmission are unknown; however, frequent interpersonal contact of nonintact skin or mucous membranes with secretions containing blood are the most likely modes of transmission.

Geographic Patterns of Transmission

The endemicity of HBV infection varies greatly worldwide (Fig.53.3) (37,38) and is influenced primarily by the predominant age at which infection occurs (Table 53.3). Endemicity of infection is considered high in those parts of

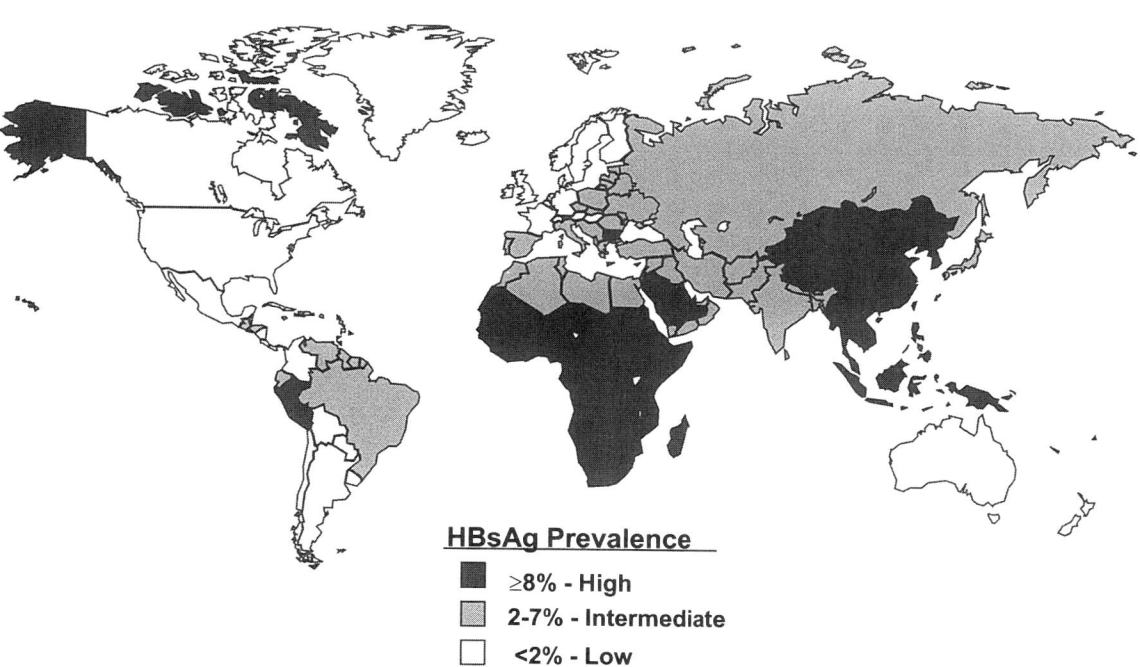

HBsAg Prevalence

- ≥8% - High
- 2-7% - Intermediate
- <2% - Low

FIGURE 53.3. Worldwide distribution and endemicity of chronic hepatitis B virus infection. *HbsAg*, hepatitis B surface antigen. (From Margolis HS, Alter MJ, Hadler SC. Viral Hepatitis. In: Evans AS, Kaslow RA, eds. *Viral Infections of Humans.* 4th ed. New York: Plenum Medical Book Co., 1997:363–418, with permission.)

the world where at least 8% of the population is chronically infected (HBsAg-positive). In these areas, 70% to 90% of the population generally have serological evidence of previous HBV infection. Almost all infections occur during either the perinatal period or early in childhood, which accounts for the high rates of chronic HBV infection in these populations. Chronic infection with HBV is strongly associated with PHC, and areas with a high endemicity of chronic HBV infection have the highest death rates from this neoplasm.

In areas of the world with an intermediate pattern of HBV infection, the prevalence of HBsAg positivity ranges from 2% to 7% and serological evidence of past infection is found in 10% to 60% of the population. In these areas there are mixed patterns of infant, early childhood and adult transmission.

In most developed parts of the world, the prevalence of chronic HBV infection is less than 1%, and the overall infection rate is 5% to 7%. Within these areas most infections occur among high-risk adult populations that include injection drug users, persons with multiple heterosexual partners, MSM, and healthcare workers (37,39).

In the U.S., an estimated 150,000 to 450,000 persons have been newly infected with HBV each year during the past two decades, of whom 39,000 to 90,000 had clinically apparent disease. Although the incidence of reported cases of acute hepatitis B has declined by 66% since its peak in 1985, an estimated 185,000 new HBV infections occurred in 1997 (CDC, unpublished data). The highest incidence of disease has occurred among young adults (20 to 29 years old), and rates are higher among blacks and Hispanics compared with whites (39). A substantial number of children become infected with HBV in well-defined settings and the epidemiology of these infections is quite different from that of infections acquired by adults (37). Since over 90% of childhood HBV infections are asymptomatic, the true incidence of childhood disease is not accurately represented by national surveillance data, which reflect reported cases of clinically apparent disease. Thus, only 1% to 3% of all acute HBV infections occurring in the U.S. are reported among children less than 5 years of age, but infec-

tions in this age group account for 20% to 30% of all chronic HBV infections (37).

National seroprevalence data indicate that the age-adjusted prevalence of HBV infection in the general population of the U.S. declined minimally during the past two decades, from 5.5% during 1976 to 1980 to 4.9% during 1988 to 1994 (40). During this latter period, the prevalence was 2.6% among non-Hispanic whites, 4.4% among Mexican-Americans, and 11.9% among non-Hispanic blacks. Among blacks, HBV prevalence increased at an earlier age (12 to 19 years old) compared with other groups, and the highest observed prevalence (21.3%) was in blacks over 50 years old. Black race, increasing number of lifetime sexual partners, and foreign birth were the factors most strongly associated with HBV infection (40).

Among reported cases of acute disease, the three predominant risk factors for infection are heterosexual exposure to an infected partner or to multiple partners (45%), injection drug use (21%), and MSM activity (15%) (Fig. 53.4) (39) (CDC, unpublished data). Exposure to an infected household contact accounts for an average of 3% of cases and healthcare-related occupational exposure to blood for an average of 1%. No recognized source for infection can be identified for about 15% of cases.

Prevention

HBV infection can be prevented by screening blood, plasma, organ, tissue, and semen donors, virus inactivation of plasma-derived products, risk-reduction counseling and services, and implementation and maintenance of infection control practices. Although such activities can reduce or eliminate the potential risk for HBV transmission, by far the single most effective prevention measure is immunization.

Preexposure vaccination generally requires three doses to induce an immune response that provides long-term protection. The recommended primary series of hepatitis B vaccine induces a protective (defined as greater than 10 milli-international units (mIU)/mL) anti-HBs response in more than 90% of healthy adults and in more than 95% of

TABLE 53.3. CHARACTERISTICS OF ENDEMIC PATTERNS OF HEPATITIS B VIRUS INFECTION

Characteristic	Endemicity of infection		
	Low	Intermediate	High
Chronic infection prevalence	0.1–1%	2–7%	8–15%
Past infection prevalence	4–15%	16–55%	40–90%
Perinatal infection	Rare (<10%)[a]	Uncommon (10–60%)[a]	Common (>20%)[a]
Early childhood infection	Rare (<10%)[b]	Common (10–60%)[b]	Very common (>60%)[b]
Adolescent/adult infection	Very common (70–90%)	Common (20–50%)	Uncommon (10–20%)

[a]Estimated percent of total infections among children up to 1 year of age.
[b]Estimated percent of total infections among children 1–5 years of age.
From Margolis HS, Alter MJ, Hadler SC. Viral Hepatitis. In: Evans AS, Kaslow RA, eds. *Viral infections of humans,* 4th ed., New York: Plenum Medical Book Co., 1997, 363–418, with permission.

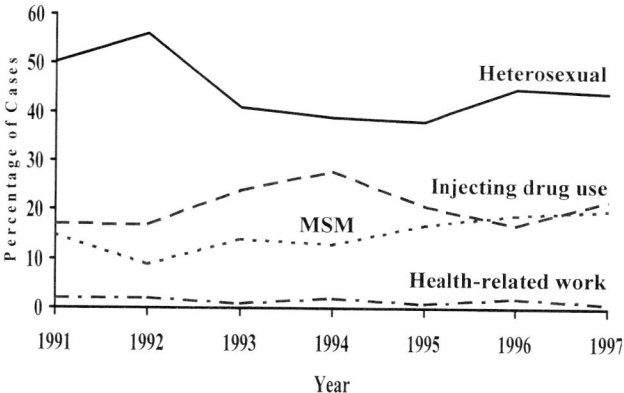

FIGURE 53.4. Trends in risk factors for reported cases of hepatitis B, Sentinel Counties, U.S., 1991–1997. *Heterosexual,* heterosexual exposure to infected sexual partner or to multiple partners; *MSM,* men who have sex with men. (From Centers for Disease Control and Prevention, unpublished data.)

infants, children, and adolescents. The major determinant of vaccine response is age with the proportion developing a protective antibody response declining to 84% in adults over 40 years old and to 75% by age 60 years (41). Other host factors that contribute to decreased immunogenicity include smoking, obesity, and immune suppression. For persons with normal immune status, protection from acute and chronic HBV infection is virtually complete among those who develop a protective antibody response following vaccination, and persists even when antibody titers become undetectable (41). In addition, infection can be effectively prevented after exposure to HBV (postexposure prophylaxis) through the passive administration of anti-HBs [hepatitis B immune globulin (HBIG)] and hepatitis B vaccine or with vaccine alone.

The primary objective of hepatitis B immunization is the prevention of chronic HBV infection and its sequelae. In areas of high and intermediate HBV endemicity, all infants should be routinely immunized against HBV infection. The strategy for elimination of HBV transmission in areas of low endemicity of HBV infection, such as the U.S., includes routine infant and adolescent vaccination; screening of pregnant women for HBsAg and administration of postexposure prophylaxis (HBIG and vaccine) to infants born to infected women; and vaccination of children, adolescents, and adults at increased risk for hepatitis B (Table 53.4) (42). Routine infant immunization ensures the prevention of HBV infections in subpopulations that have high rates of early childhood infection (i.e., Eskimos, Asian/Pacific Islanders, infants of immigrant women from high endemicity areas), assures high immunization coverage rates because of the proven vaccine delivery system, and should prevent infections in adolescents and young adults because of the proven long-term efficacy of hepatitis B immunization. However, because most clinical disease occurs in adults, the addition of routine adolescent vaccina-

tion will achieve a more rapid reduction in HBV transmission. Until the cohorts of vaccinated children reach adolescence and adulthood, efforts must be strengthened to vaccinate older adolescents and adults with high-risk behaviors or occupations (Table 53.4).

It is currently not known whether infant and childhood hepatitis B immunization will confer lifelong immunity against chronic infection, which is of particular importance where vaccination of younger persons is expected to prevent adult-acquired infection. Current data indicate that booster doses of hepatitis B vaccine are not required for at least the first decade following infant, childhood or adult immunization (38). The very long incubation period of HBV infection (40 to 120 days), coupled with the excellent anamnestic antibody response to HBsAg in previously immunized persons, would appear to limit breakthrough infections to ones that produce limited viremia and do not become persistent. For several generations to come, HBV infection will persist in the previously unimmunized population, but continued immunization of successive birth

TABLE 53.4. RECOMMENDATIONS FOR THE USE OF HEPATITIS B VACCINE AND HEPATITIS B IMMUNE GLOBULIN IN THE UNITED STATES

Preexposure protection with hepatitis B vaccine
- *Routine Vaccination of Infants*
- *Catch-up Vaccination of Children at High Risk for Infection*
  Children <11 years old residing in households of first generation immigrants from countries with an intermediate or high endemicity of HBV infection (Fig. 53.3).
- *Routine Vaccination of Adolescents*
- *Vaccination of Persons in Groups at Increased Risk for Infection*
  Heterosexual adolescents and adults with multiple sex partners in the previous 6 months or a recently acquired sexually transmitted disease.
  Adult and adolescent men who have sex with men.
  Sexual partners and household contacts of HBsAg-positive persons.
  Injection drug users.
  Persons with occupational exposure to blood.
  Clients and staff of institutions for the developmentally disabled.
  Hemodialysis patients and patients with early renal failure.
  Patients who receive clotting factor concentrates.
  International travelers staying in areas of high or intermediate HBV endemicity (Fig. 53.3) for >6 months.
  Inmates in correctional facilities.

Postexposure protection with hepatitis B vaccine and/or hepatitis B immune globulin
- *Infants born to HBsAg-positive mother*
- *Susceptible persons with percutaneous or permucosal exposure to HBsAg-positive blood*
- *Unvaccinated persons with sexual exposure to an HBsAg-positive person*

HBsAg, hepatitis B serum antigen; HBV, hepatitis B virus.

cohorts should achieve the eventual elimination of HBV transmission.

HEPATITIS C VIRUS

HCV was discovered in 1988, and was shown to be the primary etiologic agent of parenterally transmitted non-A, non-B (PT-NANB) hepatitis worldwide (43–46). PT-NANB hepatitis was first recognized in the 1970s, following development of specific serological tests to identify HBV and HAV infection. The term NANB hepatitis was applied to those cases of acute hepatitis for which other specific etiologies (HAV, HBV, Epstein-Barr virus, cytomegalovirus, and a variety of other infectious and non-infectious agents that can cause liver inflammation) could be reliably excluded. Although PT-NANB hepatitis was first recognized to be commonly associated with blood transfusion, it is now known to be an important cause of community-acquired viral hepatitis.

The characterization of HCV resulted in the development of diagnostic assays, the use of which has provided a worldwide picture of the extent of HCV infection that had previously gone unrecognized. The World Health Organization estimates that 170 million persons have been infected with HCV, most of whom are chronically infected and serve as a source for transmission to others as well as being at risk for chronic liver disease and its complications. Although the recognition of the clinical importance of HCV infection has resulted in the rapid direction of attention and resources toward developing new and improved therapies, resources for the prevention of HCV infection are still limited.

The prospects for an effective vaccine against HCV infection are disappointing. Like other RNA viruses, the substantial heterogeneity of the HCV genome is the result of mutations that occur during viral replication (47). The genetic diversity of HCV appears to prevent the development of an effective neutralizing immune response, thereby complicating efforts towards the development of a vaccine.

Natural History and Diagnosis

Like HBV infection, infection with HCV can cause a broad spectrum of disease. The incubation period for acute hepatitis C averages 6 to 7 weeks. Compared with HBV, HCV circulates in lower titers in infected serum (10^5 to 10^6) and its detection in body fluids other than serum and plasma has been highly variable. Persons with acute HCV infection typically are either asymptomatic or have a mild clinical illness. Fulminant hepatic failure following acute hepatitis C is rare.

After acute HCV infection, chronic infection develops in most persons (75% to 85%), with active liver disease developing in 60% to 70% of chronically infected persons (48). No clinical or epidemiologic features among patients with acute infection have been found to be predictive of either per-

sistent infection or chronic liver disease. The course of chronic liver disease is usually insidious, progressing at a slow rate without symptoms or physical signs in the majority of patients during the two or more decades after infection. Cirrhosis develops in 10% to 20% of persons with chronic hepatitis C over a period of 20 or more years, and hepatocellular carcinoma (HCC) in 1% to 5%, with striking geographic variations in rates of this disease. Although factors predicting severity of liver disease have not been well defined, the most convincing data show that heavy alcohol intake and age greater than 40 years at infection are associated with more severe liver disease. Extrahepatic manifestations of chronic HCV infection are considered to be of immunologic origin, and include cryoglobulinemia, membranoproliferative glomerulonephritis, and porphyria cutanea tarda (49).

The only serologic marker of HCV infection that can be detected is antibody to HCV (anti-HCV); however, anti-HCV assays do not distinguish between acute, chronic, or resolved infection. HCV infection also can be detected using qualitative and quantitative gene amplification techniques for HCV RNA, such as reverse transcriptase PCR (RT-PCR). Nucleic acid amplification and sequencing analysis of the hypervariable (HVR1) and nonstructural regions has been used to determine the relatedness of HCV isolates in studies of nosocomial transmission and differential responses to antiviral therapy (50,51).

Epidemiology

Modes of Transmission and Persons at Risk

The most efficient transmission of HCV is through large or repeated percutaneous exposures to infectious blood, such as through transfusion of blood or plasma-derived products or transplantation of organs from infectious donors, and illegal injection drug use. Hemophilia patients who have been heavily transfused with nontreated factor concentrates and injection drug users with many (more than 10) years of drug use have prevalence rates of anti-HCV exceeding 90%, higher than for any other group studied (52,53). Persons exposed to HCV through percutaneous procedures involving unsafe injection practices and use of contaminated equipment for healthcare procedures that was not adequately cleaned or disinfected are also at substantial risk for HCV infection (52). Although less efficient, small, sporadic percutaneous exposures to blood such as through accidental needlestick injuries, and inapparent percutaneous or mucosal exposures such as through perinatal and sexual exposures, also result in HCV transmission (52).

Geographic Patterns of Transmission

HCV is endemic in most areas of the world. Differences in virus- and host-specific factors are likely responsible for the individual differences observed in the natural history of HCV-related chronic disease and in responses to antiviral therapy. Differences in the frequency and extent to which various risk factors contribute to the transmission of HCV are responsible for temporal and geographic differences that have been observed in the epidemiology of hepatitis C.

For many countries in the world, no reliable data exist on prevalence of HCV infection. Using available data from seroprevalence studies among blood donors (Fig. 53.5) (52), the highest HCV prevalence (17% to 26%) by far has been reported from Egypt. Intermediate HCV prevalence (1% to 5%) has been reported from Eastern Europe, the Mediterranean, the Mideast, the Indian subcontinent, parts of Africa, and Asia. Low prevalence (0.2% to 0.5%) has been reported from Western Europe, North America, most areas of Central America, Australia, and limited regions of Africa, including South Africa. The lowest HCV prevalence (0.01% to 0.1%) has been reported from the United Kingdom and Scandinavia.

There appear to be three distinct global patterns of age-specific HCV infection prevalence that indicate geographic differences in the time periods during which there was an increased risk for acquiring HCV infection as well as different patterns of risk factor-specific disease transmission (Table 53.5) (52). In Egypt, the country with the highest reported prevalence of HCV infection, the prevalence of infection increases steadily with age, and high rates of infection are observed among persons in all age groups. This pattern indicates an increased risk for infection in the distant past followed by an ongoing high risk for acquiring infection. This high risk for infection appears to be primarily associated with transmission by unsafe injection practices

(e.g., re-use of glass syringes) and possibly by contaminated equipment used for medical procedures.

In countries with an intermediate prevalence of HCV infection, such as Japan and Italy, the age-specific prevalence of HCV infection is low in children and younger adults and increases sharply among older persons, who account for the majority of infections. This pattern indicates that the risk for HCV infection was greatest in the distant past (i.e., 30 to 50 years ago), and healthcare-related procedures and unsafe injections (including re-use of contaminated glass syringes and administration at home by nonprofessionals in which syringes were shared with other family members, neighbors, and friends) appear to have been the predominant modes of HCV transmission.

The third pattern that emerges is observed in countries with a low prevalence of infection, such as the U.S. and Australia. The age-specific prevalence is low among persons less than 20 years old, rises steadily through middle age, with the majority of infections occurring among adults 30 to 49 year old, and declines sharply among persons greater than 50 years old. This pattern suggests that most HCV transmission occurred in the relatively recent past (10 to 30 years ago) and primarily among young adults, with injection drug use being the predominant mode of transmission.

In the U.S., the estimated annual incidence was low (18 per 100,000) before 1965, increased steadily through 1980, and remained high (130 per 100,000) through 1989, corresponding to an average of 240,000 infections per year in the 1980s (54). Since 1989, the incidence of HCV infection has declined by more than 80%, primarily as a result

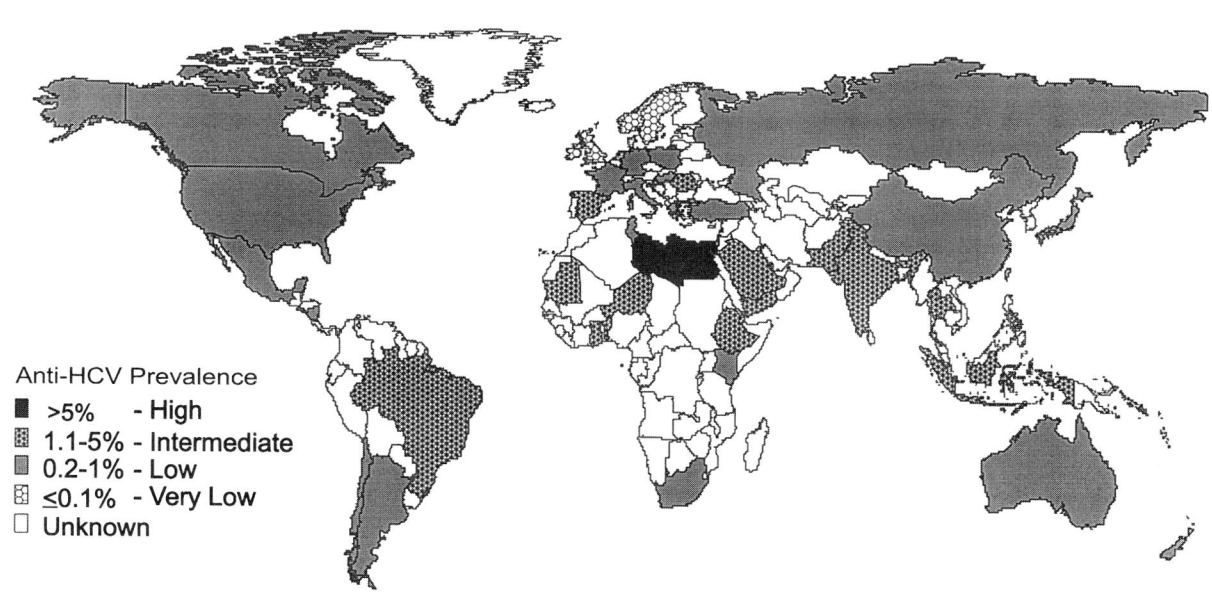

FIGURE 53.5. Worldwide distribution of hepatitis C virus (*HCV*) infection. (From Wasley A, Alter MJ. Epidemiology of hepatitis C: geographic differences and temporal trends. *Semin Liver Dis* 2000;20:1–16, with permission.)

TABLE 53.5. GLOBAL DIFFERENCES IN HEPATITIS C VIRUS TRANSMISSION PATTERNS

Characteristic	Prevalence of HCV Infection		
	Low	Moderate	High
Representative countries	United States	Japan	Egypt
	Australia	Italy	
Time period of increased incidence	Recent past	Distant past	Distant past/
	(10–30 yrs ago)	(30–50 yrs ago)	ongoing
Age with highest prevalence	Younger adults	Older adults	All ages
Relative importance of exposures among prevalent infections			
Injecting drug use	++++	++	+
Transfusions	+++	+++	+++
Medical (dental) procedures	+/−	++++	++++
Unsafe injections	+/−	++++	++++
Folk medicine	−	++	No data
Occupational	+	+	+
Perinatal	+	+	+
High-risk sex	++	+	+

From Wasley A, Alter MJ. Epidemiology of hepatitis C: geographic differences and temporal trends. *Semin Liver Dis* 2000;20:1–16, with permission.

of a decrease in cases among injection drug users (55). HCV infection occurs among persons of all ages, but the highest incidence of acute hepatitis C is found among persons 20 to 29 years old, and males predominate slightly (46,54). Non-Hispanic blacks and whites have similar incidence of acute disease; persons of Hispanic ethnicity have higher rates.

National seroprevalence data from 1988 to 1994 indicate that an estimated 3.9 million (1.8%) Americans have been infected with HCV, of whom 2.7 million are chronically infected (56). The highest prevalence of HCV infection was found among persons aged 30 to 49 years and among males. Unlike the racial/ethnic pattern of acute disease, non-Hispanic blacks had a higher prevalence of HCV infection (3.2%) than did whites (1.5%). Prevalence increased at an earlier age (12 to 19 years) among black females than among other groups, but the highest observed prevalence (9.8%) was among black males 40 to 49 years old. The risk factors most strongly associated with infection were high-risk drug and sexual behaviors (56).

In the U.S., the relative importance of the two most common exposures associated with the transmission of HCV, blood transfusion and injection drug use, has changed over time (Fig. 53.6) (189,259). Blood transfusion, which accounted for more than 20% of HCV infections acquired more than 15 years ago, accounts for less than 5% of infections acquired during the past 15 years. In contrast, injection drug use consistently has accounted for a substantial proportion of HCV infections and currently accounts for 60% of HCV transmission in the U.S. (46,53,55). An average of 20% of persons with HCV infection report sexual exposures (i.e., exposure to an infected sexual partner or to multiple partners), and other known exposures (occupational, hemodialysis, household, perinatal) together account for

about 10% of infections. In the remaining 10%, no recognized source of infection can be identified.

Prevention

Reducing the burden of HCV infection and HCV-related disease requires implementation of primary prevention activities that reduce the risks for contracting HCV infection and secondary prevention activities that reduce risks for disease progression in HCV-infected persons (53,57). There is no vaccine against HCV.

In many developing countries, donor screening and testing policies for HCV and inactivation procedures for

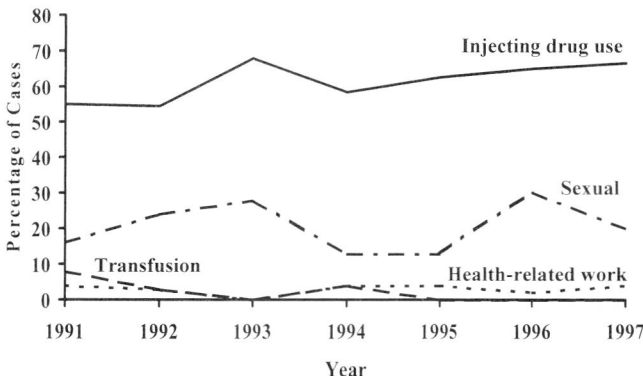

FIGURE 53.6. Trends in risk factors for reported cases of hepatitis C, Sentinel Counties, U.S., 1991–1997. *Sexual,* exposure to infected sexual partner or to multiple partners. [From Centers for Disease Control and Prevention. Recommendations for the prevention and control of hepatitis C virus (HCV) infection and HCV-related chronic disease. *MMWR* 1998;47(No. RR-19):1–39, with permission.]

plasma-derived products have not been implemented, and transfusions and organ transplants continue to be major sources for HCV infection. In these countries, improving the safety of the blood supply should be the highest priority (57). Programs also should be initiated to reduce the extent to which HCV is transmitted as a result of inadequate sterilization or disinfection of medical, surgical, and dental equipment, re-use of contaminated equipment, and unsafe injection practices (57).

Primary prevention of illegal drug injection will eliminate the greatest risk factor for HCV infection in the U.S. and other countries where this behavior plays a major role in disease transmission (53). Counseling and education to prevent initiation of high-risk drug and sexual practices is important, especially for adolescents, as is the provision of other prevention services, such as vaccination against hepatitis B and hepatitis A. To reduce the risk for HCV infection among injection drug users, communities should consider increasing access to sterile syringes and needles through services such as syringe and needle exchange programs and to drug treatment programs.

Secondary prevention activities can reduce risks for chronic disease by identifying HCV-infected persons through diagnostic testing and by providing appropriate medical management and antiviral therapy. Identification of persons at risk for HCV infection also provides infected persons the opportunity to obtain information about how they can prevent further harm to their liver and prevent transmitting the infection to others. In countries with sufficient resources, testing should be offered routinely to persons most likely to be infected with HCV and should be accompanied by appropriate counseling and medical follow-up (Table 53.6) (53,57).

TABLE 53.6. RECOMMENDATIONS FOR ROUTINE TESTING FOR HEPATITIS C VIRUS (HCV) INFECTION BASED ON RISK FOR INFECTION OR A RECOGNIZED EXPOSURE, UNITED STATES AND EUROPE

- Persons who ever injected illegal drugs.
- Persons who received plasma-derived products known to transmit HCV that were not treated to inactivate viruses;
- Persons who received transfusions or organ transplants before second generation anti-HCV testing of donors was widely implemented;
- Persons who have been on chronic hemodialysis;
- Health care, emergency medical, and public safety workers after needlesticks, sharps, or mucosal exposures to HCV-positive blood;
- Children born to HCV-positive women.

From Centers for Disease Control and Prevention. Recommendations for the prevention and control of hepatitis C virus (HCV) infection and HCV-related chronic disease. *MMWR* 1998;47(No. RR-19):1–39, and from World Health Organization. Global surveillance and control of hepatitis C. Report of a WHO Consultation organized in collaboration with the Viral Hepatitis Prevention Board, Antwerp, Belgium. *J Viral Hepatitis* 1999;6:35–47, with permission.

Immune globulin and antiviral agents are not recommended for postexposure prophylaxis of hepatitis C (53). Available data indicate that immune globulin is not effective for postexposure prophylaxis of hepatitis C (58). No assessments have been made of postexposure use of antiviral agents to prevent HCV infection. Mechanisms of the effect of interferon in treating patients with hepatitis C are poorly understood, and an established infection might need to be present for interferon to be an effective treatment (59). Furthermore, at least in the U.S., interferon (alone or combined with ribavirin) is approved only for treatment of chronic hepatitis C.

There is a large global reservoir of HCV-infected individuals who can serve as a source of transmission to others and who are at risk for HCV-related chronic diseases. To prevent new infections, public health programs should focus on ensuring a safe blood supply, implementing appropriate infection control practices, and preventing initiation of high-risk drug and sexual behaviors. In addition, more effective therapies for treatment of persons with chronic hepatitis C need to be developed, and approaches designed for treating current or former injection drug users.

HEPATITIS DELTA VIRUS

HDV was discovered by Rizzetto in 1977 (60). Studies in chimpanzees in 1979 to 1980 established that HDV was dependent on the presence of active HBV infection to cause infection (61). Serological tests for HDV and antibodies to HDV developed by the early 1980s have been used to characterize the clinical and epidemiologic aspects of infection (62,63).

Natural History and Diagnosis

The spectrum of clinical disease in acute HDV infection may vary from no illness to acute and fulminant hepatitis. In general, HDV augments the severity of both acute and chronic HBV infection. The dependence of HDV on HBV replication permits HDV infection to occur in two primary circumstances: as HDV–HBV coinfection of a person susceptible to HBV infection and as HDV superinfection of a person with chronic HBV infection. A third form of HDV infection, latent infection, may occur in persons who receive liver transplants for fulminant or chronic HBV–HDV liver disease, in which HDV infection of the new liver may occur without the recurrence of HBV infection (64). The natural course of HDV infection differs depending on whether it is a coinfection with HBV or superinfection of a person with chronic HBV infection. HDV superinfection of an HBV carrier usually leads to establishment of chronic HDV infection and chronic hepatitis, whereas coinfection usually causes self-limited hepatitis. Latent HDV infection does not cause liver disease unless HBV infection recurs, in which case both acute and chronic hepatitis usually ensue.

HDV infection is diagnosed by serological testing for HBV and HDV markers in persons with clinical symptoms of acute or chronic hepatitis. Acute HBV–HDV coinfection is verified by a positive test for IgM anti-HBc accompanied by the presence of δ-antigen or total and/or IgM anti-HDV. Delta antigen is usually present during early acute illness, whereas both IgM and IgG antibodies appear within several days to weeks after onset. The antibody response in such cases is not strong, and accurate diagnosis is best accomplished during acute illness or early convalescence. In cases of fulminant hepatitis, HDV markers in serum may be negative although δ-antigen may be demonstrable in liver. The late phase of the infection is marked by disappearance of both HBsAg and δ-antigen in liver and serum and development of specific antibodies to both viruses. The development of anti-HBs provides protection against reinfection with both HBV and HDV. Only a total anti-HDV test is commercially available in the U.S.

The diagnosis of chronic HDV infection is usually made in HBsAg-positive persons with chronic hepatitis who are also positive for anti-HDV. The most active cases can be distinguished by presence of greater degrees of liver inflammation, the presence of IgM anti-HDV and HDV RNA in the serum, and δ-antigen in the liver (65).

Epidemiology

Modes of Transmission and Persons at Risk

HDV, like HBV, is found in highest concentration in the blood of persons with acute or chronic infection. Virus titers may be extremely high (up to 10^{12} infectious doses/mL) and exceed those of HBV. HDV may be presumed to be present in serum-derived fluids such as wound exudates; however, its presence in other body fluids (semen, saliva, feces) has not been studied.

Transmission occurs by percutaneous exposure to blood containing HDV, either directly or indirectly, and by sexual contact. Direct bloodborne transmission appears highly efficient as shown by the high risk for infection in injection drug users and persons with hemophilia. However, indirect exposure to blood through open skin wounds, either directly or indirectly via contaminated environmental surfaces, has presumably been the major transmission route in outbreaks among indigent local populations in South America (66). Although less efficient than that of HBV, sexual transmission of HDV has been associated both with MSM and heterosexual activity (63). Perinatal transmission from mother to infant is uncommon, but HBsAg-positive household contacts of HBV–HDV carriers are at significant risk of infection over long periods of time (63).

Geographic Patterns of Transmission

HDV infection has been observed in all parts of the world, with the frequency generally corresponding to HBV endemicity (38). Prevalence in asymptomatic HBV carriers varies from 0% to 25%, and prevalence among persons with HBV-related chronic liver disease tends to vary more widely, from 5% to 100%. The highest HDV prevalence, that is, 20% in HBsAg-positive persons and up to 90% in persons with HBV-related chronic liver disease, has been observed in widely dispersed areas of high HBV endemicity, including the Amazon Basin and other parts of northern South America, parts of Africa, and Romania. Moderate prevalence of HDV infection, that is, 15% in HBsAg-positive persons and 30% to 50% in persons with HBV-related chronic liver disease, has been documented in southern Italy, parts of Eastern Europe, the Middle East, Africa, and in some Pacific Islands groups. Low HDV prevalence, that is, 0% to 5% in HBsAg-positive persons and 10% to 25% in persons with HBV-related chronic liver disease, is found in areas of low HBV endemicity, that is, Western Europe, North America, and Australia. The prevalence of HDV infection is very low in East and Southeast Asia despite high HBV endemicity throughout this region. The reasons for this are unclear; HDV infection is present in neighboring areas of Asia and in some Pacific Islands, and a high frequency of HDV infection has been observed among injection drug users and prostitutes in Taiwan. This virus may have been only recently introduced into ethnic Oriental populations, possibly via injection drug users.

In the U.S., HDV infection is found in about 3% of cases of acute hepatitis B and in up to 25% of cases of fulminant hepatitis (67). The most current estimates indicate that about 5,000 HDV coinfections or superinfections occur annually, about 70,000 persons are chronically infected with HDV, and about 1,000 persons die due to chronic (most) or fulminant δ-hepatitis. Prevalence studies have shown a high risk of HDV infection in HBsAg-positive injection drug users (30% to 50%) and persons with hemophilia, but much lower prevalence (less than 10%) in other high-HBV-risk groups, including MSM, persons with multiple heterosexual partners, the developmentally disabled, hemodialysis patients, and household contacts of HBV carriers (63,67).

Prevention

Measures for control and prevention of HDV infection are identical to those for HBV. General measures to prevent HBV transmission, which include sterilization of needles and instruments that penetrate the skin in a medical care setting and screening of blood for HBsAg, are effective in preventing both HBV and HDV infection. Vaccination of persons at risk of HBV infection is the best protective measure against HDV coinfection as well.

For persons chronically infected with HBV who are at risk for HDV superinfection, there is no specific prevention that can be offered, and neither hepatitis B vaccine nor HBIG is effective in preventing HDV infections. Several drug regimens may eliminate the HBV carrier state, but effectiveness is usually less than 50% and is highest in those with most recent infection. The major preventative that can be offered is counseling to avoid high-risk drug and sexual exposures. Available measures to prevent HDV superinfection are even more limited in HBV–HDV endemic areas in which poverty, crowding, insect bites, and open skin lesions facilitate disease transmission.

HEPATITIS E VIRUS

HEV was cloned and sequenced in 1990 (68), and was shown to be the etiologic agent of enterically transmitted non-A, non-B (ET-NANB) hepatitis. Large epidemics of viral hepatitis that epidemiologically resembled hepatitis A had been reported since the mid-1950s, primarily from Asia. After the development of serological tests for the diagnosis of HAV infection in the 1970s, retrospective examination of acute and convalescent serum specimens from these early outbreaks indicated that the vast majority of cases were not attributable to HAV infection (69).

Natural History and Diagnosis

The incubation period for hepatitis E is longer than for hepatitis A, with a range of 22 to 60 days and a mode of 40 days (69). Peak mean bilirubin and liver enzyme values do not differ from those observed with hepatitis A and hepatitis B. A low (0.5% to 4%) case fatality rate is associated with hepatitis E in the general population, but among pregnant women mortality has ranged from 17% to 33% (69,70). The highest rates of fulminant hepatitis and death have occurred during the third trimester. No chronic infection after hepatitis E has been documented.

During the early phase of infection, IgM anti-HEV is present and can be detected for 5 to 6 months. IgG anti-HEV has generally been detected almost simultaneously with IgM antibody. However, since a well standardized test for IgM anti-HEV is not available, the diagnosis of hepatitis E in the acutely ill patient remains somewhat problematic. Testing for IgM anti-HAV and IgM anti-HBc can exclude those causes of viral hepatitis. In parts of the world where hepatitis E has been identified and/or is considered endemic, the presence of anti-HEV can be considered diagnostic of acute infection in a symptomatic patient who is anti-HCV negative. However, in the patient who is positive for both anti-HCV and anti-HEV, the final diagnosis may depend on a history consistent with the epidemiologic features of the particular disease, including the likely source of infection, incubation period, and eventual clinical outcome. Obtaining testing for IgM anti-HEV may be required for some cases. In the U.S., tests for total and IgM anti-HEV are available only on a research-use basis.

IgG anti-HEV activity has been found for at least 1 year after acute infection in most patients, and for up to 10 years

in experimentally infected primates. The long-term persistence of IgG anti-HEV is further suggested by its detection in asymptomatic persons living in areas where HEV infection has been shown to be endemic. However, detection of antibody persistence may depend on the epitopes included in the immunoassay. Until the natural history of the antibody response to HEV infection is defined, it is difficult to determine the true frequency of HEV infection in any population. At the present time, it is not known whether the IgG anti-HEV detected by these assays represents neutralizing antibody(ies).

RT-PCR has been used to detect HEV RNA in experimentally infected animals, as well as in humans with naturally occurring infection (71). HEV RNA has been obtained by RNA extraction, or by immunoprecipitation or immunocapture of the virus prior to amplification by RT-PCR. No assays have been developed that will detect HEV antigen in stool specimens, although HEV-Ag has been detected in liver biopsies of experimentally infected animals using fluorescent antibody microscopy.

Epidemiology

Modes of Transmission and Persons at Risk

Like HAV, HEV is transmitted by the fecal-oral route. Hepatitis E occurs both in epidemic and sporadic forms and is primarily associated with the ingestion of fecally contaminated drinking water (69,70). Epidemics have occurred in a wide variety of settings including urban areas, small towns and villages, and refugee camps. In all instances there has been evidence of poor sanitary conditions with inadequate disposal of feces and contamination of water supplies with fecal material. Population-based studies during epidemic periods have demonstrated clinical attack rates ranging from 0.7% to as high as 10%. Secondary attack rates in households are low (0.7% to 2.2%).

Several epidemiologic characteristics tend to distinguish hepatitis E from hepatitis A, and these differences have not been explained even with the availability of diagnostic tests. The majority of symptomatic infections occur among young adults, and a low prevalence of infection is found among children, features which are unexpected in areas where enteric infections are highly endemic among children and adults. Furthermore, hepatitis E is associated with a low secondary attack rate among household contacts. The potential for HEV transmission from contaminated food is still under investigation, and there is no evidence of transmission by percutaneous or sexual exposures.

Geographic Patterns of Transmission

The precise worldwide distribution of HEV infection has not been determined due to the lack of well standardized and readily available serodiagnostic tests. However, the geographic distribution of countries where outbreaks and sporadic cases have been reported indicates that this disease may be endemic in developing countries (38). Epidemics and sporadic cases of hepatitis E have been reported from most of Central Asia, Southeast Asia and Indonesia, the Middle East, Northern Africa, sub-Saharan Africa, and Mexico. Outbreaks have not been recognized in Europe, the U.S., Australia, or South America.

In developed countries, including the U.S., cases of hepatitis E imported from countries with known epidemic or endemic disease have been detected, but there has been no evidence of transmission to other persons. However, unique viral strains have been isolated from two patients with acute hepatitis E in the U.S. with no history of international travel (72,73). These strains are closely related to a swine HEV, and studies are under way to investigate the possibility of a zoonotic reservoir for HEV. In some non-HEV endemic countries, anti-HEV has been detected in 1% to 20% of blood donors in contrast to the low incidence of clinically evident disease (74,75). In one of these studies, one-third of anti-HEV positive blood donors had no history of travel to HEV-endemic countries (75). However, in this and other studies, the concordance among reactive sera between different anti-HEV assays was low, indicating that seroprevalence data from non-HEV endemic countries may be unreliable (76).

Prevention

Currently the most important means of preventing hepatitis E is protection of water systems from contamination with fecal material. Epidemiologic evidence indicates that boiling water will interrupt disease transmission. Similar data concerning chlorination of water are not available, although this strategy should also be used to interrupt disease transmission in epidemic situations.

The prophylactic effect of IG has not been demonstrated. One study using IG produced in India did not show a statistically different rate of disease between exposed individuals who received IG and those who did not receive IG (77). It is unlikely that IGs prepared from parts of the world where hepatitis E is not an endemic disease would have appropriate levels of antibody. A recombinant antigen has been produced that induces antibodies in *cynomolgus* macaques, which appears to be effective in preventing infection and may prevent disease when these animals are challenged with the wild-type virus (78). Whether an effective vaccine can be produced that will prevent HEV infection and hepatitis E in humans remains to be determined.

REFERENCES

1. Feinstone SM, Kapikian AZ, Purcell RH. Hepatitis A: detection by immune electron microscopy of a virus-like antigen association with acute illness. *Science* 1973;182:1026–1028.
2. Werzberger A, Mensch B, Kuter B, et al. A controlled trial of formalin-inactivated hepatitis A vaccine in healthy children. *N Engl J Med* 1992;327:453–457.
3. Innis BL, Snitbhan R, Kunasol P, et al. Protection against hepatitis A by an inactivated vaccine. *JAMA* 1994;271:1328–1334.
4. Centers for Disease Control and Prevention. Prevention of hepatitis A through active or passive immunization: recommendations of the Advisory Committee on Immunization Practices (ACIP). MMWR 1999;48(No. RR-12):1–37.
5. Tassopoulos NC, Papaevangelou GJ, Ticehurst JR, et al. Fecal excretion of Greek strains of hepatitis A virus in patients with hepatitis A and in experimentally infected chimpanzees. *J Infect Dis* 1986;154:231–237.
6. Rosenblum LS, Villarino ME, Nainan OV, et al. Hepatitis A outbreak in a neonatal intensive care unit: risk factors for transmission and evidence of prolonged viral excretion among preterm infants. *J Infect Dis* 1991;164:476–482.
7. Bower WA, Nainan OV, Han X, et al. Duration of viremia in hepatitis A virus infection. *J Infect Dis* 2000;182:12–17.
8. Hutin YJF, Pool V, Cramer EH, et. al. A multistate, food-borne outbreak of hepatitis A. *N Engl J Med* 1999;340:595–602.
9. Robertson BH, Jansen RW, Khanna B, et al. Genetic relatedness of hepatitis A virus strains recovered from different geographical regions. *J Gen Virol* 1992;73:1365–1377.
10. Carl M, Francis DP, Maynard JP. Food-borne hepatitis A: recommendation for control. *J Infect Dis* 1983;148:1133–1135.
11. Bell BP, Shapiro CN, Margolis HS. Hepatitis A virus. In: Feigan RD, Cherry JD, eds. *Textbook of pediatric infectious diseases.* 4th ed. Philadelphia: WB Saunders, 1997:1865–1881.
12. Hadler SC, Webster HM, Erben JJ, et al. Hepatitis A in day-care centers: a community-wide assessment. *N Engl J Med* 1980;302:1222–1227.
13. Bell BP, Shapiro CN, Alter MJ, et. al. The diverse patterns of hepatitis A epidemiology in the U.S.—implications for vaccination strategies. *J Infect Dis* 1998;178:1579–1584.
14. Staes C, Schlenker T, Risk I, et al. Source of infection among persons with acute hepatitis A and no identified risk factors during a sustained community-wide outbreak, Salt Lake County, Utah, 1996. *Clin Infect Dis* 1997;25:411(abst).
15. Clemens R, Safary A, Hepburn A, et al. Clinical experience with an inactivated hepatitis A vaccine. *J Infect Dis* 1995;171:S44–S49.
16. Nalin DR. VAQTA, hepatitis A vaccine, purified inactivated. *Drugs of the Future* 1995;20:24–29.
17. Van Herck K, Beutels P, Van Damme P, et al. Mathematical models for assessment of long-term persistence of antibodies after vaccination with two inactivated hepatitis A vaccines. *J Med Virol* 2000;60:1–7.
18. Sagliocca L, Amoroso P, Stroffolini T, et al. Efficacy of hepatitis A vaccine in prevention of secondary hepatitis A infection: a randomised trial. *Lancet* 1999;353:1136–1139.
19. Lemon SM. Type A viral hepatitis: new developments in an old disease. *N Engl J Med* 1985;313:1059–1067.
20. Walter EB, Hornick RB, Poland GA, et al. Concurrent administration of inactivated hepatitis A vaccine with immune globulin in healthy adults. *Vaccine* 1999;17:1468–1473.
21. Blumberg BS, Alter HJ, Visnich S. A "new" antigen in leukemia sera. *JAMA* 1965;191:541–546.
22. Dienstag JL. Immunogenesis of the extrahepatic manifestations of hepatitis B virus infection. *Springer Semin Immunopathol* 1981;3:461–472.
23. Terazawa S, Kojima M, Yamanaka T, et al. Hepatitis B virus mutants with precore-region defects in two babies with fulminant hepatitis and their mothers positive for antibody to hepatitis Be antigen. *Pediatr Res* 1991;29:5–9.
24. McMahon BJ, Alberts SR, Wainwright RB, et al. Hepatitis B-related sequelae. Prospective study in 1400 hepatitis B surface

antigen-positive Alaskan Native carriers. *Arch Intern Med* 1990; 150:1051–1054.

25. Beasley RP, Hwang LY, Lin CC, et al. Hepatocellular carcinoma and hepatitis B virus. A prospective study of 22,707 men in Taiwan. *Lancet* 1981;2:1129–1133.
26. Hoofnagle JH, Di Bisceglie AM. Serologic diagnosis of acute and chronic viral hepatitis. *Semin Liver Dis* 1991;11:73–83.
27. Liang TJ, Hasegawa K, Rimon N, et al. A hepatitis B virus mutant associated with an epidemic of fulminant hepatitis. *N Engl J Med* 1991;324:1705–1709.
28. Harpaz R, Von Seidlein L, Averhoff FM, et al. Transmission of hepatitis B virus to multiple patients from a surgeon without evidence of inadequate infection control. *N Engl J Med* 1996;334: 549–554.
29. Alter MJ, Ahtone J, Maynard JE. Multiple-dose vial associated with transmission of hepatitis B virus in a hemodialysis unit. *Ann Intern Med* l983;99:330–333.
30. Polish LB, Shapiro CN, Bauer F, et al. Nosocomial transmission of hepatitis B virus associated with a spring-loaded fingerstick device. *N Engl J Med* 1992;326:721–725.
31. Hutin YJ, Harpaz R, Drobeniuc J, et al. Injections given in healthcare settings as a major source of acute hepatitis B in Moldova. *Int J Epidemiol* 1999;28:782–786.
32. Hutin YJ, Goldstein ST, Varma JK, et al. An outbreak of hospital-acquired hepatitis B virus infection among patients receiving chronic hemodialysis. *Infect Control Hosp Epidemiol* 1999;20: 731–735.
33. Drescher J, Wagner D, Haverich A, et al. Nosocomial hepatitis B virus infections in cardiac transplant recipients transmitted during transvenous endomyocardial biopsy. *J Hosp Infect* 1994;26:81–92.
34. Limentani AE, Elliott LM. An outbreak of hepatitis B from tattooing. *Lancet* 1979;2:86–88.
35. Kent GB, Brondum J, Keenlyside RA, LaFazia LM, Scott HD. A large outbreak of acupuncture-associated hepatitis B. *Am J Epidemiol* 1988;127:591–598.
36. Bond WW, Favero MS, Petersen NJ, et al. Survival of hepatitis B virus after drying and storage for one week. *Lancet* 1981;1: 550–551.
37. Margolis HS, Alter MJ, Hadler SC. Hepatitis B: evolving epidemiology and implications for control. *Semin Liver Dis* 1991; 11:84–92.
38. Margolis HS, Alter MJ, Hadler SC. Viral hepatitis. In: Evans AS, Kaslow RA, eds. *Viral infections of humans.* 4th ed. New York: Plenum Publishing, 1997:363–418.
39. Alter MJ, Hadler SC, Margolis HS, et al. The changing epidemiology of hepatitis B in the U.S.: need for alternative vaccination strategies. *JAMA* 1990;263:1218–1222.
40. McQuillan GM, Coleman PJ, Kruszon-Moran D, et al. Prevalence of hepatitis B virus infection in the U.S.: The National Health and Nutrition Examination Surveys 1976 through 1994. *Am J Public Health* 1999;89:14–18.
41. Hadler SC, Margolis HS. Hepatitis B immunization: vaccine types, efficacy, and indications for immunization. In: Remington JS, Swartz MN, eds. *Current clinical topics in infectious diseases.* Boston: Blackwell Science, 1992:282–308.
42. Centers for Disease Control: Hepatitis B virus: a comprehensive strategy for eliminating transmission in the U.S. through universal childhood vaccination: recommendations of the Immunization Practices Advisory Committee (ACIP). MMWR 1991;40 (No. RR-13):1–25.
43. Choo QL, Kuo G, Weiner AJ, et al. Isolation of a cDNA clone derived from a bloodborne non-A, non-B viral hepatitis genome. *Science* 1989;244:359–362.
44. Kuo G, Choo QL, Alter HJ, et al. An assay for circulating antibodies to a major etiologic virus of human non-A, non-B hepatitis. *Science* 1989;244:362–364.

45. Alter HJ, Purcell RH, Shih JW, et al. Detection of antibody to hepatitis C virus in prospectively followed transfusion recipients with acute and chronic non-A, non-B hepatitis. *N Engl J Med* 1989;321:1494–1500.
46. Alter MJ, Hadler SC, Judson FN, et al. Risk factors for acute non-A, non-B hepatitis in the U.S. and association with hepatitis C virus infection. *JAMA* 1990;264:2231–2235.
47. Bukh J, Miller RH, Purcell RH. Genetic heterogeneity of hepatitis C virus: quasispecies and genotypes. *Semin Liver Dis* 1995; 15:41–63.
48. Seeff LB. Natural history of hepatitis C. *Hepatology* 1997;26: 21S–28S.
49. Koff RS, Dienstag JL. Extrahepatic manifestations of hepatitis C and the association with alcoholic liver disease. *Semin Liver Dis* 1995;15:101–109.
50. Esteban JI, Gomez J, Martell M, et al. Transmission of hepatitis C virus by a cardiac surgeon. *N Engl J Med* 1995;334:555–560.
51. Enomoto N, Sakuma I, Asahina Y, et al. Comparison of full-length sequences of interferon-sensitive and -resistant hepatitis C virus 1b. *J Clin Invest* 1995;96:224–230.
52. Wasley A, Alter MJ. Epidemiology of hepatitis C: geographic differences and temporal trends. *Semin Liver Dis* 2000;20:1–16.
53. Centers for Disease Control and Prevention. Recommendations for the prevention and control of hepatitis C virus (HCV) infection and HCV-related chronic disease. MMWR 1998;47(No. RR-19):1–39.
54. Armstrong GL, Alter MJ, McQuillan GM, et al. The past incidence of hepatitis C virus infection: implications for the future burden of chronic liver disease in the United States. *Hepatology* 2000;31:777–782.
55. Alter MJ. Epidemiology of hepatitis C. *Hepatology* 1997;26: 62S–65S.
56. Alter MJ, Kruszon-Moran D, Nainan OV, et al. Prevalence of hepatitis C virus infection in the United States. *N Engl J Med* 1999;341:556–562.
57. World Health Organization. Global surveillance and control of hepatitis C. Report of a WHO Consultation organized in collaboration with the Viral Hepatitis Prevention Board, Antwerp, Belgium. *J Viral Hepat* 1999;6:35–47.
58. Krawczynski K, Alter MJ, Tankersley DL, et al. Effect of immune globulin on the prevention of experimental hepatitis C virus transmission. *J Infect Dis* 1996;173:822–828.
59. Peters M, Davis GL, Dooley JS, et al. The interferon system in acute and chronic viral hepatitis. *Prog Liver Dis* 1986;8:453–467.
60. Rizzetto M, Canese MC, et al. Immunofluorescence detection of a new antigen-antibody system (/anti-) associated to the hepatitis B virus in the liver and in the serum of HBsAg carriers. *Gut* 1977;18:997–1003.
61. Rizzetto M, Canese MC, Gerin JL, et al. Transmission of the hepatitis B virus associated δ-antigen to chimpanzees. *J Infect Dis* 1980;141:590–601.
62. Bonino F, Smedile A. Delta agent (type D) hepatitis. *Semin Liver Dis* 1986;6:28–33.
63. Polish LB, Gallagher M, Fields HA, et al. Delta hepatitis. Molecular biology and clinical and epidemiological features. *Clin Microbiol Rev* 1993;6:211–229.
64. Ottobrelli A, Marzano A, Smedile A, et al. Patterns of hepatitis δ reinfection and disease in liver transplantation. *Gastroenterology* 1991;101:1649–1655.
65. Bonino F, Negro F, Baldi M, et al. The natural history of δ hepatitis. *Prog Clin Biol Res* 1986;234:145–152.
66. Hadler SC, De Monson M, Ponzetto A, et al. Delta virus infection and severe hepatitis. An epidemic in the Yucpa Indians of Venezuela. *Ann Intern Med* 1984;100:339–344.
67. Alter MJ, Hadler SC. Delta hepatitis and infection in North America. In: Hadziyannis SJ, Taylor JM, Bonino F, eds. *Hepati-*

tis δ virus: molecular biology, pathogenesis, and clinical aspects. New York: Wiley-Liss, 1993:243–250.

68. Reyes GR, Purdy MA, Kim JP, et al. Isolation of a cDNA from the virus responsible for enterically transmitted non-A, non-B hepatitis. *Science* 1990;247:1335–1339.

69. Mast EE, Purdy MA, Krawczynski K. Hepatitis E. In: Alberti A, ed. *Bailliere's clinical gastroenterology.* London: Bailliere Tindall, 1996:227–242.

70. Labrique AB, Thomas DL, Stoszek SK, et al. Hepatitis E: an emerging infectious disease. *Epidemiol Rev* 1999;21:162–176.

71. Tsarev S, Emerson SU, Reyes GR, et al. Characterization of a prototype strain of hepatitis E virus. *Proc Natl Acad Sci U S A* 1992;89:559–563.

72. Kwo PY, Schlauder GG, Carpenter H, et al. Acute hepatitis E by a new isolate acquired in the United States. *Mayo Clinic Proc* 1997;72:1133–1136.

73. Schlauder GG, Dawson GJ, Erker JC, et al. The sequence and phylogenetic analysis of a novel hepatitis E virus isolated from a patient with acute hepatitis reported in the United States. *J Gen Virol* 1998;79:447–456.

74. Thomas DL, Yarbough PO, Vlahov D, et al. Seroreactivity to hepatitis E virus in areas where the disease is not endemic. *J Clin Microbiol* 1997;35:1244–1247.

75. Mast EE, Kuramoto IK, Favorov MO, et al. Prevalence of and risk factors for antibody to hepatitis E virus seroreactivity among blood donors in Northern California. *J Infect Dis* 1997;176:34–40.

76. Mast EE, Alter MJ, Holland PV, et al. Evaluation of assays for antibody to hepatitis E virus by a serum panel. *Hepatology* 1998; 27:857–861.

77. Joshi YK, Baku S, Sarin S, et al. Immunoprophylaxis of epidemic non-A, non-B hepatitis. *Indian J Med Res* 1985;81:18–19.

78. Tsarev SA, Tsareva TS, Emerson SU, et al. Recombinant vaccine against hepatitis E: dose response and protection against heterologous challenge. *Vaccine* 1997;15:1834–1838.

MOLECULAR BASES OF HEPATITIS B– AND HEPATITIS C–RELATED CHRONIC LIVER DISEASES

CHRISTIAN BRÉCHOT

Several viruses have been now identified as human hepatitis viruses (ranging from hepatitis A to G, with the recent addition of the TT virus (reviewed in ref. 1). Collectively, they are important human pathogens with an overall high prevalence worldwide. Several of them induce, after acute infection, a chronic carrier state. The common hallmark of the lesions frequently associated with this chronic carrier status is liver inflammation, which in turn induces liver fibrosis, triggers liver cell proliferation, and forms the pathogenic basis of chronic active hepatitis. The severity of chronic active hepatitis is variable but can lead to nodular fibrosis and cirrhosis and, eventually, hepatocellular carcinoma (HCC).

Hepatitis A (HAV) and E (HEV) viruses induce in some cases severe acute hepatitis but never chronic infection, and therefore will not be considered in this chapter. Other, more recently identified, agents, hepatitis G (HGV/GB-C) (2,3) and TT (TTV) (4) viruses, induce chronic infection that is highly prevalent in most geographic areas so far examined; however, their actual pathogenicity is debated and in fact likely minimal (5–7).

In contrast, hepatitis B (HBV) and C (HCV) are major pathogens given their extremely high prevalence (around

400 and 350 millions of chronically infected individuals worldwide, respectively), the high rate of chronic infection, and the significant risk of severe chronic active hepatitis and cirrhosis among chronically infected subjects. Chronic HBV infection develops in around 40% to 80% and 5% of infected neonates and adults, respectively; HCV infection is very rarely transmitted at birth but induces chronic infection in up to 60% to 80% of infected adults (Fig. 54.1). The pathogenic effects of chronic HBV and HCV infections are highly variable; some patients show only minimal liver lesions, while others (around 20%) will develop severe fibrosis and cirrhosis after 5 to 10 years. Finally, 30% to 50% of patients with cirrhosis, whatever the etiologic factor, develop HCC after 10 years. Chronic hepatitis D (HDV) infection is associated with HBV in some geographic areas and particular risk groups (such as intravenous drug users) and can significantly worsen the course of acute and chronic HBV infections (8).

Acute and chronic hepatitis induced by most hepatitis viruses clearly implicate the host immune response to viral proteins (see Chapter 52). The development of molecular biology has led to the realization that some hepatitis viruses also directly modulate liver cell proliferation and viability. This issue has important implications for understanding the molecular bases of the liver lesions and liver carcinogenesis, as well as for developing new therapeutic strategies. This chapter reviews these issues and focuses on HBV and

C. Bréchot: Institut Nacional de la Santé et de la Recherche Medical, U370, Faculte Necker E-M, 75730 Paris, France; Department of Hepatology, Necker E-M Hospital, 75015 Paris, France.

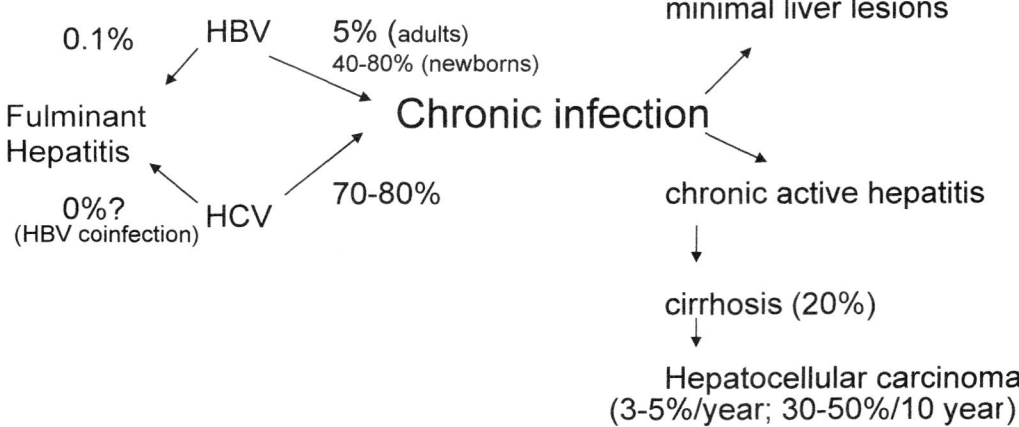

FIGURE 54.1. Schematic representation of the natural course of hepatitis B virus (*HBV*) and hepatitis C virus (*HCV*) infections. The figure emphasizes in particular the high rate of chronic HBV and HCV infection as well as the risk of chronic active hepatitis, cirrhosis, and hepatocellular carcinoma.

HCV since most of the available data have been obtained from studies of these viruses.

HEPATITIS B VIRUS

Hepatitis B Virus DNA Patterns During Acute and Chronic Hepatitis B Virus Infections

HBV DNA is a small, circular DNA with a highly compact genetic organization and overlapping open reading frames; it shares with retroviruses the use of reverse-transcription during its replication. In contrast, viral DNA integration into the cellular DNA is not necessary for viral replication (reviewed in ref. 9; see Chapter 55), but allows persistence of the viral genome in the cell. Viral DNA insertion occurs as a consequence of cellular DNA replication during liver cell proliferation, secondary to the necrosis/apoptosis of adjacent hepatocytes. HBV DNA sequences are integrated into cellular DNA in most (approx. 90%) liver tumor samples from hepatitis B surface antigen (HBsAg)-positive patients (10). Southern blotting usually suggests the monoclonal or oligoclonal proliferation of cells containing HBV DNA (11–13). Recent analyses, based on polymerase chain reaction (PCR) methodology to analyze junction HBV/cellular fragments, showed frequent multicentric occurrence of the tumor nodules (14). The restriction DNA profile differs from one tumor to another, and generally reveals several different integration sites; however, clonally expanded cells containing a single integration site are found in some cases (11). The data available to date have failed to demonstrate any preferential integration site for HBV DNA; examination of the various HBV insertion sites

reported, however, has shown a trend toward high level of integrants in chromosomes 11 and 17 (15–20); the implications of this observation are unknown.

The integration of HBV DNA is not restricted to tumor cells; clonally expanded cells containing integrated HBV DNA molecules can be identified in the nontumoral, cirrhotic livers of patients with HCC (21,22). However, the restriction profile differs from that identified in the corresponding tumors, thus suggesting the coexistence of different clones in the liver prior to tumor development; alternatively, secondary chromosomal rearrangements may have occurred during tumor growth (23). Integration has also been demonstrated in chronic HBV carriers (both adults and children) with no evidence of HCC (11,21,24–29). Some studies have even suggested that such a restriction profile, consistent with HBV DNA integration, may be observed at the acute stage of HBV infection and in subjects with a severe form of acute hepatitis (30). These data have been recently confirmed with the use of PCR-based analyses to characterize viral/cellular junction fragments (Murakami et al., personal communication). Integration therefore precedes development of the tumor, and the comparative analysis of the various restriction profiles at different times during the course of HBV infection suggests progressive clonal expansion of certain infected cells.

HBV multiplication can now be directly monitored with commercially available diagnostic kits to detect the viral DNA in serum. This has led to the description of various patterns of multiplication during the natural course of the viral infection or under therapy (reviewed in refs. 31 and 32). A frequent observation, at least in Western countries, has been the progressive decline of HBV multiplication at the time of cirrhosis development; the underlying basis of this observation is not known but it emphasizes the need for early therapy during chronic hepatitis. Interruption of HBV multiplication in a cirrhotic patient does not eliminate the risk of HCC development; still, this risk is significantly increased in patients who maintain active HBV DNA replication, likely because of the ongoing inflammation and sustained liver cell proliferation. Free viral DNA can be detected in liver cell by Southern blotting (23,30,33,34). The presence of HBV DNA replicative intermediates is generally associated with HBV viremia; in some patients, however, particularly those with HCC, replicative forms may be detected in the liver, although HBV DNA is undetectable in the serum. This suggests defective viral encapsidation and/or secretion of viral particles (35). Free monomeric HBV DNA can also be detected (mostly toward the end of viral multiplication) in acute or chronic infection. Finally, free oligomeric HBV DNA forms with complex structures have been evidenced in a few acutely infected patients; their significance is not known, but they could feasibly be intermediates in the integration process (30,35,36). Such viral oligomers have been also detected in woodchucks infected by woodchuck hepatic virus (WHV) (37,38).

A combination of immunohistochemical and *in situ* hybridization procedures has shown that HBV DNA replication, identified by HBV DNA replicative molecules, and HBsAg synthesis are generally detected in different hepatocytes; in contrast, HBV DNA replication is generally, but not systematically, shown in hepatocytes expressing hepatitis B core antigen (HBcAg) (39,40). Serum HBV DNA levels generally decline markedly by the time HCC develops, at least in Western countries, Africa, and Japan. At the time of HCC development, tumor cells generally show no or only low-level HBV DNA replication (detected by PCR tests); they usually do not express HBcAg, although HBsAg can be detected in approximately 20% of cases (41–43). Consistent with these observations, induction of HCCs by chemical carcinogens in HBsAg-expressing transgenic mice leads to decreased expression of HBsAg (44). However, as discussed below, human HCC tumor cells frequently retain expression of the HBx protein. In contrast, reports from Taiwan have shown that HBV multiplication persists frequently when HCC occurs (45,46).

These observations have led to the suggestion that different cell populations are infected by HBV; the differentiating status of certain hepatocytes may be compatible with HBV DNA replication and HBcAg expression, and such cells would therefore constitute targets for the immune response. In contrast, other liver cells may not support a complete replicative cycle, and only express HBsAg; they would be selected progressively during chronic HBV carriage (47). In Western countries and Africa, some investigators have demonstrated the persistence of replicative intermediates in tumoral liver cells from patients with HCC, and suggested that they may not normally be encapsidated (35).

Integration of viral DNA can be detected in nonhepatocytic cells; infection by HBV of peripheral blood mononuclear cells has been demonstrated using Southern blotting (48,49); free monomeric HBV DNA has been shown to associate with high molecular weight molecules, suggestive of free oligomers and possibly integrated sequences (50). The viral DNA sequences have been shown in different mononuclear cells subpopulations, including CD4- and CD8-positive lymphocytes, B lymphocytes, and monocytes (51,52). *In situ* hybridization has further supported these data (53). Whether or not mononuclear cells are really permissive for HBV DNA replication has remained unclear; several groups have failed to detect the covalently closed circular HBV DNA molecule, an intermediate in viral RNA synthesis during productive infection; this has led to challenging the reality of peripheral blood mononuclear cell (PBMNC) infection by HBV (54). Integration of the viral DNA (55) and expression of HBV transcripts (56,57), however, have now been definitely established using PCR-based techniques. Thus, collectively, the available data do support persistence of the viral DNA in mononuclear cells; the results do not distinguish, however, which cell subsets are actually infected—circulating mononuclear or bone marrow cells (58). Also, the implications of PBMNC infection on the immune response pattern during HBV infection remain unclear. Infected cells might rather be viewed as a reservoir for the virus, possibly favoring selection of some variants, and there is evidence for this hypothesis in transplanted patients (59,60). Finally, the intriguing observations of an association between HBV and some hematopoietic malignancy (61) and, in contrast, of an inhibitory action of HBV on hematopoietic cells (62) have never been followed up. HBV DNA sequences have also been found in several other tissues, including skin and pancreatic cells (reviewed in ref. 63) as well as a neuroblastoma tumor tissue (64); this nonhepatocytic tropism has been also investigated in detail in the duck model of hepadnaviral infection (65). Finally, HBV DNA sequences have been also identified in spermatozoa, a finding with potential impact on a real "vertical" HBV transmission, but the actual impact of these data have not been followed up (66).

Consequences of Hepatitis B Virus DNA Integration

Chromosomal DNA Instability

The integration of HBV DNA can directly induce chromosomal rearrangements (67) (Figs. 54.2 and 54.3); in fact, it has been suggested that viral DNA sequences encompassing the encapsidation signal may exhibit intrinsic recombinogenic activity via binding to a putative "recombinogenic" cellular protein (reviewed in ref. 68). Comprehensive allotyping and comparative genomic hybridization have recently become available, and several studies have defined

Chronic
inflammation   Genetic
Fibrosis   alterations

Clonal cell
Expansion
Transformation

Angiogenesis
Metastasis

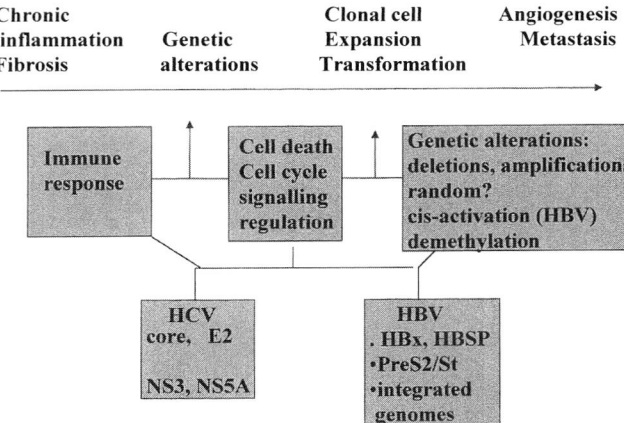

FIGURE 54.2. Schematic representation of the mechanisms involved in hepatitis B virus (*HBV*)- and hepatitis C virus (*HCV*)–related chronic liver lesions and hepatocellular carcinoma. The figure underlines the dual effects of HBV and HCV. Expression of the viral proteins stimulate the host immune response and trigger liver inflammation; some viral proteins as well as, for HBV, insertion of the viral DNA into liver cell genome also directly interfere with cell proliferation and viability and induce genetic alterations. *HBSP*, HBV splice protein.

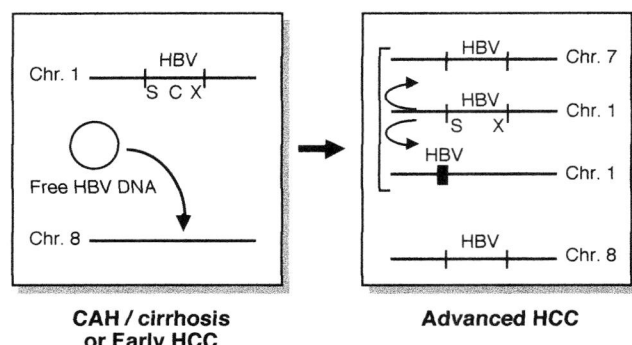

FIGURE 54.3. Schematic representation of the dynamic of hepatitis B virus (*HBV*) integrants. New integrants are generated from HBV ongoing multiplication. HBV sequences are rearranged upon integration. *CAH*, chronic active hepatitis; *HCC*, hepatocellular carcinoma.

TABLE 54.1. HEPATITIS B VIRUS INTEGRATIONS IN HEPATOCELLULAR CARCINOMA

Number of HCC	Cellular Sequence Size	Homology	Reference
1	No sequence data	Alu sequence next to viral host junction	82
1	144 bp	Retinoic acid receptor β-gene	168
1	No sequence data	Alu sequence next to viral host junction	83
1	No sequence data	hst-1 gene	87
1		Human cyclin A2 gene	172
1	1,700 bp	No homology in Genbank	84
		Poly A signal in cellular sequence	
2	43 bp	Chromosomal localization known but no information about homology	399
	39 bp		
1	1,550 bp	550 bp homology to an erbB-like gene 1 kb downstream of the junction	179
1	469 bp	Semirepetitive TBG41 (Kpn 1 family) 3 kb downstream of the β-globin gene	85
2	103 bp	No homology in Genbank	86
	98 bp	28S rRNA gene	
1	1,020 bp	Human alphoid repetitive or satellite sequence	400
1	1,060 bp	Carboxypeptidase N-like gene; expression detectable by Northern blot	80
1	4,000 bp	No homology in Genbank	401
		Some unique sequence present	
2	1,190 bp	Nonrepetitive sequence	81
		No homology in Genbank	
	1,335 bp	Nonrepetitive sequence	
		No homology in Genbank	
1		SERCA1 gene	402

bp, base pairs; kb, kilobases.

TABLE 54.2. HEPATITIS B VIRUS (HBV) INTEGRATIONS IN CELL LINES

Cell Line	Cellular Sequence Size	Homology	Reference
PLC/PRF/5	50 bp	HBV proviral insertion in human PLC cells	403
huH-7	1,342 bp	Homo sapiens chromosome 16 clone RPCI-11 Genbank accession number AC006111	404
PLC/PRF/5	120 bp	Insulin gene polymorphic region	405
	90 bp	Repetitive element in the psi-zeta globin locus	
PLC/PRF/5		Mevalonate kinase gene	406
HCC36	No sequence data	Alu and satellite sequences (shown by Southern blot)	407
ML2	No sequence data	Nonrepeated sequence next to HBV	198
ML3	No sequence data	Nonrepeated sequence next to HBV	
Hep3B	2,200 bp	L1 repeat immediately next to the junction Cellular sequence expressed in Hep3B line (Northern blot)	408

a number of commonly deleted or amplified chromosomal loci (reviewed in ref. 69) (Tables 54.1 and 54.2); interestingly, it has recently been shown that the chromosomal losses identified in HBV-positive and -negative tumors differ, suggesting some direct implication of the etiologic agent involved in altering the chromosomal patterns of HCCs. Thus, increased rates of 4q, 16q, and 11p deletions have been shown in HBV-positive HCCs. The mechanisms underlying such findings are presently unknown. HBV DNA insertion has been also identified at some loci (such as 17p13 and 4q32) that subsequently have been shown to be deleted in other tumors in the absence of detectable HBV DNA insertion in these domains (19,70–72). Integration can lead to small deletions (a few base pairs) in the cellular DNA, but several major chromosomal deletions— 11p14, 4q32, 11q13 in particular (73,74)—have been demonstrated. Translocations have been also described at the site of HBV DNA integration [chromosomes 17/X; 5/9; 17/18 (17q21-22/18q11.1-q11.2); t(3;8) (15,75–86)]. In one tumor, integrated HBV sequences were found to be coamplified with the hst-1 oncogene (87).

Synthesis of X and Truncated PreS2/S Proteins

Examination of the viral DNA sequences present in tumor cells has shown that, in a large proportion of them, sequences encoding for the HBx and/or truncated envelope PreS2/S viral proteins are retained.

HBV X(HBx)

In most integrated subviral DNAs, X-open reading frame is maintained and transcribed (88–91). Despite difficulties due to the low amount of HBx and poor quality of many anti-HBx antibodies, several studies show HBx expression in human HCC tumor cells (92,93); it is still unclear whether this also holds true for WHV-related HCCs (94). The HBx-gene is highly conserved among all mammalian hepadnaviruses and encodes a small 17-kd polypeptide that is expressed at low levels during acute and chronic hepatitis

(reviewed in refs. 95–97). The role of HBx in the viral life cycle has not clearly been defined, although genetic studies in woodchucks indicate that HBx is indispensable for the infectivity of WHV (98–100). The seminal observation that HBx transactivates cellular genes controlling cell growth suggested that HBx might participate in the transformation of hepatocytes by HBV (reviewed in refs. 95 and 96) (Figs. 54.4 and 54.5). Consistent with this notion, it has been shown that HBx can induce cell proliferation in quiescent fibroblasts (101), and deregulate cell cycle check points (102). A few *in vitro* studies have shown the transformation of certain cell types with an overexpression of HBx (103,104). Furthermore, HBx induces HCC in cer-

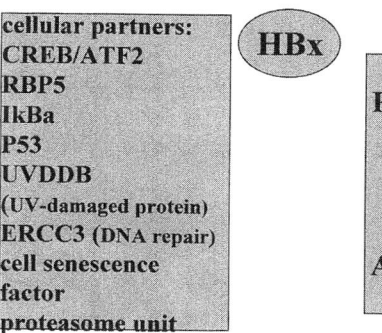

FIGURE 54.4. The different targets of HBx and the complexity of the biologic actions of HBx. **Top**: The cytoplasmic and possibly nuclear transduction cascades activated by HBx. **Bottom left**: A listing of the cellular proteins that might bind to HBx. **Bottom right**: The effect of Hbx on both apoptosis and cell proliferation. *AP*, adaptor protein; *NF-AT*, nuclear factor of activated T cells; *ras-raf-MAPK*, ras/raf/mitogen-activated protein kinase; *UVDDB*, ultraviolet-damaged DNA-binding protein.

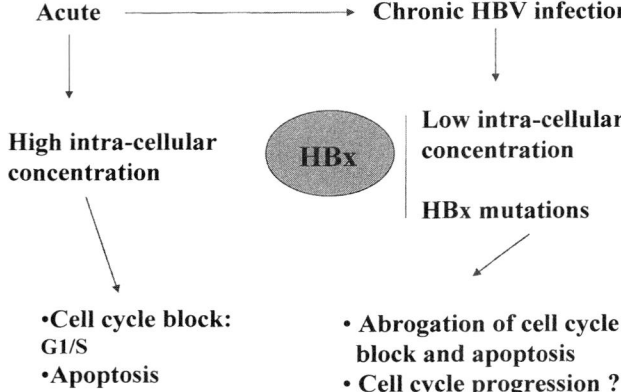

FIGURE 54.5. A model for the biologic effects of HBx on liver cells. The effects on the cell cycle of HBx might be influenced by the intracellular concentration of HBx [decreased in chronic carriers, compared to the acute stage of hepatitis B virus (*HBV*) infection] and accumulation of mutations in the HBx-encoding gene in tumor cells.

tain transgenic mice (105,106). However, in a different genetic context, HBx transgenic mice exhibit no obvious pathology (107), an increased susceptibility to chemical carcinogens (108), or an acceleration of the development of c-*myc*–induced HCC (109). These data are consistent with HBx acting as a tumor promoter during liver carcinogenesis.

The relevance of the HBx transactivation function to the viral life cycle and oncogenesis is unclear, but it is generally believed to be crucial. HBx has been shown to activate a wide variety of cellular and viral genes in *trans*, including HBV enhancers, HIV long-terminal repeats, class II and III promoters, and the proto-oncogenes c-*jun*, c-*fos*, and c-*myc* (95,96). HBx also transactivates cytokine-encoding genes such as tumor necrosis factor-α (TNF-α) (110) and transforming growth factor-β (111). The mechanisms through which HBx stimulates gene transcription in *trans* are only partially understood. The fact that HBx by itself does not bind to double-stranded DNA (dsDNA), and that genes stimulated by HBx lack any obvious consensus sequences (112), suggests that HBx stimulates transcription, presumably by interacting with cellular proteins and/or components of signal transduction pathways. The transactivation function of HBx has been shown to involve direct interaction with transcriptional factors such as RPB5 of RNA polymerases (113) and TATA-binding protein (114) or ATF/CREB (115). HBx also activates cytosolic signal transduction pathways such as ras/raf/mitogen-activated protein (MAP) kinase (MAPK), as well as Src family kinases (116,117), c-Jun N-terminal kinase (118), and Jak1-STAT (119); the effect of HBx on protein kinase C (PKC) (120) is a subject for debate. *Cis*-activating sequences have indeed been identified, and include AP-1, AP-2, nuclear factor (NF)-κB, NF-AT, and CRE sites. AP-1 and NF-κB sites are

transcriptionally activated through the ras-MAP and c-Jun N-terminal kinases pathway; however, HBx directly interacts with CREB/ATF2 factors to activate CRE elements. Finally, HBx activates Jak1-STAT (signal transducer and activator of transcription) signaling (119).

Although HBx acts in the nucleus to activate transcription, the great majority of HBx is cytosolic (121,122), strongly suggesting that it stimulates promoters bearing sites in a compartment external to the nucleus (121–124). Recent studies have analyzed in more detail the HBx–NF-κB interactions and shed some light on this issue. HBx induces nuclear translocation of NF-κB through phosphorylation, and thus degradation, of the IκB inhibitor; furthermore, HBx also directly binds IκB when it is newly synthesized as a result of NF-κB activation, and this association triggers the nuclear translocation of HBx. This mechanism may be triggered by TNF-α pathway activation during chronic hepatitis and account for a low level of nuclear HBx (125).

Other biologic activities have been described for HBx. Certain proteases and the proteasome (122,126,127) have been reported to be potential targets of HBx. HBx interacts with DNA repair factors (128,129) and the ultraviolet (UV)-damaged DNA-binding protein (UVDDB) (130), suggesting a direct link with cellular DNA repair machinery. Other potential targets have been recently suggested, such as the translation initiation factor hu-Sui1 (131) and a protein associated with senescence (132). Finally, data that are still under debate point to a direct interaction between HBx and P53 (133–135), which would lead to a functional inactivation of P53 and possibly its delocalization (136). Somatic mutations of P53 are detected in only 20% of HCCs, except in areas with a high exposure to aflatoxin B1. In this respect, it has been suggested that the association of HBx and P53 may cause the functional inactivation of P53. Some reports have suggested an inverse correlation between the detection of HBx ORF and P53 mutations, but this requires further clarification (137,138).

Overall, the final outcome of the pleiotropic effects of HBx on the cell cycle and cell viability is still the subject of much debate, and these difficulties are thought largely to be due to its heterologous and ectopic expression in various cellular environments. Several studies have recently demonstrated that HBx expression may modulate both cell proliferation and viability. In fact, according to the experimental conditions employed, HBx can abolish or, conversely, provoke apoptosis. Thus, several groups have demonstrated a reduction in cell colonies (139,140) and cell cycle arrest (119,141), an inhibition of cell transformation (140,141), and an induction (140–144) or sensitization (145) to apoptosis by HBx. On the other hand, other groups have reported the inhibition of p53-dependent apoptosis (146). The mechanisms of HBx-related control of apoptosis are not known. Colocalization of HBx and mitochondria has been recently emphasized, suggesting that it might contribute to caspase cascade activation (147; Terradillos et al., unpublished observations, 2000); HBx might also regulate fas ligand (148). Furthermore, HBx can inhibit caspase 3 activity, which is correlated with its transactivation potential (149). It is plausible that the discrepancies regarding the final outcome of HBx expression on cell viability are due to signal cascades activated in different cell types, combined with the ectopic expression level achieved. Consistent with this view, the transformation of a mouse hepatocytic cell line upon conditional expression of HBx depends on maintenance of its hepatocytic differentiation status (150).

The concept that a putative oncogene may modulate both the cell cycle and apoptosis has now been well established for several viral proteins, such as the E1A protein of adenovirus 5 (reviewed in ref. 151), the E2 protein of papillomaviruses (152), and the Tax protein of human T cell leukemia virus-1 (153). This may be interpreted as further evidence of the common pathways used by viruses to subvert cell cycle and cell death regulation. Our data suggest that an early effect of HBx expression, during infection by a nonlytic virus such as HBV, is to block the cells in the late G_1/S phases (141). It has been shown that HBV replication depends on cell cycle and differentiation status and is decreased in the S-phase (154). Thus, blocking the cells in late G_1 may favor further rounds of HBV-DNA replication by inducing the expression of liver-specific transcription and replication factors, such as increasing the pool of free dNTPs (155). In this case, the late induction of apoptosis may reflect the prolonged expression of HBx in cells blocked at the G_1/S-phase. Induction of apoptosis might favor viral particle dissemination; it might also indirectly favor persistence of selected cells expressing a low amount of the viral proteins and accumulating protective secondary genetic alterations.

In this context, we have attacked the problem from a genetic angle, and comparatively characterized the effects of HBx and its mutants from human HCC on cell growth and viability (93,141,156). We reasoned that, if the growth-suppressive effect of HBx has *in vivo* relevance, one could expect the release of such an inhibitory effect in clonally expanding tumor cells that have retained a mutated X-ORF. We characterized HBx mutants isolated from the liver tumor of patients with HBx. In sharp contrast with the wild-type HBx, we demonstrated that the HBx mutations identified in tumor cells abolished their growth suppressive and apoptotic effects. This study has therefore provided evidence of the importance of HBx mutations identified in human HCC. Abrogation of the cell cycle block will favor the selection and clonal expansion of cells containing loss of function mutations in the X-ORF. In addition to these mutations, the intracellular concentration of HBx probably constitutes an important factor. Studies of HBx-expressing transgenic mice have indeed illustrated a dual effect for HBx on cell viability; high levels of HBx, which are probably also present dur-

ing acute infection in humans, are associated with apoptosis, while low HBx levels, such as those also observed in chronically infected humans, allow liver cell proliferation (143). Consistent with this view is the low proportion of tumor cells with detectable levels of HBx and discrepancies concerning its detection (92). The mechanism by which the wild-type HBx acts to suppress the cell growth and ras-mediated transformation, as well as the biologic functions of mutants, is not clear. However, we and others have demonstrated a strict correlation between the transactivation capacity of HBx, cell cycle block, and the induction of apoptosis (141,157). In contrast, HBx-related cell transformation might not require its transactivation domains (158).

PreS2/S

Truncated forms of the PreS2/S envelope protein, generated from deleted integrated viral genomes, may also be involved in liver cell transformation (159,160). It has been reported that up to 25% of HCCs may contain viral genomes with sequences that can potentially encode for such deleted proteins (88); *in vitro* evidence is also available for a transactivating effect of PreS2/S proteins that lack their C-terminal domain on cellular genes, such as c-*myc* and c-*fos*. This transactivating effect must be indirect since truncated PreS2/S proteins are exclusively cytoplasmic, anchored into the membrane of the endoplasmic reticulum by the transmembrane domains of the S sequence. In fact, the mechanisms involved are not known, although it has been suggested that they implicate the generation of free radical oxides. More direct evidence for the role of PreS2/S comes from the demonstration of its cooperative effect with c-Ha ras in cell transformation (161).

Insertional Mutagenesis (Cis-Activation) (Fig. 54.3 and Tables 54.1 and 54.2)

The insertion of viral DNA into a cellular gene, as well as modification of its expression (i.e., *cis*-activation) is another potential consequence of HBV DNA integration. Two different situations must be distinguished: in HCCs developed in woodchucks infected by WHV, the insertion of WHV DNA into the c-*myc* or, predominantly, N-*my 2c* oncogenes is frequent (identified in at least half of the tumors so far analyzed) (162–167) (Table 54.2). Convincing evidence, both *in vitro* in cell culture and *in vivo* in transgenic mice, has been advanced in favor of the direct transforming property of constructs containing such WHV/*myc* integrants; these observations have also emphasized the fact that in these woodchuck tumors, the sites of WHV DNA integration into c-*myc* are identical to those utilized by some oncogenic retroviruses in experimentally induced animal tumors.

In contrast, in human tumors, the insertion of HBV DNA into a cellular gene has been demonstrated in only a few cases so far; furthermore, insertion of the same gene in different tumors has not been reported. In fact, a direct, *cis*-

acting promoter insertion mechanism has definitely been shown in only four cases. In the first case, HBV DNA integration occurred in an exon of the retinoic acid receptor B gene (*RAR B*) (168,169). The important contribution of retinoic acid and retinoids to cell differentiation and proliferation is well established (144,170,171).

In a second case, the human cyclin A2-encoding gene was identified by our group in early liver cancer developing on a histologically normal liver (172). Cyclin A2 plays a major role in both the S and G_2/M checkpoints of the cell cycle (173,174). The integration of HBV DNA occurred in the second intron of the cyclin A2 gene and led to the expression of hybrid PreS2/S-cyclin A2 transcripts (175). We have now demonstrated that the expression of this hybrid HBV-cyclin A2 protein does induce cell transformation (176). This study also showed the cytoplasmic delocalization of the hybrid protein inserted in the membranes of the endoplasmic reticulum because of the transmembrane topology of its PreS2/S moiety.

Other cases of the *cis*-activation of a cellular gene have been reported: *in vitro*, in the PLC/PRF/5 cell line, HBV DNA was inserted into the gene encoding human mevalonate kinase; mevalonate kinase regulates synthesis of the isoprenoid compounds, which are involved in cell proliferation (177). *In vivo*, we have recently identified using an Alu-based PCR array, insertion of the HBV DNA in the gene encoding a sarcoendoplasmic calcium adenosine triphosphatase (ATPase)-dependent pump (SERCA1). SERCAs are major regulators of endoplasmic reticulum calcium stores, and calcium homeostasis plays a major role in controlling cell proliferation and viability. We have recently demonstrated that HBV insertion *cis*-activates the SERCA1-encoding gene by amplifying previously unknown spliced transcripts, leading to the synthesis of truncated forms of the SERCA protein that regulate cell apoptosis (178).

Finally, the insertion of HBV DNA has been shown in the gene encoding for carboxypeptidase N (80) and the epidermal growth factor receptor encoding gene (179), although *cis*-activation of the cellular genes was not shown, and the impact of these findings remains unclear.

Thus, overall, it is interesting to see that study of integrated HBV DNA has led to the identification of new genes encoding proteins with a major role in cell proliferation, viability, or differentiation control (cyclin A2, RARb), or to that of new regulatory mechanisms controlling the expression of known genes (SERCA).

However, these findings have remained isolated. The reasons why insertional mutagenesis is frequent in woodchuck HCCs and rare in human tumors remain unclear. Several problems must be borne in mind when discussing this issue: (a) As pointed out above, human HCC includes a heterogeneous group of tumors; in particular, the small subgroup of patients with tumors arising on noncirrhotic livers may differ in terms of the mechanisms involved from

those with tumors developing on cirrhotic livers. (b) HBV DNA integration should be viewed as a dynamic event: as shown in Fig. 54.3, new integrants can be generated from free replicating viral genomes, and integrated viral and adjacent cellular sequences are frequently rearranged during the course of HCC. Thus, HBV integrants identified in a fully developed HCC will include both those generated during the initial integration step and those generated during secondary events. The duck hepatitis virus model provides evidence for an increase in hepadnaviral DNA integration on DNA damage induced by agents such as H_2O_2, and similar events may occur during chronic liver inflammation (180). (c) The time needed for each tumor analysis employing standard cloning strategies means that the number of tumors so far analyzed in detail is probably too small; in fact, only around 30 integrated sequences have been reported in human HCCs (Tables 54.1 and 54.2). (d) The insertion of viral DNA may occur at a distance from the activated gene, as shown in the woodchuck model for the Win locus; this further complicates such studies (181).

With these points in mind, we have developed an HBV-Alu PCR-based assay to provide a comprehensive analysis of HBV insertion sites (182). Our first screening rapidly provided around 17 new junction sequences. Interestingly, this approach has already allowed us to demonstrate at least three new cellular genes, the study of which is in progress. We therefore suggest that, given the major advances in the human genome sequencing project, the design of new methodologies to analyze large numbers of integrated sequences should enable us to challenge the concept that HBV-related *cis*-activation is a rare event; instead, we would submit that HBV DNA might be viewed as a "proviral tag" (183) capable of identifying new cellular genes or unravel new mechanisms controlling known gene expression (184); in this view, the identification of HBV insertion sites is an approach that is complementary to that based on allotyping and comparative genomic hybridization (CGH) when identifying those genes specifically involved in liver cell proliferation and viability.

Persistence of Viral Genomes in the Liver Cells

The long-term persistence of viral DNA is an absolute requirement for the development of HBV-related chronic liver disease and HCC, and is due to a combination of several factors, as discussed in the following subsections.

Hepatitis B Virus Genetic Variability

A large number of studies have led to descriptions of a complex pattern of HBV variants during all phases of the viral infection; a comprehensive review of this issue is beyond the scope of this chapter (reviewed in refs. 185–188). Mutations have been identified in all viral open reading frames and affect either the structure of the viral proteins synthesized or their amount (by modifying regulatory element structure). Mutations in the PreC sequence in particular have been described, which abrogate hepatitis B early antigen (HbeAg) secretion. There is evidence in some studies of the selection of such variants during the natural course of the viral infection and under antiviral therapy. This leads to the concept that accumulation of such mutations might modify important epitopes and favor escape from the immune system; other studies have suggested an association between infection by such variants and severe liver disease, including fulminant hepatitis. Mutations in the X-ORF have been also described, which might modulate HBV replication by altering HBx function and/or the overlapping core promoter (189,190). Of particular concern has been the identification of mutations in the "a" antigenic determinant of the envelope protein, the emergence of which might be favored by HBV vaccination or therapy based on monoclonal anti-HBs (191–193). There has been, however, no evidence so far for a real impact of these findings on the vaccination's overall efficacy.

Collectively, the interpretation of the data on HBV variants has been made difficult by several issues: (a) the polyclonal nature of the immune response to the virus, which has to be considered when discussing the concept of "escape" mutants; (b) the impact of the mutations, beside the interplay with the immune response, on the expression of the viral genomes; for example, some studies have demonstrated increased accumulation of the viral capsid in patients infected by viruses with mutations in the PreC sequence and core gene promoter; PreC mutations might also lead to accumulation of the HbeAg precursor P22 in cytoplasm and, possibly, nucleus, and might downregulate the viral genome replicative capacity (194); and (c) isolated viral ORFs, which have been generally investigated, whereas it is the interaction between all domains of this short viral genome that determines its replicative pattern (195). Thus, the new technologies that have now been made available to rapidly clone the entire viral genomes should help to clarify these important issues (196). In HCC tumor tissues, HBV integrants frequently show interruption of the core gene; in addition, viral DNA replication usually markedly decreases at the time of tumor development, leading to a reduction in HBcAg synthesis (35,48,197). In view of the role of HBc and HBe epitopes in the immune response to infected cells, it is plausible that cells containing integrated HBV DNA may "escape" immune destruction, thus conferring a selective growth advantage during the chronic course of infection. *In vivo* studies in mice inoculated with cell lines expressing different regions of the HBV genome have provided good support for this hypothesis (198). Only a few stud-

ies have addressed the questions of the rate of HBV mutations in tumor tissues (35,199). Our group has shown that mutations in PreC/C sequences that would prevent proper encapsidation can be identified in HCC tissues; nonsynonymous mutations (i.e., leading to amino acid changes) in the core gene were mostly selectively detected in either tumoral or nontumoral tissues; in contrast, most synonymous mutations were identified in both tumoral and nontumoral tissues. These observations are consistent with a selection of some HBV molecules during long-term persistence and HCC development (200). In addition, mutations have been identified on HBx-encoding sequences (141,156); as discussed above, they might reduce viral DNA replication and HBV gene expression and thus favor clonal expansion of some infected cells. They may also modify the effects of the protein on cell proliferation and viability [see HBV X(HBx), above].

Downregulation of Hepatitis B Virus Genome Expression

It has been demonstrated *in vivo* in transgenic mice that the immune response to HBV antigen will trigger the secretion of cytokines such as TNF-α, interferon-γ (IFN-γ), and interleukin-2 (IL-2), which can downregulate the accumulation of HBV RNAs (201–203) (see Chapter 52). *In vitro* studies have also shown downregulation of the core promoter by TNF-α (204). Under these conditions, cytokines released by the immune response to the virus will in turn lower the level of HBV antigen synthesis in liver cells and thus prevent elimination of the infected cells. Along the same lines, free reactive oxygen species, such as those generated during chronic inflammation, may also modulate HBV gene expression (205); the effects of such reactive oxygen species might also be relevant in those patients with alcohol-related, chronic liver disease associated with viral infection.

Recent studies have also addressed in ducks (206) and human viral infections how IFN might control viral genome replication and expression. With this view, we have been led to analyze in detail the interplay between the viral capsid and the IFN-inducible MxA cellular protein. We have demonstrated that HBV capsid inhibits the global antiviral effect of IFN on test viruses, such as the vesicular stomatitis virus (VSV), and downregulates MxA expression (207); MxA is a cellular protein induced by IFN-α and -β that shows antiviral effects on many RNA viruses. We have recently observed that MxA expression inhibits HBV genome replication, likely by diminishing cytosolic HBV RNA export (Gordien et al., in press). This is a first report of an antiviral effect of MxA on a DNA virus; it leads to the proposal of a model whereby accumulation of HBV capsid, induced in particular by dHBV expression (see below) or by some HBV core promoter variants, would counteract the inhibitory effect of MxA on HBV DNA replication.

The Role of Spliced Hepatitis B Virus (HBV) Transcripts, Encoding for a New HBV Protein (HBV Splice Protein, HBSP)

We first showed the reverse-transcription and encapsidation of a single spliced HBV RNA (207–209), leading to the secretion of defective HBV particles of which subgenomic DNA lacked the entire PreS and a part of the S sequences. A striking feature of these defective HBV particles (dHBV) is their association with chronic HBV infection. We have developed a PCR-based assay to detect them in serum; with this test, we showed a higher amount of dHBV among those patients developing a chronic carrier state after acute infection, compared with those showing resolved acute hepatitis; furthermore, dHBV was constantly found in chronic HBV carriers (210). The molecular basis of this observation is not known, but our results lead us to propose at least two complementary mechanisms: (a) We have shown that dHBV *in vitro* expression induces an important cellular accumulation of the HBV capsid protein, which, as described above, might modulate the MxA dependent IFN effects. (b) We have shown that singly spliced HBV RNA leads to the *in vivo* synthesis of a new HBV protein, referred to as HBV spliced protein (HBSP) (209); anti-HBSP antibodies have indeed been detected in about one-third of chronic HBV carriers, and the protein has been detected directly by Western blot in liver biopsies obtained from such HBV carriers. We did not see evidence of any effect on viral DNA replication. Interestingly, the *in vitro* ectopic expression of HBSP in hepatocytic cell lines leads to massive apoptosis. Thus, as for HBx, the expression of HBSP may regulate liver cell viability and favor viral particle dissemination. Liver cell apoptosis may also favor viral persistence by eliminating those cells with a high intracellular expression of HBV proteins; thus, cells with low HBV protein expression would be selected and this, in turn, would favor viral persistence.

The Molecular Bases and Implications of Hepatitis B Virus DNA Persistence in HBsAG-Negative Patients with Acute and Chronic Liver Diseases

Several studies have shown persistence of HBV DNA in serum, liver, and PBMNCs of patients with acute and chronic hepatitis (211,212), as well as in patients with HCC who lacked detectable serum HBsAG and, for some of them, all usual HBV serologic markers. This finding has been debated, but PCR-based assays have now confirmed the results obtained by Southern blotting. These observations have important implications; they suggest that the implication of HBV in liver carcinogenesis expands far beyond that predicted by classic serologic assays. They also show that improvements in the sensitivity of tests for HBsAg, together with the introduction of sensitive tests for HBV DNA, have modified the criteria for diagnosis of HBV infection.

The Molecular Bases of Hepatitis B Virus DNA Persistence

Several points should be distinguished when discussing the molecular bases of HBV DNA persistence (reviewed in refs. 10, 185, 200, 213, and 214). First, the presence of complete infectious HBV particles in such patients has been established by several complementary approaches: induction of hepatitis upon injection of such sera to chimpanzees (215,216), analysis of sera from donors and recipients of patients with posttransfusional hepatitis (217), and investigation of reinfection patterns of liver grafts after liver transplantation for HBsAg-negative cirrhosis (218). Thus, absence of HBV markers, including in some cases both anti-HBc and anti-HBs, does not formally exclude circulation in serum of HBV DNA-containing infectious HBV particles. Second, studies based on follow-up of patients with acute HBV infection have demonstrated the long-term persistence of HBV genomes, detected in serum complete HBV particles, after normalization of liver tests and detection of anti-HBs (213,219). Thus, HBV, with the availability of highly sensitive tests for HBV DNA detection, should be viewed as a virus that frequently induces persistent infection. These observations clearly also indicate, however, that HBV genomes can be detected in some individuals in the absence of liver histologic lesions. Third, the molecular bases of HBsAg-negative HBV DNA–positive infections include different, nonexclusive, mechanisms. Investigations based on careful follow-up of chronically infected patients have demonstrated that serum and liver HBV DNA frequently persists upon negativation of the usual tests for serum HBsAg detection (220–223); thus, a high proportion of the HBsAg-negative HBV DNA–positive cases simply reflect a progressive decline in HBV genome replication and expression. HBsAg might in fact be detected in such sera by using serologic tests with a higher sensitivity (224,225). These patients show in their serum anti-HBs and anti-HBc. It should be noted, however, that in rare cases, follow-up of HBV chronically infected patients can show disappearance of all HBV serologic markers despite HBV DNA persistence (C. Bréchot, personal communication, 1999). Still, other mechanisms should be envisaged when HBV DNA sequences are identified in the absence of any detectable HBV serologic markers. Although the existence of "new" hepatitis viruses was initially postulated by some authors, the results of PCR tests and sequence analyses clearly indicated that HBV was indeed present. Mutations in the envelope and capsid-encoding sequences have been described that might account for the negative serologic assays (reviewed in refs. 226 and 227). It should be emphasized, however, that in our own experience *in vitro* expression of the S gene from such genomes leads to synthesis of an HBsAg clearly recognized by conventional assays (228). Thus, although the present data do not rule out that in some cases HBV DNA mutations act by modifying the antigenicity of the viral proteins, this is not likely the main explanation for such profiles. On the other hand, a constant observation in all studies on this topic is the low amount of HBV DNA–containing particles in such sera [averaging in our experience 10 to 10^3 per milliliter (see also ref. 229)] and the low copy number per cell of HBV genomes identified in the liver; this explains the difficulties to obtain reliable results, even when using PCR. Mutations in the HBx-encoding gene have been reported that might in part account for this low HBV viremia (93,156,230,231), but this hypothesis has not yet been demonstrated. With this view, it is also important to realize that the viral load at the time of contamination is probably an important virologic factor, although very difficult to demonstrate: a low level of infectious HBV particles may lead to the infection of a limited number of hepatocytes and favor persistence of such viral infections. It is probable that an abnormal host immune response to the virus is also an important parameter, and a low or absent humoral response to the HBV proteins in patients might be considered. Finally, other environmental factors might be involved; in particular, there is evidence that chronic alcohol consumption may modulate HBV antigen expression and thus account in part for the high rate of HBV DNA–positive tests in HBsAg-negative alcoholics (232).

The Role of Hepatitis B Virus in HBsAg-Negative Hepatocellular Carcinoma

Striking geographic variations exist in terms of associations between HCC and chronic HBV infection. In Western countries (i.e., Northern Europe and the United States) and in Japan, only 15% to 20% of tumors occur in HBsAg-positive patients, and other environmental factors such as alcohol and infection with HCV are clearly major risk factors. A number of epidemiologic studies have shown a high prevalence of anti-HBs and anti-HBc antibodies in HBsAg-negative subjects (around 40% to 50% in France), indicating exposure to the virus (11,233).

The following subsections review the principal issues raised by these observations.

Prevalence of Hepatitis B Virus DNA in Liver Tumors in HBsAg-Negative Patients

The actual prevalence of these HBV DNA–positive HCCs in HBsAg-negative subjects has been a matter of debate, due to the low copy number per cell of viral DNA sequences (estimated at 0.1 to 0.01). Studies performed in different geographic regions have produced very varied results, probably because of the differences in technical conditions (specificity and sensitivity) as well as the distinct epidemiologic situations. Thanks to the sensitivity of the PCR technique, earlier observations have now been confirmed. Taken together, these studies show that HBV infection persists in a large number of subjects with HBsAg-negative HCCs, although the rate of HBV DNA positivity still varies from

one study to another, a problem principally due to difficulties in standardizing the PCR assay. These studies have led to the emphasis on the frequent co-infections by HCV and HBV in patients with HCC (see below). Interestingly, these observations have now been also made in most (234–239), although not all (240), studies from Japan (241) and Africa (242,243).

Structure of Hepatitis B Virus DNA in Tumors

With regard to the state of HBV DNA, its low copy number per cell has hampered interpretation of the results of Southern blotting. However, using our PCR test and distinct primers distributed on the S, PreS/S, C, and X HBV genes, we have been able to produce further data. In several patients, a positive result was only obtained with some of the HBV primers, a finding consistent with the presence of defective HBV DNA. In other cases, tumor DNA scored positive with all the HBV primers, which is consistent with the presence of free or integrated HBV DNA showing no gross rearrangements. Interestingly, defective HBV genomes have been identified more frequently in tumors than in non-tumor tissues. In addition, they have been demonstrated more frequently in completely seronegative individuals than in anti-HBs– and anti-HBc–positive subjects; this observation probably reflects a technical difference, since the presence of defective HBV DNA may be obscured by concomitant, complete viral genomes. The PCR profiles obtained with DNA from tumor, nontumor, and serum samples from the same European patients showed marked differences. In the serum and nontumor samples, amplification was achieved with all the primers tested; in contrast, tumoral DNA repeatedly produced negative results with at least one primer. These findings demonstrate that the HBV DNA sequences in the tumor do not derive from contaminating nontumor cells or serum-derived particles. They are also consistent with the clonal expansion of cells containing defective and integrated HBV DNA (244,245). In this view, it is interesting that a recent case of HBV-related *cis*-activation, involving the SERCA1 encoding gene, has in fact been shown in an HBsAg-negative, anti-HBc–positive, individual (178). Finally, as discussed in an earlier section, our group has identified a high rate of mutations in the HBx ORF gene in the tumor tissue from such HBsAg-negative HBV DNA–positive patients; this high rate of amino acid changes contrasted with a lower rate of mutations in PreC:C sequences (190).

Expression of Hepatitis B Virus DNA Sequences

Northern blot analysis has not proved to be sensitive enough to detect HBV RNAs in these tumors. In contrast, complementary DNA (cDNA) synthesis followed by PCR with primers on the S gene [reverse-transcription (RT)-PCR] has revealed HBV RNA sequences in most HBV DNA–positive tumors from HBsAg-negative patients. However, owing to the compact organization of the HBV genome, it is difficult to specify which viral transcripts are synthesized. Using primers located on the S, C, and X encoding sequences, our group has been able to fully demonstrate the expression of the HBx RNA in such tumors (93,246). Similar results were recently reported in Japan (235). Our study also enabled demonstration of the expression of HBx protein in both tumor and nontumor cells from such liver tissues (93).

Potential Role of Hepatitis B Virus in the Pathogenesis of HBsAg-Negative Hepatocellular Carcinoma

Taken overall, the results demonstrate a high rate of persistent HBV infection in patients with HBsAg-negative HCC, many of whom also lack detectable antibodies to the virus. They also show clonal expansion of the tumor cells containing the integrated viral DNA, and the preferential transcription in these cells of HBV RNA sequences encoding the HBx protein. The involvement of HBV in HBsAg-negative liver cancers is also reinforced by two pieces of evidence. In the woodchuck HCC model, 17% of animals infected by WHV developed primary liver cancers despite negativation of the assay for WHV surface antigen in the serum and the appearance of antibodies to surface and capsid viral antigens; furthermore, WHV DNA was detected in tumor tissue from these animals, with a much lower copy per cell number than in WHsAg-positive woodchucks (approximately 1 and 1,000 molecules per cell, respectively) (247,248), an observation fairly similar to those made in human HCCs. Ground squirrel may also prove to be an interesting model, since ground squirrel hepatic virus (GSHV) DNA sequences have been identified in HCCs developing in completely seronegative ani-

mals (249). Another piece of evidence of a direct role of HBV in liver cancer arises from the detection of HBV DNA in HCCs in HBsAg-negative patients, developing on noncirrhotic tissue, histologically very similar to normal liver; thus, cirrhosis cannot alone account for the induction of cancer in these cases (250). Finally, the increased rate of HCCs in anti-HBs positive patients observed in some studies (251) and the development of HCCs despite negativation of serum HBsAg in patients with chronic hepatitis (252) are also consistent with this hypothesis. Although these findings argue strongly in favor of a role for HBV in the development of these tumors, one paradoxical result still has to be explained: Why is the copy number of HBV DNA per cell so low if there is clonal expansion of the infected cells? It is possible to hypothesize that, after it has triggered the cascade of events that will lead to liver cell transformation, the persistence of HBV DNA is no longer necessary. Furthermore, as discussed above, there is little or no HBV replication in tumor cells, and thus no generation of new integrants from free viral genomes. Finally, chromosomal rearrangements may eliminate integrated viral DNA sequences from tumor clones. This explanation has also been put forward to account for human and bovine papillomavirus- and some retrovirus-related tumors (253–255). Interestingly, evidence has been found in the duck hepatitis (DHBV) model that supports these hypotheses (256).

Therefore, the overall data we have presented regarding HBV lead to submitting the following model to account for the multifactorial nature of liver carcinogenesis, including, in addition to HBV and HCV, other factors such as alcohol, chemical carcinogens, and hormonal factors (Fig. 54.6). A major difference between HBsAg-positive and HBsAg-negative HBV DNA–positive HCCs concerns the number of viral DNA sequences per cell and the rate of HBV DNA replication. In HBsAg-positive chronic carriers, HBV multiplication is sustained for sufficient time to induce liver cell necrosis and thus the secondary proliferation of adjacent liver cells. In these subjects, HBV may therefore act at two complementary stages of liver cell transformation: it may exert a direct role through a combination of *cis*- and *trans*-activating mechanisms; in addition, HBV may induce the promotion and clonal expansion of initiated "cells" by inducing liver cell necrosis and regeneration. In contrast, in HBsAg-negative HBV DNA–positive patients, the number of HBV DNA copy per cell is low, and viral DNA replication is barely detectable. In most of these cases, therefore, it is unlikely that HBV will be solely responsible for liver cell necrosis, chronic active hepatitis, and cirrhosis. Instead, other factors such as HCV, alcohol, or other still unrecognized agents may be responsible for cirrhosis and thus the promotion of neoplastic transformation (Fig. 54.6). On the other hand, we have presented evidence for the persistence of integrated viral DNA, which may exert a direct effect via the integration and/or synthesis of HBx. HBV, therefore, might be able to initiate liver

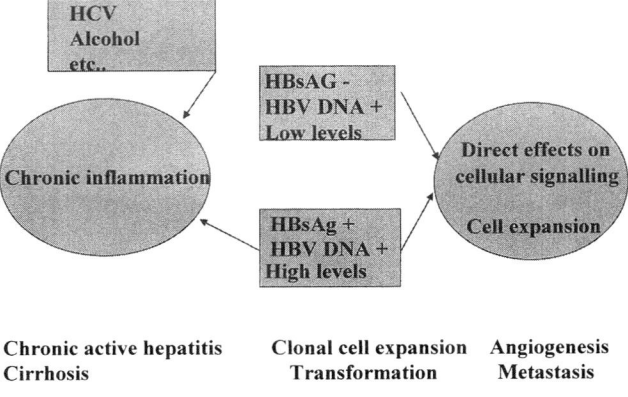

FIGURE 54.6. A hypothetical model of the implication of hepatitis B virus (*HBV*) persistence in hepatitis B surface antigen (*HBsAg*)-negative hepatocelluar carcinomas. HBV multiplication is either absent or maintained at a low level in HBsAg-negative HBV DNA–positive individuals, suggesting that HBV itself is not sufficient to induce sustained liver inflammation; other environmental factors would act synergistically and promote expansion of cells containing the viral sequences (see text). *HCV*, hepatitis C virus.

cell transformation in a limited number of clonally expanded cells; the subsequent development of an HCC would then depend on the effect of cofactors capable of promoting liver cell regeneration via the development of cirrhosis. Thus, collectively, I submit that a major implication of HBV DNA persistence is to maintain chronic HBV infection with a low replication rate, which may constitute a risk factor for liver cancer if other factors promote liver cell proliferation.

HEPATITIS C VIRUS

It is unclear whether an "asymptomatic carrier state," as defined by a strictly normal liver histology despite ongoing viral multiplication, actually exists. If so, however, it is a rare condition, as most chronically infected subjects show chronic active hepatitis of varying severity.

Hepatitis C Virus RNA Patterns During Hepatitis C Virus Infection

HCV is now recognized as a member of the Flaviviridae family, together with the pestiviruses and flaviviruses (see Chapter 55). Its genome is a positive, single-strand RNA molecule that includes two untranslated regions at the 5′ and 3′ ends, and a large open reading frame encoding for a 3,010 to 3,030 amino acid polyprotein. This polyprotein is posttranslationally processed into structural and nonstructural proteins, the cleavage being dependent on host and viral encoded enzymes. The structural proteins, encoded in the N-terminal region, include the core protein followed by two envelope glycosylated proteins: E1 and E2. The nonstructural domain encodes for six proteins: NS2, 3, 4A, 4B, 5A, and 5B.

There are still several uncertainties regarding the natural history and course of the viral infection. In particular, in the acute stage of the infection there is no strong evidence of a role for HCV in fulminant hepatitis in Western countries in the absence of HBV/HCV co-infection (257–259). This contrasts with reports from Asia that have implicated HCV in several cases in the absence of a detectable HBV infection (260,261).

HCV multiplication is sustained, showing either stable or increased (262–264) HCV RNA titers throughout the course of the chronic infection, and the long-term development of cirrhosis and HCC (262–264). The level of HCV viremia is generally low during chronic infection (around 10^5 to 10^7). However, studies of the kinetics of serum HCV RNA disappearance during IFN-α treatment suggest a high turnover rate of the viral particles (around 10^{10}) (265). Still, the influence of the viral load on the course of HCV infection has never been established, and most studies have failed to show any significant differences in plasma viral load among patients with chronic hepatitis, cirrhosis, and HCC. While this observation

contrasts markedly with other viral infections, including HIV, its interpretation should be tempered by three points. First, in most studies HCV viremia is increased in immunosuppressed subjects and correlates with the severity of the chronic hepatitis. This has been particularly well established in liver transplant recipients (257,266,267) and in HIV/HCV co-infections (268). Second, the intrahepatic viral load was not quantified in most studies, and might not strictly correlate with the levels of viremia, a technically difficult issue to address accurately. Third, other environmental factors can modify HCV viremia. In particular, chronic alcohol consumption aggravates liver cell damage in HCV-related chronic hepatitis in most series including ours. This is likely due both to its intrinsic toxic effects as well as an increase in the level of HCV viremia (269).

The pattern of HCV replication as well as its genetic variability have several important implications for understanding the potential end points of antiviral strategies:

- A complete eradication of the virus is theoretically feasible, given the absence of integrated DNA molecules. Indeed, we and others have previously demonstrated that HCV RNA is undetectable by PCR in serum, liver, and PBMNC samples in patients who show a long-term biochemical response to IFN-α (270,271).
- Since viral multiplication is ongoing during the complete course of HCV chronic infection, antivirals should be used, even though cirrhosis has already developed.
- Due to its high genetic variability, HCV develops efficient strategies to persist and escape from treatment (see below). This will significantly reduce the overall efficacy of the therapy and should prompt development of a drug combination.

The Molecular Bases of Hepatitis C Virus RNA Persistence (Fig. 54.7)

Hepatitis C Virus RNA Genetic Variability

HCV RNA shows significant genetic variability, and exhibits an estimated rate of nucleotide change of approximately 10^{-3} substitutions/site/year (272,273). This figure has been evaluated from sequential analyses of sera collected at different time points in infected humans and chimpanzees. This genetic variability can be seen in all domains of the HCV RNA but predominates in the E2 envelope protein encoding sequences where there is a hypervariable sequence (HVR 1), located in the 5′ part of this domain, with a high rate of nonsynonymous mutations (i.e., leading to amino acid changes). Some of the nonstructural (NS5A in particular) as well as the capsid-encoding sequences show a lower, yet significant, rate of variability. In contrast, the 5′ untranslated region is highly conserved among different isolates, although mutations can be identified at some sites.

814   *Chapter 54*

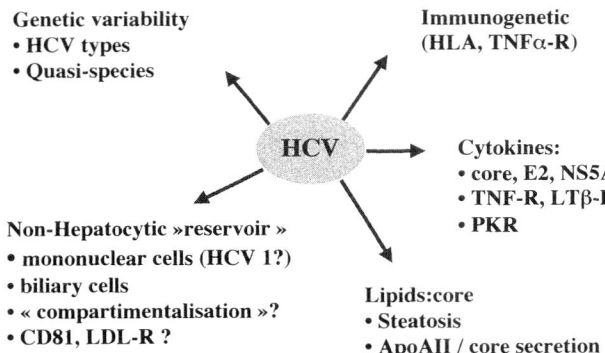

Genetic variability
• HCV types
• Quasi-species

Immunogenetic (HLA, TNFα-R)

HCV

Cytokines:
• core, E2, NS5A
• TNF-R, LTβ-R
• PKR

Non-Hepatocytic »reservoir »
• mononuclear cells (HCV 1?)
• biliary cells
• « compartimentalisation »?
• CD81, LDL-R ?

Lipids:core
• Steatosis
• ApoAII / core secretion

FIGURE 54.7. The mechanisms of hepatitis C virus (*HCV*) persistence in liver cells. Various mechanisms are employed by HCV to establish chronic infection. It shows in particular the association of mechanisms involving immune response to the virus and direct interactions with cellular signaling. *HLA*, human leukocyte antigen; *PKR*, RNA-stimulated protein kinase; *LDL*, low-density lipoprotein; *TNF*, tumor necrosis factor.

At present three major HCV types are distinguished—1, 2, and 3—as well as three to seven other types, according to the classification proposed. It is important to note the marked heterogeneity of some HCV types, such as types 2, 3, 4, and 6. The geographic distribution of these types and subtypes varies significantly. The relative prevalence of 1b is high in Japan and Europe but lower in the United States, where 1a is more prevalent. Some genotypes are predominantly found outside these areas: type 4, central Africa and the Middle East; type 5, South Africa; and type 6, Singapore. The pattern of HCV type distribution is also markedly influenced by the modes of contamination. In several geographic areas, and in particular in Europe, HCV type 3 is predominantly identified in intravenous drug users (IVDUs). In contrast, HCV 1b is primarily present in posttransfusional and so-called sporadic forms of the viral infection. HCV 1a is also associated with IVDUs in Europe. The figures regarding HCV 2 are less documented; this heterogeneous type also occurs after transfusion, but in Europe it is predominantly present in sporadic chronic infections. Sequence analysis is still the reference method to identify HCV types and subtypes, but it is obviously not possible to sequence all HCV isolates when analyzing large series of patients, in which setting PCR-based or serologic assays are necessary. The description of these assays, as well as the discussion of some pitfalls in their interpretation, has been the subject of reviews (274,275). The heterogeneity of some HCV types can modify the results, as for example for HCV 2c, which is prevalent in particular in France and Italy. It is also difficult to correctly identify mixed HCV infections (276).

The major impact on the response of virologic parameters has been recognized in virtually all studies on this topic. There is indeed a general agreement that the response to IFN therapy depends on the infecting HCV type, while the

association between certain types and liver lesion severity is highly debated [see HCV and Hepatocellular Carcinoma, below]. The particular profile of response to IFN of genotype 1b was first suggested from studies in Japan. Thus, in univariate analyses, the relative prevalence of type 1b was significantly higher among nonresponders than among responders (275,277). However, several potential biases must be considered before concluding that a given genotype is a predictive factor for poor response to treatment. In particular, the correlation between genotype and other previously established host factors, such as duration of infection, cirrhosis, etc., has to be considered, as well as the HCV viremia level. We and others have now provided evidence based on multivariate analysis of these various parameters in different geographic areas, showing that both infection by genotype 1b and high levels of HCV viremia were independent predictive factors of poor response to IFN (262,278). Further studies have now shown that HCV 1a shares a low response rate to IFN with 1b. This issue can also be addressed by analyzing the genotype distribution among long-term responders (LTRs) where types 2 and 3 predominate. Similar results have been obtained with NS4-based serotyping assays (279). This issue is further complicated by the concept of "quasi-species." HCV RNA circulates, in most cases, as a *population* of RNA molecules that also differ in serum and liver (280). These viral genomes have evolved from an original genome by point mutations and are included in the same HCV subtype. This heterogeneity of HCV RNA, referred to as "quasi-species" (by analogy with HIV), can be easily identified in the hypervariable 1 (HVR1) region of E2, and in fact HVR1 sequence shows homology in its structure with that of the V3 loop of the HIV-1 GP120 envelope protein. It has been suggested that detection of a highly heterogeneous population of HCV RNA sequences before treatment correlates with a lower rate of response to IFN (281). Our results also supported this possibility in European patients infected by types 1 or 3 (282). We have indeed shown in a multivariate analysis that the degree of HCV genome complexity is, together with HCV type 1b and a high viral load, an important and independent risk factor for a nonresponse to treatment. Such observations support the hypothesis that the high genetic variability of the HCV genome and the existence of a population of HCV RNA quasi-species favor the selection of RNA molecules that are "resistant" to antiviral factors, either during the natural course of the infection or during IFN treatment. Cloning and sequencing of the various HCV RNA genomes at different time points during the follow-up have provided evidence for time-dependent selection of some of these HCV species (reviewed in refs. 283 and 284); the actual importance of HVR1 complexity and diversity, however, is still a matter of debate (285). Selection of HCV molecules during the course of HCV infection might be partly linked to "escape mutants" or to compartmentalization of the viral genomes in different cell types (see below), but this is not demonstrated (reviewed in ref. 286).

Several studies have also analyzed in detail the kinetic and impact of HCV quasi-species during the natural course of HCV infection. Some cross-sectional studies showed a parallel between the genetic complexity and the severity of the liver disease, independently of the viremia and duration of infection (287). This observation has been challenged by the detection of molecules with the same heterogeneity in asymptomatic carriers (288,289) as well as by the finding that HVR1 variations might in fact be associated with liver lesion improvement (290). Finally it also has been suggested that HCV RNA variability might be increased in HIV/HCV co-infected patients, independently of the viral load (291). Thus, there is no clear emerging pattern on this issue so far, and the impact of the HCV quasi-species needs further investigation.

Infection by Hepatitis C Virus of Nonhepatocytic Cells

There is now evidence that HCV also infects extrahepatic cells. *In vivo*, HCV RNA sequences have been detected in fresh peripheral blood mononuclear cell (PBMC) preparations from HCV-infected patients (292,293). However, such an approach does not allow distinction between absorption of serum particles and true infection of PBMC in viremic patients. Still, several observations support this hypothesis: (a) Short-term cultures of PBMC yield a significant increase in the amount of viral RNA on stimulation by PHA and PMA (292). (b) *In situ* hybridization showed viral RNA in a limited percentage (around 1%) of circulating PBMC and lymph nodes (294,295). (c) PBMC from normal individuals can be infected by HCV (296,297). (d) There is evidence that Epstein–Barr virus–immortalized B cells and T-cell clones from HCV carriers show long-term persistence of HCV genomes (296; Bronowicki, personal communication). (e) We have presented strong evidence for the persistence of HCV RNA in PBMC obtained from HCV-positive subjects and injected into severe combined immunodeficient (SCID) mice. Artifacts due to contamination with serum particles were excluded by this approach, which showed infection of these mononuclear cells (298).

A second issue concerns the detection of replicative forms of HCV RNA in PBMC. This point has been discussed in regard to the specificity of negative HCV RNA detection. Thus, although such negative strands are clearly detected in some patients and on stimulation with mitogens, the real prevalence of this phenomenon remains unsettled (299). Interestingly, it has been suggested that HCV type 1 might show a distinct lymphotropism, in comparison to other frequent HCV types (299). Also, using a highly strand-specific method of RT-PCR, Shimizu et al. (300) were able to demonstrate HCV RNA of negative polarity in PBMC samples from infected chimpanzees. In

addition, they found that the capacity of infected PBMC and/or liver cells in chimpanzees, as well as in human lymphocyte cell lines infected *in vitro*, varied among different HCV strains, suggesting the existence of lymphotropic HCV strains. The possibility of specific cell subsets harboring HCV sequences has also been discussed. HCV negative strand RNA, possibly reflecting viral replication, was found in all cell subsets in some studies (292) and in specific cell subpopulations (monocytes and B lymphocytes) in other ones (299).

Finally, the possibility of PBMC infection by HCV has recently been confirmed in studies indicating that HCV infection of lymphoid cells may favor selection of distinctive viral variants. *In vitro* and *in vivo* studies, based on HVR1 sequence analysis, showed different quasi-species patterns between serum, liver, and PBMC (301–303). Thus, these observations support the concept of a "compartmentalization" of some HCV genomes. The differences in quasi-species composition between these tissues may arise from cellular factors in the liver and PBMC that would favor the growth of certain variants over others (302). It is not established, however, that distinct cellular tropism might be shown by some HCV variants.

Other cell types are permissive to HCV infection; we have recently demonstrated the possibility of infecting, at a low level, biliary cells in primary culture (304). Biliary lesions are frequently observed during chronic HCV infection (305), and HCV infection of the biliary cells might be involved in this phenomenon.

Overall, infection of nonhepatocytic cells might constitute a "reservoir" that would favor selection of HCV variants and viral persistence. It might also induce specific cell alterations, but this is not demonstrated; in particular, the actual impact of PBMNC infection on the quality of the immune response is unknown. Finally, PBMNC and bone marrow cell infection by HCV might be an important event in the development of cryoglobulinemia and B-cell lymphoproliferations associated with HCV infection (reviewed in refs. 296 and 306); the relative contribution of the strong polyclonal B-cell stimulation during HCV infection and of putative direct signals triggered by HCV proteins (see below) remains to be investigated.

Interactions Between Hepatitis C Virus and Major Cellular Metabolic Networks

Hepatitis C Virus Infection and Liver Lipid Metabolism

There are several observations that point out the potential importance of such association. Circulating serum HCV particles show heterogeneous density, which reflects in part the binding of a fraction of the virions to very-low-density lipoprotein (VLDL) and low-density lipoprotein (LDL) (307,308). Moreover, the LDL receptor has been proposed as one of the potential viral receptors (309,310).

A further important hallmark of chronic HCV, and not HBV, infection is its association to steatosis in at least 50% of infected subjects (305). The pathogenic importance of steatosis in the course of HCV infection is not established; however, it has been suggested by several studies that, in some patients with steatosis from various etiologies, liver lipid overload might contribute to the development of fibrosis (311,312). In addition, expression of HCV core in some transgenic mice induces steatosis (313); interestingly, these mice eventually develop HCC in the absence of detectable chronic inflammation. Consistent with this result, transgenic mice containing the complete HCV genome (314) also show steatosis followed by HCC; in contrast, however, other core-expressing transgenic mice do not show liver lesions (315), emphasizing the importance of the core expression levels, the mice genetics, and likely environmental parameters.

In this context, we have provided direct *in vitro* evidence of the role of HCV core expression in steatosis induction (316). Moreover, we have shown the association of HCV core to apolipoprotein AII (Apo AII) and the impact of this binding in the *in vitro* secretion of the viral protein (317). We have recently further investigated this issue *in vivo* by using HCV core-expressing transgenic mice as well as mice expressing both HCV core and the human ApoAII; our data demonstrate that HCV core expression does not affect beta-oxidation, but instead directly inhibits VLDL assembly and secretion. Furthermore, ectopic *in vivo* ApoAII expression induces core secretion in serum, decreases its intrahepatic level, and thus abrogates its effects on VLDL secretion. Collectively, these data lead to proposing a model whereby HCV/ApoAII interactions might regulate core accumulation, the viral protein in turn impairing liver triglyceride secretion (Fig. 54.8).

Further studies will now aim to elucidate the molecular bases of these observations and their potential impact in liver lesion development; it will also be interesting to investigate whether or not, as recently suggested (318), HCV type 3 does specifically disturb liver lipid metabolism.

Hepatitis C Virus Direct Interactions with Interferon Signaling
Chronically HCV-infected patients show an inappropriate IFN production and this has provided a rationale for the use of IFN-α in treating, now in combination with ribavirin, patients with HCV-related chronic active hepatitis. There is also emerging evidence that HCV might, as with many other viruses, evolve mechanisms to directly inhibit the IFN signaling in the infected cells. HCV polyprotein

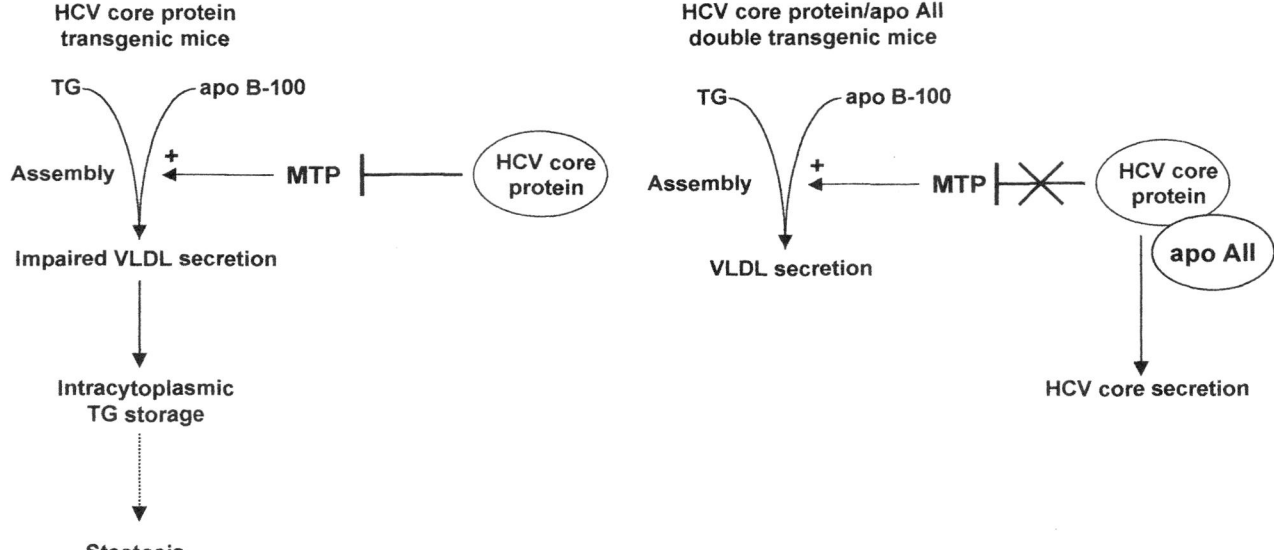

FIGURE 54.8. A model for the interactions between hepatitis C virus (*HCV*) core and liver lipid metabolism. Binding of the HCV core to apolipoprotein AII (*Apo AII*) might trigger core secretion by a presently unknown mechanism. Thus, upon translation of the core-expressing sequence, core protein might follow different pathways: (a) As described in the literature, it will be located on the cytosolic face of the endoplasmic reticulum. (b) A proportion of core will be located around triglyceride (*TG*)-containing vesicles. (c) Binding of core with AII will, in cases of high AII expression, drive core secretion. Increased expression of ApoAII, such as that obtained by fibrate treatment or, in transgenic mice, ectopic ApoAII expression, would therefore lower intracellular core concentration. The core inhibits very-low-density lipoprotein (*VLDL*), and thus triglyceride secretion and these effects are major factors in steatosis induction, the consequences of which remain to be explored. *MTP,* monosomal triglyceride transfer protein.

expression in an osteosarcoma cell line inhibits the antiviral effect of IFN-α on vesicular stomatitis (VSV) and encephalomyocarditis (EMCV) viruses, and decreases STAT3 DNA binding (319); this study did not identify, however, the viral protein(s) involved.

NS5A is a candidate HCV protein, which is possibly involved in both the inhibition of the antiviral effects of IFN and the control of cell growth and viability (see below). The pioneering studies conducted by Enomoto et al. (320,321) and Katze's group (322,323) raised the hypothesis that NS5A might directly modulate the IFN transduction pathway by associating with and inhibiting the kinase activity of the double-strand, RNA-stimulated protein kinase (PKR). In Japan, Enomoto et al. first demonstrated that mutations in a region of NS5A, which they referred to as the "IFN sensitive determining region (ISDR)," correlated with the response to IFN treatment. Thus, patients whose major circulating HCV genomes exhibited mutations in this region achieved the best response to treatment. Other (324,325), but not all (326), studies from Japan supported these findings. However, certain caveats should be borne in mind that markedly complicate the analysis of these findings. Several reports have shown that the strict correlation between ISDR mutations and treatment efficacy reported in Japan could not be demonstrated in Europe or the United States (327,328). The reasons for differences between clinical studies performed in Japan and Europe are not clear. It has been suggested that different IFN doses and regimens could affect the outcome of such comparative studies. However, this point has not been proved. It is also important to consider several virologic parameters. The impact of NS5A mutations is dependent on the HCV type. Studies in Japan have mostly been performed in patients infected with HCV 1b or, to a lesser extent, HCV type 2, but NS5A mutations are not, or only rarely, identified in HCV type 3 genomes. NS5A variability in domains located outside the ISDR, and in particular in the C terminal part of the protein, may also be implicated in the control of therapeutic efficacy (329). The conclusions of these different studies may also differ because of methodologic problems; other results have indeed been obtained when analyzing only the major form of the HCV genome or complete quasi-species complexity (330,331). Moreover, a recent study suggested that European and Japanese HCV 1b genomes could exhibit different biologic properties, a correlation between ISDR mutations, and therapeutic efficacy only being demonstrated for the Japanese isolates (332). These findings clearly need to be substantiated by further analyses. Finally, other major virologic factors, such as the viral load, should also be taken into account (324).

Several reports have now reinforced these clinical observations. *In vitro*, NS5A expression is sufficient to inhibit the antiviral effect of IFN-α on VSV and EMCV viruses (333–335). We have in particular established this point by expressing several "natural" NS5A mutants, isolated from patients with or without response to IFN, in the well-differentiated hepatocytic cell line HuH7 (Podevin et al., in press). The present data do not show, however, a correlation with the *in vivo* response to therapy.

Several important and fundamental problems remain to be solved regarding the molecular basis for the biologic effects of NS5A. NS5A is located in the perinuclear area, and is a 56- to 58-kd phosphoprotein. The kinase(s) involved are not identified, although casein-kinase II may be involved (336). Both a basal and hyperphosphorylated status of NS5A have been suggested, and expression of the complete, nonstructural HCV region is necessary in cis for the full phosphorylation of NS5A (337).

Some reports suggest that NS5A might interact with at least two major cellular signaling pathways. NS5A might bind the catalytic domain of PKR, inhibiting its dimerization and thus its activation (323,338). Furthermore, the domain involved in this interaction in NS5A might include the ISDR region and a domain adjacent to its 3' extremity. Taken together, these data suggest an elegant model whereby expression of the NS5A protein may abolish the antiviral effect of PKR on IFN stimulation, this effect being abrogated by mutations that would then favor treatment efficacy. It is important to note, however, that these data have not yet been confirmed in independent studies (Podevin et al., in press; E. Meurs, personal communication).

N-terminally deleted forms of NS5A also show transcriptional activity, but it remains to be established whether such truncated NS5A molecules exist *in vivo* and how they might participate in NS5A biologic properties. Importantly, a correlation between ISDR mutations and NS5A transcriptional activity has been recently reported (339). NS5A might bind the Grb-2 adapter protein and modulates the ERK1/2-dependent signaling (340).

Interestingly, it has also been proposed that the E2 envelope protein might also interact with PKR and inhibit its actions (341).

Hepatitis C Virus and Hepatocellular Carcinoma

A large number of studies have shown that in most parts of the world HCV constitutes a major risk factor for HCC. However, the figures remain sketchy in some regions. In Japan and Southern Europe, anti-HCV prevalence levels of 80% and 60%, respectively, have been found; in Northern Europe, recent data suggest that approximately 30% of cases of HCCs are associated with chronic HCV infection (342,343). In sub-Saharan Africa and Southeast Asia, where HBV-associated HCC is common, the impact of HCV is much less marked (around 10%). Prospective studies have also emphasized the role of HCV in various geographic areas (343).

Much data have accumulated over the past few years concerning the mechanisms that may be involved in HCV-related HCC (344,345). Clearly, chronic hepatitis, with its combination of chronic inflammation, liver cell necrosis and regeneration, and extensive fibrosis, constitutes a major step in this process (346,347). Some cases of HCV-related HCC, however, develop in the absence of associated cirrhosis and chronic hepatitis; interestingly, most of these tumors contain HCV genomes classified as 1b (348). Viral multiplication is sustained throughout the long-term course of chronic HCV infection, and the development of cirrhosis and HCC. HCV genomes persist in tumor cells and can replicate, albeit at a lower rate than in nontumoral livers (346,349,350). In contrast with HBV, the HCV genome does not integrate into cellular DNA, and replication is thus necessary for its persistence. HCV proteins can be also detected in tumor cells, testifying to HCV genome expression in these cells (B. Lebail et al., unpublished observations). A certain amount of evidence indicates that, beside inducing chronic liver inflammation, some HCV proteins may modulate liver cell proliferation and viability by interfering directly with the major cellular transduction networks. Some studies have recently focused on core, NS3, and NS5A proteins.

Hepatitis C Virus Core

In addition to its role in the packaging of viral RNA, the HCV core can indeed modulate cellular transduction pathways (reviewed in refs. 351 and 352). HCV core protein is mainly cytoplasmic, located on the endoplasmic reticulum membranes and around lipid vesicles (316,353). HCV core has been found to be associated with TNF-α receptor I and TNF-α–related lymphotoxin-β receptor, and this interaction modulates signaling by these cytokines (354,355). As discussed in a previous section, HCV core protein also associates with ApoAII. The viral core actually binds a number of cellular proteins, also including a cellular helicase (356) and a heterogeneous nuclear ribonucleoprotein K (357). However, the relevance of these various interactions is still to be fully established. The HCV core transactivates a number of cellular promoters, including c-*myc*, and activates NF-κB, AP-1, and SRE elements, interacting with c-JNK, ErK, and MAPK signaling (358). In contrast, it suppresses the P53 and P21 promoters (351,359,360). Whether or not a fraction of HCV core may also act in the nucleus during *in vivo* infection is still a matter for debate. C-terminally truncated core translocates to the nucleus and may exert distinct biologic effects (316,353,361–363); however, it has not been shown that such sequences are actually present during natural HCV infection. Some reports have nonetheless suggested that such truncated cores might be identified in tumor tissues from patients with HCC (364,365). The expression of HCV core has an impact upon cell growth and viability. In cooperation with v-Ha-ras, the HCV core can induce the transformation of immortalized Rat1 fibro-

blasts (366) and possibly primary rat fibroblasts (367). Such *in vitro* results have been substantiated by *in vivo* studies in transgenic mice, which demonstrated the induction of HCC on expression of the core sequence only (313) or of the full-length genome (368); as discussed in a previous section, the development of HCC in these animal models is preceded by steatosis in the absence of liver inflammation. However, other reports on HCV core-expressing transgenic mice did not demonstrate such changes, and the reasons for these discrepancies remain unknown (315).

In line with these results, the HCV core also modulates cell viability, although the results obtained are still under debate. It has been suggested that HepG2 cells are sensitized to Fas (369), or in contrast, there are inhibitions of the apoptosis induced in HepG2 cells by Fas, in HepG2 and MCF7 cells by TNF, and in Hela, BRK, and Chinese hamster ovary (CHO) cells by cisplatin and c-*myc* (351,370,371). Thus, the HCV core appears to be a multifunctional, cytosolic protein, capable of modulating several major cellular transduction pathways, its eventual overall effect on cell proliferation and viability being dependent on its intracellular concentration, cell differentiation, and the cellular environment.

Hepatitis C Virus NS3

The expression of NS3 may also be important, in addition to its major role in viral protein maturation and genome replication. *In vitro*, the stable expression in NIH 3T3 cells of the N-terminal part of NS3, encoding for one of the two viral serine-proteases implicated in HCV polyprotein processing, can induce a transformed phenotype (372). It has also been suggested that the N-and C-terminal moieties of NS3 may regulate the catalytic activity of protein kinase A (reviewed in ref. 373) as well as the localization of P53.

Hepatitits C Virus NS5A

This is another candidate protein that, besides its effects on the antiviral effects of IFN (see above), might also regulate cell proliferation and viability. An inhibitory effect of NS5A expression on cell apoptosis as well as a transforming effect in NIH 3T3 has recently been reported (338,374). This effect might depend on the NS5A/PKR interaction (338) and transactivation and repression of cellular promoters (334,335,374). PKR indeed does not only show antiviral activity but also regulates cell proliferation and viability (375). As stated in the previous section, however, the NS5A/PKR interactions have not yet been confirmed. Still, collectively, the interaction between HCV proteins and IFN signaling brings us back to the general and most important issue of the potential dual effect of IFN in HCV infection, which is antiviral on the one hand and antiproliferative on the other. This issue has major therapeutic implications since it would reinforce the concept raised from some clinical investigations of a protective effect of

IFN-α on HCC development, even in the absence of a detectable virologic response to therapy.

The biologic effects of HCV proteins on both antiviral and antiproliferative signaling also raise the hypothesis that the influence of some HCV types on IFN response (a well-documented observation) might not be dissociated from the potential, and highly debated, effect of some genotypes on the intensity of liver lesions and, possibly, liver carcinogenesis (reviewed in ref. 9). The impact of HCV genotypes on the risk of developing HCC is indeed an important issue to analyze. A number of recent studies point to the severity of HCV type 1–associated liver lesions, including HCC. Several, but not all, cross-sectional analyses indeed have shown higher relative prevalence of HCV 1 in patients with cirrhosis than in those with moderate chronic active hepatitis (CAH); however, these findings are difficult to interpret since the molecular epidemiology of HCV is presently changing with the recent introduction, at least in France and Italy, of other types, such as HCV 3 in intravenous drug users; in these conditions, the duration of HCV infection will differ from one type to another and markedly influence the risk of cirrhosis (262,272,376). There is still evidence for a more aggressive course of type 1–induced CAH: After liver transplantation in Europe, reinfection of the liver graft by HCV 1 induces a more rapidly progressive CAH than other HCV types, and this is not related to epidemiologic factors or to the level of viremia (377,378). In some prospective studies on the risk of developing HCC in patients with HCV-related cirrhosis, infection by genotype 1 has emerged as an independent risk factor (379,380); along the same line, HCV 1b was the most prevalent type among the patients we reported with HCV-associated HCC in the absence of cirrhosis (381). Clearly this is still indirect evidence, the interpretation of which is complicated by many intervening factors, several of them (such as alcohol and HBV co-infections) being underestimated in most studies; altogether, they are suggestive of a particular profile of HCV 1 infection. *In vitro* studies are now mandatory to analyze comparatively the different biologic properties of various HCV isolates. In particular, as discussed for HBV, a major technical limitation to these studies is the analysis of isolated domains of the viral genomes; given the size of the HCV RNA, studies on full-length clones are feasible but will require extensive efforts.

The Interactions Between Hepatitis B Virus, Hepatitis C Virus, and Alcohol in Liver Carcinogenesis

Interactions Between Hepatitis B Virus, Hepatitis C Virus, and Alcohol

HBV and HCV can interact with chronic alcohol consumption, and there is circumstantial evidence of a high incidence of HBV and HCV infection among alcoholics. The high incidence of anti-HCV in alcoholics with cirrhosis (40% to 50%), compared with that in those with minimal liver damage (around 20%), suggests that HCV infection may be involved in the development of cirrhosis in some of these patients. This might also account for the high incidence of anti-HCV (50%) among alcoholics with HCC (382–387). In contrast, there is no evidence of a role for HBV in the development of alcoholic cirrhosis, since the prevalence of anti-HBs and anti-HBc, although higher than in the general population, does not significantly differ in terms of the presence or absence of cirrhosis (diagnosed in about 20% of cases). There is, however, evidence of a role of HBV in liver cancers in alcoholics, since the incidence of serologic HBV markers is significantly higher in these patients (around 50%), and tumors frequently contain HBV DNA sequences (385,388–391).

Concomitant Infection by Hepatitis B Virus and Hepatitis C Virus Is a Major Emerging Issue

As discussed earlier, HBV DNA sequences have frequently been detected in patients with HBsAg-negative chronic liver disease. Now that anti-HCV tests are available, it is not surprising to find that such patients were in fact co-infected by HBV and HCV. Similarly, recent studies of HCV-infected subjects have confirmed the high incidence of HBV DNA persistence in the liver and/or samples. Some studies have demonstrated the clinical impact of such co-infections on the severity of chronic hepatitis (392) and possibly the efficacy of IFN (393). The high prevalence of HBV-HCV co-infections among patients with HCC has also been emphasized in Europe (394) and Japan (see previous section). HBV and HCV may interact at two levels during liver carcinogenesis: *in vivo* evidence is available for the reduced replication of both HBV DNA and HCV RNA in patients infected by the two viruses (395,396), and *in vitro* expression of HCV capsid also diminishes encapsidation of the HBV pregenome (397). In addition, it is plausible that the HBV and HCV genomes might cooperate in the carcinogenic process (398). Further molecular studies will now be needed to investigate how viral proteins might have a synergistic impact on liver cell transformation.

CONCLUSION

The combination of sensitive serologic and molecular tests for detecting viral genomes has enabled a reappraisal of the hepatitis viral infections. Studies based on these new research and diagnostic tools have led to emphasize the strong association between HBV and HCV with chronic liver diseases, including HCC; they have also provided evidence for the direct interplay between some viral proteins and major cellular transduction networks. Finally they have demonstrated that epidemiologic studies on such viral infections clearly necessitate the use of molecular markers and further reinforce the major importance of large-scale vaccination programs.

REFERENCES

1. Zuckerman AJ. Alphabet of hepatitis viruses. *Lancet* 1996;347: 558–559.
2. Simons JN, Leary TP, Dawson GJ, et al. Isolation of novel virus-like sequences associated with human hepatitis. *Nat Med* 1995; 1:564–569.
3. Linnen J, Wages J, Zhanf-Keck Z-Y, et al. Molecular cloning and disease association of hepatitis G virus: a transfusion-transmissible agent. *Science* 1996;271:505–508.
4. Miyata H, Tsunoda H, Kazi A, et al. Identification of a novel GC-rich 113-nucleotide region to complete the circular, single-stranded DNA genome of TT virus, the first human circovirus. *J Virol* 1999;73:3582–3586.
5. Alter HJ, Nakatsuji Y, Meldolder J, et al. The incidence of transfusion-associated hepatitis G virus infection and its relation to liver disease. *N Engl J Med* 1997;336:747–754.
6. Tuveri R, Jaffredo F, Lunel F, et al. Impact of TT virus in acute and chronic, viral- and non–viral-related liver diseases. *J Hepatol* 2000;33:121–127.
7. Tuveri R, Perret J, Delaporte E, et al. Prevalence hepatitis GB-C/HG and TT viruses and genetic variants in Gabon, equatorial Africa. 2001;11.
8. Rizzetto M, Rosina F. Treatment of hepatitis D. In: Zuckerman A, Thomas H, eds. *Viral hepatitis.* London: Churchill Livingstone, 1990:387–393.
9. Bréchot C. Molecular mechanisms of hepatitis B and C viruses related to liver carcinogenesis. *Hepatogastroenterology* 1998;45: 1189–1196.
10. Bréchot C. Hepatitis B virus (HBV) and hepatocellular carcinoma. HBV DNA status and its implications. *J Hepatology* 1987;4:269–279.
11. Bréchot C. Hepatitis B virus (HBV) and hepatocellular carcinoma. HBV DNA status and its implications. *J Hepatol* 1987; 4:269–279.
12. Blum HE, Offensperger W-B, Walter S, et al. Hepatocellular carcinoma and hepatitis B virus infection: molecular evidence for monoclonal origin and expansion of malignantly transformed hepatocytes. *J Cancer Res Clin Oncol* 1987;113:466–472.
13. Miller RH, Robinson WS. Common evolutionary origin of hepatitis B virus and retroviruses. *Proc Natl Acad Sci USA* 1986; 83:2531–2535.
14. Yamamoto T, Kajino K, Kudo M, et al. Determination of the clonal origin of multiple human hepatocellular carcinomas by cloning and polymerase chain reaction of the integrated hepatitis B virus DNA. *Hepatology* 1999;29:1446–1452.
15. Hino O, Shows TB, Rogler CE. Hepatitis B virus integration site in hepatocellular carcinoma at chromosome 17;18 translocation. *Proc Natl Acad Sci USA* 1986;83:8338–8342.
16. Meyer M, Wiedorn KH, Hofschneider PH. Chromosome 17:7 translocation is associated with hepatitis B virus DNA integration in human hepatocellular carcinoma DNA. *Hepatology* 1992;15:665.
17. Nagaya T, Nakamura T, Tokino T, et al. The mode of hepatitis B virus DNA integration in chromosomes of human hepatocellular carcinoma. *Genes Dev* 1987;1:773–782.
18. Rogler CE, Sherman M, Su CY, et al. Deletion in chromosome 11p associated with a hepatitis B integration site in hepatocellular carcinoma. *Science* 1985;230:319–322.
19. Slagle BL, Zhou YZ, Butel JS. Hepatitis B virus integration event in human chromosome 17p near the p53 gene identifies the region of the chromosome commonly deleted in virus-positive hepatocellular carcinomas. *Cancer Res* 1991;51:49–54.
20. Tokino T, Matsubara K. Chromosomal sites for hepatitis B virus integration in human hepatocellular carcinoma. *J Virol* 1991; 65:6761–6764.
21. Bréchot C, Hadchouel J, Scotto M, et al. State of hepatitis B virus DNA in hepatocytes of patients with HbsAg positive and HbsAg negative liver diseases. *Proc Natl Acad Sci USA* 1981;78: 3906–3910.
22. Takada S, Yaginuma K, Arii M, et al. Molecular biology of hepatitis B virus and hepatocellular carcinoma. In: Koike K, ed. *Primary liver cancer in Japan.* Tokyo: Springer–Verlag, 1992:75–87.
23. Robinson WS. Hepadnaviridae and their replication. In: Fields BN, Knipe DM, Chanock RM, et al., eds. *Fields virology.* New York: Raven Press, 1990:2137–2169.
24. Bréchot C, Hadchouel M, Scotto J, et al. Detection of hepatitis B virus DNA in liver and serum: a direct appraisal of the chronic carrier state. *Lancet* 1981;2:765–768.
25. Hadziyannis SJ, Lieberman HM, Karvountzis GG, et al. Analysis of liver disease, nuclear HBsAg, viral replication, and hepatitis B virus DNA, in liver and serum of HBeAg vs. anti-Hbe positive carriers of hepatitis B virus. *Hepatology* 1983;3:656–662.
26. Kam W, Rall LB, Smuckler EA, et al. Hepatitis B viral DNA in liver and serum of asymptomatic carriers. *Proc Natl Acad Sci USA* 1982;79:7522–7526.
27. Shafritz DA, Shouval D, Sherman H, et al. Integration of hepatitis B virus DNA into the genome of liver cells in chronic liver disease and hepatocellular carcinoma. *N Engl J Med* 1981; 305:1067–1073.
28. Yaginuma K, Kobayashi H, Kobayashi M, et al. Multiple integration site of hepatitis B virus DNA in hepatocellular carcinoma and chronic active hepatitis tissues from children. *J Virol* 1987;61:1808–1813.
29. Yasui K, Hino O, Ohtake K, et al. Clonal growth of hepatitis B virus integrated hepatocytes in cirrhotic liver nodules. *Cancer Res* 1992;52:6810–6814.
30. Lugassy C, Bernuau J, Thiers V, et al. Sequences of hepatitis B virus DNA in the serum and liver of patients with acute benign and fulminant hepatitis. *J Infect Dis* 1987;155:64–71.
31. Bréchot C. Application of molecular biology to the diagnosis of viral hepatitis. In: Zuckerman A, Thomas H, eds. *Viral hepatitis.* London: Churchill Livingstone, 1998:585–604.
32. Nowak MA, Bonhoeffer S, Hill AM, et al. Viral dynamics in hepatitis B virus infection. *Proc Natl Acad Sci U S A* 1996;93: 4398–4402.
33. Matsubara K. Chromosomal changes associated with hepatitis B virus DNA integration and hepatocarcinogenesis. In: McLachlan A, ed. *Molecular biology of the hepatitis B virus.* Boca Raton, FL: CRC Press, 1991:245–256.
34. Scotto J, Hadchouel M, Wain-Hobson S, et al. Hepatitis B virus DNA in Dane particles: evidence for the presence of replicative intermediates. *J Infect Dis* 1985;151:610–617.
35. Raimondo G, Burk R, Lieberman H, et al. Interrupted replication of hepatitis B virus in liver tissue of HBsAg carriers with hepatocellular carcinoma. *Virology* 1988;166:103–112.
36. Bréchot C, Lugassy C, Dejean A, et al. Hepatitis B virus DNA in infected human tissues viral hepatitis. In: Vyas, GN, Dienstag JL, Hoofnagle, eds. *Viral hepatitis and liver diseases.* New York: Grune and Stratton, 1984;395–409.
37. Lunel F, Abuaf N, Frangeul L, et al. Liver/kidney microsome antibody type 1 and hepatitis C virus infection. *Hepatology* 1992;16:630–636.

38. Rogler CE, Summers J. Novel forms of woodchuck hepatitis virus DNA isolated from chronically infected woodchuck liver nuclei. *J Virol* 1982;44:852–863.

39. Han KH, Hollinger FB, Noonan CA, et al. Southern-blot analysis and simultaneous in situ detection of hepatitis B virus-associated DNA and antigens in patients with end-stage liver disease. *Hepatology* 1993;18:1032–1038.

40. Bianchi L, Gudat F. Immunopathology of hepatitis B. *Prog Liver Dis* 1979;6:371–392.

41. Wang W, London T, Feitelson MA. Hepatitis B x antigen in hepatitis B virus carrier patients with liver cancer. *Cancer Res* 1991;51:4971–4977.

42. Chu CM, Liaw YF. Membrane staining for hepatitis B surface antigen on hepatocytes: a sensitive and specific marker of active viral replication in hepatitis B. *J Clin Pathol* 1995;48:470–473.

43. Chu CM, Yeh CT, Sheen IS, et al. Subcellular localization of hepatitis B core antigen in relation to hepatocyte regeneration in chronic hepatitis B [see comments]. *Gastroenterology* 1995;109:1926–1932.

44. Farza H, Dragani TA, Metzler T, et al. Inhibition of hepatitis B virus surface antigen gene expression in carcinogen-induced liver tumors from transgenic mice. *Mol Carcinogen* 1994;9:185–192.

45. Chen C, Diani A, Brown P, et al. Detection of hepatitis B virus DNA in hepatocellular carcinoma. *Br J Exp Pathol* 1986;67:1868.

46. Loncarevic I, Schrantz P, Zentgraf H, et al. Replication of hepatitis B virus in a hepatocellular carcinoma. *Virology* 1990;174:158–168.

47. London WT, Blumberg BS. Acellular model of the role of hepatitis virus in the pathogenesis of primary hepatocellular carcinoma. *Hepatology* 1982;2:105–145.

48. Pontisso P, Poon MC, Tiollais P, et al. Detection of HBV DNA in mononuclear blood cells. *Br Med J* 1984;288:1563–1566.

49. Pasquinelli C, Lauré F, Chatenaud L, et al. Hepatitis B virus DNA in mononuclear blood cells. *J Hepatol* 1986;3:95–103.

50. Lauré F, Zaguri D, Saimot A, et al. Hepatitis B virus DNA sequences in lymphoid cells for patients with AIDS and AIDS-related complex. *Science* 1985;229:561–563.

51. Calmus Y, Marcellin P, Beaurain G, et al. Distribution of hepatitis B virus DNA sequences in different peripheral blood mononuclear cells subsets in HBs antigen-positive and negative patients. *Eur J Clin Invest* 1994;75:2393–2398.

52. Yoffe B, Noonan CA, Melnick JL, et al. Hepatitis B virus DNA in mononuclear cells and analysis of cell subsets for the presence of replicative intermediates of viral DNA. *J Infect Dis* 1986;153:471–477.

53. Hadchouel M, Pasquinelli C, Fournier JG, et al. Detection of mononuclear cells expressing hepatitis B virus in peripheral blood from HBsAg positive and negative patients by in situ hybridisation. *J Med Virol* 1988;24:27–32.

54. Kock J, Theilmann L, Galle P, et al. Hepatitis B virus nucleic acids associated with human peripheral blood mononuclear cells do not originate from replicating virus. *Hepatology* 1996;23:405–413.

55. Laskus T, Radkowski M, Wang LF, et al. Detection and sequence analysis of hepatitis B virus integration in peripheral blood mononuclear cells. *J Virol* 1999;73:1235–1238.

56. Baginski I, Chemin I, Bouffard P, et al. Detection of polyadenylated RNA in hepatitis B virus-infected peripheral blood mononuclear cells by polymerase chain reaction. *J Infect Dis* 1991;163:996–1000.

57. Stoll-Becker S, Repp R, Glebe D, et al. Transcription of hepatitis B virus in peripheral blood mononuclear cells from persistently infected patients. *J Virol* 1997;71:5399–5407.

58. Romet-Lemonne JL, McLane MF, Elfassi E, et al. Hepatitis B virus infection in cultured human lymphoblastoid cells. *Science* 1983;221:667–669.

59. Feray C, Zignego A, Samuel D, et al. Persistent hepatitis B virus infection of mononuclear blood cells without concomitant liver infection: the liver transplantation model. *Transplantation* 1990;49:1155–1158.

60. Brind A, Jiang J, Samuel D, et al. Evidence for selection of hepatitis B mutants after liver transplantation through peripheral blood mononuclear cell infection. *J Hepatol* 1997;26:228–235.

61. Galun E, Ilan Y, Livni N, et al. Hepatitis B virus infection associated with hematopoietic tumors. *Am J Pathol* 1994;145:1001–1007.

62. Steinberg HS, Bouffard P, Trépo C, et al. In vitro inhibition of hemopoietic cell line growth by hepatitis B virus. *J Hepatol* 1990;64:2577–2581.

63. Dejean A, Lugassi C, Zafrani S, et al. Detection of hepatitis B virus DNA in pancreas, kidney and skin of two human carriers of the virus. *J Gen Virol* 1984;65:651–655.

64. Tagieva NE, Gizatullin RZ, Zakharyev VM, et al. A genome-integrated hepatitis B virus DNA in human neuroblastoma. *Gene* 1995;152:277–278.

65. Hosoda K, Omata M, Uchiumi K, et al. Extrahepatic replication of duck hepatitis B virus: more than expected. *Hepatology* 1990;11:44–48.

66. Hadchouel M, Scotto J, Huset CEA. Presence of HBV DNA in spermatozoa—a possible vertical transmission of HBV via the germ line. *J Med Virol* 1985;16:61–66.

67. Buendia M, Paterlini P, Tiollais P, et al. Hepatocellular carcinoma: molecular aspects. In: Zuckerman A, Thomas H, eds. *Viral hepatitis*. London: Churchill Livingstone, 1998:179–200.

68. Aoki H, Kajino K, Arakawa Y, et al. Molecular cloning of a rat chromosome putative recombinogenic sequence homologous to the hepatitis B virus encapsidation signal. *Proc Natl Acad Sci USA* 1996;93:7300–7304.

69. Ozturk M. Genetic aspects of hepatocellular carcinogenesis. *Semin Liver Dis* 1999;19:235–242.

70. Buetow KH, Sheffield VC, Zhu M, et al. Low frequency of p53 mutations observed in a diverse collection of primary hepatocellular carcinomas. *Proc Natl Acad Sci USA* 1992;89:9622–9626.

71. Debuire B, Paterlini P, Pontisso P, et al. Analysis of the p53 gene in European hepatocellular carcinomas and hepatoblastomas. *Oncogene* 1993;8:2303–2306.

72. Aguilar F, Harris CC, Sun T, et al. Geographic variation of p53 mutational profile in nonmalignant human liver. *Science* 1994;264:1317–1319.

73. Urano Y, Watanabe K, Lin C, et al. Interstitial chromosomal deletion within 4q11-q13 in a human hepatoma cell line. *Cancer Res* 1991;51:1460–1464.

74. Wang HP, Rogler CE. Deletions in human chromosome arms 11p and 13 p in primary hepatocellular carcinomas. *Science* 1988;48:72.

75. Fujimoto Y, Hampton LL, Wirth PJ, et al. Alterations of tumor suppressor genes and allelic losses in human hepatocellular carcinomas in China. *Cancer Res* 1994;54:281–285.

76. Murakami Y, Hayashi K, Hirohashi S, et al. Aberrations of tumor suppressor p53 and retinoblastoma genes in human hepatocellular carcinomas. *Cancer Res* 1991;51:5520–5525.

77. Nishida N, Fukuda Y, Kokuryu H, et al. Role and mutational heterogeneity of the p53 gene in hepatocellular carcinoma. *Cancer Res* 1993;53:368–372.

78. Tokino T, Fukushige S, Nakamura T, et al. Chromosomal translocation and inverted duplication associated with integrated hepatitis B virus in hepatocellular carcinomas. *J Virol* 1987;61:3848–3854.

79. Yeh S-H, Chen P-J, Chen H-L, et al. Frequent genetic alter-

ations at the distal region of chromosome 1p in human hepato-cellular carcinomas. *Cancer Res* 1994;54:4188–4192.

80. Pineau P, Marchio A, Terris B, et al. A t(3;8) chromosomal translocation associated with hepatitis B virus integration involves the carboxypeptidase N locus. *J Virol* 1996;70: 7280–7284.

81. Pineau P, Marchio A, Mattei MG, et al. Extensive analysis of duplicated-inverted hepatitis B virus integrations in human hepatocellular carcinoma. *J Gen Virol* 1998;79:591–600.

82. Choo KB, Liu MS, Chang PC, et al. Analysis of six distinct integrated hepatitis B virus sequences cloned from the cellular DNA of a human hepatocellular carcinoma. *Virology* 1986;154: 405–408.

83. Fowler MJF, Thomas HC, Monjardino J. Cloning and analysis of integrated hepatitis B virus DNA of the adr suntype derived from a human primary liver cell carcinoma. *J Gen Virol* 1986; 61:771–775.

84. Caselmann WH, Meyer M, Kekulé AS, et al. A trans-activator function is generated by integration of hepatitis B virus pre-S/S sequences in human hepatocellular carcinoma DNA. *Proc Natl Acad Sci USA* 1990;87:2970–2974.

85. Quade K, Saldanha J, Thomas H, et al. Integration of hepatitis B virus DNA through a mutational hot spot within the cohesive regio in a case of hepatocellular carcinoma. *J Gen Virol* 1992;73:179–182.

86. Tsuei DJ, Chen PJ, Lai MY, et al. Inverse polymerase chain reaction for cloning cellular sequences adjacent to integrated hepatitis B virus DNA in hepatocellular carcinomas. *J Virol Methods* 1994;49:269–284.

87. Hatada I, Tokino T, Ochiya T, et al. Co-amplification of integrated hepatitis B virus DNA and transforming gene hst-1 in a hepatocellular carcinoma. *Oncogene* 1988;3:537–540.

88. Schluter V, Meyer M, Hofschneider PH, et al. Integrated hepatitis B virus X and 3′ truncated preS/S sequences derived from human hepatomas encode functionally active transactivators. *Oncogene* 1994;9:3335–3344.

89. Unsal H, Yakicier C, Marçais C, et al. Genetic heterogeneity of hepatocellular carcinoma. *Proc Natl Acad Sci USA* 1994;91: 822–826.

90. Paterlini P, Poussin K, Kew MC, et al. Selective accumulation of the X transcript of hepatitis B virus in patients negative for hepatitis B surface antigen with hepatocellular carcinoma. *Hepatology* 1993;21:313–321.

91. Kairat A, Beerheide W, Zhou G, et al. Truncated hepatitis B virus RNA in human hepatocellular carcinoma: its representation in patients with advancing age. *Intervirology* 1999;42: 228–237.

92. Su Q, Schröder CH, Hofmann W, et al. Expression of hepatitis B virus X protein in HBV-infected human livers and hepatocellular carcinoma. *Hepatology* 1998;27:1109–1120.

93. Poussin K, Diennes H, Sirma H, et al. Expression of mutated hepatitis B virus X gene in human hepatocellular carcinomas. *Int J Cancer* 1999;80:497–505.

94. Jacob JR, Ascenzi MA, Roneker CA, et al. Hepatic expression of the woodchuck hepatitis virus X-antigen during acute and chronic infection and detection of a woodchuck hepatitis X-antigen antibody response. *Hepatology* 1997;26:1607–1615.

95. Yen TSB. Hepadnaviral X protein: review of recent progress. *J Biomed Sci* 1996;3:20–30.

96. Murakami S. Hepatitis B virus X protein: structure, function and biology. *Intervirology* 1999;42:81–99.

97. Klein NP, Bouchard MJ, Wang LH, et al. Src kinases involved in hepatitis B virus replication. *EMBO J* 1999;18:5019–5027.

98. Chen H, Kaneko S, Girones R, et al. The woodchuck hepatitis virus X gene is important for establishment of virus infection in woodchucks. *J Virol* 1993;67:1218–1226.

99. Zoulim F, Saputelli J, Seeger C. Woodchuck hepatitis virus X protein is required for viral infection in vivo. *J Virol* 1994;68: 2026–2030.

100. Reifenberg K, Wilts H, Lohler J, et al. The hepatitis B virus X protein transactivates viral core gene expression in vivo. *J Virol* 1999;73:10399–10405.

101. Koike K, Moriya H, Yotsuyanagi H, et al. Induction of cell cycle progression by hepatitis B virus HBx gene expression in quiescent mouse fibroblasts. *J Clin Invest* 1994;94:44–49.

102. Benn J, Schneider RJ. Hepatitis B virus HBx protein deregulates cell cycle checkpoint controls. *Biochemistry* 1995;92: 11215–11219.

103. Hohne M, Schaeffer S, Seifer M, et al. Malignant transformation of immortalized transgenic hepatocytes after transfection with hepatitis B virus DNA. *EMBO J* 1990;9:1137–1145.

104. Shirakata Y, Kawada M, Fujiki Y, et al. The X gene of hepatitis B virus induced growth stimulation and tumorigenic transformation of mouse NIH3T3 cells. *Jpn J Cancer Res* 1989;80: 617–621.

105. Kim C-M, Koike K, Saito I, et al. HBx gene of hepatitis B virus induces liver cancer in transgenic mice. *Nature* 1991;351: 317–320.

106. Yu DY, Moon HB, Son JK, et al. Incidence of hepatocellular carcinoma in transgenic mice expressing the hepatitis B virus X-protein. *J Hepatol* 1999;31:123–132.

107. Lee T-H, Finegold MJ, Shen R-F, et al. Hepatitis B virus transactivator X protein is not tumorigenic in transgenic mice. *J Virol* 1990;64:5939–5947.

108. Slagle B, Lee T, Medina D, et al. Increased sensitivity to the hepatocarcinogen diethylnitrosamine in transgenic mice carrying the hepatitis B virus X gene. *Mol Carcinogen* 1996;15: 261–269.

109. Terradillos O, Billet O, Renard CA, et al. The hepatitis B virus X gene potentiates c-myc induced liver oncogenesis in transgenic mice. *Oncogene* 1997;14:395–404.

110. Lara-Pezzi E, Majano PL, Gomez-Gonzalo M, et al. The hepatitis B virus X protein up-regulates tumor necrosis factor alpha gene expression in hepatocytes. *Hepatology* 1998;28: 1013–1021.

111. Yoo YD, Ueda H, Park K, et al. Regulation of transforming growth factor-beta 1 expression by the hepatitis B virus (HBV) X transactivator. *J Clin Invest* 1996;97:388–395.

112. Rossner MT. Hepatitis B virus X-gene product: a promiscuous transcriptional activator (review). *J Med Virol* 1992;36: 101–117.

113. Cheong JH, Yi MK, Lin Y, et al. Human RPB5, a subunit shared by eukaryotic nuclear RNA polymerases, binds human hepatitis B virus X protein and may play a role in X transactivation. *EMBO J* 1995;14:143–150.

114. Quadri I, Maguire HF, Siddiqui A. Hepatitis B virus transactivator protein X interacts with the TATA-binding protein. *Proc Natl Acad Sci USA* 1995;92:1003–1007.

115. Maguire HF, Hoeffler JP, Siddiqui A. HBV X protein alters the DNA binding specificity of CREB and ATF-2 by protein-protein interactions. *Science* 1991;252:842–844.

116. Klein NP, Schneider RJ. Activation of Src family kinases by hepatitis B virus HBx protein coupled signaling to ras. *Mol Cell Biol* 1997;17:6427–6436.

117. Benn J, Schneider RJ. Hepatitis B virus HBx protein activates Ras-GTP complex formation and establishes a Ras, MAP kinase signaling cascade. *Proc Natl Acad Sci USA* 1994;91: 10350–10354.

118. Benn J, Su F, Doria M, et al. Hepatitis B virus HBx protein induces transcription factor AP-1 by activation of extracellular signal-regulated and c-Jun N-terminal mitogen-activated protein kinases. *J Virol* 1996;70:4978–4985.

119. Lee YH, Yun Y. HBx protein of hepatitis B virus activates Jak1-STAT signaling. *J Biol Chem* 1998;273:25510–25515.

120. Kekulé AS, Lauer U, Weiss L, et al. Hepatitis B virus transactivator HBx uses a tumor promoter signalling pathway. *Nature* 1993;361:742–745.

121. Doria M, Klein N, Lucito R, et al. The hepatitis B virus HBx protein is a dual specificity cytoplasmic activator of Ras and nuclear activator of transcription factors. *EMBO J* 1995;15:4747–4757.

122. Sirma H, Weil R, Rosmorduc O, et al. Cytosol is the prime compartment of hepatitis B virus where it colocalizes with the proteasome. *Oncogene* 1998;16:2051–2063.

123. Chirillo P, Falco M, Puri PL, et al. Hepatitis B virus pX activates NF-κB dependent transcription through a Raf-independent pathway. *J Virol* 1996;70:641–646.

124. Lara-Pezzi E, Armesilla A, Majano P, et al. The hepatitis B virus X protein activates nuclear factor of activated T cells (NF-AT) by a cyclosporin A-sensitive pathway. *EMBO J* 1998;17:7066–7077.

125. Weil R, Sirma H, Giannini C, et al. Direct association and nuclear import of the hepatitis B virus X protein with the NF-cB inhibitor IcBa. *Mol Cell Biol* 1999;19:6345–6354.

126. Fischer M, Runkel L, Schaller H. HBx protein of hepatitis B virus interacts with the C-terminal portion of a novel human proteasome alpha-subunit. *Virus Genes* 1995;10:99–102.

127. Hu Z, Zhang Z, Doo E, et al. Hepatitis B virus X protein is both a substrate and a potential inhibitor of the proteasome complex [In Process Citation]. *J Virol* 1999;73:7231–7240.

128. Lee TH, Elledge SJ, Butel JS. Hepatitis B virus X protein interacts with a probable cellular DNA repair protein. *J Virol* 1995;69:1107–1114.

129. Groisman IJ, Koshy R, Henkler F, et al. Downregulation of DNA excision repair by the hepatitis B virus-x protein occurs in p53-proficient and p53-deficient cells. *Carcinogenesis* 1999;20:479–483.

130. Sitterlin D, Lee TH, Prigent S, et al. Interaction of the UV-damaged DNA-binding protein with hepatitis B virus X protein is conserved among mammalian hepadnaviruses and restricted to transactivation-proficient X-insertion mutants. *J Virol* 1997;71:6194–6199.

131. Lian Z, Pan J, Liu J, et al. The translation initiation factor, hu-Sui1 may be a target of hepatitis B X antigen in hepatocarcinogenesis. *Oncogene* 1999;18:1677–1687.

132. Sun B, Zhu X, Clayton M, et al. Identification of a protein isolated from senescent human cells that binds to hepatitis B virus X antigen. *Hepatology* 1998;27:228–239.

133. Feitelson MA, Zhu M, Duan L-X, et al. Hepatitis B x antigen and p53 are associated in vitro and in liver tissues from patients with primary hepatocellular carcinoma. *Oncogene* 1993;8:1109–1117.

134. Truant R, Antunovic J, Greenblatt J, et al. Direct interaction of the hepatitis B virus HBx protein with p53 leads to inhibition by HBx of p53 response element directed transactivation. *J Virol* 1995;69:1851–1859.

135. Wang LD, Shi ST, Zhou Q, et al. Changes in p53 and cyclin D1 protein levels and cell proliferation in different stages of human esophageal and gastric-cardiac carcinogenesis. *Int J Cancer* 1994;59:514–519.

136. Takada S, Kaneniwa N, Tsuchida N, et al. Cytoplasmic retention of the p53 tumor suppressor gene product is observed in the hepatitis B virus X gene-transfected cells. *Oncogene* 1997;15:1895–1901.

137. Unsal H, Yakicier C, Marçais C, et al. Genetic heterogeneity of hepatocellular carcinoma. *Proc Natl Acad Sci USA* 1994;91:822–826.

138. Saeki R, Jaffredo F, Takamatsu M, et al. The possible role of

HBV infection in molecular mechanisms of HCV-related hepatocarcinogenesis in Japan. In: IX Triennial International Symposium on Viral Hepatitis and Liver Disease, Rome, Italy, 1996.

139. Oguey D, Dumenco LL, Pierce RH, et al. Analysis of tumorigenicity of the X gene of hepatitis B virus in nontransformed hepatocyte cell line and the effect of cotransfection with a murine p53 mutant equivalent to human codon 249. *Hepatology* 1996;24:1024–1033.

140. Kim H, Lee H, Yun Y. X-gene product of hepatitis B virus induces apoptosis in liver cells. *J Biol Chem* 1998;273:381–385.

141. Sirma H, Giannini C, Poussin K, et al. Abrogation of cell cycle arrest and apoptosis induced by hepatitis B virus x protein by mutations present in hepatocellular carcinoma tissues. *Oncogene* 1999;18:4848–4859.

142. Chirillo P, Pagano S, Natoli G, et al. The hepatitis B virus X gene induces p53-mediated programmed cell death. *Proc Natl Acad Sci USA* 1997;94:8162–8167.

143. Terradillos O, Pollicino T, Lecoeur H, et al. p-53–independent apoptotic effects of the hepatitis B virus HBx protein in vivo and in vitro. *Oncogene* 1998;17:2115–2123.

144. Shintani Y, Yotsuyanagi H, Moriya K, et al. Induction of apoptosis after switch-on of the hepatitis B virus X gene mediated by the Cre/loxP recombination system. *J Gen Virol* 1999;80:3257–3265.

145. Su F, Schneider RJ. Hepatitis B virus HBx protein sensitizes cells to apoptotic killing by tumor necrosis factor a. *Proc Natl Acad Sci USA* 1997;94:8744–8749.

146. Elmore LW, Hancock AR, Chang SF, et al. Hepatitis B virus X protein and p53 tumor suppressor interactions in the modulation of apoptosis. *Proc Natl Acad Sci USA* 1997;94:14707–14712.

147. Takada S, Shirakata Y, Kaneniwa N, et al. Association of hepatitis B virus X protein with mitochondria causes mitochondrial aggregation at the nuclear periphery, leading to cell death. *Oncogene* 1999;18:6965–6973.

148. Shin E, Shin J, Park J, et al. Expression of fas ligand in human hepatoma cell lines: role of hepatitis-B virus X (HBX) in induction of Fas ligand. *Int J Cancer* 1999;4:587–591.

149. Gottlob K, Fulco M, Levrero M, et al. The hepatitis B virus HBx protein inhibits caspase 3 activity. *J Biol Chem* 1998;273:33347–33353.

150. Tarn C, Bilodeau ML, Hullinger RL, et al. Differential immediate early gene expression in conditional hepatitis B virus pX-transforming versus nontransforming hepatocyte cell lines. *J Biol Chem* 1999;274:2327–2336.

151. Mymryk JS. Tumour suppressive properties of the adenovirus 5 E1A oncogene. *Oncogene* 1996;13:1581–1589.

152. Goodwin EC, Naeger LK, Breiding DE, et al. Transactivation-competent bovine papillomavirus E2 protein is specifically required for efficient repression of human papillomavirus oncogene expression and acute growth inhibition of cervical carcinoma cell lines. *J Virol* 1998;72:3925–3934.

153. Chlichia K, Moldenhauer G, Daniel PT, et al. Immediate effects of reversible HTLV-1 tax function: T-cell activation and apoptosis. *Oncogene* 1995;10:269–277.

154. Ozer A, Khaoustov VI, Mearns M, et al. Effect of hepatocyte proliferation and cellular DNA synthesis on hepatitis B virus replication. *Gastroenterology* 1996;110:1519–1528.

155. Goulaoui H, Subra F, Mouscaded JF, et al. Exogenous nucleosides promote the completion of MoMLV DNA synthesis in G0-arrested Balb c/3T3 fibroblasts. *Virology* 1994;200:87–97.

156. Hsia CC, Nakashima Y, Tabor E. Deletion mutants of the hepatitis B virus X gene in human hepatocellular carcinoma. *Biochem Biophys Res Commun* 1997;241:726–729.

157. Bergametti F, Prigent S, Luber B, et al. The proapoptotic effect of hepatitis B virus HBx protein correlates with its transactiva-

tion activity in stably transfected cell lines. *Oncogene* 1999;18: 2860–2871.

158. Gottlob K, Pagano S, Levrero M, et al. Hepatitis B virus X protein transcription activation domains are neither required nor sufficient for cell transformation. *Cancer Res* 1998;58: 3566–3570.

159. Hildt E, Urban S, Lauer U, et al. ER-localization and functional expression of the HBV transactivator MHBs. *Oncogene* 1993;8: 3359–3367.

160. Lauer U, Weib L, Lipp M, et al. The hepatitis B virus PreS2/ST transactivation utilizes AP-1 and transcription factors for transactivation. *Hepatology* 1994;19:23–31.

161. Luber B, Arnold N, Stürzl M, et al. Hepatoma-derived integrated HBV DNA causes multi-stage transformation in vitro. *Oncogene* 1996;12:1597–1608.

162. Buendia MA. Hepatitis B viruses and hepatocellular carcinoma. *Adv Cancer Res* 1992;59:167–226.

163. Buendia MA, Paterlini P, Tiollais P, et al. Liver cancer. In: Zuckerman AJ, Thomas HC, ed. *Viral hepatitis: scientific basis and clinical management*. London: Churchill Livingstone, 1993: 137–164.

164. Buendia MA. Animal models for hepatitis B virus and liver cancer. In: Christian B, ed. *Primary liver cancer: etiological and progression factors*. Paris: CRC Press, 1994:211–224.

165. Etiemble J, Degott C, Renard CA, et al. Liver-specific expression and high oncogenic efficiency of a c-myc transgene activated by woodchuck hepatitis virus insertion. *Oncogene* 1994;9: 727–737.

166. Fourel G, Tiollais P, Buendia MA. Nucleotide sequence of the woodchuck N-myc gene (WN-myc1). *Nucleic Acids Res* 1990; 18:4918.

167. Fourel G, Trépo C, Bougueleret L, et al. Frequent activation of N-myc genes by hepatdnavirus insertion in woodchuck liver tumors. *Nature* 1990;347:294–298.

168. Dejean A, Bougueleret L, Grzeschik KH, et al. Hepatitis B virus DNA integration in a sequence homologous to v-erbA and steroid receptor genes in a hepatocellular carcinoma. *Nature* 1986;322:70–72.

169. Dejean A, De Thé H. Hepatitis B virus as an insertional mutagen in a human hepatocellular carcinoma. *Mol Biol Med* 1990; 7:213–222.

170. De Thé H, Chomienne C, Lanotte M, et al. The t(15;17) translocation of acute promyelocytic leukemia fuses the retinoic acid receptor alpha gene to a novel transcribed locus. *Nature* 1990;347:558–561.

171. De Thé H, Lavau C, Marchio A, et al. The PML-RAR-alpha fusion mRNA generated by the t(15,17) translocation in acute promyelocytic leukaemia encodes a functionally altered retinoic acid receptor. *Cell* 1991;66:675–684.

172. Wang J, Chenivesse X, Henglein B, et al. Hepatitis B virus integration in a cyclin A gene in a hepatocellular carcinoma. *Nature* 1990;343:555–557.

173. Desdouets C, Sobczak-Thepot J, Murphy M, et al. Cyclin A: function and expression during cell proliferation. *Prog Cell Cycle Res* 1995;1:115–123.

174. Murphy M, Stinnakre MG, Senamaud-Beaufort C, et al. Delayed early embryonic lethality following disruption of the murine cyclin A2 gene. *Nat Genet* 1997;15:83–86.

175. Wang J, Zindy F, Chenivesse X, et al. Modification of cyclin A expression by hepatitis b virus DNA integration in a hepatocellular carcinoma. *Oncogene* 1992;7:1653–1656.

176. Berasain C, Patil D, Perara E, et al. Oncogenic activation of a human cyclin A2 targeted to the endoplasmic reticulum upon hepatitis B virus genome insertion. *Oncogene* 1998;16: 1277–1288.

177. Graef E, Caselmann W, Wells J, et al. Enzymatic properties of

over-expressed HBV-mevalonate fusion proteins and mevalonate kinase proteins in the human hepatoma cell line PLC/PRF/5. *Virology* 1995;208:696–703.

178. Chami M, Gozuacik D, Saigo K, et al. New SERCA1 transcripts are revealed by hepatitis B virus-revealed by hepatitis B virus-related SERCA1 gene mutagenesis in a human hepatocellular carcinoma and control cell variability. *J Cell Biol* 2000; *in press*.

179. Zhang XK, Egan JO, Huang DP, et al. Hepatitis B virus DNA integration and expression of an Erb B-like gene in human hepatocellular carcinoma. *Biochem Biophys Res Commun* 1992; 188:344–351.

180. Petersen J, Dandri M, Burkle A, et al. Increase in the frequency of hepadnavirus DNA integrations by oxidative DNA damage and inhibition of DNA repair. *J Virol* 1997;71:5455–5463.

181. Fourel G, Couturier J, Wei Y, et al. Evidence for long-range oncogene activation by hepadnavirus insertion. *EMBO J* 1994; 13:2526–2534.

182. Minami M, Poussin K, Bréchot C, et al. A novel PCR technique using Alu specific primers to identify unknown flanking sequences from the human genome. *Genomics* 1995;2:403–408.

183. Li J, Shen H, Himmel K, et al. Leukemia disease genes: large-scale cloning and pathway predictions. *Nat Genet* 1999;23: 348–353.

184. Sanchez-Prieto R, de Alava E, Palomino T, et al. An association between viral genes and human oncogenic alterations: the adenovirus E1A induces the Ewing tumor fusion transcript EWS-FLI1 [see comments]. *Nat Med* 1999;5:1076–1079.

185. Bréchot C, Kremsdorf D, Paterlini P, et al. Hepatitis B virus DNA in HBsAg-negative patients. Molecular characterization and clinical implications. *J Hepatol* 1991;13:S49–S55.

186. Carman W, Thomas H, Domingo E. Viral genetic variation—hepatitis-B virus as a clinical example. *Lancet* 1993;341: 349–353.

187. Brunetto M, Rodriguez U, Bonino F. Hepatitis B virus mutants. *Intervirology* 1999;42:69–80.

188. Zuckerman AJ, Zuckerman JN. Molecular epidemiology of hepatitis B virus mutants. *J Med Virol* 1999;58:193–195.

189. Feitelson AM, Dunan LX, Guo J, et al. X region deletion variants of hepatitis B virus in surface antigen-negative infections and non-A, non-B hepatitis. *J Infect Dis* 1995;172:713–722.

190. Minami M, Poussin K, Kew M, et al. Precore/Core mutations of hepatitis B virus in hepatocellular carcinomas developed on noncirrhotic livers. *Gastroenterology* 1996;111:691–700.

191. Protzer-Knolle U, Naumann U, Bartenschlager R, et al. Hepatitis B virus with antigenically altered hepatitis B surface antigen is selected by high-dose hepatitis B immune globulin after liver transplantation [see comments]. *Hepatology* 1998;27:254–263.

192. Locarnini SA. Hepatitis B virus surface antigen and polymerase gene variants: potential virological and clinical significance [editorial; comment]. *Hepatology* 1998;27:294–297.

193. Hsu HY, Chang MH, Ni YH, et al. Surface gene mutants of hepatitis B virus in infants who develop acute or chronic infections despite immunoprophylaxis. *Hepatology* 1997;26: 786–791.

194. Hasegawa K, Huang J, Rogers SA, et al. Enhanced replication of a hepatitis B mutant associated with an epidemic of fulminant hepatitis. *J Virol* 1994;68:1651–1659.

195. Stuyver L, De Gendt S, Cadranel JF, et al. Three cases of severe subfulminant hepatitis in heart-transplanted patients after nosocomial transmission of a mutant hepatitis B virus. *Hepatology* 1999;29:1876–1883.

196. Gunther S, Li BC, Miska S, et al. A novel method for efficient amplification of whole hepatitis B virus genomes permits rapid functional analysis and reveals deletion mutants in immunosuppressed patients. *J Virol* 1995;69:5437–5444.

197. Loncarevic IF, Zentgraf H, Schröder CH. Sequence of a repli-

cation competent hepatitis B virus genome with a preX open reading frame. *Nucleic Acids Res* 1990;18:4940.

198. Chang PC, Hu CP, Chen SH, et al. Deletion of integrated hepatitis B virus genome and cellular flanking sequences in hepatocellular carcinoma cells in BALB/c mice. *Hepatology* 1995;21:1504–1509.

199. Clementi M, Manzin A, Paolucci S, et al. Hepatitis B virus preC mutants in human hepatocellular carcinoma tissues. *Res Virol* 1993;144:297–301.

200. Minami M, Poussin K, Kew M, et al. Precore/core mutations of hepatitis B virus in hepatocellular carcinomas developed on noncirrhotic livers. *Gastroenterology* 1996;111:691–700.

201. Koziel MJ. Cytokines in viral hepatitis. *Semin Liver Dis* 1999;19:157–169.

202. Guidotti LG, Rochford R, Chung J, et al. Viral clearance without destruction of infected cells during acute HBV infection. *Science* 1999;284:825–829.

203. Guidotti LG, Borrow P, Brown A, et al. Noncytopathic clearance of lymphocytic choriomeningitis virus from the hepatocyte. *J Exp Med* 1999;189:1555–1564.

204. Romero R, Lavine JE. Cytokine inhibition of the hepatitis B virus core promoter. *Hepatology* 1996;23:17–23.

205. Zheng Y-W, Benedict Yens TS. Negative regulation of hepatitis B virus gene expression and replication by oxidative stress. *J Biol Chem* 1994;269:8857–8862.

206. Schultz U, Summers J, Staeheli P, et al. Elimination of duck hepatitis B virus RNA-containing capsids in duck interferon-alpha-treated hepatocytes. *J Virol* 1999;73:5459–5465.

207. Rosmorduc O, Sirma H, Soussan P, et al. Inhibition of the expression of Interferon inducible MxA protein by the hepatitis B virus capsid protein. *J Gen Virol* 1999;80:1253–1262.

208. Terré S, Petit MA, Bréchot C. Defective hepatitis B virus particles are generated by packaging and reverse transcription of spliced viral RNAs *in vivo. J Virol* 1991;65:5539–5543.

209. Soussan P, Garreau F, Zylberberg H, et al. In vivo expression of a new hepatitis B virus protein encoded by a spliced RNA. *J Clin Invest* 2000;105:55–60.

210. Rosmorduc O, Petit MA, Pol S, et al. In vivo and in vitro expression of defective hepatitis B virus particles generated by spliced hepatitis B virus RNA. *Hepatology* 1995;22:10–19.

211. Bréchot C, Hadchouel J, Scotto M, et al. State of hepatitis B virus DNA in hepatocytes of patients with HbsAg positive and HbsAg negative liver diseases. *Proc Natl Acad Sci USA* 1981;78:3906–3910.

212. Bréchot C, Degos F, Lugassy C, et al. Hepatitis B virus DNA in patients with chronic liver disease and negative tests for hepatitis B surface antigen. *N Engl J Med* 1985;312:270–276.

213. Rehermann B, Ferrari C, Pasquinelli C, et al. The hepatitis B virus persists for decades after patients' recovery from acute viral hepatitis despite active maintenance of a cytotoxic T-lymphocyte response. *Nat Med* 1996;2:1104–1108.

214. Marusawa H, Uemoto S, Hijikata M, et al. Latent hepatitis B virus infection in healthy individuals with antibodies to hepatitis B core antigen. *Hepatology* 2000;31:488–495.

215. Wands JR, Fujita YK, Isselbacher KJ, et al. Identification and transmission of a hepatitis B virus-related variant. *Proc Natl Acad Sci USA* 1986;83:6608–6612.

216. Thiers V, Nakajima E, Kremsdorf D, et al. Transmission of hepatitis from hepatitis-B-seronegative subjects. *Lancet* 1988;2:1273–1276.

217. Baginski I, Chemin I, Hantz O. Transmission of serologically silent hepatitis B virus along with hepatitis C virus in two cases of posttransfusion hepatitis. *Transfusion* 1992;32:215–220.

218. Chazouillères O, Mamish D, Kim M, et al. "Occult" hepatitis B virus as source of infection in liver transplant recipients. *Lancet* 1994;343:142–146.

219. Michalak TI, Pasquinelli C, Guillot S, et al. Hepatitis B virus persistence after recovery from acute viral hepatitis. *J Clin Invest* 1994;93:230–239.

220. Mason A, Xu L, Guo L, et al. Molecular basis for persistent hepatitis B virus infection in the liver after clearance of serum hepatitis B surface antigen. *Hepatology* 1998;6:1736–1742.

221. Huo TI, Wu JC, Lee PC, et al. Sero-clearance of hepatitis B surface antigen in chronic carriers does not necessarily imply a good prognosis [see comments]. *Hepatology* 1998;28:231–236.

222. Mac Mahon B. Chronic carriers of hepatitis B virus who clear hepatitis B surface antigen: are they really "off the hook"? *Hepatology* 1998;28:265–267.

223. Loriot MA, Marcellin P, Walker F, et al. Persistence of hepatitis B virus DNA in serum and liver from patients with chronic hepatitis B after loss of HBsAg. *J Hepatol* 1997;27:251–258.

224. Shafritz DA, Lieberman HM, Isselbacher KJ, et al. Monoclonal radioimmunoassay for hepatitis B surface antigen: demonstration of hepatitis B virus DNA or related sequences in serum and viral epitopes in immune complexes. *Proc Natl Acad Sci USA* 1982;79:5675.

225. Pol S, Thiers V, Nalpas B, et al. Monoclonal anti-HBs antibodies radioimmunoassay and serum HBV-DNA hybridization as diagnostic tools of HBV infection: relative prevalence among HBsAg-negative alcoholics, patients with chronic hepatitis or hepatocellular carcinomas and blood donors. *Eur J Clin Invest* 1987;17:515–521.

226. Grethe S, Monazahian M, Bohme I, et al. Characterization of unusual escape variants of hepatitis B virus isolated from a hepatitis B surface antigen-negative subject. *J Virol* 1998;72:7692–7696.

227. Kato J, Hasegawa K, Torii N, et al. A molecular analysis of viral persistence in surface antigen-negative chronic hepatitis B. *Hepatology* 1996;23:389–395.

228. Kremsdorf D, Garreau F, Duclos H, et al. Complete nucleotide sequence and viral envelope protein expression of a hepatitis B virus DNA derived from a hepatitis B surface antigen seronegative patient. *J Hepatology* 1993;18:244–250.

229. Cacciola I, Pollicino T, Squadrito G, et al. Quantification of intrahepatic hepatitis B virus (HBV) DNA in patients with chronic HBV infection. *Hepatology* 2000;31:507–512.

230. Uchida T, Gotoch K, Shikata T. Complete nucleotide sequences and the characteristics of two hepatitis B virus mutants causing serologically negative acute or chronic hepatitis B. *J Med Virol* 1995;45:247–252.

231. Preisler Adams S, Schlayer HJ, Peters T, et al. Sequence analysis of hepatitis B virus DNA in immunologically negative infection. *Arch Virol* 1993;133:385–396.

232. Ganne-Carrié N, Kremsdorf D, Garreau F, et al. Effects of ethanol on hepatitis B virus pre-S/S gene expression in the human hepatocellular carcinoma derived HepG2 hepatitis B DNA positive cell line. *J Hepatol* 1995;23:153–159.

233. Paterlini P, Poussin K, Kew M, et al. Selective accumulation of the X transcript of hepatitis B virus in patients negative for hepatitis B surface antigen with hepatocellular carcinoma. *Hepatology* 1995;21:313–321.

234. Sugawara Y, Makuuchi M, Takada K. Detection of hepatitis B virus DNA in tissues of hepatocellular carcinomas related to hepatitis C virus which are negative for hepatitis B virus surface antigen. *Scand J Gastroenterol* 1999;34:934–938.

235. Tamori A, Nishiguchi S, Kubo S, et al. Possible contribution to hepatocarcinogenesis of X transcript of hepatitis B virus in Japanese patients with hepatitis C virus. *Hepatology* 1999;29:1429–1434.

236. Urashima T, Saigo K, Kobayashi S, et al. Identification of hepatitis B virus integration in hepatitis C virus-infected hepatocellular carcinoma tissues. *J Hepatology* 1997;26:771–778.

237. Shibata Y, Nakata K, Tsuruta S, et al. Detection of hepatitis B virus X-region DNA in liver tissue from patients with hepatitis C virus-associated cirrhosis who subsequently developed hepatocellular carcinoma. *Int J Oncol* 1999;14:1153–1156.

238. Fukuda R, Ishimura N, Niigaki M, et al. Serologically silent hepatitis B virus coinfection in patients with hepatitis C virus-associated chronic liver disease: clinical and virological significance. *J Med Virol* 1999;58:201–207.

239. Koike K, Kobayashi M, Gondo M, et al. Hepatitis B virus DNA is frequently found in liver biopsy samples from hepatitis C virus-infected chronic hepatitis patients. *J Med Virol* 1998;54: 249–255.

240. Shiratori Y, Shiina S, Zhang PY, et al. Does dual infection by hepatitis B and C viruses play an important role in the pathogenesis of hepatocellular carcinoma in Japan? *Cancer* 1997;80: 2060–2067.

241. Matsui H, Shiba R, Matsuzaki Y, et al. Direct detection of hepatitis B virus gene integrated in the Alexander cell using fluorescence in situ polymerase chain reaction. *Cancer Lett* 1997; 116:259–264.

242. Coursaget P, Le Cann P, Lebouleux D, et al. Detection of hepatitis B virus DNA by polymerase chain reaction in HBsAg negative Senegalese patients suffering from cirrhosis or primary liver cancer. *FEBS Microbiol Lett* 1991;67:35–38.

243. Dazza MC, Meneses LV, Girard PM, et al. Polymerase chain reaction for detection of hepatitis B virus DNA in HBsAg seronegative patients with hepatocellular carcinoma from Mozambique. *Ann Trop Med Parasitol* 1991;85:277–279.

244. Bréchot C. Molecular mechanisms of hepatitis B and C viruses related liver carcinogenesis. In: Rizzetto M, Purcell RH, Gerin JL, et al., eds. *Viral hepatitis and liver disease*. Rome: Edizioni Minerva Medica, 1998:490–508.

245. Paterlini P, Driss F, Pisi E, et al. Persistence of hepatitis B and hepatitis C viral genomes in primary liver cancers from HBsAg negative patients: a study of a low endemic area. *Hepatology* 1993;17:20–29.

246. Chazouillères O, Mamish D, Kim M. "Occult" hepatitis B virus as source of infection in liver transplant recipients. *Lancet* 1994; 343:142–146.

247. Gerin JL, Cote PJ, Korba BE, et al. Hepatitis B virus and liver cancer: the woodchuck as an experimental model of hepadnavirus-induced liver cancer. In: Hollinger FB, Lemon SM, Margolis H, eds. *Viral hepatitis and liver disease*. Baltimore: Williams & Wilkins, 1991:556–559.

248. Korba BE, Wells FV, Baldwin B, et al. Hepatocellular carcinoma in woodchuck hepatitis virus-infected woodchucks: presence of viral DNA in tumor tissue from chronic carriers and animals serologically recovered from acute infections. *Hepatology* 1989;9:461–470.

249. Transy C, Fourel G, Robinson WS, et al. Frequent amplification of c-myc in ground squirrel liver tumors associated with past or ongoing infection with a hepadnavirus. *Proc Natl Acad Sci USA* 1992;89:3874–3878.

250. Paterlini P, Gerken G, Khemeny F, et al. Primary liver cancer in HBsAg negative patients: a study of HBV genome using the polymerase chain reaction. In: Hollinger FB, Lemon SM, Margolis HS, eds. *Viral hepatitis and liver disease*. Baltimore: Williams & Wilkins, 1991:222–226.

251. Yu MC, Yuan JM, Ross RK, et al. Presence of antibodies to the hepatitis B surface antigen associated with an excess risk for hepatocellular carcinoma among non-asian in Los Angeles County, California. *Hepatology* 1997;25:226–228.

252. Huo T, Wu J, Lee P, et al. Sero-clearance of hepatitis B surface antigen in chronic carriers does not necessarily imply a good prognosis. *Hepatology* 1998;28:231–236.

253. Galloway DA, McDougall JK. The oncogenic potential of her-

pes simplex virus: evidence for a "hit and run" mechanism. *Nature* 1983;302:21–24.

254. Morgan D, Pecararo G, Rosenberg I, et al. Human papillomavirus type 6b DNA is required for initiation but not maintenance of transformation of C127 mouse cells. *J Virol* 1990;64: 969–976.

255. Smith KT, Campo MS. "Hit and run" transformation of mouse C127 cells by bovine papillomavirus type 4: the viral DNA is required for the initiation but not for maintenance of the transformed phenotype. *Virology* 1988;64:39–47.

256. Gong SS, Jensen AD, Rogler CE. Loss and acquisition of duck hepatitis B virus integrations in lineages of LMH-D2 chicken hepatoma cells. *J Virol* 1996;70:2000–2007.

257. Feray C, Gigou M, Samuel D, et al. Hepatitis C virus RNA and hepatitis B virus DNA in serum and liver of patients with fulminant hepatitis. *Gastroenterology* 1993;104:549–555.

258. Liang TJ, Jeffers L, Rajender K, et al. Fulminant or subfulminant Non-A, Non-B viral hepatitis: the role of hepatitis C and E viruses. *Gastroenterology* 1993;104:556–562.

259. Wright TL, Hsu H, Donegan E. Hepatitis C virus not found in fulminant non-A non-B hepatitis. *Ann Intern Med* 1991;115: 111–112.

260. Chu C, Sheen I, Liaw Y. The role of hepatitis C virus in fulminant viral hepatitis in an area with endemic hepatitis A and B. *Gastroenterology* 1994;107:189–195.

261. Yanagi M, Kaneko S, Unoura M, et al. Hepatitis C virus fulminant hepatic failure. *N Engl J Med* 1991;324:1895.

262. Nousbaum J, Pol S, Nalpas B, et al. Hepatitis C virus type 1b (II) infection in France and Italy. *Ann Intern Med* 1995;122: 161–168.

263. Gretch D, Corey L, Wilson J, et al. Assessment of hepatitis C virus RNA levels by quantitative competitive RNA polymerase chain reaction: high-titer viremia correlates with advanced stage of disease. *J Infect Dis* 1994;169:1219–1225.

264. Magrin S, Craxi A, Fabiano C, et al. Hepatitis C viremia in chronic liver disease: relationship to interferon-alpha or corticosteroid treatment. *Hepatology* 1994;19:273–279.

265. Neumann AU, Lam NP, Dahari H, et al. Hepatitis C viral dynamics in vivo and the antiviral efficacy of interferon-alpha therapy. *Science* 1998;282:103–107.

266. Feray C, Gigou M, Samuel D, et al. The course of hepatitis C virus infection after liver transplantation. *Hepatology* 1994;20: 1137–1143.

267. Chazouillères O, Kim M, Combs C, et al. Quantitation of hepatitis C virus RNA in liver transplant recipients. *Gastroenterology* 1994;109:994–999.

268. Martin P, Di Bisceglie AM, Kassianides C, et al. Rapidly progressive non-A, non-B hepatitis in patients with human immunodeficiency virus infection. *Gastroenterology* 1989;97: 1559–1561.

269. Oshita M, Hayashi N, Kasahara A, et al. Increased serum hepatitis virus RNA levels among alcoholic patients with chronic hepatitis C. *Hepatology* 1994;20:1115–1120.

270. Romeo R, Pol S, Berthelot P, et al. Eradication of HCV RNA after alpha-interferon therapy. *Ann Intern Med* 1994;121: 276–277.

271. Gil B, Qian C, Riezu-Boj JI, et al. Hepatic and extrahepatic HCV RNA strands in chronic hepatitis C: different patterns of response to Interferon treatment. *Hepatology* 1993;18: 1050–1054.

272. Bukh J, Miller RH, Purcell RH. Genetic heterogeneity of hepatitis C virus: quasispecies and genotypes. *Semin Liver Dis* 1995;15:41–63.

273. Simmonds P. Variability of hepatitis C virus. *Hepatology* 1995; 21:570–583.

274. Bréchot C, Pol S. Hepatitis C virus biology and genetic vari-

ability: implications for the management of infected patients. In: Boyer J, Ockner RC, eds. *Progress in liver diseases.* Philadelphia: WB Saunders, 1998:183–217.

275. Ohno T, Lau YN. The "gold-standard" accuracy, and the current concepts: hepatitis C virus genotype and viremia. *Hepatology* 1996;24:1312–1315.

276. Tuveri R, Rothschild C, Pol S, et al. Hepatitis C virus genotypes in French haemophiliacs: kinetics and reappraisal of mixed infections. *J Med Virol* 1997;51:36–41.

277. Bréchot C, Pol S, Hepatitis C virus biology and genetic variability: implications for the management of infected patients. In: Boyer J, Ockner RC, eds. *Progress in liver diseases.* Philadelphia: WB Saunders, 1998:183–217.

278. Martinot-Peignoux M, Marcellin P, Pouteau M, et al. Pretreatment serum hepatitis C virus RNA levels and hepatitis C virus genotype are the main and independent prognostic factors of sustained response to interferon alfa therapy in chronic hepatitis C. *Hepatology* 1995;22:1050–1056.

279. Simmonds P, Rose KA, Graham S, et al. Mapping of serotype-specific, immunodominant epitopes in the NS-4 region of hepatitis C virus (HCV): use of type specific peptides to serologically differentiate infection with HCV types 1, 2 and 3. *J Clin Microbiol* 1993;31:1493–1503.

280. Cabot B, Martell M, Esteban JI, et al. Nucleotide and amino acid complexity of hepatitis C virus quasispecies in serum and liver. *J Virol* 2000;74:805–811.

281. Okada SI, Akahane Y, Suzuki H, et al. The degree of variability in the amino terminal region of the E2/NS1 protein of hepatitis C virus correlates with responsiveness to interferon therapy in viremic patients. *Hepatology* 1992;16:619–624.

282. Le Guen B, Squadrito G, Nalpas B, et al. Hepatitis C virus genome complexity correlates with response to interferon therapy: a study in French patients with chronic hepatitis C. *Hepatology* 1997;25:1250–1254.

283. Gretch D, Polyak S, Wilson J, et al. Tracking hepatitis C virus quasispecies majour and minor variants in symptomatic and asymptomatic liver transplant recipients. *J Virol* 1996;70:7622–7631.

284. Pawlotsky JM, Germanidis G, Frainais PO, et al. Evolution of the hepatitis C virus second envelope protein hypervariable region in chronically infected patients receiving alpha interferon therapy. *J Virol* 1999;73:6490–6499.

285. Sandres K, Dubois M, Pasquier C, et al. Genetic heterogeneity of hypervariable region 1 of the hepatitis C virus (HCV) genome and sensitivity of HCV to alpha interferon therapy. *J Virol* 2000;74:661–668.

286. Cerny A, Chisari F. Pathogenesis of chronic hepatitis C: immunological features of hepatitis injury and viral persistence. *Hepatology* 1999;30:595–601.

287. Enomoto N, Kurosaki M, Tanaka Y, et al. Fluctuation of hepatitis C virus quasispecies in persistent infection and interferon treatment revealed by single-strand conformation polymorphism analysis. *J Gen Virol* 1994;75:1361–1369.

288. Naito M, Hayashi N, Moribe T. Hepatitis C viral quasispecies in hepatitis C virus carriers with normal liver enzymes and patients with type C chronic liver disease. *Hepatology* 1995;22:407–412.

289. Leone F, Zylberberg H, Squadrito G, et al. Hepatitis C virus (HCV) genomic complexity does not correlate with severity of liver disease HCV type, viral load or duration of infection. *Hepatology* 1998;28:1–6.

290. Brambilla S, Bellati G, Asti M, et al. Dynamics of hypervariable region 1 variation in hepatitis C virus infection and correlation with clinical and virological features of liver disease. *Hepatology* 1998;27:1678–1686.

291. Shermann K, Andreatta C, O'Brien J, et al. Hepatitis C in human immunodeficiency virus-coinfected patients: increased variability in the hypervariable envelope coding domain. *Hepatology* 1996;23:688–694.

292. Zignego AL, Macchia D, Monti M, et al. Infection of peripheral mononuclear blood cells by hepatitis C virus. *J Hepatology* 1992;15:382–386.

293. Zignego A, De Carli M, Monti M, et al. Hepatitis C virus infection of mononuclear cells from peripheral blood and liver infiltrates in chronically infected patients. *J Med Virol* 1995;47:58–64.

294. Moldvay J, Deny P, Pol S, et al. Detection of hepatitis C virus RNA in peripheral blood mononuclear cells of infected patients by in situ hybridization. *Blood* 1994;83:269–273.

295. Agnello V, Chung R, Kaplan L. A role for hepatitis C virus infection in type II cryoglobulinemia. *N Engl J Med* 1992;327:1490–1495.

296. Zignego A, Bréchot C. Extrahepatic manifestations of HCV infection: facts and controversies. *J Hepatol* 1999;31:1152–1154.

297. Cribier B, Schmitt C, Bingen A, et al. In vitro infection of peripheral blood mononuclear cells by hepatitis C virus. *J Gen Virol* 1995;76:2485–2491.

298. Bronowicki JP, Loriot MA, Thiers V, et al. Hepatitis C virus persistence in human hematopoietic cells injected into SCID mice [see comments]. *Hepatology* 1998;28:211–218.

299. Lerat H, Rumin S, Habersetzer F, et al. In vivo tropism of hepatitis C virus genomic sequences in hematopoietic cells: influence of viral load, viral genotype, and cell phenotype. *Blood* 1998;91:3841–3849.

300. Shimizu YK, Igarashi H, Kanematu T, et al. Sequence analysis of the Hepatitis C virus genome recovered from serum, liver, and peripheral blood mononuclear cells of infected chimpanzees. *J Virol* 1997;71:5769–5773.

301. Fujii K, Hino K, Okazaki M, et al. Differences in hypervariable region 1 quasispecies of hepatitis C virus between human serum and peripheral blood mononuclear cells. *Biochem Biophys Res Commun* 1996;225:771–776.

302. Maggi F, Fornai C, Vatteroni ML, et al. Differences in Hepatitis C virus quasispecies composition between liver, peripheral blood mononuclear cells and plasma. *J Gen Virol* 1997;78:1521–1525.

303. Afonso AM, Jiang J, Penin F, et al. Nonrandom distribution of hepatitis C virus quasispecies in plasma and peripheral blood mononuclear cell subsets. *J Virol* 1999;73:9213–9221.

304. Loriot MA, Bronowicki JP, Lagorce D, et al. Permissivity of human biliary epithelial cells to infection by hepatitis C virus. *Hepatology* 1999;29:1587–1595.

305. Goodman ZD, Ishak KG. Histopathology of hepatitis C virus infection. *Semin Liver Dis* 1995;15:70–81.

306. Zignego AL, Giannelli F, Marrocchi ME, et al. T(14;18) translocation in chronic hepatitis C virus infection [In Process Citation]. *Hepatology* 2000;31:474–479.

307. Thomssen R, Bonk S, Thiele A. Density heterogeneities of hepatitis C virus in human sera due to the binding of beta-lipoproteins and immunoglobulins. *Med Microbiol Immunol (Berl)* 1993;182:329–334.

308. Thomssen R, Bonk S, Propfe C, et al. Association of hepatitis C virus in human sera with beta-lipoprotein. *Med Microbiol Immunol* 1992;181:293–300.

309. Monazahian M, Bohme I, Bonk S, et al. Low density lipoprotein receptor as a candidate receptor for hepatitis C virus. *J Med Virol* 1999;57:223–229.

310. Agnello V, Abel G, Elfahal M, et al. Hepatitis C virus and other flaviviridae viruses enter cells via low density lipoprotein receptor. *Proc Natl Acad Sci USA* 1999;96:12766–12771.

311. Czaja AJ, Carpenter HA, Santrach PJ, et al. Host- and disease-

specific factors affecting steatosis in chronic hepatitis C. *J Hepatol* 1998;29:198–206.

312. Lettéron P, Fromenty B, Terris B, et al. Acute and chronic hepatic steatosis lead to in vivo lipid peroxidation in mice. *J Hepatol* 1996;24:200–208.

313. Moriya K, Fujie H, Shintani Y, et al. The core protein of hepatitis C virus induces hepatocellular carcinoma in transgenic mice. *Nat Med* 1998;4:1065–1070.

314. Lerat H, Honda M, Tseng CTK, et al. Hepatitis C virus transgenic mice as model for HCV associated liver disease. *Hepatology* 1998;28:498A.

315. Pasquinelli C, Shoenberger JM, Chung J, et al. Hepatitis C virus core and E2 protein expression in transgenic mice. *Hepatology* 1997;25:719–727.

316. Barba G, Harper F, Harada T, et al. Hepatitis C virus core protein shows a cytoplasmic localization and associates to cellular lipid storage droplets. *Proc Natl Acad Sci USA* 1997;94:1200–1205.

317. Sabile A, Perlemuter G, Bonbo F, et al. Hepatitis C virus core protein binds to apolipoprotein A11 and its secretion is modulated by fibrates. *Hepatology* 1999;4:1064–1076.

318. Rubbia-Brandt L, Giostra E, Quadri R, et al. Evidence that liver steatosis is virally-mediated in a subset of patients infected by hepatitis C virus (HCV) genotype 3. *J Hepatol* 1999;30(suppl 1):133.

319. Heim MH, Moradpour D, Blum HE. Expression of hepatitis C virus proteins inhibits signal transduction through the Jak-STAT pathway. *J Virol* 1999;73:8469–8475.

320. Enomoto N, Sakuma I, Asahina Y, et al. Comparison of full-length sequences of interferon-sensitive and resistant hepatitis C virus 1b. Sensitivity to interferon is conferred by amino acid substitutions in the NS5A region. *J Clin Invest* 1995;96:224–230.

321. Enomoto N, Sakuma I, Asahina Y, et al. Mutations in the nonstructural protein 5A gene and response to interferon in patients with chronic hepatitis C virus 1b infection. *N Engl J Med* 1996;334:77–81.

322. Gale MJ, Korth MJ, Tang NM, et al. Evidence that hepatitis C virus resistance to interferon is mediated through repression of the PKR protein kinase by the nonstructural 5A protein. *Virology* 1997;230:217–227.

323. Gale MJ, Blakely CM, Kwieciszewski B, et al. Control of PKR protein kinase by hepatitis C virus nonstructural 5A proteIn: molecular mechanisms of kinase regulation. *Mol Cell Biol* 1998;18:5208–5218.

324. Chayama K, Tsubota A, Kobayashi M, et al. Pretreatment virus load and multiple amino acid substitutions in the interferon sensitivity-determining region predict the outcome of interferon treatment in patients with chronic genotype 1b hepatitis C virus infection. *Hepatology* 1997;25:745–749.

325. Kurosaki M, Enomoto N, Murakami T, et al. Analysis of genotypes and amino acid residues 2209 to 2248 of the NS5A region of hepatitis C virus in relation to the response to interferon-beta therapy. *Hepatology* 1997;25:750–753.

326. Komatsu H, Fujisawa T, Inui A, et al. Mutations in the nonstructural protein 5A gene and response to interferon therapy in young patients with chronic hepatitis C virus 1b infection. *J Med Virol* 1997;53:361–365.

327. Squadrito G, Leone F, Sartori M, et al. Mutations in the nonstructural 5A region of hepatitis C virus and response of chronic hepatitis C to interferon a. *Gastroenterology* 1997;113:567–572.

328. Rispeter K, Lu M, Zibert A, et al. A suggested extension of the HCV ISDR does not alter our former conclusions on its predictive value for IFN response. *J Hepatol* 1999;30:1163–1164.

329. Duverlie G, Khorsi H, Castelain S, et al. Sequence analysis of the NS5A protein of European hepatitis C virus 1b isolates and relation to interferon sensitivity. *J Gen Virol* 1998;79:1373–1381.

330. Polyak SJ, Mac Ardle S, Liu SL, et al. Evolution of hepatitis C virus quasispecies in hypervariable region 1 and the putative interferon sensitivity-determining region during interferon therapy and natural infection. *J Virol* 1998;72:4288–4296.

331. Pawlotsky JM, Germanidis G, Neumann AU, et al. Interferon resistance of hepatitis C virus genotype 1b: Relationship to nonstructural 5A gene quasispecies mutations. *J Virology* 1998;72:2795–2805.

332. Nakano I, Fukuda Y, Katano Y, et al. Why is the interferon sensitivity-determining region (ISDR) system useful in Japan? *J Hepatol* 1999;30:1014–1022.

333. Paterson M, Laxton CD, Thomas HC, et al. Hepatitis C virus NS5A protein inhibits interferon antiviral activity, but the effects do not correlate with the clinical response. *Gastroenterology* 1999;117:1187–1197.

334. Song J, Fujii M, Wang F, et al. The NS5A protein of hepatitis C virus partially inhibits the antiviral activity of interferon. *J Gen Virol* 1999;80:879–886.

335. Polyak SJ, Paschal DM, McArdle S, et al. Characterization of the effects of hepatitis C virus nonstructural 5A protein expression in human cell lines and on interferon-sensitive virus replication. *Hepatology* 1999;29:1262–1271.

336. Ide Y, Tanimoto A, Sasaguri Y, et al. Hepatitis C virus NS5A protein is phosphorylated in vitro by a stably bound protein kinase from HeLa cells and by cAMP-dependent protein kinase A—a catalytic subunit. *Gene* 1997;201:151–158.

337. Koch J, Bartenschlager R. Modulation of hepatitis C virus NS5A hyperphosphorylation by nonstructural proteins NS3, NS4A, NS4B. *J Virol* 1999;73:7138–7146.

338. Gale M Jr, Kwieciszewski B, Dossett M, et al. Antiapoptotic and oncogenic potentials of hepatitis C virus are linked to interferon resistance by viral repression of the PKR protein kinase. *J Virol* 1999;73:6506–6516.

339. Fukuma T, Enomoto N, Marumo F, et al. Mutations in the interferon-sensitivity determining region of hepatitis C virus and transcriptional activity of the nonstructural region 5A protein. *Hepatology* 1998;28:1147–1153.

340. Tan SL, Nakao H, He Y, et al. NS5A, a nonstructural protein of hepatitis C virus, binds growth factor receptor-bound protein 2 adaptor protein in a Src homology 3 domain/ligand-dependent manner and perturbs mitogenic signaling. *Proc Natl Acad Sci USA* 1999;96:5533–5538.

341. Taylor DR, Shi ST, Romano PR, et al. Inhibition of the interferon-inducible protein kinase PKR by HCV E2 protein [see comments]. *Science* 1999;285:107–110.

342. Bréchot C, Jaffredo F, Lagorce D, et al. Impact of HBV, HCV, and GBV-C/HGV on hepatocellular carcinomas in Europe: results of an European concerted action. *J Hepatol* 1998;29:173–183.

343. Colombo M, Romeo R. Hepatitis C virus infection and hepatocellular carcinoma. In: Bréchot C, ed. *Primary liver cancer: etiological and progression factors.* Paris: CRC Press, 1994:49–55.

344. Bréchot C. Hepatitis C virus:molecular biology and clinics. In: Schmid R, Bianchi L, Blum HE, et al., eds. *Acute and chronic liver diseases. Molecular biology and clinics.* Basel: Kluwer Academic, 1996:7–27.

345. Shimotohno K. Hepatitis C virus as a causative agent of hepatocellular carcinoma. *Intervirology* 1995;38:162–169.

346. Paterlini P, Bréchot C, Hepatitis B virus and primary liver cancer in hepatitis B surface antigen-positive and negative patients. In: Bréchot C, ed. *Primary liver cancer: etiological and progression factors.* Paris: CRC Press, 1994:167–190.

347. Kew MC. Role of cirrhosis in hepatocarcinogenesis. In: Ban-

nasch P, Keppler D, Weber G, eds. *Liver cell carcinoma.* Dordrecht/Boston/London: Kluwer Academic, 1989:37–45.

348. De Mitri S, Poussin K, Baccarini P. HCV-associated liver cancer without cirrhosis. *Lancet* 1995;345:413–415.

349. Paterlini P, Driss F, Pisi E, et al. Persistence of hepatitis B and hepatitis C viral genomes in primary liver cancers from HBsAg negative patients: a study of a low endemic area. *Hepatology* 1993;17:20–29.

350. Tsuboi SO, Nagamori S, Miyazaki M, et al. Persistence of hepatitis c virus RNA in established human hepatocellular carcinoma cell lines. *J Med Virol* 1996;48:133–140.

351. Ray R, Ghosh A, Meyer K, et al. Functional analysis of a transrepressor domain in the hepatitis C virus core protein. *Virus Res* 1999;59:211–217.

352. Tsuchihara K, Hijikata M, Fukuda K, et al. Hepatitis C virus core protein regulates cell growth and signal transduction pathway transmitting growth stimuli. *Virology* 1999;258:100–107.

353. Yasui K, Wakita T, Tsukiyama-Kohara K, et al. The native form and maturation process of hepatitis C virus core protein. *J Virol* 1998;72:6048–6055.

354. Zhu N, Khoshnan A, Schneider R, et al. Hepatitis C virus core protein binds to the cytoplasmic domain of tumor necrosis factor (TNF) receptor 1 and enhances TNF-induced apoptosis. *J Virol* 1998;72:3691–3697.

355. You LR, Chen CM, Lee YHW. Hepatitis C virus core protein enhances NF-kappaB signal pathway triggering by lymphotoxin-beta receptor ligand and tumor necrosis factor alpha. *J Virol* 1999;73:1672–1681.

356. Owsianka AM, Patel AH. Hepatitis C virus core protein interacts with a human DEAD box protein DDX3. *Virology* 1999; 257:330–340.

357. Hsieh TY, Matsumoto M, Chou HC, et al. Hepatitis C virus core protein interacts with heterogeneous nuclear ribonucleoprotein K. *J Biol Chem* 1998;273:17651–17659.

358. Shrivastava A, Manna SK, Ray R, et al. Ectopic expression of hepatitis C virus core protein differentially regulates nuclear transcription factors. *J Virol* 1998;72:9722–9728.

359. Ray R, Steele R, Meyer K. Hepatitis C virus core protein represses p21 WAF1/Cip1/Sid1 promoter activity. *Gene* 1998; 208:331–336.

360. Ray RB, Steele R, Meyer K, et al. Transcriptional repression of p53 promoter by hepatitis C virus core protein. *J Biol Chem* 1997;272:10983–10986.

361. Matsuura Y, Miyamura T. The molecular biology of hepatitis C virus. *Virology* 1993;203:297–304.

362. Lo SY, Masiarz F, Hwang SB, et al. Differential subcellular localization of hepatitis C virus core gene products. *Virology* 1995;213:455–461.

363. Suzuki R, Matsuura Y, Suzuki T, et al. Nuclear localisation of the truncated hepatitis C virus core protein with its hydrophobic C-terminus deleted. *J Gen Virol* 1995;76:53–61.

364. Rüster B, Zeuzem S, Roth WK. Hepatitis C virus sequences encoding truncated core proteins detected in a hepatocellular carcinoma. *Biochem Biophys Res Commun* 1996;219:911–915.

365. Horie C, Iwahana H, Horie T, et al. Detection of different quasispecies of hepatitis C virus core region in cancerous and noncancerous lesions. *Biochem Biophys Res Commun* 1996;218: 674–681.

366. Chang S, Hu T, Hsieh TS. Analysis of a core domain in Drosophila DNA topoisomerase II. Targeting of an antitumor agent ICRF-159. *J Biol Chem* 1998;273:19822–19828.

367. Ray RB, Lagging LM, Meyer K, et al. Hepatitis C virus core protein cooperates with ras and transforms primary rat embryo fibroblasts to tumorigenic phenotype. *J Virol* 1996;70: 4438–4443.

368. Lerat H, Honda M, Tseng C, et al. Hepatitis C virus transgenic mice as model for HCV associated liver disease. *Hepatology* 1998;28:498A.

369. Ruggieri A, Harada T, Matsuura Y, et al. Sensitization to Fas-mediated apoptosis by hepatitis C virus core protein. *Virology* 1997;229:68–76.

370. Ray R, Meyer K, Steele R, et al. Inhibition of tumor necrosis factor (TNF-α)-mediated apoptosis by hepatitis C virus core protein. *J Biol Chem* 1998;273:2256–2259.

371. Marusawa H, Hijikata M, Chiba T, et al. Hepatitis C virus core protein inhibits Fas- and tumor necrosis factor alpha-mediated apoptosis via NF-kappaB activation. *J Virol* 1999;73:4713–4720.

372. Sakamuro D, Furukawa T, Takegami T. Hepatitis C virus non-structural protein NS3 transforms NIH 3T3 cells. *J Virol* 1995; 69:3893–3896.

373. Borowski P, Heiland M, Feucht H, et al. Characterisation of non-structural protein 3 of hepatitis C virus as modulator of protein phosphorylation mediated by PKA and PKC: evidences for action on the level of substrate and enzyme. *Arch Virol* 1999; 144:687–701.

374. Ghosh AK, Steele R, Meyer K, et al. Hepatitis C virus NS5A protein modulates cell cycle regulatory genes and promotes cell growth. *J Gen Virol* 1999;80:1179–1183.

375. Kaufman RJ. Double-stranded RNA-activated protein kinase mediates virus-induced apoptosis: a new role for an old actor [comment]. *Proc Natl Acad Sci USA* 1999;96:11693–11695.

376. Bréchot C. Hepatitis C virus 1b, cirrhosis, and hepatocellular carcinoma. *Hepatology* 1997;25:772–774.

377. Feray C, Gigou M, Samuel D, et al. Influence of the genotypes of hepatitis C virus on the severity of recurrent liver disease after liver transplantation. *Gastroenterology* 1995;108: 1088–1096.

378. Gane EJ, Naoumov NV, Qian KP, et al. A longitudinal analysis of hepatitis C virus replication following liver transplantation. *Gastroenterology* 1996;110:167–177.

379. Bruno S, Silini S, Crosignani A, et al. Hepatitis C virus genotypes and risk of hepatocellular carcinoma in cirrhosis: a prospective study. *Hepatology* 1997;25(3):754–758.

380. Yamauchi M, Nakahara M, Hisato N, et al. Different prevalence of hepatocellular carcinoma between patients with liver cirrhosis due to genotype II and III of hepatitis C virus. *Inter Hepatol Comm* 1994;2:328–332.

381. De Mitri MS, Poussin K, Baccarini P, et al. HCV-associated liver cancer without cirrhosis. *Lancet* 1995;345:413–415.

382. Colombo M. Hepatocellular carcinoma. *J Hepatol* 1992;15: 225–236.

383. Mendenhall CL, Seeff L, Diehl AM, et al. Antibodies to hepatitis B virus and hepatitis C virus in alcoholic hepatitis and cirrhosis: their prevalence and clinical relevance. *Hepatology* 1991;14:581–589.

384. Nalpas B, Thiers V, Pol S, et al. Hepatitis C viremia and anti-HCV antibodies in alcoholics. *J Hepatol* 1992;14:381–384.

385. Nalpas B, Driss F, Pol S, et al. Association between HCV and HBV infection in hepatocellular carcinoma and alcoholic liver disease. *J Hepatol* 1991;12:70.

386. Nalpas B, Bréchot C, ed. The role of hepatitis viruses in the genesis of hepatocellular carcinoma in alcoholic cirrhotics. In: Watson R, ed. *Alcohol and cancer.* New York: CRC Press, 1992:91–118.

387. Parés A, Barrera JM, Caballeria J, et al. Hepatitis C virus antibodies in chronic alcoholic patients: association with severity of liver injury. Hepatology 1990;12:1295–1299.

388. Attali P, Thibault N, Buffet C, et al. Les marqueurs du virus B chez les alcooliques chroniques. *Gastroenterol Clin Biol* 1981;5: 1095.

389. Nalpas B, Berthelot P, Thiers V, et al. Hepatitis B virus multiplication in the absence of usual serological markers—A study of 146 alcoholics. *J Hepatol* 1985;1:89–97.

390. Poynard T, Aubert A, Lazizi Y, et al. Independent risk factors for hepatocellular carcinoma in French drinkers. *Hepatology* 1991;13:896.

391. Saunders J, Wodak A, Morgan-Capner P, et al. Importance of markers of hepatitis B virus in alcoholic liver disease. *Br Med J* 1983;286:1851.

392. Cacciola I, Pollicino T, Squadrito G, et al. Occult hepatitis B virus infection in patients with chronic hepatitis C liver disease. *N Engl J Med* 1999;341:22–26.

393. Bonino F, Group II-AHCS. Effect of interferon-a on progression of cirrhosis to hepatocellular carcinoma: a retrospective cohort study. *Lancet* 1998;351:1535–1539.

394. Bréchot C, Jaffredo F, Lagorce D, et al. Impact of HBV, HCV and GBV-C/HGV on hepatocellular carcinomas in Europe: results of a European concerted action. *J Hepatol* 1998;29:173–183.

395. Pontisso P, Ruvoletto MG, Fattovich G, et al. Clinical and virological profiles in patients with multiple hepatitis virus infections. *Gastroenterology* 1993;105:1529–1533.

396. Ohkawa K, Hayashi N, Yuki N, et al. Long-term follow-up of hepatitis B virus and hepatitis C virus replicative levels in chronic hepatitis patients coinfected with both viruses. *J Med Virol* 1995;46:258–264.

397. Shih CM, Chen CM, Chen SY, et al. Modulation of the trans-suppression activity of hepatitis C virus core protein by phosphorylation. *J Virol* 1995;69:1160–1171.

398. Donato F, Boffetta P, Puoti M. A meta-analysis of epidemiological studies on the combined effect of hepatitis B and C virus infections in causing hepatocellular carcinoma. *Int J Cancer* 1998;75:347–354.

399. Tokino T, Tamura H, Hori N, et al. Chromosome deletions associated with hepatitis B virus integration. *Virology* 1991; 185:879–882.

400. Tsuei DJ, Chen PJ, Lai MY, et al. Inverse polymerase chain reaction for cloning cellular sequences adjacent to integrated hepatitis B virus DNA in hepatocellular carcinomas. *J Med Virol* 1994;42:287–293.

401. Sherry A, Zhou YZ, Slagle B. Frequent loss of chromosome B_p in hepatitis B virus-positve hepatocellular carcinomas from China. *Cancer Res* 1996;56:5092–5097.

402. Chami M, Gozuacik D, Saigo K, et al. Hepatitis B virus-related insertional mutagenesis implicator SERCA1 gene in the control of apoptosis. *Oncogene* 2000;19(25):2877–2886.

403. Koshy R, Koch S, von Loringhoven AF, et al. Integration of hepatitis B virus DNA: evidence for integration in the single-stranded gap. *Cell* 1983;34:215–223.

404. Yaginuma K, Kobayashi M, Yoshida E, et al. Hepatitis B virus integration in hepatocellular carcinoma DNA: duplication of cellular flanking sequences at the integration site. *Proc Natl Acad Sci USA* 1985;82:4458–4462.

405. Berger I, Shaul Y. Integration of hepatitis B virus: analysis of unoccupied sites. *J Virol* 1987;61:1180–1186.

406. Graef E, Caselmann WH, Wells J, et al. Insertional activation of mevalonate kinase by hepatitis B virus DNA in a human hepatoma cell line. *Oncogene* 1994;9:81–87.

407. Chen JY, Harrison TJ, Tsuei DJ, et al. Analysis of integrated hepatitis B virus DNA and flanking cellular sequences in the hepatocellular carcinoma cell line HCC36. *Intervirology* 1994; 37:41–46.

408. Su TS, Hwang WL, Yauk YK. Characterization of hepatitis B virus integrant that results in chromosomal rearrangement. *DNA Cell Biol* 1998;17:415–425.

55

MOLECULAR BIOLOGY OF HEPATITIS VIRUSES

MICHAEL M. C. LAI
WILLIAM S. MASON

The five human hepatitis viruses, hepatitis A to E viruses (HAV to HEV), belong to five different virus families and have distinct genomic structures and replication strategies. They also have different clinical features and outcomes in their natural infection. HAV and HEV infections are always transient and are transmitted mainly by oral–fecal routes. In contrast, HBV, HCV, and HDV infections may be either transient or chronic, and are transmitted by parenteral routes. Despite these differences, they have several important features in common. First, they all infect and replicate in hepatocytes, which are their primary target of infection. Second, they are all able to infect and replicate in resting cells, as, in the healthy liver (mitotic index ~0.0005), hepatocytes very seldom enter the cell cycle and divide. Third, infection of hepatocytes is, in general, productive but not necessarily cytolytic.

Beneath the surface of their similarity, there are substantial differences in the underlying mechanisms of viral infection and pathogenesis among the different hepatitis viruses. First, they may use different receptors to enter hepatocytes, despite their similar target cell specificity. Second, they may use different mechanisms to establish persistent infection. Third, their mechanisms of pathogenesis differ substantially. Depending on the virus, during the acute hepatitis phase, there is typically a period of 2 to 6 weeks in which many hepatocytes are infected and shedding virus, either into the bloodstream or the bile canaliculi, depending on whether virus is released from the basal or apical surface of the hepatocyte. In the meantime, the immune system attempts to eliminate the virus by a combination of cell

M. M. C. Lai: Department of Molecular Microbiology and Immunology, Howard Hughes Medical Institute, University of Southern California, Keck School of Medicine, Los Angeles, California 90033-9094.

W. S. Mason: Basic Science Division, Fox Chase Cancer Center, Philadelphia, Pennsylvania 19111.

TABLE 55.1. PROPERTIES OF HEPATITIS VIRUSES

Virus	Taxonomy (Genus, Family)	Virion Structure	Size (nm)	Genome	Virus Antigens	Transmission Route	Diseases	Laboratory Diagnosis
HAV	Hepatovirus (Picornaviridae)	Nonenveloped, icosahedral	27	7.5-kb RNA linear, ss (+)	VP1–4	Oral	Acute	IgM anti-HAV
HBV	Orthohepadnavirus (Hepadnaviridae)	Enveloped, spherical	42	3.2-kb DNA circular, ds/ss	HBsAg HBcAg HBeAg Polymerase	Parenteral	Acute and chronic	Anti-HBs Anti-HBc Anti-HBe HBsAg HBeAg Polymerase assay Virion DNA (PCR)
		Enveloped, empty spherical or tubular	22 20–200	—	HBsAg			
HCV	Hepacivirus (Flaviviridae)	Enveloped, spherical	30–80	9.5-kb RNA linear, ss (+)	Core E1 E2	Parenteral	Acute and chronic	Anti-HCV Virion RNA (RT-PCR)
HDV	Deltavirus (satellites)	Enveloped, spherical	36	1.7-kb RNA circular, ss (−)	HDAg HBsAg	Parenteral	Acute and chronic	IgM/IgG anti-HDAg
HEV	Calicivirus (Caliciviridae)	Nonenveloped, icosahedral	32–34	7.6-kb RNA linear, ss (+)	Capsid (HEV)	Oral	Acute	IgM anti-HEV (capsid)

ss, single strand; HBcAg, hepatitis B core antigen; HBeAg, hepatitis B e antigen; HBsAg, hepatitis B surface antigen; Ig, immunoglobulin; RT-PCR, reverse-transcription polymerase chain reaction; ds, double strand; (+), positive-sense; (−), negative-sense.

killing and cell curing. Liver disease may result from the direct effects of viral proteins on the cells or by cell-killing mediated by the immune system. When the immune system fails to clear the virus, chronic liver disease results. Different hepatitis viruses differ in their ability, and employ different mechanisms, to escape from the host's defense. Thus, viral hepatitis is a dynamic process of virus-host interaction.

This chapter focuses on the basic properties of the hepatitis viruses and their mechanisms of replication in the cells. A brief discussion of the molecular interactions between the virus and hosts is included to provide a basic understanding of viral pathogenesis. Additional information on this latter subject, particularly with regard to the immune defense, can be found in Chapter 52. The salient features of these five hepatitis viruses are summarized in Table 55.1.

HEPATITIS A VIRUS

Hepatitis A virus (HAV) is an enteric virus that is readily transmitted under conditions of crowding and poor sanitation. As an epidemic disease, hepatitis A has been known for thousands of years, though its viral etiology (termed "infectious hepatitis") was only established in the middle 20th century, and the virus itself was not identified until the 1970s (1–3). The primary source of transmission is ingestion of fecal material, which may contain large amounts of virus during the incubation phase of the infection (up to 10^9 virus per gram). Passive immunization (hyperimmune serum) and vaccines (inactivated virus) are now available for at-risk individuals and high-risk populations. About one-third of the United States population has a history of HAV infection, and there are approximately 100,000 to 200,000 new cases a year, with approximately 100 deaths from fulminant liver failure, mostly in the elderly. Seroprevalence rates vary significantly among socioeconomic groups in the world. Humans appear to be the only reservoirs for HAV.

Virion Morphology

HAV is the type member of the genus *Hepatovirus* in the family Picornaviridae. Like most picornaviruses (as typified by poliovirus), HAV has a nonenveloped, icosahedral structure with a diameter of about 27 nm, containing a single-stranded RNA. The virus is assembled from 12 pentamers composed of five copies each of the virion proteins VP1 (30 kd), VP2 (22 kd), VP3 (2.5 kd), and possibly VP4 (2.2 kd).

Recent reports suggested that another viral protein, 2A, which was previously thought to be a nonstructural protein, remains linked to VP1 during pentamer formation (4) and is subsequently cleaved from VP1, apparently by a host protease (5). Crude virus preparations also contain proviruses, which contain incompletely cleaved precursor proteins, and empty virus capsids lacking viral RNA. By analogy to better-studied picornaviruses, VP4 is expected to reside on the inside surface of the viral capsid, while the remaining capsid proteins are at least partially exposed. However, VP4 has so far not been unequivocally detected in the virus.

Virions are characterized by a very high degree of stability upon exposure to low pH and heat. Stability in an acid environment is probably required for the virus to reach the intestine after oral ingestion, where virus uptake into target cells is thought to occur. All human HAV isolates form a single serotype, assuring the efficacy of passive immunization and vaccination. HuHAVcr-1, a ubiquitously expressed cellular membrane protein, has been identified as a candidate cell surface receptor for HAV (6). Because this protein is not liver-specific, the hepatotropism of the virus will require additional factors.

Genome Structure

The genome organization of HAV is similar to that of other picornaviruses. HAV contains a single-stranded, positive-sense RNA of 7.5 kilobases (kb), with a 5′ noncoding region (approximately 735 nucleotides) specifying an internal ribosome entry site (IRES), followed by a coding region for the single viral polyprotein of 2,225 amino acids, a 3′ noncoding region, and a short polyA tail (Fig. 55.1). The IRES sequence

is necessary for the translation of viral proteins. A virus-encoded protein, Vpg (genome-linked viral protein), is covalently attached to the 5′ end of the genome, unlike most of the cellular messenger RNAs (mRNAs), which typically have a 5′-cap structure. This protein is involved in viral RNA replication. However, *in vitro* transcribed plus-strand RNA lacking Vpg is infectious when introduced into permissive cells, as is viral complementary DNA (cDNA). Based on available sequencing data, all human HAV isolates can be grouped into seven genotypes (differing by 15% to 25%), with multiple subtypes. The HAV RNA sequence appears to be considerably more stable than other viral RNAs, with very low mutation frequencies during serial virus passages in culture.

Virus Replication

The primary target of HAV in infected human hosts is hepatocytes. However, in tissue culture, HAV can grow in nonhepatic cells, although it usually requires extensive adaptation of the virus in culture. In contrast to many other picornaviruses, HAV does not kill the host cell during productive infection; thus, all of the HAV infections result in persistent infection in culture. Paradoxically, in HAV infections of humans, persistent infections are not observed. Typically, during the 2- to 4-week incubation phase of an infection, there is a high level of virus production by the liver, but without any overt signs of liver disease. Liver disease appears to be a consequence of the host immune response to the infection during the recovery phase, when virus production is largely shut down. Thus, alanine aminotransferase (ALT) elevation and clinical jaundice in hepatitis A usually trail the period of active virus

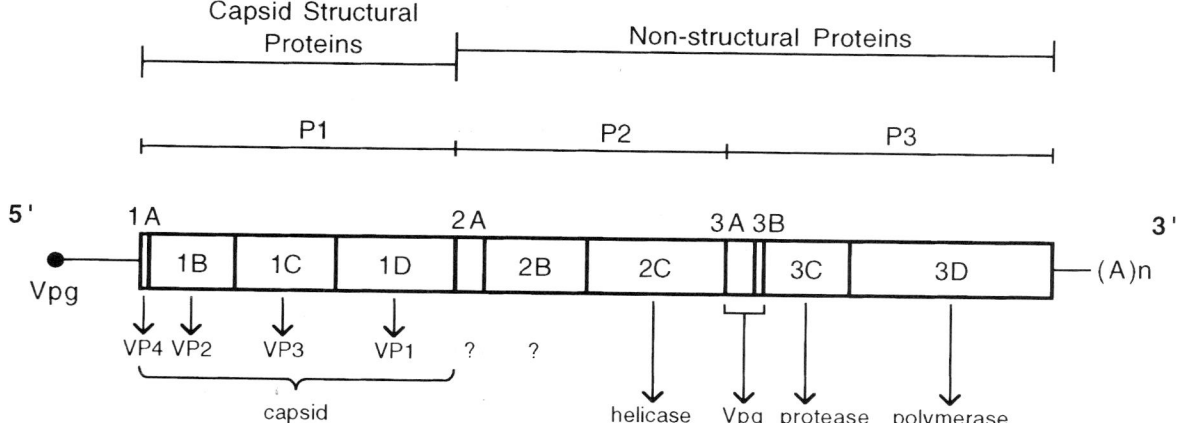

FIGURE 55.1. The hepatitis A virus (HAV) genome. The HAV genome is a 7.5-kb, single-stranded RNA of positive (coding) polarity. It has a 735-base 5′-noncoding region, which includes an internal rebosome entry site (IRES) sequence. The IRES sequence regulates translation of viral RNA. The 3′ end is a 63-base noncoding region, followed by a poly(A) tail. A viral protein (*Vpg*) is covalently linked to the 5′ end of the genome. The RNA encodes a polyprotein, which is cleaved by an autoprotease (*3C*) into viral structural proteins (*P1*) and nonstructural proteins (*P2* and *P3*), the latter of which carry out genome replication in the infected cells but are not incorporated into the virion. The biochemical functions of the individual viral proteins are indicated.

replication and production. During the incubation phase of the disease, virus is released into the bile canaliculi, from which it is ultimately transported to the intestine. Some virus is also released into the blood, though blood concentrations are generally about five logs lower than fecal concentrations.

The replication cycle of HAV, in large part, mimics that of other picornaviruses. HAV binds to a receptor molecule, HuHAVcr-1 (6), which is a ubiquitously expressed cell surface molecule. The mechanism of virus entry is not yet clear. Following virus penetration and uncoating of viral RNA in the cytoplasm, Vpg is cleaved from the RNA (7), and translation of the viral polyprotein ensues. The translation of viral proteins is by an IRES-dependent, 5′-cap–independent mechanism, which allows the ribosome to skip the 5′ end of RNA and go directly to the open reading frame (ORF) of HAV RNA. Thus, HAV protein translation is regulated by a different mechanism from translation of most of the cellular mRNAs. The viral polyprotein synthesized is then cleaved into 11 mature proteins (with the exception of the VP1-2A bond) (Fig. 55.1) by viral cysteine protease 3C in an autocatalytic process. The N-terminal portion (P1) of the polyprotein encodes the virion structural proteins, VP1-4, whereas P2 and P3 regions encode nonstructural proteins, most of which have similar functions to those of the corresponding proteins of other picornaviruses, except that 3AB of HAV may function as the Vpg without cleavage (8). The accumulation of Vpg and other nonstructural proteins leads to the initiation of RNA synthesis using the infecting RNA genome as the template. Newly made negative-strand RNA then serves as the template for the synthesis of additional positive-strand RNA. The synthesis of both strands requires the viral polymerase (3D protein) and Vpg (3A or 3AB). Presumably, Vpg primes RNA synthesis by viral polymerase from either the poly A sequence at the 3′ end of the positive-strand, or an A-A sequence at the 3′ end of the negative-strand RNA, in a mechanism similar to that of poliovirus RNA synthesis (9). Negative-strand RNA synthesis is restricted, so that most of the viral RNA in the cells is positive-stranded. As with other picornaviruses, virus replication occurs in association with the smooth endoplasmic reticulum, which may function in part to concentrate viral and cellular proteins involved in RNA synthesis. Vpg and 2BC have been shown to interact with intracellular membranes (10,11) and may facilitate the localization of replication complexes to the smooth endoplasmic reticulum (12). Once sufficient quantities of viral genomic RNA and structural proteins are made, virion assembly involving packaging of positive-strand RNA into capsids then takes place. The mechanism of HAV assembly is largely unknown.

HAV infection, in general, does not cause significant cytopathic effects, probably because of the slow replication and low level of virus production as compared to other picornaviruses, which are usually cytolytic. Moreover, HAV does not shut off host protein synthesis. Other picornaviruses have been shown to suppress cap-dependent translation of most host mRNAs, via cleavage of the p220 component of the cap-binding complex by the protease activity of 2A. The 2A protein of HAV, however, does not appear to have a protease activity (5,13). By serial passing of the virus in culture, it has been possible to select for HAV variants that are cytolytic and replicate to higher titers in cell culture. However, the possibility that the emergence of cytolytic variants might explain the rare cases of fulminant hepatitis associated with HAV infection (approximately 0.1%) has not been established. In contrary, the cell-adapted viruses often have reduced virulence in primates, thus making them candidates for the sources of vaccines. Cell-adapted strains often have point mutations in the 5′-noncoding region and 2B and 2C regions of the viral genome (14). Specifically, a single point mutation (U687G) in the 5′-noncoding region has been associated with the adaptation of HAV to growth in BSC-1 cells (15).

Infection and Pathogenesis

It is uncertain how HAV reaches the liver following oral ingestion. It is possible that the virus infects cells of the gastrointestinal tract and spreads from there to the liver. Alternatively, the ubiquitous nature of the cell-surface receptor, HuHAVcr-1, may facilitate passive binding and transport of the virus to the liver. Viral antigen expression has been detected in the cells of crypt and lamina propria in the small intestine within a few days of experimental exposure in an animal model of HAV infection, suggesting that virus might spread to the liver from primary sites of infection (16).

The long incubation period (2 to 4 weeks or longer) of HAV following exposure would seem to ensure that the virus has the opportunity to spread to the entire hepatocyte population. This raises an interesting problem, common for all the hepatitis viruses discussed below: How is the infection cleared without the liver being destroyed? Examination of liver samples collected during the incubation and subsequent clinical phases of infection revealed the importance of hepatocyte destruction in virus clearance. However, as with the other hepatitis viruses, it seems unlikely that cell death is the only mechanism for virus elimination, except, perhaps, in rare cases of fulminant hepatitis. Noncytolytic mechanisms of HAV clearance from infected hepatocytes may be inferred from studies of *in vivo* infections by lymphocytic choriomeningitis virus, another RNA virus (17). Nonetheless, direct evidence of noncytolytic clearance of HAV is still needed.

In up to 20% of patients, a relapse may follow the apparent resolution of the initial symptomatic phase of infection. Nonetheless, the duration of infection generally does not exceed 6 months. The detection of immunoglobulin M (IgM) antibody or rising titers of IgG antibodies provides reliable evidence of HAV infections.

HEPATITIS B VIRUS

Hepatitis B virus (HBV) is transmitted primarily from blood or blood-derived products. Its existence as a cause of viral hepatitis (originally termed "serum hepatitis") has been known since the 1940s, though the virus itself was not identified until the early 1970s. The virus takes its name from the fact that it was the second cause of viral hepatitis to be identified. HBV is the most prevalent of the three viruses proven to cause chronic disease of the liver (HCV and HDV being the others), with about 200 to 300 million carriers worldwide. Effective screening has nearly eliminated blood transfusion as a source of HBV infection. However, perinatal transmission from infected mothers to newborns and horizontal transmission to and among young children remain as prevalent causes of chronic HBV infection. As a result, 5% to 15% of the population is infected in certain parts of the world, including Southeast Asia and sub-Saharan Africa. An HBV vaccine has been available for two decades, but universal vaccination is only now being attempted in most parts of the world. The early vaccine was prepared using inactivated virus particles purified from the serum of chronically infected blood donors. The current vaccine is made from subviral particles [hepatitis B surface antigen (HBsAg) see Virion Morphology, below] prepared in yeast using recombinant DNA technologies.

Classification

HBV belongs to the Hepadnaviridae family, which is divided into the genera *Orthohepadnavirus* and *Avihepadnavirus*, based on differences in host species and in genome structure. The type member of the former genus is human HBV and of the latter, duck HBV (DHBV). Distinct species of orthohepadnaviruses have been found in humans, woodchucks, and ground squirrels. Virus closely related to HBV has also been found in the woolly monkey, a New World primate, and appears to be a distinct species. Hepadnaviruses have also been isolated from the great apes, but it remains unclear if these are truly distinct species from HBV. Recently, HBV-like viruses have been isolated from chimpanzees, some of which may represent virus species distinct from the human HBV (18). The *Avihepadnavirus* genus includes DHBV, heron hepatitis B virus, and Ross goose hepatitis virus. Thus, hepadnaviruses appear to be able to infect a wide range of animal species.

In addition to a lack of sequence homology between the ortho- and avihepadnaviruses, the orthohepadnaviruses contain a regulatory gene, X, which is not found in the avihepadnavirus genome (Fig. 55.2, see below).

Virion Morphology

Hepadnaviruses are enveloped viruses of 42 nm in diameter, with a double-shelled morphology under electron

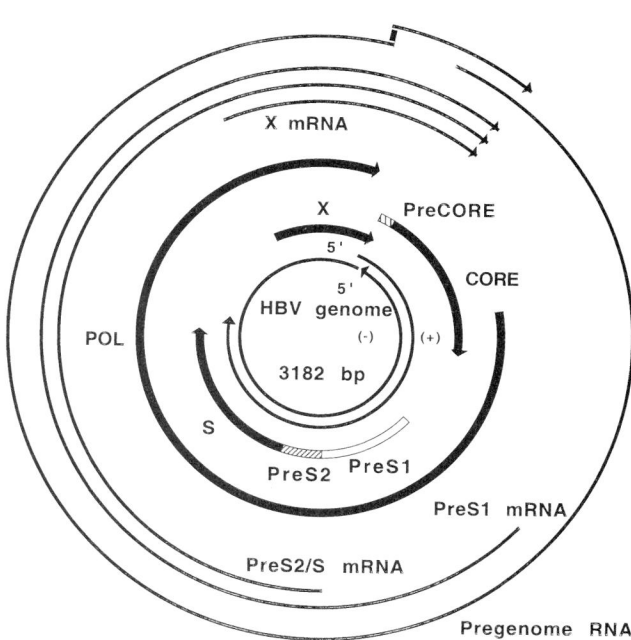

FIGURE 55.2. The genome structure of human hepatitis B virus (*HBV*). DNA strands are depicted in the center; the open reading frames (ORFs) are next, and followed by the messenger RNAs (*mRNAs*) at the outermost. The virion DNA is between 3,000 and 3,300 bases in length, partially double-stranded and partially single-stranded. It has a relaxed circular conformation maintained by a short cohesive overlap between the 5' ends of the two DNA strands (approximately 220 base pairs for HBV), neither of which are covalently closed. A 17-base, capped RNA is covalently attached to the 5' end of the plus strand, and a protein, the viral DNA polymerase, to the 5' end of the minus strand. The plus strand is always incomplete in the virions. The polymerase present in the virions will fill in the gaps in the DNA during virus replication. Four overlapping ORFs, encoding S, Core, X, and Pol, are located on the (−) strand. The core/precore ORF encodes core and e proteins, whereas the S ORF encodes three envelope proteins, S, M (S + preS2), and L (S + preS2 + pre S1). S and M are produced by distinct mRNAs (preS2/S mRNA) made from a common promoter with heterogeneous start sites around the initiation codon AUG at the 5'-end of preS2. Core and precore proteins are produced by distinct mRNAs from either a single promoter or two overlapping promoters (29). The Pol protein is produced by internal initiation of translation from the pregenomic RNA.

microscopy. The outer shell is viral envelope, consisting of HBsAg. The inner shell is the icosahedral nucleocapsid of 37 nm in diameter, consisting of the hepatitis B core antigen (HBcAg) enclosing the viral DNA genome. Virions are prevalent in the blood during transient infections and some stages of chronic infection, with titers of up to 10^{10} per milliliter. However, the most abundant virus particles in the blood are not the virions, but rather the noninfectious subviral particles made up entirely of HBsAg, without viral DNA. They are found as either spherical particles of 22 nm in diameter or filamentous structures of variable length (20 nm in width and 20 to 200 nm in length) in infected humans. Because these empty particles do not contain DNA, they are not infectious. They are generally found in at least 100-fold excess over virions and were the primary antigenic particles in the original HBV vaccine.

The envelope protein HBsAg usually consists of three protein species, large (L), middle (M), and small (S), which share the same sequence, but L and M proteins have an N-terminal extension of different lengths (L-HBsAg includes the pre-S1 and pre-S2 regions, while M-HBsAg includes pre-S2) (Fig. 2). The ratio of the three proteins in the virion is approximately 1:1:3 (L:M:S) (19). All three proteins are integral membrane proteins, with an internal hydrophobic loop, five transmembrane domains, and an external region. The external domain (the N-terminus of S protein and pre-S1 and pre-S2 regions) contains the epitopes known as HBsAg and is the common sites of mutations in the vaccine-associated HBV variants (20). The pre-S1 region, which is present only in the L-HBsAg, contains the receptor-binding domain (21).

HBcAg is a phosphoprotein and has an ability to bind RNA, probably nonspecifically. It interacts with the viral pregenome RNA to form the core particles. It is essential for both viral DNA synthesis and for virion assembly. The core particles are icosahedral in structure (22).

Genome Structure

All of the viruses within the Hepadnaviridae family contain a partially double-stranded circular DNA genome of approximately 3.2 kilobase pairs (kbp) (Fig. 55.2), neither strand being covalently closed. The minus strand is complete and has a terminal redundancy of nine nucleotides. The plus strand is always incomplete and has variable lengths; it has a constant 5′ end but a variable 3′ end. There is a short cohesive overlap between the 5′ ends of the two strands [approximately 220 base pairs (bp) for HBV]; as a result, viral DNA maintains a relaxed circular DNA structure and is partially double-stranded and partially single-stranded. Both strands also have two direct-repeat sequences (DR1 and DR2) of 10 to 11 nucleotides near the 5′ end. A 17-base RNA with a 5′-cap structure is covalently attached to the 5′ end of the plus strand (23,24), while a protein, the viral DNA polymerase, is covalently linked to the 5′ end of the minus strand (25,26). The polymerase present in virions is able to partially fill in the gap in the plus strand in *in vitro* reactions in which deoxynucleosides are added to virions partially disrupted with nonionic detergent. This fill-in reaction also occurs *in vivo* during viral replication. A small fraction of virions (about 5%) have a linear genome as a consequence of inappropriate priming of plus strand synthesis (see below) (27); these virions are also infectious, though they may give rise to aberrant replication intermediates (28).

The HBV genome is extremely compact, containing four ORFs, all of which are encoded on the minus-strand DNA and overlap each other. Furthermore, two of the ORFs encode multiple proteins: the core/precore ORF produces two proteins (the core protein and the e antigen), while the S-ORF yields three envelope proteins, including S, M (S + preS2), and L (S + preS2 + pre S1) proteins. In addition, most of these proteins are produced from different mRNAs despite the fact that some of the proteins are derived from the same ORF. S and M are translated from distinct mRNA species (preS2/S mRNA) produced by a common promoter, with heterogeneous start sites around the initiation codon AUG at the 5′ end of preS2. The shorter mRNA will synthesize S protein. L is translated from an mRNA (preS1 mRNA) starting upstream of the preS1 of the envelope ORF. Similarly, core and precore [hepatitis B early antigen (HBeAg), see below] proteins are translated from distinct mRNA species (pregenome RNA) with heterogeneous 5′

FIGURE 55.3. Hepadnavirus genome replication. Upon infection, the viral DNA is transported to the nucleus and converted to a fully double-stranded covalently closed circular (*ccc*) DNA following removal of the covalently attached protein and RNA and a 9-base terminal redundancy on the (–) strand. The cccDNA serves as the template for transcription of all of the viral RNAs, including the pregenome, which has a terminal redundancy. The pregenome serves as mRNA for the translation of the core protein and also less frequently as mRNA for the downstream pol gene (*RT*) (236–240). The newly synthesized reverse transcriptase (RT) binds to a hairpin sequence (epsilon) at the 5′ end of its own mRNA and initiates (–)-strand DNA synthesis. The primer is a tyrosine residue located near the amino terminus of the enzyme (37,38); the RT remains covalently attached to the nascent (–)-strand DNA. The initial DNA synthesis involves copying of a 4-base sequence located in a bulge in the hairpin epsilon. A translocation event then occurs so that the 4-base DNA product is annealed to its complement in an 11- to 12-base sequence, DR1, located six bases into the 3′ terminal redundancy of the pregenome. Reverse transcription then extends to the 5′ end of the pregenome, with concomitant degradation of the template by an RNase H activity located near the carboxy terminus of the RT (241). Because reverse transcription initiated in the downstream terminal redundancy (*r*), the minus strand itself acquires a short terminal redundancy. The last 17 to 18 bases of the pregenome, including the cap structure and extending through the 5′ copy of DR1, are conserved and act as the primer for plus-strand synthesis. Normally, synthesis initiates after translocation of the RNA primer to a complementary sequence, DR2, located near the 3′ end of the pregenome, but upstream of the terminal redundancy (the location of DR2 defines the length of the cohesive overlap of virion DNA) (Fig. 55.2). Circularization of DNA, which is facilitated by the terminal redundancy of the minus strand, enables the (+)-strand DNA synthesis to continue and form the relaxed circular (*RC*) DNA. However, the (+)-strand DNA synthesis never completes. Occasionally (about 5% of the time), (+)-strand synthesis begins without primer translocation, creating a linear double-stranded (*DSL*) viral DNA.

ends, which are produced from either a single core promoter or two overlapping promoters (29). The Pol protein is produced by internal initiation of translation from the same pregenome RNA as the one used for the translation of the core and precore proteins. The X mRNA produces only the X protein.

Virus Replication

Most of what is known about hepadnavirus replication has been first learned from studies of duck hepatitis B virus, and then confirmed for human hepatitis B virus. The virus replication pathway is illustrated in Fig. 55.3. Upon infection, the

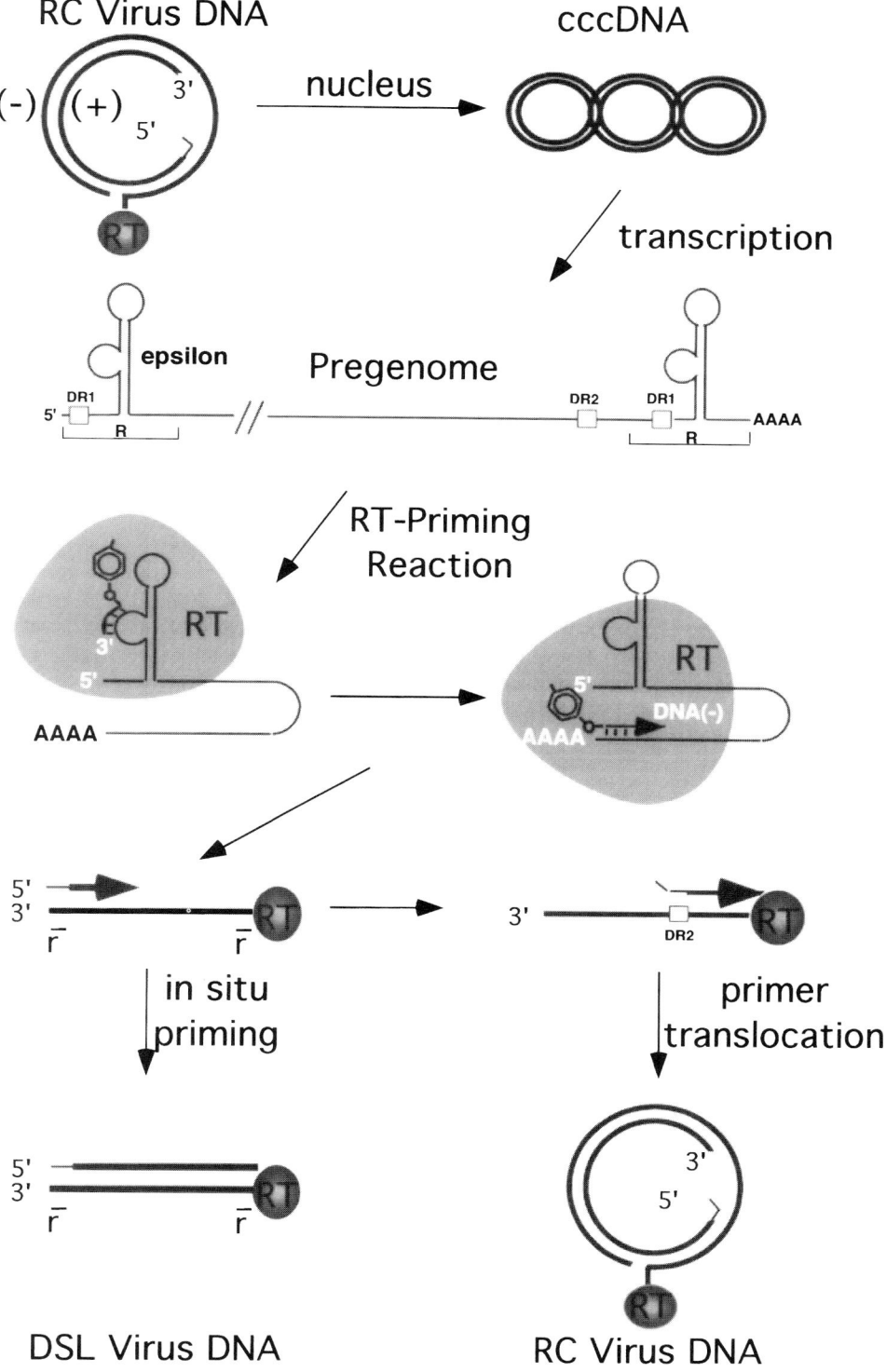

viral core particle is transported to the nucleus, the viral DNA is released, and the single-stranded gap in the DNA is filled by the viral DNA polymerase. Following the removal of the covalently attached protein and a 9-base terminal redundancy on the minus strand and the RNA on the plus strand, the DNA is converted to a fully double-stranded, covalently closed circular (ccc) DNA. The cccDNA serves as the template for transcription of all of the viral mRNAs (30), including the pregenome RNA, which is longer than the viral genomic DNA by 120 nucleotides. All of the RNAs have a common 3′-termination site and use the same polyadenylation signal, which maps to the viral core gene ORF (31) (Fig. 55.2). These mRNAs are transcribed from four promoters (core/precore, preS1, preS2/S, and X). Their transcription is controlled by two enhancers upstream of the core/precore and X promoters; the enhancers and promoters are, in turn, regulated by both general and liver-specific transcription factors. This fact explains why HBV replicates mainly in the liver. For a long time, it had been assumed that spliced RNAs were not involved in virus replication. One study, however, suggests that the large envelope protein, L, of DHBV is actually translated from two different mRNAs (32); in addition to the mRNA transcribed from the PreS1 promoter (Fig. 55.2), a second, spliced mRNA for L-HBsAg is transcribed from the core promoter. This spliced transcript is speculated to have some role in regulation of synthesis of additional copies of cccDNA in infected hepatocytes.

The early stage of infection is characterized by the translation of the pregenome mRNA into the viral nucleocapsid protein, the product of the core gene, and the viral reverse transcriptase (RT), the product of the *POL* gene (33). The nucleocapsid proteins assemble into icosahedral shells (core particles) of 240 subunits (120 dimers) (34), into which a complex of pregenome RNA and RT is packaged. The event that initiates packaging is the *cis*-binding of the RT to a stem-loop structure, epsilon, near the 5′ end of the pregenome RNA (Fig. 55.3), an event that may occur while this protein is still being translated (35,36). Within the core particle, reverse transcription initiates at a bulge on the side of the stem-loop of the pregenome, using the OH of a tyrosine residue in the amino terminal region of RT as a primer (37,38). Following copying of four nucleotides, the nascent DNA is translocated to a complementary sequence (DR1) located near the 3′ end of the pregenome, in the terminally redundant region, and reverse transcription then continues to the 5′ end of the RNA. The pregenome is degraded during reverse transcription by the RNase H activity associated with the carboxy terminal region of the RT (39,40). The last 17 to 18 nucleotides of the pregenome, including the cap, serves as the primer for second (plus) strand synthesis (23), which normally occurs after the primer is translocated to a complementary sequence near the 5′ end of the minus strand. Thus, after a short amount of plus strand synthesis, a circularization event must occur for plus strand synthesis to continue past the 5′ end of the minus strand. This is pre-

sumably facilitated by the short terminal redundancy of the minus strand (nine nucleotides) that is created because reverse transcription begins nine nucleotides into the 3′ terminal redundancy of the pregenome and continues to the end of the 5′ terminal redundancy. Plus strand synthesis is never entirely completed except during the process of cccDNA formation (33,41,42).

A second feature of the early phase of an infection is the accumulation of viral envelope proteins. These proteins are important not just for assembly of virions, which occurs by interaction of nucleocapsids with envelope proteins and budding into the endoplasmic reticulum, but also to ensure that newly made viral DNA does not all migrate to the nucleus to form more cccDNA. cccDNA formation is an early event that is quickly shut down in nondividing hepatocytes, so that cccDNA copy numbers per nucleus generally do not exceed 50. This is important for virus survival, since excessively high copy numbers can lead to cell death (43,44). Indeed, reconstruction experiments have revealed that a virus mutant that cannot shut down cccDNA synthesis is quickly replaced in the liver by a virus that can (45).

A need to negatively regulate cccDNA formation probably explains the observation that viral envelope proteins are vastly overproduced relative to what is needed to make virus. Indeed, most of the envelope protein is secreted not as part of the 42-nm virions, but as subviral 22-nm spheres and rods, which are composed exclusively of HBsAg, without core protein or viral DNA. HBsAg is generally present in serum of infected individuals at a >100-fold excess of infectious virions. The S-HBsAg, the smallest of the three envelope proteins, is the major protein component of the viral envelope in both the infectious virion and subviral HBsAg particles. The M and L proteins are present in the HBsAg preparations, of which virions constitute only a minor component, at ~5% and ~1%, respectively, of the levels of S (46).

The maturation of the viral genome (reverse transcription) takes place entirely within the core particle. Thus, unlike most other viruses, HBV nucleocapsid assembly actually begins before the replication of the viral genome. Once sufficient viral DNA synthesis has taken place, the core protein may undergo a conformational change, which triggers its association with HBsAg to form mature virions. This interaction takes place at the endoplasmic reticulum. The small form of HBsAg is required for the secretion of virus particles.

The Accessory Functions of Hepadnavirus Proteins

Among the HBV proteins, the role of two viral proteins remains unclear. One, the precore protein, is translated from an mRNA that is a few nucleotides longer at its 5′ end than the pregenome (47). These extra nucleotides encode an AUG that is in-frame with the core ORF, leading to the translation of a core protein that contains an extra 29 amino acids derived from the precore region. Part of this extra sequence serves as the signal peptide and directs the protein into the secretory pathway. After cleavage of the precore signal sequence (19 amino acids) and 34 amino acids from the carboxy terminus by cellular proteases, the protein is secreted from the cell as the so-called e antigen (HBeAg) (48,49). Thus, the e protein is longer at the N-terminus (by ten amino acids) and shorter at the C-terminus (by 34 amino acids) than the core protein. The presence of this protein in the serum is a marker of ongoing virus replication. The detection of antibodies to the e antigen, in contrast, is a good indicator that virus replication has ceased. However, the associations are not invariant, as virus variants that no longer have the capacity to make e antigen due to mutations in the precore region can become prevalent during a chronic infection. There is some evidence that the HBV e antigen may function to suppress the cellular immune response to the viral nucleocapsid subunit, thereby facilitating vertical (perinatal) transmission and chronic infection (50,51).

The second protein of uncertain function in the viral life cycle, the X protein, is exclusive to the orthohepadnaviruses (Fig. 55.2). This protein is generally believed to function as an activator of viral gene transcription, possibly by interacting with transcription factors, rather than with DNA, and its essential role in virus replication *in vivo* has been established by experiments with woodchuck hepatitis virus (52,53). However, it remains unclear if its function as an activator of transcription, only documented so far in cell culture, reflects its only function, or even one of its functions, *in vivo* (54). Cell culture studies have also suggested that X might induce cell cycle progression (55), participate in signal transduction (56), block cellular DNA repair (57), and inhibit proteasome function (58,59). Liver cancer has also been observed in some but not all strains of X transgenic mice (60,61), suggesting a similar role for X in chronically infected individuals.

Infection and Pathogenesis

As already noted, an important feature of the HBV replication cycle is the ability of the virus to sustain a chronic productive infection of hepatocytes without killing the host cells. Thus, it might be deduced that infection of the entire hepatocyte population would always result in a chronic infection; otherwise, the entire liver might be destroyed by the immune system. However, this is not the case. Infections can resolve in a very short time, probably less than 2 weeks (62–64), even after the apparent infection of every hepatocyte. Moreover, this appears to occur without a need for regeneration of the hepatocyte population from progenitor cells. On the basis of a study of transient infections of chimpanzees by HBV, one group of investigators concluded that virus may be removed without killing of the infected

cells. This work led to the inference that cytokines elaborated by the immune system are able to induce intracellular destruction of all virus replication intermediates, including cccDNA (65). There is considerable direct evidence that cytokines can induce removal of viral RNA, proteins, and replicating DNA from infected hepatocytes (66), but, as yet, no direct evidence that cytokines can induce loss of the cccDNA from an infected hepatocyte. Alternative models may therefore be necessary. These include the possibility that cccDNA is lost on cell division, as suggested for episomal Epstein–Barr virus (EBV) DNA in transformed cell lines (67), or by simple dilution of the infected cells as large numbers of infected hepatocytes are destroyed by cytotoxic T cells. These alternatives are difficult to resolve because of the lack of simple means to measure cell death rates and cumulative cell loss during the resolution of an infection. Nonetheless, as discussed in Chapter 57, these issues are critical for the rational design of antiviral therapies.

Even after infection of the entire hepatocyte population, infections usually resolve within 3 to 6 months, generally with a neutralizing antibody response (anti-HBs) that protects against reinfection. Residual virus DNA can be detected in blood and tissues years later by sensitive polymerase chain reaction (PCR) techniques, but there is so far no evidence that this residue is pathogenic. Nonetheless, individuals with a history of transient infection should be regarded as a potential source of infection (68,69).

Progression to chronic infection is assumed, then, to be inversely related to the hosts' immune response to the virus. As many as 90% of those infected before 1 year of age will become chronic carriers, a number that decreases to about 5% in adults. Chronic infection is usually defined by the presence of HBsAg in the serum for more than 1 year. [The lower cutoff of the enzyme-linked immunosorbent assays (ELISAs) currently used for HBsAg detection is between 1 and 10 ng/ml, while the blood of many carriers has titers in excess of 100 µg/ml.] Chronic infection can also be defined by the detection of viral DNA by either hybridization or PCR-based assays. Comparison of the results showed a lack of a strong correlation between HBsAg titers and HBV DNA titers in long-term carriers. One hypothesis, likely correct, is that viral DNA integrates into host DNA during the course of infection and continues to act as a template for HBsAg production, but not for pregenomic RNA, thereby dissociating HBsAg production from any dependence on ongoing virus replication. Indeed, both cell culture and animal studies suggest that the linear viral DNAs produced by *in situ* priming of plus strand synthesis (Fig. 55.3) are efficiently integrated in a collinear fashion (70,71), which would dissociate the core/precore promoter from the respective viral genes. Therefore, inhibition of viral DNA replication could occur without an effect on HBsAg production. The degree to which this transition occurs probably depends on the natural history of an infection. For instance, there is a significant difference between

HBV carriers in China and in Africa in the frequency of long-term HBsAg carriers who are also viremic (virus titers >5 × 10^5 per milliliter) (72). Thus, chronic infection may actually involve at least two different stages, an early one in which virus is produced at high titer by the liver, with virus levels as high as 10^{10} per milliliter of serum, and a later one, in which most hepatocytes have probably lost cccDNA, and technically are no longer infected, though HBsAg production, and perhaps synthesis of X protein, may continue from integrated viral DNA.

In addition, there is some evidence that peripheral blood mononuclear cells become latently infected and may have the capacity to produce virus under special circumstance. This has been deduced from cell culture studies with blood cells isolated from hosts with current or past infections, as well as from clinical studies of virus transmission routes (69,73–77). Thus, residual virus production in individuals with a history of transient infection and in HBsAg carriers, in whom virus production has virtually ceased, may arise from at least two different sources—white blood cells and hepatocytes. In addition, other tissues may also be infected and produce some virus. Early studies suggested that both exocrine and endocrine cells of the pancreas may become infected by HBV (78–80), a site of infection that is well documented in the DHBV-infected duck (81,82) and for which some evidence exists for WHV-infected woodchucks (83–85). Evidence of infection of the kidney also has been obtained for the latter species (81,84,85).

The evidence for infection of a wide variety of tissue types is surprising in view of evidence that the viral promoters/enhancers contain many elements that are generally considered liver-specific (86). The significance of this is unclear, and perhaps should be viewed with the understanding that only hepatocytes and, perhaps, cells in the kidney and pancreas of the duck appear to support virus gene expression efficiently.

Finally, there remain the issues of whether viral expression contributes directly to liver disease, including cirrhosis and hepatocellular carcinoma, or if the disease manifestations are the result of the immune response to the infection. As noted earlier, some investigators believe that the X protein may be oncogenic (87). Others have suggested that a carboxy terminus-truncated form of the M envelope protein of HBV, which functions as a general transcriptional activator in cell culture, may also be oncogenic (88–90). As for X, this effect has not been established in chronically infected individuals. On the other hand, viral gene expression may also contribute to disease progression indirectly by providing targets for the host immune response. Finally, the emergence of HBV variants during the course of a chronic infection, particularly those unable to make e antigen, may enhance pathogenicity and disease progression (91). However, some studies suggest that these mutants arise in response to, but not as a cause of, the liver disease (45,92,93).

Virus Evolution

Because hepadnaviruses replicate by reverse transcription, it might be expected that they would undergo rapid sequence evolution in and between carriers, similar to retroviruses, such as human immunodeficiency virus. However, at least two factors militate against rapid viral evolution. First, the overlap of reading frames through much of the viral genome restricts the number of viable mutations. Second, in the fully infected liver, it appears that new replication space is created only by cell death and regeneration. Therefore, many potentially viable mutants may disappear because there are no susceptible cells in the liver, and the block to intracellular cccDNA amplification restricts their stabilization through conversion to cccDNA. Although some HBV variants can escape from the antibodies induced by the current vaccines, there is still no evidence that individuals who have been successfully vaccinated are susceptible to infection by these escape mutants. Virus variation/evolution is a problem in hosts treated with the current antiviral nucleosides, as discussed in Chapters 54 and 57. It generally takes about a year or more for these drug-resistant variants to emerge as the prevalent species in the serum and liver. Quasi-species (sequence variants) are also common in long-term carriers, though their significance to, or as a reflection of, the disease course remains unclear (91).

HEPATITIS C VIRUS

After the discovery of HAV and HBV and the development of diagnostic methods for them in 1974, it was realized that a substantial number of transfusion-associated acute and chronic hepatitis cases could not be accounted for by these two viruses. These cases were termed non-A, non-B hepatitis (NANBH). The subsequently discovered hepatitis delta virus (HDV) did not fit the description of the NANBH virus. The NANBH was associated with liver cirrhosis and hepatocellular carcinoma. It was transmissible to chimpanzees, causing mild hepatitis (94); however, the etiologic agent could not be visualized or isolated. The causative agent was finally identified by cDNA expression cloning of the total nucleic acid derived from NANBH patients' sera and subsequent immunoscreening using again patients' sera (95). It was named hepatitis C virus (HCV), despite the fact that it was discovered long after HDV was identified.

Classification

HCV belongs to the *Hepacivirus* genus of Flaviviridae, which also includes the *Pestivirus* genus (e.g., bovine viral diarrhea virus, BVDV) and *Flavivirus* genus (e.g., yellow fever virus, Dengue virus, and Japanese encephalitis virus). Although there is not much primary sequence homology between HCV and other members of the Flaviviridae, they have significant similarity in their genomic structure and probably replication strategy. Therefore, the other members of Flaviviridae, in particular BVDV, are often used as models for the study of HCV. This is particularly useful for understanding HCV replication because no efficient cell culture or small animal models have been available for HCV; thus, very little information on HCV replication could be directly obtained from HCV studies. The recent creation of HCV subgenomic replicon should facilitate the studies of HCV replication in the future (95a).

Based on sequence relationship, HCV can be divided into at least six major genotypes and 11 to 12 subtypes (96). Viral sequences differing by more than 28% are considered to be in different genotypes. Different subtypes within the same genotype differ by 14% to 25%. Viral isolates differing by less than 12% are considered to be in the same clade. Genotype 1a and 1b are the predominant genotype in North America, Europe, and Asia, accounting for more than 70% of HCV isolated. Viral genotype has potentially important implications for the pathogenesis of the virus and its treatment (see Chapters 54 and 57). Genotyping usually is performed by sequencing of the selected regions (typically the 5'-untranslated region, core, or ns5b regions; see Diagnosis, below) of the viral RNA. In addition, HCV is characterized by the presence of *quasi-species* (97), a term used to describe the RNA species that differ by very minor nucleotide changes. All the HCV isolates consist of a population of virus particles, which contain a master (predominant) RNA species and other minor variants with some nucleotide changes (98,99). The complexity and evolution of quasi-species may reflect the clinical course of viral infections.

Virion Morphology

HCV is an enveloped, spherical particle of 30 to 80 nm. The variation in size of the observed particles reflects the difficulty in obtaining pure virus preparations because of the low virus titer in most sources. Virus particles have been observed in human plasma (100) and chimpanzee liver (101). They have a very low density, with a buoyant density in sucrose of 1.09 to 1.11 g/cm^3 or lower, probably because of their association with lipid and serum lipoproteins, such as lactoferrin (102), and immune complexes (103). The virus contains a 9.5-kb RNA genome. The envelope consists of two envelope proteins, E1 and E2, which probably form spikes on the virion surface, although these spikes have not been visualized. Inside the envelope is a nucleocapsid, which is likely icosahedral in structure. The nucleocapsid consists of the core (C) protein and viral RNA. The presence of the viral envelope (lipid bilayer) explains the earlier observation that infectivity of the major NANBH agent can be inactivated by treatment with chloroform or detergents (104).

Genome Structure

The viral RNA contains a single ORF, which encodes a polyprotein of approximately 3,010 amino acids. The polyprotein is processed by cellular and viral proteases into three or four structural proteins and six nonstructural proteins (Fig. 55.4). At the 5' end of the RNA is a stretch of untranslated region (5'-UTR) of 341 nucleotides, which is more conserved (more than 90% sequence homology among various HCV isolates) than most of the coding sequences. It consists of a highly conserved structure of four stem-loops and a pseudoknot structure, which together constitute the IRES (105–107). The presence of the IRES allows HCV RNA to be translated by a 5'-cap–independent translation mechanism, distinct from the mechanism of translation for most of the cellular mRNAs. Thus, this translation mechanism offers a potential target for antiviral agents. The HCV IRES includes a small part of the amino-terminus of the HCV ORF (108). Because of the conservation of the 5'-UTR sequence, it is the sequence most often used for the design of RT-PCR primers for the detection of HCV RNA in clinical settings.

At the 3' end of the RNA is another stretch of untranslated sequences (3'-UTR) of approximately 200 nucleotides. At the very 3' end is a 98-nucleotide region, termed X (109,110). This region was not present in the HCV sequences originally reported. Subsequent studies showed that this is the most conserved region of the entire viral RNA (111). It forms a three-stem-loop structure, which is conserved in all of the known virus isolates. Upstream of the X region is a stretch of poly (U) sequence of variable lengths, followed by another stretch of sequence consisting exclusively of pyrimidine residues (U and C); these regions together range approximately from 30 to 90 nucleotides. Further upstream is another stretch of sequence (approximately 30 to 40 nucleotides) that is significantly variable among different genotypes, although it is conserved within the same genotype (111). By analysis of the infectivity of the deletion mutants of the HCV RNA in chimpanzees, it has been shown that the X region and the poly-U and UC-rich sequences, but not the variable 3'-UTR sequence, are important for viral infectivity (112). The X region can stimulate the translation of viral proteins, possibly by interacting with the translation machineries at the 5'-UTR site (113). The 3'-UTR is also important for RNA replication, because it presumably contains sequences recognized by the viral polymerase for RNA replication (114). Because of its functional importance and sequence conservation, the 3'-UTR is also a potential target for antiviral agents. However, the 3'-UTR has not been a useful region for RT-PCR detection of HCV RNA, probably because of the presence of strong secondary structures. Both the 5'- and 3'-UTR interact with several cellular proteins (115–118), which may be important for translation or replication of viral RNA.

Protein Structure and Functions

The large polyprotein encoded by HCV RNA is processed by cellular and viral proteases into nine or ten different proteins (Fig. 55.4). The first protein from the N-terminus is the core protein, which constitutes the virion nucleocapsid

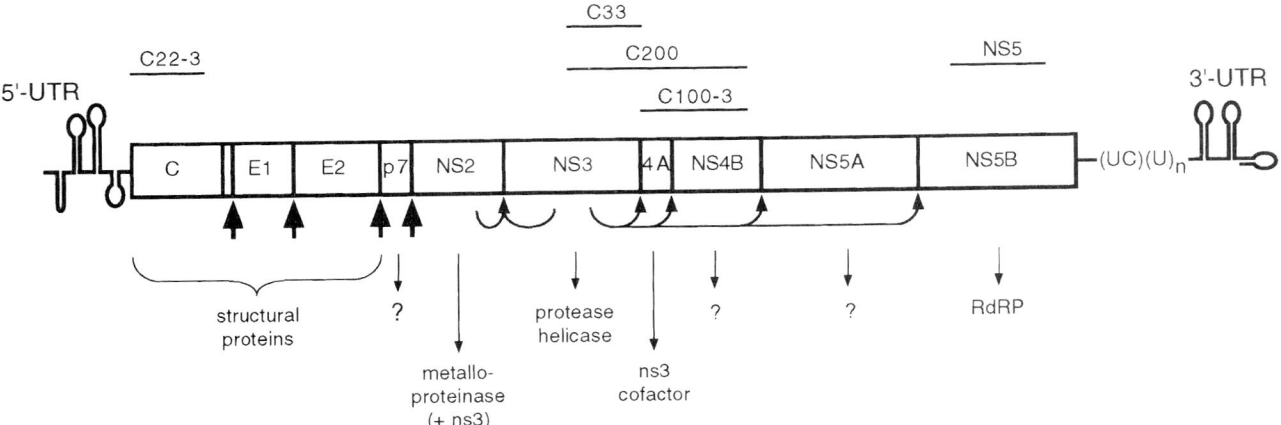

FIGURE 55.4. Hepatitis C virus (HCV) genome structure. HCV genome is a 9.5-kb, single-stranded, positive-sense RNA. It has a 341-nucleotide (nt)-long 5'-untranslated region (*UTR*), which contains an IRES sequence. Most of the length of the genome consists of an ORF, encoding a polyprotein of approximately 3,010 amino acids. The 3'-end untranslated region includes (from 5' → 3') a stretch (30 to 40 nt) of variable sequence, a U-U/C-rich region and the 98-nt conserved X region (represented by three stem-loops). The polyprotein is processed by cellular signal peptidases (*thick arrows*) into structural proteins C, E1, E2, and possibly p7, and by ns2 and ns3 proteases (*thin arrows*) into the remaining individual proteins, all of which are nonstructural proteins. The biochemical functions of the viral proteins are indicated. The *horizontal bars* on the top represent the peptides used for screening of anti-HCV antibodies in the commercial enzyme-linked immunosorbent assay (ELISA) and recombinant immunoblot assay (RIBA) screening assays.

and likely complexes with the viral RNA. The next two proteins, E1 and E2, are the envelope glycoproteins, which form a heterodimer on the surface of the virion (119). The E2 protein contains the domain important for virus binding to the receptors. It is the protein that displays the most heterogeneity, particularly in the two hypervariable regions at the very N-terminus of the protein, among various virus isolates (120,121). The function of E1 is still not clear; the E1-E2 complex appears to be the functional form of the viral envelope. E1 also interacts with the core protein (122); this interaction is important for virus assembly. The next protein is p7; whether it is a virion structural protein or not is still unclear. The cleavage of C-E1-E2-p7 from each other and from the remaining proteins is achieved by cellular signal peptidases during protein translation. The remaining proteins are all nonstructural proteins (not incorporated into the virion). The ns2 protein is a metalloproteinase, which requires Zn^{2+} ions for its activity (123). The ns2 protease activity can be demonstrated only when it is joined to the next protein ns3, and the only demonstrated function for ns2 is to autocleave the junction between ns2 and ns3. Ns3 is also a protease (a serine protease) (124), which cleaves at all the boundaries of the remaining proteins, thus releasing individual proteins. In addition, the C-terminal two-thirds of ns3 contains nucleoside triphosphatase (NTPase)/helicase activity (125), which may be important for HCV translation and/or RNA replication. The crystal structures of the ns3 protease and helicase have been determined separately (126–128), which will facilitate the future design of antivi-

ral agents. Ns4a forms a complex with ns3, and is a cofactor for the protease activity (129). The functions of ns4b and ns5a proteins are not yet clear. Ns5a is a highly phosphorylated protein. The last protein ns5b is an RNA-dependent RNA polymerase (114,130,131), which is responsible for the replication of viral RNA. Most of these proteins are probably required for viral replication. Therefore, they are potential targets for antiviral agents.

Viral Replication

Because there were no efficient cell culture systems or small animal models for HCV infection, and the virus titers in infected patients and chimpanzees are generally low, it had been difficult to study the mechanism of viral replication until recently. HCV is a hepatotropic virus, infecting primarily hepatocytes; whether HCV can infect hepatic non-parenchymal cells or extrahepatic tissues is a subject of controversy. HCV RNA can be detected by RT-PCR in many different tissues of infected patients, although the specificity of RT-PCR and the possibility of serum contamination of tissue samples have precluded firm conclusions on this issue. Nevertheless, the prevailing evidence suggests that HCV can replicate in lymphoid cells and monocytes (132). The wide range of extrahepatic manifestation of the HCV-associated diseases (e.g., type II mixed cryoglobulinemia, Sjögren's syndrome, purpura, pseudomembranous glomerulonephritis, and non-Hodgkin's B-cell lymphoma) also suggests that HCV may replicate in other tissues. Using sera from infected patients, many laboratories have demonstrated that HCV can infect and replicate in various hepatocyte cell lines, primary hepatocytes and T- and B-cell lines in tissue culture (133–137). However, the viral RNA usually persists only for a short period of time, and the viral RNA can be detected only by very sensitive RT-PCR, suggesting the inefficiency of HCV replication in cell culture.

The first step of viral infection is the attachment of the virus particles, through E2, to a surface molecule on the target cells. The cell surface molecule (i.e., viral receptor) has been reported to be CD81 (138), which is a member of the tetraspanin protein family and is widely distributed in many cell types. The function of this molecule in normal cells is not yet known. The binding of E2 to CD81 can trigger signaling pathways of CD81, resulting in aggregation of lymphoid cells and inhibition of B-cell proliferation (139). Both the antibodies against CD81 and against E2 can block the virus binding. However, CD81 does not yet qualify as a true receptor for HCV, because the binding does not trigger internalization of the virus particles into cells. Therefore, at least another molecule is likely needed for virus entry into target cells. This second molecule (or "co-receptor") may be more liver-specific, thus, explaining the hepatotropism of HCV. The identity of this molecule is still not known. Another cell surface molecule, the low-density lipoprotein (LDL) receptor, has also been implicated as an HCV receptor (140).

Once the virus enters the cell, the viral RNA is first translated into a polyprotein, from which the RNA polymerase (ns5b) is released by ns3 protease. This polymerase will then replicate viral RNA by RNA-dependent RNA synthesis into negative-sense RNA. Thus, the detection of the negative-sense RNA represents the most definitive evidence of viral replication in the cells; however, the structure of this negative-sense RNA is not yet known. The negative-sense RNA serves as the template for the synthesis of viral genomic RNA. As inferred from the replication strategy of other flaviviruses, only the full-length genomic RNA, but not subgenomic RNA, is synthesized. The mechanism of regulation of viral RNA synthesis is poorly understood. Presumably the 5′- and 3′-end sequences of viral RNA contain the *cis*-acting signal for initiation of RNA synthesis. This entire process likely takes place in the cytoplasm.

Translation of the viral polyprotein from genomic-sense RNA is mediated by an IRES-dependent mechanism (105). Translation most likely occurs on the membrane-associated ribosomes. The polyprotein synthesized is processed both during and after translation. The cleavage of the first three proteins, core, E1 and E2, is carried out by cellular signal peptidases in the endoplasmic reticulum during translation. The ns2-ns3 junction is cleaved by the autoprotease activity of these two proteins (123,141). Finally, the remaining proteins are cleaved by ns3-ns4a protease after translation. Once synthesized and released by the signal peptidase, the core protein is retained in the cytosol compartment, but is most likely

associated with intracellular membranes because its carboxyl-terminal end sequence is highly hydrophobic (142,143). In contrast, E1 and E2 (and probably p7) are translocated into the lumen of the endoplasmic reticulum, and glycosylated in the process. E1 and E2 form a heterodimer and are anchored onto the membrane of the ER because of the presence of ER-retention signal (144,145). Most of the other viral proteins are also associated with cellular membranes in the cytoplasm, where viral RNA synthesis likely takes place. Curiously, some of the viral proteins (e.g., core, ns5a, ns3) contain nuclear localization signals. Thus, some of these proteins may be translocated into the nucleus under some conditions. The significance of the potential nuclear phase in HCV infection is not known.

The newly synthesized viral genomic RNA and viral structural proteins (C, E1, and E2) then form virus particles, most likely in the ER, where the E1-E2 complex is anchored. The completed virus particles can be found in some vesicles in the cytoplasm (101). Indeed, as with many flaviviruses, proliferation of intracellular membranes is a feature of HCV infections (146,147). Virions are likely secreted into the extracellular space using cellular secretory pathways.

The Accessory Functions of Viral Proteins

Besides their functions (protease, helicase, and RNA polymerase) involved in viral replication, the various viral proteins also have other diverse accessory activities, which may not be necessary for viral replication but may affect viral pathogenesis by contributing to alterations of host cell functions. Most of these reported functions have been demonstrated only in artificial culture systems; they may occur only under special conditions.

The core protein has been demonstrated to bind to the cytoplasmic domains of tumor necrosis factor (TNF) receptor and lymphotoxin-β receptor (148–150), resulting in alterations of the cellular sensitivity to these cytokines. The precise effects of the core protein varied; both enhancement and reduction of the sensitivity to these cytokines have been reported (150–152). The core protein also binds to several cellular proteins that can serve as transcription factors, including hnRNP K and RNA helicase (153–155); correspondingly, the core protein can activate the transcription of reporter genes under the control of various promoters, including cellular promoters, such as c-*myc*, c-*fos*, and viral promoters (156,157), including retroviral long-terminal-repeat (LTR) and HBV endogenous promoters. Furthermore, the core protein has a transforming activity, capable of oncogenic transformation of rat primary embryo fibroblasts, when cooperating with c-*ras* oncogene (158). This activity may be partially caused by its ability to interact with and inhibit a bZIP protein (159) and its ability to bind to 14-3-3 protein and activate Raf-1 kinase (160). It may also suppress the cytotoxic T-cell response (161).

The E2 protein binds to CD81 molecule and may trigger the signal transduction of cells, particularly lymphocytes (139). Thus, theoretically, HCV can alter the normal functions of a cell even if HCV does not infect that particular cell type. In addition, E2 binds to and inhibits the cellular double-stranded RNA–activated protein kinase PKR (162), which is an important mediator of interferon action in the inhibition of viral translation; as a result, the antiviral effect of interferon may be blocked by E2. PKR also induces apoptosis; therefore, the inhibition of PKR by E2 may inhibit apoptosis, thus facilitating viral persistence or oncogenesis. The interaction of E2 with PKR is the result of sequence similarity between E2 and PKR as well as its natural substrate eIF-2a (162). The extent of sequence homology is particularly high for the E2 of HCV genotype 1, a fact consistent with the poor response rate of genotype 1 to interferon therapy (163). E2 also has been shown to activate transcription of stress response genes, such as glucose-regulated protein grp78 (164).

The ns5a protein also binds to PKR via a stretch of sequence termed the "interferon sensitivity determining region" (ISDR) (165). The variation of this stretch of sequences within ns5a has been shown to correlate with the sensitivity or resistance of HCV to interferon (i.e., more amino acid divergence from the prototype HCV-J strain correlates with higher sensitivity to interferon). However, this correlation appears to hold true for only Japanese HCV patients. Similar studies in the United States and Europe failed to show such a correlation (166). Nevertheless, the presence of the ISDR sequence allows the ns5a protein to bind to PKR and may confer resistance to the antiviral effects of interferon (167,168). Ns5a also binds to several other cellular proteins, including Grb2 (a growth-regulatory protein) (169) and a vesicle-associated membrane protein (a vesicle transport protein) (170). The binding of these proteins by ns5a likely contributes to perturbation of the functions of these molecules. The ns5a protein lacking the N-terminal sequences also has been shown to have a *trans*-acting activity, capable of activating transcription of cellular genes (171,172). The significance of such a finding is still unclear.

It is likely that other viral proteins may also have the ability to alter other cellular functions. Ns3 has been shown to bind to protein kinases A and C and may have oncogenic activity as well (173,174).

Viral Evolution

During chronic HCV infection, the sequences of the prevalent strains of HCV usually undergo rapid and continuous evolution. The rate of evolution has been estimated to be approximately 1 to 2×10^{-3} nucleotides per site per year (175). The most significant evolution involves the hypervariable regions of E2 protein (120,121). This region contains several antibody-binding epitopes. The variation of the E2 sequences is probably a consequence of immune selection; namely, new variants cannot be neutralized by the existing antibodies, thus allowing the new HCV variants to escape immune surveillance. This mechanism may contribute to HCV persistence. In immunocompromised patients, such as those with hypogammaglobulinemia or HIV co-infection, or bone marrow transplant recipients, the rate of RNA sequence evolution is considerably slower (176–178), suggesting that virus evolution is the result of immunoselection. The complexity of the quasi-species (as determined for the hypervariable regions) also can vary in response to interferon treatment (179).

Diagnosis

The diagnosis of HCV infection is primarily based on the detection of IgG antibodies by ELISA and recombinant immunoblot assay (RIBA) using different viral antigens (Fig. 55.4). The first commercial assay was aimed at detecting ns4 antibodies using a recombinant HCV peptide (c-100-3 peptide); subsequently, several other proteins, including ns3 (c33c and c200), core (c22-3), and ns5b, were included in the assays to increase their sensitivity and specificity. Typically, the IgG antibodies can be detected approximately 2 to 4 months postexposure at the time of ALT elevation. The presence of IgM antibodies is variable and unreliable for clinical diagnosis of acute or chronic infection (180,181). The presence of E1 and E2 antibodies, which may contain neutralizing antibodies, are also quite variable among patients. Although the detection of HCV antibodies, coupled with ALT elevation, is used as an indication of active and persistent infection (based on the assumption that most HCV infections result in persistent infection), the definitive diagnosis of HCV infection is based on the detection of viral RNA by either RT-PCR or other molecular amplification techniques. Most recent methods are capable of detecting as few as 100 copies of viral RNA. Quantitation of viral RNA in the serum is important for assessing the efficacy of treatment. Another important diagnostic test of clinical significance is the determination of viral genotype, particularly in consideration of the therapeutic options, since the genotype affects the regimen and outcome of therapy (interferon with or without ribavirin). Genotyping is typically done by sequencing the 5'-UTR, core, or ns5b regions using specific RT-PCR primers.

HEPATITIS DELTA VIRUS

Hepatitis delta virus (HDV) was first detected as a novel antigen, termed hepatitis delta antigen (HDAg), present in the nuclei of hepatocytes of some HBV carriers experiencing episodes of acute hepatitis in Italy. It was initially thought to represent a previously unidentified antigen of HBV. Later, transmission of this agent into chimpanzees, which developed acute hepatitis, and subsequent isolation of a virus particle of 36 nm (in contrast to the 42-nm HBV particles) containing an RNA genome established that HDV is a novel virus (182). HDV is classified within the satellite virus group in a floating genus, *Deltavirus* (without virus family designation). It depends on HBV for its transmission, because HDV does not encode its own envelope proteins. Nevertheless, HDV is different from other satellite viruses in that HDV does not share sequences with its helper virus HBV and can replicate autonomously even in the absence of HBV, although no virus particles are produced. For this reason, HDV has never been detected free of HBV co-infection clinically. Early reports raised the possibility of HBV-free HDV infection (in the case of reinfection of liver transplants) (183). More recently, it was discovered that these patients were infected with a low level of HBV (184).

Three genotypes of HDV have been identified so far (185). Genotype I is the most common type and has been identified in almost every part of the world. It has been associated with hepatitis of varying severity, ranging from mild to fulminant. Genotype II is detected mainly in Asia, particularly Taiwan and Japan, and has been associated with relatively milder hepatitis (186). Genotype III has been isolated only from South America so far, and is often associated with fulminant hepatitis (185). The viral RNA also exists as a quasi-species that undergoes evolution during the clinical course of infection.

Virion Structure

HDV is a 36-nm spherical particle containing an envelope made up of HBsAg (Fig. 55.5). Inside the envelope is a

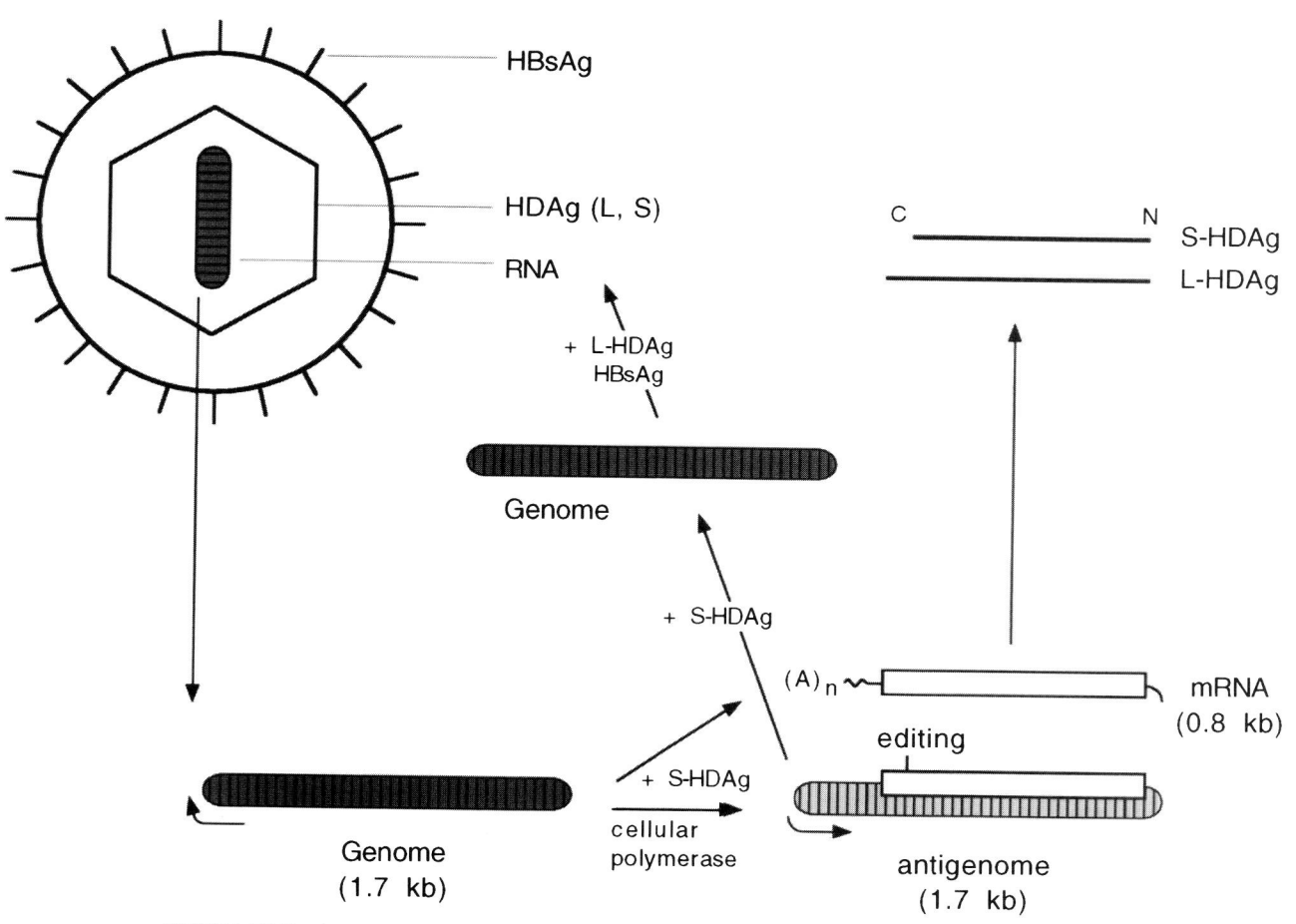

FIGURE 55.5. The genome structure and replication strategy of hepatitis delta virus (HDV). The virion contains hepatitis B surface antigen (*HBsAg*) (derived from HBV) as envelope proteins, an internal nucleocapsid consisting of hepatitis delta antigen (*HDAg*) (both the large and small forms) and a circular single-stranded RNA of 1.7 kb. The RNA genome is replicated in the presence of S-HDAg by the as-yet-undefined cellular polymerases into an antigenomic RNA of 1.7 kb and a 0.8-kb mRNA, which encodes S-HDAg. The L-HDAg is encoded from the same mRNA after an RNA editing event has extended the S-HDAg ORF. The antigenomic RNA is further replicated into genomic RNA. Together with L-HDAg and HBsAg, the genomic RNA is packaged and assembled into the virion. The S-HDAg is incorporated into the virion by interacting with L-HDAg. RNA replication takes place in the nucleus, while virus assembly occurs in the cytoplasm. *C*, carboxyl-terminus; *N*, amino-terminus.

nucleocapsid, which consists of HDAg and RNA. HDAg is the only protein encoded by HDV. The viral genome is a circular, single-stranded RNA of 1.7 kb, which is the only circular RNA and the smallest RNA genome among the human viruses (187,188). Most of the nucleotides within the RNA are complementary to each other and form intramolecular base pairing; thus, the viral RNA appears double-stranded under native conditions (189). This fact may explain the relative stability of HDV RNA in clinical samples. A small region (approximately 85 nucleotides) of the viral RNA contains a ribozyme activity, i.e., the RNA can cleave itself in the absence of any protein factors (190,191). This activity is critical for viral RNA replication. The viral RNA does not encode any protein; however, the antigenomic-sense RNA, which is replicated from the viral genome and is detected only in the infected cells, encodes a protein, namely HDAg. For this reason, HDV RNA is considered to be a negative-sense RNA.

Two forms of HDAg are usually detected in the virion, a large form (L-HDAg) of 27 kd and a small form (S-HDAg) of 24 kd. These two forms have identical sequence except that the former contains 19 additional amino acids at the C-terminus. Both the L- and S-HDAg complex with viral RNA to form the nucleocapsid of the virion. The relative ratio of these two forms is variable, but, in general, is approximately equimolar in the virion (192,193). HDAg is a phosphoprotein present in the nuclei of the infected cells and was the protein that led to the discovery of HDV. Besides its role in the formation of nucleocapsids, HDAg plays important roles in viral replication: S-HDAg is required for viral RNA replication (194), whereas L-HDAg inhibits RNA replication (195), but is required for virion assembly (196) (see Viral Replication, below). It contains sequences that mediate its nuclear localization, dimerization, and RNA binding, all of which are important for viral replication.

Viral Replication

HDV infects only hepatocytes; no extrahepatic infection has been detected. Because HDV uses HBV surface antigens as its own envelope proteins, HDV probably uses the same receptor as HBV to infect liver cells. However, the receptors for these two viruses have not been unequivocally identified. The receptor specificity most likely determines the hepatotropism of HDV. Once inside the cells, HDV can replicate in the absence of HBV, and, unlike HBV, can replicate in cell cultures of nonhepatic origin, indicating that HDV RNA replication does not require liver-specific factors.

Replication of HDV RNA takes place in the nuclei; both HDV RNA and HDAg are detected mainly in the nuclei. HDV RNA replication occurs by RNA-dependent RNA synthesis, namely, HDV RNA is first replicated into

an antigenomic-sense RNA, which is then replicated back to genomic RNA. The relative ratio of the genomic versus antigenomic RNAs is approximately 30:1, suggesting an asymmetric replication favoring the synthesis of the former RNA (197). RNA replication is thought to occur by a double rolling-circle mechanism (198): first, the antigenomic-sense RNA of multiple genomic length (e.g., 3.4 kb and 5.1 kb, etc.) is synthesized, presumably as a result of continuing rolling of the polymerase on the circular RNA template. This RNA multimer is processed by the ribozyme activity of HDV RNA into monomer-length (1.7 kb) RNA. The monomer antigenomic RNA is then ligated to form a circular RNA, which is then used for the second round of rolling circle replication to generate the monomer-length circular genomic RNA, thus completing the replication cycle. The abolition of the ribozyme activity in either the genomic or the antigenomic strand inhibited HDV RNA replication, supporting the double rolling-circle replication model (199). Ligation (circularization) of both genomic and antigenomic RNA was initially thought to be carried out by the HDV ribozyme, similar to their cleavage. But a recent study suggests that it may be mediated by cellular RNA ligases instead (200). In this replication process, no DNA intermediate is involved. Therefore, the persistent infection with HDV is not due to integration of viral genome into chromosome, but rather depends on continuous and controlled replication of HDV RNA.

Besides the 1.7-kb genomic and antigenomic RNA, HDV also synthesizes a small (0.8-kb) polyadenylated RNA of antigenomic sense, which contains an ORF encoding HDAg. This RNA is the mRNA for translation of HDAg. It appears that all of the HDAg is translated from this mRNA; the 1.7-kb antigenomic RNA, which also contains the ORF for HDAg but does not have poly(A), cannot be used for the translation of HDAg (201). The earlier literature indicated that this mRNA represents the initial product of HDV RNA replication; its synthesis is inhibited by HDAg by a feedback inhibitory mechanism (202). However, recent evidence suggests that this RNA is transcribed independently of the full-length HDV RNA and is continuously synthesized throughout the HDV replication cycle (203). The structure and coding capacity of this mRNA is different between the early and late stages of the HDV life cycle because of the occurrence of RNA editing: in the early stage the mRNA encodes S-HDAg, whereas in the late stage it encodes L-HDAg.

During HDV replication, a specific nucleotide conversion occurs at a site slightly downstream of the termination codon (on the antigenomic strand) of the ORF for HDAg, changing the termination codon for S-HDAg into a tryptophan codon, thus extending the ORF for an additional 19 amino acids (204). This extended ORF encodes L-HDAg. This mutation is termed RNA editing, because, unlike random mutations, this nucleotide conversion occurs at a specific site. This editing is carried out by a cellular double-stranded-RNA adenosine deaminase, which converts A → G at the editing site on the antigenomic strand, thus eliminating the termination codon (205). As a result of this editing, the mRNA encoding L-HDAg gradually accumulates, resulting in increasing synthesis of L-HDAg, which, in turn, inhibits further RNA synthesis and initiates virion assembly. Thus, RNA editing enables the virus to switch from the RNA replication phase into the virion assembly phase for the formation and production of virus particles. Neither the mechanism of regulation of the editing specificity nor its temporal regulation is yet known. In clinical infections, both forms of HDAg are usually detected in a variable ratio, irrespective of clinical stages. The RNA editing is likely regulated by host factors.

HDV RNA replication requires S-HDAg. Mutant HDV RNA defective in making a functional S-HDAg can be complemented by the wild-type S-HDAg supplied *in trans* (194). However, S-HDAg is not a polymerase, and HDV does not encode any other protein; therefore, HDV RNA replication is likely carried out by cellular enzymes. Precisely which cellular polymerase is responsible for HDV RNA replication is still not clear. Since *in vitro* replication studies suggested that HDV RNA replication can be inhibited by a-amanitin (an inhibitor of various DNA-dependent RNA polymerases depending on the drug concentration) at a low concentration (206), it has been suggested that RNA polymerase II may be responsible for HDV RNA replication. Recent studies suggest that cellular polymerases are also involved in HDV RNA replication (206a). In any case, these polymerases have to be converted from using DNA templates to using RNA templates. HDAg may participate in such a function by serving as a component of the transcription complex. Indeed, the abilities of S-HDAg to form protein-protein interactions and to bind RNA are required for its *trans*-activating function (207). On the other hand, L-HDAg can inhibit HDV RNA replication, probably by forming a complex with S-HDAg. Both S- and L-HDAg have been shown to either stimulate or inhibit cellular polymerase II–mediated gene expression, suggesting that HDAg may interact with cellular transcription machineries (208,209). The potential effects of HDAg on cellular transcription machineries may partially account for the pathogenesis of HDV.

Virion Assembly and Spread

HDV utilizes HBV surface antigen (HBsAg) as envelope proteins. Thus, HDV virion assembly cannot occur in the absence of HBV co-infection. The presence of both HBsAg and L-HDAg (but not S-HDAg) is sufficient to trigger the formation of virus-like particles (196), as a result of interaction between these two proteins. The last 19 amino acids, which contain a prenylation signal (210), of L-HDAg likely provide the signal that triggers virus assembly. These facts explain why RNA editing is a key event allowing HDV to start virion assembly. HDV RNA and S-HDAg are incor-

porated into virion particles by interacting with L-HDAg. The intracellular site of virion assembly is not clear; it most likely takes place in the endoplasmic reticulum, as it is the site of HBV assembly. Only the genomic RNA, but not the antigenomic RNA, is packaged into the virion. The virion particles are eventually released into the extracellular space. Similar to HBV particles, the infectivity of the HDV particles is dependent on the presence of pre-S1 sequence of HBsAg (the large form of the HBsAg).

Molecular Pathogenesis

The association of genotype III HDV with more severe hepatitis and genotype II with milder hepatitis suggests that viral genetic makeup can affect viral pathogenicity. A possible mechanism is the potential cytotoxicity of HDAg. Indeed, overexpression of HDAg in liver cell lines has been reported to cause cytotoxicity in tissue culture (211). This can be attributed to the possible effects of HDAg on the transcription machineries of host cells, as HDV will compete with host genes for the same factors for RNA synthesis. However, HDAg-expressing transgenic mice or stable cell lines, in general, are devoid of any obvious pathology. The pathogenesis of HDV may be synergistic with HBV pathogenesis, as HDV reinfection of the transplanted liver often is asymptomatic until HBV is reactivated or reinfects the transplanted liver (212). Another potential mechanism is immune-mediated pathogenesis, as CD4- and CD8-positive cells are detected in the HDV-infected liver (213). Administration of antibodies against HDAg may exacerbate HDV hepatitis in infected woodchucks (214). Therefore, humoral and cellular immune responses likely contribute to the pathogenesis of HDV.

Diagnosis

Acute delta hepatitis should be considered in every case of fulminant hepatitis and when HBV carriers develop recurrence of acute hepatitis. Since HDV/HBV co-infection and HDV superinfection of HBV carriers have different outcomes (the latter more often leads to chronic delta hepatitis), the distinction between the two modes of infection is important. This can be achieved by examining anti-HBc antibody. The detection of anti-HBc IgM antibody indicates acute HBV infection and thus HBV/HDV co-infection. HDV infection is diagnosed by detection of HDAg in the serum by enzyme-linked immunoassay (EIA) or radioimmunoassay (RIA), or of HDV RNA by dot blot hybridization or RT-PCR. The presence of IgM and IgG anti-HDAg can also be demonstrated in most cases. The detection of HDAg in the liver is considered the gold standard for diagnosis of HDV infection.

Control of HBV infections by vaccination has significantly reduced the incidence of new HDV infections in recent years.

HEPATITIS E VIRUS

Hepatitis E virus (HEV) is responsible for major outbreaks of acute food-borne hepatitis in developing tropical countries, particularly in Asia, Africa, and Central America. It was initially called enteric non-A, non-B hepatitis. A unique characteristic of HEV infection is its high mortality rate, particularly among pregnant women in the third trimester (10% to 20% mortality). The virus was originally identified by two complementary approaches: one by subtractive cloning and differential amplification of the nucleic acid material obtained from the bile of experimentally infected cynomolgus macaques (215), and the other by immunoscreening, using convalescent sera, of a cDNA expression library made from the fecal material of infected patients (216). The virus belongs to the Caliciviridae family, which are positive-stranded RNA viruses and include another human enteric virus, Norwalk virus, although HEV and Norwalk virus share no sequence homology. All of the virus isolates can be divided into two genetic groups, the Asian (type species, Burma strain) and Central American (type species, Mexican strain) groups. However, these two groups are antigenically related, and belong to the same serotype. HEV infects not only humans, but also causes prevalent infections in other animals, including pigs and rodents (217,218).

Virion Structure

HEV is a 32- to 34-nm nonenveloped spherical virus particle. The viral capsid is composed of regular arrays of cap-sid proteins, forming an icosahedral structure (219). The lack of a lipid envelope explains why the virus particle is relatively resistant to treatment with ether, chloroform, or mild detergents. Within the capsid is a 7.5-kb single-strand, positive-sense, polyadenylated RNA, with a 5′-cap structure. The RNA contains three overlapping ORFs (Fig. 55.6). ORF 1, representing approximately 5 kb from the 5′ end of RNA, encodes a polyprotein, which is likely processed into several nonstructural proteins. This polyprotein is predicted to contain several functional motifs indicative of their potential roles in protein processing and RNA replication. These motifs include methyltransferase, papain-like cysteine protease, helicase and RNA-dependent RNA polymerase (220). ORF 2 is located at the 3′ end of RNA and encodes the capsid protein, which is the protein used for the immunodetection of HEV infection (216,221). ORF 3 is localized between and overlaps the other two ORFs. It encodes an immunogenic protein of 123 amino acids of unknown functions. There is a very short stretch (27 nucleotides) of untranslated region at the 5′ end of RNA.

Viral Replication

HEV can infect various primate species, including chimpanzees, macaques, African green monkeys, tamarins, and squirrel monkeys after intravenous inoculation or oral administration. Infected animals develop viremia and shed virus in the stool; the primary target organ is the liver. HEV also infects nonprimate animal species, including pigs and rats, in natural infections. However, there is no efficient cul-

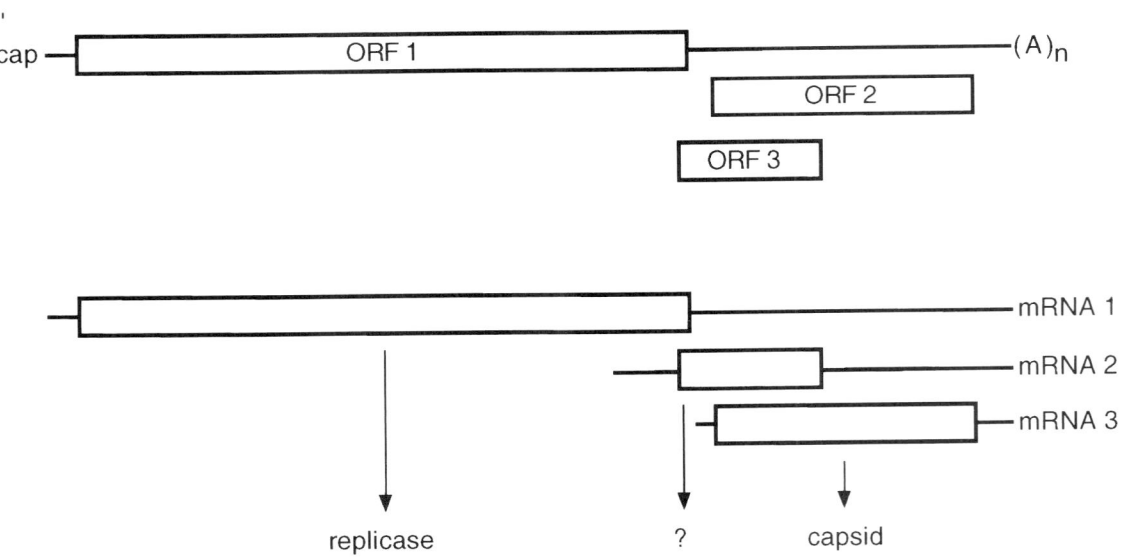

FIGURE 55.6. Hepatitis E virus (HEV) genome structure. HEV genome is a 7.5-kb single-stranded, positive-sense RNA, with a 5′-cap structure and a 3′-poly A tail. It contains three open reading frames (*ORFs*), encoding a replicase, capsid, and another protein of unknown functions. There are three corresponding genomic and subgenomic mRNAs..

ture system for HEV. Thus, the mechanisms of viral replication are largely unknown. In the infected cells, viral RNA is likely replicated by the virus-encoded RNA-dependent RNA polymerase into a negative-strand RNA, which is then used to synthesize positive-strand RNA. In addition to the 7.5-kb genomic-length RNA, two subgenomic RNA species of 3.7- and 2.0-kb, both of which are coterminal with the 3' end of the RNA genome, are detected (216,221). The full-length genomic RNA is used for the translation of ORF 1 polyprotein, which is likely processed by its own protease into multiple proteins; however, the proteolytic processing of the polyprotein has not been directly demonstrated. The two subgenomic mRNAs are used for the translation of ORF 2 and 3, respectively. Very little is known of the remaining molecular events of viral replication. Two immunodominant domains in the ORF 2 have been identified. The molecular basis of viral pathogenesis is largely unknown. The detection of widespread anti-HEV antibodies in domestic pigs and rodents suggests that these animals may serve as reservoirs for HEV infection in humans.

OTHER POTENTIAL HEPATITIS VIRUSES

The five hepatitis viruses described above still do not account for all of the sporadic and transfusion-associated acute and chronic hepatitis. So far at least two additional viruses have been identified using serum samples from non–A–E hepatitis patients by molecular cloning techniques (representational difference analysis, RDA) in recent years; these two are hepatitis G virus (HGV) and TT virus (TTV). However, the causal association of these viruses with hepatitis has not been established.

Hepatitis G Virus or GB Virus-C

The effort to identify the non–A–E virus started with serum samples that were initially obtained from a surgeon (whose initials are G.B.) with acute non–A–E hepatitis and subsequently passaged in tamarins. Using RDA techniques, two flavivirus-like sequences (GBV-A and GBV-B) were obtained from the RNA of the putative hepatitis agents in the tamarin sera (222). However, they were later found to be nonhuman (tamarin) viruses (223). Using these clones as probes, a third related virus, GBV-C, was later identified from serum of another non–A–E hepatitis patient in Africa (224). Independently, another virus, named hepatitis G virus (HGV), was directly identified by RDA techniques from another hepatitis patient (225). GBV-C and HGV were subsequently found to represent the same virus and are true human viruses (the term *HGV* is used in this chapter). Similar to HCV, HGV is a member of the Flaviviridae family and is phylogenetically most closely related to HCV (226). The genomic structure of

HGV is also very similar to that of HCV. It contains an ORF encoding a large polyprotein, which is cleaved by cellular signal peptidase and its own autoproteases (ns2 and ns3) into multiple structural and nonstructural proteins, corresponding to those of HCV. However, one striking difference between HCV and HGV is that the predicted core protein of HGV appears to be truncated and may not be translated at all. Furthermore, the initiation codon for the core protein varies drastically among different HGV isolates (227). Thus, whether HGV has a classic core protein and how the HGV particle is formed remain unknown. HGV RNA also has longer 5'- and 3'-end untranslated regions than the corresponding regions of HCV, but the terminal RNA structures at both ends appear to be very similar to those of HCV RNA (228). The translation of HGV polyprotein is also regulated by an IRES-dependent mechanism (229). Because of the poor immunogenicity of HGV proteins, no reliable immunoassay for HGV screening is available. Thus, HGV diagnosis is primarily based on the detection of HGV RNA by RT-PCR.

HGV is a blood-borne agent; thus, multiply transfused patients have a high prevalence rate of HGV infections. Even in the general population, HGV infection is very common, reaching 10% prevalence in certain normal blood donor populations (230). Although the prevalence rate of HGV in patients with various liver diseases are, in general, significantly higher than that of the normal population, various studies have failed to establish a causal relationship between HGV and hepatitis. Inoculation of HGV into chimpanzees resulted in viremia but did not cause hepatitis (231). Furthermore, HGV RNA has not been detected in the liver; nor is it in peripheral blood mononuclear cells (232). Thus, HGV most likely is not a hepatotropic virus. In contrast, GBV-B appears to be a bona fide hepatotropic virus in chimpanzees and tamarins, and can cause hepatitis after experimental inoculation in primates (223). Among the three GBV isolates, GBV-B is also the one most closely related to HCV. The role of HGV in hepatitis in humans, if any, remains to be determined.

TT Virus

This virus was originally identified by representational difference analysis of the serum samples from a Japanese patient (initials T.T.) with cryptogenic hepatitis (233). The virus sequence was subsequently detected by PCR in the sera from three of five patients with non–A–G hepatitis. The virus is a nonenveloped DNA virus, containing a single-stranded circular DNA of approximately 3,800 nucleotides (234). The viral DNA is of negative strand, meaning that the viral genomic DNA does not have a functional ORF. But the complementary DNA strand, which is present only in the infected cells, has two ORFs. The properties of these proteins and the mechanism of viral replication are largely unknown. TTV is now considered to be the first human virus member of the Circoviridae family, which otherwise infects primarily plants and nonhuman vertebrates. TTV has been shown to infect other primates, e.g., chimpanzees, as well (235).

The TT virus has been identified in a wide range of human populations, and can be classified into three genotypes, which bear no correlation with their geographic origin (234). TTV infection is particularly prevalent in multiply transfused patient populations. TTV likely has ability to replicate in the liver. However, the causal association between TTV and hepatitis in humans is questionable so far.

REFERENCES

1. Hollinger FB, Ticehurst JR. Hepatitis A virus. In: Fields BN, Knipe DM, Howely PM, eds. *Fields' virology*, 3rd ed. Philadelphia: Lippincott–Raven, 1996:735–782.
2. Zuckerman AJ, Howard CR. *Hepatitis viruses of man.* New York: Academic Press, 1979.
3. Feinstone SM, Kapikian AZ, Purceli RH. Hepatitis A: detection by immune electron microscopy of a viruslike antigen associated with acute illness. *Science* 1973;182:1026–1028.
4. Probst C, Jecht M, Gauss-Muller V. Intrinsic signals for the assembly of hepatitis A virus particles. Role of structural proteins VP4 and 2A. *J Biol Chem* 1999;274:4527–4531.
5. Graff J, Richards OC, Swiderek KM, et al. Hepatitis A virus capsid protein VP1 has a heterogeneous C terminus. *J Virol* 1999;73:6015–6023.
6. Feigelstock D, Thompson P, Mattoo P, et al. The human homolog of HAVcr-1 codes for a hepatitis A virus cellular receptor. *J Virol* 1998;72:6621–6628.
7. Dorner AJ, Rothberg PG, Wimmer E. The fate of VPg during in vitro translation of poliovirus RNA. *FEBS Lett* 1981;132: 219–223.
8. Kusov Y, Gauss-Muller V. Improving proteolytic cleavage at the 3A/3B site of the hepatitis A virus polyprotein impairs processing and particle formation, and the impairment can be complemented in trans by 3AB and 3ABC. *J Virol* 1999;73: 9867–9878.
9. Paul AV, van Boom JH, Filippov D, et al. Protein-primed RNA synthesis by purified poliovirus RNA polymerase. *Nature* 1998; 393:280–284.
10. Beneduce F, Ciervo A, Morace G. Site-directed mutagenesis of hepatitis A virus protein 3A: effects on membrane interaction. *Biochim Biophys Acta* 1997;1326:157–165.
11. Jecht M, Probst C, Gauss-Muller V. Membrane permeability induced by hepatitis A virus proteins 2B and 2BC and proteolytic processing of HAV 2BC. *Virology* 1998;252:218–227.
12. Khan NC, Hollinger FB, Melnick JL. Localization of hepatitis A virus antigen to specific subcellular fractions of hepatitis-A-infected chimpanzee liver cells. *Intervirology* 1984;21:187–194.
13. Martin A, Benichou D, Chao SF, et al. Maturation of the hepatitis A virus capsid protein VP1 is not dependent on processing by the 3Cpro proteinase. *J Virol* 1999;73:6220–6227.
14. Cohen JI, Rosenblum B, Feinstone SM, et al. Attenuation and cell culture adaptation of hepatitis a virus (HAV): a genetic analysis with HAV cDNA. *J Virol* 1989;63:5364–5370.
15. Day SP, Murphy P, Brown EA, et al. Mutations within the 5′ nontranslated region of hepatitis A virus RNA which enhance replication in BS-C-1 cells. *J Virol* 1992;66:6533–6540.
16. Asher LVS, Binn LN, Mensing TL, et al. Pathogenesis of hepatitis A in orally inoculated owl monkeys (*Aotus trivirgatus*). *J Med Virol* 1995;47:260–268.
17. Guidotti LG, Borrow P, Brown A, et al. Noncytopathic clearance of lymphocytic choriomeningitis virus from the hepatocyte. *J Exp Med* 1999;189:1555–1564.
18. Takahashi K, Brotman B, Usuda S, et al. Full-genome sequence analyses of hepatitis B virus (HBV) strains recovered from chimpanzees infected in the wild: implications for an origin of HBV. *Virology* 2000;267:58–64.
19. Heermann KH, Goldmann U, Schwartz W, et al. Large surface proteins of hepatitis B virus containing the pre-s sequence. *J Virol* 1984;52:396–402.
20. Fortuin M, Karthigesu V, Allison L, et al. Breakthrough infections and identification of a viral variant in Gambian children immunized with hepatitis B vaccine. *J Infect Dis* 1994;169: 1374–1376.
21. Neurath AR, Seto B, Strick N. Antibodies to synthetic peptides from the preS1 region of the hepatitis B virus (HBV) envelope (env) protein are virus-neutralizing and protective. *Vaccine* 1989;7:234–236.
22. Wynne SA, Crowther RA, Leslie AG. The crystal structure of the human hepatitis B virus capsid. *Mol Cell* 1999;3: 771–780.
23. Lien JM, Aldrich CE, Mason WS. Evidence that a capped oligoribonucleotide is the primer for duck hepatitis B virus plus-strand DNA synthesis. *J Virol* 1986;57:229–236.
24. Seeger C, Ganem D, Varmus HE. Biochemical and genetic evidence for the hepatitis B virus replication strategy. *Science* 1986; 232:477–484.
25. Gerlich W, Robinson WS. Hepatitis B virus contains protein covalently attached to the 5′ terminus of its complete DNA strand. *Cell* 1980;21:801–809.
26. Bartenschlager R, Schaller H. The amino-terminal domain of the hepadnaviral P-gene encodes the terminal protein (genome-linked protein) believed to prime reverse transcription. *EMBO J* 1988;7:4185–4192.
27. Staprans S, Loeb DD, Ganem D. Mutations affecting hepadnavirus plus-strand DNA synthesis dissociate primer cleavage from translocation and reveal the origin of linear viral DNA. *J Virol* 1991;65:1255–1262.
28. Yang W, Summers J. Illegitimate replication of linear hepadnavirus DNA through nonhomologous recombination. *J Virol* 1995;69:4029–4036.
29. Yu X, Mertz JE. Differential regulation of the pre-C and pregenomic promoters of human hepatitis B virus by members of the nuclear receptor superfamily. *J Virol* 1997;71:9366–9374.
30. Newbold JE, Xin H, Tencza M, et al. The covalently closed duplex form of the hepadnavirus genome exists in situ as a heterogeneous population of viral minichromosomes. *J Virol* 1995; 69:3350–3357.
31. Buscher M, Reiser W, Will H, et al. Transcripts and the putative RNA pregenome of duck hepatitis B virus: implications for reverse transcription. *Cell* 1985;40:717–724.
32. Obert S, Zachmann BB, Deindl E, et al. A spliced hepadnavirus RNA that is essential for virus replication. *EMBO J* 1996;15: 2565–2574.
33. Seeger C, Mason WS. Hepatitis B virus biology. *Microbiol Mol Biol Rev* 2000;64:51–68.
34. Bottcher B, Wynne SA, Crowther RA. Determination of the fold of the core protein of hepatitis B virus by electron cryomicroscopy. *Nature* 1997;386:88–91.
35. Hu J, Seeger C. Expression and characterization of hepadnavirus reverse transcriptases. *Methods Enzymol* 1996;275: 195–208.

36. Hu J, Seeger C. Hsp90 is required for the activity of a hepatitis B virus reverse transcriptase. *Proc Natl Acad Sci USA* 1996;93: 1060–1064.

37. Weber M, Bronsema V, Bartos H, et al. Hepadnavirus P protein utilizes a tyrosine residue in the TP domain to prime reverse transcription. *J Virol* 1994;68:2994–2999.

38. Zoulim F, Seeger C. Reverse transcription in hepatitis B viruses is primed by a tyrosine residue of the polymerase. *J Virol* 1994; 68:6–13.

39. Chen Y, Robinson WS, Marion PL. Selected mutations of the duck hepatitis B virus P gene RNase H domain affect both RNA packaging and priming of minus-strand DNA synthesis. *J Virol* 1994;68:5232–5238.

40. Summers J, Mason WS. Replication of the genome of a hepatitis B-like virus by reverse transcription of an RNA intermediate. *Cell* 1982;29:403–415.

41. Lien JM, Petcu DJ, Aldrich CE, et al. Initiation and termination of duck hepatitis B virus DNA synthesis during virus maturation. *J Virol* 1987;61:3832–3840.

42. Will H, Reiser W, Weimer T, et al. Replication strategy of human hepatitis B virus. *J Virol* 1987;61:904–911.

43. Summers J, Smith PM, Horwich AL. Hepadnavirus envelope proteins regulate covalently closed circular DNA amplification. *J Virol* 1990;64:2819–2824.

44. Summers J, Smith PM, Huang M, et al. Morphogenetic and regulatory effects of mutations in the envelope proteins of an avian hepadnavirus. *J Virol* 1991;65:1310–1317.

45. Lenhoff RJ, Luscombe CA, Summers J. Competition in vivo between a cytopathic variant and a wild-type duck hepatitis B virus. *Virology* 1998;251:85–95.

46. Heermann KH, Kruse F, Seifer M, et al. Immunogenicity of the gene S and Pre-S domains in hepatitis B virions and HBsAg filaments. *Intervirology* 1987;28:14–25.

47. Enders GH, Ganem D, Varmus H. Mapping the major transcripts of ground squirrel hepatitis virus: the presumptive template for reverse transcriptase is terminally redundant. *Cell* 1985;42:297–308.

48. Matsuda K, Satoh S, Ohori H. DNA-binding activity of hepatitis B e antigen polypeptide lacking the protaminelike sequence of nucleocapsid protein of human hepatitis B virus. *J Virol* 1988;62:3517–3521.

49. Garcia PD, Ou JH, Rutter WJ, et al. Targeting of the hepatitis B virus precore protein to the endoplasmic reticulum membrane: after signal peptide cleavage translocation can be aborted and the product released into the cytoplasm. *J Cell Biol* 1988; 106:1093–1104.

50. Milich DR, Chen MK, Hughes JL, et al. The secreted hepatitis B precore antigen can modulate the immune response to the nucleocapsid: a mechanism for persistence. *J Immunol* 1998; 160:2013–2021.

51. Milich DR, Jones JE, Hughes JL, et al. Is a function of the secreted hepatitis B e antigen to induce immunologic tolerance in utero? *Proc Natl Acad Sci USA* 1990;87:6599–6603.

52. Zoulim F, Saputelli J, Seeger C. Woodchuck hepatitis virus X protein is required for viral infection in vivo. *J Virol* 1994;68: 2026–2030.

53. Chen HS, Kaneko S, Girones R, et al. The woodchuck hepatitis virus X gene is important for establishment of virus infection in woodchucks. *J Virol* 1993;67:1218–1226.

54. Seeger C. The hepatitis B virus X protein: the quest for a role in viral replication and pathogenesis. *Hepatology* 1997;25:496–498.

55. Benn J, Schneider RJ. Hepatitis B virus HBx protein deregulates cell cycle checkpoint controls. *Proc Natl Acad Sci USA* 1995;92:11215–11219.

56. Klein NP, Schneider RJ. Activation of Src family kinases by

57. Becker SA, Lee TH, Butel JS, et al. Hepatitis B virus X protein interferes with cellular DNA repair. *J Virol* 1998;72:266–272.

58. Sirma H, Weil R, Rosmorduc O, et al. Cytosol is the prime compartment of hepatitis B virus X protein where it colocalizes with the proteasome. *Oncogene* 1998;16:2051–2063.

59. Hu Z, Zhang Z, Doo E, et al. Hepatitis B virus X protein is both a substrate and a potential inhibitor of the proteasome complex. *J Virol* 1999;73:7231–7240.

60. Kim CM, Koike K, Saito I, et al. HBx gene of hepatitis B virus induces liver cancer in transgenic mice. *Nature* 1991;351: 317–320.

61. Lee TH, Finegold MJ, Shen RF, et al. Hepatitis B virus transactivator X protein is not tumorigenic in transgenic mice. *J Virol* 1990;64:5939–5947.

62. Kajino K, Jilbert AR, Saputelli J, et al. Woodchuck hepatitis virus infections: very rapid recovery after a prolonged viremia and infection of virtually every hepatocyte. *J Virol* 1994;68: 5792–5803.

63. Jilbert AR, Wu TT, England JM, et al. Rapid resolution of duck hepatitis B virus infections occurs after massive hepatocellular involvement. *J Virol* 1992;66:1377–1388.

64. Ponzetto A, Cote PJ, Ford EC, et al. Core antigen and antibody in woodchucks after infection with woodchuck hepatitis virus. *J Virol* 1984;52:70–76.

65. Guidotti LG, Rochford R, Chung J, et al. Viral clearance without destruction of infected cells during acute HBV infection. *Science* 1999;284:825–829.

66. Guidotti LG, Chisari FV. Cytokine-induced viral purging—role in viral pathogenesis. *Curr Opin Microbiol* 1999;2:388–391.

67. Mackey D, Sugden B. The linking regions of EBNA1 are essential for its support of replication and transcription. *Mol Cell Biol* 1999;19:3349–3359.

68. Marusawa H, Osaki Y, Kimura T, et al. High prevalence of anti-hepatitis B virus serological markers in patients with hepatitis C virus related chronic liver disease in Japan [see comments]. *Gut* 1999;45:284–288.

69. Michalak TI, Pardoe IU, Coffin CS, et al. Occult lifelong persistence of infectious hepadnavirus and residual liver inflammation in woodchucks convalescent from acute viral hepatitis. *Hepatology* 1999;29:928–938.

70. Gong SS, Jensen AD, Rogler CE. Loss and acquisition of duck hepatitis B virus integrations in lineages of LMH-D2 chicken hepatoma cells. *J Virol* 1996;70:2000–2007.

71. Yang W, Summers J. Integration of hepadnavirus DNA in infected liver: evidence for a linear precursor. *J Virol* 1999;73: 9710–9717.

72. Evans AA, O'Connell AP, Pugh JC, et al. Geographic variation in viral load among hepatitis B carriers with differing risks of hepatocellular carcinoma. *Cancer Epidemiol Biomarkers Prev* 1998;7:559–565.

73. Korba BE, Wells F, Tennant BC, et al. Hepadnavirus infection of peripheral blood lymphocytes in vivo: woodchuck and chimpanzee models of viral hepatitis. *J Virol* 1986;58:1–8.

74. Korba BE, Cote PJ, Gerin JL. Mitogen-induced replication of woodchuck hepatitis virus in cultured peripheral blood lymphocytes. *Science* 1988;241:1213–1216.

75. Lieberman HM, Tung WW, Shafritz DA. Splenic replication of hepatitis B virus in the chimpanzee chronic carrier. *J Med Virol* 1987;21:347–359.

76. Laure F, Chatenoud L, Pasquinelli C, et al. Frequent lymphocytes infection by hepatitis B virus in haemophiliacs. *Br J Haematol* 1987;65:181–185.

77. Hadchouel M, Pasquinelli C, Fournier JG, et al. Detection of

mononuclear cells expressing hepatitis B virus in peripheral blood from HBsAg positive and negative patients by in situ hybridisation. *J Med Virol* 1988;24:27–32.

78. Tsukagoshi S, Shimoda T, Karasawa T, et al. Immunohistological study of the localization of hepatitis B virus associated antigens in human pancreatic tissue. *Jpn J.Gastroenterol* 1982;79:864–871.

79. Shimoda T, Shikata T, Karasawa T, et al. Light microscopic localization of hepatitis B virus antigens in human pancreas. *Gastroenterology* 1981;81:998–1005.

80. Yoshimura M, Sakurai I, Shimoda T, et al. Detection of HBsAg in the pancreas. *Acta Pathol Jpn* 1981;31:711–717.

81. Halpern MS, England JM, Deery DT, et al. Viral nucleic acid synthesis and antigen accumulation in pancreas and kidney of Pekin ducks infected with duck hepatitis B virus. *Proc Natl Acad Sci USA* 1983;80:4865–4869.

82. Halpern MS, Egan J, Mason WS, et al. Viral antigen in endocrine cells of the pancreatic islets and adrenal cortex of Pekin ducks infected with duck hepatitis B virus. *Virus Res* 1984;1:213–223.

83. Korba BE, Brown TL, Wells FV, et al. Natural history of experimental woodchuck hepatitis virus infection: molecular virologic features of the pancreas, kidney, ovary, and testis. *J Virol* 1990;64:4499–4506.

84. Korba BE, Gowans EJ, Wells FV, et al. Systemic distribution of woodchuck hepatitis virus in the tissues of experimentally infected woodchucks. *Virology* 1988;165:172–181.

85. Ogston CW, Schechter EM, Humes CA, et al. Extrahepatic replication of woodchuck hepatitis virus in chronic infection. *Virology* 1989;169:9–14.

86. Schaller H, Fischer M. Transcriptional control of hepadnavirus gene expression. In: Mason WS, Seeger C, eds. *Hepadnaviruses: molecular biology and pathogenesis*. New York: Springer-Verlag 1991:21–39.

87. Feitelson MA, Duan L-X. Hepatitis B virus X antigen in the pathogenesis of chronic infections and the development of hepatocellular carcinoma. *Am J Pathol* 1997;150:1141–1157.

88. Caselmann WH, Renner M, Schluter V, et al. The hepatitis B virus MHBst167 protein is a pleiotropic transactivator mediating its effect via ubiquitous cellular transcription factors. *J Gen Virol* 1997;78:1487–1495.

89. Luber B, Arnold N, Sturzl M, et al. Hepatoma-derived integrated HBV DNA causes multi-stage transformation in vitro. *Oncogene* 1996;12:1597–1608.

90. Hildt E, Hofschneider PH. The PreS2 activators of the hepatitis B virus: activators of tumour promoter pathways. *Recent Results Cancer Res* 1998;154:315–329.

91. Gunther S, Fischer L, Pult I, et al. Naturally occurring variants of hepatitis B virus. *Adv Virus Res* 1999;52:25–137.

92. Zhang Y-Y, Summers J. Enrichment of a precore-minus mutant of duck hepatitis B virus in experimental mixed infections. *J Virol* 1999;73:3616–3622.

93. Zhang Y-Y, Summers J. Low intercellular dynamic state of a chronic avian hepadnavirus infection. *J Virol* 2000;74: 5257–5265.

94. Bradley DW, Cook EH, Maynard JE, et al. Experimental infection of chimpanzees with antihemophilic (factor VIII) materials: recovery of virus-like particles associated with non-A, non-B hepatitis. *J Med Virol* 1979;3:253–269.

95. Choo Q-L, Kuo G, Weiner AJ, et al. Isolation of a cDNA clone derived from a blood-borne non-A, non-B viral hepatitis genome. *Science* 1989;244:359–362.

95a.Lohmann V, Korner F, Koch J-O, et al. Replication of subgenomic hepatitis C virus RNAs in a hepatoma cell line. *Science* 1999;285:110–113.

96. Simmonds P, Holmes EC, Cha TA, et al. Classification of hepatitis C virus into six major genotypes and a series of sub-

types by phylogenetic analysis of the NS-5 region. *J Gen Virol* 1993;74:2391–2399.

97. Domingo E, Martinez-Salas E, Sobrino F, et al. The quasispecies (extremely heterogeneous) nature of viral RNA genome populations: biological relevance—a review. *Gene* 1985;40: 1–8.

98. Martell M, Esteban JI, Quer J, et al. Hepatitis C virus (HCV) circulates as a population of different but closely related genomes: quasispecies nature of HCV genome distribution. *J Virol* 1992;66:3225–3229.

99. Kato N, Ootsuyama Y, Tanaka T, et al. Marked sequence diversity in the putative envelope proteins of hepatitis C viruses. *Virus Res* 1992;22:107–123.

100. Kaito M, Watanabe S, Tsukiyama-Kohara K, et al. Hepatitis C virus particle detected by immunoelectron microscopic study. *J Gen Virol* 1994;75:1755–1760.

101. Shimizu YK, Feinstone SM, Kohara M, et al. Hepatitis C virus: detection of intracellular virus particles by electron microscopy. *Hepatology* 1996;23:205–209.

102. Yi MY, Kaneko S, Yu DY, et al. Hepatitis C virus envelope proteins bind lactoferrin. *J Virol* 1997;71:5997–6002.

103. Hijikata M, Shimizu YK, Kato H, et al. Equilibrium centrifugation studies of hepatitis C virus: evidence for circulating immune complexes. *J Virol* 1993;67:1953–1958.

104. Bradley DW, Maynard JE, Popper H, et al. Posttransfusion non-A, non-B hepatitis: physiochemical properties of two distinct agents. *J Infect Dis* 1983;148:254–265.

105. Tsukiyama-Kohara K, Iizuka N, Kohara M, et al. Internal ribosome entry site within hepatitis C virus RNA. *J Virol* 1992;66: 1476–1483.

106. Honda M, Brown EA, Lemon SM. Stability of a stem-loop involving the initiator AUG controls the efficiency of internal initiation of translation on hepatitis C virus RNA. *RNA* 1996; 2:955–968.

107. Reynolds JE, Kaminski A, Carroll AR, et al. Internal initiation of translation of hepatitis C virus RNA: the ribosome entry site is at the authentic initiation codon. *RNA* 1996;2: 867–878.

108. Reynolds JE, Kaminski A, Kettinen HJ, et al. Unique features of internal initiation of hepatitis C virus RNA translation. *EMBO J* 1995;14:6010–6020.

109. Tanaka T, Kato N, Cho MJ, et al. Structure of the 3′ terminus of the hepatitis C virus genome. *J Virol* 1996;70:3307–3312.

110. Kolykhalov AA, Feinstone SM, Rice CM. Identification of a highly conserved sequence element at the 3′ terminus of hepatitis C virus genome RNA. *J Virol* 1996;70:3363–3371.

111. Yamada N, Tanihara K, Takada A, et al. Genetic organization and diversity of the 3′ noncoding region of the hepatitis C virus genome. *Virology* 1996;223:255–261.

112. Yanagi M, St. Clair M, Emerson SU, et al. In vivo analysis of the 3′ untranslated region of the hepatitis C virus after in vitro mutagenesis of an infectious cDNA clone. *Proc Natl Acad Sci USA* 1999;96:2291–2295.

113. Ito T, Tahara SM, Lai MMC. The 3′-untranslated region of hepatitis C virus RNA enhances translation from an internal ribosomal entry site. *J Virol* 1998;72:8789–8796.

114. Oh J-W, Ito T, Lai MMC. A recombinant hepatitis C virus RNA-dependent RNA polymerase capable of copying the full-length viral RNA. *J Virol* 1999;73:7694–7702.

115. Ito T, Lai MMC. Determination of the secondary structure of and cellular protein binding to the 3′-untranslated region of hepatitis C virus RNA genome. *J Virol* 1997;71:8698–8706.

116. Tsuchihara K, Tanaka T, Hijikata M, et al. Specific interaction of polypyrimidine tract-binding protein with the extreme 3′-terminal structure of the hepatitis C virus genome, the 3′X. *J Virol* 1997;71:6720–6726.

117. Ali N, Siddiqui A. Interaction of polypyrimidine tract-binding protein with the 5′ noncoding region of the hepatitis C virus RNA genome and its functional requirement in internal initiation of translation. *J Virol* 1995;69:6367–6375.

118. Ali N, Siddiqui A. The La antigen binds 5′ noncoding region of the hepatitis C virus RNA in the context of the initiator AUG codon and stimulates internal ribosome entry site-mediated translation. *Proc Natl Acad Sci USA* 1997;94:2249–2254.

119. Dubuisson J, Rice CM. Hepatitis C virus glycoprotein folding: disulfide bond formation and association with calnexin. *J Virol* 1996;70:778–786.

120. Weiner AJ, Brauer MJ, Rosenblatt J, et al. Variable and hypervariable domains are found in the regions of HCV corresponding to the flavivirus envelope and NS1 proteins and the pestivirus envelope glycoproteins. *Virology* 1991;180:842–848.

121. Hijikata M, Kato N, Ootsuyama Y, et al. Hypervariable regions in the putative glycoprotein of hepatitis C virus. *Biochem Biophys Res Commun* 1991;175:220–228.

122. Lo SY, Selby MJ, Ou JH. Interaction between hepatitis C virus core protein and E1 envelope protein. *J Virol* 1996;70:5177–5182.

123. Hijikata M, Mizushima H, Akagi T, et al. Two distinct proteinase activities required for the processing of a putative nonstructural precursor protein of hepatitis C virus. *J Virol* 1993;67:4665–4675.

124. Lin C, Pragai BM, Grakoui A, et al. Hepatitis C virus NS3 serine proteinase: trans-cleavage requirements and processing kinetics. *J Virol* 1994;68:8147–8157.

125. Tai CL, Chi WK, Chen DS, et al. The helicase activity associated with hepatitis C virus nonstructural protein 3 (NS3). *J Virol* 1996;70:8477–8484.

126. Kim JL, Morgenstern KA, Lin C, et al. Crystal structure of the hepatitis C virus NS3 protease domain complexed with a synthetic NS4A cofactor peptide. *Cell* 1996;87:343–355.

127. Yan Y, Li Y, Munshi S, et al. Complex of NS3 protease and NS4A peptide of BK strain hepatitis C virus: a 2.2 resolution structure in a hexagonal crystal form. *Protein Sci* 1998;7:837–847.

128. Love RA, Parge HE, Wickersham JA, et al. The crystal structure of hepatitis C virus NS3 proteinase reveals a trypsin-like fold and a structural zinc binding site. *Cell* 1996;87:331–342.

129. Failla C, Tomei L, De Francesco R. Both NS3 and NS4A are required for proteolytic processing of hepatitis C virus nonstructural proteins. *J Virol* 1994;68:3753–3760.

130. Behrens SE, Tomei L, De Francesco R. Identification and properties of the RNA-dependent RNA polymerase of hepatitis C virus. *EMBO J* 1996;15:12–22.

131. Lohmann V, Korner F, Herian U, et al. Biochemical properties of hepatitis C virus NS5B RNA-dependent RNA polymerase and identification of amino acid sequence motifs essential for enzymatic activity. *J Virol* 1997;71:8416–8428.

132. Laskus T, Radkowski M, Piasek A, et al. Hepatitis C virus in lymphoid cells of patients coinfected with human immunodeficiency virus type 1: evidence of active replication in monocytes/macrophages and lymphocytes. *J Infect Dis* 2000;181:442–448.

133. Nakajima N, Hijikata M, Yoshikura H, et al. Characterization of long-term cultures of hepatitis C virus. *J Virol* 1996;70:3325–3329.

134. Shimizu YK, Iwamoto A, Hijikata M, et al. Evidence for in vitro replication of hepatitis C virus genome in a human T-cell line. *Proc Natl Acad Sci USA* 1992;89:5477–5481.

135. Ito T, Mukaigawa J, Zuo J, et al. Cultivation of hepatitis C virus in primary hepatocyte culture from patients with chronic hepatitis C results in release of high titre infectious virus. *J Gen Virol* 1996;77:1043–1054.

136. Kato N, Nakazawa T, Mizutani T, et al. Susceptibility of human T-lymphotropic virus type I infected cell line MT-2 to hepatitis C virus infection. *Biochem Biophys Res Commun* 1995;206:863–869.

137. Lanford RE, Sureau C, Jacob JR, et al. Demonstration of in vitro infection of chimpanzee hepatocytes with hepatitis C virus using strand-specific RT/PCR. *Virology* 1994;202:606–614.

138. Pileri P, Uematsu Y, Campagnoli S, et al. Binding of hepatitis C virus to CD81. *Science* 1998;282:938–941.

139. Flint M, Maidens C, Loomis-Price LD, et al. Characterization of hepatitis C virus E2 glycoprotein interaction with a putative cellular receptor, CD81. *J Virol* 1999;73:6235–6244.

140. Agnello V, Abel G, Elfahal M, et al. Hepatitis C virus and other flaviviridae viruses enter cells via low density lipoprotein receptor. *Proc Natl Acad Sci USA* 1999;96:12766–12771.

141. Grakoui A, McCourt DW, Wychowski C, et al. Characterization of the hepatitis C virus-encoded serine proteinase: determination of proteinase-dependent polyprotein cleavage sites. *J Virol* 1993;67:2832–2843.

142. Santolini E, Migliaccio G, La Monica N. Biosynthesis and biochemical properties of the hepatitis C virus core protein. *J Virol* 1994;68:3631–3641.

143. Matsumoto M, Hwang SB, Jeng K-S, et al. Homotypic interaction and multimerization of hepatitis C virus core protein. *Virology* 1996;218:43–51.

144. Cocquerel L, Meunier JC, Pillez A, et al. A retention signal necessary and sufficient for endoplasmic reticulum localization maps to the transmembrane domain of hepatitis C virus glycoprotein E2. *J Virol* 1998;72:2183–2191.

145. Cocquerel L, Duvet S, Meunier JC, et al. The transmembrane domain of hepatitis C virus glycoprotein E1 is a signal for static retention in the endoplasmic reticulum. *J Virol* 1999;73:2641–2649.

146. McCaul TF, Tsiquaye KN, Tovey G, et al. A study of ultrastructural alterations in experimental non-A, non-B hepatitis by electron-beam analysis. *Br J Exp Pathol* 1982;63:325–329.

147. Spichtin HP, Eder G, Gudat F, et al. Ultrastructural alterations in hepatocytes and sinus endothelia in experimental non-A, non-B hepatitis in chimpanzees with and without immunoglobulin prophylaxis. *J Med Virol* 1983;12:215–226.

148. Chen C-M, You L-R, Hwang L-H, et al. Direct interaction of hepatitis C virus core protein with the cellular lymphotoxin-β receptor modulates the signal pathway of the lymphotoxin-β receptor. *J Virol* 1997;71:9417–9426.

149. Matsumoto M, Hsieh T-Y, Zhu N, et al. Hepatitis C virus core protein interacts with the cytoplasmic tail of lymphotoxin-β receptor. *J Virol* 1997;71:1301–1309.

150. Zhu N, Khoshnan A, Schneider R, et al. Hepatitis C virus core protein binds to the cytoplasmic domain of tumor necrosis factor (TNF) receptor 1 and enhances TNF-induced apoptosis. *J Virol* 1998;72:3691–3697.

151. Ray RB, Meyer K, Steele R, et al. Inhibition of tumor necrosis factor (TNF-alpha)-mediated apoptosis by hepatitis C virus core protein. *J Biol Chem* 1998;273:2256–2259.

152. Marusawa H, Hijikata M, Chiba T, et al. Hepatitis C virus core protein inhibits Fas- and tumor necrosis factor alpha-mediated apoptosis via NF-kappaB activation. *J Virol* 1999;73:4713–4720.

153. Hsieh T-Y, Matsumoto M, Chou H-C, et al. Hepatitis C virus core protein interacts with heterogeneous nuclear ribonucleoprotein K. *J Biol Chem* 1998;273:17651–17659.

154. Mamiya N, Worman HJ. Hepatitis C virus core protein binds to a DEAD box RNA helicase. *J Biol Chem* 1999;274:15751–15756.

155. You LR, Chen CM, Yeh TS, et al. Hepatitis C virus core protein interacts with cellular putative RNA helicase. *J Virol* 1999;73:2841–2853.

156. Shih C-M, Lo SJ, Miyamura T, et al. Suppression of hepatitis B virus expression and replication by hepatitis C virus core protein in HuH-7 cells. *J Virol* 1993;67:5823–5832.

157. Ray RB, Lagging LM, Meyer K, et al. Transcriptional regulation of cellular and viral promoters by the hepatitis C virus core protein. *Virus Res* 1995;37:209–220.

158. Ray RB, Lagging LM, Meyer K, et al. Hepatitis C virus core protein cooperates with ras and transforms primary rat embryo fibroblasts to tumorigenic phenotype. *J Virol* 1996;70:4438–4443.

159. Jin DY, Wang HL, Zhou Y, et al. Hepatitis C virus core protein-induced loss of LZIP function correlates with cellular transformation. *EMBO J* 2000;19:729–740.

160. Aoki H, Hayashi J, Moriyama M, et al. Hepatitis C virus core protein interacts with 14–3–3 protein and activates the kinase raf-1. *J Virol* 2000;74:1736–1741.

161. Large MK, Kittlesen DJ, Hahn YS. Suppression of host immune response by the core protein of hepatitis C virus: possible implications for hepatitis C virus persistence. *J Immunol* 1999;162:931–938.

162. Taylor DR, Shi ST, Romano PR, et al. Inhibition of the interferon-inducible protein kinase PKR by HCV E2 protein. *Science* 1999;285:107–110.

163. Thomas HC, Torok ME, Foster GR. Hepatitis C virus dynamics in vivo and the antiviral efficacy of interferon alfa therapy. *Hepatology* 1999;29:1333–1334.

164. Liberman E, Fong YL, Selby MJ, et al. Activation of the grp78 and grp94 promoters by hepatitis C virus E2 envelope protein. *J Virol* 1999;73:3718–3722.

165. Enomoto N, Sakuma I, Asahina Y, et al. Mutations in the nonstructural protein 5A gene and response to interferon in patients with chronic hepatitis C virus 1b infection. *N Engl J Med* 1996;334:77–81.

166. Herion D, Hoofnagle JH. The interferon sensitivity determining region: all hepatitis C virus isolates are not the same. *Hepatology* 1997;25:769–771.

167. Gale MJJ, Korth MJ, Tang NM, et al. Evidence that hepatitis C virus resistance to interferon is mediated through repression of the PKR protein kinase by the nonstructural 5A protein. *Virology* 1997;230:217–227.

168. Gale MJ, Blakely CM, Kwieciszewski B, et al. Control of PKR protein kinase by hepatitis C virus nonstructural 5A protein: molecular mechanisms of kinase regulation. *Mol Cell Biol* 1998;18:5208–5218.

169. Tan SL, Nakao H, He Y, et al. NS5A, a nonstructural protein of hepatitis C virus, binds growth factor receptor-bound protein 2 adaptor protein in a Src homology 3 domain/ligand-dependent manner and perturbs mitogenic signaling. *Proc Natl Acad Sci USA* 1999;96:5533–5538.

170. Tu H, Gao L, Shi ST, et al. Hepatitis c virus RNA polymerase and NS5A complex with a SNARE-like protein. *Virology* 1999;263:30–41.

171. Kato N, Lan K-H, Ono-Nita SK, et al. Hepatitis C virus nonstructural region 5A protein is a potent transcriptional activator. *J Virol* 1997;71:8856–8859.

172. Tanimoto A, Ide Y, Arima N, et al. The amino terminal deletion mutants of hepatitis C virus nonstructural protein NS5A function as transcriptional activators in yeast. *Biochem Biophys Res Commun* 1997;236:360–364.

173. Borowski P, zur Wiesch JS, Resch K, et al. Protein kinase C recognizes the protein kinase A-binding motif of nonstructural protein 3 of hepatitis C virus. *J Biol Chem* 1999;274:30722–30728.

174. Sakamuro D, Furukawa T, Takegami T. Hepatitis C virus nonstructural protein NS3 transforms NIH 3T3 cells. *J Virol* 1995;69:3893–3896.

175. Ogata N, Alter HJ, Miller RH, et al. Nucleotide sequence and mutation rate of the H strain of hepatitis C virus. *Proc Natl Acad Sci USA* 1991;88:3392–3396.

176. Booth JC, Kumar U, Webster D, et al. Comparison of the rate of sequence variation in the hypervariable region of E2/NS1 region of hepatitis C virus in normal and hypogammaglobulinemic patients. *Hepatology* 1998;27:223–227.

177. Ni YH, Chang MH, Chen PJ, et al. Decreased diversity of hepatitis C virus quasispecies during bone marrow transplantation. *J Med Virol* 1999;58:132–138.

178. Toyoda H, Fukuda Y, Koyama Y, et al. Effect of immunosuppression on composition of quasispecies population of hepatitis C virus in patients with chronic hepatitis C coinfected with human immunodeficiency virus. *J Hepatol* 1997;26:975–982.

179. Polyak SJ, Faulkner G, Carithers RLJ, et al. Assessment of hepatitis C virus quasispecies heterogeneity by gel shift analysis: correlation with response to interferon therapy. *J Infect Dis* 1997;175:1101–1107.

180. Brillanti S, Masci C, Ricci P, et al. Significance of IgM antibody to hepatitis C virus in patients with chronic hepatitis C. *Hepatology* 1992;15:998–1001.

181. Quiroga JA, Campillo ML, Catillo I, et al. IgM antibody to hepatitis C virus in acute and chronic hepatitis C. *Hepatology* 1991;14:38–43.

182. Rizzetto M, Hoyer B, Canese MG, et al. Delta agent: association of δ antigen with hepatitis B surface antigen and RNA in serum of δ-infected chimpanzees. *Proc Natl Acad Sci USA* 1980;77:6124–6128.

183. Rizzetto M, Macagno S, Chiaberge E, et al. Liver transplantation in hepatitis delta virus disease. *Lancet* 1987;2:469–471.

184. Smedile A, Casey JL, Cote PJ, et al. Hepatitis D viremia following orthotopic liver transplantation involves a typical HDV virion with a hepatitis B surface antigen envelope. *Hepatology* 1998;27:1723–1729.

185. Casey JL, Brown TL, Colan EJ, et al. A genotype of hepatitis D virus that occurs in northern South America. *Proc Natl Acad Sci USA* 1993;90:9016–9020.

186. Wu J-C, Choo K-B, Chen C-M, et al. Genotyping of hepatitis D virus by restriction-fragment length polymorphism and relation to outcome of hepatitis D. *Lancet* 1995;346:934–941.

187. Makino S, Chang MF, Shieh CK, et al. Molecular cloning and sequencing of a human hepatitis delta virus RNA. *Nature* 1987;329:343–346.

188. Wang KS, Choo QL, Weiner AJ, et al. Structure, sequence and expression of the hepatitis delta viral genome. *Nature* 1986;323:508–514.

189. Kos A, Dijkema R, Arnberg AC, et al. The hepatitis delta (δ) virus possesses a circular RNA. *Nature* 1986;323:558–560.

190. Wu H-N, Lin Y-J, Lin F-P, et al. Human hepatitis δ virus RNA subfragments contain an autocleavage activity. *Proc Natl Acad Sci USA* 1989;86:1831–1835.

191. Sharmeen L, Kuo MY-P, Taylor J. Self-ligating RNA sequences on the antigenome of human hepatitis delta virus. *J Virol* 1989;63:1428–1430.

192. Bonino F, Hoyer B, Ford G. The delta agent: HBsAg particles with antigen and RNA in the serum of an HBV carrier. *Hepatology* 1981;2:127–131.

193. Bergmann KF, Gerin JL. Antigens of hepatitis delta virus in the liver and serum of humans and animals. *J Infect Dis* 1986;154:702–706.

194. Kuo MY-P, Chao M, Taylor J. Initiation of replication of the human hepatitis delta virus genome from cloned DNA: role of delta antigen. *J Virol* 1989;63:1945–1950.

195. Chao M, Hsieh S-Y, Taylor J. Role of two forms of hepatitis delta virus antigen: evidence for a mechanism of self-limiting genome replication. *J Virol* 1990;64:5066–5069.

196. Chang F-L, Chen P-J, Tu S-J, et al. The large form of hepatitis

δ antigen is crucial for assembly of hepatitis δ virus. *Proc Natl Acad Sci USA* 1991;88:8490–8494.

197. Chen P-J, Kalpana G, Goldberg J, et al. Structure and replication of the genome of hepatitis delta virus. *Proc Natl Acad Sci USA* 1986;83:8774–8778.

198. Branch AD, Robertson HD. A replication cycle for viroids and other small infectious RNAs. *Science* 1984;223:450–455.

199. Macnaughton TB, Wang Y-J, Lai MMC. Replication of hepatitis delta virus RNA: effect of mutations of the autocatalytic cleavage sites. *J Virol* 1993;67:2228–2234.

200. Reid CE, Lazinski DW. A host-specific function is required for ligation of a wide variety of ribozyme-processed RNAs. *Proc Natl Acad Sci USA* 2000;97:424–429.

201. Lo K, Hwang SB, Duncan R, et al. Characterization of mRNA for hepatitis delta antigen: exclusion of the full-length antigenomic RNA as an mRNA. *Virology* 1998;250:94–105.

202. Hsieh S-Y, Taylor JM. Regulation of polyadenylation of hepatitis delta virus antigenomic RNA. *J Virol* 1991;65:6438–6446.

203. Modahl LE, Lai MMC. Transcription of hepatitis delta antigen mRNA continues throughout hepatitis delta virus (HDV) replication: a new model of HDV replication and transcription. *J Virol* 1998;72:5449–5456.

204. Luo G, Chao M, Hsieh SY, et al. A specific base transition occurs on replicating hepatitis delta virus RNA. *J Virol* 1990;64:1021–1027.

205. Polson AG, Bass BL, Casey JL. RNA editing of hepatitis delta virus antigenome by dsRNA-adenosine deaminase. *Nature* 1996;380:454–456.

206. Macnaughton TB, Gowans EJ, McNamara SP, et al. Hepatitis δ antigen is necessary for access of hepatitis δ virus RNA to the cell transcriptional machinery but is not part of the transcriptional complex. *Virology* 1991;184:387–390.

206a. Modahl LE, MacNaughton TB, Zhu N, et al. RNA-dependent replication and transcription of hepatitis delta virus RNA involve distinct cellular RNA polymerases. *Mol Cell Biol* 2000;20:6030–6039.

207. Xia Y-P, Lai MMC. Oligomerization of hepatitis delta antigen is required for both the trans-activating and trans-dominant inhibitory activities of the delta antigen. *J Virol* 1992;66:6641–6648.

208. Lo K, Sheu G-W, Lai MMC. Inhibition of cellular RNA polymerase II transcription by delta antigen of hepatitis delta virus. *Virology* 1998;247:178–188.

209. Wei Y, Ganem D. Activation of heterologous gene expression by the large isoform of hepatitis delta antigen. *J Virol* 1998;72:2089–2096.

210. Glenn JS, Watson JA, Havel CM, et al. Identification of a prenylation site in delta virus large antigen. *Science* 1992;256:1331–1333.

211. Cole SM, Gowans EJ, Macnaughton TB, et al. Direct evidence for cytotoxicity associated with expression of hepatitis delta virus antigen. *Hepatology* 1991;13:845–851.

212. Ottobrelli A, Marzano A, Smedile A, et al. Patterns of hepatitis delta virus reinfection and disease in liver transplantation. *Gastroenterology* 1991;101:1649–1655.

213. Chu C-M, Liaw Y-F. Studies on the composition of the mononuclear cell infiltrates in liver from patients with chronic active delta hepatitis. *Hepatology* 1989;10:911–915.

214. Karayiannis P, Saldanha J, Monjardino J, et al. Immunization of woodchucks with recombinant hepatitis delta antigen does not protect against hepatitis delta virus infection. *Hepatology* 1990;12:1125–1128.

215. Reyes GR, Purdy MA, Kim JP, et al. Isolation of a cDNA from the virus responsible for enterically transmitted non-A, non-B hepatitis. *Science* 1990;247:1335–1339.

216. Yarbough PO, Tam AW, Fry KE, et al. Hepatitis E virus: iden-

217. Kabrane-Lazizi Y, Fine JB, Elm J, et al. Evidence for widespread infection of wild rats with hepatitis E virus in the United States. *Am J Trop Med Hyg* 1999;61:331–335.

218. Meng XJ, Halbur PG, Shapiro MS, et al. Genetic and experimental evidence for cross-species infection by swine hepatitis E virus. *J Virol* 1998;72:9714–9721.

219. Xing L, Kato K, Li T, et al. Recombinant hepatitis E capsid protein self-assembles into a dual-domain T = 1 particle presenting native virus epitopes. *Virology* 1999;265:35–45.

220. Koonin EV, Gorbalenya AE, Purdy MA, et al. Computer-assisted assignment of functional domains in the nonstructural polyprotein of hepatitis E virus: delineation of an additional group of positive-strand RNA plant and animal viruses. *Proc Natl Acad Sci USA* 1992;89:8259–8263.

221. Tam AW, Smith MM, Guerra ME, et al. Hepatitis E virus (HEV): molecular cloning and sequencing of the full-length viral genome. *Virology* 1991;185:120–131.

222. Simons JN, Pilot-Matias TJ, Leary TP, et al. Identification of two flavivirus-like genomes in the GB hepatitis agent. *Proc Natl Acad Sci USA* 1995;92:3401–3405.

223. Schlauder GG, Dawson GJ, Simons JN, et al. Molecular and serologic analysis in the transmission of the GB hepatitis agents. *J Med Virol* 1995;46:81–90.

224. Simons NJ, Leary TP, Dawson GJ, et al. Isolation of novel virus-like sequences associated with human hepatitis. *Nat Med* 1995;1:564–569.

225. Linnen J, Wages JJ, Zhang-Keck ZY, et al. Molecular cloning and disease association of hepatitis G virus: a transfusion-transmissible agent. *Science* 1996;271:505–508.

226. Muerhoff AS, Leary TP, Simons JN, et al. Genomic organization of GB viruses A and B: two new members of the Flaviviridae associated with GB agent hepatitis. *J Virol* 1995;69:5621–5630.

227. Pickering JM, Thomas HC, Karayiannis P. Genetic diversity between hepatitis G isolates: analysis of nucleotide variation in the NS-3 and putative "core" peptide genes. *J Gen Virol* 1997;78:53–60.

228. Bukh J, Apgar CL, Yanagi M. Toward a surrogate model for hepatitis C virus: an infectious molecular clone of the GB virus-B hepatitis agent. *Virology* 1999;262:470–478.

229. Simons JN, Desai SM, Schultz DE, et al. Translation initiation in GB viruses A and C: evidence for internal ribosome entry and implications for genome organization. *J Virol* 1996;70:6126–6135.

230. Thomas HC, Pickering J, Karayiannis P. Identification, prevalence and aspects of molecular biology of hepatitis G virus. *J Viral Hepatol* 1997;4(suppl 1):51–54.

231. Bukh J, Kim JP, Govindarajan S, et al. Experimental infection of chimpanzees with hepatitis g virus and genetic analysis of the virus. *J Infect Dis* 1998;177:855–862.

232. Kao JH, Chen W, Chen PJ, et al. Liver and peripheral blood mononuclear cells are not major sites for GB virus-C/hepatitis G virus replication. *Arch Virol* 1999;144:2173–2183.

233. Nishizawa T, Okamoto H, Konishi K, et al. A novel DNA virus (TTV) associated with elevated transaminase levels in post-transfusion hepatitis of unknown etiology. *Biochem Biophys Res Commun* 1997;241:92–97.

234. Mushahwar IK, Erker JC, Muerhoff AS, et al. Molecular and biophysical characterization of TT virus: evidence for a new virus family infecting humans. *Proc Natl Acad Sci USA* 1999;96:3177–3182.

235. Abe K, Inami T, Ishikawa K, et al. TT virus infection in nonhuman primates and characterization of the viral genome: identification of simian TT virus isolates. *J Virol* 2000;74:1549–1553.

236. Chang LJ, Pryciak P, Ganem D, et al. Biosynthesis of the reverse

transcriptase of hepatitis B viruses involves de novo translational initiation not ribosomal frameshifting. *Nature* 1989;337: 364–368.

237. Schlicht HJ, Radziwill G, Schaller H. Synthesis and encapsidation of duck hepatitis B virus reverse transcriptase do not require formation of core-polymerase fusion proteins. *Cell* 1989;56:85–92.

238. Junker NM, Bartenschlager R, Schaller H. A short cis-acting sequence is required for hepatitis B virus pregenome encapsidation and sufficient for packaging of foreign RNA. *EMBO J* 1990;9:3389–3396.

239. Nassal M, Junker-Niepmann M, Schaller H. Translational inactivation of RNA function: discrimination against a subset of genomic transcripts during HBV nucleocapsid assembly. *Cell* 1990;63:1357–1363.

240. Ou JH, Bao H, Shih C, et al. Preferred translation of human hepatitis B virus polymerase from core protein- but not from precore protein-specific transcript. *J Virol* 1990;64:4578–4581.

241. Chen Y, Marion PL. Amino acids essential for RNase H activity of hepadnaviruses are also required for efficient elongation of minus-strand viral DNA. *J Virol* 1996;70:6151–6156.

LIVER TRANSPLANTATION: FACTORS AFFECTING THE BALANCE BETWEEN TOLERANCE AND REJECTION IN EXPERIMENTAL MODELS

LINA LU
SHIGUANG QIAN
ANGUS W. THOMSON

With rare exceptions, organ allograft survival in humans is dependent on the prolonged use of nonspecific immunosuppressants to prevent rejection. Despite the remarkable improvements in graft survival and quality of life that have been achieved in the past 15 to 20 years, due largely to the introduction of cyclosporine, and more recently, tacrolimus, many adverse side effects continue to be associ-

L. Lu and **A. W. Thomson:** Department of Surgery, University of Pittsburgh Medical Center, Pittsburgh, Pennsylvania 15213.

S. Qian: Thomas E. Starzl Transplantation Institute and Department of Surgery, University of Pittsburgh Medical Center, Pittsburgh, Pennsylvania 15213.

ated with the use of immunosuppressive agents, including increased risks of opportunistic infection, malignancy, and end-organ toxicities. Strenuous efforts thus continue to be made to identify protocols capable of inducing drug-free, permanent, donor-specific unresponsiveness (tolerance) that preserves overall host immunocompetence with minimal attendant side effects. Much continues to be learned from animal models. Indeed, it has been possible to induce organ transplant tolerance in rodents for many years, using a diverse range of immunosuppressive agents. Remarkably, liver allografts are accepted across major histocompatibility complex (MHC) barriers, without the need for immunosuppressive therapy in outbred pigs and in certain inbred rat and most mouse strain combinations. Why this can occur comparatively frequently with the liver, and only exceptionally for the heart and kidney, is poorly understood, but some insight has been gained into possible mechanisms. A fuller understanding of the mechanistic basis of liver allograft acceptance, and why the liver can induce systemic, donor-specific tolerance, is likely to have an important bearing on the design of future immunosuppressive strategies. This chapter focuses on recent knowledge acquired using animal models, with special reference to the mouse, in which orthotopic liver transplantation was first accomplished with consistent success in 1991 (1).

DISTINCTIVE CHARACTERISTICS OF LIVER GRAFTS AND OF THE HEPATIC MICROENVIRONMENT

Garnier et al. (2) first demonstrated that liver grafts transplanted between outbred pigs survived "spontaneously." The acceptance of pig liver allografts without immunosuppressive therapy was further shown by Calne et al. (3) in 1969 to be associated with donor-specific unresponsiveness. Similar findings have been made subsequently in rodents, both in a few rat (4,5) and in many mouse strain combinations (6). Even across species barriers (xenotransplantation), liver grafts may survive longer than other organ transplants [e.g., in hamster to rat (7) or pig to baboon (8) combinations]. In the dog, baboon, and human, immunosuppressive therapy is required to prevent liver allograft rejection, but the antidonor response is usually easier to treat than that mounted against other organs. Certain additional features distinguish the comparative tolerogenicity of hepatic allografts (Table 56.1). Thus, in humans, transplantation across ABO blood group barriers leads to the accelerated rejection of kidneys and hearts, but not liver allografts (9). Moreover, hyperacute rejection is generally not observed in liver transplantation. Unlike with the heart or kidney, a clear effect of human leukocyte antigen (HLA) haplotype matching is not apparent. Acute rejection is relatively easy to control, and irreversible acute rejection is rare. Liver graft survival curves indicate little attrition due to rejection beyond a year. In fact, there are well-documented instances of liver transplant patients from whom all immunosuppressive therapy has been withdrawn, without rejection (10).

Additional observations point to inherent liver "tolerogenicity." The liver may confer a survival advantage on other organ grafts from the same donor (strain) transplanted at the same time. Thus, simultaneous transplantation of the pancreas and liver improves the survival of the pancreas compared with the outcome for pancreas alone (11). Survival of kidney allografts is also prolonged by concomitant liver and kidney transplantation from the same donor (12). Moreover, liver allografts can prevent hyperacute rejection of renal allografts (from the same donor) in patients with preformed lymphocytotoxic antibodies (13). Many of these aspects of liver transplant tolerance have been reviewed (14,15), and the reader is directed to these articles for more exhaustive reference material. Immunologic and other factors that are thought to contribute to liver tolerance are summarized in Table 56.2. In addition, distinctive features of the liver microenvironment may influence the nature and extent of immune responses within and toward this organ. These include its potential hematopoietic activity, an unusual T-lymphocyte constituency, and a comparatively high incidence of intrahepatic T-cell death (Table 56.3).

Of related interest is portal venous tolerance. Thus, tolerance induced in animals following the oral administration of antigen [including alloantigen (16)] has been attributed, at least in part, to the role of the liver. Indeed, tolerance can be induced by the direct delivery of antigen via the portal vein (17), a route that may be more effective for tolerance induction than the conventional intravenous route. Enhanced survival of cardiac allografts with portal venous drainage (18), or after extracorporeal donor-specific liver hemoperfusion (19), also points to an important role for the liver in tolerance induction.

TABLE 56.1. FEATURES OF LIVER TRANSPLANT TOLERANCE

Transplantation across ABO barriers does not lead to accelerated liver allograft rejection
A clear effect of (HLA) haplotype matching is not apparent
Acute liver allograft rejection is relatively easy to control
Irreversible acute liver rejection is rare
The liver may confer a survival advantage on other types of organ graft from the same donor transplanted at the same time

HLA, human leukocyte antigen.

TABLE 56.2. FACTORS THAT MAY CONTRIBUTE TO LIVER TRANSPLANT TOLERANCE

Anatomic features of the liver vasculature
Regenerative ability
Low constitutive MHC antigen expression by hepatocytes
High-dose Ag-induced tolerance
Immunomodulatory effects of secreted soluble donor MHC class I molecules
Th1/Th2 cytokine imbalance
Hepatocyte cytosol and protein products (α-fetoprotein, α_2-macroglobulin, liver growth factors) are immunosuppressive
"Tolerogenic" interstitial passenger (migratory) leukocytes
In situ deletion (apoptosis) of graft-infiltrating cells

MHC, major histocompatibility complex.

TABLE 56.3. DISTINCTIVE FEATURES OF THE LIVER MICROENVIRONMENT THAT MAY CONTRIBUTE TO THE ORGAN'S "PRIVILEGED" IMMUNOLOGIC STATUS

The liver is a potential hematopoietic organ; blood from two sources, hepatic arterial and portal venous, traverses sinusoids with incomplete endothelial linings; the sinosoids, and a large macrophage bed (Kupffer cells) mixed with Ito cells, or stem cells, create an unusual nonlymphoid tissue microenvironment

There is an unusual mixture of T cells in the liver; circulating lymphocytes are not retained within conventional blood vessels, but interact with both hepatocytes and nonparenchymal cells; besides CD4+ CD8+ T cells, there are abundant NK-T cells, a special subset of CD4− CD8− TCR+ T cells, and TCRγδ T cells

The liver is a site of T-cell apoptosis; activated T cells passing through the liver may be immobilized by interactions with molecules (such as ICAM-1, VAP-1) expressed in hepatic sinusoids, or by Kupffer cells or endothelial cells; such immobilized cells may be killed through Fas-dependent or Fas-independent mechanisms by NK cells, NK-T cells, or by TNF secreted by these cells

A special cytokine environment is associated with hepatic immune responses: HGF, TGF-β, GM-CSF, and IL-6

GM-CSF, granulocyte-macrophage colony stimulating factor; HGF, hepatocyte growth factor; ICAM, intracellular adhesion molecule; IL, interleukin; NK, natural killer; TCR, T-cell receptor; TGF, transforming growth factor; TNF, tumor necrosis factor.

LIVER TRANSPLANTATION TOLERANCE AND REJECTION: THE MOUSE MODEL

Orthotopic liver transplantation in the mouse was developed at the University of Pittsburgh, with a view to gaining mechanistic insight into the regulation of liver allograft rejection, and in an effort to overcome the limitations of other models of liver transplantation. Using similar techniques to those adopted by Zimmerman et al. (4) and Kamada et al. (5) for orthotopic rat liver transplantation, Qian et al. (1) were able to achieve a technical success greater than 90% (>100-day host survival) in many mouse strain combinations. The small size of the mouse liver vessels prohibits anastomosis of the hepatic artery. As with rat liver grafts, however, this is not required for host survival or growth. The potential value of the mouse liver transplantation model reflects detailed knowledge of the mouse immune system, the existence of many congenic and recombinant strains, the development of transgenic and specific gene knockout animals, and the availability of numerous mouse-specific investigational reagents.

Tolerance to liver allografts (donor-specific graft survival in the absence of immunosuppressive therapy) is achieved in virtually all MHC (H2) incompatible mouse strain combinations tested, including outbred strains

(Qian et al., unpublished data). By contrast, skin allografts in the same strain combinations are rejected acutely. Liver allograft acceptance occurs despite early intragraft mononuclear leukocyte infiltration that is identical histologically to that observed in organ rejection, reflecting the "active" nature of liver-induced tolerance. With the acceptance of hepatic allografts, the recipients become permanently tolerant to donor strain challenge grafts, such as those of heart and even skin. Tolerance induction can be prevented by presensitization of the liver recipient to donor alloantigens. This can be achieved by skin grafting, 2 weeks or more before organ transplantation. When the host is presensitized, the liver is rejected acutely (within 4 to 5 days), providing a rejection model with which the "spontaneous" tolerance model can be compared. Other mouse models of liver allograft rejection include recipient treatment with recombinant mouse interleukin-2 (IL-2) (20) or IL-12 (21), or donor pretreatment with the hematopoietic growth factor fms-like tyrosine kinase 3 (Flt3)-ligand (FL) (22) that strikingly augments the number of potentially allostimulatory dendritic cells (DCs) within the donor liver.

SYSTEMIC, DONOR-SPECIFIC TOLERANCE

In the C57BL/10 (B10; H2b) to C3H (H2k) mouse strain combination, orthotopic liver grafts are accepted permanently, while skin or heart grafts are rejected acutely. The nature of the systemic tolerance induced by hepatic allografting is demonstrated when a B10 (donor) strain challenge heart is transplanted following liver replacement. Instead of being rejected within about 10 days, such heart grafts are protected by the transplanted liver and survive indefinitely (Table 56.4). Donor-strain (B10) skin grafts are also prolonged dramatically. By contrast, recipients of B10 livers usually reject subsequent third party (e.g., B10.D2; H2d) heart or skin grafts (Table 56.4). Hepatic tolerogenicity is so robust that ongoing skin graft rejection can be reversed by liver transplantation, thus converting sensitization to tolerance (6,23). Interestingly, significant prolongation of donor but not third-party skin allografts can be achieved in syngeneic naive irradiated mice, reconstituted with spleen cells from long-term liver allograft recipients (24,25). This suggests that these cells are capable of transferring tolerance.

Spontaneous liver transplant tolerance also occurs in a number of fully allogeneic rat strain combinations, e.g., the DA to PVG combination (26), in which livers are accepted in the absence of immunosuppression. Although tolerance may be partly MHC-associated, this is by no means a general rule. Minor histocompatibility genes do appear to play a significant role (14,15). Livers from the same donor strain, placed 100 days before challenge heart

TABLE 56.4. INDUCTION OF SYSTEMIC, DONOR-SPECIFIC TOLERANCE BY LIVER TRANSPLANTATION IN C3H (H2^K^) MICE

1st Graft	2nd Graft	2nd Graft Survival Times (Days)	Median Survival Time (Days)
None	B10 heart[d]	10, 10, 10, 11, 12	10
B10[a] liver	B10 heart	>100, >100, >100, >100, >100	>100
B10 liver	B10.D2[b] heart	12, 13, 13, 13, 13	13
None	B10 skin[c]	10, 11, 11, 12, 12	11
B10 liver	B10 skin	35, 37, 40, 45, 50	40
B10 liver	B10.D2 skin	12, 12, 13, 13, 13	13

[a]H2^b^.
[b]H2^d^.
[c]Second skin grafts transplanted 2 weeks after liver grafts.
[d]Second heart grafts transplanted immediately after liver grafts.

grafts, protect against the pathogenesis of chronic rejection (graft vessel disease) (27). Chronic rejection is also abrogated, in a donor-specific manner, in a mouse model of aortic allotransplantation by prior liver transplantation without immunosuppression (28).

HISTO- AND IMMUNOPATHOLOGIC FINDINGS

Cellular infiltration of hepatic allografts becomes apparent histologically by day 2 posttransplant, and is evident in the portal areas as a mild inflammatory infiltrate. By day 6, when the response usually peaks, there is a marked increase in the number of infiltrating leukocytes, which include T cells (predominantly), B lymphocytes, macrophages, eosinophils, and neutrophils, both in portal areas and sinusoids. Of the T-cell subsets, CD8+ cells outnumber CD4+ cells; IL-2R+ (CD25+) (activated) T cells are also evident (29). Little evidence of bile duct or hepatocyte injury is observed. Both in character and kinetics, these features resemble a rejection response, as described in detail by Demetris et al. (30) for rejecting rat liver allografts. By day 14, the graft infiltrate begins to resolve, and thereafter the graft gradually becomes relatively free of infiltrating cells. Both the hepatocytes and bile duct epithelia maintain their morphologic and functional integrity, and the animals show no signs of metabolic impairment.

The time course of the transient inflammatory reaction correlates with the T helper (Th) cell-derived cytokine messenger RNA (mRNA) profile within the graft. When compared with orthotopic syngeneic liver grafts, mouse liver allografts demonstrate upregulation of IL-2, interferon-γ (IFN-γ), IL-4, and IL-10 gene transcripts by day 2, peaking at day 6, and diminishing by day 30 (24). These observations contrast with studies in other mouse allograft models. Thus, a clear predominance of Th1 cytokines in rejecting islets (31), and of Th2 cytokines in nonrejecting cardiac grafts (32), has been reported. On the other hand, IL-6 mRNA appears to be expressed to a similar extent in syngeneic and allogeneic liver grafts, consistent with its role as a nonspecific, proinflammatory factor.

In addition to these cytokine findings, there is a rise in vascular adhesion molecule expression. Murine vascular cell adhesion molecule-1 (VCAM-1), which is not expressed on endothelium in normal liver or in liver isografts, can be detected on portal vein endothelium of mouse liver allografts by day 2 posttransplant (33). With the progression of the antiallograft response, expression of VCAM-1 is observed on liver vascular endothelium, bile duct epithelium, and sinusoids. The strong VCAM-1 expression on blood vessels and bile duct epithelium persists for at least 150 days, and is also expressed strongly on sinusoidal cells in long-surviving livers (150 days). In general terms, these observations clearly indicate that liver allograft acceptance is associated with an active immunologic response.

"PARADOXICAL" *EX VIVO* ALLOIMMUNE REACTIVITY IN TOLERANT RECIPIENTS

The spontaneous acceptance of mouse liver allografts confers permanent, systemic, donor-specific unresponsiveness to other organ grafts. Paradoxically, however, the host's immune system can readily generate vigorous *ex vivo* mixed leukocyte reaction (MLR) and cytotoxic T lymphocyte (CTL) responses within several days of culture with donor alloantigens (20,29). These tests have usually been carried out using donor splenocytes, and tumor cell lines as stimulators and targets, respectively. Very limited attention has been paid to parenchymal cells as targets, although such studies could prove insightful. This phenomenon, described as "split tolerance," has also been observed in rat liver transplantation (34) and in a number of other experimental models of alloimmune reactivity (35–37).

Nonparenchymal cells (NPCs) isolated from liver allografts up to at least 90 days posttransplant respond normally to donor or third-party stimulation in MLR (29). Freshly isolated liver NPCs, harvested during the first 2 weeks posttransplant, exhibit strong, donor-specific CTL responses. The degree of CTL activity correlates well with the extent of the histologic infiltrate, peaking between days

4 and 7, then diminishing steadily to a low, albeit still detectable, level by day 14 (Fig. 56.1). Thereafter, CTL activity in the NPC population is gradually restored to the minimal level found in normal mouse liver (20). This initially strong antidonor CTL response of liver graft-infiltrating lymphocytes, followed quickly by a fall in activity, is consistent with the histopathologic observations described above. Although other events may be involved, the death/elimination of these donor-reactive, graft-infiltrating T cells may provide a key to further understanding of mechanisms underlying liver graft acceptance.

After liver transplantation, the host's spleen cells also exhibit T-cell proliferative (MLR) responses toward both donor and third-party splenocytes, while remaining unresponsive to autologous lymphocytes. This pattern of reactivity is maintained throughout the posttransplant period. The phenomenon is not restricted to a specific mouse strain combination, as spleen cells from long-term liver graft recipients in other combinations (e.g., B10.BR → B10 or B10.BR → B10.D2) also respond normally to donor and third-party cells, but not to syngeneic stimulator cells. Spleen cells from long-term liver allograft recipients are also

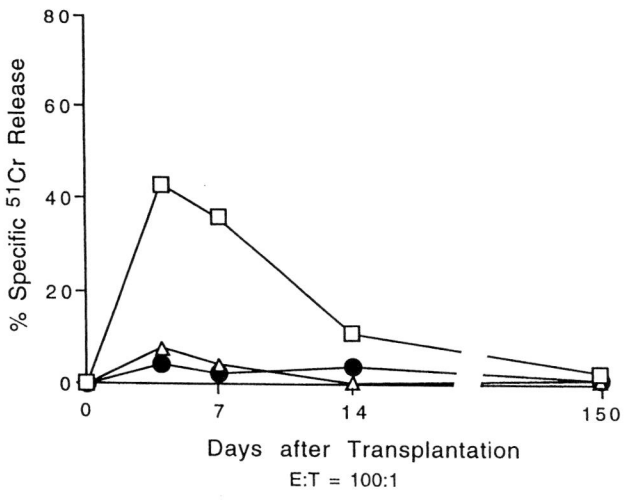

FIGURE 56.1. Cytotoxic activity of freshly isolated liver nonparenchymal cells (NPCs) from nonimmunosuppressed C3H (H2^k) recipients of B10 (H2^b) liver allografts. A 4-hour ^{51}Cr-release assay was used to determine cytotoxicity against target cells expressing donor (H2^b) alloantigen 4, 7, 14, and 150 days after transplantation. Third-party (H2^d) and syngeneic (H2^k) target cells were also used. Antidonor cytotoxic activity diminishes progressively after day 4, as donor-specific tolerance is induced.

reactive in CTL assays following restimulation with donor and third-party antigen-presenting cells (APCs).

The persistence of antidonor responsiveness in *ex vivo* assays, including the capacity to generate donor-specific CTL from the spleen, indicates that clonal deletion of CTL precursors (CTLps) does not occur. This conclusion is reinforced by observations of Vβ T-cell receptor (TCR) usage in a mouse strain combination in which the liver donor but not the recipient expresses the stimulatory endogenous super-Ag [minor lymphocyte stimulating (Mls) antigen]. In this model, no deletion or hyporesponsiveness of donor super-Ag–reactive T cells is observed (29).

DO SOLUBLE DONOR MAJOR HISTOCOMPATIBILITY COMPLEX (MHC) CLASS I ANTIGENS AND/OR ANTI-MHC CLASS II ANTIBODIES PLAY A ROLE IN TOLERANCE INDUCTION?

Although hepatocytes do not express MHC class II antigens, and express class I antigens only weakly, strongly MHC class II$^+$ DCs are located in portal areas (Fig. 56.2). Bile duct cells strongly express MHC class I (38). Following transplantation, both MHC class I and class II are induced on all liver cell types.

A role for soluble donor MHC class I antigens in the induction of liver transplant tolerance has been suggested. This argument is based on the observation that a soluble form of class I antigen is released constitutively by the liver; after liver transplantation, circulating MHC antigen switches rapidly to that of donor type (39). It has been postulated that this free class I antigen may have immunosuppressive properties, due to neutralization of donor-specific antibodies or inhibition of CTL. Several observations suggest that this contention may not be valid. First, secretion of soluble MHC class I antigens is increased during rejection episodes (39). Second, in mice, liver grafts from MHC class I (B6;β2m;H2^b)– or class II (B6;Ab^o;H2^b)–deficient donors are accepted by C3H (H2^k) recipients (40). Third, liver allografts transplanted between strain combinations matched at MHC class I and/or class II loci (i.e., no class I and/or class II antigenic differences) are all accepted spontaneously (40). These liver graft recipients are also tolerant to subsequent skin grafts of H2^b origin. Fourth, administration of soluble donor MHC class I molecules to experimental allograft recipients leads to only slight or no prolongation of organ graft survival (41).

Antidonor MHC class II antibodies have also been suggested as possible mediators of tolerance induction in liver allograft recipients. Although serum from liver-grafted rats in one strain combination (DA[RT1^a]→PVG[RT1^c]) can prolong the survival of cardiac allografts in the same combination (42), this finding has not been reproduced in other rat strain combinations (43) or in mice (44).

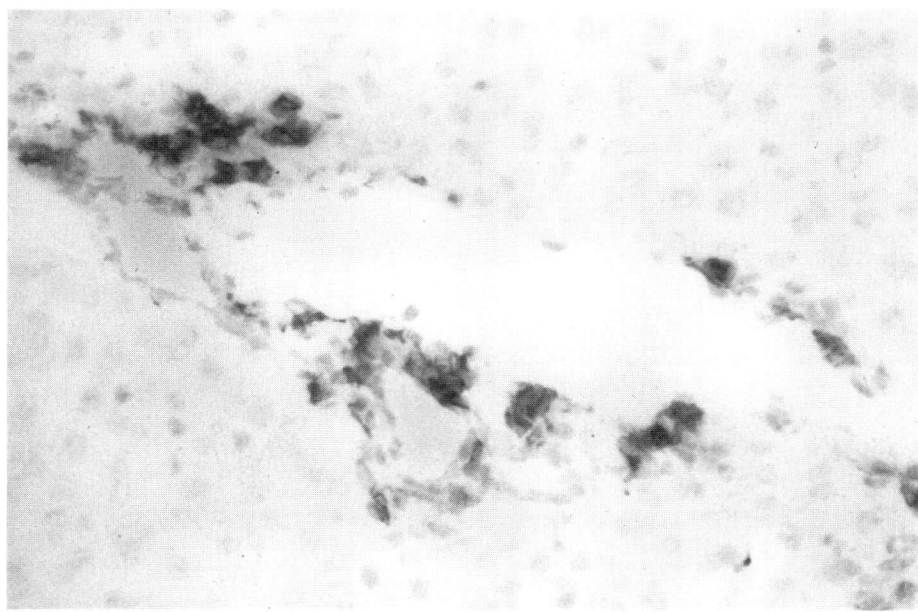

FIGURE 56.2. Cryostat section of normal B10.BR mouse (H2K^k;IE^+) liver, showing strongly major histocompatibility complex (MHC) class II–positive cells [presumptive dendritic cells (DCs)] in a portal area. All positive cells (presumptive DCs) appear to be associated with blood vessel components. There is no staining of bile duct epithelium, hepatocytes, or endothelial cells. Avidin–biotin complex (ABC) peroxidase, counterstained with hematoxylin; original magnification, ×400.

DOES T-HELPER 1 CYTOKINE DEFICIENCY ACCOUNT FOR LIVER ALLOGRAFT ACCEPTANCE?

Evidence in favor of a Th1 insufficiency theory of liver transplant tolerance has been obtained mostly from comparative studies of mouse liver allograft rejection that occurs in presensitized recipients. In this model, liver allografts are rejected acutely (within 5 days) by hosts presensitized to donor antigens by skin grafting at least 2 weeks before organ transplantation. Histologically, the liver rejection process is characterized by cell and antibody-mediated damage to parenchymal cells (hepatocyte and bile duct epithelium). This form of rejection is likely to be T-cell driven, as the adoptive transfer of splenocytes from mice presensitized to donor cells can mediate allograft rejection in otherwise naive liver transplant recipients (24). Examination of the cytokine mRNA profile within the livers of fully MHC-mismatched, presensitized recipients on days 1, 2, and 4 posttransplant reveals upregulated expression of IL-2, IFN-γ, IL-4, and IL-10 gene transcripts compared with spontaneously accepted allografts in naive recipients. The most striking difference is in IFN-γ mRNA levels, which show a 30-fold upregulation by day 2, and at least a 10-fold increase by day 4 (24).

Mouse liver allograft rejection is also linked to the deposition of immunoglobulin G2a (IgG2a), but not IgG1 or IgM alloantibodies in the graft sinusoidal, biliary, and vascular compartments. Since IFN-γ is known to promote the IgG2a isotype, these data suggest a link between an alloreactive Th1 cell response and liver rejection in presensitized recipients. A particularly interesting observation is that, in mice, IgG2a can induce complement activation, whereas the Th2-associated IgG1 antibodies cannot. Passive transfer of antibodies from mice presensitized to donor does not, however, affect the spontaneous acceptance of liver allografts. Thus, investigation of "second set" liver allograft rejection indicates that it is Th1 cell-driven, that it requires MHC class I^+ cells as lytic targets, and that it is likely to involve at least both CTL and antibody responses. These observations must be placed in the context of a large number of reports that have drawn quite diverse conclusions about the roles of Th1 and Th2 cytokines in allograft immunity.

To test directly the role of specific cytokines in liver allograft rejection, mouse recombinant (r) IL-2, IL-12, or IL-4 was administered to otherwise unmodified liver allograft recipients (B10 → C3H) (21). IL-2 is a Th1 cytokine implicated in allograft rejection, whereas IL-12 is produced primarily by APCs (DCs, macrophages, and activated B cells) and is a potent promoter of Th1 cell development. IL-4 is the cytokine most responsible for the function of Th2 cells. Administration of IL-2 or IL-12, but not IL-4, once daily from the time of transplant, resulted in liver allograft rejection between days 5 and 7. The same dose regimen of IL-2 or IL-12 was well tolerated in syngeneic liver transplantation, indicating that graft failure was not due to cytokine toxicity. In contrast to IL-2 or IL-12, high-dose IL-4 did not exacerbate the transient (histologic) rejection usually seen in mouse liver recipients. The induction of acute liver allograft rejection by IL-2 or IL-12, as well as the association of IFN-γ and IgG2a with rejection in presensitized mice, clearly indicates that Th1 cytokines are capable of mediating liver rejection, irrespective of whether this is in naive or presensitized recipients. The failure of exogenous IL-4 to induce liver rejection at high doses suggests that Th2 cytokines may not be critical in mouse liver rejection. This is supported by the absence of any correlation between message for IL-5 (eosinophil differentiation factor) and either mouse liver allograft rejection or tolerance (Thai NL, et al., unpublished observations).

Based on these recent studies, IL-2 and IL-12 appear to mediate distinct effector functions in mouse liver rejection. IL-2–mediated rejection is associated with increased intragraft infiltration, including CD4+ and CD8+ cells, and upregulated natural killer (NK) cells, lymphokine-activated killer (LAK) cells, and allospecific CTL killing. Gene transcripts for both Th1 (IFN-γ) and Th2 cytokines (IL-4, IL-10) are also upregulated in the graft. IL-12, on the other hand, induces liver allograft rejection without an increase in cellular infiltration, and by inhibiting CTL, coincident with increased IFN-γ, IL-6, IL-10 mRNA, intragraft macrophages, and complement-activating cytotoxic antibodies (21). The inhibition of cytotoxicity (CTL, NK, and LAK cell) by IL-12 is surprising, since IL-12 is also known as cytolytic T-cell maturation factor. This finding, however, has been confirmed *in vitro* by MLR.

The characterization of at least two pathways of rejection, mediated via IL-2 or IL-12/IFN-γ, provides important information for the debate about whether allograft rejection is mediated by specific T cells, or by nonspecific macrophages (delayed-type hypersensitivity, DTH). While the specific rejection of experimental allografts appears to require CTL, tolerance can also be seen in the face of strong *ex vivo* antidonor CTL activity, as observed in both mouse and rat liver transplant tolerance models ("split tolerance"). Other investigators have also shown independently the apparent absence of CTL in rejecting rodent heart allografts. In these models, the large number of macrophages and the expression of IFN-γ within the grafts suggests a DTH reaction. Rosenberg and Singer (45) have suggested that skin allograft rejection in mice requires both Th cells and CTL, but that it is the antigen-specific CTL that eventually destroys cells in the graft expressing allogeneic histocompatibility antigens. While our own work suggests that both mechanisms may be operative, and that each may be sufficient to induce rejection, it is likely that both pathways contribute to allograft rejection.

DOES APOPTOTIC DEATH OF GRAFT-INFILTRATING CELLS PLAY A ROLE IN LIVER TRANSPLANT TOLERANCE?

Liver transplant tolerance appears to be an active process. All liver grafts undergo a brisk, early episode of histologic rejection, and although donor-specific CTL activity of graft-infiltrating cells can be detected readily, there is little hepatocyte necrosis. The inflammatory response subsides within a few weeks. These observations led us to speculate that the rapid waning of the immune response *in situ* might be due to elimination, within the graft, of donor-specific CTL susceptible to programmed cell death (apoptosis). CTLps that are known to be resistant to apoptosis appear to persist, as indicated by *ex vivo* generation of CTL responses by host cells.

In normal immune responses, activation-induced cell death (AICD) may have two regulatory functions: first, to limit overexpansion of the response, and second, to eliminate potentially autoreactive T cells that have escaped intrathymic deletion. Host recognition of donor alloantigens induces activation and subsequent proliferation of T lymphocytes bearing antigen-specific receptors. In the case of mouse heart and skin grafts, this results almost invariably in graft rejection. With liver grafts, however, the initial expansion of antigen-reactive T-cell clones and graft infiltration is followed by attenuation of the CTL effector arm of the response. Rather than being rejected, the graft survives.

In vitro findings have shown that triggering of primary activated T cells via the TCR may lead to their death by apoptosis, but that resting T cells, such as CTLps, are not susceptible (46–49). In recent studies to investigate the role of apoptosis in mouse liver transplant tolerance, allograft recipients were sacrificed 4, 7, 14, 60, and 150 days after transplantation. Freshly isolated liver graft NPCs (90% of which are recipient T cells on days 4 to 14 posttransplant) exhibited high, donor-specific CTL activity initially (days 4 to 7), but this declined significantly by day 14, then decreased gradually thereafter to control levels. The fate of graft-infiltrating CTL was monitored by the detection of apoptotic activity using *in situ* transferase-mediated dUTP nick-end labeling (TUNEL) and DNA fragmentation assays. Compared with isografts, extensive apoptosis of graft-infiltrating cells was observed in portal areas of allografts (20). Apoptotic activity peaked at postoperative day 7, and declined thereafter (Fig. 56.3). The decline of CTL activity in liver grafts appeared to correlate with apoptotic activity.

The next question was whether apoptosis of the graft-infiltrating cells constituted an epiphenomenon of the alloimmune response. To further determine the relationship between apoptotic NPC and liver graft acceptance, the incidence of apoptotic, graft-infiltrating cells in nonrejecting allogeneic livers was compared to that in rejecting hepatic allografts. Acute liver rejection of B10 livers by C3H recip-

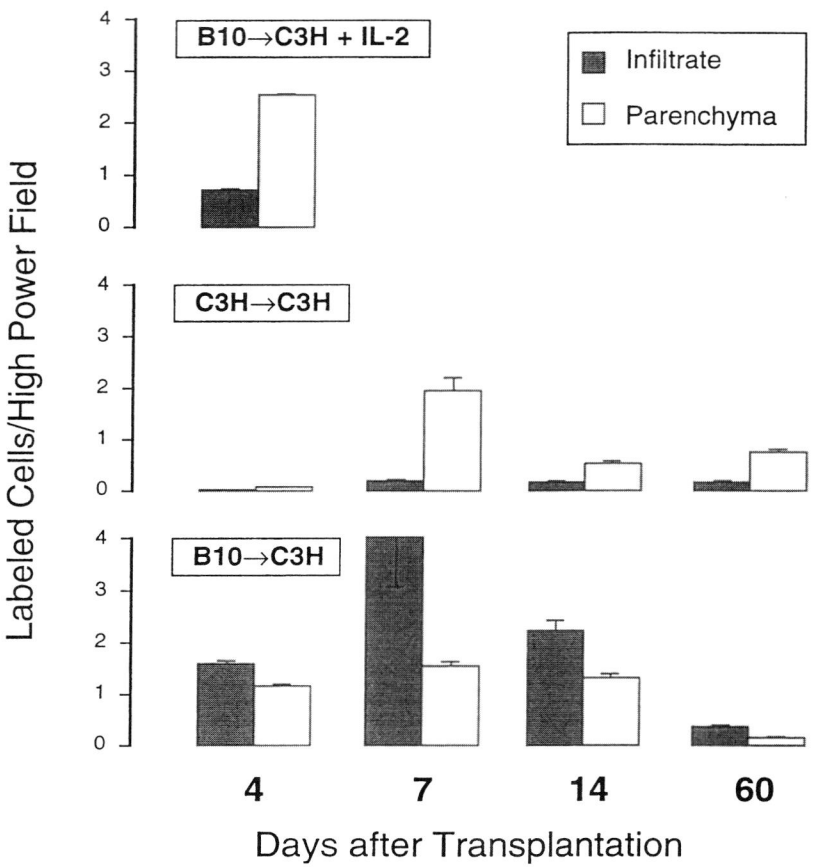

FIGURE 56.3. Incidence of apoptotic cells, determined by *in situ* transferase-mediated dUTP nick end labeling (TUNEL) within the NPC (infiltrate) and parenchymal cell populations of hepatic transplants [isografts, allografts, and allografts plus interleukin-2 (*IL-2*)] at various times after transplantation. Allograft recipients (*B10 → C3H*) given IL-2 reject their livers within 4 to 5 days. Note the comparatively high incidence of apoptotic cells in the graft infiltrate of mice that become tolerant to donor (B10 → C3H).

ients was induced by the systemic administration of mouse rIL-2 (4×10^5 U/d $\times$ 5 days from the day of transplant; median survival time 5 days). IL-2 injection (which resulted in enhanced specific CTL activity in cells isolated from the graft) was accompanied by a lower frequency of apoptotic cells within the inflammatory infiltrate. By contrast, there was a significant increase in hepatocyte death with IL-2 treatment. In liver allografts from FL-treated donors that are rejected acutely, most apoptotic cells are hepatocytes and not graft-infiltrating cells (50). These findings suggest that liver allograft survival may be the result of relatively high levels of programmed cell death within the graft-infiltrating cell population that weakens the effector arm of the host immune response.

The foregoing observations suggest that AICD may play a key regulatory role in the acceptance of MHC-disparate liver allografts in nonimmunosuppressed mice. The susceptibility of CTL to apoptosis has been linked to the interaction of FasL (CD95L) with its cell death–transducing receptor Fas (51). CTLps that lack Fas (CD95) (52) are less sensitive to apoptosis. In the liver recipient, CTLps present in host lymphoid tissue may continue to provide the basis for renewal of the potential effector CTL population. However, apoptotic death of alloreactive

CTLs, occurring predominantly within the graft, and triggered by donor alloantigens, is likely to promote graft survival unless the T cells are rescued by growth-promoting signals in the liver, such as IL-2 (53). By protecting the CTLs from apoptosis, IL-2 administration predisposes to liver graft rejection. Activated T cells may also override AICD in the case of rejection of livers from FL-treated donors (22,50). Further proof of the CTL apoptosis theory of liver acceptance requires demonstration of selective deletion of graft-infiltrating CTLs expressing TCR specific for donor MHC. This is now being investigated in mice bearing a high frequency of allospecific TCR transgenic T cells.

High levels of expression of FasL have been demonstrated on parenchymal cells within immunologically privileged sites (54), such as the mouse testis (55) and the anterior chamber of the eye (56). This has been linked to the death of specific, activated T cells, and to the maintenance of immune privilege within these sites. The normal rodent and human liver appears not to express FasL mRNA (54,57), but FasL mRNA is found within hepatocytes in inflammatory liver disease (57). Another possibility is that donor leukocytes, in particular populations of potential migratory DCs present within the graft and that may express FasL (58), or other death-inducing ligands, or secrete nitric oxide (NO) (59), could have the ability to trigger apoptosis in alloactivated T cells.

Interactions between other cell surface–expressed receptor-ligand pairs [e.g., intracellular adhesion molecule-1 (ICAM-1)/lymphocyte function–associated antigen (LFA-1), 4-1BB/4-1BBL (60)] and the role of other members of the tumor necrosis factor (TNF) family, including TNF, CD30L, CD40L, and TNF receptor apoptosis-inducing ligand (TRAIL) that may enhance or inhibit Fas-mediated AICD, are currently being tested. Specific cytokines produced by liver cells, in particular transforming growth factor-β (TGF-β) (61), which can induce T-cell apoptosis (62), may also be involved in regulation of the T-cell response. One possibility, based on other models of alloreactivity, is that deletion of high-affinity T cells may occur *in vivo* as a result of exhaustive differentiation (37,63) in the presence of large amounts of donor antigen in the liver. It is well known that tolerance can be induced by high doses of antigen, including transplantation antigens (64). This type of antigen-specific tolerance is thought to involve extrathymic T-cell exhaustion and deletion in a mature immune system of normal mice or mice with transgenic TCR (65,66). Interestingly, the induction of tolerance following rat liver transplantation can be inhibited significantly by steroid administration for the first 2 days post-transplant, suggesting that immune activation (characterized by IL-2 and IFN-γ transcripts in lymphoid tissue that are higher in tolerant compared with rejecting rats) is key to the induction of donor-specific unresponsiveness (67). Survival of low-affinity cells (that function poorly *in vivo*), however, may provide a basis for the positive response to alloantigens *in vitro*. Further investigation of the role of programmed cell death in regulating immune responses within liver and other organ allografts (including challenge grafts that are tolerated in liver recipients) may provide new insight into their comparative immune privilege and tolerogenicity.

Systemic effects of liver transplantation include the capacity of donor hematopoietic cells to migrate extensively to recipient lymphoid tissues, where donor cells can be identified indefinitely. These chimeric cells may provide not only a continuing source of allostimulation, but may also have the capacity to induce apoptosis of alloactivated T cells within the recipient lymphoid system.

MICROCHIMERISM AND LIVER ALLOGRAFT ACCEPTANCE

Several distinctive features of the liver microenvironment (Tables 56.2 and 56.3) may contribute to its immunologic privilege and inherent tolerogenicity. These include its regenerative capacity, and a comparatively heavy endowment of "passenger" leukocytes (68), including stem cells

(69,70), compared with the kidney or heart. In rodent spontaneous liver allograft acceptance models, these donor-derived leukocytes and their cytokine products appear to be essential for graft survival (71,72), and may include donor-derived "tolerogenic" or "deletional" APCs (73).

Multilineage donor hematopoietic cell microchimerism occurs in recipients of organ allografts, and is persistent and long-lasting in those animals and humans that accept their grafts, with or without the need for immunosuppressive therapy (74). It has been postulated that chimerism is an essential condition for organ allograft acceptance (71,74). The induction of tolerance to liver allografts is thought to depend both on the liver parenchyma and the NPC population (75). In rats, transplants of chimeric livers that have passenger leukocytes of recipient origin and parenchyma of donor origin do not induce tolerance to subsequent skin grafts (75). Moreover, if the number of donor leukocytes is reduced by irradiation of the rat liver donor 1 week before transplant, the outcome is rejection (76). Reconstitution of the liver leukocyte population, either by injection of liver or spleen cells, restores liver tolerogenicity (76). After liver transplantation, large numbers of donor leukocytes migrate into recipient lymphoid tissues, especially the spleen and celiac lymph nodes. Smaller numbers of donor cells are observed in the thymus (67,68,77), which does not appear to play a role in liver tolerance induction as this is not abolished by thymectomy (77). In rats, there appears to be a close relationship between the migration of donor cells to recipient lymphoid tissue, the early upregulation of IL-2 and IFN-γ production in these tissues, and tolerance induction. In rejecting rat strain combinations, there is less expression of these cytokines than in tolerant animals (67), suggesting that rapid responder T-cell activation may be an integral part of the tolerogenic process.

THE PERSISTENT DONOR-DERIVED DENDRITIC CELLS

Despite its comparative immune privilege, the liver is rich in migratory "passenger" leukocytes, including DCs, regarded traditionally as the primary antigenic component of transplanted organs and the instigators of rejection (78,79). This apparent paradox has led to recent detailed investigation of the immunobiology of DCs and other APCs within the liver, including studies of microenvironmental factors that may modify the function of these cells to confer immunologic privilege on hepatic allografts.

DCs are a consistently prominent feature of the persistent, donor-derived leukocyte populations that are observed in the tissues of tolerant mouse or rat liver allograft recipients (6,68) and in successful liver or other organ transplant patients (71,74). This phenomenon, of allogeneic donor cell persistence, can be reproduced in mice by the local or systemic infusion of *in vitro* generated, granulocyte-macrophage colony-stimulating factor (GM-CSF)–stimulated, normal liver-derived DC progenitors (80). In long-surviving tolerant rat liver allograft recipients, the persistence of donor MHC class II⁺ cells resembling DCs within challenge cardiac allografts (placed 100 days after the liver grafts) has been linked to the absence of histopathologic features of chronic rejection (graft vessel disease) (27). This contrasts with the finding in rats preconditioned with donor bone marrow cells instead of liver grafts, in which the absence of donor cells, but the presence of graft vessel disease, was observed in the challenge heart grafts (27). Thus, persistence of donor-derived cells of the DC lineage derived from a source of continuous stem/progenitor cell production (the liver) may play a key role in the inhibition of immunopathologic processes leading to acute and chronic rejection.

An important related observation is that using the myeloid lineage growth factor GM-CSF, donor-derived DCs have been grown from spontaneously tolerant mouse liver allograft recipients. The same phenomenon has been reproduced in conventionally immunosuppressed human liver transplant recipients infused with unmodified donor bone marrow cells at the time of transplant (81).

THE TOLEROGENIC POTENTIAL OF LIVER-DERIVED DENDRITIC CELLS

There is evidence that the phenotype and function of DCs may determine the balance between tolerance and immunity (73,82). DC progenitors can be propagated readily from normal mouse liver in response to GM-CSF (83), using techniques devised initially to propagate these cells from mouse bone marrow or blood. When injected either locally or systemically into allogeneic recipients, these cells migrate to T-dependent areas of lymphoid tissue, where they can readily be identified by expression of donor MHC class II antigen (80) (Fig. 56.4). Using the B10 → C3H strain combination, we have shown that donor-derived DC progenitors can be propagated from the bone marrow (isolated 14 days posttransplant) of spontaneously tolerant liver allograft recipients, but not from mice that acutely reject organ (cardiac) allografts from the same donor strain (84). Both immunocytochemical and molecular analyses were used to identify these cells. This observation raised questions about the functional significance of bone marrow–derived DC progenitors in the context of their potential *in vivo* interactions with allogeneic T cells.

Myeloid DC progenitors (DEC 205⁺, CD11c⁺, MHC class II⁺, CD80^dim, CD86⁻) propagated *in vitro* in response to GM-CSF are very weak stimulators of naive allogeneic T cells. In contrast, DCs propagated from normal bone marrow or spleen under the same conditions (MHC class II⁺, CD80^hi, CD86^hi) are potent inducers of

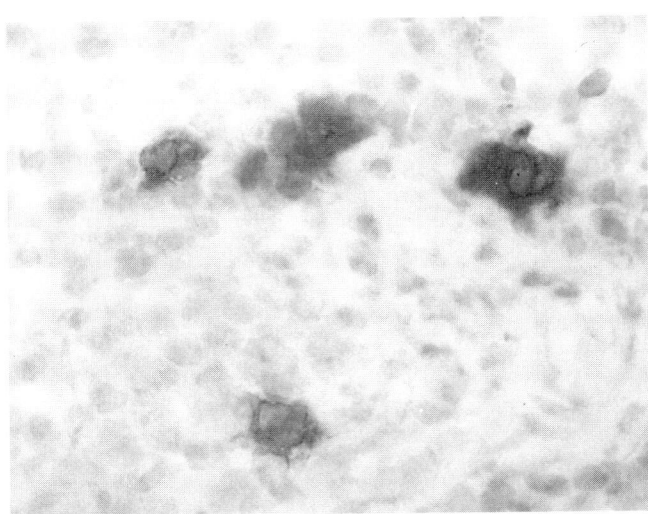

FIGURE 56.4. *In vivo* migration of *in vitro*–generated donor liver–derived dendritic cell (DC) progenitors (B10.BR;H2^k) to T-dependent areas of recipient (B10;H2^b) lymphoid tissue. The cells (2.5 × 10⁵) were injected subcutaneously and detected (IE⁺) in cryostat sections of the spleen 5 days later. The sections were stained using the amino-ethyl cabazole (ABC) peroxidase procedure, with donor-specific mouse anti-IE^k monoclonal antibody (mAb), together with appropriate controls. The fate of these liver-derived DCs recapitulates the migration of donor-derived DCs after allogeneic liver transplantation. Original magnification ×1,000.

allogeneic T-cell proliferation (85). The co-stimulatory molecule-deficient DC progenitors induce alloantigen-specific hyporesponsiveness in allogeneic T cells detected upon restimulation in secondary MLR (85). This is associated with blockade of IL-2 production. Reactivity to third-party stimulators is intact. The hyporesponsiveness induced by the co-stimulatory molecule-deficient DC progenitors is prevented by incorporation of anti-CD28 monoclonal antibodies (mAbs) in the primary MLR, and is reversed by the addition of IL-2 to restimulated T cells. These findings show that MHC class II⁺ CD86⁻ DC progenitors can induce alloantigen-specific hyporesponsiveness in T cells *in vitro*. Under the appropriate conditions, donor-derived, co-stimulatory molecule-deficient DC progenitors exhibiting these properties could contribute to the induction of donor-specific unresponsiveness to graft alloantigens *in vivo*.

The *in vivo* functional significance of these observations has been examined in mouse models of pancreatic islet and cardiac transplantation. Two days after rendering groups of B10 (H2^b) mice diabetic with streptozotocin, and 7 days before transplantation with 700 islet equivalents (99% pure) under the left renal capsule, the animals received (i.v.) either culture medium, 2.5 × 10⁶ allogeneic (B10.BR; H2^k) or syngeneic, 10-day cultured, GM-CSF–stimulated liver DC progenitors, or 10-day cultured, GM-CSF–stimulated mature (spleen) DCs. Blood glucose and body weights were recorded daily. The graft survival

TABLE 56.5. INFLUENCE OF GM-CSF STIMULATED LIVER DC PROGENITORS (MHC II⁺, CD86⁻) ON B10.BR (H-2ᴷ) PANCREATIC ISLET ALLOGRAFT SURVIVAL IN B10 (H-2ᴮ) MICE

Group	Cells Injected	Islet Graft Survival Times (Days)	Median Survival Timeᵃ (Days)
A	None (media control)	11(×4), 13(×3)	11
B	B10 DC progenitors (CD86^{dim}) (syngeneic)	15(5×), 17	15
C	B10.BR DC progenitors (CD86^{dim}) (allogeneic)	18, 19(×3), 21, 22, 27, 29, 61, 68	21*
D	B10.BR "fresh" spleen DC (allogeneic)	11(×3), 15	11

ᵃMST compared using the Kruskal–Wallis test. Pair-wise comparison by the Wilcoxon Rank Sum test.
*p <0.001 vs group B.
MST, median survival time.

times (Table 56.5) show that GM-CSF–stimulated liver DC progenitors significantly prolong allograft survival (86). Evidence has also been obtained that DC progenitors can inhibit vascularized cardiac allograft rejection. In the B10 → C3H model, 2×10^6 B10 bone marrow–derived DC progenitors given i.v. 7 days before transplantation significantly prolong heart graft survival compared with syngeneic (C3H) or third-party (BALB/c) cells (87). By contrast, and as expected, mature DC (CD86^{hi}) reduce mean graft survival time.

It must be emphasized that the DC is only one of the hematolymphopoietic lineages represented in the microchimerism of the spontaneously tolerant/successfully engrafted whole-organ recipient. This chimerism is dependent for long-term maintenance on pluripotent stem cells. The complex, two-way alloimmune reaction that ensues following liver transplantation can neither be generated nor efficiently sustained by any single lineage (88). Nevertheless, understanding the molecular regulation of MHC class II gene product expression, or that of T cell co-stimulatory and other immune regulatory molecules, such as FasL (and other TNF family members) or NO by donor bone marrow–derived APCs, and how this relates to T-cell activation or unresponsiveness (anergy/clonal deletion) is a central issue in transplantation immunology. Such insight may be key to clarifying the role of donor-derived (chimeric) DC in host responses to liver and other whole-organ transplants, and to further understanding the inherent tolerogenicity that is a feature of all organs, but most highly represented by liver.

THE ROLE OF CYTOKINES IN MODIFICATION OF LIVER DENDRITIC CELL FUNCTION

It has thus been argued that comparatively large numbers of immature, co-stimulatory molecule-deficient donor APCs (that probably include macrophages and B cells, in addition to DCs) may emanate continuously from liver allografts under the influence of GM-CSF [also a product of hepatocytes (89)]. Donor-derived DC progenitors have

been shown to migrate rapidly (within 24 hours) to T-dependent areas of recipient lymphoid tissue (80), and to induce alloantigen-specific unresponsiveness in recipient strain T cells (85). Clearly, administration of conventional T-cell directed immunosuppressive agents [cyclosporin A or tacrolimus, which inhibit production of cytokines that promote DC maturation (TNF, IL-4)] is likely not only to augment numbers of these donor cells, but also to "preserve" their immature (tolerogenic?) phenotype. Another microenvironmental cytokine that may be of importance in modulating the function of liver-derived DCs, and that has been implicated in the immunologic privilege of another tissue site (the anterior chamber of the eye) (90) is TGF-β. This cytokine is believed to confer tolerogenicity on antigen-bearing APCs that migrate from the anterior chamber of the eye to regional lymphoid tissue, and to confer systemic, antigen-specific tolerance (90). TGF-β is synthesized by hepatocytes and other liver cell types, in addition to T cells. It is mitoinhibitory for hepatocytes, and has been shown to permit the growth, but to suppress the maturation, of GM-CSF–stimulated DC (91,92). Indeed, if these TGF-β–influenced DCs are infused systemically before transplant, they prolong vascularized cardiac allograft survival in a donor-specific manner (92). Interestingly, cyclosporin A, widely used in human liver transplantation as a front-line immunosuppressant, potentiates systemic levels of TGF-β (93) that could, in turn, promote or sustain the immature DC phenotype. Other microenvironmental factors that may be important in modulating the phenotype and function of DCs and other donor liver-derived APCs, are IL-6, hepatocyte growth factor (HGF), and extracellular matrix proteins (83). Marked augmentation of the number of functional DCs in donor livers prior to transplantation, by administration of the potent DC-inducing cytokine Flt-3 ligand, renders the mouse liver more highly immunogenic (22). This results in acute liver graft rejection, with augmented antidonor CTL, NK, and LAK cell activities (50), rather than the customary tolerance induction observed in recipients of normal livers. The proposed pivotal role of DCs in determining the balance between liver transplant tolerance and rejection is depicted in Fig. 56.5.

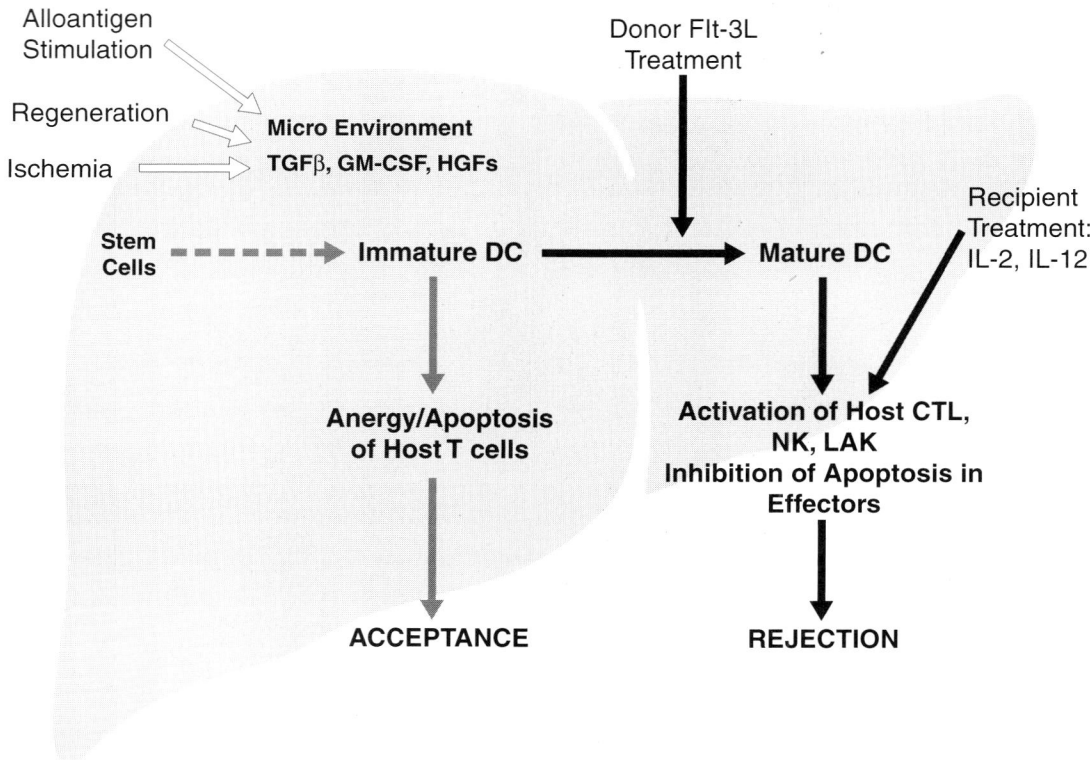

FIGURE 56.5. Proposed pivotal role of donor dendritic cells (*DCs*) in liver transplant tolerance and rejection. Growth, maturation, and function of interstitial DCs (derived from stem cells) are affected by microenvironmental factors, in particular the cytokines granulocyte-macrophage colony-stimulating factor (*GM-CSF*), transforming growth factor-β (*TGF-β*), and hepatocyte growth factors (*HGFs*), such as insulin-like growth factor. Levels of these factors are influenced by the process of liver transplantation (allogeneic environment, ischemia, hepatocyte regeneration). The interstitial DCs within the normal liver allograft that are accepted spontaneously in mice are predominantly functionally immature, with the potential to induce anergy/apoptosis of host T cells. Pretreatment of the liver donor with fms-like tyrosine kinase 3 (*Flt-3*) ligand strikingly augments numbers of functional DCs, leading to the rapid induction of host effector cells [cytotoxic T lymphocyte (*CTL*), natural killer (*NK*), and lymphokine-activated killer (*LAK*) cell activity] within the graft. Rejection can also be induced by treatment of the recipient (of a normal liver allograft) with interleukin (*IL*)-2 or IL-12.

MECHANISTIC BASIS OF LIVER-DERIVED DENDRITIC CELLS TOLEROGENICITY

Deficiency or blockade of co-stimulator molecule (CD40, CD80, CD86) expression has clearly been shown to be consistent with DC tolerogenicity, both in allograft models (73), and experimental autoimmune disease (94). DC progenitors (CD80⁻, CD86ᵈⁱᵐ) induce allogeneic T-cell anergy. An important modulator of DC maturation and function is IL-10. Treatment of DCs with IL-10 (or growth of DCs in IL-10) inhibits co-stimulatory molecule expression (95) and IL-12 production (95,96), and renders these cells capable of skewing Th cell responses toward Th2 *in vivo* (96). In a recent study, Khanna et al. (97) analyzed the T-cell stimulatory capacity, tissue trafficking, and influence of immature liver DC progenitors on allogeneic Th1 and Th2 cytokine production. The findings suggest that modulation of Th2 cytokine (IL-10) production by donor liver–derived DC progenitors might be a mechanism contributing to the capacity of liver allografts to subvert host immune responses. Interestingly, IL-10 production by hepatocytes is increased by TGF-β (98). Another regulatory molecule of interest is NO, which is produced by liver sinusoid-lining macrophages (Kupffer cells) (99) in rodents, and also by a subpopulation of myeloid DCs in response to IFN-γ, endotoxin, or interaction with allogeneic T cells (59). Its production is correlated with inhibition of T-cell proliferation, and with apoptosis both of the stimulatory DCs and the responder T-cell population (59,100). The association between inducible NO synthase expression in DCs, their apoptosis, and reduction in T-cell proliferation suggests a counterregulatory mechanism for the control of immune reactivity. Blockade of co-stimulatory molecule expression on *in vitro*–generated myeloid DCs (by CTLA4Ig) can also expose their potential to induce apoptosis in alloactivated T cells (58). This property is linked to the uniform surface expression of FasL by the DCs. Fas L is also observed on freshly isolated CD8α⁺ mouse lymphoid DCs (101) from mouse thymus or peripheral lymphoid tissue. These putative "regulatory DCs" (which share a common precursor with thymocytes) induce apoptosis in alloactivated CD4⁺ T cells (101), and inhibit cytokine (IL-2) production in CD8⁺ T cells (102).

IMPLICATIONS FOR THERAPY OF ALLOGRAFT REJECTION

Studies of possible mechanisms whereby donor-derived DCs may subvert host T-cell responses and predispose to tolerance induction are in their infancy. Those conducted to date provide pointers to novel approaches to the cell-based therapy of organ allograft rejection. One such approach is to maximize the tolerogenic signals that can be delivered to the host immune system by donor APCs. Failure of donor DCs (progenitors or mature DCs) to provide co-stimulation clearly predisposes to the induction of T-cell anergy/apoptosis *in vitro*, and to the prolongation of allograft survival. This property could be optimized in allograft recipients, and rendered longer lasting, by the administration of donor hematopoietic cells in conjunction with (a) a factor that promotes growth of the DC lineage progenitors, and (b) molecules that blockade co-stimulation, such as CTLA4Ig, or anti-CD40L (CD154) (gp 39) mAb. Although effective in rodents (103), convincing evidence has not yet been produced that co-stimulatory molecule blockade can induce organ transplant tolerance in primates. The combined approach of donor hematopoietic cells (especially immature APCs) together with blockade of co-stimulation may prove beneficial. We have shown that combination of co-stimulatory molecule-deficient donor DCs with anti-CD40L mAb given before transplant leads to long-term vascularized cardiac allograft survival (92). An attractive alternative approach may be the *ex vivo* manipulation of donor-derived APCs including genetic engineering, to augment/maximize their tolerogenicity. The liver, with its inherent capacity to produce stem/progenitor cells (69,70,83,104), and its tolerogenic potential, may be the most appropriate organ with which to embark on these studies.

ACKNOWLEDGMENTS

The authors' work is supported by National Institutes of Health grants DK49745 and AI41011, and by grants from the Roche Organ Transplantation Research Foundation. We are grateful to our many colleagues and collaborators for their input into these ongoing investigations.

REFERENCES

1. Qian S, Fung JJ, Demetris AJ, et al. Orthotopic liver transplantation in mice. *Transplantation* 1991;52:526.
2. Garnier H, Clot J, Bertrand M. Liver transplantation in the pig: surgical approach. *CR Acad Sci Paris* 1965;260:5621.
3. Calne RY, Sells RA, Pena JR, et al. Induction of immunological tolerance by porcine liver allografts. *Nature* 1969;233:472.
4. Zimmerman FA, Butcher GW, Davies HFFS, et al. Techniques for orthotopic liver transplantation in the rat and some studies of the immunologic responses to fully allogeneic liver grafts. *Transplant Proc* 1979;11:571.
5. Kamada N, Davies H, Roser B. Reversal of transplantation immunity by liver grafting. *Nature* 1981;292:840.
6. Qian S, Demetris AJ, Murase N, et al. Murine liver allograft transplantation: tolerance and donor cell chimerism. *Hepatology* 1994;19:916.
7. Monden M, Valdivia LA, Gotch M, et al. Hamster to rat orthotopic liver xenografts. *Transplantation* 1987;43:745.
8. Calne RY, White DJ, Herbertson BM. Pig to baboon liver xenograft. *Lancet* 1968;1:1176.
9. Gugenheim J, Samuel D, Reynes M, et al. Liver transplantation across ABO blood group barriers. *Lancet* 1990;336:519.
10. Ramos HC, Reyes J, Abu-Elmagd K, et al. Weaning of immunosuppression in long-term liver transplant recipients. *Transplantation* 1995;59:212.
11. Calne RY, Sells RA, Marshall VC, et al. Multiple organ grafts in the pig: techniques and results of pancreatic, hepatic, cardiac, and renal allografts. *Br J Surg* 1972;59:977.
12. Rasmussen A, Davies HF, Jamieson NV, et al. Combined transplantation of liver and kidney from the same donor protects the kidney from rejection and improves kidney graft survival. *Transplantation* 1995;59:919.
13. Fung JJ, Makowka L, Griffin M, et al. Successful sequential liver-kidney transplantation in patients with preformed lymphocytotoxic antibodies. *Clin Transplant* 1987;1:187.
14. Wood K, Farges O. Tolerance. In: Neuberger J, Adams D, eds. *Immunology of liver transplantation.* Boston: Little, Brown, 1993:139–151.
15. Kamada N. Animal models of liver transplantation and their clinical relevance. In: Neuberger J, Adams D, eds. *Immunology of liver transplantation.* Boston: Little, Brown, 1993:161–186.
16. Callery MP, Kamei T, Flye MW. The anatomic site-specificity of tolerance induction to alloantigen. *Transplantation* 1990;49:230.
17. Qian JH, Hashimoto T, Fujiwara H, et al. Studies on the induction of tolerance to alloantigens. I. The abrogation of potential for delayed type hypersensitivity responses to alloantigens by portal venous inoculation with allogeneic cells. *J Immunol* 1985;134:3656.
18. Holman JM, Todd R. Enhanced survival of heterotopic rat heart allografts with portal venous drainage. *Transplantation* 1990;49:229.
19. Gugenheim J, Charpentier B, Gigou M, et al. Delayed rejection of heart allografts after excorporeal donor-specific liver hemoperfusion. *Transplantation* 1988;45:628.
20. Qian S, Lu L, Li Y, et al. Apoptosis within spontaneously accepted mouse liver allografts: evidence for deletion of cytotoxic T cells and implications for tolerance induction. *J Immunol* 1997;158:4654.
21. Thai NL, Li Y, Fu F, et al. Interleukin-2 and interleukin-12 mediate distinct effector mechanisms of liver allograft rejection. *Liver Transplant Surg* 1997;3:118.
22. Steptoe RJ, Fu F, Li W, et al. Augmentation of dendritic cells in murine organ donors by treatment with flt3 ligand alters the

balance between transplant tolerance and immunity. *J Immunol* 1997;159:5483.

23. Kamada N, Wight DGD. Antigen-specific immunosuppression induced by liver transplantation in the rat. *Transplantation* 1984; 38:217.

24. Thai NL, Fu F, Qian S, et al. Cytokine mRNA profiles in murine orthotopic liver transplantation: graft rejection is associated with augmented Th1 function. *Transplantation* 1995;59: 274.

25. Davies HFFS, Kamada N, Roser BJ. Mechanisms of donor-specific unresponsiveness induced by liver grafting. *Transplant Proc* 1983;15:831.

26. Zimmerman FA, Davies HS, Knoll PP, et al. Orthotopic liver allografts in the rat. The influence of strain combination on the fate of the graft. *Transplantation* 1984;37:406.

27. Demetris AJ, Murase N, Ye Q, et al. Analysis of chronic rejection and obliterative arteriopathy. Possible contributions of donor antigen-presenting cells and lymphatic disruption. *Am J Pathol* 1997;150;563.

28. Subbotin V, Sun H, Aitouche A, et al. Abrogation of chronic rejection in a murine model of aortic allotransplantation by prior induction of donor-specific tolerance. *Transplantation* 1997;64: 690–695.

29. Dahmen U, Qian S, Rao AS, et al. Split tolerance induced by orthotopic liver transplantation in mice. *Transplantation* 1994; 58:1.

30. Demetris AJ, Qian S, Sun H et al. Liver allograft rejection. An overview of morphologic findings. *Am J Surg Pathol* 1990;14 (suppl 1):49.

31. O'Connell PJ, Pacheco-Silva A, Nickerson PW. Unmodified pancreatic islet allograft rejection results in the preferential expression of certain T cell activation transcripts. *J Immunol* 1993;150:1093.

32. Takeuchi T, Lowry RP, Konieczny B. Heart allografts in murine systems. *Transplantation* 1992;53:1281.

33. Dahmen U, Bergese SD, Qian S, et al. Patterns of inflammatory vascular endothelial changes in murine liver grafts. *Transplantation* 1995;60:577.

34. Murase N, Starzl TE, Tanabe M, et al. Variable chimerism, graft-versus-host disease, and tolerance after different kinds of cell and whole organ transplantation from Lewis to brown Norway rats. *Transplantation* 1995;60:158.

35. Sprent J, von Boehmer H, Nabholz M. Association of immunity and tolerance to host H-2 determinants in irradiated F_1 hybrid mice reconstituted with bone marrow cells from one parental strain. *J Exp Med* 1975;142:321.

36. Wieties K, Hammer RE, Jones-Youngblood H, et al. Peripheral tolerance in mice expressing a liver-specific class I molecule: inactivation/deletion of a T cell subpopulation. *Proc Natl Acad Sci USA* 1990;87:6604.

37. Sprent J, Hurd M, Schaefer M, et al. Split tolerance in spleen chimeras. *J Immunol* 1995;154:1198.

38. Daar AS, Fuggle SV, Fabre JW, et al. The detailed distribution of HLA-A, B, C antigens in normal human organs. *Transplantation* 1984;38:287.

39. Davies HFFS, Pollard SG, Calne RY. Soluble HLA antigens in the circulation of liver graft recipients. *Transplantation* 1989;47: 524.

40. Qian S, Fu F, Li Y, et al. Presensitization by skin grafting from MHC class I or MHC class II deficient mice identifies class I antigens as inducers of allosensitization. *Immunology* 1995;85: 82.

41. Sumimoto R, Kamada N. Specific suppression of allograft rejection by soluble class I antigen and complexes with monoclonal antibody. *Transplantation* 1990;50:678.

42. Kamada N, Shinomiya T, Takima T et al. Immunosuppressive activity of serum from liver grafted rats. Passive enhancement of fully allogeneic heart grafts and induction of systemic tolerance. *Transplantation* 1986;42:581.

43. Houssin D, Charpentier B, Gugenheim J. Spontaneous long-term acceptance of RT-1-incompatible liver allografts in inbred rats. Analysis of the immune status. *Transplantation* 1983;36: 615.

44. Dahmen U, Sun H, Li Y, et al. The role of antibody in liver allograft induced tolerance in mice: passive transfer of serum and effect of recipient B-cell depletion. *Transplant Proc* 1995;27: 511.

45. Rosenberg AS, Singer A. Evidence that the effector mechanism of skin allograft rejection is antigen-specific. *J Immunol* 1988;85: 7739.

46. Russell JH, White CL, Loh DY, et al. Receptor-stimulated death pathway is opened by antigen in mature T cells. *Proc Natl Acad Sci USA* 1991;88:2151.

47. Radvanyi LG, Mills GB, Miller RG. Relegation of the T cell receptor after primary activation of mature T cells inhibits proliferation and induces apoptotic cell death. *J Immunol* 1993;150: 5704.

48. Munn DH, Pressey J, Beall AC, et al. Selective activation-induced apoptosis of peripheral T cells imposed by macrophages: a potential mechanism of antigen-specific peripheral lymphocyte deletion. *J Immunol* 1996;156:523.

49. Ehl S, Hoffmann-Rohrer U, Nagata S, et al. Different susceptibility of cytotoxic T cells to CD95 (Fas/Apo-1) ligand-mediated cell death after activation in vitro versus in vivo. *J Immunol* 1996; 156:2357.

50. Qian S, Lu L, Fu F, et al. Donor pretreatment with Flt-3 ligand augments anti-donor CTL, NK and LAK cell activities within liver allografts and alters the pattern of intragraft apoptotic activity. *Transplantation* 1998;65:1590.

51. Lynch DH, Ramsdell F, Alderson MR. Fas and FasL in the homeostatic regulation of immune responses. *Immunol Today* 1995;16: 569.

52. Nagata S, Golstein P. The Fas death factor. *Science* 1995;267: 1449.

53. Deng G, Podack ER. Suppression of apoptosis in a cytotoxic T-cell line by interleukin 2-mediated gene transcription and deregulated expression of the protooncogene bcl-2. *Proc Natl Acad Sci USA* 1993;90:2189.

54. French LE, Hahne M, Viard I, et al. Fas and Fas ligand in embryos and adult mice: ligand expression in several immune-privileged tissues and coexpression in adult tissues characterized by apoptotic cell turnover. *J Cell Biol* 1996;133:335.

55. Bellgrau D, Gold D, Selawry H, et al. A role for CD95 ligand in preventing graft rejection. *Nature* 1995;377:630.

56. Griffith TS, Brunner T, Fletcher SM, et al. Fas ligand-induced apoptosis as a mechanism of immune privilege. *Science* 1995;270: 1189.

57. Galle PR, Hofmann WJ, Walczak H, et al. Involvement of the CD95 (APO-1/Fas) receptor and ligand in liver damage. *J Exp Med* 1995;182:1223.

58. Lu L, Qian S, Hershberger P, et al. Fas ligand (CD95L) and B7 expression on dendritic cells provide counter-regulatory signals for T cell survival and proliferation. *J Immunol* 1997;158:5676.

59. Lu L, Bonham CA, Chambers FG, et al. Induction of nitric oxide synthase in mouse dendritic cells by interferon ?, endotoxin and interaction with allogeneic T cells: nitric oxide production is associated with dendritic cell apoptosis. *J Immunol* 1996;157:3577.

60. Alderson MR, Smith CA, Tough TW, et al. Molecular and biological characterization of human 4-1BB and its ligand. *Eur J Immunol* 1994;24:2219.

61. Bissell DM, Wang S-S, Jarnagin WR, et al. Cell-specific expression of transforming growth factor-β in rat liver. Evidence for

autocrine regulation of hepatocyte proliferation. *J Clin Invest* 1995;96:447.

62. Weller M, Constam DB, Malipiero U, et al. Transforming growth factor-beta 2 induces apoptosis of murine T cell clones without down-regulating bcl-2 mRNA expression. *Eur J Immunol* 1994;24:1293.

63. Bertolino P, Heath WR, Hardy CL, et al. Peripheral deletion of autoreactive CD8+ T cells in transgenic mice expressing H-2K^b in the liver. *Eur J Immunol* 1995;25:1932.

64. Rocha B, von Boehmer H. Peripheral deletion of the T cell repertoire. *Science* 1991;251:1225.

65. Suzuki G, Kawase Y, Koyasu S, et al. Antigen-induced suppression of the proliferative response of T cell clones. *J Immunol* 1988;140:1359.

66. Moskophidis D, Lechner F, Pircher H, et al. Virus persistence in acutely infected immunocompetent mice by exhaustion of antiviral cytotoxic effector T cells. *Nature* 1993;362:758.

67. Bishop GA, Sun J, DeCruz DJ, et al. Tolerance to rat liver allografts. III. Donor cell migration and tolerance-associated cytokine production in peripheral lymphoid tissues. *J Immunol* 1996;156:4925.

68. Demetris AJ, Murase N, Fujisaki S, et al. Hematolymphoid cell trafficking, microchimerism, and GVHD reactions after liver, bone marrow, and heart transplantation. *Transplant Proc* 1993; 25:3337.

69. Taniguchi H, Toyoshima T, Fukao K, et al. Presence of hematopoietic stem cells in the adult liver. *Nat Med* 1996;2: 198.

70. Murase N, Starzl TE, Ye Q, et al. Multilineage hematopoietic reconstitution of supralethally irradiated rats by syngeneic whole organ transplantation: with particular reference to the liver. *Transplantation* 1996;61:1.

71. Starzl TE, Demetris AJ, Trucco M, et al. Cell migration and chimerism after whole organ transplantation: the basis of graft acceptance. *Hepatology* 1993;17:1127.

72. Starzl TE, Thomson AW, Murase N, et al. Liver transplants contribute to their own success. *Nat Med* 1996;2:163.

73. Thomson AW, Lu L, Murase N, et al. Microchimerism, dendritic cell progenitors and transplantation tolerance. *Stem Cells* 1995;13:622.

74. Starzl TE, Demetris AJ, Murase N et al. Cell migration, chimerism, and graft acceptance. *Lancet* 1992;339:1579.

75. Sriwatanawongsa V, Davies H, Calne RY. The essential roles of parenchymal tissues and passenger leukocytes in the tolerance induced by liver grafting in rats. *Nat Med* 1995;1:428.

76. Sun J, McCaughan GW, Gallagher ND, et al. Deletion of spontaneous rat liver allograft acceptance by donor irradiation. *Transplantation* 1995;60:233.

77. Kobayashi E, Kamada N, Delriviere L, et al. Migration of door cells into the thymus is not essential for induction and maintenance of systemic tolerance after liver transplantation in the rat. *Immunology* 1995;84:333.

78. Lechler RI, Batchelor JR. Restoration of immunogenicity to passenger cell-depleted kidney allografts by the addition of donor strain dendritic cells. *J Exp Med* 1982;155:31.

79. Larsen CP, Morris PJ, Austyn JM. Migration of dendritic leukocytes from cardiac allografts into host spleens. A novel pathway for initiation of rejection. *J Exp Med* 1990;171:307.

80. Thomson AW, Lu L, Subbotin VM, et al. In vitro propagation and homing of liver-derived dendritic cell progenitors to lymphoid tissues of allogeneic recipients. *Transplantation* 1995;59: 544.

81. Rugeles MT, Aitouche A, Zeevi A, et al. Evidence for the presence of multilineage chimerism and progenitors of donor dendritic cells in the peripheral blood of bone marrow-augmented organ transplant recipients. *Transplantation* 1997;64:735.

82. Thomson AW, Lu L, Steptoe RJ, et al. Dendritic cells and the balance between transplant tolerance and immunity. In: Schwartz R, Banchereau J, eds. *Immune tolerance.* Paris: Elsevier, 1996:173–185.

83. Lu L, Woo J, Rao AS, et al. Propagation of dendritic cell progenitors from normal mouse liver using GM-CSF and their maturational development in the presence of type-1 collagen. *J Exp Med* 1994;179:1823.

84. Lu L, Rudert WA, Qian S, et al. Growth of donor-derived dendritic cells from the bone marrow of liver allograft recipients in response to granulocyte/macrophage colony-stimulating factor. *J Exp Med* 1995;182:379.

85. Lu L, McCaslin D, Starzl TE, et al. Bone marrow-derived dendritic cell progenitors (NLDC 145+, MHC class II+, B7-1^dim, B7-2−) induce alloantigen-specific hyporesponsiveness in murine T lymphocytes. *Transplantation* 1995;60:1539.

86. Rastellini C, Lu L, Ricordi C, et al. GM-CSF stimulated hepatic dendritic cell progenitors prolong pancreatic islet allograft survival. *Transplantation* 1995;60:1366.

87. Fu F, Li Y, Qian S, et al. Costimulatory molecule-deficient dendritic cell progenitors (MHC class II+, CD80^dim, CD86−) prolong cardiac allograft survival in non-immunosuppressed recipients. *Transplantation* 1996;62:659.

88. Demetris AJ, Murase N, Rao AS, et al. The role of passenger leukocytes in rejection and "tolerance" after solid organ transplantation: a potential explanation of a paradox. In: Touraine J, Traeger J, Betuel H, et al., eds. *Rejection and tolerance.* Netherlands: Kluwer Academic, 1994:325–392.

89. Sakamoto T, Saizawa T, Mabuchi A, et al. The liver as a potential hematolymphoid organ examined from modifications occurring in the systemic and intrahepatic hematolymphoid system during liver regeneration after partial hepatectomy. *Regional Immunol* 1992;4:1.

90. Wilbanks GA, Streilein JW. Fluids from immune privileged sites endow macrophages with the capacity to induce antigen-specific immune deviation via a mechanism involving transforming growth factor-beta. *Eur J Immunol* 1992;22:1031.

91. Yamaguchi Y, Tsumura H, Miwa M, et al. Contrasting effects of TGF-beta 1 and TNF-alpha on the development of dendritic cells from progenitors in mouse bone marrow. *Stem Cells* 1997; 15:144.

92. Lu L, Li W, Fu F, et al. Blockade of the CD40-CD40 ligand pathway potentiates the capacity of donor-derived dendritic cell progenitors to induce long-term cardiac allograft survival. *Transplantation* 1997;64:1808.

93. Shin GT, Khanna A, Ding R, et al. In vivo expression of transforming growth factor-beta 1 in humans: stimulation by cyclosporine. *Transplantation* 1998;65:313.

94. Khoury SJ, Gallon L, Verburg RR, et al. Ex vivo treatment of antigen-presenting cells with CTLA4Ig and encephalitogenic peptide prevents experimental autoimmune encephalomyelitis in the Lewis rat. *J Immunol* 1996;157:3700.

95. Buelens C, Verhasselt V, De Groote D, et al. Human dendritic cell responses to lipopolysaccharide and CD40 ligation are differentially regulated by interleukin-10. *Eur J Immunol* 1997;27: 1848.

96. De Smedt T, Van Mechelen M, De Becker G, et al. Effect of interleukin-10 on dendritic cell maturation and function. *Eur J Immunol* 1997;27:1229.

97. Khanna A, Morelli AE, Zhong C, et al. Effects of liver-derived dendritic cell progenitors on Th1- and Th2-like cytokine responses in vitro and in vivo. *J Immunol* 2000;164:1346.

98. Ishizaka S, Saito S, Yoshikawa M, et al. IL-10 production in mouse hepatocytes augmented by TGF-beta. *Cytokine* 1996;8: 837.

99. Roland CR, Walp L, Stack RM, et al. Outcome of Kupffer cell

antigen presentation to a cloned murine Th1 lymphocyte depends on the inducibility of nitric oxide synthase by IFN-gamma. *J Immunol* 1994;153:5453.

100. Bonham CA, Lu L, Li Y. Nitric oxide production by mouse bone marrow-derived dendritic cells: implications for the regulation of allogeneic T cell responses. *Transplantation* 1996;62:1871.

101. Süss G, Shortman K. A subclass of dendritic cells kills CD4 T cells via Fas/Fas-ligand-induced apoptosis. *J Exp Med* 1996;183: 1789.

102. Kronin V, Winkel K, Süss G, et al. A subclass of dendritic cells regulates the response of naive CD8 T cells by limiting their IL-2 production. *J Immunol* 1996;157:3819.

103. Larsen CP, Elwood ET, Alexander DZ, et al. Long-term acceptance of skin and cardiac allografts after blocking CD40 and CD28 pathways. *Nature* 1996;381:434.

104. Drakes ML, Lu L, Subbotin VM, et al. In vivo administration of flt3 ligand markedly stimulates generation of dendritic cell progenitors from mouse liver. *J Immunol* 1997;159:4268.

The Liver: Biology and Pathobiology, Fourth Edition, edited by I. M. Arias, J. L. Boyer, F. V. Chisari, N. Fausto, D. Schachter, and D. A. Shafritz.
Lippincott Williams & Wilkins, Philadelphia © 2001.

VIRAL HEPATITIS: ANTIVIRAL THERAPY

JOSEPH TORRESI
STEPHEN LOCARNINI

Chronic viral hepatitis is a common infection, and knowledge of its etiology is important in managing and controlling its spread. The three major causes of chronic viral hepatitis include the hepatitis B virus (HBV), hepatitis C virus (HCV), and hepatitis D virus (HDV). Most infections with these viruses are acquired either parenterally or perinatally. Persistent infection can result in long-term complications including cirrhosis and hepatocellular carcinoma. HBV and HDV may produce acute and fulminant hepatitis, although HDV only produces infection in the presence of HBV infection. HCV is now the most frequent cause of parenterally acquired hepatitis in developed countries and is prevalent among injecting drug users (IDUs). In contrast to HBV and HDV, HCV is unlikely to cause severe acute hepatitis but typically results in a high rate of chronic infection. Acute hepatitis C infection is usually a mild anicteric illness that often passes unnoticed, but occasionally jaundice is a presenting feature. Under these circumstances, HCV infection is often cleared, highlighting the important role of the immune response in liver damage and viral persistence.

This chapter discusses the therapeutic approaches for managing patients with chronic viral hepatitis. Furthermore, many patients are presenting to the clinic and are multiply infected with other hepatotropic viruses and/or the human immunodeficiency virus (HIV), compounding standard therapeutic approaches.

HEPATITIS B

It is currently estimated that there are over 300 million carriers of HBV worldwide (1). Of these, 50% to 75% (150 to 225 million individuals) have active viral replication and chronic hepatitis. Cirrhosis will develop in 30% (50 to 75 million individuals) of this group and 5% to 10% (15 to 30 million) will develop hepatocellular carcinoma (HCC) (1,2). Chronic hepatitis B infection now accounts for 80% of all HCC globally. Serologic evidence of HBV can be found in 80% to 90% of cases of HCC in China and 70% of cases in Africa (1), making HBV the most frequent cause of HCC in these countries. The development of an effective vaccine has helped to control the spread of hepatitis B infection and has resulted in a reduction in the incidence of HCC (3). However, the vaccine is of no benefit to the large numbers of individuals already chronically infected with HBV. In addition, the emergence and proliferation of vaccine escape variants of HBV that fail to be neutralized by anti-HBs antibody elicited by vaccination (4) may reduce the overall efficacy of the vaccine in the long term.

J. Torresi: Department of Medicine, University of Melbourne; and Victorian Infectious Diseases Service, Royal Melbourne Hospital, Parkville, Victoria, 3050, Australia.

S. Locarnini: Department of Research and Molecular Development, Victorian Infectious Diseases Reference Laboratory, North Melbourne, Victoria, 3051, Australia.

Life Cycle

HBV is a member of the family Hepadnaviridae. It is an enveloped, partly double-stranded DNA virus containing a genome of approximately 3,200 base pairs. Virions are 42 nm in diameter, and a characteristic feature of infection is the production of a vast excess of hepatitis B surface antigen (HBsAg) envelope material in the form of 22 nm subviral particles.

The inability to grow HBV in culture has limited our understanding of the life cycle of HBV. However, the replication pathways of the animal hepadnaviruses are similar to HBV, and consequently these viruses have contributed a useful means of studying the viral life cycle. In addition, the animal viruses have provided *in vivo* models for the study of the pathogenesis of HBV and HCC (5) and for the investigation of antiviral effects of antiviral agents such as the nucleoside analogues. To understand how different therapeutic strategies aim to control chronic hepatitis B infection, it is helpful to have functional knowledge of the replicative cycle of the virus (Fig. 57.1). In the HBV replicative strategy, genomic DNA is synthesized from a pregenomic RNA template by reverse transcription (6). Another key feature in the replication cycle of HBV is the formation of a pool of covalently closed circular (CCC) or supercoiled DNA molecules (7), which exist as a viral minichromosome (8) and act as the major transcriptional template. The CCC DNA is a stable intermediate that is not affected by antiviral nucleoside analogues and accounts for the failure to eradicate infection with these agents (1).

Treatment

Under normal circumstances of infection, the HBV is not cytopathic and in both acute and chronic infections most of the liver damage seen with HBV is essentially immune-mediated. The level of inflammation varies from patient to patient and over time in individual patients. The three key components in the consideration of the outcome of the host–parasite relationship are the virus, the hepatocyte, and the host's immune response. Until recently, therapeutic management of hepatitis B has tended to focus on immune manipulation with the use of the interferons, but more recently the demonstration that nucleoside analogues could selectively inhibit viral replication and result in significant clinical benefit has heralded a renewed interest in treating chronically infected individuals.

Immune Modulating Agents

The major immune modulating agents are the interferons, thymosin-α_1, and therapeutic vaccines. Interferon-α (IFN-α) is registered for the treatment of chronic hepatitis B in most countries, while thymosin-α_1 and therapeutic vaccination with various formulations of antigen and adjuvant are still undergoing clinical trial evaluation.

Interferon-α

Biologic Properties. Interferon-α (IFN-α) has both antiviral (Fig. 57.1) and immune modulating effects and was the first agent to be licensed for the treatment of chronic hepatitis B. The administration of IFN-α leads to an induction of a cascade of intracellular host enzyme systems that inhibit viral protein synthesis (9). In addition, IFN-α enhances the human leukocyte antigen (HLA) class I display on the hepatocyte, resulting in improved host immune recognition of infected hepatocytes and their clearance (9). Natural killer T-cell function is also enhanced.

Clinical Studies. *Acute Hepatitis B.* IFN-α has been used to treat patients with acute hepatitis B, but it has not been adequately evaluated in this situation (10). Tassopoulos and colleagues (11) enrolled 100 patients with uncomplicated acute hepatitis B in a randomized controlled trial of either placebo or 3 or 10 million units (mu) of IFN-α (alfa-2b: intron A) for 6 weeks. There were no major differences in outcome between the three groups in regard to viral clearance, serum alanine aminotransferase (ALT) levels, bilirubin, or albumin. Patients in the 3-mu dose cohort reported resolution of symptoms more rapidly than those in the other cohorts, but all patients recovered within weeks and no patient developed chronic hepatitis.

There have been anecdotal reports and small case series on the use of IFN-α in severe and fulminant cases of hepatitis B, largely without evidence of benefit (10). Thus, there is little evidence to recommend the use of IFN-α in either uncomplicated or severe acute hepatitis B. Perhaps of greater promise are the second-generation nucleoside analogues such as lamivudine and adefovir dipivoxil, which have potent activity against HBV and can be taken orally and have few serious adverse side effects. The efficacy of these agents in acute hepatitis B has not been reported, but warrants careful assessment, particularly in patients with severe disease.

Chronic Hepatitis B. IFN-α therapy typically leads to a rapid decrease in serum HBV DNA levels, hepatitis B early antigen (HBeAg) seroconversion, normalization of serum ALT, and a lasting remission of disease in a proportion of patients. A large number of multiple randomized, controlled trials have shown that a 4- to 6-month course of IFN-α results in loss of serum HBeAg and viral DNA as well as long-term disease remission in 25% to 40% of treated patients (12). The response rate in children, who tolerate the drug much better than adults, is similar (13). In a meta-analysis of 15 controlled trials Wong and colleagues (14) found the overall response rate (loss of HBeAg) was 33% in treated compared to 12% in control patients, with 10% of treated and less than 2% of untreated patients becoming HBsAg negative within a year of therapy.

These studies laid the foundation for understanding the mechanism of action of IFN-α in chronic hepatitis B and defined three major types of responses to treatment:

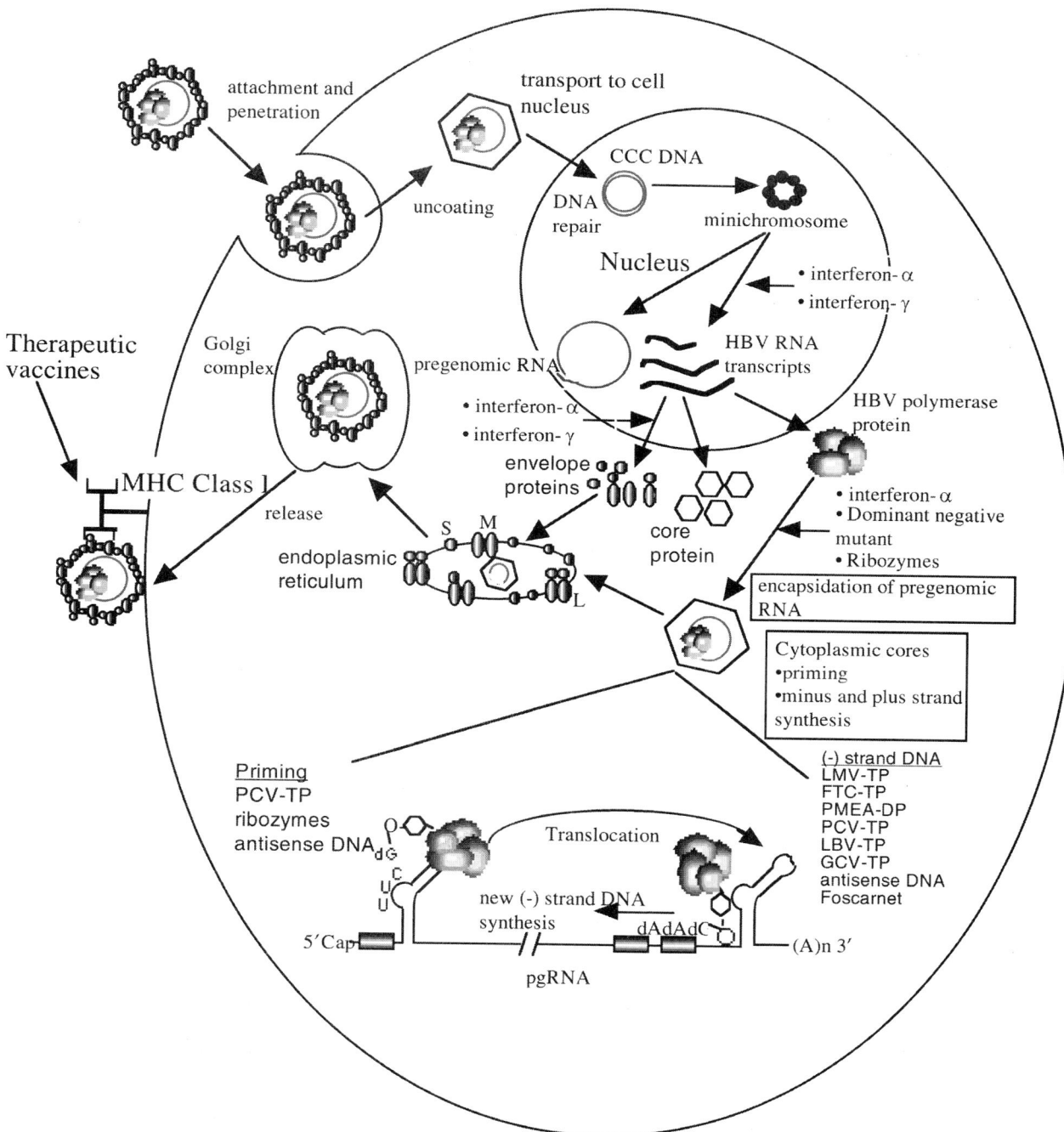

FIGURE 57.1. The life cycle of hepatitis B virus (*HBV*). Following viral attachment, penetration and uncoating the viral DNA is repaired and forms covalently closed circular (*CCC*) DNA in the cell nucleus. HBV RNA is transcribed by the host cellular RNA polymerase II and translation of viral proteins follows. Encapsidation of HBV pregenomic (*pg*) RNA occurs together with HBV polymerase and cellular proteins, including heat shock protein-90 (Hsp90). Viral assembly takes place within the endoplasmic reticulum prior to release from infected cells. The HBV genome is replicated from pgRNA within the HBV core particles by a process of reverse transcription. The initial priming step involves the synthesis of a short oligonucleotide, which is essential for translocation of the HBV polymerase-DNA complex followed by first-strand synthesis. The priming step is inhibited by penciclovir-triphosphate (*PCV-TP*), while first-strand HBV DNA synthesis can be blocked by several nucleoside triphosphates, including lamivudine-triphosphate (*LMV-TP*), fluorocytidine-triphosphate (*FTC-TP*), adefovir-diphosphate (*PMEA-DP*), lobucavir-triphosphate (*LBV-TP*), and ganciclovir-triphosphate (*GCV-TP*). The interferons generally work at the posttranscriptional level including pgRNA-core interactions and viral translation. *MHC*, major histocompatibility complex. *S*, small; *M*, middle; and *L*, large HBV envelope proteins.

1. A *transient response*, where a lowering of HBV markers (serum HBV DNA and DNA polymerase) is not sustained once therapy is stopped (Fig. 57.2). During therapy a transient decrease in serum viral DNA levels is observed, but there is no accompanying improvement in liver disease or long-term remission of hepatitis. The antiviral response is not maintained, and no HBeAg-seroconversion occurs.

2. A *partial response*, defined by the disappearance of serum HBV DNA and clearance of HBeAg, which is also associated with an improvement in the accompanying liver disease. These patients can have an exacerbation of their hepatitis (a hepatic flare) 8 to 12 weeks after commencement of therapy, coincident with the loss of HBeAg and clearance of HBV DNA from serum. Unlike the transient response group, the accompanying liver disease improves, despite serum HBsAg persistence. The patient's symptoms generally resolve, the remission in disease activity is usually sustained, and the patient has completed the transition from chronic active hepatitis B replicative phase to nonreplicative phase (15). Serum HBV DNA and liver hepatitis B core antigen (HBcAg) are no longer present and all the intrahepatic replicative intermediates of HBV DNA can no longer be found (16). Presumably, the continued HBsAg-antigenemia is derived from integrated molecules of HBV DNA (16).

3. A *complete response* to IFN therapy is heralded by a loss of HBV DNA, HBeAg, and HBsAg from serum (Fig. 57.3). As with the partial response patient, loss of markers of active hepatitis B replication coincides with the "seroconversion illness" 8 to 12 weeks after therapy has started. The loss of HBsAg and HBeAg is followed by reversal of the liver disease and a normalization of the serum aminotransferases. A substantial number of complete responders develop anti-HBs. These patients have no HBcAg or HBV DNA replicative intermediates in their follow-up liver biopsies (17).

A good response rate to IFN-α is achieved in HBeAg-positive patients with an initial high serum ALT and low HBV DNA (14,18). In these patients 6-month treatment course with IFN-α produces a 30% to 40% virologic response that is characterized by a substantial reduction of serum HBV DNA and loss of HBeAg. Seroconversion from HBeAg to anti-HBe positivity occurs in at least 20% of patients (14,18).

Relapse following completion of treatment occurs infrequently (18,19). Longer-term follow-up of patients treated with IFN-α has demonstrated that 80% of patients who lose HBeAg during therapy lose HBsAg during the decade following therapy (19), and that over 50% of patients who do not develop HBeAg seroconversion following initial treatment develop a delayed HBeAg seroconversion months to years after completion of treatment (19). Also, the cumulative incidence of the development of cirrhosis of the liver and hepatocellular carcinoma appears to be reduced in patients treated with IFN-α compared to placebo (19,20). The current treatment regi-

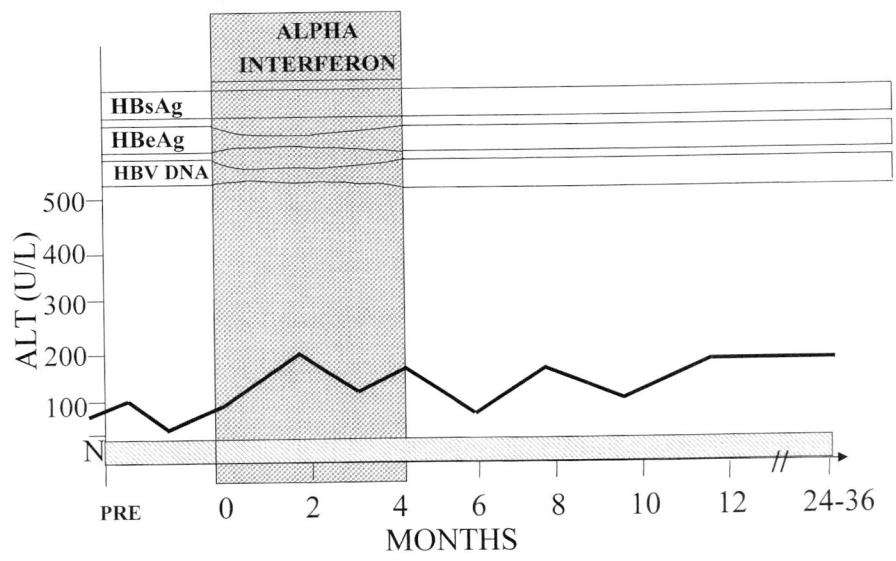

FIGURE 57.2. The serum biochemical, serologic, and virologic course of a typical patient with hepatitis B (*HBV*) early antigen (*HBeAg*)–positive chronic hepatitis B who had only a transient response to therapy with interferon-α. During treatment, a slight decrease in serum viral DNA and HBeAg levels can be observed, but hepatitis B surface antigen (*HBsAg*) persists with no change in the serum alanine aminotransferase (*ALT*) pattern. *PRE*, pretreatment virological and biochemical markers; *N*, normal range for serum ALT. (Modified from Locarnini SA, Cunningham AL. Clinical treatment of viral hepatitis. In: Jefferies DJ, DeClercq E, eds. *Antiviral chemotherapy.* New York: Wiley, 1995:441–530.)

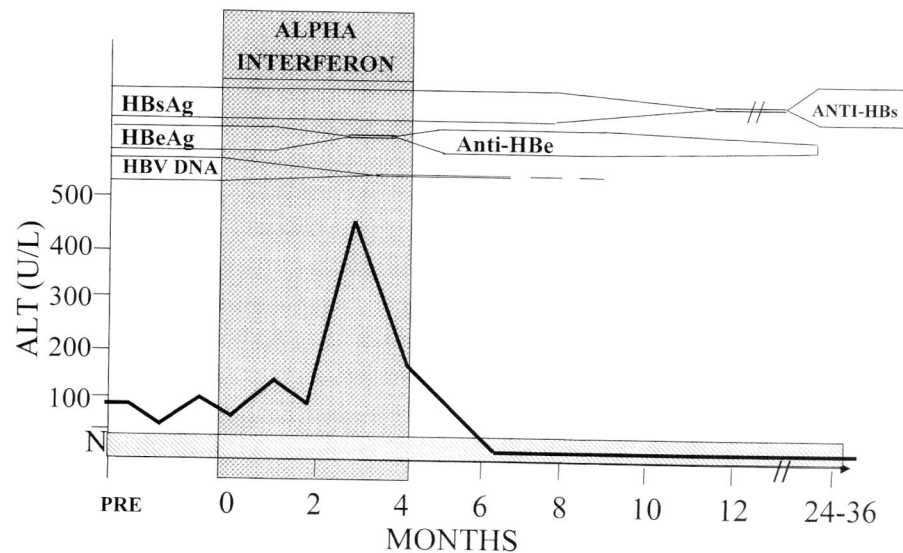

FIGURE 57.3. The serum biochemical, serologic, and virologic responses of a typical patient with hepatitis B early antigen (*HBeAg*)–positive chronic hepatitis B who had a complete response to therapy with interferon-α. During treatment, serum hepatitis B virus DNA (*HBV DNA*) and HBeAg fall steadily as in a partial response, and there is also seroconversion to anti-HBe during therapy. Following the development of anti-HBe, the titers of serum hepatitis B surface antigen (*HBsAg*) begin to fall and eventually become negative, and in some patients anti-HBs is produced. Serum HBV DNA becomes negative by polymerase chain reaction as anti-HBs develops. *ALT*, alanine aminotransferase. (Modified from Locarnini SA, Cunningham AL. Clinical treatment of viral hepatitis. In: Jefferies DJ, DeClercq E, eds. *Antiviral chemotherapy*. New York: Wiley, 1995:441–530.)

men is still individualized to the patient but typically consists of 6 months of therapy and a daily dose of 5 mu or a thrice-weekly dosage of 9 to 10 mu (14).

In patients carrying a high proportion of precore mutants of HBV, clinical relapse following IFN-α therapy is common (21) (Fig. 57.4). These patients have HBeAg-negative chronic hepatitis B, and the natural history of this disease is quite different from HBeAg-positive chronic hepatitis B. These patients often experience more severe disease with episodic exacerbations (22). Precore

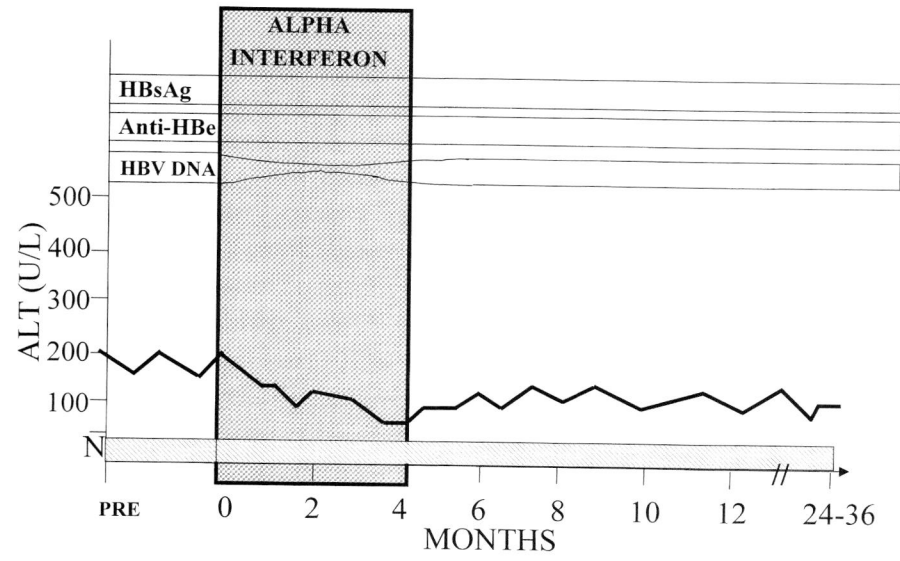

FIGURE 57.4. The serum biochemical, serologic, and virologic course of a patient with hepatitis B early antigen (HBeAg)–negative chronic hepatitis B who had a typical response to therapy with interferon-α. During treatment, a decrease in serum viral DNA and alanine aminotransferase (*ALT*) levels can be observed, but hepatitis B surface antigen (*HBsAg*) persists. However, on cessation of therapy, a relapse in viremia and disease activity are observed.

mutant HBV infection is very common in Mediterranean countries and in Asia, but rare in North America. Overall, patients with HBeAg-negative chronic hepatitis B respond less frequently to IFN-α (22). Most studies have indicated that longer courses of treatment are required with these patients, and in many cases long-term remissions in disease can be achieved. However, without HBeAg as an end point to successful therapy and with the uncertainty of what serum HBV DNA negativity by hybridization versus polymerase chain reaction (PCR) actually means clinically, the therapy of patients with HBeAg-negative chronic hepatitis B is problematic.

Thus the overall response rate to IFN-α in chronic hepatitis B is less than 50%, and retreatment of nonresponders is rarely successful. Prednisone priming before interferon therapy provides marginal if any improvement in overall response rate (23). Patients with advanced disease (24), immunodeficiencies, solid organ transplant, or other major medical problems do not generally qualify for interferon therapy.

Side effects are common with IFN-α (14). These include flu-like symptoms, granulocytopenia, alopecia,

TABLE 57.1. THE COMMON AND UNCOMMON SIDE EFFECTS EXPERIENCED BY PATIENTS TREATED WITH INTERFERON-α

Common	
Systemic	Fatigue, malaise, fever, chills, headache, backache, myalgia, arthralgia, anorexia, weight loss, vomiting, diarrhea, hair loss
Neuropsychological	Anxiety, depression, mood swings, irritability, insomnia, forgetfulness, difficulty concentrating, paresthesias, apathy, decreased libido
Hematologic	Thrombocytopenia, leukopenia, neutropenia
Autoimmune	Hyperthyroidism, hypothyroidism, psoriasis
Uncommon	
Neuropsychological	Paranoid and suicidal ideation, major depression, psychosis
Autoimmune	Hemolytic anemia, autoimmune thrombocytopenia, erythema multiforme, lupus-like syndrome, diabetes mellitus, autoimmune hepatitis
Other	Proteinuria, hypertriglyceridemia, interstitial nephritis, nephrotic syndrome, cardiac failure, cardiac arrhythmias, pneumonitis, renal and liver graft rejection in transplant recipients

Systemic side effects are especially common in the first 2 to 4 weeks of treatment, and although they are generally tolerable by patients, they are not an infrequent reason for the cessation of therapy. Severe psychiatric problems may also occur during treatment, necessitating close monitoring of patients.

weight loss, common but mild exacerbations of hepatitis, rare precipitation of liver failure especially in marginally compensated cirrhosis, acute psychiatric dysfunction, and thyroid dysfunction (Table 57.1).

Thymosin-α₁

Biologic Properties. Thymosin-α₁ (Tα₁) is a peptide that has been evaluated for its immunomodulatory activities and therapeutic potential in chronic hepatitis B, chronic hepatitis C, acquired immune deficiency syndrome (AIDS), primary immunodeficiency diseases, and cancer. Tα₁ was originally isolated from the thymus gland and is an amino-terminal acylated peptide of 28 amino acids. The basis for its mode of action is thought to be through modulation of immunologic responsiveness, as Tα₁ has effects on other immune modulators (such as IFN-α) and can increase T-cell differentiation and maturation (25).

Clinical Studies. Thymosin-α₁ has been evaluated as an adjunctive immunotherapy for chronic hepatitis B (26). The clinical responses to Tα₁ are variable, ranging from marginal benefit (27) to a complete biochemical and virologic response (26). Several randomized controlled studies have investigated the safety and efficacy of Tα₁ monotherapy for chronic hepatitis B (26,27), and a meta-analysis has been done (28). These studies have shown that Tα₁ promotes disease remission in 25% to 75% of patients treated; the results in the meta-analysis were statistically significant and showed that 6 months' treatment (1.6 mg twice weekly) almost doubled the sustained response rate (36%) compared to controls (19%). Further studies with this compound are in progress in combination with IFN-α plus the nucleoside analogues.

Therapeutic Vaccines

Vaccination of chronic HBeAg positive carriers with the prophylactic HBV vaccine containing recombinant HBsAg results in clearance of infection in up to one-fourth of patients (29). Clearance of infection may be the consequence of the stimulation of peripheral B lymphocytes with increased production of neutralizing anti-HBs antibody and/or the development of a strong cytotoxic T-cell specific response to the viral envelope protein (29).

A therapeutic vaccine for hepatitis B containing both S and pre-S2 antigens (Genhevac-B) is currently under evaluation in chronic hepatitis B and has resulted in HBeAg seroconversion (30).

Stimulation of cytotoxic T lymphocyte (CTL) responses to HBV may provide an alternative approach to clearance of chronic viral infection. A lipopeptide-based vaccine has been developed that consists of a lipidated T-helper peptide epitope covalently linked to an immunostimulant CTL epitope (tetanus toxoid), which induced HBc antigen specific major histocompatibility complex (MHC) class I memory CTL responses with the resultant clearance of HBV (29).

Such approaches have been taken into the clinic, where 90 patients with chronic hepatitis B received a therapeutic vaccine known as CY-1899 (Cytel), which comprises a CTL epitope from HBcAg (18- to 27-amino-acid residue) plus a T-helper (T_H) cell epitope and two palmitic acid residues (31). Administration of the vaccine caused no serious adverse events and initiated CTL activity, but was not associated with viral clearance.

DNA vaccination has also been explored as a potential therapeutic strategy. This method has been shown to induce neutralizing antibody responses as well as cytotoxic and helper T-cell responses against HBV. The co-delivery of cytokine genes, such as interleukin-2 (IL-2), IL-12, IFN-α, and granulocyte-macrophage colony-stimulating factor (GM-CSF) may enhance the response induced by HBV DNA vaccination (32).

Nucleoside Analogues

The nucleoside analogues, which specifically block HBV DNA replication (33), are making a significant impact on the management of HBV infections, especially in those clinical situations where the benefit of IFN-α therapy was marginal or contraindicated. Lamivudine is now registered in many countries, and phase III registration trials are under way for adefovir dipivoxil and entecavir. There are several new nucleoside analogues in phase I/II development and many undergoing preclinical evaluation.

Lamivudine

Biologic Properties. Lamivudine (LMV), the β-L-enantiomer of 2′,3′-dideoxy-3′-thiacytidine [(−) 3TC], has recently been licensed for the treatment of chronic hepatitis B. It is a potent inhibitor of HBV replication in vitro (34–36) and blocks viral DNA synthesis in HBV transfected hepatoma cell lines but has no effect on viral RNA synthesis (34,36).

The effective concentration of LMV that inhibits HBV replication by 50% (EC_{50}) in HBV-transformed HepG2 2.2.15 cells is 0.01 μM (35). The corresponding cytotoxic parameter (CC_{50}) is 50 μM (35). The initial phosphorylation of LMV to the 5′-monophosphate form is carried out by cellular deoxycytidine kinase (CdRK) (35). The subsequent conversion to the triphosphate species (LMV-TP) is by nucleoside mono- and diphosphate kinases (37).

LMV-TP inhibits HBV DNA replication by acting as a chain terminator of elongating viral DNA molecules (as it looks for 3′-OH on the ribose sugar) and competitive inhibitor of the viral polymerase (34). In the HBV-HepG2 2.2.15 cells and in hepatoma cells transiently transfected with infectious constructs of HBV, LMV has been shown to inhibit the synthesis of the first strand of HBV DNA (34). In addition, using a novel recombinant HBV baculovirus-HepG2 system, LMV has been shown to decrease intracellular levels of hepadnaviral CCC DNA, but not RNA (36).

The β-D-enantiomer of 3TC has been associated with significant cellular toxicity, while LMV (the β-L-enantiomer) lacks mitochondrial toxicity (34,35).

Clinical Studies. Clinical trials have demonstrated that LMV reduces the level of serum HBV DNA in chronic HBeAg-positive chronic carriers (38–40). Treatment of patients with chronic hepatitis B with doses of 100 to 300 mg daily for 12 to 52 weeks reduces the serum HBV DNA to undetectable levels by hybridization assays. These patients remain serum HBV DNA positive by PCR assays. Also, the relapse rate is high when therapy is stopped (38–40). A sustained loss of HBV DNA occurs in 5% to 12% of patients treated for less than 6 months; seroconversion from HBeAg to anti-HBe positivity develops in approximately 16% of patients treated for 1 year (38–40). Extended LMV therapy for up to 2 years in chronic HBV carriers with positive markers of HBeAg, HBsAg, and HBV DNA produces suppression of HBV DNA to less than 10 pg/mL (lower limit of viral DNA detection by hybridization) in 48% by week 4, in 91% by week 10, and in 100% by week 12 of treatment (38,40,41). This suppression is sustained throughout therapy in 87% of patients. Following 2 years of continuous treatment, 39% of patients lose HBeAg and 22% become anti-HBe positive (38–41). In addition, there is a correlation between the degree of elevation of the baseline serum ALT and subsequent response to LMV (42). Figure 57.5 shows a typical response during LMV therapy.

The durability of the HBeAg seroconversion is variable, with some studies indicating the HBeAg loss is indeed sustainable (39), while others have demonstrated seroreversion to HBeAg at variable time intervals after discontinuing LMV therapy (43,44). LMV treatment is also associated with a substantial decrease in hepatic necroinflammatory activity (38–40). However, it has been reported that during the course of treatment, elevations of varying severity in the serum ALT can occur in up to one-third of patients (38,41).

Importantly, LMV therapy is beneficial in chronic carriers with precore mutants of HBV. Treatment results in a marked decrease in HBV DNA, normalization of serum ALT, and histologic improvement (45). Approximately two-thirds of patients have a complete response during therapy with normalization of ALT and loss of serum HBV DNA as well as a reduction in the intrahepatic necroinflammatory markers after 52 weeks of treatment (45). Unfortunately, when treatment stops, viral replication and disease activity return.

Treatment with LMV produces a substantial clinical improvement in patients with advanced disease and decompensated liver failure. These patients experience a reduction in serum ALT, bilirubin, and HBV DNA, and stabilization of their liver failure (46). However, most patients experience a rise in HBV DNA on stopping LMV. Treatment with LMV for periods greater than 6 months results in suppression of HBV replication, with subsequent improvement

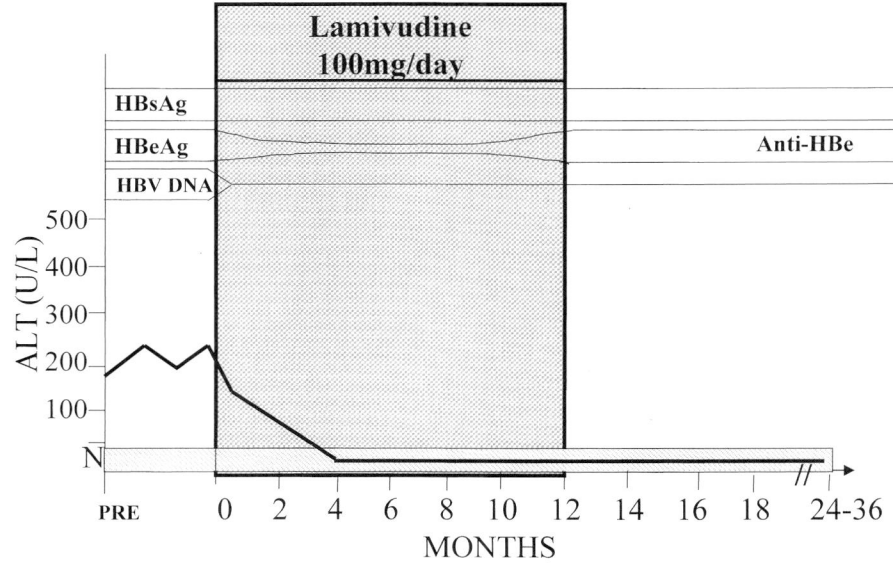

FIGURE 57.5. The serum biochemical, serologic, and virologic course of a typical patient with hepatitis B early antigen (*HBeAg*)–positive chronic hepatitis B who responded to lamivudine therapy. During treatment, the serum viral DNA levels drop rapidly, the alanine aminotransferase (*ALT*) normalizes, and HBeAg seroconversion occurs. The viral DNA becomes negative by hybridization assay, but is still positive by polymerase chain reaction. *HBsAg*, hepatitis B surface antigen; *HBV DNA*, hepatitis B virus DNA.

in liver function and liver histology associated with an increase in the serum albumin (46,47).

In patients awaiting liver transplantation, LMV inhibits HBV replication and stabilizes liver function (48). LMV has also been shown to prevent the recurrence of HBV following liver transplantation in patients with HBV-associated cirrhosis but only in combination with hepatitis B immune globulin (HBIG) (49–51). Recurrence of HBV posttransplantation occurs in 90% of patients who have a positive serum HBV DNA at the time of transplantation, compared to 30% if HBV DNA is negative, and this recurrence may be associated with the development of fibrosing cholestatic hepatitis with subsequent graft failure. Treatment with LMV results in a fall in serum HBV DNA to undetectable levels in almost every patient after 12 weeks of treatment (50). Some patients lose HBeAg, and a proportion become HBsAg negative. Liver biopsy performed at 6 months after transplantation demonstrates an improvement in necroinflammatory changes in 48% and fibrosis in 26% (50,51). However, long-term use of LMV in transplant recipients is associated with the emergence of LMV-resistant HBV mutants (52), which have been linked to subsequent graft loss (53). The combination of LMV with HBIG has significantly reduced the rate of HBV recurrence after liver transplantation in almost all patients, results in improved graft function and patient survival, and represents a most important advance in patient management (51).

The incidence of HBV associated HCC is reduced with LMV treatment. In woodchucks infected with the wood-

chuck hepatitis B virus (WHV), treatment with LMV reduces the development of HCC (54). Similarly, LMV therapy in humans is associated with a reduction in the degree of hepatic fibrosis and progression to cirrhosis and may possibly reduce the incidence of HCC (47).

LMV appears to cause minimal toxic side effects in the majority of patients. Although 17% of treated patients have been reported to experience mild elevations of serum amylase, a further 17% developed a transiently raised creatinine phosphokinase (55). Comparable changes have been observed in other studies in placebo recipients. Analysis of the effect of LMV on mitochondrial morphology and function has not demonstrated signs of mitochondrial toxicity after 6 months of therapy (56), and no clinical evidence for mitochondrial toxicity has developed in patients treated for 1 to 3 years. Other reported side effects include anorexia, nausea, vomiting, anemia and leukopenia, and peripheral neuropathy. Hepatitic flares have been documented during therapy with LMV (41), following cessation of LMV, and as a consequence of the emergence of LMV-resistant HBV mutants during therapy (41). In rare instances, hepatic decompensation has been associated with the emergence of LMV-resistant HBV mutants (41,53).

The long-term efficacy of monotherapy with nucleoside analogues such as LMV has become limited due to the emergence of HBV drug resistance. Phenotypic and genotypic resistance to LMV is now well documented (38,49,52, 53,57), and the typical responses seen are shown in Fig. 57.5. The common mutations associated with resistance to LMV occur in both the B and C domains of the viral polymerase protein. The HBV polymerase, like other reverse transcriptases, contains five conserved domains A to E (57). The LMV-resistant mutations occur predominantly within the YMDD motif (corresponding to the amino acid sequence tyrosine–methionine–aspartic acid–aspartic acid) in the major catalytic center of the enzyme (domain C) and are associated with a change of the methionine (M) to either a valine (YVDD) or isoleucine (YIDD) (52). Domain B is involved in the positioning of the template relative to the active site of the enzyme (57). The YVDD and YIDD polymerase-containing mutants demonstrate cross-resistance with emtricitabine (58) and 2′-fluoro-5-methyl-β-L-arabino-furanosyluracil (L-FMAU) (59) but remain susceptible to lobucavir (60) and adefovir dipivoxil (61) (see below). Also in patients carrying precore mutants of HBV, one-fourth of patients treated with lamivudine will develop LMV-resistant HBV mutants after week 52 of treatment (45).

Resistance to LMV is usually characterized by the reappearance of serum HBV DNA and a rise in the serum ALT (Fig. 57.6). Genotypic resistance can be detected as early as 6 months after commencing lamivudine treatment in patients with chronic hepatitis B infection, and by 12 months of therapy 27% of patients on monotherapy will have developed drug-resistant HBV mutants (41). In patients in whom the LMV-resistant mutants emerge, the rise in serum HBV DNA precedes the development of hepatic flares. These hepatitic flares are associated with HBeAg seroconversion; however, this occurs less frequently

in patients with LMV-resistant mutants (26%) as compared to patients with wild-type virus (52%) (41). In the setting of liver transplantation, however, the development of resistance to lamivudine is both more frequent and severe (50,53). In addition, reinfection of liver grafts with LMV-resistant virus (62) may result in subsequent graft dysfunction with limited treatment options.

These HBV mutants have previously been reported to be replication defective *in vitro* (63); however, the ability of these viruses to produce hepatitic flares in immunocompetent patients with chronic hepatitis B (41) challenges the clinical applicability of these findings, and patients on long-term LMV monotherapy should be monitored closely.

Adefovir and Adefovir Dipivoxil
Biologic Properties. Adefovir [9-(2-Bis[Pivaloyloxymethyl] Phosphonyl Methoxyethyl)Adenine or (PMEA)] is an acyclic analogue of deoxyadenosine monophosphate (dAMP) that has potent inhibitory activity against HBV replication (61, 64–66). In stably transfected human hepatoma cell lines, the EC_{50} of adefovir for HBV is 0.05 μM. In contrast, the CC_{50} is approximately 15 μM, giving a high selectivity index of 300 (65,66). Adefovir has poor oral bioavailability and a low cellular uptake (64). Esterification with two pivalic acid groups (bis-POM) produces the prodrug adefovir dipivoxil (bis-POM PMEA), which greatly improves oral bioavailability (64).

The diphosphate (PMEA-DP) is the active antiviral form and has a greater inhibitory effect on HBV polymerase

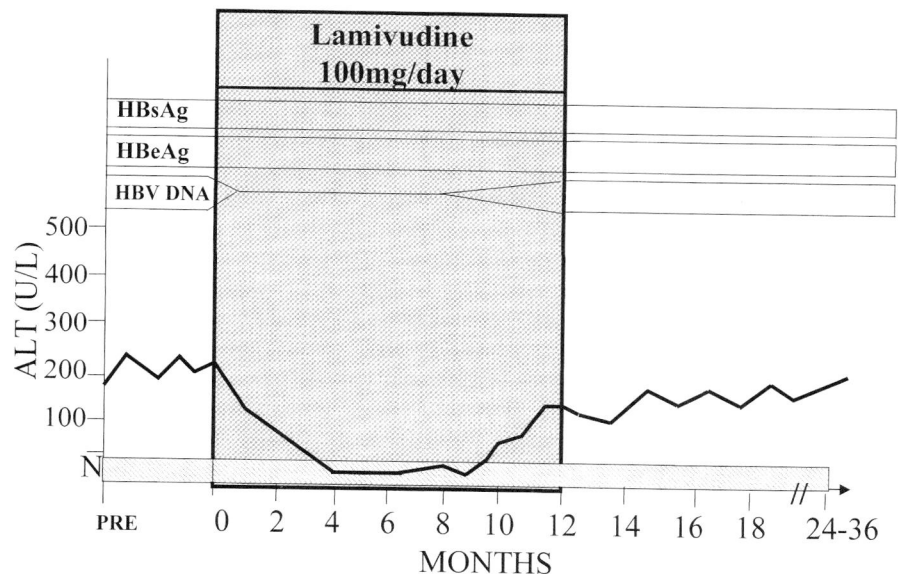

FIGURE 57.6. The serum biochemical, serologic, and virologic responses of a typical patient in whom lamivudine-resistant as hepatitis B virus (*HBV*) emerges after 6 to 9 months of monotherapy. In this patient there was an initial response to therapy with marked decrease in viremia and improvement in serum alanine aminotransferase (*ALT*), but during viral breakthrough, HBV DNA levels rise and hepatic disease activity returns. *HBeAg*, hepatitis B early antigen; *HBsAg*; hepatitis B surface antigen.

than on host cell DNA polymerase α, β, δ, and γ (64,65). PMEA is converted to the mono- and diphosphate by cellular enzymes (64); the mechanism of action of PMEA-DP includes competitive inhibition of deoxyadenosine-triphosphate (dATP) incorporation as well as chain termination of nascent viral DNA synthesis (64,65). In addition to its direct antiviral effect, adefovir may stimulate natural killer cells and promote immune responsiveness to HBV through endogenous IFN-α and other cytokine production (64).

In ducks congenitally infected with the duck hepatitis B virus (DHBV), treatment with adefovir produced a marked reduction in all markers of viral replication (67). The pregenomic RNA, preS and core proteins, as well as CCC DNA levels in the liver, were reduced (67). However, all viral parameters returned to pretreatment levels within 3 weeks of the cessation of antiviral treatment (67).

Clinical Studies. In phase I and II studies, adefovir dipivoxil (ADV) treatment has resulted in a rapid reduction in serum HBV DNA. A 97% reduction in the serum HBV DNA occurs within 1 to 2 weeks of commencing treatment (68). Up to a four-log reduction in viral load was achieved after 12 weeks of treatment at a dose of 30 to 60 mg daily of ADV (69). Some patients developed an elevated serum ALT level during treatment, but this was associated with a reduction in serum HBV DNA to undetectable levels (68).

Adefovir retains its *in vitro* and *in vivo* activity against LMV-resistant HBV (59,61). In addition, resistance to ADV has not been detected after 24 weeks of continuous treatment (69). A potential concern is the development of nephrotoxicity after prolonged treatment in patients with HIV. However, these patients received higher doses than those used in trials of patients with HBV (70).

Entecavir (BMS-200475)

Entecavir ([1S-(1α,3α,4β)]-2-amino-1,9-dihydro-9[4-hydroxy-3 (hydroxymethyl)-2-methylenecyclopentyl]-6H-purin-6-one) is a carbocyclic deoxyguanosine analogue with potent antiherpes and antihepadnaviral activity (71,72). The EC_{50} for HBV in HepG 2 2.2.15 cells is 0.00375 μM (72). In contrast, the CC_{50} is 30 μM, producing a selectivity index of greater than 8,000 (72). Treatment of woodchucks infected with WHV produced a two- to three-log reduction in serum WHV DNA, although discontinuation of treatment resulted in relapse of infection (71,72). Phase II/III clinical studies have been initiated with entecavir (ETC). Adverse events reported with ETC to date have been mainly central nervous system toxicity including headache, dizziness, and photophobia.

Emtricitabine

Emtricitabine [5-Fluoro-1-(2-Hydoxymethyl)1,3-Oxathiolan-5-yl]Cytosine, or (−) FTC] is the 5′-fluorinated derivative of LMV, and *in vitro* (−) FTC is active against HBV (73). Both enantiomers of FTC have activity against HBV, although (−) FTC is far more potent. The EC_{50} of (−) FTC

is 0.03 μM compared to 0.72 for (+) FTC (73), and (+) FTC is more cytotoxic. The intracellular phosphorylation of emtricitabine to the monophosphate and then to the triphosphate (TP) forms is carried out by cytoplasmic deoxycytidine kinase and nucleoside mono- and diphosphate kinases (73,74). The mechanism of action of (−) FTC-TP is by competitive inhibition with deoxycytidine triphosphate (dCTP) for the HBV polymerase (73). The intracellular half-life of FTC-TP in hepatoma cells has been estimated to be 2.4 hours (74). FTC has an oral bioavailability of 60% to 90% (75) and is excreted unchanged in urine (75). Antiviral cross-resistance between LMV and FTC has been reported for HBV both *in vitro* (58) and *in vivo* (76). Phase I/II studies have been completed and phase III are in progress.

Famciclovir (Penciclovir)

Biologic Properties. Famciclovir and its active form penciclovir are deoxyguanosine nucleoside analogues with inhibitory activity for hepadnaviruses (77,78). The inhibition constant (K_i) of the R-enantiomer for HBV polymerase in vitro is 0.03 μM, while the K_i for human DNA polymerase α is 175 μM, providing a substantial selectivity index (79). The likelihood of cellular toxicity is therefore low as the selectivity ratio is high (77). In Hep G2 2.2.15 cells, the EC_{90} of penciclovir-triphosphate (PCV-TP) for intracellular HBV replication is 1.6 μM, while the EC_{90} for extracellular viral release is 0.7 μM (79).

In virus-infected hepatocytes, penciclovir is phosphorylated to the triphosphate form by cellular enzymes (80). Penciclovir triphosphate competes with deoxyguanosine triphosphate (dGTP) as a substrate for HBV polymerase. Its incorporation into the HBV genome results in inhibition of HBV DNA replication by causing premature chain termination, blocking both first- and second-strand HBV DNA synthesis (78,80), and priming of first-strand HBV DNA synthesis (80).

In Peking ducks infected with DHBV (81), penciclovir treatment results in inhibition of all markers of active viral replication. The intrahepatic viral CCC DNA level is reduced, and although at the end of 6 months' treatment the CCC DNA still remained, its total level was reduced by over 50%. All viral markers of active replication returned to pretreatment levels upon withdrawal of drug (81).

Famciclovir is the oral form that is rapidly converted to 6-deoxypenciclovir after oral administration by a process of deacetylation by esterases in the small intestine. This is followed by oxidation of the purine base by aldehyde oxidase in the serum and the delivery of penciclovir to the liver (77). The half-life of the intracellular triphosphate is 12 to 18 hours (77). The bioavailability of penciclovir after oral administration of famciclovir is as high as 77% (77).

Clinical Studies. In patients with chronic hepatitis B infection, treatment with famciclovir results in a marked decrease in serum HBV DNA, although only 25% become negative by hybridization (82). Primary therapeutic failure occurs in up to 20% of patients treated with famciclovir. In responders, the serum ALT returns to normal in the majority of patients while on treatment, and seroconversion from HBeAg to anti-HBe positive develops in 15% of treated patients, while seroconversion from HBsAg to anti-HBs positive does not occur (82).

In addition, famciclovir treatment in patients with chronic hepatitis B and decompensated cirrhosis results in an improvement in liver function, and half of these patients become HBV DNA negative by hybridization assay (83).

Famciclovir has been demonstrated to be efficacious in preventing HBV recurrence following liver and bone marrow transplantation (84,85). Treatment results in marked reductions in serum HBV DNA levels and histologic improvement on liver biopsy (84,85). Famciclovir has been well tolerated in this population, and its long-term safety is excellent in patients treated for herpes virus infections (86).

Resistance to famciclovir is predominantly associated with a complex pattern of mutations in the B domain of the polymerase protein (57,87,88). Reduced sensitivity of the mutant polymerase to famciclovir has been demonstrated *in vitro* in cell culture and in the endogenous HBV DNA polymerase isolated from a patient on long-term famciclovir in whom resistance had developed (87). Generally, in patients treated for 6 to 12 months with continuous famciclovir monotherapy, resistance develops in 15% (88). As with lamivudine, the emergence of resistance to famciclovir is associated with the reappearance of serum HBV DNA and a rise in the serum ALT (87,88). In patients in whom resistance to famciclovir develops and the drug is no longer effective, treatment with LMV is able to achieve a reduction in HBV DNA levels by a mean of 99% (88).

In conclusion, famciclovir is less potent in clinical trials than LMV, and its development as a treatment for chronic hepatitis B infection has been suspended. However, the drug is occasionally used in the post–orthoptic liver transplantation (OLT) setting of multidrug resistance to LMV and HBIG, and may have a role in the development of combination regimes (see Special Groups and Challenges, below).

Ganciclovir

Ganciclovir (2-amino-1,9-{[2-hydroxy-1-{hydroxymethyl} ethoxy]methyl}-6H-purin-6-one) has excellent antiviral activity against herpes viruses including human cytomegalovirus, and only modest efficacy against the hepadnaviruses (37). Its mode of action is similar to that of penciclovir, i.e., it acts as a viral DNA chain terminator and competitive inhibitor of HBV polymerase. It has no effect against viral CCC DNA or RNA synthesis *in vitro* but potent antiviral activity has been demonstrated *in vivo* against DHBV (89).

In patients with recurrent hepatitis B infection following liver transplantation, ganciclovir treatment has produced marked reductions of serum HBV DNA and histologic improvement (90). However, parenteral ganciclovir is associated with myelotoxicity. Oral ganciclovir has also been shown to have activity against HBV in patients with chronic hepatitis B infection, with marked reductions in serum HBV DNA and normalization of serum ALT in almost half of patients (91). Administered in this way, ganciclovir was not associated with the development of myelotoxicity (91). Antiviral cross-resistance to ganciclovir is not well understood, although it may be effective in patients with severe recurrent HBV post-OTL LMV-resistant HBV (90).

Lobucavir

Biologic Properties. Lobucavir showed initial promise as an antihepadnaviral agent, but recent safety concerns have caused this compound to be suspended from further clinical development. It is included here for comparative purposes. Lobucavir (R-Bis[hydroxymethyl] cyclobutyl guanine; R-BHCG) and its congeners have antiviral activity for herpesviruses (92) and potent inhibitory activity against HBV (93). The concentration that inhibits 50% (IC_{50}) for HBV *in vitro* is 2.5 µM (92), and lobucavir retains some activity *in vitro* against LMV-resistant HBV (59). Lobucavir is phosphorylated intracellularly by cellular enzymes with an intracellular half-life of 10 hours (94).

Clinical Studies. In patients with chronic hepatitis B infection, treatment with lobucavir resulted in a two- to four-log reduction in serum HBV DNA, as assessed by branched-chain DNA hybridization (93). The serum HBV DNA returned to pretreatment levels in all patients within 4 weeks of completing therapy (93). Despite promising early results demonstrating potent antihepadnaviral activity of lobucavir, further clinical trials have now been terminated as a result of the development of malignancies in mice and rats given high doses of lobucavir for prolonged periods.

Special Groups and Challenges

Combination Chemotherapy

IFN-α and LMV are appropriate management in particular clinical subgroups (discussed in Immune Modulating Agents and Nucleoside Analogues, above). Patients who are HBeAg-positive with chronic active hepatitis and elevated serum ALT benefit from a course of either treatment. However, in patients with HBeAg-negative chronic hepatitis B, advanced disease, immunosuppression, or multiple viral co-infections, clinical management needs to be substantially improved. Several clinical trials are examining combination therapy against HBV in order to address the treatment of special groups including the management of nonresponders or drug resistance.

Viral dynamic studies obtained from short-term clinical trials of LMV and ADV in patients chronically infected with HBV have shed some light on the relationship between viral kinetics and the pathogenesis of HBV and the limited antiviral treatment success with nucleoside analogues (95,96). Estimating the half-life of free virus particles and that of virus within infected cells in persistently infected patients has allowed the theoretical estimation of the duration of antiviral treatment required to lead to complete suppression of viral replication. Nowak et al. (95) calculated that HBV particles were cleared from the serum of infected patients with a half-life of approximately 1 day. In contrast, the half-life of infected cells was longer and more variable, with an estimated range of 10 to 100 days depending on the level of hepatic necroinflammatory activity. Based on this model, the investigators predicted that during the active disease stage or elimination phase, 12 months of treatment with LMV would reduce the total body viral burden by a factor of about 10^{11}. However, to achieve this level of viral load reduction during the inactive or latent phase of chronic disease, antiviral therapy would have to be extended for many years.

Using ADV at a daily dose of 30 mg for 12 weeks, Tsiang et al. (97) extended the mathematical model of Nowak et al. (95) and described two phases of clearance of HBV. The initial phase represented clearance of free virions present at the initiation of antiviral therapy. The second, slower phase represented the loss of infected cells. Simulations and projections revealed that increasing the dose of ADV (and thus the antiviral efficacy) seemed to have no effect on the rate of virus clearance or the rate of infected cell loss, but it substantially decreased the time to clear the virus from the body from approximately 30 months for a 5-mg dose to approximately 16 months for the 30- and 60-mg doses (97). These studies do have important implications in designing therapies that maximize antiviral effect and minimize the development of drug resistance.

To date, the efficacy of combination therapy in hepatitis B with nucleoside analogues has not been fully evaluated. A recent study has shown that the combination of LMV and penciclovir *in vitro* may be more efficacious than therapy with either agent alone (98). This study examined the antiviral efficacy of LMV and penciclovir alone and in combination in primary duck hepatocytes isolated from ducks congenitally infected with DHBV (98). In this model, penciclovir resulted in greater inhibition of DHBV replication than LMV. LMV did not inhibit CCC DNA and pre-S antigen production, but penciclovir resulted in inhibition of both. In addition, penciclovir and LMV in combination produced at least additive and possibly synergistic inhibition of DHBV (98). This report supported the hypothesis that the use of combination antiviral nucleoside analogues may be more effective than single-agent therapy, and a pilot clinical study from Hong Kong has confirmed this approach (99). Lau et al. (99) compared 12 weeks of LMV monotherapy to 12 weeks of LMV plus famciclovir combination

chemotherapy in 19 Chinese patients. The mean antiviral efficacy (97) was significantly greater in the combination treatment group, which translated into a larger first-phase HBV viral load reduction of 1.9 $\log_{10}$ vs. 1.1 $\log_{10}$ for LMV monotherapy. The overall mean viral decline was also greater with 2.5 $\log_{10}$ in the combination vs 1.8 $\log_{10}$ with LMV alone (99).

Other investigators have examined the effect of combining IFN-α with Tα_1 (100), Tα_1 with famciclovir (101), Tα_1 plus famciclovir plus LMV (102), IFN-α plus famciclovir (103), IFN-α with LMV (104), and ribavirin plus IFN-α (105). The use of combination therapy for the treatment of chronic hepatitis B certainly warrants further investigation since studies are required to determine whether the use of combinations of nucleoside analogues will not only improve the therapeutic efficacy of regimens to treat chronic hepatitis B but also delay or possibly even prevent the development of resistance to single agents.

The Hepatitis B Virus–Human Immunodeficiency Virus Co-Infected Patient

The risk factors for the acquisition of HBV and the HIV are similar, and as a consequence co-infection with both viruses may occur, with over 10% of HIV-infected individuals also having chronic hepatitis B infection (106). Co-infection with HBV and HIV is associated with higher rates of chronic hepatitis B infection (107), higher levels of viral replication, lower levels of serum ALT, and milder histologic disease in the short term (108,109). HBV does not affect survival of HIV-positive patients (109). However, with the prolonged survival of HIV-infected patients in the era of highly active antiretroviral therapy (HAART), liver disease due to HBV is emerging as an important clinical problem (110).

Treatment of co-infected patients with IFN-α has been disappointing, with diminished responses to therapy and failure to clear HBV (111,112). The treatment of HIV-infected patients with HAART, and in particular regimens including LMV, has resulted in suppression of HBV replication (112). In contrast, the immune restoration produced by HAART has also resulted in the reactivation of latent HBV infection with the development of chronic hepatitis B infection (113). Exacerbations of chronic hepatitis B infection have also occurred after withdrawal of LMV or after the development of HBV resistant to LMV (114,115). These exacerbations may result in fulminant hepatitis (114), and therefore the discontinuation of LMV therapy should be monitored closely in this clinical situation.

HBV resistance to LMV in the HIV co-infected situation is associated with mutations in the YMDD motif and occurs at the rate of 20% of patients treated per year (113–115). The impact of these resistant viruses on patient survival will need to be followed closely (116). Thus, combination nucleoside analogue therapy directed at HBV may be required to control active HBV replication and prevent severe exacerbations of hepatitis.

The Hepatits B Virus–Hepatitis C Virus Co-Infected Patient

This issue is discussed below (see Hepatitis C).

Newer Therapies

In spite of the development of a range of novel nucleoside analogues that are highly effective in blocking HBV DNA replication, the development of resistance and cross-resistance requires other agents that act at alternative sites in the viral life cycle than the viral polymerase to be developed (Fig. 57.1). Recent insights into the molecular biology of HBV and HCV have led to the development of molecular therapeutic strategies that offer the potential of being the next generation of successful antiviral agents against these viruses.

Gene Therapy

Antisense Oligodeoxynucleotides. Antisense oligodeoxynucleotides (ODN) consist of DNA or RNA sequences designed to specifically bind an RNA target, resulting in the formation of an RNA-RNA (antisense RNA) or RNA-DNA (antisense DNA) hybrid, which brings about inhibition of RNA replication, reverse transcription, and translation (117). The inhibitory effects of antisense ODNs are potentiated by intracellular degradation of RNA in RNA-DNA hybrids by the cellular enzyme RNase H (117).

Antisense ODNs have been developed that inhibit HBV replication *in vitro* (117–119), and the replication of DHBV (120) and WHV (121). Phosphothiorate antisense ODNs directed to specific regions within the HBsAg and pre-S1 open reading frames (ORFs), the HBcAg gene, and the HBV ε structure all result in virtually complete inhibition of viral replication (118).

Ribozymes. Ribozymes are naturally occurring short RNA molecules with endoribonuclease activity that catalyze the sequence-specific cleavage of RNA and RNA splicing reactions (122,123). Hammerhead and hairpin ribozymes constitute two important ribozyme constructs that have been demonstrated to inhibit viral replication *in vitro* (124). Cleavage of the HBV encapsidation signal and pregenomic RNA has been demonstrated *in vitro* with hammerhead ribozymes (117) with marked reduction in HBV replication (124). However, ribozymes are relatively unstable and rapidly degraded *in vivo*, limiting the delivery of these agents. The delivery of ribozymes with activity against HBV may be improved by the use of retroviral, adenoviral, and adenovirus associated viral vectors, the last two of which are hepatotrophic, produce high titers of viral products, and can transduce cells that have not been stimulated to divide (124).

Dominant Negative Proteins. Dominant negative polypeptides and proteins are able to interact with and disrupt the function of their native counterparts intracellularly. As a consequence, these polypeptides are capable of interfering with the assembly of HBV structural and nonstructural proteins (117). The delivery of dominant negative proteins into cells by transient transfection is a relatively ineffective means of inhibiting viral replication. This can be overcome by the expression of the proteins using retroviral and adenoviral vectors (125).

HEPATITIS D

Epidemiology and Natural History

Hepatitis D, or delta, virus (HDV) is a blood-borne RNA-containing virusoid. The modes of transmission of HDV are similar to HBV and include parenteral and perinatal exposure.

Infection with HDV may occur either simultaneously with HBV (co-infection) or subsequent to HBV infection (superinfection), in either an acute or chronic illness presentation (126). The natural history of HDV/HBV superinfection can be different from that of co-infection. Patients with preexisting chronic hepatitis B infection who become superinfected with HDV are more likely to develop severe hepatitis, and have a greater likelihood of remaining chronically infected (127).

Life Cycle

Hepatitis D virus is a defective RNA virus/virusoid that generally can replicate only in the presence of HBV. The genome of HDV comprises a circular, negative-sense, single-stranded RNA of 1,700 nucleotides. Viral particles are 35 to 37 nm in diameter, with the core comprising the hepatitis delta antigen (HDAg) and the coat consisting of HBsAg (128). Thus, HDV requires HBV in order to enter and exit the hepatocyte.

Treatment

IFN-α appears to be of some benefit for patients with chronic HDV infection. Treatment involves the administration of IFN-α at doses up to 9 mu subcutaneously three times weekly for at least 12 months (129). Both the biochemical and virologic response rates are reduced if the dose is lowered to 3 million units (129). By the end of treatment up to 70% of patients receiving 9 mu three times weekly will have negative serum HDV RNA (PCR) and normal ALT (129). However, by the end of up to 12 months' follow-up at least 10% of patients will have had a virologic relapse (129). Sustained virologic responses, although infrequent, do occur and are accompanied by the simultaneous clearance of HBsAg in serum and seroconversion to anti-HBs (130).

Lau et al. (131) evaluated 12 months of LMV therapy (100 mg daily) in five patients with chronic hepatitis D. During treatment, serum HBV DNA levels fell in all patients, becoming negative by PCR. However, all patients remained HBsAg negative and HDV RNA positive, and serum ALT and liver histology did not improve. The HBV DNA levels returned to the pretreatment level without a change in disease activity when LMV was stopped.

Novel, molecular-based therapies for HDV infection are being developed. The HDV assembly and virus particle formation involves prenylation, a posttranslational lipid modification of the large HDAg (132). Several groups are examining the effects of pharmacologic agents capable of inhibiting prenylation to inhibit HDV replication (133). Until these newer therapies are evaluated and prove to be efficacious, therapy of chronic delta hepatitis will remain unsatisfactory.

Hepatitis D infection is not a contraindication to OLT of patients with HBV/HDV-associated cirrhosis. Up to 80% of patients will become reinfected with HBV/HDV, but only a proportion (40%) will redevelop hepatitis (134). The prognosis following liver transplantation in this patient population can be further improved by the long-term administration of HBIG (135). This strategy increases the 5-year survival rate to 88%, and less than 10% of patients will have reappearance of HBsAg in serum (135).

HEPATITIS C

Hepatitis C virus (HCV) accounts for the majority of cases of transfusion-acquired hepatitis and hepatitis transmitted through injecting drug use (IDU). The incidences of hepatitis C is currently reported in the United States to be 28,000 cases annually, a decrease from 170,000 annual cases before 1990 (136). This large decrease directly resulted from mandatory testing of all donor blood for HCV, and fewer infections in IDUs (136). HCV is now the most common cause of chronic liver disease in North America. HCV-related deaths are expected to increase from around 10,000 annually to nearly 30,000 annually by the year 2010 (136). In North America, advanced liver disease, specifically decompensated cirrhosis secondary to chronic HCV infection, is currently the most common indication for OLT.

Life Cycle

HCV is an RNA virus of the Flaviviridae family. Six genotypes exist, and individual isolates consist of closely related, heterogeneous populations of viral genomes (quasi-species) (137). The hepatitis C viruses are classified into six genotypes according to differences in nucleotide sequences, and this genetic heterogeneity of HCV has important clinical, diagnostic, and therapeutic implications (137).

The virus has not been reproducibly isolated *in vitro* in hepatocytes, and a number of reports have claimed successful propagation of HCV in human T-cell lymphocyte cell lines (138). A hypothetical life cycle is shown in Fig. 57.7. Following attachment, penetration, and uncoating, viral proteins are translated and viral RNA replication occurs (139) at sites at which IFN-α's antiviral action is effected (140). Interferon generally exerts its antiviral activity through the action of 2′,5′-oligo A synthetase, producing 2′,5′-oligo adenylate, which activates specific enzymes RNase L and protein kinase R (PKR). These enzymes depend on the presence of double-stranded RNA for their activity. RNase L activity results in the enzymatic digestion of RNA, while PKR phosphorylates eIF-2b, blocking initiation of any further translational events (140). In this context, the beneficial effects of interferon therapy in chronic hepatitis C can be understood to be predominately antiviral rather than immunomodulating as is the case of HBeAg-positive chronic hepatitis B (9).

Treatment

The mechanism of HCV-associated liver injury is not fully understood, but host immunologic factors are clearly important in determining the extent of hepatitis injury and ultimately, viral persistence. Importantly, the treatment of hepatitis C infection has progressed considerably since the first report describing the use of IFN-α-2b to treat chronic HCV carriers. Advances in the understanding of both the immune response to HCV and the virologic factors that help to predict a favorable treatment response have occurred, with resulting improvements in patient management. The addition of ribavirin to the treatment regimen has resulted in sustained virologic responses in up to half of select patients receiving combination treatment with IFN-α and ribavirin (141,142), as well as simplifying the approach to overall patient treatment.

Clinical Studies

Acute Hepatitis C

There have been a number of small, randomized controlled trials of IFN-α or -β in patients with acute hepatitis C (143,144). All studies have been performed in recipients of blood or blood products who were being followed prospectively posttransfusion. All studies demonstrated a decrease in the chronicity of patients treated with IFN during the acute phase of their disease, which usually occurred 1 to 2 months following serum ALT elevation. The sustained response rate ranged from 40% to 64%. From these studies, patients with acute hepatitis C should be commenced on IFN therapy if HCV RNA persists for 1 to 2 months after onset of serum ALT rises.

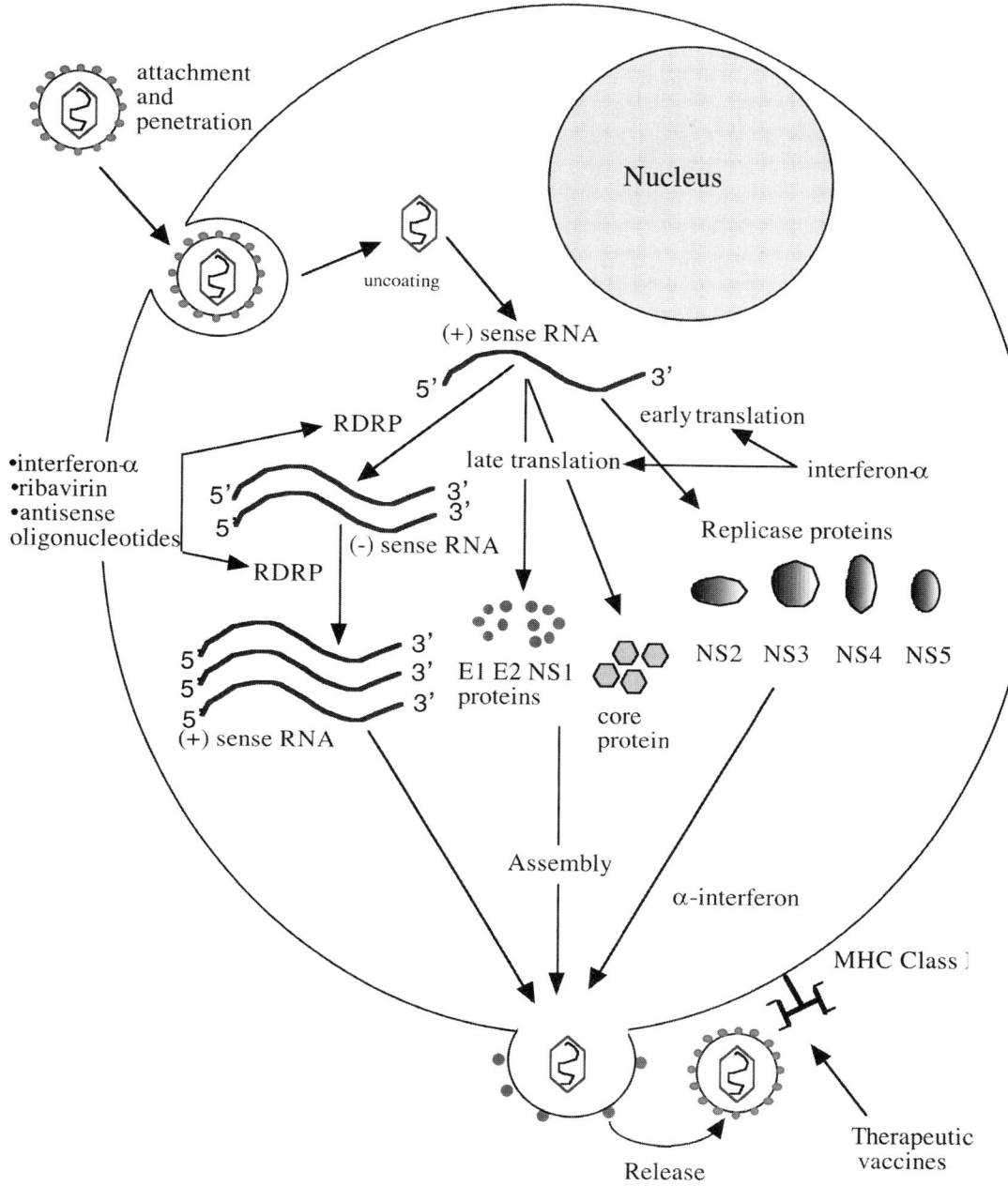

FIGURE 57.7. Hypothetical life cycle of the hepatitis C virus (HCV). Following attachment, penetration, and uncoating, the viral RNA is translated to produce a pool of replicase proteins required for genomic replication. Viral RNA replication almost certainly occurs in the smooth membrane compartment, associated with unusual tubular structures. The viral RNA is copied via the recycling of the double-stranded replicative form (RF) with the RNA-dependent RNA polymerase (*RDRP*) compromising helicase (*NS3*) and polymerase (*NS5*) activities. As the RF is unwound, a new strand is synthesized, producing the partially single-stranded, double-stranded replicative intermediate (RI). The new genomic RNA is released from RI and the RF then recycles back with the RDRP to commence the process again. In the later stages of replication more viral translation occurs, producing a pool of structural proteins that interact with the newly synthesized viral (+) RNA molecules, and complete particles are formed. The life cycle is based on the model of Chu and Westaway (139) for flaviviruses. The interferons generally are active against RNA viruses at the translational phase of replication and also reduce the amount of viral RNA formed (140). *MHC*, major histocompatibility complex. (Modified from Locarnini SA, Cunningham AL. Clinical treatment of viral hepatitis. In: Jefferies DJ, DeClercq E, eds. *Antiviral chemotherapy.* New York: Wiley, 1995:441–530.)

Chronic Hepatitis C

Interferon-α

The clinical criteria for treatment of patients with chronic hepatitis C are shown in Table 57.2. IFN-α was first demonstrated to have a beneficial effect against non-A non-B hepatitis in the mid- to late 1980s (145). Administered in a dose of 3 mu subcutaneously three times weekly for a period of 6 months, IFN-α produced a complete normalization of the serum ALT in up to 45% of patients (146,147). In patients achieving normalization of the serum ALT, it can also be shown that HCV RNA is cleared from serum in 85% (148). In addition, treatment with IFN-α alone results in histologic improvement in all patients (147).

The response to IFN-α is defined as an end of treatment response (ETR), with a normal serum ALT and negative HCV RNA at the end of the treatment course and a sustained response (SR) as a normal serum ALT and negative serum HCV RNA at least 6 months and preferably 12 months after completing treatment. Unfortunately, the relapse rate following treatment with IFN-α monotherapy alone and after having achieved a complete biochemical response is high and only 10% to 15% of patients have long-term sustained responses (147,149). In addition, up to 70% of relapses occur within the first few months after completing IFN-α (147,149). The persistence of HCV RNA in serum and liver at the end of treatment is predictive of subsequent relapse (150).

Meta-analysis of randomized trials of IFN-α has demonstrated that extended duration of therapy for between 12 and 18 months produced better response rates than 6 months (151–154). Sustained response rates of up to 30% could be achieved with extended duration of therapy. Long-term follow-up over several years in these patients has demonstrated that over 90% will maintain normal ALT and negative HCV RNA (152).

As in the case of hepatitis B, IFN-α therapy in hepatitis C is associated with a wide range of side effects (Table 57.1).

Interferon-α and Ribavirin

An important development in the treatment of HCV was the finding that ribavirin was able to normalize serum ALT

in chronically infected patients, although the drug appeared to have minimal effect on viremia (153). When combined with IFN-α, the long-term virologic response rates were markedly improved, with 40% to 59% now showing sustained responses (141,142,154).

A number of factors are associated with a higher likelihood of response to IFN-α and ribavirin therapy. The most important are pretreatment viral loads, liver histology, and viral genotype (155). Low pretreatment levels of viremia are predictive of a long-term response rather than an initial response to IFN-α (141,142,155). The sustained response rates are also higher in patients infected with non–type 1 genotypes. Genotype 1 infections are associated with a sustained response rate of 8% to 12%, while in genotypes 2 and 3 this is as high as 30% (141,142,155, 156). The presence of cirrhosis is also associated with lower end of treatment response to IFN-α and sustained response rates of 9 to 16% (149,157). In addition, the presence of cirrhosis reduces sustained virologic response rates regardless of genotypes. The sustained virologic response rates in previously untreated patients with genotype 2 or 3 infections are reduced from 65% in the absence of cirrhosis to 24% with cirrhosis, while the corresponding rates in patients with genotype 1 infections are 33% to 7%, respectively (157).

Chronic carriers with persistently normal serum ALT levels generally have mild inflammatory changes histologically and are unlikely to progress to cirrhosis of the liver (158). In these patients IFN-α treatment has not been shown to improve long-term outcome or survival and may be associated with the development of ALT flares on treatment (158,159).

Two recent important multicenter studies, one from the United States (141) and the second a collaborative international study (142), have addressed a number of important variables determining the likelihood of sustained virologic response. Both studies treated patients with IFN-α alone or IFN-α in combination with ribavirin for 24 or 48 weeks (141,142). The overall end of treatment virologic response rate was 29% following 48 weeks of IFN-α alone and 51% for IFN-α plus ribavirin (141,142). The sustained virologic response rate was highest in patients infected with genotypes 2 or 3 (65%) in contrast to genotype 1 and 4 (29%) (141,142). Of note, extending treatment from 24 to 48 weeks did not increase the sustained virologic response rate in patients infected with genotypes 2 or 3, regardless of the baseline HCV viral load (66% or 65%, respectively). In patients with genotype 1 and 4 infections, the sustained response rates were higher in patients with viral loads less than 2 million copies per milliliter (33% vs. 27%) after 48 weeks treatment (141,142). Treatment was also associated with histologic improvement (141,142). The typical events that occur in a patient with a sustained response are shown in Fig. 57.8.

TABLE 57.2. MINIMAL CRITERIA FOR TREATMENT OF PATIENTS WITH CHRONIC HEPATITIS C

Elevated ALT values for ≥6 months
Detectable serum HCV RNA
Compensated liver disease
Abstinence from drugs and alcohol
Compliant patient
Compatible liver biopsy findings
No contraindications

ALT, alanine aminotransferase; HCV, hepatitis C virus.

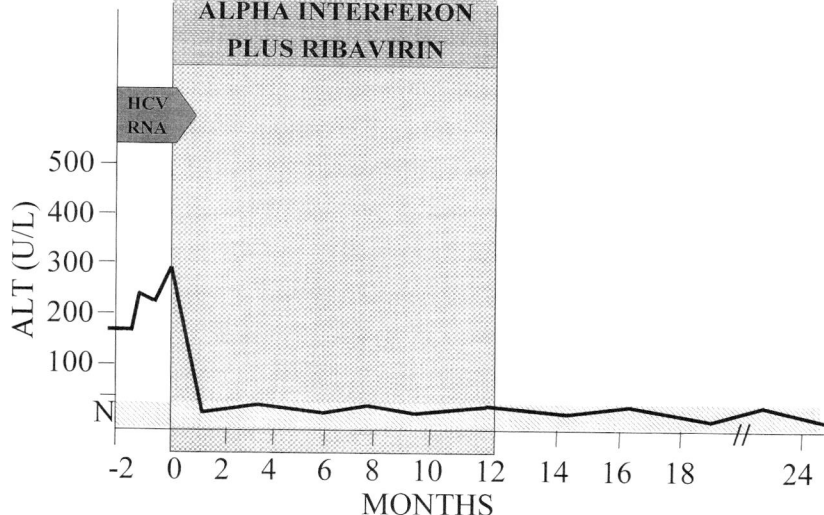

FIGURE 57.8. The serum biochemical, serologic, and virologic responses of a typical patient with chronic hepatitis C who had a complete response to therapy with interferon-α and ribavirin combination treatment. During treatment, there is rapid improvement in serum alanine aminotransferase (*ALT*), which is permanent, and a steady disappearance of hepatitis C virus RNA (*HCV RNA*) from serum as shown by polymerase chain reaction. In responders, the serum HCV RNA is mostly negative 8 to 10 weeks after commencement of therapy. When treatment is completed, the HCV RNA does not return, serum ALT remains normal, and the general clinical and histologic improvement is maintained through the follow-up period. (Modified from Locarnini SA, Cunningham AL. Clinical treatment of viral hepatitis. In: Jefferies DJ, DeClercq E, eds. *Antiviral chemotherapy*. New York: Wiley, 1995:441–530.)

Viral dynamic studies have also been carried out in hepatitis C. The serum half-life of HCV has been estimated to be 2.7 hours with a pretreatment production of 10^{12} virions per day (160). Thus the intermittent administration of IFN-α as a thrice-weekly injection may be inadequate in some patients, as the viral load may return to baseline before the administration of the next dose of IFN-α. In support of this is the finding that the administration of escalating doses of IFN-α does not increase the sustained virologic response rates (161), while the use of high-dose daily IFN-α does appear to be a more effective therapeutic strategy (162). This is currently under investigation.

Special Groups and Challenges

Treatment Relapse Patients

The virologic events that occur with relapse are shown in Fig. 57.9. Retreatment of patients who have relapsed following a previous response to IFN-α therapy results in a sustained response rate of 30% to 40% (163,164). In contrast, patients who were previously nonresponders are unlikely to achieve a sustained response with retreatment with IFN-α (163,165). The greatest sustained virologic response occurs in patients infected with a non–type 1 genotype and a serum HCV viral load of less than 2×10^6 copies/mL (164). In this setting, patients retreated with IFN-α plus ribavirin for 6 months

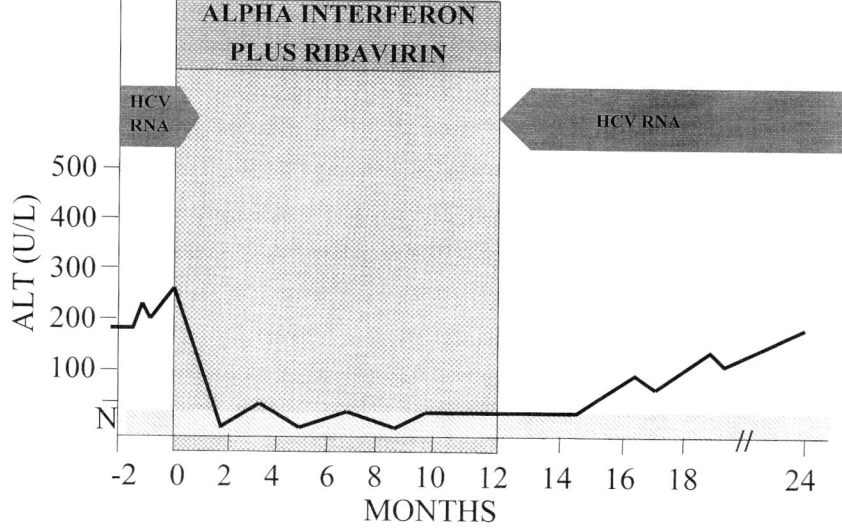

FIGURE 57.9. The serum biochemical, serologic, and virologic responses of a typical patient with chronic hepatitis C who initially had a complete response to combination therapy that was not sustained. When treatment is completed, however, the hepatitis C virus RNA (*HCV RNA*) returns almost immediately and the serum alanine aminotransferase (*ALT*) gradually rises to the pretherapy level. (Modified from Locarnini SA, Cunningham AL. Clinical treatment of viral hepatitis. In: Jefferies DJ, DeClercq E, eds. *Antiviral chemotherapy*. New York: Wiley, 1995:441–530.)

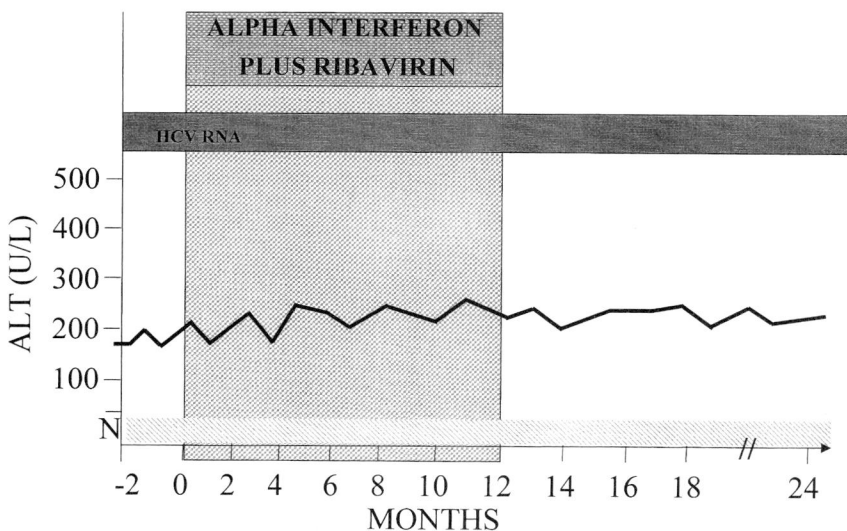

FIGURE 57.10. The serum biochemical and virologic profiles of a typical patient with chronic hepatitis C who failed to demonstrate a response to therapy. During treatment, there was no effect on serum alanine aminotransferase (*ALT*) or serum hepatitis C virus RNA (*HCV RNA*). (Modified from Locarnini SA, Cunningham AL. Clinical treatment of viral hepatitis. In: Jefferies DJ, DeClercq E, eds. *Antiviral chemotherapy*. New York: Wiley, 1995:441–530.)

had sustained virologic response rates of up to 100% compared to 40% in patients infected with genotype 1 (164). Retreatment also resulted in a histologic improvement in all patients but more so in patients treated with IFN-α plus ribavirin (67% compared to 41% for IFN-α alone) (164).

Treatment Nonresponders

The virologic events occurring in patients who do not respond to therapy are shown in Fig. 57.10.

At present, no effective regimen exists for the treatment of nonresponse patients. The use of combinations of IFN-α with multiple other agents has been generally unsuccessful in achieving a significant increase in the sustained response rate. New classes of drugs will need to be developed for this subgroup of patients with chronic hepatitis C infection (see below).

Patients Co-Infected with Other Viruses

Patients with Hepatitis C Virus and Human Immunodeficiency Virus

Co-infection with HCV and HIV is not an infrequent occurrence in the United States, with as many as 400,000 co-infected carriers (166). HCV and HIV co-infection is most frequently encountered in IDUs and hemophiliacs (166,167). In the United States, 9% of HIV-positive individuals are anti-HCV–positive compared to 1% of the general population (166,167). However, loss of HCV antibody may occur with more advanced HIV disease in 7% to 23% of HCV/HIV-positive patients (167), possibly making the seroprevalence of co-infection higher.

A number of differences exist between co-infected patients and those infected with HCV alone, some of which have important consequences for treatment outcomes. In contrast to HIV-negative patients, the HCV RNA in co-infected

patients is positive in 89% of patients rather than 50% to 70% of HIV-negative patients (167). The HCV viral load is also much higher in co-infected patients, especially in those with CD4 lymphocyte counts of less than $200 \times 10^9/mm^3$. Over 50% of co-infected patients will have HCV loads of greater than 10^9 copies/mL as compared to 1.5% of HIV-negative patients (167). Also the total viral load tends to increase at an annual rate of 0.5 log_{10}. Thus, over a 10-year period the HCV viral load will increase 58-fold as compared to threefold in HIV-negative individuals (166). As a consequence of the high viral load and infection with mixed genotypes, the response rates to IFN-α therapy may be reduced.

The rate of progression of fibrosis is higher in patients who are HIV/HCV co-infected. The prevalence of fibrosis scores of 2, 3, or 4 is 60% in HIV/HCV-infected patients as compared to 47% in patients infected with HCV alone (168). In addition, the fibrosis progression rate is higher in the subset of co-infected patients with CD4 lymphocyte counts below 200×10^9 cells/mm^3 (168). As a consequence of the higher fibrosis progression rates, the incidence of cirrhosis is 3.5-fold higher in co-infected patients (166–168). Over a 15-year period 25% of co-infected patients will develop cirrhosis of the liver compared to 6% of HIV-negative HCV-infected patients (167). The time to the development of cirrhosis is also much shorter in co-infected patients, 7 years compared to 23 years in HIV-negative patients (166). Patients infected with HCV alone and who have established cirrhosis have reduced sustained virologic response rates. Co-infected patients, therefore, may be less likely to respond to IFN-α as a consequence of more advanced disease.

Several studies of the treatment of hepatitis C infection in HIV-positive patients have now been performed, and the results of these studies have been summarized in the review by Dieterich and colleagues (166). Treatment of co-infected patients with 12 months of IFN-α produces a complete biochemical response rate that is sustained for up to 8 months after treatment in 38% of co-infected patients compared to 47% in HIV-negative patients (166). However, the sustained virologic response rates have been disappointing, with the majority of patients relapsing after 12 months of follow-up (166). In a study examining response rates to interferon in HIV/HCV–co-infected IDUs, the initial response rate was only 30% in contrast to 75% in HIV-negative HCV-infected patients. The sustained response rates 3 to 6 months after stopping treatment were 15% and 35%, respectively (167). Treatment with higher doses of IFN-α (9 mu daily for 6 to 9 months) has resulted in initial response rates of 55% and sustained response rates of 40% 6 months after stopping therapy (167). At present there is very little information regarding the efficacy of the combination of ribavirin plus IFN-α for the treatment of HCV in co-infected patients, although clinical trials are in progress (166).

Patients with Hepatitis C Virus and Hepatitis B Virus

Patients co-infected with HBV and HCV develop more severe chronic liver disease than patients infected with either HBV or HCV alone (169). The total Scheuer score, portal and lobular inflammation, and fibrosis are all worse in co-infected patients (169,170). In HBV/HCV–co-infected renal allograft recipients, a higher incidence of chronic liver disease has also been noted. Of co-infected patients, 41% developed chronic liver disease as opposed to 24% of patients infected with HBV alone and 26% infected with HCV alone (171).

In addition to the development of more severe liver disease, HBV/HCV–co-infected patients respond poorly to treatment with IFN-α (172). Both biochemical and virologic response rates are lower and relapse rates higher after cessation of treatment than those observed in patients infected with HBV or HCV alone (172). Treatment of HBV/HCV–co-infected patients with the combination of IFN-α plus ribavirin has not been assessed in the clinical trial situation, but theoretically should provide a higher virologic response for HCV.

Newer Therapies

Consensus Interferon

Consensus interferon (CIFN) is a genetically engineered molecule containing the most commonly observed amino acid residues of several natural IFN-α subtypes. Treatment of patients with chronic hepatitis C using CIFN alone has resulted in an end of treatment virologic response of 37% but a sustained virologic response rate of only 12% (173). These results are similar to those obtained with IFN-α alone. CIFN has also been used in the retreatment of chronic hepatitis C in a dose of 9 μg subcutaneously for 48 weeks (174). The sustained virologic response rates are higher after 48 weeks compared to 24 weeks. In patients

who have relapsed after prior IFN-α treatment, the sustained virologic response rate was 58% in contrast to 13% for nonresponders to prior IFN-α treatment (174).

Pegylated Interferon

A recent advance in the treatment of chronic hepatitis C infection has been the development of pegylated interferons, both 2a and 2b. Pegylated IFN-α 2a consists of IFN-α 2a covalently bound to polyethylene glycol (PEG) as a cross-linked 40-kd branched polymer, while IFN-α 2b is a 12- to 15-kd linear polymer. In comparison to standard IFN-α, pegylated IFN-α has a number of advantages, including delayed systemic clearance, with a prolonged serum half-life of 80 to 90 hours compared to 8.5 hours for IFN-α, once weekly administration, and a more consistent and sustained HCV clearance profile (175,176). Sustained virologic responses of 30% to 36% are possible with 48 weeks of treatment of pegylated IFN-α 2a alone. In combination with ribavirin, 84% of patients will have undetectable serum HCV RNA after 24 weeks of treatment, and it is anticipated that this combination will result in greater than 50% sustained virologic responses (176). Pegylated IFN-α 2a appears to be relatively well tolerated, although neutropenia may be more frequent than with IFN-α alone (176).

Gene Therapy: Antisense Oligonucleotides and RNA

Inhibition of HCV has been demonstrated using antisense ODNs directed to the 5′-noncoding region and the translational start codon of the HCV polyprotein (177). *In vitro* studies have shown that these antisense ODNs inhibited HCV RNA transcription levels and core protein translation (178). The wide sequence variability of HCV has confirmed the development of antisense ODN strategies to the 5′- and 3′-noncoding regions and to other conserved sites within the HCV genome.

Similarly, antisense RNA directed to the 5′-noncoding region has also resulted in the inhibition of HCV replication *in vitro* and in transfected cells (179).

Gene Therapy: Ribozymes

Hammerhead ribozymes designed with activity against the HCV RNA plus strand have resulted in almost complete inhibition of HCV RNA synthesis (180). Hammerhead and hairpin ribozymes that target the 5′-noncoding region and inhibit HCV RNA synthesis have also been reported to be very effective (180–182).

Therapeutic Vaccination

Vaccination of chimpanzees chronically infected with HCV genotype 1a or 1b with a vaccine containing recombinant E1 protein of HCV genotype 1b has been claimed to result in an E1 antibody seroconversion together with an improvement of liver histology and elimination of HCV antigens from the liver (183). In addition to the observed humoral E1-specific response, a T-cell proliferative response also occurs that may facilitate the clearance of HCV from the liver (183). Therapeutic vaccination may provide an alternative treatment strategy for chronic hepatitis C infection.

Other approaches for the inhibition of HCV replication based on DNA vaccination for the structural proteins have been investigated. The HCV nucleocapsid is an attractive target since it is highly conserved, and DNA vaccines targeting this region result in strong T-helper and CTL responses (184). Humoral and cellular responses can be substantially enhanced by the addition of genes encoding cytokines like GM-CSF (185). The HCV envelope proteins have also been studied in DNA immunization strategies but generally are less immunogenic (186).

Alternative and Complementary Medicines

Natural remedies including herbal preparations are classified in most countries as food supplements and are exempt from regulations on quality control and proof of efficacy that are required for standard pharmaceuticals (187). Some of these herbal products are promoted for liver disorders and contain molecules often related to flavonoids, which have proven antioxidative, antifibrotic, antiviral, or anticarcinogenic properties, including compounds such as glycyrrhizin, phyllanthin, silibinin, picroside, and baicalein (187). When patients with chronic hepatitis C take these medications in a "supervised environment," most treatments result in normalization of serum ALT, but no effect on HCV RNA levels has been demonstrated (188). Long-term use of glycyrrhizin in chronic hepatitis C has been claimed to be effective in preventing HCC (189). These studies should serve to promote interest in the development of specific hepatotropic drugs as well as novel agents active against HCV.

FUTURE DIRECTIONS

From the preceding discussion it is clear that not all the factors that can reliably predict which patients will or will not respond to a given form of therapy, which patients progress and develop complications, and what the long-term benefits and effects of therapy will actually be have been identified.

Clearly, further definition of response based on disease, stage, and patient and treatment characteristics is needed to determine the degree of benefit for particular patient subgroups. Individualization or tailoring of therapy to key response factors should become the next therapeutic approach in chronic hepatitis C (190) and chronic hepatitis B.

Attempts also need to focus on identifying predictors of clinically relevant outcomes. As the worldwide population with chronic HCV infection ages, clinicians will need to develop accurate tools that predict, and eventually prevent, adverse clinical outcomes, such as the recent report of the association between serum albumin concentration and the development of hepatic complications (191).

The future of antiviral therapy for chronic hepatitis C will be greatly facilitated by the development of a cell culture system for HCV replication. In the meantime, crystallization of the various viral enzymes (192) and successful development of modeled inhibitors (193) should help pave the way for improved treatment. Finally, cellular receptors for HCV have been putatively identified (194,195), making possible targeted strategies for possible prophylactic vaccine approaches.

REFERENCES

1. Locarnini SA, Cunningham AL. Clinical treatment of viral hepatitis. In: Jefferies DJ, DeClercq E, eds. *Antiviral chemotherapy.* New York: Wiley, 1995:441–530.
2. Beasley R. Hepatitis B virus—the major etiology of hepatocellular carcinoma. *Cancer* 1988;61:1942–1956.
3. Chang MH, Chen CJ, Lai MS, et al. Universal hepatitis B vaccination in Taiwan and the incidence of hepatocellular carcinoma in children. Taiwan Childhood Hepatoma Study. *N Engl J Med* 1997;336:1855–1859.
4. Carman WF. The clinical significance of surface antigen variants of hepatitis B virus. *J Virol Hepat* 1997;4 (suppl 1):11–20.
5. Popper H, Roth L, Purcell R, et al. Hepatocarcinogenicity of the woodchuck hepatitis virus. *Proc Natl Acad Sci USA* 1987; 84:866–870.
6. Nassal M, Schaller H. Hepatitis B virus replication—an update. *J Viral Hepat* 1996;3:217–226.
7. Summers J, Smith PM, Horwich AL. Hepadnavirus envelope proteins regulate covalently closed circular DNA amplification. *J Virol* 1990;64:2819–2824.
8. Newbold JE, Xin H, Tencza M, et al. The covalently closed duplex form of the hepadnavirus genome exists in situ as a heterogeneous population of viral minichromosomes. *J Virol* 1995; 69:3350–3357.
9. Main J, Thomas HC. Viral hepatitis. In: Galasso G, Whitley RJ, Merigan TC, eds. *Antiviral agents and human viral diseases,* 4th ed. Philadelphia: Lippincott–Raven, 1997:459–491.
10. Sanchez-Tapias JM, Mas A, Costa J, et al. Recombinant alpha-2c interferon therapy in fulminant viral hepatitis. *J Hepatol* 1987;5:205–210.
11. Tassopoulos NC, Koutelou MG, Polychronaki H, et al. Recombinant interferon-α therapy for acute hepatitis B: a randomized, double-blind, placebo-controlled trial. *J Viral Hepat* 1997;4: 387–394.
12. DiBisceglie AM, Bergasa N, Fong T-L, et al. A randomized controlled trial of recombinant alpha interferon therapy for chronic hepatitis B. *Am J Gastroenterol* 1993;88:1887–1892.
13. Sokal EM, Conjeevaram HS, Roberts EA, et al. Interferon alfa therapy for chronic hepatitis B in children: a multinational randomized controlled trial. *Gastroenterology* 1998;114:988–995.
14. Wong DK, Cheung AM, O'Rourke K, et al. Effect of alpha-interferon treatment in patients with hepatitis Be antigen positive chronic hepatitis B. A meta-analysis. *Ann Intern Med* 1993; 119:312–323.
15. Hoofnagle JH, Peters MG, Mullen KD, et al. Randomised controlled trial of recombinant human α-interferon in patients with chronic hepatitis B. *Gastroenterology* 1988;95:1318–1325.
16. Yokosuka O, Omata M, Imazeki F, et al. Changes of hepatitis B virus DNA in liver and serum caused by recombinant leukocyte interferon treatment: analysis of intrahepatic replicative hepatitis B virus DNA. *Hepatology* 1985;5:728–734.

17. Lok ASF, Ma OCK, Lau JYN. Interferon alfa therapy in patients with chronic hepatitis B virus infection: effects on HBV DNA in the liver. *Gastroenterology* 1991;100:756–761.

18. Hoofnagle JH, Di Bisceglie AM. Drug therapy: the treatment of chronic viral hepatitis. *N Engl J Med* 1997;336:347–356.

19. Lin S-M, Sheen I-S, Chein R-N, et al. Long-term beneficial effect of interferon therapy in patients with chronic hepatitis B virus infection. *Hepatology* 1999;29:971–975.

20. Brunetto MR, Oliveri F, Koehler M, et al. Effect of interferon-α on progression of cirrhosis to hepatocellular carcinoma: a retrospective cohort study. *Lancet* 1998;351:1535–1539.

21. Fattovich G, McIntyre G, Thursz M, et al. Hepatitis B virus precore/core variation and interferon therapy. *Hepatology* 1995;22:1355–1362.

22. Brunetto MR, Giarin M, Saracco G, et al. Hepatitis B virus unable to secrete e antigen and response to interferon in chronic hepatitis B. *Gastroenterology* 1993;105:845–850.

23. Lok ASF, Wu P-C, Lai C-L, et al. A controlled trial of interferon with or without prednisone priming for chronic hepatitis B. *Gastroenterology* 1992;102:2091–2097.

24. Hoofnagle JH, Di Bisceglie AM, Waggoner JG, et al. Interferon alpha for patients with clinically apparent cirrhosis due to hepatitis B. *Gastroenterology* 1993;104:1116–1121.

25. Smalley R, Talmadge J, Oldham R, et al. The thymosins—preclinical and clinical studies with fraction 5 and alpha 1. *Cancer Treat Rev* 1984;11:69–84.

26. Mutchnick MG, Appleman HD, Chung HT, et al. Thymosin treatment of chronic hepatitis B: a placebo-controlled pilot trial. *Hepatology* 1991;14:409–415.

27. Mutchnick MG, Lindsay K, Schiff E, et al. Thymosin α1 treatment of chronic hepatitis B: a multicenter placebo controlled double blind study. *Gastroenterology* 1995;108:A1127.

28. Neidzwiecki D, Luo D, Finn DS, et al. *The efficacy of thymosin alpha 1 in chronic hepatitis B: a meta-analysis.* Data on file. Sci-Clone Pharmaceuticals International Ltd.

29. Michel M. Prospects for active immunotherapies for hepatitis B virus chronic carriers. *Res Virol* 1997;148:95–99.

30. Senturk H, Tabak M, Aktogan M, et al. Therapeutic vaccination with a pre-S2 containing vaccine in chronic hepatitis B: a promising approach. *Hepatology* 1998;28:A1701.

31. Heathcote J, McHutchison J, Lee S, et al. A pilot study of the CY-1899 T-cell vaccine in subjects chronically infected with hepatitis B virus. *Hepatology* 1999;30:531–536.

32. Chow Y-H, Chiang B-L, Lee Y-L, et al. Development of Th1 and Th2 populations and the nature of immune response to hepatitis B virus DNA vaccines can be modulated by codelivery of various cytokine genes. *J Immunol* 1998;160:1320–1329.

33. Torresi J, Locarnini S. Antiviral chemotherapy for the treatment of hepatitis B virus infections. *Gastroenterology* 2000;118(suppl):83–103.

34. Doong S, Tsai C, Schinazi R, et al. Inhibition of the replication of hepatitis B virus in vitro by 2′,3′-dideoxy-3′-thiacytidine and related analogues. *Proc Natl Acad Sci USA* 1991:88;8495–8499.

35. Chang CN, Doong S, Zhou J, et al. Deoxycytidine deaminase-resistant stereoisomer is the active form of (+/−)-2′,3′-dideoxy-3′-thiacytidine in the inhibition of hepatitis B virus replication. *J Biol Chem* 1992;267:13938–13942.

36. Delaney WE, Miller TG, Isom HC. Use of the hepatitis B virus recombinant baculovirus-HepG2 system to study the effects of (−)-2′,3′ dideoxy-3′-thiacytidine on replication of hepatitis B virus and accumulation of covalently closed circular DNA. *Antimicrobial Agents Chemother* 1999;43:2017–2026.

37. Shaw T, Locarnini S. Hepatic purine and pyrimidine metabolism: implications for the antiviral chemotherapy of viral hepatitis. *Liver* 1995;15:169–184.

38. Lai C, Chien R, Leung N, et al. A one-year trial of lamivudine for chronic hepatitis B. Asia Hepatitis Lamivudine Study Group. *N Engl J Med* 1998;339:61–68.

39. Dienstag J, Schiff ER, Wright TL, et al. Lamivudine as initial treatment for chronic hepatitis B in the United States. *N Engl J Med* 1999;341:1256–1263.

40. Dienstag J, Schiff ER, Mitchell M, et al. Extended lamivudine retreatment for chronic hepatitis B: maintenance of viral suppression after discontinuation of therapy. *Hepatology* 1999;30:1082–1087.

41. Liaw Y-F, Chien R-N, Yeh C-T, et al. Acute exacerbation and hepatitis B virus clearance after emergence of YMDD motif mutation during lamivudine therapy. *Hepatology* 1999;30:567–572.

42. Chien RN, Liaw YF, Atkins M. Pretherapy alanine transaminase level as a determinant for hepatitis Be antigen seroconversion during lamivudine therapy in patients with chronic hepatitis B. *Hepatology* 1999;30:770–774.

43. Song B-C, Suh DJ, Lee HC, et al. Seroconversion after lamivudine treatment is not durable in chronic hepatitis B. *Hepatology* 1999;30:abst245.

44. Fontaine H, Driss F, Lagneau J-L, et al. Hepatitis B virus reactivation after lamivudine discontinuation. *Hepatology* 1999;30:abst754.

45. Tassopoulos NC, Volpes R, Pastore G, et al. Efficacy of lamivudine in patients with hepatitis B e antigen-negative/hepatitis B virus DNA-positive (precore mutant) chronic hepatitis B. *Hepatology* 1999;29:889–896.

46. Villeneuve JP, Condreay LD, Willems B et al. Lamivudine treatment for decompensated cirrhosis resulting from chronic hepatitis B. *Hepatology* 2000;31:207–210.

47. Goodman Z, Dhillon AP, Wu PC, et al. Lamivudine treatment reduces progression to cirrhosis in patients with chronic hepatitis B. *J Hepatol* 1999;30(suppl 1):59.

48. Honkoop P, de Man RA, Zondervan PE, et al. Histological improvement in patients with chronic hepatitis B virus infection treated with lamivudine. *Liver* 1997;17:103–106.

49. Marzano A, Debernardi-Venon W, Condreay L, et al. Efficacy of lamivudine re-treatment in a patient with hepatitis B virus (HBV) recurrence after liver transplantation and HBV-DNA breakthrough during the first treatment. *Transplantation* 1998;65:1499–1500.

50. Nery JR, Weppler D, Rodriguez M, et al. Efficacy of lamivudine in controlling hepatitis B virus recurrence after liver transplantation. *Transplantation* 1998;65:1615–1621.

51. Markowitz JS, Martin P, Conrad AJ, et al. Prophylaxis against hepatitis B recurrence following liver transplantation using combination lamivudine and hepatitis B immune globulin. *Hepatology* 1998;28:585–589.

52. Tipples GA, Ma MM, Fischer KP, et al. Mutation in HBV RNA-dependent DNA polymerase confers resistance to lamivudine in vivo. *Hepatology* 1996;24:714–717.

53. De Man RA, Bartholomeusz AI, Niesters HGM, et al. The sequential occurrence of viral mutations in a liver transplant recipient re-infected with hepatitis B: hepatitis B immune globulin escape, famciclovir non-response followed by lamivudine resistance resulting in graft loss. *Hepatology* 1998;29:669–675.

54. Peek S, Toshkov I, Erb H, et al. 3′-thiacytidine (3TC) delays development of hepatocellular carcinoma (HCC) in woodchucks with experimentally induced chronic woodchuck hepatitis virus (WHV) infection. Preliminary results of a lifetime study. *Hepatology* 1997;26:A957.

55. Dienstag J, Perrillo R, Schiff E, et al. A preliminary trial of lamivudine for chronic hepatitis B infection. *N Engl J Med* 1995;333:1657–1661.

56. Honkoop P, De Man RE, Scholte HR, et al. Effect of lamivu-

dine on morphology and function of mitochondria in patients with chronic hepatitis B. *Hepatology* 1997;26:211–215.

57. Bartholomeusz A, Schinazi RF, Locarnini SA. Significance of mutations in the hepatitis B virus polymerase selected by nucleoside analogues and implications for controlling chronic disease. *Viral Hepat Rev* 1998;3:167–187.

58. Ladner SK, Miller TJ, Otto MJ, et al. The hepatitis B virus M539V polymerase variation responsible for 3TC resistance also confers cross resistance to other nucleoside analogues. *Antiviral Chem Chemother* 1998;9:65–72.

59. Ono-Nita SK, Kato N, Shiratori Y, et al. Susceptibility of lamivudine-resistant hepatitis B virus to other reverse transcriptase inhibitors. *J Clin Invest* 1999;103:1635–1640.

60. Fu L, Liu S-H, Cheng Y-C. Sensitivity of L-(–)2′,3′-dideoxythiacytidine resistant hepatitis B virus to other nucleoside analogues. *Biochem Pharmacol* 1999;57:1351–1359.

61. Xiong X, Flores C, Yang H, et al. Mutations in hepatitis B DNA polymerase associated with resistance to lamivudine do not confer resistance to adefovir in vitro. *Hepatology* 1999;28:1669–1673.

62. Yoshida EM, Ma MM, Davis JER, et al. Post-liver transplant allograft reinfection with a lamivudine resistant strain of hepatitis B virus: long-term follow-up. *Can J Gastroenterol* 1998;12:125–129.

63. Melegari M, Scaglioni PP, Wands J. Hepatitis B virus mutants associated with 3TC and famciclovir administration are replication defective. *Hepatology* 1998;27:628–633.

64. Naesens L, Snoeck R, Andrei G, et al. HPMPC [cidofovir], PMEA [adefovir] and related acyclic nucleoside phosphonate analogues: a review of their pharmacology and clinical potential in the treatment of viral infections. *Antiviral Chem Chemother* 1997;8:1–23.

65. Heijtink R, Kruining J, de Wilde G, et al. Inhibitory effects of acyclic nucleoside phosphonates on human hepatitis B virus and duck hepatitis B virus infections in tissue culture. *Antimicrob Agents Chemother* 1994;38:2180–2182.

66. Heijtink R, De Wilde G, Kruning J, et al. Inhibitory effect of 9-[2-phosphonoyl-methoxyethyl]-adenine (PMEA) on human and duck hepatitis B virus infection. *Antiviral Res* 1993;21:141–153.

67. Nicoll A, Colledge D, Toole J, et al. Inhibition of duck hepatitis B virus replication by 9-[2 phosphonylmethoxyethyl] adenine, an acyclic phosphonate nucleoside analogue. *Antimicrob Agents Chemother* 1998;42:3130–3135.

68. Gilson R, Chopra K, Murray-Lyon I, et al. A placebo controlled phase I/II study of adefovir dipivoxil [Bis POM PMEA] in patients with chronic hepatitis B infection. *Hepatology* 1996;24:A620.

69. Jeffers L, Heathcote E, Wright T, et al. A phase II dose-ranging, placebo-controlled trial of adefovir dipivoxil for the treatment of chronic hepatitis B virus infection. *Antiviral Res* 1998;37:A197(abst).

70. Deeks SG, Collier A, Lalezra J, et al. The safety and efficacy of adefovir dipivoxil, a novel anti-human immunodeficiency virus (HIV) therapy, in HIV-infected adults: a randomised, double-blind, placebo-controlled trial. *J Infect Dis* 1997;176:1517–1523.

71. Genovesi EV, Lamb L, Medina I, et al. Efficacy of the carbocyclic 2′ deoxyguanosine nucleoside BMS-200475 in the woodchuck model of hepatitis B virus infection. *Antimicrob Agents Chemother* 1998;42:3209–3217.

72. Innaimo S, Seifer M, Bisacchi G, et al. Identification of BMS-200475 as a potent and selective inhibitor of hepatitis B virus. *Antimicrob Agents Chemother* 1997;41:1444–1448.

73. Furman PA, Davis M, Liotta DC, et al. The anti-hepatitis B virus activities, cytotoxicities, and anabolic profiles of the (–)

and (+) enantiomers of *cis*-5-fluoro-1-(2 [hydroxymethyl]-1,3-oxythiolan-5-yl)-cytosine (FTC). *Antimicrob Agents Chemother* 1992;36:2686–2692.

74. Paff MT, Averett DR, Prus KL, et al. Intracellular metabolism of (–) and (+)-cis-5-fluoro-1-[2-(hydroxymethyl) 1,3-oxathiolan-5-yl]cytosine in HepG2 derivative 2.2.15 (subclone P5A) cells. *Antimicrob Agents Chemother* 1994;38:1230–1238.

75. Frick LW, St. John L, Taylor LC, et al. Pharmacokinetics, oral bioavailability, and metabolic disposition in rats of (–)-cis-5-fluoro-1-[2-(hydroxymethyl)-1,3-oxathiolan 5-yl] cytosine, a nucleoside analog active against human immunodeficiency virus and hepatitis B virus. *Antimicrob Agents Chemother* 1993;37:2285–2292.

76. Fischer KP, Tyrrell DL. Generation of duck hepatitis B virus polymerase mutants through site-directed mutagenesis which demonstrate resistance to lamivudine ((–)-beta-L-2′, 3′-dideoxy-3′-thiacytidine) in vitro. *Antimicrobial Agents Chemother* 1996;40:1957–1960.

77. Vere Hodge R. Review: antiviral portrait series number 3. Famciclovir and penciclovir. The mode of action of famciclovir including its conversion to penciclovir. *Antiviral Chem Chemother* 1993;4:67–84.

78. Tsiquaye K, Slomka M, Maung M. Oral famciclovir against duck hepatitis B virus replication in hepatic and nonhepatic tissues of ducklings infected in ovo. *J Med Virol* 1994;42:306–310.

79. Korba BE, Boyd MR. Penciclovir is a selective inhibitor of hepatitis B virus replication in cultured human hepatoblastoma cells. *Antimicrob Agents Chemother* 1996;40:1282–1284.

80. Shaw T, Locarnini SA. Preclinical aspects of lamivudine and famciclovir against hepatitis B virus. *J Viral Hepat* 1999;6:89–106.

81. Lin E, Luscombe C, Wang Y, et al. The guanine nucleoside analog penciclovir is active against chronic duck hepatitis B virus infection in vivo. *Antimicrob Agents Chemother* 1996;40:413–418.

82. Main J, Brown L, Howells C, et al. A double blind, placebo-controlled study to assess the effect of famciclovir on virus replication in patients with chronic hepatitis B virus infection. *J Viral Hepat* 1996;3:211–215.

83. Benner K, Rosen H, Flora K. Famciclovir treatment of decompensated HBV cirrhosis. *Hepatology* 1996;24:A622.

84. Boker K, Ringe B, Kruger M, et al. Prostaglandin E plus famciclovir—a new concept for the treatment of severe hepatitis B after liver transplantation. *Transplantation* 1994;57:1706–1708.

85. Lau GK, Liang R, Wu PC, et al. Use of famciclovir to prevent HBV reactivation in HBsAg-positive recipients after allogeneic bone marrow transplantation. *J Hepatol* 1998;28:359–368.

86. Cirelli R, Herne K, McCrary M, et al. Famciclovir: review of clinical efficacy and safety. *Antiviral Res* 1996;29:141–151.

87. Aye T, Bartholomeusz A, Shaw T, et al. Hepatitis B virus polymerase mutations during antiviral therapy in a patient following liver transplantation. *J Hepatol* 1997;26:1148–1153.

88. Tillmann HL, Trautwein C, Bock T, et al. Mutational analysis of hepatitis B virus on sequential therapy with famciclovir and lamivudine in patients with hepatitis B virus reinfection occurring under HBIG immunoglobulin after liver transplantation. *Hepatology* 1999;30:244–256.

89. Luscombe C, Pedersen J, Bowden S, et al. Alterations in intrahepatic expression of duck hepatitis B viral markers with ganciclovir chemotherapy. *Liver* 1994;14:182–192.

90. Gish RG, Lau JY, Brooks L, et al. Ganciclovir treatment of hepatitis B virus infection in liver transplant recipients. *Hepatology* 1996;23:1–7.

91. Hadziyannis SJ, Manesis EK, Papakonstantinou A. Oral ganciclovir treatment in chronic hepatitis B virus infection: a pilot study. *Hepatology* 1999;31:210–214.

92. Seifer M, Hamatake RK, Colonno RJ, et al. In vitro inhibition of hepadnavirus polymerases by the triphosphates of BMS-200475 and lobucavir. *Antimicrob Agents Chemother* 1998;28: 3200–3208.

93. Bloomer J, Chan R, Sherman M, et al. A preliminary study of lobucavir for chronic hepatitis B. *Hepatology* 1996;26:A1199.

94. Yamanaka G, Tuomari A, Hagen M, et al. Selective activity and cellular pharmacology of [1R-1 alpha,2 beta,3 alpha]-9-[2,3-bis[hydroxymethyl]cyclobutyl] guanine in herpesvirus-infected cells. *Mol Pharmacol* 1991;40:446–453.

95. Nowak MA, Bornhoeffer S, Hill A, et al. Viral dynamics in hepatitis B virus infection. *Proc Natl Acad Sci USA* 1996;93: 4398–4402.

96. Zeuzem S, de Man RA, Honkoop P, et al. Dynamics of hepatitis B infection *in vivo*. *J Hepatol* 1997;27:431–436.

97. Tsiang M, Rooney JF, Toola JJ, et al. Biphase clearance kinetics of hepatitis B virus from patients during adefovir dipivoxil therapy. *Hepatology* 1999;29:1863–1869.

98. Colledge D, Locarnini S, Shaw T. Synergistic inhibition of hepadnaviral replication by lamivudine in combination with penciclovir in vitro. *Hepatology* 1997;26:216–225.

99. Lau GKK, Tsiang M, Hou J, et al. Clearance kinetics of HBV infection in Chinese patients: lamivudine versus lamivudine plus famciclovir. *Hepatology* 1999;30:A732.

100. Rasi G, Mutchnick MG, Di Virgilio D, et al. Combination low-dose lymphoblastoid interferon and thymosin alpha 1 therapy in the treatment of chronic hepatitis B. *J Viral Hepat* 1996; 3:191–196.

101. Lau G, Kwok A, Karlberg J, et al. A twenty-six weeks trial of thymosin α1 plus famciclovir in the treatment of Chinese immune tolerant adult patients with chronic hepatitis B. *Hepatology* 1998; 28(4,pt 2):216A.

102. Leung Y, So T. Treatment of chronic hepatitis B using thymosin alpha 1 and a combination of two nucleoside analogues, lamivudine and famciclovir. *Hepatology* 1998;28:A216.

103. Marques AR, Lau DT, McKenzie R, et al. Combination therapy with famciclovir and interferon-alpha for the treatment of chronic hepatitis B. *J Infect Dis* 1998;178:1483–1487.

104. Mutimer D, Naoumov N, Honkoop P, et al. Combination alpha-interferon and lamivudine therapy for alpha-interferon-resistant chronic hepatitis B infection: results of a pilot study. *J Hepatol* 1998;28:923–929.

105. Cotonat T, Quiroga JA, Lopez-Alcorocho JM, et al. Pilot study of combination therapy with ribavirin and interferon alfa for the retreatment of chronic hepatitis B e antibody-positive patients. *Hepatology* 2000;31:502–506.

106. Housset C, Pol S, Carnot F, et al. Interactions between human immunodeficiency virus 1, hepatitis delta virus and hepatitis B virus infections in 260 chronic carriers of hepatitis B virus. *Hepatology* 1992;15:578.

107. Hadler SC, Judson FN, O'Malley PM, et al. Outcome of hepatitis B virus infection in homosexual men and its relation to prior human immunodeficiency virus infection. *J Infect Dis* 1991;163:454–459.

108. Perrillo RP, Regenstein FG, Roodman ST. Chronic hepatitis B in asymptomatic homosexual men with antibody to the human immunodeficiency virus. *Ann Intern Med* 1986;105: 382–383.

109. Scharschmidt B, Held M, Hollander H, et al. Hepatitis B in patients with HIV infection: relationship to AIDS and patient survival. *Ann Intern Med* 1992;117:837.

110. Ockenga J, Tillman HL, Trautwein C, et al. Hepatitis B and C in HIV-infected patients. Prevalence and prognostic value. *J Hepatol* 1997;27:18–24.

111. McDonald JA, Caruso L, Karayiannis P, et al. Diminished responsiveness of male homosexual chronic hepatitis B virus carriers with HTLV-III antibodies to recombinant alpha-interferon. *Hepatology* 1987;7:719–723.

112. Nagai K, Hosaka H, Nakamura N, et al. Highly active anti-retroviral therapy used to treat concurrent hepatitis B and human immunodeficiency virus infections. *J Gastroenterol* 1999;34:275–281.

113. Benhamou Y, Bochet M, Thibault V, et al. Long-term incidence of hepatitis B virus resistance to lamivudine in human immunodeficiency virus-infected patients. *Hepatology* 1999;30: 1302–1306.

114. Bessesen M, Ives D, Condreay L, et al. Chronic active hepatitis B exacerbations in human immunodeficiency virus-infected patients following development of resistance to or withdrawal of lamivudine. *Clin Infect Dis* 1999;28:1032–1035.

115. Thibault V, Benhamou Y, Seguret C, et al. Hepatitis B virus (HBV) mutations associated with resistance to lamivudine in patients coinfected with HBV and human immunodeficiency virus. *J Clin Microbiol* 1999;37:3013–3016.

116. Colin JF, Cazals-Hatem D, Loriot MA, et al. Influence of human immunodeficiency virus infection on chronic hepatitis B in homosexual men. *Hepatology* 1999;29:1306–1310.

117. Weizsacker VF, Weiland S, Kock J, et al. Gene therapy for chronic viral hepatitis: ribozymes, antisense oligonucleotides, and dominant negative mutants. *Hepatology* 1997;26:251–255.

118. Korba BE, Gerin J. Antisense oligonucleotides are effective inhibitors of hepatitis B virus replication in vitro. *Antiviral Res* 1995;28:225–242.

119. Wu J, Gerber M. The inhibitory effects of antisense RNA on hepatitis B virus surface antigen synthesis. *J Gen Virol* 1997;78: 641–647.

120. Soni PN, Broen D, Saffie R, et al. Biodistribution, stability, and antiviral efficacy of liposome-entrapped phosphothiorate antisense oligodeoxynucleotides in ducks for the treatment of chronic duck hepatitis B virus infection. *Hepatology* 1998;28:1402–1410.

121. Bartholomew RM, Carmicheal EP, Findeis MA, et al. Targeted delivery of antisense DNA in woodchuck hepatitis virus-infected woodchucks. *J Viral Hepat* 1995;2:273–278.

122. Cech T. The chemistry of self-splicing RNA and RNA enzymes. *Science* 1987;236:1532–1539.

123. Haseloff J, Gerlach W. Simple RNA enzymes with new and highly specific endoribonuclease activities. *Nature* 1988;334: 585–591.

124. Welch P, Tritz R, Yei S, et al. Intracellular application of hairpin ribozyme genes against hepatitis B virus. *Gene Ther* 1997;4: 736–743.

125. Wands J, Geissler M, Putlitz J, et al. Nucleic acid-based antiviral and gene therapy of chronic hepatitis B infection. *J Gastroenterol Hepatol* 1997;12(suppl):354–369.

126. Rizzetto M. The delta agent. *Hepatology* 1983;3:729–737.

127. Lin HH, Liaw YF, Chen TJ, et al. Natural course of patients with chronic B hepatitis following acute delta virus superinfection. *Liver* 1989;9:129–134.

128. Bonino F, Heermann K-H, Rizzetto M, et al. Hepatitis delta virus: protein composition of delta antigen and its hepatitis B virus-derived envelope. *J Virol* 1985;58:945–950.

129. Farci P, Mandas A, Coinana A, et al. Treatment of chronic hepatitis D with interferon alpha-2a. *N Engl J Med* 1994;330: 88–94.

130. Rosina F, Marzano A, Garripoli A, et al. Chronic type D hepatitis: clearance of hepatitis B surface antigen during and after treatment with alfa interferon. *Hepatology* 1990;12:883.

131. Lau DT-Y, Doo E, Park Y, et al. Lamivudine for chronic delta hepatitis. *Hepatology* 1999;30:546–549.

132. Huang SB, Lai MMC. Isoprenylation mediates direct protein-protein interactions between hepatitis large delta antigen and hepatitis B virus surface antigen. *J Virol* 1993;67:7659–7662.

133. Glenn JS. Shutting the door on hepatitis Delta virus (HDV): Sensitivity to prenylation inhibition prompts new therapeutic strategy. *Viral Hepat Rev* 1999;5:13–26.

134. Ottobrelli A, Marzano A, Smedlie A, et al. Patterns of delta virus reinfection and disease in liver transplantation. *Gastroenterol* 1991;101:1649–1655.

135. Samuel D, Zignego AI, Reynes M, et al. Long-term clinical and virological outcome after liver transplantation for cirrhosis caused by chronic delta hepatitis. *Hepatology* 1995;21:333–339.

136. Alter MJ. The epidemiology of acute and chronic hepatitis C. *Clin Liver Dis* 1997;1:559.

137. Simmonds P. Variability of hepatitis C virus. *Hepatology* 1995;21:570–582.

138. Shimizu YK, Iwamoto A, Hijikata M, et al. Evidence for *in vitro* replication of hepatitis C virus genome in a human T-cell line. *Proc Natl Acad Sci USA* 1992;89:5477–5481.

139. Chu PWG, Westaway EG. Characterization of Kunjin virus RNA-dependent RNA polymerase: reinitiation of synthesis *in vitro*. *Virology* 1987;157:330–337.

140. Samuel CE. Mechanisms of the antiviral action of interferons. *Prog Nucleic Acid Res Mol Biol* 1988;35:27–72.

141. McHutchison JG, Gordon SC, Schiff ER, et al. Interferon alfa-2b alone or in combination with ribavirin as initial treatment for chronic hepatitis C. Hepatitis Interventional Therapy Group. *N Engl J Med* 1998;339:1485–1492.

142. Poynard T, Marcellin P, Lee SS, et al. Randomised trial of interferon alpha2b plus ribavirin for 48 weeks or for 24 weeks versus interferon alpha2b plus placebo for 48 weeks for treatment of chronic infection with hepatitis C virus. International Hepatitis Interventional Therapy Group. *Lancet* 1998;352:1426–1432.

143. Omata M, Yokosuka O, Takano S, et al. Resolution of acute hepatitis C after therapy with natural beta interferon. *Lancet* 1991;338:914–915.

144. Lampertico P, Rumi M, Romeo R, et al. A multicenter randomized controlled trial of recombinant interferon-α(2b in patients with acute transfusion-associated hepatitis C. *Hepatology* 1994;19:19–22.

145. Hoofnagle JH, Mullen KD, Jones DB, et al. Treatment of chronic non-A, non-B hepatitis with recombinant human alpha interferon. *N Engl J Med* 1986;315:1575–1578.

146. Marcellin P, Boyer N, Giostra E, et al. Recombinant human alpha-interferon in patients with chronic non-A, non-B hepatitis: a multicenter randomized controlled trial from France. *Hepatology* 1991;13:393–397.

147. Causse X, Godinot H, Chevallier M, et al. Comparison of 1 or 3 MU of interferon alfa-2b and placebo in patients with chronic non-A, non-B hepatitis. *Gastroenterology* 1991;101:497–502.

148. Shindo M, Di Bisceglie AM, Cheung L, et al. Decrease in serum hepatitis C viral RNA during alpha interferon therapy for chronic hepatitis C. *Ann Intern Med* 1991;115:700–704.

149. Jouet P, Roudot-Thoraval F. Comparative efficacy of interferon alfa in cirrhotic and noncirrhotic patients with non-A, non-B, C hepatitis. *Gastroenterology* 1994;106:686–690.

150. Shindo M, Arai K, Sokawa Y, et al. Hepatic hepatitis C virus RNA as a predictor of a long-term response to interferon-alpha therapy. *Ann Intern Med* 1995;122:586–591.

151. Poynard T, Leroy V, Cohard M, et al. Meta-analysis of interferon randomised trials in the treatment of viral hepatitis C: effects of dose and duration. *Hepatology* 1996;24:778–789.

152. Poynard T, Bedossa P, Chevallier M, et al. A comparison of three interferon alfa-2b regimens for the long-term treatment of chronic non-A, non-B hepatitis. Multicenter Study Group. *N Engl J Med* 1995;332:1457–1462.

153. Di Bisceglie AM, Conjeevaram HS, Fried MW, et al. Ribavirin as therapy for chronic hepatitis C. A randomized, double-blind, placebo-controlled trial. *Ann Intern Med* 1995;123:897–903.

154. Lai MY, Kao JH, Yang PM, et al. Long-term efficacy of ribavirin plus interferon alfa in the treatment of chronic hepatitis C. *Gastroenterology* 1996;111:1307–1312.

155. Martinot-Peignoux M, Marcellin P, Pouteau M, et al. Pretreatment serum hepatitis C virus RNA levels and hepatitis C virus genotype are the main and independent prognostic factors of sustained response to interferon alfa therapy in chronic hepatitis C. *Hepatology* 1995;2:1050–1056.

156. Mahaney K, Tedeschi V, Maertens G, et al. Genotypic analysis of hepatitis C virus in American patients. *Hepatology* 1994;20:1405–1411.

157. Schalm SW, Weiland O, Hansen BE, et al. Interferon-ribavirin for chronic hepatitis C with and without cirrhosis: analysis of individual patient data of six controlled trials. *Gastroenterology* 1999;117:408–413.

158. Serfaty L, Chazouilleres O, Pawlotsky JM, et al. Interferon alfa therapy in patients with chronic hepatitis C and persistently normal aminotransferase activity. *Gastroenterology* 1996;110:291–295.

159. Sangiovanni A, Morales R, Spinzi G, et al. Interferon alfa treatment of HCV RNA carriers with persistently normal transaminase levels: a pilot randomized controlled study. *Hepatology* 1998;27:853–856.

160. Neumann AU, Lam NP, Dahari H, et al. Hepatitis C viral dynamics in vivo and the antiviral efficacy of interferon-alpha therapy. *Science* 1998;282:103–107.

161. Marcellin P, Pouteau M, Martinot-Peignoux M, et al. Lack of benefit of escalating dosage of interferon alfa in patients with chronic hepatitis C. *Gastroenterology* 1995;109:156–165.

162. Bekkering FC, Brouwer JT, Leroux-Roels G, et al. Ultrarapid hepatitis C virus clearance by daily high-dose interferon in non-responders to standard therapy. *J Hepatol* 1998;28:960–964.

163. Marcellin P, Boyer N, Pouteau M, et al. Retreatment with interferon-alpha of chronic hepatitis C virus infection. *Lancet* 1994;344:690–691.

164. Davis GL, Esteban-Mur R, Rustgi V, et al. Interferon alfa-2b alone or in combination with ribavirin for the treatment of relapse of chronic hepatitis C. *N Engl J Med* 1998;339:1493–1499.

165. Bresci G, Parisi G, Banti S, et al. Re-treatment of interferon-resistant patients with chronic hepatitis C with interferon-alpha. *J Viral Hepat* 1995;2:155–158.

166. Dieterich DT, Purow JM, Rajapakasa R. Activity of combination therapy with interferon alfa-2b plus ribavirin in chronic hepatitis C patients co-infected with HIV. *Semin Liver Dis* 1999;19(suppl 1):88–94.

167. Zylberberg H, Pol S. Reciprocal interaction between human immunodeficiency virus and hepatitis C viral infections. *Clin Infect Dis* 1996;23:1117–1125.

168. Benhamou Y, Bochet M, Di Martino V, et al. Liver fibrosis progression in human immunodeficiency virus and hepatitis C virus coinfected patients. *Hepatology* 1999;30:1054–1058.

169. Weltman MD, Brotodihardjo A, Crew EB, et al. Coinfection with hepatitis B and C or B, C and delta viruses results in severe chronic liver disease and responds poorly to interferon-alpha treatment. *J Virol Hepat* 1995;2:39–45.

170. Huang EJ, Wright TL, Lake JR, et al. Hepatitis B and C coinfections and persistent hepatitis B infections: Clinical outcome and liver pathology after transplantation. *Hepatology* 1996;23:396–404.

171. Durlik M, Gaciong Z, Soulch L, et al. Clinical course of concomitant HBV and HCV infection in renal allograft recipients. *Ann Transplant* 1996;1:11–12.

172. Zignego AL, Fontana R, Puliti S, et al. Impaired response to alpha interferon in patients with an inapparent hepatitis B and hepatitis C virus coinfection. *Arch Virol* 1997;142: 535–544.

173. Tong MJ, Reddy KR, Lee WM, et al. Treatment of chronic hepatitis C with consensus interferon: a multicenter, randomized, controlled trial. *Hepatology* 1997;26:747–754.

174. Heathcote EJ, Keeffe EB, Lee SS, et al. Re-treatment of chronic hepatitis C with consensus interferon. *Hepatology* 1998;27: 1136–1143.

175. Algranati NE, Sy S, Modi M. A branched methoxy 40 kDa polyethylene glycol (PEG) moiety optimises the pharmacokinetics (PK) of PEGinterferon α-2A (PEG-IFN) and may explain its enhanced efficacy in chronic hepatitis C (CHC). *Hepatology* 1999;4:A120.

176. Sulkowski M. Combination therapy with PEG interferon α-2A (PEG-IFN) and ribavirin in the treatment of patients with chronic hepatitis C (CHC): a phase II open label study. *Hepatology* 1999;24:A145.

177. Alt M, Renz R, Hofschneider PH, et al. Specific inhibition of hepatitis C viral gene expression by antisense phosphothioate oligodeoxynucleotides. *Hepatology* 1995;22:707–717.

178. Hanecak R, Brown-Driver V, Fox MC, et al. Antisense oligonucleotide inhibition of hepatitis C virus gene expression in transformed hepatocytes. *J Virol* 1996;70:5203–5212.

179. Putlitz JZ, Encke J, Wands JR. The use of antisense and other molecular approaches to therapy of chronic viral hepatitis. *Viral Hepat Rev* 1998;4:207–227.

180. Lieber A, He CY, Polyak SJ, et al. Elimination of hepatitis C virus RNA in infected human hepatocytes by adenovirus-mediated expression of ribozymes. *J Virol* 1996;70:8782–8791.

181. Sakamoto N, Wu CH, Wu GY, et al. Intracellular cleavage of hepatitis C virus RNA and inhibition of viral protein translation by hammerhead ribozymes. *J Clin Invest* 1996;98: 2720–2728.

182. Welch PJ, Tritz R, Yei S, et al. A potential therapeutic application of hairpin ribozymes: in vitro and in vivo studies of gene therapy for hepatitis C virus infection. *Gene Ther* 1996;3: 994–1001.

183. Depla E, Priem S, Verschoor E, et al. Therapeutic vaccination of chronically infected chimpanzees with the HCV E1 protein. *Hepatology* 1999;30:408A.

184. Lagging LM, Meyer K, Hoft D, et al. Immune response to plasmid DNA encoding the hepatitis C virus core protein. *J Virol* 1995;69:5859–5863.

185. Geissler M, Geisen A, Tokushige K, et al. Enhancement of cellular and humoral immune responses to hepatitis C virus core protein using DNA-based vaccines augmented with cytokine-expressing plasmids. *J Immunol* 1997;158:1231–1237.

186. Saito T, Sherman GJ, Kurokohchi K, et al. Plasmid DNA-based immunisation for hepatitis C virus structural proteins: immune responses in mice. *Gastroenterology* 1997;112:14–20.

187. Schuppan D, Jia J-D, Brinkhaus B, et al. Herbal products for liver diseases: a therapeutic challenge for the new millenium. *Hepatology* 1999;30:1099–1104.

188. van Rossum TGJ, Vulto AG, Hop WCJ, et al. Intravenous glycyrrhizin for the treatment of chronic hepatitis C: a double-blind, randomized, placebo-controlled phase I/II trial. *J Gastroenterol Hepatol* 1999;14:1093–1099.

189. Arase Y, Ikeda K, Murashima N, et al. The long term efficacy of glycyrrhizin in chronic hepatitis C patients. *Am Cancer Soc* 1997;79:1494–1500.

190. Poynard T, McHutchison J, Goodman Z, et al. Is an "a la carte" combination interferon alfa-2b plus ribavirin regimen possible for the first line treatment in patients with chronic hepatitis C? *Hepatology* 2000;31:211–218.

191. Khan MH, Farrell GC, Byth K, et al. Which patients with hepatitis C develop liver complications? *Hepatology* 2000;31: 513–520.

192. Lesburg CA, Cable MB, Ferrari E, et al. Crystal structure of the RNA-dependent RNA polymerase from hepatitis C virus reveals a fully encircled active site. *Nat Struct Biol* 1999;6: 937–943.

193. DiMarco S, Rizzi M, Volpari C, et al. Inhibition of the hepatitis C virus NS3/4A protease. *J Biol Chem* 2000;275:7152–7157.

194. Pileri P, Uematsu Y, Campagnoli S, et al. Binding of hepatitis C virus to CD81. *Science* 1998;282:938–941.

195. Agnello V, Abel G, Elfahal M, et al. Hepatitis C virus and other flaviviridae viruses enter cells via low density lipoprotein receptor. *Proc Natl Acad Sci USA* 1999;96:12766–12771.

The Liver: Biology and Pathobiology, Fourth Edition, edited by I. M. Arias, J. L. Boyer, F. V. Chisari, N. Fausto, D. Schachter, and D. A. Shafritz.
Lippincott Williams & Wilkins, Philadelphia © 2001.

HORIZONS

TISSUE ENGINEERING OF THE LIVER

ANTONIA E. STEPHEN
ROBERT LANGER
JOSEPH P. VACANTI

The liver is a complex organ that is responsible for performing many vital functions including bile synthesis, detoxification, energy metabolism and production of proteins such as clotting factors. Lack of a certain level of liver function is not compatible with human life. Twenty-six thousand people die each year from end-stage liver disease in the United States at an estimated annual cost of $9 billion (1). Options currently available for treating patients with liver failure are limited. Patients with renal failure are placed on dialysis, and diabetics with pancreatic islet cell failure receive replacement insulin via subcutaneous injection. Although these therapies are far from perfect, they provide treatment and function as a bridge to transplantation. Unlike these organ failure support modalities, there are no options short of transplantation for treating many patients with liver failure.

Orthotopic liver transplantation is the only treatment currently in use for treating many patients with liver failure. Major advances in the development of drugs, surgical procedures, and medical equipment have improved care of these patients. Despite remarkable progress, liver transplantation has serious limitations. A major problem is the shortage of donor organs. Unfortunately, up to 25% of patients with liver failure die annually while waiting for a suitable organ. The donor shortage is particularly problematic for the pediatric patient population in which congenital diseases are a leading cause of organ failure. Even if a patient is fortunate enough to receive an organ in a timely fashion, liver transplantation has significant morbidity and mortality. Patients who receive an allograft are required to be on immunosuppression for life and remain at risk of contracting serious infections. Additional complications include graft rejection, biliary leaks, hypercoagulability, and risks associated with a major operation.

New treatments are being pursued in an attempt to meet the needs of these patients (see Chapters 56 and 57). These include transplantation of autologous or allogenic hepatocytes, *ex vivo* or *in vivo* liver-directed gene therapy, xenotransplantation, extracorporeal bioartificial liver assist devices and tissue engineering of replacement liver tissue.

INTRODUCTION TO TISSUE ENGINEERING

History

Scientific experimentation using the general concept of tissue engineering was attempted as far back as 1933, when investigators encased mouse tumor cells in a polymer mem-

A. E. Stephen: Laboratory for Tissue Engineering and Organ Fabrication, Harvard Medical School, Boston, Massachusetts 02115; Department of Surgery, Massachusetts General Hospital, Boston, Massachusetts 02114.

R. Langer: Department of Chemical Engineering, Harvard–MIT Division of Health Science and Technology, Massachusetts Institute of Technology, Cambridge, Massachusetts 02139.

J. P. Vacanti: Department of Pediatric Surgery, Harvard Medical School; and Department of Pediatric Surgery, Massachusetts General Hospital, Boston, Massachusetts 02114.

brane and inserted them in the abdominal cavity of a pig. The cells were not killed by the pig's immune system (2). During the next several years there were major advancements in cell biology and polymer chemistry which set the stage for the field of tissue engineering. In 1975, pancreatic islet cells in semipermeable membranes were used for glucose control in diabetics. In the past two decades, tissue engineering has greatly expanded to include virtually every tissue in the human body. Tissue-engineered skin substitutes are generated by seeding fibroblast cells onto a collagen scaffold which serves as a neo-dermis. The end result is a skin construct consisting of dermis and epidermis. Clinical studies of patients with skin loss from burns, diabetic ulcers or dermatologic surgery have demonstrated the usefulness of these products (2).

Tissue Engineering

Tissue engineering is an interdisciplinary field that combines principles of engineering and the life sciences toward the development of biological substitutes that restore, maintain, or improve tissue function (3). Although there are different approaches to the creation of new tissue, most investigators use cells combined with matrices. The process begins with the *in vitro* culture of isolated cells. These cells are then seeded onto a matrix consisting of polymers or collagen, the protein which forms scaffolding in normal human tissue. The matrix provides mechanical support for the cells and guides their structural development. Once the cells are seeded onto the polymer, the matrix–cell construct

is implanted into the host. The location of implantation depends upon what type of tissue is being engineered. The construct can be implanted as a closed system which is isolated from the host or as an open system which is integrated into the host. In open systems of cell transplantation, transplanted cells are in direct contact with the recipient and become incorporated into the host. Closed and open systems are depicted in Figures 58.1 and 58.2. Examples of both are described below. In the open system, the matrix degrades over time, leaving only the new tissue in place in the host. Key issues in this process include the type of matrix used and the cells chosen for implantation.

Polymer Matrices Used in Tissue Engineering

The matrix used in tissue engineering creates and maintains a space for formation of the tissue and guides its structural development. Important characteristics of the matrix include mechanical strength, biodegradability and high surface-to-volume ratio. The surface-to-volume ratio ensures

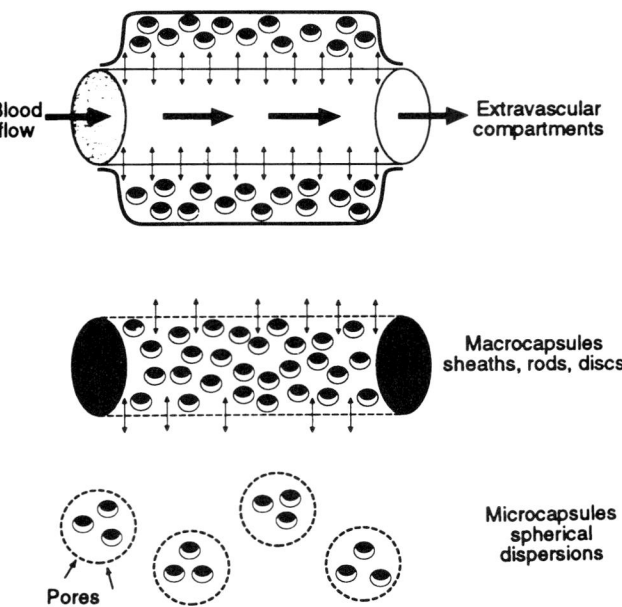

FIGURE 58.1. Three common closed system configurations for cell transplant devices. (From Langer R, Vacanti JP. Tissue engineering. *Science* 1993;260:920–926, with permission.)

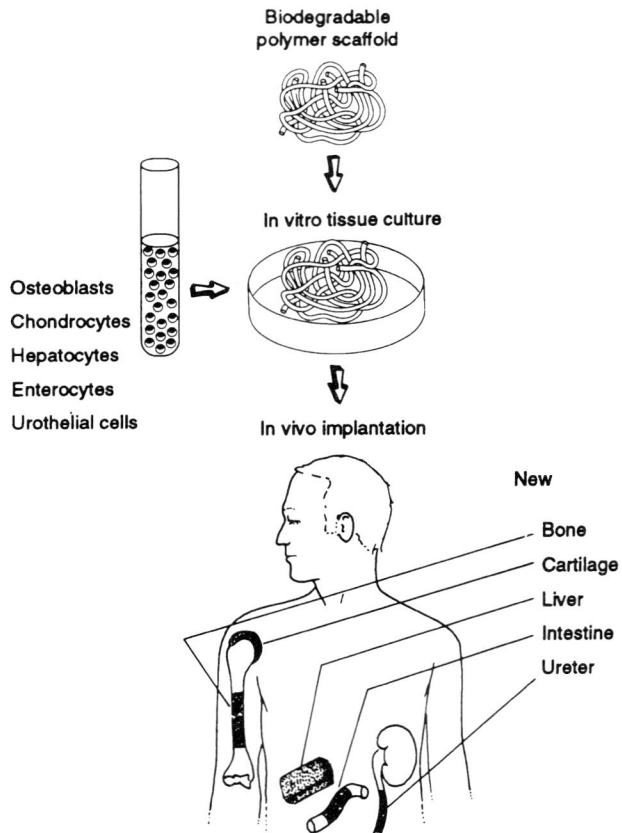

FIGURE 58.2. Three-dimensional highly porous scaffolds composed of synthetic polymers for cell transplant devices. (From Langer R, Vacanti JP. Tissue engineering. *Science* 1993;260: 920–926, with permission.)

adequate delivery of nutrients to cells as they grow and pro-liferate on the matrix. In addition, biocompatibility in the host and cell-adhesiveness are necessary to ensure survival of the mammalian cells on the matrix. The polymers are porous, allowing diffusion of oxygen and nutrients to the implanted cells. Synthetic materials such as lactic-polygly-colic acid or polyacrylonitrile-polyvinyl chloride and nat-ural materials such as collagen, hydroxyapatite or alginate are all in use, often in combination. Most early experiments in tissue engineering used polyglycolic acid polymers, a material used in surgical practice as dissolvable suture. The polymers can be fabricated into specific shapes which are designed for use in tissue engineered heart valves, blood ves-sels, or cartilage and bone. The shapes can be simple, such as a tube for manufacture of intestine or blood vessels, or more complex, such as that used to engineer a nose or ear. The use of natural materials in combination with synthetic polymers has been investigated. For example, coating poly-glycolic acid polymers with collagen increases cell adhesive-ness. The incorporation of specific growth factors into the polymer has also been investigated. Epidermal growth fac-tor, in a slow-release form, increases vascularization and engraftment of liver cells in animal models (2).

Cells Used in Tissue Engineering

The cell type chosen for use in tissue engineering is critical. In laboratory studies, progenitor cells from syngeneic ani-mals are harvested from the tissue of interest and seeded onto the polymer scaffold. This construct is then implanted into an animal of the same syngeneic strain. In clinical prac-tice, the cells are generally derived from the patient or close relatives. For example, cells could be isolated from a healthy site in a patient, expanded *in vitro*, and reimplanted. Given that such cells may not always be readily available or appro-priate, a reliable source of cells for a wide variety of clinical applications would be useful. One approach to solve the cell-source difficulty is isolation of human stem cells (see Chapters 42 and 61). These cells can potentially proliferate through multiple generations and be manipulated to differ-entiate into the desired cell types. Recent studies reveal that stem cells from human embryonic blastocysts possess these characteristics (4). In addition, cells may be modified by gene therapy before reimplantation to replace a defective gene (see Chapter 62).

HEPATOCYTE INJECTION

Tissue engineering of the liver began as an idea of cell trans-plantation. In an orthotopic liver transplant, the patient receives essentially an entire organ. This may not be neces-sary, because in many liver diseases far less liver tissue is required for sufficient function. For example, some meta-bolic deficiencies could be cured with replacement of only

5% of normal liver function. In 1985, the concept of cell transplantation was put forth in a review article written by a transplant surgeon who was well aware of the shortcom-ings of organ transplantation. It was proposed that trans-plantation of only those important functional cellular ele-ments of an organ would have many advantages over organ transplantation (5).

The liver is particularly amenable to such treatment for several reasons. Although the liver is comprised of multiple cell types, the majority of metabolic and detoxification processes are performed by a single well-differentiated cell type, the hepatocyte. However, in response to injury or sur-gical resection, hepatocytes turn off differentiation-specific genes and begin to proliferate until the liver structure is regenerated, when growth stops and normal function resumes (6) (see Chapter 42 and website chapter W-31). This enormous proliferative potential makes use of less cells to restore function, an attractive alternative to whole organ transplantation. In addition, unlike the heart or the intes-tine, the liver does not require contractile function which would make reconstruction of a new functional organ more difficult.

Early studies investigating cell transplantation for treat-ment of liver failure used injections of suspensions of hepa-tocytes (see Chapter 61). In one set of studies, hepatocytes were injected into the portal vein of Gunn rats, a strain of Wistar rat with a deficiency of uridine diphosphate glu-curonyltransferase (UDPGT) (7). Because of the enzyme deficiency, Gunn rats are unable to conjugate bilirubin. After injection of the replacement hepatocytes, the bilirubin level was followed and compared to control Gunn rats who had received a saline injection. The bilirubin level in rats that had received liver cells was significantly lower com-pared with the bilirubin level of the control animals, indi-cating that the injected cells maintained function. In other studies, hepatocytes were injected into the portal vein or peritoneal cavity of rats with liver failure induced by dimethylnitrosamine (8). Rats receiving replacement hepa-tocytes survived significantly longer than controls. In another experiment, Hepatitis B virus surface antigen (HBsAg)-producing transgenic hepatocytes were injected into the spleen. Within two days, half of the cells had migrated to the liver and the remainder were found in the lung, the pancreas, and the spleen (9,10). This suggested that there may be factors secreted from either the host liver or the injected hepatocytes directing patterns of migration (see Chapter 61).

These early studies supported the idea that cell trans-plantation could replace liver function. There were limita-tions noted, however, in particular with regard to survival of the implanted cells and the length of time the injected cells remained functional. This led to the idea of providing struc-tural support when implanting replacement cells.

An extracellular matrix (ECM) surrounds many cell types in the human body (see Chapters 32 and 33 and website chapters ⬚ W-27 and W-28). In general, most cells require an ECM for viability and function. It provides structural support for the cells and also helps regulate cell behavior. The specific composition of the ECM depends on the organ or tissue. The ECM of the native liver consists of fibronectin, collagen, heparin sulfate proteoglycan, and other molecules. The matrix provides a surface for cell attachment, allowing the adherent cells to maintain polarity. If dissociated cells are placed into mature tissue as a suspension without a support surface, cell polarity can be lost. In addition, the ECM influences growth and liver-specific function. Once the importance of the ECM was appreciated, new techniques in tissue engineering were developed which included a support structure for the living cells.

BIOARTIFICIAL LIVER SUPPORT DEVICES

Extracorporeal liver assist devices have been used in patients with fulminant hepatic failure to provide detoxification and metabolic function. The design of these devices is a closed tissue engineering system in which hepatocytes remain separate from the patient (Fig. 58.1). In these systems, cultured hepatocytes are coupled with a support matrix in a bioreactor. Plasma or blood flow is directed through the *ex vivo* device, bringing components of the patient's blood in contact with the functional hepatocytes. This design is particularly useful for providing temporary metabolic support in patients who may recover liver function. It can also be used as a bridge to transplantation by improving pretransplant management, much as kidney dialysis is used for patients awaiting renal transplantation.

Several investigators and commercial companies are developing extracorporeal liver assist devices. The systems differ in the source of hepatocytes and design of the bioreactor. In experimental models, rat and porcine hepatocytes have been evaluated for use in these systems (11,12). With regard to the support matrix and bioreactor, devices using hepatocytes within a matrix of hollow fiber membranes have been developed and investigated (13). In one that was tested clinically, cells derived from a contact-inhibited human hepatoblastoma cell line were seeded onto cartridges originally developed for hemodialysis (14). In another clinically tested device, porcine hepatocytes were attached to collagen microcarriers contained within a dialysis cartridge (15).

Preliminary clinical studies reveal the potential usefulness of extracorporeal liver support systems. They will likely be most beneficial in situations in which temporary and emergent liver support is required, providing a life-saving alternative when transplantation is not immediately available. However, as with kidney dialysis, bioartificial livers should not be considered a replacement for hepatic transplantation.

GROWING HEPATOCYTES ON POLYMER SCAFFOLDS

The observation that engrafted cells benefit from a support matrix led to the next, and perhaps most important, phase in creating replacement liver tissue. In the early 1990s, tissue engineering of the liver involved hepatocytes loaded onto biodegradable scaffolds, which were then implanted into host animals. In this model, synthetic, biodegradable polymers consisting of such substances as polylactic and polyglycolic acid are used (Fig. 58.2). These polymers have a large surface area and are highly porous in order to support maximal nutrient exchange and host tissue ingrowth. In addition, the polymer must have sufficient strength to withstand implantation into a host. Hepatocytes loaded onto the polymer are allowed to adhere in culture, after which the cell–polymer construct is implanted into the host animal. The site of implantation is often the mesentery, which provides a blood supply to the newly implanted cells. Because of its biodegradability, the artifical polymer atrophies at a controlled rate, leaving behind new tissue and no foreign material. The rate of degradation of the polymer can be controlled by altering its composition. This basic model has been extensively used in laboratory investigation of tissue engineering of the liver, and its evolution in the past two decades is described below.

The initial studies were performed using polymers consisting of polyglycolic acid fibers measuring 15 microns in diameter (16,17). Hepatocytes were isolated from Lewis rats with the use of collagenase perfusion and subsequent purification (18). The methods used in harvesting the cells is a critical component of this model; the ability to generate large numbers of viable hepatocytes is crucial. In these studies, *in situ* liver perfusion was superior to isolated organ perfusion with regard to cell yield and viability, and the composition of collagenase was the most critical variable in optimizing the perfusions. The hepatocytes obtained in the harvest were seeded onto small individual pieces of the polyglycolic acid mesh, and the cells allowed to attach for approximately one hour *in vitro*. The cell–polymer construct was implanted into the mesentery of Lewis rats and allowed to grow *in vivo*. The small bowel mesentery was chosen as the site of implantation for several reasons (19). The mesentery supplies a large surface area of well-vascularized tissue and it can be folded over such that the construct has host tissue on either side, maximizing contact with host blood vessels. Through a midline laparotomy, the construct can be sewn in place in a relatively atraumatic fashion, without jeopardizing the intraabdominal organs of the host animal. In addition, the accessibility of the mesentery with regard to its location just below the abdominal wall in the midline makes analysis of the cell–polymer implants technically feasible.

After set periods of time, animals were killed and the implants were analyzed. The initial experiments yielded encouraging results. A significant number of hepatocytes were well-engrafted onto the polymer sponge after one week *in vivo*. In addition to successful engraftment of the hepatocytes, capillary and mesenchymal ingrowth from the host into the implanted tissue was noted. This neovascularization indicated that the new tissue incorporates into the host and generates a blood supply. Immunoperoxidase studies using anti-albumin antibody demonstrated that the engrafted cells maintain liver specific function (19). In Gunn rats transplanted with hepatocyte–polymer constructs, serum bilirubin levels significantly declined once again indicating maintained hepatocyte function *in vivo*. In this same study, bromodeoxyuridine staining of the implanted tissue revealed DNA synthesis, indicating active regeneration within the grafts (14). Additional studies confirmed efficient conjugation of bilirubin by the Gunn rats which received implanted hepatocyte–polymer constructs (20) (see Chapter 20).

PREVASCULARIZATION AND HEPATOTROPHIC STIMULATION

Although the transplanted hepatocytes adhered to the matrix and demonstrated preserved function, a large number of the cells did not survive. The basic model at this stage consisted of loading cells onto biodegradable polymers and implanting the construct into a vascularized bed of a host animal. With the goal of increasing hepatocyte survival and proliferation, important developments took place which improved upon the basic model described above (Fig. 58.3).

Prevascularized Polymers

To survive and proliferate, cells of any kind require an adequate blood supply. Implanting the cell–polymer construct into the mesentery provides a well-vascularized tissue bed for the growing hepatocytes. Despite the abundant blood supply available in the mesentery, there is still an initial period when many implanted cells are not sufficiently in contact with the vessels to ensure nutrient exchange adequate for survival. This is especially true for cells seeded in the center of the three-dimensional polymer. In preliminary experiments, a significant proportion of the cell death took place in the first several hours and days, suggesting that time prior to vessel ingrowth is crucial to cell survival. Lack of oxygen and nutrients at the center of the implant caused the death of many cells. By implanting the polymer into the mesentery several days prior to cell seeding, ingrowth of fibrovascular tissue is allowed to occur (Fig. 58.3). The cells are subsequently implanted into a more vascularized environment. This technique improved the survival of hepatocytes on prevascularized polymers (20).

Hepatotrophic Factors/Stimulation

A challenge in replacing liver tissue with implanted cells is to ensure ongoing proliferation and survival of these cells. The ability to encourage proliferation should permit the initial transplantation of smaller numbers of hepatocytes.

Following resection or injury, the liver has an amazing ability to regenerate (see Chapter 42 and website chapter W-31) (21). Specific hepatotrophic factors play a key role in

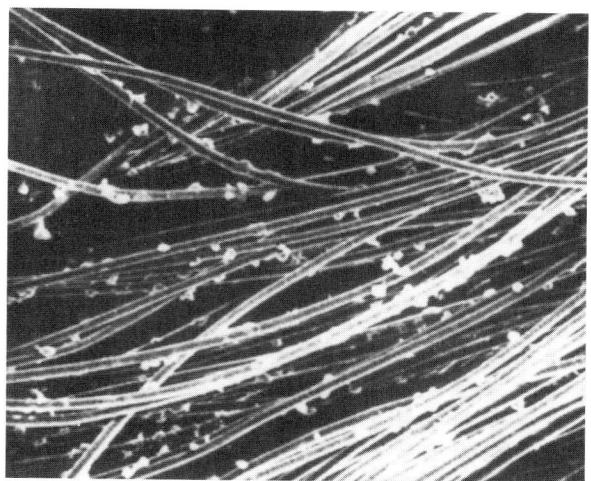
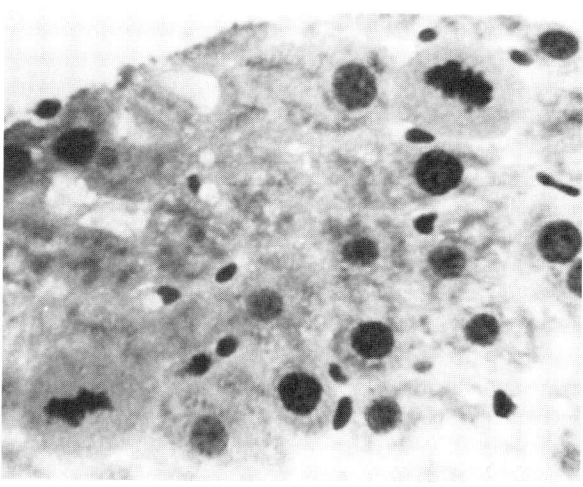

FIGURE 58.3. A: Scanning electron micrograph of polymer fibers with attached hepatocytes. **B:** Polymer-cell graft of hepatocytes 1 week after implantation in rat omentum. (From Vacanti JP. Beyond transplantation. *Arch Surg* 1988;123:547.)

the regenerative process. Some of these growth factors have been well characterized. Epidermal growth factor (EGF), hepatocyte growth factor (HGF), insulin and glucagon are hepatic mitogens (see Chapter 42 and website chapter 🖳 W-31). These trophic stimuli are present in portal blood. Providing these factors to implanted cells should increase survival and stimulate proliferation. This has been accomplished using several different techniques.

Partial Hepatectomy

Following partial liver resection, hepatocytes rapidly proliferate until the basal mass is restored. To recreate this situation in an experimental animal, partial hepatectomy was performed at the time of implantation of a hepatocyte–polymer construct. Analysis of the implants showed that the number of cells present on the polymer was increased upon addition of partial hepatectomy to the experimental protocol. As demonstrated by bromodeoxyuridine staining, partial hepatectomy stimulated a large number of transplanted hepatocytes to enter the cell cycle and proliferate (22). The addition of a portacaval shunt, described below, further improved survival and proliferation of transplanted hepatocytes.

Portacaval Shunting

Because the hepatocyte–polymer construct is implanted into the mesentery, it is not in direct contact with portal blood but is perfused by the systemic circulation. The portal flow continues to perfuse the native liver. To redirect portal blood and hepatotrophic factors toward the implanted hepatocytes, portacaval shunt was performed in experimental animals. An end-to-side portacaval shunt was created one or two weeks prior to implantation of hepatocyte-laden scaffolds. Upon implantation, the constructs were immediately perfused with blood rich in hepatotrophic factors. Previous studies revealed that portacaval shunting enhances cell survival (22–24). In animals with a p.c.s., the overall number of surviving cells was greater and the implanted hepatocytes formed a more organized liver structure. In addition, functional studies in Gunn rats demonstrated higher levels of bilirubin clearance upon addition of a portacaval shunt.

Following our studies on portacaval shunting and partial hepatic resection for hepatotrophic stimulation, the addition of these procedures to the model of implanted cell–polymer devices became standard. Combination of the two procedures had a more significant effect on cell survival and proliferation than either did alone. We postulate that partial hepatectomy stimulates production of liver-specific growth factors which are present at increased levels in the portal circulation. Both the procedures are required to maximize exposure of the newly implanted hepatocytes to hepatotrophic factors.

Microspheres

EGF is a hepatic mitogen that is incorporated into biodegradable microspheres. These microspheres are subsequently implanted onto the polymer with hepatocytes, exposing the cells to this growth factor during *in vivo* development of new liver tissue. The microspheres are composed of a copolymer of lactic and glycolic acid and measure approximately 20 microns in diameter. As they degrade, EGF is released into the surrounding tissue, thereby providing a slow, continuous source of hepatotrophic stimulation. Addition of microspheres containing EGF increased the number of surviving cells in hepatocyte–polymer implants and contributed to ongoing proliferation of these cells (24).

Cotransplantation with Islets of Langerhans

Pancreatic islet cells also release hepatotrophic stimuli into the portal blood stream (25). Hepatocytes were cotransplanted with islets of Langerhans, which provide a local source of insulin and glucagon to the growing liver cells. Studies done in our laboratory and elsewhere reveal that the addition of islet cells combined with portacaval shunting improves cell survival (24,26).

ENGINEERING VASCULARIZED TISSUE

Tissue engineered skin has been approved for clinical use. Other structures, such as cartilage and bone, are most likely not far behind. One advantage of engineering organs such as skin or bone is that their blood supply can be derived from the surrounding tissue of the host. In these tissues, vessel ingrowth from the periphery of the implanted cells provides adequate nutrient exchange for the growing cell mass. A large organ with a complex blood supply, such as the liver, would most likely not survive in this fashion. The blood supply of the liver is highly complex (see website chapter 🖳 W-32). The hepatic artery and portal vein provide inflow, branch into progressively smaller vessels and eventually into capillaries. Interaction of capillaries with hepatocytes and other liver cells is vital to liver function. Described below are two experimental approaches designed to manufacture liver tissue with intact vasculature.

Three-Dimensional Polymer Scaffolds

Three-dimensional (3D) polymer scaffolds have been designed with an intrinsic network of interconnected branching channels (27). Hepatocytes and nonparenchymal liver cells are seeded onto the polymer, and the constructs are placed in static culture or continuous flow conditions to simulate *in vivo* blood flow. Successful attachment of the cells onto the 3D polymer occurs in both static and flow conditions. When the culture media are analyzed for albumin, there is a significantly higher concentration of albumin in flow compared to static conditions. This demonstrates that the flow of nutrients through channels provides a more conducive environment for hepatocyte function and provides an experimental model for vascularized liver tissue.

Silicon Wafer Technology

To manufacture more complex vascular systems, techniques of tissue engineering have been combined with microfabrication technology (28). After careful study of the pattern of branching blood vessels in the liver, a vascular network pattern was etched into the surface of a silicon wafer. This creates an array of connected trenches into which endothelial cells are seeded, much as cells are seeded onto polymers. The endothelial cells form a confluent monolayer which lines the etched channels and essentially recreates a blood vessel network. The endothelial tissue can be lifted from the surface of the silicon wafer and folded into a three-dimensional configuration. This is a working model for engineered vasculature, and is a potential solution to the problem of manufacturing large complex organs.

CONCLUSION

Organ shortage is a major problem in health care. Tissue engineering provides a potential solution to this problem. The growth of cells on biodegradable scaffolds into new, functional organs could result in an appealing alternative to whole organ transplantation. In this chapter, we have reviewed the exciting laboratory experiments working toward this goal as it applies to the liver. Early experiments growing hepatocytes on polymers showed the potential of this technology and demonstrated survival and retained function of the cells. Further progress was made with the addition of a partial hepatectomy and portacaval shunt to the experimental model. Current investigation is focused on developing an experimental model for a vascularized liver, a challenging but hopefully attainable goal. The experimental model of a tissue engineered liver holds great promise for treatment of patients with liver failure and for application in the engineering of additional tissue for therapeutic benefit.

REFERENCES

1. American Liver Foundation, Fact sheet: hepatitis, liver and gallbladder disease in the United States. Cedar Grove, NJ: American Liver Foundation, 1996.
2. Vacanti JP, Langer R. Tissue engineering: the design and fabri-
cation of living replacement devices for surgical reconstruction and transplantation. *Lancet* 1999;354:32–34.
3. Skalak R, Fox CF, eds. *Tissue engineering.* New York: Wiley–Liss, 1988.
4. Thomson JA, Itskovitz-Eldor J, Shapiro SS, et. al. Embryonic stem cell lines derived from human blastocysts. *Science* 1998; 282:1145–1147.
5. Russell PS. Selective transplantation. *Ann Surg* 1985;201: 255–262.
6. Mooney D, Hansen L, Vacanti JP, et al. Switching from differentiation to growth in hepatocytes: control by extracellular matrix. *J Cell Physiol* 1992;151:497–505.
7. Matas AJ, Sutherland DER, Steffes MW, et al. Hepatocellular transplantation for metabolic deficiencies: decrease of plasma bilirubin in Gunn rats. *Science* 1976;192:892–894.
8. Sutherland DER, Numata M, Matas AJ, et al. Hepatocellular transplantation in acute liver failure. *Surgery* 1977;82:124–132.
9. Gupta S, Aragona E, Vemuru RP, et al. Permanent engraftment and function of hepatocytes delivered to the liver: implications for gene therapy and liver re-population. *Hepatology* 1991;14: 144–149.
10. Hansen LK, Vacanti JP. Hepatocyte transplantation using artificial biodegradable polymers. In: Hoffman MA, ed. *Current controversies in biliary atresia.* Georgetown, TX: Landes Biosciences, 1992:96–106.
11. Balis UJ, Behnia K, Dwarakanath B, et al. Oxygen consumption characteristics of porcine hepatocytes. *Meta Eng* 1999;1: 49–62.
12. Rozga J, Podesta L, LePage E, et al. A bioartificial liver to treat severe acute liver failure. *Ann Surg* 1994;219:538–546.
13. Jauregui HO, Gann KL. Mammalian hepatocytes as a foundation for treatment in human liver failure. *J Cell Biochem* 1991; 45:359–365.
14. Sussman NL, Chong MG, Koussayer T, et al. Reversal of fulminant hepatic failure using an extracorporeal liver assist device. *Hepatology* 1992;16:60–65.
15. Rozga J, Williams F, Ro M-S, et al. Development of a bioartificial liver: properties and function of a hollow-fibre module inoculated with liver cells. *Hepatology* 1993;7:258–265.
16. Mooney DJ, Kaufmann PM, Sano K, et al. Transplantation of hepatocytes using porous, biodegradable sponges. *Transplant Proc* 1994;26:3425–3426.
17. Mooney DJ, Park S, Kaufmann PM, et al. Biodegradable sponges for hepatocyte transplantation. *J Biomed Mater Res* 1995;29:959–965.
18. Aiken J, Cima L, Schloo B, et al. Studies in rat liver perfusion for optimal harvest of hepatocytes. *J Pediatr Surg* 1990; 25:140–145.
19. Johnson LB, Aiken J, Mooney DJ, et al. The mesentery as a laminated vascular bed for hepatocyte transplantation. *Cell Transplant* 1994;3:273–281.
20. Fontaine M, Schloo B, Jenkins R, et al. Human hepatocyte isolation and transplantation into an athymic rat, using prevascularized cell polymer constructs. *J Pediatric Surg* 1995;30:56–60.
21. Bucher NLR. Liver regeneration: an overview. *J Gastroenterol Hepatol* 1991;6:615–624.
22. Kaufmann PM, Sano K, Uyama S, et al. Heterotopic hepatocyte transplantation: assessing the impact of hepatotrophic stimulation. *Transplant Proc* 1994;26:2240–2241.
23. Uyama S, Kaufmann PM, Takeda T. Delivery of whole liver-equivalent hepatocyte mass using polymer devices and hepatotrophic stimulation. *Transplantation* 1993;55:932–935.
24. Sano K, Cusick RA, Lee H, et al. Regenerative signals for heterotrophic hepatocyte transplantation. *Transplant Proc* 1996; 28:1857–1858.
25. Starzl TE, Francavilla A, Halgrimson CG, et al. The origin, hor-

monal nature, and action of hepatotrophic substances in portal venous blood. *Surg Gynecol Obstet* 1973;137:179–199.

26. Ricordi C, Lacy PE, Callery MP, et al. Trophic factors from pancreatic islets in combined hepatocyte-islet allografts enhance hepatocellular survival. *Surgery* 1989;105:218–223.

27. Kim SS, Utsunomiya H, Koski JA, et al. Survival and function of hepatocytes on a novel three-dimensional synthetic biodegrad-

able polymer scaffold with an intrinsic network of channels. *Ann Surg* 1998;228:8–13.

28. Kaihara S, Borenstein J, Koka R, et al. Silicon micromachining to tissue engineer branched vascular channels for liver fabrication. *Tissue Eng* 2000;6:105–117.

29. Langer R, Vacanti JP. Tissue engineering. *Science* 1993;260: 920–926.

The Liver: Biology and Pathobiology, Fourth Edition, edited by I. M. Arias, J. L. Boyer, F. V. Chisari, N. Fausto, D. Schachter, and D. A. Shafritz.
Lippincott Williams & Wilkins, Philadelphia © 2001.

59

A GENOMIC VIEW OF HEPATOLOGY: THE EXAMPLE OF LIVER FIBROSIS

JOSÉ M. LORA
DEBORAH N. FARLOW
NADINE S. WEICH
JOSÉ-CARLOS GUTIÉRREZ-RAMOS

Since the advent of the genetics revolution initiated by the discoveries of Mendel and Morgan, modern biology has based its success in a reductionist view of the natural world and in an operational approach to tackle its mysteries. The discoveries in molecular biology and biochemistry during the twentieth century have strengthened this view. Any approach not analytical in nature would be defined as "descriptive." Biologists were trained for decades in, for example, the focused study of a particular class of proteins or on the role of a specific signal transduction pathway in a particular aspect of cell behavior. This way of looking at biology is clearly backed by an impressive array of basic discoveries with very important consequences in how we understand life and treat disease, and its continuing success in years to come is practically certain. However, one of the very foundations of this reductionist framework in the context of molecular biology, namely gene sequencing and database generation, is bringing as a consequence a new way to study biology and medicine, more interested in the "big picture" of how genes are coordinately regulated (1). It is clear that there is information in the coordinated patterns of expression of large numbers of genes. For example, by looking at the expression profile of genes in normal liver versus fibrotic liver we might find groups of genes whose expression levels are modulated in a similar way, and therefore, we can hypothesize that they might be playing a role in the course of disease. This is an important difference from the hypothesis-driven, traditional approach in which

some previous data involving a particular gene in a disease were necessary. For example, it wasn't until the generation of the Sonic hedgehog knockout mouse that a role of this gene in human holoprosencephaly was recognized (2,3). Obviously, dependence on serendipitous observations like this one poses a problem for an effective large-scale attack on a specific pathological problem.

In this Horizons chapter we present our perspective on how genomics can help us understand the basis of hepatic fibrosis, and how we are approaching this pathological process to identify potential target genes for basic research and therapeutic intervention. In the first part of the chapter we provide a very brief overview of some areas that have had an important impact on current genomics. In the second section we describe how some of these genomic techniques (especially global analysis of gene expression) can be capitalized in the study of liver fibrosis.

AN OVERVIEW OF GENOMICS

Mapping

Why is mapping necessary? Genes are arrayed in chromosomes in a definite physical way, and any sequencing effort needs to have a general framework of the entire genome to be able to locate genes with respect to each other, and operationally, to clone and order the myriad of fragmentary sequences that any such effort will yield. In other words, if a hypothetical chromosome contains 3 genes, A, B and C, we need to know the order in which they lay on that chromosome as well as the distance between each pair of them.

Historically, two major types of genomic linkage maps have been developed: genetic and physical.

J. M. Lora, D. N. Farlow, N. S. Weich, and **J.-C. Gutiérrez-Ramos:** Department of Immunobiology and Inflammation, Millennium Phamaceuticals, Inc., Cambridge, Massachusetts 02139.

Genetic Linkage Maps

Genetic linkage maps were the earliest to be constructed, and they focused on a number of model organisms, notably the bacteria *Escherichia coli* and *Salmonella typhymurium*, T4 and lambda bacteriophages, and the fruitfly *Drosophila melanogaster*. These maps are based on recombination frequencies between genes, and the main rationale is that the probability of a recombination event between any two markers or *alleles* is proportional to the distance between those two markers. In one extreme example, if we were to look at two alleles of the same gene, the recombination frequency essentially will be zero (there is no space between them to recombine), and these markers are said to be linked (4,5). When we apply this kind of linkage analysis to the whole genome, we generate a map based on recombination frequencies between genes which informs us about the relative distances between those genes in the genome.

These elegant maps have marked a golden age of genetics during the first half of the twentieth century. Genes were predicted to be physical entities and in fact they behaved as such, following definite genetic laws. The practical problem with these maps is that, as genome size and complexity increases, they become more cumbersome to obtain and utilize, and drop in useful resolution. These charts have proven to be most suitable for organisms with relatively few genes, short life cycles and large numbers of offspring. Although human genetic maps have been successfully constructed and have proven to be useful (6–9), other methods are needed to effectively chart the entire human genome.

Physical Maps

In a similar way that landmarks are key in constructing geographic maps, specific sequence landmarks can be used to generate physical genomic maps, which are as dense and as rich in resolution as necessary.

The first generation of physical maps was constructed based on restriction analysis. One can use restriction endonucleases (and combinations of them) to make *restriction maps* with as much detail as needed (10,11). By choosing the appropriate enzyme one can generate macrorestriction maps of fragments of 1 million base pairs (Mb) in average size (approximately 3,600 fragments for an intact human genome), or, when a finer map is needed, microrestriction maps, with smaller fragment sizes. Since the restriction sites are short DNA sequences randomly distributed across the genome, we can, in principle, construct maps of unbiased resolution across the entire genome, independently of gene density in specific areas.

Regardless of the method used to generate them, physical maps are collections of tags randomly and, ideally, homogeneously distributed across the genome (or the genome fragment) under study. One of the key uses of these

maps is the construction of ordered libraries that will be instrumental in any cloning and sequencing project (see Genomic Sequencing, below). In principle, we can assemble all the pieces of a restriction analysis into an ordered, linear and therefore meaningful map of the DNA fragment under study.

Sequencing

We will start this section by revisiting our reasons for supporting the sequencing of the human genome. We and others see three main reasons for this enterprise. First, there is no map with a resolution lower than the sequence itself that can give us information about true gene structure. It is only by determining the DNA sequence of the entire genome that we can infer functions of genes or that we can draw structural relationships between them. Further, by comparing related genes in different organisms we can draw evolutionary networks that not only can be fundamental *per se*, but that can be very useful for example in the field of animal modeling of disease. Solely by sequencing can we draw a clear relationship, for example, between human matrix metalloproteinase-1 (mmp-1) and rat mmp-13, enabling us to monitor mmp-13 function in an animal model of liver fibrosis. Second, having the sequence information in hand, we can manipulate genes, and study their function by generating mutations and creating transgenic animals or cell lines, and eventually utilizing them as therapeutic agents in gene therapy. For example, the complete nucleotide sequence of the Baker's yeast *S. cerevisiae* genome has been determined recently (12). As a consequence of that information, a yeast collection of deletion mutants for all yeast genes is being generated. Third, the vast amount of human sequence that is becoming available is tremendously accelerating positional cloning efforts (13). Mutations responsible for human diseases are being mapped at the nucleotide level of resolution at a pace not possible just a few years ago. We no longer need to rely on the sometimes random discovery, cloning and sequencing of specific genes in specific laboratories: we are now obtaining the sequence in an unbiased and high throughput way (5,14).

Genomic Sequencing

There are essentially two strategies to human genome sequencing. The first one makes use of the mapping information as described previously to order the material to be sequenced. In the alternative approach, there is massive random sequencing, and later the sequences generated in that way are assembled in their proper order.

Ordered Libraries

Using as starting material the high-density physical maps discussed above, we can construct ordered libraries of overlapping clones. Each of these individual clones is then sequenced and the data collected are immediately assigned a place in the genome (15,16). This is the more commonly accepted strategy, and the one preferred and implemented by the publicly funded Human Genome Project. The major drawback of this approach is the huge amount of effort and time needed to construct the appropriate and completely contiguous physical map (i.e., one without gaps).

"Shotgun" Sequencing

The principle behind this way to tackle the problem is to break the whole genome into small random fragments of DNA, sequence all those fragments, and then use bioinformatics to assemble all the sequences into a consistent and complete nucleotide sequence of the whole genome (17). This approach is, in theory, a much faster way to resolve the problem, although it relies on an immense computing power at the assembling stage. In fact, it has been criticized in the past as nonapplicable to complex genomes such as the human genome. However, very recently, this method has been applied successfully to resolve the nucleotide sequence of the *D. melanogaster* genome (18). This milestone has generated a lot of confidence in the shotgun strategy and, as this chapter is being written, scientists have applied this method to the human genome, and are at the final stages of human sequence assembly.

Expressed Sequence Tag Sequencing

Most of human DNA is junk. Not garbage, junk. As Sidney Brenner has pointed out, junk is kept, and garbage is discarded. Scientists currently cannot adequately explain the presence of the extensive amount of noncoding DNA in the human genome. Whatever its function (if any), the fact is that it does not code for genes that can make protein, and an alternative approach to sequence the human genome is plainly to sequence the coding genome. It is estimated that the human genome has between 80,000 and 110,000 genes, and there is considerable effort being put into the identification and sequencing of these genes. This goal is being accomplished by sequencing a multitude of expressed sequence tag (EST) libraries, or in other words, cDNA libraries (19). These sequences can further be used as probes for FISH (fluorescent in situ hybridization) and the genes mapped into specific regions of chromosomes, in a combination of physical mapping and sequencing techniques. There is, of course, a tremendous amount of redundancy in these libraries; many (if not most) genes are expressed in more than one tissue. The UniGene project is attacking this problem by cataloging all expressed genes, clustering this information and assigning all these ESTs to individual genes, thereby generating a compilation of nonredundant sequence information (20).

Expression Profiling

Without knowledge of its expression context, a nucleotide sequence is of limited use. Traditionally, whenever a new gene was cloned and sequenced, a limited expression profile study was attached (for example, a Northern blot of a handful of human tissues, and, if antibodies were available, a Western blot). This information has been instrumental in the further characterization of the physiological roles of these genes. However, the limited numbers of genes for which expression data were available made this approach very limited. Now, for the first time, we can start looking at the coordinated expression of thousands of genes at the same time (1,21–26). In the most widely used approach, oligonucleotides or cDNA fragments corresponding to genes are spotted onto a physical support (e.g., nylon or glass) of very small dimensions. These highly packed sets of arrayed pieces of DNA (or *microarrays*) can then be used in hybridization experiments to compare RNA populations from different cell types, different tissues with physiopathological conditions, etc. The huge datasets generated are then analyzed by powerful software into a user-friendly readout that renders, for example, complex patterns of coordinated expression changes of groups of genes during a specific pathological process.

An alternative high-throughput method of profiling is the serial analysis of gene expression (SAGE). A sequence as short as nine base pairs is enough to identify a particular transcript (27). A population of RNA is used to produce cDNA, and then cleaved to generate such short pieces, and those closest to the 3′ end of the mRNA are selected. In a subsequent step, a number of these short fragments are concatenated, and then sequenced. This system is useful to compare different populations of RNAs, and also gives a quantitative inference for each transcript, based on the number of times the same fragment is sequenced out of the entire group of mRNAs (27).

LIVER FIBROSIS MEETS GENOMICS

Fibrosis is the substitution of normal tissue by collagenous scar tissue. In the liver, fibrosis occurs as a consequence of hepatic damage by a number of different causes (alcohol consumption, viral hepatitis, autoimmune processes, genetic diseases, etc.). The end result of these injuries is hepatocyte death and activation of hepatic stellate cells (HSC) that in turn proliferate, become contractile and synthesize large amounts of fibrillar collagens (28) (for a review of stellate cell biology and liver fibrosis see Chapters 31 and 32).

In the next section we present the approach we are using to identify genes that are potential targets for therapeutic intervention, with special emphasis on the reliability of the techniques used. We proceed in a production mode, and apply high-throughput methods to the entire process, from gene discovery to, ultimately, drug discovery.

Microarrays for Gene Discovery in Liver Fibrosis

It is now firmly established that the activated hepatic stellate cell (aHSC) is the key effector of hepatic fibrosis. During their activation from the quiescent state, HSCs undergo a change in the expression patterns of a multitude of genes (28,29). The study of these dynamic changes is predicted to be of great importance, because we can hypothesize, for example, that genes upregulated during activation may be necessary for such activation, in a "guilt by association" paradigm. In fact, we know that collagen, transforming growth factor-1 (TGF-β1), tissue inhibitor of metaloproteinase 1 (TIMP-1), and many other genes with clear involvement in the activated phenotype of HSCs are upregulated during activation, and essentially silent in the quiescent state. Ideally, we would like to identify the entire set of genes whose expression levels change during HSC activation and perpetuation stages (28), and transcriptional profiling using microarray technology offers a tremendous advantage for achieving this goal.

We have completed a set of preliminary experiments in which we compared the expression profiles of aHSCs with that of normal hepatocytes, as well as tissue from fibrotic and normal livers. These experiments have revealed extensive changes in the expression profiles of many genes from these sources. We found that there are sets of genes preferentially expressed in aHSC or in hepatocytes and normal livers, while other sets of genes were observed to not change their expression profiles.

Array Construction and Hybridization

We have been working with nylon-based microarrays, built in-house by our Transcriptional Profiling Core Facility. In short, the printing process is carried out by robots developed internally with technologies adapted from those used in the computer industry for the printing of electronic microchips. A detailed description of the production process itself is beyond the scope of this overview.

Probes to be used in the hybridization procedure are generated by first isolating total RNA from the samples to be studied (aHSCs, whole fibrotic liver, purified hepatocytes, whole normal liver) and then synthesizing cDNA which is radioactively labeled to a high specific activity. Nylon filters containing fragments of thousands of genes under study are then hybridized to the radioactively labeled cDNA in duplicate and washed, and hybridization signals are digitally scanned. The raw data obtained are normalized to the mean of each dataset, allowing comparisons across different datasets.

As a critical determinant of the accuracy and reproducibility of data obtained from the many thousands of genes spotted on each array, all experiments described have been performed in replicate by using identical samples of RNA from each tissue of interest to probe two different filters. Figure 59.1 shows log–log phase scatterplots of duplicate filters probed with cDNA generated from RNA isolated from primary hepatocytes or activated stellate cells. Each colored spot on the graph represents an individual gene. Spots colored red are those whose level of expression detected on one filter is significantly similar to the equivalent spot on the replicate. Spots colored black represent those genes whose levels of expression would appear to be significantly different between the replicate filters and flagged upon analysis as representing unreliable data. Typically, we see more events of nonduplication in genes with lower levels of expression in the sample being used to probe the arrays, as is to be expected.

We have further demonstrated the reliability of data obtained utilizing the microarray technology in several ways. First, identical samples of RNA have been used to probe filter sets in several different microarray experiments. In all cases examined, similar levels and/or patterns of expression of specific genes have been detected throughout all experiments performed, independent of whether identical or dissimilar arrays were utilized. Furthermore, in all cases in the experiments described here, for each gene whose differential gene expression pattern was of sufficient interest to warrant further study, reverse transcription–polymerase chain reaction (RT-PCR) technology was used to determine concordance of the differential expression data generated through the microarray hybridization with that detected through the PCR-based strategy. Finally, as will be described in more detail in the following section, analysis of several "marker" or "control" genes present on the array was performed to assess the reliability of the data collected.

Transcriptional Profiling of Differential Gene Expression in Liver Fibrosis Using Microarray Technology

Gene Expression in Stellate Cells as Compared to Primary Hepatocytes

One possible first question to answer might be "what genes are expressed at higher levels in activated stellate cells than in normal hepatocytes?" Figure 59.2A shows a log–log phase scatterplot comparison of the average values from replicate filters for each gene on the array with respect to the level of expression in each of the samples. Each spot on the graph represents an individual gene; those colored blue are those which have a two-fold or higher differential expression in the two samples. Those located to the left of the center diagonal line are those expressed at higher levels in activated stellate cells than in normal hepatocytes, whereas those to the right show the converse pattern.

To validate these initial observations, we investigated the expression of two genes previously known to be transcribed

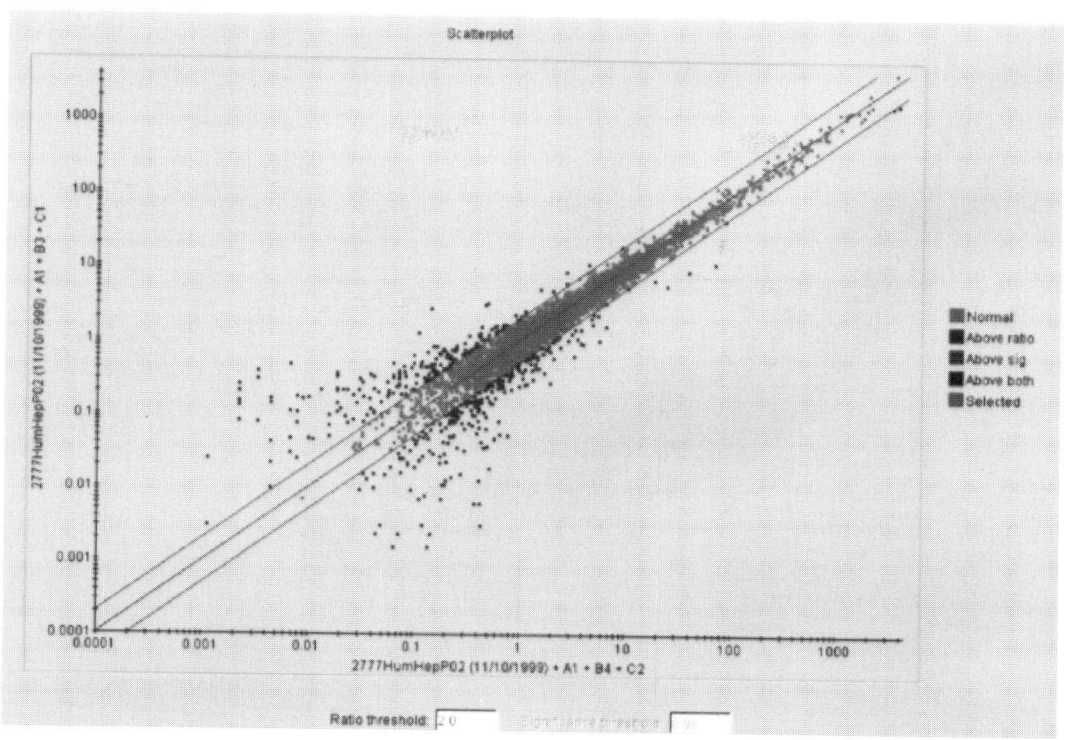

A

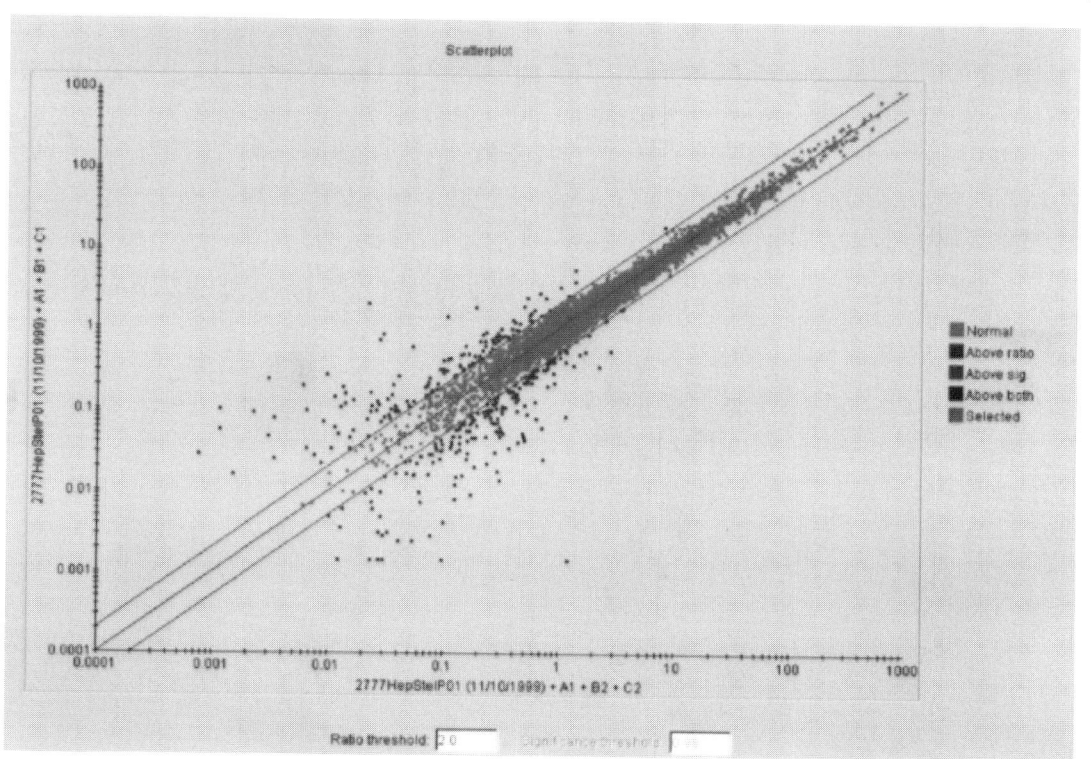

B

FIGURE 59.1. Scatterplots corresponding to filters hybridized with human hepatocyte RNA (**A**) or human activated stellate cell RNA (**B**). *Spots within the two blue parallel lines* represent those for which the absolute values did not differ more than two-fold in the duplicate filters. Genes with low expression levels (left-lower corner) tend to present a higher degree of variation, as expected. See Color Plate 15.

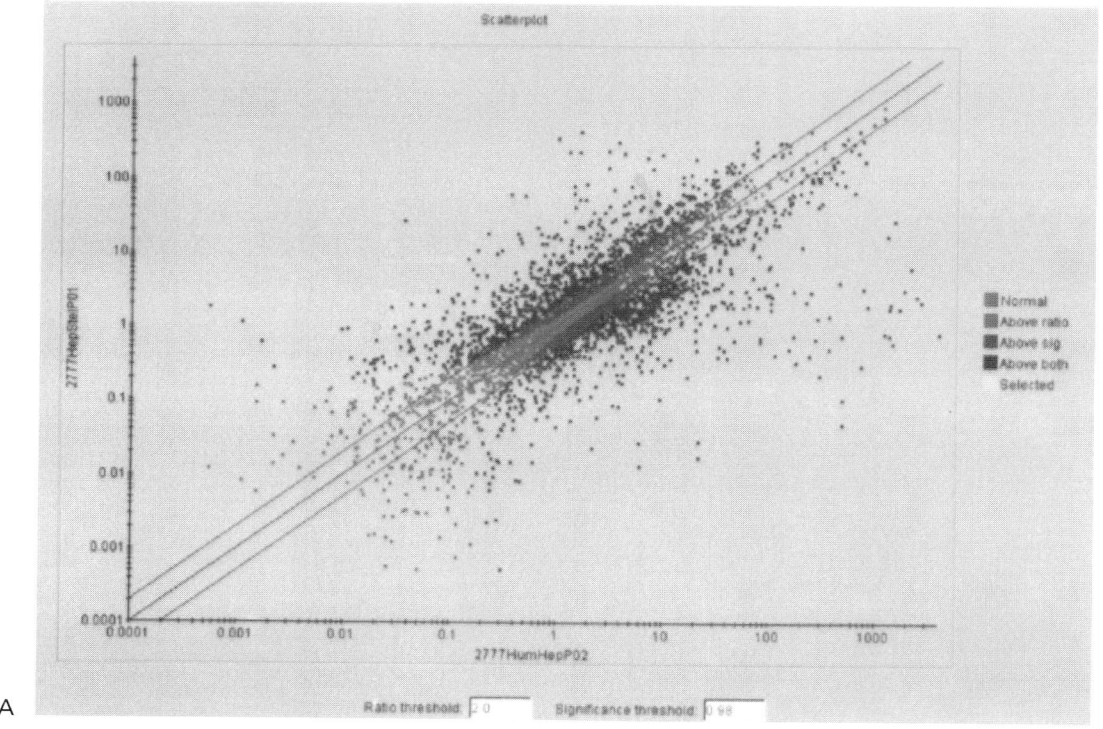

A

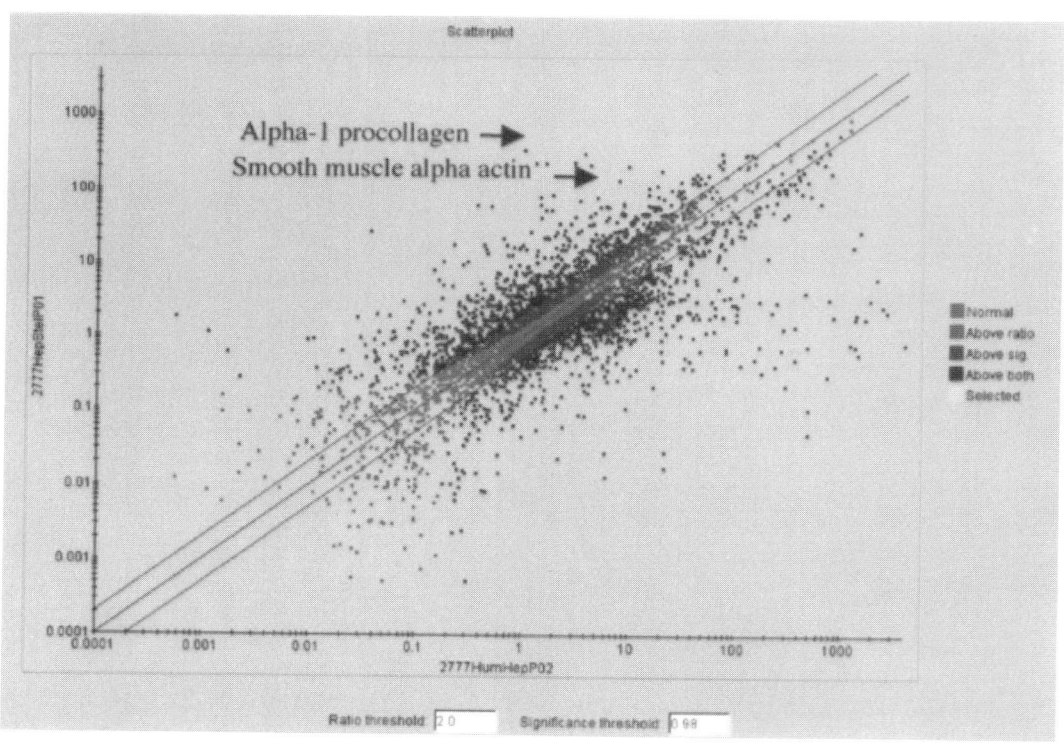

B

FIGURE 59.2. Scatterplots comparing activated hepatic stellate cells (aHSCs) with hepatocyte expression. **A:** *Spots to the left of the upper blue line* represent genes whose expression levels in aHSC compared to hepatocytes are higher than two-fold. *Spots to the right of the lower blue line* represent genes whose expression levels in hepatocytes compared to aHSC are higher than two-fold. **B:** Two representative marker genes, procollagen and smooth muscle α-actin, are indicated. See Color Plate 16.

at significantly higher levels in activated stellate cells than in primary hepatocytes: α1 procollagen and smooth muscle α-actin (28). The arrows indicate the yellow spots representing each of these two genes. The position of each of the two spots shows sharply higher levels of expression of the two marker genes in the stellate cells compared to the hepatocytes, further confirming the validity of the data collected in this experiment. Further analysis of the data produced in this experiment involved the generation of lists of large numbers of genes with annotations of interest and more detailed determination of their patterns of expression using RT-PCR analysis in an extensive panel of clinical and nonclinical samples representing diseased and normal tissues and cells.

Gene Expression in Stellate Cells as Compared to Normal and Fibrotic Liver Tissue

A second experiment involved three RNA samples, from normal liver tissue, fibrotic liver tissue and activated stellate cells. Along with direct comparison of each of these samples to each other as described for the initial experiment, we performed extensive "clustering" analyses using the self-organizing map (SOM) method (30) to arrange genes in particular groups based on their patterns of expression in *all three* samples. As described above, several methods of analysis were used to ascertain the validity of the microarray data obtained, and these data were used to identify genes for more extensive transcription analysis profiling using RT-PCR technology.

CONCLUSION

Determination of the nucleotide sequence of entire genomes, including that of *Homo sapiens*, is already a fact. However, it is necessary to study the patterns of gene expression in order to extract functional information from mere sequence. In the context of liver fibrosis, this functional genomic approach should push the field to a new level of analysis. By determining sets of genes coordinately controlled during the fibrogenic process, we will be able to dissect entire signal transduction pathways, and this very fact should help us not only to understand the biology behind hepatic fibrosis, but also to rationally design new drugs for therapeutic intervention. At this time there are only a handful of genes clearly established to be involved in liver fibrosis (28), yet our microarray experiments detect dozens of coordinately regulated genes in activated stellate cells (Fig. 59.2). It is reasonable to hypothesize that there are potential therapeutic targets among those thus far unappreciated transcripts.

On a different front, if we are able to associate a well defined change of expression pattern of groups of genes to the process of fibrosis, we will be able to use gene chips as a diagnostic (and ideally prognostic) tool.

Finally, this genomic approach to liver disease can be taken one step further and combined with pharmacogenomics, so that personalized care can be applied to each patient, based on specific marker genes analyzed in the context of global expression analysis.

As a first step, we have shown that these technologies are reliable and that they can be applied to the study of fibrogenesis in the liver. The implementation of these new approaches suggests a bright horizon in the understanding of liver disease and its rational treatment.

REFERENCES

1. Brent R. Genomic biology. *Cell* 2000;100:169–183.
2. Chiang C, Litingtung Y, Lee E, et al. Cyclopia and defective axial patterning in mice lacking Sonic hedgehog gene function. *Nature* 1996;383:407–413.
3. Roessler E, Belloni E, Gaudenz K, et al. Mutations in the human Sonic Hedgehog gene cause holoprosencephaly. *Nat Genet* 1996;14:357–360.
4. Griffiths AJF, Miller JH, Suzuki DT, et al. *An introduction to genetic analysis*. New York: Freeman, 1999:94–144.
5. Cantor CR, Smith CL. *Genomics. The science and technology behind the Human Genome Project*. New York: Wiley–Liss, 1999:165–206.
6. Churchill GA, Giovannoni JJ, Tanksley SD. Pooled sampling makes high resolution mapping practical with DNA markers. *Proc Natl Acad Sci USA* 1993;90:16–20.
7. Dib C, Fauré S, Fizames C, et al. A comprehensive genetic map of the human genome based on 5,264 microsatellites. *Nature* 1996;380:152–154.
8. Donis-Keller H, Green P, Helms C, et al. A genetic linkage map of the human genome. *Cell* 1987;51:319–337.
9. Shuler GD, Boguski MS, Stewart EA, et al. A gene map of the human genome. *Science* 1996;275:540–546.
10. Huang ME, Chuat JC, Thierry A, et al. Construction of a cosmid contig and of an EcoRI restriction map of yeast chromosome X. *DNA seq* 1994;4:293–300.
11. Wang D, Fang H, Cantor CR, et al. A contiguous NotI restriction map of band q223 of human chromosome 21. *Proc Natl Acad Sci USA* 1992;89:3222–3226.
12. Goffeau A, Barrell BG, Bussey H, et al. Life with 6000 genes. *Science* 1996;274:546–563.
13. Stubbs L. Long-range walking techniques in positional cloning strategies. *Mamm Genome* 1992;3:127–142.
14. Ansorge W, Voos H, Zimmermann J, eds. *DNA Sequencing: Automated and advanced approaches*. New York: Wiley–Liss, 1995.
15. Branscomb E, Slezak T, Pae R, et al. Optimizing restriction fragment fingerprinting methods for ordering large genomic libraries. *Genomics* 1990;8:351–366.
16. Zhu Y, Cantor CR, Smith CL. DNA sequence analysis of human chromosome 21. *Not* I linking clones. *Genomics* 1993; 18;199–205.
17. Venter JC, Smith HO, Hood L. A new strategy for genome sequencing. *Nature* 1996;381:364–366.
18. Adams MD, Celniker SE, Holt RA, et al. The genome sequence of. *Drosophila melanogaster*. *Science* 2000;287:2185–2195.
19. Hillier L, Lennon G, Becker M, et al. Generation and analysis of 280,000 human expressed sequence tags. *Genome Res* 1996; 6:807–828.
20. Wheeler DL, Chappey C, Lash AE, et al. Database resources of

the National Center for Biotechnology Information. *Nucleic Acids Res* 2000;28:10–14.

21. Lander ES. The new genomics: global views of biology. *Science,* 1996;274:536–539.
22. Lander ES. Array of hope. *Nat Genet* 1999;21:3–4.
23. Duggan DJ, Bittner M, Chen Y, et al. Expression profiling using cDNA microarrays. *Nat Genet* 1999;21:10–14.
24. Naftali K, Alard JD, Pittet JF, et al. Global analysis of gene expression in pulmonary fibrosis reveals distinct programs regulating lung inflammation and fibrosis. *Proc Natl Acad Sci USA* 2000;97: 1778–1783.
25. Zhao R, Gish K, Murphy M, et al. Analysis of p53-regulated gene expression patterns using oligonucleotide arrays. *Genes Dev* 2000; 14:981–993.

26. Khan J, Bittner ML, Chen Y, et al. DNA microarray technology: the anticipated impact on the study of human disease. *Biochim Biophys Acta* 1999;1423:M17–M28.
27. Velculescu VE, Zhang L, Vogelstein B, et al. Serial analysis of gene expression. *Science* 1995;270:484–487.
28. Friedman SL. Molecular regulation of hepatic fibrosis, an integrated cellular response to tissue injury. *J Biol Chem* 2000;75:2247–2250.
29. Lalazar A, Wong L, Yamasaki G, et al. Early genes induced in hepatic stellate cells during wound healing. *Gene* 1997;195: 235–243.
30. Tamayo P, Slonim DK, Mesirov J, et al. Interpreting patterns of gene expression with self-organizing maps: methods and application to hematopoietic differentiation. *Proc Natl Acad Sci USA* 1999;96:2907–2912.

The Liver: Biology and Pathobiology, Fourth Edition, edited by I. M. Arias, J. L. Boyer, F. V. Chisari, N. Fausto, D. Schachter, and D. A. Shafritz.
Lippincott Williams & Wilkins, Philadelphia © 2001.

AFTER PROTEOMICS COMES GLYCOMICS: HOW PROTEINS AND SACCHARIDES INTERACT AND INFLUENCE CELL BIOLOGY

RAM SASISEKHARAN
ZACHARY SHRIVER
UMA NARAYANASAMI
GANESH VENKATARAMAN

Historically, it was thought that the extracellular matrix (ECM) surrounding cells was an inert scaffold, providing a hydration sphere and a platform for cell growth and differentiation but little else. However, in recent years it has become increasingly evident that cellular function and phenotype are highly influenced by the ECM. The emerging picture is one of an active interplay between the ECM and the cell: cells synthesize their ECM in a highly regulated and specific fashion, and in turn, the ECM serves to modulate and process signals at the cell surface and hence influence cell function. Together, these observations elicit one fundamental question: *How does the ECM modulate cell function?*

Direct contact between the cells and the ECM influences cell shape and morphology, thus impinging on cell function. Numerous studies have determined that processes such as proliferation, migration, and apoptosis can be induced by cell shape. For example, elongation of a cell has been associated with increased DNA synthesis, whereas contraction and rounding results in increased apoptosis. In addition, the ECM can promote or inhibit cell-specific gene transcription, imparting the characteristic features of a particular organ. Several examples of this level of regulation are known: hepatocytes must contact the ECM to synthesize cell type-specific proteins, and only with an appropriate ECM will mammary tissue express the tissue specific protein β-casein. In addition to the direct role that the ECM plays in cell function, it indirectly impinges on a cell's processing of signals by growth factors, mitogens, and cytokines. The ECM components interact with signaling molecules at every step in their trajectory from the originating cell to the target cell. The list of signaling molecules that are known to bind to components of the ECM is growing rapidly, as is an appreciation of the roles that this interaction has on the biology of these molecules (1,2).

The major components of the ECM are fibrous proteins that provide tensile strength (e.g., collagens and elastin), adhesive glycoproteins (e.g., fibronectin, laminin, and tenascin), and proteoglycans. In global terms, the ECM is composed of two major classes of molecules — proteins and polysaccharides. The composition of each is not static; rather, both change in response to external stimuli. The emerging picture replaces the idea of the ECM as an amorphous ensemble of unrelated molecules with a model wherein the diverse players of the ECM seem to act in concert to control the physiological status of cells and tissues. A number of excellent reviews have been written on the subject of the role of the proteinaceous component of the ECM and its biological functions (3). This prospectus will focus instead on the second major component of the ECM, the

---

R. Sasisekharan and G. Venkataraman: Division of Bioengineering, Massachusetts Institute of Technology, Cambridge, Massachusetts 02139.

Z. Shriver: Division of Bioengineering and Environmental Health, Massachusetts Institute of Technology, Cambridge, Massachusetts 02139.

U. Narayanasami: Division of Hematology and Oncology, New England Medical Center, Boston, Massachusetts 02111.

complex polysaccharides, also known as glycosaminoglycans (GAGs).

The GAG component of the ECM is made primarily of the free polysaccharide hyaluronan and polysaccharides attached to a core protein known as proteoglycans (4). Proteoglycans consist of multiple GAG oligosaccharide side chains, which usually make up most of the mass of the proteoglycan. This gives most proteoglycans a "Christmas tree" appearance, where the protein core is surrounded by GAG extensions (Fig. 60.1), generally one to three oligosaccharide chains. Because of the presence of the GAG chains, the molecular mass of proteoglycans is routinely over 100 kDa and can reach 1,000 kDa. As most of the mass (and area) of a proteoglycan arises from the linear, extended conformation of the GAG chains, it might be expected that most factors that interact with a proteoglycan do so with the GAG extensions. Numerous growth factors and cytokines bind to proteoglycans, most to the polysaccharide component, thus providing the dominant example of noncovalent protein–polysaccha-

ride interactions. Proteoglycans are extruded by cells into the ECM as well as to the cell surface, thereby providing the cells with a GAG "fur coat." It appears that there is a signature associated with the GAG "fur coat" worn by divergent cell types such that each cell type responds to the repertoire of signaling molecules in different, sometimes dramatic, ways. To begin to appreciate the nature of a cell's GAG fur coat requires an understanding of the molecular structure of the oligosaccharide chains.

The family of GAGs encompasses four major members, which typically possess a dissaccharide repeat unit of a hexosamine (either glucosamine or galactosamine) linked to a uronic acid (either iduronic or glucuronic acid) (5). The first member is the aforementioned hyaluronan, which is a polymeric extension of 250 to 25,000 disaccharide units of glucosamine linked to glucuronic acid. Hyaluronan is found in synovial fluid and the vitreous humor of the eye, where its primary function is to provide a viscous hydration sphere, as suits its anionic character (4). The second member of the

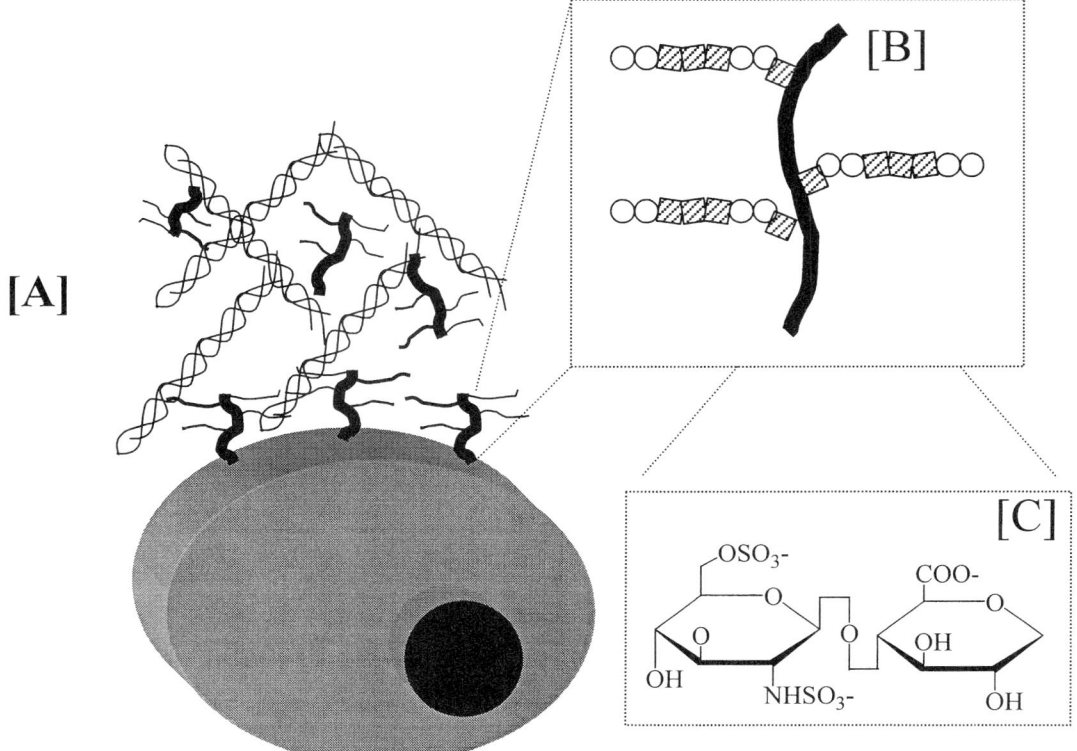

FIGURE 60.1. Macromolecular and chemical composition of heparin/heparan sulfate glycosaminoglycan (HLGAG) proteoglycans. **A:** Proteoglycans are present at the cell surface and extruded by the cell into the extracellular matrix. **B:** The structure of all proteoglycans is similar, containing a protein core (shown in *black*) and extending from the core HLGAG oligosaccharide chains (*open circles and dashed squares*). The structure of the oligosaccharide chain is such that there are regions of aggregate chemical character. In the diagram, regions of high sulfation (*NS* regions) are depicted as *open circles*, while regions of low sulfation (*NAc* regions) are shown as *dashed squares*. **C:** The basic structure of all HLGAG proteoglycans is the disaccharide repeat unit of glucosamine and uronic acid. Variability in structure comes from differential sulfation. Here the disaccharide unit is O-sulfated at the C-6 position and N-sulfated at the C-2 position.

GAG family is keratan sulfate. Keratan sulfate consists of a disaccharide repeat unit of glucosamine and galactose. Third is chondroitin/dermatan sulfate, consisting of galactosamine linked to uronic acid. Both keratan sulfate and chondroitin/dermatan sulfate can have sulfation of the disaccharide unit, the predominant source of sequence variability within the GAG chain, making them inherently more variable in structure than hyaluronan. The fourth member is the heparin/heparan sulfate-like GAGs (HLGAGs). As with other GAGs, HLGAGs are complex acidic polysaccharides that are attached to the core protein of proteoglycans such as syndecan, perlecan, or betaglycan. The length of HLGAGs ranges from approximately 20 to 200 disaccharide repeat units, and in this case, the basic repeat unit is glucosamine linked to a uronic acid (5).

Perhaps the most complex of the GAG family members is HLGAGs. HLGAGs possess the most structural diversity, due to modifications of the disaccharide repeat unit. Unlike the other members of the family (except dermatan sulfate), there are two possibilities for the uronic component of the disaccharide unit, *viz.*, α-L-iduronic acid or β-D-glucuronic acid. In addition, unique to HLGAG structure, there are three potential sites for O-sulfation, and the amine of the glucosamine can be sulfated, acetylated, or unsubstituted. Together, these modifications make HLGAGs potentially more structurally diverse than any other GAG (2). Of the ECM molecules involved in the modulation of biological processes, HLGAGs appear to be the most important based on the number of different growth factors and cytokines that they bind and regulate (1). As such, this prospectus will focus on the molecular and biological characteristics of HLGAGs. To gain an appreciation of the exact role of HLGAGs in these various processes, it is necessary to understand HLGAGs at the molecular level.

HEPARIN/HEPARAN SULFATE GLYCOSAMINOGLYCANS

Based on the number of structural modifications above, there are 48 possible disaccharide units possible for heparin/heparan sulfate glycosaminoglycans (HLGAGs) (6). This value is based on our current understanding of HLGAG structure. O-sulfation can occur at the 2-O position of the uronic acid and the 6-O and 3-O positions of the glucosamine. Thus, each site is either sulfated or unsubstituted, creating eight separate combinations. In addition, there are two possibilities for the uronic acid component, either iduronic acid or glucuronic acid, giving rise to 16 different combinations of the disaccharides. Finally, the N-position of the glucosamine can be sulfated, acetylated or unsubstituted (three possible states). Taking this final factor into account results in 48 possible disaccharide building blocks. Thus, HLGAGs have the potential to carry more information than any other biopolymer, for instance DNA

(made up of 4 bases) or proteins (made up of 20 amino acids). Consider for instance a simple polymer of each kind made up of four units. For DNA, there are 4^4 or 256 possible sequences for this 4mer. In contrast, for a tetrapeptide, there are many more possibilities, 20^4 or 160,000 permutations. However, for HLGAGs, a polymer made of four disaccharide units could have a total of over five million possible sequences, a staggering degree of variation, over 30 times as much as for polypeptides and 10,000 times that of DNA! In part due to the daunting challenge of handling this type of diversity, HLGAGs have only recently been appreciated as important biological modulators.

To obtain a handle on the chemical diversity and to begin to appreciate the biology of these complex molecules, there has been significant effort aimed at elucidating the biosynthesis of HLGAGs and delineating the sequence of events that regulate HLGAG structure at the cell surface and in the ECM.

Biosynthesis of Heparin/Heparan Sulfate Glycosaminoglycans

Recent studies have shed much light on the molecular mechanisms at work during the biosynthesis of HLGAGs. The key molecular steps are (a) synthesis of the proteoglycan core, (b) priming of the oligosaccharide chain by the addition of a tetrasaccharide linker sequence, (c) extension of the HLGAG chain by copolymerization of glucuronic acid and N-acetylglucosamine, and (d) modification of the nascent chain by O-sulfation, N-deacetylation and sulfation, and partial epimerization of glucuronic acid to iduronic acid. Even though, unlike other biopolymers like DNA or proteins, HLGAG synthesis is not directed by a template, increasing evidence indicates that synthesis is not random but rather reflects formation of regulated structures within the growing polymer. Invoking a previous analogy, the protein core of proteoglycans can be thought of as the lining of the "fur coat" providing support to the glycosaminoglycan chain, synthesis of which extends from the core to form the major component of the coat.

Synthesis of the Protein Core

The first step in proteoglycans synthesis is the creation of the protein core in the endoplasmic reticulum of cells. The protein cores for proteoglycans range in size from 10 kd (serglycin) to over 400 kd (perlecan). After synthesis of the protein core, the evolving proteoglycan is transported to the Golgi for subsequent polysaccharide addition.

Synthesis of the Tetrasaccharide Linkage Region

The first step in the synthesis of the polysaccharide chain is the addition of a tetrasaccharide unit to a serine residue of the protein core. The identity of the tetrasaccharide unit, (serine)-xylose-galactose-galactose-glucuronic acid, is common to all proteoglycan structures (4). Concomitant addition of an N-acetyl glucosamine dedicates the growing chain to become an HLGAG. Much research has been conducted to identify which serines within the primary amino acid sequence of the protein core are selected. Control of addition appears to be moderated, at least in part, by the primary amino acid sequence immediately adjacent to the attachment site in the core protein. In the case of HLGAG synthesis, clustering of acidic amino acids within ten residues of the serine is a requisite for saccharide extension.

Extension of the Polysaccharide by Copolymerization of N-acetyl Glucosamine and Glucuronic Acid

After addition of the first N-acetylglucosamine, there follows extension of the disaccharide repeat unit of glucuronic acid linked $\beta1{\rightarrow}4$ to N-acetylglucosamine. This copolymerase activity that catalyzes the formation of the nascent oligosaccharide chain is actually encoded by two genes, *EXT1* and *EXT2*, both members of the exostosin family of putative tumor suppressors. These genes were originally discovered based on their functional linkage to the hereditary bone disease multiple exostoses. Both genes encode transmembrane proteins that adopt a type II topology characteristic to most glycosyltransferases. Recent studies have demonstrated that EXT1 and EXT2 form a functional heterodimeric complex within the Golgi apparatus. Together, the complex sequentially couples monomer units of N-acetyl glucosamine and glucuronic acid, creating a chain length of 20 to 200 disaccharide units.

Sequential or Concomitant Modification

Either concomitant with extension or in a sequential manner, the HLGAG disaccharide units on the nascent chain undergo O-sulfation, N-deacetylation and sulfation, and epimerization of some of the glucuronic acid moieties to iduronic acid (7). Most of the enzymes involved in the subsequent modification of the HLGAG have been cloned, and their substrate specificities are beginning to be understood. In several cases, multiple isoforms of the enzyme exist, each of which have distinct substrate specificities. For instance, to date, five isoforms of HLGAG 3-O sulfotransferase are known, as are three isoforms of the HLGAG 6-O sulfotransferase. Interestingly, N-deacetylation and concomitant sulfation is accomplished by a single enzyme with dual, separable activities. This has led to the speculation that the presence of N-unsubstituted glucosamines within the HLGAG polymer is the result of the enzyme exercising only one activity (i.e., N-deacetylation) in absence of N-sulfation.

The net result of these modification reactions is the formation of a highly heterogeneous polymer. *In vivo*, polysaccharide sequences with different modifications are segregated into *NS* regions and *NAc* regions (Fig. 60.1) on proteoglycans, further indicative of a sequence specificity for the modification enzymes (8). The *NS* regions predominantly contain iduronic acid and a high degree of sulfation, while the *NAc* regions have a high content of glucuronic acid, a low degree of sulfation, and a high degree of N-acetylation of glucosamines. Heparin, one subset of HLGAGs, is composed primarily of *NS* regions, and accordingly, is highly sulfated. *In vivo*, heparin is primarily synthesized by mast cells, where it serves to bind and store proteases. The structure of heparin is of great interest to the scientific and medical communities, beyond its biological role, due to its pharmacological use as an anticoagulant and antithrombotic agent. Conversely, heparan sulfate, which contains both *NAc* and *NS* regions, possesses more structural variability than heparin and is ubiquitously expressed.

Thus, our current understanding of HLGAG synthesis has revealed several paradigms. First, not all disaccharide combinations are equally represented within the oligosaccharide chain; unusual sequences appear once or not at all on a given glycosaminoglycan chain. Second, it is becoming clear that cells exercise exquisite control over HLGAG composition and sequence. A large part of this control is governed by cell-specific expression of only certain isoforms of some of the biosynthetic enzymes. Finally, it appears that the polymer modification reactions colocalize to the same area of the Golgi, suggesting that these enzymes form a supermolecular complex that coordinates modification reactions. Through enzyme "cross-talk" there is an extra degree of control over the fine structure of the HLGAG chain.

After synthesis, there is yet another level of regulation: intra- and intercellular trafficking to determine the location of the completed proteoglycan, whether it is transportation to the cell surface or extrusion into the ECM. The ultimate location of a proteoglycan seems to be defined mostly by the protein core. For example, perlecan is often found anchored in the matrix, whereas syndecan and betaglycan are most often present at the surface of cells. Importantly, the properties of cell-surface HLGAGs can be very different from those of matrix HLGAGs. Highlighting the point that the ECM is a dynamic, ever-changing environment, studies have shown that the type and amount of proteoglycans shed by a cell into the extracellular milieu are highly dependent on stimuli received by the cell. Since there is tissue-specific expression of isoforms of many of the biosynthetic enzymes, the length, composition, and sequence of the HLGAGs can be unique for a given cell type or for the core protein moiety.

Biological Functions of Heparin/Heparan Sulfate Glycosaminoglycans

Increasingly, HLGAGs are found to be key modulators of fundamental biological processes including cell growth, embryonic development, angiogenesis, hemostasis, and lipid metabolism. HLGAGs modulate these processes by interacting with the growth factors, cytokines, and morphogens regulating their activity and/or bioavailability. The underlying principle is that proteins perform the biochemistry by binding cell-surface receptors and initiating intracellular signaling pathways. HLGAGs modulate a protein's activity in an orthogonal manner by regulating the diffusion, receptor on- and off-rates, and effective concentration of the protein at the cell surface. These activities become especially important at the cell–tissue–organ level rather than at a single-cell level. These diverse roles beg the question of how HLGAGs perform their important *in vivo* functions. The mechanisms by which HLGAGs modulate signaling molecules can be classified under four categories:

1. *HLGAGs in the ECM can act as a reservoir, binding and storing signaling molecules.* The prototypic example of HLGAG action as a reservoir is in mast cells of the peritoneal cavity and most connective tissues. There, highly sulfated sequences of HLGAGs (typically referred to as heparin) bind to specific granule proteases through anionic interactions, storing them in an inactive form (9,10). Other examples have also been discovered: the potent mitogen fibroblast growth factor (FGF) is stored in the basement membrane and is released upon controlled digestion of the ECM by degradation enzymes. What biological function does an ECM reservoir serve? (a) Association of signaling molecules to the matrix allows for their rapid release, for instance by selective degradation of the matrix, upon introduction of a stimulus, thus avoiding *de novo* protein synthesis. (b) The history of cellular activity in a tissue might be recorded in the composition of the ECM and the profile of growth factors associated with HLGAGs in the matrix, creating an efficient signaling network.

2. *HLGAGs modulate the bioavailability of signaling molecules. HLGAGs bind to signaling molecules, modulating bioavailability and protecting them from proteolytic degradation.* Binding of proteins to HLGAGs is known to protect them from degradation by circulating proteases. Of special note is the pharmacological delivery of proteins, where HLGAG binding can dramatically influence the halflife and bioavailability of the molecule. Several examples of this are known, including FGF and interferon-γ. By this mechanism, HLGAGs influence clearance of many exogenous and endogenous biomolecules by the liver. For instance, cell-surface HLGAGs mediate low-density lipoprotein receptor-independent clearance of lipoproteins by binding to the active dimer of lipoprotein lipase, facilitating its internalization and transport into the cell. HLGAGs participate in hepatic lipase-mediated binding and uptake of HDL. In addition, some apolipoproteins (*viz.*, B and E) are known to bind to HLGAGs (4). Thus, it is becoming evident that binding of lipoproteins to heparan sulfate on cell surfaces is an important factor for lipolysis and for receptor-mediated uptake of the remnants. This has led to the proposed use of intravenous heparin as an antiatherocelotic therapeutic.

3. *HLGAGs influence diffusion of signaling molecules.* HLGAGs mediate diffusion of potent mitogens, controlling both the time of transit and how steep a gradient is formed. However, this is not just a matter of HLGAGs providing passive resistance to free diffusion by mitogens; rather, the process is closely regulated and specific sequences of HLGAGs bind signaling molecules, dictating diffusion and gradient formation in a controlled fashion. In addition, at the cell surface, binding of growth factors to HLGAGs can serve to localize signaling molecules to the cell surface, increasing their effective concentration and promoting binding to their cognate protein receptors (11). This is especially relevant in terms of the development of a morphogen gradient in embryonic development that leads to pattern formation. Developmental studies of the common fruit fly *Drosophila* have shown that one fundamental way that cells modulate morphogen movement is by expressing specific HLGAGs in the ECM and at their cell surface that interact with morphogens and regulate their diffusion, thus defining a signal gradient. The first evidence of such a role for HLGAGs arose from investigations into the Wnt family of morphogens, specifically the *Drosophila* homologue Wingless, that controls cell proliferation and differentiation during development. In these studies, it was found that HLGAGs with specific sequences have tissue-specific effects on Wingless signaling, modulating both short- and long-range functioning of the morphogen (12,13). In addition, alteration of the fine structure of the HLGAGs involved in this process abolished gradient formation and arrested development.

4. *Formation of an Active Signaling Complex at the Cell Surface.* HLGAGs at the cell surface have been shown to be receptors for signaling molecules, influencing their presentation to protein receptors at the cell surface and modulating their activity (Fig. 60.2). HLGAGs carry out this function in a number of diverse ways: (a) Protein binding to HLGAGs can induce a conformational change in the ligand, converting it form an inactive form into an active form. For example, HLGAG binding to antithrombin III converts it into an active inhibitor of thrombin and factor Xa, serine proteases involved in the coagulation cascade. In this way, HLGAGs play an intimate role in maintaining hemostasis. (b) HLGAGs can act as a template or platform for dimerization of the ligand, leading to receptor oligomerization and phosphorylation and concomitant signaling. This is the probable role that HLGAGs play in modulating the activity of a number of growth factors, including hepatocyte growth factor (HGF) and FGF (2). For example, *in vivo*, HGF, a potent mitogen, motogen, and morphogen, is nor-

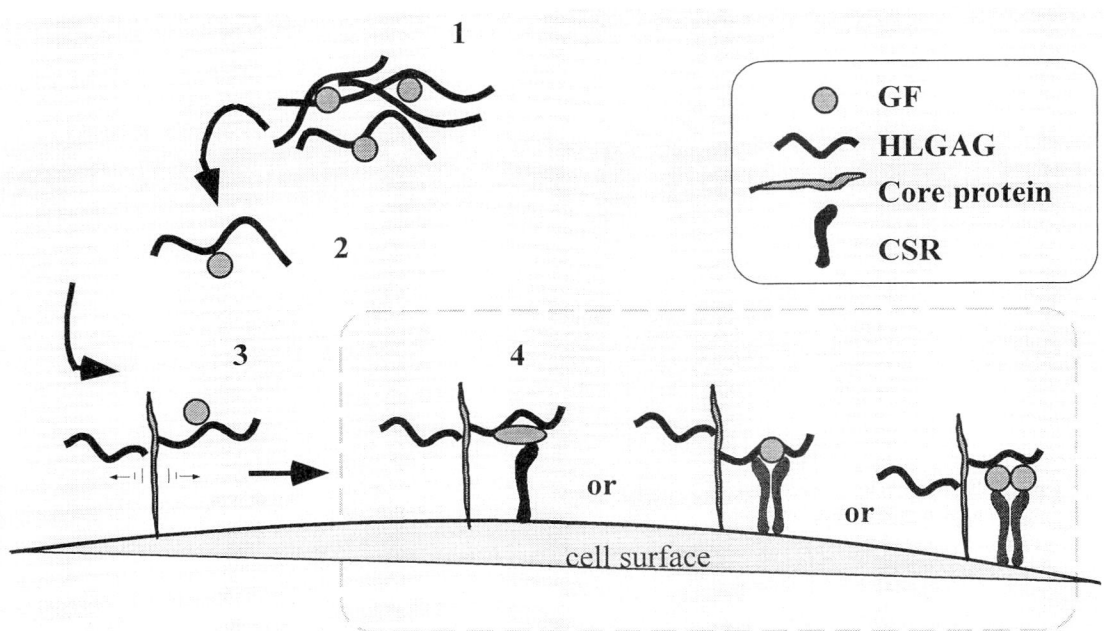

FIGURE 60.2. Heparin/heparan sulfate glycosaminoglycans (*HLGAGs*) impinge on growth factor (*GF*) functioning. At every step in the trajectory of a GF, from its release to its docking on a cell-surface receptor (*CSR*) of a recipient cell, HLGAGs can play a role in modulating GF function. *1.* HLGAGs in the extracellular matrix (ECM) can serve as a reservoir for GF storage, which can be released upon external stimulation and restructuring of the ECM. *2.* HLGAGs can bind to GFs, protecting them from degradation by circulating proteases. *3.* Binding of GFs to HLGAGs at the cell surface can increase the local effective concentration of the GF, promoting binding events at the cell surface. *4.* Finally, HLGAGs can play a direct role in the formation of an active complex at the cell surface by providing a platform for ligand and/or receptor (CSR) oligomerization or by stabilizing the formation of a ternary complex.

mally a monomer, but forms a dimer when bound to an appropriate HLGAG sequence; this dimer is the active signaling complex that promotes receptor clustering and activation of intracellular phosphorylation pathways (3). HLGAGs can stabilize an active ligand/receptor complex through the formation of a ternary complex, thereby mediating ligand–receptor specificity. For instance, consider the FGF family of growth factors. There are at least 17 family members, each of which recognizes to a greater or lesser extent four separate receptors and splice variants thereof, making for a complicated interplay. Selectivity in this case appears to be governed by HLGAG sequences that bind to both the ligand and the receptor, each of which have their own HLGAG sequence specificity. Taking FGF-2 as a representative example, it is known that certain HLGAG sequences promote binding to FGFR1, whereas other, chemically distinct, sequences are known to promote FGF-2 binding to FGFR3 (14). Similar findings have proven to be true for other members of the FGF family.

Even invoking the diverse chemical nature of HLGAGs, the range of biological functions mediated by HLGAGs is still surprising, and the list is growing daily. Investigations into the specifics of HLGAG–protein interactions using sophisticated physical chemical techniques such as nuclear magnetic resonance (NMR) and x-ray crystallography have provided much insight into how proteins pick out and interact with specific HLGAG sequences in the extracellular milieu and provide us with at least a preliminary idea of how sequence specificity is defined.

Heparin/Heparan Sulfate Glycosaminoglycan–Protein Interactions

The general observation is that most proteins that recognize HLGAG oligosaccharides bind tightly to a tetra- or hexa-saccharide. This "minimal binding size" of HLGAGs is observed in crystal structures of several protein–HLGAG complexes including FGF-1 and -2 (15,16), AT-III (17), and a virus protein, foot-and-mouth disease virus (18). What governs the specificity of binding between a particular protein and an HLGAG oligosaccharide? First, as mentioned above, not all modifications occur with equal frequency in an HLGAG chain. There are rare modifications, for instance 3-O sulfation, the presence of an unsubstituted glucosamine (formed by deacetylation of GlcNAc), or 2-O sulfation of a glucuronic acid. One or more of these might be recognized by a protein within a given sequence context and be required for high-affinity binding. The involvement of a rare modification is conceptually attractive since it provides a ready basis for selection. Indeed, this has proven to be the case for some proteins, like antithrombin III, and has facilitated identification of its HLGAG binding sequence, but it is certainly not true of many protein systems.

Specificity might also arise from spacing of binding sites. This level of specificity is most readily envisioned when one appreciates that many proteins that bind to HLGAGs are not monomeric units, but rather form oligomers. For instance, HGF has been postulated to form a dimer upon binding to an HLGAG oligosaccharide, as has FGF. In this case, selectivity does not arise from unusual modifications within the tetra- to hexasaccharide sequence recognized by the monomer; rather, specificity arises from the *spacing* of these units. Those sequences that are spaced for optimal formation of the dimer (or higher oligomer) bind with tight affinity in a cooperative manner, while those sequences that do not have optimal spacing bind with lower affinity.

A final level of specificity arises from conformational consideration of the linear HLGAG sequence. The conformational flexibility of iduronic acid affords specificity by two separate mechanisms (19). First, sampling conformational space allows for optimal topological positioning between substituents on the protein and the oligosaccharide, namely the sulfate moieties of the saccharide and the basic residues of the protein. Second, the presence of iduronic acid versus glucuronic acid within a binding sequence will dictate whether the oligosaccharide sequence can be accommodated by the protein's binding site. Both allow for a high degree of selectivity. In this manner, an analogy can be drawn between protein binding to HLGAGs and protein binding to DNA. In both cases, protein binding induces a conformational change in the helical repeat pattern of the acidic, polyanionic biopolymer, and the specificity of this "kink" provides for high-affinity binding.

Together, these three levels of specificity govern binding of a particular protein to an HLGAG chain, thereby allowing HLGAGs to orchestrate multifaceted, complex biological phenomena.

Heparin/Heparan Sulfate Glycosaminoglycans in Pathophysiological Conditions

While the vital regulatory role of HLGAGs in normal biological processes is becoming appreciated, HLGAGs also seem to play an equally important role in the development of pathogenic processes such as amyloid-associated (AA) fibril formation, Alzheimer's disease, tumor growth, metastasis and invasion, and atherosclerosis (2), to name just a few. Herein, we will outline a few of the disease processes wherein HLGAGs have been implicated as vital players in disease onset and progression.

Coreceptors for Pathogenic Invasion

Cell-surface HLGAGs serve as important host receptors for viral proteins such as cyclophilin A and TAT of the HIV virus, glycoprotein G of respiratory syncytial virus, L1 major capsid protein of human papillomavirus 11, and the gB, gC, and gD glycoproteins of herpes simplex virus-1 (HSV-1). HLGAGs also play important roles in bacterial pathogenesis (20), for instance mediating infection by *Helicobacter pylori*, *Streptococcus pyogenes*, *Neisseria* species, *Yersinia*, and certain parasitic infections.

In the case of HSV-1 gD binding, the HLGAG sequence has been partially characterized. Intriguingly, it appears that gD recognizes an unusual HLGAG structure that contains a single 3-O sulfated glucosamine. This particular 3-O sulfate is transferred to the nascent HLGAG chain by a specific isoform of 3-O sulfotransferase (3-OST-3a) that is expressed only in certain tissues (21). Thus, it appears that there is a signature associated with HLGAGs that act as docking and viral entry sites. In light of the fact that other HSV-1 cell-surface glycoproteins also bind to HLGAGs on target cells, this raises the possibility that HSV-1 infection is almost entirely mediated by HLGAGs. Whether HSV-1 is the exception or this holds true for a larger class of infectious agents remains to be seen.

Association with Amyloid-Associated Fibrils

The deposition of proteins as insoluble amyloid fibrils in the liver is marked by dramatically increased amounts of HS in the afflicted organ. Immunohistochemical studies reveal the colocalization of HLGAG proteoglycans and amyloid fibrils. Consistent with these findings, in a mouse model of AA amyloidosis, there was close temporal and spatial association between the amyloid fibrils and HLGAGs in all affected organs, while other glycosaminoglycan proteoglycans (e.g., chondroitin/dermatan sulfate proteoglycans) did not colocalize. In this model, HLGAG proteoglycans were also found in the lysosomes of hepatocytes and Kupffer cells in the liver, indicating that they were actively being produced and degraded. In a separate study, the composition of HLGAGs found in amyloid fibrils was found to be similarly independent of tissue type but distinct from HLGAGs from unaffected tissue (22). Thus, there may be "novel" amyloid-specific HLGAGs that mediate fibril formation and deposition. Drawing from parallels in the molecular events leading to the pathogenesis of AA amyloidosis and Aβ fibril formation in Alzheimer's disease, one possible role for altered HLGAG sequences in AA amyloidosis is that amyloid (monomer) binding to novel HLGAG sequences protects it from novel turnover and promotes formation of a seed complex that can rapidly generate fibrous structures, leading to amyloidosis. In this manner, HLGAGs directly impinge on the disease process, and by interfering with this interaction, it may be possible to mitigate the disease process.

Heparin/Heparan Sulfate Glycosaminoglycans in Tumor Biology

HLGAGs impinge on tumor biology in every step of its trajectory from tumor initiation to growth and recruitment of a blood supply, to tumor metastasis, including mediating sites of metastasis (23) (Fig. 60.3). As affords a molecule with the ability to form a range of possible structures, the role of HLGAGs in each step depends on the sequence context. Roughly, these roles can be divided into *potentiators* of tumor growth and metastasis and *inhibitors* of tumor growth and metastasis. Each will be discussed in turn. That HLGAGs can perform opposite actions is not without precedent; other components of the ECM have a similar action profile. For instance, degradation of ECM collagen by matrix metalloproteinases promotes tumor extravasion and metastasis, by breaking down a physical barrier. However, degradation of collagen results in the formation of endostatin, a 20-kDa fragment of collagen XVIII (24), which is a potent angiogenesis inhibitor and prevents the recruitment of blood vessels to tumor sites.

As HLGAGs are important for the formation of active signaling complex at the cell surface by multiple growth factors,

HLGAGs certainly play a role in autocrine and paracrine signaling loops, leading to dysregulation of cell growth. In addition, tissue- and vasculature-specific HLGAG sequences might provide a "signature" site for metastasis of a given tumor (25). In support of this supposition, it has been shown by many studies that the liver sinusoidal blood vessels are important sites where tumor cells extravasate and then colonize the liver. Furthermore, it has been shown that anti-proteoglycans antibodies, and not antibodies to other components of the basement membrane, such as antilaminin, antifibronectin antibodies, inhibit liver colonization of tumor cells. Similarly, use of glycosaminoglycan biosynthesis inhibitors of HLGAGs suppressed liver metastasis formation. Finally, HLGAGs are potent mediators of angiogenic signals and can serve to promote tumor angiogenesis.

On the other hand, specific HLGAG sequences can serve to *inhibit* tumor growth. HLGAGs in the basement membrane serve as a protective barrier (as does collagen), requiring degradation by heparanases before a tumor can metastasize (26,27). In addition, antitumorogenic molecules, including endostatin, bind to specific HLGAG sequences, mediating their activity and possibly their specificity. Finally, there is indirect evidence that similar to the formation of endostatin from collagen, there are cryptic HLGAG inhibitors of tumor growth that are released upon controlled degradation of the ECM.

Other Diseases

HLGAG proteoglycan expression in chronic cholestatic liver diseases may play an important role in liver fibrosis through interaction and activation of growth factors, through the mechanisms mentioned above. In addition, the clearance of chylomicron remnant lipoprotein, highly atherogenic lipid carriers, from the circulation by binding to apolipoprotein E is enhanced by HLGAGs in the space of Disse and on hepatocyte surface. As with other complex diseases, such as cancer, specific HLGAG sequences impinge on the trajectory of the disease at multiple points, such that a single role for HLGAGs in disease onset and progression is not readily definable.

Thus, these examples illustrate the point that it is no longer appropriate to simply identify the entity "HLGAGs" as being crucial modulators of a biological process without providing a context to this assertion. Subtle sequence changes can have profound, even opposing, effects with one HLGAG sequence promoting a process and another sequence inhibiting it. In many ways, this can be considered similar to concluding that "protein" or "DNA" is critical for a biological function without identifying the sequence involved, a clearly inappropriate and incomplete conclusion. Thus, as our understanding of the roles of HLGAGs in disease processes becomes more sophisticated, it becomes important to define the sequence context with which HLGAGs impinge on the onset and progression of a disease

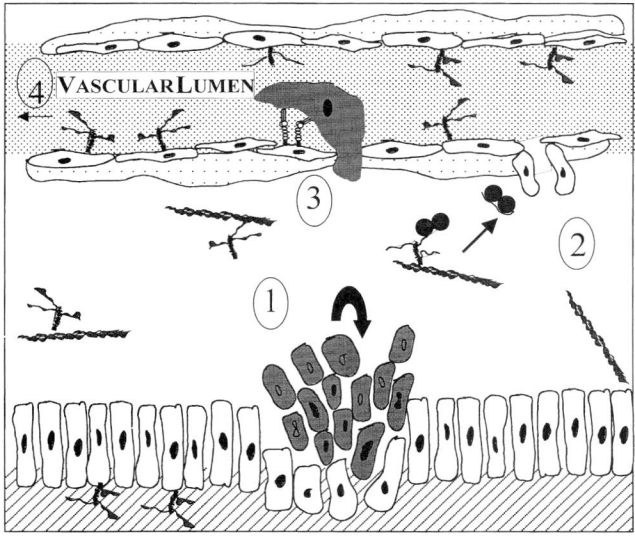

FIGURE 60.3. Heparin/heparan sulfate glycosaminoglycans (HLGAGs) impinge on cancer development in multifaceted ways. *1*. HLGAGs modulate growth factor signaling, thus affecting autocrine signaling loops. *2*. HLGAGs play an important regulatory role in regulating angiogenic signals. *3*. HLGAGs provide a barrier to tumor metastasis, requiring degradation by heparanases. *4*. HLGAGs can provide a tissue-specific "signature" for tumor metastasis.

process. Only then can a true understanding of HLGAG function be gained, thus identifying novel targets for the generation of new therapeutic modalities.

SIGNIFICANCE AND FUTURE DIRECTIONS

HLGAGs as regulators of biological function represent an important paradigm at the interface of cell–tissue–organ development and maintenance. The emerging view is that unique sequences of extracellular HLGAGs bind specifically to important proteins, including morphogens, growth factors, cytokines, chemokines and many other signaling molecules, and influence biological processes at the cell–tissue–organ interface through these interactions. However, the enormous sequence and structural diversity of HLGAGs is one of the factors that have made it difficult to study sequence–structure–function relationships. At present, structure–function studies are scratching the surface of this paradigm. Important progress is being made towards the development of much needed tools for analyzing tissue-derived HLGAGs. These include techniques for the isolation, affinity fractionation and sequencing of HLGAGs that bind to target proteins and chemical synthesis of defined HLGAG sequences. Such approaches will rapidly facilitate structure–function studies and facilitate the discovery of how HLGAGs regulate fundamental biological processes including development and morphogenesis, tissue regeneration, angiogenesis, and tumor growth and metastases.

Importantly, this paradigm opens new approaches and strategies for therapeutic intervention at the cell–tissue–organ level. For example, an understanding of how HLGAGs, in a dynamic fashion, impinge on the topological and functional organization of hepatocytes can lead to important breakthroughs in liver regeneration. In fact, a sophisticated understanding of ECM–cell interactions will revolutionize the field of organ repair and/or tissue engineering, helping herald the age of molecular medicine that will target a whole organ instead of a single cell. Also, identification of specific sequences that impinge on a particular biological process will allow for the development of novel molecular therapeutics based on polysaccharide structure. Addition of defined saccharide sequences to pharmacological protein preparations can allow for a more accurate prediction of their activity and bioavailability. Synthetic molecular mimics of HLGAG sequences may provide much needed defenses against bacterial and viral diseases, and new agents to combat atherosclerosis, cancer, and Alzheimer's disease, among other diseases.

Finally, a better understanding of the role of HLGAGs is likely to become very important for the rapid development and expansion of the field of glycomics, or the study of how proteins and saccharides interact with one another, thus impinging on cell physiology (Fig. 60.4). Especially with the maturation of the field of genomics and the sequencing of the human genome, the next stage in gaining a complete understanding of how genotype translates into phenotype is through the fields of proteomics (i.e., the study of how pro-

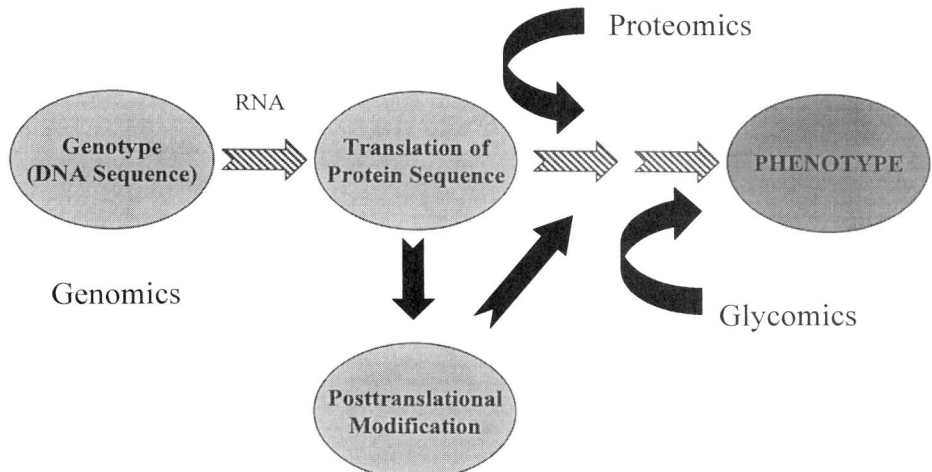

FIGURE 60.4. General paradigm of how genotype translates into phenotype. The center of the flow chart (marked with the *dashed arrows*) illustrates the central dogma of molecular biology, that is, a DNA sequence is translated into a protein through an RNA intermediary. Temporally and spatially regulated translation of proteins leads to expression of a particular phenotype. In addition, the activities of certain proteins are modulated by the addition of posttranslational modifications, including phosphorylation, glycosylation, and acetylation. Since proteins are created in the context of a cell and interact with a variety of other molecular players, the field of proteomics seeks to identify "cross-talk" between proteins. Glycomics, a relatively new field, in a similar manner to proteomics, seeks to understand the nature of "cross-talk" between polysaccharides and proteins and how this impinges on phenotype.

teins in a cell come together and interact and communicate with one another) and glycomics. Already proteomics promises to become a key tool in following the orchestration of multiple molecular players within the cell, and glycomics should do the same.

In summary, we have touched the tip of the iceberg with regard to the biological impact of these complex molecules. Just the discovery of the importance of DNA and proteins heralded the biotechnology revolution, so should the study of complex oligosaccharides such as HLGAGs herald an age of new and exciting scientific and clinical discoveries.

REFERENCES

1. Tumova S, Woods A, Couchman JR. Heparan sulfate proteoglycans on the cell surface: versatile coordinators of cellular functions. *Int J Biochem Cell Biol* 2000;32:269–288.
2. Conrad HE. *Heparin-binding proteins*. San Diego: Academic Press, 1998:183–202.
3. Piez KA. History of extracellular matrix: a personal view. *Matrix Biol* 1997;16:85–92.
4. Varki AR, Cummings J, Esko H, et al. *Essentials of Glycobiology*. New York: Cold Spring Harbor Laboratory Press, 1999:145–161.
5. Ernst SR, Langer CL, Cooney R, et al. Enzymatic degradation of glycosaminoglycans. *Crit Rev Biochem Mol Biol* 1995;30:387–444.
6. Venkataraman G, Shriver Z, Raman R, et al. Sequencing complex polysaccharides. *Science* 1999;286:537–542.
7. Rosenberg RD, Shworak NW, Liu J, et al. Heparan sulfate proteoglycans of the cardiovascular system. Specific structures emerge but how is synthesis regulated? *J Clin Invest* 1997;100:S67–S75.
8. Lindahl U, Kusche-Gullberg M, Kjellen L. Regulated diversity of heparan sulfate. *J Biol Chem* 1998;273:24979–24982.
9. Humphries DE, Wong GW, Friend DS, et al. Heparin is essential for the storage of specific granule proteases in mast cells [see comments]. *Nature* 1999;400:769–772.
10. Forsberg E, Pejler G, Ringvall M, et al. Abnormal mast cells in mice deficient in a heparin-synthesizing enzyme [see comments]. *Nature* 1999;400:773–776.
11. Perrimon N, Bernfield M. Specificities of heparan sulphate proteoglycans in developmental processes. *Nature* 2000;404:725–728.
12. Lin X, Perrimon N. Dally cooperates with *Drosophila* Frizzled 2 to transduce Wingless signalling [see comments]. *Nature* 1999;400:281–284.
13. Tsuda M, Kamimura K, Nakato H, et al. The cell-surface proteoglycan Dally regulates Wingless signalling in *Drosophila* [see comments]. *Nature* 1999;400:276–280.
14. Guimond SE, Turnbull JE. Fibroblast growth factor receptor signalling is dictated by specific heparan sulphate saccharides. *Curr Biol* 1999;9:1343–1346.
15. DiGabriele AD, Lax I, Chen DI, et al. Structure of a heparin-linked biologically active dimer of fibroblast growth factor. *Nature* 1998;393:812–817.
16. Faham S, Hileman RE, Fromm JR, et al. Heparin structure and interactions with basic fibroblast growth factor. *Science* 1996;271:1116–1120.
17. Jin L, Abrahams JP, Skinner R, et al. The anticoagulant activation of antithrombin by heparin. *Proc Natl Acad Sci U S A* 1997;94:14683–14688.
18. Fry EE, Lea SM, Jackson T, et al. The structure and function of a foot-and-mouth disease virus-oligosaccharide receptor complex. *EMBO J* 1999;18:543–554.
19. Ernst S, Venkataraman G, Sasisekharan V, et al. Pyranose ring flexibility. Mapping of physical data for iduronate in continuous conformational space. *J Am Chem Soc* 1998;120:2099–2107.
20. Duensing TD, Wing JS, van Putten JP. Sulfated polysaccharide-directed recruitment of mammalian host proteins: a novel strategy in microbial pathogenesis. *Infect Immun* 1999;67:4463–4468.
21. Shukla D, Liu J, Blaiklock P, et al. A novel role for 3-O-sulfated heparan sulfate in herpes simplex virus 1 entry. *Cell* 1999;99:13–22.
22. Lindahl B, Lindahl U. Amyloid-specific heparan sulfate from human liver and spleen. *J Biol Chem* 1997;272:26091–26094.
23. Engelberg H. Actions of heparin that may affect the malignant process. *Cancer* 1999;85:257–272.
24. O'Reilly MS, Boehm T, Shing Y, et al. Endostatin: an endogenous inhibitor of angiogenesis and tumor growth. *Cell* 1997;88:277–285.
25. Tovari J, Paku S, Raso E, et al. Role of sinusoidal heparan sulfate proteoglycan in liver metastasis formation. *Int J Cancer* 1997;71:825–831.
26. Vlodavsky I, Friedmann Y, Elkin M, et al. Mammalian heparanase: gene cloning, expression and function in tumor progression and metastasis [see comments]. *Nat Med* 1999;5:793–802.
27. Hulett MD, Freeman C, Hamdorf BJ, et al. Cloning of mammalian heparanase, an important enzyme in tumor invasion and metastasis [see comments]. *Nat Med* 1999;5:803–809.

LIVER REPOPULATION THROUGH CELL TRANSPLANTATION

DAVID A. SHAFRITZ
MARIANA D. DABEVA
MARKUS GROMPE

In the past three decades, many attempts have been made to utilize isolated hepatocytes for transplantation and treatment of liver diseases, acute and chronic liver failure, and hereditary metabolic disorders. In most cases, the number of transplanted cells retained as functioning hepatocytes has been very low and not adequate to ameliorate any of these disease conditions. Recently, however, several animal models have been developed in which more than 90% of host hepatocytes can be replaced by transplanted donor cells. This phenomenon is analogous to repopulation of the hematopoietic system after bone marrow transplantation. Liver repopulation occurs when transplanted cells have a growth advantage over endogenous hepatocytes in the setting of damage to recipient liver cells. This chapter discusses current knowledge concerning this process and implications of cell transplantation for treatment of genetically inherited and acquired liver diseases.

HEPATOCYTE TRANSPLANTATION

Currently, orthotopic liver transplantation of whole donor livers is the only mode of effective treatment for acquired and genetic hepatic disorders, especially when these diseases reach their end stages (1–3). However, the number of patients who can benefit from this procedure is limited by the availability of donor organs. In addition, liver transplantation is expensive, carries significant morbidity and mortality and requires, in most cases, long-term immunosuppressive therapy (4). Moreover, many disorders treated by liver transplantation are caused by dysfunction of hepatocytes, and in principle, it should not be necessary to replace the entire organ. This is particularly true for genetic deficiencies of proteins produced

D. A. Shafritz: Departments of Medicine and of Cell Biology and Pathology, Marion Bessin Liver Research Center, Albert Einstein College of Medicine of Yeshiva University, Bronx, New York 10461.

M. D. Dabeva: Department of Medicine, Liver Research Center, Albert Einstein College of Medicine, Bronx, New York 10461.

M. Grompe: Department of Molecular and Medical Genetics, Oregon Health Sciences University, Portland, Oregon 97201.

specifically by hepatocytes in which selective replacement by normal hepatocytes would clearly be therapeutic. Examples include hemophilia A and B, hypercholesterolemia and phenylketonuria. Thus, recent studies have begun to explore the use of hepatocyte transplantation as an alternative to transplantation of the entire organ.

Cell transplantation has the following potential advantages compared to whole liver transplantation: (a) it is less invasive (lower morbidity and cost); (b) if harvesting methods were efficient, cells from a single donor liver could be used for many recipients; (c) cells can be cryopreserved; and (d) transplantation of hepatocytes or hepatocytic cell lines may be less immunogenic than solid organs.

In addition, cell transplantation can be used in an autologous setting in which the patient's own cells are genetically manipulated *ex vivo* and then transplanted back into the liver. In the past 20 years, much has been learned about optimal methods for hepatocyte isolation and preservation, alternative routes for administration, transplantation sites and ideal dosages of cells (reviewed in ref. 5). Several clinical trials have also been performed in humans. Nevertheless, the ultimate efficacy of hepatocyte transplantation has been hampered by the fact that only a small percentage of the total hepatocellular mass can be replaced in humans using currently available methods.

CLINICAL TRIALS OF HEPATOCYTE TRANSPLANTATION

Allogeneic hepatocyte transplantation has had some limited clinical success. In a landmark report in 1998, a child with Crigler–Najjar type I, suffering from dangerous hyperbilirubinemia, was given 7.5×10^9 allogeneic donor hepatocytes by infusion via a portal vein catheter (6) (see Chapter 20). The procedure resulted in reduction, but not normalization, of serum bilirubin levels. Although the procedure was only partially effective, the patient still shows glucuronosyltransferase activity in the liver three years after cell transplantation (J. Roy Chowdhury, *personal communication,* 2000).

Allogeneic hepatocyte transplantation for the treatment of acute liver failure has been used in several centers, but generally has not been successful in significantly enhancing survival (7,8). Studies have also been conducted in patients with chronic liver disease and cirrhosis, again with only marginal, if any success (8,9).

Hepatocyte transplantation has also been used in conjunction with *ex vivo* retroviral gene therapy for five patients with a defect in the low-density lipoprotein (LDL) receptor (10). In this study, the proportion of liver cell mass replaced was estimated to be approximately 1%. This procedure resulted in a very modest decrease in plasma cholesterol in several of these patients. These results are encouraging, but also highlight another important problem of tissue replacement with standard hepatocyte transplantation protocols;

namely, that only limited (or no) division of transplanted cells takes place in the recipient liver under most circumstances. Therefore, augmented expression of the transferred gene through proliferation of transplanted cells, which is necessary for effective *ex vivo* gene therapy, does not occur.

ANIMAL MODELS TO AUGMENT PROLIFERATION OF TRANSPLANTED HEPATOCYTES

Attempts to increase the proportion of transplanted hepatocytes or transduced, transplanted hepatocytes in the liver simply by stimulating liver regeneration (for example, through the use of partial hepatectomy or CCl_4-induced hepatic necrosis) have generally failed to show significant benefit (11). This is not surprising if one considers that, on average, hepatocytes need to undergo only one or two rounds of cell division to replace the mass of liver removed by a two-thirds partial hepatectomy (12,13), and both endogenous and transplanted hepatocytes compete for this very limited proliferative response. Performing repeated partial hepatectomies is also generally not effective, since both transplanted and host hepatocytes can again respond similarly to this regenerative stimulus. Repeated cell transplantations have also been performed (14,15), but this has not significantly increased the efficacy of liver replacement by transplanted cells. Two exceptions, which remain unexplained, are liver repopulation by transplanted hepatocytes in Nagase analbuminemic rats and Gunn rats, using ligation of portal vein branches to induce atrophy of selected hepatic lobes, while other lobes containing the transplanted cells are induced to proliferate (16,17). Under these circumstances, there was preferential liver repopulation by transplanted hepatocytes (up to about 15% to 20% of parenchymal mass) with improved biochemical function for albumin synthesis (16) and UDP-glucuronyl transferase (17), respectively.

Kay and coworkers (18) have used an alternative approach by inducing temporary toxic injury to host hepatocytes prior to hepatocyte transplantation by injecting an adenovirus vector expressing a nonsecreted urokinase-plasminogen activator gene. In these experiments, 5% to 7% liver repopulation by transplanted cells was achieved with an estimated 3 to 4 rounds of cell division. Similar repopulation (10% to 16%) has been obtained by using anti-Fas antibody to induce apoptosis in the liver after transplanting transgenic hepatocytes overexpressing the *bcl-2* gene, which renders these cells resistant to apoptotic challenge (19).

SPONTANEOUS LIVER REPOPULATION

In 1991, Sandgren et al. (20) observed clonal expansion of hepatocytes involving multiple rounds of cell division in a transgenic mouse model prepared to study blood clotting disorders (see Chapter 63). The urokinase plasminogen activator (uPA) gene under control of the albumin promoter was introduced into mice with the intention that uPA would be synthesized in hepatocytes and secreted into the serum. Most of the animals died from uncontrolled bleeding, but the liver also showed unexpected pathology; namely, extensive inflammation, necrosis and a paucity of mature hepatocytes. Even more unexpected was the finding that animals in two founder lines survived and showed spontaneous development of nodular regions of liver containing normal hepatocytes (Fig. 61.1). uPA-expressing hepatocytes underwent necrosis, but the transgene had been inactivated in the healthy nodules by somatic deletion, and these revertant hepatocytes proliferated and eventually replaced nearly all of the parenchymal mass. Molecular analysis demonstrated that each nodule was clonal and derived from a single cell. In some cases, an entire liver lobe was derived from a single revertant cell. This implied that complete liver repopulation was possible, if selection conditions favored the expansion of the replacing cell population.

Kvittingen et al. (21,22) subsequently showed that this same phenomenon also occurs in human liver. They performed molecular and immunohistochemical analyses of the livers of children with hepatorenal tyrosinemia type I (HT1). These livers were obtained from patients undergoing liver transplantation. HT1 is caused by deficiency of the enzyme fumarylacetoacetate hydrolase (FAH), the last step in the tyrosine metabolic pathway (Fig. 61.2). Accumulation of fumarylacetoacetate is toxic to hepatocytes and causes liver failure. In 17 of 19 patients, large nodules consisting of healthy, FAH-positive hepatocytes were found (21). Cells in these nodules were shown to express FAH and to have reverted the disease phenotype. Again, the data were best explained by clonal expansion of single hepatocytes which had spontaneously reverted to a normal phenotype, leading to selective proliferation. The size of the nodules of normal liver tissue observed in both rodents and humans implied that expanding cells (hepatocytes) are capable of multiple rounds of cell division (20,21), which was contrary to existing dogma in the field of liver regeneration.

LIVER REPOPULATION WITH TRANSPLANTED HEPATOCYTES

In vivo selection of revertant hepatocyte nodules, as described above, raised the obvious question of whether transplanted cells could be selected in a similar fashion. To address this question, Rhim et al. (23) transplanted syngeneic wild-type hepatocytes, marked with the *E. coli* β-galactosidase gene, to identify transplanted cells, into uPA transgenic animals. As expected, transplanted hepatocytes appeared as nodules of various sizes scattered throughout the liver and significantly repopulated transgenic recipients (Fig. 61.3). The number of cells in β-galactosidase-positive nodules indicated that transplanted hepatocytes had undergone at least 12 divisions. Interestingly, repopulation was not associated with premalignant transformation of the cells, and repopulation could be achieved with transplanted

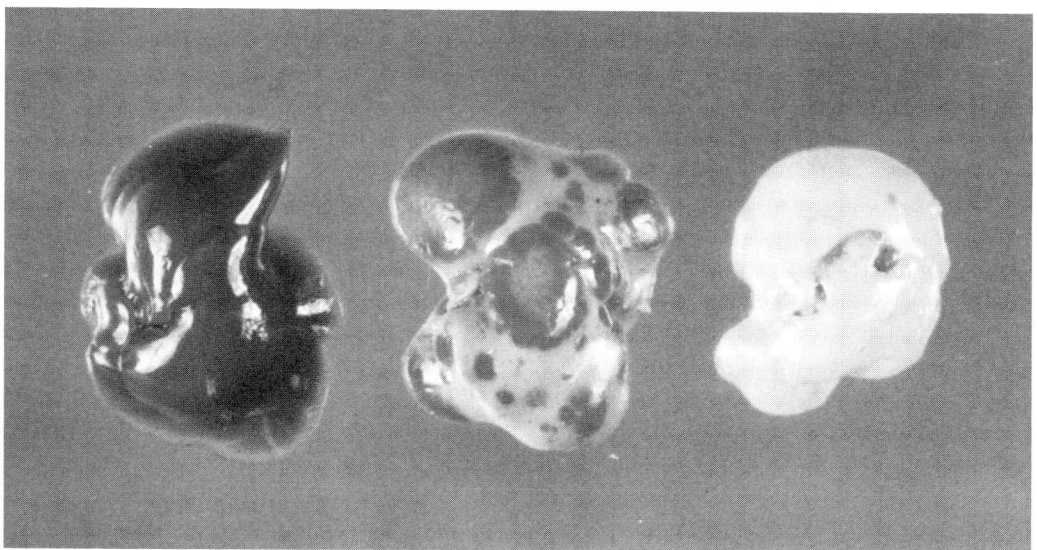

FIGURE 61.1. Spontaneous liver repopulation of urokinase plasminogen activator (uPA) transgenic mouse liver by endogenous hepatocytes that have deleted the uPA transgene. **Left,** liver from a 5-week-old nontransgenic mouse; **center,** liver from a hemizygous uPA transgenic mouse; **right,** liver from a homozygous uPA transgenic mouse. (From Sandgren EP, Palmiter RD, Heckel JL, et al. Complete hepatic regeneration after somatic deletion of an albumin-plasminogen activator transgene. *Cell,* 1991;66:245–256, with permission.) See Color Plate 17.

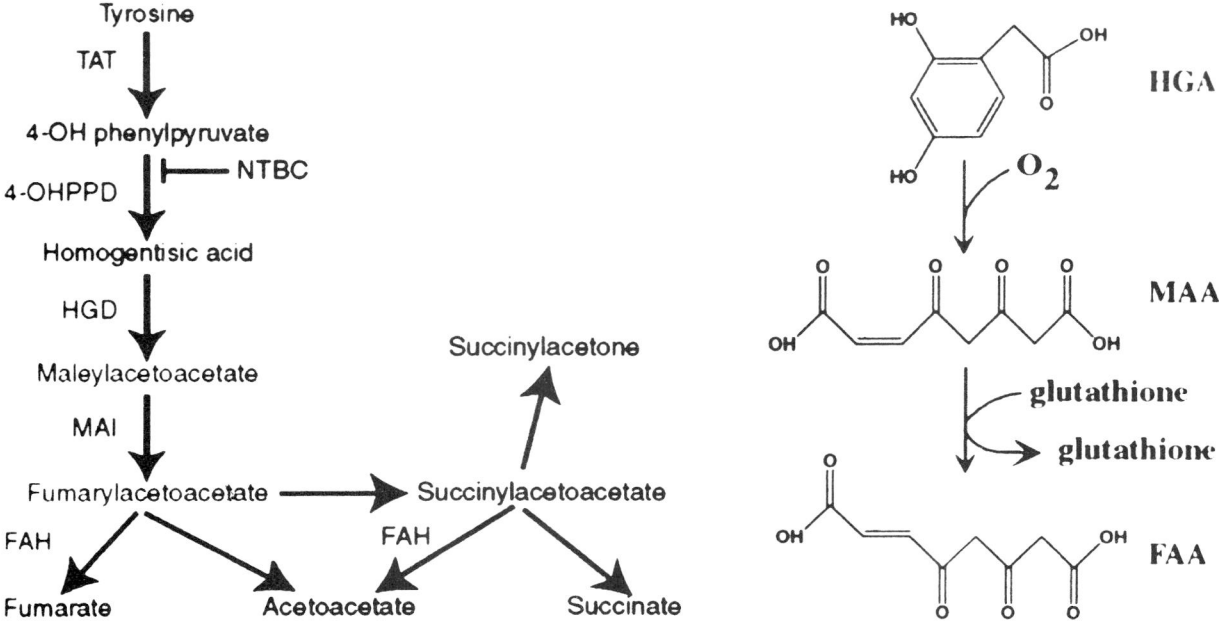

FIGURE 61.2. Tyrosine degradation pathway. *TAT*, tyrosine amino transferase; *4-OHPPD*, 4-hydroxyphenylpyruvate dioxygenase; *HDG*, homogentisic acid dioxygenase; *MAI*, maleylacetoacetate isomerase; *FAH*, fumarylacetoacetate hydrolase.

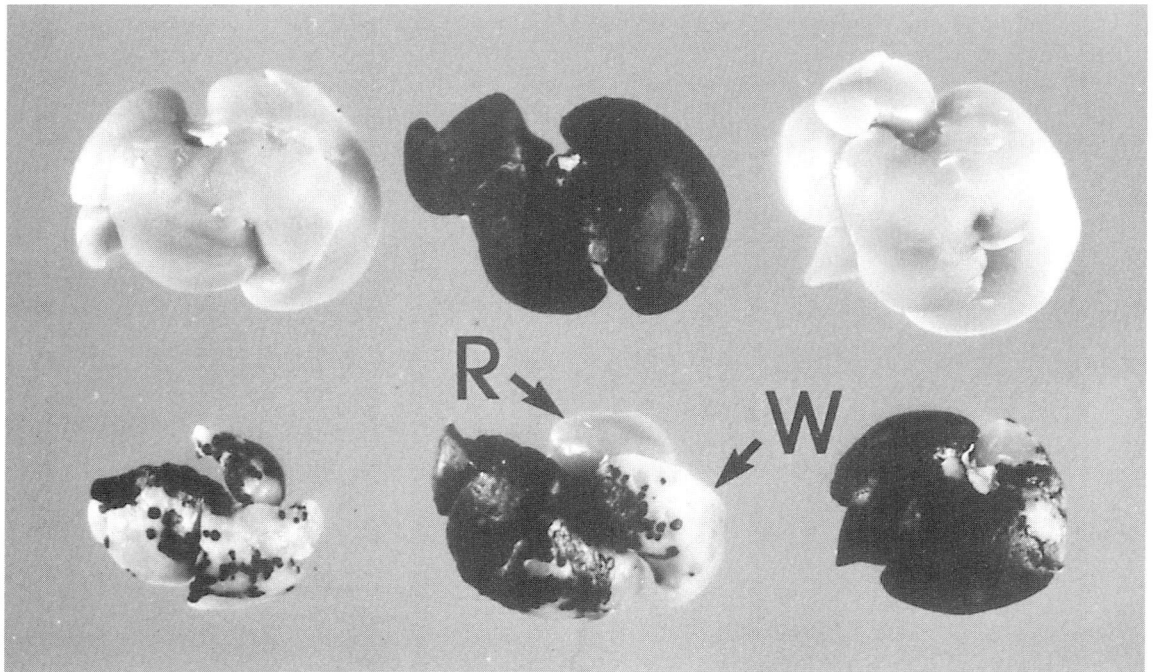

FIGURE 61.3. Repopulation of uPA transgenic mouse liver with transplanted normal mouse hepatocytes containing a lacZ marker transgene. Livers from a nontransgenic control (**top, left**), a lacZ-positive control (**top, center**), a control mouse lacking the Alb-uPA transgene and transplanted with lacZ cells (**top, right**), and three livers from Alb-uPA transgenic mice receiving lacZ cells (**bottom**). All tissues were stained with X-gal, which produces a blue color in lacZ-positive cells. Red areas (*R*) represent endogenous cells that have lost uPA transgene expression, and white areas (*W*) represent residual endogenous liver still expressing the uPA transgene. (From Rhim JA, Sandgren EP, Degen JL, et al. Replacement of disease mouse liver by hepatic cell transplantation. *Science*, 1994;263,1149–1152, with permission.) See Color Plate 18.

cells as efficiently as with endogenous revertant cells. Recently, the uPA model has been utilized to show that cryopreserved hepatocytes can effectively repopulate diseased liver (24), thus verifying one of the potential advantages of cell as compared to solid organ transplantation.

Because spontaneous revertant nodules had been observed in human HT1 (21,22), the possibility of therapeutic liver repopulation was explored in a murine model of HT1 produced by targeted gene disruption of the FAH gene in mouse embryonic stem cells (25). In this model, the accumulation of fumarylacetoacetate (FAA) and other hepatotoxic intermediates in tyrosine metabolism can be prevented by administration of 2(2-nitro-4-trifluoromethylbenzoyl)-1,3 cyclohexane dione (NTBC), a pharmacologic inhibitor of tyrosine catabolism upstream of FAH (26) (Fig. 61.2). Liver failure in FAH null mice develops only when NTBC administration is discontinued. After transplantation of syngeneic wild-type hepatocytes into FAH mutant recipients, the animals were either maintained on NTBC or taken off this agent (27). In the presence of continued NTBC treatment, only scattered transplanted cells in small clusters were observed and there was no effective liver repopulation, similar to results observed two days after hepatocyte transplantation (Fig. 61.4, upper panel). If NTBC treatment was discontinued, transplanted cells proliferated preferentially over endogenous hepatocytes and formed large clusters by 3 weeks (Fig. 61.4, middle panel). Within 6 weeks after stopping NTBC treatment in conjunction with hepatocyte transplantation, transplanted donor cells replaced more than 95% of host hepatocytes (Fig. 61.4, lower panel). Animals with repopulated livers remained healthy, had normal liver function tests and showed a relatively normal liver structure many months after cell replacement (27). These results provided proof of principle in an animal model that liver repopulation could effectively cure a metabolic disease, the mouse equivalent of HT1. Transplanted, repopulating hepatocytes completely integrated into the preexisting hepatic architecture and expressed all functions required for normal health of the animal. Similarly, a rat model of Wilson's disease can also be treated by cell transplantation (28). A recent report of partial liver repopulation by transplanting transgenic hepatocytes from mice expressing a human *MDR3* gene into mdr2 null mice represents another example of potentially how therapeutic cell transplantation might be conducted (29). Taken together, these results illustrate the principle that liver repopulation will occur if hepatocytes in the host liver are exposed to a cytotoxic disease process and if the cytotoxic effect is cell-autonomous (i.e., it does not affect other cells, host or transplanted, in the adjacent parenchyma). Table 61.1 contains a partial list of genetic liver diseases which probably fulfill these criteria and for this reason might be good candidates for treatment by hepatocyte transplantation.

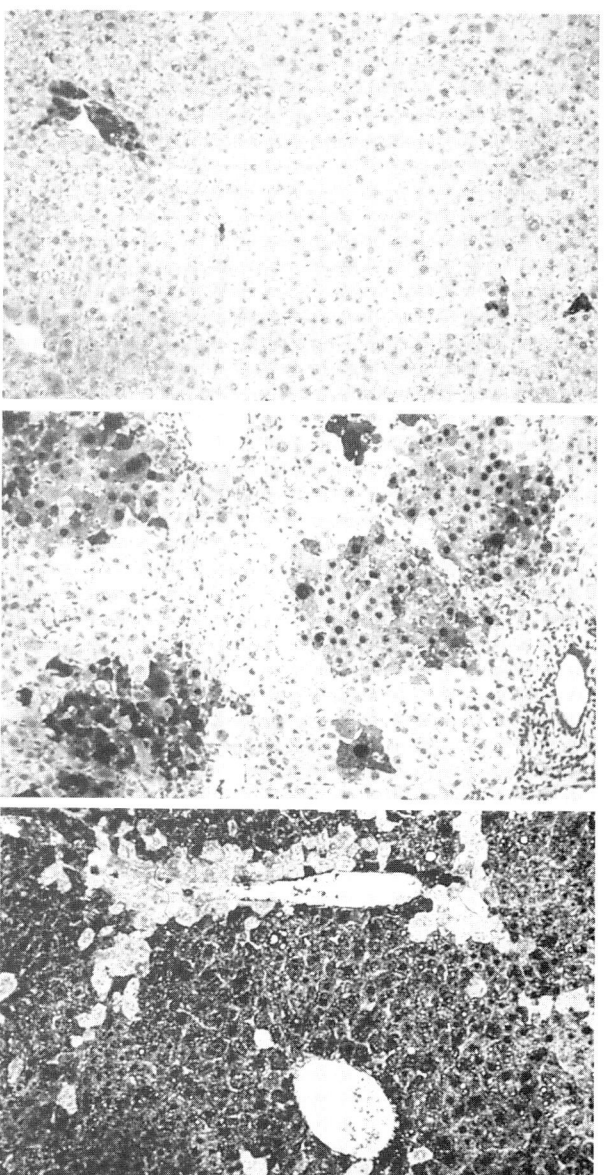

FIGURE 61.4. Liver repopulation in the fumarylacetoacetate hydrolase (FAH) null mouse 2 days (**top**), 3 weeks (**middle**) and 6 weeks (**bottom**) after transplantation of FAH⁺ hepatocytes. If FAH⁻ mice transplanted with FAH⁺ hepatocytes are taken off 2(2-nitro-4-trifluoromethylbenzoyl)-1,3 cyclohexane dione (NTBC), progressive liver repopulation occurs (see text for experimental details). See Color Plate 19.

In the FAH-deficient mouse model, only 1,000 donor cells is sufficient to produce near-complete liver repopulation after 6 to 8 weeks (27). Thus, transplantation of as few as 0.001% of the hepatic mass (1/100,000 cells) can be therapeutic, if accompanied by host selection. The replication potential of transplanted repopulating cells was also determined by serial transplantation with limiting numbers of normal hepatocytes through seven rounds of serial trans-

TABLE 61.1. CANDIDATE DISORDERS FOR LIVER REPOPULATION

Hereditary tyrosinemia type I
Wilson's disease
α_1-antitrypsin deficiency, Z-allele
Glycogen storage disease type I (Van Gierke's disease)
Glycogen storage disease type IV (Debrancher enzyme
   deficiency)
Galactosemia
Hereditary fructose intolerance
Hemochromatosis
Bile acid synthesis disorders
Progressive familial intrahepatic cholestasis types 1, 2 and 3

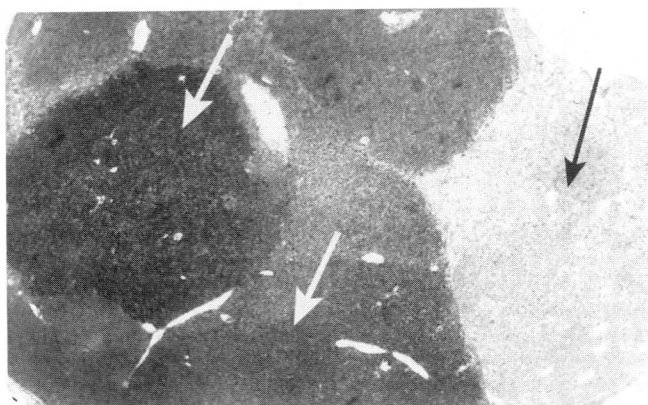

FIGURE 61.5. Repopulation of the liver in fumarylacetoacetate hydrolase (FAH) null mice with FAH-positive hepatocytes after infusion into the portal vein of a recombinant MuLV retrovirus containing the full-length human FAH coding region. Individual clusters of FAH⁺ cells, showing different levels of FAH expression (denoted by *white arrows*), are probably derived from single FAH⁻ hepatocytes transduced with h-FAH MuLV retrovirus. *Black arrow* indicates region of nontransduced FAH⁻ liver.

plantation into FAH null mice (30). Repopulating liver cells were able to double at least 100 times without loss of function and without becoming malignant. These results are analogous to findings after bone marrow transplantation.

The functional integrity of serially transplanted cells was also established. First, blood parameters of normal hepatic function were measured including levels of transaminases, bilirubin and amino acids. Second, repopulated livers showed a normal lobular architecture and a central lobular pattern of glutamine synthetase expression. Thus, adult murine liver contains cells with "stem cell-like" regenerative capacity. Using unfractionated male donor hepatocytes transplanted into female recipients, donor-derived cells were detected by Y chromosome-specific *in situ* hybridization. Interestingly, the only donor-derived cell type detected was hepatocytes, as all other hepatic cell types in the repopulated liver were of host origin, including biliary epithelium, stellate cells, Kupffer cells and endothelial cells (30). Therefore, despite their high regenerative capacity, the lineage potential of the serially transplantable repopulating liver cells used in these experiments may be restricted to hepatocytic differentiation. It was also observed unexpectedly that large hepatocytes, which contain tetraploid and octaploid cells, exhibit a much higher repopulation potential than small diploid hepatocytes in this model (31).

GENE THERAPY IN THE SETTING OF LIVER REPOPULATION

Based on successful liver repopulation with transplanted hepatocytes, studies were undertaken to determine whether hepatocytes corrected by gene therapy might also be capable of repopulating diseased liver in FAH null mice, a specific model in which the newly introduced and expressed gene provides transplanted cells with a selective advantage for survival. Mutant mice were infused through the portal vein with a retroviral vector containing the human *FAH* gene and were then taken off NTBC, allowing selection to

occur (27). Within 8 weeks, more than 90% of hepatocytes in the recipient liver were retrovirally transduced and expressed FAH (Fig. 61.5). *In vivo* selection and proliferation of transduced hepatocytes greatly enhanced the efficacy of liver gene therapy in this model. Furthermore, it has been shown in the HT1 model that hepatocytes which were explanted into tissue culture and retrovirally transduced *ex vivo* retain their ability to repopulate the liver (32) and can be serially transplanted. However, although *in vivo* selection for genetically corrected cells clearly works in HT1, most hereditary and many acquired liver diseases do not create an environment as favorable as HT1 for selection.

The FAH null mouse also provides another example of the role of selection in spontaneous liver repopulation. Mice which are FAH-deficient but also heterozygous for a mutation in homogentisic acid dioxygenase (HGD), an enzyme upstream of FAH in the pathway (see Fig. 61.2), spontaneously repopulate their liver with hepatocytes which have become homozygous for HGD deficiency (33). HGD deficiency prevents the accumulation of FAA and thus provides a selective advantage to cells which have lost the wild-type *HGD* gene. This example of an *in vivo* suppressor mutation shows that liver repopulation can occur after genetic events in second genes not directly involved in causing liver disease.

CREATING SPACE FOR TRANSPLANTED HEPATOCYTES

To achieve successful liver repopulation with transplanted cells, two conditions need to be met: (a) the transplanted cell must have a selective advantage in either proliferation or survival, as compared to endogenous hepatocytes, and (b) endogenous hepatocytes need to be removed from the liver either acutely or chronically to provide the impetus for transplanted cells to proliferate and restore the liver mass. In tyrosinemia type I, Wilson's disease and uPA transgenic mice, metabolic damage to endogenous hepatocytes is caused by the genetic disease or altered metabolic state. However, this situation is the exception rather than the rule, and more generally applicable protocols need to be found. In bone marrow transplantation, lethal whole body irradiation and chemotherapy are used to destroy the endogenous marrow. However, complete or near total eradication of the recipient's cells cannot be applied to liver repopulation, because a minimum of approximately 20% to 25% metabolic function of this organ is critical for survival, and at present only 1% to 2% of hepatocyte mass can be replaced acutely by cell transplantation.

Recent work in a rat model has pointed to a potential practical solution to this problem which may have general applicability. Laconi et al. (34) developed an approach to liver repopulation by chemically blocking the regenerative capacity of the host liver using lasiocarpine, a pyrrolizidine alkaloid that is taken up selectively by hepatocytes, where it is metabolized to its active form and alkylates cellular DNA. This causes proliferation arrest of hepatocytes in the G2 phase or G2/M boundary of the cell cycle (35,36), so that these cells cannot restore liver mass in response to a proliferative stimulus. However, adequate metabolic function is maintained by DNA-damaged hepatocytes, so that animals survive two-thirds partial hepatectomy which creates a stimulus for liver repopulation. Gross liver damage by the pyrrolizidine alkaloid is repaired within 3 to 4 months following hepatocyte transplantation (34). Gordon et al. (37) have recently shown that partial hepatectomy induces proliferation of endogenous small hepatocyte-like progenitor cells in the pyrrolizidine alkaloid model which appear to play a role in the regeneration process.

Using a less toxic pyrrolizidine alkaloid, retrorsine, Laconi and colleagues (38) demonstrated near total (up to 99%) liver repopulation by transplanting genetically marked rat hepatocytes that are positive for the bile canalicular membrane protein dipeptidyl peptidase IV (DPPIV) into the liver of a congenic strain of mutant rats not expressing DPPIV enzyme activity. Because DPPIV is expressed uniquely at the canalicular domain of mature, fully differentiated hepatocytes, it was possible to follow the structural relationship between transplanted and host hepatocytes at all stages during liver repopulation by colocalization of DPPIV with Mg^{++}/K^+ ATPase, the classical marker of the bile canaliculus (38). The general features and kinetics of liver repopulation were essentially analogous to those observed in uPA transgenic and FAH null mice. Within two months, there was 40% to 60% replacement by transplanted hepatocytes in female rats and greater than 95%

replacement in male rats. The levels of transplanted cells increased to 98% to 99% in male rats at 9 months post-hepatocyte transplantation (Fig. 61.6A,B) and remained constant at 40% to 60% in female rats at 12 months (the duration of experiments conducted).

After transplanting 1 to 2×10^6 hepatocytes, which represents about 0.1% to 0.2% of the total hepatic mass, transplanted cells began to proliferate within 24 hours, expanded rapidly and became totally integrated into the hepatic parenchyma within 4 to 7 days (38). Hybrid bile canaliculi were observed between transplanted and endogenous hepatocytes and normal hepatic cords were formed, without evidence of hyperplastic nodules, adenomatous transformation, or compression of the surrounding liver parenchyma (Fig. 61.6C,D). The entire liver structure became remodeled within 2 months and appeared normal on histologic analysis. Biochemical function of transplanted cells was demonstrated by glucose-6-phosphatase activity, glycogen synthesis and storage, and albumin synthesis (38).

Using the same experimental approach, normal albumin synthesis and normal serum albumin levels have been achieved in Nagase analbuminemic rats (NAR) by hepatocyte transplantation (39). In this case, immunosuppression of cell transplant recipients was required because the animals were not inbred. Thus, both biochemical and physiologic function of the liver can be restored by hepatocyte transplantation in the rat under selective conditions, again consistent with results observed in uPA transgenic and FAH null mice (20,23,25–27).

The above experiments illustrate that functional liver repopulation with transplanted cells can be achieved using a cell-cycle block in host hepatocytes (retrorsine) in combination with a mitotic stimulus to transplanted cells (partial hepatectomy). Although retrorsine itself may not be ideal for clinical use, other DNA-damaging agents such as X-rays or DNA cross-linkers are being studied. Guha et al. (40) have achieved 75% to 80% hepatocyte repopulation after radiotherapy with 50 Gy to the liver, followed by hepatocyte transplantation and two-thirds partial hepatectomy.

The driving force for liver repopulation in the retrorsine/PH hepatocyte transplantation model is different from that in uPA transgenic and FAH null mice; however, in all three systems, normal liver physiologic function is restored. In another transgenic mouse model for liver repopulation using the herpes simplex virus thymidine kinase (TK) gene under control of the albumin promoter, which causes hepatocyte death and an inflammatory reaction when ganciclovir is administered, variable results have been obtained following hepatocyte transplantation (41). Under the same protocol, some animals are healthy after ganciclovir treatment and wild-type hepatocyte transplantation, whereas others are sick. The healthy animals showed 74% to 84% liver repopulation with restoration of the liver lobular structure and normal biochemical function. Sick animals also showed considerable liver repopulation (up to 50% or

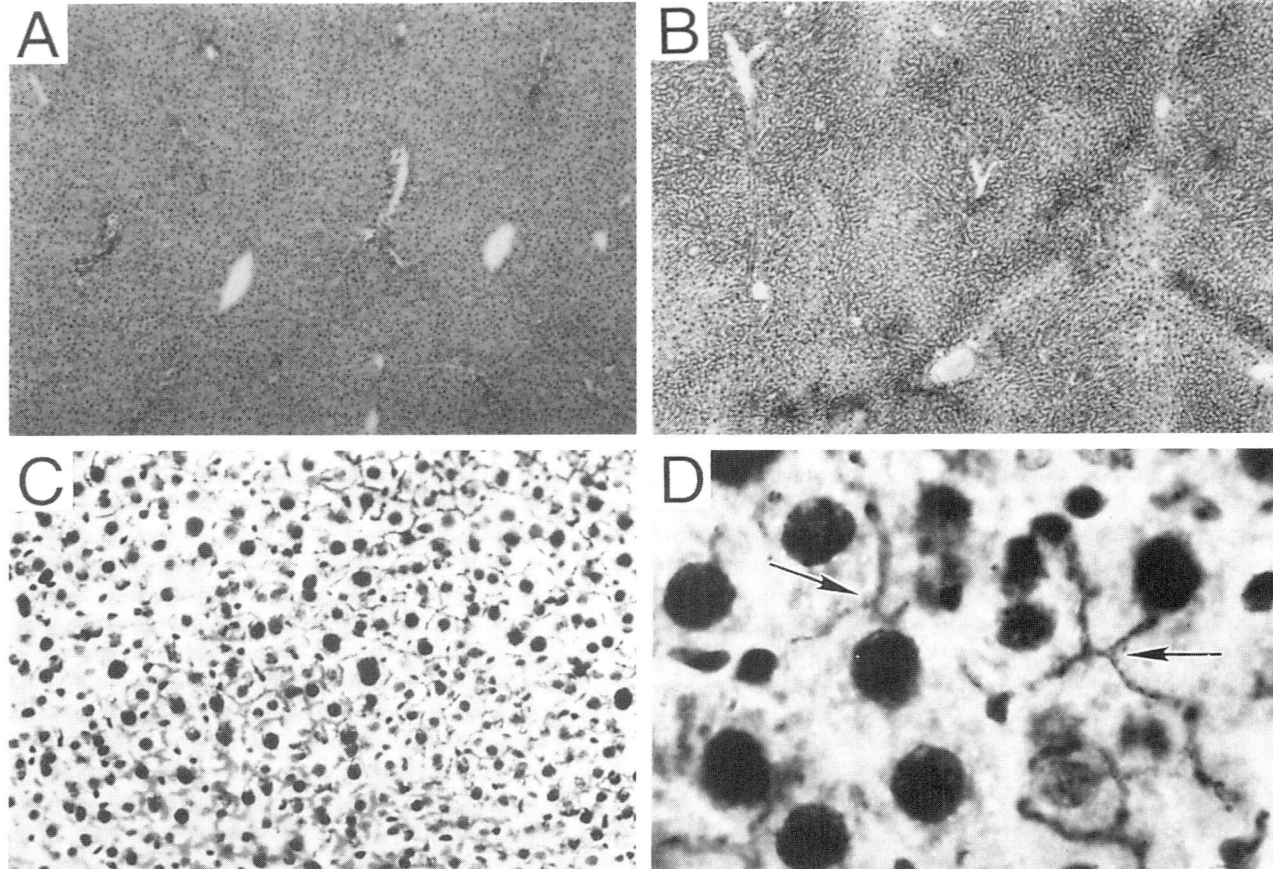

FIGURE 61.6. Liver repopulation by dipeptidyl peptidase IV (DPPIV)+hepatocytes in DPPIV⁻ mutant Fischer 344 rats in the retrorsine/partial hepatectomy model. **A:** Liver from DPPIV⁻ rat before hepatocyte transplantation. **B:** Liver from same DPPIV⁻ rat 9 months after transplantation of DPPIV⁺ hepatocytes. **C:** Expanding clusters of DPPIV⁺ hepatocytes in DPPIV⁻ rat liver two months after transplantation of DPPIV⁺ hepatocytes. **D:** Higher magnification of region from panel C showing formation of hybrid bile canaliculi between endogenous (DPPIV⁻) and transplanted (DPPIV⁺) hepatocytes as denoted by *arrows*. (From Laconi E, Oren R, Mukhopadhyay DK, et al. Long-term, near-total liver replacement by transplantation of isolated hepatocytes in rats treated with retrorsine. *Am J Pathol* 1998;153:319–329, with permission.) See Color Plate 20.

more) but without restoration of the liver lobular structure and clearly abnormal biochemical function. Thus, the restoration of normal liver architecture, which is variable in this model, is a key parameter in determining the efficacy of therapeutic liver repopulation. This has major implications in terms of methods and potential applications in humans, especially in patients with advanced cirrhosis.

In humans, methods gentler than partial hepatectomy (PH) will be necessary to stimulate liver proliferation, for example infusions of hormones, growth factors, and other agents, such as peroxisomal proliferators. The mitogenic hormone T3 has been shown in rats to partially replace PH in the retrorsine liver repopulation model (42). After initially stimulating hepatocyte proliferation, T3 augments apoptosis of megalocytic (DNA alkylated) hepatocytes in retrorsine-treated liver (42), which is also observed in this model after PH (43). In the final analysis, however, differ-

ent liver diseases will require different strategies to achieve effective liver repopulation.

ROLE OF LIVER STEM CELLS

In most liver repopulation experiments reported to date, unfractionated suspensions of liver cells were used and thus it remained unclear whether all hepatocytes or only a rare subpopulation(s) participate in this process. In addition, it may be necessary to distinguish between cells capable of short-term repopulation and cells which produce long-term repopulation and can be serially transplanted. The high regenerative capacity of serially transplantable cells in particular has raised the question of whether liver stem cells may be responsible for this process. The existence of stem cells in the adult liver has been postulated for some time, but their physiological significance remains controversial (44,45). After partial hepatectomy, virtually all hepatocytes participate in liver regeneration and stem cells are not required (46). Similarly, normal cell turnover in the adult liver is very slow and appears to be accomplished by division of differentiated hepatocytes (44–46). However, progenitor- or stem cell-dependent liver regeneration has been observed in specialized animal models. For example, when rats are given a chemical toxin which damages hepatocytes and simultaneously inhibits their ability to divide (for example D-galactosamine), regeneration occurs via cells residing in the portal area that give rise to oval cells which subsequently proliferate and differentiate into mature hepatocytes (47,48).

It would seem reasonable to hypothesize that adult liver cells are not homogeneous in their capacity for cell division and that subpopulations with high repopulation capacity might exist. If this were the case, the efficiency of liver repopulation could be enhanced by first isolating cells with higher proliferative potential and using only purified fractions for transplantation. These cells may be identical to the oval cell precursors seen during progenitor-dependent liver regeneration. In the hematopoietic system, repopulation experiments with purified fractions of total bone marrow were used to identify stem cells. Similar experiments have now been performed with liver cells.

In FAH mutant mice, three sets of experiments have been performed to address whether differentiated hepatocytes or stem cells are responsible for repopulation observed in this model (31). First, cell fractionation by centrifugal elutriation was used to identify and purify three major size fractions of hepatocytes (16, 21 and 27 μm). Each fraction was transplanted in competition with unfractionated liver cells with a distinct genetic marker, the latter serving as a baseline reference for liver repopulation. It was found that the larger hepatocytes, which represent about 70% of the population, were primarily responsible for liver repopulation. In contrast to expectation, small diploid hepatocytes were inferior to the larger cells in competitive repopulation experiments. Second, competitive repopulation was performed between naïve liver cells and those that had been serially transplanted up to seven times. Interestingly, serial transplantation neither enhanced nor diminished the liver repopulation capacity. If serial liver repopulation was stem cell-dependent, this result would suggest that the ratio of progenitors:differentiated hepatocytes was kept constant during a 10^{20}-fold cell expansion. More likely, this result means that virtually all the original input cells (more than 95% hepatocytes) were capable of serial transplantation. The third set of experiments involved retroviral marking of donor hepatocytes *in vitro* and *in vivo*. Again, no evidence of a rare stem cell responsible for liver repopulation was detected. Together, these experiments strongly suggest that fully differentiated, binucleated hepatocytes which constitute the majority of liver cells are most useful for therapeutic liver repopulation and have a stem cell-like capacity for cell division; however, other cell types are also capable of repopulating the liver (see Liver Repopulation by Oval Cells, below).

LIVER REPOPULATION BY OVAL CELLS

Hepatocyte progenitor (or oval) cells can be isolated from the liver of rats treated with D-galactosamine or the pancreas of rats treated with a copper-deficient diet, which causes atrophy of pancreatic acini and proliferation of duct-like oval cells expressing genes in the hepatocytic lineage (49,50). When either hepatic- or pancreatic-derived progenitor cells are transplanted to the liver, these cells proliferate modestly and differentiate into mature hepatocytes (51). These experiments were conducted under nonselective conditions. When a crude preparation of cells from the normal mouse pancreas was transplanted into the liver of FAH null mice, small clusters of cells with a differentiated hepatocyte phenotype were observed (52). In some animals, extensive liver repopulation occurred, indicating selection of pancreatic epithelial cells which have the capacity for massive proliferation and differentiation into hepatocytes. These combined studies suggest that progenitor cells exist in both the liver and pancreas, and under appropriate circumstances, these cells can be activated to repopulate the liver.

LIVER REPOPULATION WITH FETAL HEPATOBLASTS

Classical embryological studies have traced the proliferation and differentiation of precursor or determined stem cells into the hepatocytic and biliary epithelial lineages during normal liver development in both rodents and humans (for review, see ref. 45). This process begins at day E8.5 in the mouse, with proliferation of epithelial cells of the ventral foregut and migration of these cells into the septum transversum, where they come into contact with mesenchymal cells. These cells express α-fetoprotein and then albumin, and subsequently, the liver bud forms at day E11. Their morphology changes to characteristic hepatoblasts which begin to differentiate into hepatocytes and biliary epithelial cells between day E15 and day E16. Thus, the fetal liver contains epithelial cells that are in different stages of lineage progression, some of which might still contain the full potential of liver stem cells. Whether these cells can be isolated, cultured and transplanted for therapeutic liver repopulation and whether fetal liver stem cells or progenitor cells from adult animals will exhibit properties superior to those of mature hepatocytes in terms of durability, function and self renewal remains to be determined.

Studies with fetal rat liver cells in the retrorsine model indicate that there are at least three distinct subpopulations of hepatoblasts at days E12–14, one appearing to be bipotential on the basis of histochemical markers and the other two with either a unipotent hepatocytic or biliary epithelial cell phenotype (53). The bipotential cells proliferate in retrorsine-treated cell transplantation recipients, whereas the unipotent cells proliferate in normal rats. Both retrorsine-treated and normal liver require PH or T3 treatment to augment proliferation of transplanted day E12–14 fetal liver cells (53). In a normal host liver, up to 10% hepatocyte repopulation can be achieved with day E12–14 fetal liver cells (54). These cells have been shown by double label immunohistochemistry/*in situ* hybridization to undergo active DNA synthesis for an extended period (4 to 6 months) after their transplantation, and therefore seem to have a selective proliferative advantage over host hepatocytes. Finally, it should also be noted that with day E12–14 rat fetal liver cells, both hepatocytic cords and mature bile duct structures are derived from transplanted cells, and complete new lobules are formed (Fig. 61.7).

STEM CELLS AND LIVER REPOPULATION

Embryonic stem cells originate from the inner cell mass of the mammalian blastocyst (Chapter 2). They are totipotent and when isolated and introduced back into blastocysts which have been implanted into a female host, they contribute to the formation of all tissues of the embryo. Under certain conditions, these cells can be propagated in culture as stable, undifferentiated pluripotent stem cell lines (55). During development, embryonic stem cells give rise to somatic stem cells and primitive germ cells (reviewed in

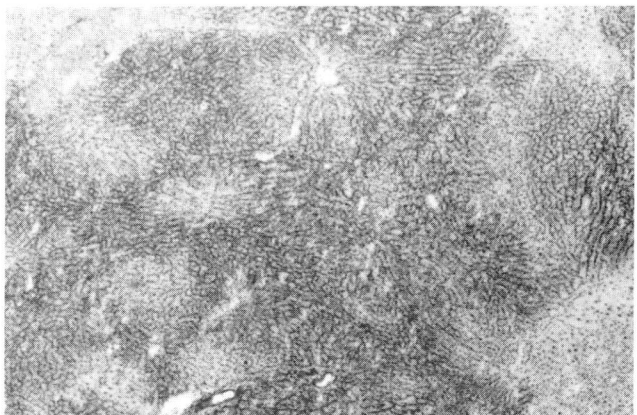

FIGURE 61.7. Repopulation of dipeptidyl peptidase IV (DPPIV)⁻ mutant rat liver by transplanted DPPIV⁺ day E13 fetal liver cells, showing completely new liver lobules containing DPPIV⁺ hepatocyte cords and DPPIV⁺ bile ducts. See Color Plate 21.

refs. 56 and 57 and references therein) and are considered self-renewing, clonogenic and pluripotent. Somatic stem cells differentiate further into multipotent tissue stem cells which have been identified and isolated from the neural crest, bone marrow and central nervous system (56–61), and these cells exhibit self-renewing properties.

It has also become evident that stem cells are very pliable, and they can change their expected phenotype when removed from the stem cell niche and transplanted into a new residence. For example, it was shown that hematopoietic stem cells from adult mouse bone marrow, when transplanted into the mouse blastocyst, begin to express fetal globin whereas in the adult spleen, they produce adult globin (62). Stem cells from adult brain, when transplanted into sublethally irradiated mice, colonize the host bone marrow and differentiate into granulocytes, macrophages and B cells (63). Highly purified hematopoeitic stem cells (HSC) transplanted into bone marrow of lethally irradiated mice repopulate the regenerating muscle of a wounded recipient animal (64) or of the dystrophin-defective mouse (65).

Prompted by these findings, recent studies have been conducted and show that transplanted bone marrow cells that engraft in the liver can differentiate into hepatocytes. Petersen et al. (66) transplanted unfractionated bone marrow cells from male rats (containing a Y chromosome) into lethally irradiated female recipients. Female rats that were successfully engrafted were then treated with 2-acetamino-fluorene (2-AAF), followed by CCl₄ to induce oval cell proliferation and liver regeneration under conditions in which hepatocyte proliferation is blocked (45). In 2-AAF/CCl₄-treated bone marrow cell transplant animals, approximately 0.1% of isolated hepatocytes in the regenerating liver were positive for expression of the Y-chromosome *sry* gene. In addition, using the mutant Fischer 344 wild-type DPPIV⁺ rat as recipient of bone marrow cells from DPPIV⁻ animals, evidence for DPPIV⁺ hepatic cells was also observed after 2-AAF/CCl₄ treatment (66). In separate studies, Theise et al. (67) reported that lethally irradiated female mice that received either unfractionated bone marrow cells or FACS-sorted CD34⁺lin⁻ cells from male donors showed Y chromosome-positive cells in the liver by fluorescence in situ hybridization (FISH). In these studies, cells with the morphologic appearance of hepatocytes and both a Y chromosome and evidence of synthesis of albumin were found up to 8 months following bone marrow transplantation (Fig. 61.8). Their estimate of total hepatocyte mass was an order of magnitude higher than that of Petersen et al. (about 1% to 2%), but in neither case was there extensive liver repopulation by transplanted cells. Lagasse, Grompe and colleagues have transplanted purified hematopoietic stem cells into FAH null mice and obtained significant liver repopulation and functional correction of HT1 liver disease (67a). Thus, "hematopoietic" stem cells have a much broader range of plasticity than previously expected. The relative efficiency of liver repopula-

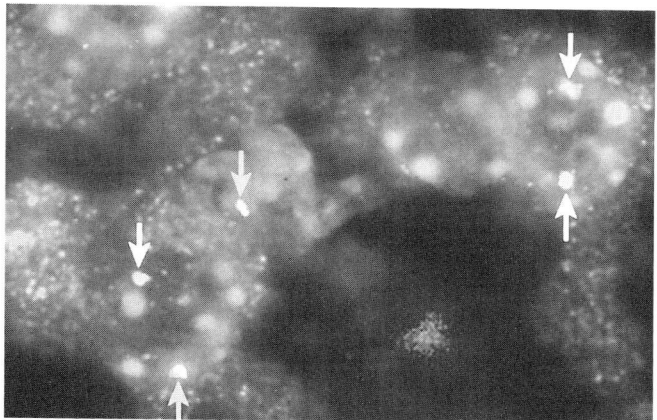

FIGURE 61.8. Detection of Y chromosome-positive hepatocytes in the liver of a female mouse after transplantation of bone marrow cells from a male donor. *Bright green dots* in blue-stained nuclei of hepatocyte (highlighted by *white arrows*) indicate transcription centers for albumin mRNA. The finely stippled, bright green staining surrounding the nuclei is cytoplasmic albumin mRNA. One hepatocyte also contains a red-labeled Y chromosome (*red arrows*), indicating that it is of male origin and derived from the transplanted bone marrow. A second cell of undetermined phenotype also contains a red-labeled Y chromosome, indicating that it also is of male bone marrow origin. See Color Plate 22.

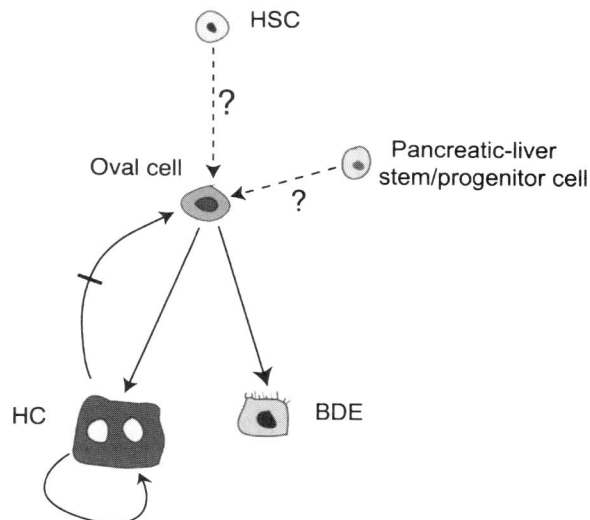

FIGURE 61.9. Schematic diagram illustrating the potential cell types capable of repopulating the liver after cell transplantation. *BDE*, bile duct epithelial cells; *HC*, hepatocytes; *HSC*, hematopoietic stem cells.

tion by bone marrow-derived stem cells compared to hepatocytes has not yet been determined. This comparison will obviously be very important in determining whether liver repopulation by stem cells has any practical applicability or remains a phenomenon of purely scientific interest. Most recently, Theise et al. (68) and Alison et al. (69) have reported the presence of Y chromosome-positive hepatocytes in the liver of human female recipients of male bone marrow cells and human male recipients of orthotopic liver transplants from female donors.

A schematic diagram depicting the various cell types that have been found to proliferate or differentiate into mature liver epithelial cell phenotypes after their transplantation is shown in Figure 61.9. In this diagram, pancreatic and liver stem/progenitor cells, as well as hematopoietic stem cells, are shown to potentially funnel into this system through formation of oval cells which can then proliferate and differentiate into mature liver phenotypes. How this occurs and the number of steps and intermediate cell types involved are currently unknown. In other studies, it has been clearly demonstrated that mature hepatocytes can proliferate and repopulate the liver without reverting to an undifferentiated or immature epithelial cell phenotype. The possibility that some hepatocytes also dedifferentiate and enter the "oval cell" pool, however, cannot be excluded at this time. Future studies will also be needed to determine the roles of these various cell types in normal liver growth control, regeneration and repopulation.

XENOGRAPHIC LIVER CELL TRANSPLANTATION

In uPA transgenic mice crossed with T cell-immunodeficient Swiss athymic nude mice, Rhim et al. (70) have achieved significant liver repopulation with xenographic rat hepatocytes. Repopulation was comparable to results obtained with syngeneic mouse hepatocytes. Similarly, Rogler and colleagues (71) have shown that woodchuck hepatocytes are able to repopulate the liver of uPA transgenic/Rag-2 knockout (T and B cell-deficient) mice, providing a convenient model to study woodchuck hepatitis virus biology. Xenographic repopulation with rat hepatocytes has also been performed successfully in Rag-1/FAH double mutants (M. Grompe, *personal communication,* 2000). Finally, in preliminary studies, human hepatocytes have been reported to yield about 10% repopulation in uPA transgenic/Rag-2 null mice (72).

ROLE OF THE LIVER MICROENVIRONMENT

An interesting aspect of liver repopulation is that the host site in which the transplanted cells are engrafted seems to play a role in their phenotypic behavior. When hepatocytes are transplanted into the dorsal fat pad, spleen, or peritoneal cavity, expression of some hepatocyte-specific genes occurs, but this is usually quite limited and a fully mature hepatocytic morphology is the exception rather than the rule. However, when mature hepatocytes, hepatocytic or pancreatic progenitor cells, hepatoblasts or most recently bone marrow cells are transplanted to the liver, cells with a mature hepatocytic phenotype are observed. With early fetal liver cells, both hepatocytes and mature bile ducts are produced (53,54). When transformed, undifferentiated hepatoma cell lines are transplanted into the liver, they assume a mature hepatocytic phenotype and become arrested in cell growth (73). Thus, the local liver environment plays an important role in determining the phenotype of transplanted cells.

PROSPECTS FOR THE FUTURE

Liver repopulation by transplanted cells has a bright future and will be applicable to the treatment of many liver diseases. Four main challenges exist for this field and will need to be addressed by future research: (a) Are human liver stem/progenitor cells superior to adult hepatocytes in therapeutic liver repopulation? (b) Can hematopoietic or embryonic stem cells be used for liver repopulation? (c) Which is the safest and clinically most useful protocol to "make space" for transplanted cells in the human liver? (d) Which gene/toxin combination(s) will work for *in vivo* expansion of genetically manipulated hepatocytes? and (e) Can hepatocytes, hepatocyte progenitor cells or stem cells be utilized for *ex vivo* gene therapy under conditions in which transplanted cells can be massively amplified? As indicated above, no single protocol is likely to be uniformly successful, and different strategies will need to be developed and implemented to meet the varying nuances of specific pathophysiologic states that exist in the progression of different liver diseases. Active research is currently being conducted to address these issues and will likely lead to human application of these methods in the not too distant future.

REFERENCES

1. Horwich AL. Inherited hepatic enzyme defects as candidates for liver-directed gene therapy. *Curr Top Microbiol Immunol* 1991; 168:185–200.
2. Le-Coultre C, Mentha G, Belli DC. Liver transplantation in children: past, present and future. *Eur J Pediatr Surg* 1997;7: 221–226.
3. Rela M, Muiesan P, Heaton ND, et al. Orthotopic liver transplantation for hepatic-based metabolic disorders. *Transpl Int* 1995;8:41–44.
4. Busuttil RW, Klintmalm GB. *Transplantation of the liver.* Philadelphia:WB Saunders, 1996: xxvii, 903.
5. Gupta S, Chowdhury JR. Hepatocyte transplantation. In: Arias IM, ed. *The liver: biology and pathobiology.* New York: Raven Publishers, 1994:1519–1536.
6. Fox IJ, Chowdhury JR, Kaufman SS, et al. Treatment of the Crigler-Najjar syndrome type I with hepatocyte transplantation. *N Engl J Med* 1998;338:1422–1426.
7. Bilir BM, Guinette D, Karrer F, et al. Hepatocyte transplantation in acute liver failure. *Liver Transpl* 2000;6:32–40.
8. Strom SC, Chowdhury JR, Fox IJ. Hepatocyte transplantation for the treatment of human disease. *Semin Liver Dis* 1999;19:39–48.
9. Mito M, Kusano M. Hepatocyte transplantation in man. *Cell Transpl* 1993;2:65–74.
10. Grossman M, Rader DJ, Muller DWM, et al. A pilot study of *ex vivo* gene therapy for homozygous familial hypercholesterolemia. *Nat Med* 1995;1:1148–1154.
11. Kay MA, Woo SL. Gene therapy for metabolic disorders. *Trends Genet* 1994;10:253–257.
12. Grisham JW. A morphologic study of deoxyribonucleic acid synthesis and cell proliferation in regenerating rat liver: autoradiography with thymidine-H3. *Cancer Res* 1962;22:842–849.
13. Bucher NLR, Swaffield MN. The rate of incorporation of labeled thymidine into the deoxyribonucleic acid of regenerating rat liver in relation to the amount of liver excised. *Cancer Res* 1964;240: 1611–1625.
14. Rozga J, Holzman M, Moscioni AD, et al. Repeated intraportal hepatocyte transplantation in analbuminemic rats. *Cell Transplant* 1995;4:237–243.
15. Rajvanshi P, Kerr A, Bhargava KK, et al. Efficacy and safety of repeated hepatocyte transplantation for significant liver repopulation in rodents. *Gastroenterology* 1996;111:1092–1102.
16. Moscioni AD, Rozga J, Chen S, et al. Long-term correction of albumin levels in the Nagase Analbuminemic Rat: repopulation of the liver by transplanted normal hepatocytes under a regeneration response. *Cell Transplant* 1996;5:499–503.
17. Ilan Y, Chowdhury NR, Prakash R, et al. Massive repopulation of rat liver by transplantation of hepatocytes into specific lobes of the liver and ligation of portal vein branches to other lobes. *Transplantation* 1997;64:8–13.
18. Vrancken Peeters MJ, Patijn GA, Lieber A, et al. Expansion of donor hepatocytes after recombinant adenovirus-induced liver regeneration in mice. *Hepatology* 1997;25:884–888.
19. Mignon A, Guidotti JE, Mitchell C, et al. Selective repopulation of normal mouse liver by Fas/CD95-resistant hepatocytes. *Nat Med* 1998;4:1185–1188.
20. Sandgren EP, Palmiter RD, Heckel JL, et al. Complete hepatic regeneration after somatic deletion of an albumin-plasminogen activator transgene. *Cell* 1991;66:245–256.
21. Kvittingen EA, Rootwelt H, Berger R, et al. Self-induced correction of the genetic defect in tyrosinemia type I. *J Clin Invest* 1994; 94:1657–1661.
22. Kvittingen EA, Rootwelt H, Brandtzaeg P, et al. Hereditary tyrosinemia type I. Self-induced correction of the fumarylacetoacetase defect. *J Clin Invest* 1993;91:1816–1821.
23. Rhim JA, Sandgren EP, Degen JL, et al. Replacement of disease mouse liver by hepatic cell transplantation. *Science* 1994; 263:1149–1152.
24. Jamal HZ, Weglarz TC, Sandgren EP. Cryopreserved mouse hepatocytes retain regenerative capacity *in vivo. Gastroenterology* 2000; 118:390–394.
25. Grompe M, Al-Dhalimy M, Finegold M, et al. Loss of fumarylacetoacetate hydrolase is responsible for the neonatal hepatic dysfunction phenotype of lethal albino mice. *Genes Dev* 1993;7: 2298–2307.
26. Grompe M, Lindstedt S, Al-Dhalimy M, et al. Pharmacological correction of neonatal lethal hepatic dysfunction in a murine model of hereditary tyrosinaemia type I. *Nat Genet* 1995;10: 453–460.
27. Overturf K, Al-Dhalimy M, Tanguay R, et al. Hepatocytes corrected by gene therapy are selected *in vivo* in a murine model of hereditary tyrosinaemia type I. *Nat Genet* 1996;12:266–273.
28. Yoshida Y, Tokusashi Y, Lee GH, et al. Intrahepatic transplantation of normal hepatocytes prevents Wilson's disease in Long-Evans cinnamon rats. *Gastroenterology* 1996;111:1654–1660.

28b. Irani AP, Mahli M, Slehria S, et al. Correction of liver disease following transplantation of normal hepatocytes in LEC rats modeling Wilson's disease. *Mol Ther* 2001;3:302–309.

29. deVree JML, Ottenhoff R, Bosma PJ, et al. Correction of liver disease by hepatocyte transplantation in a mouse model of progressive intrahepatic cholestosis. *Gastroenterology* 2000;119:1720–1730.

30. Overturf K, Al-Dhalimy M, Ou CN, et al. Serial transplantation reveals the stem-cell-like regenerative potential of adult mouse hepatocytes. *Am J Pathol* 1997;151:1273–1280.

31. Overturf K, Al-Dhalimy M, Finegold M, et al. The repopulation potential of hepatocyte populations differing in size and prior mitotic expansion. *Am J Pathol* 1999;155:2135–2143.

32. Overturf K, Al-Dhalimy M, Manning K, et al. *Ex vivo* hepatic gene therapy of a mouse model of hereditary tyrosinemia type I. *Hum Gene Ther* 1998;9:295–304.

33. Manning K, Al-Dhalimy M, Finegold M, et al. *In vivo* suppressor mutations correct a murine model of hereditary tyrosinemia type I. *Proc Natl Acad Sci USA* 1999;96:11928–11933.

34. Laconi E, Sarma DS, Pani P. Transplantation of normal hepatocytes modulates the development of chronic liver lesions induced by a pyrrolizidine alkaloid, lasiocarpine. *Carcinogenesis* 1995;16:139–142.

35. Samuel A, Jago MV. Localization in the cell cycle of the antimitotic action of the pyrrolizidine alkaloid, lasiocarpine and of its metabolite, dehydroheliotridine. *Chem Biol Interact* 1975;10:185–197.

36. Mattocks AR, Driver HE, Barbour RH, et al. Metabolism and toxicity of synthetic analogues of macrocyclic diester pyrrolizidine alkaloids. *Chem Biol Interact* 1986;58:95–108.

37. Gordon GJ, Coleman WB, Hixson DC, et al. Liver regeneration in rats with retrorsine-induced hepatocellular injury proceeds through a novel cellular response. *Am J Pathol* 2000;156:607–619.

38. Laconi E, Oren R, Mukhopadhyay DK, et al. Long-term, near-total liver replacement by transplantation of isolated hepatocytes in rats treated with retrorsine. *Am J Pathol* 1998;153:319–329.

39. Oren R, Dabeva MD, Petkov PM, et al. Restoration of normal serum albumin levels in Nagase analbuminemic rats using a newly described strategy for hepatocyte transplantation. *Hepatology* 1999;29:75–81.

40. Guha C, Sharma A, Gupta S, et al. Amelioration of radiation-induced liver damage in partially hepatectomized rats by hepatocyte transplantation. *Cancer Res* 1999;59:5871–5874.

41. Braun KM, Degen JL, Sandgren EP. Hepatocyte transplantation in a model of toxin-induced liver disease: variable therapeutic effect during replacement of damaged parenchyma by donor cells. *Nat Med* 2000;6:320–326.

42. Oren R, Dabeva MD, Karnezis AN, et al. Role of thyroid hormone in stimulating liver repopulation by transplanted hepatocytes. *Hepatology* 1999;30:903–913.

43. Gordon GJ, Coleman NB, Grisham JW. Bax-mediated apoptosis in the livers of rats after partial hepatectomy in the retrorsine model of hepatocellular injury. *Hepatology* 2000;32:312–320.

44. Sell S. Liver stem cells. *Mod Pathol* 1994;7:105–112.

45. Grisham JW, Thorgeirsson SC. Liver stem cells. In: Potten CS, ed. *Stem cells*. New York: Academic Press, 1997:233–282.

46. Michalopoulos GK, DeFrances MC. Liver regeneration. *Science* 1997;276:60–66.

47. Lemire JM, Shiojiri N, Fausto N. Oval cell proliferation and the origin of small hepatocytes in liver injury induced by D-galactosamine. *Am J Pathol* 1991;139:535–552.

48. Dabeva MD, Shafritz DA. Activation, proliferation and differentiation of progenitor cells into hepatocytes in the D-galactosamine model of liver regeneration. *Am J Pathol* 1993;143:1606–1620.

49. Rao MS, Dwivedi RS, Yeldandi AV, et al. Role of periductular and ductular epithelial cells of the adult pancreas in pancreatic hepatocyte lineage. A change in differentiation commitment. *Am J Pathol* 1989;134:1069–1086.

50. Dabeva MD, Hwang S-G, Vasa SRG, et al. Differentiation of pancreatic epithelial progenitor cells into hepatocytes following transplantation into rat liver. *Proc Natl Acad Sci USA* 1997;94:7356–7361.

51. Dabeva MD, Hurston E, Sharitz DA. Transcription factor and liver-specific mRNA expression in facultative epithelial progenitor cells of liver and pancreas. *Am J Pathol* 1995;147:1633–1648.

52. Grompe M, Al-Dhalimy M, Overturf K, et al. Hepatic repopulation by adult murine pancreatic liver stem cells. *Am J Hum Genet* 1998;63:9.

53. Dabeva MD, Petkov PM, Sandhu J, et al. Proliferation and differentiation of fetal liver epithelial progenitor cells after transplantation into adult rat liver. *Am J Pathol* 2000;156:2017–2031.

54. Dabeva MD, Petkov PM, Sandhu J, et al. Proliferation and differentiation of fetal liver epithelial progenitor cells transplanted into adult rat liver. *FASEB J* 2000;14:A285.

55. Thomson JA, Itskovitz-Eldor J, Shapiro SS, et al. Embryonic stem cell lines derived from human blastocyst. *Science* 1998;282:1145–1147.

56. Fuchs E, Segre JA. Stem cells: a new lease on life. *Cell* 2000;100:143–155.

57. Weissman I. Stem cells: units of development, units of regeneration and units of evolution. *Cell* 2000;100:157–168.

58. Whetton AD, Graham GJ. Homing and mobilization in the stem cell niche. *Trends Cell Biol* 1999;9:233–239.

59. Gage FH. Stem cells of the central nervous system. *Curr Opin Neurobiol* 1998;8:671–676.

60. Stemple DL, Anderson DJ. Isolation of a stem cell for neurons and glia from mammalian neural crest. *Cell* 1992;1:973–985.

61. Morrison SJ, White PM, Zock C, et al. Prospective identification, isolation by flow cytometry, and *in vivo* self-renewal of multipotent mammalian neural crest cells. *Cell* 1999;96:737–739.

62. Geiger H, Sick S, Bonifer C, et al. Globin gene expression is reprogrammed in chimeras generated by injecting adult hematopoietic stem cells into mouse blastocyst. *Cell* 1998;93:1055–1065.

63. Bjornson CR, Rietze RL, Reynolds BA, et al. Turning brain into blood: a hematopoietic fate adopted by adult neural stem cells *in vivo*. *Science* 1999;283:534–537.

64. Ferrari G, Cusella-DeAngelis G, Coletta M, et al. Muscle regeneration by bone marrow-derived myogenic progenitor. *Science* 1998;279:1528–1530.

65. Gussoni E, Soneoka Y, Strickland CD, et al. Dystrophin expression in the mdx mouse restored by stem cell transplantation. *Nature* 1999;401:390–394.

66. Petersen BE, Bowen WC, Patrene KD, et al. Bone marrow as a potential source of hepatic oval cells. *Science* 1999;284:1168–1170.

67. Theise ND, Badve S, Saxena R, et al. Derivation of hepatocytes from bone marrow cells in mice after radiation induced myeloablation. *Hepatology* 2000;31:235–240.

67a. Legasse E, Conners H, M-Dahling M, et al. Purified hematopoietic stem cells can differentiate into hepatocytes in vivo. *Nat Med* 2000;6:1229–1234.

68. Theise ND, Nimmakayalu M, Gardner R, et al. Liver from bone marrow in humans. *Hepatology* 2000;32:11–16.

69. Alison MR, Poulson R, Jeffrey R, et al. Hepatocytes from nonhepatic adult stem cells. *Nature* 2000;406:257.

70. Rhim JA, Sandgren EP, Palmiter RD, et al. Complete reconstitution of mouse liver with xenogeneic hepatocytes. *Proc Natl Acad Sci USA* 1995;92:4942–4946.

71. Petersen J, Dandri M, Gupta S, et al. Liver repopulation with xenogenic hepatocytes in B and T cell-deficient mice leads to chronic hepadnavirus infection and clonal growth of hepatocellular carcinoma. *Proc Natl Acad Sci USA* 1998;95:310–315.

72. Dandri M, Burda MR, Torok E, et al. Repopulation of mouse liver with human hepatocytes and in vivo inffection with hepatitis B virus. *Hepatology* 2001;33:981–988.

73. Coleman WB, Wennerberg AE, Smith GJ, et al. Regulation of the differentiation of diploid and some aneuploid rat liver epithelial (stem-like) cells by the hepatic microenvironment. *Am J Pathol* 1993;142:1373–1382.

The Liver: Biology and Pathobiology, Fourth Edition, edited by I. M. Arias, J. L. Boyer, F. V. Chisari, N. Fausto, D. Schachter, and D. A. Shafritz.
Lippincott Williams & Wilkins, Philadelphia © 2001.

62

LIVER-DIRECTED GENE THERAPY

CLIFFORD J. STEER
BETSY T. KREN
NAMITA ROY CHOWDHURY
JAYANTA ROY CHOWDHURY

In the past decade, there has been an explosive increase in the knowledge of the genetic basis of inherited and acquired diseases, DNA and RNA sequence elements that regulate their expression, as well as the mechanisms involved in endogenous repair pathways of genomic DNA. This has resulted in the development of a variety of strategies for treatment of inherited and acquired disorders using nucleic acids in place of conventional drug therapy. Despite some spectacular scientific achievements, however, unequivocal success in the treatment of genetic disorders by gene therapy has been elusive. This chapter provides an overview of the current methods of gene transfer to the liver and discusses in brief the prospects of treating liver diseases by these novel strategies.

Liver-directed gene therapy can be used for diverse therapeutic strategies. Gene therapy may be used to treat inherited disorders by replacing missing gene products that are normally expressed in the liver. Gene transfer can also be used for generating extrahepatic proteins, such as

coagulation factors or hormones. Proteins that are normally expressed in extrahepatic tissues, such as the catalytic subunit of the apolipoprotein B mRNA editing enzyme (APOBEC-1), which is expressed in the intestine, can be generated ectopically in the liver to reduce the production of low-density lipoproteins (1). Pharmacological gene products, such as vaccines, single chain antibodies, dominant negative proteins, immunomodulatory substances, and agents that induce or inhibit apoptosis could be generated in the liver for specific therapeutic purposes. Another goal of liver-directed gene therapy is to inhibit the expression of deleterious proteins, such as viral proteins or mutant α1-antitrypsin, by transferring synthetic antisense RNAs or ribozymes or genes that express antisense RNAs (2), ribozymes or dominant negative proteins (3). Recently, technologies have been developed which are designed to correct the endogenous faulty copy of the gene, either by targeted replacement of the defective gene (4,5), or by site-directed correction of a target genomic sequence (6,7). These newer approaches allow the repaired gene to remain at its native site under the control of its endogenous promoter.

Targets of liver-directed gene therapy include inherited metabolic disorders, as well as acquired conditions, such as infectious and neoplastic diseases, cirrhosis of the liver, and immune rejection of transplants. As the liver is capable of synthesizing a large amount of protein, it can also be utilized to generate proteins, such as insulin or growth hor-

C. J. Steer: Departments of Medicine and Genetics, Cell Biology, and Development, University of Minnesota Medical School, Minneapolis, Minnesota 55455.

B. T. Kren: Department of Medicine, GI Division, University of Minnesota Medical School, Minneapolis, Minnesota 55455.

N. Roy Chowdhury: Departments of Medicine and Molecular Genetics, Albert Einstein College of Medicine, Bronx, New York 10461.

J. Roy Chowdhury: Departments of Medicine and Molecular Genetics, Albert Einstein College of Medicine; Jack D. Weiler Hospital of Albert Einstein College of Medicine, Bronx, New York 10461.

mone, for treatment of diseases for which the liver is not the primary site. Table 62.1 lists some of the inherited disorders that are current targets of gene therapy.

Neoplastic diseases present a special set of challenges for the gene therapist. The goal is to eliminate the tumor cells with as little damage to the host as possible. Gene therapy strategies for the treatment of neoplastic disorders may be classified as (a) killing or inhibiting the growth of the tumor cells, (b) inducing immune response against tumor cells, (c) reducing vascular supply to tumors, and (d) enhancing the effect of conventional therapies, for example, chemotherapy and radiotherapy. Killing tumor cells is attempted by transferring "suicide genes," such as the gene for the herpes simplex virus thymidine kinase (HSV-TK), which converts a prodrug, ganciclovir, to its active phosphate derivative (8). Cytosine deaminase (9) and purine nucleoside phosphorylase (which converts fludarabine to a diffusible toxic metabolite) (10) are other genes that are being used for this purpose. p53, a sentinel gene of the cell cycle, has been used to induce apoptosis in tumor cells (11).

Because it is not possible to transfer genes to all cells even in a well-circumscribed tumor, the efficacy of tumor killing must depend on the extent of bystander effect, that is, killing of neighboring cells. Bystander effect typically depends on the exchange of toxic agents between neighboring cells. For example, ganciclovir phosphate generated in a cell by the action of HSV-TK may diffuse to surrounding

TABLE 62.1. A PARTIAL LIST OF DISEASES TARGETED FOR LIVER-DIRECTED GENE THERAPY

Inherited Liver Disorders
Crigler–Najjar syndrome type I
Familial hypercholesterolemia and other lipid metabolic
  disorders
Maple syrup urine disease
Progressive familial intrahepatic cholestasis
Phenylketonuria
Tyrosinemia
Mucopolysaccharidosis VII
α_1-antitrypsin deficiency
Ornithine transcarbamylase deficiency
Wilson's disease
Glycogen storage diseases, e.g., von Gierke's disease and
  Pompe's disease
Inherited Systemic Disorders
Hemophilia A and B
Oxalosis
Acquired Disorders
Infectious diseases, e.g., hepatitis B and C
Malignant neoplasms: hepatomas, cholangiocarcinomas,
  metastatic tumors
Extrahepatic tumors (inhibition of neovascularization)
Cirrhosis of the liver
Allograft or xenograft rejection

cells, thereby extending the zone of cell killing beyond the cells that are transduced with HSV-TK. In other cases, the contact with a tumor cell undergoing apoptosis as a result of expression of the wild-type p53 may deliver a "kiss of death" to neighboring cells (12).

The successful treatment with suicide genes is limited by the inability of currently available methods to deliver the genes to enough tumor cells to eliminate the tumor. Furthermore, it is difficult to deliver the genes in a targeted fashion to tumor cells without transducing surrounding normal cells. The toxicity to adjacent normal cells could be reduced by targeting the gene to tumor cells. Tagging the DNA to a monoclonal antibody directed against AF-20, a 180-kd tumor-specific cell surface glycoprotein, has been used to direct genes to AF-20-positive cells, such as hepatoma cell lines (13). Expression of a toxic gene could be limited to specific tumors by using tumor-specific promoters (e.g., α-fetoprotein or carcinoembryonic antigen) to drive the expression of transgene. An alternative approach utilizes E1B-mutant adenoviruses that are capable of replicating in cells that lack active p53, which includes many tumor cells (14). However, although these mutant adenoviruses have been shown to kill tumor cells effectively, their replication may not always depend on the absence of p53.

Because it is nearly impossible to kill all tumor cells, particularly those that are located at distant metastatic sites, by direct expression of toxic genes, many investigators have concentrated on immunotherapy of cancer (15). Immunotherapy is based on the fact that many tumors express antigens that are not expressed by normal adult cells. Although these "neoantigens" are, in fact, native or altered "self" proteins, administration of various cytokines or expression of these cytokines by gene transfer is being used to evoke immune response against the tumor cells. Molecular identification of tumor-associated antigens, such as those from melanoma cells, may permit gene transfer-based tumor vaccination. Isolation and genetic manipulation of antigen-presenting cells may permit the induction of a potent immune response against tumor cells. Large tumors often produce cytokines, such as TGFβ or interleukin 10 (IL10), that may suppress immune response, or stimulate the development of immune suppressor cells (16). Thus, "debulking" the tumor by surgery, radiotherapy, chemotherapy or gene therapy may augment the effect of immunotherapy.

Another interesting and effective method relies on the fact that tumor growth is dependent on the development of new blood vessels. Therefore, tumors, both primary and neoplastic, are particularly sensitive to the inhibition of neovascularization by the expression of angiostatin or endostatin (17,18).

Finally, gene therapy is likely to be effective in combination with chemotherapy or radiotherapy (19). Irradiation of tumors has been shown to enhance the number of tumor cells that can be transduced using recombinant viruses. Expression of suicide genes, driven by radiation-sensitive promoters, may be enhanced by irradiation (20). On the other hand, transferring genes such as ATM (mutated in ataxia telangiectasia) that increase the sensitivity of cells to irradiation may increase the efficacy of radiotherapy in killing tumor cells.

Gene therapy methods are being explored for the prevention or treatment of infections of the liver, particularly by viruses, such as hepatitis virus B or C. These approaches can be divided into (a) DNA-based vaccination (21) and (b) interference with the viral life-cycle by delivery of antisense RNAs, ribozymes, or DNA ribonucleases. Ribozymes, antisense RNAs or dominant negative proteins (3,22) can also be expressed within the target cells by gene transfer. Interestingly, both sense and antisense RNAs can inhibit the replication of hepatitis B virus (23,24). DNA vaccination (25) has the potential advantage over conventional vaccines in that the pure antigen is generated *in vivo*, which eliminates the possibility of contamination with microbes or other organic material. Furthermore, the DNA itself may serve as an adjuvant, enhancing the immune response. In this respect, the immunogenicity of antigens contained in viral vectors may turn into an advantage, permitting an immune response to poorly immunogenic molecules. Many antigens are presented poorly by antigen-presenting cells. In these cases, the antigenic peptides may be expressed directly in the antigen-presenting cells by gene transfer. Another approach is based on the expression of single chain antibodies or antibody fragments within the cells vulnerable to viral infections by gene transfer (26). This method, termed "intracellular vaccination," could render cells resistant to infection by specific viruses.

Although the treatment of neoplastic and infectious diseases is a major goal of liver-directed gene therapy, treatment of inherited disorders presents a special opportunity. Because many inherited disorders are caused by the abnormality of a single gene, the effect of gene therapy can be evaluated directly and precisely in these conditions. For this reason, although the inherited disorders are much less common than acquired diseases, single gene abnormalities continue to be important targets of liver-directed gene therapy.

GENE TRANSFER TO THE LIVER

Genes may be delivered to the liver via isolated hepatocytes, or by direct administration of the gene. Normal isolated hepatocytes may be transplanted without any genetic manipulation to replace missing gene products (27,28). However, as the cells are allogeneic, it is necessary to main-

tain long-term immunosuppression. Alternatively, hepatocytes isolated from the liver of the mutant may be transduced with therapeutic genes prior to transplantation. The latter method does not require immunosuppression and is termed *ex vivo* gene therapy. *Ex vivo* gene transfer may also be used to conditionally immortalize the hepatocytes (29), so that they can be expanded in culture (30), or for expression of proteins for abrogation of immune rejection of allografts or xenografts. Not unexpectedly, the development of *in vivo* gene therapy has paralleled the progress in hepatocyte transplantation and *ex vivo* gene therapy.

In vivo and *ex vivo* gene transfer into hepatocytes can be achieved using nonviral or viral vectors. A brief account of these methods follows and is summarized in Table 62.2.

RECOMBINANT VIRUSES

Many viruses have evolved mechanisms to enter mammalian cells, exit from endosomes, translocate to the nucleus and express viral genes as episomes or after integration into host chromosomes. Replication-deficient recombinant viruses that express desired transgenes, but not the viral proteins, are used commonly for gene transfer. For liver-directed gene therapy, the desirability of a recombinant virus depends on the attainable infectious titer, ability of the virus to infect nondividing cells, efficiency of integration into the host genome, repeatability of administration, and safety of the vector system. Although none of the currently available vectors satisfy all these criteria, a relatively large choice for specific applications has been developed. The commonly used recombinant viral vectors are described below.

Retrovirus-Based Vectors

Retroviruses integrate their complementary DNA into the host genome as a part of their life-cycle (31). Thus, the transgene is transmitted faithfully to the progeny of the transduced cells (32,33). The RNA genome of retroviruses encodes the major viral proteins, *gag*, *pol* and *env* (34). The coding region is flanked on the 5′ and 3′ ends by the "long terminal repeats" (LTRs) that comprise a promoter, enhancers and polyadenylation signals that are needed for viral transcription. Upstream of the 5′ LTR there are packaging sequences (ψ) that are required for incorporation of the viral RNA genome into viral particles. Moloney's murine leukemia virus (MoMuLV) has been used most extensively for generating recombinant vectors. Replication-defective retroviruses are generated by replacing most or all viral genes by target transgenes (35). The plasmid vector is transfected into "packaging cell lines" that provide the required viral proteins in *trans*, thereby generating a repli-

TABLE 62.2. SUMMARY OF FEATURES OF LIVER-DIRECTED GENE THERAPY METHODS

Method	Integration and Persistence	*In vivo* Gene Transfer Efficiency to Liver	Liver Specificity	Immunological[a] and Other Issues
RECOMBINANT VIRAL VECTORS:				
Murine leukemia-based retroviruses	Integration is required.	Requires mitosis. Low efficiency in quiescent cell types, e.g., hepatocytes.	None	Nonimmunogenic. Difficult to obtain very high titers. Envelope can be pseudotyped with other proteins to increase stability and broaden host range.
Lentivirus-based retroviruses	Integration is required.	Can infect nondividing cells, but cell cycling may be needed. Low to intermediate efficiency for liver.	None	Nonimmunogenic. Difficult to obtain very high titers. Envelope can be pseudotyped with other proteins to increase stability and broaden host range.
Adeno-associated virus	Can exist in both episomal and integrated forms.	Can infect quiescent and dividing cells. Low to intermediate efficiency for liver.	None	Causes humoral immune response. Can be grown at high titers. Site-specificity of integration of the wild type virus is lost in the absence of *rep*. Can undergo lytic cycle in the presence of helper proteins. Limited packaging space.
Simian virus 40	Can exist in both episomal and integrated forms.	Infects both quiescent and dividing cells. High efficiency.	None	No significant immune response. Can be grown at high titers. Limited packaging space.
Adenovirus	Episomal. Can persist for several months in the absence of host immune response.	Efficiently infects both dividing and nondividing cells. Very high efficiency for liver.	Liver targeted	Evokes both humoral and cell-mediated host immune response. Viral gene deletion reduces primary immunogenicity, but does not permit repeated injection. Host tolerization permits repeated gene transfer.
Hybrid viruses	Combines advantages of different viruses.	Efficiency of adenoviral vectors is combined with persistent nature of other viruses.	Liver targeted	Adenoviral proteins provided in *trans* may evoke immune response. Site-specific integration or episomal replication may be possible.
NONVIRAL VECTORS:				
Injection of naked DNA or RNA	Transient	Intermediate efficiency	Liver targeted	Probably nonimmunogenic
Receptor and/or liposome-mediated plasmid delivery	Transient	Low efficiency	Liver targeted	Probably nonimmunogenic
Oligonucleotides designed to form DNA triplex or to convert single nucleotides	Permanent	Low efficiency	Liver targeted	Nonimmunogenic

[a]In all cases, an expressed transgene is potentially immunogenic in a mutant lacking the transgene product.

cation-deficient recombinant virus (Fig. 62.1). As most of the viral coding sequences are deleted, the recombinant retrovirus can accommodate relatively large exogenous DNA segments.

Retroviruses enter mammalian cells through specific surface receptors, which limit their range of infectivity. However, the host range can be expanded, or the virus can be redirected via alternative receptors by modifying the viral envelope to contain specific proteins, such as the G-protein of the vesicular stomatitis virus (VSV). Such modifications may also increase the stability of the virus, permitting concentration by centrifugation. After entry into mammalian cells, the RNA genome is reverse-transcribed into double-stranded DNA provirus, which is incorporated into a preintegration nucleoprotein complex (PIC). The PIC must be transferred into the nucleus for integra-

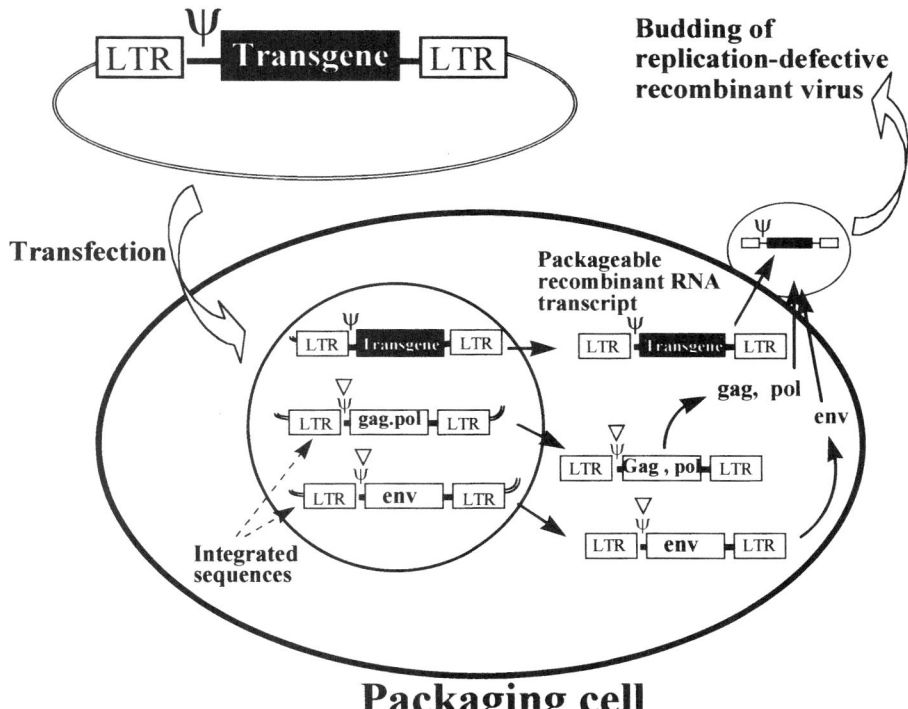

FIGURE 62.1. A schema of the construction of a typical recombinant retrovirus: The gene of interest (transgene) is cloned into a transfer plasmid. The transgene is flanked by the *cis* elements of a modified Moloney's murine leukemia virus genome, including two long-terminal repeats (LTRs) and the packaging signal (ψ). The coding sequences of the viral proteins are mostly deleted. The transfer plasmid is transfected into a packaging cell line that contains integrations of the coding regions of the viral genes, *gag*, *pol* and *env*. These integrations do not contain the ψ region and, therefore, their transcripts cannot be packaged into the recombinant virus. The recombinant RNA containing the transgene and the ψ region is packaged along with the viral proteins provided in *trans* by the packaging cells. The recombinant virus can infect other cells, but cannot replicate because of the absence of the genes for the viral proteins.

tion of the provirus into the host genome. The PIC of MoMuLV does not pass through intact nuclear membranes, and therefore, mitosis-associated dissolution of nuclear envelope is required for the integration of the MoMuLV provirus (33,36). This limits the efficiency of these viruses in transferring genes into hepatocytes, which are normally quiescent *in vivo*. Interestingly, long-term correction of hemophilia A was recently reported in newborn, factor VIII-deficient mice using retroviral vectors expressing human factor VIII (37). In contrast, lentiviruses, which are a different class of retroviruses, form PICs that can be translocated through the pores of intact nuclear membranes. They are, in fact, being explored as potential vectors for gene transfer into nondividing cells. However, lentivirus-based gene transfer in the liver *in vivo* may also require the hepatocytes to be in cell cycle (38).

Promoters and enhancers within the U3 region of the 3′ LTR are copied into the 5′ LTR during reverse transcription into double-stranded DNA. Therefore, deletions intro-

duced into this region result in the loss of functional U3 regions in both the 5′ and the 3′ LTR. These "self-inactivating" (SIN) vectors are less liable to cause insertional activation of a deleterious gene by the integrated proviral genome (39).

Recombinant Adeno-Associated Virus

Adeno-associated virus-2 (AAV-2) is a small (4.7 kb) single-stranded DNA virus of the parvovirus family that integrates preferentially on the q13.4-ter arm of human chromosome 19 (40). When infection with a "helper virus," such as adenovirus (41) or herpes simplex virus (42) occurs, AAV sequences are "rescued" from the integration site, resulting in productive lytic infection. In the absence of a helper virus, the infection becomes latent, and the viral genome remains integrated in the host chromosome for long periods. A permissive state for AAV replication can also be induced by the treatment of cells with a variety of genotoxic stimuli, such as heat shock, hydroxyurea,

UV light and irradiation (43–45). Thus, it is proposed that the helper virus proteins are not directly involved in AAV replication, but provide factors, such as adenoviral proteins E1A and E1B, that maximize the synthesis of the AAV gene products and host proteins necessary for AAV replication (46).

There are five serotypes of human AAV. Whereas AAV type 2 is used most commonly for vector development, characterization of other serotypes is under way. The AAV type 2 receptor is a membrane-associated heparin sulfate proteoglycan, which is present in many cell surfaces, thus explaining the broad host infectivity of this virus. Receptor binding is required for its internalization. The wild-type AAV is not known to cause human disease and has a broad range of infectivity. The AAV genome comprises three promoters (p5, p19, and p40), a polyadenylation signal, a nonstructural gene (*Rep*), and the structural *Cap* gene. At both ends of the viral genome are 145 bp inverted terminal repeats (ITR) that form T-shaped hairpin structures. The ITRs are needed for integration of the virus into the host genome (47). The 3′-OH end of the ITR primes second-strand synthesis, generating a double-stranded DNA with a covalently closed hairpin at one end. *Rep* mediates nicking at the terminal resolution site, thereby generating a linear duplex, which is the substrate for a new round of replication. The second-strand synthesis is needed for gene expression and integration of the virus. The ITR hairpin structures and cellular recombination pathways are required for viral integration. The viral

Rep protein also directs the site specificity of AAV integration into chromosome 19. The viral genome integrates as a head-to-tail concatamer. All viral-encoded genes, approximately 96% of the viral genome, can be replaced with foreign DNA of choice and packaged into an AAV virion. The cis-acting AAV ITRs that are retained do not appear to contain dominant enhancer/promoter activity. Thus, the expression of the transgene is determined by the transcriptional regulatory elements inserted in the expression cassette. This ability of AAV vectors to carry regulatory elements, such as tissue-specific enhancers/promoters, and splice sites, without interference from the viral genomes, allows for greater control of transferred gene expression. Tumor-specific expression of HSV-TK gene under the control of AFP/albumin promoter was obtained in hepatocellular carcinoma cell lines (48). When toxic gene products, such as suicide genes, are expressed, a tight transcriptional control of the transgene using tissue- or cell-specific promoters is critical in achieving a high therapeutic ratio.

AAV vectors are generated by cotransfecting into packaging 293 cells two plasmids, one containing the transgene, flanked by ITRs, and the other encoding *rep, cap,* and adenoviral proteins (Fig. 62.2). The 293 cells provide E1A in *trans.* The recombinant AAV is generated by infection with a helper virus (adenovirus or herpes simplex virus) or transfection with a plasmid encoding critical adenoviral proteins. When helper virus infection is utilized, the recombinant AAV needs to be purified from the helper virus.

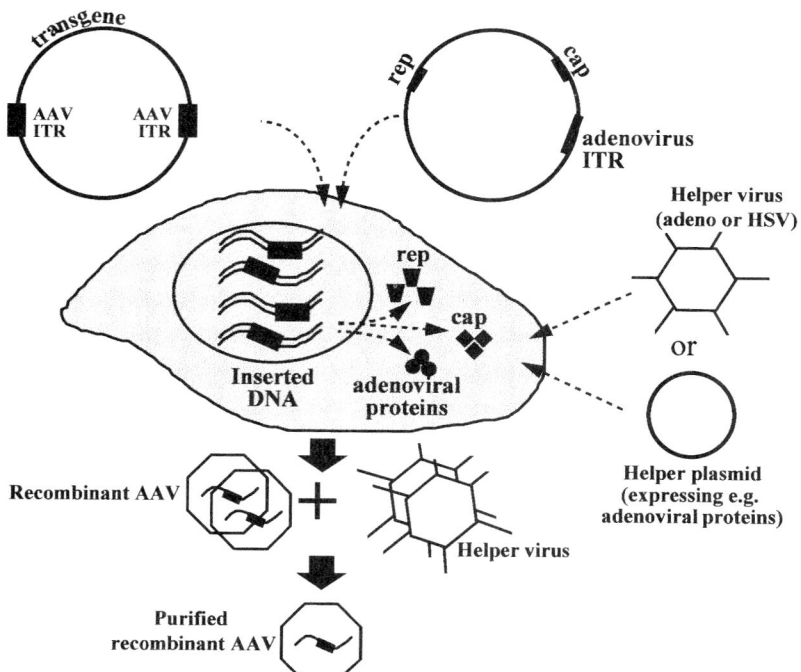

FIGURE 62.2. Production of recombinant adeno-associated virus (*AAV*): Two plasmids, one containing the transgene [flanked by inverted terminal repeats (*ITRs*)] and another encoding the helper proteins, *rep, cap* and adenoviral proteins are transfected into 293 packaging cells. AAV is generated by infecting the transfected cells with a helper virus [E1A-deleted adenovirus or herpes simplex virus (*HSV*)] or by transfecting with a plasmid encoding the critical adenoviral protein. If a helper virus is used, the recombinant AAV needs to be purified from the helper virus.

Following introduction into cells, AAV vectors are initially in an episomal form. They may persist as episomes, but normally integrate into the host genome progressively, probably in the course of days to weeks. Delayed attainment of a plateau of transgene expression is characteristic of AAV vectors. The site-specific integration of recombinant AAV should reduce the risk of insertional mutagenesis. The site-specificity is lost in recombinant AAV vectors in which the AAV coding sequences are deleted. Therefore, newer vectors that retain the *rep* gene are being developed (49). Although the initial efforts at gene transfer to the liver *in vivo* using AAV vectors resulted in modest transgene expression, improvement of viral titers has resulted in better transgene expression (50–53). Because integrations of wild-type parvoviruses occur naturally in the human genome without untoward side effects, this vector is thought to be safe for clinical use. A limitation of AAV-based vectors is the limited size of inserts that these can accommodate. Initial studies of intramuscular administration of AAV-based vectors for delivering coagulation factor IX in patients with hemophilia B resulted in low levels of protein production (54). However, infusion of 8.7×10^{13} particles of the recombinant virus into the portal vein of factor IX-deficient dogs resulted in the appearance of 5% of normal levels of factor IX activity in plasma (53). Currently, only a small fraction of hepatocytes can be transduced with AAV vectors. It is not clear at present whether only a small subset of hepatocytes is permissive to AAV-mediated gene transfer, or whether the transduction efficiency can be increased by using higher doses. Recombinant AAV causes a humoral immune response, which may be a problem if the vector needs to be readministered.

Recombinant AAV has several advantages for application in cancer gene therapy (55). The current design of AAV vectors provides an efficient DNA carrier system, free from the possibility of recombination with wild-type virus. As the vectors are integrated into the cellular genome and transmitted to the cell progeny, they are not diluted or lost upon cell division, which offers an important benefit in cancer gene therapy over episomal vectors. Unlike retroviruses, AAV vectors can infect nondividing cells, which extends their usefulness to the treatment of slow-growing tumors, although the rate of transduction of noncycling cells is much lower than that for dividing cells in culture (56). Treatment of cultured cells with agents that affect DNA metabolism, including irradiation and topoisomerase inhibitors, can improve AAV transduction of both dividing and nondividing cells (57). Thus, the efficiency of AAV-mediated cancer gene therapy could be enhanced when used in combination with conventional tumor therapies, such as irradiation or chemotherapy.

Simian Virus 40-Based Vectors

Recombinant simian virus 40 (SV40) is a nonenveloped DNA virus of the papova family with a 5.2 kb circular double-stranded genome. The large (Tag) and small (tag) T antigens, which are expressed by differential splicing of a single RNA transcript, are required for transcription of the viral structural genes VP1, VP2 and VP3. Tag is the most immunogenic protein of SV40 and is able to impart an immortalizing effect on the cell. In the recombinant viral genome, the *Tag* gene is replaced by a target transgene (Fig. 62.3). Viral particles are generated by transfecting the recombinant genome into COS-7 cells that provide Tag in *trans*. Because the recombinant virus lacks the *Tag* gene, it cannot replicate (58), and its immunogenicity is markedly reduced (59). The SV40 is a small virus, and the capacity of the recombinant SV40 to accommodate exogenous DNA is limited to 4.7 kb. SV40 vectors can be concentrated to 10^{12} infectious units per ml (60). Preliminary studies suggest that the recombinant SV40 integrates into the host chromosomal DNA. The ability of these vectors to infect nondividing cells makes them attractive for liver-directed gene therapy (61,62).

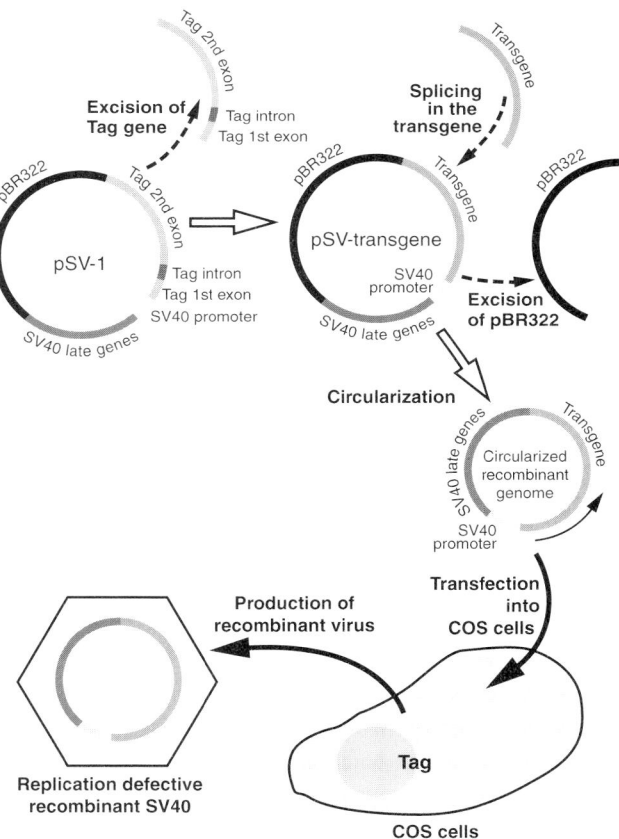

FIGURE 62.3. Generation of a replication-defective recombinant *SV40* virus: The full-length SV40 genome is cloned into a plasmid (*pSV-1*), from which the coding region of the T-antigen (*Tag*) is deleted and replaced by the transgene. The recombinant viral genome is excised and recircularized. The recircularized genome is transfected into COS cells, which provide Tag in *trans*, generating a helper-free replication-defective recombinant SV40.

Recombinant Adenovirus

Adenoviruses are large linear double-stranded DNA viruses. Vectors derived from human adenovirus type 5 and type 2 are commonly used for gene transfer. These vectors can be generated at high titers and can express transgenes in both dividing and quiescent cells (63,64). In addition, following systemic administration in animals, the virus is preferentially localized to the liver, leading to the transduction of the great majority of hepatocytes *in vivo* (65). The adenoviral receptor CAR, which is also involved in the internalization of the Coxsackie virus, is highly concentrated in rodent liver. Following infection, the virus exits from the endocytotic vesicles and translocates to the nucleus, where it persists episomally, without integration into the host genome. It is uncertain, however, whether such efficient gene transfer occurs in the human hepatocytes *in vivo*.

Recombinant adenoviral vectors are produced by disrupting the E1 domain, which encodes transcription factors required for the expression of other adenoviral genes by cloning the transgene of interest into this region. Additional adenoviral genes, for example, E3 and E4, may be deleted to increase the "stuffing space" in the vector. The recombinant virus is generated in a helper cell line that provides the viral proteins in *trans* (66).

Application of adenoviral vectors in gene therapy is limited by the highly immunogenic nature of the viral proteins. Host-neutralizing antibodies block gene transfer by repeated administration of the vector. Antiadenoviral cytotoxic lymphocytes attack the adenovirally infected host cells, causing hepatitis and rapid loss of the transgene after secondary gene transfer (67). To prevent any *de novo* expression of adenoviral genes, "gutless" vectors, devoid of viral structural genes, have been developed. Although these vectors exhibit prolonged transgene expression (68), immunogenicity can be retained because of the presence of viral proteins provided in *trans* by the packaging cells during generation of the recombinant virus (69). Therefore, repeated gene transfer requires the generation of vectors based on a different strain of adenovirus. Expression of immunomodulatory genes, such as adenoviral E3, by the recombinant vector is being explored for abrogating adenovirus-specific host immune response (70).

Alternative strategies seek to tolerize the host specifically to adenoviral antigens, leaving the general immune system intact. Injection of recombinant adenovirus *in utero* (71), to newborn rats (65), intrathymic inoculation of adenoviral proteins in young adult rats (72), or oral administration of small doses of adenoviral proteins in adult rats (73) have been used successfully to abrogate humoral- and cell-mediated immune response against adenoviral antigens in rodents. Inhibition of costimulation between antigen-presenting cells and cytotoxic lymphocytes by the administration of CTLA4-Ig and CD-40 antibodies to the host has also been explored in rodents with limited success (74). Although the tolerization methods permit repeated administration of adenoviral vectors in experimental animals, safety concerns remain regarding tolerization of human hosts to adenoviruses, which, in the wild form, are human pathogens.

Recombinant Baculovirus

The recombinant baculovirus *Autographa californica* nuclear polyhedrosis (AcNPV) is commonly used for generating recombinant proteins in insect cells (75). Among mammalian cells, hepatocytes can be infected by baculoviral vectors, and the transgene is expressed with the use of internal promoters that function in mammalian cells. Recombinant baculoviruses can accommodate large segments of exogenous DNA. Although the gene transfer efficiency and immunogenicity of recombinant baculoviruses *in vivo* have not been well-characterized, recombinant vectors consisting partly of baculoviral sequences and partly of sequences from other viruses are being evaluated for *in vivo* application.

Herpes Simplex Virus-1

Herpes simplex virus-1 (HSV-1) is a 150-kb double-stranded DNA virus with a broad host range (76,77). These vectors efficiently infect nondividing cells and are useful for gene transfer into neuronal cells and hepatocytes. However, long-term gene expression in the liver has not been achieved with the currently available HSV vectors.

NONVIRAL VECTORS

There are now well defined criteria that apply to any successful gene therapy and/or repair process. Conceptually, the approach must provide (a) efficient delivery of DNA from the extracellular environment to the cell nucleus, (b) specificity of targeting, (c) small particle size, (d) stability of both vehicle and DNA and (e) minimal toxicity to cells. The vehicles designed for gene delivery can be classified as either viral or nonviral. Viral vectors have been widely utilized in gene therapy research, owing to their efficient delivery of transgenes into cells. However, nonviral gene transfer provides an alternate and potentially superior method of transgene delivery for several reasons. First, nonviral vectors are composed largely of synthetic components. Thus, they are simpler to manufacture and do not require extensive testing for potentially contaminating infectious agents that make production of viral vectors costly. Second, as a result of their synthetic nature, nonviral delivery systems are less likely to be immunogenic. Third, they are less dependent on maintaining a strict molecular structure for the introduction of recombinant genes, thereby allowing a greater range of molecular modifications. Finally, the pharmaceutical formulation and application of nonviral delivery systems may be easier to implement, in part due to their potentially greater stability than viral vectors.

A number of different approaches have been developed for nonviral gene delivery, with varying success. Three major categories of nonviral delivery systems for systemic delivery of nucleic acids to tissues have been studied extensively over the past decade (78). Lipid-based delivery systems encompass both lipid-encapsulated and cationic lipid/nucleic acid complexes (lipoplex). These lipid-based DNA delivery systems provided some of the initial proof-of-principle experiments for systemic nonviral delivery and expression of transgenes *in vivo* (79). Polyplex systems consist of complexes formed by the addition of nucleic acid to a cationic polymer. These polycation-based delivery systems, such as poly-L-lysine (PLL) (80,81), polyethylenimine (PEI) (82), polyglucosamines (83,84), lipopolyamines (85), and cationic peptides (86) form water-soluble complexes which can provide simple but very efficient delivery systems. The presence of free amino groups on these agents makes them amenable to chemical modification for the attachment of a variety of targeting ligands. Lipopolyplex delivery systems are hybrid complexes that contain both polycationic polymers and lipids. Compaction of large molecular weight DNA with polycations prior to lipid encapsulation/complexation produces a DNA core surrounded by a lipid shell. Two major advantages of the hybrid over the lipoplex systems is the reduction in particle size and increased protection of the nucleic acid from nuclease degradation.

Regarding the major barriers to nucleic acid delivery to cells, the greatest success has been in the ability to transfer them across the plasma membrane. The cationic lipid-transfecting agents such as lipofectamine, DOTAP, and the cationic polymers, including poly-L-lysine and PEI, have significantly improved nucleic acid transfer across the plasma membrane into the cytoplasm (87,88). The substantially enhanced transfection efficacy observed with these delivery vehicles *in vitro* is associated with small, stable uniform particle size. Unfortunately, these nucleic acid/cationic complexes exhibit significant cellular toxicity and low transfection efficiency in the presence of serum.

The cellular toxicity of these cationic complexes may in part be dependent on their large particle size (89), as well as the high positive ζ potential required for efficient uptake of the complexes through nonspecific cationic-mediated endocytosis (82,90–92). The low transfection efficiency of these particles by serum proteins both *in vitro* and *in vivo* results in part by neutralization of the ζ potential required for cellular uptake (93,94). The interaction with serum proteins also dampens the transfection efficiency by increasing the size of the delivery particles to greater than 100 nm, the maximum size of the fenestrations in the hepatic sinusoids, as well as the coated pits involved in endocytosis (95,96). Thus, these cationic delivery agents have exhibited little utility for *in vivo* delivery due to their inability to deliver the therapeutic transgene effectively.

The characteristic cellular toxicity associated with the cationic-based delivery systems both *in vitro* and *in vivo* has been ameliorated by polyethylene glycol (PEG) modification of the delivery systems (97). This hydrophilic molecule prevents aggregation, stabilizes and maintains the small size required for endocytosis, and diminishes binding of serum proteins. However, the shielding of the cationic charge by the PEG has reduced the efficiency of transfection by these modified delivery systems.

To overcome these hurdles, the delivery systems have been modified with ligands to promote receptor-mediated endocytic delivery. For example, asialoorosomucoid (ASOR) (80, 81) and galactose (85,98,99) have been conjugated to PLL, lipopolyamines and PEI for targeting to the asialoglycoprotein receptor (ASGPr) on hepatocytes. Lipid-based delivery systems have utilized galactocerebrosides as the targeting moiety for the ASGPr (99–101). Receptor-mediated ligand targeting has also been exploited using transferrin-, folate-, and cell-specific antibodies conjugated to the polycations or liposomes (102–105). These ligand-targeted systems have been shown to increase hepatocyte-directed gene delivery both *in vitro* (101, 105,106) and *in vivo* (80,107). Additionally, the ligand/receptor-mediated endocytosis obviates the need for an overall net positive charge. In fact, negatively charged particles promote more effective ligand/receptor-mediated nucleic acid delivery (103). Additionally, ligand/receptor-mediated delivery systems are, unlike cationic lipids or polycations, able to efficiently transfect nonadherent cell lines (104). Finally, this route of entry of the DNA into the cells through the "normal" endosomal/lysosomal trafficking appears to improve efficient nuclear translocation of foreign DNA (108), the most difficult barrier to successful gene delivery (87,109).

In the past few years, significant progress has been made in overcoming the barrier to efficient nuclear translocation of exogenous DNA. Both PEI and other polycations have been used successfully in compacting and protecting the DNA from nuclease degradation within the endosome (104). Also, a number of disruptor peptides have been incorporated into the delivery vehicles to promote endosomal release of the nucleic acid into the cytoplasm (110). In fact, PEI exhibits a novel characteristic in its ability to disrupt the endosome by acting as a proton sponge (111). Once released from the endosome, the efficient nuclear entry of nucleic acids greater than approximately 125 nucleotides appears to be dependent on several factors. In particular, the size of the DNA particle as well as the delivery agent appear to play critical roles in effective nuclear localization and expression in both quiescent and replicating cells (88,104,112). The more compact the DNA particle, the greater the nuclear localization and increased expression of the introduced transgene. In addition, unlike the cationic lipids, polyplex delivery agents do not appear to inhibit nuclear expression of the exogenous transgene (112).

The most dramatic improvement in the effective delivery of transgenes from the cytosol to the nucleus has come from the incorporation of nuclear localization signals on the plasmid constructs (88,113,114). Thus, the translocation of the transgene into the nucleus exploits the active transport pathways used by their respective proteins, which increases nuclear localization/expression 10- to 10,000-fold depending on cell type. In one example, by including a muscle-specific transcription factor binding site in the construct, the introduced transgene demonstrated tissue-specific nuclear localization, while remaining in the cytoplasm of nonmuscle cells (114). However, nuclear localization could be reproduced in the nonmuscle cells by complementation with the muscle-specific transcription factor. This represents an important refinement in tissue-specific gene targeting by promoting nuclear localization to only the desired target cells. Taken together, there has been significant progress in improving nonviral delivery systems to overcome the known barriers for effective nucleic acid delivery to the nuclei of quiescent cells. The targeting of viral and nonviral vectors to hepatocytes via the ASGPr or other receptors (13,95) is just one example of targeted cell delivery (105).

TARGETED GENE MODIFICATION

Homologous Recombination

In many experimental systems, the successful transfer of a cloned, modified gene into the genome of the host organism is now possible (115,116). Ideally, the introduced gene is returned only to its homologous location and is integrated at the target site. The process is a precise means for repairing mutated or damaged DNA, insuring accurate chromosomal disjunction during meiosis. Our understanding of the process of homologous pairing and DNA strand exchange is predominately derived from extensive biochemical analyses of purified RecA protein from *Escherichia coli* and genetic studies carried out in bacteriophage and yeast. The transformation protocols studied in lower eukaryotes ultimately developed into the strategies for gene targeting in higher organisms. However, the observed genetic contradictions and the lack of biochemical data hindered identification of precise mechanisms to pursue experiments in higher organisms. Moreover, the lack of illegitimate integration commonly observed in higher eukaryotic systems during plasmid transformation in yeast raises certain doubts as to the ubiquity of their recombination system. However, structural homologs of yeast recombination proteins rad51 and/or rad52 as well as many of the other proteins involved in the homologous recombination pathway have been identified in higher eukaryotes (117). This suggests that fundamentally similar biological mechanisms are involved in homologous recombination from bacteria to higher animals and plants. Thus, the critical factors affecting successful gene targeting elucidated in transformation analysis of lower eukaryotes may prove to be widely applicable.

Since the precise duplication of genomic DNA is vital to the survival of a species, eukaryotic evolution has produced elaborate and redundant mechanisms to limit the effects of mutagens and exogenous genetic invaders. Unfortunately, even with the explosive increase in studies designed to characterize the various genomic DNA repair pathways in cultured cells from higher eukaryotes, successful targeted mod-

ification of genomic DNA by homologous recombination has been limited (4). Significant impediments remain to be resolved for this process to function effectively as an *in vivo* approach to gene therapy. First, the integration of exogenous DNA into the genome is extremely inefficient, and can occur in the absence of sequence homology between the introduced gene and genomic integration site (118). Second, as a defensive strategy, sequences in the chromatin are sequestered, thus promoting a low efficiency of pairing between the introduced DNA and its genomic target (119). However, the utility *in vitro* for targeted gene disruption to establish the functional activity of a particular gene has been quite successful (120,121).

With our growing understanding of how homologous recombination is regulated in mammalian cells, the process of generating only the desired integration at the target site with significant increases in the frequencies is possible. In particular, the recent report of a 1% frequency of targeted homologous replacement or generation of the 3-bp deletion associated with cystic fibrosis transmembrane conductance regulator using a short (488 nucleotide) DNA fragment indicates potential for therapeutic use (122). Ironically, many of the factors involved with improving the frequencies of targeted gene replacement require inactivation of other DNA repair proteins and/or pathways (4), which is not feasible in an *in vivo* setting. Additionally, homologous recombination is cell cycle-regulated with reduced activity outside of S-phase, precluding its effective use in many quiescent cell types, such as hepatocytes (123–125).

Triplex DNA

The use of triplex DNA to perform site-specific modification of genomic DNA is based on the formation of a three-stranded or triple-helical nucleic acid structure. In short, the exogenous third strand of nucleic acid binds in the major groove of a homopurine region of the DNA, forming Hoogsteen or reverse Hoogsteen hydrogen bonds with the purine base (126). The triplex formation can occur at physiologic pH, yet not all polypurine sites bind triplex-forming oligonucleotides with high affinity. In fact, the polypurine regions must be guanine-rich and 12 to 14 nucleotides in length for adequate triplex formation to occur. Additionally, monovalent cations such as Na+ and K+ inhibit triplex formation, rendering that complex under physiologic conditions difficult. Modified bases have been used to counteract the inhibitory effect of monovalent cations on triplex formation. For example, the thymidine purine analog 7-deaza-2′-deoxyxanthosine exhibits the ability to form triplex DNA at physiologic pH and salt conditions, as well as maintaining an all-purine backbone motif (127). The initial approach to the triple-helix site-directed modification of DNA used cross-linking agents such as psoralen or other mutagens to covalently attach to the triplex-forming oligonucleotide (126). After intercalation of the psoralen at the target $^{5'}$ApT$^{3'}$ site in the DNA, UV-irradiation results in cross-linking of the thymines in the two strands. This substrate is then repaired by the endogenous DNA repair activity in the cell, producing the characteristic T:A to A:T transversions at a low frequency.

Although this technique has been used to modify episomal DNA in mammalian cells *in vitro* (128), the target sequence constraints and requirement for cross-linking agents have limited its application in living cells. However, targeted gene knockouts of the genomic hypoxanthine phosphoribosyl transferase gene in cultured cells were successfully created using this approach (129). Interestingly, rather than the expected T to A transversions, the majority of the knockouts resulted predominately from small deletions and some insertions, suggesting that the endogenous repair pathway involved was not that of mismatch repair. Further investigation indicated that these triple-helix-forming nucleotides could be used to promote insertions and deletions at target sites without cross-linking agents to promote modification of the DNA (130). In fact, these triple-helix-forming oligonucleotides, in the absence of cross-linking agents, are able to induce recombination via a nucleotide excision repair pathway (131). Interestingly, the ability of the triplex-directed psoralen cross-linked DNA substrates to induce recombination was only partially dependent on functional nucleotide excision repair. This suggested that other endogenous DNA repair pathways are involved in processing the mutated DNAs into recombinagenic intermediates. However, it is now well established that triplex DNA-mediated recombination is not affected in mismatch repair-deficient cells.

The problem of sequence constraint for triple-helix formation, targeted single nucleotide, and homologous DNA-based gene correction has been overcome, in part, by the use of novel approaches such as bifunctional oligonucleotides (132–134). These oligonucleotides contain regions that form triple-helical structures as well as conventional Watson–Crick base pairs. These modified oligonucleotides have been used successfully to promote site-specific nucleotide correction and gene targeting in both cell-free systems and cultured cells. These exciting new advances using triple-helix-forming oligonucleotides suggest that this form of genomic modification may have therapeutic potential in treating genetic disorders.

Ribozymes, Antisense, and DNA Ribonucleases

Ribozymes are RNA enzymes that bind to specific RNA substrate sequences and catalyze endoribonucleolytic cleavage (135–137). They have become a valuable resource in both basic and translational research based on their ability to cleave a variety of target RNAs. They have been exploited to target viral RNAs in infectious diseases, dominant oncogenes in cancers, and specific somatic mutations in a variety of genetic disorders. RNA cleavage is a naturally occurring intramolecular reaction primarily involved in the processing of certain introns to form the mature RNA. However, endoribonucle-

olytic cleavage can be engineered to occur as a trans-acting event. Ribozymes hybridize to complementary RNA sequences in which the central portion forms a specific secondary structure where closely located reactive groups mediate the directed cleavage of the target RNA. The domains, or helices of ribozymes that base-pair to substrate RNAs, are functionally separable from the moieties that effect cleavage. As a result, the substrate specificity of ribozymes can be altered, within certain constraints, to allow catalytic trans-cleavage of specified sites within the target RNA.

Hairpin ribozymes require only a guanosine (G) residue immediately 3′ to the cleavage site, although a GUC sequence is optimal. The hammerhead ribozyme is even less constrained, requiring only a UN dinucleotide for cleavage where N is A, C, or U. The resulting RNA fragments are rapidly degraded, rendering the molecule nonfunctional. A potential advantage of the ribozyme over other antisense technologies is related to the catalytic nature of the cleavage. Ribozymes can be expressed either in cells or synthesized and packaged for cellular uptake. Moreover, they have been shown to remain catalytically active for weeks during expression in an intact organ after somatic gene transfer. In one study, recombinant adenoviral vectors containing human growth hormone ribozyme expression cassettes were used to ablate growth hormone in both cultured cells and livers of mice (138).

Ribozymes have been designed to cleave the RNAs of human hepatitis viruses, although studies on these viruses have proceeded slowly, in part due to inadequate tissue culture models. However, both hammerhead (139,140) and hairpin (141) ribozymes have been used successfully to inhibit viral production of both hepatitis B and hepatitis C infection in cells. The expressed hammerhead ribozymes, individually or in combination, were efficient at reducing or eliminating the respective plus- or minus-strand hepatitis C virus RNAs expressed in cultured cells and from primary human hepatocytes obtained from chronic hepatitis C-infected patients (139). In contrast, cleavage-deficient ribozymes with a point mutation in the hammerhead domain had no significant effect (140). Also, it is possible to target a variety of highly conserved hepatitis C viral RNA sequences simultaneously with multiple ribozyme genes expressed from a single vector (142). This type of gene therapy could, in fact, result in a constant and continuous supply of multiple intracellular ribozymes, thereby decreasing the potential development of drug-resistant viral variants. Hepatitis B virus, a partially double-stranded DNA virus, replicates through a pregenomic RNA intermediate, which provides a therapeutic target for a novel antiviral gene therapy based on ribozyme RNA cleavage. In fact, hairpin ribozymes have been successfully designed and formulated to disrupt hepatitis B virus replication by targeting the pregenomic RNA intermediate (143).

The 5′-nontranslated region of hepatitis C virus contains important elements which control hepatitis C virus translation. Antisense oligonucleotides bound to asialoglycoprotein-polylysine complexes were targeted to HuH-7 cells by receptor-mediated endocytosis, and they specifically inhibited the C virus-directed protein synthesis in the cells (144). Antisense oligonucleotides were also targeted via the asialoglycoprotein receptor to hepatitis B virus-infected cells, resulting in specific inhibition of viral protein synthesis and replication *in vitro* (145). A 21-mer phosphorothioate-linked oligonucleotide DNA complementary to the hepatitis B virus polyadenylation signal and 5′-upstream sequences was complexed to a targetable DNA carrier consisting of asialoglycoprotein coupled to polylysine. Preexposure of the HuH-7 cells to targeted complexed antisense DNA substantially blocked viral gene expression and viral replication after transfection of B virus DNA.

DNA ribonucleases are catalytic molecules consisting of synthetic single-stranded DNA that specifically cleave substrate RNA in a manner analogous to ribozymes with catalytic efficiencies exceeding that of comparable ribozymes (146). They are easier to prepare and deliver to cells and less sensitive to chemical and enzymatic degradation. Similar to the structure of ribozymes, the DNA ribonucleases have three domains. A catalytic domain consisting of 15 nucleotides is flanked by two substrate-recognition domains which bind target RNA through Watson–Crick base pairing. These DNA analogs of ribozymes could be prepared to inhibit hepatitis C. DNA ribonucleases directed against the hepatitis C viral genome can specifically cleave the targeted RNA. DNA ribonuclease with point mutations in the catalytic domain had significantly lower inhibitory effects; however, activity was not eliminated, suggesting the presence of some antisense contribution. DNA ribonucleases can be made to specifically cleave target hepatitis B viral RNA and substantially inhibit intracellular viral gene expression (147).

Single Nucleotide Modification

A novel approach to gene therapy has recently been developed which utilizes the endogenous repair pathways of the cell to correct single base pair mutations (6,7). The gene

repair technology, called "chimeraplasty," is based on the ability of specifically designed chimeric RNA/DNA oligonucleotides to correct point mutations in genomic DNA. The targeted correction is site-specific and permanent, thereby maintaining endogenous gene regulation. This gene alteration approach was based on studies elucidating the molecular aspects of DNA repair. It was reported that a significant increase in efficiency of pairing between an oligonucleotide approximately 50 bases long and a genomic DNA target occurred only if RNA replaced DNA in a portion of the targeting oligonucleotide (148,149).

Other modifications of the hybrid oligonucleotide, or chimeraplast, were made to increase stability and improve localization to genomic target sites in mammalian cells (Fig. 62.4) (6). In the original design, two single-stranded ends, comprised of unpaired nucleotide hairpin caps, flank the double-stranded region of the chimeric molecule. The 5′ and 3′ ends are juxtaposed and sequestered, and, together with 2′-O-methylated modification of the RNA residues, contribute to enhanced nuclease resistance of the chimeraplast. The length of the oligonucleotide dictates the extent of homology between the chimeraplast and its genomic target; a 68-mer is designed to include a 25-bp region of homology containing a single mismatch with the gene sequence. This engineered mismatch appears to initiate modification of the genomic target, with the chimeraplast acting as a template for the alteration of the DNA sequence. The sequestered 5′ and 3′ ends minimize end-to-end ligation, whereas the RNA segments, the region of homology, and the "nick" are all essential for chimeraplast activity. The physical and enzymatic stability conferred by its secondary structure and the modified RNA are important in ensuring the survival of the chimeraplast en route to and within the cell.

It is postulated that the mismatch created between the chimeraplast and its target genomic DNA creates the "illusion" of a base mutation, thus activating certain endogenous DNA repair functions (7). The process exploits the efficient, evolutionarily conserved set of enzymatic pathways used to repair mutations caused by natural and artifi-

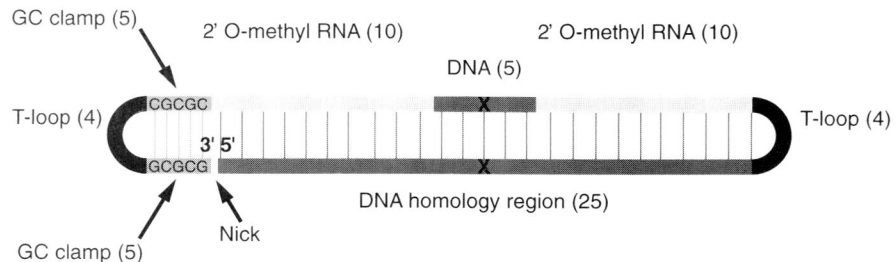

FIGURE 62.4. Key features of the chimeric RNA/DNA molecule. Chimeraplasts are typically 68 nucleotides (nt) in length and include 20 2′-O-methyl modified ribonucleotides in the 25-nt segment homologous to the target gene. The DNA and RNA residues in the homology region are shown in *dark and light gray*, respectively. They contain two hairpins caps of four T residues each (indicated in *black*), and a 5-bp GC clamp. The 25-nt region of homology is mismatched with the genomic sequence at a single nucleotide (*X*) targeted for change. The numbers of nucleotides are indicated in parentheses.

cial mutagens. These factors act as the "sensing" mechanisms in the cell leading to the identification and repair of unwanted modifications of DNA. This endogenous DNA repair activity can be harnessed for the targeted modification of genes. The double-stranded regions containing modified RNA appear to recruit endogenous repair functions by accentuating the mismatched region of the chimeraplast and the genomic DNA.

Probing the Mechanism

The machinery for homologous recombination and DNA repair is highly conserved throughout evolution (117). Thus, to investigate the process of chimeraplasty and critical aspects of their structural design, test systems in both bacteria and mammalian cell-free extracts have recently been described. These systems utilize either plasmid-based selectable systems or colorimetric identification which demonstrates chimeraplast-mediated gene conversion. The plasmid selectable system has been developed using neomycin phosphotransferase (*neo*) genes which confer either kanamycin (kanR) or tetracycline resistance (tetR) (150,151). The colorimetric assay utilizes the β-galactosidase enzymatic activity of the *lacZ* gene to cleave the synthetic substrate X-gal and produce the characteristic blue color (152). The three genes were first modified by *in vitro* site-directed mutagenesis to introduce single nucleotide changes resulting in inactive gene products. These altered genes in the plasmid-based test systems can then serve as substrates for gene repair. If site-specific nucleotide correction or insertion occurs, then the plasmids confer appropriate antibiotic resistance. Similarly, cleavage of the X-gal substrate after chimeraplasty results in blue-colored cells or colonies.

Using these bacterial systems, a variety of structural changes in chimeraplast design have been characterized for improved targeting and nucleotide conversion (150). For example, a chimeraplast with a 35-nt homology region was 10-fold more active than one containing a 25-nt region, which was approximately 40-fold more active than 15 nucleotides of homology. Thus, chimeraplasts exhibit a significant correlation of homology length with gene repair activity, similar to classical homologous targeting experiments employing cloned DNA fragments (153).

The chimeraplast is designed to be complementary to the Watson–Crick strands of the target DNA. Thus, it is expected that two pairing events could occur: one involving an RNA/DNA hybrid and the other a DNA/DNA duplex, each containing a mismatched base pair. To establish the potential contribution to the repair process of the "hybrid" or the DNA/DNA mismatched base pair, 68-mer chimeraplasts that contained only one mismatched strand with the *neo* gene were designed (150). The oligonucleotide with the mismatch on the "all-DNA" strand directed the repair at a higher efficiency than the one with the mismatch on the "RNA/DNA" strand, or even the original "double-mismatched" chimeraplast. The results suggest that mismatches created by the

DNA strand are more efficiently repaired. In addition, the primary role of the RNA/DNA hybrid strand is to increase structural stability and enhance pairing with the target DNA.

The various endogenous DNA repair pathways were investigated using *E. coli* strains deficient in specific repair proteins (150). Gene modification by chimeraplasty was either significantly reduced or undetectable in strains containing defects in RecA, a DNA pairing protein, or in the mismatch repair binding protein MutS. However, other DNA and RNA modification enzymes such as adenine (*dam*) and cytosine (*dcm*) methylases, as well as dUTPase (*dut*) and uracil N-glycosylase (*ung*) involved in base excision repair were, in fact, dispensable.

The requirement for both RecA and MutS proteins implies at least a two-step process, involving factors from homologous recombination as well as mismatch repair pathways (Fig. 62.5). It is speculated that RecA-dependent pairing of the chimeraplast with its target DNA is followed

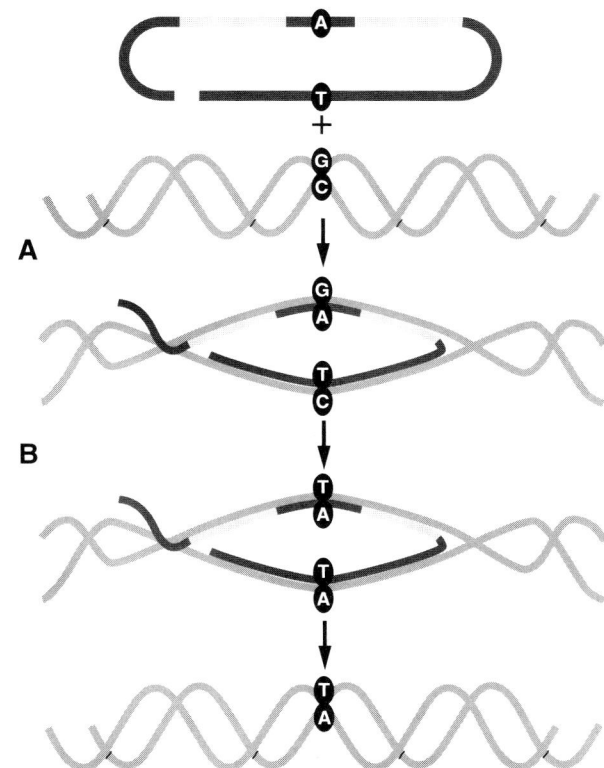

FIGURE 62.5. The process of chimeraplasty. **A:** The chimeraplast is designed to be complementary to the target gene except for a single base pair mismatch. In the initial pairing reaction, the chimeraplast aligns in perfect register using Watson–Crick base pairing with its target homologous genomic DNA except for the engineered single-bp mismatch. **B:** The endogenous DNA repair pathway(s) detect the mispaired bases, and modify the genomic sequence complementary to that of the chimeraplast. Thus, by exploiting the cell's own repair pathway(s), the genomic misspelling is precisely corrected, and the expression of the modified gene product remains under endogenous genetic regulatory controls at its native genomic site.

by the recognition of the mismatch and its repair, involving MutS and other proteins. The RNA portion of the oligonucleotide appears to provide an essential role in strand pairing, as control oligonucleotides comprised entirely of DNA with the identical sequence and structure exhibited no detectable activity. Furthermore, when the chimeraplast was modified by replacing the RNA/DNA strand with an all-RNA strand, an improvement in the targeted conversion activity of the chimeraplast was observed, supporting the role of the RNA/DNA duplex in efficient pairing.

Mammalian Studies

Both recombination and mismatch repair pathways are evolutionarily conserved, suggesting an application of chimeraplasty to mammalian systems (117,154,155). In fact, it was shown that HuH-7 cell-free extracts could support *in vitro* dose-dependent conversion of the mutant *neo* gene, as well as insertion of a deleted base pair into the tetracycline gene (151). Further, when a cell line lacking the mismatch repair protein hMSH2 was used to prepare the extracts, or an antibody to hMSH2 was included in the reaction, little chimeraplast repair activity was detected. Interestingly, using this same *in vitro* approach, rat liver mitochondrial protein extracts also supported chimeraplast conversion of a plasmid encoding a *neo* resistance gene.

Using the *lacZ* plasmid system, cell-free nuclear extracts from a variety of different cell lines efficiently catalyzed dose-dependent nucleotide conversion (152). Also, the nuclear extract from a homozygous isogenic $p53^+/p53^+$ embryonic fibroblast cell line induced 300-fold less conversion than p53 null extract. Thus, wild-type p53 may inhibit the initial pairing step in chimeraplast repair, as p53 decreases the recombination activity of RecA and its human homolog Rad51 (156–158). Overall, these data suggest a significantly conserved mechanism of nucleotide conversion in both prokaryotes and eukaryotes which appears to be distinct from that of homologous recombination in its requirement for MutS or hMSH2 protein.

Cell Culture Studies

It was originally reported that the chimeric RNA/DNA oligonucleotides were able to effect site-specific nucleotide conversion of episomal DNA in cultured cells (159). This was followed by the seminal report demonstrating targeted single nucleotide conversion to correct the sickle cell genomic DNA point mutation in cultured lymphoblastoid cells (160). Subsequently, it was shown that chimeric oligonucleotides could introduce a missense mutation in genomic DNA in cultured HuH-7 human hepatoma cells (161). Interestingly, under conditions in which RNA/DNA hybrids were active in promoting nucleotide exchange, the corresponding all-DNA duplexes, despite nuclear uptake, were essentially inactive (159–161).

These early studies, however, emphasized the need for improved delivery of chimeraplasts to hepatocytes. Moreover, the therapeutic benefit from this approach for treatment of hepatic diseases requires not only targeted delivery of chimeraplasts to the liver, but also efficient nuclear translocation and directed nucleotide exchange in quiescent G_0 hepatocytes. Thus, the galactose sugar was used as the targeting ligand for delivery of these molecules to the liver, based on previous reports of high specificity and efficiency in targeting nucleic acids to the hepatocyte asialoglycoprotein receptor (95,100,107) (Fig. 62.6). PEI was modified because it was an effective carrier of the oligonucleotides *in vitro* and was amenable to chemical modification and sugar attachment to its free amino groups. Additionally, anionic liposomes containing galactocerebroside for targeting to the asialoglycoprotein receptor were formulated to encapsulate the oligonucleotides for delivery (101,162). The specificity and efficiency of hepatocyte uptake and nuclear localization of fluorescein-labeled chimeraplasts were demonstrated by confocal microscopy.

Chimeric oligonucleotides were designed that targeted both the transcribed and nontranscribed rat factor IX genomic DNA strands (163). The molecules were identical

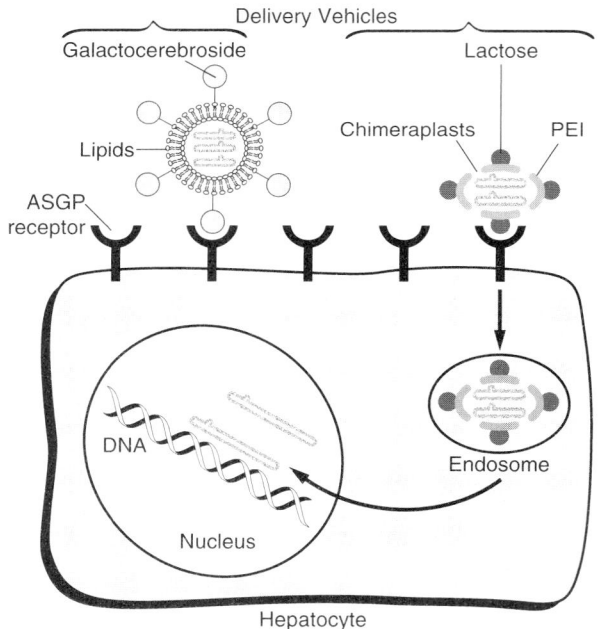

FIGURE 62.6. Asialoglycoprotein receptor (*ASGP receptor*)-mediated targeted delivery of chimeraplasts to hepatocytes. Chimeraplasts are shown encapsulated in anionic liposomes with galactocerebroside as the targeting ligand or complexed with lactosylated polyethylenimine (*PEI*). They are taken up by the hepatocytes via asialoglycoprotein receptor-mediated endocytosis of either delivery system. Following release from the endosome, the chimeraplasts enter the nucleus and form a paired intermediate with the targeted homologous genomic DNA sequence. The single-bp mismatch then activates the endogenous DNA repair machinery, which induces a nucleotide change at the target site.

in sequence to the wild-type gene except for the engineered nucleotide mismatch. The targeted nucleotide change at Ser[365] would introduce a missense mutation in the rat genomic sequence resulting in the active site Ser[365] to Arg[365], characteristic of certain human factor IX mutations. Primary rat hepatocytes were transfected with chimeraplasts using both the PEI and liposomal delivery systems. The conversion efficiency was determined by polymerase chain reaction (PCR) amplification of a 374-nt fragment spanning the targeted nucleotide change, as well as by sequence analysis. A to C conversion at Ser[365] was detected in 25% of the gene pool for factor IX, and was irrespective of the targeted strand. Similar results were obtained with correction of the missense mutation responsible for the factor IX deficiency in isolated hepatocytes from the Chapel Hill strain of hemophilia B dogs (164).

The UDP-glucuronosyltransferase (*UGT1A1*)-deficient Gunn rat animal model of Crigler–Najjar syndrome type I was tested to determine whether chimeraplasts could also correct a frameshift mutation. Insertion of a single guanosine at position 1206 in the *UGT1* coding sequence would restore the proper reading frame of the *UGT1A1* mRNA, production of the UDP-glucurosyltransferase enzyme, as well as reestablish the wild-type *Bst*N I restriction site (165). The design of the correcting chimeraplast (CN3) differed from those in previous studies in that the DNA region flanked by the modified RNA bases was increased to nine nucleotides with a central mismatched base pair. Isolated Gunn rat hepatocytes were transfected with the CN3 chimeraplasts using the targeted anionic liposome delivery system. Nucleotide insertion was determined by differential hybridization analysis of the wild-type corrected sequence (1206G) and the 1206A mutant sequence. Moreover, a double transfection of Gunn rat hepatocytes, immortalized using a temperature-sensitive SV40 T-antigen (29), resulted in a dose-dependent frameshift correction frequency of about 25%.

Site-Directed Nucleotide Conversion In Vivo

Success in the primary rat hepatocytes suggested that chimeraplasty may be a potential tool for *in vivo* gene modification. Thus, a series of experiments were performed on male rats to determine whether the chimeric oligonucleotides could mutate the factor IX gene in hepatocytes (163). The molecules were complexed to PEI and delivered by tail vein injection. After several days, liver tissue was collected and genomic DNA was isolated for analysis. The PCR-amplified products were analyzed by duplicate filter lift hybridization and indicated a dose-related genomic DNA conversion frequency of 15% to 40%. Similar results were obtained by reverse transcription (RT)-PCR analysis for RNA, suggesting a potential biological effect of the genomic DNA conversion. Sequence analysis of the cloned PCR products confirmed the specificity of the A to C conversion at Ser[365] from both the cell culture and *in vivo* studies.

The factor IX coagulant activity was determined by an activated partial thromboplastin time (aPTT) assay using human factor IX-deficient plasma. The results indicated a significant reduction (approximately 40%) in factor IX activity, which, together with the percent genomic conversion, remained unchanged through 72 weeks. Moreover, direct sequence analysis of the amplicons from random samples at 18 months confirmed the polymorphism at Ser[365] (Fig. 62.7). Thus, the site-directed conversion of the factor

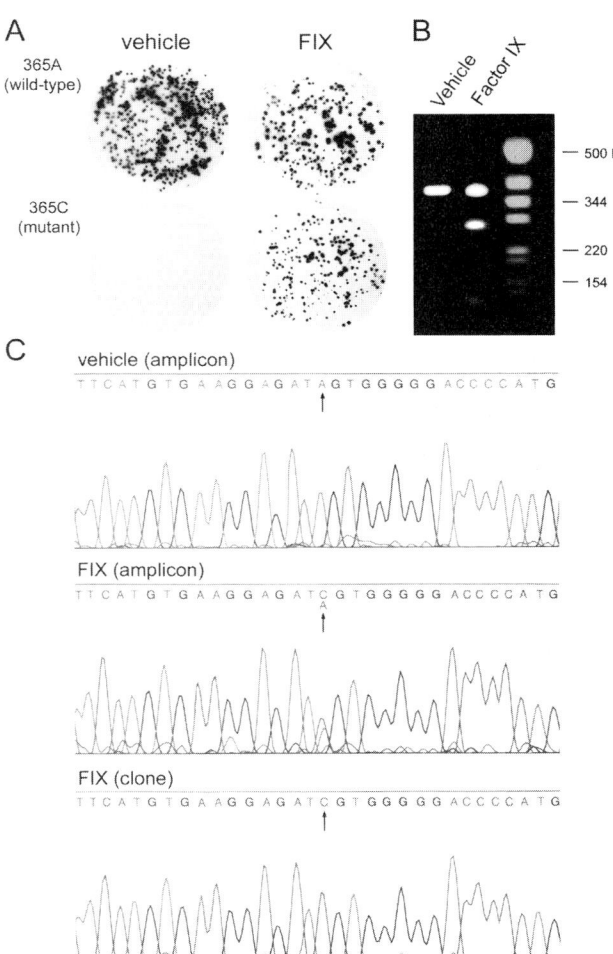

FIGURE 62.7. Filter lift hybridizations, restriction fragment length polymorphism and sequence analyses of DNA isolated from the liver. **A:** Hybridization patterns of duplicate filter lifts of the cloned polymerase chain reaction (PCR) products from liver DNA of rats 18 months postinjection with vehicle (left) or factor IX (*FIX*) chimeraplasts (**right**). **B**: PCR amplicons were subjected to *Sau*3AI restriction enzyme digestion and analyzed by agarose gel electrophoresis and ethidium bromide staining. The site-specific A to C conversion creates a new restriction site, resulting in the partial cleavage of the amplicons from the factor IX-treated animals, but not from vehicle-treated controls. **C:** Direct DNA sequencing of the PCR-amplified *factor IX* gene surrounding the targeted C insertion site at Ser[365] (*arrows*) is shown for wild-type/vehicle (**top**), factor IX amplicon (**middle**), and factor IX clone (**bottom**). See Color Plate 23.

IX gene in intact liver appears to be permanent and phenotypically stable. In addition, the replicative stability of the targeted nucleotide conversion was determined by performing a 70% partial hepatectomy after nucleotide modification. The surgical procedure induces the liver remnant to undergo compensatory regeneration, a process in which 95% of the hepatocytes replicate in two synchronous waves (166). Factor IX activity in these animals was determined periodically by aPTT assays between 9 and 78 weeks postinjection/hepatectomy. The factor IX coagulant activity in these test animals decreased to approximately 40%, while the conversion frequencies remained unchanged, indicating that the genomic mutation is stable during replication.

Experiments were then performed to establish that chimeric RNA/DNA oligonucleotides could efficiently replace a deleted nucleotide. The CN3 chimeraplast designed to insert a single base pair in the mutated *UGT1A1* gene in Gunn rat hepatocytes was administered intravenously using both delivery systems (167). DNA was isolated from liver tissue after 1 week and revealed that the targeted G was inserted at a frequency of approximately 20% in the animals. In contrast, no G insertion was observed in the vehicle control animals. This genomic alteration was unchanged after six months, and was confirmed by restriction fragment length polymorphism (RFLP) analysis and direct sequencing of the PCR-amplified region of the *UGT1A1* gene (165). Southern blot analysis of genomic DNA from these animals indicated that the *Bst*N I restriction site was also partially restored in the CN3-treated animals, while the DNA isolated from the vehicle-treated controls remained resistant to *Bst*N I digestion.

Western blot analysis confirmed that the genotypic correction reestablished expression of the 52-kd UDP-glucuronosyltransferase type I microsomal enzyme in the liver. In addition, serum bilirubin levels dropped below 50% of their pretreatment levels, and remained at these levels more than one year after treatment (Fig. 62.8). In contrast, the serum bilirubin levels of control animals treated with a nonrelevant chimeraplast increased over the same time period. Moreover, repeated administration of the correcting chimeraplasts resulted in further reductions in serum bilirubin levels. Finally, high-performance liquid chromatography (HPLC) analysis of bile from the CN3-treated animals detected both mono- and diglucuronide-conjugated bilirubin, while the bilirubin in control bile remained unconjugated. Taken together, these data suggest that the mismatch repair pathways in hepatocytes may be sufficiently active to make this strategy feasible for other liver-related disorders resulting from single base pair mutations or deletions such as hemophilia B and α_1-antitrypsin deficiency.

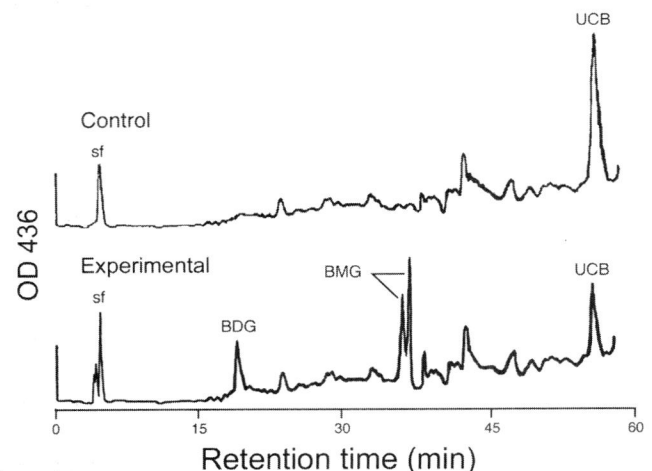
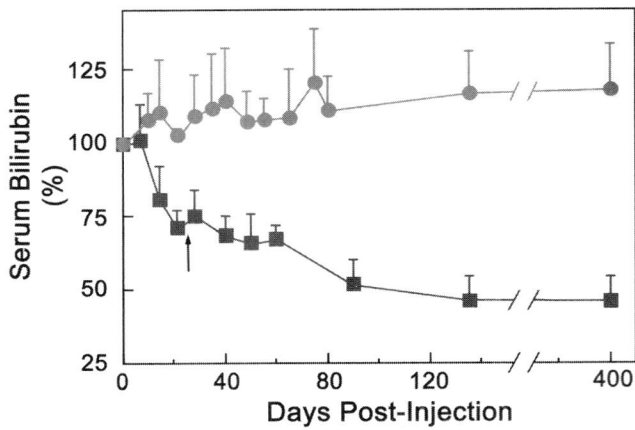

FIGURE 62.8. Bilirubin conjugation and serum levels in Gunn rats treated with chimeraplasty. **A:** High-performance liquid chromatography (HPLC) analysis of bile pigments from Gunn rat livers. Bile ducts were cannulated and the bile collected and analyzed for bilirubin conjugation. Both mono- (*BMG*) and diglucuronidated bilirubin (*BDG*) were detected in the bile of CN3-treated rats. In contrast, bilirubin from the control animals remained unconjugated. **B:** Rats treated with CN3 (*squares*) complexed with lactosylated polyethylenimine (PEI) or encapsulated in targeted anionic liposomes exhibited an approximately 25% drop in serum bilirubin levels. Readministration of CN3 (*arrow*) resulted in a further decrease to <50% of the initial bilirubin levels. In contrast, animals treated with a nonrelevant chimeraplast (*circles*) exhibited no change or an increase in serum bilirubin levels. Each data point is the mean ± SD. $P < 0.001 \geq 14$ days for the CN3-treated animals. CN3, chimeraplast designed to correct the *UGT1A1* genetic defect in Gunn rats. *sf*, solvent front; *UCB*, unconjugated bilirubin.

FUTURE DIRECTIONS

The chimeric RNA/DNA oligonucleotides are capable of promoting site-specific base conversion or insertion in intact liver, resulting in sustained phenotypic changes associated with modification of the genomic DNA. The introduction of a missense mutation *in vitro* in primary rat hepatocytes was independent of the genomic strand of targeted DNA, suggesting that transcriptional activity does not affect the conversion rate. This result confirmed studies in transformed cell lines, indicating that transcription of the β-globin locus was not required to effect a missense site-directed nucleotide conversion (160,161). However, structural aspects of the targeted nucleotide in the DNA loci may influence conversion efficiency, as repair of mismatched DNA has been shown to be bidirectional and strand-specific and also dependent on nucleosomal position (168–170). Moreover, the site-directed genomic DNA modifications observed in hepatocytes and intact liver suggest that the endogenous DNA repair pathway(s)/proteins required are sufficiently active in nonreplicating and quiescent cells. In fact, unlike proteins involved in homologous recombination, the hMSH2 protein levels remain constant throughout the cell cycle (171).

The ability to induce targeted nucleotide exchange in the absence of selection or cell replication provides an extremely powerful tool for *ex vivo* hepatocyte gene therapy. This approach might allow incremental repair of lesions greater than one nucleotide, thus expanding the repair capacity of this technology. To this end, a novel eukaryotic transposon system called *Sleeping Beauty* has recently been characterized and may provide the capacity to insert much larger fragments of DNA (up to 5 kb) (172). Although still in its infancy as a gene therapy approach, this transposon-based system may offer an alternative to viral-mediated gene augmentation, as well as mediating genomic integration in the absence of cell replication.

Vector systems have also been created exploiting the bacteriophage T7 RNA polymerase and its promoter. In this system, the transgene is expressed in the cytoplasm using the T7 RNA polymerase supplied by the transfected plasmid (173). This system bypasses the requirement for nuclear localization of the transgene for efficient transfection, as well as providing only transient expression of the transgene. In fact, this approach may provide great utility in ameliorating the consequences of certain types of liver diseases by providing expression of the telomerase activity required to sustain the regenerative capacity of hepatocytes (174). This ability to efficiently modify the genomic DNA of hepatocytes *in vitro* may prove to be an effective method of gene therapy, as transplantation of normal hepatocytes has been shown to provide effective treatment for Crigler–Najjar syndrome type I (27). Moreover, the recent report of successfully generating conditionally immortal-ized human hepatocytes using the cre/lox targeting system suggests the possibility of now expanding genetically modified hepatocytes to provide sufficient numbers for transplantation (175).

The efficient chimeraplast-mediated site-directed alteration of genomic DNA *in vivo* is an exciting prospect for not only treating genetic disorders of the liver, but also potentially modifying gene expression to suppress oncogenesis. As we begin to better understand the role of telomerase overexpression in the genesis of cancers such as hepatomas (176), the potential for chimeraplasty to introduce nonsense mutations may provide an effective method of disabling the telomerase gene, and thereby reversing the phenotype. As we characterize the process of chimeraplasty, identify the players, and further refine and improve the delivery systems to hepatocytes, hepatomas, and other tissues, this technology may provide a significant advance in gene therapy to liver and other target organs.

There have been a number of additional successful applications of chimeric oligonucleotides for the modification of genomic sequences. For example, chimeric RNA/DNA oligonucleotides have been used to correct the carbonic anhydrase II nonsense mutation in nude mouse primary kidney tubular cells (177,178), and the missense mutation in the tyrosinase gene responsible for melanin production in albino mouse melanocytes (179,180) both in cell culture and *in vivo*. Chimeraplasty has also been used *in vivo* to correct the *mdx* point mutations responsible for muscular dystrophy in both mice and dogs (181). Finally, it has been reported that chimeraplasts can efficiently induce targeted genomic DNA nucleotide changes in plants for improved herbicide resistance (182–184). Collectively, these studies suggest that numerous cell types are capable of performing chimeraplast-mediated modifications of their genomic sequences. Thus, as we enter the new millennium, the potential of this new technology presents us with the prospect of obtaining unequivocal success in gene therapy for treating liver-based genetic disorders.

CONCLUSION

Although an "ideal" gene therapy vector has not been developed yet, the availability of various options suitable for specific applications assures that liver-directed gene therapy will be successful during the next few years. In view of the rapid development in the area of recombinant viruses, particularly hybrid vectors utilizing components of different viral genomes, it can be predicted safely that the gene transfer methods that will be in common use a decade from now have not yet been developed. Nonviral gene delivery vehicles are less popular at this time because long-term gene expression *in vivo* has been difficult using plasmid DNA or synthetic nucleic acids. However, the advent of targeted gene modification, using RNA-DNA chimeraplasts or strand-invasion techniques, offers the opportunity of effecting permanent genetic alterations in the liver, without the need to use recombinant viruses. The concerted efforts of many laboratories across the world make it very likely that, despite initial disappointments, gene therapy will find an important niche in the treatment of both inherited and acquired liver diseases.

ACKNOWLEDGMENTS

The authors acknowledge the important contributions by many investigators in the field of liver-directed gene therapy who were not cited because of limited space.

REFERENCES

1. Greeve J, Jona VK, Roy Chowdhury N, et al. Hepatic gene transfer of the catalytic subunit of the apolipoprotein B mRNA editing enzyme results in a reduction of plasma LDL levels in normal and Watanabe heritable hyperlipidemic rabbits. *J Lipid Res* 1996;37:2001–2017.
2. Ozaki I, Zern MA, Liu S, et al. Ribozyme-mediated specific gene replacement of the α1-antitrypsin gene in human hepatoma cells. *J Hepatol* 1999;31:53–60.
3. Ji W, St CW. Inhibition of hepatitis B virus by retroviral vectors expressing antisense RNA. *J Viral Hepatitis* 1997;4:167–173.
4. Yañez RJ, Porter ACG. Therapeutic gene targeting. *Gene Ther* 1998;5:149–159.
5. Lanzov VA. Gene targeting for gene therapy: prospects. *Mol Genet Metab* 1999;68:276–282.
6. Yoon K. Single-base conversion of mammalian genes by an RNA-DNA oligonucleotide. *Biogenic Amines* 1999;15:137–167.
7. Kmiec EB, Kren BT, Steer CJ. Targeted gene repair in mammalian cells using chimeric RNA/DNA oligonucleotides. In: Friedman T, ed. *Development of human gene therapy*. Cold Spring Harbor, NY: Cold Spring Harbor Laboratory Press, 1999;643–670.
8. Kokoris MS, Sabo P, Adman ET, et al. Enhancement of tumor ablation by a selected HSV-1 thymidine kinase mutant. *Gene Ther* 1999;6:1415–1426.
9. Mullen CA, Coale MM, Lowe R, et al. Tumors expressing the cytosine deaminase suicide gene can be eliminated *in vivo* with 5-fluorocytosine and induce protective immunity to wild type tumor. *Cancer Res* 1994;54:1503–1506.
10. Mohr L, Shankara S, Yoon S-K, et al. Gene therapy of hepatocellular carcinoma *in vitro* and *in vivo* in nude mice by adenoviral transfer of the *Escherichia coli* purine nucleoside phosphorylase gene. *Hepatology* 2000;31:606–614.
11. Roth JA, Nguyen D, Lawrence DD, et al. Retrovirus-mediated wild-type p53 gene transfer to tumors of patients with lung cancer. *Nat Med* 1996;2:985–991.
12. Frank DK, Frederick MJ, Liu TJ, et al. Bystander effect in the adenovirus-mediated wild-type p53 gene therapy model of human squamous cell carcinoma of the head and neck. *Clin Cancer Res* 1998;4:2521–2528.
13. Mohr L, Schauer JI, Boutin RH, et al. Targeted gene transfer to hepatocellular carcinoma cells *in vitro* using a novel monoclonal antibody-based gene delivery. *Hepatology* 1999;29:82–89.
14. Harada JN, Berk AJ. p53-Independent and -dependent requirements for E1B-55K in adenovirus type 5 replication. *J Virol* 1999;73:5333–5344.
15. Paillard F. Immunosuppression mediated by tumor cells: a challenge for immunotherapeutic approaches. *Hum Gene Ther* 2000,11:657–658.
16. Fakhrai H, Dorigo O, Shawler DL, et al. Eradication of established intracranial rat gliomas by transforming growth factor β antisense gene therapy. *Proc Natl Acad Sci USA* 1996;93:2909–2914.
17. Tanaka T, Cao Y, Folkman J, et al. Viral vector-targeted anti-angiogenic gene therapy utilizing an angiostatin complementary DNA. *Cancer Res* 1998;58:3362–3369.
18. Blezinger P, Wang J, Gondo M, et al. Systemic inhibition of tumor growth and tumor metastases by intramuscular administration of the endostatin gene. *Nat Biotechol* 1999;17:343–348.
19. Heise C, Sampson-Johannes A, Willams A, et al. ONYX-015, an E1B gene-attenuated adenovirus, causes tumor-specific cytolysis and antitumoral efficacy that can be augmented by standard chemotherapeutic agents. *Nat Med* 1997;3:639–645.
20. Kawashita Y, Ohtsuru A, Kaneda Y, et al. Regression of hepatocellular carcinoma *in vitro* and *in vivo* by radiosensitizing suicide gene therapy under the inducible and spatial control of radiation. *Hum Gene Ther* 1999;10:1509–1519.
21. Encke J, zu Putlitz J, Wands JR. DNA vaccines. *Intervirology* 1999;42:117–124.
22. Scaglioni P, Malegari M, Takahashi M, et al. Use of dominant negative mutants of the hepadnaviral core protein as antiviral agents. *Hepatology* 1996;24:1010–1017.
23. zu Putlitz J, Wands JR. Specific inhibition of hepatitis B virus replication by sense RNA. *Antisense Nucleic Acid Drug Dev* 1999;9:241–252.
24. zu Putlitz J, Wieland S, Blum HE, et al. Antisense RNA complementary to hepatitis B virus specifically inhibits viral replication. *Gastroenterology* 1998;115:702–713.
25. Encke J, zu Putlitz J, Geissler M, et al. Genetic immunization generates cellular and humoral immune responses against the nonstructural proteins of the hepatitis C virus in a murine model. *J Immunol* 1998;161:4917–4923.
26. zu Putlitz J, Skerra A, Wands JR. Intracellular expression of a cloned antibody fragment interferes with hepatitis B virus surface antigen secretion. *Biochem Biophys Res Commun* 1999;255:785–791.
27. Fox IJ, Roy Chowdhury J, Kaufman SS, et al. Treatment of Crigler-Najjar syndrome type I with hepatocyte transplantation. *N Engl J Med* 1998;333:1422–1426.
28. Roy Chowdhury J, Strom SC, Roy Chowdhury N, et al. Hepatocyte transplantation in humans: gene therapy and more. *Pediatrics* 1998;102:647–648.
29. Fox IJ, Roy Chowdhury N, Gupta S, et al. Conditional immortalization of Gunn rat hepatocytes: an *ex vivo* model for evaluating methods for bilirubin-UDP-glucuronosyltransferase gene transfer. *Hepatology* 1995;21:837–846.
30. Tada K, Roy Chowdhury N, Prasad VR, et al. Long-term amelioration of bilirubin glucuronidation defect in Gunn rats by transplanting genetically modified immortalized autologous hepatocyes. *Cell Transplant* 1998;7:607–616.
31. Miller AD. Development of applications of retroviral vectors. In: Coffin JM, Hughes SH, Varmus HE, eds. *Retroviruses*. Cold Spring Harbor, NY: Cold Spring Harbor Press, 1997;437–473.
32. Verma IM, Somia N. Gene therapy—promises, problems and prospects. *Nature* 1997;389:239–242.
33. Kalpana GV. Retroviral vectors for liver-directed gene therapy. *Semin Liver Dis* 1999;19:27–37.
34. Robbins PD, Ghivizzani SC. Viral vectors for gene therapy. *Pharmacol Ther* 1998;80:35–47.
35. Anderson WF, McGarrity GJ, Moen RC. Report to the NIH

Recombinant DNA Advisory Committee on murine replication-competent retrovirus (RCR assays). *Hum Gene Ther* 1993; 4:311–321.

36. Roe T, Reynolds TC, Yu G, et al. Integration of murine leukemia virus depends on mitosis. *EMBO J* 1993;12:2099–2108.

37. Park F, Ohashi K, Chiu W, et al. Efficient lentiviral transduction of liver requires cell cycling *in vivo*. *Nat Genet* 2000;24:49–52.

38. VandenDriessche T, Vanslembrouck V, Goovaerts I, et al. Long-term expression of human coagulation factor VIII and correction of hemophilia A after *in vivo* retroviral gene transfer in factor VIII-deficient mice. *Proc Natl Acad Sci USA* 1999;96:10379–10384.

39. Yee JK, Moores JC, Jolly DJ, et al. Gene expression from transcriptionally disabled retroviral vectors. *Proc Natl Acad Sci USA* 1987;84:5197–5201.

40. Samulski RJ, Zhu X, Xiao X, et al. Targeted integration of adeno-associated virus (AAV) into human chromosome 19. *EMBO J* 1991;10:3941–3950.

41. Atchison RW, Casto BC, Hammon WMcD. Adenovirus-associated defective virus particles. *Science* 1965;149:754–756.

42. Buller RM, Janik JE, Sebring ED, et al. Herpes simplex virus types 1 and 2 completely help adeno-associated virus replication. *J Virol* 1981;40:241–247.

43. Yakinoglu AO, Heilbronn R, Burkle A, et al. DNA amplification of adeno-associated virus as a response to cellular genotoxic stress. *Cancer Res* 1988;48:3123–3129.

44. Yakobson B, Hrynko TA, Peak MJ, et al. Replication of adeno-associated virus in cells irradiated with UV light at 254 nm. *J Virol* 1989;63:1023–1030.

45. Walz C, Schlehofer JR, Flentje M, et al. Adeno-associated virus sensitizes HeLa cell tumors to gamma rays. *J Virol* 1992;66: 5651–5657.

46. Bartlett RJ, McCue JM. Adeno-associated virus based gene therapy in skeletal muscle. *Methods Mol Biol* 2000;133:127–156.

47. Berns KI, Giraud C. Biology of adeno-associated virus. *Curr Top Microbiol Immunol* 1996;218:1–23.

48. Su H, Lu R, Chang JC, et al. Tissue-specific expression of herpes simplex virus thymidine kinase gene delivered by adeno-associated virus inhibits the growth of human hepatocellular carcinoma in athymic mice. *Proc Natl Acad Sci USA* 1997; 94:13891–13896.

49. Recchia A, Parks RJ, Lamartina S, et al. Site-specific integration mediated by a hybrid adenovirus/adeno-associated virus vector. *Proc Natl Acad Sci USA* 1999;96:2615–2620.

50. Snyder RO, Miao CH, Patijn GA, et al. Persistent and therapeutic concentrations of human factor IX in mice after hepatic gene transfer of recombinant AAV vectors. *Nat Genet* 1997;16: 270–276.

51. Herzog RW, Yang EY, Couto LB, et al. Long-term correction of canine hemophilia B by gene transfer of blood coagulation factor IX mediated by adeno-associated viral vector. *Nat Med* 1999;5:56–63.

52. Snyder RO, Miao C, Meuse L, et al. Correction of hemophilia B in canine and murine models using recombinant adeno-associated viral vectors. *Nat Med* 1999;5:64–70.

53. Wang L, Nichols TC, Read MS, et al. Sustained expression of therapeutic level of factor IX in hemophilia B dogs by AAV-mediated gene therapy in liver. *Mol Ther* 2000;1:154–158.

54. Kay MA, Manno CS, Ragni MV, et al. Evidence for gene transfer and expression of factor IX in hemophilia B patients treated with an AAV vector. *Nat Genet* 2000;24:257–261.

55. Guha C, Roy Chowdhury N, Roy Chowdhury J. Recombinant adenoassociated virus in cancer gene therapy. *J Hepatol* 2000; 32:1031–1034.

56. Russell DW, Miller AD, Alexander IE. Adeno-associated virus vectors preferentially transduce cells in S phase. *Proc Natl Acad Sci USA* 1994;91:8915–8919.

57. Alexander IE, Russell DW, Miller AD. DNA-damaging agents greatly increase the transduction of nondividing cells by adeno-associated virus vectors. *J Virol* 1994;68:8282–8287.

58. Lane DP, Crawford LV. T antigen is bound to a host protein in SV40-transformed cells. *Nature* 1979;278:261–263.

59. DeCaprio JA, Ludlow JW, Figge J, et al. SV40 large tumor antigen forms a specific complex with the product of the retinoblastoma susceptibility gene. *Cell* 1988;54:275–283.

60. Strayer DS, Zern MA. Gene delivery to the liver using simian virus 40-derived vectors. *Semin Liver Dis* 1999;19:71–81.

61. Kondo R, Feitelson MA, Strayer DS. Use of SV40 to immunize against hepatitis B surface antigen: implications for the use of SV40 for gene transduction and its use as an immunizing agent. *Gene Ther* 1998;5:575–582.

62. Botchan M, Stringer J, Mitchison T, et al. Integration and excision of SV40 DNA from the chromosome of a transformed cell. *Cell* 1980;20:143–152.

63. Prevec L, Schneider M, Rosenthal KL, et al. Use of human adenovirus-based vectors for antigen expression in animals. *J Gen Virol* 1989;70:429–434.

64. Jaffe HA, Danel C, Longenecker G. Adenovirus-mediated *in vivo* gene transfer and expression in normal rat liver. *Nat Genet* 1992;1:372–378.

65. Takahashi M, Ilan Y, Sengupta K, et al. Induction of tolerance to recombinant adenoviruses by injection into newborn rats: long term amelioration of hyperbilirubinemia in Gunn rats. *J Biol Chem* 1996;271:26536–26542.

66. Horwitz MS. Adenovirudae and their replication. In: Fields BN, Knipe DM, eds. *Virology*. New York: Raven Press, 1990: 1679–1721.

67. Yang Y, Li Q, Ertl HCJ, et al. Cellular and humoral immune responses to viral antigen create barriers to lung-directed gene therapy with recombinant adenoviruses. *J Virol* 1995;67: 2004–2015.

68. Morrel N, O'Neil W, Rice K, et al. Administration of helper-dependent adenoviral vectors and sequential delivery of different vector serotype for long-term liver-directed gene transfer in baboon. *Proc Natl Acad Sci USA* 1999;96:12816–12821.

69. Ghosh SS, Takahaski M, Thummala NR, et al. Liver-directed gene therapy: promises, problems and prospects at the turn of the century. *J Hepatol* 2000;32:238–252.

70. Ilan Y, Droguett G, Roy Chowdhury N, et al. Insertion of the adenoviral E3 region into a recombinant viral vector prevents antiviral humoral and cellular immune responses and permits long-term gene expression. *Proc Natl Acad Sci USA* 1997;94:2587–2592.

71. Lipshutz GS, Sarkar R, Flebbe-Rehwaldt L, et al. Short-term correction of factor VIII deficiency in a murine model of hemophilia A after delivery of adenovirus murine factor VIII *in utero*. *Proc Natl Acad Sci USA* 1999;96:13324–13329.

72. Ilan Y, Attavar P, Takahashi M, et al. Induction of central tolerance by intrathymic inoculation of adenoviral antigens into the host thymus permits long term gene therapy in Gunn rats. *J Clin Invest* 1996;98:2640–2647.

73. Ilan Y, Prakash R, Davidson A, et al. Oral tolerization to adenoviral antigens permits long term gene expression using recombinant adenoviral vectors. *J Clin Invest* 1997;99:1098–1106.

74. Kay MA, Meuse L, Gown AM, et al. Transient immunomodulation with anti-CD40 ligand antibody and CTLA4Ig enhances persistence and secondary adenovirus-mediated gene transfer into mouse liver. *Proc Natl Acad Sci USA* 1997;94:4686–4691.

75. Hoffmann C, Sandig V, Jennings G. Efficient gene transfer into human hepatocytes by baculovirus vectors. *Proc Natl Acad Sci USA* 1995;92:10099–10103.

76. Frenkel N. Defective interfering herpes virus. In: Nahmias AJ, Dowdel WR, eds. *The human herpes viruses: an interdisciplinary perspective*. New York: Elsevier Science, 1981:91–121.

77. Fung Y, Federoff HG, Brownlee M, et al. Rapid and efficient gene transfer in human hepatocytes by herpes viral vectors. *Hepatology* 1995;22:723–729.
78. Felgner PL, Barenholz Y, Behr J-P, et al. Nomenclature for synthetic delivery systems. *Hum Gene Ther* 1997;8:511–512.
79. Nicolau C, Le Pape A, Soriano P, et al. *In vivo* expression of rat insulin after intravenous administration of the liposome-entrapped gene for rat insulin I. *Proc Natl Acad Sci USA* 1983; 80:1068–1072.
80. Findeis MA, Wu CH, Wu GY. Ligand-based carrier systems for delivery of DNA to hepatocytes. *Methods Enzymol* 1994;247: 341–351.
81. Martinez-Fong D, Mullersman JE, Purchio AF, et al. Nonenzymatic glycosylation of poly-L-lysine: a new tool for targeted gene delivery. *Hepatology* 1994;20:1602–1608.
82. Boussif O, Lezoualc'h F, Zanta MA, et al. A versatile vector for gene and oligonucleotide transfer into cells in culture and *in vivo*: Polyethylenimine. *Proc Natl Acad Sci USA* 1995;92: 7297–7301.
83. Goldman CK, Soroceanu L, Smith N, et al. *In vitro* and *in vivo* gene delivery mediated by a synthetic polycationic amino polymer. *Nat Biotechnol* 1997;15:462–466.
84. Erbacher P, Zou S, Bettinger T, et al. Chitosan-based vector/DNA complexes for gene delivery: biophysical characterization and transfection ability. *Pharm Res* 1998;15:1332–1339.
85. Remy JS, Kichler A, Mordvinov V, et al. Targeted gene transfer into hepatoma cells with lipopolyamine-condensed DNA particles presenting galactose ligands: a stage toward artificial viruses. *Proc Natl Acad Sci USA* 1995;92:1744–1748.
86. Murphy JE, Uno T, Hamer JD, et al. A combinatorial approach to the discovery of efficient cationic peptoid reagents for gene delivery. *Proc Natl Acad Sci USA* 1998;95:1517–1522.
87. Zabner J, Fasbender AJ, Moninger T, et al. Cellular and molecular barriers to gene transfer by a cationic lipid. *J Biol Chem* 1995;270:18997–19007.
88. Subramanian A, Ranganathan P, Diamond SL. Nuclear targeting peptide scaffolds for lipofection of nondividing mammalian cells. *Nat Biotechnol* 1999;17:873–877.
89. Fischer D, Bieber T, Li Y, et al. A novel non-viral vector for DNA delivery based on low molecular weight, branched polyethylenimine: effect of molecular weight on transfection efficiency and cytotoxicity. *Pharm Res* 1999;16:1273–1279.
90. Lappalainen K, Jaaskelainen I, Syrjanen K, et al. Comparison of cell proliferation and toxicity assays using two cationic liposomes. *Pharm Res* 1994;11:1127–1131.
91. Friend DS, Papahadjopoulous D, Debs RJ. Endocytosis and intracellular processing accompanying transfection mediated by cationic liposomes. *Biochim Biophys Acta* 1996;1278:41–50.
92. Labat-Moleur F, Steffan A-M, Brisson C, et al. An electron microscopy study into the mechanism of gene transfer with lipopolyamines. *Gene Ther* 1996;3:1010–1017.
93. Li S, Rizzo MA, Bhattacharya S, et al. Characterization of cationic lipid-protamine-DNA (LPD) complexes for intravenous delivery. *Gene Ther* 1998;5:930–937.
94. Ogris M, Brunner S, Schüller S, et al. PEGylated DNA/transferrin-PEI complexes: reduced interaction with blood components, extended circulation in blood and potential for systemic gene delivery. *Gene Ther* 1999;6:595–605.
95. Steer CJ. Receptor-mediated endocytosis: mechanisms, biological function, and molecular properties. In: Zakim D, Boyer TD, eds. *Hepatology: a textbook of liver disease.* Philadelphia: WB Saunders, 1996:149–214.
96. Hara T, Tan Y, Huang L. *In vivo* gene delivery to the liver using reconstituted chylomicron remnants as a novel nonviral vector. *Proc Natl Acad Sci USA* 1997;94:14547–14552.
97. MacLachlan I, Cullis P, Graham RW. Progress towards a synthetic virus for systemic gene therapy. *Curr Opin Mol Ther* 1999;1:252–259.
98. Perales JC, Grossmann GA, Molas M, et al. Biochemical and functional characterization of DNA complexes capable of targeting genes to hepatocytes via the asialoglycoprotein receptor. *J Biol Chem* 1997;272:7398–7407.
99. Bandyopadhyay P, Ma X, Linehan-Stieers C, et al. Site-directed nucleotide exchange in genomic DNA of rat hepatocytes using RNA/DNA oligonucleotides. Targeted delivery of liposomal systems and lactosylated polyethylenimine to the asialoglycoprotein receptor. *J Biol Chem* 1999;274:10163–10172.
100. Spanjer HH, Scherphof GL. Targeting of lactosylceramide-containing liposomes to hepatocytes *in vivo*. *Biochim Biophys Acta* 1983;734:40–47.
101. Bandyopadhyay P, Kren BT, Ma X, et al. Enhanced gene transfer into HuH-7 cells and primary rat hepatocytes using targeted liposomes and polyethylenimine. *BioTechniques* 1998;25:282–292.
102. Mislick KA, Baldeschwieler JD, Kayyem JF, et al. Transfection of folate-polylysine DNA complexes: evidence for lysosomal delivery. *Bioconjug Chem* 1995;6:512–515.
103. Lee RJ, Huang L. Folate-targeted, anionic liposome-entrapped polylysine-condensed DNA for tumor cell-specific gene transfer. *J Biol Chem* 1996;271:8481–8487.
104. Kircheis R, Kichler A, Wallner G, et al. Coupling of cell-binding ligands to polyethylenimine for targeted gene delivery. *Gene Ther* 1997;4:409–418.
105. Cotten M, Wagner E. Receptor-mediated gene delivery strategies. In: Friedman T, ed. *Development of human gene therapy.* Cold Spring Harbor, New York: Cold Spring Harbor Laboratory Press, 1999:261–277.
106. Wu GY, Wu CH. Receptor-mediated gene delivery and expression *in vivo*. *J Biol Chem* 1988;263:14621–14624.
107. Chowdhury NR, Wu CH, Wu GY, et al. Fate of DNA targeted to the liver by asialoglycoprotein receptor-mediated endocytosis *in vivo*. Prolonged persistence in cytoplasmic vesicles after partial hepatectomy. *J Biol Chem* 1993;268:11265–11271.
108. Coonrod A, Li FQ, Horwitz M. On the mechanism of DNA transfection: efficient gene transfer without viruses. *Gene Ther* 1997;4:1313–1321.
109. Brisson M, Huang L. Liposomes: conquering the nuclear barrier. *Curr Opin Mol Therapeut* 1999;1:140–146.
110. Mahato RI, Monera OD, Smith LC, et al. Peptide-based gene delivery. *Curr Opin Mol Therapeut* 1999;1:226–243.
111. Godbey WT, Wu KK, Hiraski GJ, et al. Improved packing of poly(ethylenimine)/DNA complexes increases transfection efficiency. *Gene Ther* 1999;6:1380–1388.
112. Pollard H, Remy JS, Loussouarn G, et al. Polyethylenimine but not cationic lipids promotes transgene delivery to the nucleus in mammalian cells. *J Biol Chem* 1998;273:7507–7511.
113. Zanta MA, Belguise-Valladier P, Behr J-P. Gene delivery: a single nuclear localization signal peptide is sufficient to carry DNA to the cell nucleus. *Proc Natl Acad Sci USA* 1998;96:91–96.
114. Valcik J, Dean BS, Zimmer WE, et al. Cell-specific nuclear import of plasmid DNA. *Gene Ther* 1999;6:1006–1014.
115. Thomas KR, Folger KR, Capecchi MR. High frequency targeting of genes to specific sites in the mammalian genome. *Cell* 1986;44:419–428.
116. Capecchi MR. Altering the genome by homologous recombination. *Science* 1989;244:1288–1292.
117. Aravind L, Walker DR, Koonin EV. Conserved domains in DNA repair proteins and evolution of repair systems. *Nucleic Acids Res* 1999;27:1223–1242.
118. Roth DB, Wilson JH. Relative rates of homologous and nonhomologous recombination in transfected DNA. *Proc Natl Acad Sci USA* 1985;82:3355–3359.

119. Rubnitz J, Subramani S. The minimum amount of homology required for homologous recombination in mammalian cells. *Mol Cell Biol* 1984;4:2253–2258.

120. Cohen-Tannoudji M, Babinet C. Beyond 'knock-out' mice: new perspectives for the programmed modification of the mammalian genome. *Mol Hum Reprod* 1998;4:929–938.

121. Müller U. Ten years of gene targeting: targeted mouse mutants, from vector design to phenotype analysis. *Mech Dev* 1999;82: 3–21.

122. Goncz KK, Kunzelmann K, Xu Z, et al. Targeted replacement of normal and mutant CFTR sequences in human airway epithelial cells using DNA fragments. *Hum Mol Genet* 1998;7: 1913–1919.

123. Wong EA, Capecchi MR. Homologous recombination between coinjected DNA sequences peaks in early to mid-S phase. *Mol Cell Biol* 1987;7:2294–2295.

124. Thyagarajan B, Cruise JL, Campbell C. Elevated levels of homologous recombination activity in the regenerating rat liver. *Somat Cell Mol Genet* 1996;22:31–39.

125. Yamamoto A, Taki T, Yagi H, et al. Cell cycle-dependent expression of the mouse Rad51 gene in proliferating cells. *Mol Gen Genet* 1996;251:1–12.

126. Chan PP, Glazer PM. Triplex DNA: fundamentals, advances, and potential applications for gene therapy. *J Mol Med* 1997; 75:267–282.

127. Faruqi AF, Krawczyk SH, Matteucci MD, et al. Potassium-resistant triple helix formation and improved intracellular gene targeting by oligodeoxyribonucleotides containing 7-deazaxanthine. *Nucleic Acids Res* 1997;25:633–640.

128. Wang G, Levy DD, Seidman MM, et al. Targeted mutagenesis in mammalian cells mediated by intracellular triple helix formation. *Mol Cell Biol* 1995;15:1759–1768.

129. Majumdar A, Khorlin A, Dyatkina N, et al. Targeted gene knockout mediated by triple helix forming oligonucleotides. *Nat Genet* 1998;20:212–214.

130. Vasquez KM, Wang G, Havre PA, et al. Chromosomal mutations induced by triple helix-forming oligonucleotides in mammalian cells. *Nucleic Acids Res* 1999;27:1176–1181.

131. Faruqi AF, Datta HJ, Carroll D, et al. Triple-helix formation induces recombination in mammalian cells via a nucleotide excision repair-dependent pathway. *Mol Cell Biol* 2000;20:990–1000.

132. Broitman S, Amosova O, Dolinnaya NG, et al. Repairing the sickle cell mutation. I. Specific covalent binding of a photoreactive third strand to the mutated base pair. *J Biol Chem* 1999;274:21763–21768.

133. Chan PP, Lin M, Faruqui AF, et al. Targeted correction of an episomal gene in mammalian cells by a short DNA fragment tethered to a triplex-forming oligonucleotide. *J Biol Chem* 1999;274:11541–11548.

134. Culver KW, Hsieh W-T, Huyen Y, et al. Correction of chromosomal point mutations in human cells with bifunctional oligonucleotides. *Nat Biotechnol* 1999;17:989–993.

135. Kruger K, Grabowski PJ, Zaug AJ, et al. Self-splicing RNA: autoexcision and autocyclization of the ribosomal RNA intervening sequence of Tetrahymena. *Cell* 1982;31:147–157.

136. Symons RH. Small catalytic RNAs. *Annu Rev Biochem* 1992; 61:641–671.

137. Welch PJ, Barber JR, Wong-Staal F. Expression of ribozymes in gene transfer systems to modulate target RNA levels. *Curr Opin Biotechnol* 1998;9:486–496.

138. Lieber A, Kay MA. Adenovirus-mediated expression of ribozymes in mice. *J Virol* 1996;70:3153–3158.

139. Lieber A, He CY, Polyak SJ, et al. Elimination of hepatitis C virus RNA in infected human hepatocytes by adenovirus-mediated expression of ribozymes. *J Virol* 1996;70:8782–8791.

140. Sakamoto N, Wu CH, Wu GY. Intracellular cleavage of hepatitis C virus RNA and inhibition of viral protein translation by hammerhead ribozymes. *J Clin Invest* 1996;98:2720–2728.

141. Welch PJ, Tritz R, Yei S, et al. A potential therapeutic application of hairpin ribozymes: *in vitro* and *in vivo* studies of gene therapy for hepatitis C virus infection. *Gene Ther* 1996;3:994–1001.

142. Welch PJ, Yei S, Barber JR. Ribozyme gene therapy for hepatitis C virus infection. *Clin Diagn Virol* 1998;10:163–171.

143. Welch PJ, Tritz R, Yei S, et al. Intracellular application of hairpin ribozyme genes against hepatitis B virus. *Gene Ther* 1997;4: 736–743.

144. Wu CH, Wu GY. Targeted inhibition of hepatitis C virus-directed gene expression in human hepatoma cell lines. *Gastroenterology* 1998;114:1304–1312.

145. Nakazono K, Ito Y, Wu CH, et al. Inhibition of hepatitis B virus replication by targeted pretreatment of complexed antisense DNA *in vitro. Hepatology* 1996;23:1297–1303.

146. Oketani M, Asahina Y, Wu CH, et al. Inhibition of hepatitis C virus-directed gene expression by a DNA ribonuclease. *J Hepatol* 1999;31:628–634.

147. Asahina Y, Ito Y, Wu CH, et al. DNA ribonucleases that are active against intracellular hepatitis B viral RNA targets. *Hepatology* 1998;28:547–554.

148. Kotani H, Kmiec EB. Transcription activates RecA-promoted homologous pairing of nucleosomal DNA. *Mol Cell Biol* 1994;14:1949–1955.

149. Kotani H, Kmiec EB. A role for RNA synthesis in homologous pairing events. *Mol Cell Biol* 1994;14:6097–6106.

150. Kren BT, Metz R, Kumar R, et al. Gene repair using RNA/DNA oligonucleotides. *Semin Liver Dis* 1999;19:93–104.

151. Cole-Strauss A, Gamper H, Holloman WK, et al. Targeted gene repair directed by the chimeric RNA/DNA oligonucleotide in a mammalian cell-free extract. *Nucleic Acids Res* 1999;27:1323–1330.

152. Igoucheva O, Peritz AE, Levy D, et al. A sequence-specific gene correction by an RNA-DNA oligonucleotide in mammalian cell characterized by transfection and nuclear extract using a lacZ shuttle system. *Gene Ther* 1999;6:1960–1971.

153. Thomas KR, Capecchi MR. Site-directed mutagenesis by gene targeting in mouse embryo-derived stem cells. *Cell* 1987; 51:503–512.

154. Eisen JA. A phylogenetic study of the MutS family of proteins. *Nucleic Acids Res* 1998;26:4291–4300.

155. Marra G, Schar P. Recognition of DNA alterations by the mismatch repair system. *Biochem J* 1999;338:1–13.

156. Lee S, Elenbaas B, Levin A, et al. p53 and its 14 kDa C-terminal domain recognize primary DNA damage in the form of insertion/deletion mismatches. *Cell* 1995;81:1013–1020.

157. Stürzbecher H-W, Donzelmann B, Henning W, et al. p53 is linked directly to homologous recombination processes via RAD51/RecA protein interaction. *EMBO J* 1996;15: 1992–2002.

158. Duddenhoffer C. Specific mismatch recognition in heteroduplex intermediates by p53 suggests a role in fidelity control of homologous recombination. *Mol Cell Biol* 1998;18: 5332–5342.

159. Yoon K, Cole-Strauss A, Kmiec EB. Targeted gene correction of episomal DNA in mammalian cells mediated by a chimeric RNA•DNA oligonucleotide. *Proc Natl Acad Sci USA* 1996; 93:2071–2076.

160. Cole-Strauss A, Yoon K, Xiang Y, et al. Correction of the mutation responsible for sickle cell anemia by an RNA-DNA oligonucleotide. *Science* 1996;273:1386–1389.

161. Kren BT, Cole-Strauss A, Kmiec EB, et al. Targeted nucleotide exchange in the alkaline phosphatase gene of HuH-7 cells mediated by a chimeric RNA/DNA oligonucleotide. *Hepatology* 1997;25:1462–1468.

162. Templeton NS, Lasic DD, Frederik PM, et al. Improved DNA: liposome complexes for increased systemic delivery and gene expression. *Nat Biotechnol* 1997;15:647–652.

163. Kren BT, Bandyopadhyay P, Steer CJ. *In vivo* site-directed mutagenesis of the factor IX gene by chimeric RNA/DNA oligonucleotides. *Nat Med* 1998;4:285–290.

164. Evans JP, Brinkhous KM, Brayer GD, et al. Canine hemophilia B resulting from a point mutation with unusual consequences. *Proc Natl Acad Sci USA* 1989;86:10095–10099.

165. Roy-Chowdhury J, Huang TJ, Kesari K, et al. Molecular basis for the lack of bilirubin-specific and 3-methylcholanthrene-inducible UDP-glucuronosyltransferase activities in Gunn rats. The two isoforms are encoded by distinct mRNA species that share an identical single base deletion. *J Biol Chem* 1991;266:18294–18298.

166. Higgins GM, Anderson RM. Experimental pathology of the liver. I. Restoration of the liver of the white rat following partial surgical removal. *Arch Pathol* 1931;12:186–202.

167. Kren BT, Parashar B, Bandyopadhyay P, et al. Correction of the UDP-glucuronosyl-transferase gene defect in the Gunn rat model of Crigler-Najjar syndrome type I with a chimeric oligonucleotide. *Proc Natl Acad Sci USA* 1999;96:10349–10354.

168. Fang WH, Modrich P. Human strand-specific mismatch repair occurs by a bidirectional mechanism similar to that of the bacterial reaction. *J Biol Chem* 1993;268:11838–11844.

169. Klungland A, Lindahl T. Second pathway for completion of human DNA base excision-repair: reconstitution with purified proteins and requirement for DNase IV (FEN1). *EMBO J* 1997:3341–3348.

170. Wellinger RE, Thoma F. Nucleosome structure and positioning modulate nucleotide excision repair in the non-transcribed strand of an active gene. *EMBO J* 1997:5046–5056.

171. Meyers M, Theodosiou M, Acharya S, et al. Cell cycle regulation of the human DNA mismatch repair genes hMSH2, hMLH1, and hPMS2. *Cancer Res* 1997;57:206–208.

172. Ivics Z, Hackett PB, Plasterk RH, et al. Molecular reconstitution of Sleeping Beauty, a Tc-1-like transposon from fish, and its transposition in human cells. *Cell* 1997;91:501–510.

173. Brisson M, He Y, Li S, et al. A novel T7 RNA polymerase autogene for efficient cytoplasmic expression of target genes. *Gene Ther* 1999;6:263–270.

174. Rudolph KL, Chang S, Millard M, et al. Inhibition of experimental liver cirrhosis in mice by telomerase gene delivery. *Science* 2000;287:1253–1258.

175. Kobayshi N, Fujiwara T, Westerman KA, et al. Prevention of acute liver failure in rats with reversibly immortalized human hepatocytes. *Science* 2000:287:1258–1262.

176. Suda T, Isokawa O, Aoyagi Y, et al. Quantitation of telomerase activity in hepatocellular carcinoma: a possible aid for a prediction of recurrent diseases in the remnant liver. *Hepatology* 1998;27:402–406.

177. Lai L-W, O'Connor HM, Lien Y-H. Correction of carbonic anhydrase II mutation in renal tubular cells by chimeric RNA/DNA oligonucleotide. Conference Proceedings: 1st Annual Meeting of the American Society of Gene Therapy, Seattle WA 1998:183a.

178. Lai L-W, Chau B, Lien Y-HH. *In vivo* gene targeting in carbonic anhydrase II deficient mice by chimeric RNA/DNA oligonucleotides. Conference Proceedings: 2nd Annual Meeting of the American Society of Gene Therapy, Washington, DC 1999:236a.

179. Alexeev V, Yoon K. Stable and inheritable changes in genotype and phenotype of albino melanocytes induced by an RNA/DNA oligonucleotide. *Nat Biotechnol* 1998;16:1343–1346.

180. Alexeev V, Igoucheva O, Domashenko A, et al. Localized *in vivo* genotypic and phenotypic correction of the albino mutation in skin by RNA-DNA oligonucleotide. *Nat Biotechnol* 2000;18:43–47.

181. Bartlett RJ, Denis MM, Kornegay JN, et al. Can genetic surgery be used to revert muscular dystrophy mutations in live animals? Conference Proceedings: 1st Annual Meeting of the American Society of Gene Therapy, Seattle, WA 1998, 1998:153a.

182. Zhu T, Peterson DJ, Tagliani L, et al. Targeted manipulation of maize genes *in vivo* using chimeric RNA/DNA oligonucleotides. *Proc Natl Acad Sci USA* 1999;96:8768–8773.

183. Beetham PR, Kipp RB, Sawycky XL, et al. A tool for functional plant genomics: chimeric RNA/DNA oligonucleotides cause *in vivo* gene-specific mutations. *Proc Natl Acad Sci USA* 1999;96:8874–8778.

184. Zhu T, Mettenburg K, Peterson DJ, et al. Engineering herbicide-resistant maize using chimeric RNA/DNA oligonucleotides. *Nat Biotechnol* 2000;18:555–558.

63

NOVEL STRATEGIES FOR MANIPULATING HEPATIC GENE EXPRESSION *IN VIVO*

MARXA L. FIGUEIREDO
ERIC P. SANDGREN

TRANSGENESIS AND GENE TARGETING

For the past two decades, molecular genetic advances have been applied to manipulate the mouse genome with increasing specificity. The first breakthrough involved the development of transgenic mouse technology. Transgenic mice are generated by introducing specifically constructed gene sequences into the germline that target expression of this foreign DNA to one or more cell types (Fig. 63.1). Most commonly, pronuclear microinjection is used to introduce purified double-stranded DNA sequences of up to 50 kilobases (kb) in length into one of the two pronuclei in the fertilized mammalian egg. The exogenous DNA, a *trans*ferred *gene*tic material (*transgene*), may be of prokaryotic or eukaryotic origin, and typically becomes integrated into the mammalian genome by an incompletely characterized mechanism (1). Resulting animals are born with one to many copies of the transgene in each of their cells, although if the transgene integrates into the zygote DNA after cell division has commenced, a mosaic animal can be generated that lacks transgene DNA in some cells. The mouse that develops from the microinjected egg is referred to as the *founder* transgenic mouse. If the germ cells of the founder

transmit the transgene to its offspring, then all descendants of this animal are members of a unique lineage or line of mice. All animals within a line will possess the transgene at the same location within the genome, and typically display the same pattern of transgene expression. Interestingly, many copies of the transgene can be joined together and integrated as a single linear array or *concatamer* through what is thought to be a homologous recombination process. However, the number of copies of the transgene present within the genome (*copy number*) may not be correlated with the level of transgene expression in the animal.

A large number of enhancer/promoters have been employed to target transgene expression to hepatocytes with variable specificity, and the resulting transgenic mice have been used to study basic mechanisms of hepatic metabolism, growth regulation and carcinogenesis (reviewed in refs. 2–7). However, for some studies, transgene targeting strategies have limitations. For example, targeting expression of mutant H-*ras* to hepatocytes using the albumin enhancer/promoter (which is activated in fetal hepatoblasts) induces fetal liver hyperplasia and death of most transgenic mice shortly after birth, precluding a thorough analysis of the role of this oncogene in hepatocarcinogenesis (8). To address this limitation, it becomes crucial to have an inducible transgene expression system that can be turned on and off at will.

A second, more recently developed methodology involves gene targeting by modification or "knockout" of endogenous genes. By using this technique, endogenous genes can

---

M. L. Figueiredo: Department of Pathobiological Sciences, University of Wisconsin–Madison, Madison, Wisconsin 53706.

E. P. Sandgren: Department of Pathobiological Sciences, School of Veterinary Medicine, University of Wisconsin–Madison, Madison, Wisconsin 53706.

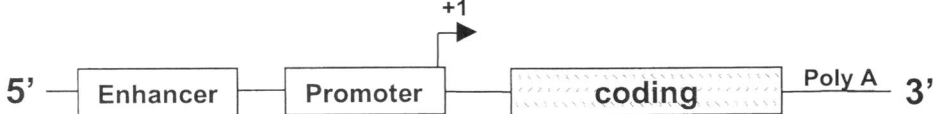

FIGURE 63.1. Molecular components of a typical transgene (double-stranded DNA). "Enhancer" and "Promoter" are gene regulatory elements that direct cell type- and developmental stage-specific gene expression. (*+1*) transcriptional start site; "coding," coding sequence for a gene of interest; polyadenylation (*polyA*) signal, sequence directing addition of polyA tract and often important for mRNA stability. Transgenes also may contain flanking locus control regions to enhance expression (reviewed in refs. 61 and 62). These regions are believed to mediate formation and maintenance of a more "open" conformation of surrounding DNA, thus favoring binding of transcription factors and enhancing transgene expression.

be deleted or inactivated following homologous recombination with gene targeting vectors in embryonic stem (ES) cells (9–12). ES cell lines are derived from the inner cell mass of the blastocyst (embryonic stage corresponding to day 4 post-fertilization), and have the capacity to generate any cell in the mammalian body (totipotency). DNA fragments designed to undergo homologous recombination at selected DNA target sites are introduced into ES cells by electroporation. A gene targeting construct can be designed that is homologous to an endogenous gene but that contains one or more genetic modifications, such as deletions or mutations. Following homologous recombination between the targeting construct and the endogenous gene, these gene differences will be introduced into the ES cell (Fig. 63.2). Cultured ES cells with the appropriate genetic modification then are selected using one of several available selection

schemes (reviewed in ref. 11). These ES cells are injected back into a blastocyst, and they can become incorporated into the recipient inner cell mass and subsequently colonize the embryo. ES cell-injected blastocysts are surgically transferred into the uterus of a surrogate mother, in which they resume development. Resulting animals are chimeras, composed of exogenously-derived ES cells and endogenous blastocyst cells. If the introduced ES cells have colonized the recipient mouse germline, some offspring of the chimeric mouse derived from these germ cells will be of the ES cell genotype. ES cell-derived offspring are mated to each other to generate animals that are homozygous for the gene modification (typically only one allele of the target gene will be altered in the ES cell). The strength of this system is that it allows for selection and expansion in culture of the small fraction of ES cells undergoing homologous recombination.

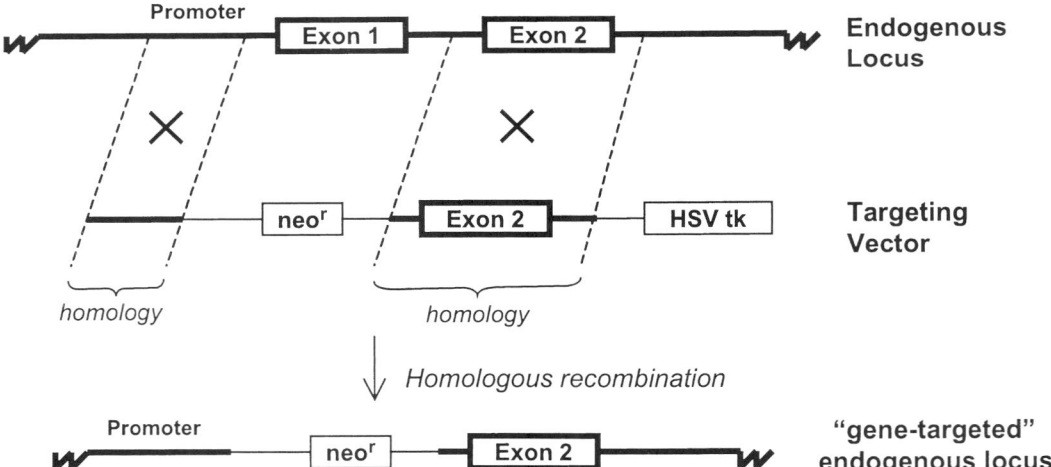

FIGURE 63.2. Targeting modifications to an endogenous locus in embryonic stem (ES) cells. A targeting vector that contains areas of homology to an endogenous gene is introduced into ES cells. The horizontal bold lines indicate endogenous DNA or regions of the vector that are homologous to the endogenous gene. The *X* indicates crossing-over between ES cell genomic DNA and the targeting vector. The most frequent selection scheme employed uses ganciclovir (GCV) and G418. GCV is a substrate rendered toxic by the enzyme thymidine kinase of the Herpes Simplex Virus (*HSV tk*). Following exposure to GCV, cells with nonhomologous integration of the whole targeting vector will be destroyed (negative selection). The cytotoxic antibiotic G418 is detoxified by the neo resistance gene product. Following exposure to G418, cells without the targeting vector will be destroyed, while cells containing the neo[r] gene will survive (positive selection).

Despite the importance of this approach, the inability to manipulate the timing of gene deletion or the specific cell type undergoing gene deletion has limited its usefulness. Certain gene deletions are lethal during fetal development, making it difficult to determine the function of the gene at later developmental stages. In the remainder of this chapter, we describe recently developed methodologies that permit temporal and spatial control of gene expression or deletion, and thereby extend our power to understand the genetic basis of development and function *in vivo*.

INDUCIBLE SYSTEMS

The Evolution of Inducible Systems: Past and Present

Over the last few years, several systems have been developed that permit activation and/or repression of transgene expression by an inducer molecule. Four general categories of regulatory systems have been tested. These include: (a) inducible promoters (responsive to heat shock, inflammatory mediators, or heavy metal ions); (b) ligand-regulated systems (antibiotic-regulated); (c) hormone-regulated systems (steroid hormone regulation); and (d) dimeric ligands (rapamycin-induced dimerization of effectors) (reviewed in refs. 13–15). Most inducible systems are binary, containing as basic elements an *activator protein* and a *target gene*. The activator protein regulates target gene expression by binding to regulatory sequences linked to the target gene (i.e., regulation occurs in *trans*). Therefore, the activator protein is termed a *trans*activator. Expression of the activator protein is targeted to a specific cell type by a tissue-specific promoter. Target transgenes have three elements: a nucleotide sequence to which the transactivator protein binds, a minimal promoter that cannot stimulate transcription initiation on its

own, and the coding sequence of a gene whose expression is to be turned on. To function appropriately, an optimal inducible system must possess several characteristics: (a) a nontoxic inducer; (b) production of high levels of transactivator protein; (c) restriction of transactivator protein production to the desired cell type; (d) minimal target gene expression in the absence of transactivator protein or inducer; (e) high-level induction of target gene expression in the presence of transactivator protein and inducer; and (f) no pleiotropy (i.e., nontarget endogenous genes should not be activated or repressed). Not all systems are practical for use in mice due to inducer cost, toxicity, or effects on expression of endogenous genes (commonly upregulation); uneven inducer distribution in tissues; or high background expression of a target gene in the absence of the inducer. Most successful experimental studies in mice have employed the tetracycline-inducible system, which is described in detail below.

Tetracycline-Based Regulatory Systems

The Original Tetracycline Responsive System: Tet-responsive Transactivator Protein

In 1992, Bujard and colleagues demonstrated the ability of the antibiotic tetracycline (Tet) to modulate gene expression in mammalian cells engineered to carry the Tet transactivator system (Tet system) (16). Mechanistically, the Tet system is a binary system based on cell type-specific expression of a Tet-responsive transactivator protein (tTA), and a target gene under the control of a tTA-responsive promoter element. tTA binding to the target gene is regulated by the antibiotic tetracycline or one of its derivatives (doxycyline or anhydrotetracycline, for example), which function as inducer molecules (Fig. 63.3). The tTA protein contains two functional elements: a DNA binding domain from the Tet repressor protein (TetR) of the *Escherichia coli (E. coli) tet* operon, and a

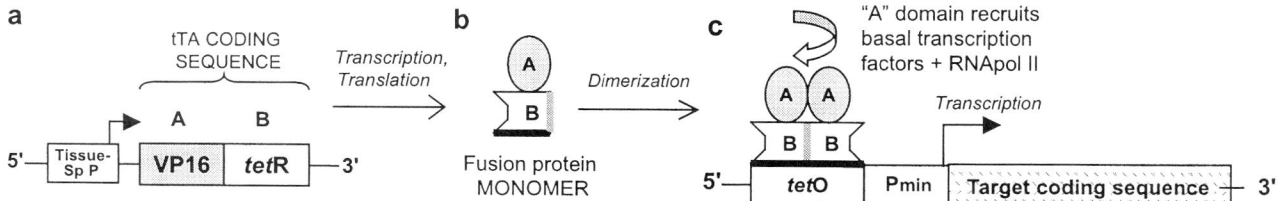

FIGURE 63.3. The original tetracycline transactivator (*tTA*) fusion protein. **(a)** tTA was generated by fusing two distinct functional domains: the transactivation domain of the Viral Protein 16 (*VP16*) from Herpes Simplex Virus (HSV), here depicted as *A* (Activates), and the DNA-binding domain of the TetR repressor protein from the *E. coli* Tn10 *tet* operon, here shown as *B* (Binds DNA). tTA is expressed in a specific cell type due to the presence of a tissue-specific promoter (*tissue-Sp P*). **(b)** The tTA gene is transcribed and translated to generate a monomer, with "A" and "B" domains. **(c)** the tTA protein functions as a dimer, binding to tet operator (*tetO*) sequences on DNA and activating transcription from the minimal promoter (P_min) of the target gene in the *absence* of inducer (Tet or Dox). For convenience, only one of the seven *tetO* repeats is depicted. Shown as a *gray vertical line* is the region that corresponds to the dimerization domain of tTA and as a *black horizontal line* the DNA-binding domain of tTA. (Modified from Kistner A, Gossen M, Zimmermann F, et al. Doxycycline-mediated quantitative and tissue-specific control of gene expression in transgenic mice. *Proc Natl Acad Sci USA*, 1996;93:10933–10938.)

transactivation domain from the viral protein 16 (VP16, from Herpes Simplex Virus). This fusion protein binds DNA specifically as a dimer at a 19 base-pair (bp) DNA sequence, the *tet* operator (*tet*O). The tTA-responsive target transgene contains *tet*O sequences fused to a minimal promoter upstream of the coding region of the gene of interest. To limit target gene expression in the uninduced state, it is important that the tTA-responsive target gene regulatory element has low or no background expression. For this purpose, a "minimal" promoter is used, which consists of a regulatory element that cannot recruit all necessary transcription proteins on its own. Most often, a human cytomegalovirus minimal promoter (hCMV P_{min}) is employed. It is cloned adjacent to multimerized *tet*O sequences (seven were most efficient). Binding of tTA to the *tet*O element brings the VP16 activation domain next to the minimal promoter, thereby producing a fully active gene regulatory element capable of mediating expression of the linked coding sequence. Binding of Tet to the TetR domain of tTA induces a conformational change that eliminates tTA binding to the *tet*O sequence, thereby turning off target gene expression (Fig. 63.4a). This Tet-responsive system proved to be a breakthrough in inducible gene expression in mammalian cells, since tTA was shown to activate gene expression up to five orders of magnitude in the absence of Tet in cultured cells. Importantly, Tet and its derivatives are relatively inexpensive, and are not toxic to mammalian cells at levels that efficiently turn off gene expression. Furthermore, Tet is widely distributed in tissues (including the central nervous system), and passes from mother to offspring through the placenta and in milk. Use of the inducible transgene expression system in mice requires that both target and transactivator transgenes are present in the same animal. In a typical experiment, separate lines of transgenic mice are generated that carry only one of the transgene pair, and these lines are crossed to generate bitransgenic mice carrying both constructs. A principal limitation of this system involves target gene induction kinetics: it may take several days before *in vivo* clearance of Tet (or Dox) sufficiently reduces inducer concentration so that tTA can bind to *tet*O sequences and initiate target gene expression. This system is available commercially as the Tet-off system (Clonetech, Palo Alto, CA, U.S.A.).

The Reverse Tetracycline Responsive System: Reverse Tetracycline Transactivation (rtTA)

The reverse tetracycline transactivation (rtTA) system, which provides a "reverse" transactivator binding phenotype relative to tTA, was first described in 1995 (17). The rtTA protein was derived from tTA by random mutagenesis, and contains four amino acid substitutions in the TetR moiety that allow rtTA to bind *tet*O sequences only in the *presence* of Tet or its analogs (Fig. 63.4b). However, the binding affinity of rtTA for Tet is 100X lower than that of tTA; therefore it becomes important to use the more avidly-binding Tet derivative doxycycline (Dox) (17). This system is useful when animals need to be maintained in the

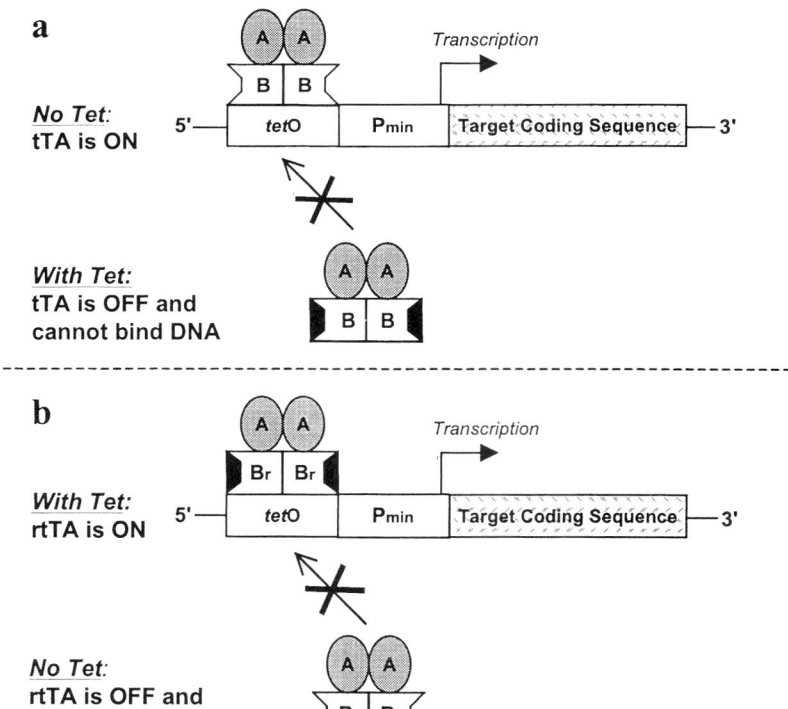

FIGURE 63.4. Mechanism of action of tetracycline transactivator (*tTA*) and reverse tTA (*rtTA*). **(a)** The tTA. The *symbol in black* represents the inducer [tetracycline (*Tet*) or doxycycline (*Dox*)]. Each dimer of tTA binds to one *tet*O sequence (19 bp) in the *absence* of Tet and recruits the transcriptional machinery to a TATA box-containing minimal promoter via the VP16 transactivation domain. This system is described commercially as the Tet-off system. **(b)** The rtTA. Following binding of Dox or Tet to rtTA, the conformation of the TetR (DNA-binding) domain changes, rtTA now is able to bind DNA at the *tet*O sequence, and transcription can be initiated. This system is described commercially as the Tet-on system. *A*, activator; *B*, binding; *Br*, reverse binding. (Modified from Kistner A, Gossen M, Zimmermann F, et al. Doxycycline-mediated quantitative and tissue-specific control of gene expression in transgenic mice. *Proc Natl Acad Sci USA*, 1996;93: 10933–10938.)

repressed state for long periods of time, or when rapid target gene induction is desired (which for tTA is limited by the rate of disappearance of Tet from the cell or body). Using the rtTA system, Kistner et al. reported a steady-state 10^5-fold induction of reporter gene activity in the liver of transgenic mice receiving Dox in drinking water, although high background expression was observed in other organs (18). The principal limitation of this system in mice is the frequent presence of significant background target gene expression in the absence of Dox. This system is available commercially as the Tet-on system (Clonetech).

Modifications of the Tetracycline-based Regulatory Systems

Bidirectional vectors for gene expression

Bidirectional vectors have been developed that permit regulation of expression of multiple coding regions simultaneously (Fig. 63.5) (19–20). In this system, the target contains seven *tet*O sequences flanked by two minimal promoters (in opposite orientation to one another). Each minimal promoter directs expression of a separate coding sequence. This unit forms a *bidirectional promoter* (P_{bi-1}), allowing coordinated regulation of two transcriptional units from the centrally located *tet*O sequences. If one coding sequence encodes an easily detected reporter protein, expression of a nonassayable protein encoded by the other target gene can be monitored via the reporter function. Baron et al. described the successful use of this system in cultured HeLa cells, and suggested that the system also worked in transgenic mice (20).

Mutually exclusive two-gene expression system

Baron et al. also have described a mutually exclusive inducible gene expression system (21). This approach combines the tTA and rtTA systems, although with several modifications. Alterations were introduced into both transactivator proteins and into the *tet*O DNA sequence. DNA binding sites were altered by changing nucleotides at different locations in the *tet*O sequence. This produced novel *tet*O sequences, termed *tet*O$_{4C}$ and *tet*O$_{6C}$, that differed in their

TetR moiety binding specificities. Amino acid changes in the regulator proteins (tTA and rtTA) consisted of (a) modifications in the TetR domains that conferred new DNA binding specificities; (b) shortened VP16 transactivation domain, which remained active but was tolerated in higher concentrations by cells (reviewed in ref. 22); and (c) replacement of the class B by a class E dimerization domain in tTA but not rtTA (class B and E domains are naturally occurring dimerization region variants that cannot form heterodimers; Fig. 63.6). The latter modification eliminated the possibility of heterodimerization between tTA and rtTA. These alterations produced tTA2$^E_{4C}$ and rtTA2$^B_{6C}$, which bound to *tet*O$_{4C}$ and *tet*O$_{6C}$, respectively. Although their DNA-binding specificities were altered, these tTA and rtTA mutants maintain their original capacity to bind Tet and turn target genes off or on. When used *in vitro* with a graded concentration of an inducer, they provide a system to regulate the expression of two target genes in a mutually exclusive manner (Fig. 63.6). This system has not yet been demonstrated in mice.

Combining a transcriptional activator (rtTA) and a transcriptional repressor (tTR)

In contrast to other Tet system modifications, the Tet-controlled transcriptional repressor system provides the option of specifically repressing basal target gene transcription. This tet-silencing system requires three transgenes. The first is the target transgene, containing the typical *tet*O multimer, minimal promoter, and gene coding sequence. The two remaining genes produce fusion proteins that bind to *tet*O sequences. The first is rtTA, with the original type B dimerization domain. The second is a new fusion protein that we will refer to as the tet-controlled transrepressor (tTR; 23,24). tTR was derived from the original tTA protein by performing the following two modifications: replacing the type B by the type E dimerization domain in the TetR moiety, and fusing this modified TetR domain to a silencer domain (the N-terminus KRAB repressor domain from the mammalian Kox-1 or Kid-1 protein) (Fig. 63.7; reviewed in ref. 25). The KRAB domain is a Krüpel-associated box (KRAB) present in one-third of all human zinc finger proteins, and is a potent

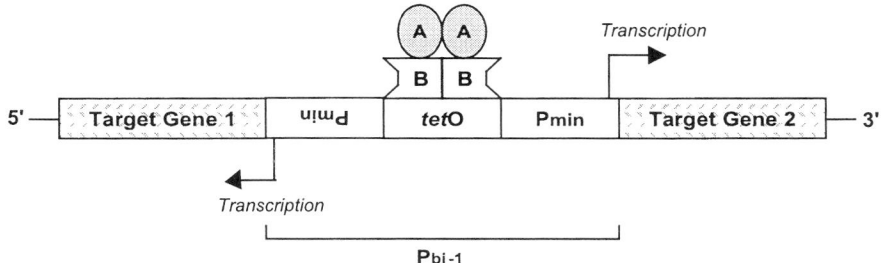

FIGURE 63.5. The bidirectional promoter P_{bi-1}. Tetracycline transactivator (tTA) activates two minimal promoters by binding to a central *tet*O multimer sequence. The *arrows* indicate direction of transcription for each target gene. *A*, activator; *B*, binding. (Modified from Baron U, Freundlieb S, Gossen M, et al. Co-regulation of two gene activities by tetracycline via a bidirectional promoter. *Nucleic Acids Res*, 1995;23:3605–3606.)

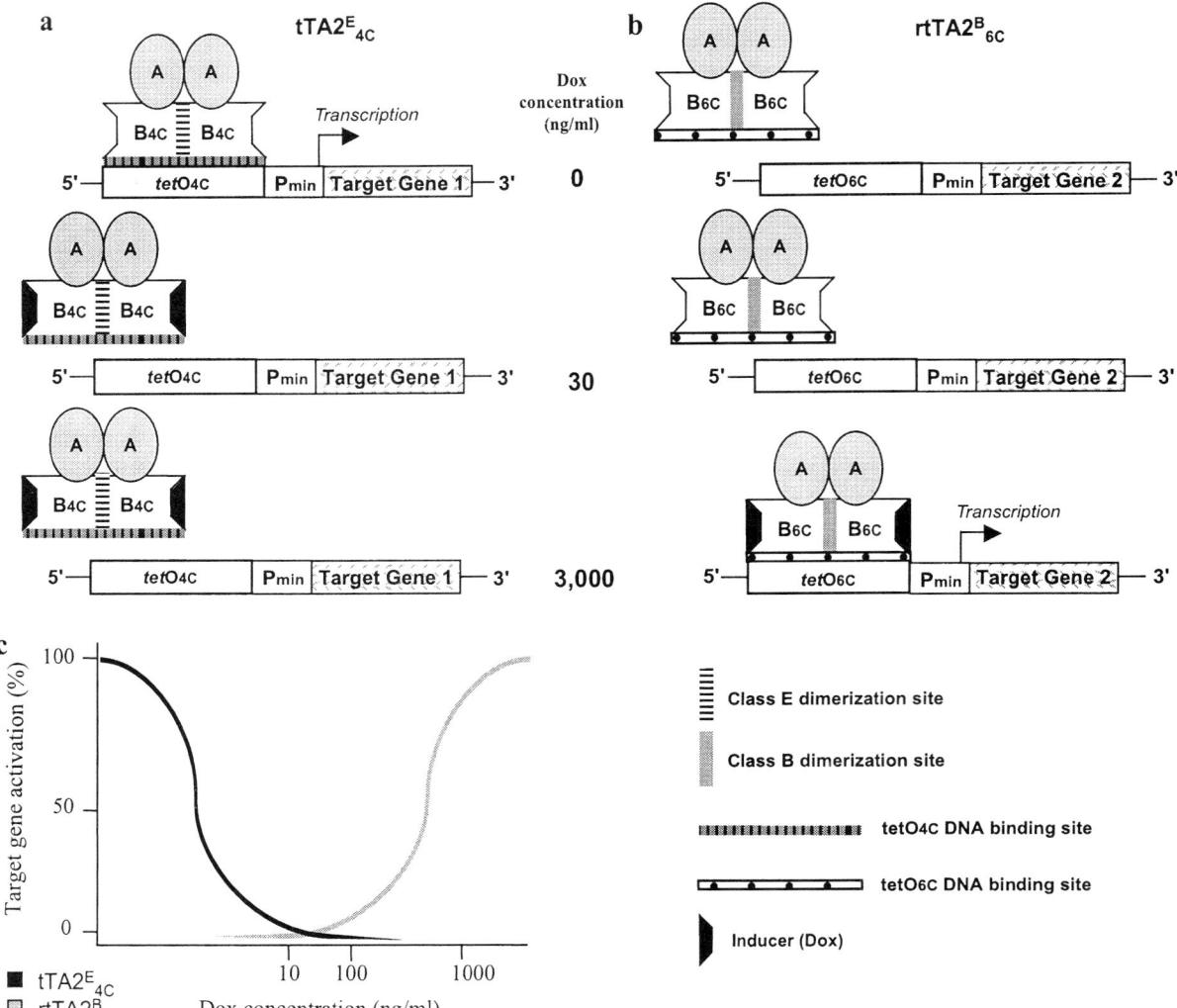

FIGURE 63.6. Mutually exclusive regulation of two target genes by doxycycline (Dox). The transactivator tTA2$^E_{4C}$ binds tetO-P$_{4C}$ in absence of Dox **(a)**, whereas rtTA2$^B_{6C}$ binds tetO-P$_{6C}$ in the presence of Dox (3,000 ng/ml) **(b)**. At intermediate Dox levels (30ng/ml), neither target gene is activated. Transcriptionally activated genes are indicated by the presence of an *arrow*. tTA2$^E_{4C}$ contains the class E dimerization domain, whereas rtTA2$^B_{6C}$ contains the class B dimerization domain; therefore, these proteins cannot form heterodimers. The inducer used in this system must be Dox, since rtTA is 100 times more sensitive to Dox than it is to Tet (18). **c:** Graph indicating the independent expression of two different target genes, turned on by either tTA2$^E_4$ (*black line*), or rtTA2$^B_{6C}$ (*gray line*). *A*, activator. (Modified from Baron U, Schnappinger D, Helbl V, et al. Generation of conditional mutants in higher eukaryotes by switching between the expression of two genes. *Proc Natl Acad Sci USA*, 1999;96:1013–1018 and Blau HM, Rossi FM. Tet B or not tet B: advances in tetracycline-inducible gene expression. *Proc Natl Acad Sci USA*, 1999;96:797–799.)

transcriptional repressor (26). Because of these changes, rtTA and tTR cannot form heterodimers, and in the absence of Dox there is reduced basal expression from the target transgene because it now binds a potent repressor molecule. The result can be a 6-fold reduced level of basal transcription, coupled with high-level activation of gene expression by rtTA upon addition of Tet (23). Dox must be used in this system since rtTA has a 100X higher affinity for Dox than it has for Tet. This system overcomes one of the major limitations of regulated gene expression in mammalian systems: low-level

background expression. This system is available commercially as the transcriptional silencer system or tTS (Clonetech). *In vivo* use of these systems has not yet been described.

Novel Mutations in rtTA: the rtTA2^S-M2 Transactivator

Recently, five new rtTAs have been identified in a random mutagenesis screen by Urlinger et al. (27). The most promising new transactivator, rtTA2^S-M2, functions at a 10-fold lower Dox concentration than the original rtTA, is more stable in eukaryotic cells, is associated with no

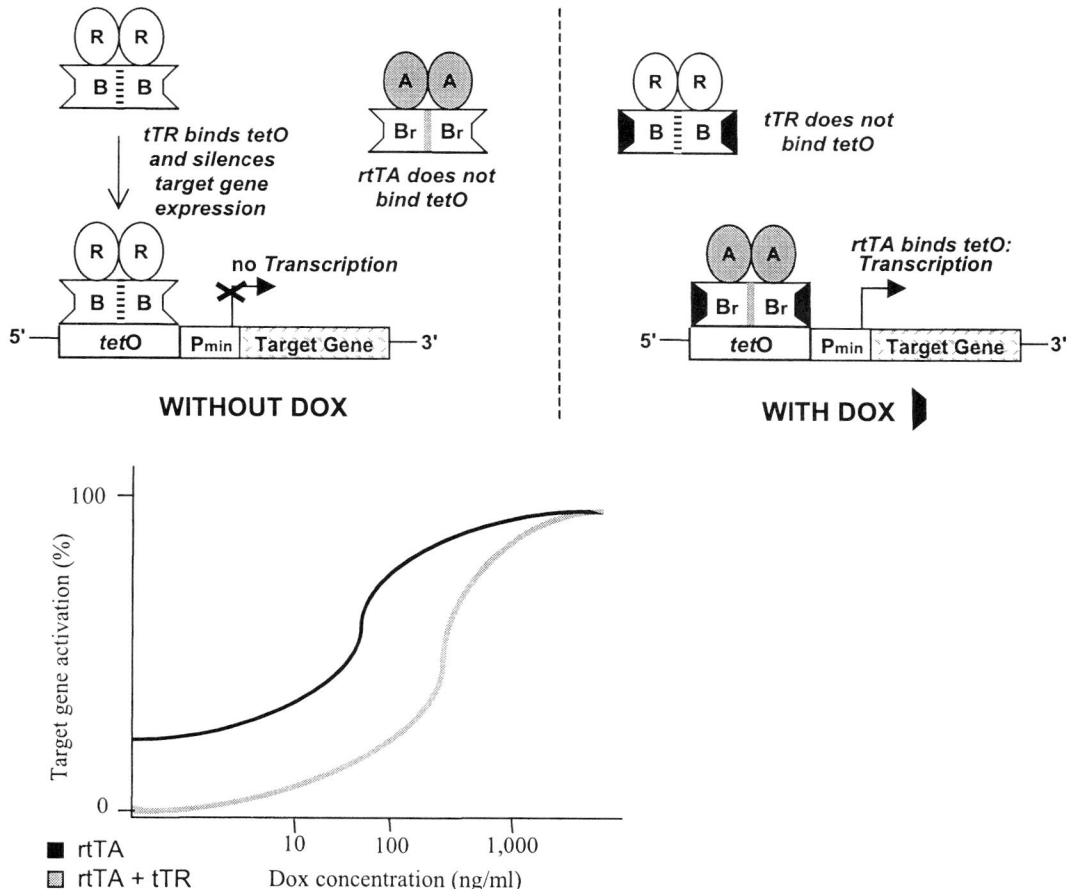

FIGURE 63.7. The "silencing" system: transcriptional transrepressor (*tTR*) and reverse transcriptional activator (*rtTA*) proteins work together to reduce background expression. The "silencing" system is composed of a tTR and an rtTA, both inducer-responsive. The inducer used in this system must be doxycycline (*Dox*), since rtTA is 100 times more sensitive to Dox than to tetracycline (Tet) (17). In the absence of inducer, tTR binds to *tet*O and inhibits target gene expression. In the presence of Dox, rtTA binds to *tet*O and induces target gene expression. tTR and rtTA have different dimerization domains, (*vertical striped* or *gray lines*, respectively), which prevents heterodimer formation. The graph indicates how the basal level of target gene expression can be reduced without affecting the fully induced expression level. (Modified from Blau HM, Rossi FM. Tet B or not tet B: advances in tetracycline-inducible gene expression. *Proc Natl Acad Sci USA*, 1999;96:797–799.)

detectable background expression in the absence of inducer, and allows stringent regulation of target genes over a range of 4 to 5 orders of magnitude in stably transfected HeLa cells. These new versions of rtTA combine tightness of expression control with a broad regulatory range and likely will be used widely in future experimental studies.

THE CRE/LOX SYSTEM

The Cre protein is a 38-kd site-specific recombinase encoded by the bacteriophage P1 genome that mediates intramolecular (excisive or inversional) and intermolecular (integrative) site-specific recombination between specific nucleotide sequences termed *lox*P sites. Its function in phage is to resolve dimeric lysogenic P1 plasmids that arise by general recombination, a process that facilitates the effective partition of the P1 prophage. A *lox*P site (locus of crossing-over) consists of two 13-bp inverted repeats separated by an 8-bp asymmetric spacer region. One molecule of Cre binds per inverted repeat, so that two Cre molecules bind at each *lox*P site. Recombination with a second *lox*P sequence occurs in the asymmetric spacer. Thus, when Cre binds to *lox*P sites engineered to flank part of a gene, there is deletion of the gene sequence that lies between them (Fig. 63.8). The Cre system can be used for two basic purposes: tissue-specific gene deletion or gene activation. This opens up possibilities for elegant control of alterations of gene expression in animals.

The effect of loss of certain genes cannot be investigated fully in mice because the null state causes early embryonic

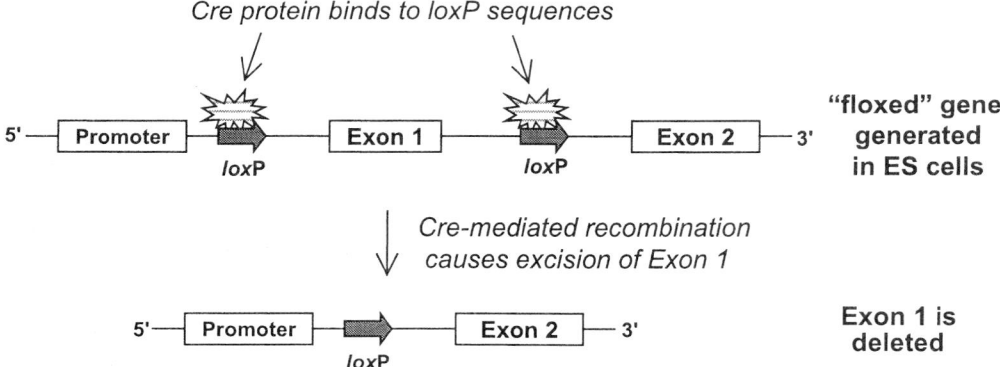

Cre protein binds to loxP sequences

FIGURE 63.8. Knocking out a gene using the Cre/lox system. A selected "floxed" (flanked by *lox*P sites) locus must be introduced into the genome via homologous recombination in embryonic stem cells. The resulting gene-targeted animal then can be mated to a transgenic mouse expressing Cre in a specific cell type. In these cells only, Cre recombinase will bind to the *lox*P sites and excise the intervening DNA. *ES*, embryonic stem.

lethality. To overcome this limitation, these genes can be "knocked out" in adult tissues using Cre/lox. Two mouse lines are required for this "conditional" gene deletion: first, a conventional transgenic line with Cre expression targeted to the cell type of interest, and second, a mouse line carrying the target gene flanked by two *lox*P sites (a "floxed" gene). The latter is generated in ES cells. Cre-mediated recombination occurs only in cells expressing the recombinase, and excision of the target gene ensues (Fig. 63.8). This approach first was demonstrated by deleting a DNA polymerase β gene segment in lymphocytes (28), and has been

used since to study gene deletion in hepatocytes (29–31) and other tissues (reviewed in ref. 12). Activation of gene expression also can be accomplished using Cre. In this approach a transgene or an endogenous gene is engineered to contain a floxed sequence that interrupts transcription or translation of the chosen target gene. Cre expression removes the interrupting sequence, thereby "activating" gene expression (Figs. 63.9 and 63.10). This approach has been shown to work in transgenic mice (32–34).

The Tet-inducible and Cre-controlled systems can be combined (Fig. 63.10) (35–37). In this approach, tTA can

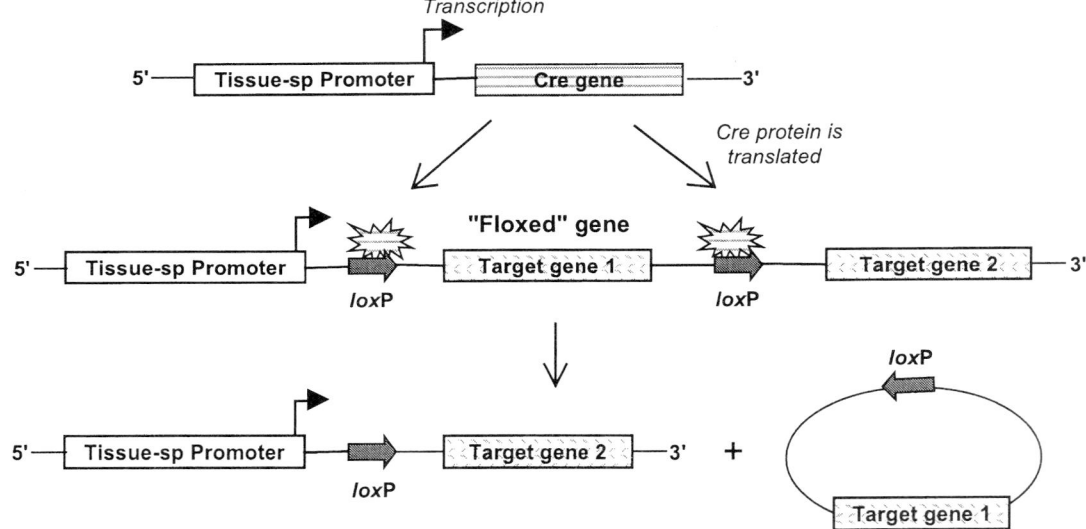

FIGURE 63.9. Activation of gene expression by Cre-mediated gene rearrangement. Cre, represented as a *star*, binds to lox sites in a target transgene. The result is a deletion of Gene 1, bringing Gene 2 under control of the promoter. The circular piece of DNA containing Gene 1 is degraded. Transcription termination sequences could be substituted for Gene 1 as a means to block transcription of Gene 2 in the unrearranged transgene. A complication of this approach is the fact that transgenes typically integrate in multiple copies. Thus, multiple deletion intermediates may be observed.

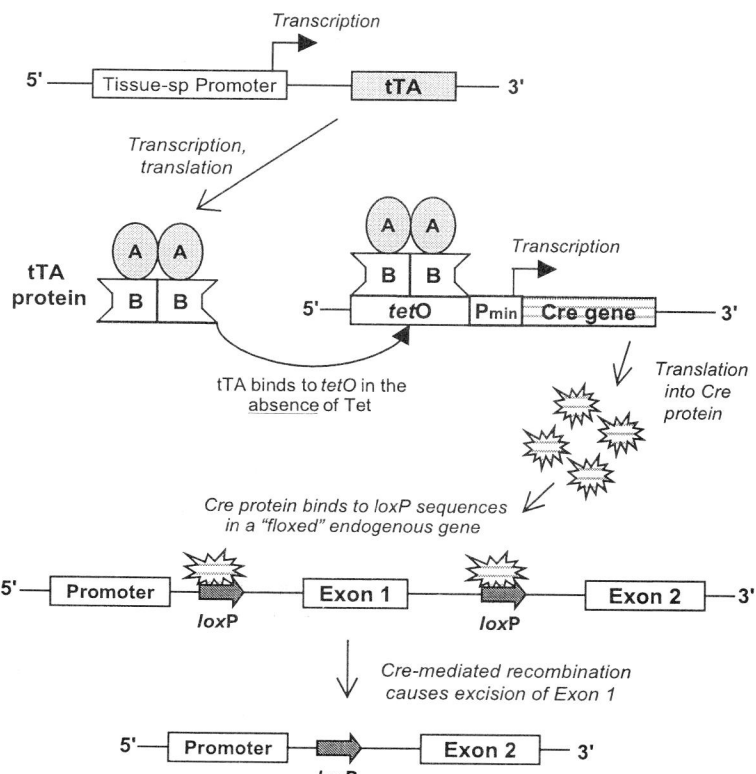

FIGURE 63.10. Inducible Cre/lox: an overview of the combined Cre/lox and Tet systems. Tet-responsive transactivator protein (*tTA*) is expressed in a specific cell type due to the presence of a tissue-specific promoter (*tissue-sp promoter*). In the absence of the inducer Tet, the tTA transactivator binds to the target construct containing *tetO* sequences and a minimal promoter (P_{min}). The Cre gene is transcribed, translated, and mediates deletion of the target gene only in the Cre-expressing cells. *A*, activator; *B*, binding.

regulate expression of the Cre gene from a promoter containing *tet*O sequences. In the absence of Tet, the Cre gene is expressed and induces site-specific recombination between two *lox*P sites in a target gene. In the presence of Tet, the Cre gene is not expressed and recombination does not occur. By establishing inducible expression of the recombinase, which then permanently activates other transgenes, knocks out specific genes, or even switches between the expression of two genes, this combined approach greatly increases the available experimental flexibility.

APPLICATIONS OF TET AND CRE/LOX SYSTEMS TO THE STUDY OF LIVER GROWTH AND DISEASE

Experiments employing traditional approaches to modifying the mouse genome have provided important information about regulation of liver growth and metabolism (2–7). Transgenic technology has been used to identify the effects of overexpression of growth factors and/or oncogenes on liver development, regeneration, and cancer, and to assess the metabolic consequences of changing patterns of gene expression. Gene-targeted mice have been used to identify developmental and pathobiological effects of the deletion of single or multiple genes in liver and many other tissues. Nevertheless, questions that can be answered by

these models are limited, principally due to the constitutive nature of transgene expression, which must follow the expression pattern dictated by its gene regulatory element, and the global nature of gene knockouts, which are present in all cells throughout all stages of development. These obstacles can be overcome by employing an inducible transgene system or a conditional gene targeting system. The remainder of this chapter discusses potential applications of these methodologies to studies of liver biology and disease.

Liver Development

The ability to knock out activity of specific genes has provided an extremely powerful tool to identify genes whose expression is essential for tissue development and to assess how these genes influence development (see chapter 2). In mouse, liver development initiates at day 9.5 of the 19.5 day gestation period, thus inactivation of genes that are essential for mouse development at an earlier gestational stage will be lethal before liver development begins. To bypass this limitation, an essential part of the target gene can be flanked by *lox*P sites (Fig. 63.8), and expression of Cre can be targeted to the early hepatoblasts. Both albumin (AL) and α-fetoprotein (AFP) genes are expressed in hepatoblasts from the earliest stages of liver development (38,39); either can be used to direct Cre expression, although AFP also is expressed in yolk sac and developing gut and so provides less cell-type specificity. (Unfortunately, cell-specific promoters to target other liver cell types have not been identified). Cre-expressing cells then undergo deletion of floxed DNA, leading to loss of target gene activity. Typically, experiments are designed so that mice carry the Cre-expressing transgene, one null allele of the target gene, and one floxed allele of the target gene. In this way, fetal survival is ensured (since usually, though not always, the floxed allele will be expressed normally), and the likelihood of target gene deletion is maximized (because only one allele needs to undergo Cre-mediated DNA deletion). Target gene inactivation is restricted to Cre-expressing cells, and the consequences can be assessed without the complication of gene loss in other cell types.

This approach still has limitations. The most important relates to the efficiency of Cre-mediated target gene deletion. Any variation in Cre transgene expression in the target cell population also will affect the kinetics of deletion, since binding of the Cre protein to the *lox*P sites is influenced by intracellular Cre concentration. Thus, target gene rearrangement may not display identical kinetics in all target cells. In fact, if gene deletion kills or injures target cells, a selective process may favor survival and outgrowth of cell populations with inefficient Cre-mediated deletion, and experimental interpretation must recognize this possibility.

Inducible transgene approaches can be employed to identify the effects of upregulated gene expression on liver development. To study developmental gene effects, gene induction must be rapid, as provided by the Tet-on system. Gene induction kinetics in the converse Tet-off system are far too slow following removal of inducer (and likely variable among individual mice) to permit reliable transgene modulation during fetal liver development. Candidates for inducible transgene expression to study fetal liver development include genes active in growth or metabolic pathways, genes encoding dominant-negative proteins that may interfere with these pathways, or even toxins to selectively damage or ablate liver cell populations at specific stages of development. A second important use of inducible systems in this context will be to suppress expression of transgenes in fetal liver. As noted earlier, fetal hepatoblast-targeted expression of mutant H-*ras* induces diffuse hepatic hyperplasia and perinatal death of transgenic mice (8). Keeping transgene expression turned off in fetal and young mouse hepatocytes should permit identification of mutant H-*ras* effects in adult mouse liver.

Liver Regeneration

Liver regeneration, particularly after two-thirds partial hepatectomy, is a highly studied process for which many changes in the pattern of gene expression have been identified (reviewed in refs. 7,40,41) (see Chapter 42 and website chapter 🖳 W-31). Following surgical removal of two-thirds of the liver mass, most remaining hepatocytes synchro-nously enter the cell cycle, replicate DNA, and divide, restoring liver mass within a week to 10 days. Non-parenchymal cells also replicate within days of hepatectomy. During this process, the liver continues to function. Despite our knowledge of gene expression changes occurring throughout this process, the critical regulatory pathways remain incompletely defined. Recent progress in identifying these pathways has relied upon use of gene-targeted mice. For example, mice lacking functional interleukin-6 (IL-6) or tumor necrosis factor receptor type I (TNFR-I) display markedly attenuated liver growth responses to partial hepatectomy, implicating IL-6 and TNFα pathways as important determinants of liver regeneration (42,43). Fausto has reviewed in detail recent studies of liver regeneration in gene-targeted mice (44). He concluded that further progress will require selective deletion of candidate regulatory genes in subsets of cells or after completion of fetal development to avoid the lethality associated with global deletion of certain genes. For example, hepatocyte growth factor (HGF) is believed to be a key regulatory molecule in liver regeneration, but the effect of its loss on regeneration cannot be assessed because HGF-null mice die before or shortly after birth (45,46). Conditional HGF gene deletion in appropriate target cells of adult mice should permit evaluation of its role in this process.

This example also illustrates several of the current limitations of this approach. HGF is expressed by non-parenchymal cells in liver. Efficient delivery of Cre to these target cells, using transgenic or viral vector approaches, is not currently possible due to lack of characterized targeting elements. To address this problem, target gene deletion can be engineered to be less tissue-specific but more developmental stage-specific. A ubiquitously expressed transactivator can be designed to regulate an inducible Cre transgene (such as *tetO*-P_{min}-Cre). The ROSA 26 gene regulatory element (R26) is expressed in all cells of the body in fetal and adult mice (47,48). Mice expressing R26-rtTA can be administered doxycycline as adults, activating rtTA binding to *tetO*-P_{min}-Cre. In theory, all cells in these adult mice should express Cre protein and delete the floxed target sequence. If ubiquitous deletion of the target gene in adults is not lethal, the resulting mice can be used to study the role of that gene in hepatic regeneration.

Furthermore, whichever Cre delivery system is employed, excision of HGF may not occur in all relevant target cells. Thus, interpreting experiments using cell-specific deletion methodology will require evaluation of deletion efficiency in the target cell population. To address this problem, floxed target gene loci can be engineered so that deletion of the floxed DNA segment activates expression of a previously silent marker gene, such as the bacterial *lacZ* gene, thereby permanently identifying cells that no longer can express the target gene. Using the example of HGF, an experiment may suggest that deletion of the HGF gene in adult mice does not affect liver regeneration. However, if deletion occurred only in 50% of liver nonparenchymal cells, this finding would not support a conclusion that HGF produced in liver had no role in regeneration.

Tet-inducible transgene approaches may be useful in additional ways to define the effects of genes that influence hepatic regeneration. Expression of putative growth stimulatory or inhibitory genes can be induced prior to or at defined times during posthepatectomy regeneration. This approach may be particularly effective in mice receiving a one-third partial hepatectomy, which is reported to "prime" or induce replication competence in hepatocytes without inducing widespread passage through the G_1-S boundary (49–51). Tet-induced genes or gene combinations can be assessed for their "sufficiency" to promote cell cycle progression in one-third hepatectomized mice. Past approaches to defining sufficiency have involved intravenous infusion of growth modulatory substances, often into the portal vein; the inducible transgene approach would complement these studies by permitting localized production within the tissue microenvironment. The potential usefulness of this approach would be influenced by the kinetics of transgene induction.

In certain forms of liver disease, parenchymal regeneration may depend upon activation of a nonhepatocytic progenitor or "stem" cell lineage (52). This type of regeneration is proposed to follow hepatic injury in which replication of surviving hepatocytes is inhibited. The Tet-inducible transgene approach could be used to ablate putative precursor cell populations, using, for example, targeting of the cytotoxic diphtheria toxin gene, thereby identifying the effect on regeneration of loss of that cell type. A gene regulatory element expressed in target cells but not in other cell types would be needed to direct transgene expression. The AFP gene is one candidate: in adult liver, AFP expression normally is low, but in several rat models of severe hepatic injury AFP expression is reactivated in a subset of cells that are proposed to represent hepatocyte progenitors. A noninducible AFP-diphtheria toxin transgene could not be used for this purpose because it would cause fetal death secondary to transgene-mediated destruction of fetal yolk sac, gut, and liver.

Liver Growth Disorders and Cancer

Cancer is largely a genetic disease, although its course has many environmental influences. Typically, multiple genetic changes collaborate during carcinogenesis to produce a fully malignant cell, and malignant cells from different neoplasms may be genetically distinct. Identifying and characterizing causative genetic changes represents at least as complex a task as characterizing liver regeneration after partial hepatectomy, and the approaches to identifying relevant growth signaling pathways in each context will be similar.

Deletions of one or more growth inhibitory or DNA protective genes, termed "tumor suppressor genes," is a universal theme in cancer genetics. In some cases, inheritance of one defective copy of a tumor suppressor gene predis-

poses an individual to cancer in one or more tissues. Actual development of the disease is associated with loss or inactivation of the remaining allele. Examples include childhood retinoblastoma (the pRb gene) and Li-Fraumani syndrome (the p53 gene). These conditions can be modeled in gene-targeted mice (reviewed in refs. 53,54), but often deletion of both copies is lethal during fetal development (as for pRb) (55), or produces a spectrum of cancers that may not include the tissue of interest (p53 null mice do not typically develop liver cancer) (56,57). These concerns can be addressed by restricting conditional gene knockouts to hepatocytes (or any other cell type to which Cre protein can be delivered). Although it remains important to assess penetrance of Cre-mediated deletions in the target cell population, incomplete penetrance is not as great a concern in this experimental context, since loss of both copies of a cancer-relevant tumor suppressor gene may produce a selective growth advantage in, and subsequent amplification of, affected cells.

Inducible transgene strategies may become critical for *in vivo* study of growth stimulatory oncogenes. Fetal hepatoblast-targeted expression of mutant H-*ras* induces diffuse hyperplasia, not neoplasia (8). Restricting expression to adult hepatocytes will be necessary to identify the effects of this oncogene in the adult tissue context. Perhaps even more exciting, availability of inducible gene expression systems (including inducible cell type-specific Cre transgenes) provides the means to conduct a detailed analysis of interactions between oncogenes, tumor suppressor genes, and growth factors during hepatocarcinogenesis. Analysis can include assessing (a) the combined effects of two or more genetic changes (already established for some combinations without inducibility); (b) the phenotypic consequences of the relative timing or order of expression or deletion of cancer genes; and (c) the effect of turning on and off expression of specific oncogenes, to determine whether persistent expression is necessary for maintenance of the neoplastic state or whether neoplastic cells can progress to a state of independence from the initiating neoplastic stimulus. The latter has been accomplished for skin in a study demonstrating that down-regulation of mutant H-*ras* expression in papillomas caused these lesions to regress (58). The tremendous flexibility of experimental design provided by this technology will dramatically improve our understanding of the complex genetic underpinnings of abnormal liver growth.

Other Conditions

The liver has primary functional roles in detoxifying endogenous and exogenous toxins and in regulating metabolism (see website chapters 🖳 W-14 and W-15). Proper functioning requires the concerted actions of multiple genes. Gene deletion experiments can address the role of specific genes in each process. Restricting gene deletion to hepatocytes improves the accuracy of this assessment when the target gene also influences the development or function of cell types in multiple tissues. Global deletion of the aryl hydrocarbon receptor (AhR) gene, which is involved in metabolic breakdown of chlorinated hydrocarbons such as dioxin, produces a spectrum of abnormalities in the mouse liver but also in the immune system (59,60). Hepatocyte-specific deletion will help to clarify the specific functions of this gene in liver. The importance of cytoskeletal and other structural molecules to hepatocyte function and viability similarly can be determined using conditional, cell type-specific gene deletion, without complications introduced by alterations in other tissues. The genetic basis of any process specific to mouse liver can be addressed with ever-increasing sophistication using the tools of conditional gene targeting and inducible transgene expression.

Future Directions

Relatively few reports describing the use of inducible and conditional deletion methodology have been published, but this condition will change dramatically during the next few years. Several trends are likely to be observed. First, as experimental design catches up with currently available technology, studies more frequently will employ methodological refinements such as the tet-transrepressor system, new-generation transactivator molecules, and combined inducible/conditional deletion systems. Second, the technology itself will change rapidly, permitting increasingly precise control of gene expression and deletion. This change will include refinement of current and development of new systems that will become efficient, practical, and cost-effective for use in animal models. Third, with the availability of multiple, independently regulatable systems, researchers will begin to manipulate simultaneously or sequentially the expression and/or deletion of large collections of genes, permitting mechanistic study of multigenic traits. These experiments will provide a more thorough understanding of the genetic basis of health and disease in mice, improving our knowledge of the corresponding conditions in humans.

ACKNOWLEDGMENTS

We thank T. Weglarz and K. Braun for editorial assistance and R. Szakaly for assistance with figures. M.L.F. was supported by a National Institutes of Health (NIH) Molecular Biosciences Training Grant (5T32GM07215). Work in this area in the authors' laboratory is supported by NIH grant R01-CA76361 (to E.P.S.).

REFERENCES

1. Brinster RL, Chen HY, Trumbauer ME, et al. Factors affecting the efficiency of introducing foreign DNA into mice by microinjecting eggs. *Proc Natl Acad Sci USA* 1985;82:4438–4442.

2. Merlino G. Transgenic mice: designing genes for molecular models. In: Arias IM, et al., eds. *The liver: biology and pathobiology* 3rd ed. New York: Raven Press, 1994:1579–1589.

3. Sandgren E.P. Transgenic models of hepatic growth regulation and hepatocarcinogenesis. In: Jirtle RL, ed. *Liver regeneration and carcinogenesis, molecular and cellular mechanisms*. San Diego: Academic Press, 1995:257–300.

4. Nizielski SE, Lechner PS, Croniger CM, et al. Animal models for studying the genetic basis of metabolic regulation. *J Nutr* 1996;126:2697–2708.

5. Bosch F, Pujol A, Valera A. Transgenic mice in the analysis of metabolic regulation. *Annu Rev Nutr* 1998;18:207–232.

6. Fausto N. Mouse liver tumorigenesis: models, mechanisms, and relevance to human disease. *Semin Liver Dis* 1999;19:243–252.

7. Fausto N. Liver regeneration. *J Hepatol* 2000;32:19–31.

8. Sandgren EP, Quaife CJ, Pinkert CA, et al. Oncogene-induced liver neoplasia in transgenic mice. *Oncogene* 1989;4:715–724.

9. Kuhn R, Schwenk F, Aguet M, et al. Inducible gene targeting in mice. *Science* 1995;269:1427–1429.

10. Sauer B. Inducible gene targeting in mice using the Cre/lox system. *Methods* 1998;14:381–392.

11. Muller U. Ten years of gene targeting: targeted mouse mutants, from vector design to phenotype analysis. *Mech Dev* 1999;82:3–21.

12. Nagy A. Cre recombinase: the universal reagent for genome tailoring. *Genesis* 2000;26:99–109.

13. Yarranton GT. Inducible vectors for expression in mammalian cells. *Curr Opin Biotechnol* 1992;3:506–511.

14. Burcin MM, O'Malley BW, Tsai SY. A regulatory system for target gene expression. *Front Biosci* 1998;3:1–7.

15. Harvey DM, Caskey CT. Inducible control of gene expression: prospects for gene therapy. *Curr Opin Chem Biol* 1998;2:512–518.

16. Gossen M, Bujard H. Tight control of gene expression in mammalian cells by tetracycline-responsive promoters. *Proc Natl Acad Sci USA* 1992;89:5547–5551.

17. Gossen M, Freundlieb S, Bender G, et al. Transcriptional activation by tetracyclines in mammalian cells. *Science* 1995;268:1766–1769.

18. Kistner A, Gossen M, Zimmermann F, et al. Doxycycline-mediated quantitative and tissue-specific control of gene expression in transgenic mice. *Proc Natl Acad Sci USA* 1996;93:10933–10938.

19. Hofmann A, Nolan GP, Blau HM. Rapid retroviral delivery of tetracycline-inducible genes in a single autoregulatory cassette. *Proc Natl Acad Sci USA* 1996;93:5185–5190.

20. Baron U, Freundlieb S, Gossen M, et al. Co-regulation of two gene activities by tetracycline via a bidirectional promoter. *Nucleic Acids Res* 1995;23:3605–3606.

21. Baron U, Schnappinger D, Helbl V, et al. Generation of conditional mutants in higher eukaryotes by switching between the expression of two genes. *Proc Natl Acad Sci USA* 1999;96:1013–1018.

22. Shockett PE, Schatz DG. Diverse strategies for tetracycline-regulated inducible gene expression. *Proc Natl Acad Sci USA* 1996;93:5173–5176.

23. Forster K, Helbl V, Lederer T, et al. Tetracycline-inducible expression systems with reduced basal activity in mammalian cells. *Nucleic Acids Res* 1999;27:708–710.

24. Freundlieb S, Schirra-Müller C, Bujard H. A tetracycline controlled activation/repression system with increased potential for gene transfer into mammalian cells. *J Gene Med* 1999;1:4–12.

25. Blau HM, Rossi FM. Tet B or not tet B: advances in tetracycline-inducible gene expression. *Proc Natl Acad Sci USA* 1999;96:797–799.

26. Ryan RF, Schultz DC, Ayyanathan K, et al. KAP-1 corepressor protein interacts and colocalizes with heterochromatic and

euchromatic HP1 proteins: a potential role for Kruppel-associated box-zinc finger proteins in heterochromatin-mediated gene silencing. *Mol Cell Biol* 1999;19:4366–4378.

27. Urlinger S, Baron U, Thellmann M, et al. Exploring the sequence space for tetracycline-dependent transcriptional activators: novel mutations yield expanded range and sensitivity. *Proc Natl Acad Sci USA* 2000;10:1–6.

28. Gu H, Marth JD, Orban PC, et al. Deletion of a DNA polymerase β gene segment in T cells using cell type-specific gene targeting. *Science* 1994;265:103–106.

29. Stec DE, Davisson RL, Haskell RE, et al. Efficient liver-specific deletion of a floxed human angiotensin transgene by adenoviral delivery of Cre recombinase *in vivo*. *J Biol Chem* 1999;274:21285–21290.

30. Imai T, Chambon P, Metzger D. Inducible site-specific somatic mutagenesis in mouse hepatocytes. *Genesis* 2000;26:147–148.

31. Kellendonk C, Opherk C, Anlag K, et al. Hepatocyte-specific expression of Cre recombinase. *Genesis* 2000;26:151–153.

32. Lakso M, Sauer B, Mosinger B Jr, et al. Targeted oncogene activation by site-specific recombination in transgenic mice. *Proc Natl Acad Sci USA* 1992;89:6232–6236.

33. Orban PC, Chui D, Marth JD. Tissue- and site-specific DNA recombination in transgenic mice. *Proc Natl Acad Sci USA* 1992;89:6861–6865.

34. Grieshammer U, Lewandoski M, Prevette D, et al. Muscle-specific cell ablation conditional upon Cre-mediated DNA recombination in transgenic mice leads to massive spinal and cranial motoneuron loss. *Dev Biol* 1998;197:234–247.

35. St-Onge L, Furth PA, Gruss P. Temporal control of the Cre recombinase in transgenic mice by a tetracycline responsive promoter. *Nucleic Acids Res* 1996;24:3875–3877.

36. Utomo AR, Nikitin AY, Lee WH. Temporal, spatial, and cell type-specific control of Cre-mediated DNA recombination in transgenic mice. *Nat Biotechnol* 1999;17:1091–1096.

37. Holzenberger M, Zaoui R, Leneuve P, et al. Ubiquitous postnatal LoxP recombination using a doxycycline auto-inducible Cre transgene (DAI-Cre). *Genesis* 2000;26:157–159.

38. Zaret K. Early liver differentiation: genetic potentiation and multilevel growth control. *Curr Opin Genet Dev* 1998;8:526–531.

39. Spear BT. Alpha-fetoprotein gene regulation: lessons from transgenic mice. *Semin Cancer Biol* 1999;9:109–116.

40. Taub R. Liver regeneration 4: transcriptional control of liver regeneration. *FASEB J* 1996;10:413–427.

41. Taub R, Greenbaum LE, Peng Y. Transcriptional regulatory signals define cytokine-dependent and -independent pathways in liver regeneration. *Semin Liver Dis* 1999;19:117–127.

42. Cressman DE, Greenbaum LE, DeAngelis RA, et al. Liver failure and defective hepatocyte regeneration in interleukin-6-deficient mice. *Science* 1996;274:1379–1383.

43. Yamada Y, Kirillova I, Peschon JJ, et al. Initiation of liver growth by tumor necrosis factor: deficient liver regeneration in mice lacking type I tumor necrosis factor receptor. *Proc Natl Acad Sci USA* 1997;94:1441–1446.

44. Fausto N. Lessons from genetically engineered animal models. V. Knocking out genes to study liver regeneration: present and future. *Am J Physiol* 1999;277:G917–G921.

45. Schmidt C, Bladt F, Goedecke S, et al. Scatter factor/hepatocyte growth factor is essential for liver development. *Nature* 1995;373:699–702.

46. Uehara Y, Minowa O, Mori C, et al. Placental defect and embryonic lethality in mice lacking hepatocyte growth factor/scatter factor. *Nature* 1995;373:702–705.

47. Zambrowicz BP, Imamoto A, Fiering S, et al. Disruption of overlapping transcripts in the ROSA β geo 26 gene trap strain leads to widespread expression of β-galactosidase in mouse embryos and hematopoietic cells. *Proc Natl Acad Sci USA* 1997;94:3789–3794.

48. Kisseberth WC, Brettingen NT, Lohse JK, et al. Ubiquitous expression of marker transgenes in mice and rats. *Dev Biol* 1999;214:128–138.

49. Mead JE, Braun L, Martin DA, et al. Induction of replicative competence ("priming") in normal liver. *Cancer Res* 1990;50:7023–7030.

50. Webber EM, Godowski PJ, Fausto N. *In vivo* response of hepatocytes to growth factors requires an initial priming stimulus. *Hepatology* 1994;19:489–497.

51. Liu ML, Mars WM, Zarnegar R, et al. Collagenase pretreatment and the mitogenic effects of hepatocyte growth factor and transforming growth factor-α in adult rat liver. *Hepatology* 1994;19:1521–1527.

52. Sell S, Ilic Z. Liver stem cells, R.G. Landes Company, Austin, Texas, 1997.

53. Ghebranious N, Donehower LA. Mouse models in tumor suppression. *Oncogene* 1998;17:3385–3400.

54. Attardi LD, Jacks T. The role of p53 in tumour suppression: lessons from mouse models. *Cell Mol Life Sci* 1999;55:48–63.

55. Jacks T, Fazeli A, Schmitt EM, et al. Effects of an Rb mutation in the mouse. *Nature* 1992;359:295–300.

56. Donehower LA, Harvey M, Slagle BL, et al. Mice deficient for p53 are developmentally normal but susceptible to spontaneous tumours. *Nature* 1992;356:215–221.

57. Jacks T, Remington L, Williams BO, et al. Tumor spectrum analysis in p53-mutant mice. *Curr Biol* 1994;4:1–7.

58. Chin L, Tam A, Pomerantz J, et al. Essential role for oncogenic Ras in tumour maintenance. *Nature* 1999;400:468–472.

59. Fernandez-Salguero P, Pineau T, Hilbert DM, et al. Immune system impairment and hepatic fibrosis in mice lacking the dioxin-binding Ah receptor. *Science* 1995;268:722–726.

60. Schmidt JV, Su GH, Reddy JK, et al. Characterization of a murine Ahr null allele: involvement of the Ah receptor in hepatic growth and development. *Proc Natl Acad Sci USA* 1996;93:6731–6736.

61. Bulger M, Groudine M. Looping versus linking: toward a model for long-distance gene activation. *Genes Dev* 1999;13:2465–2477.

62. Dillon N, Sabbattini P. Functional gene expression domains: defining the functional unit of eukaryotic regulation. *Bioessays* 2000;22:657–665.

The Liver: Biology and Pathobiology, Fourth Edition, edited by I. M. Arias, J. L. Boyer, F. V. Chisari, N. Fausto, D. Schachter, and D. A. Shafritz.
Lippincott Williams & Wilkins, Philadelphia © 2001.

REGULATION OF THE EUKARYOTIC CELL CYCLE

DAVID F. CRAWFORD
HELEN PIWNICA-WORMS

The cell division cycle is the process by which cells duplicate their genetic material and then segregate this genetic material equally to two daughter cells. Cells coordinate their growth with the cell division cycle such that the resulting daughter cells are equal in size, as well as in genetic makeup, to the original parental cell. Regulation of the cell division cycle is critical for controlling cellular proliferation and therefore for maintaining the health of the organism. Human malignancies have genetic defects that lead to deregulated cellular proliferation. Most of these mutations activate proteins that promote cellular proliferation, inactivate proteins that suppress cellular proliferation, or make cells less susceptible to death. While each of these types of mutations may indirectly regulate cell proliferation, a large percentage of tumors bear mutations in genes whose protein products directly regulate the cell division cycle (1,2). The role of cell cycle regulatory mechanisms in liver regeneration and deregulation of these processes in hepatic malignances provide excellent examples of these principles.

Cell cycle regulation is critical to liver regeneration (see Chapter 42 and website chapter 💻 W-31). The normal state of hepatocytes within the adult liver is a quiescent or nonproliferative one. This is not to say that these cells are dormant. In contrast, hepatocytes are highly active in terms of metabolic and differentiation-specific functions; they are just not proliferating. However, upon partial hepatectomy, the remaining hepatocytes reenter the cell cycle and proliferate until the liver is completely restored (both in terms of cell number and structure), and at precisely this point, hepatocytes exit the cell cycle and again become quiescent. The interesting question arises as to the nature of the signal transduction pathway that regulates both the entry and the exiting of hepatocytes from the cell cycle in this highly controlled and orchestrated fashion (3). In this chapter, our current understanding of the cell division cycle is reviewed and its relevance to liver homeostasis is discussed.

BACKGROUND

The eukaryotic cell cycle has emerged as an exciting field of study over the last decade, in part due to the discovery that the molecules that regulate cell cycle progression have been conserved throughout evolution. General principles and themes have been derived from seemingly disparate disciplines using a variety of model systems (frogs, marine invertebrates, yeast, cultured mammalian cells, and transgenic and knockout mice) and approaches (genetic, biochemical, cell biological, and physiological). Many of the regulatory

D. F. Crawford: Departments of Pediatrics and of Cell Biology and Physiology, Washington University School of Medicine; Department of Pediatrics, St. Louis Children's Hospital, St. Louis, Missouri 63110.

Helen Piwnica-Worms: Department of Cell Biology and Physiology, Howard Hughes Medical Institute, Washington University School of Medicine, St. Louis, Missouri 63110-1093.

mechanisms are shared among different organisms, so it is often the case that what is learned from cell cycle studies conducted in yeast and frogs is generally applicable to humans. However, for the purposes of this chapter, the specifics of regulation of the mammalian cell cycle will be discussed, unless another organism is specifically mentioned.

A typical cell division cycle in somatic cells consists of four phases: the G1- (*G*ap phase *1*) which follows mitosis and precedes the onset of DNA synthesis, S- (DNA *S*ynthesis phase), G2- (*G*ap phase *2*) which follows the completion of DNA synthesis and precedes the onset of mitosis, and M-phase (*M*itosis) (4). While the duration of the cell cycle and its phases varies widely among organisms and cell types, a typical proliferating mammalian cell divides about once every 24 hours (5). The ultimate goal of the cell division cycle is to generate two daughter cells that are equal in size and genetic makeup to the original parental cell. A schematic representation of a typical somatic cell cycle is shown in Figure 64.1.

Cells have evolved regulatory mechanisms that control the onset and completion of cell-cycle events under normal growth conditions. In addition, cells can delay cell-cycle progression when previous cell-cycle events have not been completed or if a problem is detected. This chapter focuses on the regulatory mechanisms that control the cell cycle, rather than the actual mechanics of DNA replication, mitosis, and cytokinesis.

PROTEIN KINASE COMPLEXES REGULATE THE CELL CYCLE

The passage of cells through the cell cycle is controlled by protein kinase complexes composed of cyclins and cyclin-dependent protein kinases (Cdks) (6). These complexes are inhibited by cyclin-dependent protein kinase inhibitors (CKIs), and modulated by the action of protein kinases and protein phosphatases (7). Cdks control progression through

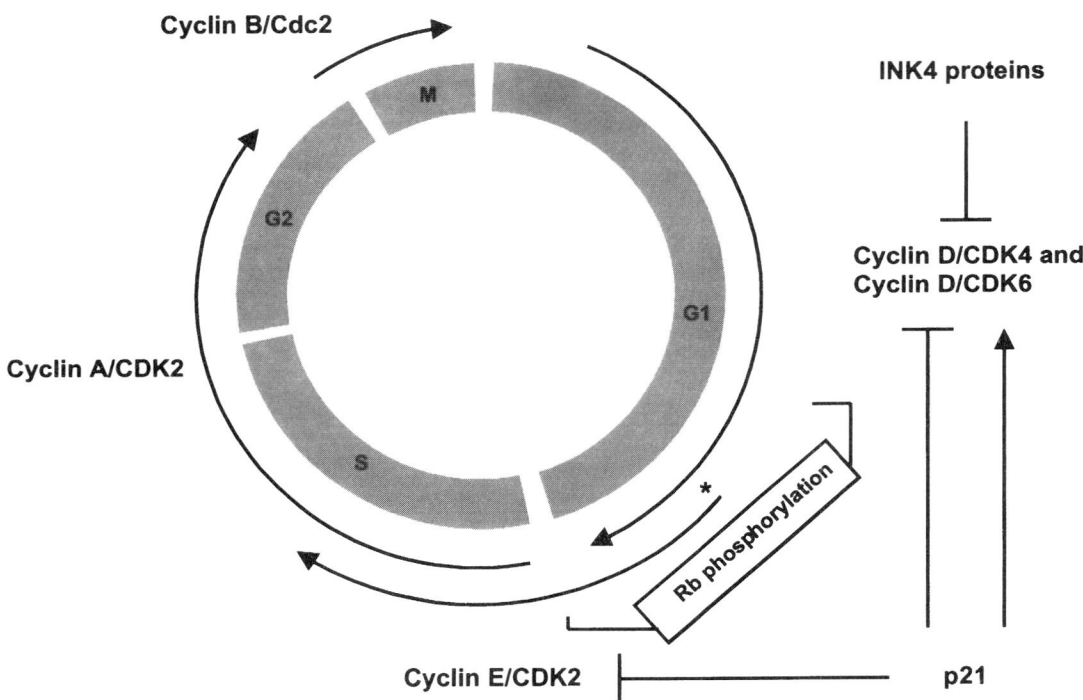

FIGURE 64.1. The eukaryotic cell cycle: A schematic representation of a typical somatic cell cycle. Cells duplicate their DNA during S-phase and partition it equally between the two daughter cells during mitosis [M-phase (*M*)]. G1 and G2 phases (*G1* and *G2*, respectively) intervene between periods of DNA synthesis and mitosis. The cyclin/Cdk complexes that control progression through the cell division cycle are shown schematically, and *thin arrows* indicate the place in the cell cycle where they exert their effect. RB phosphorylation occurs during G1 (shown with a *box and brackets*). The *asterisk* represents the Restriction Point, after which Rb phosphorylation and entry into S-phase (*S*) are no longer dependent on the presence of growth factors in the extracellular environment. Cyclin/Cdk complexes are inhibited by two classes of cyclin-dependent protein kinase inhibitors (CKIs) (p21 and INK4 families). The p21 family functions to negatively regulate cyclin D/Cdk complexes in certain contexts and to positively regulate these complexes by promoting assembly in other contexts (17,18).

particular cell-cycle phases by phosphorylating other proteins, leading to the activation or inactivation of these target proteins. There are distinct Cdks that function in particular cell-cycle transitions. For example, Cdk1 (more commonly known as Cdc2) is critical in promoting the transition from G2 into mitosis, while Cdk2 is required for progression from G1- into S-phase (Fig. 64.1).

A complex set of regulatory mechanisms modulates the action of the Cdks (6). First, the Cdks are inactive as protein kinases unless they are complexed to a cyclin molecule. Specific cyclins serve as partners (and thereby as activators) of each Cdk. For example, cyclin B1 functions as the partner for Cdc2 in promoting entry into mitosis, while the D-type cyclins complex with either Cdk4 or Cdk6 to promote passage through G1. Regulated synthesis and degradation of the cyclins lead to their cyclical abundance throughout the cell cycle, hence the origin of the name for this family of proteins.

Another important mechanism that controls Cdk activity is reversible phosphorylation (8). For example, phosphorylation of Cdc2 at one amino acid residue (threonine 161) is required for full activation, while phosphorylation at other residues (threonine 14 and tyrosine 15) leads to inactivation of Cdc2. Other key regulators of the cyclin/Cdk complexes are the CKIs (7), which inhibit the activity of cyclin/Cdk complexes that regulate the G1- to S-phase transition. Upregulated expression of CKIs is often associated with cell-cycle arrest and cellular differentiation (7). To date, seven CKIs have been identified. These CKIs fall into two families, the p21 and INK4 families. Finally, Cdks are also regulated at the level of subcellular localization. For example, the cyclin B1/Cdc2 complexes shuttle between the nucleus and the cytoplasm throughout interphase and begin to accumulate in the nucleus during prophase (9–11). Similarly, cyclin D1 accumulates in the nucleus as cells progress through G1 but exits the nucleus as cells enter S-phase (12).

THE G1- TO S-PHASE TRANSITION

Passage through G1 and entry into S-phase requires cyclin D/Cdk and cyclin E/Cdk complexes. Levels of the D-type cyclins are tightly linked to the presence of growth factors in the extracellular environment, and withdrawal of growth factors leads to their rapid proteolysis (13). Both proteolysis and subcellular localization contribute to the regulation of G1 cell-cycle progression. The degradation of cyclin D1 and its subcellular localization are both dependent on the activity of glycogen synthase kinase -3β(GSK-3β) (12). When activated, the cyclin D/Cdk complexes phosphorylate target proteins, including Rb (the product of the gene that is mutated in the hereditary form of retinoblastoma). Phosphorylation of Rb relieves Rb-mediated transcriptional repression and also frees the E2F1 transcription factor to allow activation of E2F1-specific promoters (14,15). This allows transcription of genes important for S-phase entry (16). In this way, the presence of mitogens is linked to the cell cycle through the D-type cyclins and Rb in a signaling pathway referred to as the RB pathway (Fig. 64.2). Whereas the INK4 family of CKIs function as specific inhibitors of cyclin D/Cdk complexes, the p21 family of inhibitors has been shown to positively regulate cyclin D/Cdk activity in certain contexts by promoting assembly of the complex (17,18). There is sequential activation of cyclin/Cdk complexes that drives cells through G1 and into S-phase. Early in G1, cells are dependent on the D-type cyclins which complex with either Cdk4 or Cdk6 to promote progression through G1. Late in G1, cyclin E is synthesized, and when complexed with Cdk2, promotes entry into S-phase. Thereafter, cyclin A begins to accumulate, and in complex with Cdk2, it promotes progression through the S- and G2 phases of the cell cycle.

THE G2- TO M-PHASE TRANSITION

Just like the G1- to S-phase transition, passage from G2 into mitosis is controlled by cyclin/Cdk complexes. Entry into mitosis requires the activity of the Cdc2 kinase. Cdc2 is subject to multiple levels of regulation including periodic association with the B-type cyclins, reversible phosphorylation and intracellular compartmentalization (for reviews see refs. 6,8,19). Accumulation of cyclin B1 occurs during the S- and G2 phases of the cell cycle due to transcriptional upregulation of the cyclin B1 gene (20) and stabilization of the cyclin B1 protein (21). Cyclin B1 binding induces conformational changes in Cdc2, which in turn allows Cdc2 to be phosphorylated on three regulatory sites: threonine 14, tyrosine 15, and threonine 161 (22–25). Cdc2 is retained in an inactive state throughout the S- and G2 phases of the cell cycle by threonine 14 and tyrosine 15 phosphorylation (26–31). The Wee1 protein kinase phosphorylates Cdc2 on tyrosine 15, whereas the Myt1 protein kinase phosphorylates Cdc2 on both threonine 14 and tyrosine 15 (30–40). In late G2, the Cdc25C phosphatase dephosphorylates Cdc2 on both threonine 14 and tyrosine 15, leading to the activation of Cdc2/cyclin B complexes (41–45). In addition to cyclin binding and reversible phosphorylation, Cdc2 is also regulated at the level of intracellular compartmentalization. Throughout interphase, Cdc2/cyclin B1 complexes shuttle between the nucleus and the cytoplasm (9–11). The apparent cytoplasmic localization of Cdc2/cyclin B1 complexes (46) is due to a nuclear export sequence (NES) in cyclin B1 which facilitates rapid export of Cdc2/cyclin B1 complexes from the nucleus. Phosphorylation of the NES in late prophase is proposed to both promote the nuclear import and block the nuclear export of cyclin B1

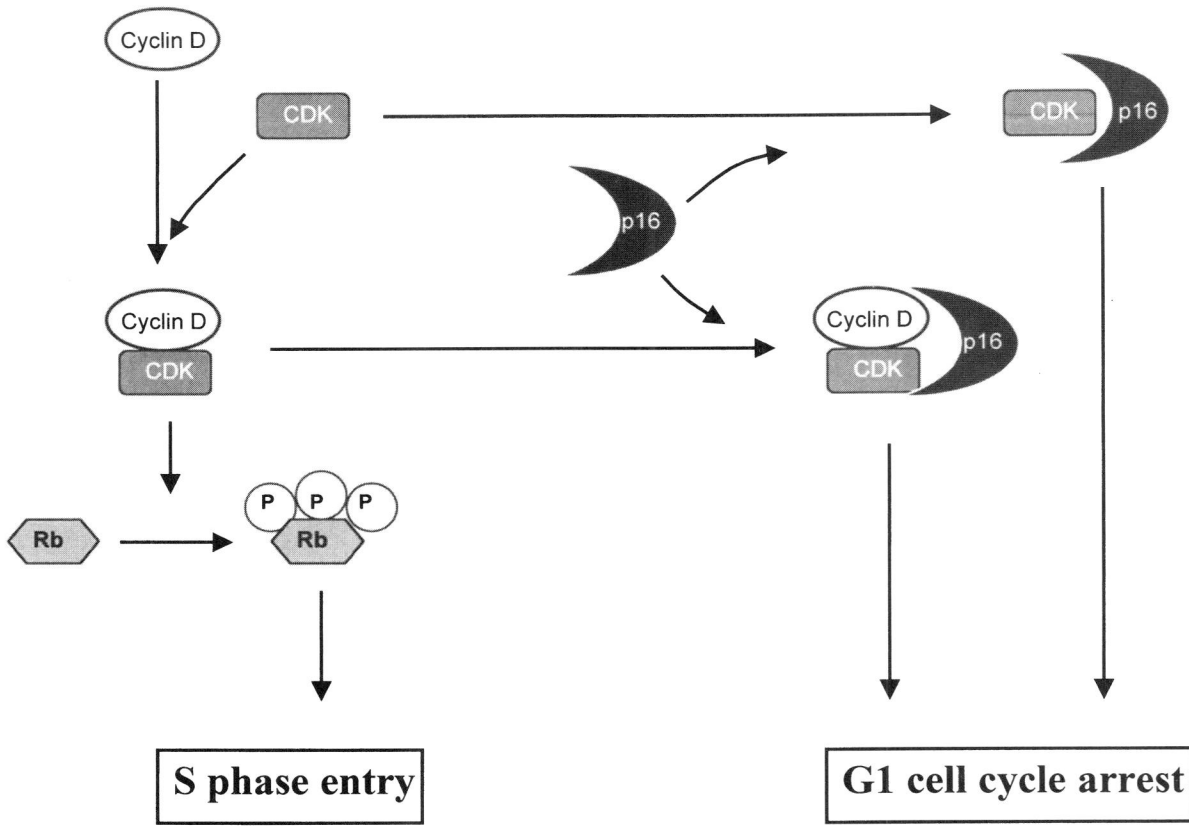

FIGURE 64.2. The RB pathway: The sequence of events leading to S-phase entry and the action of p16INK4a (and other INK4 proteins) in blocking entry into S-phase. Cyclin D synthesis requires growth factors in the extracellular environment. Cyclin D associates with Cdk4 (or 6), which leads to activation of the protein kinase function of the complex. This protein complex initiates sequential phosphorylation of Rb, which relieves the transcriptional repression imposed by Rb, thereby promoting S-phase entry. p16 is capable of binding Cdks in the absence or presence of their cyclin partners, inhibiting both the formation of the cyclin/Cdk complex and the activity of the protein complex. p16 binding prevents cyclin/Cdk complexes from phosphorylating Rb, which in turn prevents entry into S-phase. *CDK*, cyclin-dependent protein kinases; *P*, phosphorylation of the Rb protein.

(10,11,47). Thus, entry into mitosis requires not only the activation of Cdc2 by Cdc25C but also the accumulation of active Cdc2/cyclin B1 complexes in the nucleus.

CELL-CYCLE CHECKPOINTS MAINTAIN THE INTEGRITY OF THE GENOME

Cell-cycle progression is dependent on the completion and fidelity of previous steps in the cell cycle. Signaling pathways that regulate the order, the timing and the fidelity of the cell division cycle are referred to as cell-cycle checkpoints. Checkpoints are signal transduction cascades that recognize a problem (such as damaged or incompletely replicated DNA) and transmit the signal to the cell-cycle machinery, to cause a cell-cycle arrest (48). Checkpoints are essential for maintaining genomic stability. The checkpoints that have been best characterized include the DNA damage check-

point, the DNA replication checkpoint, and the spindle assembly checkpoint. Defective checkpoints allow cells to divide when DNA is damaged or incompletely replicated or when chromosomes are incorrectly partitioned, resulting in increased genetic damage. Defective checkpoint pathways are a common feature of human cancer (1).

In response to DNA damage, eukaryotic cells delay progression of the cell cycle in the G1, S- and G2 phases of the cell cycle to avoid passing mutations on to the daughter cells. DNA-damaging agents include environmental and therapeutic radiation, environmental toxins, and chemotherapeutic agents. Detection of DNA damage during G1 requires several proteins, including ATM (ataxia-telangiectasia mutated) (49), which is the protein encoded by the gene mutated in ataxia-telangiectasia. Following recognition of DNA damage, the protein kinase function of ATM is activated, leading to phosphorylation of other proteins. This signal leads to accumulation of a transcription factor known as p53 (50). p53 upregulates the expression of many genes, including the CKI known as p21 (51). Increased expression of p21 inactivates cyclin/Cdk complexes that regulate the G1- to S-phase transition, leading to a G1 cell-cycle arrest. In this way, ATM, p53, and p21 regulate entry into S-phase following DNA damage, in a signaling pathway referred to as the p53 pathway (Fig. 64.3).

During the G2 phase of the cell cycle, just as in G1, DNA damage is detected and the signal is transmitted by way of ATM and possibly the related protein, ATR (52,53). The mechanisms by which DNA damage is detected and then relayed to the cell-cycle machinery in the G2 phase of the cell cycle are not completely understood. DNA damage leads to the accumulation of p53, but the G2 arrest following DNA damage can occur in the absence of p53. The G2 DNA damage checkpoint prevents activation of Cdc2/cyclin B complexes by preventing Cdc25C from dephosphorylating Cdc2 (54). This signal transduction pathway is known as the Cdc25C regulatory pathway (Fig. 64.4). This signaling cascade culminates in the phosphorylation and functional inactivation of Cdc25C by mediating

the binding of 14-3-3 proteins to Cdc25C (54,55). 14-3-3 proteins prevent Cdc25C from accumulating in the nucleus (55–59). In the absence of DNA damage, Cdc25C accumulates in the nucleus, where it presumably dephosphorylates and activates Cdc2 to drive cells into mitosis. Thus, the cell-cycle arrest that occurs in both the G1 and G2 phases of the cell cycle following DNA damage is due to the inability of cells to activate cyclin/Cdk complexes.

The DNA replication checkpoint prevents the onset of mitosis until DNA replication is complete. This ensures that each daughter cell gets a full complement of genetic material. Some components of this pathway are shared with the G2 DNA damage checkpoint. The DNA replication checkpoint can be demonstrated experimentally by treating cells with hydroxyurea, which prevents the completion of DNA synthesis. As with the G2 DNA damage checkpoint, the DNA replication checkpoint prevents activation of Cdc2 by maintaining Cdc25C in a 14-3-3-bound form (54,55,60,61).

The spindle assembly checkpoint arrests mitotic progression if the spindle is not assembled or if all the chro-

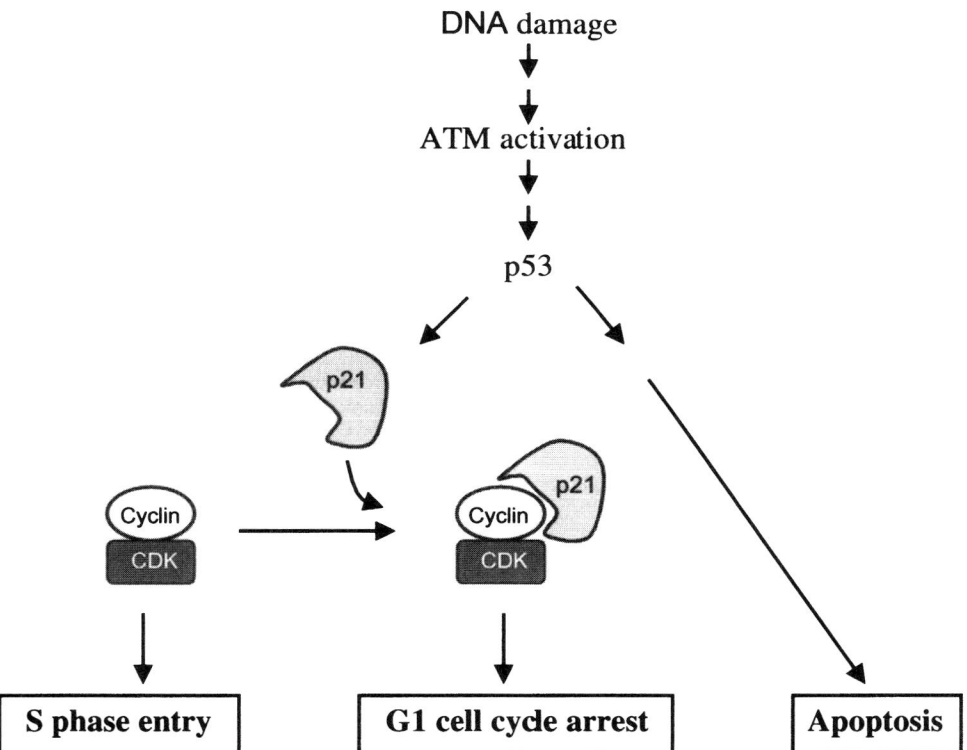

FIGURE 64.3. The p53 pathway: If the DNA of cells is damaged, the p53 pathway is activated. Through a mechanism that is not yet fully understood, DNA damage leads to activation of ataxia–telangiectasia mutated (*ATM*), a protein kinase. Activation of ATM in turn leads to upregulation of p53 through stabilization of p53 protein. The mechanism employed by ATM to achieve this is also not fully characterized. p53 regulates both cell-cycle arrest and programmed cell death (apoptosis). In its role as a mediator of cell-cycle arrest, p53 serves as a transcription factor, promoting the expression of several proteins, including p21. p21 binds to the cyclin/Cdk complexes that promote entry into S-phase, inactivating their protein kinase function and causing a G1 cell-cycle arrest.

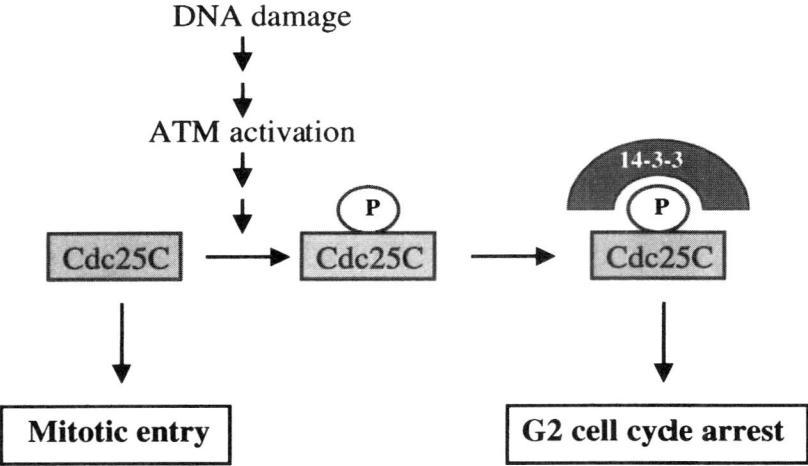

FIGURE 64.4. The Cdc25C pathway. In addition to the p53 pathway, DNA damage leads to the activation of another signal transduction pathway known as the Cdc25C pathway. Although the ataxia–telangiectasia mutated (*ATM*) protein is thought to play a role in this signal transduction pathway, the mechanism by which it is activated and the way by which it transmits the signal are not well understood. However, activation of the Cdc25C pathway leads to phosphorylation of Cdc25C on a critical regulatory site, serine-216. Phosphorylation of serine 216 promotes the binding of 14-3-3 proteins to Cdc25C. 14-3-3 binding prevents Cdc25C from activating Cdc2/cyclin B complexes, and this leads to a G2 cell-cycle arrest. *P*, phosphorylation of the Cdc25C protein.

mosomes are not properly oriented and attached to the spindle. The spindle assembly checkpoint was identified by showing that when a chromosome is displaced from the spindle, cells block mitotic progression, and also by isolating yeast mutants that continue to divide in the absence of a fully functional spindle (62–64). This checkpoint ensures the accurate segregation of sister chromatids to the two daughter cells, thereby preventing aneuploidy. The spindle assembly checkpoint prevents activation of a complex known as the anaphase-promoting complex, or APC (65). Activation of the APC leads to the ubiquitin-mediated proteolysis of proteins that inhibit the metaphase to anaphase transition.

CELL-CYCLE REGULATORY MECHANISMS CONTRIBUTE TO HEPATIC REGENERATION

Following partial hepatectomy, the remaining hepatocytes reenter the cell division cycle to regenerate the liver to its original size and proportions (Chapter 42 and website chapter 🖳 W-31). Reentry into the cell cycle occurs in a synchronous fashion, so partial hepatectomy has been used as a model system to study cell-cycle control *in vivo*. Furthermore, liver regeneration also serves as a useful model system for studying the signal transduction pathway that leads to cell-cycle resumption from quiescence. Some of the details of the pathway between growth factor stimulation and reinitiation of the cell division cycle are addressed in reviews (3,66) and in Chapter 36.

Transient increases in the expression and activity of several cell-cycle regulatory molecules have been observed in livers in the hours following partial hepatectomy. One of the most pronounced changes in protein expression is observed for cyclin D1 (67,68). A strong upregulation of cyclin D1 protein is observed in mouse liver following partial hepatectomy, usually peaking at about 48 hours after

partial hepatectomy. Upregulation of the cyclin D1 protein is also noted in rat liver following partial hepatectomy and in mitotically active human liver following transplantation (67), but the change is less dramatic. Increased expression of cyclins D2, D3, E, and A have also been reported in some studies (68–70), consistent with the role of the cyclin D, E, and A molecules in promoting progression through G1 and entry into S-phase in hepatocytes that have reinitiated the cell division cycle. Modest increases in the expression of Cdks 2 and 4 following partial hepatectomy have also been reported (67–69,71), consistent with their role as binding partners for the G1-S cyclins. More importantly, these studies have also demonstrated that partial hepatectomy leads to a large increase in active cyclin D1/Cdk4 and cyclin E/Cdk2 complexes. Substantial increases in Cdc2 protein levels following partial hepatectomy have also been observed, usually at a later time following partial hepatectomy (67,68).

An increase in the expression of p21 has also been observed following partial hepatectomy (69,70,72,73). Increased binding of p21 and p27 to complexes containing cyclin D1 has been observed in this setting (71,72) and may reflect a role for p21 and p27 in promoting the assembly of cyclin D/Cdk complexes (17,18). A role for p21 in controlling cell-cycle reentry is supported by experiments using transgenic and knockout animals as well. In animals with forced overexpression of p21, hepatic regeneration following partial hepatectomy is markedly impaired (74). Overexpression of p21 in this context likely inhibits cyclin E/Cdk2 and perhaps cyclin D/Cdk complexes as well. Finally, animals with targeted deletion of the p21 gene demonstrate a more rapid reentry into the cell cycle following partial hepatectomy, perhaps due to more rapid activation of cyclin E/Cdk complexes (72). Once the liver has been restored to its original size and proportions, hepatocytes exit the cell cycle and stop proliferating. The mechanisms regulating cell-cycle exit are not known but may involve one or more CKIs.

MUTATIONS IN CELL-CYCLE REGULATORY PROTEINS ARE COMMON IN HEPATIC MALIGNANCIES

Defects in checkpoint proteins and cell-cycle regulatory proteins are common in cancer cells, including hepatic malignancies (Chapter 68). These alterations allow cancer cells to grow with decreased dependence on mitogens, proliferate in the presence of damaged DNA, and display genomic instability. While mutations of many different genes have been shown to play a role in hepatic malignancies, large proportions of these tumors have mutations in some component of the cell-cycle regulatory machinery.

In nontransformed cells, the RB pathway serves as a regulator of cellular proliferation, and mutations in components of this signaling pathway are common in cancer cells (13). One of the INK4 cyclin-dependent kinase inhibitors (CKIs), p16INK4a, is frequently mutated in human malignancies. Germline mutations in p16INK4a have been linked to the hereditary form of melanoma (75,76), and somatic mutations of the gene have been noted in many sporadic malignancies, including some hepatocellular carcinomas (77–79). Mutations that lead to overexpression of one of the cyclin D genes, cyclin D1, are commonly found in human malignancies, including about 10% of hepatocellular carcinomas (80,81), and may be correlated with a worse prognosis (82,83). Mutations that lead to an overexpression of cyclin A have also been noted in a fraction of hepatocellular carcinomas, and this may also predict a worse prognosis (84). Recent data suggest that cyclin D1, Cdk4, or both may also be overexpressed in a majority of hepatoblastomas (85), while another study showed decreased cyclin D1 expression and increased expression of cyclins D2 and D3 in these tumors (86). Mutations leading to a loss of RB expression have also been noted in many different sporadic human malignancies including a substantial portion of hepatocellular carcinomas (87–90).

The majority of human tumor cells have mutations in the p53 pathway, which transmits the DNA damage signal to either the cell-cycle or cell-death machinery. ATM, a protein that functions early in this pathway, is a tumor suppressor protein. When ATM is mutated in the germline, the result is a disease known as ataxia-telangiectasia, which is characterized by a predisposition to lymphoid malignancies (leukemia and lymphoma), immunodeficiency, and ataxia. However, mutations in this gene are uncommon in sporadic human malignancies, and have not been reported in hepatocellular carcinomas. Mutations in p53 are the most common genetic alteration in human malignancies (91), and are frequently found in hepatocellular carcinomas (92–97). In regions of the world where aflatoxin exposure is common, a surprisingly large proportion of mutations in p53 are found at a specific amino acid (R249S). In one report, p53 mutations were also noted in hepatoblastomas (98), but this finding was not confirmed in other studies (99–101). Occasional mutations of p21 (about 5%) have also been noted in hepatocellular carcinomas (102). On the other hand, decreased p21 expression is common in hepatocellular carcinomas, since p21 expression is dependent on a normally functioning p53 gene, which is frequently mutated in these tumors.

Chronic infection with hepatitis B virus (HBV) or hepatitis C virus (HCV) can lead to neoplastic transformation (Chapters 54–56). While the mechanism of virus-induced transformation is probably due to multiple factors, a contributory role for deregulation of the cell division cycle has been suggested. HBV and HCV encode proteins that bind to and transcriptionally suppress the expression of p53, respectively (103,104). This might interfere with the action of p53 in regulating the cell division cycle or apoptosis. The mechanisms by which hepatitis viruses contribute to oncogenesis are poorly understood at present. However, proteins encoded by these viruses may follow the paradigm established by other viral oncoproteins; that is, they may exert their effect by interfering with the action of proteins that regulate cellular proliferation or cell death.

While the majority of hepatocellular carcinomas have mutations in proteins involved in regulating the cell division cycle, there are many other mutations that play a role in hepatocellular carcinogenesis. For example, mutations in the β-catenin gene are common in hepatocellular carcinomas (105,106), while mutations in APC are common in hepatoblastoma (98,107,108). Interestingly, β-catenin and APC function in the same intracellular signal transduction pathway.

CONCLUSION

Despite the complexity of higher eukaryotes, the mechanisms for controlling cell-cycle progression are remarkably similar to those employed by simple eukaryotes such as yeast. As a more complete understanding of the cell-cycle regulatory mechanisms in simple and higher eukaryotes has been obtained, it has generally been observed that basic mechanisms are conserved, but higher eukaryotes often make use of multiple proteins to accomplish what requires only a single protein in yeast. For example, yeast makes use of a single Cdk to regulate progression through the cell cycle, while mammals have distinct Cdks for each cell-cycle phase. Much remains to be learned about the regulation of the action of cyclin/Cdk complexes, and model organisms will continue to be used for many of these studies. However, the additional complexities of the cell division cycle in higher eukaryotes will require studies in whole animals (wild-type, transgenic, and knockout) and in cultured mammalian cells. The ultimate goal of these studies will be a complete elucidation of how extracellular and intracellular signals are integrated to control the expression and regulation of cell-cycle proteins which in turn serve to control the cell division cycle.

ACKNOWLEDGMENTS

Research from the author's (H.P.-W.) laboratory was supported by National Institutes of Health (NIH) grant GM 47017. H.P.-W. is an Investigator of the Howard Hughes Medical Institute.

REFERENCES

1. Hartwell LH, Kastan MB. Cell cycle control and cancer. *Science* 1994;266:1821–1828.
2. Hunter T, Pines J. Cyclins and cancer. II: Cyclin D and CDK inhibitors come of age. *Cell* 1994;79:573–582.
3. Fausto N, Laird AD, Webber EM. Liver regeneration. 2. Role of growth factors and cytokines in hepatic regeneration. *FASEB J* 1995;9:1527–1536.
4. Pardee AB. G1 events and regulation of cell proliferation. *Science* 1989;246:603–608.
5. Murray A, Hunt T. *The cell cycle: an introduction*. New York: WH Freeman and Company, 1993.
6. Morgan DO. Cyclin-dependent kinases: engines, clocks, and microprocessors. *Annu Rev Cell Dev Biol* 1997;13:261–291.
7. Harper JW, Elledge SJ. Cdk inhibitors in development and cancer. *Curr Opin Genet Dev* 1996;6:56–64.
8. Atherton-Fessler S, Hannig G, Piwnica-Worms H. Reversible tyrosine phosphorylation and cell cycle control. *Semin Cell Biol* 1993;4:433–442.
9. Toyoshima F, Moriguchi T, Wada A, et al. Nuclear export of cyclin B1 and its possible role in the DNA damage-induced G2 checkpoint. *EMBO J* 1998;17:2728–2735.
10. Yang J, Bardes ES, Moore JD, et al. Control of cyclin B1 localization through regulated binding of the nuclear export factor CRM1. *Genes Dev* 1998;12:2131–2143.
11. Hagting A, Karlsson C, Clute P, et al. MPF localization is controlled by nuclear export. *EMBO J* 1998;17:4127–4138.
12. Diehl JA, Cheng M, Roussel MF, et al. Glycogen synthase kinase-3β regulates cyclin D1 proteolysis and subcellular localization. *Genes Dev* 1998;12:3499–3511.
13. Sherr CJ. Cancer cell cycles. *Science* 1996;274:1672–1677.
14. Weintraub SJ, Chow KN, Luo RX, et al. Mechanism of active transcriptional repression by the retinoblastoma protein. *Nature* 1995;375:812–815.
15. Zhang HS, Postigo AA, Dean DC. Active transcriptional repression by the Rb-E2F complex mediates G1 arrest triggered by p16INK4a, TGFβ, and contact inhibition. *Cell* 1999;97:53–61.
16. Hatakeyama M, Weinberg RA. The role of RB in cell cycle control. *Prog Cell Cycle Res* 1995;1:9–19.
17. Cheng M, Olivier P, Diehl JA, et al. The p21(Cip1) and p27(Kip1) CDK 'inhibitors' are essential activators of cyclin D-dependent kinases in murine fibroblasts. *EMBO J* 1999;18:1571–1583.
18. LaBaer J, Garrett MD, Stevenson LF, et al. New functional activities for the p21 family of CDK inhibitors. *Genes Dev* 1997;11:847–862.
19. Yang J, Kornbluth S. All aboard the cyclin train: subcellular trafficking of cyclins and their CDK partners. *Trends Cell Biol* 1999;9:201–210.
20. Hwang A, Maity A, McKenna WG, et al. Cell cycle-dependent regulation of the cyclin B1 promoter. *J Biol Chem* 1995;270:28419–28424.
21. King RW, Deshaies RJ, Peters J-M, et al. How proteolysis drives the cell cycle. *Science* 1996;274:1652–1659.
22. Draetta G, Piwnica-Worms H, Morrison D, et al. Human cdc2 protein kinase is a major cell-cycle regulated tyrosine kinase substrate. *Nature* 1988;336:738–744.
23. Draetta G, Beach D. Activation of cdc2 protein kinase during mitosis in human cells: cell cycle-dependent phosphorylation and subunit rearrangement. *Cell* 1988;54:17–26.
24. Morla AO, Draetta G, Beach D, et al. Reversible tyrosine phosphorylation of cdc2: dephosphorylation accompanies activation during entry into mitosis. *Cell* 1989;58:193–203.
25. Krek W, Nigg EA. Differential phosphorylation of vertebrate p34cdc2 kinase at the G1/S and G2/M transitions of the cell cycle: identification of major phosphorylation sites. *EMBO J* 1991;10:305–316.
26. Gould KL, Nurse P. Tyrosine phosphorylation of the fission yeast cdc2+ protein kinase regulates entry into mitosis. *Nature* 1989;342:39–45.
27. Krek W, Nigg EA. Mutations of p34cdc2 phosphorylation sites induce premature mitotic events in HeLa cells: evidence for a double block to p34cdc2 kinase activation in vertebrates. *EMBO J* 1991;10:3331–3341.
28. Norbury C, Blow J, Nurse P. Regulatory phosphorylation of the p34cdc2 protein kinase in vertebrates. *EMBO J* 1991;10:3321–3329.
29. Solomon MJ, Lee T, Kirschner MW. Role of phosphorylation in p34cdc2 activation: identification of an activating kinase. *Mol Biol Cell* 1992;3:13–27.
30. Parker LL, Piwnica-Worms H. Inactivation of the p34cdc2-cyclin B complex by the human wee1 tyrosine kinase. *Science* 1992;257:1955–1957.
31. Liu F, Stanton JJ, Wu Z, et al. The human Myt1 kinase preferentially phosphorylates Cdc2 on threonine 14 and localizes to the endoplasmic reticulum and Golgi complex. *Mol Cell Biol* 1997;17:571–583.
32. Honda R, Ohba Y, Yasuda H. The cell cycle regulator, human p50wee1, is a tyrosine kinase and not a serine/threonine kinase. *Biochem Biophys Res Commun* 1992;186:1333–1338.
33. Igarashi M, Nagata A, Jinno S, et al. Wee1+-like gene in human cells. *Nature* 1991;353:80–83.
34. McGowan CH, Russell P. Human Wee1 kinase inhibits cell division by phosphorylating p34cdc2 exclusively on Tyr 15. *EMBO J* 1993;12:75–85.
35. McGowan CH, Russell P. Cell cycle regulation of human WEE1. *EMBO* 1995;14:2166–2175.
36. Parker LL, Sylvestre PJ, Byrnes MJ III, et al. Identification of a 95-kDa WEE1-like tyrosine kinase in HeLa cells. *Proc Natl Acad Sci U S A* 1995;92:9638–9642.
37. Watanabe N, Broome M, Hunter T. Regulation of the human WEE1Hu CDK tyrosine 15-kinase during the cell cycle. *EMBO J* 1995;14:1878–1891.
38. Mueller PR, Coleman TR, Kumagai A, et al. Myt1: a membrane-associated inhibitory kinase that phosphorylates Cdc2 on both threonine-14 and tyrosine-15. *Science* 1995;270:86–90.
39. Mueller PR, Coleman TR, Dunphy WG. Cell cycle regulation of a Xenopus Wee1-like kinase. *Mol Biol Cell* 1995;6:119–134.
40. Booher RN, Holman PS, Fattaey A. Human myt1 is a cell cycle-regulated kinase that inhibits cdc2 but not cdk2 activity. *J Biol Chem* 1997;272:22300–22306.
41. Lee MS, Ogg S, Xu M, et al. cdc25+ encodes a protein phosphatase that dephosphorylates p34cdc2. *Mol Biol Cell* 1992;3:73–84.
42. Dunphy WG, Kumagai A. The cdc25 protein contains an intrinsic phosphatase activity. *Cell* 1991;67:189–196.
43. Gautier J, Solomon MJ, Booher RN, et al. cdc25 is a specific tyrosine phosphatase that directly activates p34cdc2. *Cell* 1991;67:197–211.

44. Strausfeld U, Labbe JC, Fesquet D, et al. Dephosphorylation and activation of a p34cdc2/cyclin B complex *in vitro* by human cdc25 protein. *Nature* 1991;351:242–245.

45. Sebastian B, Kakizuka A, Hunter T. Cdc25M2 activation of cyclin-dependent kinases by dephosphorylation of threonine-14 and tyrosine-15. *Proc Natl Acad Sci U S A* 1993;90:3521–3524.

46. Pines J, Hunter T. The differential localization of human cyclin A and B is due to a cytoplasmic retention signal in cyclin B. *EMBO J* 1994;13:3772–3781.

47. Li J, Meyer AN, Donoghue DJ. Requirement for phosphorylation of cyclin B1 for Xenopus oocyte maturation. *Mol Biol Cell* 1995;6:1111–1124.

48. Hartwell LH, Weinert TA. Checkpoints: controls that ensure the order of cell cycle events. *Science* 1989;246:629–634.

49. Savitsky K, Bar-Shira A, Gilad S, et al. A single ataxia telangiectasia gene with a product similar to PI-3 kinase. *Science* 1995;268:1749–1753.

50. Morgan SE, Kastan MB. p53 and ATM: cell cycle, cell death, and cancer. *Adv Cancer Res* 1997;71:1–25.

51. el-Deiry WS, Tokino T, Velculescu VE, et al. WAF1, a potential mediator of p53 tumor suppression. *Cell* 1993;75:817–825.

52. Tibbetts RS, Brumbaugh KM, Williams JM, et al. A role for ATR in the DNA damage-induced phosphorylation of p53. *Genes Dev* 1999;13:152–157.

53. Cliby WA, Roberts CJ, Cimprich KA, et al. Overexpression of a kinase-inactive ATR protein causes sensitivity to DNA-damaging agents and defects in cell cycle checkpoints. *EMBO J* 1998;17:159–169.

54. Peng C-Y, Graves PR, Thoma RS, et al. Mitotic and G2 checkpoint control: regulation of 14-3-3 protein binding by phosphorylation of Cdc25C on serine-216. *Science* 1997;277:1501–1505.

55. Zeng Y, Piwnica-Worms H. The DNA damage and replication checkpoints in fission yeast require nuclear exclusion of the Cdc25 phosphatase via 14-3-3 binding. *Mol Cell Biol* 1999;19:7410–7419.

56. Kumagai A, Dunphy WG. Binding of 14-3-3 proteins and nuclear export control the intracellular localization of the mitotic inducer Cdc25. *Genes Dev* 1999;13:1067–1072.

57. Dalal SN, Schweitzer CM, Gan J, et al. Cytoplasmic localization of human Cdc25C during interphase requires an intact 14-3-3 binding site. *Mol Cell Biol* 1999;19:4465–4479.

58. Lopez-Girona A, Furnari B, Mondesert O, et al. Nuclear localization of Cdc25 is regulated by DNA damage and 14-3-3 protein. *Nature* 1999;397:172–175.

59. Yang J, Wonkler K, Yoshida M, et al. Maintenance of G2 arrest in the *Xenopus* oocyte: a role for 14-3-3-mediated inhibition of Cdc25 nuclear import. *EMBO J* 1999;18:2174–2183.

60. Zeng Y, Forbes KC, Wu Z, et al. Replication checkpoint in fission yeast requires Cdc25p phosphorylation by Cds1p or Chk1p. *Nature* 1998;395:507–510.

61. Kumagai A, Yakowee PS, Dunphy WG. 14-3-3 Proteins act as negative regulators of the mitotic inducer Cdc25 in *Xenopus* egg extracts. *Mol Biol Cell* 1998;9:345–354.

62. Nicklas RB. How cells get the right chromosomes. *Science* 1997;275:632–637.

63. Hoyt MA, Totis L, Roberts BT. *S. cerevisiae* genes required for cell cycle arrest in response to loss of mitotic apparatus. *Cell* 1991;66:507–517.

64. Li R, Murray AW. Feedback control in mitosis in budding yeast. *Cell* 1991;66:519–531.

65. Morgan DO. Regulation of the APC and the exit from mitosis. *Nat Cell Biol* 1999;1:E47–E53.

66. Zhang BH. Growth signals in liver regeneration. *J Gastroenterol Hepatol* 1997;12:44–46.

67. Albrecht JH, Hu MY, Cerra FB. Distinct patterns of cyclin D1 regulation in models of liver regeneration and human liver. *Biochem Biophys Res Commun* 1995;209:648–655.

68. Ehrenfried JA, Ko TC, Thompson EA, et al. Cell cycle-mediated regulation of hepatic regeneration. *Surgery* 1997;122:927–935.

69. Jaumot M, Estanyol JM, Serratosa J, et al. Activation of cdk4 and cdk2 during rat liver regeneration is associated with intranuclear rearrangements of cyclin-cdk complexes. *Hepatology* 1999;29:385–395.

70. Albrecht JH, Rieland BM, Nelsen CJ, et al. Regulation of G(1) cyclin-dependent kinases in the liver: role of nuclear localization and p27 sequestration. *Am J Physiol* 1999;277:G1207–G1216.

71. Kato A, Ota S, Bamba H, et al. Regulation of cyclin D-dependent kinase activity in rat liver regeneration. *Biochem Biophys Res Commun* 1998;245:70–74.

72. Albrecht JH, Poon RY, Ahonen CL, et al. Involvement of p21 and p27 in the regulation of CDK activity and cell cycle progression in the regenerating liver. *Oncogene* 1998;16:2141–2150.

73. Crary GS, Albrecht JH. Expression of cyclin-dependent kinase inhibitor p21 in human liver. *Hepatology* 1998;28:738–743.

74. Wu H, Wade M, Krall L, et al. Targeted *in vivo* expression of the cyclin-dependent kinase inhibitor p21 halts hepatocyte cell-cycle progression, postnatal liver development and regeneration. *Genes Dev* 1996;10:245–260.

75. Kamb A, Shattuck-Eidens D, Eeles R, et al. Analysis of the p16 gene (CDKN2) as a candidate for the chromosome 9p melanoma susceptibility locus. *Nat Genet* 1994;8:23–26.

76. Hussussian CJ, Struewing JP, Goldstein AM, et al. Germline p16 mutations in familial melanoma. *Nat Genet* 1994;8:15–21.

77. Kita R, Nishida N, Fukuda Y, et al. Infrequent alterations of the p16INK4A gene in liver cancer. *Int J Cancer* 1996;67:176–180.

78. Chaubert P, Gayer R, Zimmermann A, et al. Germ-line mutations of the p16INK4(MTS1) gene occur in a subset of patients with hepatocellular carcinoma. *Hepatology* 1997;25:1376–1381.

79. Lin YW, Chen CH, Huang GT, et al. Infrequent mutations and no methylation of CDKN2A (P16/MTS1) and CDKN2B (p15/MTS2) in hepatocellular carcinoma in Taiwan. *Eur J Cancer* 1998;34:1789–1795.

80. Nishida N, Fukuda Y, Komeda T, et al. Amplification and overexpression of the cyclin D1 gene in aggressive human hepatocellular carcinoma. *Cancer Res* 1994;54:3107–3110.

81. Zhang YJ, Jiang W, Chen CJ, et al. Amplification and overexpression of cyclin D1 in human hepatocellular carcinoma. *Biochem Biophys Res Commun* 1993;196:1010–1016.

82. Nishida N, Fukuda Y, Ishizaki K, et al. Alteration of cell cycle-related genes in hepatocarcinogenesis. *Histol Histopathol* 1997;12:1019–1025.

83. Sato Y, Itoh F, Hareyama M, et al. Association of cyclin D1 expression with factors correlated with tumor progression in human hepatocellular carcinoma. *J Gastroenterol* 1999;34:486–493.

84. Chao Y, Shih YL, Chiu JH, et al. Overexpression of cyclin A but not Skp 2 correlates with the tumor relapse of human hepatocellular carcinoma. *Cancer Res* 1998;58:985–990.

85. Kim H, Ham EK, Kim YI, et al. Overexpression of cyclin D1 and cdk4 in tumorigenesis of sporadic hepatoblastomas. *Cancer Lett* 1998;131:177–183.

86. Iolascon A, Giordani L, Moretti A, et al. Analysis of CDKN2A, CDKN2B, CDKN2C, and cyclin Ds gene status in hepatoblastoma. *Hepatology* 1998;27:989–995.

87. Zhang X, Xu HJ, Murakami Y, et al. Deletions of chromosome 13q, mutations in Retinoblastoma 1, and retinoblastoma protein state in human hepatocellular carcinoma. *Cancer Res* 1994;54:4177–4182.

88. Nakamura T, Iwamura Y, Kaneko M, et al. Deletions and rearrangements of the retinoblastoma gene in hepatocellular

carcinoma, insulinoma and some neurogenic tumors as found in a study of 121 tumors. *Jpn J Clin Oncol* 1991;21:325–329.

89. Fujimoto Y, Hampton LL, Wirth PJ, et al. Alterations of tumor suppressor genes and allelic losses in human hepatocellular carcinomas in China. *Cancer Res* 1994;54:281–285.

90. Nishida N, Fukuda Y, Kokuryu H, et al. Accumulation of allelic loss on arms of chromosomes 13q, 16q and 17p in the advanced stages of human hepatocellular carcinoma. *Int J Cancer* 1992;51:862–868.

91. Hollstein M, Sidransky D, Vogelstein B, et al. p53 mutations in human cancers. *Science* 1991;253:49–53.

92. Ozturk M. Genetic aspects of hepatocellular carcinogenesis. *Semin Liver Dis* 1999;19:235–242.

93. Murakami Y, Hayashi K, Hirohashi S, et al. Aberrations of the tumor suppressor p53 and retinoblastoma genes in human hepatocellular carcinomas. *Cancer Res* 1991;51:5520–5525.

94. Li D, Cao Y, He L, et al. Aberrations of p53 gene in human hepatocellular carcinoma from China. *Carcinogenesis* 1993;14:169–173.

95. Unsal H, Yakicier C, Marcais C, et al. Genetic heterogeneity of hepatocellular carcinoma. *Proc Natl Acad Sci U S A* 1994;91:822–826.

96. Hsu IC, Metcalf RA, Sun T, et al. Mutational hotspot in the p53 gene in human hepatocellular carcinomas. *Nature* 1991;350:427–428.

97. Ozturk M. p53 mutation in hepatocellular carcinoma after aflatoxin exposure. *Lancet* 1991;338:1356–1359.

98. Oda H, Nakatsuru Y, Imai Y, et al. A mutational hot spot in the p53 gene is associated with hepatoblastomas. *Int J Cancer* 1995;60:786–790.

99. Kusafuka T, Fukuzawa M, Oue T, et al. Mutation analysis of p53 gene in childhood malignant solid tumors. *J Pediatr Surg* 1997;32:1175–1180.

100. Ohnishi H, Kawamura M, Hanada R, et al. Infrequent mutations of the TP53 gene and no amplification of the MDM2 gene in hepatoblastomas. *Genes Chromosomes Cancer* 1996;15:187–190.

101. Chen TC, Hsieh LL, Kuo TT. Absence of p53 gene mutation and infrequent overexpression of p53 protein in hepatoblastoma. *J Pathol* 1995;176:243–247.

102. Furutani M, Arii S, Tanaka H, et al. Decreased expression and rare somatic mutation of the CIP1/WAF1 gene in human hepatocellular carcinoma. *Cancer Lett* 1997;111:191–197.

103. Feitelson MA, Zhu M, Duan LX, et al. Hepatitis B x antigen and p53 are associated *in vitro* and in liver tissues from patients with primary hepatocellular carcinoma. *Oncogene* 1993;8:1109–1117.

104. Ray RB, Steele R, Meyer K, et al. Transcriptional repression of p53 promoter by hepatitis C virus core protein. *J Biol Chem* 1997;272:10983–10986.

105. de La Coste A, Romagnolo B, Billuart P, et al. Somatic mutations of the β-catenin gene are frequent in mouse and human hepatocellular carcinomas. *Proc Natl Acad Sci U S A* 1998;95:8847–8851.

106. Miyoshi Y, Iwao K, Nagasawa Y, et al. Activation of the β-catenin gene in primary hepatocellular carcinomas by somatic alterations involving exon 3. *Cancer Res* 1998;58:2524–2527.

107. Giardiello FM, Petersen GM, Brensinger JD, et al. Hepatoblastoma and APC gene mutation in familial adenomatous polyposis. *Gut* 1996;39:867–869.

108. Kurahashi H, Takami K, Oue T, et al. Biallelic inactivation of the APC gene in hepatoblastoma. *Cancer Res* 1995;55:5007–5011.

The Liver: Biology and Pathobiology, Fourth Edition, edited by I. M. Arias, J. L. Boyer, F. V. Chisari, N. Fausto, D. Schachter, and D. A. Shafritz.
Lippincott Williams & Wilkins, Philadelphia © 2001.

MOLECULAR AND CELLULAR CONTROL OF ANGIOGENESIS

PATRICIA A. D'AMORE
IRA M. HERMAN

HEPATIC VASCULAR DEVELOPMENT

The vascular system is formed via a combination of vasculogenesis and angiogenesis. Vasculogenesis is the *de novo* formation of vessels via the assembly of angioblasts or endothelial precursors. In angiogenesis, new vessels are formed by the migration and proliferation of endothelial cells (EC) from preexisting vessels. From the limited lineage data that have been gathered, liver vascularization appears to result from a combination of vasculogenesis and angiogenesis (1) (see Chapter 2 and website chapter 🖳 W-32). In humans, hepatic angiogenesis is initiated as the vitelline plexus extends from the early yolk sac blood vessels. At roughly the same time (approximately five weeks postconception), hepatic cords grow into the mesenchymal tissue of the transverse septum and primitive sinusoidal structures form between the hepatic cords. Almost immediately thereafter, the umbilical veins lose their connection to the sinus venosus as the ductus venosus becomes a shunt, conducting umbilical blood to the heart via the hepatic veins and the vena cava. By the fifth and sixth weeks of life, the paired post hepatic vitelline veins form a complex anastomosis around the gut prior to their degeneration and coalescence into what will become a portal vein, which receives the splenic and mesenteric veins, distally.

P. A. D'Amore: Departments of Ophthalmology and Pathology, Harvard Medical School, Boston, Massachusetts 02115; Schepens Eye Research Institute, Boston, Massachusetts 02114.

I. M. Herman: Department of Cell and Molecular Physiology, Tufts University School of Medicine, Boston, Massachusetts 02111.

These descriptions of early intrahepatic angiogenesis, while incomplete, help to emphasize several essential aspects of hepatic angiogenesis as well as identify how organogenesis is intimately linked to microvascular morphogenesis. The molecular and cellular mechanisms that underlie these pivotal events represent some of the key areas of basic and clinical research today. In this chapter, we describe recent work in the fields of vascular cell and molecular biology that have provided insight into some of the signaling cascades responsible for the recruitment and remodeling of the hepatic vasculature. While many of these basic studies of vascular cell biology have been studied in extrahepatic models, it is reasonable to believe that these general principles apply to hepatic angiogenesis as well.

HEPATIC SINUSOIDS

Although it is likely that the general mechanisms that regulate liver vascular growth and function are similar to those of other microvascular beds, it is also important to point out the distinct differences in structure that exist between hepatic sinusoids and the microvasculature in other tissue beds. The sinusoids are the site of the majority of the blood–tissue interface in the liver. The liver cells are organized into acinar-like structures with blood entering the sinusoidal space from the portal venule, surrounding both surfaces of the hepatic plate, and exiting via hepatic venules. The sinusoids interconnect via fenestrations, forming a labyrinth of vessels closely associated with the liver parenchyma. The sinusoids are larger in caliber than the average capillary and are more closely associated with the tissue parenchyma (hepatocytes) than the typical EC (see Chapter 30 and website chapters ⌨ W-26 and W-32). The EC and hepatocytes are separated by the space of Disse, the extracellular space of the liver. The liver parenchyma cells, under the space of Disse, have surfaces characterized by extensive microvillar structures that serve as an accessible site for materials that are circulating in the plasma (2).

The composition of the sinusoidal lining has long been a subject of controversy, with some believing that there are two distinct cell types, the EC and the Kupffer cells, and others postulating that the EC could "transform" into phagocytic Kupffer cells. Although lineage analysis will have to be conducted to definitively address this issue, there are studies that describe a population of mesenchymal cells that appear to be "trapped" in the subendothelial space of the growing liver primordia (at about 5 weeks of gestation in the human) that are stellate cell progenitors (3). Recent analysis using immunohistochemistry, classic staining methods, and ultrastructural analysis demonstrate the sinusoidal wall to consist of EC, Kupffer cells, dendritic cells, natural killer (NK) cells, and stellate cells (4).

Endothelial Cells

Sinusoidal EC differ phenotypically from the EC that comprise the more topical continuous capillaries in that they lack PECAM-1, CD34, and 1F10 but exhibit CD4, ICAM-1, CD-32, and CD-14 (see Chapter 30 and website chapter ⌨ W-26). Two stages of sinusoidal differentiation have been identified during human fetal liver development (5). During the first 5 to 12 weeks of development as the EC are acquiring the classic sinusoidal architecture, they lose the markers of continuous EC and reduce their production of laminin, thrombospondin, and fibronectin. The second phase of differentiation, which occurs in weeks 10 to 20, is characterized by the expression of the markers of the adult sinusoidal EC.

The nature of the local signals that govern these tissue-specific changes in EC phenotype are unknown. Evidence for hepatocyte influence on EC phenotype comes from an analysis of sinusoidal EC organization using a monoclonal antibody (SE-1) that is specific for sinusoidal EC. The first SE-1 positivity, noted in 15-day-old rat embryos, was randomly distributed throughout the liver parenchymya and was not associated with the large vessels (6). The immunoreactive cells increased in number and became interconnected during development. Furthermore, the intensity of the staining increased from the weakest in the most primitive EC to the strongest levels in the adult sinusoidal EC, suggesting that SE-1 antigen expression in the EC might be controlled by association of the EC with the hepatocytes.

Stellate Cells

Characterization

For the purposes of this discussion of angiogenesis, we will focus on the roles that the stellate cells (see Chapter 31 and website chapter ⌨ W-26) may play as the liver equivalent of the pericyte. The Kupffer cells, largely phagocytic in nature, are distinct from the hepatic stellate cells, which are located perisinusoidally and are more abundant in the intermediate and peripheral portions of the hepatic lobule than the central zone (7). Although the functions of the stellate cells have not been entirely elucidated, their isolation and establishment in culture (8) has provided significant insight into the range of their contributions to hepatic function (for review see ref. 9). Stellate cells store retinol, participate in extracellular matrix metabolism and are the source of a variety of effector molecules.

Contractility of the Stellate Cells

Viewing the stellate cells as the liver counterpart of the pericytes or smooth muscle cells (SMC) leads to a consideration of their potential contractile functions. One of us (IMH) has demonstrated that collagen IV-enriched endothelial-synthesized extracellular matrix supports pericyte proliferation (10). In these growth-stimulated pericytes, smooth muscle (SM) contractile proteins cannot be detected. Similarly, when pericytes are stimulated to proliferate under the control of exogenously added basic fibroblast growth factor (bFGF)-2 and heparin (both of which are components of the endothelial-derived matrix), SM actin, SM myosin, and calponin expression are also repressed. However, transforming growth factor (TGF)β-1 causes growth-arrest and the induction of the SM phenotype *in vitro* (see Endothelial Cell–Stellate Cell Interactions, below, for a more extensive discussion). In light of the low numbers of SMC in hepatic vessels, stellate cells have become a candidate for regulating sinusoidal diameter and therefore influencing blood flow (11). Accordingly, examination of the effect of stellate cell contraction on portal pressures in injured livers revealed that endothelin-1 and angiotensin administration led to a significant increase in portal pressure (12). The pressure increases were greatest in injured livers where the increase was shown to correlate to the activation of the stellate cells as measured by the increased expression of SM-actin.

REGULATION OF VESSEL ASSEMBLY AND GROWTH

Growth Factors and Their Receptors

Vascular Endothelial Growth Factor, Flk-1 and Flt-1

There is a large body of compelling evidence that points to vascular endothelial growth factor (VEGF)-A as a key regulator of vasculogenesis and angiogenesis (for review see ref. 13). The isoforms of VEGF-A, which are produced by alternative splicing from a single gene, are potent mitogens and chemoattractants for EC. Tyrosine kinase receptors for VEGF include Flt-1 (VEGFR-1) and Flk-1/KDR (VEGFR-2), receptors expressed primarily but not only by the endothelium (14,15). VEGF is produced by a variety of mesenchymal and stromal cells, and the receptor–ligand pair shows a coordinate pattern of expression during development. In most developing organs, the forming vasculature stains positively for both VEGF receptors, while the stromal cells immediately surrounding the nascent vessels express VEGF (16,17).

The central role of VEGF in vascular development is well demonstrated in the embryonic lethality of mice deficient in VEGF (18,19) or either of its receptors (20,21). In particular, Flk-1-deficient mice die between embryonic day (E)8.5 and E9.5, and have virtually no vascular structures (20). On the other hand, Flt-1 null mice are also embryonic-lethal, with a vascular defect that appears to be at the level of remodeling (21).

Angiopoietins and Tie-2

Tie-2 receptors, like the VEGF receptors, appear to be relatively specific to the vascular endothelium. Tie-2 (also known as Tek) is expressed at high levels in the vasculature of developing mouse embryos but is greatly reduced in endothelium of adult animals (17). Mice lacking tie-2 die *in utero* by E9.5. These mice display defects that include engorged and distended yolk sac vessels, a ruptured and disorganized dorsal aorta, and uniformly sized vessels, suggesting abnormal vascular remodeling (22).

The ligands for Tie-2 are the angiopoietins (ang), with ang-1 acting as an activating ligand (i.e., it promotes tyrosine phosphorylation of the receptor) (23) and ang-2 acting as an antagonist of the action of ang-1 (24). Ang-1-deficient mice have a phenotype similar to the Tie-2 −/− mice with limited remodeling of the primary vascular plexus (25). Ultrastructural analysis of microvessels in the ang-1 null mice reveal a lack of pericytes and scattered, disorganized collagen fibers. The EC appear detached and seem to have defective matrix.

Fibroblast Growth Factor

There is extensive evidence to indicate that acidic (aFGF; FGF-1) and basic (bFGF; FGF-2) fibroblast growth factor (FGF) are potent mitogens and angiogenic factors (for review see ref. 26), and while it has been established that bFGF (FGF-2) is a component of select subendothelial basement membranes *in vivo* and *in vitro*, its mode of release and function in the matrix remain somewhat equivocal (27). Since matrix (heparan sulfate)-bound FGF is found in the basement membrane of quiescent endothelial cells, it has been suggested to act as a wound healing or survival agent, being released following tissue injury (27,28).

Unlike VEGF, targeted disruption of the bFGF genes does not result in any obvious vascular phenotypes (29).

Platelet-Derived Growth Factor

The platelet-derived growth factor (PDGF) family consists of homodimers (PDGF-AA or -BB) or heterodimers (PDGF-AB) made from the pairwise assembly of the two related PDGF chains, A and B. The effects of PDGF isoforms on a particular cell type is a function of the cell's repertoire of PDGF receptors, which consist of dimers of the α and β subtypes of the PDGF tyrosine kinase receptor. The α receptor binds both PDGF chains, whereas the β receptor is specific for the PDGF-B chain.

The main involvement of PDGF in vessel assembly appears to be the recruitment of mural cell precursors to forming vessels. The patterns of PDGF ligand and receptor expression are consistent with this role with developing capillaries expressing PDGF BB mRNA, while the nearby mesenchyme expresses the PDGF β receptor (30). This hypothesis was supported by tissue culture studies in which vascular EC induced the directed migration and proliferation of pericyte precursors via the secretion of PDGF BB (31). As has been reported for SMC in culture (32), PDGF-BB downregulates the expression of αSM-actin in mesenchymal cells that have been induced to differentiate toward a pericyte/SMC lineage (33), suggesting that once mesenchymal cells are recruited to the forming vessel, PDGF expression must be suppressed so that the cells can differentiate into mural cells.

As is the case for the other growth factors and receptors, the phenotypes of PDGF- and PDGF-receptor-null mice have provided valuable insight into its role in vascular development. Mice lacking PDGF-B or the PDGF β receptor exhibit similar phenotypes, with the most relevant defect for this discussion being the absence of mesangial cells in the kidney phenotypes (34,35). Since mesangial cells are the renal correlate of the capillary pericyte (36), it is not surprising to find that these animals also lack pericytes throughout their vascular beds (37).

These heterotypic interactions, if out of balance, may also be a source of pathology. In cholestatic liver disease there is an accumulation of myofibroblasts with accompanying fibrosis in the vicinity of the proliferating bile ducts. Although fibroblasts have historically been implicated in this process, there is evidence to suggest that stellate cells may also be involved. Studies using stellate cells from normal rats and bile ducts from rats with cholestasis revealed that the bile ducts secreted PDGF BB, which acted as a chemoattractant for the stellate cells (38). These results lead to the suggestion that this interaction may also contribute to periductular fibrosis in cholestatic pathologies.

Endothelial Cell–Stellate Cell Interactions

The interaction between hepatocytes and nonparenchymal cells of the liver is likely to influence liver function. These interactions are two-way communications with the hepatocytes impacting the nonparenchymal cells such as EC and the EC modulating the function of the hepatocytes (Figure 65.1).

Activation and Function of Transforming Growth Factor-β

Tissue culture (39) and *in vivo* observations (37) indicate that the EC can recruit the undifferentiated mesenchymal cells to the vicinity of the EC. Once this has occurred, differentiation of the mesenchymal cell to the pericyte (and presumably stellate cell) phenotype occurs. Using a system in which microvascular EC are cocultured with undifferentiated mesenchymal (10T1/2) cells, we have shown that contact between the EC and mesenchymal cells induces the expression of SM-specific proteins including αSM-actin, SM myosin, SM22 α, and calponin (39). Previous studies using coculture of EC with SMCs or pericytes had indicated that this heterotypic contact leads to the activation of transforming growth factor (TGF)β-1 in a plasminogen activator-dependent process (40). Evidence of a role of TGF-β *in vivo* comes from the analysis of mice with targeted disruption of TGFβ-1 in which 50% of TGF-β1 null mice died as a result of defects in yolk sac vasculogenesis, inadequate capillary tube formation, and matrix deformities (41). TGFβ-1 is the prototypic member of the TGFβ gene family and coordinates a variety of activities such as the regulation of growth, "differentiation," and extracellular matrix production (42). Thus, the local activation of TGF-β in the microvasculature is likely to have multiple effects including the inhibition of endothelial proliferation (43) and migration (44), the induction of pericyte/stellate cell differentiation (39) and the stimulation of basement membrane synthesis (45). Interestingly, recent work has demonstrated that

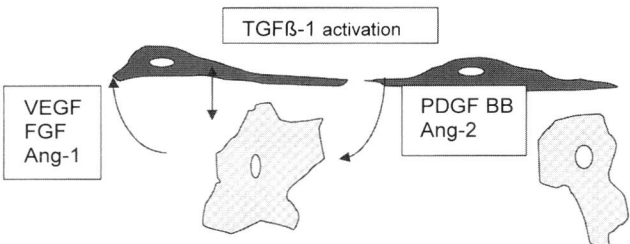

FIGURE 65.1. Schematic of possible paracrine interactions between sinusoidal endothelial cells (EC) and stellate cells. Sinusoidal EC release platelet-derived growth factor BB (*PDGF BB*), which acts to recruit mesenchymal cells to the forming sinusoids. Upon contact between the EC and the mesenchymal cells, transforming growth factor β-1 (*TGFβ-1*) is activated. The TGF-β acts to induce stellate cell differentiation, inhibit EC proliferation and stimulate matrix production. Stellate cells (as well as the liver parenchyma) secrete vascular endothelial growth factor (*VEGF*) and fibroblast growth factor (*FGF*), which act as mitogens and/or survival factors for the sinusoidal EC. *Ang-1*, angioprotein 1.

TGFβ-1 activation may be mediated by interaction between EC and stellate cells. A novel Kruppel-like factor called Zf9 is upregulated in stellate cells in response to injury and upregulates urokinase plasminogen activator, leading to an increase in activated TGFβ-1 (46). Excess synthesis of matrix proteins by the sinusoidal EC in response to injury may lead to conversion of the hepatic EC from a sinusoidal phenotype in which there is little basement membrane material to a continuous endothelium (47).

Cell–Cell Interactions in Cell Survival

As an example of hepatocyte effects on the EC, there is increasing evidence that newly formed vessels require the continued presence of VEGF for their survival. As has been well documented, the pericyte (48) (and perhaps by analogy the stellate cell) is in close association with the EC. The strategic locations of these cell populations place them in a position capable of participating in unique heterocellular signaling, events that may be essential for their sustained growth and/or survival. This was elegantly demonstrated in a prostate tumor model in which VEGF expression was under hormonal control (49). Reduction of VEGF levels led to regression of the forming blood vessels.

Tissue culture studies suggest that sinusoidal EC may be similarly dependent on exogenous factors, with VEGF as a candidate. Media conditioned by adult rat hepatocytes can substitute for the addition of other factors such as bFGF in supporting the survival of cultured sinusoidal EC (50). Although VEGF was one component of the conditioned media, there was no clear demonstration that VEGF was the active molecule in the conditioned media. A role for VEGF in the survival of liver vascular EC *in vivo* is indicated by the results of studies in which VEGF was inactivated in postnatal mice either by gene targeting or by administration of a soluble VEGF receptor (51). In both cases, impaired liver development was a primary finding, and increased apoptosis of EC led to the conclusion that "VEGF is required not only for proliferation but also for survival of endothelial cells." When a VEGF-neutralizing reagent was administered four weeks postnatally, there was no effect on liver EC. However, adult mouse liver does make significant levels of VEGF with no active vessel growth. Thus, it is possible that the lack of effect in adult animals is due to the fact that the exogenously added soluble receptor is unable to access the VEGF and that the constitutively produced VEGF is necessary for the survival of the sinusoidal EC. Results of studies in which dominant negative VEGF receptors are expressed in an inducible manner will begin to address the role of VEGF in normal adult murine liver.

Vessel stabilization is also influenced by the angiopoietins (see the section above entitled Angiopoietins and Tie-2), although the mechanisms underlying the stabilization have not been elucidated. A protein called hepatic fibrinogen/angiopoietin-related protein that has homology to the angiopoietins, but does bind tie-2, has been identified in human and murine liver as well as in the circulation and has been shown to act as a survival factor for the endothelium (52).

POSTNATAL ANGIOGENESIS

In general, vascular endothelium in the adult human seldom divides (53). The exceptions to this include new vessel growth as part of reproduction, wound healing and tumor growth.

Tumor Angiogenesis

It is now well accepted that solid tumors are dependent on an ever-increasing vascular supply for continued tumor growth (54). In addition to the role of the vasculature in nourishing the primary tumor, the vasculature provides a means for tumor cell metastases. A strong correlation between microvascularity and prognosis was initially demonstrated to be an independent predictor of metastatic disease in invasive breast cancer (55). Similar analysis of vessel density in hepatocellular carcinoma (HCC) found microvessel density of be an independent predictor of disease-free survival in small (less than 5 cm) HCC, whereas in larger tumors, tumor size was the sole predictor (56).

As a result of the acknowledgment of the angiogenesis dependence of tumors, there has been a tremendous interest in elucidating the regulators of tumor vessel induction and growth, and in identifying developing agents that can block vascular growth. The role of VEGF in HCC was investigated in a murine xenograft model using a tetracycline-regulated retroviral system (57). VEGF overexpression resulted in an increase in tumor growth with accompanying angiogenesis, whereas suppression of VEGF production led to reduced tumor growth. The interaction between hepatic EC and stellate cells may also make an important contribution in hepatocarcinogenesis as well as under circumstances of injury and repair. Although hepatocarcinoma cells expressing VEGF (assayed alone) did not have altered migration, their coculture with EC led to a significant increase in the invasive ability of the tumor cells.

Incubation of cultured stellate cells under hypoxic conditions such as might occur in pathology led to increased levels of VEGF mRNA and elevated levels of VEGF protein in the conditioned media. Not only did the stellate cells produce VEGF, they also displayed Flk-1 and Flt-1, and hypoxia induced expression of Flt-1 mRNA, but not Flk-1 (58). Hypoxia plays an important role in tumor vascularization by directly inducing VEGF (59–61). In addition, investigations into the role of hepatitis B virus-encoded transcription factor HBV-X have revealed that the transcriptional activated HBV-X protein (HBx) itself stimulates the transcription of VEGF, and that the levels of HBx were increased by hypoxia (62). Thus, VEGF production by hepatitis B-induced hepatocarcinoma can be induced by multiple mechanisms.

The identification by O'Reilly et al. (63) of the endogenous angiogenesis inhibitors angiostatin and endostatin as cleavage products of liver proteins plasminogen and collagen XVIII, respectively, has led to the concept that a novel liver function may be to regulate extrahepatic EC proliferation (64). How these "precursor" molecules are cleaved to their biologically active forms is not clear, and it has been hypothesized that the activation may be local and mediated by proteases that are cell-associated (65).

Liver Regeneration

Because of the ubiquitous role of VEGF in developmental, postnatal, physiologic, and pathologic angiogenesis, there has been significant interest in the role that VEGF might play in liver regeneration (see Chapter 42 and website chapter 🖫 W-31). In rats with a 70% liver resection, there was an increase in VEGF mRNA, which peaked at 3 days after the resection, followed by elevation in flt-1 and flk-1 at 72 to 168 hours (66). Administration of exogenous VEGF to rats following partial hepatectomy led to an increased labeling index of hepatocytes in the treated animals (67).

CONCLUSION

During the past decade, the molecular and cellular mechanisms that regulate vascular cell "differentiation" have come under close scrutiny (for review see refs. 68 and 69). In light of the important role that cell–cell and cell–matrix interactions play in the regulation of morphogenesis during development and disease in other systems, these areas have also become fruitful areas of investigation in the study of the vasculature. Whereas significant inroads have been made into understanding the early steps in vessel assembly, little is known about the molecular and cellular events that regulate vascular morphogenesis. Further, the growth and function not only of the EC but also the pericytes (stellate cells in the liver) are influenced by paracrine signals that pass between the cells and by juxtacrine communication with the associated matrix. Acute or chronic perturbations in these signaling pathways would likely play instrumental roles in altering the organ function. These are essential gaps in our knowledge, and results of future experimentation should provide important new insights into our understanding of the molecular mechanisms regulating microvascular morphogenesis during development and disease.

ACKNOWLEDGMENTS

The authors are supported by National Institutes of Health (NIH) grants CA45548 (P.A.D.), EY05318 (P.A.D.),

GM55110 (I.M.H.), and GM/EY9033. P.A.D. is a Jules and Doris Stein Research to Prevent Blindness Professor.

REFERENCES

1. Pardanaud L, Dieterlen-Lièvre F. Emergence of endothelial and hemopoietic cells in the avian embryo. *Anat Embryol (Berl)* 1993; 187:107–114.
2. Goresky C, Groom A. Microcirculatory events in the liver and the spleen. In: Renknin E, Michel C, eds. *The Cardiovascular System.* Bethesda: American Physiological Society, 1984: 689–780.
3. Enzan H, Himeno H, Hiroi M, et al. Development of hepatic sinusoidal structure with special reference to the Ito cells. *Microsc Res Tech* 1997;15:336–349.
4. Wake K. Cell–cell organization and function of 'sinusoids' in liver microcirculation system. *J Electron Microsc (Tokyo)* 1999;48: 89–98.
5. Couvelard A, Scoazed J, Dauge M, et al. Structural and functional differences of sinusoidal endothelial cells during liver organogenesis in humans. *Blood* 1996;87:4568–4580.
6. Morita M, Qun W, Watabane H, et al. Analysis of the sinusoidal endothelial cell organization during the developmental stage of the fetal rat liver using a sinusoidal endothelial cell specific antibody, SE-1. *Cell Struct Funct* 1998;23:341–348.
7. Bloom W, Fawcett D. *A textbook of histology.* Philadelphia: WB Saunders, 1975.
8. Knook D, EC S, Preparation and characterization of Kupffer cells from rat and mouse liver. In: Wisse E, Knook E, eds. *Kupffer cells and other liver sinusoidal cells.* Amsterdam: Elsevier/North Holland Biomedical, 273–288.
9. Kawada N. The hepatic perisinusoidal stellate cell. *Histol Histopathol* 1997;12:1069–1080.
10. Newcomb P, Herman IM. Pericyte growth and contractile phenotype: modulation by endothelial-synthesized matrix and comparison with aortic smooth muscle cells. *J Cell Physiol* 1993;155: 385–393.
11. McCuskey R. Morphological mechanisms for regulating blood flow through hepatic sinusoids. *Liver* 2000;20:3–7.
12. Rockey D, Weisiger R. Endothelin induced contractility of stellate cells from normal and cirrhotic rat liver: implications for regulation of portal pressure. *Hepatology* 1996;24:233–240.
13. Klagsbrun M, D'Amore PA. Vascular endothelial growth factor and its receptors. *Cytokine Growth Factor Rev* 1996;7:259–270.
14. Terman BI, Dougher-Vermazen M, Carrion ME, et al. Identification of the KDR tyrosine kinase as a receptor for vascular endothelial cell growth factor. *Biochem Biophys Res Commun* 1992;187:1579–1586.
15. Barleon B, Hauser S, Schllman C, et al. Differential expression of the two VEGF receptor flt and KDR in placenta and vascular endothelial cells. *J Cell Biochem* 1994;54:56–66.
16. Millauer B, Wizigmann-Voos S, Schnürch H, et al. High affinity VEGF binding and developmental expression suggest Flk-1 as a major regulator of vasculogenesis and angiogenesis. *Cell* 1993; 72:835–846.
17. Dumont DJ, Fong G-H, Puri MC, et al. Vascularization of the embryo: a study of flk-1, tek, tie, and vascular endothelial growth factor expression during development. *Dev Dyn* 1995; 203:80–92.
18. Ferrara N, Carver-Moore K, Chen H, et al. Heterozygous embryonic lethality induced by targeted inactivation of the VEGF gene. *Nature* 1996;380:439–442.
19. Carmeliet P, Ferriera V, Breier G, et al. Abnormal blood vessel development and lethality in embryos lacking a single VEGF allele. *Nature* 1996;380:435–439.
20. Shalaby F, Rossant J, Yamaguchi TP, et al. Failure of blood-island formation and vasculogenesis in Flk-1-deficient mice. *Nature* 1995;376:62–66.
21. Sato T, Tozawa Y, Deutsch U, et al. Distinct roles of the receptor tyrosine kinases Tie-1 and Tie-2 in blood vessel formation. *Nature* 1995;376:70.
22. Dumont DJ, Gradwohl G, Fong G-H, et al. Dominant-negative and targeted null mutations in the endothelial receptor tyrosine kinase, tek, reveal a critical role in vasculogenesis of the embryo. *Genes Dev* 1994;8:1897–1907.
23. Davis S, Aldrich TH, Jones PF, et al. Isolation of angiopoietin-1, a ligand for the TIE2 receptor, by secretion-trap expression cloning. *Cell* 1996;87:1161–1169.
24. Maisonpierre PC, Suri C, Jones PF, et al. Angiopoietin-2, a natural antagonist for Tie2 that disrupts *in vivo* angiogenesis. *Science* 1997;277:55–60.
25. Suri C, Jones PF, Patan S, et al. Requisite role of angiopoietin-1, a ligand for the TIE2 receptor, during embryonic angiogenesis. *Cell* 1996;87:1171–1180.
26. Gerwins P, Skoldenberg E, Claesson-Welsh L. Function of fibroblast growth factors and vascular endothelial growth factors and their receptors in angiogenesis. *Crit Rev Oncol Hematol* 2000;34:185–194.
27. D'Amore PA. Modes of FGF release *in vivo* and *in vitro. Cancer Metastasis Rev* 1990;9:227–238.
28. Healy MA, Herman IM. Density-dependent accumulation of basic fibroblast growth factor in the subendothelial matrix. *Eur J Cell Biol* 1992;59:56–67.
29. Ortega S, Ittmann M, Tsang S, et al. Neuronal defects and delayed wound healing in mice lacking fibroblast growth factor. *Proc Natl Acad Sci USA* 1998;95:5672–5677.
30. Holmgren L, Glaser A, Pfeifer-Ohlsson S, et al. Angiogenesis during human extraembryonic development involves the spatiotemporal control of PDGF ligand and receptor gene expression. *Development* 1991;113:749–754.
31. Hirschi KK, Rohovsky SA, Beck LH, et al. Endothelial cells modulate the proliferation of mural cell precursors via platelet-derived growth factor-BB and heterotypic cell contact. *Circ Res* 1999;84:298–304.
32. Corjay MH, Thompson MM, Lynch KR, et al. Differential effect of platelet-derived growth factor-versus serum-induced growth on smooth muscle α-actin and nonmuscle β-actin mRNA expression in cultured rat aortic smooth muscle cells. *J Biol Chem* 1989;264:10501–10506.
33. Rohovsky SA, Hirschi KK, D'Amore PA. Growth factor effects on a model of vessel formation. *Surg Forum* 1996;47:390–391.
34. Leveen P, Pekny M, Gebre-Medhin S, et al. Mice deficient for PDGF B show renal, cardiovascular, and hematological abnormalities. *Genes Dev* 1994;8:1875–1887.
35. Soriano P. Abnormal kidney development and hematological disorders in PDGF β-receptor mutant mice. *Genes Dev* 1994;8: 1888–1896.
36. Schlondorff D. The glomerular mesangial cell: an expanding role for a specialized pericyte. *FASEB J* 1987;1:272–281.
37. Lindahl P, Johansson BR, Leveen P, et al. Pericyte loss and microaneurysm formation in PDGF-β-deficient mice. *Science* 1997;277:242–245.
38. Kinnman N, Hultcrantz R, Barbu V, et al. PDGF-mediated chemoattraction of hepatic stellate cells by bile duct segments in cholestatic liver injury. *Lab Invest* 2000;80:697–707.
39. Hirschi K, Rohovsky SA, D'Amore PA. PDGF, TGF-β and heterotypic cell–cell interactions mediate the recruitment and differentiation of 10T1/2 cells to a smooth muscle cell fate. *J Cell Biol* 1998;141:805–814.
40. Sato Y, Tsuboi R, Lyons R, et al. Characterization of the activation of latent TGF-β by co-cultures of endothelial cells and per-

icytes or smooth muscle cells: a self-regulating system. *J Cell Biol* 1990;111:757–763.

41. Dickson MC, Martin JS, Cousins FM, et al. Defective haematopoiesis and vasculogenesis in transforming growth factor-β1 knock-out mice. *Development* 1995;121:1845–1854.

42. Bonewald L. Regulation and regulatory activities of transforming growth factor β. *Crit Rev Eukaryot Gene Expr* 1999;9:33–44.

43. Antonelli-Orlidge A, Saunders KB, Smith SR, et al. An activated form of transforming growth factor β is produced by cocultures of endothelial cells and pericytes. *Proc Natl Acad Sci USA* 1989;86:4544–4548.

44. Sato Y, Okada F, Abe M, et al. The mechanism for the activation of latent TGF-β during co-culture of endothelial cells and smooth muscle cells: cell-type specific targeting of latent TGF-β to smooth muscle cells. *J Cell Biol* 1993;123:1249–1254.

45. Basson CT, Kocher O, Basson MD, et al. Differential modulation of vascular cell integrin and extracellular matrix expression *in vitro* by TGF-β1 correlates with reciprocal effects on cell migration. *J Cell Physiol* 1992;153:118–128.

46. Kojima S, Hayashi S, Shimokado K, et al. Transcriptional activation of urokinast by the Kruppel-like factor Zf9/COPEB activates TGF-β1 in vascular endothelial cells. *Blood* 2000;95:1309–1316.

47. Neubauer K, Kruger M, Quondametteo F, et al. Transforming growth factor-β1 stimulates the synthesis of basement membrane proteins laminin, collagen type IV and entacin in rat liver sinusoidal endothelial cells. *J Hepatol* 1999;1999:692–702.

48. Cogan DG, Kuwabara T. The mural cell in perspective. *Arch Ophthalmol* 1967;78:133–139.

49. Benjamin LE, Golijanin D, Itin A, et al. Selective ablation of immature blood vessels in tumors follows vascular endothelial growth factor withdrawal. *J Clin Invest* 1999;103:159–165.

50. Krause P, Markus PM, Schwartz P, et al. Hepatocyte-supported serum-free culture of rat liver sinusoidal endothelial cells. *J Hepatol* 2000;32:718–726.

51. Gerber H-P, Hillan KJ, Ryan AM, et al. VEGF is required for growth and survival in neonatal mice. *Development* 1999;126:1149–1159.

52. Kim I, Kim HG, Kim H, et al. Hepatic expression, synthesis and secretion of a novel fibrinogen/angiopoietin-related proetin that prevents endothelial-cell apoptosis. *Biochem J* 2000;15:603–610.

53. Hobson B, Denekamp J. Endothelial proliferation in tumours and normal tissues: Continuous labelling studies. *Br J Cancer* 1984;49:405–413.

54. Folkman J. Tumor angiogenesis. In: Holland JF, Bast RC, Morton DL, et al., eds. *Cancer Medicine,* 4th ed. Baltimore: Williams & Wilkins, 1996;1:181–204.

55. Weidner N, Semple JP, Welch WR, et al. Tumor angiogenesis and metastasis—correlation in invasive breast carcinoma. *N Engl J Med* 1991;324:1–8.

56. Sun H, Tang Z, Li X, et al. Microvessel density of hepatocellular carcinoma: its relationship with prognosis. *J Cancer Res Clin Oncol* 1999;125:419–426.

57. Yoshihi H, Kuriyama S, Yoshi J, et al. Vascular endothelial growth factor tightly regulates *in vivo* development of murine hepatocellular carcinoma cells. *Hepatology* 1998;28:1489–1496.

58. Ankoma-Sey V, Wang Y, Dai Z. Hypoxic stimulation of vascular endothelial growth factor expression in activated rat hepatic stellate cells. *Hepatology* 2000;31:141–148.

59. Shweiki D, Itin A, Soffer D, et al. Vascular endothelial growth factor induced by hypoxia may mediate hypoxia-initiated angiogenesis. *Nature* 1992;359:843–845.

60. Shima DT, Deutsch U, D'Amore PA. Hypoxic induction of vascular endothelial growth factor (VEGF) in human epithelial cells is mediated by increases in mRNA stability. *FEBS Lett* 1995;370:203–208.

61. Liu Y, Cox SR, Morita T, et al. Hypoxia regulates vascular endothelial growth factor expression in endothelial cells: identification of a 5′ enhancer. *Circ Res* 1995;77:638–643.

62. Lee S, Lee Y, Bae S, et al. Human hepatitis B virus X protein is a possible mediator of hypoxia-induced angiogenesis in hepatocarcinogenesis. *Biochem Biophys Res Commun* 2000;268:456–461.

63. O'Reilly MS, Holmgren L, Shing Y, et al. Angiostatin: a novel angiogenesis inhibitor that mediates the suppression of metastases by a Lewis lung carcinoma. *Cell* 1994;79:315–328.

64. Clement B, Musso O, Lietard J, et al. Homeostatic control of angiogenesis: a newly identified function of the liver. *Heptatology* 1999;29:621–623.

65. O'Reilly M, Wiederschain D, Stetler-Stevenson W, et al. Regulation of angiostatin production by matrix metalloproteinase-2 in a model of concomitant resistance. *J Biol Chem* 1999;274:29568–29571.

66. Mochida S, Ishidawa K, Inao M, et al. Increased expressions of vascular endothelial growth factor and its receptors, flt-1 and KDR/flk-1, in regenerating rat liver. *Biochem Biophys Res Commun* 1996;4:176–179.

67. Assy N, Spira G, Paizi M, et al. Effect of vascular endothelial growth factor on hepatic regenerative activity following partial hepatectomy in rats. *J Hepatol* 1999;30:911–915.

68. Risau W. Differentiation of endothelium. *FASEB J,* 1995;9:926–933.

69. Beck L Jr, D'Amore PA. Vascular development: cellular and molecular regulation. *FASEB J* 1997;11:365–373.

DYNAMICS OF HEPATITIS B VIRUS INFECTION

MARTIN A. NOWAK

Mathematicians can contribute to understanding the dynamics of viral replication *in vivo* and thereby predict optimal timing of drug treatment and immunotherapy. This chapter provides a current example and illustrates the value of this type of analysis. Treatment of chronic hepatitis B virus (HBV) infections with the reverse transcriptase inhibitor lamivudine leads to a rapid decline in plasma viremia. Analysis of this decline provides estimates for the crucial kinetic constants of HBV replication in patients.

Worldwide, more than 250 million people are chronically infected with HBV, and 25% to 40% of these will die from liver cirrhosis or primary hepatocellular carcinoma (1,2). Chronic HBV infection is often the result of exposure early in life, leading to viral persistence in the absence of strong antibody or cellular immune responses (3). Therapy of HBV carriers can aim to inhibit viral replication and/or to enhance immunological responses against the virus (4).

The nucleoside analogue, (−)-2′-deoxy-3′-thiacytidine (lamivudine), originally developed as an anti-human immunodeficiency virus (HIV) drug, has potent inhibitory effects on HBV replication *in vivo* (5,6). Chronic HBV carriers were treated with various doses of lamivudine. Plasma virus load was quantified at frequent time points before, during, and after treatment using quantitative methods for determining viral DNA. In the first study, 45 patients were treated for 28 days; in a subsequent study, 50 patients were treated for 24 weeks. Figure 66.1 shows the plasma virus changes in six patients treated for 28 days. After the onset of therapy, the viral levels declined rapidly, but as soon as the drug was withdrawn, the virus returned. Figure 66.2 shows the changes in plasma viremia in six patients treated for 24 weeks. Again we observed a rapid decline in the plasma virus load, which fell below the detection limit in almost all patients within 2 to 4 weeks, and again in most patients the virus resurged rapidly as soon as the drug was withdrawn.

M. A. Nowak: Institute for Advanced Study, Princeton, New Jersey 08540.

Both hepatitis B e-antigen (HBeAG) and serum alanine aminotransferase (ALT) decline slowly during long-term lamivudine treatment. HBeAg is a viral protein produced by infected cells; its production is not directly inhibited by lamivudine (7), and changes in the serum concentration can therefore reflect changes in infected liver cell mass. ALT is released from damaged liver cells; thus it is an indicator of the level of cell damage and death.

For a quantitative analysis of these observations, we designed a simple but natural mathematical model based on ordinary differential equations for uninfected cells, x, infected cells, y, and free virus, v:

$$dx/dt = \lambda - dx - bvx$$
$$dy/dt = bvx - ay$$
$$dv/dt = ky - uv \tag{1}$$

Uninfected, susceptible cells are produced at a rate, λ, which may be constant or depend on the total population size of uninfected and infected cells. Uninfected cells die at rate dx, and become infected at rate bvx, where b is the rate constant describing the infection process. Infected cells are produced at rate bvx and die at rate ay. Free virions are produced from infected cells at rate ky and are removed at rate uv. Strictly speaking, the decay rate of free virus should also be a function of the uninfected (and infected) cell population, but we expect the leading term of viral decay to be independent of changes in the host cell population. Therefore, it is a reasonable assumption to treat u as a constant. The magnitude of the parameters a, b, k, and u will be determined by antiviral immune responses. In the absence of treatment, the system converges to a steady state of persistent infection, provided the basic reproductive ratio of the virus, $\lambda b (k - a)/(adu)$, is larger than 1. This condition is likely to be fulfilled if patients have weak immune responses against free virus (low u) or against infected cells (low a). Hence, in our simple model, weak immune responses predispose to the carrier state.

In the replication cycle of HBV, the viral reverse transcriptase is responsible for the synthesis of new HBV DNA from the pregenomic mRNA template (8,9). Therefore,

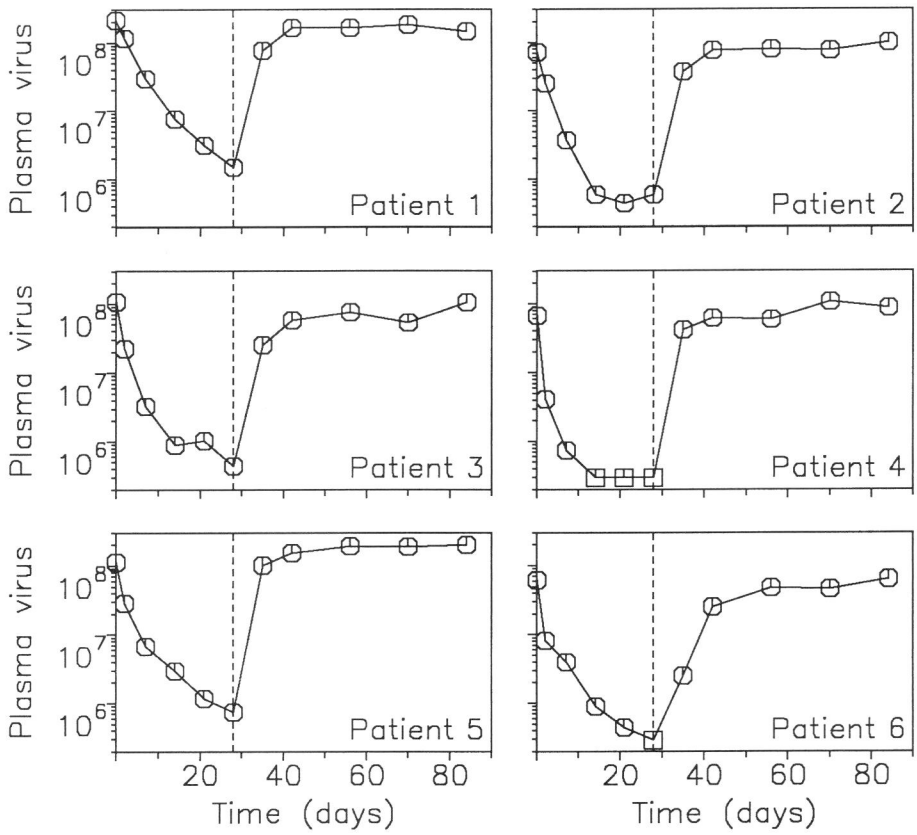

FIGURE 66.1. Rapid decline in plasma virus in six hepatitis B virus (HBV)-infected patients receiving lamivudine. After 28 days, the treatment was stopped and virus load returned rapidly to pretreatment levels. Plasma virus is shown in copies of viral DNA per ml. *Squares* indicate that virus load was below the detection limit.

lamivudine can prevent the production of new virus particles from already infected cells ($k = 0$). However, the viral polymerase is also essential for completing the double-stranded circular DNA before migration to the cell nucleus (10), and hence there is some evidence that lamivudine can prevent the infection of new cells ($b = 0$) (11). This implies that during treatment free virus is decaying exponentially according to $v(t) = v_0 e^{-ut}$. Similarly, infected cells are decaying exponentially according to $y(t) = y_0 e^{-at}$. Here v_0 and y_0 indicate free virus and infected cells at the beginning of therapy. If lamivudine does not effectively prevent infection of new cells, then the above equations are still very good approximations, provided u is substantially larger than a. Therefore, our analysis does not rely on the assumption that lamivudine also blocks new infection. From the decline of free virus we can estimate the decay rate u. Before treatment, the steady state of free virus implies $k y_0 = u v_0$. We know v_0, hence we can estimate $k y_0$, which is the total virus production per day.

From the one-month study, we can estimate the initial rate of virus decline during the first 2 days of treatment. We

obtain an average of $u = 0.67$ per day (standard deviation $\sigma = 0.32$, sample size $n = 23$), which corresponds to a half-life time ($T_{1/2}$) of 1.0 days. Hence, in the absence of treatment, about 50% of the plasma virus is replenished every day. The total serum virus load (for 3 liters of serum) before treatment varies in different patients, ranging from 10^{10} to 10^{12} particles with an average of 2.2×10^{11} ($\sigma = 2.6 \times 10^{11}$, $n = 45$). Consequently, the total amount of virus production (release into the serum) follows a wide distribution with an average of 1.3×10^{11} particles per day ($\sigma = 8.2 \sigma 10^{10}$, $n = 23$). These differences are likely to reflect different population sizes of virus-infected cells in individual patients. Plasma virus levels usually correlate with abundance of infected cells as determined by histological examination of the liver (12).

Virus decline during treatment is not strictly exponential (Fig. 66.1). This can be explained by the assumption that the efficacy of the drug is not 100%. Assuming a certain efficacy ρ, viral decay occurs according to $v(t) = v_0 (1 - \rho + \rho e^{-ut})$. Fitting this function provides an estimate for the efficacy of the drug at various doses. We find that for daily

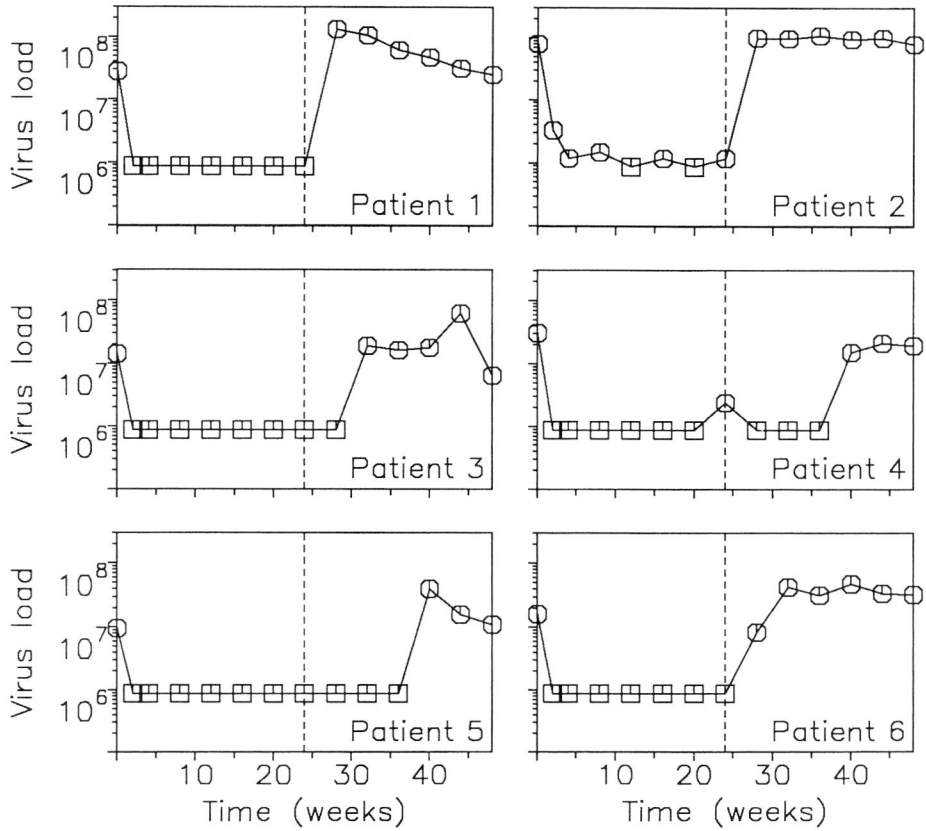

FIGURE 66.2. Hepatitis B virus (HBV) plasma virus load in six patients receiving lamivudine for 24 weeks. In most patients, the virus load declined rapidly below the detection limit (*square symbols*). In all patients, the virus load returned rapidly to pretreatment levels when the treatment was stopped.

doses of 20, 100, 300 and 600 mg, viral replication is inhibited by 87%, 97%, 96%, and 99%, respectively.

When therapy is withdrawn, virus resurges according to $dv/dt = ky - uv$. Hence, the initial virus growth rate can be approximated by

$$v(t) = v_1 e^{-ut} + (ky_1/u)(1 - e^{-ut}) \qquad (2)$$

where v_1 and y_1 indicate the levels of free virus and infected cells at the end of therapy. We know v_1 by direct measurement, we have determined the decay rate, u, and hence we can estimate ky_1, which is the rate of virus production from infected cells at the end of therapy. Comparing ky_0 and ky_1 gives an estimate for the decay rate of infected (virus-producing) cells, a, and consequently their half-life. This method requires the *initial* growth rate of virus after therapy has stopped, since y is treated as a constant. The approximation is accurate if the virus load is determined early after the end of treatment. In our study, treatment was withdrawn after 28 days, and the virus load was determined at days 28 and 35. For the different patients we obtained a broad distribution with an average decline of

$a = 0.043$ per day ($\sigma = 0.035$, $n = 20$), corresponding to a $T_{1/2}$ of 16 days.

The broad distribution of turnover rates of infected cells may be a consequence of heterogeneity of the immune response against infected cells in different patients (13,14). Damaged liver cells release ALT, and hence plasma ALT levels should provide some crude estimate for the amount of cell death in the liver. If most cell damage is caused by immune responses directed to infected cells (15), then ALT levels provide some estimate for the strength of the immunological response against HBV. We find a positive correlation between the decay rate of infected cells and the pretreatment ALT level among different patients (16). This supports our hypothesis that the variability of cell decay rates reflects different strengths of anticellular immune responses and is not simply caused by fluctuations in measurement or inaccurate approximation.

In the subsequent study, treatment continued for 24 weeks, but sampling was less frequent (the first timepoints were after 2 and 4 weeks, then every 4 weeks), and we cannot obtain accurate estimates of the viral or cellular decay rates with the above methods. However, we can obtain an independent estimate of the turnover of infected cells from the initial decay of HBeAg. Reverse transcriptase inhibitors such as lamivudine have no direct effect on the synthesis and secretion of HBeAg, which derives from mRNA transcribed from existing covalently closed circular DNA (cccDNA) molecules of HBV within infected cells. The capacity of the infected host to synthesize this protein is dependent on the rate of infection of cells (inhibited by lamivudine) and the rate of lysis of infected cells (not inhibited by lamivudine) and dependent on immune recognition of these cells. Hence, the initial decay of HBeAg in patients taking lamivudine should reflect the decay of infected hepatocytes. During the first 8 weeks of treatment we observed an average decline of $a = 0.053$ per day ($\sigma = 0.039$, $n = 29$), which corresponds to a $T_{1/2}$ of 13 days. This is in agreement with our previous estimate. Again we find a strong correlation between decay of infected cells and ALT levels among different patients.

It is likely that HBV infects and replicates at different rates in a number of cell types (17,18). Therefore, the estimated viral production rates and turnover rates of infected cells have to be interpreted as average values. Similarly the rate of production of viral particles and HBeAg from an infected cell may depend on the number of cccDNA molecules of HBV in the nucleus of an infected cell. During drug treatment the cccDNA copy number per infected cell may decline, which could lead to less viral and HBeAg production independent of the death of infected cells. Therefore, the decline of viral production and HBeAg could overestimate the actual rate of clearance of infected cells and instead reflect the decay of cccDNA. However, for practical purposes, the most important figure is the decay of potential virus "production units" during treatment, independent of whether this reflects cell death or decay of viral cccDNA. Patients with high ALT levels, however, clear virus-producing units faster.

A half-life of 10 days for infected, virus-producing hepatocytes implies that about 7% of this cell population is removed per day. These cells may either be lysed or cured from viral cccDNA by anticellular immune responses (19–23).

The HBV data provide an interesting comparison with HIV dynamics. In HIV-1 infection, most patients have a turnover rate of infected cells of approximately 2 days, and free virus is cleared faster than this (24–28). In HBV infections, decay of plasma virus occurs with a half-life of about 1 day in patients who generally seem to have no antibody against free virus. Interestingly, there is a much wider distribution of half-lives of virus-producing cells in HBV-infected patients, ranging from 10 to 100 days and a viral decay half-life of about 1 day. HBV is believed to be largely noncytopathic, and therefore the turnover rates of infected cells can be due to different anticellular immune responses. HIV, on the other hand, can probably kill an infected cell within 2 days, and the rather uniform turnover rate of infected (virus-

producing) cells could be the consequence of a tight struggle between viral cytopathicity and the strong cytotoxic T lymphocyte (CTL) response found in most HIV patients.

The total amount of virus production (release into the periphery) is larger for HBV: on average about 10^9 HIV particles are generated every day, compared to about 10^{11} HBV particles. Thus, chronic HBV infection emerges also as a rapid dynamic process with vast amounts of virus and infected cells produced and removed every day. However, with respect to accumulation of genetic diversity and escape from drug treatment and immune responses, a relevant figure is the generation time of viral replication, which is largely determined by the turnover rate of virus-infected cells, and is much larger in HIV.

Treatment of chronic HBV infections with lamivudine leads to a rapid and sustained decline of plasma virus levels, but clinical benefit with a reduced risk of cirrhosis and development of liver cancer will greatly depend on the decline of infected cells (29–31). In patients where infected cells decline with a half-life of 10 days, treatment for one year could potentially reduce the number of infected cells to approximately 10^{-11} of its initial value. Eradication of the virus infection depends on whether the efficacy of the drug is sufficiently high to reduce the basic reproductive ratio of the virus below unity (in analogy to epidemiological theory) (32). In patients with an infected cell half-life of 100 days, one year of treatment could reduce the number of infected cells to approximately 8% of its initial value. Thus, lamivudine could be used over a prolonged period as single-agent therapy or to reduce the number of infected cells prior to immunotherapy designed to eradicate infected cells. Immunotherapy without antiviral treatment could be problematic because of the very large number of infected liver cells in the typical HBV carrier. A quantitative understanding of HBV dynamics will make it possible to devise optimal treatment strategies for individual patients.

REFERENCES

1. Weissberg JI, et al. Survival in chronic hepatitis B. *Ann Intern Med* 1984;101:613–616.
2. Beasley RP, et al. Hepatocellular carcinoma and hepatitis B virus. *Lancet* 1981;2:1129–1133.
3. Ferrari C, et al. Cellular immune response to hepatitis B virus-encoded antigens in acute and chronic hepatitis B virus infection. *J Immunol* 1990;145:3442–3449.
4. Regenstein F. New approaches to the treatment of chronic viral-hepatitis-B and viral-hepatitis-C. *Am J Med* 1994;96:47–51.
5. Doong SL, et al. Inhibition of the replication of hepatitis B virus *in vitro* by 2′,3′-dideoxy-3′-thiacytidine and related analogues. *Proc Natl Acad Sci USA* 1991;88:8495–8499.
6. Dienstag JL, et al. Double-blind, randomized, 3-month, dose-ranging trial of lamivudine for chronic hepatitis-B. *Hepatology* 1994;20:199–205.
7. Chang CN, et al. Biochemical pharmacology of (+)- and (−)-2′,3′-dideoxy-3′-thiacytidine as antihepatitis B virus agents. *J Biol Chem* 1992;267:22414–22420.

8. Ganem D, Varmus HE. The molecular biology of the hepatitis B viruses. *Annu Rev Biochem* 1987;56:651–693.
9. Tiollais P, Buendia MA. Hepatitis B virus. *Sci Am* 1991;264: 116–123.
10. Ganem D, et al. Hepatitis B virus reverse transcriptase and its many roles in hepadnaviral genomic replication. *Infect Agents Dis* 1994;3:85–93.
11. Severini A, et al. Mechanism of inhibition of duck hepatitis B virus polymerase by (−)-β-L-2′,3′-dideoxy-3′-thiacytidine. *Antimicrob Agents Chemother* 1995; 39:1430–1435.
12. Di Bisceglie AM, et al. Correlation between hepatic and serologic markers of HBV infection in patients with chronic hepatitis-B. *Hepatology* 1994;20:A296.
13. Bertoletti A, et al. Natural variants of cytotoxic epitopes are T-cell receptor antagonists for antiviral cytotoxic T cells. *Nature* 1994; 369:407–410.
14. Nayersina R, et al. HLA A2 restricted cytotoxic T-lymphocyte responses to multiple hepatitis-B surface-antigen epitopes during hepatitis-B virus-infection. *J Immunol* 1993;150:4659–4671.
15. Moriyama T, et al. Immunobiology and pathogenesis of hepatocellular injury in hepatitis-B virus transgenic mice. *Science* 1990; 248:361–364.
16. Nowak MA, et al. Viral dynamics in hepatitis B virus infection. *Proc Natl Acad Sci USA* 1996; 93:4398–4402.
17. Mason A, et al. Hepatitis-B virus-replication in diverse cell-types during chronic hepatitis-B virus-infection. *Hepatology* 1993;18: 781–789.
18. London WT, Blumberg BS. A cellular-model of the role of hepatitis-B virus in the pathogenesis of primary hepatocellular-carcinoma. *Hepatology*, Suppl, 1982;2:S10–S14.
19. Chisari FV, Ferrari C. Hepatitis-B virus immunopathogenesis. *Annu Rev Immunol* 1995;13:29–60.
20. Guidotti LG, Chisari FV. To kill or to cure: options in host-defense against viral infection. *Curr Opin Immunol* 1996;8: 478–483.
21. Bianchi L, Gudat F. Viral antigens in liver tissue and type of inflammation in hepatitis-B. In: Bianchi L, Gerok W, Sickinger K, et al, eds. *Virus and the liver.* Lancaster, England: MTP Press, 1980;197–204.
22. Sherlock S, Dooley J. *Diseases of the liver and biliary system,* 9th ed. Oxford: Blackwell Scientific, 1991.
23. Payne RJH, et al. A cellular model to explain the pathogenesis of infection by the hepatitis B virus. *Math Biosci* 1994;123:25–58.
24. Wei X, et al. Viral dynamics in human immunodeficiency virus type 1 infection. *Nature* 1995;373:117–122.
25. Ho DD, et al. Rapid turnover of plasma virions and CD4 lymphocytes in HIV-1 infection. *Nature* 1995;373:123–126.
26. Coffin JM. HIV population dynamics *in vivo*: implications for genetic variation, pathogenesis, and therapy. *Science* 1995;267: 483–488.
27. Nowak MA, et al. Antigenic oscillations and shifting immunodominance in HIV-1 infections. *Nature* 1995;375:193.
28. Schuurman R, et al. Rapid changes in human immunodeficiency virus type 1 RNA load and appearance of drug-resistant virus populations in persons treated with lamivudine (3TC). *J Infect Dis* 1995;171:1411–1419.
29. Mason WS. The problem of antiviral therapy for chronic hepadnavirus infections. *J Hepatol* 1993;17:S137–S142.
30. Mason WS, et al. Characterization of the antiviral effects of 2′ carbodeoxyguanosine in ducks chronically infected with duck hepatitis B virus. *Hepatology* 1994;19:398–411.
31. Jacyna MR, Thomas HC. Pathogenesis and treatment of chronic infection. In: Zuckerman, A, Thomas HC, eds. *Viral hepatitis.* Edinburgh, New York: Churchill Livingstone, 1993:185–205.
32. Anderson RM, May RM. *Infectious diseases of humans.* Oxford: Oxford University Press, 1991.

The Liver: Biology and Pathobiology, Fourth Edition, edited by I. M. Arias, J. L. Boyer, F. V. Chisari, N. Fausto, D. Schachter, and D. A. Shafritz.
Lippincott Williams & Wilkins, Philadelphia © 2001.

TELOMERES AND TELOMERASE IN EXPERIMENTAL LIVER CIRRHOSIS

KARL LENHARD RUDOLPH
RONALD A. DEPINHO

In humans, continual hepatocyte destruction by a diverse array of hepatotoxins, ranging from chronic viral hepatitis to alcohol, stimulates abnormal patterns of hepatocyte regeneration, ultimately culminating in liver fibrosis after many years of ongoing injury. The resulting compromise in liver function due to loss of hepatocytes, coupled with distortion of organ architecture, leads to a cascade of pathophysiological events with potentially life-threatening complications. Left unchecked, these pathological processes culminate in extensive fibrotic replacement, diminished hepatocyte reserve, and fatal end-stage liver failure (1–3).

Regardless of its etiology, cirrhosis evolves slowly over many years. Chronic hepatocyte death and renewal is one of the major predisposing factors for cirrhosis, whereas acute self-limited episodes of hepatic necrosis generally do not elicit a cirrhotic response even following severe bouts of hepatitis (4). Therapeutic methotrexate use for psoriasis has provided a minimal time estimate required for the development of cirrhosis in humans, averaging 48 months (5–7). In more common forms of liver injury, such as chronic viral hepatitis or alcohol abuse, this time interval is 4 to 7 times longer.

On the cellular level, the conversion of hepatic stellate cells into myofibroblast-like cells, as well as a marked decrease in hepatocyte proliferative activity, characterize cirrhosis. Activated stellate cells are the principal source of extracellular matrix during chronic liver injury. Notable features of the activated stellate cell include an increase in cell volume, loss of retinoid droplets, modest focal proliferation, acquisition of smooth muscle-like features, and enhanced fibrogenic activity (1–3). One current hypothesis proposes that hepatocyte destruction itself serves as an activation signal, possibly via the release of insulin-like growth factor or lipid peroxides generated from apoptotic cell membranes (8). It therefore follows that factors governing the survival of hepatocytes could potentially influence stellate cell activation and fibrogenesis. The other key aspect of end-stage cirrhosis, hepatocellular proliferative arrest (9–12), is not well understood and may relate to altered hepatocyte–matrix interactions (13–16) and/or abundant transforming growth factor β 1 (TGF-β1), a known potent inhibitor of hepatocyte growth in culture (17–20).

Whereas many studies have addressed the common endpoints of cirrhosis, little is known about the molecular lesions governing the progressive induction of cirrhosis during its long latency. Classical explanations propose that long-standing organ-architectural changes induced by processes such as chronic inflammation, cytokine production, and extracellular matrix reorganization, among others,

K. L. Rudolph: Department of Gastroenterology and Hepatology, Medical School Hannover, Hannover 30623, Germany.

R. A. DePinho: Departments of Adult Oncology, Medicine and Genetics, Dana-Farber Cancer Institute, and Harvard Medical School, Boston, Massachusetts 02115.

become irreversible at some point. Another, not mutually exclusive thesis has proposed that sustained cellular turnover in chronic liver disease precipitates cellular senescence and/or crisis as a result of telomere attrition.

Telomeres are specialized structures at the ends of eukaryotic chromosomes consisting of simple repeat elements (TTAGGG) that are coated with telomere binding proteins (21–23). Normal telomere lengths measure 8 to 15 kb in humans. With each cell division telomeres shorten due to incomplete replication of chromosomal ends by DNA polymerase (24,25). The telomere synthesizing enzyme telomerase solves this "end replication problem" of DNA polymerase by adding TTAGGG repeats to the shortened telomere (26). In humans, telomerase activity is stringently regulated and restricted to tissue stem cells and germ cells, while most somatic cells and tissues exhibit little or no telomerase activity (27–30). Extensive experimental support has led to the concept that telomere shortening functions as a mitotic clock limiting the growth of normal somatic cells in culture (24 and 31–34). Telomere-associated cellular senescence could provide a plausible explanation for the lengthy period of chronic liver damage (often clinically silent) preceding the onset of impaired hepatocyte growth and survival, and ultimately overt cirrhosis. The telomere hypothesis of liver cirrhosis proposes that chronic liver injury induces continual waves of liver destruction and regeneration, resulting in critical telomere shortening, in turn cumulating in hepatocyte replicative senescence or death, and ultimately liver cirrhosis. Furthermore, as telomeres generally cannot be lengthened in hepatocytes due to a lack or insufficient levels of telomerase, this model provides a rational explanation for the irreversible nature of end-stage cirrhosis. This chapter focuses on recent experimental evidence that supports the hypothesis that telomere shortening plays a central pathogenic role in most forms of cirrhosis.

TELOMERE SHORTENING AND CELLULAR SENESCENCE

Primary human cells grow for a limited number of cell divisions in culture before they undergo replicative senescence, a state characterized by large flattened cell morphology and irreversible loss of the capacity for cell division (35). That telomere length governs the replicative capacity of cultured cells has been clearly demonstrated in studies showing that ectopic expression of telomerase sustains telomere length and endows certain cell types (e.g., fibroblasts and endothelial cells) with apparently unlimited growth potential (36,37). Nevertheless, immortalization of other cell types (e.g., keratinocytes or mammary epithelial cells) requires, under certain culture conditions, inactivation of the p16/Rb pathway (38,39), in addition to telomerase reactivation, suggesting that telomerase-independent mechanisms can under certain instances induce senescence in these cells.

A great deal of debate and speculation has surrounded the issue of whether significant telomere attrition occurs *in vivo* and whether such shortening contributes to the pathogenesis of age-related disorders and diseases of chronic cell turnover (e.g., immunosenescence in advanced human immunodeficiency virus (HIV) infection (40,41), and bone marrow exhaustion in myeloproliferative diseases (42,43), among others). Although the role of telomere dynamics in aging is controversial, a variety of studies described age-dependent telomere shortening in high-proliferative cell compartments (44–49). For example, fibroblasts, lymphocytes, and vascular endothelial cells (especially in areas of hemodynamic stress) demonstrated telomere shortening, whereas quiescent organ systems (brain) were found to maintain stable telomeres (48). In contrast, other studies did not find a correlation between donor age and telomere length in fibroblasts and osteoblasts (50–51). Moreover, telomeres in lymphocytes seem to shorten with varying dynamics during life, where rapid telomere loss is observed in young children, followed by an apparent plateau between age 4 and young adulthood, and moderate telomere shortening later in life (52). Together these data indicate that regulation of telomere length is complex *in vivo*, likely involving factors other than the number of cell divisions. That telomere shortening can have an impact on organismal functions has been shown in the telomerase-deficient mouse, where telomere attrition is associated with diminished capacity to respond to acute and chronic stresses that require robust proliferative responses (53,54, see also Defective Liver Regeneration in Telomerase-Deficient Mice, below). It is conceivable that such deficiencies could contribute to certain aspects of the aging process in humans.

The mechanisms by which critically short telomeres signal cell-cycle withdrawal are not understood. One hypothesis suggests that critically short telomeres can no longer fulfill their capping function at the chromosomal termini. While telomeres are not detected as abnormal DNA ends, uncapped chromosomes may be sensed as broken chromosome ends or double-strand breaks. The telomeric complex consisting of telomere repeats and telomere-binding proteins has been shown to form t-loop structures in which the terminus of the telomere is buried in more proximal telomere sequences (55). One possible uncapping mechanism might be that loss of telomere repeats could at some point inhibit t-loop formation of telomeric ends, which in turn are sensed by the double-strand break repair pathway. Alternatively to the uncapping hypothesis, telomere shortening may result in altered chromatin structure and altered gene expression of gene loci immediately proximal to the telomere. This telomere position effect is a well established phenomenon in yeast but has not been verified in mammals.

The senescence signal has been shown to engage the tumor suppressor pathways p53 and Rb (56–58), and inactivation of Rb and/or p53 by either viral oncoproteins (59) or antisense neutralization (60) can extend the replicative lifespan of primary human cells *in vitro*. Unless telomere maintenance mechanisms are activated in such cells, further telomere shortening culminates in a period of massive cell death and genomic instability, termed crisis (32,61). Rare surviving clones emerging from crisis have always activated mechanisms of telomere maintenance, predominantly by reactivation of telomerase (62,63).

The telomerase holoenzyme consists of several essential components required for enzyme activity: the catalytic subunit, which functions as a reverse transcriptase (27–29), *te*lomerase *r*everse *t*ranscriptase (TERT), and the telomerase RNA component (TERC), which serves as a template for the synthesis of telomere repeats (64–66). TERC is expressed ubiquitously in human tissues, whereas expression of TERT is restricted to germ cells, early progenitor cells of the stem cell compartments, and activated lymphocytes (28,29,67,68). Expression of TERT seems to be a major determinant governing the level of telomerase activity in any given cell type and is found to be markedly upregulated in the majority of human cancers.

THE REPLICATIVE PROPERTIES OF HEPATOCYTES

The growth of mature adult hepatocytes in culture has been difficult and requires optimized tissue culture conditions such as cocultivation with epithelial cells, growth in collagen gel systems, and growth factor supplementation. Under such conditions, human hepatocytes can be maintained in culture over long periods of time, but generally these cultures lose liver-specific functions or undergo terminal differentiation after a very short period of time in culture (69,70). Telomere shortening is not the cause of this growth-arrested terminally differentiated state, since its induction occurs in primary hepatocytes of different species possessing widely varying telomere lengths (71). Rather, this premature senescence phenotype is consistent with the observation that a variety of telomere-independent stimuli, such as activated RAS, can induce a senescent-like state in cultured cells (72,73). Along these lines, it is tempting to speculate that activation of the RAS pathway may result from the release of hepatocytes from their physiological milieu and exposure to serum growth factors (74). In contrast to the early growth arrest of mature hepatocytes, some studies have demonstrated that under certain conditions hepatocytes possess moderate cell division capacity (10 to 37 population doublings) before they reach senescence (75,76). In addition, ectopic expression of the oncogenic SV40 large T antigen (which inhibits p53 and Rb function) has been shown to facilitate continuous hepatocyte proliferation in culture (77,78). To what extent telomere shortening limits the growth of hepatocytes has not yet been established. Moreover, experiments assessing the capacity of ectopic telomerase expression to extend the replicative

capacity of human hepatocytes have not been reported. *In vivo* experiments on serial transplantation of mouse hepatocytes revealed a stem cell-like regenerative potential, capable of at least 69 population doublings (79). Similar experiments have not been performed with human hepatocytes, but several factors would predict a shorter replicative lifespan for human hepatocytes compared to those of mouse. The telomere length of human hepatocytes is approximately 8 kb (see Fig. 67.1), whereas telomeres in different mouse strains are 10 to 80 kb in length with high interchromosomal variations (80,81). If telomere shortening is the critical stimulus of cellular senescence in hepatocytes, it is conceivable that the longer telomeres and modest levels of telomerase activity in mice could account for the observed longer replicative potential of mouse hepatocytes.

TELOMERE SHORTENING AND PROLIFERATIVE DISORDERS IN HUMAN CIRRHOSIS

The normal liver is a quiescent organ with low mitotic activity; thus, telomere lengths are not expected to shorten with advancing age. Indeed, comparative measurement of mean telomere lengths in human livers from healthy control groups across multiple independent studies does not show detectable age-dependent telomere shortening (82–84, Fig. 67.1). In sharp contrast, telomere shortening has been documented in age-matched chronic hepatitis B and C virus-infected livers, where the shortest telomeres are found in cirrhotic livers (82–84, Fig. 67.1). Specifically, three independent studies have demonstrated that the mean telomere length of hepatitis B and C virus-induced cirrhosis averaged 5.7 kb compared with 8.2 kb in age-matched control samples. Whether comparable degrees of telomere shortening takes place in cirrhosis brought about by other agents of hepatocyte destruction has not yet been established.

The shortened telomere length observed in cirrhotic liver approaches the range of telomere lengths associated with the onset of cellular senescence in primary human cells in culture (33). Consistent with the hepatocyte senescence concept is the presence of a variety of morphological and molecular signatures of senescence in the cirrhotic liver. Those correlates include increasing p53 expression (85) and an accumulation of p21[CIP/WAF] (86), a downstream target of p53 and inhibitor of cyclin-dependent kinases. Another prominent feature of cirrhosis is the development of large cell changes (LCC), a cytological finding characterized by hepatocyte enlargement and nuclear pleomorphism with hyperchromasia and multinucleation (87). Such morphological changes are reminiscent of the cytological changes associated with senescence of other cell types following passage in culture (35). Finally, a decrease in hepatocyte proliferation is evident as chronic liver disease evolves into cirrhosis (9–12). During active hepatic injury, the precirrhotic

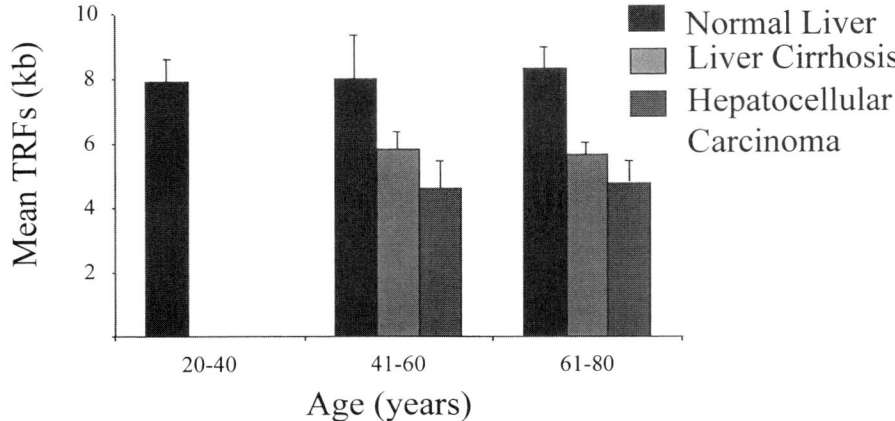

FIGURE 67.1. Depicted are the results of three separate studies on telomere length as a measure of the size of terminal restriction fragments (*TRFs*) in normal liver samples, cirrhotic liver samples, and hepatocellular carcinomas (HCC) (82–84). Since the liver is a quiescent organ, telomeres do not shorten in the normal liver during aging. Cirrhotic liver samples show significantly shorter telomere lengths in contrast to age-matched normal liver samples. The decreased telomere length in cirrhosis seems to be disease-specific, because short telomeres are seen in all cirrhotic samples independent of the age of the patient. None of the studies showed significant differences in telomere length between cirrhotic samples of different origins. In most cases cirrhosis was induced by chronic hepatitis C and/or B virus infections, but telomere shortening was also present in virus negative cirrhotic samples. Since more than 80% of hepatocellular carcinomas develop in cirrhotic livers, short telomeres are also correlated to HCC. In addition, the telomere length in HCC is often significantly shorter than in the surrounding noncancerous tissue, suggesting that telomere shortening and genomic instability might promote hepatocarcinogenesis.

liver exhibits an up to 16-fold increase in the numbers of cycling cells compared to the healthy, quiescent liver (11). In contrast, hepatocyte proliferation decreases in advanced stages of chronic liver diseases, correlating with the onset and progression towards cirrhosis (9–12). Altogether, these data on telomere shortening, activated DNA-damage responses, and decreased hepatocyte proliferation in cirrhotic livers are consistent with the view that telomere shortening plays a key role in limiting the regenerative capacity of hepatocytes and may presage the development of cirrhosis. The correlative nature of these data prompted a series of studies in the telomerase knockout mouse designed to fortify the causal link between telomere attrition and the cirrhotic process.

THE TELOMERASE-DEFICIENT MOUSE AS A MODEL SYSTEM FOR LIVER CIRRHOSIS

Mice homozygous null for the gene encoding the essential telomerase RNA component (mTERC−/−) lack telomerase activity (88). mTERC−/− mice exhibit progressive telomere shortening with each successive generation arising from mTERC−/− intercrosses (G1 to G6) (88). While early generations (G1 to G3) of mTERC−/− mice have long telomeres and are phenotypically normal, severe telomere shortening in late generations (G4 to G6) is associated with end-to-end chromosomal fusions, growth arrest, and apop-

tosis (53,89). These findings are more pronounced in organ systems with high rates of renewal (e.g., germ cells, epidermis, hematopoietic system, and intestinal tract). Moreover, as phenotypically normal midgeneration mTERC−/− mice advance in age, progressive telomere attrition leads to impaired organ function with a diminished capacity to respond to acute and chronic stress. Such mice exhibit impaired wound healing, diminished hematopoietic reserve and a shortened lifespan (53,54). The mTERC−/− mouse therefore permits the study of telomere attrition and its biological impact on long-term organ homeostasis under conditions of accelerated cellular turnover, including those encountered in diseases typified by chronic cellular turnover such as the regenerating liver.

DEFECTIVE LIVER REGENERATION IN TELOMERASE-DEFICIENT MICE

mTERC−/− mice exposed to three different hepatocyte ablation protocols (genetic ablation in the albumin-directed urokinase plasminogen activator (Alb-uPA) transgenic mouse, surgical ablation by partial hepatectomy, or chemical ablation with CCl4 treatment) exhibit defects in liver regeneration as telomeres become critically short (90). The first system, the Alb-uPA transgenic mouse, provides a means to explore factors governing hepatocyte regenerative capacity. Alb-uPA expression has been shown to cause widespread hepatocyte death and liver failure in newborn mice (91). However, approximately 60% of transgenic mice do survive as a result of spontaneous transgene deletion in rare hepatocytes that then clonally expand (formation of regenerative nodules) to reconstitute the entire organ by 3 months of age (92). The growth of regenerative liver nodules in the Alb-uPA system has been estimated to require approximately 20 cell doublings of a single transgene-negative hepatocyte (92). Using this model, decreased survival of transgene carriers was observed in mice with short telomeres as compared to mice with long telomeres (transgene transmission: 16% vs. 31%, respectively). In addition, the few surviving midgeneration mTERC−/− mice exhibited reduced fitness and poor weight gain relative to control mice with long telomeres. Impaired growth of regenerative nodules in mice with short telomeres correlated with increased apoptosis and decreased proliferation of hepatocytes.

The second approach used to determine liver regenerative capacity in mTERC−/− mice was partial hepatectomy (PH): surgical removal of two-thirds of the liver (93,94). In this setting greater than 50% of the remaining hepatocytes follow a highly synchronized cell cycle reentry pattern, reaching peak S-phase activity at 24 to 48 hours, maximal mitosis at 72 hours, and cessation of cell division at 96 hours post-PH. After this regenerative wave, normal organ histology is reestablished within 1 week (93,94). Consistent with the shorter telomeres in mTERC−/− mice, the liver mass at 72 hours after PH was reduced relative to wild-type mice. Cell cycle analysis of post-PH livers showed a normal reentry into the cell cycle at 24 hours after PH in both groups. In contrast, at 72 hours post-PH, flow cytometry of cells from the regenerating liver front revealed a decreased progression through mitosis in mice with short telomeres, which showed a 2- to 3-fold increase in the G2/M fraction relative to wild-type mice. This effect correlated microscopically with an increase in the number of mitotic figures in mice with short telomeres at 48 to 96 hours post-PH, specifically with an increase in the metaphase and anaphase fractions of the mitotic cells. These findings are consistent with the hypothesis that telomere loss may interfere with progression through mitosis due to the generation of end-to-end chromosomal fusions, opposing kinetochore alignment, and anaphase bridges (95–96, 23). Indeed, at 48 to 96 hours post-PH, H&E-stained liver sections showed many aberrant mitotic figures and anaphase bridges only in liver samples of mice with short telomeres. Together, these findings indicate that telomere dysfunction delays the mitotic progression of regenerating hepatocytes and in turn delays the restoration of liver mass after surgical hepatectomy.

The third approach used to assess the impact of telomere dysfunction on liver regeneration was toxin-mediated chronic liver injury. Repeated administration of the hepatotoxin carbon tetrachloride (CCl_4) is a commonly employed method designed to produce many cycles of destruction–regeneration and ultimately some features of cirrhosis after prolonged alternate day treatments (97). In wild-type mice it usually takes 2 to 3 months of continuous applications of CCl_4 to generate fibrosis and impairment of liver function. The long telomeres and promiscuous telomerase activity in wild-type mouse livers (see The Replicative Properties of Hepatocytes, above) may account for the delayed cirrhotic response in the CCl_4 system. The generation of mTERC−/− mice with short telomeres afforded the opportunity to directly assess whether telomere reserve and maintenance is protective against development of cirrhosis. When mTERC−/− mice are exposed to repeated chemically induced liver damage, pathological signs of liver cirrhosis develop more rapidly and are more pronounced compared with control mice with long telomeres (90, Fig. 67.2). Specifically, centrilobular fibrosis emerges after 2 or 4 weeks of alternate-day CCl_4 exposure in mice with short telomeres, whereas wild-type mice show minimal changes at 4 weeks. In addition to accelerated fibrosis, mice with shortened telomeres show enhanced steatosis, enlarged hepatocytes, and nuclear pleomorphism in response to chronic liver damage. This accelerated development of cirrhosis correlated with decreased hepatocyte proliferation, increased TGF-β 1 expression, and activation of stellate cells (90). On the organismal level, accelerated cirrhosis formation in mTERC−/− mice with short telomeres was accompanied by impaired gain of body weight, increased ascites, elevated bilirubin, and decreased albumin levels relative to wild-type mice.

TELOMERASE THERAPY INHIBITS EXPERIMENTAL LIVER CIRRHOSIS IN MICE

To determine whether somatic restoration of telomerase activity could block the development of cirrhosis in mice with dysfunctional telomeres, an adenoviral vector was constructed that directed the expression of mTERC to the livers of mTERC−/− mice (90). These studies established that mTERC gene delivery conferred a growth advantage to hepatocytes of mice with short telomeres in the setting of chronic liver injury induced by CCl_4. The restoration of telomerase activity via adenovirus-mediated mTERC gene transfer delayed the pace of cirrhosis development in mTERC−/− mice with short telomeres (see Defective Liver Regeneration in Telomerase-Deficient Mice, above) to levels seen in wild-type mice. This attenuated cirrhotic response correlated with a rescue of telomere dysfunction as evidenced by a reduction of abnormal mitotic figures, particularly anaphase bridges. In addition, mTERC gene delivery was associated with lowered TGFβ-1 expression, improved hepatocyte proliferation, increased serum albumin, and near complete elimination of ascites formation.

Together, these data underscore the importance of hepatocyte-regeneration in the pathogenesis of liver cirrhosis and forge a pathogenetic link between telomere dysfunc-

mTERC+/+   G3 mTERC-/-   G6 mTERC-/-

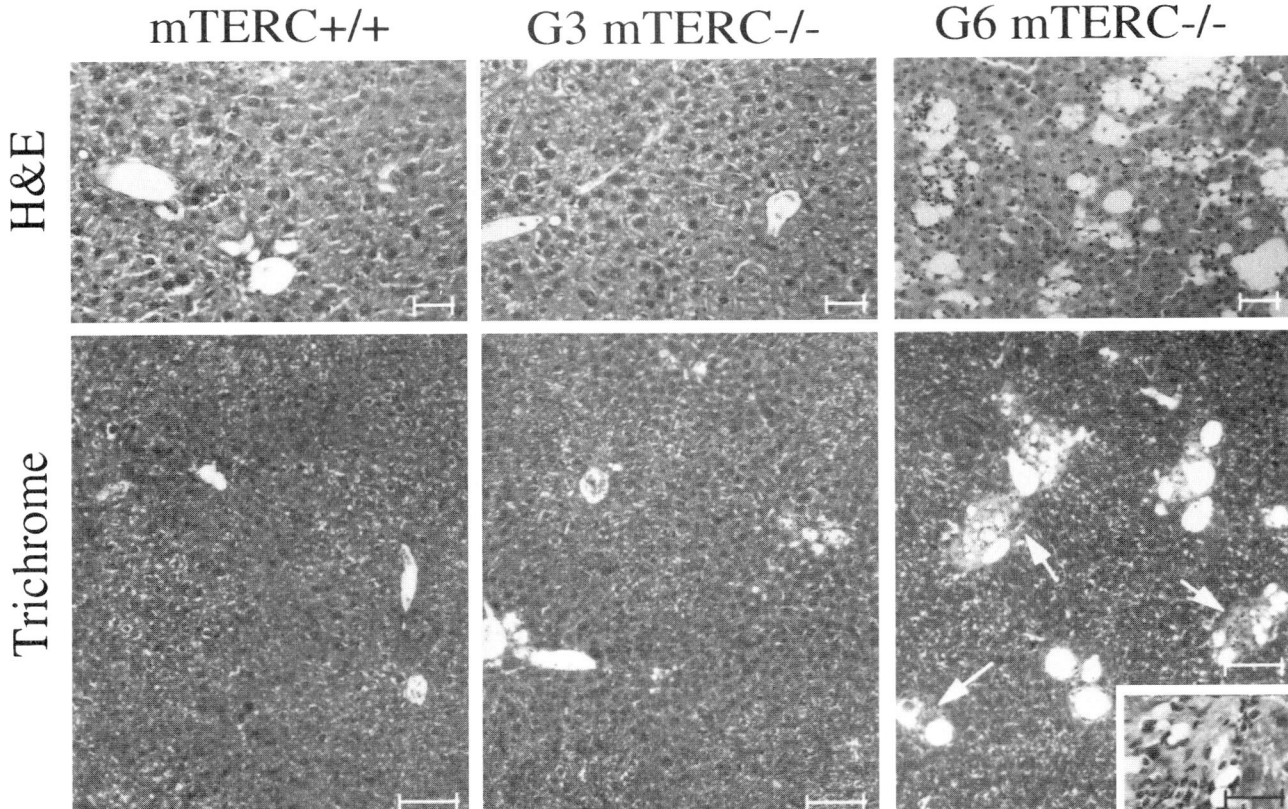

H&E

Trichrome

FIGURE 67.2. Telomere shortening in the essential telomerase RNA component (*mTERC–/–*) mice correlates with accelerated induction of liver cirrhosis by repeated CCl₄ injections. mTERC+/+ (telomerase activity, long telomeres), G3 mTERC–/– (no telomerase activity, intermediate telomere length), and G6 mTERC–/– mice (no telomerase activity, short telomeres) were treated with six intraperitoneal injections of CCl₄. No obvious liver damage was present in mice with long telomeres, but increased centrilobular fibrosis (*blue areas* in Trichrome stain, *bar:* 100 µm. **Inset:** *bar:* 50 µm) and steatosis [Hematoxilin–Eosin-stain (*H&E*), *bar:* 50 µm] were present in liver sections of mice with short telomeres. In addition, serum bilirubin levels were increased and serum albumin levels were decreased in mice with short telomeres. These features of accelerated cirrhosis were rescued in G6 mTERC–/– mice, which were pretreated with a telomerase-expressing adenovirus. (From Rudolph KL, Chang S, Millard M, et al. Inhibition of experimental liver cirrhosis in mice by telomerase gene delivery. *Science* 2000;287:1253–1258, with permission.) See Color Plate 24.

tion, anaphase bridges, increased hepatocyte apoptosis, and impaired liver regeneration. It remains speculative as to whether liberation of lipid peroxides (formed by dying hepatocytes) and/or activation of cell-cycle inhibitors such as TGF-β1 promote stellate cell activation and increased fibrosis in this model of accelerated cirrhosis development. Another, not mutually exclusive possibility is that telomere shortening alters the ability of cells to cope with various stresses (e.g., diminished oxidative stress capacity), possibly resulting in increased hepatocyte death. Moreover, these data imply that telomerase reactivation could eventually delay the progression of chronic high-turnover diseases, such as cirrhosis, a supposition that is now testable.

GENOMIC INSTABILITY, TELOMERASE, AND LIVER CANCER

The observations that the replicative potential of human cells is determined by their amount of telomeric DNA, and that the vast majority of human cancers express telomerase activity (27,61), have led to the hypothesis that the repression of telomerase activity in most somatic human tissues serves as a tumor suppressor mechanism. Investigation of mTERC–/– mice revealed that the effects of telomerase deficiency and telomere shortening on tumorigenesis *in vivo* are more complex. The reader is directed to several papers and reviews that detail this subject (53,61,88,

98–100). In brief, tumor suppression associated with the lack of telomerase and increased telomere dysfunction is governed largely by the integrity of p53-dependent DNA damage responses (98,99). While clearly in some settings it can serve as a barrier to cancer, in the setting of defective DNA-damage responses (p53−/−), telomere dysfunction actually promotes end-to-end fusions, increased genomic instability, and enhanced cancer initiation (98).

It is a matter of current debate whether telomere shortening induces genomic instability and cancer formation in humans, especially during aging or in the setting of high-turnover diseases. In hepatocellular cancer (HCC), a tight correlation between cirrhosis and cancer formation has long been recognized with over 80% of HCCs emerging from cirrhotic livers (101–103). The current hypothesis states that chronic inflammation, continuous cellular proliferation, and direct oncogenic action of viruses/toxins finally produce genetic lesions, which cause cellular transformation. Given the short telomere length in cirrhosis and HCC (82–84), it is also possible that telomere shortening itself participates in this transformation process by induction of genomic instability. In line with this hypothesis, a variety of studies revealed cytogenetic abnormalities in HCC, describing chromosomal losses as well as gains in virtually all cancers investigated (104–112). Nevertheless, it remains a point of debate whether karyotypic alterations represent a secondary event in genetically unstable cancer cells, or presage and directly promote tumorigenesis.

The other key aspect of human hepatocellular carcinoma is the frequent upregulation of telomerase in more than 80% of the cancers (113–121), which is consistent with high rates of telomerase reactivation in other human cancer types. These studies imply a prominent role for telomere maintenance in tumor progression, as opposed to the potential impact of telomere shortening on genomic insta-

bility and early stages of cancer development. To understand the dual role of telomerase in cancer initiation and progression (Fig. 67.3), it will be important to characterize at what time of cancer progression telomerase is activated and whether genomic instability induced by critical telomere shortening precedes telomerase reactivation and cancer growth. Several investigations have revealed a correlation between HCC progression and telomerase activity (120,121); that is, robust telomerase activity was found to be common in larger, moderate to poorly differentiated HCC as opposed to smaller, well-differentiated HCC. While these results suggest that telomerase reactivation occurs as a late event during hepatocarcinogenesis, there is also evidence for telomerase activity in precancerous hepatic lesions (118,119), such as large dysplastic nodules and hepatocellular adenoma. The frequent upregulation of the myc oncogene in hepatocarcinogenesis (122,123) and the role of myc in the activation of transcription of TERT (124,125) might explain the early detection of high levels of telomerase activity in some precancerous hepatic lesions.

PROSPECTS

The telomere hypothesis of liver cirrhosis provides a rational explanation for two prominent clinical features of cirrhosis: the decrease in hepatocyte proliferation following prolonged hepatocyte turnover and the irreversibility of cirrhosis. The studies using mTERC−/− mice provide strong genetic evidence for the concept that telomere shortening and associated dysfunction promotes the development of cirrhosis in the setting of chronic liver damage. It will be crucial to prove, however, that similar mechanisms are at work in the development of human cirrhosis. Along these lines, it will be important to elucidate whether telomerase

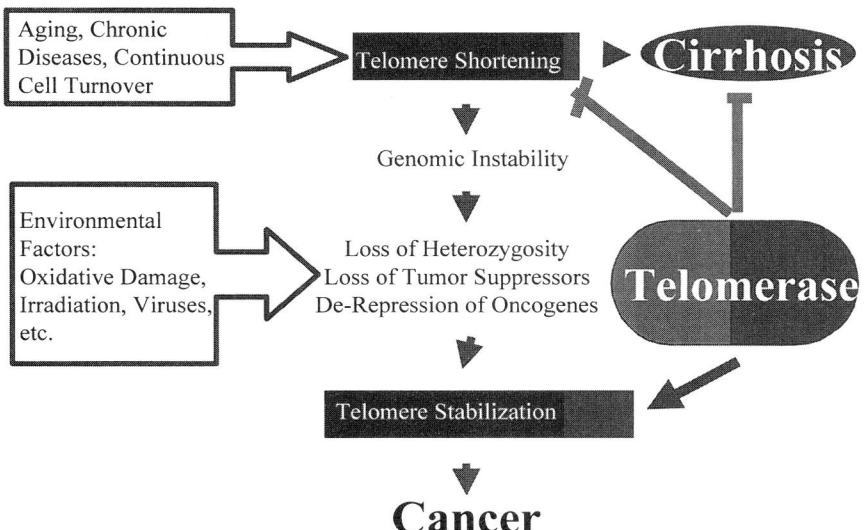

FIGURE 67.3. Telomerase may have a dual role in carcinogenesis. Restricted telomerase expression in somatic tissues will limit the growth of transformed cells to a certain number of cell doublings, thus inhibiting cancer growth. In contrast, telomere shortening in nontransformed cells as a function of cell turnover during aging and chronic diseases eventually fuels genomic instability. This instability in turn enhances the rate of genomic alterations required for cellular transformation. In the liver these complex relationships are evident. Hepatocellular carcinomas (HCCs) develop in over 80% in underlying cirrhosis, when telomeres are critically short indicating that telomere shortening and genomic instability might play a role in the initiation of HCC. In contrast, more than 80% of HCC have reactivated telomerase, supporting the hypothesis that telomere maintenance is required for cancer growth and progression.

expression and telomere maintenance can extend the lifespan of primary human hepatocytes in culture or improve hepatocyte transplantation efficiency *in vivo*. Another key aspect of future studies is to understand how telomere shortening signals hepatic growth arrest and whether telomere shortening induces genetic alterations involved in fibrogenesis. The studies of mTERC−/− mice suggest that telomerase gene delivery could potentially delay the progression of cirrhosis when telomeres become critically short. However, to evaluate the potential use of telomerase in the treatment of cirrhosis, it will be necessary to understand the consequences of telomerase in cancer initiation and progression. Since enforced telomerase expression could abrogate an important barrier to cancer in cirrhotic livers, development of HCC might be a limiting side effect of "telomerase therapy." On the other hand, it is also conceivable that early telomerase reactivation long before the onset of cirrhosis could prevent telomere dysfunction and genetic instability and thus diminish the rate of HCC development. The telomerase-deficient mouse should prove useful in exploring the effects of telomere shortening on tumor initiation as well as the necessity of telomere maintenance for tumor progression. Given the fact that cirrhosis is the seventh leading cause of death worldwide, and that the only potentially life saving treatment—liver transplantation—is unavailable for the majority of patients, a careful evaluation of telomerase treatment for cirrhosis should prove to be an active area of future investigation.

ACKNOWLEDGMENTS

We thank Drs. C. Harley, I. Arias, L. Chin, N. Sharpless, S. Chang, N. Bardesy, G. David, G. Morgan, M. Millard, D. Castrillon, S. Artandi, K. Wong, and M. Watabe for critical reading of the manuscript. Supported by Deutsche Forschungsgemeinschaft Grant Ru 745/1-1 (to K.L.R), and the Dana-Farber Cancer Institute (DFCI) Cancer Core Grant (to R.A.D.). R.A.D. is funded by National Institutes of Health (NIH) Grants (R01HD34880 and R01HD28317), an American Heart Association Grant-in-Aid, and the American Cancer Society.

REFERENCES

1. Friedman SL. The cellular basis of hepatic fibrosis. *N Engl J Med* 1983;328:1828-1835.
2. Williams EJ, Iredale JP. Liver cirrhosis. *Postgrad Med J* 1998;870:193–202.
3. Alcolado R, Arthur MJP, Iredale JP. Pathogenesis of liver fibrosis. *Clin Sci* 1997;92:103–112.
4. Karvountzis GG, Redeker AG, Peters RL. Long term followup studies of patients surviving fulminant viral hepatitis. *Gastroenterology* 1974;67:870–877.
5. Ashton RE, Millward-Sadler GH, White JE. Complications in methotrexate treatment of psoriasis with particular reference to liver fibrosis. *J Invest Dermatol* 1982;79:229–232.
6. Dahl MGC, Gregory MM, Scheuer PJ. Methotrexate hepatoxicity in psoriasis: comparison of different dose regimens. *Br Med J* 1972;1:654–656.
7. Millward-Sadler GH, Ryan TJ. Methotrexate induced liver disease in psoriasis. *Br J Dermatol* 1974;90:661–667.
8. Friedman SL. Stellate cell activation in alcoholic fibrosis—an overview. *Alcohol Clin Exp Res* 1999;23:904–910.
9. Delhaye M, Louis H, Degraef C, et al. Relationship between hepatocyte proliferative activity and liver functional reserve in human cirrhosis. *Hepatology* 1996;23:1003–1011.
10. Delhaye M, Louis H, Degraef C, et al. Hepatocyte proliferative activity in human liver cirrhosis. *J Hepatol* 1999;30:461–471.
11. Kaita KD, Pettigrew N, Minuk GY. Hepatic regeneration in humans with various liver disease as assessed by Ki-67 staining of formalin-fixed paraffin-embedded liver tissue. *Liver* 1997;17:13–16.
12. Rudi J, Waldherr R, Raedsch R, et al. Hepatocyte proliferation in primary biliary cirrhosis as assessed by proliferating cell nuclear antigen and Ki-67 antigen labeling. *J Hepatol* 1995;22:43–49.
13. Arthur MJ. Fibrosis and altered matrix degradation. *Digestion* 1998;59:376–380.
14. Friedman SL. Cellular networks in hepatic fibrosis. *Digestion* 1998;59:368–371.
15. Schuppan D, Cho JJ, Jia JD, et al. Interplay of matrix and myofibroblasts during hepatic fibrogenesis. *Curr Top Pathol* 1999;93:205–218.
16. Martinez-Hernandez A, Amenta PS. The hepatic extracellular matrix. II. Ontogenesis, regeneration and cirrhosis. *Virchows Arch A Pathol Anat Histopathol* 1993;423:77–84.
17. Fausto N, Mead JE, Gruppuso PA, et al. Effects of TGF-β in the liver: cell proliferation and fibrogenesis. *Ciba Found Symp* 1991;157:165–174.
18. Milani S, Herbst H, Schuppan D, et al. Transforming growth factors β 1 and β 2 are differentially expressed in fibrotic liver disease. *Am J Pathol* 1991;139:1221–1229.
19. Roulot D, Sevcsik AM, Coste T, et al. Role of transforming growth factor β type II receptor in hepatic fibrosis: studies of human chronic hepatitis C and experimental fibrosis in rats. *Hepatology* 1999;6:1730–1738.
20. Bedossa P, Peltier E, Terris B, et al. Transforming growth factor-β 1 (TGF-β 1) and TGF-β 1 receptors in normal, cirrhotic, and neoplastic human livers. *Hepatology* 1995;21:760–766.
21. Blackburn EH. Structure and function of telomeres. *Nature* 1991;350:569–573.
22. McElligott R, Wellinger RJ. The terminal DNA structure of mammalian chromosomes. *EMBO J* 1997;16:3705–3714.
23. van Steensel B, Smogorzewska A, de Lange T. TRF2 protects human telomeres from end-to-end fusions. *Cell* 1998;92:401–413.
24. Harley CB, Futcher AB, Greider CW. Telomeres shorten during ageing of human fibroblasts. *Nature* 1990;345:458–460.
25. Greider CW. Telomere length regulation. *Annu Rev Biochem* 1996;65:337–365.
26. Lingner J, Cooper JP, Cech TR. Telomerase and DNA end replication: No longer a lagging strand problem? *Science* 1995;269:1533–1534.
27. Kim NW, Piatyszek MA, Prowse KR, et al. Specific association of human telomerase activity with immortal cells and cancer. *Science* 1994;266:2011–2015.
28. Nakamura TM, Morin GB, Chapman KB, et al. Telomerase catalytic subunit homologs from fission yeast and human. *Science* 1997;277:955–959.
29. Meyerson M, Counter CM, Eaton EN, et al. hEST2, the puta-

tive human telomerase catalytic subunit gene, is up-regulated in tumor cells and during immortalization. *Cell* 1997;90:785–795.

30. Kolquist KA, Ellisen LW, Counter CM, et al. Expression of TERT in early premalignant lesions and a subset of cells in normal tissues. *Nat Genet* 1998;19:182–186.

31. Allsopp RC, Vaziri H, Patterson C, et al. Telomere length predicts replicative capacity of human fibroblasts. *Proc Natl Acad Sci USA* 1992;89:10114–10118.

32. Sedivy JM. Can ends justify the means? Telomeres and the mechanisms of replicative senescence and immortalization in mammalian cells. *Proc Natl Acad Sci USA* 1998;95:9078–9081.

33. Wright WE, Shay JW. The two-stage mechanism controlling cellular senescence and immortalization. *Exp Gerontol* 1992;27:383–389.

34. De Lange T. Telomeres and senescence: ending the debate. *Science* 1998;279:334–335.

35. Hayflick L, Moorhead PS. Serial cultivation of human diploid cell strains. *Exp Cell Res* 1961;25:585–621.

36. Bodnar AG, Ouellette M, Frolkis M, et al. Extension of lifespan by introduction of telomerase into normal human cells. *Science* 1998;279:349–352.

37. Yang J, Chang E, Cherry AM, et al. Human endothelial cell life extension by telomerase expression. *J Biol Chem* 1999;274:26141–26148.

38. Dickson MA, Hahn WC, Ino Y, et al. Human keratinocytes that express hTERT and also bypass a p16(INK4a)-enforced mechanism that limits life span become immortal yet retain normal growth and differentiation characteristics. *Mol Cell Biol* 2000;20:1436–1447.

39. Kiyono T, Foster SA, Koop JI, et al. Both Rb/p16INK4a inactivation and telomerase activity are required to immortalize human epithelial cells. *Nature* 1998;396:84–88.

40. Pommier JP, Gauthier L, Livartowski J, et al. Immunosenescence in HIV pathogenesis. *Virology* 1997;231:148–154.

41. Nichols WS, Schneider S, Chan RC, et al. Increased CD4+ T-lymphocyte senescence fraction in advanced human immunodeficiency virus type 1 infection. *Scand J Immunol* 1999;49:302–306.

42. Ohyashiki JH, Ohyashiki K, Fujimura T, et al. Telomere shortening associated with disease evolution patterns in myelodysplastic syndromes. *Cancer Res* 1994;54:3557–3560.

43. Ball SE, Gibson FM, Rizzo S, et al. Progressive telomere shortening in aplastic anemia. *Blood* 1998;91:3582–3592.

44. Lindsey J, McGill NI, Lindsey LA, et al. In vivo loss of telomeric repeats with age in humans. *Mutat Res* 1992;256:45–48.

45. Slagboom PE, Droog S, Boomsma DI. Genetic determination of telomere size in humans: a twin study of three age groups. *Am J Hum Genet* 1994;55:876–882.

46. Vaziri H, Schachter F, Uchida I, et al. Loss of telomeric DNA during aging of normal and trisomy 21 human lymphocytes. *Am J Hum Genet* 1993;52:661–667.

47. Vaziri H, Dragowska W, Allsopp RC, et al. Evidence for a mitotic clock in human hematopoietic stem cells: loss of telomeric DNA with age. *Proc Natl Acad Sci USA* 1994;91:9857–9860.

48. Allsopp RC, Chang E, Kashefi-Aazam M, et al. Telomere shortening is associated with cell division *in vitro* and *in vivo*. *Exp Cell Res* 1995;220:194–200.

49. Chang E, Harley CB. Telomere length and replicative aging in human vascular tissues. *Proc Natl Acad Sci USA* 1995;92:11190–11194.

50. Kveiborg M, Kassem M, Langdahl B, et al. Telomere shortening during aging of human osteoblasts *in vitro* and leukocytes *in vivo*: lack of excessive telomere loss in osteoporotic patients. *Mech Ageing Dev* 1999;106:261–271.

51. Mondello C, Petropoulou C, Monti D, et al. Telomere length in fibroblasts and blood cells from healthy centenarians. *Exp Cell Res* 1999;248:234–242.

52. Frenck RW Jr, Blackburn EH, Shannon KM. The rate of telomere sequence loss in human leukocytes varies with age. *Proc Natl Acad Sci USA* 1998;95:5607–5610.

53. Rudolph KL, Chang S, Lee HW, et al. Longevity, stress response, and cancer in aging telomerase-deficient mice. *Cell* 1999;96:701–712.

54. Herrera E, Samper E, Martin-Caballero et al. Disease states associated with telomere deficiency appear earlier in mice with short telomeres. *EMBO J* 1999;18:2950–2960.

55. Griffith JD, Comeau L, Rosenfield S, et al. Mammalian telomeres end in a large duplex loop. *Cell* 1999;97:503–514.

56. Vaziri H, Benchimol S. Alternative pathways for the extension of cellular life span: inactivation of p53/pRb and expression of telomerase. *Oncogene* 1999;18:7676–7680.

57. Reddel RR. Genes involved in the control of cellular proliferative potential. *Ann N Y Acad Sci* 1998;854:8–19.

58. Vaziri H, West MD, Allsopp RC, et al. ATM-dependent telomere loss in aging human diploid fibroblasts and DNA damage lead to the post-translational activation of p53 protein involving poly (ADP-ribose) polymerase. *EMBO J* 1997;16:6018–6033.

59. Shay JW, Pereira-Smith O, Wright WE. A role for both RB and p53 in the regulation of human cellular senescence. *Exp Cell Res* 1991;196:33–39.

60. Hara E, Tsurui H, Shinozaki A, et al. Cooperative effect of antisense-Rb and antisense-p53 oligomers on the extension of life span in human diploid fbroblasts, TIG-1. *Biochem Biophys Res Commun* 1991;179:528–534.

61. Artandi SE, DePinho RA. A critical role for telomeres in suppressing and facilitating carcinogenesis. *Curr Opin Genet Dev* 2000;10:39–46.

62. Bryan TM, Reddel RR. Telomere dynamics and telomerase activity in *in vitro* immortalised human cells. *Eur J Cancer* 1997;33:767–773.

63. Counter CM, Botelho FM, Wang P, et al. Stabilization of short telomeres and telomerase activity accompany immortalization of Epstein-Barr-virus-transformed human B lymphocytes. *J Virol* 1994;68:3410–3414.

64. Blackburn E. The telomere and telomerase: How do they interact? *Mt Sinai J Med* 1999;66:292–300.

65. Lingner J, Cech TR. Telomerase and chromosome end maintenance. *Curr Opin Genet Dev* 1998;8:226–232.

66. Nugent CI, Lundblad V. The telomerase reverse transcriptase: components and regulation. *Genes Dev* 1998;12:1073–1085.

67. Feng J, Funk WD, Wang SS, et al. The RNA component of human telomerase. *Science* 1995;269:1236–1241.

68. Harley CB. Human ageing and telomeres. *Ciba Found Symp* 1997;211:129–39; discussion 139–144.

69. Kono Y, Yang S, Letarte M, et al. Establishment of a human hepatocyte line derived from primary culture in a collagen gel sandwich system. *Exp Cell Res* 1995;221:478–485.

70. Ferrini JB, Pichard L, Domergue J, et al. Long-term cultures of adult human hepatocytes. *Chem Biol Interact* 1997;107:31–45.

71. Block GD, Locker J, Bowen WC, et al. Population expansion, clonal growth, and specific differentiation patterns in primary cultures of hepatocytes induced by HGF/SF, EGF and TGF α in a chemically defined (HGM) medium. *J Cell Biol* 1996;132:1133–1149.

72. Serrano M, Lin AW, McCurrach ME, et al. Oncogenic ras provokes premature cell senescence associated with accumulation of p53 and p16INK4a. *Cell* 1997;88:593–602.

73. Ridley AJ, Paterson HF, Noble M, et al. Ras-mediated cell cycle arrest is altered by nuclear oncogenes to induce Schwann cell transformation. *EMBO J* 1988;7:1635–1645.

74. de Lange T, DePinho RA. Unlimited mileage from telomerase? *Science* 1999;283:947–949.

75. Gibson-D'Ambrosio RE, Crowe DL, Shuler CE, et al. The establishment and continuous subculturing of normal human adult hepatocytes: expression of differentiated liver functions. *Cell Biol Toxicol* 1993;9:385–403.

76. Hino H, Tateno C, Sato H, et al. A long-term culture of human hepatocytes which show a high growth potential and express their differentiated phenotypes. *Biochem Biophys Res Commun* 1999;256:184–191.

77. Liao WS, Ma KT, Woodworth CD, et al. Stimulation of the acute-phase response in simian virus 40-hepatocyte cell lines. *Mol Cell Biol* 1989;9:2779–2786.

78. Kobayashi N, Fujiwara T, Westerman K, et al. Prevention of acute liver failure in rats with reversibly immortalized human hepatocytes. *Science* 2000;287:1258–1262.

79. Overturf K, al-Dhalimy M, Ou CN, et al. Serial transplantation reveals the stem-cell-like regenerative potential of adult mouse hepatocytes. *Am J Pathol* 1997;151:1273–1280.

80. Kipling D, Cooke HJ. Hypervariable ultra-long telomeres in mice. *Nature* 1990;347:400–402.

81. Zijlmans JM, Martens UM, Poon SS, et al. Telomeres in the mouse have large inter-chromosomal variations in the number of T2AG3 repeats. *Proc Natl Acad Sci USA* 1997;94:7423–7428.

82. Kitada T, Seki S, Kawakita N, et al. Telomere shortening in chronic liver diseases. *Biochem Biophys Res Commun* 1995;211:33–39.

83. Miura N, Horikawa I, Nishimoto A, et al. Progressive telomere shortening and telomerase reactivation during hepatocellular carcinogenesis. *Cancer Genet Cytogenet* 1997;93:56–62.

84. Urabe Y, Nouso K, Higashi T, et al. Telomere length in human liver diseases. *Liver* 1996;16:293–297.

85. Livni N, Eid A, Ilan Y, et al. p53 expression in patients with cirrhosis with and without hepatocellular carcinoma. *Cancer* 1995;75:2420–2426.

86. Albrecht JH, Meyer AH, Hu MY. Regulation of cyclin-dependent kinase inhibitor p21(WAF1/Cip1/Sdi1) gene expression in hepatic regeneration. *Hepatology* 1997;25:557–563.

87. Lee RG, Tsamandas AC, Demetris AJ. Large cell change (liver cell dysplasia) and hepatocellular carcinoma in cirrhosis: matched case-control study, pathological analysis, and pathogenetic hypothesis. *Hepatology* 1997;26:1415–1422.

88. Blasco MA, Lee HW, Hande MP, et al. Telomere shortening and tumor formation by mouse cells lacking telomerase RNA. *Cell* 1997;91:25–34.

89. Lee HW, Blasco MA, Gottlieb GJ, et al. Essential role of mouse telomerase in highly proliferative organs. *Nature* 1998;392:569–574.

90. Rudolph KL, Chang S, Millard M, et al. Inhibition of experimental liver cirrhosis in mice by telomerase gene delivery. *Science* 2000;287:1253–1258.

91. Heckel JL, Sandgren EP, Degen JL, et al. Neonatal bleeding in transgenic mice expressing urokinase-type plasminogen activator. *Cell* 1990;62:447–456.

92. Sandgren EP, Palmiter RD, Heckel JL, et al. Complete hepatic regeneration after somatic deletion of an albumin-plasminogen activator transgene. *Cell* 1991;66:245–256.

93. Diehl AM, Rai RM. Liver regeneration 3: Regulation of signal transduction during liver regeneration. *FASEB J* 1996;10:215–227.

94. Rudolph KL, Trautwein C, Kubicka S, et al. Differential regulation of extracellular matrix synthesis during liver regeneration after partial hepatectomy in rats. *Hepatology* 1999;30:1159–1166.

95. McClintock B. The stability of broken ends of chromosomes in Zea mays. *Genetics* 1941;26:234–282.

96. Kirk KE, Harmon BP, Reichardt IK, et al. Block in anaphase chromosome separation caused by a telomerase template mutation. *Science* 1997;275:1478–1481.

97. Tamayo RP. Is cirrhosis of the liver experimentally produced by CCl$_4$ an adequate model of human cirrhosis? *Hepatology* 1983;3:112–120.

98. Chin L, Artandi SE, Shen Q, et al. p53 deficiency rescues the adverse effects of telomere loss and cooperates with telomere dysfunction to accelerate carcinogenesis. *Cell* 1999;97:527–538.

99. Greenberg RA, Chin L, Femino A, et al. Short dysfunctional telomeres impair tumorigenesis in the INK4a δ cancer-prone mouse. *Cell* 1999;97:515–525.

100. de Lange T, Jacks T. For better or worse? Telomerase inhibition and cancer. *Cell* 1999;98:273–275.

101. Curry GW, Beattie AD. Pathogenesis of primary hepatocellular carcinoma. *Eur J Gastroenterol Hepatol* 1996;8:850–855.

102. Chung RT, Jaffe DL, Friedman LS. Complications of chronic liver disease. *Crit Care Clin* 1995;11:431–463.

103. Kew MC, Popper H. Relationship between hepatocellular carcinoma and cirrhosis. *Semin Liver Dis* 1984;4:136–146.

104. Tsuda H, Oda T, Sakamoto M, et al. Different pattern of chromosomal allele loss in multiple hepatocellular carcinomas as evidence of their multifocal origin. *Cancer Res* 1992;52:1504–1509.

105. Nasarek A, Werner M, Nolte M, et al. Trisomy 1 and 8 occur frequently in hepatocellular carcinoma but not in liver cell adenoma and focal nodular hyperplasia. A fluorescence in situ hybridization study. *Virchows Arch* 1995;427:373–378.

106. Kuroki T, Fujiwara Y, Tsuchiya E, et al. Accumulation of genetic changes during development and progression of hepatocellular carcinoma: loss of heterozygosity of chromosome arm 1p occurs at an early stage of hepatocarcinogenesis. *Genes Chromosomes Cancer* 1995;13:163–167.

107. Marchio A, Meddeb M, Pineau P, et al. Recurrent chromosomal abnormalities in hepatocellular carcinoma detected by comparative genomic hybridization. *Genes Chromosomes Cancer* 1997;18:59–65.

108. Zimmermann U, Feneux D, Mathey G, et al. Chromosomal aberrations in hepatocellular carcinomas: relationship with pathological features. *Hepatology* 1997;26:1492–1498.

109. Lin YW, Sheu JC, Huang GT, et al. Chromosomal abnormality in hepatocellular carcinoma by comparative genomic hybridisation in Taiwan. *Eur J Cancer* 1999;35:652–658.

110. Huang SF, Hsu HC, Fletcher JA. Investigation of chromosomal aberrations in hepatocellular carcinoma by fluorescence in situ hybridization. *Cancer Genet Cytogenet* 1999;111:21–27.

111. Keck CL, Zimonjic DB, Yuan BZ, et al. Nonrandom breakpoints of unbalanced chromosome translocations in human hepatocellular carcinoma cell lines. *Cancer Genet Cytogenet* 1999;111:37–44.

112. Guo L, Xiao S, Guo Y. [The correlation between t(14;18) chromosomal translocation and hepatocarcinoma]. *Chung Hua I Hsueh I Chuan Hsueh Tsa Chih* 1999;16:164–166.

113. Erlitzki R, Minuk GY. Telomeres, telomerase and HCC: the long and the short of it. *J Hepatol* 1999;31:939–945.

114. Nouso K, Urabe Y, Higashi T, et al. Telomerase as a tool for the differential diagnosis of human hepatocellular carcinoma. *Cancer* 1996;78:232–236.

115. Tahara H, Nakanishi T, Kitamoto M, et al. Telomerase activity in human liver tissues: comparison between chronic liver disease and hepatocellular carcinomas. *Cancer Res* 1995;55:2734–2736.

116. Nakayama J, Tahara H, Tahara E, et al. Telomerase activation by hTRT in human normal fibroblasts and hepatocellular carcinomas. *Nat Genet* 1998;18:65–68.

117. Nagao K, Tomimatsu M, Endo H, et al. Telomerase reverse transcriptase mRNA expression and telomerase activity in hepatocellular carcinoma. *J Gastroenterol* 1999;34:83–87.

118. Nishimoto A, Miura N, Oshimura M. [Clinical significance of telomerase activity in precancerous lesion of the liver]. *Nippon Rinsho* 1998;56:1244–1247.

119. Hytiroglou P, Kotoula V, Thung SN, et al. Telomerase activity in precancerous hepatic nodules. *Cancer* 1998;82:1831–1838.

120. Kanamaru T, Yamamoto M, Morita Y, et al. Clinical implications of telomerase activity in resected hepatocellular carcinoma. *Int J Mol Med* 1999;4:267–271.

121. Nakashio R, Kitamoto M, Nakanishi T, et al. [Telomere length and telomerase activity in hepatocellular carcinoma]. *Nippon Rinsho* 1998;56:1239–1243.

122. Himeno Y, Fukuda Y, Hatanaka M, et al. Expression of oncogenes in human liver disease. *Liver* 1988;8:208–212.

123. Tiniakos D, Spandidos DA, Kakkanas A, et al. Expression of ras and myc oncogenes in human hepatocellular carcinoma and non-neoplastic liver tissues. *Anticancer Res* 1989;9:715–721.

124. Wang J, Xie LY, Allan S, et al. Myc activates telomerase. *Genes Dev* 1998;12:1769–1774.

125. Greenberg RA, O'Hagan RC, Deng H, et al. Telomerase reverse transcriptase gene is a direct target of c-Myc but is not functionally equivalent in cellular transformation. *Oncogene* 1999; 18:1219–1226.

The Liver: Biology and Pathobiology, Fourth Edition, edited by I. M. Arias, J. L. Boyer, F. V. Chisari, N. Fausto, D. Schachter, and D. A. Shafritz. Lippincott Williams & Wilkins, Philadelphia © 2001.

MECHANISM(S) OF HEPATOCARCINOGENESIS: INSIGHT FROM TRANSGENIC MOUSE MODELS

SNORRI S. THORGEIRSSON

During the last two decades, important advances have been made in research on the mechanisms of hepatocarcinogenesis by employing transgenic animals, including transgene overexpression and more recently gene knockout techniques. Both these approaches have been extremely valuable and important in defining *in vivo* the role and impact of genes thought to either favor or suppress normal and neoplastic cell growth. Applying these methodologies it is possible to generate animal models to dissect out genetic alterations associated with different stages of neoplastic development, and it is also possible to assess the impact of environmental risk factors.

Human hepatocellular carcinoma (HCC) is one of the most common cancers worldwide with an estimated 0.25 to 1 million newly diagnosed cases each year (1). In addition, the survival rate is less than 3% over 5 years, which reflects

limited and rather ineffective treatment. A serious, and perhaps the major, problem for both treatment and prognostic evaluation of HCC is the incomplete understanding of the molecular basis for the pathogenesis of this tumor. It is therefore appropriate at this time to ask whether the transgenic mouse models of liver cancer have yielded information that is useful for a better understanding of the pathogenesis of human liver cancer.

In this review, data from transgenic mouse models that examine the interaction of c-myc and transforming growth factor (TGF)-α in liver carcinogenesis will be used to analyze the possible usefulness of these models for understanding human liver cancer. Hepatic transgene expression has traditionally been achieved by targeting hepatocytes with constitutive or inducible gene regulatory sequences expressed in these cells. This subject has been extensively reviewed (2). For a more comprehensive discussion of transgenic and knockout mouse models used in studying experimental liver carcinogenesis, the reader is referred to a recent review of this topic (5).

S. S. Thorgeirsson: Laboratory of Experimental Carcinogenesis, National Cancer Institute, National Institutes of Health, Bethesda, Maryland 20892-4255.

ETIOLOGY OF HUMAN HEPATOCELLULAR CARCINOMA

The most important risk factors associated with the development of HCC are chronic infections with hepatitis B virus (HBV) and/or hepatitis C virus (HCV) (see Chapters 53–55). Chemical carcinogens are also known to be associated with HCC. Perhaps the best known of the potential and known human liver carcinogens is aflatoxin B1 (AFB1), which forms adducts with DNA and protein, and causes mutation of the p53 codon 249 (6). Alcohol, and in particular alcoholic cirrhosis, are also important risk factors for HCC, although it is still uncertain whether alcohol is a complete hepatocarcinogen (7). In fact, cirrhosis associated with chronic liver disease (CLD) is one of the most important risk factors for development of HCC. Whether this is due to errors made during DNA replication, or DNA damage that may originate from immune responses or alcohol that give rise to elevated levels of reactive oxygen intermediates (ROI), which are mutagenic (8), has not been clarified. There is, however, evidence that HCC may develop from hepatic adenomas, and once the tumor forms, its morphology gradually shifts from a more- to a less-differentiated phenotype (9). What appears to be common to all the major risk factors of human HCC is the capacity to induce a substantial and sustained increase in the proliferation of a fraction of hepatocytes, leading to the development of multiple hepatocyte populations, many of which may be monoclonal (10). Expansion of these monoclonal populations that frequently display altered phenotypes may therefore afford the opportunity to accumulate genetic alterations that eventually result in the development of HCC.

INTERACTION OF C-MYC AND TRANSFORMING GROWTH FACTOR-α IN LIVER CARCINOGENESIS

In light of the central role that the proto-oncogene c-myc plays in cell replication, differentiation and apoptosis, it is not surprising that aberrant expression of c-myc has been implicated in a wide variety of both experimentally induced and naturally occurring tumors (12) including HCC (13–15). In addition, c-myc is frequently found to be coexpressed with TGF-α, a ligand for the epidermal growth factor receptor (EGFR) tyrosine kinase, in human tumors including HCC (16), suggesting that their interaction may represent a critical step in malignant growth. Indeed, data from *in vitro* experiments suggest that c-myc overexpression may sensitize clonally derived liver epithelial cells to the TGF-α/EGFR autocrine growth signaling, thereby favoring malignant transformation, once c-myc and TGF-α are coexpressed in these cells (17). Consistent with these observations, the preneoplastic phase in c-myc/TGF-α mice is characterized by uniform expression of the c-myc transgene in the liver, while TGF-α is predominantly expressed in perivascular dysplastic regions, basophilic foci, and single cells in clear-cell foci, concomitant with high proliferating cell nuclear antigen index labeling in all these areas (18,19). In addition, tumors in both c-myc and c-myc/TGF-α mice display overexpression of both the TGF-α transgene and of the endogenous TGF-α and c-myc genes. However, EGFR expression is mostly unchanged or diminished compared with nontumorous tissues and control livers (19).

Takagi et al. (20) also showed induction of the TGF-α transgene and in tumors of TGF-α single-transgenic mice, while Sandgren et al. (21) demonstrated overexpression of both transgenes in tumors of their c-myc/TGF-α mice. Expression of EGFR is unchanged in both these transgenic models (20–22). Taken together, these observations emphasize the collaborative role of c-myc and TGF-α in promoting a selective growth advantage to liver tumor cells. Also, the data suggest that one of the mechanisms by which c-myc can promote oncogenic transformation via TGF-α/EGFR autocrine signaling may simply be the induction of TGF-α ligand. TGF-α, in turn, is able to amplify this loop, as suggested by the overexpression of c-myc in TGF-α and c-myc/TGF-α mice.

SEQUENTIAL CHANGES DURING C-MYC/TRANSFORMING GROWTH FACTOR-α INDUCED HEPATOCARCINOGENESIS

There are essentially two theories that have been proposed to explain carcinogenesis; the somatic mutation theory, and tissue organization field theory. The evidence accumulated over the last two decades appears to support the validity of the somatic mutation theory. It is therefore generally accepted that neoplastic development is a multistep process in which the steps represent gene mutations or epigenetic changes such as methylation, leading to either activation of a dominant oncogene or inactivation of a tumor suppressor. These mutations appear to occur in a time-dependent sequence that constitutes a genetic pathway characteristic for a particular cancer (23). Furthermore, the precursor lesions and subsequent histological features characteristic of neoplastic development culminating in a malignant tumor are posited to be the phenotypic reflections of the genetic pathway. Indeed, the molecular pathology of and the proposed genetic pathway in colorectal cancer appear to strongly support the somatic mutation theory of cancer development (23,24). These observations have highlighted the importance of establishing, in an experimental carcinogenesis model, a well defined histological feature for each step in the neoplastic process.

In light of the dominance of the somatic mutation theory in current cancer research, is it time to completely abandon the tissue organization field theory of carcinogenesis? This theory basically states that carcinogens disrupt the flow of information between the stroma and the parenchyma and/or among cells within those tissues. Consequently, although the effect of carcinogens on the intracellular structures is deleterious, it is not directly responsible for the development of neoplasia (25,26). The central tenet of the theory is that neoplastic development may occur entirely via incipient phenomena once the signals that maintain normal tissue organization are disrupted. While it is certainly true that development of cancer always disrupts the structure of the tissue in which it develops, it is equally true that mutations and/or methylation changes are central characteristics of the early (pre)neoplastic cell populations. Nevertheless, the issue of disruption of tissue environment is particularly important in viral-induced liver cancer. Both HBV and HCV induce drastic changes in the tissue environment of the liver (inflammatory reaction, cell death, regeneration, fibrosis, and development of cirrhosis) prior to the appearance of neoplastic lesions (27). It is therefore possible that the mutational events, as well as chromosomal aberrations observed in liver cancer, are sec-

ondary events to the "tissue disruption" caused by, in this case, HBV or HCV. In any event, even under these conditions, the validity and the importance of the genetic pathway concept in neoplastic development would not be diminished.

HISTOLOGICAL LESIONS DURING LIVER CARCINOGENESIS IN C-MYC/TRANSFORMING GROWTH FACTOR-α MICE

The incidence and time course of the major morphological changes observed in c-myc/TGF-α mice are summarized in Figure 68.1. The sequence of these morphological changes proceeds via early dysplastic and focal lesions to benign hepatocellular adenoma (HCA) and finally hepatocellular carcinoma (HCC). This chain of events is very similar to that seen during chemically induced liver cancer in mice, suggesting that this transgenic mouse model (5) may portray events common in the neoplastic development of the liver induced by a variety of etiological agents. Since the

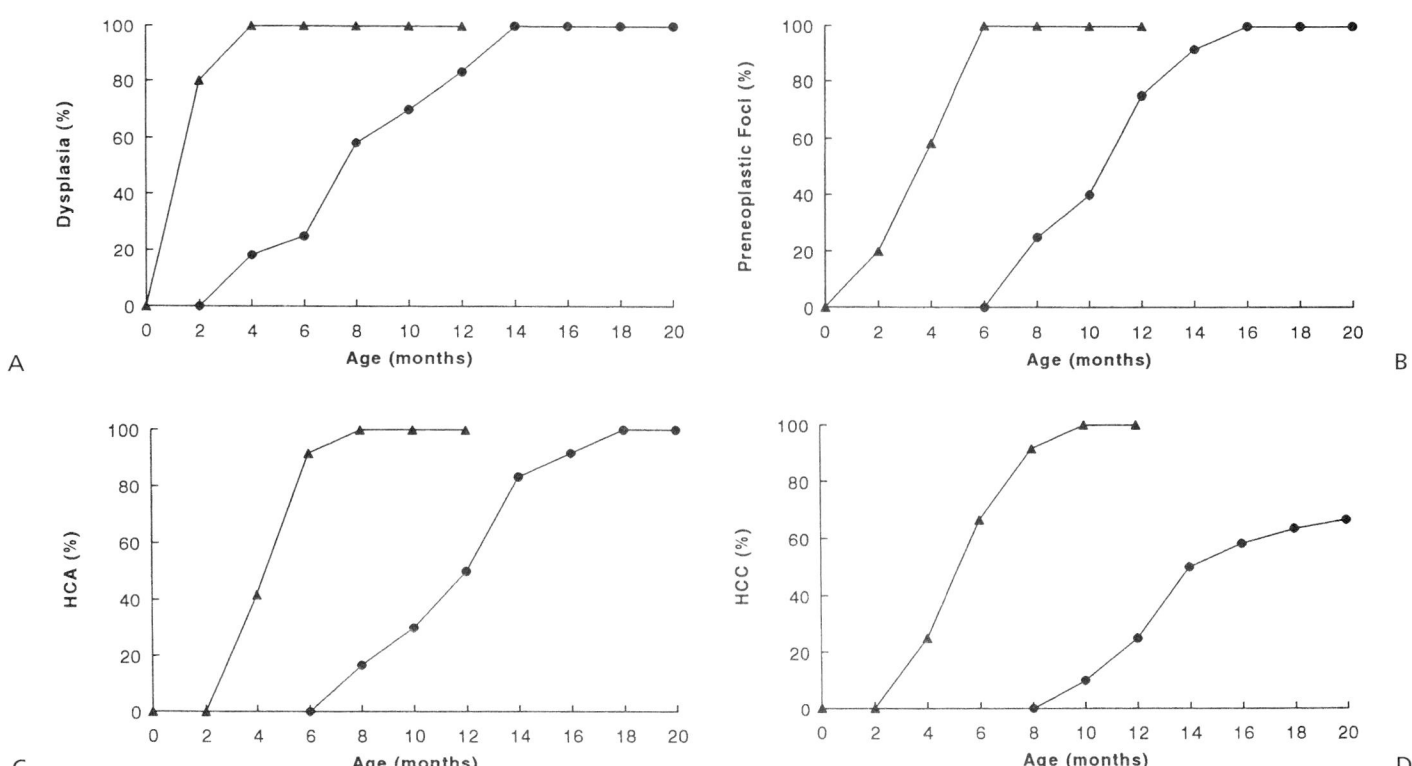

FIGURE 68.1. Incidence and time course of hepatic lesions in c-myc (*circles*) and c-myc/transforming growth factor (TGF)-α (*triangles*) transgenic mice. **A:** Dysplasia. **B:** Preneoplastic foci. **C:** Hepatocellular adenoma (*HCA*). **D:** Hepatocellular carcinoma (*HCC*). Values are percentages of animals affected at each time. (From Santoni-Rugiu E, Nagy P, Jensen MR, et al. Evolution of neoplastic development in the liver of transgenic mice coexpressing c-*myc* and transforming growth factor-α. *Am J Pathol* 1996;149:407–428, with permission.)

c-myc/TGF-α model offers a rare opportunity to examine the early stages during liver carcinogenesis, considerable effort has been devoted to characterize these events (18,19,29,30–32). Most of the remainder of this review is devoted to discussing these early events and the potential relevance of these conditions for cellular and molecular aspects of human liver carcinogenesis.

LIVER CELL DYSPLASIA: AN EARLY EVENT IN HEPATOCARCINOGENESIS

The earliest and indeed the primary effect of overexpressing c-myc and TGF-α either alone or together in the liver is to induce continuous proliferation of the hepatocytes and thereby disrupt the normal process of the gradual mitogenic silencing of the liver that occurs during the first few weeks of life (19) (see Chapter 2). The earliest morphological consequence of forcing continuous replication of hepatocytes via the c-myc/TGF-α transgenes is the appearance of perivascular dysplastic hepatocytes prior to the emergence of preneoplastic lesions (18,19) (Fig. 68.2). These lesions then expand rapidly into the hepatic lobules and the central veins by the second month of age and accompany thereafter the development of neoplastic lesions (19).

Liver cell dysplasia (LCD) was first described by Anthony, Vogel, and Barker (1973) as cellular and nuclear pleomorphism and enlargement, multinucleation, hyperchromatism, and prominent nucleoli of human cells in cirrhotic nodules. Anthony et al. (33) further proposed a progression from cirrhosis to LCD and ultimately to HCC, considering LCD a premalignant condition because it was associated with increased risk of HCC. Since the original observations by Anthony et al. (1973), a number of studies have attempted to more precisely define the role of dysplasia in human HCC (34–38). Although morphometric studies have resulted in subdivision of dysplastic cells into large and small types, it has been difficult to determine which one is the preferred tumor precursor (39,40). This is perhaps not surprising as the differentiation of high-grade dysplasia from neoplastic lesions is admittedly difficult and still based on arbitrary morphological criteria without the support of molecular genetic analysis (41).

Occurrence of hepatic dysplasia resembling the one originally described by Anthony et al. (1973) in the human liver is a common characteristic of early stages in hepatocarcinogenesis seen in a number of transgenic models. Although the extent and severity of the dysplastic lesions may differ, transgenic mice in which the c-myc, TGF-α, mutated H-*ras*, HBsAg, HBx gene, and especially the SV40 Large T antigen (SV40Tag) are targeted to the liver, all show early signs of hepatic dysplasia (21,42–46). Data obtained in transgenic mice harboring liver-specific expression of SV40Tag have resulted in two major proposals for the cell kinetics that provoke the multistep process culminating in

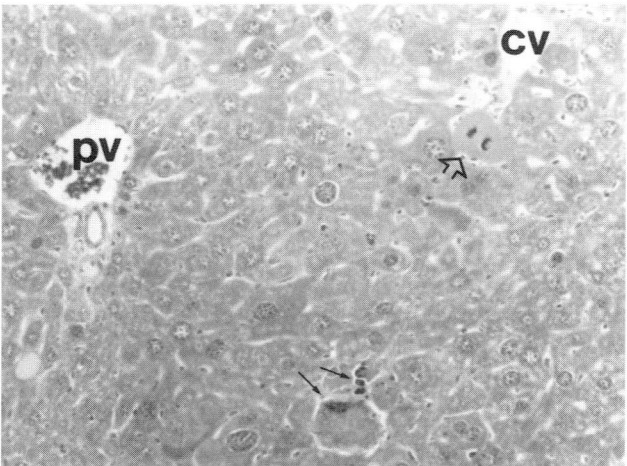

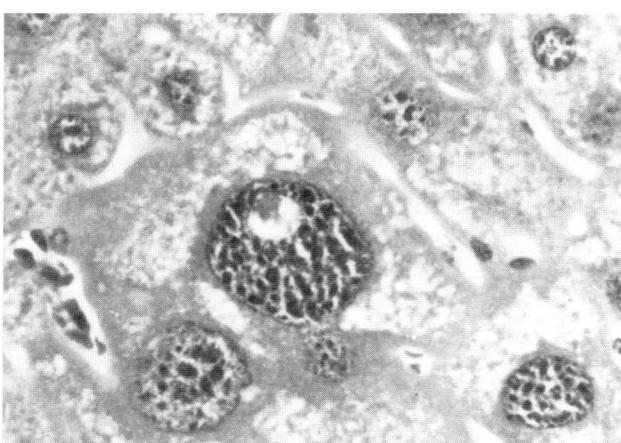

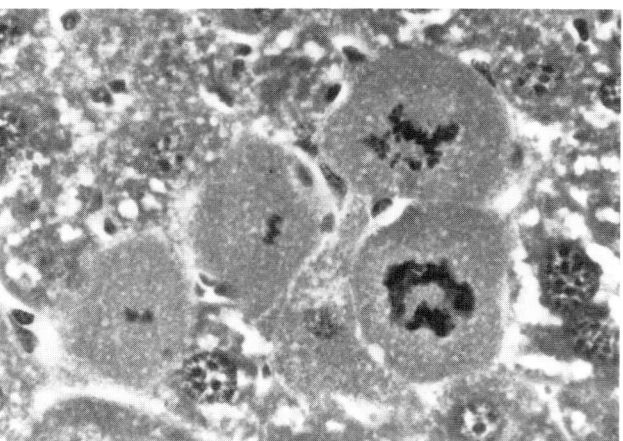

FIGURE 68.2. Patterns of dysplastic lesions in c-myc/transforming growth factor (TGF)-α transgenic mice. **A:** widespread liver dysplasia in a 2-month-old male animal. Some dysplastic hepatocytes are undergoing apoptosis (*thin arrow*) or mitosis (*open arrow*). *pv*, portal vein; *cv*, central vein. **B:** typical large dysplastic hepatocyte characterized by cellular and nuclear pleomorphism and hypertrophy, multiple prominent nucleoli, and nuclear pseudoinclusions. **C:** atypical mitosis in dysplastic hepatocytes. H&E; original magnification, ×150 (**A**), ×2000 (**B**), and (**C**). (From Santoni-Rugiu E, Nagy P, Jensen MR, et al. Evolution of neoplastic development in the liver of transgenic mice co-expressing c-*myc* and transforming growth factor-α. *Am J Pathol* 1996;149:407–428, with permission.)

tumor formation. Sepulveda et al. (46), using transgenic mice in which the regulatory elements of the human α-1-antitrypsin gene was used to control the expression of the SV40Tag, described the kinetics consisting of four distinct stages: (a) embryonal/fetal stage, no recognizable histological changes; (b) newborn to 2 weeks of age, hyperplastic hepatocytes with reduced amounts of cytoplasm but no nuclear alterations; (c) between 3 and 8 weeks of age, diffuse liver cell dysplasia without observable tumor nodules; and (d) 8 weeks of age and older, formation of HCCs in a background of liver dysplasia. Highly proliferative large and small cells with normal or increased nuclear/cytoplasmic ratios, respectively, constituted the population of dysplastic hepatocytes in this transgenic model. In contrast, Schirmacher et al. (47), employing the major urinary protein (MUP) gene promoter to direct the expression of the SV40Tag to the liver, described a step-wise progression towards HCC formation involving (a) early large cell-type dysplasia with abnormal mitoses, resulting in apoptotic cell death of most and possibly all of the original hepatocyte population, and (b) appearance and expansion of periportal transitional hepatocytes leading to multifocal hyperplasia and formation of hepatic tumors. The step-wise progression leading to HCCs in the c-myc/TGF-α mice is quite similar to that seen in the MUP-SV40Tag transgenic mice, in particular, the early appearance of the dysplastic hepatocytes prior to disruption of the liver structure or any morphological evidence (e.g., foci and nodules) of preneoplastic lesions. Also, the extensive proliferation and the frequent apoptotic death of these dysplastic hepatocytes at early stages of the neoplastic process are strikingly similar. The SV40Tag is expressed at high levels in the dysplastic hepatocytes in the MUP-SV40Tag mice, and may cause the apoptotic death in these cells by inducing abnormal DNA replication via interaction with both Rb and p53 proteins (47). In the c-myc/TGF-α mice, the dysplastic hepatocytes, particularly those located pericentrally, expressed the highest level of the TGF-α transgene, whereas the expression of c-myc transgene was not selectively increased in these cells. In addition, the dysplastic hepatocytes also expressed high levels of TGF-β1 and uPA transcripts and proteins. Upregulation of TGF-β1 has been reported in human and experimentally induced HCCs (48–52). The question of whether generation of initiated cell population would occur in the liver during the early dysplastic phase in c-myc/TGF-α mice was addressed by Santon-Rugui et al. (19). The results from the transplantation of the dysplastic liver pieces onto nude mice demonstrated that livers containing the combination of dysplasia and the apparent vascular invasion yielded more tumors than those having only dysplastic lesions (Table 68.1). All the tumors derived from the transplanted liver were trabecular hepatocellular carcinomas composed almost entirely of small diploid cells considerably different from the large dysplastic cells. Despite the low number of donors, the conclusion that can be drawn from these experiments is that the initiated cell population is generated during the early dysplastic stage of the neoplastic process. Furthermore, the data suggest that the initiated cell population may be able to progress to hepatocellular carcinomas without going through focal and nodular stages. Although the nature and derivation of the initiated cell population have still not been defined, it seems unlikely that the large dysplastic hepatocytes, including those displaying vascular invasion, are the precursors. These cells are extremely vulnerable to apoptosis and account for almost all apoptotic cells in the transgenic livers (53).

MECHANISM OF LIVER DYSPLASIA IN C-MYC/TRANSFORMING GROWTH FACTOR-α TRANSGENIC MICE

The close association of dysplasia and development of liver tumors in a number of different transgenic mouse models that all have chronic nontoxic stimulation of hepatocyte replication in common provides important clues to the cellular and molecular bases of the neoplastic process in this organ. Hepatic dysplasia presented as nuclear pleomor-

TABLE 68.1. TRANSPLANTATION OF DYSPLASTIC LIVER TISSUE INTO NUDE MICE

Histological Diagnosis in Donors	Number of Donors[a]	Age of Donors (mo)	Number of Recipients with Tumors	Number of Tumors in Recipient/Number of Transplanted Pieces
Dysplasia without vascular invasion	4	1.5	1/4 (25%)	2/12 (17%)
Dysplasia with vascular invasion	5	2.5	3/5 (60%)	5/12 (42%)
				2/6 (33%)
				6/8 (75%)
Dysplasia with carcinoma	1	5.0	1/1 (100%)	9/10 (90%)

[a]Six to 12 pieces from each transgenic liver were transplanted.
From Santoni-Rugin E, Nagy P, Jensen MR, et al. Evolution of neoplastic development in the liver of transgenic mice co-expressing c-myc and transforming growth factor-α. *Am J Pathol* 1996;149:407–428, with permission.

phism, multiple nucleoli, and the presence of abnormal mitotic figures is the manifestation of an abnormal cell cycle progression of the hepatocytes. The facts that SV40Tag is an effective inducer of tumors in a variety of tissues in transgenic mice, and that the same type of progression to neoplasia occurs in different types of tissues, are almost certainly due to a powerful disruption of Rb and p53 functions leading to proliferation and genomic instability, respectively (54). In contrast, neither TGF-α nor c-myc have the same capacity as SV40Tag to transform a wide variety of cell types in the transgenic mouse models. It is therefore possible, despite a type of progression similar to that of hepatic neoplasia seen in the SV40Tag and c-myc/TGF-α mice, that the molecular mechanisms responsible for neoplastic development in these two transgenic models may differ. A possible explanation may have to do with the DNA repair capacity of mouse hepatocytes. The only pathology detected in mice with DNA repair gene (ERCC-1) deficiency is in the liver (55). The livers of ERCC-1 knockout mice were populated by dysplastic hepatocytes characterized by increased nuclear size and varying degrees of polyploidy and aneuploidy, and the mice died of liver failure before weaning (55). Since the liver was the only organ affected in these DNA repair-deficient mice at a time when most organs, including the liver, are rapidly growing, it seems that proliferating hepatocytes are subjected to high levels of endogenous DNA damage. It is therefore reasonable to hypothesize that a possible mechanism for the genesis of the large dysplastic hepatocytes in c-myc/TGF-α mice may be due to a functional deficiency of hepatic DNA repair as a consequence of a chronic proliferative stimulus induced by the transgenes. The widespread and prolonged liver dysplasia seen in these mice is consistent with this view. Also, a similar mechanism has been proposed for the MUP promoter/SV40Tag transgenic mice, where the transgene overexpression in the original hepatocyte population induces multiple rounds of DNA replication without normal cytokinesis, resulting in the formation of giant nucleated cells undergoing apoptosis (47). Studies in human liver have also indicated the large dysplastic cells as the product of an abnormal or altered liver regeneration, and the small dysplastic cell population (with a high nuclear:cytoplasmic ratio similar to liver cancer cells) as a more likely candidate for the pretumorous cell type in the liver (39,40). It is important to note regarding this point that both the SV40Tag (46,47) and the c-myc/TGF-α transgenic models, and to a lesser extent the c-myc mice, display, after the formation of large dysplastic cells, the emergence of a population of small cells. In the SV40Tag mice these small cells are represented by periportal transitional cells, forming multifocal hyperplasia, showing arrangement and structure abnormalities, and preceding the appearance of frank tumors. In the c-myc/TGF-α transgenic livers, small dysplastic cells constitute part of the peritumorous tissue and are mostly local-ized around portal areas. In addition, in the tumors and adjacent tissues oval cells were also detectable. The latter cells were described in hepatocarcinogenesis of SV40Tag mice (56), but not in TGF-α single transgenic mice, and whether they participate in tumor formation or are simply a regenerative response to the liver damage remains to be defined. It is also noteworthy that in the livers of 6- to 8-month-old TGF-α monotransgenic mice, Webber et al. (57) described, besides large dysplastic cells with low proliferative activity, clusters of small replicating cells without, however, a preferential periportal location (57). Those authors proposed that in this model tumors may originate from the small cells.

PLOIDY AND KARYOTYPE ALTERATION DURING EARLY DYSPLASIA

In order to define the extent and the nature of early genomic lesions during dysplasia, Sargent et al. (31) analyzed ploidy and karyotype alterations associated with early events in c-myc/TGF-α mice. At three weeks of age the liver of c-myc/TGF-α mice revealed normal histology and euploid karyotype. In contrast, the early dysplastic phase analyzed at 10 weeks was associated with a dramatic increase in aneuploidy, chromosome breakage and translocations. The breakage was not high enough to account for the 80% chromosome loss and gain observed in hepatocytes from the c-myc/TGF-α mice, suggesting a possible aberration of the spindle formation or a block in the synthesis of DNA. Also, the occurrence of endoreduplications provides further evidence of a spindle disruption or DNA synthesis block (58,59). The association of aneuploidy and chromosome damage with the transition from a benign to malignant state has been observed in a number of experimental systems. For example, Danielsen and colleagues (60) observed an increased aneuploidy and translocations in chemically induced mouse liver nodules. Also, a similar increase in aneuploidy and chromosome damage was observed in rat liver harboring neoplastic nodules with cellular atypia (61–64). In addition, similar chromosomal abnormalities were observed during multistage carcinogenesis in mouse skin and salivary gland (65,66). Frequently broken regions of chromosomes are designated as fragile sites. These regions have been demonstrated to be tissue-specific and consist of G-light bands that are actively transcribed, possibly due to local decondensation of the chromosome (67). Genes regulating growth such as oncogenes, suppressor genes, and growth factors are often located in G-light bands (68,69). These actively transcribed regions are frequently altered during carcinogenesis (68–70). Specific breakages on chromosomes 1, 4, 7, and 12 occurred at high frequency in the c-myc/TGF-α mice during the dysplastic phase. These chromosomal regions contain both tumor susceptibility genes and demonstrate loss of heterozygosity in

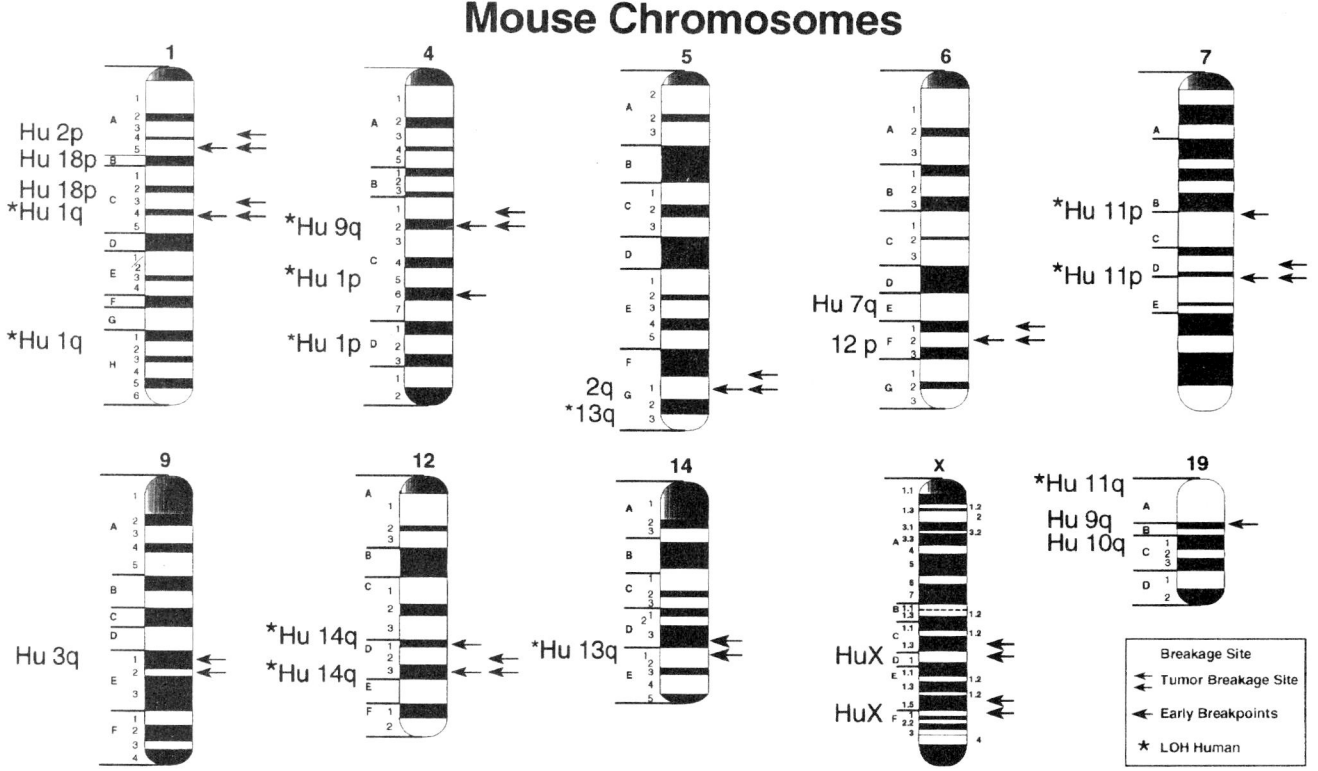

FIGURE 68.3. Idiograms of chromosomes 1, 4, 5, 6, 7, 9, 12, 14, X and 19. The *single arrows* indicate regions that were found to have a statistically significant number of chromosome breaks in 10-week-old c-myc/transforming growth factor (TGF)-α double transgenic mouse livers. The *double arrows* indicate regions that were found to have statistically significant chromosome breakage in metaphase spreads isolated from hepatocellular carcinoma prepared from 30-week-old double transgenic c-myc/TGF-α mice. The homologous region of the human chromosome is indicated at the left. *LOH*, loss of heterozygosity. (From Sargent LM, Zhou X, Keck CL, et al. Nonrandom cytogenetic alterations in hepatocellular carcinoma from transgenic mice overexpressing c-myc and transforming growth factor-α in the liver. *Am J Pathol* 1999;154:1047–1055, with permission.)

mouse tumors (31). The break points on mouse chromosomes 1, 4, 7, and 12 correspond to human 1q, 1 p, 11 p15.5, 11 p13, and 14q32 (70,71) (Fig. 68.3). Human 1q, 1 p, 11p, and 14q are also rearranged in human liver tumors. Due to the highly conserved genetic linkage groups between human and mouse (70), further examination of these fragile regions may provide critical information about tumor susceptibility genes in human HCC.

DISRUPTION OF REDOX HOMEOSTASIS DURING DYSPLASIA

Compelling evidence suggests that endogenous oxidants generated by multiple intracellular pathways may constitute an important class of naturally occurring carcinogens (72,73). Reactive oxygen species (ROS) are endogenous oxygen-containing molecules generated during aerobic metabolism (74). ROS represent many species that include superoxide ($O_2^{\bullet}$), hydroxyl ($HO^{\bullet}$), peroxyl ($RO_2^{\bullet}$), and alkoxyl ($RO^{\bullet}$) radicals, as well as nonradical molecules such as singlet oxygen ($^1O_2$) and hydrogen peroxide (H_2O_2) that can be easily converted into radicals. ROS can induce genetic mutations as well as gross chromosomal alterations and thus contribute to cancer development at all stages (75,76). Furthermore, there is a considerable body of evidence suggesting that oxidative damage to DNA may play a critical role in aging (77,78).

As pointed out earlier, the characteristic features of hepatocarcinogenesis in the c-myc/TGF-α transgenic mice are early and widespread dysplasia (19), as well as profound chromosomal abnormalities (31) associated with marked cellular enlargement, upregulation of TGF-β1 gene expression, and selective growth cessation indicative of premature senescence (79,80). Also, the presence of nonrandom chromosomal breaks prior to tumor development and persistent enhancement of chromosomal damage in HCC suggested that c-myc/TGF-α hepatocytes exhibited a mutator phenotype (75). Given the known carcinogenic properties of ROS, Factor et al. (29) examined the possibility that enhanced metabolic generation of oxygen radicals in rapidly

proliferating c-myc/TGF-α transgenic hepatocytes might be responsible for the genetic instability and acceleration of liver cancer in this animal model. To clarify the biochemical events that may be responsible for the genotoxic and carcinogenic effects observed in this transgenic model, several parameters of redox homeostasis in the liver were examined prior to the development of hepatic tumors. By two months of age, the production of ROS, determined by the peroxidation-sensitive fluorescent dye, 2′,7′-dichlorofluorescin diacetate (DCFH-DA), was significantly elevated in c-myc/TGF-α transgenic hepatocytes versus either wild-type or c-myc single-transgenic cells, and occurred in parallel with an increase in lipid peroxidation (Figs. 68.4 and 68.5). Concomitant with a rise in oxidant levels, antioxidant defenses were decreased, including total glutathione content and the activity of glutathione peroxidase (GPx), whereas thioredoxin reductase (TR) activity was not changed. However, hepatic tumors which developed in c-myc/TGF-α mice exhibited an increase in TR activity and a very low activity of GPx. In addition, specific deletions were detected in mtDNA as early as five weeks of age in the transgenic mice (Fig. 68.6).

A close correlation exists between the degree of ROS overproduction and the occurrence of liver tumors in the transgenic mice. The increase in the cellular oxidative stress was more pronounced and sustained in c-myc/TGF-α than c-myc mice, consistent with the carcinogenic data (18,19). Although constitutive expression of c-myc alone was sufficient to increase intracellular ROS, albeit to a lesser extent, c-myc expression did not result in an

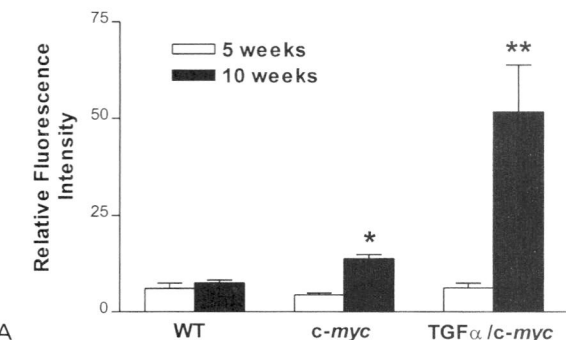

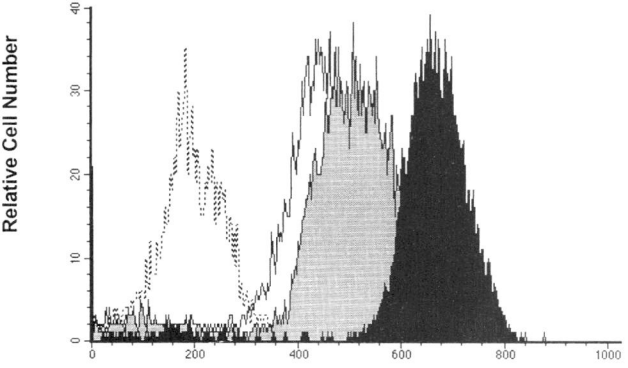

FIGURE 68.4. Changes in intracellular generation of peroxides in c-myc and c-myc/transforming growth factor (*TGF*)-α transgenic hepatocytes as measured by 7′-dichlorofluorescin (DCF)-fluorescence. Hepatocytes isolated from 5- and 10-week-old wild-type (*WT*) c-myc and c-myc/TGF-α mice by collagenase perfusion were incubated in the absence or presence of 5 μM of the oxidative-sensitive probe DCF diacetate (DCFH-DA) for 30 min at 37°C and subjected to flow cytometry. **A:** Relative DCF-fluorescence intensity measured as difference between DCF fluorescence and autofluorescence in unstained cell suspensions for each cell preparation analyzed. Values were converted from log fluorescence to linear fluorescence intensity by appsplication of the equation for which every 256 channels of separation represent a 10-fold difference. Data are shown as mean ± S.E., n = 5 in each group of mice. * p<0.01, ** p<0.05 when compared with wild-type and c-myc mice, respectively, using Student's *t* test; **B:** comparative flow cytometry distributions of DCF-fluorescence intensity. The histograms represent the number of cells as a function of fluorescence intensity expressed as channel number (log-fluorescence intensity). The panel represents the overlay of four representative flourescence activated cell sorting (FACS) analysis performed on 10-week-old wild-type (*white area*), c-myc (*gray area*), and c-myc/TGF-α (*black area*) hepatocytes. The *dashed histogram* shows the autofluorescence profile in unstained wild-type hepatocytes. (From Factor VM, Kiss A, Woitach JT, et al. Disruption of redox homeostasis in transforming growth factor α/c-myc transgenic mouse model of accelerated hepatocarcinogenesis. *J Biol Chem* 1998;273:15846–15853, with permission.)

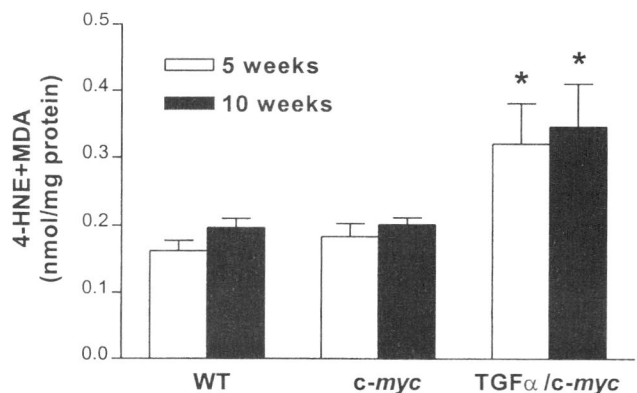

FIGURE 68.5. Levels of lipid peroxidation in c-myc and c-myc/transforming growth factor (*TGF*)-α livers. The data were generated using the Calbiochem Lipid Peroxidation Kit, which assays both malondialdehyde (MDA) and 4-hydroxyalkenals (4-HNE). The data are shown as mean ± S.E., n = 5 in each age group. * p<0.05 when compared with age-matched wild-type (WT) and c-myc mice by Student's *t* test. (From Factor VM, Kiss A, Woitach JT, et al. Disruption of redox homeostasis in transforming growth factor a/c-myc transgenic mouse model of accelerated hepatocarcinogenesis. *J Biol Chem* 1998;273:15846–15853, with permission.)

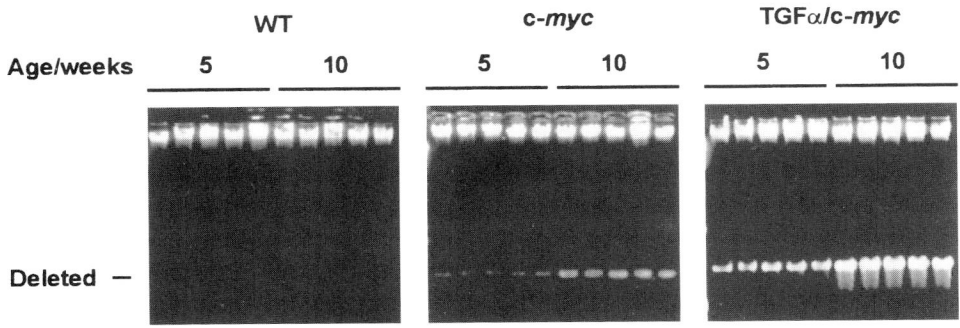

FIGURE 68.6. Polymerase chain reaction (PCR) detection of deletion in liver mitochondrial DNA (mtDNA). Total hepatic DNAs from wild-type (WT), c-myc and c-myc/transforming growth factor (*TGF*)-α mice at 5 and 10 weeks of age were subjected to PCR amplification and separated using a 1% Tris-acetate-EDTA-agarose gel electrophoresis. The position of PCR deletion product of 851 bp is indicated. (From Factor VM, Kiss A, Woitach JT, et al. Disruption of redox homeostasis in transforming growth factor α/c-myc transgenic mouse model of accelerated hepatocarcinogenesis. *J Biol Chem* 1998;273:15846–15853, with permission.)

increase in lipid peroxidation or specific chromosomal damage at 10 weeks (31). However, in the c-myc as well as c-myc/TGF-α livers, there were significantly increased amounts of mitochondrial DNA (mtDNA) deletion starting from 5 weeks of age. MtDNA is known to be 10- to 15-fold more sensitive to oxidative damage than nuclear DNA (81,82). Enhanced ROS generation associated with progressive accumulation of mtDNA damage is frequently described in aging rodent and human livers, as well as in degenerating diseases associated with oxidative liver damage (83–90). Further characterization of double transgenic hepatocytes revealed the presence of lipofuscin granules, a pigment ascribed to the aging process and thought to be a byproduct of lipid peroxidation (78). The data reported by Factor et al. (29) suggest that increased ROS generation in c-myc and c-myc/TGF-α hepatocytes may lead to premature oxidative damage of hepatic mtDNA. Although it remains to be determined, it seems possible that overexpression of the TGF-α transgene alone might also promote ROS production. However, a considerably lower level of chromosomal damage (31) and a longer latency of liver tumor development are observed in TGF-α (91) and in c-myc single-transgenic mice (19). These observations suggest that coexpression of TGF-α and c-myc transgenes may cause synergistic augmentation of ROS production and also decrease the antioxidant defense, resulting in the acceleration of hepatic carcinogenesis in c-myc/TGF-α double-transgenic mice.

The source(s) of ROS generation in c-myc and c-myc/TGF-α remains to be determined and appear to be multiple. Recent evidence suggests the presence of a plasma membrane-bound H_2O_2-generating system in nonphagocytic cells linked to the Ras family of small GTP-binding proteins that can function as a universal effector system for growth factors, hormones, and cytokines

(92–96). The possibility that H_2O_2 might be a naturally occurring intracellular product of the proliferative stimulus provided by c-myc has been discussed (97). Although it cannot be determined conclusively from the studies of c-myc and c-myc/TGF-α transgenic mice, DNA damage could be produced by hydroxyl radical and other oxidizing species such as lipid hydroperoxides, and hydrogen peroxides (98–100).

The data discussed here provide the first biochemical evidence that coexpression of TGF-α and c-myc transgenes in mouse livers results in overproduction of ROS. These data support the hypothesis that chronic stimulation of cell proliferation in the liver facilitates the creation of an environment of oxidative stress leading to massive DNA damage and acceleration of hepatocarcinogenesis in this animal model. Further studies are necessary to elucidate the signaling pathways that regulate ROS generation and the nature of the specific ROS responsible for genetic damage.

IMPACT OF ANTIOXIDANT TREATMENT ON NEOPLASTIC LESIONS IN C-MYC/TRANSFORMING GROWTH FACTOR-α TRANSGENIC MICE

Antioxidants, including vitamin E (VE), have been reported to initiate a wide range of physiological responses that lower cancer risk (101). One of the best characterized functions of VE, an integral component of plasma lipoproteins, is the scavenging of lipid peroxyl radicals in biological membranes, thus preventing the formation of highly reactive lipid peroxidation products (102), which have been shown to have both mutagenic and carcinogenic properties (98,99). More recent work has shown that VE can also directly reduce ROS production by interfering with the assembly of membrane-bound NADPH-oxidase complexes (103). Furthermore, new evidence indicates that VE, in addition to its well-characterized antioxidant function, can protect against cancer formation by enhancing immunological surveillance, as well as by affecting signal transduction pathways involved in the regulation of cell proliferation and apoptosis (104–106). Consistent with these observations, VE has been found to negatively regulate protein kinase C (107), implicated as an endogenous tumor promoter (108–109).

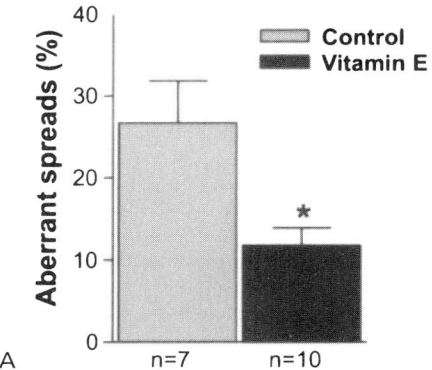

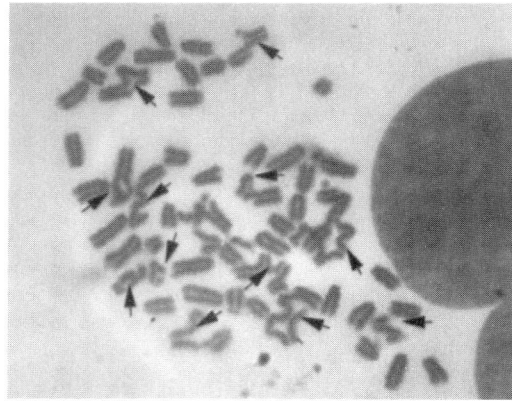

Factor et al. (110) have used the c-myc/TGF-α model to test the potential of VE to increase genetic stability and protect against the development of liver cancer. To address these objectives, 3-week-old c-myc/TGF-α transgenic mice were divided into two groups, one receiving a control diet with (2000 IU/kg diet) and one without VE supplementation. The effect of VE treatment on liver tumorigenesis was assessed at both the early stage (10 weeks of age) and end stage (26 weeks) of tumor development. The results showed that VE is able to protect liver tissue against oxidative stress and suppress the tumorigenic potential of c-myc oncogene. Dietary supplementation with VE, starting from weaning, decreased ROS generation and increased the chromosomal as well as mtDNA stability in the liver (Figs. 68.7 and 68.8). Similarly, dietary VE reduced the rate of hepatocyte proliferation, the extent of liver dysplasia, and increased viability of hepatocytes (Fig. 68.9). At six months of age, VE treatment decreased the incidence of adenomas by 65% and prevented malignant conversion (Fig. 68.10 and Table 68.2). These data support an etiological role for ROS in the c-myc/TGF-α mouse model of accelerated carcinogenesis and establish the importance of VE in suppressing the tumorigenic process in the liver. In this *in vivo* system, VE given at concentrations achievable via diet supplementation is able to modulate oncogenic activity of c-myc and TGF-α and reverse the biochemical, cellular, and cytogenetic characteristics associated with both tumor initiation and progression (19,29,31). Most significantly, VE dietary supplementation restored the cellular redox balance prior to the development of preneoplastic lesions and decreased the rate of hepatocyte proliferation. Inhibition of mitogenesis occurred concurrent with enhanced chromosomal stability, suggesting "a cause and an effect relationship." These results indicate that ROS generated by overexpression of c-myc and TGF-α in the liver are the primary carcinogenic agents in this animal model. Furthermore, the data demonstrate that dietary supplementation with VE can effectively inhibit liver cancer development.

FIGURE 68.7. Vitamin E (VE) dietary supplementation reduced chromosomal damage. **A:** Percentage of cells with chromosomal alterations. The histogram shows that the cumulative frequency of aberrant metaphases as measured by the presence of chromatid and chromosome gaps, and/or breaks, and/or exchanges was significantly lower in c-myc/transforming growth factor (TGF)-α mice fed with VE-supplemented diet (*p< 0.05). The cytogenetic analysis was performed on primary hepatocyte cultures established from 10-week-old c-myc/TGF-α mice fed with control or VE-supplemented diet. Fifty to 100 metaphase spreads were scored for each individual mouse according to the international nomenclature. Values are expressed as the mean percentage ± SE. **B and C:** Representative examples of chromosomal aberrations in c-myc/TGF-α mouse fed with control **(B)** or VE-supplemented diet **(C)**. Note extensive breakage and chromosomal rearrangements in c-myc/TGF-α mouse fed with control diet. *Arrows* indicate gaps, breaks, triradial and quadroradial exchanges. (From Factor VM, Laskowska D, Jensen MR, et al. Vitamin E reduces chromosomal damage and inhibits hepatic tumor formation in a transgenic mouse model. *Proc Natl Acad Sci USA* 2000;97:2196–2201, with permission.)

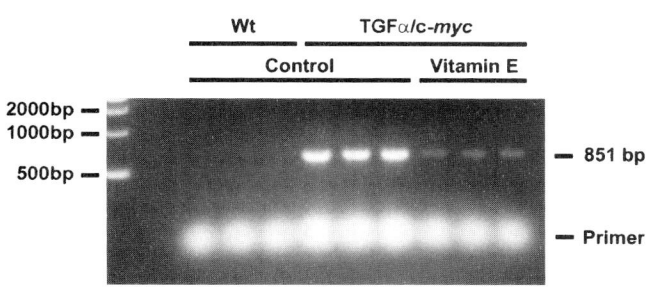

FIGURE 68.8. Polymerase chain reaction (PCR) detection of deletion in liver mtDNA. Total hepatic DNA samples from 10-week-old wild-type, and c-myc/transforming growth factor (TGF)-α mice fed with control or vitamin E (VE)-supplemented diet were subjected to PCR amplification and separated using a 1% Tris-acetate-EDTA-agarose gel electrophoresis. The position of PCR deletion product of 851 bp is indicated. The deletion was undetectable in 10-week-old wild-type livers in the absence of oxidative stress. In contrast, the deletion was readily detectable in the age-matched c-myc/TGF-α mice. The deletion product was more abundant in c-myc/TGF-α mice fed with control diet, which manifest increased reactive oxygen species generation. (From Factor VM, Laskowska D, Jensen MR, et al. Vitamin E reduces chromosomal damage and inhibits hepatic tumor formation in a transgenic mouse model. *Proc Natl Acad Sci USA* 2000;97:2196–2201, with permission.)

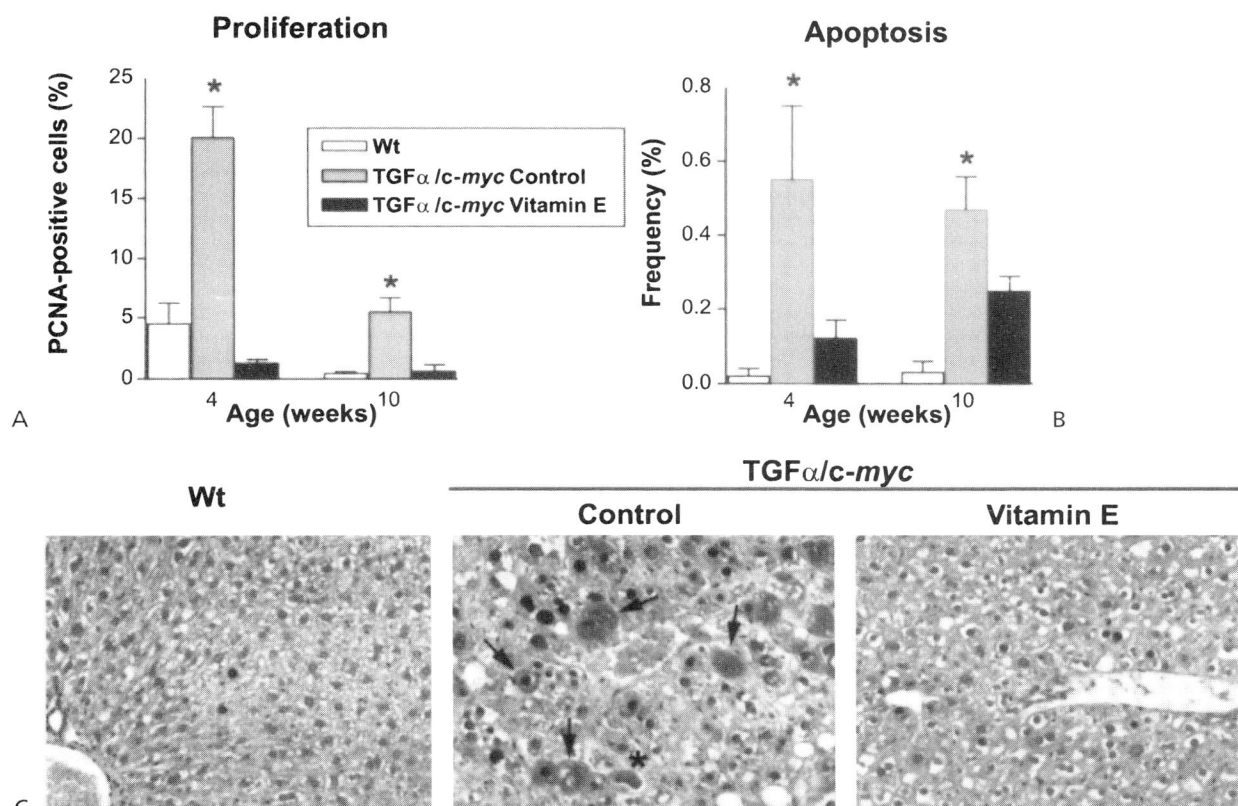

FIGURE 68.9. Vitamin E (VE) dietary supplementation reduced the rate of hepatocyte proliferation and apoptosis in c-myc/transforming growth factor (*TGF*)-α transgenic livers. **A:** Labeling index of PCNA-positive hepatocytes. Histograms show a significantly higher labeling index in c-myc/TGF-α mice fed with control diet than in c-myc/TGF-α mice fed with VE-supplemented diet (*p=7.1E-05, p=0.01 at four and ten weeks of age, respectively). Values are expressed as mean percentage ± SE (n=5 in each group of mice). **B:** Apoptotic index of hepatocytes. Histograms show that the apoptotic index is significantly higher in c-myc/TGF-α mice fed with control diet than in c-myc/TGF-α mice fed with VE-supplemented diet (*p<0.05 at both four and 10 weeks of age). **C:** Representative proliferating cell nuclear antigen (PCNA) immunoperoxidase staining of liver samples illustrating a decreased percentage of nuclei exhibiting PCNA-immunoreactivity in 10-week-old c-myc/TGF-α mice fed with VE-supplemented diet. Note the high frequency of mitotic cells (*arrows*) and the presence of apoptotic cells (*asterisk*) in control c-myc/TGF-α livers. Paraffin-embedded sections were counterstained with hematoxylin, ×150 original magnification. (From Factor VM, Laskowska D, Jensen MR, et al. Vitamin E reduces chromosomal damage and inhibits hepatic tumor formation in a transgenic mouse model. *Proc Natl Acad Sci USA* 2000;97:2196–2201, with permission.)

Multi-Stage Hepatocarcinogenesis

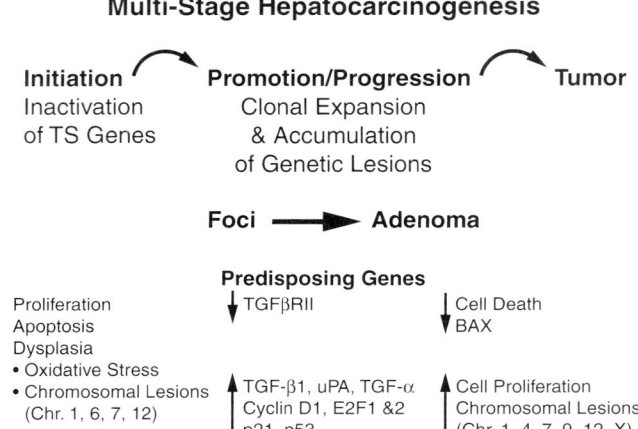

FIGURE 68.10. Summary of cellular and genetic changes during development of hepatic neoplasia in c-myc/transforming growth factor (*TGF*)-α transgenic mice. *TS,* tumor suppressor.

SUMMARY OF NEOPLASTIC EVENTS DURING HEPATOCARCINOGENESIS IN C-MYC/TRANSFORMING GROWTH FACTOR-α TRANSGENIC MICE

Severe LCD, characterized by hypertrophic and polymorphic hepatocytes, develops rapidly in c-myc/TGF-α mice and becomes widespread throughout the liver parenchyma by the second month of age, accompanying thereafter the development of neoplastic lesions (19). However, it has also been demonstrated that many of the large dysplastic cells, after an initial period of replication mostly driven by overexpression of the transgenes and of the urokinase-type plasminogen activator, undergo apoptotic cell death closely associated with the autocrine upregulation and activation of TGF-β1 (19), a potent growth inhibitor and apoptosis inducer for hepatocytes (reviewed in ref. 111).

These observations strongly indicated that the mechanisms controlling cell proliferation and survival, which are considered critical targets in oncogenesis, are profoundly perturbed by overexpression of the transgenes in the liver. Also, a large body of evidence indicates that oncogene overexpression can lead to malignant transformation by disrupting mechanisms regulating G1/S transition (112–114). These observations prompted Santoni-Rugiu et al. (53) to identify which components of the pathway that governs G1-progression and entry into the S phase are targeted by constitutive expression of c-myc and TGF-α and may result in neoplastic growth in the liver. The results obtained from these studies showed that coexpression of c-myc and TGF-α transgenes leads to neoplastic growth in the liver by targeting distinct members of the pRb/E2F pathway, resulting in a deregulation of cell cycle progression. Furthermore, the reduced apoptotic rates in c-myc/TGF-α tumors, in which TGF-α is expressed at higher levels than in noncancerous tissues (18,19), suggest that this growth factor may act as a survival factor for hepatic (pre)neoplastic cells. These and other relevant data are summarized in the context of the multistep process of neoplastic development of the liver shown in Figure 68.10.

CONCLUSION

Despite the existence of considerable information regarding the etiological factors and the cellular biology of human liver cancer, a comprehensive description of the molecular events occurring during the multistep process of human hepatocarcinogenesis does not currently exist. There are notable similarities between the initial cellular events during HBV- and/or HCV-initiated human liver carcinogenesis and those observed in c-myc/TGF-α mice. These early changes predominantly involve disruption of the cell-cycle control mechanism(s) for the hepatocytes. Although the transgenic mouse model does not suffer the

TABLE 68.2. VITAMIN E DIETARY SUPPLEMENTATION INHIBITS HEPATOCARCINOGENESIS IN C-MYC/TGFα TRANSGENIC MICE

| Diet group | Incidence% | | Multiplicity | Maximum Tumor Size | LBW% |
	Adenomas	Carcinomas	Mean ± SE	mm, Mean ± SE	Mean ± SE
Control diet	100 (15/15)[a]	27 (4/15)	4.3 ± 0.6	6.7 ± 0.8	7.91 ± 0.34
Vitamin E, 2,000 units	35 (7/20)	0 (0/20)	0.4 ± 0.3	3.2 ± 0.6	4.56 ± 0.14
P	1.7E-07	0.03	2.3E-07	0.026	1.2E-07

[a]In parentheses, the number of mice with adenomas/carcinomas per total number of mice.
LBW, liver body weight; P, probability.
From Factor VM, Laskowska D, Jensen MR, et al. Vitamin E reduces chromosomal damage and inhibits hepatic tumor formation in a transgenic mouse model. *Proc Natl Acad Sci USA* 2000;97:2196–2201, with permission.

intense inflammatory response seen in the virally inflamed human liver, the consequences appear to be similar, namely, the appearance of abnormal mitosis reflected in the emergence of dysplastic cell populations concomitant with reduced capacity of DNA repair and apoptosis control. In addition, the early genetic damage observed in the transgenic mice is syntenic (orthologous) with lesions known to be associated with human hepatocellular carcinomas. It therefore seems reasonable to suggest that the early events observed in the c-myc/TGF-α mice represent a realistic model of human hepatocarcinogenesis. Furthermore, the discovery that the major consequence of inducing unregulated proliferation of hepatocytes is the disruption of redox homeostasis in the liver, which results in extensive genetic damage, may have therapeutic implications.

It is evident that to acquire a full understanding of the neoplastic process, all of the genetic pathways involved in this multistep process must be identified. A complete genetic "blueprint" of the cancer development would include a sequential description of all of the genes, whether mutated or functionally altered, that are involved in the process. Furthermore, the identity and description of the modifier genes and their impact on each step of the neoplastic development are also required. Acquisition of this data set will then form the basis for achieving a complete description of the neoplastic process, including the functional effects and interactions of the genes to reveal the evolution of the tumor. Moreover, this data set would provide a source for identifying potential therapeutic targets for intervention, as well as prognostic predictions.

From the genetic viewpoint, animal models, as exemplified by the c-myc/TGF-α transgenic mouse, that provide a useful model of the human disease may provide the best hope to achieve, within a reasonable time-frame, the complete genetic description of the neoplastic process. Essentially, an unlimited quantity of tumors of a specific stage can be acquired from genetically identical mice raised in a closely controlled environment. Furthermore, it is possible to construct transgenic mice carrying a specific gene addition or deletion and to study the consequences in a defined genotype. Due to the conservation of genetic linkage groups between mouse and human, the identification of genetic alterations in mouse liver carcinogenesis should be useful for the identification of critical genetic alterations in human hepatocarcinogenesis.

REFERENCES

1. Parkin DM. The global burden of cancer. *Seminars in Cancer Biology* 1998;8:219–235.
2. Macri P, Gordon JW. Delayed morbidity and mortality of albumin/SV40 T-antigen transgenic mice after insertion of an α-fetoprotein/herpes virus thymidine kinase transgene and treatment with ganciclovir. *Human Gene Therapy* 1994;5:175–182.
3. Merlino G. Transgenic mice: designing genes for molecular models. In: Arias IM, Boyer JL, Fausto N, et al, eds. *The Liver: Biology and Pathbiology,* 3rd ed. New York: Raven Press, 1994; 1579–1589.
4. Sandgren EP. Transgenic models of hepatic growth regulation and hepatocarcinogenesis. In: Jirtle RL, ed. *Liver regeneration and carcinogenesis: cellular and molecular mechanisms.* New York: Academic Press, 1994;257–300.
5. Santoni-Rugiu E, Thorgeirsson SS. Transgenic animals as models for hepatocarcinogenesis. In: Strain A, Diehl A, eds. *Liver Growth and Repair.* London: Chapman & Hall, 1998:100–142.
6. Liang TJ. P53 protein and aflatoxin B1: the good, the bad, and the ugly. *Hepatology* 1995;22:1330–1332.
7. Nalpas B, Feitelson M, Brechot C, et al. Alcohol, hepatotropic viruses and hepatocellular carcinoma. *Alcohol Clin Exp Res* 1995;19:1089–1095.
8. Guyton KZ, Kensler TW. Oxidative mechanisms in carcinogenesis. *Br Med Bull* 1993;49:523–544.
9. Beasley RP, Hwang LY. Epidemiology of hepatocellular carcinoma. In: Vyas GN, Dienstag, JL, Hoofnagle JH, eds. *Viral Hepatitis and Liver Disease.* New York: Grune & Stratton, 1984; 209–224.
10. Shafritz DA, Shouval D, Sherman HI, et al. Integration of hepatitis B virus DNA into the genome of liver cells in chronic liver diseases and hepatocellular carcinoma. Studies on percutaneous liver biopsies and postmortem tissue specimens. *N Engl J Med* 1981;305:1067–1073.
11. Amati B, Land H. Myc-Max-Mad: a transcription factor network controlling cell cycle progression, differentiation and death. *Curr Opin Genet Dev* 1994;4:102–108.
12. DePinho RA, Schreiber-Agus N, Alt FW. MYC family oncogenes in the development of normal and neoplastic cells. *Adv Cancer Res* 1991;57:1–46.
13. Su TS, Lin L-H, Liu WY, et al. Expression of c-*myc* gene in human hepatoma. *Biochem Biophys Res Commun* 1985;132: 264–268.
14. Zhang XK, Huang DP, Chin DK, et al. The expression of oncogenes in human developing liver and hepatomas. *Biochem Biophys Res Commun* 1987;142:932–938.
15. Tabor E. Tumor suppressor genes, growth factor genes, and oncogenes in hepatitis B virus-associated hepatocellular carcinoma. *J Med Virol* 1994;42:357–365.
16. Grisham JW. Interspecies comparison of liver carcinogenesis: implications for cancer risk assessment. *Carcinogenesis* 1997;18: 59–81.
17. Collins Presnell S, Thompson MT, Strom SC. Investigation of the cooperative effects of transforming growth factor-α and c-*myc* overexpression in rat liver epithelial cells. *Mol Carcinog* 1995;13:233–244.
18. Murakami H, Sanderson N, Nagy, P, et al. Transgenic mouse model for synergistic effects of nuclear oncogenes and growth factors in tumorigenesis: interaction of c-*myc* and transforming growth factor α in hepatic oncogenesis. *Cancer Res* 1993;53: 1719–1723.
19. Santoni-Rugiu E, Nagy P, Jensen MR, et al. Evolution of neoplastic development in the liver of transgenic mice co-expressing c-*myc* and transforming growth factor-α. *Am J Pathol* 1996; 149:407–428.
20. Takagi H, Sharp R, Hammermeister C, et al. Molecular and genetic analysis of liver oncogenesis in transforming growth factor α transgenic mice. *Cancer Res* 1992;52:5171–5177.
21. Sandgren EP, Luetteke NC, Qiu TH, et al. Transforming growth factor alpha dramatically enhances oncogene-induced carcinogenesis in transgenic mouse pancreas and liver. *Mol Cell Biol* 1993;13:320–330.
22. Takagi H, Sharp R, Takayama H, et al. Collaboration between

growth factors and diverse chemical carcinogens in hepatocarcinogenesis of transforming growth factor α transgenic mice. *Cancer Res* 1993;53:4329–4336.

23. Bodmer WF. The somatic evolution of cancer. The Harveian Oration of 1996. *J R Coll Physicians Lond* 1997;31:82–89.

24. Fearon E, Vogelstein B. A genetic model for colorectal tumorigenesis. *Cell* 1990;61:759–767.

25. Orr JW. The early effects of 9:10-dimethyl-1:2-benzanthracene on mouse skin, and their significance in relation to the mechanism of chemical carcinogenesis. *Br J Cancer* 1995; 9:623–632.

26. Kaufman DG, Arnold JT. Stromal-epithelial interactions in the normal and neoplastic development. In: Sirica AE, ed. *Cell and molecular pathogenesis.* Philadelphia: Lippincott-Raven Publishers, 1996:403–432.

27. Ishak KG. Chronic hepatitis: morphology and nomenclature. *Mol Pathol* 1994;7:690–713.

28. Frith CH, Ward JM, Turosov VS. Tumors of the liver. In: Turosov V, Mohr U, eds. *Pathology of tumours in laboratory animals* Vol. 2. Lyon: IARC Scientific Publications, 1994: 223–270.

29. Factor VM, Kiss A, Woitach JT, et al. Disruption of redox homeostasis in transforming growth factor α/c-myc transgenic mouse model of accelerated hepatocarcinogenesis. *J Biol Chem* 1998;273:15846–15853.

30. Santoni-Rugiu E, Jensen MR, Factor VM, et al. Acceleration of c-myc-induced hepatocarcinogenesis by coexpression of transforming growth factor (TGF)-α in transgenic mice is associated with TGFβ1 signaling disruption. *Am J Pathol* 1999;154: 1693–1700.

31. Sargent LM, Sanderson ND, Thorgeirsson SS. Ploidy and karyotypic alterations associated with early events in the development of hepatocarcinogenesis in transgenic mice harboring c-myc and transforming growth factor α transgenes. *Cancer Res* 1996;56:2137–2142.

32. Sargent LM, Zhou X, Keck CL, et al. Nonrandom cytogenetic alterations in hepatocellular carcinoma from transgenic mice overexpressing c-myc and transforming growth factor-α in the liver. *Am J Pathol* 1999;154:1047–1055.

33. Anthony PP, Vogel CL, Barker LF. Liver cell dysplasia: a premalignant condition. *J Clin Pathol* 1973;26:217–223.

34. Cohen C, Berson SD, Geddes EW. Liver cell dysplasia: association with hepatocellular carcinoma, cirrhosis and hepatitis B antigen carrier status. *Cancer* 1979;44:1671–1676.

35. Roncalli M, Borzio M, De Biagi G. Liver cell dysplasia and hepatocellular carcinoma: a histological and immunohistochemical study. *Histopathology* 1985;9:209–221.

36. Cohen C, Berson SD. Liver cell dysplasia in normal, cirrhotic and hepatocellular carcinoma patients. *Cancer* 1986;57: 1535–1538.

37. Roncalli M, Borzio M, De Biagi G, et al. Liver cell dysplasia in cirrhosis. A serologic and immunohistochemical study. *Cancer* 1986;57:1515–1521.

38. Lefkowitch JH, Apfelbaum TF. Liver cell dysplasia and hepatocellular carcinoma in non-A, non-B hepatitis. *Arch Pathol Lab Med* 1987;111:170–173.

39. Watanabe S, Okita K, Harada T, et al. Morphologic studies of the liver cell dysplasia. *Cancer* 1983;51:2197–2205.

40. Roncalli M, Borzio M, Tombesi MV, et al. A morphometric study of liver cell dysplasia. *Hum Pathol* 1988;19:471–474.

41. International Working Party. Terminology of nodular hepatocellular lesions. *Hepatology* 1995;22:983–993.

42. Sandgren EP, Quaife CJ, Pinkert CA, et al. Oncogene-induced liver neoplasia in transgenic mice. *Oncogene* 1989;4:715–724.

43. Lee GH, Merlino G, Fausto N. Development of liver tumors in transforming growth factor α transgenic mice. *Cancer Res* 1992; 52:5162–5170.

44. Toshkov I, Chisari FV, Bannasch P. Hepatic preneoplasia in hepatitis B virus transgenic mice. *Hepatology* 1994;20: 1162–1172.

45. Koike K, Moriya K, Iino S, et al. High-level expression of hepatitis B virus HBx gene and hepatocarcinogenesis in transgenic mice. *Hepatology* 1994;19:810–819.

46. Sepulveda AR, Finegold MJ, Smith B, et al. Development of a transgenic mouse system for the analysis of stages in liver carcinogenesis using tissue specific expression of SV-40 large T antigen controlled by regulatory elements of a human α-1 antitrypsin gene. *Cancer Res* 1989;49:6108–6117.

47. Schirmacher P, Held WA, Yang D, et al. Selective amplification of periportal transitional cells precedes formation of hepatocellular carcinoma in SV 40 large Tag transgenic mice. *Am J Pathol* 1991;139:231–241.

48. Carr BI, Huang TH, Itakura K, et al. TGFβ gene transcription in normal and neoplastic liver growth. *J Cell Biochem* 1989;39: 477–487.

49. Nagy P, Evarts RP, McMahon JB, et al. Role of TGFβ in normal differentiation and oncogenesis in rat liver. *Mol Carcinog* 1989;2:345–354.

50. Nakatsukasa H, Evarts RP, Hsia C-H, et al. Expression of transforming growth factor-β1 during chemical hepatocarcinogenesis in the rat. *Lab Invest* 1991;65:511–517.

51. Ito N, Kawata S, Tamura S, et al. Elevated levels of transforming growth factor β messenger RNA and its polypeptide in human hepatocellular carcinoma. *Cancer Res* 1991;51: 4080–4083.

52. Bedossa P, Peltier E, Terris B, et al. Transforming growth factor-beta 1 (TGF-β1) and TGF-β1 receptors in normal, cirrhotic, and neoplastic human livers. *Hepatology* 1995;21:760–766.

53. Santoni-Rugiu E, Jensen MR, Thorgeirsson SS. Disruption of the pRb/E2F pathway and inhibition of apoptosis are major oncogenic events in liver constitutively expressing c-myc and transforming growth factor α. *Cancer Res* 1998;58:123–134.

54. Liu J, Li H, Nomura K, et al. Frequent spontaneous sister chromatid exchange in hepatocytes of transgenic mice harboring the SV40-T antigen gene. *J Cancer Res Clin Oncol* 1992;118: 601–605.

55. McWhir J, Selfridge J, Harrison DJ, et al. Mice with DNA repair gene (ERCC-1) deficiency have elevated levels of p53, liver nuclear abnormalities and die before weaning. *Nat Genet* 1993;5:217–224.

56. Bennoun M, Rissel M, Engelhardt N, et al. Oval cell proliferation in early stages of hepatocarcinogenesis in simian virus 40 large T transgenic mice. *Am J Pathol* 1993;143:1326–1336.

57. Webber EM, Wu JC, Wang L, et al. Overexpression of transforming growth factor-α causes liver enlargement and increased hepatocyte proliferation in transgenic mice. *Am J Pathol* 1994; 145:398–408.

58. Paweletz N, Ghosh S, Vig BK. Mitosis and the induction of aneuploidy. *Prog Clin Biol Res* 1989;318:217–229.

59. Brinkley BR, Tousson A, Valdivia MM. The kinetochore of mammalian chromosomes: structure and function in normal mitosis and aneuploidy. *Basic Life Sci* 1985;36:243–267.

60. Danielsen HE, Brogger A, Reith A. Specific gain of chromosome 19 in preneoplastic mouse liver cells after diethylnitrosamine treatment. *Carcinogenesis* 1988;12:177–180.

61. Becker FF, Fox RA, Klein LM, et al. Chromosome patterns in rat hepatocytes during N-2-fluorenylacetamide carcinogenesis. *J Natl Cancer Inst* 1971;46:1261–1269.

62. Sargent LM, Settler GL, Roloff B, et al. Ploidy and specific karyotypic changes during promotion with phenobarbital,

2,5,12′,5′-tetrachlorobiphenyl, and/or 3,4,3′,4′-tetra-chloro-biphenyl in rat liver. *Cancer Res* 1992;52:955–962.

63. Dragan YP, Sargent L, Xu YH, et al. The initiation-promotion-progression model of rat hepatocarcinogenesis. *Proc Soc Exp Biol Med* 1993;202:16–24.

64. Herens C, Gonzalez ML, Barbason H. Cytogenetic changes in hepatomas from rats treated with chronic exposure to diethyl-nitrosamine. *Cancer Genet Cytogenet* 1992;60:45–52.

65. Aldaz CM, Conti CJ, Klein-Szanto AJP, et al. Progressive dysplasia and aneuploidy are hallmarks of mouse skin papillomas: relevance to malignancy. *Proc Natl Acad Sci USA* 1987;84: 2029–2032.

66. Cowell JK, Wigley CB. Chromosome changes associated with the progression of cell lines from preneoplastic to tumorigenic phenotype during transformation of mouse salivary gland. *J Natl Cancer Inst* 1982;69:425–433.

67. Popescu NC. Chromosome fragility and instability in human cancer. *Crit Rev Oncog* 1994;5:121–140.

68. Hecht DF. Fragile sites, cancer chromosome breakpoints and oncogenes all cluster in light G bands. *Cancer Genet Cytogenet* 1988;31:17–20.

69. Glover TW, Stein CK. Chromosome breakage and recombination at fragile sites. *Am J Hum Genet* 1988;43:265–273.

70. Searle AG, Peter J, Lyon MF, et al. Chromosome maps of man and mouse, III. *Genomics* 1987;1:3–18.

71. Copeland NG, Jenkins NA, Gilbert DJ, et al. A genetic linkage map of the mouse, current applications and future prospects. *Science* 1993;262:57–66.

72. Cerutti PA, Trump BF. Inflammation and oxidative stress in carcinogenesis. *Cancer Cells* 1991;3:1–7.

73. Dreher D, Junod AF. Role of oxygen free radicals in cancer development. *Eur J Cancer* 1996;32A:30–38.

74. Chance B, Sies H, Boveris A. Hydroperoxide metabolism in mammalian organs. *Physiol Rev* 1979;59:527–605.

75. Cerutti PA. Oxy-radicals and cancer. *Lancet* 1994;344:862–863.

76. Wiseman H, Halliwell B. Damage to DNA by reactive oxygen and nitrogen species: role in inflammatory disease and progression to cancer. *Biochem J* 1996;313:17–29.

77. Ames BN, Shigenaga MK. Oxidants are a major contributor to aging. *Ann N Y Acad Sci* 1992;663:85–96.

78. Martin GM, Austad SN, Johnson TE. Genetic analysis of ageing: role of oxidative damage and environmental stresses. *Nat Genet* 1996;13:25–34.

79. Kao CY, Factor VM, Thorgeirsson SS. Reduced growth capacity of hepatocytes from c-myc and c-myc/TGF-alpha transgenic mice in primary culture. *Biochem Biophys Res Commun* 1996; 222:64–70.

80. Factor VM, Jensen MR, Thorgeirsson SS. Coexpression of c-myc and rransforming growth factor alpha in the liver promotes early replicative senescence and diminishes regenerative capacity after partial hepatectomy in transgenic mice. *Hepatology* 1997; 26:1434–1443.

81. Lee CM, Weindruch R, Aiken JM. Age-associated alterations of the mitochondrial genome. *Free Radic Biol Med* 1997;22:1259–1269.

82. Shigenaga MK, Hagen TM, Ames BN. Oxidative damage and mitochondrial decay in aging. *Proc Natl Acad Sci USA* 1994;91: 10771–10778.

83. Hagen TM, Yowe DL, Bartholomew JC, et al. Mitochondrial decay in hepatocytes from old rats: membrane potential declines, heterogeneity and oxidants increase. *Proc Natl Acad Sci USA* 1997;94:3064–3069.

84. Yen TC, King KL, Lee HC, et al. Age-dependent increase of mitochondrial DNA deletions together with lipid peroxides and superoxide dismutase in human liver mitochondria. *Free Radic Biol Med* 1994;16:207–214.

85. Sastre J, Pallardo FV, Pla R, et al. Aging of the liver: age-associated mitochondrial damage in intact hepatocytes. *Hepatology* 1996;24:1199–1205.

86. Filser N, Margue C, Richter C. Quantification of wild-type mitochondrial DNA and its 4.8-kb deletion in rat organs. *Biochem Biophys Res Commun* 1997;233:102–107.

87. Cahill A, Wang X, Hoek JB. Increased oxidative damage to mitochondrial DNA following chronic ethanol consumption. *Biochem Biophys Res Commun* 1997;235:286–290.

88. Mansouri A, Gaou I, Fromenty B, et al. Premature oxidative aging of hepatic mitochondrial DNA in Wilson's disease. *Gastroenterology* 1997;113:599–605.

89. Mansouri A, Fromenty B, Berson A, et al. Multiple hepatic mitochondrial DNA deletions suggest premature oxidative aging in alcoholic patients. *J Hepatol* 1997;27:96–102.

90. Fromenty B, Grimbert S, Mansouri A, et al. Hepatic mitochondrial DNA deletion in alcoholics: association with microvesicular steatosis. *Gastroenterology* 1995;108:193–200.

91. Jhappan C, Stahle C, Harkins RN, et al. TGF alpha overexpression in transgenic mice induces liver neoplasia and abnormal development of the mammary gland and pancreas. *Cell* 1990;61:1137–1146.

92. Sundaresan M, Yu ZX, Ferrans VJ, et al. Regulation of reactive-oxygen-species generation in fibroblasts by Rac1. *Biochem J* 1996;318:379–382.

93. Meier B, Radeke HH, Selle S, et al. Human fibroblasts release reactive oxygen species in response to interleukin-1 or tumour necrosis factor-alpha. *Biochem J* 1989;263:539–545.

94. Meier B, Jesaitis AJ, Emmendorffer A, et al. The cytochrome b-558 molecules involved in the fibroblast and polymorphonuclear leucocyte superoxide-generating NADPH oxidase systems are structurally and genetically distinct. *Biochem J* 1993;289: 481–486.

95. Jones SA, Wood JD, Coffey MJ, et al. The functional expression of p47-phox and p67-phox may contribute to the generation of superoxide by an NADPH oxidase-like system in human fibroblasts. *FEBS Letters* 1994;355:178–182.

96. Krieger-Brauer HI, Medda PK, Kather H. Insulin-induced activation of NADPH-dependent H_2O_2 generation in human adipocyte plasma membranes is mediated by Galphai2. *J Biol Chem* 1997;272:10135–10143.

97. Xu Y, Nguyen Q, Lo DC, et al. c-myc-Dependent hepatoma cell apoptosis results from oxidative stress and not a deficiency of growth factors. *J Cell Physiol* 1997;170:192–199.

98. Dianzani MU. Lipid peroxidation and cancer. *Crit Rev Oncol Hematol* 1993;15:125–147.

99. Halliwell B, Aruoma OI. DNA damage by oxygen-derived species. Its mechanism and measurement in mammalian systems. *FEBS Letters* 1991;281:9–19.

100. Retel J, Hoebee B, Braun JE, et al. Mutational specificity of oxidative DNA damage. *Mutat Res* 1993;299:165–182.

101. Ames BN. Micronutrients prevent cancer and delay aging. *Toxicol Lett* 1998;102-103:5–18.

102. Traber M, Sies H. Vitamin E in humans: demand and delivery. *Annu Rev Nutr* 1996;16:321–347.

103. Cachia O, Benna JE, Pedruzzi E, et al. Alpha-tocopherol inhibits the respiratory burst in human monocytes. Attenuation of p47(phox) membrane translocation and phosphorylation. *J Biol Chem* 1998;273:32801–32805.

104. Meydani M, Lipman RD, Han SN, et al. The effect of long-term dietary supplementation with antioxidants. *Ann N Y Acad Sci* 1998;854:352–360.

105. Brigelius-Flohe R, Traber MG. Vitamin E: function and metabolism. *FASEB J* 1999;13:1145–1155.

106. Prasad KN, Kumar A, Kochupillai V, et al. High doses of multi-

ple antioxidant vitamins: essential ingredients in improving the efficacy of standard cancer therapy. *J Am Coll Nutr* 1999;18: 13–25.

107. Ricciarelli R, Tasinato A, Clement S, et al. Alpha-Tocopherol specifically inactivates cellular protein kinase C alpha by changing its phosphorylation state. *Biochem J* 1998;334:243–249.

108. Blobe GC, Obeid LM, Hannun YA. Regulation of protein kinase C and role in cancer biology. *Cancer Metastasis Rev* 1994; 13:411–431.

109. Livneh E, Dull TJ, Berent E, et al. Release of a phorbol ester-induced mitogenic block by mutation at Thr-654 of the epidermal growth factor receptor. *Mol Cell Biol* 1988;8:2302–2308.

110. Factor VM, Laskowska D, Jensen MR, et al. Vitamin E reduces chromosomal damage and inhibits hepatic tumor formation in a transgenic mouse model. *Proc Natl Acad Sci USA* 2000;97: 2196–2201.

111. Schulte-Hermann R, Grasl-Kraupp B, Bursch W. Apoptosis and hepatocarcinogenesis. In: Jirtle RL, ed. *Liver regeneration and carcinogenesis: cellular and molecular mechanisms*. New York: Academic Press, 1995:141–178.

112. Weinberg RA. The retinoblastoma protein and cell cycle control. *Cell* 1995;81:323–330.

113. Bartek J, Bartkova J, Lukas J. The retinoblastoma protein pathway and the restriction point. *Curr Opin Cell Biol* 1996;8: 805–814.

114. Sherr CJ. Cancer cell cycles. *Science* 1996;274:1672–1677.

The Liver: Biology and Pathobiology, Fourth Edition, edited by I. M. Arias, J. L. Boyer, F. V. Chisari, N. Fausto, D. Schachter, and D. A. Shafritz.
Lippincott Williams & Wilkins, Philadelphia © 2001.

ORPHAN NUCLEAR RECEPTORS AND THE REGULATION OF CHOLESTEROL AND BILE ACID METABOLISM

JOYCE J. REPA
MAKOTO MAKISHIMA
TIMOTHY T. LU
DAVID J. MANGELSDORF

Cholesterol is an essential component of biological membranes, as well as the sole precursor of bile acids, certain vitamins, and steroid hormones. However, excessive unesterified cholesterol can be toxic to cells, and conditions resulting in elevated cholesterol levels have been implicated in several disease states including atherosclerosis and gallstone formation. Cholesterol homeostasis is maintained by a series of regulatory pathways to control the synthesis of endogenous cholesterol, the absorption of dietary sterol and the elimination of cholesterol and its catabolic end products, bile acids (See Chapter 16). Research over the last decade has revealed that many of these regulatory pathways rely on the ability of lipid-sensitive transcription factors to alter the expression of key enzymes and transport proteins to control cholesterol and bile acid metabolism. The regulation of intracellular cholesterol synthesis is mediated by

membrane-bound transcription factors of the basic helix-loop-helix-leucine zipper family, called sterol regulatory element-binding proteins (SREBPs). Under low-sterol conditions, SREBPs are proteolytically cleaved to release these transcription factors from their membrane anchor and allow them to enter the nucleus, where they activate genes encoding key enzymes in cholesterol biosynthesis (reviewed in refs. 1–3). Recently, members of another family of transcription factors, the nuclear hormone receptors, have also been found to play key roles in cholesterol homeostasis, particularly in the regulation of cholesterol elimination through increased bile acid production and excretion, enhanced cellular cholesterol efflux, and inhibition of intestinal cholesterol absorption. The study of these nuclear hormone receptors suggests their potential as targets for new drug therapies aimed at alleviating hypercholesterolemia.

ORPHAN NUCLEAR HORMONE RECEPTORS INVOLVED IN CHOLESTEROL HOMEOSTASIS

Introduction to Nuclear Hormone Receptors

Nuclear hormone receptors comprise a large superfamily of ligand-activated transcription factors that regulate the

J. J. Repa, M. Makishima, and **D. J. Mangelsdorf:** Department of Pharmacology, Howard Hughes Medical Institute, University of Texas Southwestern Medical Center, Dallas, Texas 75390-9050.

T. T. Lu: Department of Pharmacology, University of Texas Southwestern Medical Center, Dallas, Texas 75390-9041.

expression of numerous genes involved in development and adult physiology (4–6). These proteins contain a highly conserved central approximately 70-amino-acid DNA-binding motif consisting of two zinc finger modules that defines this receptor superfamily. In addition, the carboxyl half of these receptors contains a less-conserved ligand-binding domain responsible for hormone binding, dimerization, and ligand-dependent activation. With few exceptions, these receptors reside in the nucleus of cells and are bound to specific DNA sequences located in the 5′-flanking region of receptor-regulated genes. In the absence of ligand, the receptors are associated with corepressor proteins that maintain the adjacent gene in a transcriptional "off" state. Upon binding their respective lipophilic ligand or hormone, these nuclear receptors undergo a conformational change to release their corepressor and recruit a coactivator protein that allows interaction with the general transcription machinery to regulate target gene expression (7,8).

Analysis of early members of the nuclear hormone receptor superfamily revealed structure/activity characteristics that were exploited to discover novel receptor proteins. These new family members, termed 'orphan receptors' because their cognate ligands are unknown, have been the subjects of intense study over the last decade (reviewed in refs. 5,9–11). The goal of this research has been to identify (a) the physiologic and synthetic ligands of an orphan receptor; (b) the target genes regulated by the ligand-activated orphan receptor; and (c) the biological role of the orphan receptor, often facilitated by the analysis of mouse strains that either lack or overproduce the receptor of interest. Rapid progress in this field of research has recently revealed that several orphan nuclear hormone receptors play important roles in cholesterol and bile acid metabolism (reviewed in refs. 12–16). These findings offer the exciting opportunity to develop novel therapeutic agents that target these receptors and regulate various aspects of cholesterol metabolism in hopes of alleviating lipid disorders.

The Liver X Receptors, LXRα and LXRβ

Liver X receptor (LXRα) (NR1H3, also known as RLD-1 in the rat) was so named based on its initial isolation from a human liver cDNA library (6,17,18). The tissue distribution of LXRα was determined by Northern blot analyses revealing that LXRα is present in liver, adipose, intestine, kidney, lung, spleen, adrenal gland, and macrophage (12,17–20). The *LXRα* gene is located on human chromosome 11 (11). LXRβ (NR1H2, also known as NER, UR, RIP15, and OR-1) is ubiquitously expressed, being found in nearly every tissue tested (12,19–22). The human *LXRβ* gene has been localized to chromosome 9q13.3 (22). To investigate the expression patterns and regulation of the LXRs, the promoter regions of these genes in the mouse have been identified and characterized (20,23,24). Evidence suggests that LXRα expression is enhanced by activators of

the peroxisome proliferator activated receptors (PPARs), particularly PPARγ (20,25). The LXR proteins are highly related and share approximately 77% amino acid sequence identity in both their DNA- and ligand-binding domains. This would suggest that they are likely to be activated by a common set of ligands to regulate an overlapping array of target genes. However, the dissimilarity inherent in these proteins may also allow for the development of receptor-selective ligands that could target specific genes, particularly when the differential tissue distribution of the LXRs is considered.

The LXRs form obligate heterodimers with the retinoid X receptor (RXR), an orphan nuclear receptor bound and activated by 9-*cis*-retinoic acid (26). The RXR/LXR complex belongs to the class of permissive heterodimers since RXR ligands, or rexinoids, can elicit transcriptional activity of this complex in the absence of LXR agonists (17). Interestingly, rexinoid activity requires the LXR, but not the RXR, activation motif located in the LXR ligand-binding domain, suggesting that ligand binding by one receptor induces a conformational change in its partner to elicit a transcriptional response (27). The RXR/LXR heterodimer preferentially binds to a direct repeat DNA sequence consisting of two conserved hexanucleotides (AGGTCA) separated by four bases (a DR-4 motif referred to as an LXRE) (Fig. 69.1) (17,21). Such DR-4 motifs have been identified in a number of RXR/LXR target genes and are critical to LXR-mediated gene regulation (described below). A recent study utilizing biochemical and molecular techniques also suggests that LXRα may function on certain gene targets as a monomer, although this finding still awaits substantiation in biological systems and animal models (28).

The search for ligands of the LXRs began by testing fractions of organic extracts prepared from animal tissues using a cell-based reporter assay (29). In this assay, cultured cells are transiently transfected with the orphan receptor cDNA and a luciferase reporter gene. Cells are then exposed to candidate ligands and monitored for ligand-dependent luciferase activity (30). This analysis identified the first activators of both LXRα and LXRβ as a unique class of oxysterols, some of which are derived from cholesterol. This finding was not too surprising as ligands of other nuclear receptor family members are lipophilic derivatives of acetyl CoA, and several are also cholesterol metabolites (vitamin D_3 and steroid hormones). Structure/activity analysis of LXR ligands revealed the most potent physiologic activators to be 22(R)-hydroxycholesterol (22HC), 24(S)-hydroxycholesterol (24HC) and 24(S),25-epoxycholesterol (24,25EC) (29,31,32). Further analysis demonstrated that only the naturally occurring stereoisomer of each oxysterol is an effective activator of LXRs. The development of a scintillation proximity assay to directly measure ligand/receptor interaction firmly demonstrated that these oxysterols bind LXRs with affinities of 0.1 - 0.4 μM, a concentration range that is consistent with those reported in various tissues (31).

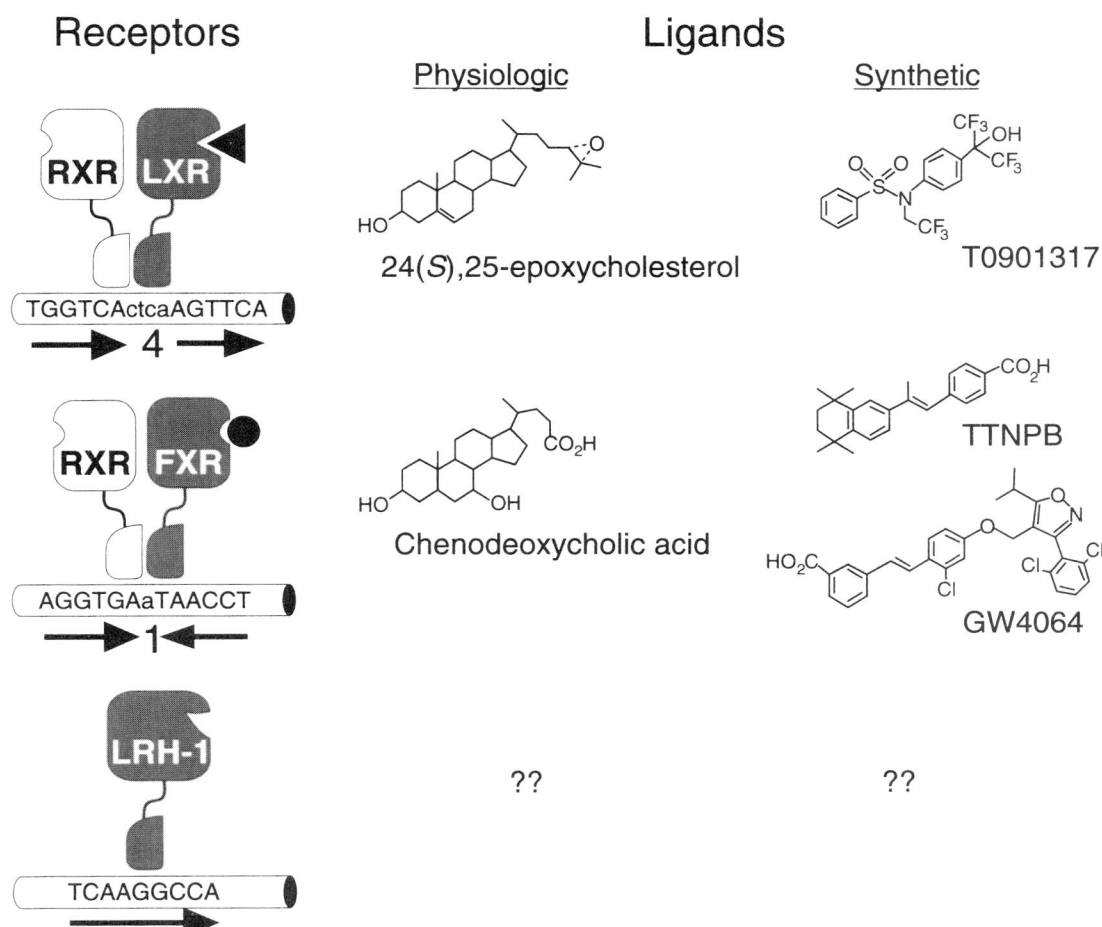

FIGURE 69.1. Characterization of the orphan nuclear receptors, liver X receptor (*LXR*), farnesoid X receptor (*FXR*) and liver receptor homologue (*LRH*)-1. The dimerization preference and DNA-binding motif recognized by each receptor is illustrated on the **left**. The DR4 (LXRE) depicted is derived from the rat cholesterol 7α-hydroxylase (CYP7A1) gene promoter (32). The IR1 (FXRE) shown for the retinoid X receptor (RXR)/FXR heterodimer is from the murine *ibabp* gene (44). This LRHRE is found in the human CYP7A1 gene (57). The synthetic ligands shown are described in references 41, 136, and 137. Note, TTNPB (a synthetic retinoid) is not selective for FXR, as it also binds and activates the retinoic acid receptors (RARs).

24HC is found in brain, where LXRβ is abundant, due to the tissue-specific activity of a cholesterol 24-hydroxylase (CYP46) (33–35). 24,25EC is present in liver, where LXRα expression is greatest (36). In contrast to other oxysterols which are derived from cholesterol, 24,25EC is synthesized in liver directly from squalene in a shunt pathway that bypasses the final steps of cholesterol biosynthesis (37). 22HC has been detected in bovine adrenal gland and human meconium (38,39). The analysis of synthetic analogs of these oxysterols demonstrated that monooxidation of the side-chain is required for LXR binding and activation, that sterols with a 24-oxo group have improved activity, and that introduction of an oxygen on the sterol B-ring results in a ligand that is selective for the LXRα recep-

tor isoform (31). Recently, a high-affinity, nonsteroidal synthetic LXR agonist has been also been described (40,41).

The Farnesoid X Receptor (Bile Acid Receptor)

The farnesoid X receptor (FXR) (NR1H4, also known as RIP14) was initially isolated from liver cDNA libraries by a variety of techniques (6,42,43). Northern analyses and *in situ* hybridization have shown that FXR expression is restricted to adrenal cortex, intestine, colon, kidney and liver (12,42). Like the LXRs, FXR binds DNA as a heterodimer with RXR, and is permissive to rexinoid activation. However, the DNA sequence recognized by the RXR/FXR heterodimer is an inverted hexanucleotide repeat separated by a single base (an IR-1 motif referred to as an FXRE; Fig. 69.1).

FXR is most closely related to the insect ecdysone receptor, and early studies revealed that this orphan receptor can be weakly activated by supraphysiological concentrations of ligands structurally similar to ecdysone (farnesoids and synthetic retinoids), hence the original nomenclature, farnesoid X receptor. Recently, however, three laboratories have independently identified bile acids as the bona fide ligands of FXR, prompting some investigators to rename this orphan the bile acid receptor, BAR (44–46). Cell-based reporter assays revealed that the primary dihydroxy bile acid chenodeoxycholic acid (CDCA) is the most active ligand for human, mouse and rat FXR (44–46). FXR is also weakly activated in this cell reporter system by the secondary bile acids lithocholic acid and deoxycholic acid. In this assay, no activation was observed with other bile acids (muricholic acid, ursodeoxycholic acid, cholic acid) or initially with conjugated bile acids. The failure of conjugated bile acids to function as ligands in the cell-based assay was vexing, as these make up the vast majority of bile acids in tissues. However, while conjugation with taurine and glycine makes bile acids more soluble, it also reduces their ability to passively diffuse through the cell membrane. Cells of the enterohepatic system harbor membrane transporters to actively take up conjugated bile acids. Therefore, when the cell-based reporter assay was modified to introduce either the liver sodium taurocholate cotransporter polypeptide (NTCP) or the enterocyte apical sodium-dependent bile acid transporter (ASBT) into the transfected cells, it was found that the conjugated forms of CDCA were capable of inducing FXR-mediated gene expression (45,46). Thus, the physiologically relevant ligands are the conjugated bile acids which show activity well within the range of reported intracellular concentrations (47–49). Indeed, several of *in vitro* biochemical binding assays have confirmed that a number of both conjugated and unconjugated bile acids directly bind to FXR (44,45,50). The unequivocal confirmation of the role of FXR as the bile acid receptor was obtained by analyzing *fxr*-knockout mice which fail to upregulate FXR-target genes following bile acid administration (51).

The Liver Receptor Homologue-1

The liver receptor homologue-1 (LRH-1) (NR5A2, also known as PHR-1, FTZ-F1b1, FTF, FFR1A, OR2.0, hB1F, FFLR and CPF) was isolated by a variety of molecular cloning methods and found to be the homolog of the *Drosophila fushi tarazu F1* gene (6,52–57). LRH-1 expression is limited to liver, intestine, colon, ovary and pancreas (12,54,58). The gene for human LRH-1 has been mapped to chromosome 1q32.1 (54,56). This orphan receptor binds DNA as a monomer to an extended version of the hexanucleotide recognized by most nuclear hormone receptors (called an LRHRE; Fig. 69.1). No ligand has yet been identified for LRH-1.

LRH-1 is highly related to the mammalian orphan receptor steroidogenic factor-1 (SF-1). SF-1 expression is restricted to steroidogenic tissues and is essential for both the development of these organs as well as the expression of key enzymes responsible for the conversion of cholesterol to steroid hormones in adult tissues (reviewed in ref. 59). It is tempting to speculate that LRH-1 plays a similar role in the liver, exocrine pancreas and intestine, tissues all derived from gut endoderm. Preliminary reports support the hypothesis that LRH-1 plays an essential role in development, as LRH-1 gene ablation in the mouse is embryonic lethal (T. Kerr and D. W. Russell, 2001, *personal communication*). Furthermore, LRH-1 regulates α-fetoprotein and the transcription factor HNF-3β, two gene products involved in early liver development (54,60). In the adult liver, LRH-1 appears to be essential for the liver-specific expression of key enzymes responsible for the conversion of cholesterol to bile acids [(57,61) discussed in Genes Encoding Key Enzymes of Bile and Biosynthesis, below)].

The Small Heterodimer Partner

The small heterodimer partner (SHP) was isolated by molecular cloning techniques that identify proteins which associate with nuclear hormone receptors (62,63). This atypical orphan receptor lacks a DNA-binding domain, and appears to repress gene transcription through its interaction with other nuclear hormone receptors (64–66). Northern blotting revealed that SHP is abundantly expressed in the liver, and present at lower levels in adrenal gland, heart, pancreas and intestine (12,63,67). The SHP gene is localized to human chromosome 1p36.1 (67). Recently, mutations in the human SHP gene have been linked to a mild form of obesity (67), further supporting a role for this protein in lipid metabolism.

SHP is closely related to the orphan receptor DAX-1. DAX-1 interacts with SF-1 to regulate steroidogenesis. In a similar manner, SHP has been shown to associate with LRH-1 to affect the expression of key enzymes in bile acid biosynthesis [(68,69) discussed in Genes Encoding Key Enzymes of Bile Acid Biosynthesis, below].

Other Nuclear Hormone Receptors Implicated in Cholesterol Metabolism

Numerous diet and drug studies have implicated several additional nuclear hormone receptors in the control of cholesterol conversion to bile acids, particularly in the regulation of cholesterol 7α-hydroxylase (CYP7A1), the rate-limiting enzyme in the neutral pathway of bile acid biosynthesis (reviewed in 12,70). Fibrates, ligands of PPARα, strongly repress *CYP7A1* in humans and rodents (71–74). Agonists of the murine xenobiotic receptor PXR also produce a decrease in CYP7A1 levels (75,76). Cell reporter assays to investigate CYP7A1 promoter regulation have also suggested roles for COUP-TFII and HNF4 (77). All of these receptors have been localized to tissues of the enterohepatic circulation, which further supports their role in bile acid metabolism, but their molecular mechanisms of action have yet to be fully elucidated.

Very recently antidiabetic drugs of the thiazolidinedione class that activate PPARγ have been shown to increase LXRα levels, and hence LXR target genes involved in cholesterol metabolism (20,25). PPARγ is not present at significant levels in liver or intestine (being found only in the very proximal duodenum: Repa and Mangelsdorf, 2000, *unpublished observations*). Therefore, PPARγ probably does not modulate bile acid biosynthetic genes. However, in other tissues, particularly macrophages, this PPARγ/LXRα cascade initiates "reverse cholesterol transport" and thereby redistributes peripheral cholesterol to the liver, where it can be converted to bile acids or excreted directly into bile [(20,25) discussed in Genes Affecting Cholesterol and Bile Acid Transport, below)].

HEPATIC GENES AFFECTING CHOLESTEROL AND BILE ACID METABOLISM THAT ARE REGULATED BY NUCLEAR HORMONE RECEPTORS

An expanding number of genes involved in cholesterol homeostasis are being discovered that are transcriptionally regulated by orphan nuclear receptors. For the most part, these genes appear to control the catabolism of cholesterol to bile acids and the intracellular transport and efflux of sterols and bile acids. In addition, nuclear receptors have been implicated in the gene regulation of apolipoproteins and transfer proteins [cholesterol ester (CETP) and phospholipid transfer proteins (PLTP)] involved in the systemic transport of cholesterol and other lipids (78–82). Growing evidence suggests that these orphan nuclear receptors serve as intracellular lipid sensors that coordinately regulate genes to alleviate high lipid concentrations. In particular, as sterol sensors, the LXRs have been implicated in the control of reverse cholesterol transport (RCT) (reviewed in ref. 15). The RCT hypothesis, first proposed by Glomset in 1980, holds that cholesterol is effluxed from peripheral cells to produce high-density lipoprotein (HDL), which mediates the movement of cholesterol back to the liver, where it is excreted into bile (83). The RXR/LXR heterodimer appears to upregulate a number of genes that are involved in RCT (see Genes Affecting Cholesterol and Bile Acid Transport, below).

Genes Encoding Key Enzymes of Bile Acid Biosynthesis

Bile acids are exclusively synthesized in the liver. This results from the fact that the genes of the bile acid biosynthetic pathways are abundantly (e.g., cholesterol 27-hydroxylase,

CYP27) or exclusively (e.g., sterol 12α-hydroxylase, CYP8B1 and cholesterol 7α-hydroxylase, CYP7A1) expressed in this organ (84,85). The reader is referred to Chapter 16 and website chapters 🖳 W-22 through W-24 in this volume for a complete description of the bile acid metabolic pathways. The liver-specific expression of CYP7A1 and CYP8B1 results from transcriptional regulation by the orphan receptor LRH-1 (57,61). The extended DNA half-site sequence recognized by LRH-1 has been identified in the promoters of the CYP7A1 and CYP8B1 genes, and is conserved in several animal species (57,61) (Fig. 69.1).

As the rate-limiting enzyme of the classic bile acid synthesis pathway, CYP7A1 has been the subject of intense study over the last decade and was found to be transcriptionally regulated by a number of dietary, hormonal and drug treatments (reviewed in refs. 12, 70, 86, and 87). It appears that CYP7A1 is controlled by at least five orphan nuclear receptors, including RXR, LXR, FXR, LRH-1, and SHP. *CYP7A1* was the first target gene identified for the RXR/LXR heterodimer, and a DR4 binding motif was found in the promoter of the murine *cyp7a1* gene (32,88). Under conditions of elevated hepatic cholesterol and hence oxysterol concentration, CYP7A1 expression is induced in the liver of rodents (88–90). In the mouse, this induction requires the presence of LXRs (particularly LXRα), RXRs (particularly RXRα) and a functional LXRE in the *cyp7a1* gene promoter (32,88,91). The LXRE of the human *CYP7A1* gene promoter contains a two-nucleotide change from the rodent, making it a relatively poor RXR/LXR binding site. This finding may explain why humans do not increase bile acid synthesis as robustly as rodents when fed high levels of dietary cholesterol (92). Interestingly, hamsters also fail to exhibit increased CYP7A1 transcription following cholesterol feeding (90). However, the hamster CYP7A1 LXRE is identical to that of the mouse and rat, and the hamster LXRα is bound and activated by the same array of oxysterols that activate mouse and human LXRs, suggesting that some other component of the LXR/oxysterol signaling pathway is impaired in this species (93; Repa and Mangelsdorf, 2000, *unpublished observation*). Recently, synthetic LXR agonists have been shown to upregulate CYP7A1 expression in the hamster, which points to the possibility that hamsters are incapable of producing adequate cholesterol-derived LXR ligands (41).

CYP7A1 expression is strongly repressed by bile acids (reviewed in refs. 12, 70, 86, and 87). The molecular basis for this feedback regulation has recently been elucidated and involves the orphan nuclear receptors FXR, LRH-1 and SHP (68,69). Feedback repression of CYP7A1 is achieved by the binding of bile acids to FXR, which leads to increased transcription of the FXR target gene *SHP*. SHP, which is a potent transcriptional repressor, then forms a heterodimeric complex with LRH-1 and thereby reduces expression of LRH-1-dependent genes (including *CYP7A1*, *CYP8B1*, and *SHP* itself). Various steps of this regulatory cascade have been confirmed in animal studies: hepatic SHP expression is increased in mice fed bile acids, and decreased in mice with diminished bile acid pools (e.g., *cyp7a1*- and *cyp27*-knockout mice) (69,94); bile acid-mediated upregulation of SHP requires FXR and a functional FXRE in the promoter of the SHP gene (51,68,69); and SHP and LRH-1 have been shown to functionally interact by a variety of methods (68,69). Further verification of the FXR/SHP/LRH-1 regulatory cascade awaits the analyses of *shp*- and *lrh-1*-knockout mouse strains.

Agonists of other orphan nuclear receptors have also been found to transcriptionally repress CYP7A1 gene expression. Activators of the xenobiotic receptor PXR (also known as SXR) have been shown to decrease the levels of CYP7A1 (40,76). Ligands of PPARα, such as fibrates, have also been reported to repress CYP7A1 gene transcription (40,72,74). However, the precise molecular mechanisms for PXR- and PPARα-mediated CYP7A1 regulation have not yet been fully elucidated.

Genes Affecting Cholesterol and Bile Acid Transport

Members of three families of proteins responsible for lipid transport have been found to be regulated by orphan nuclear hormone receptors: the lipocalin family of small, cytosolic binding proteins responsible for sequestration and cellular translocation of lipids; the cholesterol ester transfer protein (CETP) and phospholipid transfer protein (PLTP) which are involved in the blood-borne transport of lipids; and the adenosine triphosphate (ATP)-binding cassette (ABC) family of membrane-bound transporters involved in cellular trafficking and efflux of lipids.

Cytosolic Lipid-Binding Proteins

Some of the earliest, and most profoundly, upregulated target genes identified for nuclear hormone receptors were members of the lipocalin family of cytosolic lipid-binding proteins. Exposing cells to high levels of vitamin A and its derivatives causes a rapid increase in the transcription of cellular retinoid-binding proteins (CRABPs and CRBPs) mediated by the retinoic acid receptors (RARs) (95). Likewise, activation of the PPAR family of nuclear hormone receptors results in increased transcription of cytosolic fatty acid-binding proteins: liver-FABP regulated by PPARα, and adipocyte lipid-binding protein (ALBP/aP2) regulated by PPARγ (96,97). Under these circumstances, lipid/ligand activation of the nuclear hormone receptor results in increased cytosolic binding protein expression and a reduction of the free lipid/ligand concentration within the cell. In a similar manner, bile acids were found to transcriptionally upregulate the expression of the ileal bile acid-binding protein (IBABP) (98,99). Analysis of the IBABP gene promoter revealed the presence of an IR-1 binding motif recognized

by FXR and responsible for bile acid-mediated gene transcription (44,51,100). IBABP is abundantly, and exclusively, expressed in the ileal enterocyte, a cell exposed to millimolar concentrations of bile acids (49). Feeding mice a diet containing additional cholic acid or chenodeoxycholic acid does not result in further upregulation of IBABP expression, presumably because FXR is already saturated with bile acids present at levels far exceeding its apparent dissociation constant (approximately 10 to 50 μM) (44,45). However, treating mice with a potent, synthetic RXR agonist results in a modest (about 2-fold) increase in IBABP mRNA levels, most likely through RXR/FXR-mediated activation (Repa and Mangelsdorf, 2000, *unpublished observation*). Furthermore, in the *fxr*-knockout mouse the basal level of IBABP is completely repressed and is not upregulated by FXR/RXR agonists (51). Based on this apparent pattern of nuclear receptor-mediated regulation of lipocalin protein expression, it will be interesting to see if transcription of a hepatic bile acid-binding protein is likewise mediated by FXR, or if expression of any of the expanding family of oxysterol-binding proteins is regulated by the oxysterol/LXR signaling pathway (101,102).

Cholesterol Ester Transfer Protein and Phospholipid Transfer Protein

Blood-borne transport of cholesterol and other lipids is affected by the liver production and secretion of CETP and PLTP, which ultimately contribute to HDL maturation (103). CETP has been identified as a target gene of LXRs, and contains an LXRE in its gene promoter essential for oxysterol-mediated upregulation of gene transcription (80). Testing this finding in the mouse model is complicated by the fact that mice do not produce CETP. However, studies using cell reporter assays and transgenic mice suggest that LXR-mediated upregulation of CETP may favor cholesterol transfer from the periphery to the liver (80,104). PLTP expression is regulated by bile acids and FXR through an IR-1 motif identified in the 5′-flanking region of that gene (82). Long-term feeding of a cholic acid-containing diet to mice indeed results in a modest increase in hepatic PLTP RNA levels (81).

Adenosine Triphosphate (ATP)–Binding Cassette Transporters

Most recently, several members of the ATP-binding cassette (ABC) transporter family of proteins have been found to be transcriptionally regulated by orphan nuclear receptors. ABC transporters comprise a large superfamily of membrane-bound proteins containing two six-transmembrane spanning domains and two nucleotide binding folds that hydrolyze ATP to provide energy for the transport of various substrates (the reader is referred to the excellent website http://www.med.rug.nl/mdl/humanabc.htm, and the reviews in refs. 105–107). These four protein domains can be provided by a single gene product (a full-transporter), or by the dimerization of two half-transporters each providing a transmembrane domain and ATP-binding cassette. Based upon a rather limited assessment of the subcellular localization of these transporters, it appears that the full-transporters are most often integral proteins of the cell plasma membrane, and half-transporters are associated with membranes of intracellular organelles. In addition, several full-transporters exhibit a distinct cellular polarity being localized selectively to the basolateral, apical or in the case of hepatocytes, the canalicular membrane (107,108).

Great strides have been made in the understanding of ABC transporter function with the identification of several human genetic disorders arising from mutations in ABC genes. *ABCA1* was recently identified as the genetic locus responsible for Tangier disease, a rare autosomal recessive disorder characterized by a lack of circulating HDL cholesterol and the appearance of cholesterol-engorged macrophages and other reticuloendothelial cells (109–111). This phenotype, along with results obtained in cell-based assay systems, suggest that ABCA1 plays a pivotal role in cellular cholesterol and phospholipid efflux to apoAI in the formation of HDL to initiate RCT (reviewed in ref. 112). This phenotype was recapitulated in *abca1*-knockout mice, which also exhibit an increase in the intestinal absorption of cholesterol (113–115). ABCA1 is a full-transporter expressed in a wide variety of tissues that appears to be localized to the plasma membrane, although its distribution in particular membranes of polarized cells is still undetermined (116,117). *ABCA1* was first identified as a transcriptionally upregulated gene in sterol-loaded macrophages (116). However, recent studies support the hypothesis that sterol-loading *per se* is not responsible for ABCA1 gene induction, but rather it is the generation of sterol-derived LXR agonists that drives transcription of this gene (40). Administration of physiologic or synthetic ligands of the RXR/LXR heterodimer to mice results in a rapid, robust upregulation of ABCA1 expression in enterocytes and isolated macrophages, which requires the presence of LXR (40). Macrophages and enterocytes share the distinction that they are two cell types that can experience a large surge in intracellular sterol levels by the nonsaturable uptake of free cholesterol from phagocytosis or exposure to oxidized LDL, and from the intestinal lumen, respectively. As such, these cells may be more reliant on LXR-mediated efflux of cholesterol by increased ABCA1 expression. An LXRE has been identified in the promoter region of the mouse and human ABCA1 genes (118,119). Several independent laboratories have confirmed and extended the observation that *ABCA1* is an LXR target gene responsible for increased cholesterol efflux from the macrophage (20,25,120,121). In addition, the LXR-mediated upregulation of ABCA1 expression in the enterocyte is associated with decreased cholesterol absorption efficiency, which implies that this transporter effluxes cholesterol back from the intestinal cell to the lumen (40) (Fig. 69.2).

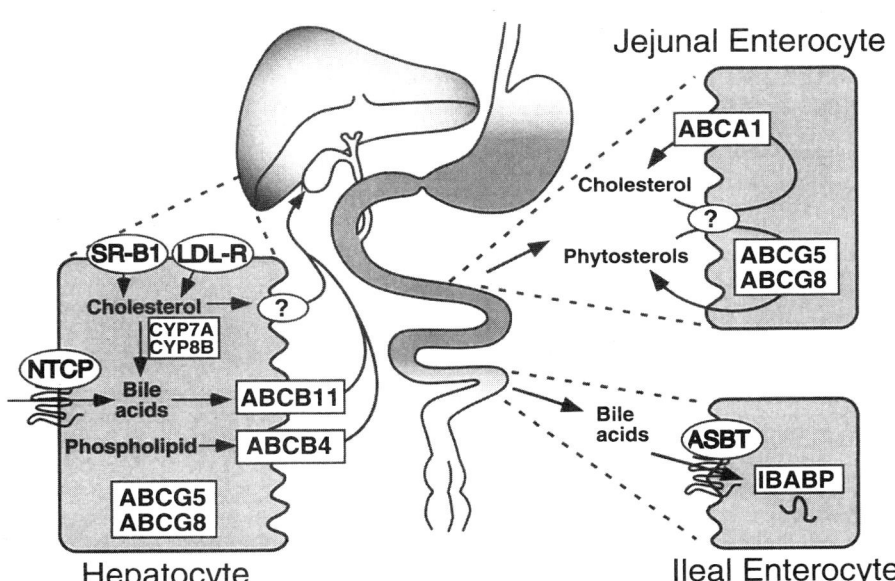

FIGURE 69.2. Orphan nuclear receptor regulation of genes involved in cholesterol and bile acid metabolism. Gene products shown in *boxes* are target genes of orphan nuclear receptors as described in the text. The subcellular location of ATP-binding cassettes (*ABCs*) A1, G5 and G8 are tentative. *ASBT*, apical sodium-dependent bile salt transporter; *IBABP*, ileal bile acid-binding protein; *LDL-R*, low-density lipoprotein receptor; *NTCP*, sodium taurocholate cotransporter polypeptide; and *SR-B1*, scavenger receptor type B1 (an HDL receptor).

Analysis of sterol-loaded macrophages led to the discovery of another LXR-regulated ABC transporter, ABCG1 (formerly called ABC-8 or white). Northern analyses revealed that ABCG1 expression is restricted to macrophages, spleen, brain, thymus, lung, and adrenal gland (122,123). ABCG1 has also been implicated in lipid efflux from macrophages, although being a half-transporter it may be involved in the intracellular trafficking of cholesterol and phospholipid preceding efflux (124). Studies have demonstrated that *ABCG1* is a direct target gene of the RXR/LXR heterodimer (19), although the precise molecular mechanism of action has yet to be determined. No human genetic disorder has yet been attributed to mutations in ABCG1, nor has another half-transporter dimer partner been identified.

Mutations in the gene encoding ABCB11 (also called the bile salt efflux pump, bsep) are responsible for progressive familial intrahepatic cholestasis type 2 (PFIC2), a genetic disorder that causes markedly abnormal hepatic bile salt secretion and liver failure (125). This full-transporter exhibits a liver-specific expression pattern, and has been localized to the hepatocyte canalicular membrane (108,125,126) (Fig. 69.2). The analyses of *fxr*-knockout mice strongly support the notion that ABCB11 is a target gene of the RXR/FXR heterodimer. The expression level of ABCB11 in *fxr*−/− mice is reduced and is not upregulated following cholic acid feeding as is observed in wild-type mice (51). The presence of a potential RXR/FXR DNA binding motif in the promoter of the human *BSEP* gene has been reported (107).

PFIC3 results from mutations in the ABC transporter responsible for phospholipid secretion at the canalicular membrane (127). This transporter, ABCB4, is also called MDR3 in humans, and mdr2 in the mouse and rat. Elimination of ABCB4 in a mouse strain by targeted gene ablation, revealed that the bile of *mdr2*−/− mice contains no phospholipid and essentially no cholesterol, yet normal bile salt concentrations (128). This demonstrated the importance of phosphatidylcholine in the solubilization and flow of cholesterol into bile. ABCB4 has been found to be regulated at the level of transcription by a wide variety of peroxisome proliferators that serve as ligands of PPARα in the liver (129). Likewise, short-term oral administration of synthetic RXR and PPARα agonists to mice results in increased levels of ABCB4 mRNA in liver (Repa and Mangelsdorf, 2000, *unpublished observation*). Further analysis of the ABCB4 gene is necessary to determine whether it is a direct target of RXR/PPARα regulation.

Subtractive cloning techniques to identify LXR target genes in liver and intestine resulted in the recent discovery of a novel ABC half-transporter, ABCG5 (130). Further analysis revealed that this gene was located on human chromosome 2p21 in a head-to-head orientation with a second half-transporter, ABCG8 (130). This same region had previously been identified as the possible genetic locus for sitosterolemia, a rare genetic disorder characterized by hyperabsorption of plant sterols and increased cholesterol absorption (131,132). Indeed, mutations in ABCG5 and/or ABCG8 have now been linked to the development of sitosterolemia (130,133). The fact that a mutation in either gene results in the same phenotype strongly suggests that these two half-transporters form a functional dimer. The ABCG5 and ABCG8 genes are expressed exclusively in liver and intestine, and show coordinate changes in expression by dietary cholesterol and agonists of RXR and LXR (130; Repa et al., 2001, *unpublished observation*). Additional studies are necessary to delineate the molecular mechanism of RXR/LXR regulation, and to ascertain the relative roles of ABCs A1, G5, and G8 in cholesterol absorption and biliary cholesterol secretion.

The emerging pattern of orphan nuclear receptor regulation of ABC transporters suggests that under high lipid/ligand concentrations an orphan receptor will upregulate the expression of the corresponding ABC transporter to efflux that lipid/ligand. It will be interesting to see if regulated ABC proteins can be identified for other nuclear hormone receptors. This pattern of regulation has been extended to a nonmammalian organism, with the finding that the only nuclear hormone receptor in *Drosophila* for which a ligand has been identified, the ecdysone receptor, also regulates the transcription of an ABC transporter that controls the cellular efflux of ecdysone (134).

ORPHAN NUCLEAR HORMONE RECEPTORS AS LIPID SENSORS THAT COORDINATELY REGULATE GENES TO CONTROL INTRACELLULAR LEVELS OF LIPIDS/LIGANDS

The small, lipophilic endogenous ligands being described for the orphan nuclear receptors play essential roles in physiology. Cholesterol, the precursor of LXR oxysterols, is integral to cell membrane function, and is necessary for the production of bile acids, and certain vitamins and hormones. Yet, at high intracellular concentrations it can elicit cell death. Bile acids, the ligands of FXR, are detergent-like molecules necessary for the solubilization of dietary lipids and fat-soluble vitamins for absorption, and for promoting cholesterol outflow into bile. Again, high concentrations of FXR ligands can lead to cell death and cholestatic disorders. LXR and FXR appear to respond to rising concentrations of their ligands by turning on a set of genes encoding proteins to reduce those intracellular ligand levels, thus serving as intracellular lipid sensors. Three families of target genes have been identified to achieve this goal (Table 69.1). Cytosolic binding proteins levels are increased in order to sequester the lipid and reduce the intracellular concentration of ligand. The production of cytochrome P450 genes are altered to increase catabolism of the ligand (e.g., LXR inducing CYP7A1), or reduce synthesis of the ligand (e.g.,

TABLE 69.1. NUCLEAR ORPHAN RECEPTORS AS LIGAND SENSORS

Ligand	Receptor	Cytosolic Binding Protein	Cytochrome P450	ABC Transporter	Confirmed in Receptor KO Mouse
Oxysterols	LXRs	?	↑CYP7A1	ABCA1, ABCG1	(88)
				ABCG5, ABCG8	(40)
Bile acids	FXR	IBABP	↓CYP7A1	ABCB11 (bsep)	(51)
			↓CYP8B1		
Fatty acids, fibrates	PPARs	L-FABP	↑CYP4A	ABCB4 (mdr2)	
Xenobiotics	PXR/SXR	?	↑CYP3A	?	(138)
Xenobiotics	CAR	?	↑CYP2B	?	(139)

Proteins shown in italics are present in liver.
IBABP, ileal bile acid binding protein; L-FABP, liver fatty acid binding protein; CYP7A1, cholesterol 7α-hydroxylase; CYP8B1, sterol 12α-hydroxylase; bsep, bile salt efflux pump; mdr2, multidrug resistance gene 2 (MDR3 in humans).

FXR repressing CYP7A1) (135). Finally, the new family of ABC transporters have been identified as targets, whereby an activated orphan nuclear receptor will increase the expression of the respective ABC transporter that can efflux the lipid/ligand from the cell. It will be interesting to see if additional target genes of these three protein families will be identified for other orphan receptors. It may also be possible that the characteristics of an ABC transporter, cytosolic binding protein, or cytochrome P450 enzyme, may lead to the identification of a ligand for another orphan receptor.

CONCLUSION

The last several years have seen an explosion of new discoveries that have revitalized the fields of cholesterol, bile acid and fatty acid metabolism. These discoveries are highlighted by the finding of a set of coordinate transcriptional regulatory systems that are mediated by the orphan nuclear receptors. Because of the historical importance other members of this family of receptors have had in the pharmaceutical industry (i.e., the steroid hormone receptors), it is likely that an entirely new set of therapeutic drugs, based on the pharmacology of the orphan receptors, is on the horizon. In addition, since the breakthroughs in this field have just begun, it is clear that a number of important new avenues still remain to be explored.

ACKNOWLEDGMENTS

Support was provided by the Howard Hughes Medical Institute, The Robert A. Welch Foundation, and the Human Frontier Science Program.

REFERENCES

1. Brown MS, Goldstein JL. The SREBP pathway: regulation of cholesterol metabolism by proteolysis of a membrane-bound transcription factor. *Cell* 1997;89:331–340.
2. Brown MS, Goldstein JL. A proteolytic pathway that controls the cholesterol content of membranes, cells, and blood. *Proc Natl Acad Sci USA* 1999;96:11041–11048.
3. Horton JD, Shimomura I. Sterol regulatory element-binding proteins: activators of cholesterol and fatty acid biosynthesis. *Curr Opin Lipidol* 1999;10:143–150.
4. Mangelsdorf DJ, Thummel C, Beato M, et al. The nuclear receptor superfamily: the second decade. *Cell* 1995;83:835–839.
5. Giguère V. Orphan nuclear receptors: from gene to function. *Endocr Rev* 1999;20:689–725.
6. Nuclear Receptors Nomenclature Committee. A unified nomenclature system for the nuclear receptor superfamily. *Cell* 1999;97:161–163.
7. McKenna NJ, Lanz RB, O'Malley BW. Nuclear receptor coregulators: cellular and molecular biology. *Endocr Rev* 1999;20:321–344.
8. Glass CK, Rosenfeld MG. The coregulator exchange in transcriptional functions of nuclear receptors. *Genes Dev* 2000;14:121–141.
9. Kliewer SA, Lehmann JM, Willson TM. Orphan nuclear receptors: shifting endocrinology into reverse. *Science* 1999;284:757–760.
10. Sladek R, Giguère V. Orphan nuclear receptors: an emerging family of metabolic regulators. *Adv Pharmacol* 2000;47:23–87.
11. Willy PJ, Mangelsdorf DJ. Nuclear orphan receptors: the search for novel ligands and signaling pathways. In O'Malley B, ed. *Hormones and signaling* Vol. 1. San Diego: Academic Press, 1998;1:307–358.
12. Repa JJ, Mangelsdorf DJ. The role of orphan nuclear receptors in the regulation of cholesterol homeostasis. *Annu Rev Cell Dev Biol* 2000;16:459–481.
13. Russell DW. Nuclear orphan receptors control cholesterol catabolism. *Cell* 1999;97:539–542.
14. Gustafsson J-Å. Seeking ligands for lonely orphan receptors. *Science* 1999;284:1285–1286.
15. Tall AR, Costet P, Luo Y. 'Orphans' meet cholesterol. *Nat Med* 2000;6:1104–1105.
16. Schoonjans K, Brendel C, Mangelsdorf D, et al. Sterols and gene expression: control of affluence. *Biochim Biophys Acta* 2000;1529:114–125.
17. Willy PJ, Umesono K, Ong ES, et al. LXR, a nuclear receptor that defines a distinct retinoid response pathway. *Genes Dev* 1995;9:1033–1045.
18. Apfel R, Benbrook D, Lernhardt E, et al. A novel orphan receptor specific for a subset of thyroid hormone-responsive elements and its interaction with the` retinoid/thyroid hormone receptor subfamily. *Mol Cell Biol* 1994;14:7025–7035.

19. Venkateswaran A, Repa JJ, Lobaccaro J-MA, et al. Human White/murine ABC8 mRNA levels are highly induced in lipid-loaded macrophages: a transcriptional role for specific oxysterols. *J Biol Chem* 2000;275:14700–14707.

20. Chawla A, Boisvert WA, Lee C-H, et al. A PPARγ-LXR-ABCA1 pathway in macrophages is involved in cholesterol efflux and atherogenesis. *Mol Cell* 2001;7:161–171.

21. Teboul M, Enmark E, Li Q, et al. OR-1, a member of the nuclear receptor superfamily that interacts with the 9-*cis*-retinoic acid receptor. *Proc Natl Acad Sci USA* 1995;92: 2096–2100.

22. Song C, Kokontis JM, Hiipakka RA, et al. Ubiquitous receptor: a receptor that modulates gene activation by retinoic acid and thyroid hormone receptors. *Proc Natl Acad Sci USA* 1994;91: 10809–10813.

23. Alberti S, Steffensen KR, Gustafsson J-Å. Structural characterisation of the mouse nuclear oxysterol receptor genes *LXRα* and *LXRβ*. *Gene* 2000;243:93–103.

24. Tobin KAR, Steineger HH, Alberti S, et al. Cross-talk between fatty acid and cholesterol metabolism mediated by liver X receptor-α. *Mol Endocrinol* 2000;14:741–752.

25. Chinetti G, Lestavel S, Bocher V, et al. PPAR-α and PPAR-γ activators induce cholesterol removal from human macrophage foam cells through stimulation of the ABCA1 pathway. *Nat Med* 2001;7:53–58.

26. Mangelsdorf DJ, Evans RM. The RXR heterodimers and orphan receptors. *Cell* 1995;83:841–850.

27. Willy PJ, Mangelsdorf DJ. Unique requirements for retinoid-dependent transcriptional activation by the orphan receptor LXR. *Genes Dev* 1997;11:289–298.

28. Tamura K, Chen YE, Horiuchi M, et al. LXRα functions as a cAMP-responsive transcriptional regulator of gene expression. *Proc Natl Acad Sci USA* 2000;97:8513–8518.

29. Janowski BA, Willy PJ, Devi TR, et al. An oxysterol signalling pathway mediated by the nuclear receptor LXRα. *Nature* 1996;383:728–731.

30. Heyman RA, Mangelsdorf DJ, Dyck JA, et al. 9-Cis retinoic acid is a high affinity ligand for the retinoid X receptor. *Cell* 1992;68:397–406.

31. Janowski BA, Grogan MJ, Jones SA, et al. Structural requirements of ligands for the oxysterol liver X receptors LXRα and LXRβ. *Proc Natl Acad Sci USA* 1999;96:266–271.

32. Lehmann JM, Kliewer SA, Moore LB, et al. Activation of the nuclear receptor LXR by oxysterols defines a new hormone response pathway. *J Biol Chem* 1997;272:3137–3140.

33. Dhar AK, Teng JI, Smith LL. Biosynthesis of cholest-5-ene-3β, 24-diol (cerebrosterol) by bovine cerebral cortical microsomes. *J Neurochem* 1973;21:51–60.

34. Lütjohann D, Breuer O, Ahlborg G, et al. Cholesterol homeostasis in human brain: evidence for an age-dependent flux of 24S-hydroxycholesterol from the brain into the circulation. *Proc Natl Acad Sci USA* 1996;93:9799–9804.

35. Lund EG, Guileyardo JM, Russell DW. cDNA cloning of cholesterol 24-hydroxylase, a mediator of cholesterol homeostasis in the brain. *Proc Natl Acad Sci USA* 1999;96:7238–7243.

36. Spencer TA, Gayen AK, Phirwa S, et al. 24(*S*),25-epoxycholesterol. Evidence consistent with a role in the regulation of hepatic cholesterogenesis. *J Biol Chem* 1985;260:13391–13394.

37. Spencer TA. The squalene dioxide pathway of steroid biosynthesis. *Acc Chem Res* 1994;27:83–90.

38. Dixon R, Furutachi T, Lieberman S. The isolation of crystalline 22R-hydroxycholesterol and 20α,22R-dihydroxycholesterol from bovine adrenals. *Biochem Biophys Res Commun* 1970; 40:161–165.

39. Lavy U, Burstein S, Gut M, et al. Bile acid synthesis in man. II. Determination of 7α-hydroxycholesterol, (22R)-22-hydroxy-

cholesterol, and 26-hydroxycholesterol in human meconium. *J Lipid Res* 1977;18:232–238.

40. Repa JJ, Turley SD, Lobaccaro J-MA, et al. Regulation of absorption and ABC1-mediated efflux of cholesterol by RXR heterodimers. *Science* 2000;289:1524–1529.

41. Schultz JR, Tu H, Luk A, et al. Role of LXRs in control of lipogenesis. *Genes Dev* 2000;14:2831–2838.

42. Forman BM, Goode E, Chen J, et al. Identification of a nuclear receptor that is activated by farnesol metabolites. *Cell* 1995;81: 687–693.

43. Seol W, Choi H-S, Moore DD. Isolation of proteins that interact specifically with the retinoid X receptor: two novel orphan receptors. *Mol Endocrinol* 1995;9:72–85.

44. Makishima M, Okamoto AY, Repa JJ, et al. Identification of a nuclear receptor for bile acids. *Science* 1999;284:1362–1365.

45. Parks DJ, Blanchard SG, Bledsoe RK, et al. Bile acids: natural ligands for an orphan nuclear receptor. *Science* 1999;284: 1365–1368.

46. Wang H, Chen J, Hollister K, et al. Endogenous bile acids are ligands for the nuclear receptor FXR/BAR. *Mol Cell* 1999;3: 543–553.

47. Akashi Y, Miyazaki H, Nakayama F. Correlation of bile acid composition between liver tissue and bile. *Clin Chim Acta* 1983;133:125–132.

48. Setchell KDR, Rodrigues CMP, Clerici C, et al. Bile acid concentrations in human and rat liver tissue and in hepatocyte nuclei. *Gastroenterology* 1997;112:226–235.

49. Mallory A, Kern F, Smith J, et al. Patterns of bile acids and microflora in the human small intestine. *Gastroenterology* 1973; 64:26–33.

50. Bramlett KS, Yao S, Burris TP. Correlation of farnesoid X receptor coactivator recruitment and cholesterol 7α-hydroxylase gene repression by bile acids. *Mol Genet Metab* 2000; 71:609–615.

51. Sinal CJ, Tohkin M, Miyata M, et al. Targeted disruption of the nuclear receptor FXR/BAR impairs bile acid and lipid homeostasis. *Cell* 2000;102:731–744.

52. Becker-André M, André E, DeLamarter JF. Identification of nuclear receptor mRNAs by RT-PCR amplification of conserved zinc-finger motif sequences. *Biochem Biophys Res Commun* 1993;194:1371–1379.

53. Ellinger-Ziegelbauer H, Hihi AK, Laudet V, et al. FTZ-F1-related orphan receptors in *Xenopus laevis*: transcriptional regulators differentially expressed during early embryogenesis. *Mol Cell Biol* 1994;14:2786–2797.

54. Galarneau L, Paré J-F, Allard D, et al. The α1-fetoprotein locus is activated by a nuclear receptor of the *Drosophila* FTZ-F1 family. *Mol Cell Biol* 1996;16:3853–3865.

55. Kudo T, Sutou S. Molecular cloning of chicken FTZ-F1-related orphan receptors. *Gene* 1997;197:261–268.

56. Li M, Xie Y-H, Kong Y-Y, et al. Cloning and characterization of a novel human hepatocyte transcription factor, hB1F, which binds and activates enhancer II of hepatitis B virus. *J Biol Chem* 1998;273:29022–29031.

57. Nitta M, Ku S, Brown C, et al. CPF: An orphan nuclear receptor that regulates liver-specific expression of the human cholesterol 7α-hydroxylase gene. *Proc Natl Acad Sci USA* 1999;96: 6660–6665.

58. Boerboom D, Pilon N, Behdjani R, et al. Expression and regulation of transcripts encoding two members of the NR5A nuclear receptor subfamily of orphan nuclear receptors, steroidogenic factor-1 and NR5A2, in equine ovarian cells during the ovulatory process. *Endocrinology* 2000;141:4647–4656.

59. Parker KL, Schimmer BP. Steroidogenic factor 1: a key determinant of endocrine development and function. *Endocr Rev* 1997;18:361–377.

60. Rausa FM, Galarneau L, Bélanger L, et al. The nuclear receptor fetoprotein transcription factor is coexpressed with its target gene HNF-3β in the developing murine liver intestine and pancreas. *Mech Dev* 1999;89:185–188.

61. del Castillo-Olivares Ad, Gil G. α₁-Fetoprotein transcription factor is required for the expression of sterol 12α-hydroxylase, the specific enzyme for cholic acid synthesis. *J Biol Chem* 2000;275:17793–17799.

62. Masuda N, Yasumo H, Tamura T, et al. An orphan nuclear receptor lacking a zinc-finger DNA-binding domain: interaction with several nuclear receptors. *Biochim Biophys Acta* 1997; 1350:27–32.

63. Seol W, Choi H-S, Moore DD. An orphan nuclear hormone receptor that lacks a DNA binding domain and heterodimerizes with other receptors. *Science* 1996;272:1336–1339.

64. Johansson L, Thomsen JS, Damdimopoulos AE, et al. The orphan nuclear receptor SHP inhibits agonist-dependent transcriptional activity of estrogen receptors ERα and ERβ. *J Biol Chem* 1999;274:345–353.

65. Lee Y-K, Dell H, Dowhan DH, et al. The orphan nuclear receptor SHP inhibits hepatocyte nuclear factor 4 and retinoid X receptor transactivation: two mechanism for repression. *Mol Cell Biol* 2000;20:187–195.

66. Seol W, Chung M, Moore DD. Novel receptor interaction and repression domains in the orphan receptor SHP. *Mol Cell Biol* 1997;17:7126–7131.

67. Nishigori H, Tomura H, Tonooka N, et al. Mutations in the small heterodimer partner gene are associated with mild obesity in Japanese subjects. *Proc Natl Acad Sci USA* 2001;98: 575–580.

68. Goodwin B, Jones SA, Price RR, et al. A regulatory cascade of the nuclear receptors FXR, SHP-1, and LRH-1 represses bile acid biosynthesis. *Mol Cell* 2000;6:517–526.

69. Lu TT, Makishima M, Repa JJ, et al. Molecular basis for feedback regulation of bile acid synthesis by nuclear receptors. *Mol Cell* 2000;6:507–515.

70. Chiang JYL. Regulation of bile acid synthesis. *Frontiers Biosci* 1998;3:176–193.

71. Bertolotti M, Abate N, Loria P, et al. Regulation of bile acid synthesis in humans: studies on cholesterol 7 α-hydroxylation *in vivo*. *Ital J Gastroenterol* 1995;27:446–449.

72. Marrapodi M, Chiang JYL. Peroxisome proliferator-activated receptor α (PPARα) and agonist inhibit cholesterol 7α-hydroxylase gene (*CYP7A1*) transcription. *J Lipid Res* 2000;41: 514–520.

73. Cheema SK, Agellon LB. The murine and human cholesterol 7α-hydroxylase gene promoters are differentially responsive to regulation by fatty acids mediated via peroxisome proliferator-activated receptor α. *J Biol Chem* 2000;275:12530–12536.

74. Hunt MC, Yang Y-Z, Eggertsen G, et al. The peroxisome proliferator-activated receptor α (PPARα) regulates bile acid biosynthesis. *J Biol Chem* 2000;275:28947–28953.

75. Li YC, Wang DP, Chiang JYL. Regulation of cholesterol 7α-hydroxylase in the liver. *J Biol Chem* 1990;265:12012–12019.

76. Ståhlberg D. Effects of pregnenolone-16α-carbonitrile on the metabolism of cholesterol in rat liver microsomes. *Lipids* 1995; 30:361–364.

77. Stroup D, Chiang JYL. HNF4 and COUP-TFII interact to modulate transcription of the cholesterol 7α-hydroxylase gene (*CYP7A1*). *J Lipid Res* 2000;41:1–11.

78. Andersson Y, Majd Z, Lefebvre A-M, et al. Developmental and pharmacological regulation of apolipoprotein C-II gene expression. *Arterioscler Thromb Vasc Biol* 1999;19:115–121.

79. Laffitte BA, Repa JJ, Joseph SB, et al. LXRs control lipid-inducible expression of the apolipoprotein E gene in macrophages and adipocytes. *Proc Natl Acad Sci USA* 2001;98:507–512.

80. Luo Y, Tall AR. Sterol upregulation of human *CETP* expression *in vitro* and in transgenic mice by an LXR element. *J Clin Invest*, 2000;105:513–520.

81. Urizar NL, Dowhan DH, Moore DD. The farnesoid X-activated receptor mediates bile acid activation of phospholipid transfer protein gene expression. *J Biol Chem* 2000;275: 39313–39317.

82. Laffitte BA, Kast HR, Nguyen CM, et al. Identification of the DNA binding specificity and potential target genes for the farnesoid X-activated receptor. *J Biol Chem* 2000;275: 10638–10647.

83. Glomset JA. High-density lipoproteins in human health and disease. *Adv Intern Med* 1980;25:91–116.

84. Andersson S, Davis DL, Dahlbäck H, et al. Cloning, structure, and expression of the mitochondrial cytochrome P-450 sterol 26-hydroxylase, a bile acid biosynthetic enzyme. *J Biol Chem* 1989;264:8222–8229.

85. Eggertsen G, Olin M, Andersson U, et al. Molecular cloning and expression of rabbit sterol 12α-hydroxylase. *J Biol Chem* 1996;271:32269–32275.

86. Princen HMG, Post SM, Twisk J. Regulation of bile acid biosynthesis. *Curr Pharm Des* 1997;3:59–84.

87. Vlahcevic ZR, Pandak WM, Stravitz RT. Regulation of bile acid biosynthesis. *Gastroenterol Clin North Am* 1999;28:1–25.

88. Peet DJ, Turley SD, Ma W, et al. Cholesterol and bile acid metabolism are impaired in mice lacking the nuclear oxysterol receptor LXRα. *Cell* 1998;93:693–704.

89. Jelinek DF, Andersson S, Slaughter CA, et al. Cloning and regulation of cholesterol 7α-hydroxylase, the rate-limiting enzyme in bile acid biosynthesis. *J Biol Chem* 1990;265:8190–8197.

90. Horton JD, Cuthbert JA, Spady DK. Regulation of hepatic 7α-hydroxylase expression and response to dietary cholesterol in the rat and hamster. *J Biol Chem* 1995;270:5381–5387.

91. Wan Y-JY, An D, Cai Y, et al. Hepatocyte-specific mutation establishes retinoid X receptor α as a heterodimeric integrator of multiple physiological processes in the liver. *Mol Cell Biol* 2000;20:4436–4444.

92. Chen J, Cooper AD, Levy-Wilson B. Hepatocyte nuclear factor 1 binds to and transactivates the human but not the rat CYP7A1 promoter. *Biochem Biophys Res Commun* 1999;260: 829–834.

93. Crestani M, Galli G, Chiang JYL. Genomic cloning, sequencing, and analysis of the hamster cholesterol 7α-hydroxylase gene (*CYP7*). *Arch Biochem Biophys* 1993;306:451–461.

94. Repa JJ, Lund EG, Horton JD, et al. Disruption of the sterol 27-hydroxylase gene in mice results in hepatomegaly and hypertriglyceridemia: reversal by cholic acid feeding. *J Biol Chem* 2000;275:39685–39692.

95. Mangelsdorf DJ, Umesono K, Evans RM. The retinoid receptors. In: Sporn MB, Roberts AB, Goodman DS, eds. *The retinoids: biology, chemistry, and medicine* 2nd ed. New York: Raven Press, 1994:319–349.

96. Schoonjans K, Staels B, Auwerx J. Role of the peroxisome proliferator-activated receptors (PPAR) in mediating the effects of fibrates and fatty acids on gene expression. *J Lipid Res* 1996;37: 907–925.

97. Tontonoz P, Hu E, Graves RA, et al. mPPAR γ 2: tissue-specific regulator of an adipocyte enhancer. *Genes Dev* 1994;8: 1224–1234.

98. Kanda T, Niot I, Foucaud L, et al. Effect of bile on the intestinal bile-acid binding protein (I-BABP) expression. *In vitro* and *in vivo* studies. *FEBS Lett* 1996;384:131–134.

99. Kanda T, Foucand L, Nakamura Y, et al. Regulation of expression of human intestinal bile acid-binding protein in Caco-2 cells. *Biochem J* 1998;330:261–265.

100. Grober J, Zaghini I, Fujii H, et al. Identification of a bile acid-

responsive element in the human ileal bile acid-binding protein gene. *J Biol Chem* 1999;274:29749–29754.

101. Bahar RJ, Stolz A. Bile acid transport. *Gastroenterol Clin North Am* 1999;28:27–58.

102. Laitinen S, Olkkonen VM, Ehnholm C, et al. Family of human oxysterol binding protein (OSBP) homologues: a novel member implicated in brain sterol metabolism. *J Lipid Res* 1999;40: 2204–2211.

103. Bruce C, Chouinard RA, Tall AR. Plasma lipid transfer proteins, high-density lipoproteins, and reverse cholesterol transport. *Annu Rev Nutr* 1998;18:297–330.

104. Tall AR, Jiang X-C, Luo Y, et al. Lipid transfer proteins, HDL metabolism, and atherogenesis. *Arterioscler Thromb Vasc Biol* 2000;20:1185–1188.

105. Klein I, Sarkadi B, Váradi A. An inventory of the human ABC proteins. *Biochim Biophys Acta* 1999;1461:237–262.

106. Borst P, Zelcer N, van Helvoort A. ABC transporters in lipid transport. *Biochim Biophys Acta* 2000;1486:128–144.

107. Müller M. Transcriptional control of hepatocanalicular transporter gene expression. *Semin Liver Dis* 2000;20:323–337.

108. Kipp H, Arias IM. Newly synthesized canalicular ABC transporters are directly targeted from the Golgi to the hepatocyte apical domain in rat liver. *J Biol Chem* 2000;275:15917–15925.

109. Brooks-Wilson A, Marcil M, Clee SM, et al. Mutations in *ABC1* in Tangier disease and familial high-density lipoprotein deficiency. *Nat Genet* 1999;22:336–345.

110. Rust S, Rosier M, Funke H, et al. Tangier disease is caused by mutations in the gene encoding ATP-binding cassette transporter 1. *Nat Genet* 1999;22:352–355.

111. Bodzioch M, Orsó E, Klucken J, et al. The gene encoding ATP-binding cassette transporter 1 is mutated in Tangier disease. *Nat Genet* 1999;22:347–351.

112. Yokoyama S. Release of cellular cholesterol: molecular mechanism for cholesterol homeostasis in cells and in the body. *Biochim Biophys Acta* 2000;1529:231–244.

113. Orsó E, Broccardo C, Kaminski WE, et al. Transport of lipids from Golgi to plasma membrane is defective in Tangier disease patients and *Abc1*-deficient mice. *Nat Genet* 2000;24: 192–196.

114. McNeish J, Aiello RJ, Guyot D, et al. High density lipoprotein deficiency and foam cell accumulation in mice with targeted disruption of ATP-binding cassette transporter-1. *Proc Natl Acad Sci USA* 2000;97:4245–4250.

115. Christiansen-Weber TA, Voland JR, Wu Y, et al. Functional loss of *ABC1* in mice causes severe placental malformation, aberrant lipid distribution, and kidney glomerulonephritis as well as high-density lipoprotein cholesterol deficiency. *Am J Pathol* 2000;157:1017–1029.

116. Luciani MF, Denizot F, Savary S, et al. Cloning of two novel ABC transporters mapping on human chromosome 9. *Genomics* 1994;21:150–159.

117. Wang N, Silver DL, Costet P, et al. Specific binding of apoA-I, enhanced cholesterol efflux and altered plasma membrane morphology in cells expressing ABC1. *J Biol Chem* 2000; 275: 33053–33058.

118. Costet P, Luo Y, Wang N, et al. Sterol-dependent transactivation of the ABC1 promoter by LXR/RXR. *J Biol Chem* 2000;275:28240–28245.

119. Schwartz K, Lawn RM, Wade DP. ABC1 gene expression and apoA-I-mediated cholesterol efflux are regulated by LXR. *Biochim Biophys Res Commun* 2000;274:794–802.

120. Venkateswaran A, Laffitte BA, Joseph SB, et al. Control of cellular cholesterol efflux by the nuclear oxysterol receptor LXRα. *Proc Natl Acad Sci USA* 2000;97:12097–12102.

121. Claudel T, Leibowitz MD, Fiévet C, et al. Reduction of atherosclerosis in apolipoprotein E knockout mice by activation of the retinoid X receptor. *Proc Natl Acad Sci USA* 2001;98: 2610–2615.

122. Savary S, Denizot F, Luciani M-F, et al. Molecular cloning of a mammalian ABC transporter homologous to *Drosophila white* gene. *Mamm Genome* 1996;7:673–676.

123. Croop JM, Tiller GE, Fletcher JA, et al. Isolation and characterization of a mammalian homolog of the *Drosophila white* gene. *Gene* 1997;185:77–85.

124. Klucken J, Büchler C, Orsó E, et al. ABCG1 (ABC8), the human homolog of the *Drosophila white* gene, is a regulator of macrophage cholesterol and phospholipid transport. *Proc Natl Acad Sci USA* 2000;97:817–822.

125. Strautnieks SS, Bull LN, Knisely AS, et al. A gene encoding a liver-specific ABC transporter is mutated in progressive familial intrahepatic cholestasis. *Nat Genet* 1998;20:233–238.

126. Gerloff T, Stieger B, Hagenbuch B, et al. The sister of P-glycoprotein represents the canalicular bile salt export pump of mammalian liver. *J Biol Chem* 1998;273:10046–10050.

127. de Vree JML, Jacquemin E, Sturm E, et al. Mutations in the *MDR3* gene cause progressive familial intrahepatic cholestasis. *Proc Natl Acad Sci USA* 1998;95:282–287.

128. Oude Elferink RPJ, Groen AK. Mechanisms of biliary lipid secretion and their role in lipid homeostasis. *Semin Liver Dis* 2000;20:293–305.

129. Miranda S, Vollrath V, Wielandt AM, et al. Overexpression of mdr2 gene by peroxisome proliferators in the mouse liver. *J Hepatol* 1997;26:1331–1339.

130. Berge KE, Tian H, Graf GA, et al. Accumulation of dietary cholesterol in sitosterolemia caused by mutations in adjacent ABC transporters. *Science* 2000;290:1771–1775.

131. Patel SB, Salen G, Hidaka H, et al. Mapping a gene involved in regulating dietary cholesterol absorption. The sitosterolemia locus is found at chromosome 2p21. *J Clin Invest* 1998;102: 1041–1044.

132. Salen G, Shefer S, Nguyen L, et al. Sitosterolemia. In: Bittman R, ed. *Cholesterol: its functions and metabolism in biology and medicine.* New York: Plenum Publishing, 1997;28:453–476.

133. Lee M-H, Lu K, Hazard S, et al. Identification of a gene, *ABCG5*, important in the regulation of dietary cholesterol absorption. *Nat Genet* 2001;27:79–83.

134. Hock T, Cottrill T, Keegan J, et al. The *E23* early gene of *Drosophila* encodes an ecdysone-inducible ATP-binding cassette transporter capable of repressing ecdysone-mediated gene activation. *Proc Natl Acad Sci USA* 2000;97:9519–9524.

135. Waxman DJ. P450 gene induction by structurally diverse xenochemicals: central role of nuclear receptors CAR, PXR, and PPAR. *Arch Biochem Biophys* 1999;369:11–23.

136. Zavacki AM, Lehmann JM, Seol W, et al. Activation of the orphan receptor RIP14 by retinoids. *Proc Natl Acad Sci USA* 1997;94:7909–7914.

137. Maloney PR, Parks DJ, Haffner CD, et al. Identification of a chemical tool for the orphan nuclear receptor FXR. *J Med Chem* 2000;43:2971–2974.

138. Xie W, Barwick JL, Downes M, et al. Humanized xenobiotic response in mice expressing nuclear receptor SXR. *Nature* 2000;406:435–439.

139. Wei P, Zhang J, Egan-Hafley M, et al. The nuclear receptor CAR mediates specific xenobiotics induction of drug metabolism. *Nature* 2000;407:920–923.

The Liver: Biology and Pathobiology, Fourth Edition, edited by I. M. Arias, J. L. Boyer, F. V. Chisari, N. Fausto, D. Schachter, and D. A. Shafritz.
Lippincott Williams & Wilkins, Philadelphia © 2001.

SUBJECT INDEX

Page numbers in italics refer to illustrations; page numbers followed by t refer to tables